CLINICAL
PREVENTIVE
MEDICINE

CLINICAL PREVENTIVE MEDICINE

RICHARD N. MATZEN, M.D.

Emeritus Physician, The Cleveland Clinic Foundation
First and Former Chairman, Department of Preventive Medicine
and Emil Buehler Scholar in Preventive and Aviation Medicine
The Cleveland Clinic Foundation
Cleveland, Ohio

RICHARD S. LANG, M.D., M.P.H., F.A.C.P.

Head, Section of Preventive Medicine
The Cleveland Clinic Foundation
Cleveland, Ohio
Assistant Professor, Department of Internal Medicine
The Ohio State University College of Medicine
Columbus, Ohio
Clinical Associate Professor of Medicine
College of Medicine of the Pennsylvania State University
Hershey, Pennsylvania

with 223 illustrations

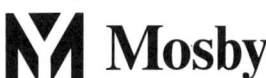 Mosby

St. Louis Baltimore Boston Chicago London Philadelphia Sydney Toronto

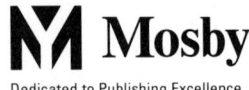

Editor: Stephanie Manning
Developmental Editor: Carolyn Malik
Project Manager: John Rogers
Production Editor: Chris Murphy
Designer: David Zielinski

Copyright © 1993 by Mosby–Year Book, Inc.

All rights reserved. No part of this publication may be reproduced, stored in a retrieval system, or transmitted, in any form or by any means, electronic, mechanical, photocopying, recording, or otherwise, without prior written permission from the publisher.

Permission to photocopy or reproduce solely for internal or personal use is permitted for libraries or other users registered with the Copyright Clearance Center, provided that the base fee of $4.00 per chapter plus $.10 per page is paid directly to the Copyright Clearance Center, 27 Congress Street, Salem, MA 01970. This consent does no extend to others kinds of copying, such as copying for general distribution, for advertising or promotional purposes, for creating new collected work, or for resale.

Printed in the United States of America

Mosby–Year Book, Inc.
11830 Westline Industrial Drive
St. Louis, Missouri 63146

Library of Congress Cataloging in Publication Data
Clinical preventive medicine/editors, Richard N. Matzen, Richard S. Lang.
  p. cm.
    Includes bibliographical references and index.
    ISBN 0-8016-3176-9
    1. Medicine, Preventive. I. Matzen, Richard N. II. Lang,
Richard S.
    [DNLM: 1. Preventive Medicine, WB 108 C641 1993]
RA427.9.C55 1993
613—dc20
DNLM/DLC
for Library of Congress
                                93-17186
                                   CIP

93 94 95 96 97 C / MV 9 8 7 6 5 4 3 2 1

CONTRIBUTORS

Denise V. Abe, M.D.
Clinic Preceptor
Internal Medicine Residency Training Program
Virginia Mason Clinic and Hospital
Seattle, Washington

Ronald T. Acton, Ph.D.
Professor, Departments of Medicine, Microbiology and Epidemiology
Director, Immunogenetics/DNA Diagnostic Laboratory
University of Alabama Health Services Division
University of Alabama at Birmingham
Birmingham, Alabama

David Ray Baines, M.D., F.A.A.F.P.
Chairman
Ad hoc Committee for Minority Populations
National Heart, Lung and Blood Institute
National Institutes of Health
Bethesda, Maryland

Richard Bamberg, Ph.D., MT (ASCP) SH, CLD (NCA)
Professor and Chair
Department of Special Programs
School of Health Related Professions
University of Alabama at Birmingham
Birmingham, Alabama

Tamsen Bassford, M.D.
Assistant Professor
Department of Family and Community Medicine
University of Arizona College of Medicine
Tucson, Arizona

Gerald J. Beck, Ph.D.
Acting Chairman
Department of Biostatistics and Epidemiology
The Cleveland Clinic Foundation
Cleveland, Ohio

Jerome L. Belinson, M.D.
Chairman
Department of Gynecology
Vice Chairman
Division of Surgery
The Cleveland Clinic Foundation
Cleveland, Ohio
Professor of Gynecology
The Ohio State University
Columbus, Ohio

Michael P. Bennetts, M.D.
Medical Director
Adult Inpatient Psychiatric Service
Department of Psychiatry
The Cleveland Clinic Foundation
Cleveland, Ohio

Andres W. Bhatia, M.D.
Department of Hematology and Medical Oncology
The Cleveland Clinic Foundation
Cleveland, Ohio

Ronald Bialek, M.P.P.
Director
Health Program Alliance
The Johns Hopkins University School of Hygiene and Public Health
Baltimore, Maryland

Linda D. Bradley, M.D.
Department of Gynecology
The Cleveland Clinic Foundation
Cleveland, Ohio

G. Thomas Budd, M.D.
Department of Hematology and Medical Oncology
The Cleveland Clinic Foundation
Cleveland, Ohio

Enrico G. Camara, M.D.
Associate Professor
Department of Psychiatry
University of Hawaii at Manoa
John A. Burns School of Medicine
Honolulu, Hawaii

John P. Campbell, M.D.
Section of Preventive Medicine
Department of Internal Medicine
The Cleveland Clinic Foundation
Cleveland, Ohio
Associate Professor of Internal Medicine
College of Medicine of the Pennsylvania State University
Hershey, Pennsylvania

Kirste L. Carlson, N.D., M.S.N., R.N.C.S.
Clinical Nurse Specialist
Psychiatric Nursing
The Cleveland Clinic Foundation
Cleveland, Ohio

Sue Shu-Kwan Chan, M.D., M.P.H.
Clinical Faculty
Department of Pediatrics
University of California
San Francisco, California
Department of Pediatrics
Children's Hospital
Oakland, California

Arif Zafar Chaudhry, M.D., M.B., B.S., DTM&H
Department of Internal Medicine
Cleveland Clinic, Florida
Consultant Physician
Internal Medicine, Infectious Disease
North Beach Hospital
For Lauderdale, Florida

C. Patrick Chaulk, M.D., M.P.H.
Department of Health Policies and Management
Division of Public Health
The Johns Hopkins School of Hygiene and Public Health
Baltimore, Maryland

Arthur Mason Chen, M.D.
Clinical Faculty
Department of Family and Community Medicine
University of California
San Francisco, California
Chief Medical Consultant
Association of Asian Pacific Community Health Organizations
Special Programs Director
Asian Health Services
Oakland, California

Todd Cohen, M.D.
Resident
Department of Urology
The Cleveland Clinic Foundation
Cleveland, Ohio

Gregory B. Collins, M.D.
Section Head, Alcohol and Drug Recovery Center
Department of Psychiatry
The Cleveland Clinic Foundation
Cleveland, Ohio

Jack T. Collins, M.D., F.A.C.P.
Section of Preventive Medicine
Department of Internal Medicine
The Cleveland Clinic Foundation
Cleveland, Ohio

Roslyn S. Collins, B.A.
Medical Writer

Teresa A. Conroy, B.S.N., M.S.N.C., R.N.C., C.C.D.C.II
Staff Nurse
Coordinator, Outpatient Codependency Program
Alcohol and Drug Recovery Center
Department of Psychiatry
The Cleveland Clinic Foundation
Cleveland, Ohio

Michael D. Cressman, D.O.
Director, The Lipid Research/Referral Clinic
Department of Heart and Hypertension Research
The Cleveland Clinic Foundation
Cleveland, Ohio

Garland Y. DeNelsky, Ph.D.
Director
Cleveland Clinic Smoking Cessation Program
Head, Section of Psychology
Department of Psychiatry and Psychology
The Cleveland Clinic Foundation
Cleveland, Ohio

Jacob W. E. Dijkstra, M.D.
Director, Cutaneous Care Center
Department of Dermatology
The Cleveland Clinic Foundation
Cleveland, Ohio

Robert J. Dimeff, M.D.
Medical Director
Section of Sports Medicine
Department of Orthopaedic Surgery
The Cleveland Clinic Foundation
Assistant Clinical Professor
Department of Family Medicine
Case Western Reserve University School of Medicine
Cleveland, Ohio

Dudley Dinner, M.D.
Director, Sleep Disorders Center
Department of Neurology
The Cleveland Clinic Foundation
Cleveland, Ohio

Richard L. Dunn, M.D.
Section of Preventive Medicine
Department of Internal Medicine
The Cleveland Clinic Foundation
Cleveland, Ohio

Salvatore J. Esposito, D.M.D.
Chairman, Department of Dentistry
The Cleveland Clinic Foundation
Cleveland, Ohio

Kathleen H. FitzSimons, B.A., M.A.
Training Consultant
Department of Training and Development
The Cleveland Clinic Foundation
Cleveland, Ohio

Gregory J. Forstall, M.D.
Clinical Associate
Department of Infectious Disease
The Cleveland Clinic Foundation
Cleveland, Ohio

Ora Frankel, M.D.
Instructor, Department of Psychiatry
Washington University
Outpatient Director
Child Psychiatry Clinic
Department of Child Psychiatry
St. Louis Children's Hospital
St. Louis, Missouri

Karen-Rae Friedman-Kester, M.S., R.D., L.D.
Partner, Friedman-Kester & Kleiner
Specialists in Nutrition
Gates Mills, Ohio

Richard Garcia, M.D.
Department of Pediatrics
The Cleveland Clinic Foundation
Cleveland, Ohio

Robert W. Gerlach, M.P.A.
Administrator
Cancer Center
The Cleveland Clinic Foundation
Cleveland, Ohio

Gita P. Gidwani, M.D.
Department of Gynecology
The Cleveland Clinic Foundation
Cleveland, Ohio

David Scott Golden, B.S., R.N.
Alcohol and Drug Recovery Center
The Cleveland Clinic Foundation
Cleveland, Ohio

Lilian Gonsalves, M.D.
Head, Consultation Liaison Section
Department of Psychiatry and Psychology
The Cleveland Clinic Foundation
Cleveland, Ohio

Giesele Robinson Greene, M.D.
Assistant Clinical Professor
Department of Internal Medicine
Division of Geriatric Medicine
Case Western Reserve University School of Medicine
Cleveland Ohio,
Director of Medical Services
Personal Physician Care Incorporated Health Plan

Phillip Hall, M.D.
Department of Nephrology
The Cleveland Clinic Foundation
Cleveland, Ohio
Professor of Medicine
The Ohio State University College of Medicine
Columbus, Ohio
Professor of Medicine
College of Medicine of the Pennsylvania State University
Hershey, Pennsylvania

Stephen P. Hayden, M.D., F.A.C.P.
Department of General Internal Medicine
The Cleveland Clinic Foundation
Cleveland, Ohio
Assistant Clinical Professor
Department of Medicine
Case Western Reserve University School of Medicine

Göran Hellers, M.D., Ph.D.
Assistant Professor
Karolinska Institute Medical School
Chairman
Department of Surgery
Huddinge University Hospital
Huddinge, Sweden

L. Sunday Homitz, B.A., B.F.A., B.S.P.T.
Physical Therapist
Dance Medicine Specialist
Section of Dance Medicine
Department of Sports Medicine/Orthopaedic Surgery
The Cleveland Clinic Foundation
Cleveland, Ohio

Gordon B. Hughes, M.D., F.A.C.S.
Director of Education
Department of Otolaryngology and Communicative Disorders
The Cleveland Clinic Foundation
Cleveland, Ohio

Ruth Imrie, M.D.
Department of Pediatrics and Adolescent Medicine
The Cleveland Clinic Foundation
Cleveland, Ohio
Clinical Instructor of Pediatrics
Faculty of Medicine
Case Western Reserve University School of Medicine
Cleveland, Ohio

Loretta Roach Isada, M.D.
Assistant Professor of Clinical Internal Medicine
Department of Internal Medicine
Northeastern Ohio University School of Medicine
Rootstown, Ohio
Akron General Medical Center
Department of Cardiology
Akron, Ohio

Dennis W. Jahnigen, M.D.
Head, Section of Geriatric Medicine
Department of Internal Medicine
The Cleveland Clinic Foundation
Cleveland, Ohio

Kurt W. Jensen, Psy.D.
Director
SOLUTIONS
Cleveland, Ohio

Vanessa K. Jensen, Psy.D.
Head, Section of Pediatric Psychology
Department of Pediatric and Adolescent Medicine
The Cleveland Clinic Foundation
Cleveland, Ohio

George Kanoti, S.T.D.

F.J. O'Neill Chairman
Department of Bioethics
The Cleveland Clinic Foundation
Cleveland, Ohio

Martin Keller, M.D., Ph.D.

Professor Emeritus
Department of Preventive Medicine
The Ohio State University College of Medicine
Columbus, Ohio

Donald Thurman Kirkendall, Ph.D.

Associate Professor
Health, Physical Education, Recreation, and Dance
Illinois State University
Normal, Illinois

Eric A. Klein, M.D.

Department of Urology
The Cleveland Clinic Foundation
Cleveland, Ohio

Susan M. Kleiner, Ph.D., R.D.

Partner, Friedman-Kester & Kleiner
Specialists in Nutrition
Gates Mills, Ohio
Adjunct Member
Sarah W. Stedman Center for Nutritional Studies
Duke University Medical Center
Durham, North Carolina

Milton Lakin, M.D., F.A.C.P.

Head, Section of Male Sexual Medicine
Department of Urology
The Cleveland Clinic Foundation
Cleveland, Ohio
Clinical Assistant Professor of Medicine
College of Medicine of the Pennsylvania State University
Hershey, Pennsylvania

Richard S. Lang, M.D., M.P.H., F.A.C.P.

Head, Section of Preventive Medicine
Department of Internal Medicine
The Cleveland Clinic Foundation
Cleveland, Ohio
Assistant Professor of Medicine
The Ohio State University College of Medicine
Columbus, Ohio
Clinical Associate Professor of Medicine
College of Medicine of the Pennsylvania State University
Hershey, Pennsylvania

Richard J. Lederman, M.D., Ph.D.

Department of Neurology
Director, Medical Center for Performing Artists
The Cleveland Clinic Foundation
Cleveland, Ohio

Waldon Lim, M.D.

Assistant Professor of Clinical Medicine
University of California-San Francisco
District Medical Director
Health Center #4
Department of Public Health
San Francisco, California

David Longworth, M.D.

Chairman
Department of Infectious Diseases
The Cleveland Clinic Foundation
Cleveland, Ohio
Associate Professor of Medicine
The Ohio State University College of Medicine
Columbus, Ohio

Peter L. Lubs, M.S.

Industrial Hygiene Consultant
Department of Pulmonary Medicine
The Cleveland Clinic Foundation
Cleveland, Ohio
Corporate Director of Occupational Health
The Lubrizol Corporation
Wickliffe, Ohio

Donald A. Malone, Jr., M.D.

Department of Psychiatry
The Cleveland Clinic Foundation
Cleveland, Ohio

Richard N. Matzen, M.D.

Emeritus Physician, The Cleveland Clinic Foundation
First and Former Chairman, Department of Preventive Medicine
and Emil Buehler Scholar in Preventive and Aviation Medicine
The Cleveland Clinic Foundation
Cleveland, Ohio

Daniel J. Mazanec, M.D., F.A.C.P.

Director, Center for the Spine
Education Program Director
Department of Rheumatic and Immunologic Disease
The Cleveland Clinic Foundation
Cleveland, Ohio

Michael G. McKee, Ph.D.

Head, Section of Applied Psychophysiology and Biofeedback
Department of Psychiatry and Psychology
The Cleveland Clinic Foundation
Cleveland, Ohio

Howard P. Moliff, B.S.N., R.N.

Alcohol and Drug Recovery Center
The Cleveland Clinic Foundation
Cleveland, Ohio

Drogo K. Montague, M.D.

Head, Section of Prosthetic Surgery
Department of Urology
Director, Center for Sexual Function
The Cleveland Clinic Foundation
Cleveland, Ohio
Professor of Surgery
The Ohio State University College of Medicine
Columbus, Ohio

Douglas Moodie, M.D.
Chairman
Department of Pediatric and Adolescent Medicine
The Cleveland Clinic Foundation
Cleveland, Ohio
Professor of Pediatrics
The Ohio State University College of Medicine
Columbus, Ohio

Don C. Ng, M.D.
Assistant Clinical Professor of Medicine
Division of General Internal Medicine
Medical center
University of California-San Francisco
San Francisco, California

Peter Ng, M.D.
San Francisco Department of Public Health
Health Center #4
San Francisco, California

Jeffrey W. Olin, D.O.
Head, Section of Atherosclerosis and Lipids
Department of Vascular Medicine
The Cleveland Clinic Foundation
Cleveland, Ohio
Associate Professor of Medicine
The Ohio State University College of Medicine
Columbus, Ohio

Rosalinda J. Ott, M.D.
Assistant Professor
Pediatrics and Community Medicine
Tufts University School of Medicine
Associate Staff
Department of Pediatrics
New England Medical Center
Boston, Massachusetts

Barbara Gould Pelowski, Ph.D.
Director of the The Upper School
The Laurel School
Shaker Heights, Ohio

Thomas L. Petty, M.D.
Professor of Medicine and Associate Dean
Denver Campus
Rush, Presbyterian-St. Luke's Medical Center
Chicago, Illinois
President
Presbyterian–St. Luke's Center for Health Sciences Education
Denver, Colorado

David G. Pietz, M.D.
Department of Gastroenterology
Department of Internal Medicine
Caylor Nickel Medical Center
Bluffton, Indiana
Retired, 1991

Thomas L. Plesec, Ph.D.
Co-Director
Cleveland Clinic Smoking Cessation Program
Section of Psychology
Department of Psychiatry and Psychology
The Cleveland Clinic Foundation
Cleveland, Ohio

Jeffrey M. Roseman, M.D., Ph.D., M.P.H.
Associate Professor of Epidemiology
Director, Center for Health Risk Assessment and Disease Prevention
University of Alabama at Birmingham
Birmingham, Alabama

Peter Sam, M.D.
Clinical Instructor
Department of Family and Community Medicine
University of California
San Francisco, California
Clinic Physician, Asian Health Services
Oakland, California

Joan D. Shainoff, R.N., B.S.N., B.A.
Section of Preventive Medicine
Department of Internal Medicine
The Cleveland Clinic Foundation
Cleveland, Ohio

Steven W. Siegel, M.D.
St. Paul Urologic Systems
St. Paul, Minnesota

Cathy A. Sila, M.D.
Associate Medical Director
Cerebrovascular Program
Department of Neurology
The Cleveland Clinic Foundation
Cleveland, Ohio

Michael V. Sivak, Jr., M.D.
Chief, Division of Gastroenterology
University Hospitals of Cleveland
Professor of Medicine
Case Western Reserve University School of Medicine
Cleveland, Ohio

Martin L. Smith, S.T.D.
Associate Bioethicist
Department of Bioethics
The Cleveland Clinic Foundation
Cleveland, Ohio

Glen D. Solomon, M.D., F.A.C.P.
Associate Professor of Medicine
Department of Internal Medicine
The Ohio State University College of Medicine
Director of Research and Education
The Headache Center of Cleveland Clinic
The Cleveland Clinic Foundation
Cleveland, Ohio

Geza T. Terezhalmy, D.D.S., M.A.
Head, Section of Oral Medicine
Department of Dentistry
The Cleveland Clinic Foundation
Cleveland, Ohio

Holly L.Thacker, M.D.

Clinical Assistant Professor of Medicine
The College of Medicine of the Pennsylvania State University
Hershey, Pennsylvania
Staff Physician, Diagnostic Section
Department of General Internal Medicine
Medical Consultant
The Mature Woman's Program
Department of Gynecology
The Cleveland Clinic Foundation
Cleveland, Ohio

Kristin Thorisdottir, M.D.

Department of Dermatology
The Cleveland Clinic Foundation
Cleveland, Ohio

Kenneth J. Tomecki, M.D.

Department of Dermatology
The Cleveland Clinic Foundation
Cleveland, Ohio

Richard Troy, M.D.

Fellow
Department of Urology
The Cleveland Clinic Foundation
Cleveland, Ohio

Andrew M. Tucker, M.D.

Section of Sports Medicine
Department of Orthopaedics
The Cleveland Clinic Foundation
Assistant Professor
Department of Family Medicine
Case Western Reserve University School of Medicine
Cleveland, Ohio

Harvey M. Tucker, M.D.

Chairman
Department of Otolaryngology
The Cleveland Clinic Foundation
Cleveland, Ohio

Donald B. Underwood, M.D.

Head, Section of Cardiography
Department of Clinical Cardiology
The Cleveland Clinic Foundation
Cleveland, Ohio

Jacques Van Dam, M.D., Ph.D.

Instructor of Medicine
Harvard Medical School
Director, Endoscopic Gastrointestinal Oncology
Associate Director, Gastrointestinal Endoscopy
Brigham and Women's Hospital
Boston, Massachusetts

Frederick Van Lente, Ph.D.

Chairman
Department of Biochemistry
Clinical Pathology
The Cleveland Clinic Foundation
Cleveland, Ohio

Gary A. Varley, M.D.

Department of Ophthalmology
The Cleveland Clinic Foundation
Cleveland, Ohio

William O. Wagner, M.D.

Head, Section of Allergy and Immunology
Department of Pulmonary and Critical Care Medicine
The Cleveland Clinic Foundation
Cleveland, Ohio

Winston F. Wong, M.S., M.D.

Clinical Faculty
Family and Community Medicine
University of California-San Francisco
San Francisco, California
Medical Director
Asian Health Services
Oakland, California

William B. Zuti, Ph.D.

Professor and Chair
Department of Physical and Health Education
Radford University
Radford, Virginia

FOREWORD

The next time you make hospital rounds, ask yourself how many of your patients would need to be there if the knowledge we have today about disease prevention and health promotion could have been brought to bear in their lives 10 or 20 years ago. Just today, in my rounds, I saw patients with terminal squamous cell carcinoma of the lung, multi-infarct dementia, intractable congestive heart failure from ischemic cardiomyopathy, and end-stage renal disease from nephrosclerosis.

How many patients are we going to see in our office this week who will have a preventable disease or injury in the next 20 years if we don't take time now to identify their risk factors and educate them about what they should do to minimize them?

Are we so busy in our daily practices treating sniffles and hemorrhoids that we ignore the opportunity to prevent cancer of the lung or stroke 15 years from now? We can no longer be. Patients now demand information from their physicians about prevention. They seek direction about preventive interventions that often get much media attention.

My colleagues, Drs. Richard Matzen and Richard Lang, have co-edited a practical and comprehensive textbook on *clinical* preventive medicine, written by noted authorities on the subject, especially for practicing physicians.

This book is unique in many respects. An entire section is devoted to mental wellness and the seminal role of the psychologist and psychiatrist in maintaining mental health and enhancing quality of life. Another chapter emphasizes the importance of career choice in the happiness and hence well-being of the individual.

Because nutrition obviously plays a pivotal role in maintaining health and preventing many diseases, physicians will appreciate the five chapters in this book that are devoted to this subject.

This book also addresses racial, ethnic, and cultural differences, which must be taken into consideration in optimizing the effectiveness of preventive health care. Special attention is given to women's needs, including the stresses faced by the two-career woman.

Perusal of the table of contents of this text makes it apparent that virtually every practicing physician, irrespective of his or her specialty, has an opportunity if not an obligation to discuss preventive measures with his or her patients.

Unfortunately, educating a patient about the evils of tobacco, alcohol, and saturated fats is not as glamorous or exciting as treating a patient for acute myocardial ischemia with tPA and balloon angioplasty, nor is it as rewarding monetarily.

The medical education system is more oriented to diagnosis and treatment of disease that already exists than it is to prevention. In fact, preventive medicine is often relegated to electives if it is offered at all. Teachers of preventive medicine are in short supply because the programs to train the specialists in preventive medicine are poorly funded and under-subscribed.

This book points out the enormous opportunity for physicians to prevent human suffering, economic dislocation, and mental anguish by prolonging useful life.

The surgeon who performs a triple bypass operation to prevent a myocardial infarction is practicing preventive medicine, albeit tertiary prevention, and gets instantaneous gratification from his or her efforts by seeing the patient recover and resume full activities. The adulation of the grateful patient and family is exhilarating.

What gratification, what reward does the family physician get from repeatedly persuading patients to stay on low-fat diets, stop smoking, and take their blood pressure pills so that they won't have to have a coronary bypass 20 years later? Inner self-satisfaction of a job well done!

Evidence is accumulating that preventive medicine is paying big dividends in promoting health and prolonging life. Nowhere is it more apparent than in the field of cardiovascular disease. In the last 20 years, control rates for hypertension have gone up from 16% to 55% while consumption of saturated fat and cigarettes has sharply decreased, which explains, at least partially, why the mortality rate from coronary disease has decreased by 50% and from stroke by 58%. The unsung heroes of this battle are the primary care physicians and motivated specialists who have persuaded thousands of their patients to adopt more healthful life-styles. It is very exciting, not very lucrative, but enormously satisfying to realize that hundreds of thousands of people are alive today who wouldn't be here if it weren't for family physicians and others practicing preventive medicine.

With few exceptions, the major breakthroughs that have added materially to human longevity have come from preventing disease, not treating it.

The bottom line of this book is that every physician can and should practice preventive medicine. This is a clinically oriented textbook that provides scientific information and practical guidelines in preventive medicine for all clinicians.

Ray W. Gifford, Jr., M.D.

PREFACE

This text is designed for the office use of practitioners who see patients daily in a clinical setting and have the opportunity to apply preventive medical principles. Use of the text will supplement the knowledge of all primary care physicians in clinical preventive medicine, even in some areas where perhaps it has not heretofore been perceived to play a role. By continual awareness of the place of preventive medicine in all our practices and in the well_being and health of our patients, clinical prevention should become a part of applied office practice on an equal footing with treatment, and addressed just as routinely.

Our intent also has been to supply a tool to be used both in medical school and residency training, particularly in those disciplines of primary care. This text will also be useful in the specialty training of preventive medicine board candidates in the portion of their postgraduate years devoted to clinical preventive medicine.

In the evolution of this book, the subjects covered were given a great deal of thought to produce a volume that addresses the perceived needs of physicians in practice. To that end, more than 100 physicians commented on the proposed table of contents, resulting in valuable suggestions that were incorporated and addressed. It was rewarding to find a high degree of enthusiasm for the book and anticipation by the medical community of its publication. Following that first year, authors were sought to represent their fields, but most importantly, also to be in clinical practice themselves. We felt it important to define the term *preventive medicine* in a subspecialty context, as well as in its crossspecialty definition, role, and application. Preventive medicine as delivered in other countries was felt to be important too, particularly as this country is now in the throes of redefining its health care delivery system. Teaching clinical preventive medicine in its basic units of screening, cost effectiveness, epidemiology, counseling, and the implementation of its use in the office have been addressed as well. As the editors feel that this opportunity to employ prevention as a pervasive practice is universal and transcends disciplines, and that quality of life and happiness are a part of the prevention of morbid states, a conscious effort has been made to include subjects that traditionally have not been addressed. An example is the appropriate selection of a career or one's life work as important to health, happiness, and job satisfaction, hence quality of life. A quote from the contemporary naval historian and novelist, Patrick

O'Brien, alluding to medical practice in the British Navy of the early 1800's , is illustrative:

"Dr. Harrington, the physician of the fleet, an old and esteemed acquaintance, a learned man with very sound ideas on hygiene and preventive medicine...talked of the squadron's remarkable good state of health...'I put it down largely to the use of wind sails to bring at least some fresh air below '(and)' to the continual serving-out of antiscorbutics, and to the provision of wholesome wine instead of the pernicious rum; although it must be admitted that happiness, comparative happiness, is a most important factor."[1]

Prevention is by no means "new," but in the years since World War II the general public has adopted an attitude of physical fitness, diet, and proactive health that has demanded of medicine an increasing response and knowledge base. The individuals in medicine too, being a part of that greater public, have evolved such that leaders in preventive medicine have emerged from fields other than the subspecialty of preventive medicine per se. There nevertheless continues to be an onus placed on these efforts, notably by some corporations (but by no means all) to prove that preventive efforts are "cost effective" in a time of limited resources. These proofs are difficult (and impossible in the short term) but are increasingly published. A quote from a recent article by William H. Crosby illustrates that as long ago as ancient Rome the "cost effectiveness" of preventive medicine was believed in and indeed proven:

"Once in service, soldiers were insured a healthy environment by the safe water supply, varied diet, regular health inspections, preventive medical measures (such as mosquito netting), monitoring of food, cremation of dead outside the city and camp walls, sanitary public latrines, and construction of sewers...The general conditions of military life were so good that the Roman soldier lived almost five years longer than the average Roman civilian."[2]

Indeed, the United States as a nation has expressed a belief in the necessity and rewards of prevention through the establishment of Healthy People 2000: National Health Promotion and Disease Preventive Objectives.[3] This document outlines a national strategy for improving the health of the American public. James L. Mason states in that work that "we can no longer afford not to invest in prevention...and the 1990's should be the decade of prevention in the United States."

Another effort underscoring the shift to prevention was the convening of the U.S. Preventive Services Task Force and the subsequent publication of the Guide to Clinical Preventive Services.[4] Our text was "in the writing" at the time this guide appeared and works well with it by expanding on some issues, supplementing others, and exploring a number of areas that were not addressed.

Whatever practice one is in, the individual physician must recognize that prevention is an important aspect of current and future medical care. It therefore behooves us to become knowledgeable about prevention. Clinical prevention is clearly the only way that the health objective of our nation can hope to be met. Both the Healthy People 2000 and Guide to Clinical Preventive Services documents are referred to repeatedly throughout our text. We sincerely hope that the contribution of this volume will assist in achieving the announced health care goals and objectives for the nation and complement the working guide to provision of clinical preventive services.

REFERENCES

1. O'Brian P: *The Ionian Mission*, New York and London, 1992, W .W. Norton & Co.

2. Crosby WH: The medical legacy of the Roman legions, *MD* 37(2):79-90, 1993.

3. U.S. Department of Health and Human Services Public Health Service: *Healthy People 2000: National Health Promotion and Disease Prevention Objectives*, Boston, 1992, Jones & Bartlett.

4. Report of the U.S. Preventive Services Task Force: *Guide to clinical preventive services*, Baltimore, 1989, Williams & Wilkins.

To my parents Annie Andersen Matzen and Christian F. Matzen; Ragnhild Matzen Cushing and Dr. Edward Cushing, Anne Matzen Mann and Joseph R. Mann, Dagmar Matzen Close and Herbert S. Close, C. Frederick Matzen and his wife Dorothy; and my wife Patricia and our children.

Richard N. Matzen, Sr.

To my parents "Jack" and Margaret Lang who with their generation have taught me the need for prevention; to my sister Margaret Ann, and my extended family; and most importantly to my wife Lisa and our children Jonathan, Katherine, William, and Daniel, whose generation will benefit most from the principles contained herein.

Richard S. Lang

Acknowledgements

There are so many persons both known and unknown to us, particularly the staff at the Mosby–Year Book and individual authors' support staff, that it is impossible to be complete in listing everyone who deserves our sincere thanks.

Thanks must be expressed to Thomas Manning who approached us four years ago to see if we had interest in such a text. Tom was the prime mover in the early days of getting us off the mark and building a table of contents. His energy and foresight are very much appreciated. We are indebted also to George Stamathis for having the faith to pick up the option for Mosby–Year Book to publish this work, and for talented editors Carolyn Malik, Chris Murphy, Stephanie Manning, and James Shanahan for their close support, daily assistance, and insights.

A grant from the Emil Buehler Trust enabled Dr. Matzen not to only afford more time for this effort but to fund the gathering and execution of materials. The interest and encouragement of their board is deeply appreciated.

We are indebted of course to our contributing authors whose efforts make this text possible. We trust they will find reward in its culmination and in their contribution in this field.

This work could not have been easily accomplished without the close support, understanding, and talents of an excellent secretarial staff. Theresa Bloom and Sharon McFadden have been indispensable in this regard. The staff of the Cleveland Clinic Foundation Library has gone far afield in their very direct and personal assistance, as has the other preventive medicine section support staff.

Lastly, and perhaps most importantly, we appreciate the devotion and support of our spouses, E. Patricia Matzen and Lisa R. Kraemer who have shielded us from interruptions both social and otherwise and have been a continual source of encouragement in the most difficult times. And to our children Prudence, Annie, Richard, Katherine, and Patricia, and Jonathan, Katherine, William, and Daniel, our thanks for the support and understanding of our preoccupation they have shown.

CONTENTS

Part I

PRINCIPLES OF PREVENTIVE MEDICINE AND CLINICAL PREVENTION

Chapter 1

PREVENTIVE MEDICINE TODAY—DEFINITION, MISSION, AND MANPOWER

Richard N. Matzen, Sr.

"One day while listening to Beethoven's Ninth Symphony, I suddenly realized that maybe you can't tell someone what preventive medicine is, just like you can't teach someone to compose beautiful music. You just give people the basic tools and hope with years of practice that they are able to master the concepts."

T.W. GRACE[5]

OVERVIEW

The term *preventive medicine* several decades ago brought to mind the traditional School of Public Health, infectious disease control, sanitary engineering, occupational health, and all those disciplines that have been the concerns of governmental agencies and, to a lesser extent, volunteer groups. The term now is used in almost all the specialties of medicine by the public and government (legislative bodies) in a much broader context, addressing those illnesses, diseases, and conditions that are seen in the practice of medicine in the office on a daily basis as well as in the "traditional" sense. With the widespread use of the term by persons of different concerns and views of the world, the term has become personalized so that one person's meaning may not be another's. This results in a lack of understanding between people trying to communicate, and indeed it has been difficult to define the evolving term *preventive medicine*. Everyone has a general sense of what it is, but it lacks clear definition, much like the phrase "motherhood and apple pie." We will define the term more specifically in this chapter and see where we are in this expanding discipline, a discipline that is the appropriate concern of *all* practicing physicians regardless of specialty and not just the few who devote all their professional time to it.

The chapters that follow go on to address prevention in a practical sense so that this book may be useful for the practicing physician, medical school faculty, and educators in various residencies. We have attempted to address issues and fields of medicine that even by today's standards have been unaddressed or underdeveloped regarding prevention, and we hope this creative thinking will be both apparent and useful. Prevention must become a part of the philosophy of the practitioner, all practitioners, if it is to succeed as a discipline. This book has specifically and intentionally not been designed to cover those areas that are traditionally in the domain of what is generally called "public health." Those areas have a large body of sophisticated literature extant already. The definition of *clinical preventive medicine* cited below is probably as specific a one as exists and for our purposes of clarification, a very good one in regard to the purpose of this text—the delivery of preventive medicine in the office of the physician who is not a preventive medicine specialist.

On January 9 and 10, 1989, a special meeting of representatives to the House of Delegates of the AMA from various preventive medicine organizations was held at the Carter Center in Atlanta, Georgia. The organizations represented were the American College of Preventive Medicine, Aerospace Medical Association, American College of Occupational Medicine, American Association of Public Health Physicians, and Association of Preventive Medicine Residents. One of the purposes of that meeting was to develop a definition of *clinical preventive medicine (CPM)*. This was accomplished using as a basis for that definition one that appeared as a part of a clinical preventive medicine survey conducted by the Board of Preventive Medicine. This board certifies candidates by examination as having completed the required training and proven to be competent in this field just as other medical specialty boards certify in their respective fields, e.g., internal medicine. A candidate can now select a particular track within preventive medicine to concentrate his or her studies, be examined, and certified (more than one examination can be taken for certification). Preventive medicine board examinations are now given in aerospace medicine, occupational medicine, and public health and general preventive medicine. This "summit" meeting forwarded the definition to the board, recommending that the board develop an additional examination to demonstrate special competence in CPM as another of the examinations offered for certification. The examination could be taken by a current board certified individual in preventive medicine as well to demonstrate special competence in CPM in addition to his or her original field of concentration (e.g., occupational medicine). The summit meeting also recommended that physicians certified by other boards with an MPH (Master of Public Health) and 1 year of residency in CPM be eligible for that examination. Although the definition was devised for this purpose, it is quite clearly one that could be applied, with minor change of emphasis, to *all* clinical practice. Therefore we propose to use this definition to define the "field of play" on which all the players may perform: obstetrics/gynecology and pediatrics (both long-time practitioners of prevention), cardiology, endocrinology, psychiatry, etc., and of course foremost those specialists in internal and family medicine who are so fundamental to health care delivery. No one is excluded from the game, and all specialties can be said to be "in play."

Clinical preventive medicine defined

"Clinical preventive medicine (CPM) is an integral part of preventive medicine concerned with the maintenance and promotion of health and the reduction of risk factors which result in injury and disease. CPM is practiced in the clinical setting through the assessment of risk factors to disease and injury and the application of preventive interventions. The CPM practitioner may be involved in risk reduction programs for individuals, communities, employees, or other populations.

Clinical preventive medicine specialists have the knowledge and skills necessary to accomplish the following:

A. Assess risk of individuals for disease, using techniques such as screening and health risk assessment tools.

B. Implement interventions to modify or eliminate individuals' risk for disease/injury, using biologic, behavioral, and environmental approaches.

C. Organize and manage practice settings to facilitate the integration and monitoring of personal preventive services and be an advocate for health promotion activities for the individual.

D. Apply risk assessment, risk reduction, and media techniques to communities and populations including employee groups: be an advocate for health promotion and a resource for information about prevention strategies in the community.

E. Evaluate the effectiveness of individual and community risk reduction techniques and be a consultant to physicians, industry, and government for program development and evaluation."[1]

Delivery of preventive medical care

One should not infer from the foregoing that there are no physicians trained in, capable of, or practicing in CPM, because there are many. They are the current board-certified preventive-medicine physicians, those who, in addition, hold another board certification (e.g., internal medicine), and those who, by virtue of philosophy of practice and dedication to the field, have accumulated this knowledge and experience. The recommendations emphasize the *clinical* aspect of preventive medicine and recognize it as a particular (and enlarging) preventive medicine board subset, as is the case, for example, with aerospace medicine. Many pioneers in the clinical application of preventive skills used in office practice and primary care are from other disciplines. The cadre of certified specialists in preventive medicine is very small, however, and probably will remain so for the next decade.

As suggested previously, all physicians regardless of discipline can and should practice CPM. These skills may be gained by reading, attending courses, etc., and can be learned not only while in training but also while in practice. The primary care physician, for example, may learn these skills to employ in his practice even to the degree that he or she could become board eligible if not certified. This physician's practical goal would be to apply the appropriate preventive concepts to his or her particular practice. *CPM practitioner* is also used to refer to the preventive medicine specialist who receives "macro training" in formal residency programs to fulfill board qualification requirements. That training includes in-depth training generic to the boards, such as in statistics, which may not be necessary to applied prevention as employed by the generalist. In the latter case the physician has picked certain parts of the total training program of the board-qualified specialist to become skilled in order to deliver the best care to his patient group. Both are included in the term *CPM practitioner*.

Not all persons certified by the Board of Preventive

Medicine are members of the College of Preventive Medicine, but the number of certified college members and their distribution in the several fields of employment illustrate the relative paucity of specialists in this field. The number of certified college members in each field of primary interest is: aerospace medicine, 252; general preventive medicine, 328; occupational medicine, 318; public health, 179; and general preventive medicine and public health, 233. The total is 1,310. Contrast this with your own specialty organization size.

Of the college members, 385 were working in government, 219 were working in universities, industry and business employed 216, 89 were in the military services, and 401 gave no answer as to primary site of employment. The office of the college believes that the number of the military may be inaccurate and some of the government employees may actually be military.* Manpower issues will be further explored at the end of this chapter. If preventive medicine is to be delivered to patients in their day-to-day care, it falls to the training programs of other disciplines to incorporate into those residency years an overlying philosophy of prevention, if not discrete blocks of time in the discipline. More clinically oriented preventive medicine specialists must be trained to interact with their clinical colleagues to facilitate this training.

The key players must be the primary care deliverers, whether they be in "general practice," certified in family practice, or in internal medicine. These are the care givers most people expect to meet their needs and their families' needs. Because preventive medicine by definition suggests the discovery of disease *potential* or a disease or condition at an *asymptomatic stage,* the person in medicine most likely to do this is the physician who knows the patient (and, one hopes, the family) for a long time. Their genetic history, social/economic circumstances, and folk ways affect the individual's predisposition and susceptibility to clinical conditions. The paradigm would be the late nineteenth and early twentieth century family physician in a small rural town. The industrial age unsettled the family of the twentieth century, and society now finds the family not only unstable as a unit, but also unstable in its geographic location and social/financial security.

To replace that old paradigm we must cultivate acute quick-read primary care givers who are better trained than ever before and are renaissance people skilled not only in medicine, but also in economics and culture, for example, to appreciate and evaluate all these forces that affect the patient's life, may produce illness and, by modification, facilitate prevention. What an exceedingly "complete physician" he or she must be! This core of primary care givers is asked to undertake the traditional physician's role and a "preventist," not to mention gate-keeper, humanist, and

spiritual adviser. This demands the best and brightest. It is up to those bodies of governance to ensure that the reward is equal to the task asked of these people. In addition, the medical schools and those of us engaged in residency training in *all* fields must ensure that the physician graduating to patient care responsibility is up to the task.

It is here, at the training level, that the qualified or certified specialist in preventive medicine could be employed to maximize the use of the talents of a group still in short supply. This specialist may also be responsible for research, such as to determine whether certain screening is cost effective, to learn whether certain vaccines hold promise in eradicating disease, to weigh the role of genetics in disease prevention, or to determine whether career counseling at an early age results in happier, more productive, and healthier individuals.

To date, the financial rewards to the practitioner of preventive medicine have been relatively low on the scale of physician remuneration, turning aside many who might otherwise find satisfaction in this field. Reimbursement to the primary care giver for delivery of preventive medicine is also minimal at best. For society's good (perhaps even financial well-being), we must increase the incentive for today's medical graduates to enter this discipline. Government may find that supporting an increased number of slots in preventive medicine training programs would support the common good. We need to increase the numbers of specialists in this field to produce the educators of the next generation of physicians as soon as possible.

Primary, secondary, and tertiary prevention

There are levels of positive interference in the evolution of a morbid state or disease:

Primary prevention. The prevention of the occurrence of a disease, condition, or injury. Examples: the use of polio or measles vaccine; the control of pollution or exposures that would result in morbidity.

Secondary prevention. The early detection of the potential for the development of a disease or condition or the existence of a disease while asymptomatic to allow positive interference to prevent, postpone, or attenuate the symptomatic clinical state. Example: the prophylactic use of INH in tuberculosis in a person recently converted to a tuberculin-positive state.

Tertiary prevention. The treatment of an existing symptomatic disease process or condition to ameliorate its effects, delay or prevent its progress, and prevent complications of the underlying process. Example: the close control of diabetes to prevent its complications.

Screening

Prevention implies detection, and the discussion of detection immediately leads to consideration of the means of detection. Screening is an important tool in detection.

---

*From data supplied by Denise Cohen, membership coordinator, American College of Preventive Medicine, Spring, 1992.

Screening can be done on an individual basis over a period of years, tailoring that screening to the particular needs of the individual patient. Screening can be done with a subset of patients with similar characteristics and risks. It can be done on a practice-wide basis, or it can address units of population (so-called mass screening). Whatever the need or the case, certain principles should be applied to the planning of that screening. These principles were documented in a World Health Organization paper by Wilson and Jungner in 1968.[14] The physician concerned with screening should keep this reference at hand. This statement is directly quoted from their work, as it is so well stated it could only suffer by abstraction:

"The central idea of early disease detection and treatment is essentially simple. However, the path to its successful achievement (on the one hand, bringing to treatment those with previously undetected diseases and, on the other, avoiding harm to those persons not in need of treatment) is far from simple, though sometimes it may appear deceptively easy. For this reason we have devoted this section to a reasonably full discussion of a number of points that might be regarded as guides to planning case-finding. This is especially important when case-finding is carried out by a public health agency, where the pitfalls may be more numerous than when screening is performed by a personal physician. For ease of description rather than from dogma we have called these points collectively 'principles.' The following is an attempt to elaborate on at least some of these principles:

World Health Organization Definition

1. The condition sought should be an important health problem.
2. There should be an accepted treatment for patients with recognized disease.
3. Facilities for diagnosis and treatment should be available.
4. There should be a recognizable latent or early symptomatic stage.
5. There should be a suitable test or examination.
6. The test should be acceptable to the population.
7. The natural history of the condition, including development from latent to declared disease, should be adequately understood.
8. There should be an agreed policy on whom to treat as patients.
9. The cost of case-finding (including diagnosis and treatment of patients diagnosed) should be economically balanced in relation to possible expenditure on medical care as a whole.
10. Case-finding should be a continuing process and not a 'once and for all' project."

Their text goes on to elaborate each of the principles listed. This small book (or large pamphlet) is difficult to obtain but is in university libraries. Despite its date, it is *not* dated material, and the principles remain as relevant as ever. If you are concerned with screening, this work, *Principles and Practice of Screening for Disease,* is well worth consulting.

Selective vs. mass screening

Selective screening is much more desirable than mass screening. An example of this superiority is the National Tuberculosis Association's (NTA's) use of the mobile chest x-ray screening program as a mass screening method in the first half of this century. The goal of the NTA was to eradicate tuberculosis in our society by finding cases to isolate and treat, and thus remove the risk of further communication of the disease. Along with the patch test, generally used in the schools, the mobile van with x-ray equipment was stationed at target locations and brought to businesses for screening. Annual x-ray examinations were encouraged, and the association waged an effective and massive campaign of public education about the disease over many decades. In its early years, by most measures, it could be said to be cost effective in waging war on the personal and financially devastating drain imposed on the individual, the family, and society as a whole by the "white plague."

As nutrition, sanitary conditions, housing, and effective treatment improved, especially after World War II, when the modern antituberculous antibiotics became available, cases became more and more sparse. In the 1960s the NTA found that the yield of this program was minimal and the cost appreciable, but that there were pockets of people in the general population where the disease still existed to a greater degree. The mass screening of the mobile van was abandoned in favor of selective screening of this population subset. This group was found in the less fortunate, poor, homeless, and derelict members of our society, and screening (by x-ray examination) therefore was limited to prisons, city hospitals serving the poor, and programs aimed at the indigent. The mobile unit program of state and local societies was given up only against fierce resistance by members of the "TB Society." This is a testament not only to the devotion of the members, but to the thoroughness of the educational campaign the association waged over the years.

Each practicing physician must examine selective screening and apply it to his or her patient population with discrimination. One physician's needs may differ considerably from his or her colleague's practice and needs in the same city. A target subset within a practice may not differ by age alone but by race as well. For example, in our practice, which tends to be international, the subset of Japanese who are here for a limited time in various manufacturing enterprises is not only subject to the high incidence of gastric cancer, to which this group is genetically and culturally predisposed, but this group also demands continuation of the screening program they receive at home. We do not even consider such screening for our average patient. A similar example is the Arab from the Middle East who may well be considered to have a kidney stone unless proven otherwise. As the world gets smaller, many of us even now are living in a global village, a trend that can only accelerate. Not only an awareness, but also a knowledge of geographic, ethnic, and racial predispositions are becoming necessities to practice medicine well (see Part

VII, Chapters 33-37).

The private clinical practice also provides a setting for making good decisions about cost effectiveness to the individual. The personal physician is in the best position to know that a patient, by virtue of his genetic makeup, personality, stresses, behavioral characteristics, and financial resources, is best served with particular interval screening procedures. Ideally the physician not only will advise the patient about the continuing screening process, but also will ask the patient for input and his or her perception of needs.

Cost effectiveness becomes a critical issue when the common good is considered in our time of shrinking resources. Many practitioners therefore use the random care visit to address a preventive care concern, such as by taking blood pressure, often without charge. Screening must be done with circumspection and logic, weighed not only for cost but also for effectiveness—has the proposed screen proven to be of worth in your experience with the particular use to which you wish to put it?

A guide to screening and positive preventive interventions

In 1989 a landmark guide was published as the result of 4 years of intense work on the part of 22 expert panelists and the supportive work of hundreds of people, public and private agencies, professional organizations, and others in medicine and related health care fields. The panelists made up the U.S. Preventive Services Task Force, which was commissioned in 1984 by the Department of Health and Human Services to examine not only the merits of the periodic health examination, but also the available methods of screening for disease, and advise about the use, effectiveness, and positive clinical intervention that might result from such examinations and screening. The resulting publication, *A Guide to Clinical Preventive Services,* Report of the U.S. Preventive Services Task Force, is now readily available (see Resources at the end of the chapter) and should be a part of every physician's library.[13]

This milestone report provides a discussion of 169 preventive interventions targeting 60 clinical conditions. The conclusions reached in evaluating each intervention are of course "panel opinions," and the report acknowledges and cites the opinions of other bodies that at times vary from its own. In addition, each conclusion is meant to be a "best opinion" of the task force in light of medical knowledge as it existed at the time of its convening, with full recognition that there would be new evidence on the subjects regarding screening, positive intervention, treatment, and so on. In recognition of this continual evolution of knowledge and in a continuing effort to place an educated opinion at the disposal of the practicing physician, a panel has been appointed to continue to monitor all the issues addressed, as well as new developments in other diseases that could be added to the original target group.[15]

Just as various medical colleges at times adhere to screening principles contrary to these guidelines, the individual practitioner may vary his practice to suit the circumstances of his own patients in light of his clinical experience. Some of the authors of the chapters that follow express their own opinions, at times in agreement and at times at variance with other sources. It is up to each physician to be an "informed consumer" and employ these interventions as well as possible to his or her patients' circumstances. Nonetheless, we all should appreciate and be familiar with the work of the authors of "the guide" (see Chapter 5 regarding practices in other countries).

Some of the issues addressed in this text are not addressed by the guide, and others in the guide are addressed here in more detail based on the author's experience. Still others are cited as areas of concern that are not particularly considered to relate to prevention. These issues are presented to stimulate the practitioner to think of prevention in relation to *all* conditions and diseases, and to contemplate their etiologies, which, through evolution and with time, often after a long time, result in a symptomatic condition.

The guidelines given by this textbook, the previously discussed recommendations, and the recommendations of the various colleges and volunteer health associations should be used to screen your patients in an organized way.

Devising an office screening program

All the recommendations regarding screening are useful only if they are used by those in practice. Patients and society increasingly consider prevention, just as much as diagnosis and treatment, to be the responsibility of the physician. Indeed, education of the patient, directly or by a designated physician extender or other professional (e.g., dietitian, registered nurse, etc.), is a part of total patient care, and in the specialty of preventive medicine it assumes a vital role in the delivery of health care.

To deliver such care in a consistent manner in office practice requires establishing histories, physicals, and check-off sheets of reminders for screens, and making this a basic part of the patient record. Some references are listed in "Resources" at the end of this chapter that can be used to help you address your own system and risk assessment, and to help in the upgrading, updating, or total revision of it. This entire matter is explored in depth in Chapter 8, Integrating Clinical Preventive Services into Office Practice, and in Chapter 9, The Preventive History and Physical Examination.

The Regenstrief Institute for Health Care and the Department of Medicine of Indiana University School of Medicine with the Department of Statistics of Purdue University have devised a computer medical record system that provides for reminders on request to initiate screening procedures on a schedule.[12] This particular system also was designed to be a reminder of tertiary prevention steps. One might consider this approach, depending on personal computer sophistication and comfort level as well as existing or planned office systems. If such a record system is attractive, a search of the literature on stored systems and reminders would be appropriate.

In the Section of Primary Care of the Department of Internal Medicine at the Cleveland Clinic Foundation, a flow sheet or checklist of reminders to the physician is a part of the chart of all employee patients of the foundation. These physicians find it useful not only as a reminder but also because it eliminates the onerous task of searching the chart to determine when something was last done. One could easily devise such a sheet (see Chapters 8 and 9).

Healthy People 2000

A second major work published in the last few years under the auspices of the U.S. Department of Health and Human Services, Public Health Service (the first being the *Guide to Clinical Preventive Services*) that deserves a place on your office bookshelf is *Healthy People 2000 — National Health Promotion and Disease Prevention Objectives*.[8] This report is available as the full report (a reference tome) or in a summary form of 153 pages (see Resources). This book documents a national strategy for significantly improving the nation's health and quality of life in this decade by the year 2000. The objectives are thought to be both important and attainable but obviously cannot be attained unless all of us involved in the delivery of health care have agreed to these goals and are aware of the need to implement them. The document sets a splendid vision of how things could be. This book is important to those of us involved with preventive medicine, not only for what it says, but also for the unstated message it (and the guide) delivers. That message is overriding concern among our nation's leaders in health care and our elected representatives with prevention.

The reader will find in many subsequent chapters reference to the document's contents. Consider the summary list of objectives by title to determine where your interest lies and whether these issues pertain.

Healthy People 2000: Summary List of Objectives

---

1. Physical activity and fitness
2. Nutrition
3. Tobacco
4. Alcohol and other drugs
5. Family planning
6. Mental health and mental disorders
7. Violent and abusive behavior
8. Educational and community-based programs
9. Unintentional injuries
10. Occupational health and safety
11. Environmental health
12. Food and drug safety
13. Oral health
14. Maternal and infant health
15. Heart disease and stroke
16. Cancer
17. Diabetes and chronic disabling conditions
18. HIV infection
19. Sexually transmitted diseases
20. Immunization and infectious diseases
21. Clinical preventive services
22. Surveillance and data systems

Each of these objectives includes health-status objectives, risk-reduction objectives (as related to cited present baselines), and services and protection objectives. The goals to be reached by these strategies are the following:

1. Increase the span of healthy life for U.S. citizens.
2. Reduce health disparities among citizens.
3. Achieve access to preventive services for all.

Not only are all these issues addressed by age group (child, adolescent, adult, etc.), but also by races — notably the large groups in our diverse society (black Americans, Hispanic Americans, Asian and Pacific Islander Americans, and native Americans). Finally, a host of useful references accompany the document on these subjects; the references alone are of great use. (See Part VI: Specific Approaches to Different Patient Groups (Ages) and Part VII: Racial and Ethnic Considerations in Clinical Prevention, Chapters 27-37).

Preventive medicine as a specialty

Preventive medicine is one of the 24 recognized medical specialties represented in the American Board of Medical Specialties. Preventive medicine has been defined as a specialized field of medical practice:

". . . focusing on the health of defined populations in order to promote and maintain health and well being and prevent disease, disability, and premature death." [Task Force definition, National Conference on Graduate Education in Preventive Medicine, adopted in April 1980].

Working with large populations, as well as with individual patients, physicians trained in preventive medicine aim to preserve and promote good health, to prevent disease, injury and disability, and to facilitate early diagnosis and treatment of illness. Traditionally, physicians in preventive medicine have served as health planners and administrators, teachers of preventive medicine, researchers in preventive medicine, and clinicians applying preventive medicine in health care. The American Board of Preventive Medicine has certified physicians in this specialty since 1949.

Preventive medicine comprises four specialties: general preventive medicine, public health, occupational medicine, and aerospace medicine. However, there are only three board examinations, with general preventive medicine and public health being combined.

General preventive medicine. General preventive medicine is characterized by the study of, and intervention in, health and disease processes as they occur in communities or in other defined populations. These specialists develop strategies to assess risk factors, to promote health-enhancing behavior (primary prevention), to facilitate early diagnosis and treatment of disease and injury (secondary prevention), and to foster rehabilitation of persons with disabilities (tertiary prevention).[4]

Public health. The practice of public health is characterized by participation in activities designed to organize community-based strategies of health promotion and disease prevention for individuals and populations. Specialists in public health and general preventive medicine work in many settings, including private clinics, local, state, and federal departments of health; academic and health care institutions, group practice, and research organizations.

Occupational medicine. Occupational medicine focuses on the health of workers, their ability to perform work, and the physical and chemical environments in the workplace. These specialists also consider specific health-promotion and disease-prevention programs in their workplace activities. Physicians in occupational medicine have specialized knowledge of toxicology, radiation, mechanical stresses, and the psychologic effects of the workplace.[10] The majority of board-certified occupational medicine physicians are employed by large corporations or are affiliated with universities. Some are employed as epidemiologists, and others work as medical directors, responsible for the administration of health services and health-promotion programs in industrial settings.[2]

Aerospace medicine. Aerospace medicine is oriented toward special or hazardous environments associated with aviation and space. Specialty training for physicians in this field addressed the diagnosis, prevention, and treatment of disorders associated with these environments and with the adaptive systems designed to support life under such conditions. Many physicians in aerospace medicine work for the military, airline medical departments, federal agencies, or major aerospace companies.

In addition to the knowledge of basic and clinical sciences and the skills common to all physicians, distinctive aspects of preventive medicine include knowledge of and competence in the following:

- Epidemiology and biostatistics
- Administration (including planning, organization, management, financing, and evaluation of health programs)
- Environmental and occupational health
- Application of social and behavioral factors in health and disease
- Application of primary, secondary, and tertiary preventive measures within clinical medicine[3]

Preventive medicine is one of the few specialties in which a shortage of physicians is projected; a number of studies have supported this prediction. The Graduate Medical Education National Advisory Committee predicted a 25% shortage into the 1990s.[6] This continuing shortage of physicians trained in preventive medicine and public health has been recognized in studies by HRSA[7] and the Institute of Medicine.[11] Indeed, the shortage is with us now. The fact that "preventists" are likely to drive older Chevies is certainly not the only reason. There simply are not enough training programs or students within existing programs to meet current *clinical* needs, much less to meet the shortage that will be upon us if a serious effort is made to meet the goals of Healthy People 2000. Many of those certified in preventive medicine are immediately absorbed into the teaching and research programs of the schools of public health, governmental posts (city, county, state, national, and armed forces), and industry as already noted. It is not yet apparent to graduating medical students that there is a *clinical* application to preventive medicine and that indeed these clinicians often actually *do* practice medicine as do internists and others (See Manpower, Training, and Career Issues for the Specialist in Preventive Medicine, p. 10).

Clinical decision making is a rapidly growing "specialty" or skill with identifiable, excellent training programs. Those who use the computer tools of clinical decision making represent a mix of specialists (surgeons, internists, preventists, etc.) who employ prevention in their specialties. Appropriately skilled persons strive to make correct clinical decisions and hence prevent untoward sequelae that result from a "less than best" decision. This field requires clinical knowledge and skill, computer knowledge, and, what has so long been the core of the traditional MPH-trained specialist in preventive medicine, statistics and probabilities. It is not hard to imagine a future board certification in clinical decision making that requires an additional year or more of training as the field expands, knowledge accrues, and expectations increase.

There are more than 70 preventive medicine training programs in the United States and Canada, but these programs are small and graduate only approximately 120 specialists per year.[2] Board certification requires 3 years: a clinical year, an academic year, and a practicum year. A fourth year of training, teaching, research, or practice is needed before a board examination in preventive medicine can be taken.

The clinical year may be in internal medicine, pediatrics, family practice, or another field of primary care. It may also be a traditional rotating internship or transitional year. The academic year may lead to an MPH (Master of Public Health) or other advanced degree and is spent in a school of public health, medical, or other graduate school. The academic year gives the preventive medicine physician a foundation in epidemiology, biostatistics, health services administration, environmental health, and social and behavioral medicine. It is possible at this point to branch off into study leading to a PhD, DrPH. (Doctor of Public Health), or ScD (Doctor of Science).[2]

The practicum year gives residents supervised practical experience and continued education in their field of specialty. The year of practicum could be spent in occupational health, aerospace medicine, or general preventive medicine in a hospital, health department, or ambulatory care setting.

The specialty examinations leading to board certification are given by the American Board of Preventive Medicine. Any (or more than one) of three specialty examinations may be taken: (1) a combined exam in public health and general preventive medicine, (2) aerospace medicine, or (3) occupational medicine.

Professional organizations

There are seven major organizations in this field: the American College of Preventive Medicine, the Association of Teachers of Preventive Medicine, the Aerospace Medical Association, the American College of Occupational and Environmental Medicine, the American Public Health Association, the American Association of Public Health Physicians, and the American Occupational Medical Association. Their journals may be found in any medical library, and annual meeting announcements are listed in the meeting issue of the *Journal of the American Medical Association*. Programs can be obtained to determine whether the meeting will address areas of your particular interest. Other associations involved with preventive medicine are the American Board of Preventive Medicine, the American Council of Graduate Medical Education, the American Association of Medical Colleges, the American Medical Association, the Association of Preventive Medicine Residents, the Association of Schools of Public Health, and the Association of State and the Territorial Health Officers.

MANPOWER, TRAINING, AND CAREER ISSUES FOR THE SPECIALIST IN PREVENTIVE MEDICINE

This chapter previously stated that there is and will continue to be a shortage of specialists in preventive medicine, and that many such specialists are absorbed by the universities and the government, leaving fewer to practice clinical preventive medicine in the area of primary care. The concern was also put forth that too few were engaged in teaching nonpreventive medicine board candidates and that the specialists in the field were unavailable because of the manpower shortage to assist in the instruction of primary care specialists in an organized program to be integrated with the residency training of the latter.

The purpose of this part of the chapter is to present data and to provide information on the careers available in preventive medicine so that students early in their medical training may intelligently consider the option of making this field a career. It is certainly one of the frontiers of medicine with great opportunity. It remains to be seen whether the government will perceive that funding the expansion of training programs is vital to providing the infrastructure that will produce a truly "healthy" health care

system to evolve in this era of sparse resources. Many have projected that preventive medicine will decrease medical care costs in the future, the caveat being that it will require a large up-front investment or "front loading."

Hersey, Boudreau, and Zeid[9] at Battelle recently completed a manpower study for the Centers for Disease Control (CDC) and the Health Resources and Services Administration (HRSA) Bureau of Health Professions. The CDC and bureau are to be applauded for their commission. The material presented is important to their missions, but it also deserves wider dissemination.

A review of selected representative data from this source makes up this section of the chapter, and the factual data and all charts and graphs in this section are from this source, *Practicing Preventive Medicine: A National Survey of Preventive Medicine Residency Graduates*.

Two subsets of preventive medicine, aerospace medicine and occupational medicine, have been studied previously so they were not included in the manpower study. The subject groups were public health and general preventive medicine. The latter group included both those who are involved in traditional preventive medicine and those involved in clinical preventive medicine. The general preventive medicine group makes up more than two thirds of the graduates of residency programs in preventive medicine.

The objectives of the study were to describe the professional activities of graduates, identify the training perceived as important, examine the training grant program (HRSA Title VII PMR) effect, and help improve priorities for the training of graduates.

The study was conducted in the spring and summer of 1991. The methodology was to take a census of preventive medicine residency (PMR) graduates from 43 U.S. PMR programs in general preventive medicine (GPM) and public health (PH) and combined programs by questionnaire. These programs were from the CDC, university programs (both with and without schools of public health), and programs that were affiliated with health departments. The response rate was 75% among PMR graduates. In these 10 years, there were 1070 PMR graduates from these 43 PMR programs, or roughly only 107 in any year on average.

The CDC PMR is the largest single program and represented 13.8% of graduates receiving questionnaires. (1979-1989). Eight public health school PMRs represented 37.4% of residents, 23 medical school PMRs graduated 32.3% of residents, 9 health department PMRs 12.1%, and 2 military PMRs 4.4%. To control for career maturation, the analysis was of two groups, those graduating between 1979 and 1984 and those graduating between 1985 and 1989.

The size of the CDC program has been noted. Of the large university-based programs, there were only two graduating 10 or more residents a year. Both are affiliated with schools of public health; they are Johns Hopkins Uni-

Table 1-1. Distribution of PMRs in the study

Program	Earlier 1979-84 n	Recent 1985-89 n	Total 1979-89 n	% of total
CDC PMR	54	64	118	14.8
School of public health (8 PMRs)	128	170	298	37.4
Medical school PMR (23 PMRs)	73	175	248	31.1
Health dept. PMR (9 PMRs)	41	50	91	11.4
Military PMR (2 PMRs)	14	28	42	5.3
Non-CDC PMRs	256	423	679	85.2
All PMR (includes CDC PMR)	310	487	797	100

Adapted from Hersey J, Boudreau C, Zeid A: *Practicing preventive medicine: a national survey of preventive medicine residency graduates,* Arlington, Va, 1992, Battelle.

versity and the University of Washington. They produce a quarter of all graduates. There are seven moderate-size university programs; three are affiliated with schools of public health (University of California-Berkeley, University of Hawaii, and Tulane University). The other four are affiliated with medical schools (Loma Linda University, University of Maryland, Mt. Sinai (NYC), and University of North Carolina). They graduate four to nine residents per year and represent 21.6% of the total. There were 21 PMR programs in the small-program group, with three affiliated with schools of public health (University of Michigan, University of California-San Diego, and University of California-Los Angeles). The remaining 18 were affiliated with medical schools. *These smaller university programs graduated 23.8% of the total, but most importantly represented the fastest-growing programs.*

The total number of respondents from the training programs that make up the study group, and their percentage of graduates, is given in Table 1-1.

The study team found that even if nonrespondents were included, the findings would not be altered greatly.

Involvement in public health, teaching, research, and clinical care of PMR graduates

The first part of this chapter projected that many graduates were absorbed into universities, government, and activities other than clinical preventive medicine. In addition, it was presumed that there is and would be a shortage in teachers of preventive medicine in particular for students in nonpreventive medicine residencies. This study defines where graduates have spent their career time and the percentage of that time devoted to different activities, such as clinical care or research. The study indicates that individuals do perform *several* services, such as teaching,

research, *and* patient care.

It might be presumed that *where* one trained would predispose him or her toward a career site, and it did; 71.4% of 1979-1984 graduates of a military PMR continued to work in the military. A medical school, school of public health, or university was the work site of a quarter of university-based PMRs; 48.8% of health department PMRs worked in state or local government facilities. Finally, of the CDC graduates, 68.5% of the early graduates worked in the federal government, and the great majority of those at CDC. (This must attest to the fact that these graduates found work there fulfilling and that the CDC program was highly successful in training persons to fill its own needs.)

In the area of clinical preventive medicine or patient care, 68.2% of non-CDC graduates provide patient care. A quarter of medical school PMRs and public health school PMRs worked primarily in a patient care setting, and most often this was in *private practice.* Table 1-2 shows the primary work affiliation of PMR graduates from different programs. In Table 1-3 the site of the practice of medical care is broken down into private practice and hospital, and public clinic and hospital, with the great majority in private practice. (However, the total in medical care is only about 18.5% or roughly 146 graduates in 10 years.)

As noted previously, a response in a particular category does not mean that the respondent confines his or her effort to only that category, such as clinical or public health. In Table 1-6, the amount of time spent in patient care of various PMR graduates is given. Again CDC PMR graduates are less involved in patient care than graduates of other programs. This table also shows that health department persons are as involved in patient care as other non-CDC groups.

There are two pie charts listed as Figs. 1-1 and 1-2 that show the mean work allocation of both recent and earlier PMR graduates. Whether the differences in the two groups are due to stage of career (earlier graduates tend to do more administration) or change in career aims (later graduates are more engaged in research) is not obvious. Overall the time spent in different activities is interesting, and the table shows that non-CDC PMRs are contributing most to direct clinical patient care.

Similar tables in this report address time spent in research and in administration, but that is less of our concern in this text. A clue to the magnitude of these endeavors is provided in the pie charts.

Without going into the extensive data also provided in the text, we can conclude that *graduates are satisfied or very satisfied with their positions and work, at a rate of 85% to 95%.* With the CDC PMRs, the figure is above 90%.

Income

The Battelle Report also presents three tables of income, which may interest those considering this field as a

Table 1-2. Primary work affiliation of PMR graduates

Group		N	CDC	Other federal government	State or local health department	University	Medical care	Other/military
CDC PMR 1979-84	N	54	31	6	3	6	4	4
	%		57.4	11.1	5.6	11.1	7.4	7.4
CDC PMR 1985-89	N	64	43	4	11	6	0	0
	%		67.2	6.2	17.2	9.4	0	0
School of public health PMR 1985-89	N	126	6	11	16	36	33	24
	%		5.8	8.7	12.7	28.6	26.2	19.1
School of public health PMR 1985-89	N	170	12	17	33	43	32	33
	%		11.5	10.0	19.4	25.3	18.8	19.4
Medical school PMR 1979-84	N	72	1	6	15	18	19	13
	%		1.4	8.3	20.8	25.0	26.4	18.1
Medical school PMR 1985-89	N	171	9	15	32	49	40	26
	%		8.7	8.8	18.7	28.7	23.4	15.2
Health department PMR 1979-84	N	41	0	2	20	3	9	7
	%		0	4.9	48.8	7.3	21.9	17.1
Health department PMR 1985-89	N	50	2	1	29	5	6	7
	%		4.0	2.0	58.0	10.0	12.0	14.0
Military PMR 1979-84	N	14	0	0	2	0	2	10
	%		0	0	14.3	0	14.3	71.4
Military PMR 1985-89	N	28	0	0	1	0	1	26
	%		0	0	3.6	0	3.6	92.9

Adapted from Hersey J, Boudreau C, Zeid A: *Practicing preventive medicine: a national survey of preventive medicine residency graduates*, Arlington, Va, 1992, Battelle.

Table 1-3. Primary work affiliation of PMR graduates in medical care settings

Group		N	All medical care	Private practice	Private hospital	Public clinic/hospital	HMO
CDC PMR 1979-84	N	54	4	2	2	0	0
	%		7.4	3.7	3.7	0.0	0.0
CDC PMR 1985-89	N	64	0	0	0	0	0
	%		0	0.0	0.0	0.0	0.0
School of public health PMR 1979-84	N	126	33	17	5	5	6
	%		26.2	13.5	4.0	4.0	4.8
School of public health PMR 1985-89	N	170	32	10	6	11	5
	%		18.8	5.9	3.5	6.5	2.9
Medical school PMR 1979-84	N	72	19	16	0	1	3
	%		26.4	22.2	0.0	1.4	4.2
Medical school PMR 1985-89	N	171	40	12	17	2	9
	%		23.4	7.0	9.9	1.2	5.3
Health department PMR 1979-84	N	41	9	6	1	2	0
	%		21.9	14.6	2.4	4.9	0.0
Health department PMR 1985-89	N	50	6	4	2	0	0
	%		12.0	8.0	4.0	0.0	0.0
Military PMR 1979-84	N	14	2	1	0	1	0
	%		14.3	7.1	0.0	7.1	0.0
Military PMR 1985-89	N	28	1	1	0	0	0
	%		3.6	3.6	0.0	0.0	0.0

Adapted from Hersey J, Boudreau C, Zeid A: *Practicing preventive medicine: a national survey of preventive medicine residency graduates*, Arlington, Va, 1992, Battelle.

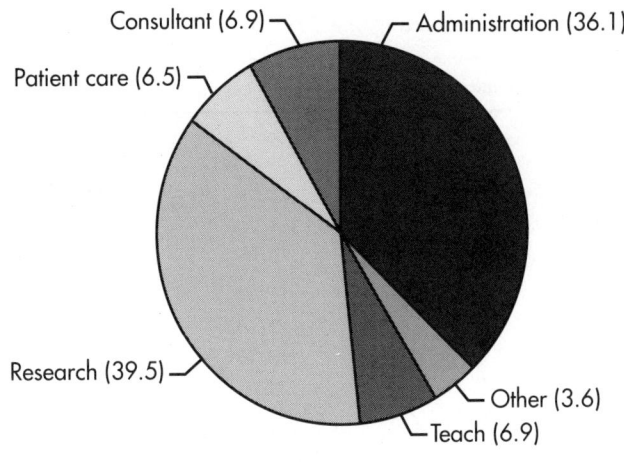

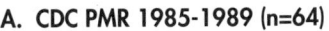

A. CDC PMR 1985-1989 (n=64)

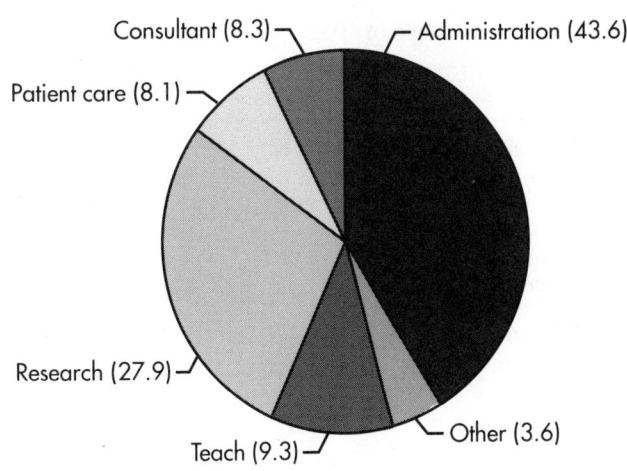

A. CDC PMR 1979-1984 (n=54)

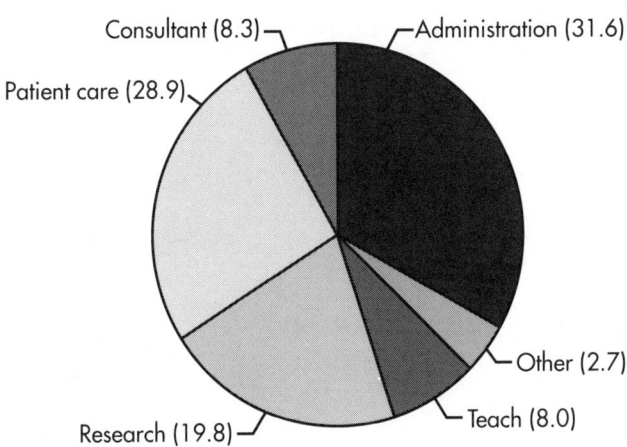

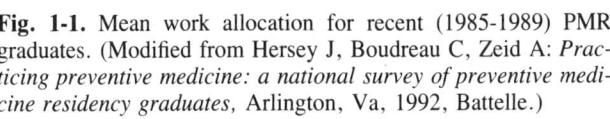

B. OTHER PMR 1985-1989 (n=420)

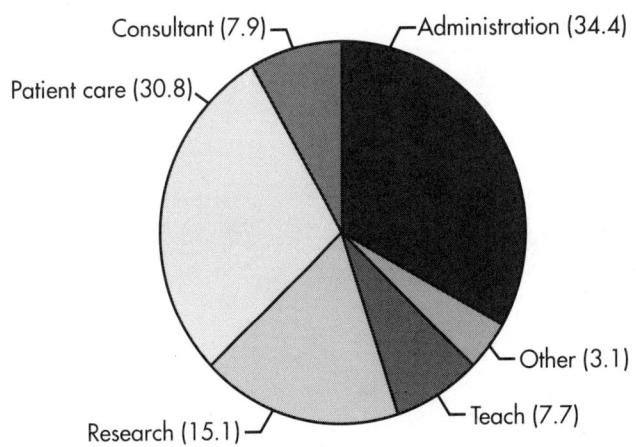

B. NON-CDC PMR 1979-1984 (n=250)

Fig. 1-1. Mean work allocation for recent (1985-1989) PMR graduates. (Modified from Hersey J, Boudreau C, Zeid A: *Practicing preventive medicine: a national survey of preventive medicine residency graduates,* Arlington, Va, 1992, Battelle.)

Fig. 1-2. Mean work allocation for earlier (1979-1984) PMR graduates. (Modified from Hersey J, Boudreau C, Zeid A: *Practicing preventive medicine: a national survey of preventive medicine residency graduates,* Arlington, Va, 1992, Battelle.)

career. There does not appear to be a linear correlation between income and job satisfaction. Income, of course, partly depends on one's employer/certification. In Tables 1-4 and 1-5 this is documented. Those in medical care showed the highest income. This may account for the groups trained at university public health departments doing better financially as they gravitate toward patient care.

Contributions to national health objectives

Job satisfaction appears to be high in this field, as previously noted. The reasons cannot be determined from this data, but certainly having time for one's family and the income levels play a role. Having a sense of mission and

contributing to the common good may play a part in that satisfaction, because this group of specialists contributes heavily to attaining the national health objectives as outlined in *Healthy People 2000.* This satisfaction comes from the role of the specialty: addressing the health problems, producing solutions, and delivering health care to large groups of people rather than to individuals. As shown in Table 1-6, however, these physicians often balance that broader mission ("macro" preventive medicine) with some time devoted to individual health care ("micro" preventive medicine), and each activity may help make the other more rewarding.

The Battelle report describes the contributions to na-

Table 1-4. Percentage of PMR graduates in different income categories by work setting

Gross annual income		Federal government	Health department	Academic setting	Medical care	Other/military
1979-84 graduates	N	**62**	**55**	**61**	**64**	**50**
Less than $50,000	%	1.6	3.6	14.8	14.1	22.0
$50,000 or more	%	98.3	96.4	85.2	85.9	78.8
$75,000 or more	%	80.6	63.6	65.6	71.9	64.0
$100,000 or more	%	17.7	5.5	39.3	48.4	34.0
$125,000 or more	%	0.6	0.0	16.4	29.7	20.0
1985-89 graduates	N	**102**	**104**	**101**	**77**	**88**
Less than $50,000	%	7.8	6.7	29.7	10.4	12.5
$50,000 or more	%	92.2	92.3	70.3	89.6	81.8
$75,000 or more	%	49.0	44.0	31.7	66.2	69.3
$100,000 or more	%	5.9	1.9	8.9	33.8	29.6
$125,000 or more	%	0.0	0.0	5.0	19.5	11.4

Table 1-5. Percentage of PMR graduates in various income groups by certification status

Board certification	N	Less than $50,000	$75,000 or more	$100,000 or more	$125,000 or more
1979-84 graduates					
No board	52	21.2	53.9	17.3	7.7
PM board only	94	9.6	67.0	19.2	8.5
PM + clinical board	56	7.1	76.7	41.1	17.9
Clinical board only	93	7.5	77.4	39.8	19.4
1985-89 graduates					
No board	127	22.8	43.3	13.4	6.3
PM board only	131	9.2	52.7	16.8	6.1
PM + clinical board	71	4.2	62.0	21.1	8.5
Clinical board only	147	13.6	50.3	10.9	5.4
All graduates					
No board	179	22.3	46.4	15.1	6.7
PM board only	225	9.3	58.7	17.8	7.1
PM + clinical board	127	3.1	68.5	29.9	12.6
Clinical board only	240	11.2	60.8	22.1	10.8

Adapted from Hersey J, Boudreau C, Zeid A: *Practicing preventive medicine: a national survey of preventive medicine residency graduates,* Arlington, Va, 1992, Battelle.

tional health objectives of physicians trained in preventive medicine. Two summary tables are included here. Table 1-7 shows both the number of physicians and percentage of the sample involved in various objectives, such as mental health, infectious disease, or chronic disease. Table 1-8 on p. 16 presents the number and percentage of those contributing to one or more national health objectives.

Motivation and training

This report provides insight into the motivation for entering preventive medicine and the training received at the various programs. Not surprisingly the single greatest reason for entering the field was to prevent disease. Of recent graduates, 81.3% of the CDC PMRs and 74.2% of the non-CDC PMRs gave this as a primary reason. Of the former, three fourths cited the opportunity to do research as well; of the latter, a little over half. The desire to influence policy was cited by a similar number in each group. A desire to help others, to teach, and to gain opportunities in international health were other significant but less dominant reasons given. Finally, a desire to administer public health programs and dissatisfaction with primary care were mentioned; these were mentioned most often by non-CDC trainees.

The respondents also rated the strengths and weaknesses of the various programs in detail. A good to excellent rating was given to training in clinical preventive medicine by the following percentage of recent graduates of each program: military, 71.4%; schools of public health, 57.8%; medical schools, 54.9%; health depart-

Table 1-6. Patient care involvement of PMR graduates

Group	N	Patient care involvement		Type of care		
		Percent engaged	Percent of time	Clinical preventive medicine	Primary care	Specialty care
CDC PMR 1979-84	54	38.9	8.1 (18.2)	11.2 (18.2)	44.8 (44.2)	39.5 (40.5)
CDC PMR 1985-89	64	39.1	6.9 (13.1)	21.6 (36.2)	35.8 (45.7)	42.6 (47.8)
School of public health PMR 1979-84	128	69.5	30.9 (33.9)	23.5 (27.5)	41.0 (38.4)	31.8 (41.0)
School of public health PMR 1985-89	170	63.5	25.4 (31.1)	32.7 (30.4)	51.8 (34.6)	13.3 (29.7)
Medical school PMR 1979-84	73	72.6	33.4 (32.3)	40.2 (35.7)	34.2 (33.9)	22.1 (36.9)
Medical school PMR 1985-89	175	69.7	35.7 (34.4)	34.4 (31.4)	46.5 (35.4)	18.3 (32.3)
Health department PMR 1979-84	41	51.2	35.1 (42.6)	29.3 (33.1)	52.8 (40.3)	17.9 (36.7)
Health department PMR 1985-89	50	66.0	24.5 (29.9)	35.1 (34.8)	41.8 (37.3)	18.6 (34.2)
Military PMR 1979-84	14	50.0	9.1 (14.8)	47.8 (49.5)	25.7 (42.8)	14.3 (37.8)
Military PMR 1985-89	28	82.1	17.2 (20.5)	63.0 (37.1)	28.0 (37.9)	8.9 (21.5)

Adapted from Hersey J, Boudreau C, Zeid A: *Practicing preventive medicine: a national survey of preventive medicine residency graduates,* Arlington, Va, 1992, Battelle.
Note: The first part of this table shows (1) the percentage of respondents who reported that they spend part of their average work week providing direct patient care; and (2) the mean percentage of the average work week that respondents spend in patient care. The last three columns of the table show (for those respondents who provide patient care) the mean allocation of total patient care time spent in the following patient care activities: (1) clinical preventive medicine (e.g., screening, immunization, behavioral counseling), (2) primary care, or (3) specialty or tertiary care. Standard deviations for these means are shown in parentheses.

Table 1-7. Contributions of PMR graduates to national health objectives

Contributions	All PMRs 1979-84		All PMRs 1985-89		Total 1979-89	
	N	%	N	%	N	%
Sample size	**310**	**100.0**	**487**	**100.0**	**797**	**100.0**
AIDS/STDS	106	34.2	208	42.7	318	39.4
Infectious disease	98	31.6	206	42.3	304	37.6
Chronic disease	93	30.0	182	37.4	275	34.5
Maternal and child health	89	28.7	141	29.0	230	28.9
Occupational health	60	19.4	109	12.4	169	21.2
Environmental health	63	20.3	89	18.3	152	19.1
Mental health	24	7.7	51	5.6	51	6.4
Other prevention	64	20.6	95	19.5	159	20.0
Epidemiology/surveillance	155	50.0	290	60.0	445	55.8
International health	67	21.6	94	19.3	161	20.2
Public primary care	60	19.4	121	24.9	181	22.7
Teaching preventive medicine	64	20.6	114	23.4	178	22.3

Adapted from Hersey J, Boudreau C, Zeid A: *Practicing preventive medicine: a national survey of preventive medicine residency graduates,* Arlington, Va, 1992, Battelle.
Note: Contributions include respondents who: (1) worked 25% or more, (2) initiated a program, (3) directed a program, or (4) published in an area.

Table 1-8. PMR graduates contributing to one or more national health objectives

| | | Number of health objectives | | |
Group		One or more	Two or more	Three or more
CDC PMR				
1979-84	N	51	35	15
(n=54)	%	94.4	64.8	27.8
CDC PMR				
1985-89	N	64	40	17
(n=64)	%	100.0	62.5	26.6
Non-CDC PMR				
1979-84	N	208	24	68
(n=248)	%	83.9	50.0	27.5
Non-CDC PMR				
1985-89	N	376	260	141
(n=420)	%	89.5	61.9	33.3

Adapted from Hersey J, Boudreau C, Zeid A: *Practicing preventive medicine: a national survey of preventive medicine residency graduates,* Arlington, Va, 1992, Battelle.
Contributions include respondents who: (1) worked 25% or more, (2) initiated a program, (3) directed a program, or (4) published in an area. Information about contributions was obtained for each of eight areas: AIDS/STDs, infectious disease, chronic disease, environmental health, maternal and child health, mental health, occupational health, and other prevention.

ments, 46.7%; and CDC, 18.9%. Each program had its strengths and weaknesses, but all appeared to be strong in epidemiology and biostatistics, with the military and CDC in the forefront. One's goals should be considered when selecting a training program. The original report may be helpful to those who are interested and should be consulted. One might assume that the respondents' suggestions for improving the programs would focus on the weaknesses but this is not true. The two military programs that were strongest in teaching clinical preventive medicine drew suggestions for further improving the program in that aspect. Conversely, one graduate of a medical school program stated that his residency should place greater emphasis on epidemiology and administrative skills and that clinical preventive medicine should be left to the fields of family practice and internal medicine "where it belongs."

The effect of training grants

One cannot read the report's Chapter 6, on the effect of the Health Resources and Services Administration Grants for Preventive Medical Training under title VII, section 788(c) of the Public Health Service Act, without being impressed that these grants are very important to training an expanding corps of specialists in preventive medicine. The number of PMR residencies that receive HRSA PMR training grants has decreased from 20 in 1983 to 13 in 1992, which is very few.

Two quotes from graduates of schools of public health are worth citing to emphasize this need:

"Today, with less tuition support, fewer traineeship dollars, higher costs and loans from medical schools which need to be repaid, and a lifetime of earning half of average MD incomes, it seems *very difficult* financially to go into public health. I don't think I could go through the same training today."

"Had financial support been available during my academic year, I wouldn't have had to work three afternoons per week, which prevented me from taking some classes and participating in some residency programs. Without traineeship money in my second year, I would have had to leave the program. More financial support is needed if the nation wants to have physicians trained in preventive medicine."

Legislation for the HRSA PMR training grant program was enacted in 1981; the program was implemented in 1983. These grants were planned to increase the number of persons trained in preventive medicine. They were successful, because the total number of graduates in the years 1987-1989 was 68% higher than before the grants were implemented. More than 75% of that growth is attributable to the grants. Among programs receiving grants, the graduates have doubled; unfortunately, among programs where grants were discontinued, the number of graduates has decreased. Although the grants are used to plan and develop programs, the report cites HRSA information that 65% to 75% of the grant monies were used in alleviating the trainees' expenses, such as tuition. Thus the grants supported the individual and enabled the program to expand to accommodate more students. In 1989-1990 the 11 participating programs received 31.9% of their support from this source.

Funding for the program in its first year of 1983 was $990,000. From fiscal 1984 to 1989, $1.5 to $1.6 million was disbursed per year, and in 1990, although $2.5 million was authorized, only $1.7 million was appropriated. The program size by applicants and awards is given in Table 1-9.

Programs operated by state and local health agencies are not eligible for HRSA grants. Comparing the years of 1980-1982 and 1987-1989, the number of graduates from 17 PMR programs that received grants after 1985 increased 138.2%. In other PMR programs, there was only a 21.8% increase. Unfunded programs did increase in students, albeit at a slower rate. The fact that they increased in students suggests that the granted programs did not take away residents from the others, which, of course, would not accomplish the goal. These figures, showing the increase in resident graduates in funded and unfunded programs, are listed in Table 1-10.

Chapter 7 of the report, "Improving the Match Between Training and Practice," is not reviewed here because it does not pertain to our subject. However, this chapter enables the PMR to compare the strengths of his or her program with others. It also enables the programs themselves to compare their strengths, and the physician contemplat-

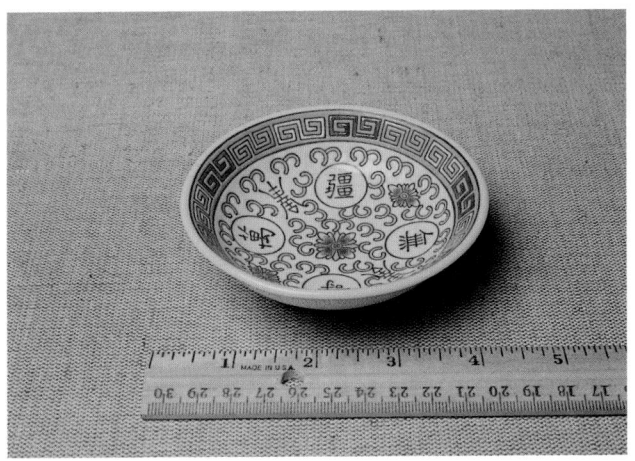 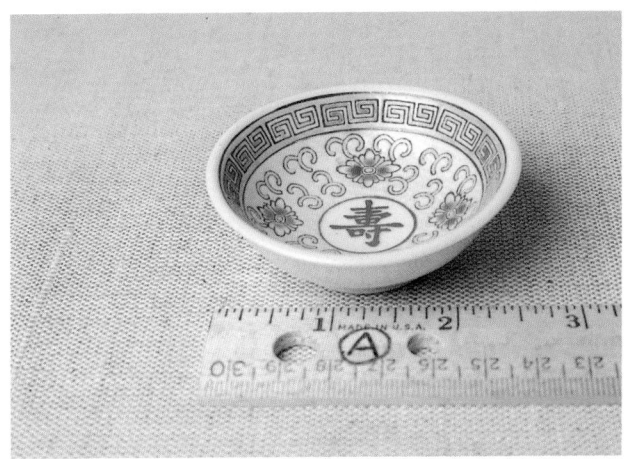

Plates 1 and 2. Lead-leaching dishes. Courtesy of Norman Shapiro, Hawaii Department of Health, Food & Drug Branch. A brochure showing many poisonous ceramics may be obtained by contacting this organization as listed in Chapter 37 Resources.

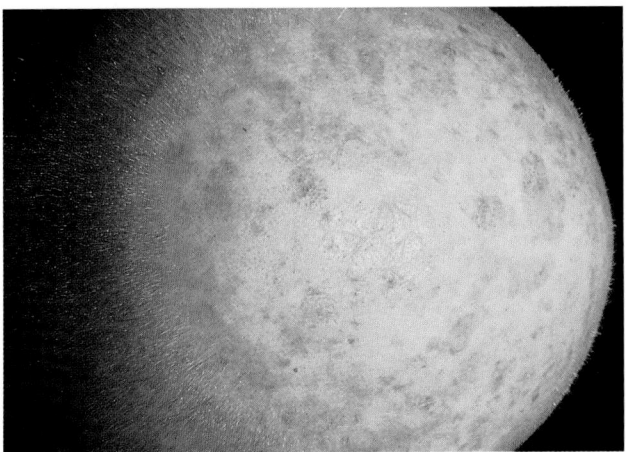

Plate 3. Actinic or solar keratosis.

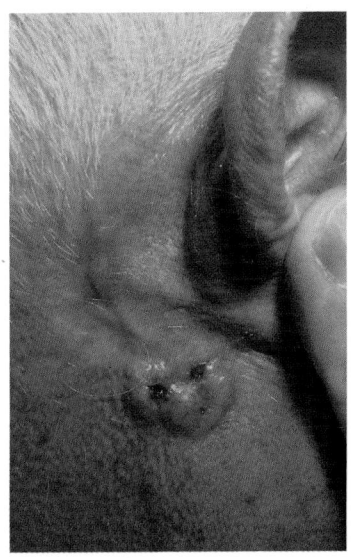

Plate 4. Basal cell skin carcinoma.

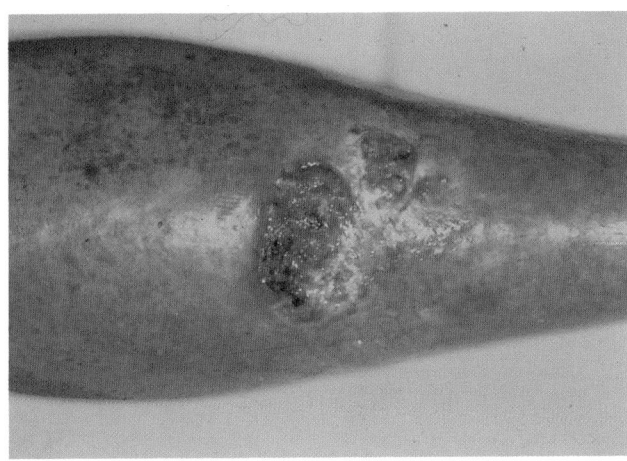

Plate 5. Squamous cell carcinoma of the skin.

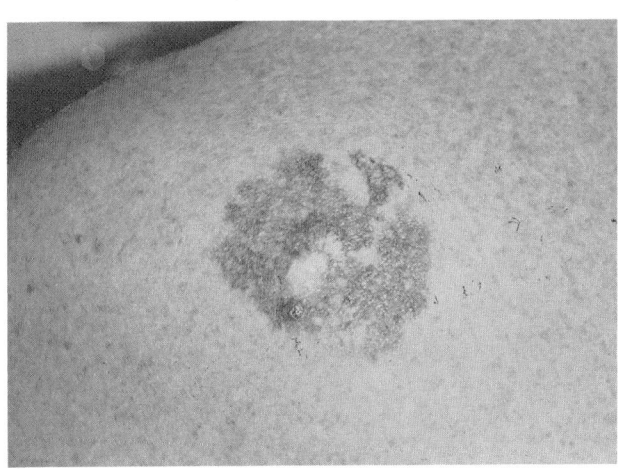

Plate 6. Malignant melanoma.

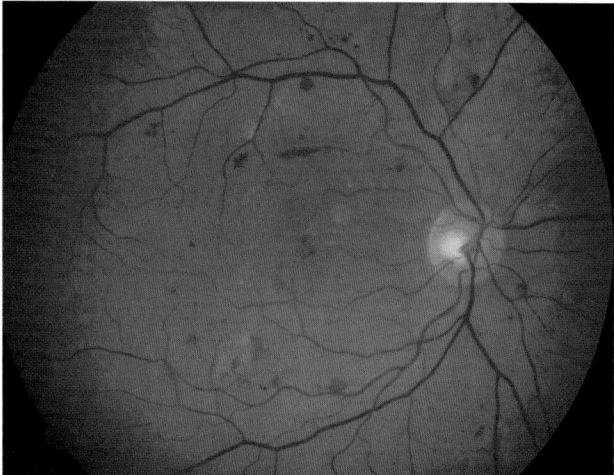

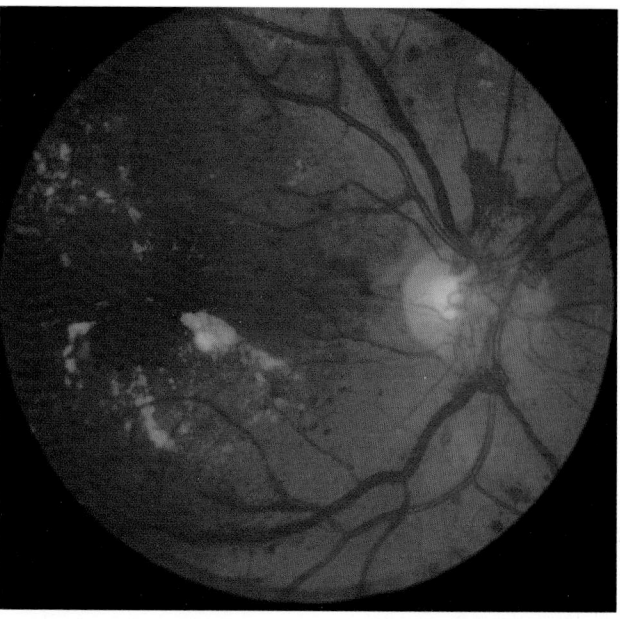

Plate 7. Retinal photograph demonstrating retinal hemorrhages, microaneurysms, and hard exudates typically seen with background diabetic retinopathy.

Plate 8. Retinal photograph demonstrating retinal hemorrhages and hard exudates consistent with milder stages of diabetic retinopathy. However, the presence of disc neovascularization defines this as proliferative diabetic retinopathy.

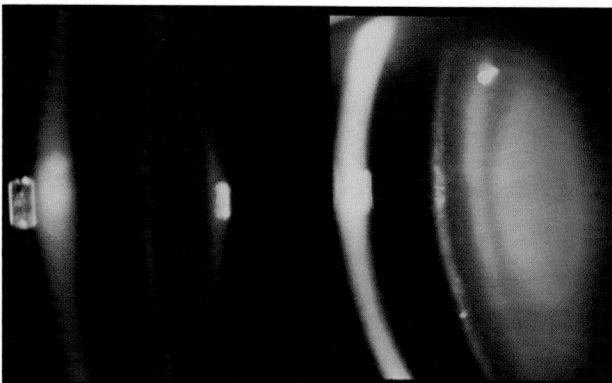

Plate 9. The slit lamp photograph *(left)* demonstrates a clear lens. The slit beam through the lens *(right)* demonstrates a yellowish opacity typical of the aging nuclear sclerotic cataract.

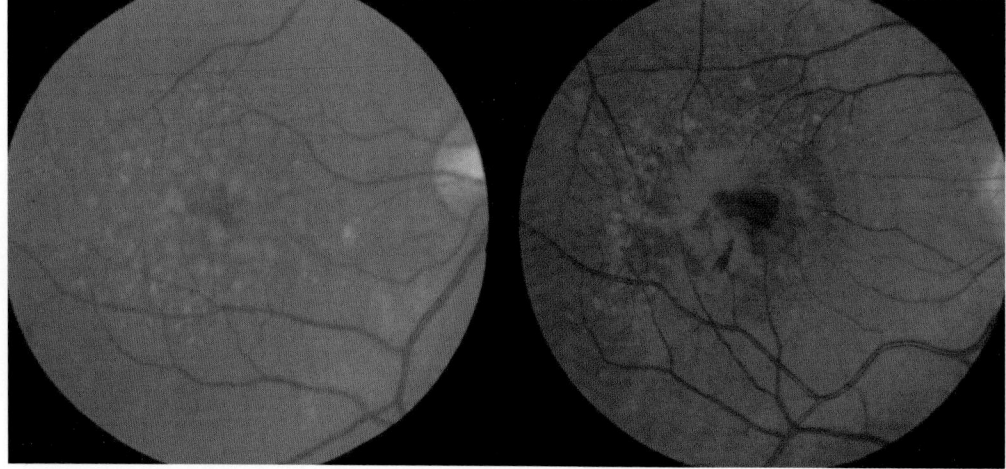

Plate 10. Age-related macular degeneration (ARMD). Retinal photographs demonstrating drusen seen in "dry" nonproliferative ARMD *(left)* and subretinal hemorrhage and exudation consistent with choroidal neovascular proliferation as seen in "wet" or proliferative ARMD *(right)*.

Table 1-9. Summary of HRSA PMR training grants

Cycle	Year	Program applicants	Program awards	Percent funded	Average award/year
Cycle 1	1983-85	31	20	64.5%	$ 69,700
Cycle 2	1986-88	40	14	35.0%	$110,800
Cycle 3	1989-91	26	11	42.3%	$134,800
Cycle 4	1992-94	25	13	52.0%	$115,800

Adapted from Hersey J, Boudreau C, Zeid A: *Practicing preventive medicine: a national survey of preventive medicine residency graduates,* Arlington, Va, 1992, Battelle.

Table 1-10. Number of PMR graduates in 1979-1981 and in 1987-1989 depending on HRSA PMR training grant status

HRSA PMR training grant status	1980-1982 (a)	1987-1989 (b)	Net gain (b − a)	Percent change (b ÷ a)
HRSA PMR grant after 1986 (17 programs)*	76	181	105	138.2%
No HRSA PMR grant after 1986 (15 programs)†	70	86	16	22.9%
Health dept. PMR (9 programs)	29	40	11	37.9%
Federal PMR‡ (3 programs)	48	53	5	10.4%
Subtotal: no HRSA grant (26 programs)	147	179	32	21.8%
Total PMRs (44 programs)§	223	360	137	61.4%

Adapted from Hersey J, Boudreau C, Zeid A: *Practicing preventive medicine: a national survey of preventive medicine residency graduates,* Arlington, Va, 1992, Battelle.
*University-based PMRs that received HRSA funding in either the 1986-88 grant cycle (14 programs) or the 1989 grant cycle (3 PMRs received new HRSA funding in 1989).
†University-based PMRs that did not receive HRSA funding in the 1986-88 or 1989 grant cycle. Nine of these 15 programs received HRSA grants only from 1983-85 and six never received HRSA PMR training grants.
‡Federal PMRs included the CDC PMR and PMRs at Madigan Army Medical Center and Walter Reed Army Institute of Research.
§Includes the now inactive programs at the University of Illinois College of Medicine and the University of Michigan School of Public Health.

ing application for a residency to consider which might be best for his or her particular needs and goals. The graduates cited epidemiology, biostatistics, and infectious disease as the greatest common strengths of all the programs. This might be expected, because these program ingredients were the foundation of public health. In most, but not all, programs, the next most common strengths were in clinical preventive medicine and chronic disease. Surprisingly, occupational medicine and environmental health received the fewest "good to excellent" ratings in most programs. There are residency programs that address these fields in particular. However, as a part of residencies addressing the entire field, these fields are weaker.

REPORT CONCLUSIONS

In Chapter 8 of the report, the strengths in PMR programs were noted, challenges enumerated, and recommendations made by the authors.

LEADERSHIP IN PUBLIC HEALTH

Strengths. There were obvious strengths in the field, notably in *initiating and developing programs,* and in *management* (where graduates strongly urged increased training). To illustrate the magnitude of the responsibilities assumed, earlier PMR graduates handled a mean budget of $22.3 million and supervised a staff of 160. A total of

58.8% of respondents conducted *research* in preventing/controlling disease, and 55.8% conducted research in epidemiology and disease surveillance. The subject areas or diseases studied displayed a wide range and are fascinating. They are not confined to the original area of interest and activity of the discipline (infectious disease) but range from identifying the cause of toxic shock syndrome to the effect of diet in cancer. It is rewarding to note that fully two thirds of graduates are involved in patient care from non-CDC PMR programs, and almost 80% of that group is in an activity of primary care and/or *clinical preventive medicine.*

CHALLENGES

Identify. We previously noted that most physicians in other areas do not completely understand what the specialty of preventive medicine is. Indeed, many do not understand that it is *not* a subdivision of internal medicine and that it has its own board certification structure. Still fewer appreciate that within that certification there are three elections: general preventive medicine and public health, aerospace medicine, and occupational medicine. The Batelle authors note that within the specialty there is confusion about definition and mission too. (This is contrary, the author suspects, to 40 to 50 years ago, when the mission was basically infectious disease.) Because of their talents, peculiar to the field, preventive medicine specialists were likely to expand their role to other diseases, as in the study of the epidemiology of cancer. With this expertise applied to an expanded role, the borders of the specialty inevitably became blurred. With this growth in scope, areas such as chronic disease, environmental health, mental health, and injury prevention have been brought into the sphere of preventive medicine. It really is a field that knows no bounds in its application.

In addition, as each training program has developed with its own definition of mission, the uniformity of training seen in most other residency programs (e.g., surgery) is lacking. This may not necessarily be bad, but it does mean that graduates of these programs reflect the strengths and weaknesses of their programs and probably view themselves and their field (preventive medicine) somewhat differently. For example in the minds of the residents (not those studied) the practicum year is possibly the least well defined by the board and the most varied in practice.[4]

The report notes that 43.3% of PMR graduates are certified in another clinical specialty as well, and this author suspects that this too may affect how that individual sees the mission and definition of the field of preventive medicine.

Low rates of board certification. A low rate of board certification after PMR training may stem partly from the fact some are already board certified in another field, but also from two other reported causes given by graduates. The first is a perception that certification is not needed, not an advantage, and costs additional money. (Grace[4] also suggests that the lack of definition of the year of experience required to take the boards makes students unsure of their ability to pass the board of choice.) Second, in some cases financing is unavailable for the year in a school of public health, the year is not taken, and a certification requirement is missed.

Limited funding. The evidence accumulated shows that lack of funds in the sponsoring institution limits the size and scope of the PMR program. When funds are provided to both the institution and the candidates, the number of graduates grows enormously. (The growth seems to result from a modest investment.) Presently there are only 13 supported PMR programs, compared with 20 in 1983, although the need with increasingly tight budgets is greater. Nowhere is this more evident than in state and local health department programs, which are ineligible for the federal funding cited.

Strengthening public health infrastructure. The vital role played by these physicians in the infrastructure of public health, the nation's health, and the ability to accomplish the nation's health care goals is clear. They are valuable not only to the general population, but increasingly to the medically underserved and those without access to many forms of care, particularly through state and local health departments.

One possible source of continued and increased funding is the federal government (per HRSA Title VII), but other sources must be approached as well. For example, the growing HMO industry has a vested interest in preventists. Private individuals and foundations too should not be counted out.

Toward the future. Whether the members of the field are capable of meeting the challenges is not in question but is a function of the number in the field and the number training to enter the field. Those already in the field are occupied with their own problems of program funding and meeting their current responsibilities. (For example, imagine the effect on the infectious disease program of health departments, in manpower and budget, of one disease, AIDS.).

The diversity of training is both a handicap and a blessing in this author's opinion. Whereas most residencies are found in free-standing hospitals and universities, the PMR programs are found in schools of public health, universities, local and state health programs, and the governmental arms such as CDC and the armed forces. Thus there are currently multiple funding sources for graduates and programs, limited though they may be. Efforts to address these common challenges must be by the cooperation and consultation with all of the organizations previously listed that are involved with preventive medicine.

RECOMMENDATIONS

Clarification of identity. The authors of the study conclude that there is a lack of knowledge about the contributions and accomplishments of PMR graduates and that this needs to be disseminated widely, emphasizing their contributions to national health objectives. This information about training and career opportunities needs to be transmitted to medical students, and the authors suggest several ways to do this. In addition, the authors suggest that a task force of experts (including program directors) clarify the scope of the field and competencies required in light of the changing demands on the field. This information, too, should be disseminated to medical students, those in training, funding sources (including members of Congress and concerned governmental agencies), and present and potential employers. As a great number of graduates rendering clinical care have noted, experience in the clinical application of preventive medicine during residency training needs to be studied.

Funding. The HRSA PMR Training Grant Program needs to be funded up to authorized levels. Additional funding outside of government needs to be aggressively sought.

Board certification. The American Board of Preventive Medicine should communicate the advantages of certification to PMR residents as well as all the groups just noted.

Recommendations to various PMR training programs

CDC PMR. Developing ways for those trainees without an MPH to obtain it should be explored. In light of the graduates' suggestions and the considerable administrative responsibilities they assume, training and experience in program management should be strengthened.

Health department PMRs. Creative approaches to reverse the decline in these programs must be undertaken. This might be done by (1) linking training to relevant local health needs, (2) affiliating with existing programs in medical schools and public health programs, and statewide public health initiatives, and (3) demonstrate the need for increased funding of these PMRs to city, county, or state governments.

Public health and medical school PMRs. No important difference was demonstrated in the training and subsequent careers of graduates of these two programs, and they have common goals; therefore they should work closely together in coordinating programs and initiatives to achieve their goals.

SUMMARY

The term *preventive medicine* is defined. To be available to all, preventive care is best delivered by all physicians, regardless of specialty. The primary care givers, led by the specialists, will determine the future of preventive medicine as an applied discipline. The shortage of "specialists" in preventive medicine is documented. One important role, at least in the near future, is to teach the next generation of physicians (as well as conduct research, etc.). Primary, secondary, and tertiary preventive medicine is defined and related to the mission of the preventist and others. In that relationship, screening and positive early prevention is assigned to the "preventist," and appropriate screening is defined by established WHO guidelines. The importance of screening in the office is considered. Finally, the training necessary for certification in the field is reviewed and the manpower shortage discussed.

Preventive medicine graduates from a 10-year period were surveyed, and their careers were documented in a report by Battelle, which was reviewed in some detail. The survey presents a telling picture of the roles assumed by the current manpower pool in this field. The accomplishments of this group and their various training and rewards, are reviewed, and some conclusions and proposals for the field are considered.

Acknowledgment

The author wishes to thank Dr. James Hersey of Batelle for early access to the manuscript, "Practicing Preventive Medicine: A National Survey of Preventive Medicine Residency Graduates," and his constructive suggestions and additions to this chapter.

REFERENCES

1. ACPM News, the Newsletter of the American College of Preventive Medicine 1:3, 1989.
2. American College of Preventive Medicine: *Careers in Preventive Medicine* (pamphlet), Washington, DC, 1989, ACPM.
3. American College of Preventive Medicine: *Directory of preventive medicine residency programs in the United States and Canada,* Washington D.C., 1991, ACPM.
4. Crowley AE, Etzes SI, editors: *Directory of graduate medical education programs accredited by the accreditation council for graduate medical education,* Chicago, 1989, American Medical Association.
5. Grace TW: Special contribution: a resident's adventures in preventive medicine wonderland, *Am J Prev Med* 8:66, 1992.
6. Graduate Medical Education National Advisory Committee: *Volume II: Modeling, research and data technical panel,* Washington, DC, 1980, US Government Printing Office (DHHS Pub. No. (HRA) 81-652), 229-333.
7. Health Services and Resources Administration (HRSA), Bureau of Health Professions: *Seventh report to the president and congress on the status of health personnel,* Washington, DC, 1990, US Government Printing Office (DHHS Pub. No. HRS-P-OD-90-1).
8. Healthy People 2000 Consortium: *Healthy people 2000: national health promotion and disease prevention objectives (full report and summary report),* Washington, DC, 1990, Government Printing Office.
9. Hersey J, Boudreau C, and Zeid A: *Practicing preventive medicine: a national survey of preventive medicine graduates. Final report to the Centers for Disease Control and the Health Resources and Services Administration, Bureau of Health Professions,* Arlington, Va, 1992, Battelle.
10. Lawrence SV: Changing times focus attention on medicine in the workplace, *Forum Med* 3:476, 1979.
11. Institute on Medicine, Committee on the Study of the Future of Public Health, National Academy of Sciences: *The future of public health,* Washington, DC, 1988, National Academy Press.
12. McDonald CJ et al: Reminders to physicians from an introspective computer medical record, *Ann Intern Med* 100:130, 1984.
13. Report of the U.S. Preventive Services Task Force: *Guide to clinical preventive services,* Baltimore, Maryland, 1989, Williams & Wilkens.
14. Wilson JMG, Jungner G: *Principles and practice of screening for disease,* Geneva, 1968, The World Health Organization (printed in France).
15. Woolf SH, Sox HC Jr: The expert panel on preventive services: continuing the work of the US preventive services task force, *Am J Prev Med* 7:326, 1991.

▬▬▬▬▬▬▬ RESOURCES ▬▬▬▬▬▬▬

Directory of preventive medicine residency programs in the United States and Canada (general preventive medicine, occupational medicine, public health, aerospace medicine), American College of Preventive Medicine, 1015 15th St. NW, Washington, D.C., 2005.

Guide to clinical preventive services, An assessment of 169 interventions, Report of the United States Preventive Services Task Force, 1989, Williams & Wilkins, 428 E. Preston St., Baltimore, Maryland 21202. *Guide to clinical preventive services* is an authoritative collective opinion of the Preventive Services Task Force on screening, counseling, and positive intervention for 60 target conditions by 169 techniques.

Healthy people 2000: national health promotion and disease prevention objectives. It is published as a full report and a summary report and were priced at $31 and $9 respectively through January, 1991. For updated information and prices write the superintendent of documents order and information desk, Washington, D.C. *Healthy people 2000* is a working document of goals, ways to achieve them in the present decade, and a statement by the U.S. Department of Health and Human Services, Public Health Service. It represents the combined collective opinions of all government levels, 300 national organizations, some 10,000 interviews, expert consortiums, and the National Academy of Science. It is of value to appraise your personal practice goals in the light of your own community situation and as a rather specific reading of national directions in health.

How to practice prospective medicine, ed 2, 1979, J.H. Hall and J.D. Zwemer, Methodist Hospital of Indiana. To order, contact: Prospective Medical Center, 6220 Lawrence Drive, Indianapolis, Indiana 46226. *How to practice prospective medicine* was first published in 1970. The word prospective was used like "preventive." This volume was designed for the teaching program of internal medicine residents. It approaches disease from the standpoint of risk. It has multiple health hazard appraisal charts and a complete set of Geller-Gestner tables for the appraisal of risks in male, female, black, and white patients from "entry age" of 5 to 9, to 70 to 74. This is a very valuable and too-little-known work eminently suited to office practice.

Hayward RSA et al: *Preventive care guidelines: 1991, Ann Intern Med* 114:758, 1991. *Preventive care guidelines* is a critique and very fine comparison of the recommendations of the American College of Physicians, the Canadian Task Force on the Periodic Health Examination, U.S. Preventive Services Task Force, and other authorities. It is an article well worth keeping in hand while reading the *Guide to clinical preventive services,* both as a balance and for the philosophy it presents. There can be dissenting opinions of equal merit and jus-

tification at any point in the evolution of medical knowledge.

Primary care clinics in office practice, volume 16, number 1, March 1989, Prevention in Practice, WB Saunders Co., The Curtis Center, Independence Square West, Philadelphia, PA 19106-3399. *Primary care clinics* presents a very concise pair of flow sheets for the patient's chart that could be modified for your practice. These charts are on the last two pages of this small volume.

Public health and preventive medicine, Maxcy-Rosenau, ed 12, John M. Last, MD, DPH, Appleton-Century-Crofts, Norwalk, Conn. *Public health and preventive medicine* is a comprehensive tome and reference work for the serious student, particularly in schools of public health and other training programs. The first edition was in 1913.

Teaching preventive medicine in primary care, William H. Barker, MD, 1983, Springer Series on Medical Education, volume 5, Springer Publishing, 200 Park Ave South, New York, NY 10003. In chapter four of *Teaching preventive medicine in primary care,* Drs. R.S. Thompson and J.R. Miller address prevention in a health maintenance organization and present a basic innovative flow chart/cumulative decision tree of interaction of receptionist, nurse, and physician. It is a good introduction to the reader's own practice and needs, particularly as more of us are participating in HMOs. In Chapter five, another early and authoritative "preventist," Dr. Paul Frame, discusses delivering health care in a totally different setting: "Prevention in a rural family practice." It includes clinical chart flow sheets, assessments, or forms that can easily be updated and modified even yearly as knowledge changes. (Also see Dr. Frame's, "A Critical Review of Adult Health Maintenance," in four parts, *J Fam Pract,* vols. 22-23, 1986.)

1992-1993 Directory of graduate medical education programs by the American Medical Association. Copies may be purchased from: Order Department OP416792, AMA, P.O. Box 109050, Chicago, IL 60610.

Chapter 2

THE PERIODIC HEALTH EXAMINATION

Richard S. Lang

In this century, the periodic health examination has evolved from the efforts of individuals and organizations who have recognized that the promotion of good health and prevention of disease and injury are possible and important to the overall goals of an effective health care system. Only in relatively recent years, however, have those interventions incorporated under the umbrella term *preventive health services* been evaluated in a scientific and consistent fashion to define those of most benefit, those of least benefit that should be eliminated, and those to be targeted for further evaluation and study to determine efficacy. Healthy People 2000, the National Health Promotion and Disease Prevention Objectives outlined by the Department of Health and Human Services in late 1990, further emphasizes the role of prevention in the future of this country's health care system.[50] This chapter reviews the evolution of the periodic medical examination to illustrate what is known, what is not known, and how best we should apply this examination to the individual patients we examine in our offices.

DEFINITIONS

The term *periodic health examination* is now used to describe a set of health prevention and promotion services offered to an individual at intervals in his or her life. These services are based on consideration of age, sex, inheritable and life-style risk factors, and other circumstances such as occupation and environment. The term has several synonyms, such as *health maintenance examination* and *well adult care,* and includes screening studies and maneuvers, risk determination, immunizations, and counseling. The purposes of the periodic health examination are to identify disease at an early or presymptomatic stage, determine the individual risk of a person, prevent or postpone the onset of a detected disease or the serious sequelae of existing disease, and maintain health.

Prevention is defined as the act of hindering or averting the occurrence of disease or injury. *Primary prevention* pertains to reducing the likelihood of a disease or injury; immunization and risk factor modification are examples of primary prevention. *Secondary prevention* refers to detecting a condition in its earliest stage to facilitate intervention to stop or retard the progression of that condition; screening and intervention programs are examples of secondary prevention. Primary prevention aims to reduce *incidence* of disease, whereas secondary prevention tries to affect *prevalence.* To date, practitioners and researchers have placed greater emphasis on secondary prevention (screening and intervention) than on primary prevention (alteration of risk factors), although a shift of emphasis toward primary prevention is under way.

Inherent in the goals of the periodic health examination is the concept of *health:* a state of complete physical, mental, and social well-being, not merely the absence of disease and infirmity. The primary health care provider addresses some aspect of all of these areas during interactions with patients. For a variety of reasons, the traditional primary care doctor–patient interaction has often emphasized the physical aspect of this definition more than the mental and social. Primary prevention by way of health education and health promotion helps to address the mental and social aspects of maintaining "health." *Health education* refers to those "learning experiences designed to predispose, enable, and reinforce voluntary adaptations of individual or collective behavior conducive to health."[40] *Health promotion* is the "combination of health education and related organizational, economic, and environmental supports for behavior conducive to health."[40] In the broad sense, health promotion is those activities designed to alter behavior, environment, or heredity in order to improve health.

Maintaining health has come to mean staying well. In the periodic health examination the concept of "wellness" has meant the absence of symptoms and has been equated with "asymptomatic," which is defined as "one who does not have symptoms or does not recognize the symptoms as being related to the disease."[28] In the Canadian literature the term *noncomplainant* is used to define "an individual who undergoes a health examination without having specific complaints or concerns about his or her health."[6] This term is broadened by the concept of *case finding* or screening for a disease when patients are being seen for unrelated symptoms. The concept of the well, asymptomatic, or noncomplaining individual causes difficulty for many practitioners because perceptions vary. Patient and physician (observer) perceptions differ regarding what wellness is and how complaints or concerns can be expressed. Patients run the spectrum from the stoic individual to the chronic complainer or hypochondriac. The stoic individual may be seen as asymptomatic when in fact symptoms are present but disregarded. The chronic complainer may be judged symptomatic when in fact he or she is experiencing his or her own normal state of health. Similarly, the physician defines health, wellness, or symptoms in the framework of his or her own perceptions and biases. These variations in perceptions and expression cloud the concept of the periodic health examination for the practitioner. Other problems arise from anecdotal experience of physicians. A missed diagnosis or a new diagnosis made in a late stage of a disease often causes a physician to be overly cautious about that diagnosis in future patient encounters. The practitioner may tend to "overscreen" future patients for the condition he or she overlooked in the earlier patient, disregarding screening guidelines and the scientific evidence pertaining to them. Conversely, lack of knowledge about a disease process or techniques of prevention for that disease may cause a physician to overlook a given test or intervention and "underscreen" an individual. The periodic health examination can provide an important framework for physicians in their approach to the variety of patients who enter the office on any given day and assist in overcoming these problems of perception, bias, anecdote, and lack of knowledge. The foundation of the periodic health examination is based on the following precepts:

1. Patients without symptoms can harbor organic disease.
2. Disease can be detected at an "early" stage.
3. Discovery of disease can lead to arrest, reversal, retardation, or cure of that disease and thereby reduce morbidity and/or mortality.[26]

ORIGINS OF THE PERIODIC HEALTH EXAMINATION

The concept of the periodic health examination was brought to the United States by Dr. G.M. Gould at the turn of the century in an address to the American Medical Association, "A System of Personal Biological Examination: The Condition of Adequate Medical and Scientific Conduct of Life."[39] This idea was soon taken up and further developed by life insurance companies, spearheaded by Dr. E.L. Fisk in the first quarter of this century.[26] He created the Life Extension Institute, where policyholders would undergo periodic health examinations. It was felt that these examinations would prolong life expectancy of the policyholders, ultimately resulting in financial savings to the company. The concepts and benefits of this program would be accepted and unchallenged for many years.

In 1923 the American Medical Association (AMA) officially endorsed the periodic health examination in the publication *Periodic Health Examination: A Manual for Physicians*.[3] In the same year, a nationwide campaign promoting having a health examination "on your birthday" took place. Over the next two decades, as the United States struggled with the Depression, little was written about the periodic health examination.[26] In 1940, the AMA book on the periodic health examination was revised and re-emphasized as being important. The AMA indicated that physicians were "indifferent to the concept of examining healthy persons" and that "only certain categories of workers were undergoing periodic examinations."[3] This 1940 manual emphasized and advised the use of "simple" procedures and advocated discussion of the subject of the periodic examination at medical conferences. In 1947 the AMA manual again was revised and included such forward thinking concepts as awareness of the effect of patients' religious preferences on preventive intervention, variability of diet among individuals, assessment of psychologic status and interpersonal relationships, exposures as cause of disease, and written prescriptions for healthful living such as "walk at least 3 miles each day" and "add an orange or cereal at breakfast." The periodic examination continued to evolve in the next several years, but not until the mid-1970s was the practice challenged in a serious way.[3,47] From the 1970s until today, individuals and groups working independently as well as together have brought forward the science of the periodic health examination by establishing principles for the critical evaluation of preventive and periodic interventions.

THE CANADIAN TASK FORCE ON THE PERIODIC HEALTH EXAMINATION

The Canadian Task Force on the Periodic Health Examination was established in 1976 at the request of the Conference of Deputy Ministers of Health of Canada to "determine how the periodic health examination might enhance or protect the health of the population."[6] They were challenged to provide a plan for a lifetime program of periodic health assessment for all persons living in Canada. This landmark undertaking contributed mightily to the preventive health literature and the foundation for establishing preventive care guidelines. The task force deliberated for

Effectiveness of intervention

The effectiveness of intervention was graded according to the quality of the evidence obtained, as follows:

I: Evidence obtained from at least one properly randomized controlled trial.

II-1: Evidence obtained from well designed cohort or case-control analytic studies, preferably from more than one centre or research group.

II-2: Evidence obtained from comparisons between times or places with or without the intervention. Dramatic results in uncontrolled experiments (such as the results of the introduction of penicillin in the 1940s) could also be regarded as this type of evidence.

III: Opinions of respected authorities, based on clinical experience, descriptive studies or reports of expert committees.

From Canadian Task Force on the Periodic Health Examination: The periodic health examination, *Can Med Assoc J* 121:1193-1254, 1979.

Research priority questions

1. Efficacy: Does early detection lead to better outcome?
2. Effectiveness: Does early detection benefit those screened?
3. Efficiency: Is the maneuver or procedure available with optimal use of resources?
4. Frequency: When should maneuvers be repeated?
5. What is the effectiveness of health promotion, education, and counseling?
6. What are the effects of labeling persons with disease?
7. What are the statistical performance characteristics of detection maneuvers?

From Canadian Task Force on the Periodic Health Examination: The periodic health examination, *Can Med Assoc J* 121:1193-1254, 1979.

over 3 years and filed their initial document in 1979. They established that the periodic health examination has two goals: prevention of specific disease and promotion of health.[6] The task force first sought to identify those conditions of importance to specific age groups that were preventible. They suggested that the annual physical examination be abandoned and replaced by a selective approach directed at specific important conditions and determined by a person's age and sex.[6]

The criteria the task force used for assessing the importance of a condition included the mortality and morbidity caused by the condition, the validity and acceptability of maneuvers to identify the risk for a condition, and the effectiveness of the resulting intervention. The impact of a condition on the individual, the individual's family, and society were all considered in defining its importance.[6]

The effectiveness of the intervention was weighted depending on the kind of evidence supporting that intervention (see box above). The weighing of that evidence in classifying maneuvers and interventions into a framework in a standardized fashion is probably the most important accomplishment of the Canadian task force.[49]

The task force went on to outline health protection packages for age and sex groups to replace the annual physical examinations so long used in medical care in North America. They recommended that procedures be carried out on a case finding basis when patients consulted a practitioner for unrelated symptoms. They cautiously recommended counseling, noting the lack of evidence supporting the effectiveness of such intervention. The report also addressed and recognized barriers of cost, public expectation, time, and incentives to the provision of preventive interventions and outlined the need for research to fill gaps in the medical literature pertinent to preventive interventions.[6] The research priorities they identified are outlined (see box, above right).

Since their initial undertaking the Canadian task force has continued to review the evolving medical literature, and update their recommendations.[7-25,49] These updates have used the same methods and criteria for evidence to define the effectiveness of an intervention. Battista et al. in reviewing the periodic health examination as an "evolving concept" noted that "any doctor-patient encounter is an opportunity for prevention" and that "although the mandate of the task force is to formulate guidelines for preventive practice rather than implementation strategies, the latter has always been of great concern to its members."[4] They noted three areas of importance for integration of preventive care into primary health care, knowledge, attitudes, and behavior, and cited as most critical the behavior of the health care provider.[4] Barriers to implementation relate not only to health care providers but also to patients and to organization of practice settings. These issues are addressed in Chapter 8.

The work of the Canadian task force has served as a model for the United States government and other health care organizations for evaluation of preventive programs in the establishment of "packages," "guidelines," "interventions," and "services" that together serve as the framework for individual physicians and individual patients to make decisions. The box on p. 24 lists selected recommended preventive maneuvers of the Canadian task force that are also endorsed by other major health groups. Of note is the relatively low number of screening interventions that these groups agree should be applied to asymptomatic adults of normal risk.

FRAME AND CARLSON

In 1975, two family physicians in the United States, Paul S. Frame and S.J. Carlson, pioneered major changes in the way screening examinations would be viewed. Their work preceded by a few years that of Breslow and Somers and of the Canadian Task Force. They undertook a critical review of the medical and scientific evidence to support

---

Summary of selected preventive care interventions for asymptomatic adults recommended by major expert groups*

Screening

Nonfasting cholesterol measurement
Blood pressure measurement
Clinical breast examination
Mammography
Cervical Pap smear

Counseling

Tobacco use, alcohol and substance use, exercise, diet, sexual practices, injury prevention, dental health promotion

Vaccinations

Tetanus-diphtheria toxoid
Influenza (age 65+ or persons at risk)
Pneumococcus (age 65+ or persons at risk)

---

*Ages for and intervals of interventions vary among expert groups. Expert groups considered include the U.S. Preventive Services Task Force, the Canadian Task Force on the Periodic Health Examination, and the American College of Physicians. Other interventions are advised in selected populations on the basis of consideration of risk. Other interventions are not agreed on by the groups considered.

Criteria to evaluate a condition for inclusion in a health maintenance protocol

1. The condition must have a significant effect on the quality or quantity of life.
2. Acceptable methods of treatment must be available.
3. The condition must have an asymptomatic period during which detection and treatment significantly reduce morbidity or mortality.
4. Treatment in the asymptomatic phase must yield a therapeutic result superior to that obtained by delaying treatment until symptoms appear.
5. Tests that are acceptable to patients must be available at reasonable cost to detect the condition in the asymptomatic period.
6. The incidence of the condition must be sufficient to justify the cost of screening.

From Frame PS: A critical review of health maintenance. Part I. Prevention of atherosclerotic diseases, *J Fam Pract* 22:341-346, 1986.

---

screening for specific diseases in asymptomatic healthy adults.[30-33] In doing so they established specific criteria to evaluate whether or not a screening procedure for a disease was justified. These criteria, outlined in the box, are similar to those used by Breslow and Somers and the Canadian task force. And like these other groups, Frame and Carlson advocated replacing the traditional annual complete physical examination with a "rational selective longitudinal health maintenance program." During the decade that followed, this selective approach to health maintenance became accepted; it continues to be today.

In 1986 Frame updated his recommended protocol for adult health maintenance.[34-37] He warned that "the best health maintenance protocol is worthless unless it is used on a day to day basis by primary care physicians on a large percentage of their patients."[34] He sought to provide a concise protocol, noting that "including marginal tests of uncertain benefit wastes precious time and money and makes it less likely that physicians and patients will comply with the program."[34] In updating his recommendations, he made comparisons with the Canadian recommendations and evaluated the scientific evidence. Frame's recommendations serve as a reasonable basic guide for physicians, who can then individualize health maintenance protocols for individual patients on the basis of risk factors and ongoing medical problems. Frame advocates a complete physical examination at the outset of patient interac-

tion to establish a data base and a flow sheet to assist the practitioner in incorporating the principles of the health maintenance process.

More recently, Frame has directed efforts at the practical application of the health maintenance concept for the individual practitioner by outlining barriers to implementation and providing strategies for overcoming those barriers.[29]

BRESLOW AND SOMERS

About the same time as Frame and Carlson's work and the recommendations of the Canadian task force, Dr. Lester Breslow and Ann R. Somers outlined what they termed "The Lifetime Health-Monitoring Program," a schedule over the lifetime of an individual of "packages" of effective individual preventive procedures.[5] They divided the human lifespan into 10 periods: infancy, preschool, school age, adolescence, young adulthood, young middle age, older middle age, elderly, and old age. They based these divisions on consideration of "changing lifestyle, health needs, and problems."[5] They then sought to bring together the epidemiologic and clinical approaches to clinical prevention for each of these groups. As Frame and Carlson and the Canadian task force continued their work, Breslow and Somers also applied criteria to determine the appropriateness of a preventive intervention (see box). For each of the 10 life periods outlined, health goals were established and appropriate services outlined. Like the other pioneers of the periodic health examination of this period, they recommended abandoning the "annual ritual" of the yearly examination, relied also on "prudent" interpretation in the absence of scientific evidence for a given procedure, and included educational and counseling procedures as part of the overall program.

Breslow and Somers' criteria for preventive interventions

1. Procedure is appropriate to the health goals of the relevant group and acceptable to that population.
2. Procedure is directed to primary or secondary prevention of an identified disease or condition that has a definite effect on the length or quality of life.
3. The natural history of the disease or condition is understood sufficiently.
4. For a screening intervention, the disease or condition has an asymptomatic period when intervention can take place and reduce morbidity or mortality.
5. Acceptable methods of effective treatment are available for the condition discovered.
6. The prevalence and seriousness of the disease justify the cost of intervention.
7. The procedure is easy to administer and reasonable in cost.
8. Resources are available for follow-up diagnostic or therapeutic intervention.

From Breslow L, Somers AR: The lifetime health-monitoring program: a practical approach to preventive medicine, *N Engl J Med* 296:601-608, 1977.

Personal risk factors to review in the cancer related examination

1. Tobacco use
2. Sun exposure
3. Sexual practices
4. Environmental or occupational exposures
5. Diet and nutrition

Included also in Breslow and Somers's discussion are a consideration of cost of preventive measures and the belief that cost should be covered by health insurance systems. They correctly recognize the difficulties of measuring cost and benefit in preventive intervention of this kind:

There is reason to hope that such a program of preventive medicine would eventually reduce the amount of expensive curative care now needed, although it would be misleading to claim that any such savings could be achieved in the short run. By definition, the potential savings, if any, from preventive medicine—to the individual and to society—should show up in future years. Even so, the amount is problematical. Those who are saved by good preventive services from heart attacks and cancer in their 40's and 50's will eventually die of something else. It has been rightly said that life itself is the one fatal condition that cannot be avoided. The primary object of preventive care is not to save money but to save lives, to avoid premature death, and to improve the quality of life.[5]

Furthermore, Breslow and Somers point out that the doctor-patient relationship would be enhanced by incorporating these kinds of preventive principles into day to day patient care. They note that greater emphasis on counseling of an individual within an epidemiologic framework can replace routine testing and mechanical and depersonalizing aspects of screening and testing.[5]

THE AMERICAN CANCER SOCIETY

In 1980 the American Cancer Society (ACS) conducted a comprehensive review of the medical literature leading to revised guidelines for the cancer related examination.[1] These guidelines were organized to help individual physi-

cians and patients determine the best detection protocol for that person's individual needs in searching for early detection of cancer. Two significant conclusions of the review were that (1) early detection is effective in reducing morbidity and mortality of several cancers and (2) changes in the recommendations provide greater benefit to the population as a whole at greatly reduced risk, cost, and inconvenience.[1] The review went on to emphasize that the benefit of the cancer related check-up and consultation for modification of personal cancer risk factors was particularly important in the early adult age groups because so many personal health habits are established at that time. This revised set of guidelines recognized that tests in persons without symptoms that had been accepted as routine, such as the performance of chest radiographs on an annual basis for detection of lung cancer, were not justified on a cost-benefit basis and therefore should be abandoned.[1] This change in policy by a respected organization devoted to prevention of cancer clearly illustrates the shift from accepted opinion to careful evaluation of effectiveness of interventions by review of scientific evidence.[43]

Since 1980, as new knowledge has been accumulated, components of the American Cancer Society guidelines have been revised.[28,45] Again, these changes have been based on the principles that evidence should indicate that the recommended testing is medically effective, that medical benefits outweigh the risk of the procedure, that the cost is reasonable, and that the actions are practical and feasible. More importantly these guidelines emphasize that the cancer related examination should *always* include health counseling about personal risk factors.[28] The box above lists those personal risk factors the American Cancer Society advocates be reviewed as part of the cancer related examination. They note that these guidelines are "simply advice, not commands" and have provided evidence that despite practitioners' finding this framework helpful, the guidelines are not being followed.[43] Table 2-1 summarizes the current American Cancer Society Guidelines.

THE AMERICAN COLLEGE OF PHYSICIANS

Following the lead of Frame and Carlson, Breslow and Somers, the Canadian task force, and the American Cancer Society, the American College of Physicians (ACP) set forth in 1981 guidelines for "an individualized plan for

Table 2-1. Summary of American Cancer Society recommendations for the early detection of cancer in asymptomatic people

Test or procedure	Population		
	Sex	Age	Frequency
Sigmoidoscopy, preferably flexible	M & F	50 and over	Every 3 to 5 years
Fecal occult blood test	M & F	50 and over	Every year
Digital rectal examination	M & F	40 and over	Every year
Pap test	F	All women who are or who have been sexually active, or have reached age 18, should have an annual Pap test and pelvic examination. After a woman has had three or more consecutive satisfactory normal annual examinations, the Pap test may be performed less frequently at the discretion of her physician.	
Pelvic examination	F	18-40 Over 40	Every 1-3 years with Pap test Every year
Endometrial tissue sample	F	At menopause, women at high risk*	At menopause
Breast self-examination	F	20 and over	Every month
Clinical breast examination	F	20-40 Over 40	Every 3 years Every year
Mammography†	F	40-49 50 and over	Every 1-2 years Every year
Health counseling and cancer checkup‡	M & F M & F	Over 20 Over 40	Every 3 years Every year

From Levin BI, Murphy GP: Revision in American Cancer Society guidelines for the early detection of colorectal cancer, *CA-A Journal for Physicians* 42:296-299, 1992.
*History of infertility, obesity, failure to ovulate, abnormal uterine bleeding, or estrogen therapy.
†Screening mammography should begin by age 40.
‡To include examination for cancers of the thyroid, testicles, prostate, ovaries, lymph nodes, oral region, and skin.

preventive health care" for patients to replace the traditional annual physical examination.[2] As their predecessors had, they outlined that these recommendations were *minimal* preventive measures "for asymptomatic persons at low medical risk." The guidelines were produced by the Medical Practice Committee of the ACP after critical review of the medical literature pertaining to the periodic health examination. Their efforts summarize the recommendations of Frame and Carlson, Breslow and Somers, the Canadian task force, and the American Cancer Society in a graphic format to demonstrate consistency and areas of disagreement.

Since this summary, the ACP has sought to further the science of the use of common diagnostic and screening tests. Sox et al. addressed the routine use of chest radiographs, electrocardiograms, and laboratory studies both as baseline studies and in ambulatory screening.[48] In collaboration with the Blue Cross and Blue Shield Association's Medical Necessity Program, the ACP produced guidelines in 1991 outlining their own preventive care guidelines.[27,42,48] Their summary attempts to highlight areas of agreement as well as disagreement among the major guideline recommendations that have been made and to point out those recommendations that need most clarification.

They distinguished between "general interventions" that should be offered to persons who have neither symptoms nor risk factors of the target condition and "selective interventions" that should be applied to persons without symptoms who have one or more risk factors for their target condition.[42] They note that agreement among the American College of Physicians, Canadian task force, and U.S. Preventive Services Task Force are for the most part consistent in "general intervention" guidelines but differ in definition of risk and thereby application of "selective interventions."[42] The box on p. 27 includes selected recommendations of these guidelines for "general intervention" where agreement among the major expert groups exists. Importantly, the ACP review of preventive care guidelines outlines reasons for disagreement or differences in preventive care guidelines by the major groups. These are outlined in the box. The efforts of the ACP provide another step in the process of promoting a consistent standard for periodic health examinations and preventive care.

THE AMERICAN MEDICAL ASSOCIATION

The American Medical Association (AMA) first advocated the concept of the periodic medical examination of healthy persons in 1923. In 1983 the Council on Scientific

---

Proposed reasons for differences in preventive care guidelines among major authoritative groups

Different evidence was available at the time the guidelines were made.

Different methods were used to construct the recommendations.

Different value judgments of the potential outcomes of preventive interventions were made.

Different considerations of economic costs of preventive strategies were made.

Summarized from Hayward RS et al: Preventive care guidelines: 1991, *Ann Intern Med* 114:758-783, 1991.

Aspects of cardiovascular risk factor evaluation addressed by an Ad Hoc Committee of the American Heart Association

Cardiac history including symptoms and risk factors
Family history of cardiac disease and risk factors
Diet survey
Physical examination
Smoking
Blood pressure
Cholesterol and blood lipids
Plasma glucose
Body weight and body fat
Exercise
Behavioral considerations

Grundy SM et al: Cardiovascular risk factor evaluation of healthy American adults, American Heart Association, *Circulation* 75:1340A-1362A, 1987.

Affairs of the AMA readdressed the principles of the periodic health examination and in doing so considered the recommendations of previously published authoritative reports that had developed predominantly in the previous 10 years.[3] They concluded that the periodic evaluation was important in the early detection of disease and in the recognition and correction of risk factors; that the optimal frequency of the examination varied among individuals; that recommendations by the AMA and other groups serve as a framework that should be individually modified; that testing of individuals should be pursued only when adequate treatment or intervention and follow-up observation can be ensured; that continued investigation is needed to determine the usefulness of screening tests; and most importantly that "physicians need to improve their skills in fostering patients' good health and in dealing with long recognized problems such as hypertension, obesity, anxiety, and depression, as well as the excessive use of alcohol, tobacco, and drugs."[3] In compiling their report, the council recognized that physicians and physician groups are unlikely to agree on all of those procedures that should be undertaken and when they should be undertaken for a given individual, and that recommendations frequently change as new data and evidence accumulate. They indicated that recommendations should be viewed only as "informed guidelines," and that in applying these guidelines the practitioner must assume the "obligation" for follow-up monitoring of a potentially harmful condition.[3] They emphasized the building of mutual trust and knowledge in the doctor-patient relationship, the merit of using anniversaries or birthdays as reminders for persons to assess health periodically, and the consideration of cost.

More recently, the American Medical Association has assisted the U.S. Preventive Services Task Force in disseminating the conclusions of their efforts. The *Journal of the American Medical Association* was hailed as an important vehicle for helping to break down the barriers to widespread adoption of preventive practices outlined by the preventive services task force.[44] In commenting on the journal's joining with the U.S. Preventive Services Task Force, Lawrence noted that "many physicians perceive a lack of consensus among recommending groups regarding appropriate clinical preventive services," indicating that the joining of the *Journal of the American Medical Association* with the task force was a step toward functional consensus.[44]

THE AMERICAN HEART ASSOCIATION

In 1987, an ad hoc committee of the American Heart Association (AHA) chaired by Scott Grundy issued a position statement regarding cardiovascular and risk factor evaluation of healthy American adults.[41] The association established their position that "prevention is the greatest need in cardiovascular medicine."[41] As the American Cancer Society had recognized that prevention of cancer was possible, the American Heart Association noted that "many cardiovascular diseases, particularly atherosclerotic heart disease, can be prevented."[41] Their statement reviews the relationships between primary risk factors (hypercholesterolemia, smoking, and hypertension) and coronary heart disease as well as secondary risk factors such as obesity, diabetes mellitus, and reduced concentration of high-density lipoproteins. This effort by the AHA helped to establish prevention of coronary heart disease as a major goal of persons practicing cardiology and to heighten public awareness of risk factors and their relationship to this major cause of death in U.S. adults. The box above lists those aspects of evaluation and screening pertinent to cardiovascular disease addressed by the American Heart Association in the 1987 document.

OBOLER AND LAFORCE

Following the framework that had been established in the previous 15 years, in 1989 Sylvia Oboler and Mark

Table 2-2. Recommendations for screening asymptomatic adults of average risk

Procedure by age group	Frequency
Men	
Age 20 to 59	
Blood pressure measurement	Every 2 years
Weight	Every 4 years
Dental screening	Annually
Cardiac auscultation for valve disease	Once
Skin examination for dysplastic nevi	Once
Age 60 or older	
Blood pressure measurement	Every 2 years
Weight	Every 4 years
Visual acuity	Annually
Hearing	Annually
Dental screening	Annually
Cardiac auscultation for valve disease	Once
Abdominal palpation for aortic aneurysm	Annually
Women	
Age 20 to 39	
Blood pressure measurement	Every 2 years
Weight	Every 4 years
Dental screening	Annually
Cardiac auscultation for valve disease	Once
Skin examination for dysplastic nevi	Once
Pelvic exam with Papanicolaou smear	Every 3 years†
Age 40 to 59	
Blood pressure measurement	Every 2 years
Weight	Every 4 years
Dental screening	Annually
Breast palpation*	Annually
Pelvic examination with Papanicolaou smear	Every 3 years
Age 60 or older	
Blood pressure measurement	Every 2 years
Weight	Every 4 years
Visual acuity	Annually
Hearing	Annually
Dental screening	Annually
Cardiac auscultation for valve disease	Once
Breast palpation*	Annually
Pelvic examination with Papanicolaou smear	Every 3 years

From Oboler SK, LaForce FM: The periodic physical examination in asymptomatic adults, *Ann Intern Med* 110:214-226, 1989.
*Includes mammography.
†After two negative test results, 1 year apart.

LaForce critically evaluated the components of the physical examination applied to asymptomatic adults.[46] They noted that "internists have generally not applied the same standards to the physical examination as they have to other diagnostic tests."[46] They then set out to review the medical literature and scientific evidence for the various components of the physical examination applied to the periodic evaluation of adult patients. They cited trials that had shown that applying the general medical examination to patients without symptoms was a "medically unproductive exercise." They did recognize, however, that the examination conveyed "a special sense of caring," helped to establish "friendship and trust" in defining mutual expectations with patients, and provided the reassurance that patients often seek.[46] They concentrated their efforts on evaluation of the physical maneuvers of the periodic examination; their conclusions are outlined in Table 2-2. They caution that these are minimal standards that should be modified with respect to individual risk, presence of symptoms, and need for reassurance. Their work serves to break down the dogma of accepted practice by consideration of scientific evidence.

THE U.S. PREVENTIVE SERVICES TASK FORCE

In 1984, stimulated by the example and success of the Canadian task force, the U.S. Preventive Services Task Force was organized under the U.S. Department of Health and Human Services. Like the Canadian task force, the U.S. group was charged with outlining recommendations for the appropriate use of preventive interventions based on a critical review of scientific evidence of clinical effectiveness of those interventions for medical clinicians. This task force worked in concert with the Canadian group and used common methods for evaluating the quality of evidence and formulating recommendations. The rules for classifying scientific evidence used by the U.S. task force were adopted from the Canadian rules with minor modifications.[51] A similar classification system for grading the strength of recommendations was likewise used.

In 1989, the U.S. Preventive Services Task Force published the *Guide to Clinical Preventive Services: an Assessment of the Effectiveness of 169 Interventions*.[51] This monumental document has helped to focus the attention of government, physicians, and the public on the importance of preventive intervention in clinical practice. This effort also serves as a means of establishing consensus not only among physicians practicing in the United States but in Canada as well. The sense of cooperation between the Canadian and U.S. task forces is evident in this work.[38] This report provides summaries of evidence and comprehensive recommendations for preventive care in children, adults, and pregnant women (see Chapter 1). Together with the work of the Canadian task force, this guide provides a comprehensive review of the medical literature and helps to define research needs and priorities.

The task force divides their recommendations into screening, counseling, and immunizations and chemoprophylaxis.[51] The greater portion of their recommendations relates to screening interventions. Selected services from the guidelines, which the ACP and the Canadian task force also recommend, are outlined in the box on p. 24.

In our experience, the size and depth of the work provide an excellent reference for the practitioner rather than a practical and easy to use day-to-day desktop guide to use in the care of the individual office patient. The guide serves to remind clinicians of the many areas of accepted clinical practice that are not well founded in scientific evidence and clear efficacy. In pointing out "gray" areas and at times being neutral in either recommending or not recommending a given intervention, the guidelines may disappoint some practicing clinicians, who must in these instances rely on their own knowledge and experience for application to their own unique patient base. On the other hand, recommendations for patient education and counseling given in the text outline methods to assist clinicians, particularly those early in their educational process, to become better educators and counselors.[51] These are highlighted in the box at right and discussed further in Chapter 8.

When the Preventive Services Task Force project ended in 1989 with the publication of the *Guide,* the need for an ongoing program of reevaluation and revision became clear. Some of the areas outlined in the guide had already become outdated at the time of publication because of accumulation of new data. The U.S. Public Health Service therefore established the expert panel on preventive services to continue the work begun by the task force and to update recommendations with revised versions of the *Guide to Clinical Preventive Services.*[52] The stated mission of the expert panel preventive services is "to evaluate the efficacy and effectiveness of clinical preventive services not examined by the U.S. Preventive Services Task Force" and "to re-evaluate clinical preventive services examined by the U.S. Preventive Services Task Force and for which there are new scientific evidence, new technologies that merit consideration, or other reasons to re-evaluate the U.S. Preventive Services Task Force recommendations."[52] The focus of their efforts is to be on primary and secondary prevention for patients in traditional primary care settings. This prioritization is based on the burden of suffering, uncertainty about appropriate practice, timeliness, cost, availability of evidence, and feasibility.[52]

SUMMARY AND CONCLUSIONS

The evolution of the periodic health examination serves as a case in point of replacing accepted dogma with scientific evidence. The current dilemma for physicians is the distillation of this mountain of information into a practical approach to patient care. How then does the physician consider the many and sometimes varied recommendations of guidelines by individual experts, organizations, societies, and governments? How does the physician provide both a short- and a long-term plan for individual patients? How are these plans affected by reimbursement for preventive services and the expectations of patients? Like the now accepted components of the history and physical examination generally used in medical education (chief complaint, history of present illness, social history, family history, review of medical symptoms, vital signs, physical examination, and laboratory studies leading to a problem

---

Recommendations for patient education and counseling

1. Develop a therapeutic alliance.
2. Counsel all patients.
3. Ensure that patients understand the relationship between behavior and health.
4. Work with patients to assess barriers to behavior change.
5. Gain commitment to change from patients.
6. Involve patients in selecting risk factors to change.
7. Use a combination of strategies.
8. Design a behavior modification plan.
9. Monitor progress through follow-up contact.
10. Involve office staff.

From U.S. Preventive Service Task Force: *Guide to clinical preventive services: an assessment of the effectiveness of 169 interventions,* Baltimore, 1989, Williams & Wilkins.

---

list and plan) the approach to preventive care similarly needs to be ingrained into the primary practitioner's mind. The practitioner must consider prevention an important component of the service he or she provides. The practitioner needs to envision every patient encounter as an opportunity for institution of preventive care. The common threads of the recommendations reviewed in this chapter are the consideration of risk factors and the application of proven interventions. Ideally assessment of risk factors for common and important conditions, institution of screening interventions of proven efficacy, and application of immunizations for appropriate and proven chemoprophylaxis will become priorities for health care providers. It is hoped that an evolution toward greater emphasis on effectiveness, benefit, and implementation of counseling by physicians, replacing the current concentration, of both time and monetary resources, on screening alone. will take place. Box 2-3 provides a guideline for the practitioner to consider in practice as a beginning framework for the institution of preventive services in the asymptomatic patient of low risk. As risk factor profiles for patients are constructed, preventive services become targeted at those conditions of greatest concern.

REFERENCES

1. American Cancer Society: Report on the cancer-related health checkup, *CA—A Journal for Physicians* 30:194-240, 1980.
2. American College of Physicians: Periodic health examination: a guide for designing individualized preventive health care in the asymptomatic patients, *Ann Intern Med* 95:729-732, 1981.
3. American Medical Association Council on Scientific Affairs: Medical evaluation of healthy persons, *JAMA* 249:1626-1633, 1983.
4. Battista RN et al: The periodic health examination: an evolving concept, *Can Med Assoc J* 130:1288-1292, 1984.
5. Breslow L, Somers AR: The lifetime health-monitoring program: a practical approach to preventive medicine, *N Engl J Med* 296:601-608, 1977.

6. Canadian Task Force on the Periodic Health Examination: The periodic health examination, *Can Med Assoc J* 121:1193-1254, 1979.

7. Canadian Task Force on the Periodic Health Examination: The periodic health examination. 2. 1984 update, *Can Med Assoc J* 130:1278-1285, 1984.

8. Canadian Task Force on the Periodic Health Examination: The periodic health examination. 2. 1986 update, *Can Med Assoc J* 134:721-729, 1986.

9. Canadian Task Force on the Periodic Health Examination: The periodic health examination. 2. 1987 update. *Can Med Assoc J* 138:618-626, 1988.

10. Canadian Task Force on the Periodic Health Examination: The periodic health examination. 2. 1989 update, *Can Med Assoc J* 141:209-216, 1989.

11. Canadian Task Force on the Periodic Health Examination: The periodic health examination, 1989 update. 3. Preschool examination for developmental, visual and hearing problems, *Can Med Assoc J* 141:1136-1140, 1989.

12. Canadian Task Force on the Periodic Health Examination: The periodic health examination, 1989 update. 4. Intrapartum electronic fetal monitoring and prevention of neonatal herpes simplex, *Can Med Assoc J.* 141:1233-1240, 1989.

13. Canadian Task Force on the Periodic Health Examination: The periodic health examination, 1990 update. 1. Early detection of hyperthyroidism and hypothyroidism in adults and screening of newborns for congenital hypothyroidism, *Can Med Assoc J* 142:955-961, 1990.

14. Canadian Task Force on the Periodic Health Examination: The periodic health examination, 1990 update. 2. Early detection of depression and prevention of suicide, *Can Med Assoc J* 142:1233-1238, 1990.

15. Canadian Task Force on the Periodic Health Examination: The periodic health examination, 1990 update. 3. Interventions to prevent lung cancer other than smoking cessation, *Can Med Assoc J* 143:269-272, 1990.

16. Canadian Task Force on the Periodic Health Examination: The periodic health examination, 1990 update. 4. Well-baby care in the first 2 years of life, *Can Med Assoc J* 143:867-872, 1990.

17. Canadian Task Force on the Periodic Health Examination: The periodic health examination, 1991 update. 1. Screening for cognitive impairment in the elderly, *Can Med Assoc J* 144:425-431, 1991.

18. Canadian Task Force on the Periodic Health Examination: The periodic health examination, 1991 update. 2. Administration of pneumococcal vaccine, *Can Med Assoc J* 144:665-671, 1991.

19. Canadian Task Force on the Periodic Health Examination: The periodic health examination, 1991 update. 3. Secondary prevention of prostate cancer, *Can Med Assoc J* 145:413-428, 1991.

20. Canadian Task Force on the Periodic Health Examination: The periodic health examination, 1991 update. 4. Screening for cystic fibrosis, *Can Med Assoc J* 145:629-635, 1991.

21. Canadian Task Force on the Periodic Health Examination: The periodic health examination, 1991 update. 5. Screening for abdominal aortic aneurysm, *Can Med Assoc J* 145:783-789, 1991.

22. Canadian Task Force on the Periodic Health Examination: The periodic health examination, 1991 update. 6. Acetylsalicylic acid and the primary prevention of cardiovascular disease, *Can Med Assoc J* 145:1091-1095, 1991.

23. Canadian Task Force on the Periodic Health Examination: The periodic health examination, 1992 update. 1. Screening for gestational diabetes, *Can Med Assoc J* 147:435-443, 1992.

24. Canadian Task Force on the Periodic Health Examination: The periodic health examination, 1992 update. 2. Routine prenatal ultrasound screening, *Can Med Assoc J* 147:627-633, 1992.

25. Canadian Task Force on the Periodic Health Examination: The periodic health examination, 1992 update. 3. HIV antibody screening, *Can Med Assoc J* 147:867-876, 1992.

26. Charap MH: The periodic health examination: genesis of a myth, *Ann Intern Med* 95:733-735, 1981.

27. Eddy DM, editor: *Common screening tests,* Philadelphia, 1991, American College of Physicians.

28. Fink DI: Guidelines for the cancer related checkup. In *American Cancer Society textbook of clinical oncology,* Atlanta, 1991, American Cancer Society.

29. Frame PS: Health maintenance in clinical practice: strategies and barriers, *Am Fam Physician* 45:1192-1200, 1992.

30. Frame PS, Carlson SJ: A critical review of periodic health screening using specific screening criteria. Part 1. Selected diseases of respiratory, cardiovascular, and central nervous systems, *J Fam Pract* 2:29-36, 1975.

31. Frame PS, Carlson SJ: A critical review of periodic health screening using specific screening criteria. Part 2. Selected endocrine, metabolic, and gastrointestinal diseases, *J Fam Pract* 2:123-129, 1975.

32. Frame PS, Carlson SJ: A critical review of periodic health screening using specific screening criteria. Part 3. Selected diseases of the genitourinary system, *J Fam Pract* 2:189-194, 1975.

33. Frame PS, Carlson SJ: A critical review of periodic health screening using specific screening criteria. Part 4. Selected miscellaneous diseases, *J Fam Pract* 2:283-289, 1975.

34. Frame PS: A critical review of adult health maintenance. Part 1. Prevention of atherosclerotic diseases, *J Fam Pract* 22:341-346, 1986.

35. Frame PS: A critical review of adult health maintenance. Part 2. Prevention of infectious diseases, *J Fam Pract* 22:417-422, 1986.

36. Frame PS: A critical review of adult health maintenance. Part 3. Prevention of cancer, *J Fam Pract* 22:511-520, 1986.

37. Frame PS: A critical review of adult health maintenance. Part 4. Prevention of metabolic, behavioral, and miscellaneous conditions, *J Fam Pract.* 23:29-39, 1986.

38. Goldbloom RB, Lawrence RS: Preface. In *Preventing disease: beyond the rhetoric,* New York, 1990, Springer-Verlag.

39. Gould GM: A system of personal biological examination: the condition of adequate medical and scientific conduct of life, *JAMA* 35:134-138, 1900.

40. Green LW: Prevention and health education. In *Maxcy-Rosenau public health and preventive medicine,* Norwalk, Conn, 1986, Appleton-Century-Crofts.

41. Grundy SM et al: Cardiovascular and risk factor evaluation of healthy American adults. A statement for physicians by an ad hoc committee appointed by the Steering Committee. American Heart Association, *Circulation* 75:1340A-1362A, 1987.

42. Hayward RS et al: Preventive care guidelines: 1991, *Ann Intern Med* 114:758-783, 1991.

43. Holleb AI: Guidelines for the cancer related checkup: five years later, *CA—A Journal for Physicians* 35:194-196, 1985.

44. Lawrence RS, Mickalide AD: Preventive services in clinical practice: designing the periodic health examination, *JAMA* 257:2205-2207, 1987.

45. Levin BI, Murphy GP: Revision in American Cancer Society recommendations for the early detection of colorectal cancer, *CA—A Journal for Physicians* 42:296-299, 1992.

46. Oboler SK, LaForce FM: The periodic physical examination in asymptomatic adults, *Ann Intern Med* 110:214-226, 1989.

47. *Periodic health examination: a manual for physicians,* Chicago, 1947, American Medical Association.

48. Sox HC, editor: *Common diagnostic tests: use and interpretation,* Philadelphia, 1987, American College of Physicians.

49. Spitzer WO: The periodic health examination: introduction. *Can Med Assoc J* 130:1276-1278, 1984.

50. U.S. Department of Health and Human Services Public Health Service: *Healthy People 2000—national health promotion and disease prevention objectives,* US Government Printing Office, 1991, DHHS Pub No (PHS) 91-50213.

51. U.S. Preventive Services Task Force: *Guide to clinical preventive*

services: an assessment of the effectiveness of 169 interventions, Baltimore, 1989, Williams & Wilkins.

52. Woolf SH, Sox HC: The expert panel on prevention services: continuing the work of the US Preventive Services Task Force. *Am J Prev Med* 7:326-330, 1991.

RESOURCES

Healthfinder, C/O National Health Information Clearing House (NHIC), P.O. Box 1133, Washington, DC 20013-1133. Provides a summary of health risk appraisals that may be used as tools to help people recognize health risk.

Guide to Clinical Preventive Services: an assessment of the effectiveness of 169 interventions. Report of the U.S. Preventive Services Task Force, Wilkins & Wilkins, 428 E. Preston Street, Baltimore, MD 21202. Full report of the U.S. Preventive Services Task Force assessing the effectiveness of preventive intervention and providing a comprehensive bibliography for these interventions.

Common Screening Tests, Edited by David M. Eddy, American College of Physicians, Philadelphia, PA, 19175. Comprehensive review of the use of common screening tests.

Health Services Directorate, Health Services and Promotion Branch, Department of National Health and Welfare, Tunney's Pasture, Ottawa, Ontario, Canada KIA 1B4. Provides Canadian Task Force reports on the periodic health examination.

Chapter 3

TEACHING PREVENTIVE MEDICINE

Martin D. Keller

In 1983 the Association of Teachers of Preventive Medicine sponsored the publication of a monograph on *Teaching Preventive Medicine in Primary Care,* edited by William H. Barker.[4] Although published nearly a decade ago, this book remains the most comprehensive discussion of the teaching of what is currently termed "clinical preventive medicine." Therefore this chapter will avoid duplication of this work and draw largely on the author's experience in teaching preventive medicine to medical students, graduate students, and residents.

SCOPE

Preventive medicine and public health are often termed social medicine or population medicine. Rosenau's book was first titled *Preventive Medicine and Hygiene,* renamed *Preventive Medicine and Public Health,* and later renamed *Public Health and Preventive Medicine.* The shift in emphasis, as Last reported in the preface to the eleventh edition, is an acknowledgment that the larger context is public health, to which the disciplines of preventive medicine are the major contributors. The American Board of Preventive Medicine includes the specialties of general preventive medicine/public health, occupational medicine, and aerospace medicine, all of which deal primarily with the protection of the health of groups. During the past 2 decades, with the growth of interest and specialization in primary health care, new emphasis has been placed on clinical preventive medicine, a subspecialty that brings closer together the preventive care of the individual and the prevention of disease in the community. Some have suggested that clinical preventive medicine may be a fourth subspecialty under the American Board of Preventive Medicine (see Chapter 1). This chapter is concerned primarily with education in clinical preventive medicine.

BACKGROUND

Preventive medicine, as a distinct field, had its beginnings early in the twentieth century, in the wake of advances in bacteriology. As preventive medicine demonstrated the successful application of medical measures in the control of infectious diseases, the conviction grew that the disciplines associated with preventive medicine could be successfully applied as well in the control of noninfectious diseases. The development of information and thought in the field of preventive medicine may be traced through changes in the sequence of editions of key textbooks in this field. This is particularly true of the first major textbook on preventive medicine, by Milton J. Rosenau, issued in 1913,[11] which is now in its thirteenth edition, edited by John M. Last, and published in January, 1992.[9] Rosenau's words in the preface to the first edition are instructive:

Exact knowledge has taken the place of fads and fancies in hygiene and sanitation; the capable health officer now possesses facts concerning infections which permit their prevention and even their suppression in some instances. Many of these problems are complicated with economic and social difficulties, which are given due consideration, for preventive medicine has become a basic factor in sociology.

In 1953 Leavell and Clark[10] employed a model of the "natural history of disease" as a framework for the presentation of available information on the prevention of specific diseases and for revealing gaps in our knowledge regarding the interaction of disease-causing agents with populations at risk and the role of environmental factors in this interaction. The model illustrates how preventive measures may be applied throughout the natural history of a disease: from the period before the disease occurs, through its early or inapparent stages, to its clinical manifestations, and to the progression to recovery or to chronicity, disability, and death. At each stage, there are measures that may be taken to prevent the occurrence or to detect the presence of the disease and to intervene early enough to allow the greatest chance of reversal or favorable modification to achieve the best possible outcome.

The natural history model remains a compelling way of presenting the basic principles of preventive medicine to medical students, physicians, and allied health professionals. The model may suffer, however, from its global nature, as it appears to encompass all of medical care and public health, without clearly delineating "prevention."

Salive[12] points out that the field of preventive medicine is beset by an identity crisis that seriously affects the content and structure of preventive medicine education. In many instances, the purposes of preventive medicine are stated so broadly as to include all things that are associated with the prevention and control of disease and the promotion of health in individuals and in populations. Salive refers to the view that the strength of preventive medicine resides in its ability to redefine its role in medical education as our social structures and the needs of the population change. However, he sees the specialty at risk of becoming "a chameleon," continually altering its coloration to suit changing social, economic, educational, and technical environments. There appears to be no consensus regarding the essential nature of this field. Perhaps this characterization of preventive medicine education is extreme, but it reflects a lack of distinction between the needs of medical students, those of practitioners of medicine, and those of specialists in preventive medicine. How broadly the field is defined is mostly conditioned by the interests and enthusiasms of the teachers, often without regard to the needs and interests of students at different levels of development and specialization.

THE PRECLINICAL YEARS OF THE MEDICAL CURRICULUM

With very few exceptions, students arrive in medical schools with a vision of themselves as healers in one-to-one relationships with patients. To be confronted with demands to learn the abstract principles of epidemiology and biostatistics often seems a surprising diversion, if not an outright shock. These subjects appear out of place, particularly in the medical schools that have introduced clinical encounters into the early phases of the curriculum. Even in the relatively few medical schools that provide significant time and persuasive teachers of preventive medicine in the "preclinical" years of the curriculum, little attention is given to building on this early education to integrate the

concepts and skills of preventive medicine into the "clinical" years that follow. As a result, nearly all medical students are graduated with little positive feeling toward epidemiology and biostatistics and little recognition of the importance of these disciplines to them as physicians.

In addition, many of the principles of preventive medicine that are imparted are not so labeled. For example, medical students generally learn about immunizations and well-child examinations in pediatrics; prenatal care in obstetrics; risk reduction of heart disease and cancer in internal medicine; and a variety of similar topics in the other clinical departments. Medical students have little opportunity to work with specialists in preventive medicine, except in a few specifically devised electives, and there is generally little time in the medical curriculum for more than cursory exposure to preventive medicine, as such.

With the advent of departments of family and community medicine, new opportunities appeared to interweave clinical service, usually based in ambulatory medical care, with the teaching of preventive medicine. For the medical student, the primary care clinics can offer a natural setting for learning how physicians apply preventive measures in the care of individual patients. In such settings, medical students can also gain appreciation of the value for clinicians of information derived from health surveys, case-control studies, cohort studies, clinical trials, and community trials. Students can be helped to recognize how such information, appearing in medical journals, is utilized in the development of practice guidelines and the assessment of clinical efficacy. The general subject of medical decision making can bridge preventive medicine and clinical care, illustrating the place of epidemiology and biostatistics in clinical problem solving. Of course, this is only in part the province of departments of family and community medicine. Such teaching has for many years been provided by departments of preventive medicine and, to some extent, by other clinical departments. However, with continuing emphasis on narrow specialization in most clinical services, and in preventive medicine as well, fewer and fewer models for teaching clinical preventive medicine can be found in colleges of medicine and university hospitals. In many colleges of medicine, both primary care and preventive medicine have been relegated to second-class status.

What then is the role, within colleges of medicine, of specialists in the disciplines of preventive medicine? These disciplines generally include epidemiology, biostatistics, occupational and environmental health, health care studies, behavioral sciences, and health education. It is unlikely that any of these can, in the near future, find a proper place and sufficient time in the medical curriculum. Painful as it may be for dedicated specialists in departments of preventive medicine, much of their teaching efforts must be directed to strengthening the teaching of the principles of their specialties in other departments (as was suggested in Chapter 1). As a trade-off for such labor in the vineyards of others, perhaps they can acquire more time in the curriculum and more faculty resources for lectures, conferences, and planned experiences for students in the key areas of preventive medicine. This would be an affirmation of the importance of their disciplines in the preparation of effective physicians.

It is possible to take advantage of the early rush to "clinical exposure" that often duplicates, in an elementary way, the later and more extensive experience with patients on the clinical services. From the point of view of education, many of these early patient encounters are equivalent to eating a sandwich before going to a banquet. However, by recognizing and building on the keen interest of medical students in patients, it is possible to introduce the principles of epidemiology and biostatistics in terms of the

practice of medicine: the medical history, concepts of risk, screening for inapparent diseases, and the evaluation of diagnostic procedures and treatment. From the outset, such teaching can build a framework for the continuation of preventive medicine education as an integral part of the study of pathophysiology and clinical care. The interaction of specialists in preventive medicine with basic scientists and clinicians throughout the medical curriculum can have other salutary effects. Bringing such faculty members together in teaching efforts allows them to become better acquainted with the expertise of their cross-disciplinary colleagues and prepares them for collaboration in research and scholarly activity as well as in teaching.

The box below presents a model for a preclinical course in preventive medicine. It is the product of the experience of one faculty of preventive medicine attempting to build a

---

Model for a preclinical course in preventive medicine

1. **What does this case or disease represent in the community?**
   Concepts of causality
   Agents of disease
   Persons-at-risk, profile of high-risk persons
   Interaction of agent, host, and environment
   The course of the disease
   Strategies of intervention
     Primary prevention
     Secondary: early detection and care
     Tertiary: diagnosis and treatment of overt disease
   Illustration of the natural history of selected diseases of current concern

2. **Who is normal?**
   How do we determine the "normal range" of test results?
   Selecting screening tests: Sensitivity, specificity, predictive value, and the effect of prevalence on predictive value
   Ruling-in and ruling-out
   Serial and parallel testing
   Current thinking regarding routine screening tests

3. **How well do you know the odds?**
   How do we make decisions from data?
   The role of probability in medical decision-making
   Descriptive statistics: mean, median, mode, standard deviation, and standard error
   Testing hypotheses: comparing means and proportions; and correlations
   Type I and type II errors
   How to understand statistical statements in the medical literature
   Examples of the use of statistics in medicine

4. **How long do I have? Thoughts on prognosis.**
   Distinction between risk factors and prognostic factors
   Survival analysis
   Cohort studies to assess prognosis
   Biases that may affect cohort studies
   Combinations of factors affecting prognosis

5. **What shall we do for the patient?**
   Thoughts on the choice of treatments
   Clinical trials
     Selection of a study population
     Allocation of patients to treatment and control groups
     Randomization
     Double-blind studies
   Types of biases and methods of reducing bias
   Ethical considerations
   Examples of past and present clinical trials

6. **There is a lot of it going around!**
   Description of the occurrence of a disease
     Incidence
     Prevalence
     Secular trends
     Crude rates
     Cause-specific rates
     Proportional and standard mortality ratios
   Relative and attributable risks
   Methods of rate adjustment
   Investigating an outbreak of a disease, including examples of such investigations

7. **Are you a case or a control?**
   Retrospective and prospective studies, advantages and disadvantages
   Odds ratio and relative risk
   Concurrent and historical cohort studies
   Illustrative examples of case-control and cohort studies

basis for the continuation of preventive medicine teaching throughout the medical curriculum. Teaching is likely to be best when the teachers are most comfortable with the method and the content. This model, if utilized, must be modified and adapted to the interests and needs of other departments and student bodies.

A seven-part series of lectures and discussions is designed to illustrate how the concepts of preventive medicine relate to questions of human health and disease and to the provision of medical care. Usually, a brief presentation of a case is used to introduce the subject of each lecture or discussion.

Dr. Richard Matzen offered a very useful suggestion for an additional unit in the series in the box on p. 34, to be titled "Who is the patient?" This unit would emphasize the concept that every patient represents one or more very specific subsets of the general population (genetic, cultural, occupational, and other demographic subsets). These variables, together with age and sex, affect the probability of the occurrence of certain diseases, as well as affecting health knowledge, attitudes, and behaviors. Such considerations not only help in history taking and medical decision making, but they also lend additional intrigue and intellectual stimulation to the practice of medicine.

The listing of topics to be covered at each of the lectures (see box) may resemble the table of contents of a book but actually represents a set of readings and handouts distributed to medical students in preparation for the aforementioned sessions. This approach seeks to make the concepts of preventive medicine meaningful to the students in terms that relate to their interest in patients and medical care. Wherever possible, basic scientists and clinicians are involved in preparing and reviewing the material and participating in the presentations. As may be seen from the sequence of topics presented above, the curriculum emphasizes the importance of epidemiology and related biostatistical methods, not only in preventive medicine, but also in the entire scope of the health and medical sciences, and their application and importance to individual patients.

This overall approach appears to be effective in presenting introductory material and preparing for continuation of preventive medicine education later in the curriculum. However, like many other approaches, this has not been adequately evaluated. It is difficult to do so without a specifically designed experiment utilizing more than one method of instruction, allocating students at random, and determining the effectiveness of alternative methods, not only immediately after the presentations but in the later years of the medical curriculum, postgraduate years, and during the practice of medicine.

THE CLINICAL YEARS OF THE MEDICAL CURRICULUM

The clinical setting, in which medical students, interns, and residents acquire experience in treating patients, gives further opportunity to present the patient as an indicator of the health of the community. Each case can illustrate the natural history of a disease and the strategies of intervention that may prevent the disease, detect it at an early stage, and provide proper medical diagnosis and treatment in a timely fashion. In this context, the principles of epidemiology and health statistics can come alive for the medical student. For example, a patient with AIDS represents an instance of the pandemic of HIV infection. We can look back at how this disease was first recognized in the United States, how our present knowledge and understanding unfolded, how the combined efforts of clinical, laboratory, epidemiological, and public health professionals have made important contributions, and how they will continue to do so.

Similarly, although perhaps less dramatically, the discussion may focus on a case of coronary heart disease. What does this case represent in the community at large? How well are we controlling this serious health problem? To the degree that we appear to be making progress, to what do we owe our success? Can we really explain the decline in coronary disease mortality over the last 2 to 3 decades? What are we doing that is right, if anything? If we could know, perhaps we could do more. On the other hand, to the degree that we are not succeeding, what are the reasons for this lack of success? To what extent is the failure due to lack of knowledge, insufficient resources, mixed-up priorities, or problems of policy, planning, organization, and management? Finally, what must we do now; what are the logical next steps in controlling the disease presented by the patient? Where does this disease stand in the overall hierarchy of our medical and social priorities? These are essentially the questions asked by specialists in preventive medicine. Such questions can be introduced effectively in the teaching of clinical medicine through cases. In this endeavor, an alliance of preventive medicine faculty, basic scientists, and clinicians will benefit faculty and students alike.

Another approach to instruction in preventive medicine, during the clinical years, involves the application of the principles and techniques of prevention to individual patients. The educational objective is the inculcation of the habit of thinking about the special preventive or prospective medical care needs of each patient. Most physicians recognize that a given complaint may not be of great consequence to the patient's health in comparison with other health risks often unknown to the patient. The patient's complaint must be addressed, but the patient would be poorly served if this is where it ended. Consider, for example, a young person who seeks advice regarding the appearance of red blood in the stool. The blood may be found to originate in a small hemorrhoid. However, the patient may also have hypertension, hyperlipidemia, and any number of other health hazards that need attention. The patient's lifestyle may be the most serious health hazard. The armamentarium of the physician therefore must include an understanding of the questions to be asked, the tests to be performed, and the counseling to be offered in relation to the patient's age, sex, medical history, family history, occupational history, habits, and so forth. Although these ideas are often presented in the history-taking course, they tend to fade into the background as medical students encounter patients with serious and dramatic illnesses, and therefore they must be reinforced.

One of the problems of preventive medicine is its all-inclusiveness. For example, at some stage in adolescence, the most important preventive intervention may be the effective presentation of information regarding contraception, responsible sexual behavior, and preparation for parenthood. Similarly, there is need for a progression of effective preventive measures through prenatal care, the care of parents and infants, the preschool and school years, and into adult life. Often overlooked are the so-called "sandwich" years in which adults face the pressures of both children and aging parents. In our society, with the rapid growth of the elderly population, preventive measures in the later years to retain functional capacity, prevent infirmity, and assure comfort and dignity become an essential part of preventive medicine. No single specialty can hope to address all of these problems. Even the specialists in family medicine do not generally deal with all members of the family and with the multitude of generational problems and needs. Preventive medicine may appear so comprehensive that the medical student, as well as the practitioner, will despair of learning where to start and where to end. Yet, the physician is perhaps in the best position to lend strength to all other avenues of health promotion and disease prevention. Through the interaction of the preventive medicine faculty and teachers of clinical care, medical students can gain a sense of security in carrying out the preventive measures indicated for the patients they treat. The *Guide to Clinical Preventive Services*,[13] issued by the U.S. Preventive Services Task Force in 1989, can serve as a valuable resource for instruction in the application of specific screening and diagnostic tests.

In most medical schools, in the junior or senior years, students are allowed to pursue a number of electives. In some schools, these are designated as "selectives," a set of approved assignments that somewhat restrict the scope of the electives. In our experience, dating to 1970, assignment to preventive medicine in the senior year was at first mandatory and later selective. The mandatory program was an overwhelming task for the faculty of preventive medicine and seemed overly restrictive to a significant number of the medical students. Each medical student was required to spend at least 1 month on a full-time special assignment in preventive medicine. It proved exceedingly difficult to accomodate all the students within the Department of Preventive Medicine. Consequently arrangements were made for field experience in a variety of aspects of preventive medicine and public health. The faculty members, who were well acquainted with health and health-related organizations in Ohio, were able to identify agencies and preceptors for medical students throughout the state. In addition, a number of organizations and persons were identified in other parts of the United States and abroad who were willing to accept a medical student for 1 or more months of assignment. The basic requirements of the program were:

1. Selection of a topic deemed by a faculty advisor to be relevant to preventive medicine
2. Determination of a location in which the student could carry out the approved assignment
3. A prospectus, developed by the student and approved by the faculty advisor, specifying the activities to be carried out and their relevance to the medical curriculum
4. Identification of a preceptor at the site of the assignment who agreed to supervise the student
5. Agreement by the student to prepare a paper on a selected aspect of the assignment, with the agreement of the preceptor
6. Oral presentation of the paper at a seminar for faculty and students at a designated date after the end of the assignment

Students who were assigned to locations within the United States spent at least 1 month, full time in this elective, and students who were assigned outside of the United States spent at least 2 months. Since the inception of the program, several changes have been made. Most important, in the early 1980s, the assignments in preventive medicine were made part of the "selective" arrangement and were no longer mandatory for all students. This change allowed the faculty to be more selective in approving student requests and removed the restrictiveness of the program from students who wished to pursue other assignments. Despite this, well over one third of all the students have continued to request assignment in preventive medicine each year. The basic format of the assignments has been retained.

At about the time that the preventive medicine assignments became "selectives," an additional opportunity was developed. Following the initiative of the American Medical Student Association, a program of "Medical Education and Community Organization" was introduced for students at all levels of the medical curriculum. Students have taken advantage of this primarily at the end of the first year of the curriculum and at the end of the second year. The format for this assignment is similar to that of the more traditional preventive medicine assignment. However, instead of the student preparing a prospectus, a format is provided to the student for the study of a selected community, emphasizing the structure and function of the health-care system. Most of the communities to which students have been assigned are in rural areas or small towns. Stipends are provided to defray some of the students' expenses. Students generally spend 1 month interacting with physicians, health departments, other health-related agencies, hospitals, voluntary health agencies, organizations, medical societies, and any other organizations that relate to the structure and function of health care in the selected community. A seminar is held at the close of each assignment period, at which the students are required to present illustrative cases and speak on the utilization of community resources and referral patterns in the care of specific patients. Emphasis is placed on social and economic factors as well as medical interventions.

The field assignment, as previously described, gives students an opportunity to examine the principles of preventive medicine in actual communities. Students have an opportunity to discuss these matters with a variety of health professionals in the communities to which they are assigned and to develop a sense of how the overall health-care system operates. We found this to be an important capstone to the instruction in preventive medicine that is presented in the preclinical and clinical years.

POSTGRADUATE EDUCATION IN CLINICAL PREVENTIVE MEDICINE

On May 11, 1992, an article titled "Prevention Tries to Break into Medicine's Mainstream" appeared in the *American Medical News*. I had the distinct feeling of revisiting arguments that have been made over and over for at least 3 decades. The high cost of health care and the high incidence of chronic diseases, many of which are associated with poor health habits, should be a challenge to all physicians to practice anticipatory, preventive care. Yet there are many barriers to such practice, including the traditional "medical model" based on repair rather than prevention, and existing reimbursement practices that do not include preventive services. All this is well known, and one might ask why one should renew the call to prevention. The answer may lie in the realization that ever greater numbers of Americans are being enrolled in managed care programs and, sooner or later, some form of universal health care system will be instituted in which all Americans will be enrolled. Considering that 250 million or more persons will be covered in a coordinated health insurance program, investments in prevention can be distributed over a large enough population that the investments constitute an actual cost-containment advantage.

Primary care physicians, in particular, will be charged with responsibility for the provision of health promotion and disease prevention measures for their patients. Therefore preventive medicine undoubtedly should be included in the postgraduate education of primary physicians. However, all of the medical specialties need such education, as do all of the allied health-professional programs.

In this section, the basic requirements for residency training in general preventive medicine/public health will be presented as a basis for the education of specialists in clinical preventive medicine, as well as for the infusion of preventive medicine concepts, information, and skills into the postgraduate education of all medical specialties.

Residency training in preventive medicine is the recognized process by which physicians may be certified in one or more of the specialties covered by the American Board of Preventive Medicine: general preventive medicine/public health, occupational medicine, and aerospace medicine. The following discussion deals primarily with general preventive medicine, as this is currently the main route to specialization in clinical preventive medicine.

At a meeting of the Council of Preventive Medicine Residency Programs in March, 1992, preventive medicine as a specialty was characterized by[1]:

1. The study of disease processes as they occur in communities and in defined population groups,
2. The stimulation of practices with respect to the community and the individual that will advance health by promoting health-enhancing environments and behaviors, preventing disease and injury, making possible early diagnosis and treatment, and fostering habilitation and rehabilitation of persons with disabilities

This definition appears to be almost as broad as medical science itself. Somewhere within it resides the specialty of clinical preventive medicine.

There is a set of common components that make up the speciality of preventive medicine, independent of particular subspecialties or fields of practice. Various areas of research or practice may emphasize one or more of these components, but an understanding of all of these is considered essential to specialization in preventive medicine. For the most part, these subjects are included in the curricula of preventive medicine residencies[1]:

1. Application of biostatistical principles and methodology
2. Recognition of epidemiological principles and methodology
3. Planning, administration, and evaluation of health and medical programs and the evaluation of outcomes of health behavior and medical care
4. Recognition, assessment, and control of environmental hazards to health, including those of occupational environments
5. Recognition of the social, cultural, and behavioral factors in medicine
6. Application and evaluation of primary, secondary, and tertiary prevention
7. Assessment of population and individual health needs

To achieve eligibility for certification by the American Board of Preventive Medicine, residents are required to have at least 1 year of postgraduate clinical internship or residency, to pursue an academic program that includes a curriculum approved by the Preventive Medicine Residency Review Committee, and to have a supervised practicum year in which the principles, knowledge, and skills of preventive medicine are applied in a field of special study.

Among the areas of special study and subspecialization, clinical preventive medicine stands as the link between preventive medicine and the other clinical specialties. Specialists in preventive medicine are considered population-based physicians, but the clinical preventive medicine specialist is concerned with both the individual patient and the group from which the patient is drawn. The clinical preventive medicine specialist brings to the clinical setting the skills of epidemiology, biostatistics, and the other components of preventive medicine. An example of clinical preventive medicine training is presented by Crucetti et al.,[5] referring to the program at the Johns Hopkins School of Hygiene and Public Health. Residents obtain the Master of Public Health degree in the first year and pursue clinical rotations in the second and third years. At the end of that time, the residents are eligible for certification in general preventive medicine/public health. Courses are presented on risk assessment, the public health aspects of various risk factors, behavioral aspects of chronic diseases, and the principles and application of preventive measures and health education in primary medical care. Residents also pursue courses in the management of office medical practice and rotations in a variety of clinics, such as preventive cardiology, behavioral medicine, hypertension, and exercise physiology/rehabilitation. Because there are as yet relatively few programs of this sort, each program tends to develop a set of courses and rotations to suit the particular setting, the available faculty, and the interests of students and faculty. As is the case at Johns Hopkins, such programs generally include research training, particularly in regard to clinical trials and the evaluation of outcomes. In the residency program in general preventive medicine/public health at Ohio State University, we have not developed a formal subspecialty area in clinical preventive medicine but rather have individualized elective programs and practicum experience in this area to serve the particular interests and career aspirations of each resident.

Specialists in preventive medicine, in collaboration with other clinical specialists, conduct research to provide scientific bases for clinical preventive medicine. For example, the *Guide to Clinical Preventive Services*[13] assesses the effectiveness of 169 interventions in preventive health care. The Expert Panel on Preventive Services[14] examines the application of preventive practices such as screening, counseling, immunization, and chemoprophylactic regimens. In each instance, specific preventive interventions are rated according to the quality of the available evidence and the support such evidence gives the recommendations that may be made. Such work provides an approach and a rationale for the utilization of scientific information in the practice of clinical preventive medicine. It also highlights the areas in which additional research is required to pro-

vide new information and to clarify ambiguities. Mastery of such information and, where possible, participation in the accumulation of additional knowledge is at least in part the province of the specialist in clinical preventive medicine.

In my own experience as an attending physician in internal medicine and a faculty member in preventive medicine, I found it rewarding to introduce the principles of preventive medicine into clinical rounds. The topics mentioned earlier, as part of the medical curriculum, serve well in this setting. Asking what a specific case may represent in the community leads to a set of epidemiologic and biostatistical considerations:

1. Who are the persons at risk of this disease?
2. How is this disease detected?
    Screening and diagnostic tests, and the "normal range"
3. How have we obtained our knowledge regarding this condition?
    Case series, case-control studies, cohort studies, and clinical trials
4. What do we know about incidence, prevalence, and secular trends in this disease?
5. How can we utilize the concepts of probability in medical decision making?

The objective is to so inculcate these ideas in the residents' experience that they become part of the natural way they think about patients. This takes time, and these ideas must be continually reinforced.

Specialists in clinical preventive medicine function at at least three different levels.

1. The application of epidemiologic and biostatistical techniques in the definition of risk factors, in risk assessment, and in trials of interventions to prevent, detect, or modify the effects of specific illnesses in selected samples of patients. This may result in the promulgation of preventive medicine guidelines, akin to clinical trials of treatment modalities in specific diseases, and the development of clinical practice guidelines.
2. Development of strategies for applying available knowledge and techniques to the implementation of preventive medicine guidelines.
3. Application of risk assessment methods and preventive interventions in individual patients or groups of patients.

In health risk assessments or appraisals, the objective is to develop individualized prescriptions for prevention, based on the best available data. In a sense, this seeks to avoid "shotgun" prevention measures, in the same way that refinements in the treatment of disease seek to eliminate "shotgun" therapeutic measures. Methods are available for the use of health risk appraisals, with specifically designed forms and computer entry and analysis, in physicians' offices, clinics, hospitals, and large managed care programs.[7] Specialists in clinical preventive medicine are in a position to help in the further development of such methods and in fostering their general use in medical care.

The parallels to clinical medical care in general are apparent. The differences lie in the reliance on epidemiologic and biostatistical methods, and the emphasis on health promotion, disease prevention, and early detection. In general, primary physicians do not have the knowledge, equipment, or time to carry out adequate individualized health risk appraisals or to develop patient-specific prescriptions for prevention. Specialists in clinical preventive medicine, particularly in managed care programs, likely will conduct special services to carry out the aforementioned tasks. As the size of the patient population increases, such services not only will improve overall health care but also will prove to be cost effective.

As in all developing fields, specialists in clinical preventive medicine will continually find the rules of the game changing and consequently will need to master new techniques and new bodies of knowledge. The road to progress is perpetually under construction. One area that is particularly suited for specialists in clinical preventive medicine is quality assurance. Although this is not as yet generally included in the preventive medicine curriculum, it is likely to become an essential feature in the near future. The field of quality assurance has grown rapidly in the past decade, and many medical and allied disciplines have contributed to it. Specialists trained in epidemiology and biostatistics are well prepared for the study and implementation of quality assurance programs and outcomes studies. Quality assurance to date primarily has been applied in hospital settings and may be characterized best as an aspect of hospital epidemiology. Just as in the control of hospital infections, quality assurance is a form of surveillance, collection of data, analysis, interpretations, interventions to improve health care, and evaluation of the effects of such interventions.[8] Physicians who specialize in clinical preventive medicine may be particularly suited to oversee quality assurance programs, infection control programs, and risk management programs, all of which share some of the characteristics of epidemiologic surveillance, investigation, and analysis. Recently, a Committee on Quality Improvement was formed in the Medical Care Section of the American Public Health Association. The objective was to create a gathering point for the clinicians, epidemiologists, biostatisticians, health services researchers, and others who are concerned with this rapidly growing area of research and practice.

As reported previously, specialists in clinical preventive medicine are concerned with the individual and the community. This is clearly expressed in a paper by Greenlick,[6] based on Greenlick's experience in a prepaid group practice and a medical school department of public health in preventive medicine. Greenlick states that the traditional one-to-one relationship of physician and patient can and should be extended to include other concerns, such as the allocation of resources, the epidemiologic bases of clinical practice, and the needs of persons who do not regularly receive physician care. Thus the one-to-one orientation is extended to include the health of the community from which the patients are drawn, namely, a "one-to-n" orientation. This certainly fits the basic curriculum for residents in preventive medicine and is appropriate to the rapidly increasing coverage of the United States population in prepaid, managed care programs.

There are many other areas of endeavor that are open to physicians in general and to specialists in clinical preventive medicine in particular. The field of medical informatics is growing rapidly, and the physicians of the future will practice in health care organizations in which medical information systems are an essential part of daily operation. Preventive medicine residencies are responding by making medical informatics a key part of the curriculum. This is becoming increasingly feasible as new medical students and residents are computer literate and new information networks become more user friendly. The ability to aggregate data on patients, medical procedures, outcomes, quality measures, and other related variables opens new areas of operational research for institutions and large health care systems.

Changes in the technology, organization, and financing of health care also open new career paths for preventive medicine residents. The American Medical Association recently published a book titled *Leaving the Bedside: The Search for a Non-Clinical Medical Career*.[2] This book explores the reasons physicians leave patient care and the opportunities in alternative careers in medicine. Actually, specialists in clinical preventive medicine can have the best of both careers; they can continue to serve individual patients while directing a considerable portion of their efforts to the scientific and administrative matters concerned with the health of patient groups and communities. Appendix 2 of this AMA publication lists many nonpractitioner positions held by medical school graduates. Many of these are relevant to the education and training received by preventive medicine residents who specialize in clinical preventive medicine.[3]

SUMMARY

The health care system of the United States, despite its many strengths, has serious deficiencies in access to health care and in the structure of the system itself. Whatever proposals may be attempted for improving health care, the boundaries between personal health and public health are likely to become less distinct. In this process, clinical preventive medicine will offer an avenue for the incorporation of preventive medical care into medical practice and into the health care of the community in general. There is no consensus on the ways preventive medicine may best be incorporated into the medical school curriculum and postgraduate medical education. This chapter has suggested some educational initiatives for the existing medical education system and an outlook for the future.

REFERENCES

1. American College of Preventive Medicine, Council of Preventive Medicine Residency Programs: *Special requirements common to residency education in preventive medicine,* from the minutes of the March, 1992, council meeting.
2. American Medical Association, Department of Physician Licensure and Career Resources: *Leaving the bedside: the search for a nonclinical medical career,* 1992, AMA.
3. American Medical Association, Department of Physician Licensure and Career Resources: Appendix 2, Non-practitioner positions held by medical school graduates. In Rucker TD, Keller MD, editors: *Careers in medicine: traditional and alternative opportunities,* Garret Park, Md., 1986, Garret Park Press.
4. Barker WH, editor: *Teaching preventive medicine in primary care,* New York, 1983, Springer.
5. Crucetti JB, Klag MJ, and McBean AM: Clinical preventive medicine: can it be taught? *Perspect Prevention* 2:8, 1988.
6. Greenlick MR: Educating physicians for population-based clinical practice, *JAMA* 267:1645, 1992.
7. Hutchins EB: *Healthier people: health risk appraisal program* (5 volumes), Carter Center, Emory University, Atlanta, 1988.
8. Keller MD: Quality assurance: a new role for the hospital epidemiologist, *Qual Assur Util Rev* 5:127, 1990.
9. Last JM, editor: *Maxcy-Rosenau-Last, public health and preventive medicine,* ed 13, E. Norwalk, Conn., 1992, Appleton and Lange.
10. Leavell HR, Clark EG: *Preventive medicine for the doctor and his community: an epidemiologic approach,* St. Louis, 1953, McGraw-Hill.
11. Rosenau MJ: *Preventive medicine and hygiene,* 1913, Appleton.
12. Salive ME: Preventive medicine residency training: a resident's perspective, *Am J Prev Med* 7:248, 1991.
13. U.S. Preventive Services Task Force: *Guide to clinical preventive services: an assessment of the effectiveness of 169 interventions,* Baltimore, 1989, Williams and Wilkins.
14. Woolf SH, Sox HC: The Expert Panel on Preventive Services: continuing the work of the U.S. Preventive Services Task Force, *Am J Prev Med* 7:326, 1991.

RESOURCES

Clinical preventive medicine: can it be taught? by Crucetti JB, Klag MJ, and Bean AM, *Perspect prevention* 2:8, 1988.

Directory of preventive medicine residency programs in the United States and Canada (General Preventive Medicine, Occupational Medicine, Public Health, Aerospace Medicine), American College of Preventive Medicine, 1015 15th St. NW, Washington, DC 20005.

Guide to clinical preventive services, An assessment of 169 interventions, Report of the United States Preventive Services Task Force, Williams & Wilkins, 428 E Preston St., Baltimore, MD 21202.

Healthier people: health risk appraisal programs (5 volumes), E.B. Hutchins, 1988, Carter Center, Emory University, PO Box 109050, Chicago, IL 60610.

Teaching preventive medicine in primary care, William H. Barker, M.D., editor, 1983, Springer Series on Medical Education, volume 5, Springer Publishing, 200 Park Ave South, New York, NY 10003.

1992-1993 Directory of graduate medical education programs, The American Medical Association; copies may be purchased from: Order Dept. OP416792, AMA, P.O. Box 109050, Chicago, IL 60610.

Chapter 4

ETHICAL CONSIDERATIONS AND THE QUALITY OF LIFE

George A. Kanoti
Martin L. Smith

"There is nothing permanent except change."

HERACLITUS

THE CASE OF MRS. JEREMY

Today physicians practice clinical preventive medicine in an environment replete with thickets, brambles, and blind pathways. A physician can easily become lost in the forest of options and risks and can be stung by the nettles of government or third-party payers or patient rights. Many physicians use their technology and the objectivity of their science as a compass to avoid these pitfalls and hazards. The following scenario illustrates some of the hazards of medical practice in the 1990s.

Mrs. Jeremy apologized to the receptionist for her tardiness. The babysitter for her two toddlers arrived late, and, because she recently moved to the city, she took the wrong bus to get to the doctor's office. She brought Matthew, her 8-year-old son, to be seen by the doctor.

She wrote on the intake form that Matthew's asthma had been diagnosed by a family practice doctor in a neighboring city. Matthew's prescribed medications of albuterol and cromolyn sodium, both delivered by inhalers, were about to run out. Mrs. Jeremy brought along Matthew's inhalers. Matthew's medical history was unremarkable aside from his asthma. His health care insurance coverage was through Medicaid.

The nurse charted that Mrs. Jeremy was a single parent and that she and her three children recently changed their residence to be closer to her parents. Mrs. Jeremy volunteered that she is currently dating several men. One is a frequent visitor, and she sees the relationship as promising. Mrs. Jeremy was pleasant and cooperative when answering questions about Matthew's medical history and asthma symptoms. His asthmatic attacks occur almost exclusively in their apartment and never in school.

A few minutes after the nurse finished her interview and examination, Dr. Hilary entered the examination room. When she entered she detected a strong odor of stale tobacco smoke. As she reviewed Matthew's medical history and symptoms with Matthew and Mrs. Jeremy, Mrs. Jeremy provided responses that were consistent with the nurse's charted notes. With prompting from Mrs. Jeremy, Matthew described two recent asthma attacks. Both occurred in the evening after he returned to their apartment. His symptoms, satisfactorily relieved by the inhalers, included shortness of breath, coughing, audible wheezing, and minor chest tightness. Stethoscopic examination of Matthew's lungs revealed some slight wheezing. Dr. Hilary concluded that the diagnosis of asthma was reasonable based on the presence of appropriate and authorized prescriptions and the information provided by Mrs. Jeremy and Matthew.

"Before I write a new prescription for Matthew, let's talk about things that might aggravate Matthew's asthma," Dr. Hilary said. "Does anyone at home smoke?" Matthew began to answer but stopped when his mother shot him a disapproving look.

A delicate ethical moment in the nascent relationship between Dr. Hilary, Mrs. Jeremy, and Matthew has occurred. Dr. Hilary faces a practical moral choice: Should she pursue Matthew's ambiguous signal or should she respect Mrs. Jeremy's exercise of parental authority and not intervene further with questions?

This moment also raises a series of ethical questions for Dr. Hilary: As a professional dedicated to fostering preventive medicine, what are her ethical responsibilities in this situation? If Mrs. Jeremy is a smoker, how far should

41

Dr. Hilary pursue this issue, as Matthew, not the mother, is the patient? How much attention should be given to the societal issue of getting one more person to stop smoking, with the potential health benefits for numerous persons?

The answers to these questions are not simple. They are influenced by many subtle but forceful unknown factors in the relationship between Dr. Hilary, Mrs. Jeremy, and Matthew. It can be presumed that Dr. Hilary is dedicated to a responsible and effective use of her skills and expertise to treat Matthew's asthma and to prevent further complications and exacerbations.

Mrs. Jeremy also has certain assumptions and expectations of Dr. Hilary as a physician. Does she expect Dr. Hilary merely to prescribe a continuation of Matthew's drugs? Does she expect Dr. Hilary to "stay out of her private affairs?" Does she want the doctor's advice about how to prevent further asthma attacks? What would be in Matthew's best interests?

CHANGING EXPECTATIONS

One reason that these questions are difficult to answer is that the expectations, roles, responsibilities, and ethical standards for physician behavior are changing. These changes are due in part both to the changes in medical practice that have led to medicine's success and to changes in the cultural climate. Physicians' ability to alleviate effectively the symptoms of the ill and injured and to postpone their death has led subtly but forcibly to a reshaping of perceived roles, responsibilities, and expectations of physicians. Furthermore, physicians find patient autonomy, economic and legal concerns, and third-party payer involvement necessary, if unwelcome, partners in every decision they make.

Although the basic concepts of health, disease, and quality of life are also changing, the most elemental of all these changes is the nature of the physician-patient relationship. The implications of this change on the identification of physicians' roles and ethical responsibilities are profound.

NEW ETHICAL STANDARDS

A shift is occurring in the ethical standards by which the quality of the physician-patient relationship is judged.[3] Traditionally, physicians were motivated and judged by their ability to make decisions that were in the patient's best interest. This benevolent parental or paternalistic model was suitable and effective for years. It was built on trust and nurtured by continuous attention to patient needs. Patients tended to be passive and accepting of "doctor's orders" because they had confidence in the physician's knowledge, believed in the physician's commitment to care for them, and trusted that the physician was motivated by their best interest.

This environment has changed. The age of patient autonomy and the rise of patient rights and numerous malpractice suits have replaced the previous benevolent ethical standard with a new ethical standard: Act according to patient wishes and directives. Furthermore, the standards for physician-patient relations have been influenced by third-party payer involvement and the adaptation of a business model for medicine. Informed consent[8] and informed refusal[2] are two phrases that describe this ethical and paradigm shift. The result, at times, is an atmosphere of mistrust and an adversarial emphasis on patient rights and patient autonomy.

Perhaps the most perplexing question for the physician in this new environment is how to achieve the goals of preventive medicine (i.e., to promote and protect the health of the patient as well as prevent the occurrence of disease by interventions and recommendations to improve the patient's quality of life) while being respectful of patient autonomy. What are a physician's responsibilities, and how should a physician respond to a patient's noncompliance or refusal of a clearly medically indicated treatment?

The appropriate response by physicians to this change is not to long for a return to the "golden age" of paternalism. Rather, they should develop strategies and techniques to educate, motivate, and empower patients to use their autonomy with their physician's help to maintain and protect their health and experience a quality of life consistent with their goals and values. This response is not merely an accommodation to the winds of change; its roots are in an ethical analysis that demonstrates the value of mutual identification of personal goals and values and shared decision making.

QUALITY OF LIFE

The goal of preventive medicine is to foster the quality of life of patients by maintaining and promoting their health and preventing disease. Defining quality of life[16] is difficult because the concept contains general and vague abstract elements.

Quality of life can be described as a personalized vision of values and goals that reflects a patient's life-style and ambitions, philosophic and religious beliefs about the purpose of living, and the moral requirements of living. Knowledge of these "visions of values and goals" is subjective, individual, and personal. In contrast, the assumption often is made that the descriptive term "preventive" in preventive medicine refers to what "objectively" is good and desirable, and that what is being prevented is clearly understood as deleterious to patients. The targets of prevention, however, are not so clear or easily stated as "objective" fact when a patient enters the physician's office. Disease, disability, injury, and trauma clearly are not desirable concepts when viewed as abstract phenomena. But defining these abstract phenomena in a concrete situation is problematic because each person may have a different concept of disability and undesirability.

One of the results of the "subjectivizing" of what may have been thought to be clear and objective concepts (i.e., disease, disability, injury) is the creation of an additional challenge for preventive medicine. The clinical process must now incorporate exploration of the individual patient's definition of "quality of life."

PHYSICIAN ROLES

The traditional roles of a physician include not only healer, but also teacher, counselor, and advisor. The autonomous environment of modern medicine forces physicians to combine and include all of these roles in clinical encounters with patients.

Although the physician's power and significance may have been lost in recent years, these roles of teaching, advising, and counseling are intrinsic to the physician's identity. This is especially noticeable in the field of preventive medicine where health and disease are individualized and must be explored with each patient. The physician, therefore, needs to discover (if hidden) or acquire (if absent) these skills to fulfill these roles.

One major skill is the ability to ask questions that will reveal a patient's personal perspective on personal goals and values.[15] Physician questions that encourage the confidence of the patient or family will of necessity address personal and even philosophic or religious ideas. Physicians usually are not comfortable with this line of questioning. Instead of inquiring about historic or physiologic "facts" and encouraging patients to describe the onset of symptoms or disease, the physician will need to use imagination, metaphors, and images to evoke patient and family assessment of their personal values and goals. Open-ended questions are good vehicles for these discussions. Potential areas for exploration with a patient include feelings and attitudes about current health status, perception of the physician's role, thoughts about independence and control, the importance of specific personal relationships, overall attitudes toward life and death and disability, the significance of religious background and beliefs, and a description of the patient's physical and social environment.

To fulfill the teaching role, the physician must be able to translate medical information and concepts into language and images that the "student-patient" can understand,[4] as well as reinforce ideas by various oral, written, visual, and even tactile means. Counselor or advisor roles require the ability to help the patient weigh options and assess circumstances in view of the goals of preventive medicine and those of the patient and family. Counseling also requires a database of supportive and educational services to which the patient can be referred when appropriate.

One of the challenges of acting as teacher, counselor, and advisor is to avoid any semblance of coercion (either subtle or overt) as well as manipulation and deception. Respect for patients and their autonomy requires open dialogue, truthfulness, and assisting patients to choose freely from various options.[14] Respect for patients does not exclude making medical recommendations or using persuasive logic. The temptation to use coercion, manipulation, and deception to attain a good end may be strongest when patients are noncompliant or medically unsophisticated or when they require more time than usually allotted in a busy schedule.

Not all patients respond to instruction. The physician's obligation has been fulfilled if a genuine attempt is made to educate and advise patients. In the mutual decision-making model, each party is expected to contribute to the decision; even if one party does not contribute, the other party can still fulfill the responsibilities of a shared decision maker.

THE CASE OF MRS. JEREMY REVISITED

A return to the original case will illustrate some useful techniques to elicit parental and patient confidence and to promote patient health.

Dr. Hilary asked "Does anyone at home smoke?" This direct question is logical and prompted both by the presence of the odor of stale smoke in the examination room and the reported pattern of Jeremy's asthma attacks. Nevertheless, a direct question about potentially sensitive or socially questionable behavior could easily prompt a defensive attitude and even an obstinate stance from Matthew's mother. A direct question could evoke negative emotions in Mrs. Jeremy and create a barrier to Dr. Hilary's primary objectives: to educate and to engage Mrs. Jeremy and Matthew in the creation of strategies that will lead to increased health for Matthew (and even, perhaps, for Mrs. Jeremy and her other children).

An alternative approach could avoid the negative emotion and elicit cooperation from Mrs. Jeremy and Matthew. Dr. Hilary could first explore the pattern of asthma attacks reported by Matthew (i.e., the asthma attacks seem to occur primarily in the home environment). With this focus, Dr. Hilary could emphasize the value of reviewing various agents or allergens in the apartment that might cause or aggravate the asthma. Or, Dr. Hilary could ask if Matthew's former physician identified the asthma as allergic and, therefore, precipitated by inhaled pollens, molds, smoke, dust, or animal dander. She could ask whether there is a correlation between Matthew's asthma attacks and his exercise routines or exposure to cold air.

Dr. Hilary also could explain that the inhalers only counter the symptoms of the asthma, not the initiating factor(s). If these initiating factors could be identified and avoided, recurrent asthma attacks might be prevented. Dr. Hilary could give examples from her medical practice of common initiators of asthma attack, including passive smoking, and successful strategies her patients used to prevent or diminish symptoms. In this inquiry, Dr. Hilary could begin to educate and motivate Mrs. Jeremy and Matthew to look for initiating factors in their environment.

Even if tobacco smoke is identified as a probable causative factor for Matthew's asthma and Mrs. Jeremy reveals that she or her friends or visitors are smokers, Dr. Hilary probably would not be able to help Matthew by taking a confrontational moralistic stance on the evils of smoking. Instead, negotiation, compromise, and counseling might be necessary. Dr. Hilary might ask the following questions: Do Mrs. Jeremy and her friends want to quit smoking? Have they attempted to quit? Are they aware of the community resources and programs for smoking cessation?[9] If the desire to quit smoking is not present, would Mrs. Jeremy be willing to create a smoke-free environment in her apartment by insisting that smoking take place outside? Or, could specific areas in her apartment (e.g., Matthew's bedroom) be kept as smoke free as possible? Finally, it would be appropriate for Dr. Hilary to give information about the current scientific evidence about the health dangers for Matthew and her other children from "secondary" smoke.

The goals of preventive medicine are applicable to Dr. Hilary's goals in this encounter: to promote and protect Matthew's health and to prevent the recurrence of his asthma as much as possible by offering recommendations to improve the quality of his life. The achievement of these goals, although not easy, is not impossible. The ethical moment requires Dr. Hilary's time, sensitivity, imagination, and even negotiation. To meet this challenge Dr. Hilary needs the skills not only of a scientist and physician, but also those of an educator, advisor, and counselor.

ADVANCE DIRECTIVES

As this book illustrates, preventive medicine is concerned with health promotion, health protection, and preventive services. But even the best efforts and achievements in preventive medicine for individual patients ultimately cannot prevent death. This unavoidable reality that someday will meet all patients (and their physicians) creates an additional responsibility for physicians, especially those in general practice. The responsibility is to initiate conversation with patients about their wishes regarding end-of-life decisions and to educate patients about advance directives (e.g., living wills,[6] durable powers of attorney for health care,[1] patient value histories,[11] medical directives[7]) in the event that patients lose the ability to participate in their own health care choices.

Living wills commonly anticipate two medical situations: terminal illness and permanent unconsciousness. In advance of either of these prognoses, the living will directs physicians and family about the patient's wishes regarding life-supporting or death-prolonging treatments. A durable power of attorney for health care allows the patient to designate a proxy or surrogate to make health care decisions when the patient is unable to do so. In the United States most states have legislatively recognized the legal validity of at least one of these written advance directives.

Because living wills tend to be nonspecific about medical eventualities, additional advance directive tools have been recommended. The first is a patient values history, which elicits, through a series of structured interviews with the patient, various values from the patient that can be used as guides for decision making on behalf of the patient. Examples of interview questions are the following: How important is it for you to be independent and self-sufficient? What goals do you have for the future? What will be important to you when you are dying (e.g., physical comfort, no pain, family members present)?

A second advance directive tool aimed at specifying and making concrete patient wishes about life-supports is the medical directive. The patient is asked to imagine being in a coma, unconscious, or sustaining brain damage with various prognoses and then to indicate wishes concerning possible life-supports and treatments such as cardiopulmonary resuscitation, a ventilator, artificial nutrition and hydration, and major and minor surgery. Neither the medical directive nor the patient values history has been legislatively approved in any state.

The Patient Self-Determination Act[10,12,13] mandates, as part of a provider's agreement with Medicare, that during the admission process hospitals, health maintenance organizations, skilled nursing facilities, home health agencies, and hospice programs provide written information to adult patients about advance directives and inquire whether a patient has executed such directives. This federal act undoubtedly has increased public awareness about patients' rights for informed consent and refusal and their role in end-of-life decision making. There is a general perception that the time of hospital or nursing home admission is not the optimum moment for appropriate and substantive discussion about such issues. During the admission process patients frequently are seriously or acutely ill, mentally debilitated, or even unconscious. Many of these discussions on admission are carried out as an administrative task (e.g., between admissions clerk and the patient) rather than as a part of a clinical process (e.g., in the context of a physician-patient relationship).

The context of a physician-patient dialogue and identification of general health care goals, values, and quality of life (usually in the outpatient setting) is better suited for soliciting a patient's wishes about life-supporting or death-prolonging therapies should these become necessary.[5] In this less stressful setting, patients can be educated about various options and therapies if they are unable to make decisions because of a life-threatening illness. Over a series of office visits patients will reflect on these issues and raise questions. Confusion, fears, and misunderstandings can be addressed. Actual documents (according to specific state statute) can be reviewed or provided, discussed, and incorporated into the patient's medical record.

Physicians may tend to reserve conversations about advance directives for geriatric patients or those with degenerative diseases. This approach is not realistic. Anyone can experience life-threatening illness, trauma, and loss of mental capacity. If patient autonomy is a value to be honored, then all adult patients should be given the opportunity to express their wishes, values, and directives before end-of-life choices must be made.

Some physicians may be reluctant to initiate such conversations with patients, especially the young and the healthy, for fear of needlessly scaring or upsetting patients. In fact, the reverse may be true. Many patients wait for their physicians to initiate these discussions and welcome and are even relieved when such discussions occur.[17]

CONCLUSION

Although change is rapidly affecting medicine, commitment to the goals of preventive medicine will provide the stability and the resources to meet these changing times. Good medicine like good wine stands the test of time. Ethically, the physician faces the challenge to develop, if necessary, or to perfect the traditional roles of physician: teacher, advisor, and counselor. The responsibilities of a physician include more than the responsibility to cure when possible and to care always. It also includes the responsibility to teach and to advise.

REFERENCES

1. Annas GJ: The health care proxy and the living will, *N Engl J Med* 324:1210-1213, 1991.
2. Annas GJ, Densberger JE: Competence to refuse medical treatment: autonomy versus paternalism. In Friedman E, editor: *Making choices: ethical issues for health care professionals*, Chicago, American Hospital Publishing, 1986.
3. Brody H: The physician/patient relationship. In Veatch RM, editor: *Medical ethics*, Boston, Jones and Bartlett Publishers, 1989.
4. Cousins N: The physician as communicator, *JAMA* 248:587-589, 1982.
5. Emanuel L: PSDA in the clinic, *Hastings Cent Rep* 21:S6-S7, 1990.
6. Emanuel EJ, Emanuel LL: Living wills: past, present and future, *J Clin Ethics* 1:9-19, 1990.
7. Emanuel LL, Emanuel EJ: The medical directive, a new comprehensive advance care document, *JAMA* 261:3288-3293, 1989.
8. Faden RR, Beauchamp R, King NMP: *A history and theory of informed consent*, New York: Oxford University Press, 1986.
9. Glynn TJ: Methods of smoking cessation—finally, some answers, *JAMA* 263:2795-2796, 1990.
10. Greco PJ et al: The patient self-determination act and the future of advance directives, *Ann Intern Med* 115:639-643, 1991.
11. Lambert P, Gibson JM, Nathanson P: The values history: an innovation in surrogate medical decision-making, *Law Med Health Care* 18:202-212, 1990.
12. LaPuma J, Orentlicher D, Moss RJ: Advance directives on admission, clinical implications and analysis of the patient self-determination act of 1990, *JAMA* 266:402-405, 1991.
13. McCloskey EL: The patient self-determination act, *Kennedy Inst Ethics J* 1:163-169, 1991.
14. Quill TE: Recognizing and adjusting to barriers in doctor-patient communication, *Ann Intern Med* 111:51-57, 1989.
15. Smith RC, Hoppe RB: The patient's story: integrating the patient- and physician-centered approaches to interviewing, *Ann Intern Med* 115:470-477, 1991.
16. Walter JJ, Shannon TA, editors: *Quality of life, the new medical dilemma*, New York: Paulist Press, 1990.
17. Wolf SM et al: Sources of concern about the Patient Self-Determination Act, *N Engl J Med* 325:1666-1671, 1991.

RESOURCES

Advance directives

Choice in Dying (Formerly Concern for Dying/Society for the Right to Die), 250 West 57th Street, New York, NY 10107 (212) 246-6962. Provides information and forms for each state's Living Will and/or Durable Power of Attorney for Health Care.

State Medical Associations. Numbers are available from local hospital or physician.

End-of-life decisions

Radey C: *Choosing wisely: How patients and their families can make the right decisions about life and death*, New York, 1992, Doubleday.

Anderson P: *Affairs in order: a complete resource guide to death and dying*, New York, Macmillan, 1991.

Sankar A: *Dying at home: a family guide for caregiving*, Baltimore, The Johns Hopkins University Press, 1991.

Ethics Committees and Ethics Consultants. Contact local hospital.

Hospice Programs. Numbers are available through local hospital's Social Work Department.

Physician-patient communications

Scheller MD: *Building partnerships in hospital care: empowering patients, families & professionals*. Palo Alto, Bull Publishing Company, 1990.

Chapter 5

A SEVEN COUNTRY PERSPECTIVE OF CLINICAL PREVENTIVE MEDICINE

C. Patrick Chaulk
Ronald Bialek

The preventive services provided to the populations in the countries discussed in this chapter reflect a range of health care systems and cultures among the industrialized nations. Preventive services are described in one of the least densely populated and largest countries in the world, Canada, as well as in one of the most densely populated countries in the world, Japan. Canada uses a predominantly publicly financed health care system, whereas Japan uses both employer-based financing and public insurance. In both countries, essentially no one is uninsured.

The preventive services reviewed include primary preventive services such as immunization practices and prenatal care as well as prevention counseling and education, and secondary preventive services such as screening mammography and Papanicolaou smears.

The health care systems that deliver these services include a wide range of financing and delivery structures: centralized, state-financed systems such as Great Britain and Canada; decentralized state-financed systems such as Sweden; and mixed systems with varying combinations of employer-based funding coupled with national/local funding such as France, Japan, and Germany.

Finally, the U.S. health care system is described. The U.S. system has the greatest mix of public and private payers. Policy making traditionally has been highly decentralized. Although there are no restrictions on provider salaries, some fees for certain hospital and ambulatory services (Medicare) have most recently been established.

Overall, the countries presented display a wide diversity in utilization patterns for preventive and certain curative services, health care cost-containment strategies, and in the way they provide health insurance for various segments of their country's respective populations.

Countries examined:

a. Countries using employer-based systems

- Japan
- France
- Federal Republic of Germany (formerly West Germany)

b. Countries using government-based single payer systems

- Great Britain
- Canada
- Sweden

c. Mixed: employer, individual, and government-funded system

- United States

JAPAN: HEALTH POLICY AND HEALTH INSURANCE ISSUES

Geographically small and composed of essentially four main islands, Japan is the third most populated nation in the world. Although the 124 million citizens (1990) of Japan are roughly half the number of people in the United States, they are crowded into an area about the size of California. Since about 70% of Japan is uninhabitable because of forests and rugged mountains, and another 27% is used for farming and industry, only 3% of the country is actually habitable. About 326 persons reside on each square kilometer of land.[6] A culturally homogeneous people, the Japanese speak principally one language and are predominantly Buddhists or Shintoists.[127]

The government is a constitutional monarchy with a multiparty democracy led by the Liberal Democratic Party since 1955.[127,70] Japan is composed of 47 prefectures (states), 32 large municipal governments, over 850 health centers at the state and local level, and 1106 community health centers (1991).[88]

Modern Japanese health care can be traced to the incremental introduction of Western medicine into Japan by Dutch traders during the two centuries before the mid-1800s. Because of Japan's strict policy of isolationism, contact with any other Western or Eastern cultures was excluded.[88]

Perhaps the earliest evidence of the penetration of Western medical services into Japan was the introduction of smallpox vaccine in 1858 and with it the establishment of a vaccination clinic in Edo, now known as Tokyo. With the enactment of the Medical Code in 1874, the adoption of other Western medical practices began to accelerate. The Japanese expressed an early interest in the German medical system, and, in fact, the teaching faculty at the newly established Tokyo University Medical School in 1874 was reportedly almost entirely composed of Germans. A series of national level reforms in 1938 began a process of centralizing health policy making, including the establishment of the Ministry of Health and Welfare and the enactment of the National Health Insurance Law. This law established health insurance societies in each municipality to expand medical care to self-employed workers such as farmers and fishermen.[98]

In 1938 the Rockefeller Foundation, as part of its rich history of public health philanthropy, funded the establishment of the Institute of Public Health. Through this Institute the Western approach to training public health professionals was formally introduced in Japan. Today the Institute is recognized as the only formal school of public health in Japan.[88]

These public health advancements, however, were dealt a severe setback as a result of the destructive social and economic consequences of World War II. Fortunately, several postwar developments rapidly reinvigorated the Japanese health care system. Fundamentally, the passage of a new constitution declared, in part, that public health improvement and health promotion were henceforth to be national responsibilities.[82] In addition, the postwar industrial transformation of Japan has resulted in its rise as a major economic power whose capitalistic economy now rivals the United States. Both the constitutional focus on health and the economic growth of the past several decades have facilitated the development of a health care system that provides health insurance and medical care to all Japanese citizens while restraining health care expenditures far better than most other countries.[70]

Unlike the British and Swedish systems, which rely on one public insurance program, Japan's system of compulsory public health insurance uses several different programs with employer-based plans for workers and their dependents, as well as strictly public programs targeting the elderly.[60]

Approximately 63% of the population, generally workers and their dependents, are covered through one of nearly 1800 public health insurance societies linked to employment, so-called Health Insurance for Employees (HIE). HIE policies are funded through equal payroll tax contributions of 4.15% made by both employees and their employers. In addition, company bonuses are taxed at 0.5% for employers and 0.3% for employees to fund HIE policies.[42] HIE programs include government-managed insurance for smaller firms (less than 300 employees), insurance societies under joint management-labor control, and associations of public employees.[70] Although Japan has no true private health insurance, HIE plans occasionally offer supplementary benefits.[42,59,70]

For self-employed workers and their dependents, insurance is provided through a system of national health insurance (NHI) financed by municipalities or through national health insurance associations. Approximately 37% of the Japanese are enrolled in this manner.[70]

Finally, health insurance is provided to certain elderly Japanese as a result of the Geriatric Health Act enacted in 1983. Financed by contributions from the other plans, the Geriatric Health Act uses these funds to pay for health care for all Japanese over age 70.[70]

Copayments for the three programs range from 10% to 30% of the negotiated fee schedule. The co-pays are higher under the NHI program (as much as 30%, and they are capped at approximately $400 per month for a single illness; for low-income individuals, out-of-pocket expenses are capped at $200 per month).*[59] Only recently, however, have the elderly been required to make co-payments for either medical services or prescription drugs.

System capacity and use of medical services

Japanese health policy is highly centralized. The most striking consequence of this is the establishment of a uniform fee schedule for services regardless of the point of service (hospital or clinic) or experience of the provider (novice or highly experienced physician). Although the fees are the same for the same service, the economic consequences of payment are widely different for the physician depending on whether care is provided in a hospital or in a free-standing clinic. In the case of hospital-based care, the hospital is paid directly by the patient (or insurer); and the hospital-based physician, in turn, is paid a salary. The hospital-based physician, therefore, has little economic incentive to treat more patients or to provide more or less

*All financial figures in this chapter are expressed in terms of U.S. dollars.

care. The physician is paid the same salary regardless of the volume of patients treated or intensity of services provided.[67,68,70]

On the other hand, nonhospital-based physicians are paid on a fee-for-service basis. The more patients seen and the more services provided, the greater the physician's income.* There is economic incentive, therefore, for young physicians to choose primary care careers. Because clinic-based physicians do not have hospital admitting privileges, the emphasis is on nonhospital-based careers over hospital-based careers. Medical consultation is preferred to hospitalization. Japanese physicians average nearly 13 consultations per patient each year, versus 5.3 in the United States.[70] Fewer Japanese are hospitalized (7.8%) than in the United States (12.8%), and consequently far fewer surgical procedures are performed in Japan per capita (22.0/1000) than in the United States (91.0/1000).[70,110] Thus, even without a global budget, cost containment is addressed through economic incentives that stimulate delivery of primary and preventive rather than hospital-based care or inpatient diagnostic procedures.[68,70]

The Japanese are free to choose their own physician, although there are fewer physicians per capita to choose from than in most other nations—only 1.6 physicians per 1000 population.[109] As a result, Japanese physicians spend less time with patients. One observer found that Japanese physicians in one clinic were on average seeing between 40 and 50 patients per physician in a single morning. Because physicians generally do not take appointments, patients are commonly seen on a first-come, first-served basis, which results in waiting times of 1 hour or more.[67]

Even though Japan has no shortage of pharmacists (0.6 per 1000 population), Japanese physicians prescribe *and* dispense medications in their clinics. Partly because of this dual pharmaceutical role of the physician, Japan spends more than $330 per capita on drugs, one of the highest levels of spending on drugs in the world.[109]

Hospital care in Japan is unique. A hospital in Japan is defined according to bed size: facilities with more than 20 beds are designated as hospitals; those with fewer beds are designated as clinics. In addition, hospitals are commonly used as long-term care facilities. On the other hand, clinics not only do not provide long-term care, but patients, at least technically, must be discharged from a clinic within 48 hours of the admission.[68] Excluding smaller facilities, which are likely to provide short-term care, and shifting long-term care to hospitals in part account for the extremely long average length of stay for hospital patients: nearly 53 days, by far the longest in the world.[70] The hospital staffing ratio per bed (0.77) in Japan is one of the lowest among industrialized countries.[42]

*The difference in income between clinic-based and salaried hospital-based physicians may be substantial. Ikegami states that clinic-based physicians may earn twice as much as hospital-based specialists. (Ikegami N: Japanese health care: low cost through regulated fees, *Health Affairs* 10(3):87-109, 1991.)

Medical economics and expenditures

Despite the high number of physician encounters, drug prescriptions, and lengthy hospital stays, Japan has managed to contain its health care expenditures. In 1990, according to the Organization for Economic Cooperation and Development (OECD),* for example, health care expenditures totaled 6.5% of the Gross Domestic Product (GDP), roughly half that of the United States (Table 5-1). In part, this low percentage is due to an economy that has experienced considerable growth over the past two decades. Japan's per capita spending of $1113 on health care in 1990 was well behind the United States ($2566) and Canada ($1795), as well as Sweden ($1421), France ($1379), and Germany ($1287).[60] Public spending accounts for the majority (73%) of health care expenditures in Japan.[109] In contrast to other countries such as Great Britain and Canada, Japan does not have a global health care budget; however, it does have other spending controls. These mechanisms include negotiated physician fees for office-based and hospital-based services, hospital per diem rates, salaried incomes for hospital-based physicians, and caps on hospital construction and capital improvements.

For example, hospital and physician fee schedules are established by the central government in consultation with the Central Social Insurance Medical Council, a body composed of providers, insurers, and consumers.[59] In addition to establishing fee limits, the Council prohibits balance billing of patients. Some expenditures for hospital-related (less than 20 beds) capital purchases must receive approval from the local government, although this approval is sporadic, not unlike the Certificate of Need process used in the United States to control capital expenditures. Similar expenditures for clinics (greater than 20 beds) are unregulated, which has promoted the duplication of certain technology and services. For example, Japan has the highest number of computerized axial tomography (CT) units per capita in the world.[70] Japan also has 2078 cardiac catheterization laboratory centers, 1.7 times as many as in the United States, and roughly the same number of open heart

*The Organization of Economic Cooperation and Development (OECD) was formed in 1961 by twenty countries: Austria, Belgium, Canada, Denmark, France, the Federal Republic of Germany, Greece, Iceland, Ireland, Italy, Luxembourg, the Netherlands, Norway, Portugal, Spain, Sweden, Switzerland, Turkey, the United Kingdom and the United States. Four additional countries, Japan (1964), Finland (1969), Australia (1971), and New Zealand (1973), subsequently joined the OECD. According to the treaty establishing the OECD and signed by these nations, OECD seeks to promote policies designed: (1) "to achieve the highest sustainable economic growth and employment and a rising standard of living in Member countries, while maintaining financial stability, and thus contribute to the development of the world economy"; (2) "to contribute to sound economic expansion in Member as well as non-member countries in the process of economic development; and" (3) "to contribute to the expansion of world trade on a multilateral, non-discriminatory basis in accordance with international obligations."

Table 5-1. A comparison of health system capacity and utilization of medical services between the United States and Japan: circa 1989

	1 United States	2 Japan	Ratio 1:2
Percent GDP on health care	12.4	6.5	1.90
Per capita on health care	$ 2,566	$ 1,113	2.30
Percent public funding	42	73	0.57
Hospitals*			
Beds†	3.8	15.6	0.24
Average length of stay (ALOS) (days)	7.2	52.1	0.13
Occ. rate	65.5	84.1	0.77
Admission rate‡	12.8	7.8	1.64
Physicians			
Number†	2.3	1.6	1.41
Average no. visits	5.3	12.9	0.41
% Primary care§	34	—	—
MD expenditure‖	183,281	183,761	0.99

From OECD Health Data File.

*Data based on acute care hospitals only, i.e., hospitals in which the ALOS is less than 30 days (1988). However, data for Japan may exclude some short-term hospitals.

†Per 1000 population.

‡Percent of total populations.

§Percent of physicians identifying themselves as general practitioners, pediatricians, internists.

‖Physician expenditures per physician (i.e., total physician spending for outpatient and inpatient services per number of active practicing physicians. Figures expressed in U.S. dollars 1988. (Source, HCFA calculations of OECD data.)

ALOS, average length of hospital stay; *Occ. Rate,* hospital patient occupancy rate; *Average no. visits,* Average number of visits made to physicians (may include telephone contacts).

surgical centers as the United States (3.2 per million population versus 3.4 per million, respectively). With 11.2 adult cardiologists per 100,000 population, Japan has 2.3 times as many per 100,000 as in the United States, far more than any other country[30] (Table 5-2). Nonetheless, evidence by Collins-Nakai et al. suggests that far fewer invasive cardiac procedures are performed in Japan than in the United States.

Other reasons given for lower medical expenditures in Japan include lower administrative costs due to a uniform fee schedule (administrative costs estimated at 2.5%), simplified billing procedures and no competitive insurance marketing expenses; fewer surgical procedures, due to an emphasis on ambulatory care; fewer medical malpractice law suits because of fewer attorneys (roughly one tenth as many attorneys in Japan as in the United States); less specialization because of preference for training primary care physicians.[70,93]

Japan's health profile

By certain measures, Japan has one of the best health profiles in the world.[84] Life expectancy at birth in 1989 for men was 75.9 years and for women it was 81.8 years[60] (Table 5-3). Both are well above the U.S. average. In 1986 about 1851 Japanese were over 100 years old, with women outnumbering men in this venerable group approximately 4 to 1. In that same year, the world's oldest reliably documented human was a 120-year-old Japanese man living in southern Japan.[98] Japanese longevity has been attributed in part to a very low-fat Japanese diet. The per person consumption of fat in Japan has been estimated to be roughly 82 grams per day, less than half the estimated amount of fat consumed per person per day in the United States, Canada, and Germany.[28] Another source suggests that the fat content may be as low as 57 grams per day.[93] The Ministry of Health estimates that roughly 26% of all calories in the daily Japanese diet are derived from fats.[70]

Japan has the lowest infant mortality rate in the world: 4.59 per 1000 live births (1989)[87] (Table 5-3). Japanese women have ready access to early, free, and continuous prenatal care; home visiting services if needed; rubella vaccination for young women of childbearing age; and family planning services. In addition, only 5% of Japanese infants are classified as low birth weight, and the rate of cesarean section births is about one third that of the United States.[90] Immunization rates for Japanese children are estimated to be 83% for DPT, 95% for OPV, 73% for MMR.[116]

In other more contemporary areas, such as communicable diseases, however, Japan has the greatest number of reported cases of AIDS in Asia. This dubious distinction may be short-lived, however, as unpublished reports of other less developed Asian countries suggest that major increases in the incidence of this infection in those countries is anticipated. Nonetheless, the number of patients with AIDS in 1990 was still far below the number in the United States.

Clinical preventive services: a population profile

Through the establishment of a large number of publicly funded clinics and health centers, Japan has demonstrated a commitment to public and preventive health measures.[56] In 1987, 1.5% of all government health care expenditures were used to fund public preventive screening programs. Approximately 15.1% of national government expenditures were for public welfare assistance. Most local government health expenditures went to public hospitals (51.5%), a smaller portion (6.1%) went to fund local health centers.[69]

Perinatal preventive services and maternal disability. Maternal disability eligibility criteria and cash maternity benefits in Japan are treated the same as other short-term disabilities. Pregnant women, however, not only receive

Table 5-2. A comparison of cardiovascular mortality rates and cardiovascular services among six countries (circa 1990)*

	United States	Canada	Sweden	Germany	Japan	Great Britain
CV mortality†	369.2	329.6	428.8	422.7 (1989)	214.9	429.7
CV surgeons (no.)	2,459	112	—	340	1,701	150
Adult† cardiologists	4.82	2.54	—	2.90	11.2	3.48
Cath labs (no.)	1259 (1988)	49	16	179	2078	51
Caths†	373.5 (1988)	236.0 (1989)	113.0	255.0	—	102.0
PTCAs†	84.7	39.0	12.8	14.4	16.2	14.8
Open heart surgical centers (no.)	826	33	7	40	400	46
Open heart operations†	261.8 (1988)	63.0 (1989)	75.0	48.9	16.2	42.0 (1989)
CABG procedures†	141.8 (1988)	—	50.6	33.0	—	26.6 (1989)
Valve procedures†	23.3	—	17.9	9.6	—	8.3 (1989)

From Collins-Nakai RL, Huysman HA, Scully HE: Task force 5: access to cardiovascular care: an international comparison, *J Am Coll Cardiol* 19:1477-1485, 1992.
*Figures for France unavailable.
†Rate per 100,000 population.
CV, Cardiovascular; *PTCA*, percutaneous transluminal coronary angioplasty; *CABG*, coronary artery bypass graft surgery.

cash benefits but also a lump sum maternity grant of roughly $1400.[43] Maternity cash benefits are provided for a total of 14 weeks.[43]

Ironically, Japan's extremely low infant mortality rate has been achieved despite the fact that normal pregnancies are not a routine health insurance benefit in Japan. Instead, pregnancy services are fully covered under public programs administered and financed through the Ministry of Health. If the pregnancy results in complications, such as the need to perform a cesarean section, insurance covers the condition.[43]

Substantial improvements in pregnancy outcomes and pediatric care have been made in Japan over the past 40 years. These improvements are the result of strong public support for healthy infants and children, which began shortly after World War II during the early 1950s. In 1950, the infant mortality rate (IMR) in Japan was 60.1/1000 live births (compared to 29.2/1000 in the United States). Maternal mortality rates were 176/100,000 and 83.3/100,000, respectively.[83] With growing concern over these statistics, the Japanese government promulgated national guidelines in 1958, which recommended the establishment of Maternal and Child Health Clinics (MCHCs) throughout the country. By 1965 when these guidelines were formally codified through enactment of the Maternal and Child Health Law, there were more than 400 such clinics. As a result, the infant mortality rate (4.6/1000 live births) and the maternal mortality rate (8.5/100,000) have been reduced 13- and 20-fold, respectively, since 1950 (Table 5-4). Today, a wide range of preventive and health promotion services is provided throughout Japan in Health Centers administered by the prefectures and in Community Health Centers (CHC) and MCHCs administered locally.

Pregnant women are encouraged to register their preg-

Table 5-3. A comparison of health status measures between the United States and Japan: circa 1989

	1 United States	2 Japan	Ratio 1:2
Life expectancy (years at birth)			
Men	71.8	75.9	0.94
Women	78.5	81.8	0.95
% Population >65 yr	12.6	11.5	1.09
Mortality rate*			
Crude	827	—	—
Circulatory disease	365	—	—
Cancer	195	—	—
Infant mortality rate (IMR)†	9.8	4.59	2.13
Low birth rate (%)	7	5	1.40
Maternal mortality‡	6.6	8.5	0.78

From OECD Health Data File.
*Rate per 100,000 population.
†*IMR*, Infant mortality rate per 1000 live births.
‡Rate per 100,000 live births, 1987. From Rowland D: Health status in Eastern European countries, *Health Affairs* 10(3):202-215, 1991.

nancy with a local health authority. At that time the woman receives a maternal and child health handbook *(Boshi Kenko Techo)* in which she will maintain a detailed record of her maternity progress, clinical evaluations, findings, and recommendations made throughout her pregnancy. She is expected to take the handbook with her for all prenatal visits. A comprehensive record of her child's birth and development is later added to this handbook.

Unlike women in the United States and in many other countries, most Japanese women remain in the hospital for up to a week postpartum, even for uncomplicated deliver-

Table 5-4. Perinatal health trends in Japan: 1950-1990

Year	IMR*	NMR†	MMR‡	Births§ to female <15 yr	Births§ to female 15-19 yr	Birth‖ rate female >20 yr
1950	60.1	27.4	176.1	49	56,316	13.3
1960	30.7	17.0	130.6	5	19,734	4.3
1970	13.1	8.7	52.1	12	20,165	4.5
1980	7.5	4.9	20.5	14	14,576	3.6
1990	4.6	2.6	8.5	18	17,477	3.6

From *Maternal and child health statistics of Japan,* Maternal and Child Health Division, Children and Families Bureau, Ministry of Health and Welfare, Japan, 1991.
*IMR, Infant mortality rate per 1000 live births.
†NMR, Neonatal mortality rate per 1000 live births.
‡MMR, Maternal mortality rate per 100,000 live births.
§Reported as total number of births.
‖Births per 1000 females.

ies. After their hospital discharge, a public health nurse makes a routine home visit to evaluate the new infant and mother for potential problems during this postpartum period. Breast-feeding appears to be more common in Japan than in the United States. An estimated 90% of new mothers were reported to be breast-feeding, at least initially, in 1985, and nearly half continued to breast-feed for a longer period.[83]

In addition to a comprehensive system of maternal care, Japan's low infant mortality rate may be attributed in part to a variety of other characteristics of Japanese culture. First, the adolescent pregnancy rate is very low: four times lower than in Canada, Sweden, and Great Britain, and ten times lower than in the United States.[28] In 1990, for example, only 1.4% of all births were to teenaged mothers.[83] Furthermore, among all births to adolescents in Japan, only 18 (less than 0.1%) were to teens under age 15.[83] In the vast majority of cases, teenagers who become pregnant terminate their pregnancy.

Second, young Japanese women appear to be less sexually active than in other countries. One survey has suggested that adolescent women in the United States are nearly four times as likely to have been sexually active before the age of 20 compared to Japanese females. Consequently, the age-specific fertility rate for young Japanese women is one of the lowest in the world. For women under 20 the recorded fertility rate has never been above 4.1/1000 women during the 1980s and was 3.6/1000 women in 1990.[83]

Third, there are very few single mothers in Japan. In 1982, less than 1% of all mothers were unmarried, compared to over 25% in the United States.[28]

Nonetheless, among women who do become pregnant, early prenatal care is encouraged and made readily available through public clinics. In addition, pregnant women can receive publicly financed comprehensive physical examinations at a clinic or hospital during the early and late trimesters of their pregnancy. Public clinics offer a special medical aid program that addresses important prenatal conditions or complications during pregnancy, such as toxemia, gestational diabetes, anemia, or obstetric bleeding.[83]

Pediatric preventive services. Preventive services for Japanese children are a major concern for Japanese society. This focus is facilitated by a declining fertility rate, which dropped from 3.7 children/woman in 1950 to 1.7/woman in 1985. Greater family planning has resulted in smaller families, fewer children, and a greater opportunity for more careful attention and nurturing of children's needs and development.[115]

Significantly, the various public health clinics, including school-based programs, are linked and integrated to facilitate a system of coordinated and continuous care from early pregnancy throughout childhood. As a result of this coordinated system, Japan has ensured the delivery of a wide range of preventive and health promotion services to women and children, as well as adults. Today, more than 1100 clinics provide virtually all preventive services for preschool-aged children.[100]

For children these services include the following:

- Newborn screening for five metabolic diseases, hypothyroidism, hepatitis B, and neuroblastoma
- Special formula for children with congenital metabolic conditions
- Childhood vaccinations
- Infant screening and developmental examinations on four separate occasions during the first year of life, and twice a year thereafter until they enter school
- Management and special assistance programs for disabled children, including nurse visitation services
- Continued services and evaluation for families with low-birth-weight infants
- Medical aid programs for children with chronic diseases
- Access to child care classes for parents
- Home visiting services by public health nurses for needy families

For adolescents these services include the following:

- Counseling for the prevention of obesity in children
- Premarital and family planning classes targeted to adolescents
- Rubella vaccination for girls in secondary school
- Postexamination counseling after all health examinations

Once children enter school, school-based clinics administered through the Ministry of Education continue to provide preventive and health promotion services. School-based health promotion programs involve content-specific instruction in injury and disease prevention and normal physical and psychologic development (elementary school), injury prevention, environmental health and disease prevention (junior high school), with contemporary health issues involving the community and national health and environmental problems added during the senior high school years. Complete dental services are also available through MCHCs and school-based clinics. Other specific screening services provided for both preschool- and school-aged groups include vision, speech, and hearing evaluation, and periodic urinalysis.

Adult preventive services. Because of public attention to mass screening and attendant funding, preventive screenings have become popular in Japan. It has been estimated that nearly every Japanese undergoes on average one screening per year.[69] Although insurance does not cover routine physical examinations,[42] for a small fee, Japanese over age 40 may receive annual screening services consisting of limited physical examination, selected laboratory studies (liver function, serum cholesterol, hematocrit, and urinalysis), and blood pressure measurement. As many as one third of these adults choose to receive more intensive screening including electrocardiogram and ocular fundus examination. Separate cancer screening examinations (lung, gastric, breast, and cervix) are available for selected age groups.[69]

Japanese tradition places high regard for the elderly, who frequently live with their adult children. In 1975, for example, 75.8% of all Japanese over age 65 were estimated to be living with their children. Although this living pattern has been declining in recent years, it nonetheless remains much more prevalent than in Western countries.

Although free medical care was introduced for the elderly in Japan in 1973, the enactment of the Health and Medical Services for the Elderly Act in 1982 has amended this service somewhat because of concern over excessive use of services by a growing elderly population. In addition, the Elderly Act seeks to coordinate health services and activities for the elderly, including sickness prevention programs and rehabilitation services. Prevention and health promotion services are implemented locally, including annual health screenings, development of health education programs targeting the elderly, and distribution of a health diary for elderly citizens in which to record medical and health problems. Discretion is given to local health authorities to achieve these goals.

FRANCE: COMBINING SICKNESS FUNDS AND SOCIAL SECURITY

This vastly Catholic country (approximately 90% of France is Roman Catholic) with about 56.1 million people has a rich history of multiparty politics and constitutional revision.[36,125] Despite this Catholic tradition, birth control is publicly financed in France, and the controversial abortifacant, RU-486, was first developed and marketed here.[36,125]

Although historically divided on many issues, the French appear to be in general agreement over the quality of their health care system. Forty-one percent of French people in a recent poll responded that they believed that "only minor changes were necessary to make [their health care system] work better."[10]

Health insurance in France is compulsory. Financing is derived from sickness funds (caisses d'insurance maladié), which are part of the national Social Security Program (Sécurité Sociale). Employers and employees pay contributions into the sickness funds, which are managed by representatives of labor and management. This system finances approximately 73% of all health care expenditures. Health care charges are reimbursed by the funds, directly for hospital care and indirectly to patients for ambulatory care after they have first paid their physician directly. The level of physician fees is set through negotiations between Social Security administrators and physician associations and result in the establishment of some degree of cost sharing for patients.[91]

There are few insurers in France, and virtually all French are insured through one of three types of sickness funds. One insurer, Regime General, a network of more than 100 sickness funds for workers, insures approximately 80% of the population.[59] Another set of funds insures farmers and rural commercial businessmen. A third fund (so-called "No-No" fund by some because it insures neither salaried nor rural workers) insures the self-employed. Public assistance insures the poor and unemployed.[91]

Like Germany, France relies on central-government-regulated sickness funds to finance health insurance for workers and their dependents. Virtually all insurers are nonprofit, and so-called Mutuelles (friendly societies) provide supplemental benefits not covered under the sickness fund. On the other hand, for-profit insurers are rare and serve essentially to supplement or replace mandated health coverage under the nonprofit plans or to help meet cost-sharing requirements.[59] Private insurers account for only a small percentage of health care expenditures.

Table 5-5. A comparison of health system capacity and utilization of medical services between the United States and France: circa 1989

	1 United States	2 France	Ratio 1:2
Percent GDP on health care	12.4	8.9	1.39
Per capita on health care	$ 2566	$ 1379	1.86
Percent public funding	42	75	
Hospitals*			
Beds†	3.8	5.4	0.70
Average length of stay (ALOS) (days)	7.2	7.3	0.98
Occ. rate	65.5	76.4	0.85
Admission rate‡	12.8	20.1	0.63
Physicians			
Number†	2.3	2.6	0.88
Average no. visits	5.3	7.1	0.74
% Primary care§	34	53	0.64
MD expenditure‖	183,281	57,270	3.2

From OECD Health Data File.

*Data based on acute care hospitals only, i.e. hospitals in which the ALOS is less than 30 days. (1988)

†Per 1000 population.

‡Percent of total populations.

§Percent of physicians identifying themselves as general practitioners, pediatricians, internists.

‖Physician expenditures per physician (i.e., total physician spending for outpatient and inpatient services per number of active practicing physicians). Sums expressed in U.S. dollars 1988. Source: HCFA calculations of OECD data.

System capacity and use of medical services

Consumers are free to choose from a relative abundance of physicians, some 2.6/1000 population, slightly above the U.S. rate of 2.3/1000 population[60] (Table 5-5). Approximately 53% (76,673 in 1989) are general practitioners; the remaining 47% (63,398) are various specialists.[59] The French visit their physicians often, averaging 7.1 visits per year, which is second only to Japan and Germany.[109] In 1989 French physicians made roughly 7.8 consultations per person, compared to 10.8 for Germany and 5.2 in Great Britain.[62] The average annual income for French physicians is around $64,606 (1990).[60] (Incomes may be substantially greater, however, for some private physicians.) There are more than 3700 hospitals, including acute, long-term care and psychiatric facilities in France. Although only approximately 28% of the hospitals are public facilities, they contain roughly 65% of all hospital beds. The remainder are private commercial and private nonprofit institutions. Hospital planning is guided by the use of a health map, which defines hospital service needs for specific areas. The health map governs new hospital construction and expansion for both public and private hospitals.[91]

A much higher percentage of the French are hospitalized as compared to U.S. citizens. In 1988 the hospital admission rate was roughly 20.1%,* and the average length of stay was 7.3 days. Both are greater than in the United States.[109]

Medical economics and expenditures

France spent approximately 8.9% of its GDP on health, or $1379 per person in 1990, 86% less than the United States.[60] It has been estimated, however, that only a small proportion of the French people (an estimated 10% of the population) consumes approximately 75% of total health care expenditures. Approximately half of all health care expenditures is spent for hospital-related care, some 30% is spent for ambulatory physician care. The remainder is spent for medical goods and drugs.[91]

In 1983 France instituted a program of global budgeting for hospitals. This program established national expenditure targets (ETs) for hospital and sickness funds, by which specific budgets were developed for public hospitals. The program was first implemented at the regional level and later expanded to include local hospitals. These targets include expenditures for public, hospital-based physician services.[59,91]

Budget controls on hospitals have managed to restrain hospital spending. In an analysis of hospital expenditures in France, the U.S. Government Accounting Office estimates that annual growth in spending on inpatient care was reduced approximately 9% between 1984 and 1987.[59] During a similar period (1985-1987) the percentage of GDP devoted to health care remained unchanged at 8.5%. This percentage compares with steady increases experienced before this period. In 1975 the percentage of GDP was 7.0%; during the 1980s it rose to 7.6%, peaking in 1985 at 8.5%.[110]

The French engage in limited cost-sharing for medical care, depending on the type of service provided. Ambulatory physician visits require 25% co-pays, hospitalizations require a 20% co-pay for the first 30 hospital days, and dental care has a 30% co-pay. Prescription drugs have very limited coverage: 30% to 70% cost-sharing depending on the nature of the drug, and some drugs require full consumer payment. Cost-sharing for the poor is provided through the social welfare system.[59]

The portion of hospitalizations extending beyond 30 days is covered fully if the admission is on an approved list developed by the *Securité Sociale*. For the first 30 days, the coverage is 80%.[91]

Public, hospital-based physicians are salaried, whereas private hospital-based physicians are paid on a fee-for-service basis. Although private for-profit hospitals (*cliniques*)

*Percent of total population.

do not pay their physicians salaries, the rates physicians charge are fixed on a fee-for-service basis. This rate is independent of the volume of services provided to that patient. While the per diem rates permitted may differ among *cliniques,* each *clinique* must charge each sickness fund the same rate. Ambulatory care physicians and physicians in private hospitals are reimbursed on a uniform fee-for-service basis; however, the reimbursement is established by the government, and physicians are in certain instances allowed to balance bill patients beyond the established fee schedule.[59,91]

Three basic categories of physicians encompass both general practitioners and specialists and are defined according to the fees charged and level of reimbursement. For one category (Sector I) fees are established by the *Sécurité Sociale*. Physicians are reimbursed at 75% of the established fee. A second category of physicians (Sector II) charge fees in excess of those approved by the *Sécurité Sociale,* but patients are reimbursed at the same levels established for the first category of physicians. Finally, a third category of physicians—those who choose not to participate in the *Sécurité Sociale*—charge rates that are essentially unregulated and patients, usually the more affluent, receive no reimbursement from the insurance funds.[91] To encourage acceptance of Sector I fees, physicians are given incentives, including greater government contributions to their benefits programs and lower taxes if they agree to accept this fee schedule.

France's health profile

Of the 56 million people living in France, approximately 10 million are more than 60 years old.[60,91] Approximately 14% of the population is over age 65.[60] Overall life expectancy at birth is 80.9 years for French women, and 72.7 years for French men (1990)[60] (Table 5-6). The fertility rate for young French women is roughly 1.8/1000 women. Approximately 22% of all births in France are to unmarried women.[28] The infant mortality rate of 7.36/1000 live births is the eighth lowest among the developed countries. Only 5.0% of all births produce low-birth-weight infants.[87]

The French have an extremely low risk of cardiovascular disease. According to 1987 WHO data, the French had, by far, the lowest age-adjusted mortality rate for circulatory disease (224/100,000) among Western European countries.[106] On the other hand, France had one of the highest rates of age-adjusted mortality related to injuries. Approximately 40% of deaths in children less than 14 years in 1985 were caused by motor vehicle injuries.[81] Overall, however, motor vehicle injuries (4.2/1000 population) are relatively low compared to the other countries.[60] With a total of 9718 cases, France had the highest number of reported case of AIDS among all eastern European countries.

Table 5-6. A comparison of health status measures between the United States and France: circa 1989

	1 United States	2 France	Ratio 1:2
Life expectancy (years at birth)			
Men	71.8	72.7	0.98
Women	78.5	80.9	0.97
% Population >65 yr	12.6	14.0	0.90
Mortality rate*			
Crude	827	715	1.16
Circulatory disease	365	224	1.62
Cancer	195	205	0.95
IMR†	9.8	7.36	1.33
Low birth rate (%)	7	5	1.40
Maternal mortality‡	6.6	9.3	0.70

From OECD Health Data File.
*Rate per 100,000 population.
†Rate per 1000 live births.
‡Rate per 100,000 live births, 1987. From Rowland D: Health status in eastern European countries, *Health Affairs* 10(3):202-215, 1991.

Clinical preventive services: a population profile

In France many preventive services are well covered. For example, government funding reimburses providers for immunizations, and pediatric preventive services are well covered under both public and private insurance programs.[59]

Perinatal preventive services and maternal disability. Perinatal care and well-baby care are fully covered, and pregnant women with uncomplicated pregnancies are urged to make at least seven prenatal visits for evaluation and care. On average, however, they probably make less than six visits.[112] Prenatal care is provided by family practitioners, midwives, and obstetricians. Obstetricians and some 10,356 (1989) midwives appear to manage most of the newborn deliveries, with family practitioners attending a small portion (less than 5%) of all deliveries. Frequently, maternal management is provided through a "shared-care system" involving combinations of providers such as an obstetrician and a midwife.

Health workers also make antenatal visits to women considered to be at high risk or who otherwise have failed to make prenatal visits.[112] Postpartum home visitations are optional locally.

In France women are eligible for maternal disability benefits, although they are slightly less generous than in several other countries discussed in this analysis (Canada, Sweden, and Great Britain). Pregnant women must meet certain eligibility requirements such as being insured for at least 10 months before delivery of the infant to qualify for disability benefits. Cash benefits may reach 84% of salaried earnings, up to $63 per day (regular disability benefits are capped at 50% of earnings). Payment of benefits may begin as early as 6 weeks before the child's birth and continue for 10 weeks after delivery, or for a total of 16 weeks.[42,59]

Other social benefits for young families include additional protected leave time to care for young children and priority placement in public housing. They also are eligible for financial assistance (birth subsidies).[91] For example, a new mother may take a job-protected leave for up to 3 years with retention of her pension rights, but usually without any remuneration. Occasionally, however, she may receive a minimal salary. France also guarantees a family allowance of between 10% and 13% of the woman's average monthly wage. Finally, families of two or more children have priority for any available public housing.[64]

Pediatric preventive services. Since 1945 federal law permitted children to receive preventive evaluations from birth to 6 years. In 1970 compulsory examinations were required for children 8 days postpartum, and thereafter at 9 months and at 2 years of age. Information is collected and forwarded to the appropriate maternal and child health bureau.[80]

France has an extensive publicly funded preschool system called maternal school (ecole maternelle) for children 3 years and older.[27] Although the program is noncompulsory, virtually all (90%) 3 year olds attend maternal school. In addition to a range of educational and social experiences for the children, they receive extensive preventive health examinations by a team composed of a physician, a nurse, a child psychologist, and a social worker. This examination includes assessment of language skills, developmental screening, psychomotor assessment, hearing and vision testing, and a physical examination. Parents are urged to participate and receive advice and counseling about any pertinent findings. Children are referred to their family physician if additional examination or treatment is recommended (e.g., immunizations or additional laboratory testing), and the MCH team ensures that such follow-up is obtained in most cases.[27] Thus the preschool setting becomes a natural encounter site for providing essential preventive screening and health promotion for children. Immunization rates for 1 year olds are high for DPT (96%) and polio (97%), but much lower for measles (41%).[121] In the United States, except for childhood immunization requirements, the preschool/day care setting becomes a missed opportunity for preventive care.

A second preventive opportunity for children occurs when they enter elementary school at approximately age 5 to 6 years. At this encounter, a school health team replaces the MCH team and performs additional developmental screening focusing on abnormalities that might lead to school difficulties. This school health team, which works full time, is salaried.[27]

Examination of both groups of children is free and is designed to provide additional points of preventive care between the perinatal period and the time of entry into the primary school system.[137] School health services provide preventive services and are coordinated with other services in the school system to address environmental issues, nutrition, and health education.

Adult preventive services. Adults are eligible for free comprehensive annual preventive examinations every 5 years, and women may undergo free mammography beginning at age 45. Physicians do not need a clinical justification for such services: They may be provided and reimbursed as preventive screening. Eye examinations and preventive dental care are fully covered and include dentures and eyeglasses.[59] Influenza vaccinations are available for individuals over age 65 as a primary preventive service. Public clinics also provide comprehensive mental health services by psychologists, psychiatrists, and psychiatric nurses, including substance abuse treatment, for individuals of all ages.[91]

SWEDEN: LOCAL PLANNING, FINANCING, AND UNIVERSAL COVERAGE

The Nordic Region comprises Sweden, Denmark, and Norway, Finland, Iceland and three other autonomous territories, the Faeroes, Aland, and Greenland. With a population of more than 8.4 million people, Sweden is the most populous Nordic country, nearly double the population of Denmark, the next largest country.[36,128]

Sweden is a predominantly Protestant constitutional monarchy. About 17% of the population is over the age of 65, a greater percentage than any of the other Nordic countries. Its unemployment rate in 1986 was 2.4%, one-third the rate of the United States.

Sweden's health care system is characterized by compulsory public insurance, which is only supplemented by private insurance.[42] Private health insurance is purchased by approximately 7% of the population, mostly business executives and their dependents.[42] Because public health insurance benefits are comprehensive, private insurance has only a supplemental role, providing coverage for elective procedures and more generous hospital accommodations.

The people of Sweden have mixed views on their health care system. In a recent poll, as many as 58% of the people polled responded that "fundamental changes (were) needed to make (the system) work better." Only 32% were generally satisfied with their current health care system.[10]

With enactment of the Health and Medical Services Act in 1983, local county councils were given greater autonomy in health planning and construction of medical facilities.[55] Consequently, the central government's role increasingly is limited to setting broad policy, and the actual development and administration of the system occurs locally.[42]

For example, issues related to health planning, services,

and efficiency are handled at the national level by the Ministry of Health and Social Affairs, the National Board of Health and Welfare, and the Swedish Planning and Rationalization Institute. Although broad policy and planning are centralized, the responsibility for the financing and delivery of health services resides in some 23 county councils and three large municipalities, not in the council areas. These 26 authorities are responsible for the delivery of both hospital care and primary health care, as well as levying a proportional income tax, which finances roughly 65% of the total health care expenditures. Additional funding is derived from payroll taxes (roughly 10.1%) plus a national tax of 6.5%.

Because funding is primarily raised at the county level, the trend in recent years has been toward more decentralization so that health policy decision making, unlike in Great Britain, is shared between the national government and county councils.

System capacity and use of medical services

In general, concern over the need to control health expenditures has contributed to a deemphasis on hospital-based care and a focus stressing health promotion, prevention, and primary care.[55,73,74]

With 3.1 physicians per 1000 population, Sweden has more physicians per capita than any other Scandinavian country and all other European countries except Belgium (3.3), Greece (3.2), and Spain (3.6) (Table 5-7).[60] Approximately one fourth of Swedish physicians practice outside the hospital setting.[74] On average, Swedish patients make 2.8 physician contacts per year, which is the lowest among the Scandinavian countries (Denmark, 5.2; Finland, 3.7; Iceland, 4.9; and Norway, 5.7), and nearly half the number of physician visits per year in the United States. With 1.1 dentists per 1000 population, Sweden has more dentists per capita than the other countries analyzed here.[60]

Regarding use of inpatient services, the acute care hospital admission rate of 16.8%* and occupancy rate of 78.4% are, among the Scandinavian countries, second only to Denmark. The average length of acute care hospital stay (7.1 days) is the lowest of all Scandinavian countries.[109]

Medical economics and expenditures

In 1990 Sweden spent $1421 per person, about 8.7% of GDP, on health care. This level of spending was 81% less than in the United States. Public spending accounts for approximately 90% of all health care expenditures.[60]

Unlike the other countries discussed in this analysis, Sweden has reduced its health expenditures as a percentage of GDP from 9.5% (1980-1985) to 9.0% (1986-1988)

*Percent of total population.

Table 5-7. A comparison of health system capacity and use of medical services between the United States and Sweden: circa 1989

	1 United States	2 Sweden	Ratio 1:2
Percent GDP on health care	12.4	8.7	1.42
Per capita on health care	$2566	$1421	1.80
Percent public funding	42	90	0.46
Hospitals*			
Beds†	3.8	4.1	0.92
Average length of stay (ALOS) (days)	7.2	7.1	1.01
Occ. rate	65.5	78.4	0.83
Admission rate‡	12.8	16.8	0.76
Physicians			
Number†	2.3	3.1	0.74
Average no. visits	5.3	2.8	1.89
% Primary care§	34	—	—
MD expenditure‖	183,281	—	—

From OECD Health Data File.
*Data based on acute care hospitals only, i.e., hospitals in which the ALOS is less than 30 days (1988).
†Per 1000 population.
‡Percent of total populations.
§Percent of physicians identifying themselves as general practitioners, pediatricians, internists.
‖Physician expenditures per physician (i.e., total physician spending for outpatient and inpatient services per number of active practicing physicians). Sums expressed in U.S. dollars 1988. From HCFA calculations of OECD data).

to 8.7% (1990).[60,110] Approximately 15% of the 9.2% of GNP spent on health care in 1986 was for primary health care services, most of which are preventive services. Hospitals have global budgets. There are physician fee schedules, and physicians may not balance bill patients.[42]

Sweden's health profile

As is the case with some other Scandinavian countries, Sweden's health profile is one of the best in the world. Among the Scandinavian countries, the people of Sweden in 1989 had the longest life expectancy at birth both for men (74.8 years) and women (80.6 years)[60] (Table 5-8). Sweden also has more people over age 65 (17.7%) than any other Scandinavian country. The crude mortality rate in 1990 was 11.1/1000.[60]

Sweden has the second lowest infant mortality rate (5.77) in the world. Only 4.0% of all births are low birth weight.[87] Sweden's adolescent pregnancy rate of 11/1000 women is one of the lowest; however, the percentage of births to unmarried mothers (48.4%) is the highest among the Nordic countries and over double the rate in the United States.[28,74]†

†This may be due in part to certain tax advantages for single versus married individuals. (Personal communication, Anne Johansen, 1992.)

Table 5-8. A comparison of health status measures between the United States and Sweden: circa 1989

	1 U.S.	2 Sweden	Ratio 1:2
Life expectancy (years at birth)			
Men	71.8	74.8	0.95
Women	78.5	80.6	0.97
% Population >65 yr	12.6	17.7	0.71
Mortality rate*			
Crude	827	741	1.11
Circulatory disease	365	373	0.97
Cancer	195	166	1.17
IMR†	9.80	5.77	1.69
Low birth rate (%)	7	4	1.75
Maternal mortality‡	6.6	4.8	1.37

From OECD Health Data File.
*Rate per 100,000 population.
†Rate per 1000 live births.
‡Rate per 100,000 live births, 1987. (From Rowland D: Health status in Eastern European countries, *Health Affairs* 10(3):202-215, 1991.)

Sweden's rates of certain preventable injury-related deaths for adolescents are 30/100,000 population for motor vehicle accidents, 19.5/100,000 for suicide, and 2.3/100,000 for homicide.[28] The World Health Organization (WHO) estimates that the likelihood of dying from motor vehicle injuries in Sweden is one of the lowest in Europe. Motor vehicle safety is important and reflected in the safety record of Swedish-made automobiles and highway safety legislation such as laws requiring automobile headlights to be on during the daytime.[92]

In 1991 Sweden reported 487 cases of AIDS, second to Denmark in the number of reported AIDS cases in Scandinavia.

Clinical preventive services: a population profile

An emphasis on ambulatory care. Both hospital and ambulatory health care are covered 100% under public insurance, but both levels of care require a $10 per day user fee (capped at 15 user fees per year). There are no additional out-of-pocket expenses for prescription drugs.[42]

Since the 1970s, Sweden has tried to redirect its health care system away from hospital and medical specialty health care toward increased primary and preventive health care services.[55,73,74] In 1969 and 1979 the National Board of Health established a national policy affecting preventive services, especially for women and children. In addition to emphasizing preventive health care, the Board has encouraged parents to take an active role in creating an environment that fosters the development of their children.[73]

Perinatal services and maternal disability. Free prenatal care is accessible to most women; thus virtually all pregnant women receive adequate prenatal care. In fact, although 12 to 13 prenatal examinations are recom-

mended, one study suggests that women make closer to 14 prenatal visits.[112] It is recommended that two or three of these prenatal visits be made to a physician and the other 10 to 12 to a midwife.[74] To enhance pregnancy outcomes, parents are permitted time off work to attend (as many as eight) prenatal and postnatal parenting classes.[64]

Prenatal visitation rates are believed to be near 100%, and less than 1% of all deliveries occur outside the hospital.[74] The consequences of such nonepisodic care is reflected in the country's exceptionally low infant mortality rate. In 1989 the IMR was 5.77/1000 live births, making it the lowest rate among the Scandinavian countries and the second lowest in the world. Sweden's proportion of low-birth-weight infants (4.0%) is comparable to Norway and Finland, but better than Denmark (6.0%).[87]

Midwives in Sweden and in most other Scandinavian countries play a significant role in providing prenatal care. Most prenatal services are provided through health clinics, where midwives provide the majority of care for nearly all of the 14 prenatal visits made by Swedish women. Midwives attend all normal deliveries in Sweden, as they do in Finland and Norway. To enhance pregnancy outcomes, Sweden, like France, has an outreach program for pregnant women, using a home visiting system with health workers who make home prenatal visits to women considered to be at high risk or to women who have failed to make their recommended prenatal visits.[112] Maternity disability is treated equal to other short-term disabilities, and cash benefits are paid for up to 13 weeks postpartum.

Sweden is recognized as having one of the most liberal parental leave policies in Europe. For example, in addition to the cash benefits under maternal disability, fathers are entitled to take up to 10 days parental leave at 90% of their salary after their child's birth. Overall, parents who have worked continuously for 6 months before delivery are eligible to take as many as 450 days of job-protected leave between them at 90% of their salaries to care for their child. Beyond this period, parents are allowed as many as 90 days per year for child care matters (e.g., illness) during which time they will receive an additional $10 per day. Parents can divide this leave time equally between themselves, or one parent may take it all. Beyond the preschool period, parents may reduce the number of hours worked per week to 75% of normal until their children reach the age of 10 years.[42,64] During any periods of leave, parents receive full job protection and retention of their pension rights.[64]

Pediatric preventive services. Sweden has the largest population of children under 15 years, and the largest number of pediatricians per capita (3.3) in the Nordic region.[74] Long a leader in children's health, Sweden has a well-developed system of child health centers staffed by a range of health care providers who perform screening examinations, conduct development assessments of preschool-aged children, and provide free immunizations to preschoolers.[73] Frequent visits to the physician are encouraged, and the range of routine preventive screening services provided to children has steadily broadened in recent years. These services include screening for inborn errors of metabolism; preschool assessments of vision, hearing, and speech; counseling on nutrition and child development; and routine childhood immunizations. Over 95% of infants and only slightly fewer older children receive these preventive services.[74] Consequently, most of Sweden's children are fully immunized. Immunization rates for 1 year olds are among the highest in the world: 99% for DPT, 98% for polio, and 93% for measles.[121]

Once in the education system, children are eligible for continued preventive care through the country's extensive school health services system, which continues to provide screening and regular examinations.[74] Health education, developed at the federal government level, includes programs that have led to a decrease in the use of tobacco and alcohol among schoolchildren. The school serves as the focus for a variety of preventive education programs directed at reducing teen smoking and alcohol use, as well as sex education programs. For example, Sweden is participating in an international project directed at the health of schoolchildren. The results of this project indicate that Swedish schoolchildren use tobacco and alcohol much less than schoolchildren in the other European countries participating in the project.[73]

The Swedish Board of Education conducts surveys to determine alcohol, drug, and tobacco use among schoolchildren. Some startling results have been found. Earlier surveys found that approximately one third of the country's ninth-graders drink alcohol at least once a month. On the other hand, tobacco use has been declining steadily, and the percentage of students identifying themselves as regular smokers appears to be the lowest among the Nordic countries.[74]

One measure of Sweden's success in attempting to encourage primary and preventive care over hospital care has been the decrease in the number of hospital days for children. In 1960 the mean number of hospital days for children was 14; by 1980 it fell to 4.6 days.[74]

During the 1970s Sweden began an aggressive dental services program for children. As a result, virtually all children and adolescents undergo regular dental examination and receive any necessary care. Preventive care also includes counseling families about oral hygiene, the role of diet in dental health, and the need for fluoride supplements. Evaluations of this effort revealed a marked decrease in dental caries among children. Between 1973 and 1983 the prevalence of caries-free children doubled from 35% to 70%.[74]

Adult preventive services. PAP smear examinations and mammography are widely available for Swedish women as part of an established program of cervical and breast cancer screening. In particular, as in Finland, Iceland, and Great Britain, Sweden has instituted a systematized cervical cancer screening program. Begun more than two decades ago, this nationwide program has as its target achieving 100% PAP smear testing among eligible women between the ages of 30 and 49 years. Written notification is generated by a centralized computer program, which monitors at-risk age groups and notifies them periodically of the need, time, and place for a cervical PAP smear.[54,75] This program of aggressive outreach to notify women has achieved over 70% compliance among the target population.

GREAT BRITAIN: CAPITATED FEES, CENTRALIZED CONTROL, AND A PRIMARY HEALTH CARE FOCUS
The National Health Service

An island nation of approximately 57 million citizens off the north European coast, Great Britain is governed under a centuries-old system of constitutional monarchy and representative democracy.[36,129] The British health care system is administered through the National Health Service (NHS), one of the three main branches of the British social welfare system.

Introduced as legislation in 1946, the NHS was ultimately enacted into law in 1948. The NHS provides comprehensive health care coverage to virtually all citizens of England. The administration of health services under the NHS is delegated to 14 Regional Health Authorities (RHA), each with between 2 and 5 million citizens. RHAs recently were charged with conducting health assessments and health improvement goals for regional constituents. These regions, in turn, are further divided into 191 District Health Authorities (DHA), each with approximately 300,000 people. The DHAs, which contain a range of medical care and public health administrative units, including the Family Health Service Authorities, are responsible for the direct administration and delivery of medical services by contracting with district hospitals and physicians, and for monitoring quality of care.[42]

Great Britain's highly nationalized system of public health insurance is compulsory for all residents. Private health insurance, which plays only a minor supplementary role as it does in Japan and Sweden, is purchased by the more affluent and covers private hospital care and certain types of elective surgery.[42] In fact, only about 10% of the population has private health insurance.[42] Public insurance provides comprehensive financial coverage for hospital and ambulatory care, and prescriptions require modest copayments. Individuals with certain limiting conditions such as epilepsy, however, are not required to meet cost-sharing requirements.[94]

Generally speaking, everyone registers with a general practitioner for their primary health care; unlike the Germans, British patients may not consult directly a medical specialist without a general practitioner's referral. Timeliness of some services has been criticized. Waiting times of 1 to 2 years are not unusual for nonemergent surgery, and the decisions regarding access to certain expensive medical procedures result in extended waits for organ transplants and kidney dialysis.[42]

As in Sweden, most hospitals are government owned as a result of nationalization of facilities under the 1948 law. Each of the roughly 1700 hospitals within the NHS is allocated a specific budget by the DHA so that hospital expenditures fall within global budgets. Expenditures for physician services are controlled through negotiated fee schedules that use a system of capitated payment. Although hospital-based GPs are salaried government employees, non-hospital-based physicians are paid through a capitated payment system established by the government. Balance billing of patients by providers is strictly prohibited. Thus physicians are reimbursed through a combination of capitated fees, allowances, and sporadic fee-for-service.[137]

Rationing of services, extended waits for certain procedures, and limited consumer choice probably explain to a great extent the apparent dissatisfaction among some with the health care system. A 1988 Louis Harris survey revealed that as many as 52% of the British polled believed that their health care system required fundamental change to make it work better. Approximately 17% of the respondents agreed with the statement that the ". . . health care system has so much wrong with it that we need to completely rebuild it."[11]

System capacity and utilization of medical services

Virtually all hospitals are government owned as a result of enactment of the NHS. As part of its national effort to control health care spending, Great Britain controls the number of physicians trained, the number of hospital beds available, and medical technology. For example, Great Britain has reduced the number of acute-care hospital beds to 2.8 per 1000 population, well below Canada (4.5) and the United States (3.8) (Table 5-9). Its average length of hospital stay of 7.8 days per admission is less than in most other industrialized countries, yet its hospital occupancy rate at 76.4% is comparatively high.[109]

Great Britain has a relatively low ratio of physicians per capita (1.4 per 1000 people) among the OECD countries. On average, the British appear to make relatively fewer physician visits per year (4.5) than most other Europeans.[109]

Medical economics and expenditures

Partially as a result of low use of health care services and partially as a result of national controls on health care spending, Great Britain has managed to keep its health care expenditures one of the lowest among the developed nations. During the 1980s, health care spending as a percentage of GDP has remained between 5.8% and 6.0%. In

Table 5-9. A comparison of health system capacity and use of medical services between the United States and Great Britain: circa 1989

	1 United States	2 Great Britain	Ratio 1:2
Percent GDP on health care	12.4	6.1	2.03
Per capita on health care	$ 2566	$ 909	2.82
Percent public funding	42	87	0.48
Hospitals*			
Beds†	3.8	2.8	1.35
Average length of stay (ALOS) (days)	7.2	7.8	0.92
Occ. rate	65.5	76.4	0.85
Admission rate‡	12.8	12.9	0.99
Physicians			
Number†	2.3	1.4	1.64
Average no. visits	5.3	5.7	0.92
% Primary care§	34	63	0.53
MD expenditures‖	183,281	34,823	5.26

From OECD Health Data File.
*Data based on acute care hospitals only, i.e., hospitals in which the ALOS is less than 30 days (1988).
†Per 1000 population.
‡Percent of total population.
§Percent of physicians identifying themselves as general practitioners, pediatricians, internists.
‖Physician expenditures per physician (i.e., total physician spending for outpatient and inpatient services per number of active practicing physicians.) Sums expressed in U.S. dollars 1988. (From HCFA calculations of OECD data.)

1990 it reached 6.1%, or approximately $909 per capita.[60,110] This level is much less than in Canada and about half the level in the United States.

The NHS is financed through public taxes, out-of-pocket fees, and other taxable contributions. As in Sweden, the financing of health care in Great Britain is centralized. Approximately 87% of financing is obtained nationally from general funds; the remainder is obtained from employer and employee contributions to the National Insurance Fund.[42] With national control over health expenditures, the NHS budget, capital construction funds, and appointments over regional and district health authorities, most major health policy decisions and health initiatives are established at the national level.[55]

Private health insurance is available but primarily covers services provided by medical specialists in private practice. Additionally, private insurance is preferred by large employers as supplemental coverage to ensure timely medical care of their employees as well as more comprehensive coverage for elective or procedural-oriented care. Typically, private insurance is not purchased as the primary source for payment of primary medical care.[42]

Physicians still maintain incomes comparable to physicians in many other countries despite tight national controls on health expenditures. Physicians are paid on a capitated fee basis for each patient they have a contract to serve; however, they may obtain additional income through selected fees for providing maternal care, preventive pediatric care, and cancer screening. Thus British general practitioners earn on average about $42,641 annually from service in the NHS, although additional fees may raise their incomes another 20% to 30%. Specialists (consultants) are salaried and generally earn slightly less than general practitioners.

Britain's health profile

Despite aggressive cost containment and the low use of medical services, the health profile of citizens in Great Britain is better in some respects than in the United States. Life expectancy at birth is better for men (72.8 years) than in the United States (71.8) but about the same for women (78.4 years versus 78.5 years in the United States). Compared to the other countries discussed here, Great Britain has one of the largest over-65 populations (15.6%)[109] (Table 5-10).

The infant mortality rate is 8.42 per 1000 live births. Approximately 7% of all births are low birth weight (less than 2500 grams).[87] About 21% of all births are to unmarried women, and the adolescent pregnancy rate (29.5/1000) is half the rate in the United States (50.9/1000).[28]

Compared to the other countries discussed here, Great Britain has the lowest adolescent and young adult injury-related mortality rates for motor vehicle accidents, suicide (9.9/100,000 young men and 2.3/100,000 young women), and homicide.[28] The low motor vehicle-related death and injury rates are due in part to compulsory seat belt use throughout Great Britain. Great Britain ranks fifth among the European nations in the number of reported cases of AIDS (3884).

Clinical preventive services: a population profile

A general practitioner's focus. General practitioners, in conjunction with district nurses, health visitors, and usually a midwife, serve together in the general practitioner's clinic as the main focus for the delivery of health care.[46] Physicians are either reimbursed on a per capita basis (for ambulatory care) or are salaried (for hospital-based care). Family Practitioner Committees let contracts for primary health care with a full range of providers including physicians, dentists, optometrists, and pharmacists.[52,96] The British are free to choose their family practitioner depending on the physician's capacity for new patients; but, unlike in Germany, patients may not self-refer to a specialist. General practitioners are reimbursed predominantly through a system of capitation, although they may qualify for additional income through reimbursement for certain expenses or through fees for selective services to the el-

Table 5-10. A comparison of health status measures between the United States and Great Britain: 1989

	1 United States	2 Great Britain	Ratio 1:2
Life expectancy (years at birth)			
Men	71.8	72.8	0.98
Women	78.5	78.4	1.00
% Population >65 yr	12.6	15.6	0.80
Mortality rate*			
Crude	827	854	0.96
Circulatory disease	365	389	0.93
Cancer	224	195	1.14
IMR†	9.80	8.42	1.16
Low birth rate (%)	7	7	1.00
Maternal mortality‡	6.6	6.4	1.03

From OECD Health Data File.
*Rate per 100,000 population.
†Rate per 1000 live births.
‡Rate per 100,000 live births, 1987. (From Rowland D: Health status in eastern European countries, *Health Affairs* 10(3):202-215, 1991.)

derly or for delivering preventive services such as immunizations and family planning.[52,94]

Recent national initiatives have been based on improving the delivery of preventive services, including immunizations and cancer screening, as well as increasing provider awareness of health promotion and disease prevention practices. Despite the use of financial incentives, these initiatives have been criticized by many providers as too intrusive in the practice of medicine.[94]

Perinatal preventive services and maternal disability. Obstetric care is provided by obstetricians, general practitioners, and midwives. Most deliveries appear to be managed by midwives in hospitals, with general practitioners and obstetricians supervising less than one fourth of all deliveries.[94,112] The Maternity Advisory Committee (MAC) was established in 1981 to advise the NHS with respect to obstetric care. Prenatal care clinics also provide family planning services and free pharmaceuticals.[52] The most recent MAC report recommended regionalizing neonatal intensive care services to improve quality of care and reduce costs.[52]

As a reflection of the country's attitude toward comprehensive perinatal health care, community midwives attached to general practitioner clinics are scheduled to visit all women during their first 2 weeks postpartum, and the new mother is visited once again by a community nurse (health visitor).[137] Because of limited funding and staff, however, actual visitation services may vary from those recommendations according to region.[52,112] For these reasons, preference is given, when possible, to families with existing health problems.

Depending on their prior employment status, pregnant

women are eligible for maternity disability benefits, so-called Statutory Maternity Pay (SMP). For example, women employed at least 6 months, but no longer than 2 years, before childbirth are entitled to weekly cash benefits of approximately $60 per week for up to 14 weeks. If the woman was employed longer than 2 years, her SMP benefits are raised to 90% of her average weekly salary for the first 6 weeks, and then reduced to $60 per week the last 8 weeks. Families with children receive additional benefits. Families with two or more children often are given priority for public housing. Single mothers are eligible for income maintenance allowances.[64]

Pediatric preventive services. General practitioners provide most pediatric care and do not receive any special fees for conducting developmental assessments on children. UNICEF estimates that roughly 22% of all mothers breast-feed their infants for up to 6 months.[28] Newborns are routinely screened for hypothyroidism and phenylketonuria. Ninety-five percent of infants under 1 year of age receive well-child care, and about 70% of children ages 1 to 5 receive recommended well-child examinations.[137] Generally, prescriptions are free for children and adolescents.

A unique preventive service provided for children and families in Great Britain is the Health Visiting Service (HVS). The HVS, which is over a century old, provides preventive health care and health promotion services to residents in specified geographic regions. Historically, the principal focus of the HVS had been maternal and child health services in an attempt to reduce the country's infant mortality rate. This system of local preventive and primary care services for children and families is provided by registered nurses who also receive training in public health. Services provided through HVS include periodic home visits during an infant's first year of life, and less frequently thereafter until the child enters school. For the most part, home visitations do not entail direct medical care but focus instead on identifying potential problems and providing anticipatory guidance and other counseling to parents. However, HVS nurses do immunize children in families with limited access to conventional immunization services.

Limited studies evaluating the impact of the HVS program have identified several benefits, including broad dissemination of home safety information, increased immunization rates, participation in postpartum breast-feeding, and reductions in pediatric hospital admissions.[28]

Most pediatric health care is provided at community child health clinics staffed by community health physicians and nurses. These clinics are publicly funded and staffed by salaried physicians. Services provided through the child health clinics include information on preventive services, free dental care, and immunizations. In addition, the vast majority of DHAs also use multidisciplinary health care teams (Child Development Teams or District Handicap Teams) composed of a pediatrician, a psychologist, a family physician, and a public health nurse who screen and advise families regarding children with physical and educational disabilities.

Childhood immunizations are voluntary. Nonetheless, the DHAs are using WHO's European goal of 90% immunization of all 2 year olds. In 1985 the national Health Education Council launched a major television advertising campaign to increase childhood immunizations.[52,53,94] Due in part to this campaign, immunization rates in 1989 for 2 year olds had increased to 87% for DT and polio, 80% for measles, and 75% for pertussis.[53]

Despite these national figures, rates of childhood immunization vary significantly by region. For example between 1987 and 1988, roughly 7% of all DHAs reported achieving between only 35% and 65% immunization rates among children for measles and pertussis. Similar variations also were reported for DPT vaccination. More than 10% of the DHAs had immunization rates under 77%, and only 50% of the DHAs reported immunization rates of 90% or more for polio. In an effort to achieve the WHO childhood immunization goals, the Family Practitioner Committees have begun to offer financial incentives to providers. General practitioners are scheduled to receive sliding-scale-based bonuses for achieving specific immunization rates among their 2-year-old pediatric populations. If they immunize 90% of their eligible patients, they will receive an end-of-the-year bonus of about $3000 (£1700). If an immunization rate of over 70% of all eligible children is achieved, a bonus of approximately $1,000 (£579) will be given.[53]

During later years, school nurses provide extensive screening and examination of school-aged children. When problems are identified, children are referred to their physician for further evaluation and treatment. School nurses also provide health education and counseling services, immunize children, and conduct various screening services. School nurses play a particularly important role in identifying children with special educational needs and in assisting children with disabilities.[53]

Adult preventive services. During 1988 Great Britain launched a major cervical cancer screening program with the assistance of the Family Practice Committee. The program, similar to Sweden's, is based on a computerized notification system to alert women between the ages of 20 and 64 about the need to obtain a PAP smear. To increase provider participation, general practitioners are given bonuses for achieving specific levels of screening among female patients.

Recently, breast cancer screening was added to the country's cancer screening program. This program also involves a computerized notification system to encourage age-eligible women to undergo mammography.[94] Finally, incentives also are available to providers who conduct other health education and promotion programs for groups of individuals.[94]

Table 5-11. Expansion of coverage under the German sickness funds: 1883-1986

Year	No. insured (millions)	% Population insured	No. sickness funds
1885	4.7	10.0	18,942
1911	10.0	21.5	22,000
1914	16.0	23.0	13,500
1932	18.7	30.0	6600
1951	20.0	48.1	1992
1960	27.1	85.0	2028
1970	30.6	88.0	1827
1976	33.5	90.0	1425
1982	35.8	89.8	1286
1986	36.5	90.2	1184

From Henke K: *The Federal German Republic, advances in health economics and health services research,* Suppl 1, 1990, pp 145-168.

Table 5-12. Distribution of sickness funds and membership: Jan. 1, 1986

Type of fund	Number of funds	Membership (in thousands)
Local sickness funds	269	9394
Industrial funds	743	2371
Crafts funds	155	1398
Sailor's fund	1	28
Miner's fund	1	262
Blue collar workers' funds	8	372
White collar workers' funds	7	6283
All funds*	1175	20,180

From Henke K: *The Federal Republic of Germany, advances in health economics and health services research,* Suppl 1, 1990, pp 145-168.
*Without rural funds.

Regional Health Authorities have been encouraged to establish within their regions health promotion and disease prevention targets including cardiovascular and cholesterol screening goals, as well as smoking cessation campaigns. In addition, HVS nurses are scheduled to make an annual home visit to the very elderly and homebound.

GERMANY: FROM SICKNESS FUNDS TO SICKNESS CERTIFICATES

Germany, a country of about 61 million people, insures its people through a means-tested compulsory system of employer-based sickness funds, or *Krankenkassen*.[126] Established over a century ago, these funds have evolved over time with the express purpose of protecting workers and their employers from the economic consequences of illness (Table 5-11). Numbering approximately 1200 today, these public, nonprofit sickness funds have emerged through associations with a variety of trade and employment organizations, including professional associations, trade unions, blue collar and white collar workers' funds, and special maritime funds (Table 5-12). Consequently, German workers and employers have had an influential role in shaping their health care system. Germans appear to be generally satisfied with the results of this arrangement. Only a small minority (13%) of German citizens surveyed in 1990 appear to believe any significant reform of health care is necessary.[10]

Today the sickness funds, managed by boards of trustees, collect payroll contributions from employers and employees. These contributions are then submitted to physician associations to be distributed as payment for medical services. The sickness funds, however, do more than simply indemnify physicians and hospitals; they manage benefits, set premium contributions for both employers and employees (which range from a combined contribution of 8% to 16% of a worker's gross salary), and negotiate fee

schedules for physician services and hospital care.[42,65] As a result of the negotiated fee schedules, all physicians and hospitals receive essentially identical fees for identical services.

Participation in the sickness funds is compulsory depending on an individual's income. Workers earning more than $35,580 per year (1990) are exempted from compulsory participation in a sickness fund.[65] Instead, they can enroll either in a sickness fund or one of a handful of private insurance plans. Some wealthier Germans opt for private insurance. This decision is driven largely by the health insurance tax. Because the taxable salary is uncapped, the tax is very progressive.[42] The higher one's income, the more money paid into the sickness fund. Thus individuals with incomes above certain income levels benefit by purchasing private health insurance rather than contributing to a sickness fund.[65] Some higher-income individuals, however, choose to be insured by a public sickness fund because they provide family rather than individual coverage.

Approximately 90% of Germany's population is insured through the sickness funds, and 8% to 9% are privately insured.[42,65] Public-funded welfare plans insure the remaining 2% of the population. Of the 8.08% of GDP spent on health care in 1989, sickness funds accounted for 62% and private health insurance 8% of those expenditures.[63,110]

Whether health insurance derives from a sickness fund or a private insurer, all health insurance plans are required to cover a minimum level of health benefits.[59] Thus benefits are quite similar under both public and private insurance, although private plans include coverage for additional benefits such as private hospital rooms. Insurers employ a community-type rate, which results in more uniform premiums.[42]

System capacity and use of medical services

Under the German health care system, patients are free to choose their physician. Although physician fees are ne-

Table 5-13. A comparison of health system capacity and utilization of medical services between the United States and Germany: circa 1989

	1 United States	2 Germany	Ratio 1:2
Percent GDP on health care	12.4	8.1	1.53
Per capita on health care	$ 2566	$ 1287	1.99
Percent public funding	42	72	0.58
Hospitals*			
Beds†	3.8	7.3	0.52
Average length of stay (ALOS) (days)	7.2	12.7	0.56
Occ. rate	65.5	85.5	0.76
Admission rate†	12.8	18.7	0.68
Physicians			
Number†	2.3	3.0	0.76
Average no. visits	5.3	11.5	0.46
% Primary care§	34	55-60	0.68
MD expenditures‖	183,281	67,067	2.73

Source: OECD Health Data File.
*Data based on acute care hospitals only, i.e., hospitals in which the ALOS is less than 30 days (1988).
†Per 1000 population.
‡Percent of total populations.
§Percent of physicians identifying themselves as general practitioners, pediatricians, internists.
‖Physician expenditures per physician (i.e., total physician spending for outpatient and inpatient services per number of active practicing physicians.) Sums expressed in U.S. dollars 1988. HCFA calculations of OECD data.

gotiated and regulated, physicians are otherwise free to practice as they desire.[59,66]

Germany has 3.0 physicians and 7.3 acute-care hospital beds per 1000 population (1989), more than in most of the other countries in this analysis[60] (Table 5-13). In fact, the number of acute-care hospital beds is nearly double the number in the United States. With only a nominal co-payment for hospital care, restricted to the first 2 weeks of hospitalization, and no co-payment for ambulatory services, Germans have little disincentive to use their health care system, although physicians serve as gatekeepers to hospital-based services.[42,59]

For example, Germans make on average 11.5 physician contacts per year, well above physician contact rates for other European countries, and more than double the rate in the United States.*[109] Primary care specialties (e.g., gen-

*Physician contact data in this chapter should be interpreted with caution. Some countries may include hospital inpatient physician visits or telephone contacts with physicians. These may differ, therefore, from rates of physician "visits." See, for example, Health care systems in twenty-seven countries, Schieber GJ, Poullier JP, Greenwald LM: *Health Affairs* 10(3):22-38, 1991.

eral practitioners, pediatricians, and internists) account for 55% to 60% of all German physicians.[15] Specialists *(Gebietsärzte)* compose a smaller but growing number of physicians in Germany. However, the percentage of physicians identified as general practitioners has declined from a high of 62% to the current level of 43%.[57]

Public hospitals operated by state and local governments account for roughly half of all acute-care hospital beds. Churches and other nonprofit hospitals house nearly 41% of all acute-care beds, whereas private commercial hospitals house only about 4% of all acute-care beds.[57]

With respect to hospital use, both the average length of stay (12.7 days) and the average occupancy rate (85.5%) for acute-care hospitals are higher than in any other OECD country, again well above U.S. averages (7.2 days and 65.5%, respectively.)[109]

With such high use patterns involving a fee-for-service payment arrangement, physician incomes in Germany are relatively high compared to other European countries. The 1988 average net income (after expenses but before taxes) for German physicians was $98,624, ($81,759 average real income in 1986)[58] ranging from $80,979 for general practitioners to $111,378 for specialists.[66]

Medical economics and expenditures

Despite this pattern of high health care use, health care spending as a percentage of GDP has remained relatively stable in Germany since 1980. In that year health expenditures accounted for 7.9% of GDP. Since then the percentage has varied little, rising to a high of 8.46% in 1988, only to drop to 8.1% in 1990.[110] In 1989 the laws governing the sickness funds were amended as a result of enactment of the Health Care Reform Act of 1989. The impact of this reform may partially explain the decline in percentage of GDP spent on health care, as the percentage of GDP spent on sickness funds declined from 5.52% in 1988 to 5.00% in 1989.[110,113] Overall, health care expenditures in Germany for 1990 were $1287 per capita, about 99% less than in the United States.[60]

Germany's health profile

A profile of Germany's health status reveals a population with a life expectancy at birth of 72.6 years for men and 79.0 for women, both slightly higher than in the United States[60] (Table 5-14). Approximately 15.4% of the German population is over age 65 years, compared to 12.6% in the United States. Germany's infant mortality rate is substantially lower than the U.S. rate. In 1989 the infant mortality rate in Germany was 7.44 per 1000 live births, 31.7% below the U.S. rate.[87] The percent of low-birth-weight infants born in Germany in 1989 was 6.0% lower than in Canada, Great Britain, and the United States.[87] Overall, the fertility rate for adolescent women (9/1000 15- to 19-year-olds) is one of the lowest among the developed countries.[28]

Clinical preventive services: a population profile

Sickness and preventive service certificates. As in Japan, German physicians providing care in the hospital setting are salaried, whereas non-hospital-based physicians are reimbursed on a fee-for-service basis at government negotiated rates.[59] Most privately insured patients pay at the time of service, and in turn are reimbursed later by their insurance company. Patients enrolled in sickness funds are provided *Krankenscheine* or "sickness certificates" on a quarterly calendar basis to be presented at each physician encounter. The physician submits the certificate to the sickness fund for reimbursement. A similar certificate is issued for hospital care. To counter the economic problems with a fee-for-service system, a cap exists on the quarterly amount that can be paid to the physician for services rendered to any patient. A separate "preventive services certificate" to cover services such as mammography and PAP smears is also distributed to patients, and physicians are thus reimbursed separately for certain preventive services.[59]

The commonly accepted practice in Germany of seeking specialists without a referral from the general practitioner has probably decreased the number of opportunities for more widespread preventive screening and counseling by primary care physicians. Specialists, therefore, are likely to provide some degree of primary and preventive care.

Perinatal care and maternal disability. Most insurance plans provide comprehensive coverage for prenatal care. Pregnant women are provided a special "sickness certificate," which entitles them to unlimited prenatal visits, free pharmaceuticals, and home nursing services for women confined to bed rest.[59]

Although the recommended number of prenatal visits for uncomplicated pregnancy in Germany is 10, on average women probably make only 8.5 visits.[64] Most women who do not obtain timely prenatal care typically are considered high risk for health problems and are often sought out through a program using home visitations.[64] To encourage timely prenatal care, women are given a financial stipend to obtain early prenatal care, as well as a maternity bonus to help defray expenses during pregnancy.[90a]

Pregnant women who have been employed and insured 1 to 2 months before delivery are eligible for maternity disability benefits, which are equal to 100% of regular earnings. (This is more generous than the 80% of earnings allowed for regular sickness and disability.) Women continue to receive cash benefits for 8 weeks postpartum (12 weeks in the case of a pregnancy involving twins or a premature infant). Pregnant women are entitled to a total of 14 weeks of cash benefits before and after delivery of their baby.[42]

In addition to the maternity cash benefits, any parent living or employed in Germany is entitled to additional government-funded cash benefits of roughly $360 per month if he or she remains home to care for a child. Pre-

Table 5-14. A comparison of health status measures between the United States and Germany: circa 1989

	1 United States	2 Germany	Ratio 1:2
Life expectancy (years at birth)			
Men	71.8	72.6	0.98
Women	78.5	79.0	0.99
% Population >65 yr	12.6	15.4	0.81
Mortality rate*			
Crude	827	817	1.01
Circulatory disease	365	382	0.95
Cancer	195	211	0.92
IMR†	9.80	7.44	1.31
Low birth rate (%)	7	6	1.16
Maternal mortality‡	6.6	8.9	0.74

From OECD Health Data File.
*Rate per 100,000 population.
†Rate per 1000 live births.
‡Rate per 100,000 live births, 1987. (From Rowland D: Health status in eastern European countries, *Health Affairs* 10(3):202-215, 1991.)

viously, this benefit was limited to parents caring for children under the age of 15 months. Since 1991, however, these cash benefits were expanded to parents caring for their children up to the age of 3 years. During this time the parents have job-protected leave with cash benefits, in addition to the maternity benefits paid during the 14-week postpartum period. Beyond this time, parents are entitled to 5 days annual leave per child to be paid from the Sickness Fund to care for sick children under age 8.[42]

Pediatric preventive services. Germany has about 1000 pediatricians, approximately 6% of all physicians nationwide (1986-1987),[15] as compared with about 7% in the United States.[4]

Newborns routinely undergo screening for congenital problems such as hypothyroidism, phenylketonuria, and galactosemia. Child health care, which is usually provided by office-based physicians rather than public health clinics, typically includes a set number of free comprehensive screening exams during the child's preschool years, plus any additional preventive care as indicated up to the age of 6 years.[137] During these preventive examinations, free immunizations are administered. As a result, immunization rates for 1-year-olds were high (1987), averaging 94% for DPT, 94% for polio, and about 47% for measles.[59,121]

Adult preventive services. Beyond adolescence, public and private health insurance plans provide coverage for preventive medical examinations, which include PAP smears and mammography for women over the age of 20. Preventive screenings are available for men over the age of 45.[59] Other preventive services covered by health insurance for both men and women include stool testing for occult blood to screen for colon cancer, administration of influenza vaccine, routine eye examinations, and complete dental examinations from the age of 12 to 20, with coverage that includes partial payment for dentures and other restorative work.[59]

CANADA: UNIVERSAL HEALTH CARE IN THE SHADOW OF LALONDE
The seeds of prevention

This large country, bordered by two oceans, is inhabited by only 26 million people. Most declare themselves to be of French and British heritage; about 2% are native Indians. Although it is the second largest country in the world, it is one of the least populated countries, with fewer than three people per square kilometer.[36,124] Only 11.5% of the population is over the age of 65.[60]

Canada is governed under a parliamentary democracy, and its 10 provinces provide complete coverage for comprehensive hospital and medical care through provincial public health plans. This plan is consistent with the Canadian government's historical role in providing a broad range of other social services such as education, unemployment insurance, and welfare.

Canada can be viewed as one of the leaders in the contemporary field of clinical preventive services. Beginning with the publication of the LaLonde Report in 1974, a new focus was given to clinical health care. Then Secretary of Health and Welfare, Marc LaLonde, published *A New Perspective on the Health of Canadians,* in which he highlighted the relative importance of life-style, environmental exposures, human biology, and medical care as the primary determinants of human health.[76] Among these, he argued, the first three were the most important. In part, because of the LaLonde Report, the Health Promotion Directorate, a national organization that funds a variety of locally based health promotion projects aimed at risk factor reduction among Canadian populations, was subsequently established in 1978. Other major prevention activities initiated in part at least by the LaLonde Report included holding the First International Conference on Health Promotion in 1986 in Ottawa, establishing the Canadian Healthy Communities Project, convening the Canadian Task Force on the Periodic Health Examination, and developing a major health promotion survey of Canadians. In addition, several landmark prevention documents have been published in Canada such as *Achieving Health For All: A Framework For Health Promotion,* and the *Canadian Task Force Report on the Periodic Health Examination,*[17-24,119] both of which stimulated federal activity in prevention policy in the United States.

Many cities and provinces have proactive agencies charged with designing and implementing health promotion programs. Toronto houses the Metropolitan Toronto District Health Council while the provincial government of Ontario has established the Premier's Council on Health

Strategy, which provides advice and guidance on health policy. The Toronto District Health Council's activities are important because Toronto consumes about one third of the provincial health budget.

Whatever their preferences regarding prevention, Canadians, by and large, are pleased with their health care system. In a recent 10-nation survey to assess the level of satisfaction with their respective health care systems, Canadians were the most satisfied. (The United States was the least satisfied with its health care system.)[10]

System capacity and use of medical services

Despite significant cost containment of physician fees, Canada still has about the same ratio of physicians to population as the United States, which has little fee regulation. Canada has 2.2 physicians per 1000 population and has chosen to maintain an adequate supply of general practitioners over specialists (Table 5-15). For example, Ontario has a policy that establishes a general practitioner/specialists ratio of 55:45. And although physicians are not assigned to patients as in Great Britain, virtually all Canadians can identify a personal physician.[119]

U.S. physicians earn on average about 60% more than Canadian physicians, $132,200 compared to $82,740 in

Table 5-15. A comparison of health system capacity and use of medical services between the United States and Canada: circa 1989

	1 United States	2 Canada	Ratio 1:2
Percent GDP on health care	12.4	9.0	1.37
Per capita on health care	$ 2566	$ 1795	1.42
Percent public funding	42	75	0.56
Hospitals*			
Beds†	3.8	4.5	0.84
Average length of stay (ALOS) (days)	7.2	8.9	0.80
Occ. rate	65.5	80.3	0.81
Admission rate‡	12.8	13.3	0.96
Physicians			
Number†	2.3	2.2	1.04
Average no. visits	5.3	6.6	0.80
% Primary care§	34	53	0.64
MD expenditures‖	183,281	112,035	1.64

From OECD Health Data File.

*Data based on acute care hospitals only, i.e. hospitals in which the ALOS is less than 30 days. (1988)

†Per 1000 population.

‡Percent of total populations.

§Percent of physicians identifying themselves as general practitioners, pediatricians, internists.

‖Physician expenditures per physician (i.e., total physician spending for outpatient and inpatient services per number of active practicing physicians.) Sums expressed in U.S. dollars 1988. (From HCFA calculations of OECD data.)

Canada in 1987. Much of this variation can be explained by unregulated physician fees and a more specialty-rich medical profession in the United States.[16] In addition, administrative and professional liability costs are much greater in the United States. Annual medical malpractice premiums in the United States average $15,000 compared to $1470 in Canada: a 10-fold difference.[16,33] Whatever the relative attractiveness of practicing in the United States versus Canada, the U.S. Government Accounting Office reports that the number of physicians emigrating from Canada to the United States actually decreased each year from 663 physicians in 1978 to 386 physicians in 1985. In addition, the number of applications for medical school in Canada were 2.5 times greater in 1988-1989 than in the United States.[16]

Canadians average about 6.6 physician visits a year (1987). They may choose their family physician, but in most provinces are required to obtain a referral to visit a specialist.[16] Canada has 4.5 hospital beds per 1000 population. The admission rate for Canadians is 13.3%*, and the acute-care hospital occupancy rate is 80.3%. The average length of hospital stay in Canada is 8.9 days, approximately 24% longer than in the United States. There are 0.8 pharmacists per 1000 population in Canada, about 20% more than in the United States, and 0.5 dentists per 1000 population. Nonetheless, Canadians spend roughly the same per capita ($187) on pharmaceuticals as do Americans ($182).[109]

In Canada, capital expenditures are regulated. Consequently, medical technology is considerably less available than in the United States, which has substantially more cardiac catheterization units, open-heart surgery units, radiation therapy units, and magnetic resonance imaging (MRI) units than Canada.[16] For example, in 1989 Canada had 1.2 open-heart surgery units per million persons compared to 3.3 in the United States. In that same year, Canada had 0.5 MRI per million persons compared to 3.7 MRI units per million population in the United States.[104]

Although there are no restrictions on access to physician care, there may be waiting periods for access to certain technology and diagnostic procedures, which vary among the provinces. For example, a study of Newfoundland in 1989 identified waiting periods of 2 months for CT scanning and a 6- to 10-month wait for surgical hip replacement. Even mammography screening may entail a 2- to 3-month wait.[104]

Medical economics and expenditures

Canada spends more money on health care than all other countries except the United States: in 1990, 9.0% of its GDP, about $1795 per capita, which is about 43% less than the United States.[60] Public spending accounts for approximately 75% of these expenditures.[109]

Of the total 1987 Canadian health care budget, 16% was consumed by physician services compared to 19% in the United States. Only 1.2% of all health care spending was attributed to overhead in Canada, compared to nearly 5% of the U.S. health care budget.[16]

Canada has established expenditure targets for health care. Provincial budgets are negotiated between the federal government and the provinces. If these targets are exceeded, fees are lowered during the next fiscal cycle. Physician fees are established between the province and local physician associations, guided by the federal-provincial set global budgets.[104] Physician fees in the United States are comparable in the nonsurgical or diagnostic areas; but fees for surgical services, anesthesiology, and radiology were from 3.3 to 3.7 times greater in the United States than in Canada.[48] Such a reimbursement schedule may encourage surgery and diagnostic evaluation over primary and preventive care.

Provinces also negotiate global budgets with hospitals. To further pressure the provinces, federal contributions to health care budgets are capped; thus increases in health care expenditures are borne disproportionately by the provinces.[104] Although financing may be well controlled, there are concerns about the coordination and planning aspects of the Canadian health care system, which vary from province to province and even within provinces.[119]

Canada's health profile

Life expectancy for Canadians is longer than for U.S. citizens. In 1986 the life expectancy at birth was 73.0 years for Canadian men and 79.7 years for Canadian women[60] (Table 5-16). The crude mortality rate in Canada

Table 5-16. A comparison of health status measures between the United States and Canada: circa 1989

	1 United States	2 Canada	Ratio 1:2
Life expectancy (years at birth)			
Men	71.8	73.0	0.98
Women	78.5	79.7	0.98
% Population >65 yr	12.6	11.5	1.09
Mortality rate*			
Crude	827	—	—
Circulatory disease	365	—	—
Cancer	195	—	—
IMR†	9.8	7.2	1.36
Low birth rate (%)	7	6	1.16
Maternal mortality‡	6.6	—	—

From OECD Health Data File.
*Rate per 100,000 population.
†Rate per 1000 live births.
‡Rate per 100,000 live births, 1987. (From Rowland D: Health status in eastern European countries, *Health Affairs* 10(3):202-215, 1991.)

Percent of total population.

(7.3/1000 population) is lower than in the United States (8.7/1000 population).

The infant mortality rate of 7.2 per 1000 live births in 1989 also is substantially better than the U.S. rate.[87] Only 6% of all Canadian births in 1989 were low birth weight compared to 7% in the United States.[87] The country's adolescent pregnancy rate of 24.4/1000 is less than half that of the U.S. rate.

Adolescent suicide rates in 1985 in Canada (23.7/100,000) were 25% higher than in the United States. On the other hand, adolescent deaths caused by motor vehicle accidents were 22% lower than in the United States.[28]

In Toronto, much the center of prevention activity, age-adjusted mortality rates have declined by nearly one third between 1977 and 1987. Mortality rates declined about 45% for cardiovascular disease, 50% for injuries, and nearly 40% for cirrhosis. Although the lung cancer mortality rate for men declined by approximately one fourth, it increased by more than two thirds for women.[116,119]

Other indices, however, suggest problem areas with respect to health status.[120] With a total of 4427 cases of AIDS, Canada ranks fourth among the Americas for this disease. Inequities exist for certain ethnic and economic groups within Canada. Native Indian populations have significantly higher infant mortality rates than whites. Low income men, in the lowest quintile for income, have a life expectancy that is 14.3 years shorter than for men in the highest quintile.[119] Thus despite what is billed to be universal health care, vulnerable populations appear to have limited access to timely health care, much like the situation in the United States.

Clinical preventive services: a population profile

In accordance with Federal standards codified in the Canada Health Act of 1984, local provincial officials have some flexibility in designing health insurance benefits packages for provincial residents. Provincial health benefits plans are required to cover all medically necessary services and procedures; but they are not required to reimburse providers for eyeglasses, certain prescription drugs, and general dental care.[16]

As a result, the delivery of certain preventive services varies throughout Canada if only because insurance coverage for adult preventive services may vary from province to province. For example, certain types of counseling, such as family planning and regular eye examinations, have been removed from the payment schedule in Alberta or reduced to one per year.[16] In Nova Scotia, annual physical examinations are no longer reimbursable. On the other hand, the residents of Ontario receive benefits beyond the minimum federal guarantee, including broader mental health services, pharmaceutical coverage for the elderly, reimbursement for certain types of physiotherapeutic services, and coverage for certain services provided by a wide range of nonphysician providers such as chiroprac-

tors, osteopaths, and chiropodists.[16] Finally, many provinces consider certain preventive services such as sphygmomanometry and clinical breast examinations routine parts of the periodic health examination. It is argued, therefore, that these services should not be unbundled and billed independently.

Regardless of the benefits covered, there are no cost-sharing requirements for covered services. Those preventive benefits covered, like all other covered medical services, involve neither a deductible nor a co-payment, which eliminates any indirect financial barriers to care.[59]

Nonetheless, despite the generally broad coverage of most preventive services, utilization of preventive services, while not universal, is probably higher than in the United States given the absence of any significant financial barriers to care.[119]

Perinatal preventive services and maternal disability. The infant mortality rate in Canada is 7.2 per 1000 live births, about 28% less than the U.S. rate. Canada has one of the most generous maternal disability benefits programs, allowing women a total of 25 weeks disability for pregnancy, including 8 weeks before delivery and 17 weeks postpartum. The level of payment is the same as for other short-term disabilities.[43]

Pediatric preventive services. Despite its overall interest in health promotion and disease prevention, Canada lacks a formal prevention policy for children. Unlike the objectives set forth in *Healthy People 2000*[38] in the United States, which includes specific maternal and child health objectives, Canada has yet to develop a similar public policy. Nor does Canada have a system of targeted programs addressing maternal and child health issues. Given the universality of Canada's health care system and a widespread system of public health departments and in some provinces, community health centers, however, pediatric services are readily accessible.[95] Because there are more primary care physicians than specialists, primary and preventive health care receive considerable attention.

Although family physicians provide much preventive care, community health centers and school clinics also serve as primary preventive centers for certain services such as immunizations. Immunization rates for 1-year-olds are approximately 85% for all routine childhood vaccines.[121] As with certain other countries, however, Canada has experienced increases in the incidence of both measles and pertussis: for example, 2816 cases of measles in 1985 compared with 15,136 cases in 1986. Even accounting for underreporting in 1985, it would appear that immunization patterns vary from published reports. On the other hand, improper vaccine storage may have resulted in vaccine failures among those children who were inoculated.[1,50,131]

Adult preventive services. The vast majority of Canadians report that they have a personal family physician who delivers virtually all preventive care.[5] Although data are limited, the delivery of many adult preventive services appears to vary among provinces. One survey of general practitioners by Battista[7] suggests that at least in New Brunswick and Quebec, cancer screening may be conducted routinely. Ninety-five percent of the physicians in that survey reported that they performed clinical breast examinations, obtained PAP smears, and conducted smoking cessation counseling for patients. On the other hand, these same physicians reported much lower rates of mammography (3% in New Brunswick, 20% in Quebec) and occult blood screening (8% in New Brunswick, 15% in Quebec), the latter not a recommended screening procedure.[5] Another study found that physicians in Quebec who performed breast examinations had a high likelihood (95%) of also performing a PAP smear.[7]

UNITED STATES: TECHNOLOGIC OPULENCE AND FRAGMENTED HEALTH CARE

In the United States, health insurance, or the lack thereof, is essentially a consequence of an individual's place of employment, family status, income, age, health status, or serendipity. Of all the countries described in this analysis, the U.S. health care financing system is by far the most complicated. And despite the enormous expenditures for health care in the United States, it is the only industrialized country in the world, besides South Africa, to have a significant population of uninsured citizens.

In 1990 about 35.7 million people in the United States, 1.4 times the entire population of Canada, were uninsured.[41] These individuals comprise nearly 17% of the U.S. population under age 65, and their numbers reflect a

steady rise in the percent of uninsured Americans. As recently as 1988, 15.9% of the population was uninsured; by 1990, the number had increased to 16.6%.[41]

The percentage of uninsured individuals varies considerably from state to state. According to the Employee Benefits Research Institute (EBRI), in Connecticut, North Dakota, and Wisconsin, approximately 8.5% of the population was uninsured as of March 1991. On the other hand, New Mexico (26.4%), Texas (24.1%) Mississippi (22.9%), and Florida (22.9%) all had substantially higher percentages of uninsured people[41] (Table 5-17).

Principles of U.S. health insurance

In the United States, health insurance has evolved historically to protect individuals against the economic consequences of large and unforeseen medical expenses. Insurance seeks to provide economic protection against those medical events that are both expensive and unpredictable. To achieve this goal, insurers use the principle of risk spreading. Maximum risk spreading occurs when individuals in a large group, such as a community, each pay insurance premiums based on the possible high claims of a few in that group. As a result, the high costs generated by a few are shared by all to provide insurance protection for everyone and to prevent any one member from paying inordinately large sums of money because of severe illness.

On the other hand, there is less sharing of risk when an insurer charges premiums to an individual based on the best estimates of medical expenses the *individual* will incur. In this instance there is less risk sharing, as individu-

Table 5-17. Percentage of uninsured within states, March 1991

New England	10.9	**East North Central**	11.8	**Mountain**	18.0
Maine	13.2	Ohio	12.1	Montana	16.4
New Hampshire	11.5	Indiana	12.7	Idaho	18.0
Vermont	11.1	Illinois	13.2	Wyoming	14.4
Massachusetts	11.1	Michigan	11.0	Colorado	17.3
Rhode Island	13.9	Wisconsin	8.6	N. Mexico	26.4
Connecticut	8.5	**West North Central**	11.9	Arizona	19.8
Mid Atlantic	13.2	Minnesota	10.2	Utah	10.2
New York	14.4	Iowa	9.8	Nevada	19.2
New Jersey	11.9	Missouri	14.6	**Pacific**	20.1
Pennsylvania	12.4	N. Dakota	—	Washington	13.4
South Atlantic	19.1	S. Dakota	14.3	Oregon	15.8
Delaware	16.4	Nebraska	10.3	California	22.1
Maryland	16.0	Kansas	12.6	Alaska	17.9
District of Columbia	23.9	**East South Central**	18.3	Hawaii	9.2
Virginia	18.9	Kentucky	15.6	**West South Central**	23.4
W. Virginia	16.6	Tennessee	16.0	Arkansas	21.1
N. Carolina	16.2	Alabama	20.5	Louisiana	22.5
S. Carolina	18.9	Mississippi	22.9	Oklahoma	22.3
Georgia	17.7			Texas	24.1
Florida	22.9				

From Employee Benefits Research Institute: *Sources of health insurance and characteristics of the uninsured, analysis of the March 1991 current population survey,* EBRI Issue Brief, No. 122, February 1992.

als pay larger premiums as their health status deteriorates. The first example uses the principle of *community rating,* whereas the latter uses the strategy of *underwriting* in establishing premiums. Risk spreading based on the workplace as the community or denominator for insuring Americans is common because most Americans receive their health insurance through the workplace.[41] Over time, however, community rating has become less common, and increasingly sophisticated underwriting techniques have enabled certain insurers to engage in selective underwriting activities whereby "low-risk" individuals are "creamed" from larger groups, and charged lower premiums, and "high-risk" individuals are left to face the possibility of going uninsured or being charged inordinately high premium rates. Whether an insurer uses a community rate or underwrites policies individually, insurance actuaries determine the premium rates charged based on the degree of risk spreading the insurer is seeking to achieve.

Currently, the marketing of health insurance, particularly to small groups, has come under considerable scrutiny by state legislatures, and reform measures have been enacted to redirect the insurance market back toward a philosophy of community rating and to limit underwriting practices that limit or exclude individuals from coverage because of preexisting illnesses.[86]

Employer-sponsored health insurance

Since the 1940s, most Americans have received their health insurance as an employment benefit, even though no one in the continental United States, including both employers and employees, is required to purchase health insurance.

Because employment-based health insurance in the United States is not portable, employees changing jobs automatically lose coverage (although they are eligible for extended workplace coverage for 18 to 36 months through the Consolidated Omnibus Budget Reconciliation Act [COBRA] of 1985) and must seek coverage anew either independently or through their new employer.

In recent years, however, the percent of individuals receiving their health insurance through their employer has declined. In 1988 about 66.2% of all Americans had private employer-sponsored health insurance; by 1990 this number declined to 64.2%[41]

During the 1980s rapidly rising health insurance premium rates and overall increases in health care costs forced many employers to pare down benefits, to eliminate coverage for dependents, or drop entirely employer-sponsored plans. Several additional factors have contributed to this steady growth in the uninsured population. First, rising health care costs have been coupled with a general economic downturn, forcing more workers and their dependents into uninsured status. Second, the U.S. economic base has shifted from its historic manufacturing emphasis, with a strong union influence that pushed for broader

worker health benefits, to a service economy, which has led to more limited health insurance coverage.

The increase in the percent of uninsured then is due largely to declines in employment-based insurance coverage, as a result of shifts in unemployment, termination of coverage by the employer, or eventual loss of coverage as a result of job switching. Thus in stark contrast to other industrialized nations, changes in employment status, particularly loss of employment, may jeopardize an individual's ability to remain or become insured in the United States.

Even among the employed, however, the probability of being insured and the extent of health benefits an employee might receive varies according to the size of the firm in which they work. As was evident earlier, firm size plays little if any role in determining whether individuals in other industrialized countries are insured. In the United States, however, employees in larger firms are much more likely to be insured than employees in smaller firms. For example, in 1990 roughly 86% of employees in firms with at least 100 employees were reported to be insured compared to 64% of employees in firms with fewer than 25 employees.[41] Roughly half of the uninsured in 1990 were either self-employed or employed in firms of less than 25 employees, or were dependents of such employees.[41] Although most people are insured as a result of their employment status, most of the uninsured are employed as well; they are likely to work in small firms (less than 25 employees) or work in part-time or seasonal jobs that do not offer employer-sponsored health plans.[41]

Employees in small firms are likely to be uninsured for several reasons, some independent of any lack of an employer-sponsored plan. One reason relates to health insurance premiums and their renewal for both individuals and groups. Although premiums are established at the time of initial purchase from the insurer, the rate may undergo substantial upward adjustment at renewal time (usually annually) if the group has submitted several claims or one large claim during the coverage period. In some cases groups may experience premium increases so large that over the course of several renewal periods they are unable to afford the policy and they become uninsured and very likely uninsurable under any other plan. This problem occurs most frequently in smaller firms.

Second, unlike in many other countries, insurance companies in the United States for the most part no longer use community rating to establish insurance premiums. Instead, insurers frequently engage in underwriting practices whereby individuals and smaller groups are charged premiums based on the individual's previous medical claims history, on the identification of existing medical problems, or, through the use of health risk appraisal techniques, identify potential medical problems that might result in large medical claims. Such premium rates often are established independent of the health status or experience of other individuals in the community. On the other hand, premiums for larger groups are established based in part on the number of individuals through whom the risk is to be shared. Because one large claim in a small group can quickly offset profit and contingency margins of the insurer, this practice of underwriting is most commonly applied to employees in small firms to identify potential sources of large claims and where the risk-spreading base is very limited. Once identified, these "high-risk" individuals could be either charged higher premiums, excluded from coverage for that particular medical condition, or refused coverage altogether.[86]

Finally, insurers also pass through to employees in small firms the costs associated with the underwriting process itself, the concomitant marketing to compete for insurance sales in this highly volatile small group market, as well as the other administrative expenses that accrue to the sale of health insurance to small businesses. Together, these other factors may drive the costs of a policy up as much as 40% for employees in small firms and substantially enhance the probability that health insurance will be unaffordable.[58]

Another unique practice for insuring U.S. workers involves businesses that self-insure. As a result of the Federal Employee Retirement Income Security Act of 1974 (ERISA), businesses that self-insure, (i.e., assume the risk of insuring their employees and/or their dependents) avoid compliance with a variety of state insurance regulations. ERISA permits a self-insuring employer to provide health insurance as an employee benefit without benefit guarantees provided by an insurance company. As a result, self-insured businesses avoid state insurance requirements such as mandated health benefits, premium rate restrictions, and limitations on underwriting employees and their dependents for selected medical conditions, and are able to generate additional cost savings by avoiding the administrative expenses, risk charges, and taxes associated with the purchase of health insurance from private insurers. Because the risk-spreading base for self-insurance is actuarially insufficient for smaller firms, usually only larger firms (i.e., bigger than 1000 employees) find it financially feasible to self-insure. More moderate-sized firms (between 100 and 500 employees) are typically unable to predict claims securely or to spread risk adequately; and if they do elect to self-insure, they generally purchase excess insurance to cover larger, unanticipated claims.

Public-sponsored health plans

Public-sponsored health insurance programs in the United States provide limited, categorical coverage to certain poor, disabled, and elderly individuals.

For example, the joint federal-state program, Medicaid, enacted in 1965 as Title XIX of the Social Security Act, is the principal source of health insurance for the poor. The program finances health care for certain low-income populations: the aged, blind, disabled, and families with dependent children. Incomes and resources (assets) must meet qualifying standards, which are determined by each state within broad federal guidelines. But because of the categorical qualifying standards, not all poor individuals receive support through Medicaid. Medicaid provides health insurance coverage for only 47% of the poor, and even less coverage for the near-poor.[41,58]

Medicaid fails to cover all the poor because being poor alone is not a sufficient criterion. For example, categorical eligibility requirements essentially exclude single men, unless permanently disabled, as well as poor couples without children from coverage. These criteria may work together to limit one's eligibility. Furthermore, there is considerable variability among the states regarding the income eligibility requirements, as well as the range of optional benefits covered from state to state. For example, it is not unusual for states to set the income eligibility threshold of less than 60% of the federal poverty level. Thus Medicaid is not one uniform program. Because of the discretion given to the states in the administration, design of optional benefits, and criteria for qualifying individuals for coverage there effectively are 50 different programs throughout the United States.

Medicaid also fails as the safety net for certain vulnerable populations such as children and pregnant women. Approximately 15% of all U.S. children were uninsured in 1990. These 9.8 million children under the age of 19 years were more likely to be in families where the head of household worked in a small firm (less than 25 employees) or was self-employed.[41]

On the other hand, Medicare, also enacted in 1965, is a more inclusive federal public health insurance program with presumptive eligibility for the elderly over age 65 and, through legislative amendment, permanently disabled and renal dialysis patients under age 65. Nevertheless, Medicare provides hospital and medical coverage only if those eligible have been employed for at least 40 quarters. To qualify for the Medicare disability provision, that disability must have existed for 24 consecutive months. In addition, beneficiaries are required to pay certain enrollment fees, co-payments, and deductibles, which may be additional barriers to health care for Medicare beneficiaries. Finally, Medicare does not cover prescription drugs, dental services, hearing aides, or long-term care.

Because the elderly tend to experience high rates of poverty and disability, Medicaid often supplements Medicare in providing health care coverage for this population. In fact, Medicaid is the principal source of assistance for purchasing long-term care for the elderly.

Finally, under both public programs, but especially under Medicaid, physician fees are regulated so that participating physicians typically are paid less than the rate private commercial and nonprofit insurers pay to physicians caring for similar non-Medicare or non-Medicaid patients.

Table 5-18. Medicaid reimbursement rates for screening mammography by states and District of Columbia as of December 1990

State	Reimbursement Rate[*]
Alabama	0
Alaska	0
Arizona	$ 69.39
Arkansas	$ 46.44
California	$ 50.42
Colorado	$ 28.28
Connecticut	—
Deleware	$ 35.00
District of Columbia	$ 53.36
Florida	$ 90.00[†]
Georgia	$ 44.00
Hawaii	—
Idaho	$ 40.61
Illinois	$ 70.65
Indiana	$ 88.90
Iowa	$ 85.40[†]
Kansas	$115.00
Kentucky	$ 22.00 inpatient/$28.60 outpatient
Louisiana	0
Maine	$ 30.00
Maryland	$ 30.00
Massachusetts	$ 49.00
Michigan	0
Minnesota	$ 82.50
Mississippi	$ 56.00
Missouri	$ 33.00
Montana	$ 96.70
Nebraska	$ 75.00
Nevada	0
New Hampshire	$ 50.00
New Jersey	—
New Mexico	$ 7.48
New York	$ 30.00
North Carolina	0
North Dakota	$ 75.00
Ohio	$ 20.00
Oklahoma	0
Oregon	$ 41.92
Pennsylvania	$ 6.00
Rhode Island	$ 35.00
South Carolina	$ 64.00
South Dakota	—[‡]
Tennessee	$ 48.37
Texas	@$150.00[§]
Utah	$ 30.77
Vermont	$ 51.00
Virginia	0
Washington	—[‡]
West Virginia	$ 31.50
Wisconsin	$ 63.99
Wyoming	$ 66.84

0, state does not reimburse for this procedure; —, no rate reported.
*CPT Code 76092, screening mammography, bilateral (two film study of each breast).
†Rate reported is for CPT Code 76091, diagnostic mammography, bilateral.
‡State reimburses a percentage of physician's usual and customary fee.
§State reimburses physicians on a profile system.

Even reimbursement rates for established secondary preventive services such as mammography and PAP smears vary considerably from state to state. For example, a survey by the American College of Obstetricians and Gynecologists in 1990 revealed that Medicaid reimbursement rates for mammography ranged from a low of $6.00 in Pennsylvania to a high of $150.00 in Texas[85] (Table 5-18). Lower reimbursement tends to discourage physician participation in the delivery of medical services.[114] This tendency is particularly relevant for new physicians, who are generally willing to accept new patients but whose startup costs make it prohibitive for them to serve a large number of patients whose insurer reimburses at a rate considerably lower than privately insured patients. Thus public health insurance in the United States, unlike in the other countries described in this analysis, plays a more limited role in meeting its citizens' health care needs.

What it means to be uninsured in the United States

Unlike other industrialized countries, the United States has a significant number of uninsured individuals, many of whom are also poor. For example, of all the uninsured in March 1991 EDRIA survey, 28.0% were in families below the federal poverty level (FPL), and another 32.1% were below 200% of the FPL. Thus 60.1% of the uninsured resided in families at or below 200% of the FPL.[41] Poverty is an additional barrier to their being able to obtain either curative or preventive services, which compromises their health status.

Uninsured persons in the United States are more likely than insured persons to report their health status as fair or poor. Among Americans surveyed in the 1977 National Medical Care Expenditure Survey (NMCES), a higher percentage of the uninsured (15%) reported their health status as "fair/poor" compared to insured respondents (11%).[35] This finding was supported by a 1986 national survey by the Robert Wood Johnson (RWJ) Foundation, which found that 12% of uninsured respondents (compared to only 9% of insured respondents) reported their health status as "fair/poor."[47] Poverty, as well as lack of health insurance, has been associated with poor health status.[39,117,133] In the absence of a national health insurance system, these findings are significant because the poor are less able to afford health insurance.

The uninsured are at greater risk than the insured for a variety of preventable diseases.[118] Regardless of ethnicity, income, or health status, the uninsured receive fewer preventive services than the insured.[6,107] An analysis of the 1982 National Health Interview Survey revealed that lack of health insurance was the strongest predictor of whether individuals received preventive screening such as blood pressure, glaucoma, PAP smear, and clinical breast examinations[137] (Table 5-19).

The uninsured, even those reporting their health status as "fair/poor," tend to use ambulatory and inpatient ser-

Table 5-19. Proportion of women inadequately screened for preventive services by selected characteristics: 1982 health interview survey

Characteristic	Blood pressure	PAP smear	Clinical breast examination	Glaucoma
Overall	12	27	38	30
Insured*	11	25	36	28
Uninsured	18	39	50	43
Education <12 yr	13	33	45	38
Education >12 yr	12	23	34	27
Poverty	10	34	45	42
Nonpoverty	13	26	38	30
Black race	7	21	32	32
White race	13	27	38	29

From Woolhandler S, Himmelstein D: Reverse targeting of preventive care due to lack of health insurance, *JAMA* 259:2872-2874, 1988. Copyright 1988, American Medical Association.
*Health insurance was the strongest predictor of the use of these preventive services.

vices at rates considerably lower than the insured. According to the NMCES, the uninsured had lower rates of physician visits (5.2 visits) compared to insured respondents (9.5 visits).[134] The RWJ survey in 1986 also found that the uninsured had fewer physician visits (3.2) compared to the insured (4.4), even among those reporting poorer health status. As individuals become insured, however, their use of services typically increases. Wilensky et al.[134] have shown that previously uninsured persons consume more medical services during periods when they are insured than during periods when they are uninsured.

The uninsured are also less likely to have a regular source of medical care.[9] One study demonstrated that the uninsured are twice as likely as the insured to be without a regular source of health care.[35] This fact is important because continuity of health care has been associated with more efficient use of medical services, fewer emergency room admissions, shorter lengths of hospital stay, and better health outcomes.[29,132] A regular source of care is likely to be more appropriate, less costly, and more thorough because the patient's history and problems are more familiar to the provider and will be factored more effectively into the patient's evaluation and treatment.[40] According to data from the National Access Survey many uninsured were twice as likely to use emergency rooms or outpatient clinics for medical care than insured patients.[2] Similarly, according to the 1986 National Health Interview Survey, the uninsured are more likely than insured patients to visit a physician in an emergency room (6.9% vs. 4.1%).[26]

When individuals lose their health insurance, especially when they are poor, they run the risk of substantial adverse health outcomes. Lurie et al.[79] have shown that when poor people lose public health insurance (Medicaid) they undergo an important decrease in medical encounters,

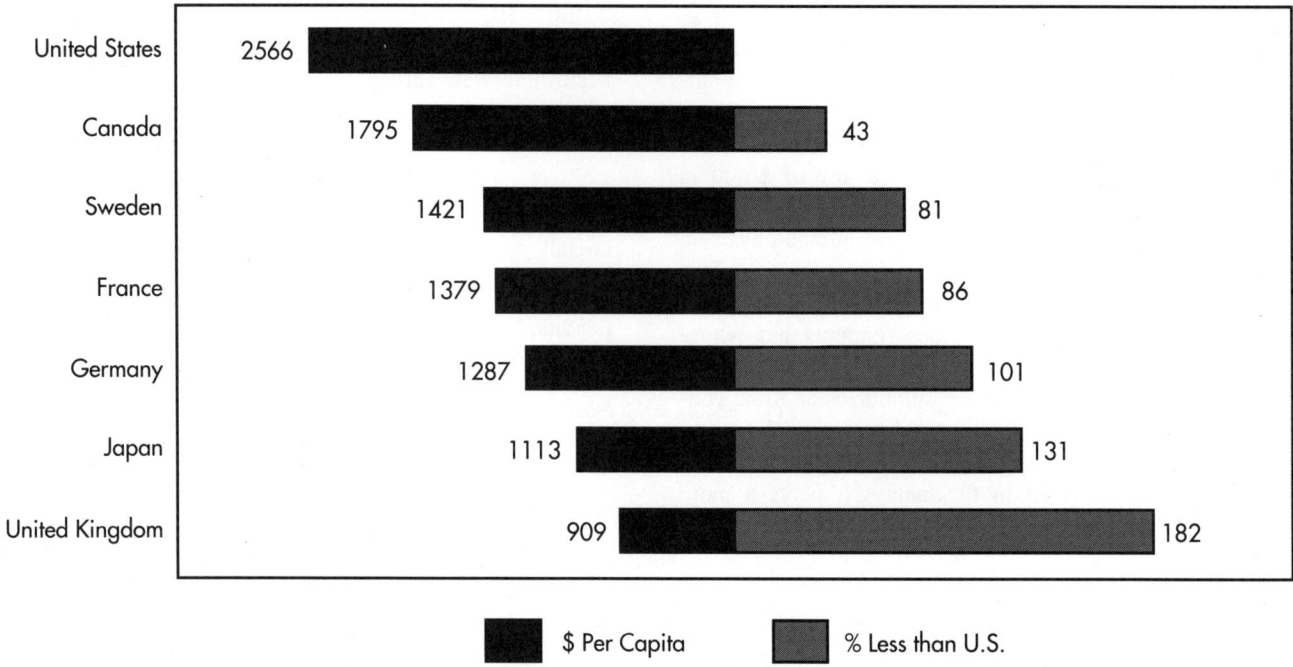

Fig. 5-1. Health care spending among six nations compared with the United States. (From Health Data File, Organization of Economic Cooperative Development, 1991.)

including physician visits, and an increase in rates of morbidity and mortality.[79] Individuals terminated from California Medicaid (Medi-Cal) experienced an increase in uncontrolled hypertension among previously hypertensive patients and a deterioration in blood glucose control among diabetic patients. In addition, four patients in this group died from non-injury-related causes, compared to no deaths among patients in the insured group. Another patient died after failing to seek medical care, believing that he would not be cared for if he could not pay for needed heart medicine. Finally, 6 months after termination from Medi-Cal, self-perception of health status among those dropped from coverage deteriorated significantly compared to the insured group.

Lack of insurance is particularly important for pregnant women and children. Data suggest that birth outcomes are worse for uninsured compared to privately or publicly insured women.[14] A U.S. Government Accounting Office study of prenatal care among women between 1986 and 1987 found that 84% of uninsured women, compared to only 36% of women on Medicaid, reported that money was a major financial barrier to prenatal care.[99] Other studies indicated that as many as one sixth of all women giving birth in the United States had no insurance, while another 9% were underinsured because they had no maternity insurance, and as many as 17% of women of child-bearing age may be uninsured.[12,44] Lack of health insurance is financially risky for pregnant women and their families, as hospital maternity costs average over $4300.

Uninsured children face similar problems. National data indicate that uninsured children use less medical care than insured children. Analysis of the 1980 NMCES reveals that uninsured children average 40% fewer physician visits than children with either private insurance or Medicaid. The percentage of children with only one physician visit was highest among uninsured children (36.3%), followed by privately insured children (31.0%) and children receiving Medicaid coverage (29.0%).[49] Lack of insurance means less continuity of care for children. On the other hand, a regular source of care results in greater medication compliance by children, fewer missed appointments, and more opportunity to provide broader preventive care such as mental health.[8,25]

Thus even though the uninsured appear to be in worse health, they use fewer timely medical and preventive services than do insured individuals. The consequences include greater economic and human suffering because of delayed diagnosis and treatment.

Medical economics and expenditures

The United States spends, by virtually any measure, more on health care than any other nation. In 1990, the most recent year for comparative international spending data, the United States spent $2566 per person on health care, 43% more per capita than the next highest spending country, Canada[60] (Fig. 5-1). Similarly in 1990, the United States spent 12.4% of its GDP on health care,[60] compared with 9.0% of GDP spent by Canada, the next

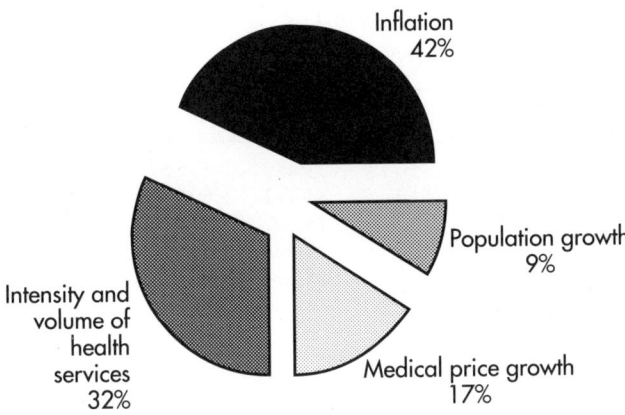

Fig. 5-2. Factors contributing to increased health spending: 1988-1989. (From CRS analysis of National Health Expenditure data.)

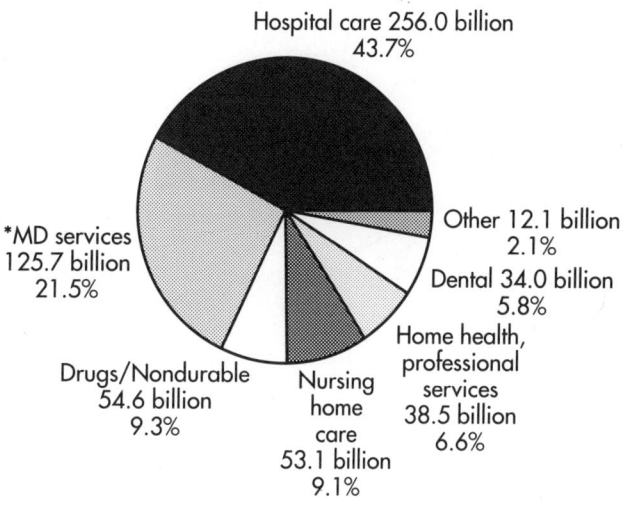

Total = $585.3 billion
*Excludes hospital-based physicians (e.g. anesthesiologists, radiologists, pathologists, and medical residents).

Fig. 5-3. Distribution of personal health care spending, 1990. (From CRS analysis of National Health Expenditure data.)

highest country. The Health Care Financing Administration (HCFA) recently projected that by the year 2000, U.S. health care spending will equal $1.615 billion, or 16.4% of GDP.[77]

If health expenditures continue to rise at their current pace, health care spending in the United States will double approximately every 7 years.[72] This rate, however, is comparable to increases in other countries between 1965 and 1988.[122]

Increases in health care spending in the United States have been due to medical price inflation (17%), as well as the volume and the intensity of medical services provided to patients (32%) (Fig. 5-2). Other factors contributing to rising health care costs are general inflation (42%) and population growth (9%), especially growth in the nation's elderly population.[58] The last factor is particularly significant. The elderly are more likely to be hospitalized and, therefore, more likely to use health care resources. In 1987 for example, HCFA estimated that health care expenditures, on average, were $745 per capita for children under the age of 19, $1535 per capita for adults between the ages of 19 and 65, and $5360 per capita for those over 65.[71] In 1987 those over 65 consumed 35% of all hospital expenditures.[71,72]

Personal health care: hospitals and physicians. Of the $666.2 billion in national health expenditures in 1990, personal health care accounted for $585.3 billion, or 88% of all health care expenditures. Administrative expenses, including marketing and profits associated with private insurance companies, accounted for $38.7 billion (5.8%), government public health activities accounted for $19.3 billion (2.9%), noncommercial research accounted for another $12.4 billion (1.8%), and construction spending totaled $10.4 billion (1.6%).[77]

The largest portion of personal health care expenditures

was attributed to hospital care, which accounted for $256.0 billion (43.7%). Physician services accounted for $125.7 billion (21.5%), nursing home care consumed $53.1 billion (9.1%), and drugs and supplies consumed another $54.6 billion (9.3%). Dental services accounted for only $34.0 billion (5.8%). Together these expenditures accounted for 89.4% of all personal health care spending in 1990[77] (Fig. 5-3).

Between 1960 and 1990, national spending on hospital care grew from $9.3 billion to $256 billion.[122] Furthermore, hospital margins—the difference between the revenues received by hospitals and costs—more than doubled between 1965 and 1989, increasing from 2.35% to 5.9%.[122]

Not only hospital expenditures but also physician expenditures per physician rose substantially in the United States in recent years. Physician incomes for U.S.-based physicians, regardless of medical specialty, far exceed those of physicians in other countries. For example, the average real income in 1987 for U.S. physicians was $132,200, up from $104,744 (1987 constant dollars) in 1969. By comparison, the average real income for physicians was $82,764 in Canada, $81,759 in the former West Germany (1986), $44,571 in Japan (1986), and $42,641 in Great Britain.[122] Income for French physicians was approximately $64,606 (1990).[60]

However, such data may be very misleading. Because of definition and reporting differences, these figures may understate actual physician incomes. The German and French figures, for example, do not consistently include hospital-based physician incomes because such data are

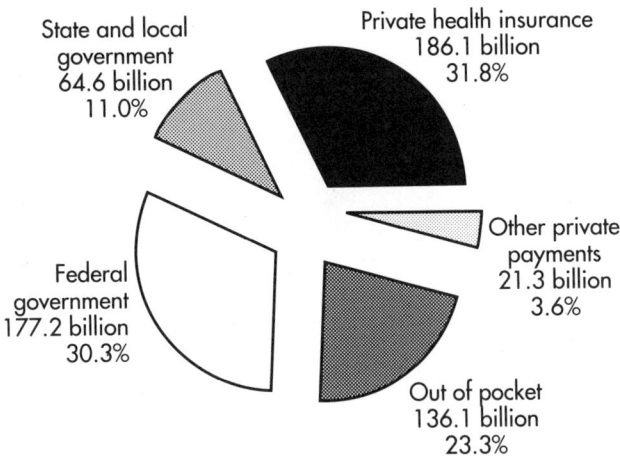

Fig. 5-4. U.S. personal health care expenditures by payer: 1990. (From CRS analysis of National Health Expenditure data.)

Table 5-20. Distribution of U.S. primary care physicians: 1963-1986

Specialty	1963	1986	% Change
General/family practice	73,489	67,687	− 7.9%
General internal medicine	34,742	69,996	+ 101.5%
General pediatrics	14,207	33,364	+ 134.8%
Total primary care	122,438	171,047	+ 39.7%
Total physicians*	248,818	499,197	+ 100.6%
% Primary care	49.2%	34.3%	− 14.9%

From Barnett PG, Midtling JE: Public policy and the supply of primary care physicians, *JAMA* 262:2864-2868, 1989.
*Excludes 27,657 (1963) and 69,963 (1986) physicians with specialties unknown.

not reliably disaggregated from total hospital expenditure data. Another approach is to use physician expenditures per physician as a surrogate for income. This approach provides the following amount per physician: $183,281 (United States); $112,035 (Canada); $67,062 (former West Germany); $183,261 (Japan); $34,823 (United Kingdom); $52,270 (France). This approach may be only slightly better, but the relative differences between countries may be more valid. Nonetheless, both approaches suffer from other denominator difficulties because they do not consistently exclude non-active physicians that might lower average income estimates among active physicians.

The biggest purchaser of personal health care: government. The biggest single purchaser of personal health care in the United States is government. In 1990 the federal government accounted for 30.3% ($177.2 billion), and state and local governments accounted for another 11.0% ($64.6 billion) of all U.S. personal health care spending. The remainder of personal health care spending was attributed to private insurance, including both employer and employee spending ($186.1 billion or 31.8%), out-of-pocket consumer spending ($136.1 billion or 23.3%), and other nongovernment sources such as philanthropy and investment income ($21.3 billion or 3.6%)[77] (Fig. 5-4).

Health care programs funded by government sources, especially programs funded by the federal government such as Medicare, have been the source of much of the rapid growth in health care spending. Medicare pays for both physician services (Medicare Part B) and hospital services (Medicare Part A). Only in limited situations does Medicare provide financial coverage for nursing home care. Medicare pays a substantial portion of all hospital costs and, for the elderly, is the principal payer of health

care for both physician and hospital services. Medicare is a major payer for diagnostic services, as these services are most frequently used by the elderly. Among the top 10 most frequently used inpatient radiologic procedures in 1990, Medicare was the principal payer for all but one procedure (pregnancy ultrasound).[61]

In recent years, however, attempts have been made to reduce the reimbursement levels paid to hospitals and physicians receiving Medicare funds. Between 1980 and 1985, for example, Medicare spending per enrollee grew 6.1% annually, whereas national health care spending grew only 4.3% annually. After federal enactment in 1983 of the prospective payment system, reimbursement for hospital services billed to Medicare was capped per diagnosis. As a result, federal hospital spending between 1985 and 1988 grew at only 2.9% annually compared to national spending, which grew 4.0% annually.[122]

Recently, fees also have been capped for physician services financed by Medicare (Part B). To achieve this limit, the fee schedule was decoupled from the traditional payment philosophy of "customary, prevailing, and reasonable" charges billed by physicians and made uniform from state to state. The new reimbursement rates are based on a Resource-Based Relative Value Scale (RBRVS) system incorporating considerations for factors such as time spent with the patient, medical training, and degree of difficulty. Additional adjustments are made for certain geographic variations.

Medicaid spending trends have shown considerable growth over the past decade. Although the total number of beneficiaries has remained relatively unchanged, the mix of recipients has changed with changes in eligibility.* This growth, however, has been most dramatic in recent years. Between 1980 and 1990 Medicaid spending grew by

*Between 1975 and 1991 the number of Medicaid recipients has fluctuated from as few as 21.6 million (1980) to as many as 26.2 million (1991). (From *1990 HCFA Statistics*, US Department of Health and Human Services, HCFA Pub. No. 03313, September 1991).

Table 5-21. Health expenditure and physician indices of seven industrialized countries—1989*

Country	1 1990 per capita†	2 1990 % GDP‡	3 % Public funded§	4 Percentage physicians who are generalists‖	1988 Average expenditures per physician (US $)**	Physicians per 1000 pop. (1988)
United States	2566	12.4	42	33	$183,281	2.3
Canada	1795	9.0	75	52	$112,035	2.2
Sweden	1421	8.7	90	—	—	2.9
France	1379	8.9	75	53	$ 52,270	2.6
Germany	1287	8.1	72	54	$ 67,067	2.9
Japan	1113	6.5	73	—	$183,261	1.6
Great Britain	909	6.1	87	63	$ 34,823	1.4

*OECD Health Data File.
†1990 Per capita: Per capita spending on health care.
‡1990 %GDP: Percent of GDP devoted to health care.
§% Public: Percent of all health expenditures publicly financed.
‖Source: US Public Health Service, 1992.
**Health Care Finance Administration calculation based on 1988 OECD data.

nearly 23%, compared to overall state budget growth of only 9.8%. Medicaid expenditures now constitute the largest share of many state budgets, and the National Association of State Budget Officers has estimated that Medicaid consumed as much as 14% of state expenditures in 1991.

Cost containment. From a health policy standpoint, cost containment efforts directed at federal programs are likely to have a substantial impact on national health care expenditures. For example, the federal share of all spending on hospital services has grown from about 15% in 1965 to approximately 41% in 1990.[122] Conversely, out-of-pocket spending by Americans on hospital care declined nearly 20% to 5%, and private insurance spending on hospital services dropped from 41% to 35% during this time.[122]

A similar trend can be seen with physician services. Federal spending in 1965 amounted to only 1.4% of all spending on physician services that year, but by 1990 grew to 28%. On the other hand, out-of-pocket spending saw a significant drop during this period. Consumer out-of-pocket spending accounted for 61% of all spending on physician services in 1965, but dropped to 19% by 1990,[122] as compared to 7% in West Germany (1985) and 3% in Great Britain (1987).[24] Thus altering the degree to which the federal government pays for health care would likely produce significant changes in the rate of health care spending in the United States. This effect has significant import because projections indicate continued increases in total as well as government-based spending on health care during the 1990s. HCFA estimates that spending on health care will rise to more than $1.6 trillion by the year 2000. This amount would equal 16.4% of GDP. HCFA also predicts that the federal share will total $534.9 billion (33.1%) and the state/local government share will total another $238.8 billion (14.8%). By the year 2000, total government spending on health care will nearly equal all

forms of private sector spending on health care unless substantial cost containment is achieved.

System capacity and use of medical services

The United States has 2.3 physicians per 1000 persons, more than in Great Britain and Japan, and slightly more than in Canada. However, compared to other countries, the United States has far more specialists than generalists[97] and the percentage who are categorized as primary care physicians is declining. In 1963 primary care physicians, including general practitioners, family physicians, general internists, and general pediatricians constituted 49.2% of all physicians with declared specialties. By 1986 this number declined 14.9% so that primary care physicians were 34.3% of all U.S. physicians (Table 5-20). Among all physician specialties, family physicians and general practitioners declined nearly 8%, whereas all other specialties increased during this period.[4] Overall the United States has comparatively fewer primary care physicians, but higher physician expenditures than the other countries described in this analysis (Table 5-21).

Americans average 5.3 physician contacts per year, fewer contacts than in Great Britain (5.7), Canada (6.6), France (7.2), Germany (11.5), and Japan (12.9), but more than in Sweden (2.8).[60] Public programs such as Medicare and Medicaid, however, have substantially increased access to medical care for the poor and the elderly in the United States. In 1964 before enactment of these two major public insurance programs, 21.0% of the US population over age 65 and 28.2% of poor families (annual incomes less than $10,000) reported no physician visit during that year. By 1987, however, nearly 25 years after enactment of these programs, the percentages dropped to 9.5% and 12.8%, respectively.[37]

Regarding hospital resources, the United States appears to have substantial unused hospital capacity. The hospital

Table 5-22. Biomedical research and development (BMRD) funding: amount per country and percent of total for all countries (1980)*

Country	Amount of BMRD funding (millions in 1975 U.S. dollars)	Percentage of all funding for all countries
United States	5256	48.18
Japan	1523	13.96
Germany	1271	11.65
France	712	6.53
Great Britain	495	4.54
Sweden	251	2.30
Canada	176	1.62
All other countries	1225	11.22
Total	10,909	100.00

*From Shepard DS, Durch JS: In *Assessing medical technologies*, Washington DC, 1985, National Academy of Sciences, Institute of Medicine.

admission rate for the U.S. population is 12.8%*, the lowest among the countries discussed here. The U.S. hospital occupancy rate (65.5%) and average length of hospital stay (7.2 days) also are comparatively low, suggesting substantial unused hospital capacity.[60]

Without global budgets or national cost-containment programs directed at capital purchases and construction, the U.S. health care system has considerably more medical technology than other countries.[3] The United States funds more than 48% of the world's biomedical research, nearly 3.5 times more than in Japan, which ranks second. In 1980 the United States, Japan, and Germany funded 74% of all biomedical research in the world (Table 5-22). For example, the Congressional Budget Office (CBO) has estimated that the United States has 7.4 MRI machines for every 2 million people, compared to 1.9 in Germany and 0.9 in Canada.[24]

Radiologic imaging procedures are performed at high rates in the United States, partially because there is more technology to perform such procedures. The United States ranks second to Japan in the number of CT scans, which has contributed to the fact that CT scanning of the head was one of the most common inpatient radiologic procedures performed in the United States in 1990. Medicare paid for 54.2% of the nearly 1.4 million CT scans of the head performed in that year.[61]

The United States has substantially greater technologic capacity to deliver cardiovascular services than most other countries except Japan. Although it has only 1.4 times as many cardiovascular surgeons (2459) as the next highest country, Japan (1990), the rate of open heart procedures in the United States was 16.2 times greater than in Japan, 6.2 times greater than in Great Britain, 5.4 times greater than

in Germany, 4.2 times greater than in Canada, and 3.5 times greater than in Sweden in 1990 (see Table 5-2).

A study comparing coronary artery bypass surgery (CABG) in the United States and two Canadian provinces found there were 2.3 times more CABG procedures in the United States than in the Canadian provinces. Furthermore, the U.S. rate was four times greater for patients over age 75.[89]

Although international comparisons are not readily available, the National Center for Health Statistics (NCHS) has compiled various utilization data regarding medical care in the U.S. short-stay hospitals. Four of the five most common surgical procedures performed in the United States as reported by the Health Insurance Association of America (HIAA) are related to pregnancy.[61] The vast majority of nonmaternity hospital care involves treatment for cardiovascular conditions (3641), genitourinary tract disease (2204), or malignancies (1670) (all in thousands).[61] However, length of stay in U.S. hospitals for most medical conditions is far less than in many other OECD countries.[61]

Gaps in the insurance net. Given the patchwork system of health insurance, utilization of services in the United States, although high overall, varies according to an individual's insurance status and income. Thus uninsured individuals and, to a lesser extent, individuals receiving Medicaid obtain fewer medical services than those with private health insurance. They are more likely not to have a regular physician or routine source of health care, which leads to more episodic and less comprehensive medical care. The uninsured are less likely to obtain timely preventive services such as mammography and PAP smears and are more likely than insured patients to experience complications caused by chronic conditions. Both the lack of insurance and the failure of most insurance plans to cover immunization accounts in large part for the fact that the United States has fewer young children immunized that most other industrialized nations.

In the absence of universal health insurance coverage, utilization of medical services places health care providers in the unique position of providing free (uncompensated) care when treating the uninsured. Contrary to the arrangement in most other industrialized countries, physicians, and especially hospitals, who provide health care to patients without health insurance face the risk of going unpaid. In 1981, 5.0% of all hospital care was uncompensated. By 1988 this number had increased to 6.1%. The burden of uncompensated care, however, varies considerably by type and location of hospital. Uncompensated care falls disproportionately on those hospitals located in regions with higher concentrations of poor and uninsured persons. Thus for urban, inner-city public hospitals, the percentage of uncompensated care has been more than double the national average, increasing from 12.8% in 1981 to 14.7% in 1988. To a lesser extent, teaching hos-

*Percent of total population.

Table 5-23. Infant mortality and low-birth-weight distribution in the United States by race/ethnicity: 1989

Race	Infant mortality rate			Low birth weight		
	Nonwhite	White	Ratio NW/W	Nonwhite	White	Ratio
Black	17.7	8.2	2.2	13.2	5.7	2.3
Puerto Rican	11.2	8.2	1.4	9.5	5.7	1.7
Native American	10.3	8.2	1.3	6.3	5.7	1.1
Mexican American	7.9	8.2	0.9	6.7	5.7	1.2
Asian American	6.9	8.2	0.8	6.7	5.7	1.2
Chinese American	6.1	8.2	0.7	5.0	5.8	0.9

From *Troubling trends persist: shortchanging America's next generation,* a report of the National Commission to Prevent Infant Mortality, March, 1992.

pitals assume a disproportionate share of uncompensated care as well. In 1981, 9.8% of care in major teaching hospitals was uncompensated care. This rate increased to 10.0% by 1988. Nonteaching hospitals reported only 3.9% uncompensated care in 1981 and 5.1% in 1988.[122]

Thus the health insurance system in the United States may be described as a patchwork system of health care coverage, buttressed by technologic opulence, which provides extremely high quality health care for those with adequate health insurance or otherwise sufficient financial resources. Public health insurance, either Medicare or Medicaid, provides less than comprehensive coverage for the poor and the elderly, leaving many economically vulnerable to expensive medical care. Absent this or private health insurance, many individuals, most of whom work or are members of working families, must forego preventive care as well as essential curative care. This arrangement is truly unique among the industrialized nations.

U.S. health profile

The quality of health in the United States, as measured by selected morbidity and mortality rates, stands in stark contrast to its enormous expenditures devoted to health care. Despite spending more on health care than any other country, the United States has one of the highest infant mortality and low-birth-weight rates, as well as rates of cancer and heart disease, which exceed those of other countries that spend considerably less.

In 1989 the United States ranked twenty-second among all countries in the world in infant mortality.[87] For certain populations such as certain racial and ethnic minorities, infant mortality rates are much higher (Table 5-23). The infant mortality rate for black children in 1989 was 17.7, compared to 8.2 for white children: a rate more than twofold higher. For Puerto Ricans it was 11.2. On the other hand, the rates for Asian Americans (Japanese, Filipino, and Chinese Americans) was lower. In 1983 approximately 6.8 percent of all births were low birth weight; a rate higher than that for Canada, France, West Germany, and Sweden.[28] In 1989 this percentage had not changed substantially (7.0%). Again, this rate was lowest for white

infants (5.7%) compared to black (13.2%) or Puerto Rican (9.5%). Virtually all races, except Chinese American infants (5.0%), had higher percentages of low-birth-weight infants than whites.[87] Nearly 62% of all legal abortions in 1985 in the United States were performed on women under the age of 24, the highest rate in a nine-nation survey.[28]

Life expectancy at birth is 71.8 years for men and 78.5 for women, the shortest among the countries described in this analysis. Only 12.6% of the U.S. population is over age 65.[60]

About one fourth of U.S. children live in single-parent families, up from 19.7% in 1980 and 11.9% in 1970. This rate far exceeds those for Canada, France, Germany, Sweden, Japan, and Great Britain. Births to unmarried women have been steadily increasing. More than 23% of all births in 1986 were to unmarried women, half the percentage for Sweden, but slightly higher than in France and Great Britain. Along with higher infant mortality and low-birth-weight rates, the adolescent fertility rate is also higher than in the other six countries[28] (Table 5-24).

Preventable injuries are a major cause of morbidity and mortality in the United States and the single leading cause of death for children and adolescents. Intentional injuries (homicide [13.7%] and suicide [12.8%]) along with motor vehicle injuries (37.7%) compose the majority of deaths in U.S. youth between the ages of 15 and 24. In 1986 these and other forms of violence and intentional injury accounted for 77.8% of all deaths for young adults in this age category. The U.S. rate is higher than the other six nations (Table 5-25). The percentage of deaths caused by homicide among U.S. adolescents is nearly five times greater than any of the other countries reviewed.[28,48]

Despite aggressive campaigns and legislation to increase use of passenger restraint systems among children, motor vehicle injuries remain the chief cause of childhood injury-related deaths.[105] Overall, the greatest number of years of productive life lost before age 65 in the United States is due to motor vehicle accidents.[105]

Unintentional injuries are the leading cause of death (1988) for children ages 1 to 4 (19.6/100,000), 5 to 9 (11.7/100,000), 10 to 14 (12.7/100,000), and 15 to 19

Table 5-24. Perinatal characteristics of seven industrialized nations

Nation	Per cap* 1989	Infant mortality rate 1989†	% Low birth weights 1989†	Maternal disability (weeks)‡	Maternal disability finances§	Births (%) unmarried mother 1986‖	Adolesc. fertility rate 1985**	Cesarean section rate (1985)††
United States	2354	9.80	7	—	—	23.4	50.9	23
Canada	1683	7.20	6	25	60%	23.4	23.7	19
Sweden	1361	5.77	4	22.5	90%	48.4	11.0	12
France	1276	7.36	5	16	$63 per day maximum	21.9	12.9	—
Germany	1232	7.44	6	14	100%	9.6	9.0	—
Japan	1035	4.59	5	14	60% + $1374 one time sum	>1.0	4.1/E (1989)	7
Great Britain	836	8.42	7	18	$60 per day	21.0	29.5	10

*Per cap, Per capita spending on health care, 1989, OECD data.

†Deaths per 1000 live births. From *Troubling trends persist: shortchanging America's next generation,* a report of the National Commission to Prevent Infant Mortality, March, 1992.

‡Disability for total weeks (before and after the birth of the infant). From *Issue brief: employee benefits research institute,* November, Institute, 1990, No. 108.

§Reported as percentage of regular salary, or as maximum per day.

‖From *Children's well-being: an international comparison,* A Report of the Select Committee on Children, Youth, and Families, March 1990,

**From *Children's well-being: an international comparison,* A Report on the Select Committee on Children, Youth, and Families, March 1990. Births per 1000 adolescents ages 15 to 19.

††Cesarean sections per 100 hospital deliveries. From Notzon FC: International differences in the use of obstetric interventions, *JAMA* 263:3286-3291, 1990.

Table 5-25. Adolescent mortality due to injuries: ages 15-24 (circa 1986)

Country	Total youth % male	Deaths % female	Violent deaths (%)	Motor vehicle accidents (%)	Suicide (%)	Homicide (%)
United States	74.7	25.3	77.8	37.7	12.8	13.7
Canada	75.3	24.7	76.2	37.5	19.8	2.9
Sweden	74.8	25.2	75.8	33.8	25.0	2.9
France	73.6	26.4	70.0	40.4	12.3	1.3
Germany	73.5	26.5	68.7	40.5	17.4	1.9
Japan	72.8	27.2	66.5	37.5	18.8	1.0
Great Britain	73.5	26.5	62.3	32.3	11.1	2.3

From *Children's well-being: an international comparison,* Select Committee on Children, Youth, and Families, USGPO 27-883, March, 1990.

Table 5-26. Percentage of nongovernment-sponsored U.S. health plans providing select clinical preventive services: 1990*

Clinical preventive service	Conventional insurance plan	PPO plan	HMO IPA plan	HMO staff plan	Point of service plan
Physical examination, adult	30	49	94	97	87
Well-child examination	39	58	96	97	98
Well-baby examination	48	68	98	98	93
Mammogram	57	70	95	96	92
PAP smear	55	70	97	99	93
Childhood immunization	47	65	97	99	90
Preventive diagnostic examination	67†	NA	94†	100†	NA
General dental	39	37	24	21	32
Eye care	24	28	52	62	40

*From *Source book of health insurance data,* Washington D.C., 1991, Health Insurance Association of America, p 34.

†Percentages are for 1989.

Table 5-27. Mandatory and Optional Medicaid Coverage, 1992

Mandatory: Federally determined covered populations	
Covered population	**Income level**
Cash assistance	
AFDC families	State determined Average is 44% of poverty
SSI—individual (aged, blind and disabled)	75% of poverty
Other targeted populations	
Pregnant women and infants up to 1 year	133% of poverty
Children aged one to five	133% of poverty
Children aged six to nine[*]	100% of poverty
Children aged 10 to 18[*]	State AFDC Level (will be phased in to 100% of poverty by the year 2001)
Elderly and disabled Medicare beneficiaries	100% of poverty with limited benefits (120% in 1995)

Optional: State may cover and still receive federal matching funds	
Medically needy	Level is state determined but may not exceed 133% of state's AFDC level Average is 53% of poverty
Pregnant women and infants up to 1 year	Up to 185% of poverty
Ribicoff children—those up to age 21 who meet state income thresholds for AFDC but do not meet categorical requirements	State AFDC level
Elderly and disabled living in the community	Up to 100% of poverty
Elderly and disabled in nursing homes	Up to 222% of poverty (three times the SSI level)

Optional: State may cover, but no federal matching funds	
General assistance population	State determined
Other indigent persons	State determined

From National Governors' Association 1992

*Coverage is being phased in for all children born after September 30, 1983. By 2001 all children under 19 years living his households with incomes below poverty will be covered by Medicaid.

Note: The 1992 federal poverty level is $6,810 for an individual and $11,570 for a family of three.

(46.7/100,000). Homicide increasingly becomes a major cause of death from childhood to adolescence, growing from the fourth leading cause for children ages 1 to 9 and the second leading cause for adolescents ages 15 to 19. The homicide death rate for black adolescents (ages 15 to 19) is eight times higher than for whites. On the other hand, the suicide rate in this age group is two times higher for whites than for blacks.[36] In a six-nation survey, the United States had the highest injury-related mortality rates for motor vehicles, firearms, and homicide, (two and three times, respectively, higher than the next highest country, Canada).[136]

The lifetime costs (both direct and indirect) of injury-related morbidity and mortality to children in 1985 amounted to $4.1 billion for children ages 1 to 4 years old, $9.7 billion for children 5 to 14 years old, and $39.1 billion for 15- to 24-year-olds. This amount was 33.5% of the lifetime costs of injuries to all Americans in 1985.[123]

The U.S. mortality rate for ischemic heart disease is comparatively high, 44% greater than the rate for Western European nations.[106] Diet has been linked as an important factor related to the development of subsequent heart disease. Caloric intake for Americans is probably the highest in the world. According to the United Nations Food and Agriculture Organization (UNFAO), between 1983 and 1985 Americans consumed on average more than 3600 calories per person per day. Many of these calories, however, were attributed to a diet that contains 167.2 grams of fat per person per day, more per capita than virtually any other nation.[28]

Clinical preventive services: a population profile

Because health insurance in the United States is not a social program and does not typically provide economic coverage for predictable events, many preventive services traditionally have not been covered. For example, according to 1990 data from the Health Insurance Association of America, conventional insurance plans offered only spotty coverage for adult physical examinations (30%), well-child care (39%), and well-baby care (48%), and only slightly better coverage for mammography screening (57%) and PAP smears (55%)[61] (Table 5-26). Mandatory and optional medical coverage as of 1992 is shown in Table 5-27.

Regardless of financing basis, health insurance, in most other industrialized nations, provides economic protection for virtually all necessary curative and preventive medical services, whether or not they are predictable or expensive.

Perinatal preventive services and maternal disability. In 1989, 24.5% of all pregnant women in the United States did not obtain prenatal care during their first trimester. Approximately 6.5% of all pregnant women did not receive *any* prenatal care that year.

Utilization of prenatal care varies considerably by race/ethnicity. Only 21.2% of all white women compared to

Table 5-28. Prenatal care characteristics and outcomes for U.S. women by race, 1987

Race	No early prenatal care (%) (1989)	Adolescent births (%) (1989)*	Unmarried teen births (1989)*	Unmarried mothers (1987)†	Preterm births (%) <37 weeks (1987)†	Low birth weight (%) <2500 grams (1987)†
White	21.1	10.8	28.4	13.9	8.2	5.6
Black	40.1	23.5	103.4	63.1	18.3	12.9
Hispanic	43.0	19.0	NA	32.6	11.0	6.2
Puerto Rican	37.3	21.9	NA	53.0	12.6	9.3

*National Center for Health Statistics: *Advance Report of Final Natality Statistics*, 1989.
†National Center For Health Statistics: *Advance Report of Final Natality Statistics*, 1987.

40.1% of black women and 43.0% of Hispanic women did not obtain early prenatal care in 1989 (Table 5-28).

Maternal disability benefits vary somewhat according to place of employment and state of residence. For the most part, maternity benefits have rather limited legal protection at the federal level compared to other countries. According to federal law (the Pregnancy Discrimination Act of 1978), any employer providing short-term disability benefits for employees must include in those benefits maternity benefits for women employees during periods of medical disability associated with pregnancy and childbirth, but this law applies only to employers with more than 15 employees. Generally speaking, however, women working full time are permitted under this law a minimum of 8 weeks of maternity leave (usually only postpartum) with full pay for a normal or uncomplicated delivery. Maternity leave and pay extending beyond this arrangement vary considerably among employers. This benefit is substantially less than those in the other countries discussed[43] (Table 5-25).

The United States has no federal family leave policy, although Congress has made several efforts to enact such legislation. In 1992, President Bush vetoed a bill that would have provided family leave. Nonetheless, several states have mandated unpaid job-protected leave for parenting and family illness reasons.[43]

With respect to infant health, the percent of mothers breast-feeding their newborns, another perinatal preventive practice, began rising after 1970 and reached a high of 62% in 1982. Since then, however, participation has declined dramatically. Roughly 58% of white women and 23% of black women initiated breast-feeding in the immediate postpartum period; however, after 6 months these rates fell to 20% and 6%, respectively.[26]

Pediatric preventive services. Since the United States does not regulate the number of physicians entering medical specialties, specialty choice is governed by personal preference, clinical interest, and pecuniary reward. Among the primary care physician specialties, pediatricians are the fewest in number. Traditionally, median income for pediatricians in the United States is among the lowest for physicians. In 1989 the median income for all pediatricians (including subspecialists) was $93,000. Other generalists such as family physicians do not earn significantly more. On the other hand, the median income for all surgical specialties, radiology, and anesthesiology was $180,000.[51]

Early pediatric screening for newborn congenital problems in the United States varies somewhat from state to state. For the most part, however, virtually all states require newborn screening for hypothyroidism and phenylketonuria; however, state interests vary regarding other newborn screenings.

Because there is no universal health insurance for children, the use of childhood medical evaluations and screenings vary according to insurance coverage, socioeconomic status, and education of the parent(s). The public school system provides some screening and evaluation services for students, but clinical services are very limited (e.g., typically no immunizations are provided through school-based clinics), and nurses, but rarely physicians, provide only emergency triage for ill students.

Federally funded community and migrant health centers provide services to poor and uninsured children and their families. Demand for their services, however, often far outpaces their resources, and funding may vary over time. Great stress is being put on these clinics because of the increasing numbers of uninsured families and their children, shrinking Medicaid funding for the very poor, coupled with rapidly growing health problems such as the spread of HIV disease and assorted mental health and substance abuse treatment needs.[31]

Virtually all industrialized nations provide full coverage for childhood immunizations; however, as few as 47% of conventional U.S. plans cover immunizations.[61] Immunization rates compiled by the Centers for Disease Control (CDC) in 1985 indicate that only two thirds to three fourths of children ages 1 to 4 years are adequately immunized. These rates vary by location (inner city, urban, and rural) and by race. Thus inner city and nonwhite children have considerably lower rates of immunization.[37,135] On the other hand, hospital and surgical care, often associated

Table 5-29. Vaccine-preventable diseases: incidence and national U.S. immunization goals

Vaccine	Infection cases					Immunizations			
	No. for select years					Case reductions 1990 objectives for nation	No. deaths	Rates for children <age 2 yr W/NW*	Goals 1990 objectives for nation
	1979	1987	1988	1989	1990	By 1990	1989/1990	1985	% Children <2
Polio†	26	6	9	5	7	< 10	—	58.9/40.1	90
Diphtheria	59	3	2	3	4	< 50	—	68.7/48.7	90
Pertussis	1623	2823	3450	4157	4570	<1000	8/10	68.7/48.7	90
Tetanus	81	48	53	55	64	< 50	—	68.7/48.7	90
Measles‡	13,597	3655	3396	18,193	27,786	< 500	32/89	63.6/48.8	90
Mumps	14,225	12,848	4866	5712	5292	<1000	—	61.8/47.0	90
Rubella	11,795	306	225	396	1125	<1000	—	61.6/47.7	90

From Centers for Disease Control (incidence data). United States Immunization Survey, division of Immunization, Centers for Disease Control in Health United States, 1988. National Center for Health Statistics, DHHS Pub. No. PHS, 89-1232 (immunization rates). *Healthy people: the Surgeon General's report on health promotion and disease prevention*, USPHS, 1979 (goals).
*Percentages are for whites (W) and nonwhites (NW). From *Child Health USE '91*, US Department of Health and Human Services, Public Health Service, HRSA, Maternal and Child Health Bureau, November 1991, DHHS Pub. No. HRS-M-CH- 91-1.
†No US polio due to wild-type virus during the 1980s.
‡Centers for Disease Control estimates that 81 of the 89 deaths in 1990 occurred in persons who were unvaccinated for measles.

with less predictable and more expensive medical conditions, are typically covered comprehensively. At the same time, prepaid group practices (HMOs, for example) provide more comprehensive coverage for the preceding services at rates approaching 98% to 99%, whereas commercial and nonprofit plans provide limited coverage for well-child care (39%) and well-baby care (48%).[61]

Immunization rates for children under 2 years in 1985 were estimated to be between 59% and 69% for the routine childhood series of immunizations.* The low rates of immunization have paralleled increasing trends in the incidence of various childhood diseases otherwise preventable through vaccination. Between 1987 and 1990 the number of pertussis cases has increased 1.6-fold, and the number of cases of measles has increased 7.6-fold. Deaths caused by these infectious diseases have increased as well (Table 5-29). Based on the 1990 Health Objectives for the Nation, the incidence of certain vaccine-preventable childhood infections is well above those objectives: Pertussis cases in 1990 were 4.5 times higher than the 1990 objectives, the incidence of mumps was 5.3 times higher, and the incidence of measles was 56 times higher.

Public programs for women and children are based chiefly on the joint federal-state Medicaid program. Categorical eligibility enables certain poor children and pregnant women to qualify for public medical insurance. Because of the dual state-federal nature of the program, funding for services, income eligibility, and covered pharma-

ceuticals varies from state to state (Table 5-30). In 1967 a comprehensive children's program, Early and Periodic Screening Development and Testing (EPSDT), was enacted, which requires coverage for a broad range of services, unlike conventional insurance plans. However, enrollment has been variable, and one study by the American Academy of Pediatrics estimated that only 22% of eligible children were enrolled and receiving EPSDT services.

Despite the patchwork coverage through a diversity of health insurance programs, the percentage of children reporting no physician visits over the past 25 years has steadily declined. Before the enactment of Medicaid, the principal insurer of poor children, 21.4% of children ages 5 to 14 reported no physician visit in the preceding 2 years. By 1984, less than 20 years after Medicaid programs were instituted, this percentage fell to 11.8% and by 1987 declined further to 10.4%.[37]

Similar increases in utilization of dental services were seen for the poor. Between 1964 and 1983 the average number of dental visits for children under the age of 18 years and below the federal poverty level increased from 0.6 to 1.0 visit per year, an increase of 66.6% compared to an increase of only 37.5% for children above the poverty level.[37] Overall, however, according to 1982 survey data, nearly one third of all school-aged children did not receive a physical examination or an eye examination at recommended intervals, whereas more than 55% did not receive a dental examination. Medicaid, however, increased the use of these preventive services (Table 5-31).

Adult preventive services. Because of the diversity of insurance plans and the number of uninsured people in the United States, adult preventive service use varies considerably. For example, traditional insurance coverage is lim-

*These rates have been estimated to be considerably lower for certain populations such as nonwhite and inner-city children and well below the goals set by the 1990 Health Objectives for the Nation.

Table 5-30. Medicaid coverage of pregnant women and children[*]

	Pregnant women and infants		Children younger than 21		
State	Maximum Medicaid income eligibility level(%FPL)	Coverage of pregnant women and infants above 133%	Coverage of all financially needy children	Maximum age for financially needy children	Age maximum for children below the poverty level
Alabama	133%	No	No	N/A	6
Alaska	133	No	Yes	21	6
Arizona	140	Yes	Yes	18	8
Arkansas	133	No	Yes	18	7
California	185	Yes	Yes	21	8
Colorado	133	No	No	N/A	8
Connecticut	185	Yes	Yes	21	6
Delaware	133	No	No	N/A	6
District of Columbia	185	Yes	Yes	21	8
Florida	150	Yes	Yes	21	7
Georgia	133	No	Yes	18	6
Hawaii	185	Yes	Yes	18	8
Idaho	133	No	No	N/A	6
Illinois	133	No	Yes	18	6
Indiana	133	No	No	N/A	6
Iowa	185	Yes	Yes	21	8
Kansas	150	Yes	Yes	18	6
Kentucky	185	Yes	Yes	18	6
Louisiana	133	No	No	N/A	8
Maine	185	Yes	Yes	21	8
Maryland	185	Yes	Yes	21	6
Massachusetts	185	Yes	Yes	21	6
Michigan	185	Yes	Yes	21	6
Minnesota	185	Yes	Yes	21	8
Mississippi	185	Yes	Yes	18	6
Missouri	133	No	No	N/A	6
Montana	133	No	Yes	19	6
Nebraska	133	No	Yes	21	6
Nevada	133	No	No	N/A	7
New Hampshire	133	No	No	N/A	6
New Jersey	100	No	No	N/A	2
New Mexico	133	No	No	N/A	6
New York	185	Yes	Yes	21	6
North Carolina	185	Yes	Yes	21	7
North Dakota	133	No	Yes	21	6
Ohio	133	No	Yes	21	6
Oklahoma	133	No	Yes	21	6
Oregon	133	No	No	N/A	6
Pennsylvania	133	No	Yes	21	6
Rhode Island	185	Yes	No	N/A	8
South Carolina	185	Yes	Yes	18	7
South Dakota	133	No	No	N/A	6
Tennessee	150	Yes	No	N/A	7
Texas	133	No	Yes	18	6
Utah	133	No	Yes	18	6
Vermont	185	Yes	Yes	21	8
Virginia	133	No	No	N/A	6
Wahington	185	Yes	No	N/A	8
West Virginia	150	Yes	No	N/A	8
Wisconsin	155	Yes	Yes	21	6
Wyoming	133	No	No	N/A	6

From Children's Defense Fund telephone survey, September 1990.

*Reflects all authorized expansions effective by January 1, 1991.

Table 5-31. Use of preventive care services among U.S. school-aged children: 1982

	No PE in recommended interval (%)	No eye examination last year (%)	No dental examination last year (%)	Frequent use of preventive services (%)
All children	30.9	32.9	55.3	—
Above poverty	31.5	32.5	51.0	73.2
Below poverty	30.2	35.4	80.5	83.0
With Medicaid	17.3	32.5	64.5	77.6
Without Medicaid	37.8	37.1	83.4	86.3

From Newacheck PW, Halfon N: Preventive care use by school-age children: differences by socioeconomic status, *Pediatrics* 82:462-468, 1988.
PE, Physical examination.

Table 5-32. Percentage of women reporting never having been screened with mammography for breast cancer, by age and ethnic status: 1987

Age	White	Black	Hispanic
All ages	61.6	70.3	73.8
40-49	57.7	64.0	76.5
50-59	53.7	69.9	63.0
60-69	61.4	71.7	75.5
70+	71.8	82.4	86.7

From 1987, US Health Interview Survey. Estimates are weighted to reflect the US Census population estimates for 1987.

Table 5-33. Use of clinical preventive services during the preceding 12 months among U.S. women by income, race, and employment status

Preventive service	No PAP smear examination (%)	No clinical breast examination (%)	No blood pressure screen (%)
Income < $10,000	62.6	56.6	11.6
Income > $50,000	47.4	40.0	9.6
White	55.3	50.5	11.6
Black	47.1	43.0	8.8
Hispanic	52.9	50.5	14.1
Employed	49.0	46.1	11.0
Unemployed	50.1	48.8	12.0

From 1987 US Health Interview Survey.

ited with respect to adult physical examinations (30%) and only slightly better coverage is provided for mammography screening (57%) and PAP smears (55%).[61] In the absence of universal coverage, a variety of women's preventive services appear underused: Most women do not receive screening mammography as recommended by either the American Cancer Society or the National Cancer Institute. According to data from the 1987 National Health Interview Survey (HIS), 63.1% of all women over the age of 40 have never received mammography screening, 19.5% have never had a clinical breast examination by a health professional, and 11.3% of all women over age 18 have never had a PAP smear.[37] In fact, regardless of age group and ethnic states, the majority of U.S. women have never undergone mammography (Table 5-32). Furthermore, a higher percentage of lower income and nonwhite women reported never having received a variety of preventive screenings including mammography, PAP smear testing, and blood pressure screening (Table 5-33). The HIS survey also suggests that women are not receiving preventive screening on a timely basis. Most women reported that they had not undergone PAP smear testing, a clinical breast examination, or blood pressure screening in the year preceding the survey. Nonwhite women, low-income women, and unemployed women were more likely not to have been screened in the preceding 12 months (Table 5-33).

Other adult services such as occult stool testing and blood pressure screenings show a similar pattern of underuse for men. According to the 1987 HIS, 41.9% of all men over age 40 had never had a digital rectal examination, and 63.9% had never received blood stool testing. Finally, although there are recommendations regarding proctoscopy for men, HIS data indicate that 77.6% of men over age 40 had never had this procedure. Rates of preventive screening based on these services were considerably lower for nonwhites (Table 5-34).

Prepaid group health plans such as Health Maintenance Organizations (HMOs), which have been in existence in the United States since the 1930s, have attracted considerable interest because of rising health care costs. HMOs and other prepaid arrangements and managed care systems are drawing increasing attention from employers seeking to find alternatives for addressing rising health care costs. Typically, preventive services are more common benefits under these arrangements.

Preventive services were given impetus after the passage of the Federal HMO Act of 1973, which required HMOs to offer specified services to participate in caring for Medicare patients. As a result, adult and pediatric ex-

Table 5-34. Use of secondary clinical preventive services in the United States, percentage of men never screened: 1987*

	Digital rectal examination (%)†	Blood stool examination (%)†	Proctoscopy (%)†	Blood pressure screening (%)‡
All races	41.9	63.9	77.6	19.3
White	39.2	62.3	75.9	19.1
Black	54.6	72.6	86.1	18.1
Hispanic	57.8	73.1	86.1	29.4

*1987 Health Interview Survey.
†Men over age 40.
‡Men over age 18.

aminations, immunizations, PAP smears, and mammography are routine HMO benefits.[61]

Overall, participation in prepaid group plans and managed care has risen dramatically during the 1980s. By 1988 for example, more than half of all individuals insured through traditional plans (about 60 million people) were also participating in some form of managed care.[104]

In light of growing evidence that preventive services can be cost efficient, reduce the burden of personal suffering, improve the quality of life, and be less expensive than certain curative interventions, a wider range of preventive services is being incorporated into traditional indemnity, prepaid group, and self-insured plans. These arrangements are so diverse, however, that reliable generalizations are difficult to make. Nonetheless, their attraction appears to be lasting and they will continue to play an increasing role in the foreseeable future as a means of affecting employee-generated health care costs, particularly in the absence of any national health reform measure.

Medicare, the largest insurer of the elderly in the United States, has begun to expand eligible benefits to include preventive services. Based on cost-effectiveness studies, Medicare now provides reimbursement for mammography, PAP smears, pneumococcal vaccination, and hepatitis B vaccination of high-risk populations.[82,101,102,108] Further studies are being conducted to examine the cost-effectiveness of other services.

Clinical preventive services and public health: federal policy initiatives in the 1990s

Public sector initiatives

Federal initiatives. Because government spending, both federal and state, is responsible for a major portion of all U.S. health care expenditures, government policy with respect to preventive services has the potential to affect significantly the level of preventive services provided to Americans. Preventive services have been the focus of several major government reports (see accompanying box on p. 87).

The future of public health. In 1988 the Institute of Medicine (IOM) released *The Future of Public Health,* which focused attention on the need to redirect public health agencies to improve their performance through a variety of recommendations and to deemphasize specialty medical training over preventive medicine. This document pointed out the need to train substantially greater numbers of public health professionals overall and to increase the number of minority-trained public health professionals in particular. The IOM report also recommended the development of relevant agendas for public health agencies based on an improved public health infrastructure.

The guide to clinical preventive services. In 1979 the Canadian Task Force on the Periodic Health Examination issued its first in a series of recommendations for a variety of clinical preventive services.[17] These recommendations were framed around the philosophy of a periodic health examination over the traditional yearly physical examination. Six additional updates have followed the first report, the most recent in 1991.[18-23]

Pursuant to the early publications, the U.S. Public Health Service through the Office of Disease Prevention and Health Promotion (ODPHP) issued the *Guide to Clinical Preventive Services* in 1989 under the direction of a 20-member panel of experts, the U.S. Preventive Services Task Force.[130] The Guide, a product of 4 years of intensive analysis and debate with respect to the medical literature on the effectiveness of some 169 preventive interventions, has been disseminated widely throughout the United States. A user-friendly version for health professionals is commonly sold in medical university bookstores and contains convenient pocket reference cards, which can be used in the clinical setting.

The Task Force applied a scientific approach to its analysis. First, the objectives of the review process were defined, including defining the types of interventions to be examined and the nature of recommendations that followed. Thus a target condition was selected only if it fulfilled two requirements: (1) It must be responsible for a substantial burden of suffering (i.e., conditions with only minor clinical significance were excluded) and (2) it must be a condition for which a potentially preventive intervention can be performed by clinicians. Second, explicit criteria, "rules of evidence," for recommending or excluding interventions were developed and applied to each topical

---

Chronology of recent federal health promotion/disease prevention publications and activities: 1979-1991

1979 Surgeon General's Report on Health Promotion and Disease Prevention*

1980 Promoting Health/Preventing Disease: Objectives for the Nation†

1983 Promoting Health/Preventing Disease: Public Health Service Implementation Plans for Attaining the Objectives for the Nation‡

1985 Model Standards: A Guide for Community Preventive Health Services (ed. 2)‡

1986 The 1990 Health Objectives for the Nation: A Midcourse Review†

1988 Future of Public Health, Report of the Institute of Medicine‡

1989 Guide to Clinical Preventive Services: An Assessment of the Effectiveness of 169 Interventions

1990 Healthy People 2000: National Health Promotion and Disease Prevention Objectives†

1991 Healthy Communities 2000: Model Standards. Guidelines for Community Attainment of the Year 2000 National Health Objectives (ed. 3)‡

*Publication of the U.S. Department of Health and Human Services.
†Publication of the American Public Health Association.
‡Publication of the Institute of Medicine.

Clinical preventive services to be evaluated by the EPPS

1. Adolescent idiopathic scoliosis screening
2. Routine iron supplementation during pregnancy
3. Vaccination services: measles, *Hemophilus influenza* Type B*
4. Hormone replacement therapy*
5. Home monitoring for premature labor
6. Prostate cancer screening*
7. HIV screening*
8. Abdominal aortic aneurysm screening

From Woolf SH, Sox HC: The expert panel on preventive services: continuing the work of the U.S. preventive services task force, *Am J Prev Med* 7(5):326-332, 1991.
*Topics being assessed in light of new evidence, preventive technologies, or interventions.

---

area studied. The interventions recommended for the three services—screening, counseling, and immunization/chemoprophylaxis—must demonstrate efficacy regarding clinical outcomes. Delivery of services is based on an individual's age, sex, and other related risk factors. Third, comprehensive literature searches were conducted, and the evidence in the literature was rigorously assessed using a predetermined set of criteria. Thus three types of studies, randomized controlled trials, cohort studies, and case-control studies, were given special emphasis and ranked in order of quality of evidence. Finally, specific guidelines were adopted to translate these findings into sound clinical practice. Some interventions were recommended strongly, some were recommended as "clinically prudent," and others were not recommended. Once the recommendations were developed by the Task Force, they were further reviewed by more than 300 experts in government, academic medical centers, and medical organizations in the United States, Canada, and Great Britain. After release of the Guide, the Task Force was disbanded. ODPHP continues its involvement in clinical preventive services by serving the successor to the Task Force, the Expert Panel on Preventive Services (EPPS).

In the fall of 1992 ODPHP began "Put Prevention Into Practice," a national prevention campaign to educate primary care providers about incorporating prevention into their practice. A kit containing a variety of materials

geared to increasing the office-based use of preventive services was disseminated to primary care providers. By 1994 ODPHP plans to have an updated and expanded version of the Guide to Clinical Preventive Services.

U.S. Preventive Services Task Force. The USPSTF was reorganized in 1989 after completing its initial mission to develop and publish the Guide to Clinical Preventive Services. To carry on its philosophical mission of expanding knowledge of clinical preventive services, the Expert Panel on Preventive Services (EPPS), as it was briefly renamed, was reorganized in 1990 by the Secretary of Health and Human Services. The new task force was established to provide ongoing evaluation of preventive services in light of new knowledge about their effectiveness, and to address additional topics not examined by the original USPSTF (see box above). Ongoing study was seen as critical, as new data and new technologies would require further study and evaluation.

The mission of the new task force is to study and evaluate preventive services not explored by the USPSTF and to reevaluate the services in the Guide in light of new information. As a result of these activities, the new USPSTF will issue new and updated editions of the Guide. It will continue to maintain working relationships with other important agencies and organizations involved in developing practice guidelines with respect to preventive services, such as the federal Agency For Health Care Policy and Research, the CDC, the National Institutes of Health, various medical specialty organizations, the American Medical Association, the American College of Physicians, and private organizations such as the RAND Corporation.[137]

In addition, the ODPHP will examine barriers to preventive services, especially financial barriers. Data indicate that a variety of factors affect the delivery of preventive services: insurance coverage, other ability to pay, and awareness and agreement among providers and consumers about the need for certain services. Financial barriers appear to be particularly important, as the few studies on the topic point to the importance of insurance or ability to pay for preventive services as the one of the most if not the most important barrier.[34] The issue, however, certainly extends beyond financing, as Canadian utilization of preventive services is not universal despite the generally good coverage among the provinces for many preventive services. Thus insurance coverage is likely to be found to be a necessary but not fully sufficient factor leading to the use of preventive services.

Healthy People 2000. Healthy People 2000 (and its predecessor, the *1990 Health Objectives for the Nation*) was compiled by the U.S. Public Health Service and established more than 226 specific health objectives for the nation.[38] It established additional objectives, which, like the earlier document, seek to reduce preventable death and disability and to direct the nation toward improving the health status of Americans. Included among these are objectives encompassing clinical preventive services.

Healthy People 2000 seeks to achieve three broad goals for Americans: (1) to increase healthy life spans; (2) to reduce health disparities between populations of differing ethnicity, income, and age; and (3) to improve access to preventive services. The program has 22 objectives; the first 21 address specific goals regarding health promotion, health protection, and preventive services. The last objective focuses on the need to conduct disease surveillance and establish data systems. Objectives also are presented for each of four age groups: children, adolescents/young adults, adults, and the elderly.

In addition to objectives related to increasing the use of individual preventive services, *Healthy People 2000* also contains specific objectives to reduce barriers to the use of preventive services. Among the barriers to preventive services identified in *Healthy People 2000* are absent or inadequate health insurance coverage, inadequate provider reimbursement, inadequate access to primary care providers (including inadequate numbers of primary care providers versus specialists, geographic maldistribution of primary care providers, and practice restrictions on other primary care providers—physician assistants, nurse practitioners), geographic barriers (rural and inner city regions), language and cultural barriers, limited or inconvenient hours available for obtaining services, and transportation barriers. Other barriers include uncertainty among providers about the selection and timing of preventive services that should be provided to patients, practice organization characteristics of providers (time restraints, data capacity limitations for tracking preventive services among individual patients, and too few nonphysician providers to assist in the delivery of preventive services). Finally, frequently there is inadequate consumer demand.

Among the objectives to reduce these barriers are the following:

- Increase to at least 50% the proportion of individuals who receive the appropriate screening, counseling,

and immunizations services recommended by the U.S. Preventive Services Task Force.
- Increase to at least 95% the proportion of individuals who have a regular source of primary care for coordinating and delivering their clinical preventive services.
- Improve both the financing and delivery of clinical preventive services so that virtually no American has a financial barrier to receiving, at a minimum, the recommendations of the USPSTF.
- Increase the delivery of clinical preventive services through federally funded primary care programs such as Maternal and Child Health programs, Community and Migrant Health Centers, the National Health Service Corps, and the Indian Health Service.
- Increase to at least 50% the proportion of primary care providers who provide clinical preventive services as recommended by the USPSTF.
- Increase to at least 90% the proportion of individuals served by local health departments that assess and ensure access to essential clinical preventive services.

Other recommendations focus on research needs, including evaluating the impact of clinical preventive services on quality of life; evaluating the efficacy, effectiveness, optimal frequency, and efficiency of clinical preventive services; studying use patterns of preventive services; and evaluating the impact of various incentives and reimbursement strategies on the delivery of clinical preventive services within primary care.

National Coordinating Committee on Clinical Preventive Services. Originally known as the U.S. Preventive Services Coordinating Committee, this committee, established in 1989 by the Secretary of Health and Human Services, is composed of members from some 30 medical organizations, federal agencies, and medical specialty societies and financing organizations to explore ways of putting preventive services into more widespread practice. Among the barriers to implementation that the committee is focusing on are reimbursement barriers, provider and public education issues, and access to preventive care. In addition, the Committee is the advisory group that helps implement the clinical preventive services objectives of *Healthy People 2000* and participates in the "Put Prevention Into Practice" campaign.

Model Standards: A guide for community preventive health services. Model Standards was developed and published by the American Public Health Association to serve as the implementation tool for state and local health agencies seeking to achieve the 1990 and *Year 2000 Health Objectives*. Model Standards incorporates all the objectives of Healthy People 2000 that involve communities. Many states have now incorporated most of the 1990 and Year 2000 health objectives into their operating agendas, and *Model Standards* offers states community implementation strategies for achieving these objectives.

The Secretary's Council On Health Promotion and Disease Prevention, 1990. The Secretary's Council was established to explore ways in which the prevention documents described earlier might be better financed and integrated into the U.S. health care system. The Council, after identifying a variety of problems and barriers to the delivery of clinical preventive services, released its recommendations in May 1990. They made several recommendations, some of which were related to clinical preventive services. In addition, the Council is exploring public-private partnerships to influence prevention activities and to develop recommendations on health information technology.

State and local health agency initiatives. State health departments and local health agencies are the backbone of the U.S. public health infrastructure. These agencies implement federal initiatives, while developing and initiating their own targeted programs guided by state and local needs.

Most of the budgets for state and local health agencies are derived from state sources. In 1988, for example, of the $10.6 billion comprising the budgets for state and local health agencies, 45% was derived from state revenues, 30% was obtained from federal grants and contracts, and only 13% was provided through local funding. Fees and other revenue generated contributed only 10%.[103]

A substantial portion of federal contributions to state health expenditures are tied to MCH activities. Of the $8.3 billion in state health expenditures in 1988, 36% are derived from federal sources, including MCH block grant funds (5%), U.S. Department of Agriculture, Women, Infants, and Children (WIC) funds (20%), and other federal funds and preventive block grants (11%).[103] Federal MCH block grants ($429 million in 1988) target a variety of preventive population-based programs: genetic screening services, lead poisoning prevention programs, MCH services, adolescent pregnancy programs, and programs directed at crippled children and children with special needs.[103] In addition to the role played by the private sector in the delivery of personal health care, the vast majority (74%, 1986) of state and local health expenditures in the United States are consumed by either institutional (17%) or noninstitutional (57%) personal health care.[103]

Private sector initiatives. Although government policy can have substantial influence on the practice of medicine in the United States, private sector activities also have been driven by concerns over cost containment and health outcomes for workers. Skyrocketing health care costs have eroded corporate profits and added substantially to the price of products, making American industry more vulnerable to international competition based on medical expenses alone.[13] Because most Americans under age 65 receive their health insurance through their place of employment, these rising expenditures have considerable importance for employers as well.

It has been estimated that the total health care costs for each active employee rose 43% between 1986 and 1988, increasing from $1358 to $1944 per active employee.[78] There are no indications that this trend will reverse or even slow. As a result, corporate America is focusing on health care and exploring ways to contain cost and raise health outcomes for workers. Increasingly, corporations are finding innovative ways to bring prevention to their employees. Benefits managers, corporate medical directors, and labor leaders all are focusing on the cost and type of health care workers receive, which increasingly involve managed care activities and preventive services. Given the pressure to control rising corporate health care costs, the private sector will continue to give greater attention to preventive services that can reduce avoidable morbidity and mortality among the workforce.

SUMMARY OF THE INTERNATIONAL EXPERIENCE

International comparisons, especially in the area of health care, are fraught with potential pitfalls. Denominators for rates and reported practices may differ in definition, fiscal budgets may be grouped and reported differently from country to country, and services may be provided by seemingly different divisions of government, thereby masking both their presence and their magnitude. Given these caveats, the comparisons made between countries in this analysis draw on the more commonly accepted international data sources such as those compiled by the OECD and the WHO. These data are most useful to compare the relative rather than the absolute differences between countries. Focusing on relative differences is likely to provide more firm footing for those seeking to study the significance of different health care systems with respect to preventive services and primary care.

With these reservations exposed, we move on to make some observations about preventive services in these countries.

It is not possible to give a precise ranking among these countries with respect to their performance in the delivery of preventive services. However, strong themes resonate throughout this analysis. It is clear that a diverse array of cultures, economies, and health care systems can deliver a wide range of essential preventive and primary care services to entire populations. However, the United States stands apart from these countries in having failed to develop an integrated and coordinated health care system that provides basic primary and preventive care for all its citizens. This anomaly exists despite spending vastly more sums on health care than any other nation. The countries described in this chapter have found different ways to provide comprehensive health care for all their citizens, using either employer-financed systems independent of or in conjunction with varying degrees of public financing. Although all use greater public funding than the United

States, they have developed health care systems that are culturally in step with other aspects of their respective countries. In spending less and instituting a variety of cost containment strategies, these countries do not appear to have jeopardized the provision of preventive and primary care services.

A recurrent theme among all the countries except the United States is that they place a high priority on preventive services for mothers and children. Prenatal care is comprehensive and accessible, often involving outreach when necessary, completely free, and convenient in all the countries discussed. For mothers working outside the home, all countries provide generous maternity disability benefits that far exceed those typically provided in the United States. Sweden, an extreme in this regard, provides liberal flexibility to enable parents to make their children's health and welfare a meaningful priority throughout a child's early years and on into school. All six countries have much lower infant mortality and low-birth-weight rates than those in the United States. Prenatal care and childbirth involve a wide range of providers, frequently nonphysicians.

Another strong theme among these countries is that most provide many preventive services, either through public clinics or through school-based programs. As a result virtually all children through adolescence receive at least basic preventive services: immunizations, vision, hearing and speech evaluation, prevention counseling (injuries, nutrition and fitness), and physical examinations.

Although some preventive services are less widespread for adults, certain primary (prenatal care, dental care, and immunizations) and secondary (mammography, PAP smears) clinical services are common in all countries. Colorectal screening and blood pressure screening are not usually independent services but instead are part of routine physical examinations and thus are not billed as separate preventive services ("unbundled").

Despite the universality of health insurance to all citizens in these countries, use of preventive services is still less than universal. Data are sparse, but several essential screening activities in Canada, for example, are still not provided by many Canadian physicians in accordance with the guidelines of the Canadian Task Force. Other countries, implicitly recognizing this fact, have developed aggressive outreach programs, especially for breast and cervical cancer, and financial incentives directed at providers to raise primary prevention participation rates for immunizations, prenatal care, and certain secondary preventive services such as cancer screening (mammography and PAP smears). Some countries have begun to electronically track traditional screening patterns for various cancers for adults (mammographies and PAP smears), as well as immunization practices for children. This approach allows resources to be redirected to infrequent users of preventive services.

The countries in this analysis have been able to provide more comprehensive preventive services than the United States because they have recognized the importance of insurance coverage in promoting prevention. Preventive and health promotion services are viewed as necessary benefits under their health insurance systems. This approach is less common under traditional indemnity plans in the United States, although managed care systems are a departure from this practice. Cost sharing is minimized for preventive services (especially primary services—prenatal care, immunizations) and typically waived for the needy and the elderly.

Another theme that results in greater preventive and health promotion services is the fundamental focus of the health care system. The foundation for these health care systems is intrinsically based on preventive and primary care. A wide range of providers is involved in the delivery of care: nurse midwives, public health nurses, school nurses, and physicians. Each country has emphasized the need for more primary care physicians rather than for specialists. In terms of both pay and prestige, they have maintained this balance.

Based on the experiences of the countries in this analysis, the following strategies appear to promote preventive and primary care services:

- Remove financial barriers, whether insurance or health benefits provisions, and cost-sharing, particularly for women and children, the poor, and the elderly.
- Encourage delivery of preventive services through financial incentives and other means directed at both providers and patients. This approach includes reimbursement for preventive services, as well as financial incentives to achieve certain levels of population-based preventive services.
- Educate providers and patients about the timeliness of various preventive services. This strategy may involve outreach efforts targeting certain services (PAP smears and mammography screening) or certain populations (through home visiting services).
- Emphasize prevention and primary care rather than curative, hospital-based care. To achieve this goal, the medical education and training system recruits, trains, and rewards primary care providers over specialists. This approach contributes to the delivery of more primary and preventive care, as well as less hospital-based care.
- Use public clinics and school-based clinics to deliver a wide range of preventive services. This strategy also draws on reimbursement arrangements and relative mixes of more generalists than specialists, and the inclusion of a wider range of primary care nonphysician providers.

Much needs to be learned about the relative importance of these strategies and how they operate independently and together to influence the delivery of preventive and primary care. The current fiscal pressures on our health care system provide an important incentive to reassess the U.S. health care system, its performance in improving our health status, and its untapped potential for delivering preventive and primary care that reaches all populations, including the most vulnerable.

Addendum

CHANGES IN THE SWEDISH HEALTH CARE SYSTEM

EDITOR'S NOTE: The authors in Chapter 5, while describing the Swedish health care system and the delivery of preventive care, note that 58% of persons polled felt that "fundamental changes (were) needed to make (the system) work better." This was one of the causes for a dramatic change in the election of 1991 that replaced a decades long reign of a liberal party with a more conservative government and is leading to major change in the Swedish health care system. The change lies not in its goals or the existence of a national health care insurance but in its method of delivery, with strong emphasis on incentives to health care deliverers. An updated note on these recent changes still in evolution is worth appending because of our own present national health care debate, and relative to this text because of the implications to preventive care. This will likely impact preventive medicine in the occupational health specialty more than any other. It is highly unlikely that the excellent preventive medicine delivered to the expectant mother, the pre-school and school-aged child will change. The contributor of this addendum is Dr. Gören Hellers, Assistant Professor of Surgery at the Karolinska Institute Medical School and Chairman of the Department of Surgery at the Huddinge University Hospital. In addition to his specialty of surgery, he has a deep interest not only in prevention but also in efficient and cost-effective health care delivery. The editors, aware that the Swedish election of 1991 might have had some impact on the concerns of our text, requested his observations late in the production of this book.

As mentioned in Chapter 5, Sweden (along with Canada and the United Kingdom) has been one of the most typical examples of a public health care system outside the socialist countries. Health care has primarily been financed and provided by the 24 counties of the country. The National Board of Health and Welfare has a supervising but not regulating function. The overwhelming majority of health care institutions in the country are owned and run by the counties. Private medicine has traditionally played a very minor role. Less than 5% of health care is private.

The financing of providers has been on a fixed budget basis with a complete disregard more or less for the actual level of production. This has not surprisingly led to a steady decrease in productivity over the years. There have been various figures given for the decreasing productivity, but a fair estimate is that it has been around 1.5% to 2% per year between 1970 and 1990. The total number of employees in the health care sector was approximately 200,000 in 1970 and 425,000 in 1990. The number of surgeries, admissions, outpatient visits and so forth during the same period of time remained constant, or in some cases even decreased slightly. As in every other budget based system, this led to increasing and eventually huge waiting lists. During the late 1980s there was an intense public debate about the apparently inefficient health care system and the long waiting lists. In many parts of the country, patients had to wait several years to undergo a simple hernia repair procedure. During 1989 and 1990 many counties decided to change from a budget based to a prospective payment type reimbursement. On the left political field, the intention was to keep the health care system public but build a kind of internal market to create incentives and increase productivity. On the right side of the political spectrum, many politicians argued that large scale privatization was necessary to create incentive. These differences of opinion prevented the politicians to go from debate to action for some time. In 1991 however there was a general election, which resulted in a significant swing from left to right. There is now a clear conservative/liberal majority. Therefore the Swedish health care system, will change fundamentally within the next few years. Stockholm County was the first county to implement these changes. For the surgical specialties, the changes were introduced January 1, 1992.

The present public debate is about future financing in principle. Many politicians seem to prefer that the system remain on the county level, although there is an increasing number of politicians arguing in favor of a compulsory national health insurance plan. This is a sensitive issue since 90% of county business is health care. If a national insurance is introduced, the counties will probably disappear as organizational bodies. Hundreds of polititians have their livelihood based on county seats so they oppose a change. A public investigation however has been initiated, and a report on the principles of a national insurance system is expected during the fall of 1993. Until then, and probably sometime beyond, the system will remain on the county level.

The following is an account of some changes that have already taken place and how these have affected the various parts of the health care service so far.

HOSPITAL CARE

In Stockholm County a prospective payment plan based on a Swedish version of diagnosis related groups (DRGs) was introduced January 1, 1992. When the new system was introduced, about 25,000 patients were on various waiting lists for various types of surgery in the county. After 6 months of prospective payment, all waiting lists have disappeared. Production has gone up by 15% to 20%, but the overall cost has increased only by approximately 4%. This is because the DRG rates were reduced by 10% from the start. The rates were calculated according to 1989 and 1990 production and the average cost at that time. Before introducing the rates in the prospective payment plans, the county made a 10% reduction of the rates since increased production was anticipated. This was done to avoid the windfall that occurred over the first couple of years when the DRGs were introduced in the United States. This assumption was apparently correct.

In 1993 the remaining specialties, except psychiatry and geriatrics, have changed to the prospective payment plan. It has not yet been decided how these specialities will be reimbursed, and until then, they will keep the old budget type system.

PRIMARY CARE

Primary care is still budget based. The primary care system however will change into a British type GP system in which every citizen has to be listed with a GP of his or her own choice. Patients may change their listing once a year. The user's fee will be low if the patient sees the GP first and then, if necessary, gets a referral to a specialist. Patients who choose to see a specialist directly without a referral will be "punished" by a much higher user's fee. Each GP will be allowed to have a minimum of 1000 patients and a maximum of 2500 on his or her list. The reimbursement for the GP will be a combination of capitation and prospective payment. It has not yet been decided how much will be capitation and how much will be prospective payment. Suggestions varying from 50-50 to 80-20 have been discussed. The system was introduced in Stockholm County on January 1, 1993 and probably nationally according to a national plan some years later.

OCCUPATIONAL HEALTH

In Sweden every company has been encouraged to provide health care service for its employees. The service should be work oriented and mainly preventive. This means that the company doctors should not see patients to take care of common colds but should care for health hazards related to the employees' working situation. More than 2000 physicians in the country are specialized in occupational health. The federal government has subsidized this type of health care by paying one third of the cost out of government funds. As of January 1, 1993, the government no longer pays. There has been a heated debate about the cessation of government contributions. Critics have argued that this will lead to decreasing quality of a very elaborate and popular service for employees; the government has argued that occupational health is, in fact, profitable for companies. A good health care program leads to decreasing health problems among the employees and hence less sick leave. Because the programs are profitable

for the companies, it is, in the days of universal deregulation, logical that the companies pay the whole cost themselves. Whether these changes will lead to a reduction in occupational health programs remains to be seen. Currently, the companies are under financial strain because of the recession, and this may lead to reduction of these programs.

SUMMARY

These are just some of the very fundamental changes that have occurred and will take place during the next few years. The system is changing toward more market orientation and increasing privatization. Hopefully the changes will lead to a more timely service with increased productivity and better quality for the Swedish health care system.

REFERENCES

1. Acres SE: Measles in Canada—1986, *Can Med Assoc J* 136:1183-1186, 1987.
2. Aday L, Anderson GM: The national profile of access to medical care: where do we stand? *Am J Public Health* 74:1331-1339, 1984.
3. *Assessing Medical Technologies,* Washington DC, 1985, Institute of Medicine.
4. Barnett PG, Midtling JE: Public policy and the supply of primary care physicians, *JAMA* 262:2864-2868, 1989.
5. Bass MJ, Elford RW: Preventive practice patterns of Canadian primary care physicians, *Am J Prev Med Suppl* 17-23, 1988.
6. Bassett MT, Krieger N: Social class and black-white differences in breast cancer survival, *Am J Public Health* 76:1400-1403, 1986.
7. Battista RN: Adult cancer prevention in primary care: patterns of practice in Quebec, *Am J Public Health* 73(9):1036-1041, 1983.
8. Becker MH, Drachman RH, Kirscht JP: Continuity of pediatrician: new support of an old shibboleth, *J Pediatr* 84:599-605, 1974.
9. Billings J, Teicholz N: Uninsured patients in District of Columbia hospitals, *Health Affairs* 9(4):158-165, 1990.
10. Blendon RJ, Leitman R, Morrison I, Donelan K: Satisfaction with health systems in ten nations, *Health Affairs,* 9:185-192, 1990.
11. Blendon RJ, Taylor H: Views on health care: public opinion in three nations, *Health Affairs* 8:149-157, 1989.
12. *Blessed events and the bottom line: financing maternity care in the United States,* Washington, DC, 1987, The Alan Guttmacher Institute.
13. Bowsher CA: Rising health care outlays are a major problem for business, *GAO,* GAO/HRD-91-102:8-10, June 1991.
14. Braveman P, Oliva G, Miller MG, et al: Adverse outcomes and lack of health insurance among newborns in an eight-county area of California, *N Engl J Med* 321:508-513, 1989.
15. Brenner G, Rublee DA: The 1987 revision of physician fees in Germany, *Health Affairs* 10(3):147-156, 1991.
16. *Canadian health insurance—lessons for the United States,* Washington DC, 1991, US General Accounting Office.
17. Canadian Task Force on the Periodic Health Examination: The periodic health examination, *Can Med Assoc J* 121:1194-1254, 1979.
18. Canadian Task Force on the Periodic Health Examination: The periodic health examination: 1984 update, *Can Med Assoc J* 130:1278-1285, 1984.
19. Canadian Task Force on the Periodic Health Examination: The periodic health examination: 1986 update, *Can Med Assoc J* 134:721-729, 1986.
20. Canadian Task Force on the Periodic Health Examination: The periodic health examination: 1988 update, *Can Med Assoc J* 138:617-626, 1988.

21. Canadian Task Force on the Periodic Health Examination: The periodic health examination: 1989 update, *Can Med Assoc J* 141:205-216, 1989.

22. Canadian Task Force on the Periodic Health Examination: The periodic health examination: 1990 update, *Can Med Assoc J* 142:955-961, 1990.

23. Canadian Task Force on the Periodic Health Examination: The periodic health examination: 1991 update, *Can Med Assoc J* 144:425-431, 1991.

24. *Congressional Budget Office Testimony: Statement of Robert D. Reischauer,* Washington DC, 1991, US Government Printing Office.

25. Charney E, et al: How well do patients take oral penicillin? A collaborative study in private practice, *J Pediatr* 40:188-195, 1967.

26. *Child Health USA '91,* US Department of Health and Human Services, Public Health Services, Health Resources and Services Administration, Maternal and Child Health Bureau, DHHS Pub No. HRS-M-CH 91-1, November, 1991.

27. *Child health: lessons from developed nations,* Hearing Before the Select Committee on Children, Youth, and Families, U.S. House of Representatives, 101st Congress, Second Session, March 20, 1990, Washington DC, 1990, US Government Printing Office.

28. *Children's well-being: an international comparison:* A Report of the Select Committee on Children, Youth, and Families, 101st Congress, Second Session, March, 1990, Washington DC, 1990, US Government Printing Office.

29. Citizens Commission on Graduate Medical Education: *The graduate education of physicians,* Chicago, 1966, Chicago, 1966, American Medical Association.

30. Collins-Nakai RL, Huysmans HA, Scully HE: Task Force 5: Access to cardiovascular care: an international comparison, *J Am Coll Cardio* 19:1477-1492, 1992.

31. Community and Migrant Health Centers: *MCH related federal programs: legal handbooks for program planners,* Association of Maternal and Child Health Programs, 1991.

32. Congressional Research Service, Insuring the uninsured: options and analysis, Oct., 1988.

33. Coyte PC, Dewees DN, Trebilcock MJ: Medical malpractice—the Canadian experience, *Am J Public Health* 324(2):89-93, 1991.

34. Davis K, et al: Paying for preventive care: moving the debate forward, *Am J Prev Med* 6(4):7-30, 1990.

35. Davis K, Rowland D: Uninsured and underserved: inequities in health care in the United States, *Milbank Q* 61(2):149-176, 1983.

36. Goetz PW, McHenry R, editors: *Encyclopedia Britannica,* Chicago, 1990.

37. *Health status of minorities and low-income groups,* ed 3, US Department of Health and Human Services, Public Health Service, Health Resources and Services Administration, Bureau of Health Professions, Division of Disadvantaged Assistance, Washington, DC, 1990.

38. *Healthy people 2000: national health promotion and disease prevention objectives,* conference edition, Washington DC, 1990, US Department of Health and Human Services,

39. *Health United States 1989,* US Department of Health and human Services DHHS Pub No (PHS) 90-1232, 1990.

40. Dutton DB: Explaining the low use of health services by the poor: costs, attitudes, or delivery systems? *Am Sociol Rev* 43:348, 1978.

41. *Employee Benefit Research Institute,* Sources of Health Insurance and Characteristics of the Uninsured, An analysis of the March 1991 Current Population Survey. Issue Brief No 122, February 1992.

42. *Employee Benefit Research Institute,* International benefits. Part 1: health care, *EBRI Issue Brief,* 106, 1990.

43. *Employee Benefit Research Institute,* International benefits: Part 3: disability, parental leave, and unemployment benefits. *EBRI Issue Brief* 108, 1990.

44. *Financing maternity care in the United States,* New York, 1987, The Alan Guttmacher Institute.

45. Fingerhut LA, Kleinman JD: International and interstate comparisons of homicide among young males, *JAMA* 263(24):3292-3295, 1990.

46. Fowler E: *Survey of the British National Health Service,* The Wesley Foundation, 1991, unpublished report.

47. Freeman HE, et al: Americans report on their access to health care, *Health Affairs,* 6(1):6-18, 1987.

48. Fuchs VR, Hahn AB: How does Canada do it? *N Engl J Med* 323(13):884-890, 1990.

49. Garfinkel S, Cordis L, Dobson A: Health services utilization in the US population by health insurance coverage. US Department of Health and Human Services, national medical care utilization and expenditure survey. Series B, descriptive report no 13. Washington DC, 1986, US Government Printing Office.

50. Gold R: Pertussis and pertussis vaccine, *Can Med Assoc J* 132(9):1043-1044, 1985.

51. Gonzalez ML: Socioeconomic characteristics of medical practice 1990/1991, Chicago, 1991. American Medical Association Center for Health Policy Research.

52. Goodwin S: Child health services in England and Wales: an overview, *Pediatrics* Suppl 86(6):1032-1037, 1990.

53. Goodwin S: Preventive care for children: immunization in England and Wales, *Pediatrics* Suppl 86(6):1056-1060, 1990.

54. Greza G: The right to prevention, early detection and medical rehabilitation under national and international aspects, *Int J Rehabil Res* 10(3):267-275, 1987.

55. Ham C: Governing the health sector: power and policy making in the English and Swedish health services, *Milbank Q* 66(2):389-414, 1988.

56. *Health and welfare in Japan,* Japanese International Corporation of Welfare Services, The Ministry of Health and Welfare, 1989, Tokyo, Japan.

57. *Health for all: the health care system in the Federal Republic of Germany,* Issued by the Federal Ministry for Youth, Family Affairs, Women and Health, Godesburg, Federal Republic of Germany, February, 1988, The Institute for Health-Systems-Research.

58. *Health care resource book,* Committee Print, Committee on Ways and Means, US House of Representative, 102nd Congress, First Session, April 16, 1991, Washington DC, 1991, US Government Printing Office.

59. *Health care spending control: the experience of France, Germany, and Japan,* US General Accounting Office, November 1991, GAO/HRD-92-9.

60. Health Data File, Organization of Economic Cooperative Development, 1991.

61. Health Insurance Association of America. *Source Book of Health Insurance Data,* Washington DC, 1991.

62. Hurst JW: Reforming health care in seven European nations, *Health Affairs* 10(3):7-21, 1991.

63. Hurst JW: Reform of health care in Germany, *Health Care Financ Rev* 12(3):73-86, 1991.

64. Ierodiaconou E: Maternity protection in 22 European countries. In Phaff JML, editor: *Perinatal health services in Europe: searching for better childbirth,* Geneva, 1986, WHO.

65. Iglehart JK: Germany's health care system, part 1, *N Engl J Med* 324(7):503-509, 1991.

66. Iglehart JK: Germany's health care system, part 2, *N Engl J Med* 324(7):1750-1756, 1991.

67. Iglehart JK: Japan's medical care system, *N Engl J Med* 319(12):807-812, 1988.

68. Iglehart JK: Japan's medical care system—part 2, *N Engl J Med* 319(17):1166-1172, 1988.

69. Ikegami N: The Japanese health care financing and delivery system: its experiences and lessons for other nations. Presented at the Inter-

national Symposium on Health Care Systems, Taiwan, December 18-20, 1989.

70. Ikegami N: Japanese health care: low cost through regulated fees, *Health Affairs* 10(3):87-109, 1991.

71. King KM: *Health care costs at the end of life,* CRS Report for Congress, Washington, DC, July 25, 1990.

72. King KM, Rimkunas RV: *National health expenditures: trends from 1960-1989: CRS Report for Congress, July 29, 1991,* Washington, DC, 1991.

73. Köhler L, Jakobsson G: *Children's health in Sweden, Socialstyrelsen,* National Board of Health and Welfare, Stockholm, 1991.

74. Köhler L, Jakobsson G: Children's health and well-being in the Nordic countries, *Clin Develop Med* No. 98, Oxford, 1987.

75. Laara E, Day NE, Hakama M: Trends in mortality from cervical cancer in the Nordic countries: association with organized screening programmes, *Lancet* :1247-1249, 1987.

76. Lalonde M: *A new perspective on the health of Canadians: a working document,* Ottawa, 1974, Health and Welfare Canada.

77. Levit KR, Lazenby HC, Cowan CA, Letsch SW: National Health Expenditures, 1990, *Health Care Financ Rev* 13:29-54, 1991.

78. *Health care outlook 1989: survey I corporate health plans: past, present, and future.* New York, 1989, Louis Harris & Associates.

79. Lurie N, et al: Termination from Medi-Cal—does it affect health? *N Engl J Med* 311:480-484, 1984.

80. Manciaux M, et al: Child health care policy and delivery in France, *Pediatrics* (Suppl) 86(6):1037-1044, 1990.

81. Manciaux M, Tursz A: Unintended injuries in children: the French situation, *Pediatrics* (Suppl) 86(6):1077-1084, 1990.

82. Mandelblatt JS, Fahs MC: The cost-effectiveness of cervical cancer screening for low-income elderly women, *JAMA* 259(16):2409-2413, 1988.

83. *Maternal and child health statistics of Japan,* Maternal and Child Health Division, Japan, 1991, Ministry of Health and Welfare.

84. *Annual report on health and welfare for 1989,* Japan, 1990, Ministry of Health & Welfare.

85. Moore KG: A survey of state medicaid policies for coverage of screening mammography and pap smear services, *Legis-Letter (ACOG)* 10(2):1-6, 1991.

86. Nadel MV (testimony): Private health insurance: problems caused by a segmented market, Statement Before the Subcommittee on Health, Committee on Ways and Means, US House of Representatives. US General Accounting Office, May 2, 1991, GAO/T-HRD-91-21.

87. *Troubling trends persist: shortchanging America's next generation,* March 1992, National Commission to Prevent Infant Mortality.

88. National health administration in Japan, *JIPA/HITC* 1:23-37, 1991.

89. Naylor CD: A different view of queues in Ontario, *Health Affairs* 10(3):110-128, 1991.

90. Notzon FC: International differences in the use of obstetric interventions, *JAMA* 263(24):3286-3291, 1990.

90a. Briskhorn H: Personal communication, 1992.

91. Chevit P: Personal communication, 1992.

92. Johansen A: Personal communication, 1992.

93. Naoko Y: Personal communication, 1992.

94. Welsby S: Personal communication, 1992.

95. Pless IB: Child health in Canada, *Pediatrics* (Suppl) 86(6):1027-1032, 1990.

96. Porter AMW, Porter JMT: Anglo-French contrasts in medical practice, *Br Med J* 26:1109-1112, 1980.

97. Politzer R, et al: Primary care physician supply and the medically underserved: a status report and recommendations, *JAMA* 226(1):104-109, 1991.

98. Powell M, Anesaki M: *Health care in Japan,* London, 1990, Routledge.

99. *Prenatal care: medicaid recipients and uninsured women obtain in-*sufficient care, U.S. Washington DC, 1987, General Accounting Office.

100. Prevention and health centers, *Community Health National Health Administration in Japan,* vol 1, Japan Interantional Cooperation Agency, Hachioji International Training Center, 1990.

101. *Preventive health services for medicare beneficiaries: policy and research issues,* US Congress, Office of Technology Assessment, February 1990.

102. *Preventive health services under medicare: the use of preventive services by the elderly,* US Congress, Office of Technology Assessment, January 1989.

103. *1988 Public health chartbook,* June 1988, Public Health Foundation.

104. *Rising health care costs: causes, implications, and strategies,* Washington DC, 1991, Congressional Budget Office.

105. Rosenberg ML, Rodriguez JG, Chorba TL: Childhood injuries: where we are, *Pediatrics* (Suppl) 86(6):1084-1091, 1990.

106. Rowland D: Health status in East European countries, *Health Affairs* 10(3):202-215, 1991.

107. Rudov MH, Santangelo N: *Health status of minorities and low income groups,* Department of Health, Education, and Welfare (Publication HPA 79-627), 1979.

108. Russell LB: *Is prevention better than cure?* Washington DC, 1986, Brookings Institution.

109. Schieber GJ, Poullier J, Greenwald L: Health care systems in twenty-four countries, *Health Affairs* 10(3):22-38, 1991.

110. Schieber GJ, Poullier J: International health spending: issues and trends, *Health Affairs* Spring:106-116, 1991.

111. Schieber GJ, Poullier J: International health care expenditure trends: 1987, *Health Affairs* Fall:169-177, 1989.

112. Schmidt E: Some characteristics of antenatal care in 13 European countries. In Phaff JML, editor: *Perinatal health services in Europe: searching for better childbirth,* Geneva, 1986, WHO.

113. Schneider M: Health care cost containment in the Federal Republic of Germany, *Health Care Financ Rev* 12(3):87-101, Spring 1991.

114. Schwartz A, Colby DC, Reisinger AL: Variation in Medicaid physician fees, *Health Affairs* 10(1):131-139, 1991.

115. Sonoda K: *Health and illness in changing Japanese society,* Tokyo, 1988, University of Tokyo Press.

116. Spasoff RA: Current trends in Canadian health care: disease prevention and health promotion, *J Public Health Policy* 11:161-168, 1990.

117. Starfield B: Effects of poverty on health status, *Bull NY Acad Med* 68(1):17-24, 1992.

118. Subcommittee on Cancer in the Economically Disadvantaged: *Cancer in the economically disadvantaged: a special report,* New York, 1986, American Cancer Society.

119. Tarimo E, Creese A, editors: *Achieving health for all by the year 2000,* Midway Reports of Country Experiences, Geneva, 1990, World Health Organization.

120. Terris M: Newer perspectives on the health of Canadians: beyond the Lalonde report, *J Publ Health Policy* 5(3):327-337, 1984.

121. *The state of the world's children 1991, UNICEF,* New York, 1991, Oxford University Press.

122. *Trends in health expenditures by Medicare and the nation,* CBO Papers, Washington, DC, January, 1991, Congressional Budget Office.

123. US Centers for Disease Control: Cost of injury, *MMWR* 38(43):743-746, 1989.

124. US Department of State, Bureau of Public Affairs: *Background notes: Canada,* January, 1991.

125. US Department of State, Bureau of Public Affairs: *Background notes: France,* November, 1990.

126. US Department of State, Bureau of Public Affairs: *Background notes: France,* June, 1991.

127. US Department of State, Bureau of Public Affairs: *Background notes: Japan,* December, 1990.

128. US Department of State, Bureau of Public Affairs: *Background notes: Sweden,* July 1989.

129. US Department of State, Bureau of Public Affairs: *Background notes: United Kingdom,* October, 1990.

130. US Preventive Services Task Force: *Guide to clinical preventive services: an assessment of the effectiveness of 169 interventions.* Baltimore, 1989, Williams & Wilkins.

131. Varughese P: Incidence of pertussis in Canada, *Can Med Assoc J* 132:1041-1042.

132. Wasson JH et al: Continuity of outpatient medical care in elderly men: a randomized trial, *JAMA* 252:2413-2417, 1984.

133. Wilensky GR: Poor, sick, and uninsured, *Health Affairs* 2:91-95, 1983.

134. Wilensky GR, Walden DC, Kasper JA: The uninsured and their use of health services. Paper presented at annual meeting of the American Statistical Association, August 10-14, 1981.

135. Williams BC: Immunization coverage among preschool children: the United States and selected European countries, *Pediatrics* (Suppl) 86(6):1052-1056, 1990.

136. Williams BC, Kotch JB: Excess injury mortality among children in the United States: comparison of recent international statistics, *Pediatrics* (Suppl) 86(6):1067-1073, 1990.

137. Williams BC, Miller CA: *Preventive health care for young children: Findings from a 10-country study and directions for United States policy,* Chapel Hill, NC, 1991, National Center for Clinical Infant Programs.

138. Woolhandler S, Himmelstein DU: Reverse targeting of preventive care due to lack of health insurance, *JAMA* 259:2872-2874, 1988.

139. Woolf SH, Sox HC: The expert panel on preventive services: continuing the work of the US preventive services task force, *Am J Prev Med* 7(5):326-332.

Chapter 6

THE CLINICAL APPLICATION OF EPIDEMIOLOGY AND THE INTERPRETATION OF DIAGNOSTIC TESTS

Gerald J. Beck

Epidemiologic studies are used to investigate the association of risk factors with disease. These studies are useful in contrast to interventional or experimental studies because the latter are often impossible or difficult to carry out as one cannot randomly assign subjects to risk or exposure factors such as smoking and asbestos. It is important, therefore, to understand the various types of epidemiologic studies and the ways in which they are used to identify and measure the effect of risk factors. This chapter describes the advantages and disadvantages of each type of study, as well as the biases that may occur. Epidemiologic studies are compared with experimental studies where the randomized controlled clinical trial is the gold standard.

A key concept in the interpretation of results from either epidemiologic or experimental studies is risk. The importance of a risk factor may differ depending on whether one interprets it from a population point of view or from the view of a single individual. This distinction will be discussed because the practicing physician is often most interested in advising a single patient on whether to change his or her exposure to a risk factor.

The usefulness and proper interpretation of a diagnostic test for a given disease must also be understood from both a population and individual point of view. Measures of the accuracy of a test are defined along with the predictive values of a test for an individual (see Chapter 9). Possible test biases that can affect the evaluation of a diagnostic test also are described.

Concepts in this chapter underlie the specific examples given in later chapters and should help the reader understand how to interpret diagnostic tests and better evaluate published epidemiologic and medical studies. Further discussion of these issues is contained in statistical or epidemiologic textbooks.* See also references listed at the end of the chapter in Resources.

TYPES OF RESEARCH DESIGNS

To interpret properly epidemiologic or medical research studies, it is important to understand the different types of research designs. Each type has advantages and disadvantages. A randomized controlled clinical trial is generally subject to less bias than other types of studies. As Sackett[33] has described, the majority of biases occur in the design phase of the investigation. The type of design also dictates what statistical analyses are appropriate. The study design needs to be appropriate for the goals of the study, whether it be identifying risk factors for a disease or assessing the effectiveness of an intervention for preventing a disease or slowing its progression.

There are two major classes of research design: observational studies and experimental studies. In an observational study individuals are observed in their natural state, whereas in an experimental study the investigator has control over an individual's exposure to an intervention or risk

*References 1, 6, 14, 16, 20, 22, 34.

Types of research designs

   I. Observational studies
      A. Cross-sectional
      B. Prospective
      C. Retrospective (case-control)
  II. Experimental studies
      A. Clinical trials
         1. Therapeutic
         2. Intervention
      B. Special designs
         1. Cross-over
         2. Factorial

---

factor. The accompanying box lists specific types of observational and experimental studies discussed in this section.

Observational studies

The three classes of observational studies are the cross-sectional, prospective (longitudinal, cohort, follow-up), and retrospective studies.

The cross-sectional study classifies the disease and exposure status of each individual in a group at a given time. This design does not consider changes that occur over time. If repeated cross-sectional studies in different groups of individuals are conducted, some evidence of temporal changes could be made. Sampling is a key issue in any cross-sectional study. Is the group being studied representative of the population of interest? Proper inference to the population is greatly facilitated by obtaining a random sample where each individual has a known chance of being selected. Often, in clinical research, only a presenting sample, such as patients available at a given hospital, is available for study. This presenting sample may not be representative of the target population of interest so that inferences to this population cannot be drawn.

Cross-sectional studies can give estimates of association between diseases or between risk factors and diseases. If the risk factor does not change over time (such as sex or race), the cross-sectional survey can provide a valid estimate of the statistical association between the factor and disease, although causality cannot necessarily be established. For a risk (exposure) factor that changes over time, the cross-sectional study may not be able to determine whether the exposure or the disease came first.

The primary summary measure from a cross-sectional study is prevalence. Prevalence is the proportion of persons sampled who have the disease or characteristic of interest. If the survey was conducted at a single point in time this estimate is called the point prevalence. If disease occurrence is calculated over a short period of time, a period prevalence can be calculated. Cross-sectional studies are particularly suited to measure the health status, needs, and

attitudes of a population. The representative samples of the U.S. population chosen for the national surveys conducted by the National Center for Health Statistics (Health Interview Survey and Health and Nutritional Examination Survey) are examples of such studies.

The second major type of observational study is the prospective study. This is also referred to as a longitudinal, cohort, or follow-up study. All of these terms imply that individuals are followed over time. A prospective study may begin with a group of individuals who are without disease and follow them until they develop disease to study the risk factors that may be associated with a disease. Alternatively, a prospective study may begin with persons who already have disease and follow them until they reach an endpoint such as death. This type of study would describe the natural history of the disease process.

A classic example of a prospective study that examines the etiology of coronary heart disease is the Framingham Heart Study,[11] which selected a sample of 5127 men and women, ages 30 to 59 years, from Framingham, Massachusetts who were free of coronary heart disease in 1952. These individuals have been reexamined periodically since that time. Much of what we know about the predictors of cardiovascular disease (e.g., smoking, hypertension, and cholesterol) has been derived from this study. Another example of a prospective study is the Harvard Six City Study,[13] which examined the association of outdoor (and indoor) air pollution with the respiratory health of individuals living in six different U.S. cities. A summary measure of disease frequency that can be calculated from a prospective study is the cumulative incidence, which is the proportion of individuals free of disease who develop the disease during a given time. Another measure of incidence is the incidence rate, the number of new cases of disease during a given time period relative to the total person-time (e.g., person-years) of observation. This measure is more appropriate if individuals are followed for different lengths of time.

The third type of observational study is the retrospective study. The distinction between this type of study and a prospective study is shown in Fig. 6-1. In the prospective study, persons are classified on their exposure or etiologic characteristic of interest and followed over time to development of disease. In the retrospective study, the opposite approach is taken.[35] Individuals are usually classified by their disease status (cases have disease, controls do not have disease), and one looks retrospectively to determine whether cases and controls differ with respect to a given exposure or etiologic characteristic. Therefore this is called a case-control study. A recent case-control study examined the association of fluorescent light exposure and cutaneous malignant melanoma.[42] It is also possible to define a retrospective cohort study where an investigator examines retrospectively data from a cohort study on disease occurrence in individuals who have had a particular exposure or etiologic characteristic of interest.[20] In this case, individuals may be selected on their exposure status, whereas in the case-control study, individuals are selected on the basis of their disease status. A case-control study can also be nested within a prospective study. An example of this type of study is the prospective study of mortality from colon cancer and the benefit of low-dose aspirin use.[38]

In carrying out a case-control study, several important issues must be considered, including selection of cases, selection of controls, and measurement of the risk factor. First, with respect to selection of cases, one major source of bias is avoided if only newly diagnosed cases are included. If cases of varying disease duration are used, the association of the risk factor with disease is clouded by the influence of the duration of exposure to the risk factor. In addition, to avoid having a heterogeneous group of cases that might weaken the association between exposure and disease, as well as to be able to replicate the study, the diagnostic criteria for defining a case must be clearly specified. As in other designs, having a representative sample of cases is important. Patients with disease from a single hospital may not be representative of all cases of that disease. Excluding individuals with a concurrent disease other than the one of interest can make the interpretation of the results more straightforward.

Second, the selection of controls is a crucial and difficult part of carrying out a case-control study.[41] The two major concerns in selecting controls are the source of the controls and the method of selection. It is also important that the information about cases and controls is of similar quality and quantity. To achieve this goal, controls may be selected from the same medical facility as the cases rather than from the general population. On the other hand, hospital controls, while easier to obtain, may not be representative of the general population, leading to a biased conclusion about the association of the risk factor and the disease. The problem arises if the cases and controls (who have some disease other than the one of interest) are admitted to the hospital with different rates depending on the disease. This problem, first recognized by Berkson[5] at the Mayo Clinic, is called Berkson's bias.

It is also important to consider how the controls are selected from the source. Although the controls should be a random sample from this source population, this method alone does not ensure that the controls and the cases are the same with respect to variables related to exposure to the risk factor or to the development of the disease. Such a variable is called a *confounder* and would affect the perceived association between exposure and disease. Common confounders include demographic factors such as age and sex. To control for known confounders, cases and controls can be matched so that the groups are comparable. Matching on a variable such as age, however, makes it impossible to compare the cases and controls on that

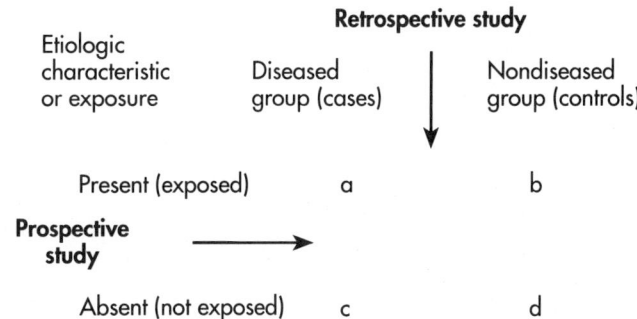

Fig. 6-1. Distinction between retrospective and prospective studies.

variable. A single (or multiple) control can be matched to each case. Alternatively, the cases and controls can be matched on a frequency basis so that the distribution of, for example, age, is the same in the controls as in the cases but individual matches are not made. The feasibility of matching is limited to a few factors unless a large number of controls is available compared to cases. Another consideration is that the person selecting the controls should not know the nature of the risk factor(s) being studied. This approach helps avoid any bias in the exposure history of the controls being selected.

The third important issue in carrying out a case-control study is the measurement of the risk factor or exposure in the cases and controls. This information can be obtained from the study subjects themselves, from family members, or from medical or work records. The information should be obtained in a similar way for both cases and controls and, ideally, it should not be known whether the individual is a case or control. This approach avoids bias in obtaining or interpreting the information. Using preexisting records for exposure information reduces the likelihood of bias because of knowledge of the disease outcome but may lead to the use of incomplete information that varies in quality.

After exposure information is determined, the definition of whether a control and a case are considered exposed must be determined. Will such determination be based on cumulative exposure or current exposure? Depending on the disease, either one may be more appropriate. For example, cumulative exposure may be most important for smoking as a risk factor for cancer, whereas current use may be more appropriate for smoking related to myocardial infarction.

Prospective versus case-control studies. The advantages and disadvantages of prospective and case-control studies are outlined in the box on p. 100. Some have already been mentioned or discussed. The prospective study is best suited for evaluating temporal relationships in a manner that can provide direct measurement of disease and the risks from various exposure or etiologic factors. This

---

Comparison of prospective and retrospective studies

	Advantages	*Disadvantages*
Prospective study	Evaluate temporal relationships	Large sample sizes
	Direct measurement of disease and risks	Long follow-up may be needed
	Uniformity of measurement	Losses to follow-up can bias results
	Minimizes bias in determining exposure	Expensive
	Valuable when exposure is rare	
	Evaluation of multiple endpoints	
Case-control study	Small sample sizes	Bias in measurement of risk factors
	Less expensive and quick	Choosing controls difficult
	Valuable when disease is rare or has long latent period	One endpoint
	Evaluation of multiple etiologic factors for a single disease	Temporal relationship difficult to establish
		Evaluation of only a few risk factors

---

can be done in a manner that minimizes bias in determining exposure, and the quality and uniformity of measurements can be better obtained than in a retrospective or case-control study. The prospective study is also valuable when the exposure is rare, as a sufficient number of exposed individuals could be found and targeted for follow-up. This is not possible in a case-control study unless the study is very large or the exposure is common among those with disease. Finally, a prospective study can be used to evaluate multiple outcomes or endpoints, whereas a case-control study is targeted to a specific disease.

Prospective studies are expensive because they often require large sample sizes and a long period of follow-up to allow the disease to develop. For example, the newly proposed Women's Health Initiative Study will examine factors relating to coronary heart disease, breast cancer, fractures, and total mortality in postmenopausal women in the United States and is expected to have a sample size of 100,000.[39] In addition, losses to follow-up, particularly when there is a long follow-up period, can lead to biased results.

The disadvantages of a prospective study become advantages of a case-control study. Case-control studies can be carried out rapidly and usually with smaller sample sizes. When the disease is rare, a case-control study would be able to start with those identified with disease and look retrospectively at their exposure history. In situations where the exposure is also rare, however, a case-control study also needs to be quite large unless the exposure is common in those with disease. Examples of this type of study are the investigations of mesothelioma in persons exposed to asbestos[9] and the development of vaginal cancer in the offspring of women who used diethylstilbestrol during pregnancy.[21]

The main disadvantage of a case-control study is the difficulty in finding appropriate controls. The possible biases that can arise in this type of study have already been discussed; even with careful planning, these biases may not be totally eliminated. One use of a case-control study is to decide whether a large prospective study should be performed. In both prospective and case-control studies, a broad enough range of exposures must be present to allow detection of any effect. Studies of dietary fat may be flawed because the population being studied may be too homogeneous.[43]

Experimental studies

In contrast to observational studies, in an experimental study the intervention or treatment assignment is under the control of the investigator. There are three major classes of experimental studies in medicine: the primary and secondary prevention trial and the therapeutic trial. In the primary prevention trial, persons free of disease are given some intervention to prevent the disease or condition from occurring. Examples are immunization or smoking cessation. In a secondary prevention trial, the treatment or intervention is given to persons who already have the disease or condition to improve their prognosis by preventing or delaying recurrences or death. Examples are treatment of cancer patients or persons with cardiovascular disease such as angina. In the therapeutic trial, persons with the disease are treated to cure the disease. Antihypertensive trials to reduce blood pressure are examples of this type of study.

In all these situations, the investigator can manipulate the intervention or the therapy. To evaluate whether an intervention or therapy works, the results must be compared to a group who received no treatment or who received standard or usual therapy. That is, if a treatment is being evaluated, it must be compared to a control group. Controls can be studied either concurrently with the treated group or historically. Historical controls are a group of subjects similar to those who are currently being studied but who were studied in the past using the previous standard treatment or no intervention. Use of historical controls allows the assignment of all new cases to the new treatment and avoids problems in obtaining informed consent; however, this approach greatly increases the potential for bias caused by different characteristics between the two groups.

The best way to avoid many biases, both known and unknown, is to use concurrent controls whereby patients are randomized to receive either the new treatment or no treatment (or the usual care) treatment. This type of study is called a randomized controlled clinical trial.[15,26,31] It is a special case of the prospective study described earlier and has the additional advantage of having a comparable control group to contrast to the treated or intervention group(s). Use of concurrent controls avoids possible biases in the patient population, diagnostic methods, and details of treatment and care that can change over time, making questionable use of historical controls.

Randomization ensures that each person has the same chance of being assigned to each of the possible treatments and that the probability of a person receiving a given treatment does not depend on what treatment another person receives. If the sample size is large enough, the major advantage of randomization is that study groups will likely be similar with respect to every factor except for the one being investigated. The actual randomization process can be unrestricted or restricted. For example, in a multicenter clinical trial, treatment balance would be desirable within each clinical center separately. Therefore, each center would have a separate randomization. This approach is an example of stratified randomization, which could also be performed to ensure balance on some known factor that might influence the results of the study, such as age, sex, or stage of disease. This approach is particularly important if the sample size is not large.

Another feature of the randomized study that can avoid possible biases, both in the selection of patients and their follow-up and assessment, is blinding or masking. In a *double-blind study,* both the investigator or treating physician and the patient do not know the treatment assignment. This approach is often possible in drug trials where placebo pills can be given to patients but is less feasible with surgical or nutritional interventions. In a *single-blind study,* the investigator, but not the patient, knows the treatment assignment. If there is some subjectivity in determining the study endpoint, neither the investigator nor the patient should know the treatment assignment. If the outcome is objective, as with a laboratory measurement or with death, then blinding of the investigator is less important.

Two special cases of clinical trial designs worth noting are the cross-over study and the factorial design study. In the cross-over study, each person acts as his or her own control by receiving both treatments, but at different times. Because this design ensures that the treatment groups being compared are identical on patient characteris-

tics, it can be performed with a smaller sample size. This study design is only feasible, however, if the treatment effect is immediate and there is no carry-over effect from having received one treatment before the other. Louis et al[25] discuss the advantages and disadvantages of the cross-over study.

The second type of special design is a factorial design, which allows simultaneous study of more than one type of treatment or intervention factor. An example of such a study is the recent Physicians' Health Study,[36] which used a 2 by 2 factorial design to study the effect of aspirin on cardiovascular endpoints and beta carotene on cancer endpoints. More often, the two factors being studied are in relationship to a single outcome such as in the Modification of Diet in Renal Disease Trial (MDRD Study Group, 1991), which is examining the influence of both a low protein and phosphorus diet and blood pressure control on the progression of renal disease in patients with chronic renal disease. The primary advantage of a factorial design is that two hypotheses can be addressed at once, thus reducing the sample size unless there is an interaction between the two factors being studied. *Interaction* means that the effect of one treatment on outcome depends on the other treatment. If there is an interaction, each treatment must be evaluated separately for each level of the other treatment factor. This reduces the sample size available for each comparison, which will also reduce the statistical power of detecting a difference.[7]

EVIDENCE FOR RISK FACTORS

This section defines how the association between exposure or risk factors and disease or outcome can be quantified for the different types of studies previously described.

As discussed in Observational Studies, the prospective study is best suited for determining the risk of disease after some exposure. The association of exposure with disease can be measured by comparing the incidence of disease in the exposed group to the incidence of disease in the unexposed group. There are several ways to summarize this comparison into a single measure of association. The relevant data for this calculation are the frequencies of exposed and unexposed individuals who develop the disease and those who do not develop the disease. These frequencies are listed in the illustration on p. 99 and are labeled a, b, c, and d in the 2 × 2 table relating exposure status to disease status. In a prospective study, a + b individuals who are exposed are selected and followed over time, and c + d individuals without exposure are selected and followed over time to determine whether disease develops. Thus the incidence of disease in exposed individuals is a/(a + b) and in the unexposed group c/(c + d). The most common measure of association between exposure and disease status is to take the ratio of these two incidences. This ratio is called the *relative risk* (or *risk ratio*). If the risk of disease is the same in the exposed and unexposed groups, the relative risk equals 1. If the relative risk is greater than 1, the risk of disease is greater in the exposed than in the unexposed groups. If the relative risk is less than 1, the exposure reduces the risk of disease (i.e., protective).

A second summary measure of the association of exposure and disease is the difference between the incidence in the exposed and unexposed groups. This difference is called the *attributable risk*. The attributable risk is of particular interest to the health planner, as it gives the absolute percentage of individuals who develop the disease after exposure after subtracting out the underlying disease rate in those not exposed. Perhaps an even more meaningful summary is to divide the attributable risk by the risk in the exposed group and express this number as a percentage called the *attributable risk percent*. In other words, if the exposure could be discontinued, the risk of disease would be reduced by this percentage.

Because persons in a prospective study may be followed for different lengths of time, incidence would be better computed with a denominator of person-time units (e.g., person-years) summed over all persons in each exposure group. The relative risks and attributable risks also could be computed using these incidences. This approach highlights that the relative risk likewise can change, depending on the length of the follow-up from exposure to the evaluation of disease status. This interpretation makes sense because if death were the outcome, in the long term, regardless of exposure status, the incidence of death would be 100% in each group, which would yield a relative risk of 1.0.

An illustration of these measures of risk is given in Table 6-1. It has been suggested that there is an association between cigarette smoking and facial wrinkling.[18] Hypothetical data showing this possible association are given in the table where smokers and nonsmokers are followed in a

prospective study to determine whether facial wrinkling appears. For the hypothetical data, the incidence of wrinkling is 80% in smokers and 20% in nonsmokers. Therefore the relative risk is 80%/20% or 4.0. Thus smokers have four times the risk of developing facial wrinkling than do nonsmokers. The attributable risk is 80% minus 20%, which equals 60%. The attributable risk percent is 60%/80% or 75%. Thus if all smoking ceased, the percentage of persons with facial wrinkling would be reduced by 75%. In the case-control study, the calculation of disease incidence is not possible; however, an approximation to the relative risk can be obtained.

For the case-control study, the absolute risks of exposed and unexposed individuals developing a disease can be calculated because the sampling is with respect to the cases and the controls and not the exposed and unexposed individuals as in a prospective study (see Fig. 6-1). That is, the incidence of disease cannot be calculated, which should be obvious, because if two controls for each case had been selected, a different answer would be obtained for the incidences in the 2 × 2 table. Under certain conditions, however, it is possible to obtain an estimate of their relative risk, which is called the *odds ratio*. The odds ratio is calculated by taking the ratio of two odds: the odds that an exposed individual will develop the disease divided by the ratio that an unexposed individual will develop the disease. That is, a/b divided by c/d, which is equivalent to ad/bc, which is sometimes called the *cross-product ratio*.

The individual odds computed in a case-control study, like the relative risk, are not meaningfully computed, but their ratio is an estimate of the true ratio of the odds and does not depend on the number of controls taken per case. Like the relative risk, an odds ratio equal to 1 indicates that there is no association between the exposure (or risk factor) and the disease or outcome. Values greater than 1 indicate an increased risk of disease with exposure, and values less than 1 indicate a decreased risk of disease with exposure. If a case-control study is population based, it is possible to calculate the incidence rates of disease. Thus in a specific population, all or a known proportion of cases

Table 6-1. Measures of risk in a prospective study: the association of cigarette smoking and facial wrinkling (hypothetical data)

| Cigarette smoking | Facial wrinkling | | |
	Yes	No	Total
Yes	80	20	100
No	40	160	200
Total	120	180	300

Incidence of wrinkling:

Smokers   80/100 = 80%
Nonsmokers 40/200 = 20%

Comparing incidences:

Relative Risk =   80%/20% = 4.0
Attributable Risk =   80% − 20% = 60%
Attributable Risk Percent = 60%/80% = 75%

Table 6-2. An unmatched case-control study: the association of cigarette smoking and facial wrinkling (hypothetical data)

| Cigarette smoking | Facial wrinkling | | |
	Cases	Controls	Total
Yes	100	60	160
No	50	90	140
Total	150	150	300

$$\text{Odds ratio} = \frac{100(90)}{60(50)} = 3.0$$

are identified and then a random sample of controls is selected.

An example of the calculation of an odds ratio is given in Table 6-2 for hypothetical data on evaluating the association of cigarette smoking and facial wrinkling. In this example, 150 individuals are selected who have facial wrinkling (cases), and 150 unmatched (independent) controls are selected without facial wrinkling. For each person, the history of cigarette smoking is then documented and the frequencies of each combination of facial wrinkling and cigarette smoking are determined as shown in Table 6-2. The odds ratio as described earlier is equal to 3.0. Thus it is estimated that a smoker is at three times the risk of a nonsmoker to develop facial wrinkling.

The accuracy of the approximation of the relative risk by the odds ratio depends on whether the disease is rare.[10] Miettinen,[29] however, has shown that the odds ratio is a valid estimate of the relative risk under the typical conditions of most case-control studies. That is, cases and controls are selected on the basis of their exposure status and only newly diagnosed cases of disease are used.[10,29]

When the cases and controls are matched on a one-to-one basis, the calculation of the odds ratio is different. This difference is illustrated in Table 6-3 where risk factor status must be determined for each case-control pair. The odds ratio that approximates the relative risk is the ratio of the number of pairs where the case and not the control is exposed to the risk factor compared to the number of pairs in which the control and not the case is exposed to the risk factor. That is, only the pairs where cases and controls differ on exposure status are used in the calculation. In the example, the odds ratio equals 3.67. Note that in this example, the 150 pairs of cases and controls have the same frequencies of exposure to smoking and occurrence of facial wrinkling as in the unmatched example in Table 6-2. Thus taking into account the matching can yield a different estimate of the odds ratio.

Significance of effect

The relative risk and odds ratio estimate the size of the effect of the association between a risk factor and disease. The statistical significance of the effect depends on the size of the effect relative to the sampling variability that arises from estimating the effect in a sample. Estimates of the variability or standard error of the relative risk and odds ratio estimates can be obtained but are beyond the scope of this chapter.[23]

The significance of the effect can be evaluated in two ways. A test of hypothesis can be performed to determine whether the relative risk or odds ratio is different from the null hypothesis where it is equal to 1 (meaning that there is no association between the risk factor and disease). The significance of the test of the null hypothesis is summarized in the p-value. The *p-value* is the probability of obtaining a result equal to or more extreme than the observed sample value given that the null hypothesis is true. The p-value is not the probability that the null hypothesis is true. Inglefinger et al.[22] discuss p-values in depth. The second method of evaluating the significance of an effect is by calculating a confidence interval on the relative risk or odds ratio.[23] The size of the confidence interval gives a measure of the precision of the estimate of the relative risk or odds ratio. If the confidence interval includes the value 1.0, we can conclude that there is no significant effect (no association between the risk factor and the disease). The significance level would be equal to 1 minus the confidence level that is used in the calculation.

A key issue in interpreting the results of a test of hypothesis or setting a confidence interval is the concept of statistical *power*, the probability of rejecting the hypothesis when it is really false. If the sample size is too small, no statistical significance may be found even in the presence of a medically important relationship. On the other hand, if the sample size is too large, a very small (but not medically important) association could be determined to be statistically significant. An important consideration in interpreting an association between a risk factor or exposure and disease or outcome is whether the association is biologically plausible. If there is some biologic mechanism that would link the risk factor or exposure to the disease, then any association found would have increased validity.

Biases and confounders

Whether or not an association is found to be significant, many biases can occur during the research process that might invalidate the result. A bias occurs if some factor produces a result that differs systematically from the truth. Many potential sources of bias can occur, many of them during the design phase of a study. Sackett[33] lists and discusses 56 types of biases. Two main types are *selection bias* and *information bias*. An example of selection bias has already been discussed in the context of a case-control study using hospital-based cases and controls (i.e., Berkson's bias).[33] Selection bias also can occur in a prospective study if patients consenting to the study are not representative of the exposed and unexposed populations. A notable example in which the representativeness of the study

Table 6-3. A matched case-control study: the association of cigarette smoking and facial wrinkling (hypothetical data)

| | | Facial wrinkling | | |
		Smoking	Nonsmoking	Total
No facial wrinkling	Smoking	45	15	60
	Nonsmoking	55	35	90
	Total	100	50	150

Odds ratio = 55/15 = 3.67.

group was questioned occurred in the randomized clinical trial of extracranial-intracranial arterial bypass surgery to reduce ischemic stroke in patients with symptomatic atherosclerotic disease of the internal carotid artery.[3,17] In this study many patients eligible (and ineligible) for the study were operated on outside the trial. Information or measurement bias occurs when the method of data collection causes the groups being compared to differ in some misleading way. This problem was already discussed in a case-control study where the recall of exposure may differ between cases and controls. In a prospective study, nonresponse or missing information during follow-up may cause the groups being compared to differ in some biased manner.

In addition to biases, there may be one or more confounding factors that could either account for the observed association between exposure and disease or mask this association. A *confounding factor* is one that is associated with both the exposure and the risk of developing the disease, independent of that exposure. An example would be the apparent association between coffee drinking and myocardial infarction. In fact, this association may be due to the effect of cigarette smoking, as smoking, the confounder, is associated with coffee drinking and is also an independent risk factor for myocardial infarction. If one has knowledge or suspects a particular factor is a confounder, the study may be designed to prevent this factor from confounding the results. In a case-control study, for example, the cases and controls could be matched on that factor. A confounder may also be controlled through data analysis, depending on the degree of the confounding. For example, if all men received one treatment and all women received another treatment, any differences between the two treatments may be due to gender rather than the treatment and this would not be possible to determine from the analysis.

Individual risk versus population risk

The measures of risk described in the previous section pertain to the population as a whole. The population risk is the average of the individual risks of persons within that population. Individuals are not homogeneous, even if they have exactly the same level of exposure to a risk factor. Therefore an individual's risk and the population risk are not the same. Zeger[44] has discussed this distinction between clinical medicine and epidemiology from a statistical point of view. He points out that newer statistical modeling methods (e.g., random effects models and empirical Bayes estimates) are now available to quantify the degree of heterogeneity in the population and take into account the characteristics of an individual.

When there is an association between a risk factor and disease, clinicians need to decide what this association means for their patients and individuals need to decide what it means for themselves. Angell[2] has discussed this concept in a recent editorial. This article cites the example of the risk of cardiovascular disease death in men depending on their cholesterol levels.[30] For men aged 40 to 69 years of age without cardiovascular disease at baseline, the 10-year risk of death from cardiovascular disease is 4.9% in those with total cholesterol levels over 240 mg/dl compared to 1.7% in those with levels under 200 mg/dl. The difference of risk among the two cholesterol level groups is only 3.2% in absolute terms but represents a relative risk of 2.9. Because the risk of death is rather small, even in those with high cholesterol, an individual may decide not to reduce their cholesterol level to lower their risk even further.

Another consideration is that even if the reduction in risk resulting from changing a risk factor is small in the population as a whole (as well as in individuals), when these effects are considered in a large population, they may have a large public health benefit, particularly if the disease is common. Angell[2] has discussed an example of this effect from the Lipid Research Clinics Trial. This "trial showed that using cholestyramine to lower serum cholesterol about 9% in middle-aged men with high cholesterol levels reduced their 7-year risk of coronary events from 8.6% to 7.0%.[24] Although such a reduction may not seem worthwhile to an individual, when spread over the estimated one to two million Americans with similar cholesterol levels, it could account for up to 32,000 fewer coronary events over the first seven years."[2] Thus in interpreting the results of epidemiologic studies or clinical trials, it is important to consider viewpoints with respect to the individual, the population, and the public health consequence. In addition, even if risk factors have large effects, they still may not be important to the individual or the population if the disease rarely occurs.

INTERPRETATION OF DIAGNOSTIC TESTS

As has been discussed, epidemiology investigates the association between risk factors and disease or outcome. The same approach can be used to investigate the association between an individual's medical history, clinical examination, signs or symptoms, laboratory or other tests, and disease status. Is the diagnostic test or criterion related to the individual's disease status? To evaluate the validity of a diagnostic test, one needs to know the true disease status. This truth may be based on a more invasive or definitive test, which is considered to provide the most accurate information on the presence or absence of disease. This test becomes the gold standard for diagnosis. From a preventive medicine point of view, the usefulness of a diagnostic test is in its ability to detect disease at an earlier stage to reduce the severity of the disease when it is detected. This approach can lead to improved prognosis assuming a treatment is available. In this case the diagnostic test is used as a screening tool rather than to confirm disease in individuals with clinical symptoms. This section

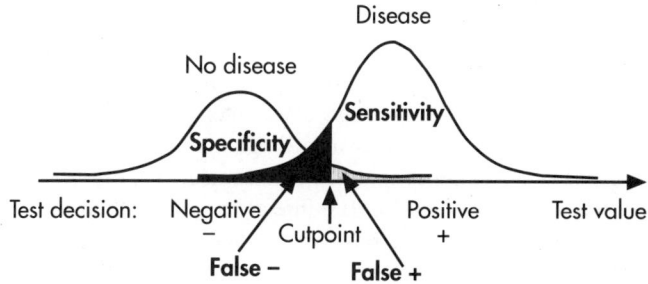

Fig. 6-2. Continuous outcome for a diagnostic test.

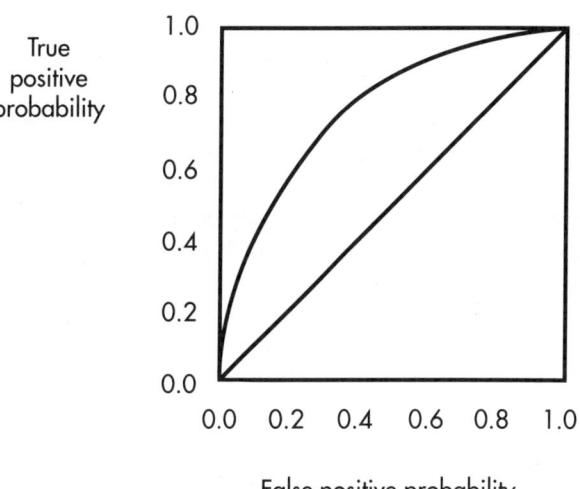

Fig. 6-3. An ROC curve.

briefly discusses the concepts used to define the accuracy of a diagnostic test as well as its usefulness in a given individual in predicting disease. These concepts are further discussed in Chapter 9 and in Galen and Gambino.[16] In addition, the section describes various test biases that affect the evaluation of the performance of diagnostic tests.

Accuracy of a diagnostic test

The accuracy of a screening or diagnostic test relates to its ability to correctly identify whether individuals have or do not have disease. Because some individuals may be misclassified on the basis of the diagnostic test, reducing the rate of these misclassifications is crucial. Two types of errors can be made. A false-positive result indicates the presence of disease when in fact there is none; a false-negative result indicates no disease when in fact there is disease.

A test can also make the correct decision in two different ways. First, among those individuals with disease, the test can correctly identify the disease. A proportion or rate of such correct decisions is called the *sensitivity* of the test. Second, among those with no disease, the test can correctly reflect that no disease is present. The proportion of individuals with such correct classifications is called the *specificity* of the test. The sensitivity of the test is equal to 1 minus the proportion of false negatives, and the specificity of a test is equal to 1 minus the proportion of false positives.

Many diagnostic tests are based on a continuous measurement such as serum creatinine or cholesterol level. In such cases, one needs to specify a single value that would separate disease from no disease or abnormal from normal. Chapter 9 contains a discussion of the limitations and difficulties of defining a normal range and hence a cutpoint between normal and abnormal. Fig. 6-2 illustrates the influence of choosing a cutpoint on the sensitivity, specificity, and false-positive and false-negative rates for a diagnostic test. The two curves in the figure represent the frequency distribution of the test value in the no-disease and disease populations. Typically, as shown, there is an overlap in these distributions, as no test perfectly discriminates between normals and abnormals. The different areas under

the curves define the proportions of individuals that are correctly or incorrectly classified within the no-disease and disease groups. The areas, then, represent proportions or probabilities of correctly or incorrectly classifying individuals based on their disease status.

It is clear that moving the cutpoint will affect all the different areas. If it is moved to the left (lower test value), the sensitivity of the test would be increased but the specificity would be decreased. Thus changing the cutpoint cannot simultaneously increase both the sensitivity and specificity or reduce both the false-positive and false-negative rates. Where the cutpoint should be placed may depend on the purpose of the diagnostic test. For example, with a screening test for HIV infection, if one uses the test for screening blood donors, the cutpoint should be moved left so that the false-negative rate is as low as possible. If one uses the test to determine whether an individual has the infection, however, one may want to move the cutpoint to the right so that there are few false-positive results, because a false report of HIV infection could be devastating. This quandary also points out the limitations of using a single diagnostic test for making a definitive diagnosis. Often if one test is positive, it is either repeated for confirmation or a second type of test is used to confirm the diagnosis. A discussion and an example of how multiple tests are useful are given in Chapter 9.

Because the accuracy of a diagnostic test measured by the sensitivity and specificity depends on the cutpoint, a better method of summarizing the overall accuracy of a test regardless of the cutpoint is needed. Such a method uses the receiver operating characteristic (ROC) curve.[27] The ROC curve plots the true positive probability versus the false positive probability that arises from every possible cutpoint (Fig. 6-3). If the diagnostic test is no better than chance in determining disease versus no disease, in which case the true positive rate equals the false-positive rate, the ROC curve would follow the 45-degree angle line of identity shown in the figure. Ideally, one would like the true positive rate to be close to 1 and the false-positive rate to be very small. In this case the ROC curve would rise steeply toward the upper left hand corner of the graph. A measure of the diagnostic accuracy of the test based on the ROC curve is the area underneath the curve. The maximum of this area is equal to 1, indicating perfect accuracy, whereas an area equal to 0.5 (the line of identity) would indicate that the accuracy of a diagnostic test is no better than flipping a fair coin to determine the presence of disease. Hence, the larger the area, the better the test. The area under the curve, therefore, can be used as a basis for comparing two different diagnostic tests on their ability to discriminate between those with and without disease. An example of such a comparison has been described for the Somogyi-Nelson Glucose Tolerance Test for diabetics to determine which time point after a meal should be used for diagnosing diabetes.[12]

Predictive value of a test

Although the sensitivity and specificity of a test are useful to determine its accuracy, what is most important from an individual or clinician's view is how well the test does in the absence of knowing the true disease status. That is, if the test is positive, what is the probability that the individual really has disease, and if the test is negative what is the probability that the individual truly does not have disease? These two probabilities are referred to as the *positive* and *negative predictive values*. The predictive value of a test, however, not only depends on the sensitivity and specificity but also on the prevalence of disease in the population to which the test is being applied. If the population has a high disease prevalence, the positive predictive value approaches 100% (assuming a high sensitivity and specificity), and the negative predictive value approaches 0. The reverse situation is true if the disease prevalence is low. An example of the effect of prevalence on predictive value is given in Chapter 9.

How the predictive value depends on sensitivity, specificity, and prevalence is derived from Bayes' theorem and is given below.

Positive PV =
$$\frac{\text{(Prevalence) (Sensitivity)}}{\text{(Prevalence) (Sensitivity)} + (1-\text{Prevalence}) (1-\text{Specificity})}$$

Negative PV =
$$\frac{(1-\text{Prevalence}) \text{(Specificity)}}{(1-\text{Prevalence}) \text{(Specificity)} + \text{(Prevalence)} (1-\text{Sensitivity})}$$

If the sensitivity and specificity of a test are known, various prevalences can be used to determine their effect on the predictive values. As can be seen, the positive predictive value of a test can be increased either by increasing the specificity or by supposing a higher prevalence for the disease in the population being tested. For the negative predictive value, it can be increased by increasing the sensitivity or by supposing a reduced prevalence of disease. The clinician must understand these interrelationships before interpreting the results of a diagnostic test or implementing a screening program. For instance, if the general population is screened for HIV infection (where the prevalence is very low), the positive predictive value can be very low despite an extremely high sensitivity and specificity of the test. Applying such a test in this situation could lead to many more false-positive results than identification of true cases of disease.[28]

Evaluating a diagnostic test

In addition to calculating the accuracy of a diagnostic test and determining its predictive value, both positive and negative, the impact of possible test biases on these measures and the test performance should be assessed as well. In addition, after the test has been accepted, its efficacy in reducing morbidity or mortality from the disease should be evaluated.

Many potential biases can occur when diagnostic tests are being evaluated.[4] First, referral or verification bias relates to which individuals are further evaluated by the gold standard or reference test. This can affect the diagnostic test's performance or perceived performance. For example, only a subset of individuals given the diagnostic test may have the disease assessed by a more invasive test such as biopsy. If the evaluation of the test is limited to these individuals, the accuracy of the test may be biased since these individuals were selected for biopsy because they are suspected to have more advanced disease. Thus reliability of the test in a more general population is not fairly assessed. This bias is also referred to as work-up bias. The best way to avoid this bias is to use a prospective study where all subjects receive the gold standard test.

Second, the gold standard, or reference test, may itself be imperfect. That is, the gold standard test may also misclassify individuals as to their true disease status. If the diagnostic test and the gold standard make errors independently of one another, the observed sensitivity and specificity (as well as the predictive values) would be lower than the actual rates. When the diagnostic test and the gold standard tend to misclassify the same patients, the observed sensitivity and specificity (and predictive values) are higher than the actual rates. Thus when the gold standard is imperfect, the bias on the perceived sensitivity and specificity may be in either direction, depending on how the test and gold standard misclassify the patients.[40]

Third, the case mix or spectrum of individuals being evaluated also can affect how well the diagnostic test performs.[32] If only individuals with more advanced disease are evaluated, such as those with Dukes stage C colon cancer, the test may appear to perform well compared with when persons with earlier stages of disease are studied.

Finally, bias in the accuracy of a diagnostic test also can occur when individuals with uninterpretable tests are excluded from the evaluation. It is important to document the number of these cases because, when the test is applied in practice, persons with uninterpretable tests need to be retested either by the same or a different method. Whether the test produces the same answer when it is repeated is also an important factor in evaluating its usefulness.

After the accuracy of a diagnostic test has been evaluated, its effectiveness in practice on reducing morbidity or mortality also must be assessed. The same types of research designs as discussed in the section, Types of Research Designs, can be used for such an assessment. The previously described advantages and disadvantages of each type of design are also present when examining the association between undergoing the test and developing the disease or dying from it. In a prospective study the death rate from a disease can be compared in those who have had the diagnostic test compared to those who have not. In a case-control study, persons with and without the disease can be compared on the basis of whether or not they have had the test. The comparability of cases and controls, as well as those selecting to have the test done or not in a cohort design, can lead to biases that can affect a comparison. To avoid these problems, the best way of evaluating a diagnostic test is to carry out a prospective randomized trial. Persons would be randomized either to receive or not receive the diagnostic test. Such trials, however, may not be possible because of the length of time needed to carry them out, costs, and ethical considerations. Thus the possible biases in the nonexperimental approaches must be recognized.

SUMMARY

The goal of research studies, both observational and experimental, is to identify risk factors for disease. Once identified, the importance of the risk factor needs to be evaluated both in terms of impact on populations as well as on individuals. Different measures of risk (relative risk, odds ratio, and attributable risk) have been defined. A key point in the evaluation of the accuracy and usefulness of diagnostic tests is that the predictive value of the test is dramatically affected by the population to which it is applied. The usefulness of a diagnostic test also depends on the presence of any biases during comparison of the test to the gold standard and application of the test in a new population.

The principles discussed in this chapter should assist the clinician in interpreting diagnostic tests and assessing the credibility of published epidemiologic and medical studies.

REFERENCES

1. Altman DG: *Practical statistics for medical research,* London, 1991, Chapman and Hall.
2. Angell M: The interpretation of epidemiologic studies, editorial, *N Engl J Med* 323:823-825, 1990.
3. Barnett HJM, et al: Are the results of the extracranial-intracranial bypass trial generalizable? Special report, *N Engl J Med* 316:820-824, 1987.
4. Begg CB: Biases in the assessment of diagnostic tests, *Stat Med* 6:411-423, 1987.
5. Berkson J: Limitations of the application of fourfold table analysis to hospital data, *Biometrics Bull* 2:47-53, 1946.
6. Bourke GJ, Daly LE, McGilvary J: *Interpretation and uses of medical statistics,* ed 3, Oxford, 1985, Blackwell Scientific Publications.
7. Brittain E, Wittes J: Factorial designs in clinical trials: the effects of non-compliance and subadditivity, *Stat Med* 8:161-171, 1989.
8. Campbell MJ, Machin D: *Medical statistics: a commonsense approach,* New York, 1990, John Wiley and Sons.
9. Churg A, et al: Lung asbestos content in chrysotile workers with mesothelioma, *Am Rev Respir Dis* 130:1042-1045, 1984.
10. Cornfield J: A method of estimating comparative rates from clinical data. Applications to cancer of the lung, breast and cervix, *J Natl Cancer Inst* 11:1269-1275, 1951.
11. Dawber TR: *The Framingham Study: the epidemiology of atherosclerotic disease,* Cambridge, 1980, Harvard University Press.
12. Erdreich LS, Lee ET: Use of relative operating characteristic analysis in epidemiology, *Am J Epidemiol* 114:649-662, 1981.
13. Ferris Jr BG, et al: Effects of sulfur oxides and respirable particles on human health: methodology and demography of populations in study, *Am Rev Respir Dis* 120:767-779, 1979.
14. Fletcher RH, Fletcher SW, Wagner EH: *Clinical epidemiology: the essentials,* Baltimore, 1981, Williams & Wilkins.
15. Friedman LM, Furberg CD, DeMets DL: *Fundamentals of clinical trials,* ed 2, Littleton, Mass, 1985, PSG Publishing Company.
16. Galen RS, Gambino SR: *Beyond normality: the predictive value and efficiency of medical diagnosis,* New York, 1975, John Wiley and Sons.
17. Goldring S, Zervas N, Langfitt T: The extracranial-intracranial bypass study: a report of the committee appointed by the American Association of Neurological Surgeons to examine the study, *N Engl J Med* 316(13):817-820, 1987.
18. Grady D, Ernster V: Does cigarette smoking make you ugly and old? *Am J Epidemiol* 135(8):839-842, 1992.
19. Griner PF, et al: Selection and interpretation of diagnostic tests and procedures: principles and applications. *Ann Intern Med* 94:553-600, 1981.
20. Hennekens CH, Buring JE: *Epidemiology in medicine,* Boston, 1987, Little, Brown.
21. Herbst AL, Ulfelder H, Poskanzer DC: Adenocarcinoma of the vagina: association of maternal stilbestrol therapy with tumor appearance in young women, *N Engl J Med* 284:878, 1974.
22. Ingelfinger JA, et al: *Biostatistics in clinical medicine,* ed 2, New York, 1987, MacMillan.
23. Kahn HA, Sempos CT: *Statistical methods in epidemiology,* New York, 1989, Oxford University Press.
24. Lipid Research Clinics Program: The Lipid Research Clinics Coronary Primary Prevention Trial results. I. Reduction in incidence of coronary heart disease, *JAMA* 251:351-364, 1984.
25. Louis TA, et al: Crossover and self-controlled designs in clinical research, *N Engl J Med* 310:24-31, 1984.
26. Meinert CL: *Clinical trials: design, conduct and analysis,* New York, 1989, Oxford University Press.
27. Metz CE: Basic principles of ROC analysis, *Semin Nucl Med* 8:283-298, 1978.
28. Meyer KB, Pauker SG: Screening for HIV: can we afford the false positive rate? *N Engl J Med* 317:238-241, 1987.
29. Miettinen OS: Estimability and estimation in case-referent studies, *Am J Epidemiol* 103:226-235, 1976.
30. Pekkanen J, et al: Ten-year mortality from cardiovascular disease in relation to cholesterol level among men with and without preexisting cardiovascular disease, *N Engl J Med* 322:1700-1707, 1990.

31. Peto R, et al: Design and analysis of randomized clinical trials requiring prolonged observation of each patient. I. Introduction and design, *Br J Cancer* 34:585-612, 1976. II. Analysis and examples, *Br J Cancer* 35:1-39, 1977.

32. Ransohoff DF, Feinstein AR: Problems of spectrum and bias in evaluating the efficacy of diagnostic tests, *Med Decis Making* 2:285-302, 1982.

33. Sackett DL: Bias in analytic research, *J Chronic Dis* 32:51-63, 1979.

34. Sackett DL, Haynes RB, Tugwell P: *Clinical epidemiology: a basic science for clinical medicine,* Boston, 1985, Little, Brown.

35. Schlesselman JJ: *Case-controlled studies: design, conduct, analysis,* New York, 1982, Oxford University Press.

36. Steering Committee of the Physicians' Health Study Research Group: Final report on the aspirin component of the ongoing Physicians' Health Study, *N Engl J Med* 321:129-135, 1989.

37. The Modification of Diet in Renal Disease Study Group, prepared by: Beck GJ et al: Design and statistical issues of the Modification of Diet in Renal Disease Trial, *Controlled Clin Trials* 12:566-586, 1991.

38. Thun MJ, Namboodiri BS, Heath Jr CW: Aspirin use and reduced risk of fatal colon cancer, *N Engl J Med* 325(23):1593-1596, 1991.

39. US Department of Health and Human Services: Vanguard Clinical Centers for the Clinical Trial and Observational Study of the Women's Health Initiative (RFP NIH-WH-92-19), *NIH Guide Grants Contracts* 21(15):1-2, 1992.

40. Valenstein PN: Evaluating diagnostic tests with imperfect standards, *Am J Clin Pathol* 93:252-258, 1990.

41. Wacholder S, et al: Selection of controls in case-control studies. I. Principles, *Am J Epidemiol* 135:1019-1028, 1992; II. Types of controls, *Am J Epidemiol* 135:1029-1041, 1992; III. Design options, *Am J Epidemiol* 135:1042-1050, 1992.

42. Walter SD, et al: The association of cutaneous malignant melanoma and fluorescent light exposure, *Am J Epidemiol* 135:749-762 1992.

43. Wynder EL, Stellman SD: The "over-exposed" control group. Review and commentary, *Am J Epidemiol* 135:459-461, 1992.

44. Zeger SL: Statistical reasoning in epidemiology, *Am J Epidemiol* 134:1062-1066, 1991.

RESOURCES

Altman DG: *Practical statistics for medical research,* London, 1991, Chapman and Hall.

Bourke GJ, Daly LE, McGilvary J: *Interpretation and uses of medical statistics,* ed 3, Oxford, 1985, Blackwell Scientific Publications.

Campbell MJ, Machin D: *Medical statistics: a common-sense approach,* New York, 1990, John Wiley and Sons.

Fletcher RH, Fletcher SW, Wagner EH: *Clinical epidemiology: the essentials,* Baltimore, 1981, Williams & Wilkins.

Galen RS, Gambino SR: *Beyond normality: the predictive value and efficiency of medical diagnosis,* New York, 1975, John Wiley and Sons.

Hennekens CH, Buring JE: *Epidemiology in medicine,* Boston, 1987, Little, Brown.

Ingelfinger JA, et al: *Biostatistics in clinical medicine,* ed 2, New York, 1987, MacMillan.

Kahn HA, Sempos CT: *Statistical methods in epidemiology,* New York, 1989, Oxford University Press.

Meinert CL. *Clinical trials: design, conduct and analysis,* New York, 1989, Oxford University Press.

Peto R, et al: Design and analysis of randomized clinical trials requiring prolonged observation of each patient. I. Introduction and design, *Br J Cancer* 34:585-612, 1976. II. Analysis and examples, *Br J Cancer* 35:1-39, 1977.

Sackett DL: Bias in analytic research, *J Chronic Dis* 32:51-63, 1979.

Sackett DL, Haynes RB, Tugwell P: *Clinical epidemiology: a basic science for clinical medicine,* Boston, 1985, Little, Brown.

Schlesselman JJ: *Case-controlled studies: design, conduct, analysis,* New York, 1982, Oxford University Press.

Chapter 7

PROACTIVE AND PREVENTIVE LABORATORY MEDICINE

Frederick Van Lente

The role of the clinical laboratory in the practice of preventive medicine can be defined in relation to two major goals: (1) to assess the risk of future disease and (2) to detect occult disease not evident by history or physical examination. Smaller yet important roles are the confirmation of suspected disease and the monitoring of chronic disease and the medications used to treat them.

The correct assessment of laboratory test performance requires a review of the statistical tools used to quantify test diagnostic efficiency and the concepts of informational content. These concepts will enhance any rational approach to the use of laboratory resources.

TEST PERFORMANCE CRITERIA

The ability of a given laboratory test to effectively yield the diagnostic information asked of it varies dramatically by test, disease, and clinical setting. The five principal concepts involved are the following:

1. Sensitivity—The positivity of a test in the presence of the disease under consideration.
2. Specificity—The negativity of a test in the absence of the disease under consideration.
3. Positive predictive value—The probability that a positive test result indicates that the patient has the disease under consideration.
4. Negative predictive value—The probability that a negative test result indicates that the patient does not have the disease under consideration.
5. Efficiency—The percentage or fraction of test results that correctly indicates the presence or absence of disease.

These concepts have become central to any discussion of the value of a given laboratory test and are particularly important when tests are used in screening and outpatient settings. Clearly, it is desirable for a test to be sensitive and

to detect all cases of a disease that it is meant to signal and to be specific to that disease and thus not confusing or confounding. The corresponding predictive values are derived from sensitivity and specificity:

$$\text{positive predictive value} = \frac{\text{true positives}}{\text{true positives} + \text{false positives}}$$

$$\text{negative predictive value} = \frac{\text{true negatives}}{\text{true negatives} + \text{false negatives}}$$

These equations introduce another factor, prevalence. Prevalence refers to the actual prevalence of the disease in question in the population being tested—that is, the ratio of the sum of true positives and false negatives to the total number of individuals tested.

The prevalence of disease is the major determinant of test effectiveness when laboratory analyses are used in the outpatient or preventive health setting. This point cannot be overemphasized because many users of laboratory tests do not distinguish the various testing environments—outpatient symptomatic, outpatient asymptomatic, elective surgery screen, or emergent. It would seem both obvious and highly desirable to use different test batteries in various populations, depending on their characteristics.

The prevalence of disease in the preventive health setting is naturally low and in some cases extremely low. This testing is equivalent to finding the "needle in the haystack." Despite some variation in these prevalence rates by location and ethnicity, they still more than suffice as guides.

The influence of prevalence on the effectiveness of laboratory tests is best illustrated by example. Let us assume that a given laboratory test exhibits both a sensitivity and specificity of 0.95 for detecting disease D when the test value is above the upper limit of the reference interval (normal range). This type of evaluation is actually a simple 2 × 2 table. Table 7-1, A shows these results at a prev-

Table 7-1. Effect of prevalence in laboratory test effectiveness

A.

	Test positive	Test negative	Total
Diseased	475	25	500
Nondiseased	25	475	500
Total	500	500	1000

B.

	Test positive	Test negative	Total
Diseased	9	1	10
Nondiseased	50	940	990
Total	59	941	1000

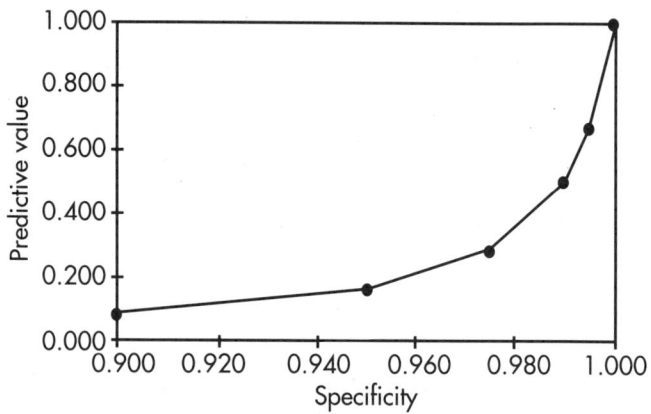

Fig. 7-1. The effect of specificity on predictive value. The prevalence of disease = 0.01, and the test sensitivity = 0.95.

alence of disease of 0.5. That is, half of the patients tested suffer from the disease. It can be seen that of the positive results, 475 are true positives but 25 are false-positive results. This test also failed to detect 25 patients with disease. A patient who presents with a test value above our discriminating limit as shown in the table, therefore, will have a 0.95 probability of having the disease in question, whereas an individual with a normal result will have a 0.95 probability of not having the disease. These numbers do not appear unreasonable and show the equivalency of sensitivity and predictive value when the disease prevalence = 0.5.

Table 7-1, *B* illustrates the use of the same test and interpretations used in Table 7-1, *A* with the exception that the prevalence of disease in the tested clinical population has decreased to 1%. Here it can be seen that of the total of 59 positive or abnormal results, 9 are true positives and 50 are false positives. Thus only 15% of the abnormal results indicate disease. If the prevalence of disease decreases to 0.1%, then only 2% of abnormal results are true positives. The percentage of abnormal results that are true positives is the predictive value of that test result.

The preceding examples illustrated the devastating effect low disease prevalence has on the true effectiveness of laboratory testing at a given degree of sensitivity and specificity. This effect is dominated by the effect of specificity. That is, specificity is the dominant concern in the majority of situations where laboratory tests are used to screen for significant pathology, especially cancer. Fig. 7-1 illustrates the effect of specificity on predictive value at a given prevalence rate of 1%. As disease prevalences approach those seen in the preventive medicine setting, the test specificity must approach perfection (1.0) before predictive values approach comfortable levels. This concept will be developed later in this chapter when specific tests and screening programs are discussed.

The information contained in the laboratory test results obtained in the preventive health setting can be improved by other means as well. These intuitive approaches, used by many in clinical practices, are still underemphasized in formal treatments of the subject. They include the strength of the signal, confirmatory testing, and pattern analysis.

When a patient presents with a given laboratory test result, it is often interpreted on an "asterisk basis," that is, normal or abnormal (positive or negative). In fact, most of the predictive value concepts just reviewed are actually designed for qualitative, positive/negative, binary classification of results. Most laboratory results, however, are continuous and can demonstrate a strength of signal. Thus some test results are worse or more abnormal than others. Stated another way, the sensitivity, specificity, and predictive value of laboratory findings change with the degree of abnormality. Fig. 7-2 shows the predictive value (probability) of a patient having suffered a myocardial infarction after open heart surgery as a function of how high the creatine kinase MB activity was on the morning after surgery.

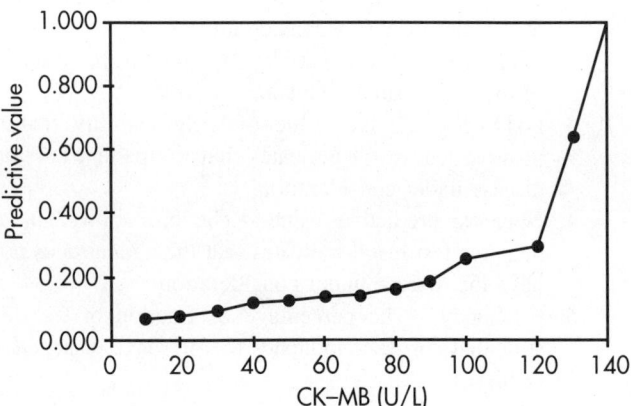

Fig. 7-2. The predictive value of creatine kinase MB isoenzyme for myocardial infarction as a function of activity or strength of signal.

It can be seen clearly that the likelihood of disease increases significantly as the laboratory "signal" for infarction increases. This same relationship exists for most laboratory tests in most circumstances. In particular, test results that reflect pathologic alteration of, or release from, reserves can signal the severity of disease by their degree of change from normality. This pattern holds true for enzymes, hemoglobin, and electrolytes.

The lack of specificity of a relatively sensitive test can be overcome by efficient confirmation by a relatively specific test. This approach to "combination testing" is a variation on combining probabilities; that is, as more indicators become "positive," the likelihood of disease increases. This concept is illustrated in Table 7-2 using a hypothetical screening test with a sensitivity/specificity of 0.99/ 0.80, a confirming test with a sensitivity/specificity of 0.80/0.99, respectively, and a disease prevalence of 0.01 or 1%. The probability that a patient with positive results for the screening test has a given disease is 0.048, but climbs to 0.80 if the confirmatory test is also positive. This approach fails to detect disease in two individuals while correctly classifying 196 initial positive healthy individuals.

The preceding discussion raises the question of why both tests are not performed simultaneously in this type of situation. The answer is multifactorial. First, the confirmatory test is often elaborate, expensive, and inaccessible. The cited criteria for testing in a screening context will be discussed in further detail later, but economics and logistics are major factors. The delay in result availability can also affect adversely the medical decision-making process. If the laboratory test is used to detect a significant disease, such as cancer, knowledge of an initial false-positive result before knowledge of a subsequent true negative confirmatory result can cause great anxiety for the patient. These issues are currently paramount in certain screening con-

Table 7-2. Combination testing: the effect on test result predictability

	Test pos	Test neg	Total
Diseased	10	0	10
Nondiseased	198	792	990
Total	208	792	1000

Plus confirmatory test sensitivity/specificity = 0.80/0.99

	Both tests pos	Second test neg	Total
Diseased	8	2	10
Nondiseased	2	196	198
Total	10	198	208

Screening test sensitivity/specificity = 0.99/0.80.
Number of individuals = 1000.
Prevalence of disease = 0.01.

Screening: the confirmatory pairs of laboratory tests

Screen	Confirm
HIV* antibody	Western blot
Metanephrines	VMA*/catecholamines
LDH*	LDH* isoenzymes
Total protein	Protein electrophoresis
Thyroxin	Thyroid stimulating hormone
Zinc protoporphyrin	Lead
Drugs—immunoassay	Drugs—GC/MS*

*HIV, human immunodeficiency virus; VMA, vanillylmandelic acid; LDH, lactate dehydrogenase; GC/MS, gas chromatography/mass spectrometry.

texts and will be discussed later in this chapter, but the above box lists examples of combinations of screening/ confirmatory tests.

Another variation of the combination testing theme is the use of multiple organ/system specific test results to arrive at a more specific diagnosis. This constellation of findings is often referred to as a pattern of results that is consistent with a certain disease state. This approach was promulgated in the late 1960s by advocates of the multitest automated clinical laboratory analyzers now in general use in both clinical chemistry and hematology. As will be discussed later, it remains doubtful if this modality is really useful in the asymptomatic patient using one test panel other than in the differential diagnosis of anemia. Nonetheless, some of these patterns have become part of the medical jargon including "microcytic anemia" or "macrocytic anemia."

NORMAL RANGE

Much of what has been discussed in the previous section assumed that a given laboratory result was compared to a reference limit of values given for apparently healthy individuals. The adequacy of the normal range concept is often criticized. Several factors affect the accuracy of these ranges as provided by many laboratories. They are often gleaned from textbooks or manufacturer's information sheets by laboratories without the resources to validate their own ranges. This practice may be restricted by new federal laboratory regulations. They also may have been derived from populations with markedly different demographics than the population being tested. They may not be current with respect to the laboratory methods in use (i.e., historical ranges). Finally, they may have been derived using the wrong statistical tools.

There seem to be no rules for normal range derivation. In the first place, who is actually normal? There are elegant lists of multiple definitions for normal, even in the medical context, but these are not totally satisfying when trying to decide the correct application of laboratory tests in a preventive health setting. In fact, in this context, the use of the word *normal* is entirely misplaced because these individuals are often used to generate the ranges in the first place. Most experts have advocated the use of the term *reference interval* instead of *normal range*. In the outpatient setting this is quite appropriate because in the absence of overt disease detected independently, the screening population's inherent laboratory test result distribution is used to identify those individuals whose results are unusual. These *outliers* are just that, and their results have little to do with the detection of disease in their cohort population. Instead, the possibility of existent pathology is inferred from other cohort populations who have a higher prevalence of disease. Sometimes this works; sometimes it doesn't.

The distribution of laboratory results obtained in individuals without disease depends on several factors. The clinician using the clinical laboratory should be aware of these factors in order to initiate informed dialogue with the provider of services when questions arise regarding these ranges. The most important factors, age and sex, strongly influence many metabolic parameters such as hemoglobin, uric acid, phosphorus, bilirubin, alkaline phosphatase, urea nitrogen, creatinine, and creatinine clearance. Genetics may influence other parameters, often between ethnic groups.

The adequate delineation of reference intervals into even age/sex groups is rare outside of the largest laboratory facilities. The reason is simple. It requires an extremely large population and database to establish ranges with confidence (150 or more individuals) when categorizing by sex and age decade (27,000 results). Even these numbers would not suffice for the pediatric population when significant changes occur within decades. It is not surprising, therefore, that these ranges are often estimations at best.

The distribution of data in reference and, therefore, in health maintenance populations exhibits many forms. Occasionally, data conform to the infamous normal (gaussian) distribution and usually reflects passive forces that dictate the usual values found in individuals. Examples include many diet-dependent analytes such as potassium. More often the distribution is either kurtotic (peaked) or skewed (trailing) because of various factors. Fig. 7-3 shows a distribution of serum bilirubin values obtained in a male preventive health population without obvious evidence of liver disease or hemolysis. This distribution is clearly skewed to higher values. Kurtotic distributions are often seen in blood analytes, which are under hormonal or neurologic control. Total calcium concentration and osmolality in serum demonstrate this type of distribution.

Data distributions can significantly affect the use of laboratory tests in the outpatient setting when the upper limit of normal is not established properly. The infamous mean plus and minus two standard deviations range (parametric method) is only accurate for normally distributed data. If, for example, the data are strongly skewed to higher values

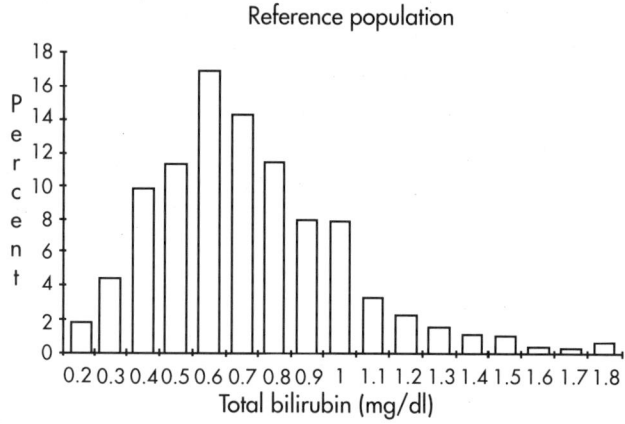

Fig. 7-3. The distribution of total bilirubin values in an apparently healthy male population.

and parametric methods are used to set the upper limit, then an inordinate number of healthy individuals will be classified by testing as abnormal because the statistical method will underestimate the upper limit. Only ranking methods (nonparametric) should be used whenever the distribution of values in the reference population is unusual.

What does the reference (normal) range dictate about the other individuals tested by the same method and whose data are compared with the original distribution? The answer depends on what the range describes (or is thought to describe). The apparent absolute standard is that because the range was calculated as mean $\pm$ 2 SD, the range encompasses the central 95% of the population. Thus 2.5% of the population must be not sick above and below this range. This criterion automatically results in a test specificity of not greater than 0.975 when the upper limit of this range is used to discriminate diseased from nondiseased patients. This statistical fact has led to the widely accepted practice of ignoring "slightly abnormal" test results. In addition, individuals exhibiting initial laboratory values at or near the limit of the reference range will often retest within the range.[22,30] This phenomenon is also well known and results from both the imprecision of the method and the statistical reality of regression to the mean.

A more controversial concept is the potential value of the normal result in many clinical settings. To the extent that a given laboratory test has an acceptable diagnostic sensitivity and, therefore, an acceptable negative predictive value, this concept has merit. In this interpretation of normal or negative laboratory results, the probability of disease is low, which allows the physician to make more effective medical decisions, especially if faced with multiple problems or possible diagnoses. In other words the normal result can allow ruling out and focus.

STANDARD LABORATORY INVESTIGATIONS

The evolution of the standard practice in most current medical situations has resulted in the widespread application of well-accepted panels of laboratory tests, a process aided immensely by the development of medical technology. The commonly available test groupings used in general outpatient testing environments include the ubiquitous chemistry panel, the complete blood count, and urinalysis. These tests are often used in an unselective, surveillance manner in populations where the prevalence of most diseases is quite low. Given the previous discussion of test efficiency, it is worthwhile to extend these principles to the specific application of multicomponent chemistry test panels. It has been stated that if the normal range for a component of a test panel has been established using a central 95th percentile technique (mean $\pm$ 2 standard deviations), then 5% of healthy individuals will be outside this range or abnormal. If n tests in a panel are assumed to be statistically independent, then the probability that a normal person will exhibit at least one abnormality is $(0.95)^n$. This statistical fact can have dramatic results. On a 20-test panel, this probability is 64%. On a six-test panel, the probability is 26%. In other words, the more tests performed, the greater the chance of a false-positive result. For this reason unnecessary tests should not be performed regardless of the economics. The fact that this effect may not be as evident is a reflection of the application of wider normal ranges and the fact that not all analytes behave randomly.

The use of these test panels in a screening mode is assumed to be valuable to detect physiologic aberrations that signal pathologic conditions. This approach, however, should satisfy effectiveness criteria, including the detection of otherwise latent disease, cost effectiveness, effectiveness of early treatment, cost/risk of misclassification, and the societal burden of targeted diseases.[6]

These concerns should be kept in mind during the following discussion, which considers the value of testing of an ambulatory asymptomatic population. Although the rationale and problems associated with selected examples of components of these standard test packages are described, an exhaustive discussion of all possible test components will not be attempted. Several useful resource references pertaining to the use of a wide variety of laboratory tests are listed at the end of this chapter.

Much of the data presented here were gathered during a joint project between the Departments of Biochemistry and Preventive Medicine at The Cleveland Clinic Foundation.[36] The patient population consisted of persons (principally executives) seen for periodic health examinations in preventive medicine who "presumed themselves well." One goal of the project was to determine the most cost-effective screening panel that could be used and accepted by patients and client corporations.

The automated chemistry profile

This section focuses on the chemistry panel as an example of the limitations of this type of laboratory testing. The box lists the usual components of chemistry test panels and

---

Common components of the chemistry panel	
Test	*System*
Total protein	Plasma cell
Albumin	Liver/kidney
Bilirubin	RBC/liver
Uric acid	Joints/kidney
Urea nitrogen	Vascular/kidney
Creatinine	Kidney
Sodium	Kidney/hormonal
Potassium	
Carbon dioxide	
Chloride	
Calcium	Kidney/bone/hormonal
Enzymes*	
CK	Muscle
LD	Muscle, liver, bone
AST	Muscle, liver
ALT	Liver
Alk Phos	Liver/bone

*CK, creatine kinase; LD, lactate dehydrogenase; AST, aspartate aminotransferase; ALT, alanine aminotransferase; Alk Phos, alkaline phosphatase.

the systems evaluated. These tests exhibit a variety of organ specificities and degrees of overlap with each other. This chapter does not review extensively the general medical uses for all of these tests but rather emphasizes appropriate expectations of the usual practice of representative tests. The tests offered are grouped together usually as a result of history and technology.

The evaluation of test performance in the health maintenance environment can be directly addressed by examining the abnormality rates in a typical executive health setting (Table 7-3). If a central 95% range of normal has

Table 7-3. Abnormality rates for standard tests in 5285 unselected executive outpatients

Test	Limit	No.	%
Bilirubin	1.5 mg/dl	218	4.1
Potassium	5.0 mmol/L	322	6.1
Glucose	120 mg/dl	292	5.5
AST*	40 U/L	153	2.9
Sodium	145 mmol/L	21	0.4
Uric Acid	8.0 mg/dl	275	5.2
Urea nitrogen	2.5 mg/dl	90	1.7
Creatinine	1.4 mg/dl	58	1.1
LD*	190 U/L	110	2.1
Alk Phos*	110 U/L	25	0.5
Total Protein	8.0 g/L	100	1.9
Calcium	10.5 mg/dl	29	0.6
	8.5	18	0.3

*AST, aspartate phosphatase; LD, lactate dehydrogenase; Alk Phos, alkaline phosphatase.

been used, the expected rate of abnormality should approach 2.5% at each limit. The degree of abnormality shown in Table 7-3 varies, but only a few tests reflect an abnormality rate expected given the 95% assumption. In fact, the limits could be thought to be both too restrictive and too generous.

When the frequency of abnormality approaches that seen in the reference population, the justification of the testing program becomes difficult. It can still be argued that the disease in question, for example myeloma, is significant enough that the single case found could justify the testing of thousands of nondiseased individuals if it led to an improved outcome, financial considerations notwithstanding. Some credence can be given these arguments provided a concerted effort is made to remove tests from panels when they simply provide no incremental information. From Table 7-3, this judgment could be made for sodium and other electrolytes except potassium, urea nitrogen, calcium, alkaline phosphatase, total protein, and creatinine.

The discovery of occult disease has become the standard for including some tests, and their exclusion from standard test panels cannot be easily defended regardless of the incidence of abnormalities and the prevalence of disease.[19] The best example of this situation is serum total calcium. It has been well documented that the discovery of incidence cases of primary hyperparathyroidism is affected by biochemical screening alone. This basic fact has remained unaltered since the community study reported by investigators at the Mayo Clinic in 1980.[15] Recently, a surgical study reemphasized the role of total calcium when compared with the confirmatory assay of parathyroid hormone.[5]

Glucose. Glucose remains a generally accepted component of the chemistry assessment profile. Provided that the individual has fasted sufficiently, this assay does provide information concerning the presence of diabetes. The prevalence of undiagnosed type II diabetics in the general adult population is about 3%, and this frequency warrants general testing.[7,31] The criteria for confirming the diagnosis of diabetes or impaired glucose tolerance using laboratory tests are straightforward.[14]

We have found that single, increased fasting serum glucose determination to be of unpredictable significance in an unselected, adult outpatient population. Repeat determinations of fasting serum glucose were in the same range as the initial value in only 55% of individuals with borderline high values and 61% of those with high screening values. The probability that the repeat value would be within the reference interval, however, was only 14% to 38%. In those with a borderline high screening value, there was a nearly equal distribution between normal, impaired, and diabetic glucose tolerance. Of those with a high screening value, only 75% showed confirmatory diabetic glucose tolerance.[13] Not surprisingly, use of just an initial value as a

guide to diagnosis would lead to misclassification of both diabetics and nondiabetics. Approximately 30% of those with borderline high initial glucose values are found to be diabetic by performance of a subsequent oral glucose tolerance, and 25% of patients with high initial values subsequently exhibited a normal oral glucose tolerance (false positives).

Hemoglobin A_{1c} concentrations have limited utility as an adjunct to the diagnosis of diabetes.[13,31] Although statistically significant differences on Hgb A_{1c} concentrations have been found in patients with initially high versus normal glucose values, there is a generally low incidence of abnormally increased values in these populations. Of patients with borderline high initial values, only 3% have increased concentrations of Hgb A_{1c}.[13] This percentage contrasts with the much higher rate of diabetic glucose tolerance in these patients.

Bilirubin. Total bilirubin is a common component of biochemical profiles. Screening for hyperbilirubinemia is further complicated by the relatively common benign Gilbert's syndrome. Fig. 7-3 shows the distribution of total bilirubin values from the reference population. It is evident that total bilirubin fails to exhibit a gaussian distribution and is skewed toward higher values. The reference interval for this population was found to be 0.3 mg/dl to 1.5 mg/dl using a nonparametric rank numbers procedure.

Of 3641 male subjects tested in a study of bilirubin values, 137 exhibited an increased total bilirubin concentration on their biochemical profile. Bilirubin values ranged from 1.6 mg/dl to 3.7 mg/dl. The distribution frequency appeared to be an extension of that shown in Fig. 7-3, and there was no evidence for a bimodal distribution. None of these subjects had an elevation of conjugated bilirubin (> 0.4 mg/dl), and the majority had nondetectable levels.

More than 80% of subjects with hyperbilirubinemia on a chemistry profile had Gilbert's syndrome. Mean values for serum haptoglobin, reticulocyte count (percent and absolute), hemoglobin, and hematocrit did not differ significantly from the remainder of the screening population. About three fourths of these individuals had exhibited additional elevations of total bilirubin within the previous 2 years. The mean difference between consecutive bilirubin determinations was 0.18 ± 0.5 mg/dl. These findings are consistent with the chronic hyperbilirubinemia associated with Gilbert's syndrome. It is noteworthy that individuals only rarely state a history consistent with chronic hyperbilirubinemia.

An increased total bilirubin in a health maintenance population can also indicate intravascular hemolysis often due to a malfunctioning prosthetic heart valve, but these patients do not usually exhibit anemia. Since reticulocytosis is not uniformly present, these individuals are either fully compensated or the haptoglobin depression is falsely positive.

A small percentage of individuals exhibited abnormality

in at least one liver enzyme activity, but rarely exhibited clinical findings consistent with liver dysfunction. Some of the others reported a history of alcohol ingestion. The clinical significance of the majority of these laboratory abnormalities was doubtful.

Based on the laboratory test result classification of individuals, the predictive value of an elevated total bilirubin on a screening biochemical profile for Gilbert's syndrome, hemolysis, or liver dysfunction is about 81%, 5%, and 14%, respectively. In our experience, clinically apparent symptomatology (hepatomegaly) related to hyperbilirubinemia was present in less than 2% of patients with an elevated total bilirubin.

Investigation of elevated total bilirubin in sera of individuals undergoing health examination has demonstrated that the majority apparently have Gilbert's syndrome by diagnosis of exclusion (i.e., no evidence for liver or hemolytic disease or other cause). The apparent prevalence of Gilbert's syndrome has been reported to be up to 6%.[3,28] We have found it to be about 3%. The variation in prevalence is undoubtedly a result of variations in reference intervals applied for total bilirubin because these patients do not exhibit signs or symptoms of disease and are easily included in "normal" populations used to determine reference intervals. Other chronic, unconjugated hyperbilirubinemia syndromes, Grigler-Najjar types I and II, are rare, less benign, and detected clinically. It has been argued that Gilbert's syndrome should not be considered a "condition" but rather an extension of normality.[3] Interestingly, bilirubin has recently been shown to exhibit potentially beneficial antioxidant activity.[33] Extrapolating this finding would suggest that individuals with Gilbert's syndrome may be at lower risk for free-radical-induced pathology than those with bilirubin levels within the reference interval. It is not obvious, therefore, what advantage accrues in screening for this condition. Clinically significant causes for hyperbilirubinemia are less common.

Aspartate aminotransferase. As can be seen in Table 7-3, there is a small yet definitive rate of abnormality in the enzyme aspartate aminotransferase (AST) on profiles run on an outpatient population. If the upper limit of the reference interval has been set at a conservative value—99th percentile limit—then these abnormalities may be clinically significant. The nature of these abnormalities may relate to more commonly occurring conditions such as obesity or alcohol abuse, both of which are known to increase aminotransferase activity in serum. In addition, a slight abnormality in AST may signal significant muscle insult secondary to sustained exercise, which is easily confirmed by measuring creatine kinase (CK) activity in serum.

Our studies also have shown that slightly increased AST activity in an apparently healthy outpatient may indicate past exposure to hepatitis B.[35] These patients do not necessarily report a history of hepatitis or jaundice, but they compose about 6% of individuals who present with increased AST activity in a health maintenance setting.

Including a wider selection of serum enzymes on profiles does not seem justified, as fewer abnormalities are discovered than those described earlier. The inclusion of lactate dehydrogenase (LD), for instance, primarily signals any hemolysis of the blood specimen that occurs during sample collection and rarely provides incremental information.

Total protein. Total protein is a component of biochemical test panels used to test an ambulatory population for occult paraproteinemia secondary to plasma cell dyscrasias. Other potential abnormalities of either increased or decreased total protein are essentially consistent with symptoms and case-finding testing. The prevalence of plasmacytomas in the general population is no more than 0.1%. Our investigation of all increased total protein values (>8.0 g/dl) in 5000 consecutive health maintenance visits discovered paraproteinemia by serum protein electrophoresis in two individuals (0.04%). This yield was not improved by also using albumin to calculate the albumin/globulin ratio as an indicator for paraproteinemia. Both cases were found subsequently to have had incipient paraproteins in their serum in previous years, although both their total protein and albumin/globulin ratio values were normal. It remains unclear to what extent patient outcome is improved by the detection of these abnormalities before patients become symptomatic.

BUN/creatinine. The effectiveness of screening for renal dysfunction using blood urea nitrogen (BUN) and creatinine values is unclear. Unfortunately, 50% of an individual's initial glomerular function must be lost before serum creatinine values increase above normal. This insensitivity restricts creatinine's ability to reflect any early negative change in glomerular filtration rate (GFR), which is reflected in the fact that creatinine demonstrates complete diagnostic sensitivity for detecting a GFR of less than 70 ml/min at a concentration of 1.2 mg/dl, albeit at a specificity of 0.85.[37] Of 7947 men seen in a health maintenance setting, only one exhibited a creatinine value above 2.0 mg/dl who was not known to have renal insufficiency. The inclusion of creatinine in biochemical profiles has been justified on the basis of evidence that suggests that early specific therapies are effective in slowing progression of renal dysfunction.[29] Urea nitrogen has not been shown to be superior to creatinine either singly or in combination.[6] Nonetheless, the value of serum creatinine measurement in an ambulatory, healthy population has yet to be verified.

Electrolytes. The inclusion of comprehensive electrolyte testing in chemistry panels used for health maintenance is problematic. The clinical conditions assessed during preventive health encounters are unlikely to involve electrolyte imbalance in any form. Abnormality rates are extremely low, with the possible exception of potassium

(Table 7-3). Potassium alterations are primarily due to the influence of diuretic therapy and are useful in the monitoring of these drug regimens. Nonetheless, if the economics were different, it would make more sense to perform this determination only when warranted by the medical history, that is, when the individual is on potassium-wasting diuretic therapy or presents with muscle pain or weakness. Uric acid abnormalities are secondary to medication in the absence of overt symptoms but also are seen in individuals with a past or familial history of gout. This abnormality may also signal the risk for nephrolithiasis. As discussed earlier, the usual pricing strategies offered by clinical laboratories place a major premium on discrete analyses that are also components of chemistry panels. This problem can discourage appropriate test utilization and, if present, should be a subject of negotiation between the clinical and laboratory services.

Complete blood count

Much of the discussion regarding chemistry panels applies to hematologic panels as well. Again, it is important to keep in mind the diagnostic goals in a low disease prevalence population. The usual expected outcome is the detection of anemia, particularly iron deficiency, and inflammatory processes. The salient parameters evaluated to achieve these goals are the erythrocyte and leukocyte counts, hemoglobin concentration, and red cell indices.

Table 7-4 lists abnormality rates found in an executive health practice for several common hematologic components. The hemoglobin and hematocrit levels were below the lower limit at a frequency expected for a central 95th percentile range. As expected in this type of population, neither the white blood cell count (WBC) nor the mean corpuscular value (MCV) exhibits a significant incidence of abnormal results. Although 75% of decreased MCV was confirmed to represent either thalassemia or iron deficiency, only 15% of increased MCV represented megaloblastic anemias. It would appear that the remainder of cases is a result of toxic changes secondary to alcohol intake or drug regimens. The experience in the preventive health setting is that the entry for investigation of the complete blood count (CBC) was more significantly triggered by a clear abnormality of the MCV because a marked decrease in hemoglobin was rarely seen in an asymptomatic population.

Urinalysis

Urinalysis is one of the major groups of laboratory tests, ranking behind only chemistry profiles and CBCs in the number of tests performed annually in the United States. These urine parameters, measured easily by the "dipstick" method, provide information about the status of the genitourinary system.

Urine is a complex biologic fluid whose composition depends on many factors, some of which are totally unrelated to the presence or risk of pathology. The contents of urine in both healthy and diseased individuals depends on body mass, fluid intake, dietary intake, exercise status, and time of day. Therefore, knowledge of the individual's habits just before collection of either a random or morning void specimen is helpful in interpreting results.

The laboratory examination of urine may now be performed by a wide variety of techniques. These vary from the historical manual techniques of dipstick, centrifuge, and microscope to totally automated, computer-controlled instruments; the latter methods are used in most large laboratories. Discussion of the diagnostic and surveillant uses of urinalysis in the preventive care setting focuses on the diagnosis of urinary tract infections, evaluation of hematuria, and evaluation of proteinuria.

Urinary tract infection. Up to 6% of women are affected by urinary tract infections each year.[10] The first line of evaluation is often urinalysis. If the infection is suspected clinically, the patient should be instructed to collect a midstream clean voided specimen for which appropriate supplies are readily available. The microscopic confirmation of infection includes the presence of red cells, white cells, and bacteria seen under the high-power microscopic field. The finding of bacteria in this examination corresponds to more than 10 organisms/ml of urine upon culturing of the urine, which is the obvious confirmation test procedure.

The screening of asymptomatic individuals for urinary tract infections can be more problematic. A recent review noted that school-aged boys and girls exhibit a prevalence of bacteremia of 0.03% and 1% to 2%, respectively. During mid-life these prevalences rise to 3% to 4% for women and increase further to as high as 10% at age 50. Geriatric patients may have an even higher incidence due to prostate and bladder dysfunction, with an incidence approaching 20% after age 65. These disease prevalences are substantially higher than many that are "screened" by other laboratory tests discussed in this chapter.

Hematuria. Although the presence of as few as 10 red blood cells in urine can signal clinically significant conditions, their presence also can result just from exercise.[4] In

Table 7-4. Abnormality rates for standard hematology tests seen in an executive health program (N = 7919)

Test	Limit	No	%
Hemoglobin	13.5*	173	2.2
Hematocrit	40.0*	194	2.5
WBC	11.0†	139	1.8
RBC	4.5*	586	7.4
MCV	100†	107	1.4
	80*	58	0.7

*Lower lower limit.
†Upper limit.

children 9% to 22% of cases of hematuria were found to be without apparent cause; in adults up to 50% of cases were found to be without apparent cause. Conditions associated with the presence of hematuria include neoplasm, stones, inflammation, and benign prostate hypertrophy.[4]

A well-thought-out diagnosis algorithm has been developed for the investigation of hematuria.[4] Central to this workup is a thorough history and physical examination to rule out specific causes, such as acute glomerulonephritis and abdominal and pelvic masses.

Proteinuria. Healthy adults excrete up to 150 mg of urine each day. About 60% is derived from normal plasma proteins and the remaining 40% is derived from the kidney and genitourinary tract. A variety of proteins are in the urine, including albumin, transferrin, amylase, urokinase, immunoglobin, and mucoprotein. The major components are albumin, mucoprotein, and immunoglobins, which account for about 95% of the total.[20,26]

The presence of excessive proteinuria must be distinguished from the transient proteinuria that results from strenuous exercise, stress, and hypothermia. As implied by its name, transient proteinuria resolves in the absence of the insult. Persistent proteinuria, which may result from either tubular or glomerular renal disease, should be evaluated completely.

The initial finding of proteinuria in the health maintenance setting should be investigated, especially if the individual is asymptomatic. Repeat urinalysis is indicated to determine whether the proteinuria is transient. If proteinuria is persistent and nonorthostatic, then further testing is warranted. Presumably a patient with significant decrement of plasma albumin would not present as an outpatient, but this result is often readily available and can be checked easily. It is also likely that plasma urea and creatinine concentrations are available for review to assess grossly the patient's renal function. Additional laboratory tests can be performed to assess the nature of the proteinuria more precisely. These tests include urine protein electrophoresis and urinary light chains; the latter should always be evaluated when an individual also exhibits an increased serum total protein and proteinuria. Twenty-four-hour urine collection to determine both total daily protein output and creatinine clearance are more useful than the initial random or morning void specimen measurements.

Other possible tests

Several laboratory parameters not usually included in the standard panels may have value in the preventive health setting. The possible selection of these tests for inclusion in a laboratory profile depends on the goals of the clinical service.

Thyroid function tests. Although thyroid disorders are among the more prevalent conditions encountered in the preventive health setting,[16] the inclusion of total thyroxin in standard chemistry profiles has been advocated by only a minority of laboratory scientists. Prevalence of nodular goiter is about 4%. Up to 2% of geriatric women are hypothyroid, and about 0.5% of the general population will contract Grave's disease. The standard explanation for exclusion of thyroxin from chemistry panels is the expense of including an immunoassay in a group of tests that are otherwise relatively inexpensive to perform. There is some truth to this argument, and the cost may justify the exclusion of thyroid testing in the absence of a case-finding scenario, that is, when a patient presents with complaints or exhibits abnormalities at examination or in other laboratory tests. An evaluation of thyroid status using total thyroxin concentrations in serum as part of a chemistry profile to assess a predominantly male population found that 1.4% of individuals exhibited thyroxin values less than 5.0 $\mu g/dl$, and 64% of these were confirmed by increased thyroid-stimulating hormone (TSH) concentrations.[36] That is, they were patients with subclinical hypothyroidism. An additional 1.5% of individuals had thyroxin values greater than 11.2 $\mu g/dl$. Although these abnormality rates are slightly less than expected using a central 95th percentile range, it is clear that thyroid dysfunction can be identified in this type of screening. The typical list price for a thyroid profile without TSH, if ordered when clinically indicated, is about $50.00. The value of not missing an occult case and confirming the thyroid status of all patients is difficult to quantify.[25]

C-reactive protein. C-reactive protein is one of the acute-phase proteins present in serum. Its concentration increases from almost undetectable levels to one-thousand-fold the original concentration in the presence of acute inflammation secondary to many conditions. It is increased abnormally in a wide variety of conditions.[8] Because of this lack of specificity, it is useful only in defined situations. Some have advocated that, similar to the sedimentation rate, C-reactive protein is useful to discriminate the presence of an inflammatory process in otherwise normal individuals.[8] In this regard, C-reactive protein is a test for disease.[8]

Unfortunately, this application of C-reactive protein has not been tested prospectively in studies on an outpatient population. The concentration of C-reactive protein also has been shown to correlate with the clinical course of infectious disease. The success of antimicrobial therapy also can be followed by repeated measurement of C-reactive protein. Nonetheless, the current tests for C-reactive protein are immunoassays and are relatively expensive.

Iron. The incidence of hereditary or idiopathic hemochromatosis is estimated to be 0.3% in the American population, but the carrier or heterozygote frequency is 10%.[27] It is more frequently found in men, who are up to 10 times more likely to have the gene than women, Several laboratory tests can identify the iron overload associated with this condition. The simplest approach is to measure total serum iron as part of the surveillance chemistry profile. In our investigation of the distribution of iron values in a male executive health population, 16 of 2000 (0.8%) patients exhibited serum iron concentrations greater than 200 μg/dl. Of these, eight had repeat measurement that also exceeded 200 μg/dl, and one had clear evidence for hemochromatosis. It has not been demonstrated that unselected screening for hemochromatosis is effective.

Reflex testing

The concept of what has become known as accelerated laboratory investigation was first described by a community hospital pathologist over 15 years ago.[1,2] This approach to profile testing expanded the role of the laboratory profession in an effort to maximize the information that could be provided to the clinician. The process involved simply the performance of additional tests at the discretion of the laboratory or pathologist when certain aforementioned standard chemistry panel tests were abnormal.[1,2] The justifications for this approach are as follows:

- It maximizes the use of blood samples—no need to redraw the patient.
- It accelerates the testing process—does not require completing the total process loop.
- It allows the use of standardized testing algorithms specific for each test and for each diagnostic goal.
- It stimulates professional interactions between clinicians and laboratorians.
- The cost of extra testing can be amortized across all tests—laboratory insurance.
- The program is particularly suited to outpatient settings where the interval between visits is usually prolonged and/or patients must travel significant distances to the site of care.
- The reflex testing algorithms are well suited to computer application and can be easily refined with experience. That is, it is a self-learning system.
- The laboratory can use available clinical information to decide what additional tests to perform.

We have had extensive experience with this type of program, which is termed Programmed Accelerated Laboratory Investigation (PALI), the name coined by the originator.[2] Our system was developed to serve an executive health program whose clientele were seen infrequently, traveled some distance to be seen, and had high expectations of service.[36] In fact, this program initially was seen by patients as a valuable attribute from which they did not wish to be excluded.

Initially, the reflex testing or PALI program was designed to use the institution's generally accepted general laboratory survey as the beginning test basis with the objective of eliminating tests subsequently shown to provide ineffective information. Tests are selected for inclusion in the algorithm test based on the following criteria:

- There are additional tests that can provide incremental information about possible diseases present.
- Abnormalities can be observed in the test in diseases that could be present in the tested (executive outpatient) population.
- Specimens collected allowed the accurate measurement of reflex tests.
- They were indicated by clinical information.

The coordination of the possible diagnostic endpoints and the knowledge of clinicopathologic correlations for the initial tests provide a starting point for the development of an expert computer model to direct the additional reflex test performance. Although this exercise is useful, the process is, in fact, easily accomplished without the use of computers or software provided the algorithms are well thought out. It is the regular and expected constellation of laboratory findings that provides the ultimate benefit in this testing program.

The development of testing algorithms is based on concepts discussed earlier. That is, the initial chemistry and hematology tests are de facto considered to be the most sensitive, and the combinations of confirmatory tests with the initial finding increase the specificity of the laboratory diagnosis. Additional tests are performed sequentially until all possible (reasonable) tests have been performed, the available specimen is exhausted, or a definitive conclusion is reached. The tests on the initial panels deemed unsuitable for reflex testing were characterized by low abnormality rates, absence of confirmatory tests, and limited association with a defined group of diagnoses.

Total bilirubin. The suggested reflex testing and diagnostic algorithm for an increased total bilirubin is shown in Fig. 7-4. This approach is designed to identify the benign hyperbilirubinemia of Gilbert's syndrome, liver dysfunction, or a hemolytic process. The presence of Gilbert's syndrome is suggested by the subsequent finding of both a normal haptoglobin and reticulocyte count. Liver disease is indicated by an increase in any accompanying liver function test, as the number of specific conditions that

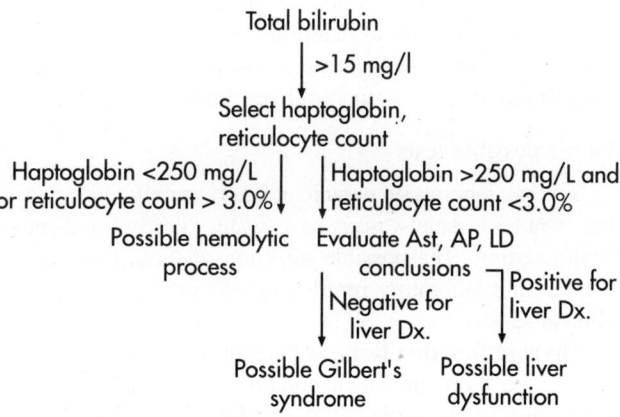

Fig. 7-4. Total bilirubin reflex testing algorithm.

could result in jaundice is substantial.

Total thyroxin. The suggested approach to the abnormal thyroid screen is based on well-accepted thyroid testing algorithms.[16,34] An increased thyroxin concentration is followed by the determination of the free thyroxin index—a decreased thyroxin by thyrotropin measurement. These two arms give reasonable confirmation of the presence of hyperthyroidism and hypothyroidism. Sensitive thyrotropin assay could also be substituted, or added to, for the free thyroxin index to confirm hyperthyroidism. Adequacy of thyroid replacement therapy should be assessed by thyrotropin determinations in patients with a history of hypothyroidism.

Aspartate aminotransferase (SGOT, AST). The testing algorithm for this enzyme determination, often considered just another of the "liver function tests," is shown in Fig. 7-5. As can be seen, this scheme is designed to evaluate the presence of a variety of conditions, not all of which concern the liver. The confirmatory testing is directed toward the identification of conditions that could exist in an ambulatory patient population, including early or late viral hepatitis, alcohol-related liver dysfunction, muscle insult, and unclassified liver inflammation.

The ratio of AST to its companion enzyme alanine aminotransferase (SGPT, ALT) can be used as a differential logic branch for determining what testing direction to take. Quite often ALT is also included on the original chemistry profile, and this step would not require additional testing.

An ALT/AST ratio greater than 1 is consistent with the liver inflammation accompanying viral hepatitis. Although this type of pathology is not at all specific for hepatitis A, B, or C, it is a convenient basis on which to evaluate outpatients, particularly those without symptoms. This approach is also used for surrogate screening of donated blood for the presence of hepatitis C. An AST/ALT ratio of less than 1 indicates the presence of more chronic liver insult, most commonly alcohol-induced, if both parameters are increased abnormally and the confirming enzyme gamma-glutamyl transferase (GT) is also increased. If neither ALT nor GT is increased, then muscle insult must be considered as a source of the increased AST; and the corresponding laboratory tests, including creatine kinase, must be performed to confirm this possibility. It should be noted that hemolysis can increase serum AST activities as well, but is noticeable only in severe hemolytic conditions requiring hospitalization.

Glucose. Increased glucose concentrations should be investigated for the presence of diabetes mellitus. The algorithm required is simple and accounts for the few questions that must be answered. Was the patient fasting? The nonfasting glucose of a normal individual can be increased to above 160 mg/dl. Has the individual exhibited a previously increased serum glucose value? Does the individual have a history of diabetes? This information allows application of the straightforward rules for the diagnosis of dia-

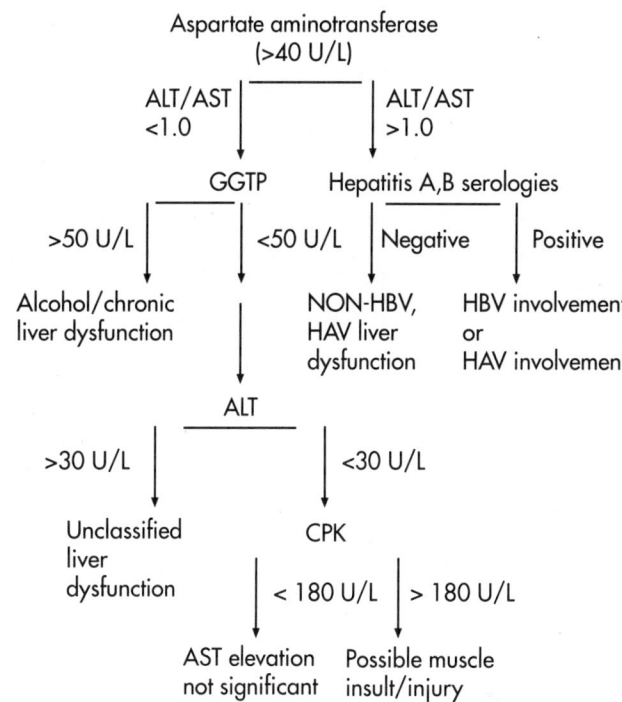

Fig. 7-5. Aspartate aminotransferase reflex testing algorithm.

betes promulgated by the National Diabetes Data Group or the World Health Organization[14] as discussed earlier. It is appropriate to include reflex determination of hemoglobin A_{1c} values in patients with known diabetes mellitus to assess control of hyperglycemia.

Algorithms for assessing hypoglycemia are based on criteria for the diagnosis of insulinoma and should include both the insulin concentration and the insulin/glucose ratio. Other causes of decreased glucose concentrations, such as severe alcoholism, are usually associated with significant disease and are not often encountered in preventive medicine populations.

Total calcium. The association of increased calcium values with primary hyperthyroidism has been previously discussed, and the algorithm of laboratory tests that should be used to confirm the presence of this disease follows.[23,24] The subsequent measurement of ionized calcium will confirm the presence of true hypercalcemia, i.e., not a result of an increased serum albumin. This measurement should be followed by the determination of intact parathyroid hormone measurement for final confirmation. On the negative side, several other conditions can result in an increased total calcium concentration in serum. These conditions include sarcoidosis, malignancy, thiazide diuretics, and hypervitaminosis D. The latter condition usually results from administration of preparations containing both 1,25-hydroxyvitamin D and calcium.

Total protein. Increased total protein values should be investigated using serum protein electrophoresis to rule out dysproteinemias. Of these, by far the most important are the multiple myelomas or plasmacytomas. The finding of a paraprotein band on the initial electrophoresis can be followed by immunoelectrophoresis, quantitative immunoglobin analysis, and determination of light chains in urine. The majority of other findings are without significant, specific importance.

Lactate dehydrogenase. Increased lactate dehydrogenase (LDH) activity in serum can result from many causes due to its wide tissue distribution. The significance of an abnormality of this enzyme varies. It is worthwhile to note whether the abnormality is isolated or accompanies increased activities of other enzymes. Thus a testing algorithm follows this logic along with performance of LDH isoenzymes to determine the tissue distribution of activity. It is important to remember that erythrocytes contain considerable amounts of LDH, and a blood sample that is hemolyzed upon collection or handling will exhibit an increased activity. If determination of LDH isoenzymes reveals an increase in the LD-1 or LD-5 fraction, the determination of CK and CK isoenzymes is required in order to determine if either heart or skeletal muscle insult is present. In the absence of a CK abnormality, increased LD-1 requires determination of haptoglobin and reticulocyte count to rule out a hemolytic process, and an increased LD-5 requires evaluation of other liver enzymes (some liver enzyme tests may already be available).

Alkaline phosphatase. An increase in this commonly performed analyte is reputed to be the most false-positive of chemistry profile components. This result is because of historically poor understanding of reference intervals and their appropriate use. As shown in Table 7-3, alkaline phosphatase in our experience was increased abnormally in only 0.5% of individuals when a 99th percentile range was used. Thus although alkaline phosphatase activity in serum can arise from many tissue sources, the laboratory can confirm only two useful conclusions from isoenzyme analysis—bone and liver. Therefore, sequential testing includes this single determination.

Mean corpuscular volume. Investigation of an increased or decreased MCV is based on well-accepted evaluation of anemias. Investigation of either an increased or decreased MCV is based on the traditional evaluation of macrocytic or microcytic anemia.[9,21] Decreased MCV with an increased distribution of erythrocyte widths prompts the confirmation of iron deficiency with measurements of total iron and iron-binding capacity, or ferritin. Decreased MCV with an erythrocyte width distribution less than 15% prompts assessment of thalassemia by determination of hemoglobin A_2 concentration and hemoglobin electrophoresis. An increased MCV can be investigated by determinations of "true" vitamin B_{12} and folic acid concentrations. Interpretations are based on results of all required supplemental determinations plus the hemoglobin concentration. Patients with decreased hemoglobin and normal MCV are assessed in light of serum haptoglobin

Results of monitoring tests in a health maintenance setting		
Diabetes		
Hemoglobin A_{1c}	>6.5%	48
	<6.5%	29
	Total	77
Hypothyroidism		
Thyrotropin [TSH]	>5.5 MU/L	4
	<5.5 MU/L	27
	Total	31
Diuretic therapy		
Potassium	<3.5 mmol/L	16
	>3.5 mmol/L	89
	Total	105
Drug monitoring		
Optimal		9
Suboptimal		14
Supraoptimal		1
Total		24

concentration and reticulocyte count.

Treatment monitoring. If an individual is receiving maintenance medication for a chronic condition, the serum concentration of that drug should be evaluated whenever the desired goals of the medication regimen are not achieved. The medications for which testing is usually available include theophylline, digoxin, and phenytoin. However, the successful evaluation of compliance and therapeutic efficacy by laboratory measurement requires careful assessment of the patient's medication status as part of the history and physical examination.

Treatment of diabetes mellitus and thyroid disease can be followed by the measurement of hemoglobin A_{1c} and thyroid stimulating hormone, respectively. The box above illustrates typical findings of such laboratory monitoring in a health maintenance setting. Although the findings may be consistent with a clinical evaluation, inappropriate values could be overlooked in the absence of testing. These tests are underutilized.

Other profile components. Several components of laboratory test panels do not indicate performance of additional, confirmatory tests. These components include those already in that capacity, such as red cell indices, and those that indicate defined circumstances that other tests do not confirm and those without informational value. Serum uric acid will indicate gout, renal insufficiency, and malignancy; but no additional tests will confirm, for example, the presence of malignancy or gout effectively. The determination of albumin serves little purpose if total protein is also measured. As already mentioned, determination of the albumin/globulin ratio does not improve detection of incipient paraproteinemia.

A listing of observed possible diagnostic yields from these algorithms from 5285 individuals tested is found in Table 7-5. The apparent success of these testing schemes is quite variable due primarily to the determination of the true abnormality rates that occurred once data were collected, retained, and analyzed. This general approach is now used widely for quality assurance purposes and indicates the advantage of retrospective analysis.

It is worthwhile to evaluate the cost of reflexive testing in terms of the testing cost required to identify an individual with a condition that can be identified in the absence of clinical signs or symptoms, that is, based on the laboratory test results alone. The cost of identifying cases of hyperparathyroidism in a health maintenance population by reflex, investigative laboratory testing can be readily determined. Total calcium exceeded 10.5 mg/dl in 33 of 6759 individuals. Normalized ionized calcium or repeat calcium determinations were increased in 20 of these 33 individuals, 5 of whom had increased intact parathyroid hormone values. The total testing cost for finding these cases was $471.20 per case of hyperparathyroidism or $0.35 per screening. At least two of the detected cases subsequently underwent successful surgery for removal of a parathyroid adenoma.

A similar analysis can be formulated for the use of the laboratory investigation of increased AST activity with the intent to identify individuals with occult exposure to hepatitis B. Of 6760 individuals tested, 205 had increased AST activities (above 40 U/L), 114 had AST/ALT ratios less than 1, and nine were hepatitis-serology positive. This testing cost $243 per case identified or $0.32 per screening.

The evaluation of total cost for identifying individuals with thyroid disease includes both cases of hypothyroidism and hyperthyroidism. Of 5267 individuals screened by

Table 7-5. Reflex testing interpretations determined in 5285 executive health patients

Interpretation	No.	% Total
Gilbert's syndrome	193	3.6
Glucose intolerance	160	3.0
Nonviral liver dysfunction	73	1.4
Possible diabetes	59	1.1
Uric acid consistent with thiazide	44	0.8
Alcohol-related liver disease	32	0.6
Possible hemolysis	16	0.3
Muscle insult	14	0.3
Thalassemia minor	11	0.2
Hepatitis B	7	0.1
B_{12}/folate deficiency	6	0.1
Iron deficiency	4	0.08
Hyperparathyroidism	4	0.08
Monoclonal gammopathy	2	0.04

measurement of total thyroxin, 141 exhibited abnormally decreased values and 34 had increased values. Of the former, 15 (0.28%) had increased TSH concentrations, and 27 (0.51%) of the latter had increased free thyroxin values. The cost per case of apparent thyroid disease was $228.14 or $1.82 per initial screening. It is unlikely that the use of newer "sensitive" TSH assays for screening for thyroid disease in apparently healthy populations will be particularly cost effective. Nonetheless, these yields are not striking in light of the potential individual testing cost associated with this type of screening approach.

RECOMMENDATIONS—CHEMISTRY PANELS FOR PREVENTIVE CARE

The combination of rationales and outcomes described in the preceding sections provides a basis for an appropriate "standard laboratory panel" of tests that could be applied in an adult preventive health population (see box below).

These tests offer the greatest information at the lowest cost. Uric acid and potassium are included due to the prevalence of abnormalities found in men. Both calcium and AST allow appropriate reflex, investigative testing on the same blood sample. Neither creatinine nor urea nitrogen were included, as their abnormality rates are too low in a health maintenance population, and no effective reflex testing regimen is available.

Of the tests listed, only glucose fulfills most consensus criteria as an appropriate test in this medical context. The current prevailing Medicare rate for a 6-test automated chemistry panel is $5.68, as compared with $16.54 for a 20-test panel. The difference in list price is $20.00 between the two panels. Tests used primarily for monitoring purposes could be obtained on an "as-needed" basis.

No studies supporting broad-based laboratory screening have been published. Only recommendations have been made, such as those of the American College of Physicians, that such screening not be routinely used for preadmission or preelective surgery screening.[7] The use of fewer tests reduces the number of false-positives results generated in a population with a low disease prevalence. The addition of a reflex testing program would add less than $0.70 to the cost of testing per individual when investigating the cause for an abnormal AST or calcium. These testing algorithms are a highly cost-effective supplement to a health screening program, especially if cost-based.

The rational chemistry profile

1. Uric acid   4. Potassium
2. Calcium   5. AST
3. Glucose

LABORATORY SCREENING PROGRAMS

In addition to the use of standard groups of laboratory tests, other specific tests are used to detect one condition only in a given population. The indication for this testing is purely demographic, and the screening goals are well defined and widely accepted. Actual differences between these testing programs and the panel tests discussed previously are few, if any. The perceived differences are a result of the public health focus on defined goals and the potential impact on the health of the population as a whole. They are often supported by professional groups or governmental agencies and require large investments of resources. Screening programs require laboratory tests that are highly sensitive without being extremely nonspecific. These programs usually use measurement of glucose and cholesterol, and as glucose screening has already been discussed in detail, the focus here is on cholesterol.

Cholesterol and cardiovascular risk

Heart disease is a major concern of the general public because it is the leading cause of death in the United States. It is also well known that a high serum cholesterol, along with other modifiable risk factors such as hypertension and smoking, are linked with an increased risk of cardiac disease. The screening population could be considered to be all adult men and women without cardiovascular symptomatology whose history does not include other risk factors.[12] The current practice, however, is to measure cholesterol in just about everyone.

The National Heart, Lung, and Blood Institute (NHLBI) of the National Institutes of Health originated the National Cholesterol Education Program in 1985 to address the issue of cholesterol and cardiac disease risk as a major public health program. Its goal was to reduce the prevalence of increased blood cholesterol in the country and, as a consequence, reduce the incidence of coronary artery disease (CAD). The basis of this approach was the results of the Lipid Research Clinics Coronary Primary Prevention Trial, which indicated that a reduction of serum cholesterol reduced the risk of CAD. This program has resulted in a national "normal range" for serum cholesterol and LDL-cholesterol based on the goals for cholesterol reduction (Table 7-6). The cholesterol value of 200 mg/dl represented the 50th percentile of the adult male population at the time this program was begun and, therefore, a major portion of the population was abnormal. This classification was without precedent in laboratory medicine, as it ignored differences in methodology for the measurement of cholesterol. Thus the program also allowed for the national standardization of serum cholesterol measurement and set goals for analytic precision and accuracy.

The emphasis on total cholesterol is a mass screening optimization, however, and should not be considered the sole parameter to assess an individual's risk for CAD. The Framingham Study demonstrated clearly the association of the HDL-cholesterol and the ratio of total cholesterol/HDL-cholesterol and the ratio of LDL-cholesterol/HDL-cholesterol with the relative risk of CAD.[12] These parameters were superior to total cholesterol. In addition, they provide for age- and sex-specific interpretations.

There are several additional pitfalls in the use of total cholesterol alone in the laboratory assessment of cardiac risk. Minority populations and women have not been studied sufficiently. Both of these issues are being addressed by current mandates for the study of African-Americans and women. Several major lipid-lowering studies have been published recently, which provide additional insight to attempts to modulate cardiac disease risk factors. The most important conclusion appears to be that although reduction of cardiac morbidity and mortality is possible by the reduction of serum cholesterol with drug regimens, the overall mortality was not reduced.[32] This result was clearly demonstrated in the Helsinki Heart Study.[11]

With these precautionary provisos, the following recommendations concern the use of laboratory tests to assess risk for CAD. The use of just total cholesterol is inappropriate in the formal medical setting, even if the medical goal is preventive. This approach can be justified only in its use outside the formal medical health setting as a means to increase awareness of health issues. Instead, total cholesterol should be performed in conjunction with determination of both triglycerides and HDL-cholesterol with calculation of LDL-cholesterol. These values should allow rational monitoring of an individual's cardiovascular risk related to the metabolism of lipids. The cholesterol methodology used by the laboratory must be standardized to the National Reference System in order to apply any recommendations of the National Cholesterol Education Program.

The intense focus on an individual's serum cholesterol value has also led to an overestimation of the reliability of a single value for indicating the individual's true mean

Table 7-6. Cholesterol: the coronary heart disease risk classifications and recommended follow-up

	Desirable	Borderline-high	High
Cholesterol	Less than 200 mg/dl	200-239 mg/dl	Greater than 240 mg/dl
LDL-Cholesterol	Less than 130 mg/dl	130-159 mg/dl	Greater than 160 mg/dl
Follow-up	Repeat within 5 years	Repeat annually	Investigate further action

cholesterol concentration. This is another example of the relevance of statistical reality in the application of numbers in the practice of medicine. The intraindividual variation in cholesterol concentration can exceed 5%, even when a highly standardized cholesterol method is used. Just as with any other laboratory test result, the physician should not base classification or treatment decisions on single values.

Recommendations for use of laboratory in preventive medicine

1. Use large test panels sparingly. Negotiate with the provider to allow smaller profiles when testing populations with a very low prevalence of disease.[18]
2. Use reflex testing for selected tests—AST, calcium, or hemoglobin—if patient recall is problematic or the cause for the abnormality is not obvious.
3. Do not base classification, diagnostic, or treatment decisions on single laboratory values without corroboration.
4. Use a complete lipid profile for the assessment of cardiovascular risk. Use a provider with a standard cholesterol method. Do not ignore the potential for variability in results not related to treatment.[17]
5. Beware of the false-positive result. The further the application of laboratory tests from the presence of disease, the more the abnormal result will not indicate significant pathology.

REFERENCES

1. Altshuler CH: Use of comprehensive laboratory data as a management tool, *Clin Lab Med* 5:673, 1985.
2. Altshuler CH, Bareta J, Cafaro AF, et al: The PALI and SLIC systems, *Crit Rev Clin Lab Sci* 3:379, 1972.
3. Bailey A, Robinson D: Does Gilbert's disease really exist? *Lancet* 1:931, 1977.
4. Bloom JK: An algorithm for hematuria, *Clin Lab Med* 8:577, 1988.
5. Broughan TA, Jaroch MT, Esselstyn CB: Parathyroid hormone assay, *Arch Surg* 121:841, 1986.
6. Cebul RD, Beck JR: Biochemical profiles. In Sox HC, editor: *Common diagnostic tests*, Philadelphia, 1987, American College of Physicians.
7. Cebul RD, Beck JR: Biochemical profiles: applications in ambulatory screening and preadmission testing of adults, *Ann Intern Med* 106:403, 1987.
8. Deodhar SD: C-reactive protein: the best laboratory indicator available for monitoring disease activity, *Cleve Clin J Med* 56:126, 1989.
9. Djulbegovic B, Hadley T, Pasic R: A new algorithm for diagnosis of anemia, *Postgrad Med* 85:119, 1989.
10. Fang LST: Urinalysis in the diagnosis of urinary tract infections, *Clin Lab Med* 8:567, 1988.
11. Frick MH, Elo O, Haapa K, et al: Helsinki Heart Study: primary-prevention trial with gemfibrozil in middle-age men with dyslipidemia: safety of treatment, changes in risk factors, and incidence of coronary heart disease, *N Engl J Med* 317:1237, 1987.
12. Garber AM, Sox HC, Littenberg B: Screening asymptomatic adults for cardiac risk factors: the serum cholesterol level, *Ann Intern Med* 110:622, 1989.
13. Gerken KL, Van Lente F: Effectiveness of screening for diabetes, *Arch Pathol Lab Med* 114:201, 1990.
14. Harris MI, Hadden WC, Knowler WC, et al: International criteria for the diagnosis of diabetes and impaired glucose tolerance, *Diabetes Care* 8:562, 1985.
15. Heath H, Hodgson SF, Kennedy MA: Primary hyperparathyroidism; incidence, morbidity and potential economic impact in a community, *N Engl J Med* 302:189, 1980.
16. Helfand M, Crapo LM: Screening for thyroid disease, *Ann Intern Med* 112:840, 1990.
17. Irwig L, Glasziou P, Wilson A, Macaskill P: Estimating an individual's true cholesterol level and response to intervention, *JAMA* 266:1678, 1991.
18. Johnson HA: Diminishing returns on the road to diagnostic certainty, *JAMA* 265:2229, 1991.
19. Kaplan EB, Sheiner LB, Boeckmann AJ, et al: The usefulness of preoperative laboratory screening, *JAMA* 253:3576, 1985.
20. Kim MS: Proteinuria, *Clin Lab Med* 8:527, 1988.
21. Klee GG, Ackerman E, Elveback LR, et al: Investigation of statistical decision rules for sequential hematologic laboratory tests, *Am J Clin Pathol* 69:375, 1978.
22. Koch DD, Hassemer DJ, Wiebe DA, Laessig RH: Testing cholesterol accuracy, *JAMA* 260:2252, 1988.
23. Lacher DA, Baumann RR, Boyd JC: Comparison of discriminant analysis procedures in laboratory differentiation of hypercalcemia, *Am J Clin Pathol* 89:753, 1988.
24. Lum G, Deshotels SJ: The clinical usefulness of an algorithm for the interpretation of biochemical profiles with hypercalcemia, *Am J Clin Pathol* 78:479, 1982.
25. Nolan JP, Tarsa NJ, Dibenedetto G: Case finding for unsuspected thyroid disease: costs and health benefits, *Am J Clin Pathol* 83:346, 1985.
26. Pesce A, First MR: *Proteinuria: an integrated review*, New York, 1979, Marcel Dekker.
27. Powell LW, Isselbacher KJ: Hemochromatosis. In Braunwald E, Isselbacher KJ, Petersdorf RG, et al, editors: *Harrison's principles of internal medicine*, ed 11, New York, 1987, McGraw-Hill.
28. Reichen J: Familial unconjugated hyperbilirubinemia syndromes, *Semin Liver Dis* 3:24, 1983.
29. Rosman JB, Ter Wee PM, Meijer S, et al: Prospective randomized trial of early dietary protein restriction in chronic renal failure, *Lancet* 2:1291, 1984.
30. Sackett DL: The usefulness of laboratory tests in health screening programs, *Clin Chem* 19:366, 1973.
31. Singer DE, Coley CM, Samet JH, Nathan DM: Tests of glycemia in diabetes mellitus, *Ann Intern Med* 110:125, 1989.
32. Smith GD, Shipley MJ, Marmot MG, Rose DM: Plasma cholesterol concentration and mortality, *JAMA* 267:70, 1992.
33. Stocker R, Yamamoto Y, McDonagh AF, et al: Bilirubin is an antioxidant of possible physiological importance, *Science* 235:1043, 1987.
34. Surks MI, Chopra IJ, Mariash CN, et al: American Thyroid Association guidelines for use of laboratory tests in thyroid disorders, *JAMA* 263:1529, 1990.
35. Van Lente F, Galen RS, Castellani W, et al: Sequential investigation of aspartate aminotransferase elevation in outpatients, *Clev Clinic J Med* 54:171, 1987.
36. Van Lente F, Castellani W, Chou D, et al: Application of the EXPERT consultation system to accelerated laboratory investigation, *Clin Chem* 32:1719, 1986.
37. Van Lente F, Suit P: Assessment of renal function by serum creatinine and creatinine clearance: glomerular filtration estimated by four procedures, *Clin Chem* 35:2326, 1989.

━━━━━━━━ **RESOURCES** ━━━━━━━━

College of American Pathologists, 325 Waukegan Road, Northfield, IL 60093-2750. Information on accredited laboratories, regulations, and proficiency.

American College of Physicians, 4200 Pine Street, Philadelphia, PA 19104. Guidelines for laboratory test screening.

National Cholesterol Education Program, National Heart, Lung, and Blood Institute, C-200, Bethesda, MD 20892. Information for patient about cholesterol; information regarding standardization of cholesterol methods.

General reference resource materials

Sox HC, editor: *Common diagnostic tests,* Philadelphia, 1987, American College of Physicians.

Statland BE: *Clinical decision levels for lab tests,* Oradell, NJ, 1987, Medical Economics.

Galen RS, Gambino SR: *Beyond normality: the predictive value and efficiency of medical diagnoses,* New York, 1975, John Wiley & Sons.

Lundberg GD: *Using the clinical laboratory in medical decision-making,* Chicago, 1983, American Society of Clinical Pathologists.

Speicher CE, Smith JW: *Choosing effective laboratory tests,* Philadelphia, 1984, WB Saunders.

Part II

THE CLINICIAN'S APPROACH TO THE WELL PATIENT AND PREVENTIVE CARE

Chapter 8

INTEGRATING CLINICAL PREVENTIVE SERVICE INTO OFFICE PRACTICE

Richard S. Lang
Joan D. Shainoff

OVERVIEW

Clinical preventive services incorporate both primary and secondary preventive interventions. Functionally, these services can be organized into three categories: screening procedures, immunization/chemoprophylaxis, and health education/counseling as in the *Guide to Clinical Preventive Services* provided by the U.S. Preventive Services Task Force.[45] As the methodology for identification of effective preventive services advanced beginning with the work of Frame and Carlson, Breslow and Somers, the Canadian Task Force on the Periodic Health Examination, and others in the 1970s and 1980s, and has continued with the Preventive Services Task Force joining this effort in the late 1980s, the benefit of clinical preventive services to the health of the population has been recognized and become more prominent and emphasized. Louis W. Sullivan, secretary of the U.S. Department of Health and Human Services, has said "Health promotion and disease prevention comprise perhaps our best opportunity to reduce the ever-increasing portion of our resources that we spend to treat preventable illness and functional impairment." He went on to say that "We would be terribly remiss if we did not seize the opportunity presented by health promotion and disease prevention to dramatically cut health care costs, to prevent the premature onset of disease and disability, and to help all Americans achieve healthier, more productive lives."[27]

The high cost of hospital care makes preventive services attractive to corporate America as well (see Chapter 63).[41] Studies have also shown that a strong health check program starting in middle age can reduce the demand for in-patient care of the elderly population.[42] *Healthy People 2000: National Health Promotion and Disease Prevention Objectives* has outlined specific goals for clinical preventive services by the year 2000. These include increasing years of "healthy life" from 62 years estimated in 1980 to at least 65 years by the year 2000, increasing to at least 50% the proportion of primary care providers who provide their patients with clinical preventive services recommended by the U.S. Preventive Services Task Force, and increasing to at least 95% the proportion of people "who have a specific source of ongoing primary care for coordination of their preventive and episodic health care."[27]

Chapter 2 reviews the evolution of the periodic health examination. We have seen the previously unchallenged benefits of the yearly examination replaced by an objective evaluation of clinical preventive services to identify those initiatives that are most effective. Unfortunately physicians have not been as successful in following recommendations for preventive services that have been proven to be beneficial and effective. The process of incorporating preventive services into clinical practice has appeared to be slow and difficult. Why has this been the case when effective interventions have been identified and major health care groups and organizations as well as the government have shifted their focus to prevention? This chapter will review the success or lack thereof of physicians in carrying out preventive interventions, review the barriers to the implementation of preventive services, and provide a plan for the individual physician to overcome those barriers to better provide and integrate clinical preventive services into office practice.

BARRIERS TO THE IMPLEMENTATION OF CLINICAL PREVENTIVE SERVICES

A useful classification of the barriers to implementation of clinical prevention has been constructed by Frame and is outlined in the box below.[20] He divides barriers into issues related to the health care delivery system, issues related to the individual patient, and issues related to the physician or health care provider. Any preventive intervention may have many barriers, some of which will be more important than others. Immunizations, for example, may be underutilized because of cultural issues and perceptions about immunization. This is discussed in the chapters of Section VII, Racial and Ethnic Considerations in Clinical Prevention. Other patient barriers to immunizations may include discomfort or lack of understanding about the benefits. Physician barriers may be present as well, such as the physician not considering the value of immunization, having disorganized medical records, or lacking knowledge about the value of the immunization. The barriers to a counseling intervention, on the other

hand, may be the time necessary for counseling (a physician barrier) or the lack of appropriate reimbursement for the time taken (a health care delivery system barrier). Therefore the practitioner must consider not only these groups of barriers, but also which of the categories are most important to the clinical prevention intervention to be undertaken. Successful implementation of immunizations, screening, and health education/counseling will be affected by differing profiles of barriers.

Belcher has pointed out that we have moved from an initial period of research devoted to the effective evaluation of the content of preventive care, to a second period of evaluating whether that care is carried out, and now to a third period of evaluation and identification of those barriers that have slowed the process of clinical prevention.[6] A review of studies since 1979 of preventive activities in practices of primary care physicians in the United States found a variable success rate, a limited number of studies, and the need for well-designed studies of physicians' preventive practices.[32] Bass has looked at the preventive practice patterns of Canadian primary care physicians who, because of the benefit of the National Health Care System of Canada and the time frame in which the Canadian Task Force has been operating, shed light on the difficulties the United States will face as greater emphasis is placed on clinical prevention.[2] He reports many successes in Canada in the implementation of the preventive guidelines proposed by the task force. At the same time, he notes some of the failures, such as the low rate of mammography usage or the continued use of chest x-rays for lung cancer screening, an activity not recommended in the Canadian Task Force report. He postulates that the slow change from the concept of the annual checkup to the periodic preventive health examination is in part due to the ease of timing of the annual examination and some confusion because of disagreement over guidelines by expert groups.[2] To understand this problem of implementation and be able to develop a successful plan for preventive services in the office practice, one must review the obstacles to implementation related to the patient, to the physician or provider, and to the health care system or organization.

Patient barriers

Battista states:

"The health care system has traditionally been viewed by the public as offering curative services, and the attitude of patients seeking alleviation of illness has essentially been passive. . . . A patient role that is appropriate for an illness-based encounter might not be optimal for prevention; therefore, a more participatory role for the patient should be encouraged. The assumption of responsibility and initiative in determining the course of one's health is essential for individuals to become more aware of prevention and more exacting in their expectations of preventive care from health care providers."[3]

Barriers to clinical prevention*

I. Patient barriers

Ignorance of benefits
Doubts about the physician's ability to detect a hidden disease
Cost of procedures
Discomfort
A conscious or unconscious desire not to change unhealthy habits
Social and cultural norms

II. Health system barriers

Inadequate reimbursement
Lack of health insurance
Population mobility
Patients with multiple physicians
Categoric, sporadic screening programs such as health fairs

III. Physician barriers

Knowledge
Uncertainty about conflicting recommendations
Uncertainty about the value of tests or interventions
Disorganized medical records
Delayed and indirect gratification from screening
Lack of time
Attitudes and personal characteristics

*Modified from Frame PS: Health maintenance in clinical practice: strategies and barriers, *Am Family Phys* 45:1192-1200, 1992.

Barriers to an individual undergoing an immunization include cultural and social norms (Are those around me being immunized?), perceived threat of the disease (I never get the flu!), discomfort (I hate needles!), cost, potential side effects (Doesn't Guillain-Barré syndrome occur with flu shots? Will the shot give me the flu?), and forgetting the appointment.

Barriers to screening interventions include social and cultural norms, perceptions of the likelihood of getting the disease, fear of finding a disease, discomfort, cost, and the implications should a problem be found. At the same time, many of these factors also are reasons why a person seeks a screening intervention. Patients often want to be reassured about a condition or to address a condition at an early stage to prevent an outcome similar to that of a friend or acquaintance who has end-stage disease or has died of a condition.

The most difficult patient barrier to overcome in preventive practice is behavior. Preventive health-related behavior includes diet, exercise, sexual practices, alcohol consumption, and other personal habits. The health belief model implies that behavior to prevent a disease is influenced by a person's perception of the personal threat of the disease or condition.[28] That is, the more severe the disease and the more susceptible the patient perceives himself or herself to the disease, the more likely he or she is to change a behavior that can influence the outcome of that condition. At the same time, changing a behavior is influenced by the ease of making the change, the perceived effectiveness of making the change, and particularly the social group influence of the change.[29] The social group differs for individuals and may involve family, friends, peers, and/or community. Identifying the influential people of a person's social group and, where possible, using them as allies can assist in getting a person to change a "negative" health-related behavior. Understanding how a specific "negative" health behavior has arisen in an individual gives insight into the difficulties ahead in trying to motivate the person to make a change. Often these behaviors are longstanding and ingrained into the upbringing, cultural background, and social norms of the individual.

The health care cost crisis in the United States, the efforts of the media, and the emphasis on preventive services via the work of the Canadian Task Force, the U.S. Preventive Service Task Force, and other major groups have helped push the responsibility for wellness and health back to the individual patient. As good preventive habits, such as not smoking, eating a low-fat diet, and exercising regularly, become more popular, people will become more motivated to seek appropriate and specific preventive advice for themselves and their families. Until then, overcoming the philosophy, "If it ain't broke, don't fix it!" will continue to be a difficult task for the practicing physician.

Health system barriers

The mobility of the population, leading many patients to encounter multiple physicians over their lifetime, causes difficulties for tracking and assuring clinical preventive services. As computer technology advances and the issue of basic health insurance for all people in the United States is addressed, problems of tracking and assuring clinical preventive services such as immunizations or proven screening tests should decline. The challenge for clinical preventive medicine in the future will likely be the provision of appropriate reimbursement for risk assessment and counseling.

Another aspect of health care delivery that affects the opportunity for preventive intervention is recognized by Battista: "A considerable amount of primary care is delivered in walk-in clinics and emergency rooms where prevention is not a priority. When preventive activity such as blood pressure measurements are done, linkage of the results to a regular source of care and follow up is both difficult and infrequent."[4] Likewise, he recognizes that the consideration of any medical encounter as an opportunity to invoke preventive activity is idealistic and not realistic.[4] The difficulty here lies in that patients come to physicians with a prioritized list of problems that need to be addressed. Prevention may not be high on that list, and even the best-intentioned provider therefore may be unable to invoke prevention. At the same time, the busy practitioner may be overtaxed by the activities of the day and thereby not allow time for effective preventive counseling, which may be time intensive. Delegating responsibility for preventive services to a nonphysician health care provider can be helpful. Nurses are an appropriate group to provide such services.[7,43]

In considering organizational barriers, one might consider a more "global" view: inadequate reimbursement to physicians for provision of preventive services, lack of health insurance for such activities by many people, and mobility of the population both geographically and individually from one health insurance provider to another. However, a more useful view is to look at the physician's individual practice setting and evaluate the barriers to the ongoing provision of preventive services. These barriers may include some of the same global factors, such as inadequate reimbursement and population mobility, but also barriers that are more easily changeable for the individual physician. These may include organization of medical records and delegation of responsibility for these services to nonphysicians in the practice. Crucial questions to ask are: What is the organizational design of the practice? and What are the resources, both individual and otherwise, within the practice that can promote preventive clinical services? In the current health care system in the United States, primary health care is provided in a variety of settings (see the box on p. 130). Within each practice setting,

---

Types of primary health care practice in the United States

Solo or individual physician
Group practice
Primary care centers
Public health units
Walk-in clinics
Preferred provider organizations (PPOs)
Health maintenance organizations (HMOs)
Occupational health programs
Hospital-based ambulatory care clinics

---

a variety of individuals may be available to provide service to the individual. This may include physicians, nurses, and other ancillary personnel within the practice, as well as resources outside the practice, such as hospital patient education programs and community and professionally sponsored programs, which can provide a variety of counseling services and education to the individual.[31] Professional societies such as the American Cancer Society, the American Heart Association, and the American Lung Association can provide much useful information.

Physician barriers

Are physicians a problem or a solution to providing better preventive care? This question, posed by Belcher et al.,[6] is best answered "both." Physicians provide some barriers to the provision of clinical preventive services but also hold the key in many ways to overcoming the barriers to the provision of these services. The box on p. 128 summarizes physician-related barriers to preventive services. Preventive services have not been traditionally a focus of the basic medical school education curriculum. Additionally, much of residency training has predominantly been inpatient, and only recently has training shifted to the outpatient and ambulatory care area. Education is also focused on diseases after they have occurred, and the medical literature has a paucity of texts concerning the science and value of clinical prevention and its delivery. Preventive medical information has also been contradictory at times, and only recently have consensus efforts been made to establish criteria for the evaluation of preventive interventions and consistent recommendations on their application.

The role of the physician in providing preventive care has often been ambiguous. The physician trained in the curative approach to medical problems and faced with a patient with a specific problem or symptom is hard pressed to spend time on prevention of other medical issues that occur much later in a patient's life. Faced with busy practice and time constraints, the time required by counseling and changing habits again presents as a barrier, particularly when reimbursement is not provided in a meaningful

way. Another issue is that the practitioner does not see the "positive" health outcomes from prevention in the same patient in a mobile population. Counseling an individual who succeeds in smoking cessation in his or her early 20s to prevent the occurrence of a lung cancer or a myocardial infarction 20 or 30 years down the road may be analogous to putting money aside early in life and planning for funds to be available at retirement. Human nature makes immediate gratification more attractive and thereby provision of preventive services less attractive to the physician who has worked through many years of medical school and postgraduate training to attain a level of expertise in the provision of curative care.

Physicians vary in their attitudes and feelings about prevention. The application of those beliefs and opinions varies as well.[1,21,39] Physicians often do not comply, even with their own recommendations.[46] Physicians also vary in the organization within their office. Integrating prevention into a practice when the practice is established is far easier than changing an already-established practice. A disorganized practice or one not organized for preventive services may be difficult to change, particularly when incentives for doing so are limited.

Key factors for overcoming these physician barriers then are (1) consensus of clinical prevention recommendations, (2) appropriate reimbursement for preventive services, (3) education about the necessity of delivering appropriate services, (4) advancement of computer applications to ease recording and tracking patients and to provide reminders about clinical preventive services, and (5) planning and organization within the practice. The first step is for the physician to establish prevention as a priority. He or she must next recognize that both the physician and patient face obstacles of time, attitudes, beliefs, cultural norms, experience and anecdotes encountered in practice, ability to record and track interventions, delayed and indirect gratification, and dealing with perceived "more serious" symptoms and diseases that are more immediately life threatening. The next step is to plan and organize the practice setting so that clinical prevention becomes systematic.[30]

INTEGRATING PREVENTIVE SERVICES
The individual: Changing behavior and habits

The Canadian Task Force, the U.S. Preventive Services Task Force, and the American College of Physicians help identify those issues most important for counseling: diet, exercise, smoking, alcohol and substance abuse, sexual practices, injury prevention, and dental care.[9-12,26,45] Establishing with the patient which of these issues are most important can be delegated to someone in the office other than the physician. The physician, however, needs to demonstrate to the patient an interest in addressing these issues. The physician's power as an authority figure and change motivator cannot be overestimated. At the same time, physicians should recognize that they are different from the individual patient socially, culturally, and in other ways that influence how the advice and counseling may be perceived. A middle-aged, overweight, physically inactive, smoking physician likely will have a difficult time persuading a young adult to engage in regular physical exercise or to stop smoking. The physician therefore should serve as much as possible as a role model.

The U.S. Preventive Services Task Force outlines a simple list of guidelines to assist clinicians to induce behavioral change in patients (see Chapter 2, p. 29). First and foremost is to convince the patient that the physician is interested in his or her health. Next is to talk to the patient, anticipate questions, and encourage a frank discussion of risk factors and preventive behavior. The physician should be knowledgeable about exercise, exercise equipment, practical low-fat diet information, smoking cessation methods, substitutes for alcoholic beverages, and other easy and practical preventive information that may be useful to patients. Educating patients about relationships between habits and outcome requires reinforcement over time. An individual's understanding of his or her own habits and the relationship of those habits to health outcomes changes over the patient's life. We become motivated to change those habits at various times in our life for a variety of reasons. A common scenario is what might be called the "age 30 syndrome." Patients often present for the first time to review their overall health some time between the ages of 25 and 35. This encounter is often motivated by several factors that seem to come together in that age group, such as finishing the educational or job training process and moving into a more permanent job, taking on financial responsibilities, getting married, having children, buying a house, buying a life insurance policy, having parents or other family members with health care problems, and recognizing that mortality is real. Before this age, people are generally not as motivated to address these issues because of a sense of "immortality." Seeking those "windows of opportunity" in the patient's life when the patient may more easily change an "unhealthy" habit produces the most success. At the same time, the physician needs to anticipate obstacles to changing behavior. Patients often do not follow physician advice concerning medication usage or lifestyle changes.[22] Initiating and maintaining behavioral change are influenced by (1) susceptibility to continuing problems if the advice is not followed, (2) severity of problems associated with not following the advice; and (3) the benefits of adopting the advice weighed against potential risk, cost, side effects, and barriers.[28] *The physician's ability to understand from the patient's viewpoint why the unhealthy behavior exists and continues may help to identify ways of changing that behavior.* To gain commitment from a patient, physicians should understand the agenda that the patient brings to the office. Preventive counseling may be better left to another

day if the patient's problem is significant in the patient's eyes. At other times, preventive intervention is possible even when another problem is being handled. Ranking and discussing alternatives to behaviors that merit change and not trying to do too much too quickly can improve the success of the overall program. Counseling a patient to lose weight, start an exercise program, stop smoking, and reduce alcohol consumption all at the same time will likely result in changing none of those behaviors. A better strategy may be to establish a set of goals over a longer time course, changing one behavior or factor at a time. Assessing the person's experience in changing behaviors may give insight into the likelihood of success and the best methods for changing a given health problem. A variety of resources should be used in developing a strategy for an individual. These may include individual counseling, group and community classes, written handouts, videotapes, and family intervention. Educational materials can strengthen recommendations but cannot substitute for the verbal and personal communication by the physician. The clinician's individual empathy, attention, and feedback are critical to changing the patient's behavior. Monitoring progress and providing follow-up contact are necessary to both communicate and reinforce the importance of preventive behavioral change, as well as to track the success of the endeavor.

Inherent in targeting appropriate prevention is the concept of risk assessment. Risk assessment is further described in Chapters 2 and 9. Several well-designed computer-based risk assessment tools have been developed to allow a practitioner to easily and quickly gather information from an individual to outline those conditions and causes of morbidity and mortality the patient is most likely to encounter. These tools are also called health hazard appraisals or health risk profiles (see Resources of this chapter and Chapter 9). These can be easily administered, computerized, and given to the patient in the office or by mail. One such use of health risk appraisal has been termed *prospective medicine,* whose purpose is to extend concern for the patient "beyond crisis oriented episodic care to comprehensive continuing concern for the apparently well patient before and after risk."[24] The book *Prospective Medicine* serves as a manual to identify and quantify health risks for an individual so as to rank priorities for reducing risk and thereby improving overall survival.[24] Risk appraisal tools can facilitate development of a priority list of deleterious health habits for an individual patient in need of change. Once this list is established, the physician can evaluate the individual's motivation and personal barriers. A model protocol for this assessment is outlined in Fig. 8-1. Key points in applying this model are identifying what might be the patient's motivation, surveying the barriers faced by the patient in making a change and participating in the process, overcoming the barriers, providing reinforcement to comply with the program, and allowing

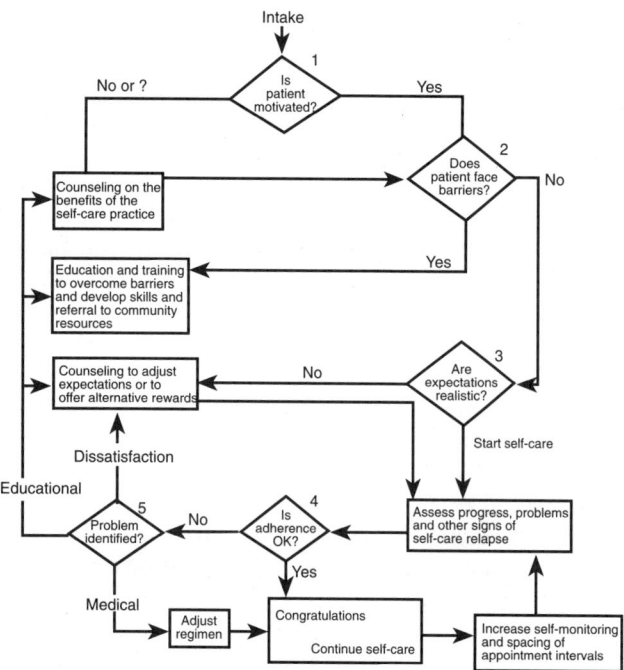

Fig. 8-1. Protocol for stepped-care approach to counseling patients in managing their medical regimen. The flow chart was prepared for a National Heart, Lung, and Blood Institute working group and benefitted from comments by Donald Fedder, DrPH, David Levine, MD, William McClelland, MD, Patricia Mullen, DrPH, Edward Roccella, PhD, and Scott Simonds, DrPH. ◇, decision node; ☐, recommended intervention. (From Green LW: How physicians can improve patients' participation and maintenance in self-care, *West J Med* 147:346-349, 1987.)

for self-monitoring and ongoing program assessment.[23] Self-monitoring is important to the success of the program but often is overlooked. Green summarizes that "feedback from self monitoring can over time become the most powerful source of reinforcement for positive behavior. If a patient continues to depend on the physician for this reinforcement, the patient can fail to make the conversion to self reliance that is so essential to long term maintenance and control coincident with chronic or compulsive disorders."[23]

The important factors, then, in implementation and integration of preventive services that the physician should consider for the individual patient are (1) determination of risk for important and likely causes of morbidity and mortality in both the short and the long term, (2) outline of a priority list and plan for clinical preventive services specific for that individual, (3) assessment of the motivation and individual barriers for successful implementation of the plan, and, (4) as the plan is carried out, provision of mechanisms for self-monitoring.

The physician

Prevention is difficult and time consuming, and must be continuous. The most important factor in the individual

physician's success in implementing a clinical preventive practice is his or her own motivation. The physician must make prevention a priority, otherwise he or she is unlikely to provide it effectively. Frame states that the physician at every visit should ask the question, "Is this patient's health maintenance up to date?"[20] Prevention should be included in every encounter if possible.[30]

After the physician decides that prevention is a priority, the next step is to attain appropriate knowledge about effective clinical prevention. The physician should learn the criteria to evaluate the effectiveness of a clinical preventive service used by the Canadian and U.S. task forces (see Chapter 2). The physician should understand both effective services and those found to be ineffective. At the same time, the practitioner must become comfortable and skilled in counseling about regular exercise, weight reduction, alcohol intake reduction, smoking cessation, injury prevention, and other preventive issues. Continuing medical education (CME) programs and seminars can teach these skills to practitioners, and medical schools can provide this kind of education to medical students and residents. This kind of education can improve health-related behavior of patients.[33]

A study by Osborn et al. showed that variance in cancer screening performance is in part related to the gender of the physician (female physicians being more likely to provide screening services), number of medical journals read by the physician (more medical journals read indicating better screening performance), and visits scheduled for prevention (better screening performance when visits are specifically scheduled for preventive services).[38] This study supports the need for physicians to increase their medical knowledge and face some of their own biases. Checklists and weekly seminars addressing clinical prevention can help improve compliance of physicians in a clinical practice.[13]

In summary, physician barriers can be overcome by (1) deciding that clinical prevention is a priority, (2) learning the criteria for evaluating the effectiveness of preventive services, (3) learning concepts of prevention and becoming skilled at counseling necessary for changing the complicated behaviors that fall under the umbrella of health-related behaviors, (4) asking the question, "Is this patient's health maintenance up to date?" at every patient visit, (5) scheduling specific visits as needed for clinical preventive services, and (6) continually exploring the biases and beliefs that may be preventing the physician from providing proven clinical prevention.

The practice organization

Despite physicians' good intentions, the implementation of clinical preventive services or health maintenance recommendations into practice settings has been less than ideal. Computer technology is adding tools, such as reminder systems, that the clinician may use in the practice setting to turn physician intentions into physician actions in the prevention arena. Reminder systems have been shown to improve the level of preventive services,[5,44] especially when properly addressed.[36] McDonald et al. showed computer-generated reminder messages to heighten the usage of preventive care by at least twofold.[35] Computer reminder messages "improved the fidelity between a physician's actions and his/her intentions." They compare this to a pilot's use of a preflight checklist in that physicians busy in practice despite the best intentions need a mechanical aid to perform according to ideals. They note that, although at the time of their analysis (1984) the cost of this technology was high, computer advances would make it less costly, which is proving to be true.[35] Ornstein has also suggested the use of computer-generated physician and patient reminders, finding that reminding both the patient and the physician improved the adherence to the recommendations for preventive services.[37] A nurse-initiated health maintenance reminder system is an effective method for implementing clinical preventive services and has the added advantage of improving the self-esteem of the nurse and the credibility of the nurse in the eyes of the physician and the patients.[14] The use of appropriate personnel in the office is a key factor that will affect whether preventive services are provided effectively. The physician should delegate some of these responsibilities to nurses and other skilled ancillary personnel as a first priority. Involving these people in the development and outline of the system increases their investment in the process and thereby the likelihood of success of the services.

Establishing a clinical preventive service in an established practice requires an investment of both time and energy at the outset by the physician, nurses, ancillary staff, and clerical staff, as well as by the patients. Implementing a new system brings change for all of these people. This process should include the development of flow sheets for tracking, reminders to both patients and physicians, the disbursement of educational material, counseling, provision of feedback, and keeping of medical records. The physician must consider all of these issues as a group to put together a comprehensive program that can then be implemented in the practice setting. Designating a nurse to oversee this process can help to assure the appropriate organization of the services. Health education and counseling will need to be a shared responsibility. All staff members should be responsible for teaching health promotion methods and, where appropriate, make the patient aware of personal responsibilities. To promote the health of individuals, one must teach health promotion skills to patients. Nursing staff should be actively involved in assembling and presenting health education material.[15] Giving information does not guarantee that learning takes place. For health education to be effective, one must assess the cognitive abilities of the patient so that expectations and plans can be set at an appropriate level. Any health education offering should be presented clearly in a comfortable environment with appropriately selected materials. Materials

such as pamphlets and booklets, printed cards, posters, and attractively designed bulletin boards are effective aids when chosen appropriately and presented without clutter. These materials, however, do not substitute for clear communication by a knowledgeable professional for establishing a therapeutic relationship that provides effective counseling about behavioral changes related to smoking, exercise, alcohol, weight control, injury, and stress management. A skilled staff can communicate the initial messages about benefits of and strategies for change, and can adapt to the special and often complex needs of each patient.[6] The physician can then build on this framework. Progress can and should be evaluated in follow-up visits and reinforced through positive feedback from the nurse and physician.

Another tool in the office setting is the flow sheet or age-specific checklist, which is commonly used for tracking periodic health maintenance services. Flow sheets outline screening guidelines, can trigger reminders, and can consolidate clinical preventive services on a single page. Flow sheets should be a maximum of one page (back and front), contain a minimum of writing, and be prominently placed in the medical record.[20] An example is provided in Fig. 8-2. An important step in the design of the flow sheet is to involve the staff in the planning and design process.[40] The responsibility for maintaining and updating the flow sheet should be assigned to responsible personnel, usually the nursing staff. Continuity of care is a necessary ingredient for using a health maintenance flow sheet. If patients are not likely to return to the practice over a long term, the usefulness of this effort is diminished.[20] Using a flow sheet does not automatically ensure clinical preventive services in a practice, although its use can be increased by concomitant education of physicians about preventive services.[34] In a well-organized practice, properly designed flow sheets can help retrieve data from medical records so that a person's preventive service needs at any time can be easily ascertained.[25]

Another tool that can be helpful is the patient-held minirecord. These have been used to promote pediatric preventive care and are now being applied to adult preventive services. The use of minirecords can be acceptable to patients and can improve knowledge and performance of clinical preventive services and provider compliance.[17] The minirecord can build cooperation between patients, physicians, and nurses in the provision of preventive care.[17] A patient-held minirecord can serve to track and remind patients of necessary preventive services.[16]

In summary, practice organization for provision of clinical preventive services includes the following: (1) identification of clinical preventive services to be provided, (2) involvement of nursing and other ancillary personnel in the design of the implementation and tracking process, (3) designation of an individual to carry out and oversee the clinical preventive services program, (4) identification of resources in the practice, including personnel and com-

Health Maintenance Flow Sheet (✓ = Performed)

Initials																										
Date Mo. / Yr.																										
PROCEDURE¹ Age	20	21	22	23	24	25	26	27	28	29	30	31	32	33	34	35	36	37	38	39	40	41	42	43	44
PHYSICAL EXAMINATION																									
Blood pressure	•		•		•		•		•		•		•		•		•		•		•		•		•
Height and weight																									
LAB TESTS																									
RPR[2]	•			•			•			•			•			•			•				•		
Gonococcal cultures[2]	•			•			•			•															
PPD Test[2]	•			•			•			•			•			•			•				•		
Thal., Sickle, Tay-Sachs[3]	•																								
Cholesterol	•					•					•					•					•				
CANCER SCREENING																									
Pelvic exam	•			•			•			•			•			•			•				•		
Pap Test[4]	•			•			•			•			•			•			•				•		
Digital rectal exam																									
Stool for occult blood																									
Mammography																									•
Breast Exam																					•	•	•	•	•
IMMUNIZATION	•										•														
Tetanus-Diptheria	•																				•				
Rubella[5] (Rubella Screenig)	•																								
Measles[6]	•																								
Mumps[7]																									
Pneumovax																									
Influenza																									
Polio[8]	•																								
COUNSELING[9]																									

Patient name:
Patient number:

1. For patients over 70 years of age, do the same procedures at the frequency shown for patients 65 to 70 years old.
2. In high-risk groups (may be performed more often if needed).
3. As part of premarital screening in high-risk groups.
4. After two initial tests 1 year apart yield negative results.
5. If screening test for immunity is negative.
6. If born after 1956 and no prior history of immunization.
7. If born after 1957 and no prior history of immunization.
8. Intervention if history of inadequate immunization.
9. Includes diet, smoking, exercise, alcohol, drugs, safety, safe sex, seat belts, violence, guns

Other maneuvers that might be performed at the discretion of the examiner are sigmiodoscopy, CBC, urinalysis, multichannel screening, general physical exam, thyroid screening, tonometry.
(These can be filled in blank spaces)

Fig. 8-2. Health maintenance flow sheet. (Modified from Primary Care Section, Department of Internal Medicine, Cleveland Clinic Foundation, Cleveland, Ohio.)

puter technology, for provision of such services, (5) design of a one-page (front and back) flow sheet with minimum writing to be placed in a prominent place in the patient record, (6) development of a reminder system, either nurse-initiated or computer-generated, to remind both patients and physicians of the need for ongoing clinical preventive services, (7) development of educational materials, including posters, pamphlets, and videos, to be displayed in the office and distributed to patients, (8) implementation of patient-held minirecords to record clinical preventive services given and outline a timetable for future services, and (9) continuous reassessment of the clinical prevention to ensure that the most current proven services are provided.

Put prevention into practice

An important program will become available in the fall of 1993 from the Public Health Service of the U.S. Department of Health and Human Services called "Put Prevention into Practice." This program was developed to help achieve the health-promotion and disease-prevention objectives for the nation established in *Healthy People 2000*, and to improve the delivery of clinical preventive services. Major health-related volunteer groups and provider organizations are joining the "Put Prevention into Practice" campaign. This comprehensive campaign will target physicians, physicians' office systems and staff, and patients. The program will include a clinician handbook that will discuss the burden of suffering caused by target

Health Maintenance Flow Sheet – Cont'd

Initials																										
Date Mo. Yr.																										
PROCEDURE[1] Age	45	46	47	48	49	50	51	52	53	54	55	56	57	58	59	60	61	62	63	64	65	66	67	68	69	70
PHYSICAL EXAMINATION																										
Blood Pressure		•		•		•		•		•		•		•		•		•		•		•		•		•
Height and weight														⌐												
LAB TESTS																										
RPR[2]		•				•				•				•				•				•				•
Gonococcal cultures [2]																										
PPD Test[2]		•				•				•				•				•				•				•
Thal., Sickle, Tay-Sachs[3]																										
Cholesterol	•					•					•					•					•					•
CANCER SCREENING																										
Pelvic exam		•				•				•				•				•				•				•
Pap Test[4]		•				•				•				•				•				•				•
Digital rectal exam		•				•				•				•				•				•				•
Stool for occult blood		•	•	•	•	•	•	•	•	•	•	•	•	•	•	•	•	•	•	•	•	•	•	•	•	•
Mammography		•		•		•	•	•	•	•	•	•	•	•	•	•		•		•		•		•		•
Breast Exam	•	•	•	•	•	•	•	•	•	•	•	•	•	•	•	•		•		•		•		•		•
IMMUNIZATION																										
Tetanus-Diptheria						•										•										•
Rubella[5] (Rubella Screening)																										
Measles[6]																										
Mumps[7]																										
Pneumovax																					•					
Influenza																					•	•	•	•	•	•
Polio[8]																										
COUNSELING[9]																										

Fig. 8-2. Health maintenance flow sheet,—cont'd.

conditions, prevention recommendations of major authoritative groups, basic techniques for providing preventive services, resources, and references. Office system materials will include patient cards for tracking preventive services and reminding patients of needs, chart alert stickers to identify specific interventions for particular patients such as the need for smoking cessation, a preventive prescription pad that will enable providers to "prescribe" needed preventive services, and reminder postcards. Patient materials will include a personal health guide, which will be a pocket-sized booklet to help the patient identify personal risk factors and also to schedule and record appropriate preventive services. The *Handbook of Preventive Services* will be updated regularly and will be divided into age-group sections: children up to age 18, adults over 18, and older adults over the age of 65. Oversight of the campaign has been provided by the National Coordinating Committee on Clinical Preventive Services. This campaign can be contacted by writing to the address listed in the Resources at the end of this chapter.

SUMMARY

The practitioner can best incorporate prevention into clinical practice by considering the obstacles the patient, the practice organization, and the physician must overcome. Utilizing the resources now available, such as "Putting Prevention into Practice" and the information provided by the U.S. Preventive Services Task Force, the individual practitioner can find the process of clinical prevention easier and more rewarding. As our health care system evolves, incentives for prevention likely will be established. These incentives, which may come through regulation or subsidy, are likely to motivate behavioral change for patients and practitioners alike.[8,18] In this way, expert recommendations, practitioner intentions, and actual practice by physicians may converge.[19]

REFERENCES

1. American Cancer Society: 1989 survey of physicians' attitudes and practices in early cancer detection, *CA Cancer J Clin* 40:77-101, 1990.
2. Bass MJ, Elford RW: Preventive practice patterns of Canadian pri-

mary care physicians. In Battista RN, Lawrence RS, editors: *Implementing preventive services,* New York, 1988, Oxford University Press.

3. Battista RN et al: The periodic health examination: 3. An evolving concept, *Can Med Assoc J* 130:1288-1292, 1984.

4. Battista RN, Fletcher SW: Making recommendations on preventive practices: methodological issues. In Battista RN, Lawrence RS, editors: *Implementing preventive services,* New York, 1988, Oxford University Press.

5. Becker DM et al: Improving preventive care at a medical clinic: how can the patient help? *Am J Prevent Med* 5:353-359, 1989.

6. Belcher DW, Berg AO, and Inui TS: Practical approaches to providing better preventive care: are physicians a problem or a solution? In Battista RN, Lawrence RS, editors: *Implementing preventive services,* New York, 1988, Oxford University Press.

7. Bigbee JL, Jansa N: Strategies for promoting health protection, *Nurs Clin Am* 26:895-913, 1991.

8. Breslow L, Somers AR: A lifetime health-monitoring program: a practical approach to preventive medicine, *N Engl J Med* 296:601-608, 1977.

9. Canadian Task Force on the periodic health examination: The periodic health examination, *Can Med Assoc J* 121:1193-1254, 1979.

10. Canadian Task Force on the periodic health examination: The periodic health examination: 2. 1985 update, *Can Med Assoc J* 134:724-727, 1985.

11. Canadian Task Force on the periodic health examination: The periodic health examination: 2. 1987 update, *Can Med Assoc J* 138:618-626, 1987.

12. Canadian Task Force on the periodic health examination: The periodic health examination: 2. 1989 update, *Can Med Assoc J* 141:209-216, 1989.

13. Cohen DI et al: Improving physician compliance with preventive medicine guidelines, *Med Care* 20:1040-1045, 1982.

14. Davidson RA et al: A nurse-initiated reminder system for the periodic health examination: implementation and evaluation, *Arch Intern Med* 144:2167-2170, 1984.

15. DeMuth JS: Patient teaching in the ambulatory setting, *Nurs Clin North Am* 24:645-654, 1989.

16. D'Souza M: Discussion of preventive practice patterns of Canadian primary care physicians. In Battista RN, Lawrence RS, editors: *Implementing preventive services,* New York, 1988, Oxford University Press.

17. Dickey LL, Petitti D: A patient-held minirecord to promote adult preventive care, *J Fam Pract* 34:457-463, 1992.

18. Evans RG: Economic barriers to preventive services: clinical obstacles or fiscal defense. In Battista RN, Lawrence RS, editors: *Implementing preventive services,* New York, 1988, Oxford University Press.

19. Fletcher SW, Siscovick DS, and Inui TS: Research on the periodic health examination: opportunities for the general internist, *J Gen Intern Med (suppl)* 1:S45-S49, 1986.

20. Frame PS: Health maintenance in clinical practice: strategies and barriers, *Am Fam Physician* 45:1192-1200, 1992.

21. Gemson DH, Elinson J: Prevention in primary care: variability in preventive practice patterns in New York City, *Am J Prev Med* 1:225-234, 1986.

22. Green LW, Eriksen MP, and Schor EL: Preventive practices by physicians: behavioral determinants and potential interventions. In Battista RN, Lawrence RS, editors: *Implementing preventive services,* New York, 1988, Oxford University Press.

23. Green LW: How physicians can improve patients' participation and maintenance in self-care, *West J Med* 147:346-349, 1987.

24. Hall JA, Zwemer JD: *Prospective medicine,* Indianapolis, 1979, Methodist Hospital of Indiana.

25. Hahn DL, Berger MG: Implementation of a systematic health maintenance protocol in a private practice, *J Fam Pract* 31:492-504, 1990.

26. Hayward RS, et al: Preventive care guidelines: 1991, *Ann Intern Med* 114:758-783, 1991.

27. US Department of Health and Human Services: *Healthy people 2000: National health promotion and disease prevention objectives,* Boston, 1992, Jones and Bartlett Publishers.

28. Janz NK, Becker MH: The health belief model: a decade later, *Health Educ Q* 11:1-47, 1984.

29. Jenkins DC: Diagnosis and treatment of behavioral barriers to good health. In Last JM, editor: *Maxcy-Rosenau public health and preventive medicine,* Norwalk, Conn, 1986, Appleton-Century-Crofts.

30. Kamerow DB: Prevention: how to practice what we preach, *J Fam Pract* 32:461-462, 1991.

31. Leatt P, Frank J: Organizational issues related to integrating preventive services into primary care. In Battista RN, Lawrence RS, editors: *Implementing preventive services,* New York, 1988, Oxford University Press.

32. Lewis CE: Disease prevention and health promotion practices of primary care physicians in the United States. In Battista RN, Lawrence RS, editors: *Implementing preventive services,* New York, 1988, Oxford University Press.

33. Logsdon DN, Lazaro CM, and Meier RV: The feasibility of behavioral risk reduction in primary medical care, *Am J Prev Med* 5:249-256, 1989.

34. Madlon-Kay DJ: Improving the periodic health examination: use of a screening flow chart for patients and physicians, *J Fam Pract* 25:470-473, 1987.

35. McDonald CJ et al: Reminders to physicians from an introspective computer medical record system: a two-year randomized trial, *Ann Intern Med* 100:130-138, 1984.

36. Norman P, Fitter M: Patients' views on health screening in general practice, *Fam Pract* 8:129-132, 1991.

37. Ornstein SM et al: Computer-generated physician and patient reminders. Tools to improve population adherence to selected preventive services, *J Fam Pract* 32:82-90, 1991.

38. Osborn EH et al: Cancer screening by primary care physicians: can we explain the differences? *J Fam Pract* 32:465-471, 1991.

39. Romm FJ, Fletcher SW, and Hulka BS: The periodic health examination: comparison of recommendations and internists' performance, *South Med J* 74:265-271, 1981.

40. Shank JC, Powell T, and Llewelyn J: A five year demonstration project associated with improvement in physician health maintenance behavior, *Fam Med* 21:273-278, 1989.

41. Stifler LT: Preventive health programs attract industry, *Hospitals* 65:68, 1991.

42. Tatara K et al: Relation between use of health check ups starting in middle age and demand for inpatient care by elderly people in Japan, *Br Med J* 302:615-618, 1991.

43. Thier SO: The future of disease prevention, *J Gen Intern Med* 5(suppl): S136-S137, 1990.

44. Turner RC, Waivers LE, and O'Brien K: The effect of patient-carried reminder cards on the performance of health maintenance measures, *Arch Intern Med* 150:645-647, 1990.

45. U.S. Preventive Services Task Force: *Guide to clinical preventive services: an assessment of the effectiveness of 169 interventions,* Baltimore, 1989, Williams and Wilkins.

46. Woo B et al: Screening procedures in the asymptomatic adult, comparison of physicians' recommendations, patients' desires, published guidelines, and actual practice, *JAMA* 254:1480-1484, 1985.

━━━━━━━ **RESOURCES** ━━━━━━━

Put Prevention into Practice, US Public Health Service, Office of Disease Prevention and Health Promotion (ODPHP), ODPHP National Health Information Center, P.O. Box 1133, Washington, DC 20013-1133. (This prevention implementation program for practicing physicians will be available to physicians in 1993. Physicians can be placed on the mailing list by writing to this address.)

Prevention report, ODPHP National Health Information Center. (This newsletter is provided by the Office of Disease Prevention and Health Promotion and outlines key information, new literature, activities, and resources relative to clinical prevention.)

Prospective medicine, by Hall JH and Zwemer JD, Methodist Hospital of Indiana (1979), 1604 N. Capital Ave., Indianapolis IN 46202. (This book outlines methods for establishing 10-year health risk profiles and preventive health priorities for individual patients.)

Directory of health risk appraisals, The Society of Prospective Medicine, P.O. Box 55110, Indianapolis IN 46205-0110. (Details descriptions of major health risk appraisals available and where to find them.)

Chapter 9

THE PREVENTIVE HISTORY AND PHYSICAL EXAMINATION

Richard S. Lang
Richard L. Dunn

In the patient who perceives himself or herself to be well, the preventive history and physical examination are designed to assist the physician and patient to focus on diseases or conditions that are present but unknown to the patient or may be reasonably expected to be encountered by the patient by virtue of inheritance, life-style, or other risks at some point in time. In the patient who presents with symptoms, the purpose of the preventive history and physical examination is the same, but in addition, one may serve the patient well by employing the preventive examination at the same time as addressing the complaint, hence, altering the course of unrecognized disease in a positive way. This approach differs from the traditional physician-patient encounter that often is directed at evaluating existing medical problems or complaints alone at the time of treatment or monitoring of an existing disease. The *challenge* to the preventive practitioner is to convey to the patient the need for action now and to *motivate* him or her to carry out these changes to effect a longer, or at least healthier, happier life. The attitude of the preventist might be described as considering the patient as harboring multiple latent conditions until proven otherwise.

Inherent in this endeavor is the concept of risk. Webster defines *risk* as "possibility of loss, injury, disadvantage or destruction; a dangerous element or factor, or peril."[9] In preventive medicine, risk implies the statistical likelihood of encountering a condition or disease based on a variety of factors including family or genetic medical history, race, sex, age, environment, social habits, occupation, and other medical conditions. Amalgamating these factors for an individual in order to stratify that person into a general

framework of overall risk is an important goal of the preventive interview. To do so requires a working knowledge of causes of morbidity and mortality. The preventive history should consider causes of morbidity and mortality a person is most likely to encounter in the near and distant future. Based on this history, the preventive plan should act to assist the patient in not only potentially lengthening his or her life span but also in improving quality of life during that time.

CAUSES OF MORTALITY

Understanding the common causes of mortality for patients of a given age group assists the practitioner in the discussion of preventive issues facing the patient in the near future and also in mapping out common conditions to be thought about later in life. Table 9-1 depicts "all cause" mortality in the United States. Heart disease and cancer account for more than half of total deaths. Stroke and accidents account for another 11%. Chronic obstructive lung disease, pneumonia, and influenza make up an additional 7.4%. Table 9-2 depicts causes of death among children. Almost half of total deaths in this age group relate to accidents or homicide. Cancer, although an important cause of death, is less frequent than in the overall population. Table 9-3 stratifies mortality by age group and sex. This information is helpful to the practitioner to educate the patient about the most common causes of death in his or her age group. Teenagers and young adults are often unaware of accidents, homicide, and suicide being such frequent causes of death in their own age group. Likewise, the elderly may be unaware of the importance of pneumonia and

Table 9-1. Mortality for leading causes of death in the United States—1988

Rank	Cause of death	Number of deaths	Death rate per 100,000 population*	Percent of total deaths
	All causes	**2,167,999**	**725.4**	**100.0**
1	Heart diseases	765,156	246.6	35.3
2	Cancer	485,048	170.4	22.4
3	Cerebrovascular diseases	150,517	46.9	6.9
4	Accidents	97,100	36.2	4.5
5	Chronic obstructive lung diseases	82,853	27.5	3.8
6	Pneumonia and influenza	77,662	23.5	3.6
7	Diabetes	40,368	13.6	1.9
8	Suicide	30,407	11.1	1.4
9	Cirrhosis of liver	26,409	9.9	1.2
10	Diseases of arteries	23,185	7.6	1.1
11	Nephritis	22,392	7.1	1.0
12	Atherosclerosis	22,086	6.4	1.0
13	Homicide	22,032	8.1	1.0
14	Septicemia	20,925	6.7	1.0
15	Diseases of infancy	18,220	8.3	0.8
	Other and ill-defined	283,639	95.5	13.1

From Boring CC, Squires TS, Tong T: Cancer statistics, 1992, *CA Cancer J Clin* 42(1):19-38, 1992.
*Age-adjusted to the 1970 U.S. standard population.
Source: Vital Statistics of the United States, 1988.

Table 9-2. Leading causes of death among children aged 1-14, both sexes: United States—1988

Rank	Cause of death	Number of deaths	Death rate per 100,000 population*	Percent of total deaths
	All causes	**16,354**	**32.1**	**100.0**
1	Accidents	7073	14.0	43.2
2	Cancer	1638	3.3	10.0
3	Congenital anomalies	1412	2.6	8.6
4	Homicide	840	1.7	5.1
5	Heart diseases	676	1.3	4.1
6	Pneumonia and influenza	313	0.6	1.9
7	Cerebral palsy	275	0.5	1.7
8	Suicide	243	0.6	1.5
9	Meningitis	182	0.3	1.1
10	Benign neoplasms	172	0.3	1.1
11	HIV infection	168	0.3	1.0
12	Diseases of infancy	151	0.3	0.9
13	Chronic obstructive lung diseases	147	0.3	0.9
14	Septicemia	140	0.3	0.9
15	Cerebrovascular diseases	127	0.3	0.8
	All others	2797	5.4	17.1

From Boring CC, Squires TS, Tong T: Cancer statistics, 1992, *CA Cancer J Clin* 42(1):19-38, 1992
*Age-adjusted to the 1970 U.S. standard population.
Source: Vital Statistics of the United States, 1988.

influenza as a cause of death in their age group and consequently may be more willing to undergo appropriate vaccination for these diseases. Of particular note is the marked increase in the last few years of HIV infection as a cause of death in the male 15-34 and 35-54 age groups and in the female 15-34 age group pointing to the need for continued emphasis on prevention of this disease in these and all groups.[2,7] The role of accidents in all age groups is generally under-recognized by both patients and physicians. The physician's role in prevention of accidents is under-recognized as well (see Chapters 20, 27, 35, 64, 65). For example, a physician review of whether or not an adult wears a seat belt may motivate a person to use this preventive intervention. The patient is often surprised that this is discussed and important in a general medical history. Suicide

and homicide are also causes of death common to many of the age groups listed and often unrecognized as important causes of death by practitioners. Again, assessment and counseling by the physician regarding these issues may help to reduce these important causes of death.

In addition to knowledge of causes of death stratified by age and sex, the practitioner should be aware of similar information for the race or races of the persons seen in his or her practice. For example, Table 9-4 depicts ratios of age-adjusted death rates for causes of death for black and white races in the United States. Homicide, HIV infection, diseases of the kidney, and diabetes take on a greater importance as causes of death in the black population.[7] Hall and Zwemer have developed a table of multiple risk factors for all decades ages 5-74 in male and female, black and white

Table 9-3. Mortality, 10 leading causes of death, by age group and sex, United States, 1988

All Ages		Ages 1-14		Ages 15-34	
Male	**Female**	**Male**	**Female**	**Male**	**Female**
All causes 1,125,540	**All causes 1,042,459**	**All causes 9702**	**All causes 6652**	**All causes 71,516**	**All causes 25,788**
1. Heart diseases 385,402	Heart diseases 379,754	Accidents 4520	Accidents 2553	Accidents 27,297	Accidents 7938
2. Cancer 258,088	Cancer 226,960	Cancer 925	Cancer 713	Homicide 10,065	Cancer 3434
3. Accidents 65,821	Cerebrovascular diseases 90,758	Congenital anomalies 797	Congenital anomalies 615	Suicide 9606	Homicide 2698
4. Cerebrovascular diseases 59,759	Pneumonia and influenza 40,828	Homicide 485	Homicide 355	HIV infection 5726	Suicide 2033
5. Chronic obstructive lung diseases 48,939	Chronic obstructive lung diseases 33,914	Heart diseases 371	Heart diseases 305	Cancer 3671	Heart diseases 1491
6. Pneumonia and influenza 36,834	Accidents 31,279	Suicide 181	Pneumonia and influenza 147	Heart diseases 3174	HIV infection 845
7. Suicide 24,078	Diabetes 23,393	Pneumonia and influenza 166	Cerebral palsy 136	Cirrhosis of liver 739	Cerebrovascular diseases 570
8. Cirrhosis of liver 17,196	Atherosclerosis 13,759	Cerebral palsy 139	Benign neoplasms 87	Cerebrovascular diseases 665	Pneumonia and influenza 447
9. Diabetes 16,975	Septicemia 11,793	Meningitis 99	Meningitis 83	Pneumonia and influenza 664	Congenital anomalies 422
10. Homicide 16,712	Nephritis 11,512	HIV infection 96	HIV infection 72	Congenital anomalies 517	Cirrhosis of liver 371

From Boring CC, Squires TS, Tong T: Cancer statistics, 1992, *CA Cancer J Clin* 42(1):19-38, 1992.
Source: Vital Statistics of the United States, 1988.

Continued.

Table 9-3, cont'd. Mortality, 10 leading causes of death, by age group and sex, United States, 1988.

Ages 35-54		Ages 55-74		Ages 75+	
Male	Female	Male	Female	Male	Female
All causes 126,349	All causes 68,577	All causes 449,269	All causes 309,025	All causes 446,280	All causes 615,344
Heart diseases 32,555	Cancer 27,889	Heart diseases 168,058	Cancer 109,063	Heart diseases 180,693	Heart diseases 270,675
Cancer 26,458	Heart diseases 11,273	Cancer 139,417	Heart diseases 95,582	Cancer 87,555	Cancer 85,808
Accidents 14,395	Accidents 4670	Chronic obstructive lung diseases 22,523	Cerebrovascular diseases 18,748	Cerebrovascular diseases 35,029	Cerebrovascular diseases 68,022
HIV infection 7870	Cerebrovascular diseases 3271	Cerebrovascular diseases 20,142	Chronic obstructive lung diseases 15,321	Chronic obstructive lung diseases 24,501	Pneumonia and influenza 33,216
Suicide 6528	Cirrhosis of liver 2330	Accidents 10,718	Diabetes 9349	Pneumonia, and influenza 24,414	Chronic obstructive lung diseases 16,928
Cirrhosis of liver 6013	Suicide 2209	Pneumonia and influenza 9137	Accidents 5916	Accidents 8240	Atherosclerosis 12,248
Homicide 4349	Diabetes 1700	Cirrhosis of liver 8572	Pneumonia and influenza 5700	Diabetes 6453	Diabetes 12,002
Cerebrovascular diseases 3782	Chronic obstructive lung diseases 1358	Diabetes 7852	Cirrhosis of liver 4674	Diseases of arteries 6364	Accidents 9785
Diabetes 2197	Homicide 1212	Diseases of arteries 6615	Nephritis 3106	Nephritis 6228	Septicemia 7960
Substance abuse 2110	Pneumonia and influenza 1053	Suicide 5198	Diseases of arteries 2981	Atherosclerosis 6108	Nephritis 7635

From Boring CC, Squires TS, Tong T: Cancer statistics, 1992, *CA Cancer J Clin* 42(1):19-38, 1992.
Source: Vital Statistics of the United States, 1988.

populations so that pertinent risk factors may be appraised at any entry age. (see Chapter 1 Resources) Consequently, interventions by the practitioner should be particularly attentive to these causes of death and their prevention.

Subdivision may be necessary within each category listed as a cause of death. This is particularly true for cancer, as evidenced by Tables 9-5 and 9-6 depicting cancer mortality for age group and sex in the United States.

Cancer incidence differs from cancer mortality, reflecting the differences in clinical course and effectiveness of treatment for the various cancer types. Figs. 9-1 and 9-2 from the American Cancer Society[2] graphically depict this difference. In men, cancers of the prostate, lung, colon and rectum, and urinary tract account for about two thirds of cancer incidence and death. Whereas the incidence rate of lung cancer is only 18%, more than one third of cancer

death is attributed to lung cancer. This reflects the poor prognosis and relative ineffectiveness of treatment for lung cancer compared with other cancers. In women, cancers of the breast, lung, colon and rectum, and uterus and ovary account for about two thirds of cancer incidence and a little less than two thirds of cancer deaths. Again, lung cancer accounts for a greater proportion of cancer mortality than cancer incidence.

Knowledge of this information helps to establish a general framework to discuss both short- and long-term preventive intervention. A young male may present with concerns about preventing cancer, motivated by cancer occurring in a friend or family member. He may be unaware of common causes of death in his own age group such as accidents, homicide, suicide, and HIV infection. His inquiry about cancer can lead to a general discussion of causes of

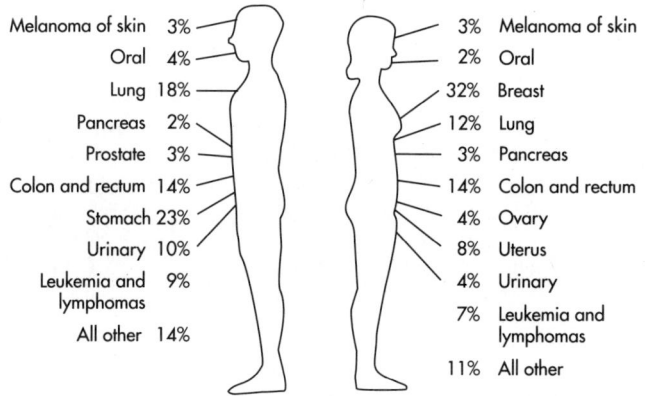

Fig. 9-1. 1992 estimated cancer incidence by site and sex. (From Boring CC, Squires TS, Tong T: Cancer Statistics 1992, *CA Cancer J Clin* 42:19-38, 1992.

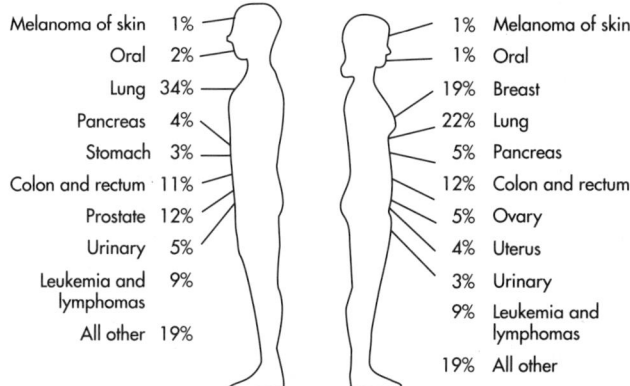

Fig. 9-2. 1992 estimated cancer deaths by site and sex. (From Boring CC, Squires TS, Tong T: Cancer Statistics 1992, *CA Cancer J Clin* 42:19-38, 1992.

Table 9-4. Ratio of age-adjusted death rates for leading causes of death by race: United States, 1989

Cause of death	Ratio of black to white
All causes	1.58
Heart disease	1.43
Cancer	1.33
Cerebrovascular diseases	1.89
Accidents	1.30
Chronic obstructive pulmonary disease	0.84
Pneumonia and influenza	1.52
Diabetes mellitus	2.30
Suicide	0.59
Chronic liver disease and cirrhosis	1.67
Homicide	6.61
Human Immunodeficiency Virus infection	3.27
Nephritis, nephrotic syndrome, and nephrosis	3.08
Atherosclerosis	1.03
Septicemia	2.67
Perinatal conditions	2.93

From *Monthly Vital Statistics Report*. National Center for Health Statistics; USDHHS, Bethesda, MD; Vol. 40(8):(supplement 2), 1992.

Table 9-5. Mortality for the five leading cancer sites for males by age group, United States, 1988

All ages	Under 15	15-34	35-54	55-74	75+
All cancer **258,088**	**All cancer** **971**	**All cancer** **3671**	**All cancer** **26,458**	**All cancer** **139,417**	**All cancer** **87,555**
Lung 88,059	Leukemia 362	Leukemia 685	Lung 8903	Lung 55,092	Lung 23,877
Prostate 28,982	Brain and CNS 234	Non-Hodgkin's Lymphomas 459	Colon and rectum 2369	Colon and rectum 14,451	Prostate 17,303
Colon and rectum 28,111	Endocrine 114	Brain and CNS 438	Brain and CNS 1360	Prostate 11,339	Colon and rectum 11,086
Pancreas 11,722	Non-Hodgkin's lymphomas 76	Skin 250	Non-Hodgkin's lymphomas 1354	Pancreas 6558	Pancreas 3845
Leukemia 9724	Connective tissue 38	Hodgkin's disease 241	Pancreas 1269	Esophagus 4299	Leukemia 3483

From Boring CC, Squires TS, Tong T: Cancer statistics, 1992, *CA Cancer J Clin* 42(1):19-38, 1992.

Table 9-6. Mortality for the five leading cancer sites for females by age group, United States, 1988

All ages	Under 15	15-34	35-54	55-74	75 +
All cancer 226,960	All cancer 756	All cancer 3434	All cancer 27,889	All cancer 109,063	All cancer 85,808
Lung 45,225	Leukemia 262	Breast 675	Breast 8757	Lung 27,473	Colon and rectum 15,021
Breast 42,172	Brain and CNS 200	Leukemia 413	Lung 5216	Breast 20,333	Lung 12,409
Colon and rectum 28,997	Endocrine 88	Uterus 34	Colon and Rectum 1969	Colon and Rectum 11,852	Breast 12,403
Ovary 12,397	Connective Tissue 46	Brain and CNS 313	Uterus 1819	Ovary 6677	Pancreas 5833
Pancreas 12,126	Kidney 33	Non-Hodgkin's lymphomas 205	Ovary 1641	Pancreas 5579	Ovary 3914

From Boring CC, Squires TS, Tong T: Cancer statistics, 1992, *CA Cancer J Clin* 42(1):19-38, 1992.

mortality both in the near future and later in his life. This presents an opportunity for counseling about interventions to prevent those causes of death most likely to occur sooner, while at the same time modifying risk factors for cancer and heart disease in order to attain long-term benefit. As the preventive interview proceeds, further data specific for the individual will help to narrow the risk factor profile for that individual and direct prioritization and specific discussion of preventive interventions.

CAUSES OF MORBIDITY

Morbidity refers to "the condition of being diseased."[9] This comes from the Latin *morbidus,* which means sick or not in good health. It contrasts with mortality, which equates to death. More "significant" conditions or causes of morbidity have usually been those that ultimately lead to death. Morbidity, however, also includes conditions that affect quality of life but may not directly influence death. Causes of morbidity may be viewed as either chronic or acute. The box at right depicts selected chronic conditions occurring in the United States for all ages.

Recognizing these conditions as being common and several as having preventive components will allow the practitioner in the preventive interview to consider appropriate counseling and education pertinent to these conditions. Table 9-7 depicts a more detailed analysis of selected chronic conditions in the United States stratified by age and sex.

This information allows the practitioner to focus on chronic conditions often affecting the quality of life of an individual but frequently overlooked by the practitioner

---

Number of selected reported chronic conditions per 1,000 persons, United States, 1990, all ages

1. Chronic sinusitis	131.3
2. Arthritis	125.3
3. Hypertension	110.2
4. Hearing impairment	94.7
5. Hay fever or allergic rhinitis	90.2
6. Back impairment	70.3
7. Chronic bronchitis	51.1
8. Deformity or orthopaedic impairment of the lower extremities	47.4
9. Asthma	41.9
10. Migraine headache	39.8

From National Center for Health Statistics, USDHHS, *Vital and Health Statistics* 10(181):82-83, 1992.

until the problem has run its course and requires treatment. The preventive medical examination also is directed to these common conditions, looking for early signs that may portend problems later in life. The frequent occurrence of bunions, corns, calluses, and ingrown toenails is an example of often overlooked conditions that can be prevented with attention to early signs of these problems.

Similarly, a working knowledge of the frequency of acute conditions may be helpful to the practitioner. Table 9-8 depicts a few of the acute conditions and their relative occurrence in the various age groups. Of note is the common occurrence of influenza in younger age groups in contrast to a less frequent occurrence in the elderly population. As noted earlier, however, influenza is a common

Table 9-7. Number of selected reported chronic conditions per 1,000 persons, by sex and age: United States, 1990

Type of chronic condition	Male					Female				
	Under 45	45-64	65 years and over			Under 45	45-64	65 years and over		
			Total	65-74	75+			Total	65-74	75+
Selected conditions of the genitourinary, nervous, endocrine, metabolic, and blood and blood-forming systems										
Goiter or other disorders of the thyroid	2.0	9.5	10.8	8.8	14.5	12.2	44.9	45.0	56.0	29.9
Diabetes	5.6	48.6	96.5	102.0	86.3	7.4	52.4	91.1	102.3	75.9
Anemias	4.6	2.5	9.5	8.9	10.8	25.9	22.5	29.5	28.1	31.4
Migraine headache	20.9	23.9	3.3	4.7	0.7	55.8	87.3	33.6	37.0	28.9
Kidney trouble	6.0	19.6	17.6	18.6	15.9	10.9	19.7	28.7	34.2	21.2
Bladder disorders	1.7	3.4	13.9	4.5	31.8	14.5	24.6	48.2	42.3	56.1
Diseases of prostate	2.9	22.8	78.5	68.0	98.0					
Selected circulatory conditions										
Ischemic heart disease	4.2	84.3	199.5	173.2	248.6	1.8	34.9	111.5	106.5	118.4
Heart rhythm disorders	17.5	26.7	55.3	48.3	68.3	23.7	44.4	70.9	69.8	72.5
High blood pressure (hypertension)	38.1	221.9	291.7	285.0	304.2	32.3	215.1	424.3	409.8	444.1
Cerebrovascular disease	1.6	19.0	73.5	60.9	96.9	1.1	14.5	55.5	40.8	75.5
Varicose veins of lower extremities	4.8	17.6	38.7	27.5	59.7	25.8	73.6	99.2	99.5	98.7
Hemorrhoids	22.7	71.1	46.2	53.4	32.7	28.9	70.8	68.1	73.4	60.8
Selected respiratory conditions										
Chronic bronchitis	40.4	31.6	58.0	62.0	50.5	51.7	81.1	79.3	87.8	67.8
Asthma	43.4	28.8	34.1	28.6	44.3	44.1	47.7	38.0	35.6	41.2
Hay fever or allergic rhinitis without asthma	89.1	80.6	66.0	65.1	67.6	96.3	108.4	68.9	83.5	49.0
Chronic sinusitis	99.9	162.7	136.9	132.2	145.5	127.7	199.5	162.3	171.7	149.6
Selected skin and musculoskeletal conditions										
Arthritis	25.8	204.9	374.5	373.3	376.8	35.8	289.7	538.4	472.2	628.6
Gout, including gouty arthritis	3.2	26.5	44.6	48.3	37.8	1.1	12.8	24.4	20.8	29.4
Intervertebral disc disorders	12.2	51.3	30.7	40.9	11.8	11.5	35.1	24.5	24.4	24.8
Trouble with bunions	2.1	10.4	6.0	3.2	11.1	8.9	43.1	55.0	56.8	52.7
Bursitis, unclassified	7.9	26.7	37.1	39.2	33.0	8.6	47.5	47.2	46.7	47.8
Trouble with dry (itching) skin, unclassified	12.9	19.7	30.4	30.6	30.4	20.7	25.3	43.5	46.4	39.5
Trouble with ingrown nails	20.1	33.0	38.3	34.3	45.7	14.9	35.0	58.4	56.2	61.6
Trouble with corns and calluses	10.0	22.7	25.0	23.0	28.6	13.7	41.9	62.9	65.1	59.9
Impairments										
Visual impairment	30.3	49.5	86.0	73.3	109.8	11.7	28.4	63.8	33.9	104.5
Cataracts	1.2	17.4	98.0	81.2	129.4	2.5	26.3	193.8	137.2	271.0
Glaucoma	1.1	11.5	53.7	44.1	71.7	0.7	12.3	49.1	41.5	59.5
Hearing impairment	49.7	197.8	395.5	350.1	480.2	29.6	106.0	269.1	194.9	370.3
Tinnitus	12.6	59.6	98.1	101.3	92.3	9.8	48.2	87.9	88.4	87.2
Selected digestive conditions										
Ulcer	11.0	31.6	38.2	38.3	38.1	14.3	25.8	29.6	29.2	29.9
Hernia of abdominal cavity	6.7	35.1	55.5	42.7	79.3	6.4	24.0	58.2	56.5	60.4
Gastritis or duodenitis	7.6	14.6	17.6	15.8	20.8	10.6	20.9	24.5	27.1	21.1
Frequent indigestion	16.6	36.5	35.2	29.2	46.4	18.9	29.1	45.8	57.0	30.6
Spastic colon	1.9	3.2	9.3	9.3	9.5	7.2	18.5	18.0	12.7	25.2
Frequent constipation	4.9	5.6	30.5	17.3	55.1	15.5	22.3	69.7	47.3	100.2

From National Center for Health Statistics, USDHHS, *Vital and health statistics* 10(181):84-85, 1992.

Table 9-8. Number of acute conditions per 100 persons per year, by age and type of condition: United States, 1990

Type of acute condition	All ages	Under 5	5-17	18-24	25-44	45 Years and over		
						Total	45-64	65+
All acute conditions	171.9	365.0	238.4	174.8	145.1	111.1	114.4	105.8
Common cold	25.0	65.8	32.2	27.2	20.3	14.6	14.0	15.4
Influenza	43.4	60.3	61.8	46.3	43.0	27.6	33.0	19.3
Digestive system conditions	5.3	4.2	7.3	6.6	4.9	4.3	4.3	4.4
Injuries	24.4	27.6	29.7	28.8	25.2	18.3	19.9	15.9

From National Center for Health Statistics, USDHHS, *Vital and health statistics* 10(181):13, 1992.

cause of death in the elderly age group. Therefore influenza vaccination becomes increasingly important in households in which an elderly person resides with young children. Injuries occur throughout all age groups but are more common in younger persons. The common cold occurs most often in children. This information will guide the practitioner to discuss preventive issues related to a person's specific home situation. An example may be the counseling of soon-to-be parents regarding injury prevention in children and hygiene in the prevention of spread of infections. Similarly, inquiry into personal and family history of digestive disease conditions may guide the practitioner to specific counseling about over-the-counter preparations in the young adult when these symptoms increase in frequency.

For the practitioner, each patient visit represents an opportunity for preventive intervention. Simply by knowing the general age of the patient, this mortality and morbidity framework easily narrows the issues. The interview then allows for further focusing of preventive interventions.

THE INTERVIEW

The key to a successful preventive interview involves several factors. First, the patient should feel comfortable. The patient may feel guilty or inhibited about certain issues. Therefore establishing rapport, first by working through questions that most patients have come to expect as being part of the practitioner/patient interview and later discussing more difficult areas for which the person may be less likely to be as open, is often helpful. Another factor is ease of communication. Interpreters may be helpful and necessary if language is a problem. Family members may help but at other times may hinder good communication. The practitioner is encouraged to see any patient presenting with family present both alone, and *if* the person wishes, with the family members. An initial meeting with the patient alone is often useful in making the patient feel more at ease. In other situations, the opposite may be true and visiting first with the patient and his or her family may be helpful. Another factor is the attention of the physician

or practitioner. The physician should convey his or her interest in the patient. He or she should be attentive to the patient, listen, provide eye contact, and convey empathy. The patient should feel that the health care provider is interested in his or her specific problems. Therefore, interruptions and distractions should be avoided. Likewise the patient must feel that information discussed is confidential.

An organized sequence for the interview is preferable but may not always be possible. The physician is encouraged to allow the patient to express his or her concerns fully and openly. Time constraints may require continuation of a discussion at a later visit. Patients may need to be re-directed, but caution should be exercised not to interrupt too frequently. The purpose of the preventive interview is to obtain information but also to provide counseling. Counseling should be considered and offered at anytime during the encounter with the patient including during the physical examination and after the history and physical examination have been completed. Care should be given also to convey to the patient a sense of personal responsibility to implement change in his or her own life that can favorably alter disease risk factors. Thereby, emphasis is on future rather than past habits. The patient is encouraged to learn from the past and change the present in order to affect the future.

The physician's appearance and image are often helpful in providing preventive advice. The physician as a role model is a powerful tool in changing a person's preventive behavior. Exercise habits, diet, and personal habits such as smoking and alcohol consumption reflect on the reliability of the physician providing advice to the patient.

Patients go to a preventive examination with a variety of emotions and agendas. Eliciting exactly what motivated the person to seek an examination often will point to the opportunities the physician has to modify risk factors. The concern of a loved one, the death of a friend or another family member, a symptom, or fear of a disease are often reasons for patient requesting a preventive examination. These reasons, however, may not be obvious or easily volunteered by the patient unless the practitioner specifically searches and asks. Hostility may mask the true concerns of a patient, and guilt may override a person's ability to change behavior. Comfort and attention by the practitioner will often help to circumvent these emotions. With experience, the preventive physician can become adept at identifying the true concerns of patients and capitalize on the opportunities for preventive intervention presented by each patient encounter.

HEALTH HISTORY QUESTIONNAIRE

A health history or preventive history questionnaire serves as a useful tool to prepare both the patient and physician for the discussion and examination. A questionnaire such as that depicted in Table 9-9 can be submitted to the patient by mail or presented to the patient in person by ancillary personnel in the office before the physician interview and examination.

Table 9-9 can be developed for a practitioner's unique practice setting. The kinds of questions asked, the manner in which they are asked, and the emphasis of the questionnaire depends on the unique population served by the practitioner. The questionnaire depicted in Table 9-9 has been developed for and serves well in a patient population that is urban, middle class, high school or college educated, middle age and older, and Caucasian or black. The manner in which these questions are asked may not be as useful in persons of other cultures or educational and socioeconomic groups. The components of the questionnaire involve demographic data, medications, prior medical history, vaccination history, family history, occupational history, social history, and review of organ systems.

Demographic data

This should include the name, address, and phone number to allow future contact with the patient. Age will help to stratify causes of mortality and morbidity. Education, employer, job, and job title should be listed. Reviewing these questions verbally serves as a way of showing the interest of the physician in the individual and allowing the individual to become more comfortable with the physician-patient interaction.

Patient problems and concerns

This portion of the questionnaire allows the patient to write down the reasons why he or she seeks an evaluation. As noted above, the true reasons why a person comes in for an examination may not always be apparent. Discussing this portion of the questionnaire in detail can serve as a means of finding those true reasons. Helpful questions include "What caused you to come in for an examination today?" or "Are you here today for a particular question or concern, or because you or your spouse, child, etc. are worried about you?" Many factors may motivate a person to go in for an examination including friends, family, symptoms, birthday, illness or death of acquaintances, me-

dia, or fears. Uncovering these reasons is an important goal of the initial part of patient interview, as the encounter should be directed at the reason the person sought an evaluation.

Medications

All medications, dosages, and length of time used should be listed. This should include substances not often thought of by patients as being true medications such as vitamins, pain relievers, birth control pills, antacids, laxatives, antihistamines, inhalers, eye drops, skin preparations, and other over-the-counter substances. Many of these medications may cause side effects or interact with prescription medications (see Chapter 14). Comprehensive recording of these medications allows for prevention of these kinds of interactions. The Medical Letter provides a good source for drug interactions (see Resources section), listing numerous drugs and the possible adverse interactions, and recommendations for preventing such occurrences.[6] Table 9-10 depicts a few selected drugs and their potential interactions from this handbook.

Patients may also list prescription drugs that have been prescribed but are not taken in the way they were prescribed. Reviewing each drug and how often the person actually takes the drug is important to know about all medications used by the individual. Requesting patients to bring all medications with them so that the prescription listed on each bottle can be reviewed is a helpful way of knowing what the patient is actually taking. Looking at the date of the prescription and the number of pills in the bottle can demonstrate the compliance level of the patient. Other questions that help to outline all medications taken by a patient are to ask the patient whether he or she takes any prescription medications of other family members and whether or not he or she uses sleeping aids. This kind of information is often not volunteered electively by patients.

Previous medical history

Previous medical history includes listing of prior operations, hospitalizations, broken bones, serious illnesses, allergic reactions, and ongoing medical conditions. Some patients will be compulsive about listing all previous illnesses and injuries, whereas others will frequently forget hospitalizations or prior surgeries. During the physical examination, any scars present that are not accounted for in the listing on the questionnaire should be asked about and that data recorded. Drug reactions should likewise be specified as many people feel they are "allergic" to a given medication, whereas in fact they had a side effect of the medication that would thereby not necessarily preclude use of another medication in that class of drugs any time in the future. Asking the patient about specific diseases such as diabetes or heart disease as outlined in question 4 in Table 9-9 draws attention to major disease categories that the patient may have overlooked in listing serious illnesses.

Table 9-9. Preventive medicine medical history

Name _____ Date_____
Address_____
Home phone _____ Business phone_____
Employer_____ Job _____
Age_____ Place of birth_____ Date of birth _____
Education (highest level attained) _____

1. Please list all **present problems and concerns:**
    1. _____
    2. _____
    3. _____

2. Please list all *medications* taken regularly, dosage, and length of time each has been used. *Include over-the-counter* medications, vitamins, aspirin, birth control pills, antacids, nasal sprays, eye drops, injections, and topical (skin) preparations.

Medication months taking medication	Dosage	Number of years or
_____	_____	_____
_____	_____	_____
_____	_____	_____
_____	_____	_____
_____	_____	_____

3. Please list all *past* operations, hospitalizations, broken bones, serious illnesses, and allergies:

	Year	Reason or Problem
Hospitalizations:	____	_____
	____	_____
	____	_____
Fractures or broken bones:	____	_____
	____	_____
Prior blood transfusions	____	_____
	____	_____
Serious illnesses:	____	_____
	____	_____
	____	_____

Drug allergies or reactions	Name of Drug	Reaction
	_____	_____
	_____	_____
	_____	_____

4. Have you had any of the following? (Please circle)
   Diabetes, heart disease, cancer, emphysema, bronchitis, migraine, gout, colon polyps or disease, stroke, kidney disease, gallbladder disease, high blood pressure, vascular disease, neurologic disease, serious infection

5. **Vaccinations**
   Please list approximate year of last vaccination for the following—if known:
   Tetanus and diphtheria_____
   Pneumovax (pneumococcal vaccine)_____
   Flu vaccine_____
   Hepatitis B_____
   Measles _____
   Mumps_____
   Rubella_____

6. **Family Medical History**

	Living?	Age(s) now or age at death	Significant medical problems and/or cause of death
Father	___ yes ___ no	_____	_____
Mother	___ yes ___ no	_____	_____
Spouse	___ yes ___ no	_____	_____
Brothers	___ yes ___ no	_____	_____
Sisters	___ yes ___ no	_____	_____
Sons	___ yes ___ no	_____	_____
Daughters	___ yes ___ no	_____	_____
Grandparents			
Maternal GF	___ yes ___ no	_____	_____
GM	___ yes ___ no	_____	_____
Paternal GF	___ yes ___ no	_____	_____
GM	___ yes ___ no	_____	_____

Uncles and aunts with significant diseases _____
_____
_____

Table 9-9, cont'd. Preventive medicine medical history.

Is there any family history of (please circle):
Ulcers, tuberculosis, alcoholism, heart disease, cancer, stroke, diabetes, emphysema, high blood pressure, high cholesterol, kidney disease, colon polyps, ulcers, gout, Alzheimer's disease, congenital disorders, or other serious illness

7. Tobacco:
   Have you ever smoked? ___ yes ___ no
   Do you smoke now? ___ yes ___ no
   a. _____ cigarettes a day?
   b. _____ cigars a day?
   c. _____ ounces or pouches a week? (pipe)
   Total years you have smoked in your life _____
   Do you chew tobacco or use snuff? ___ yes ___ no
   If you have quit tobacco, what year did you quit? _____

8. Do you use alcohol? ___ yes ___ no
   a. _____ ounces liquor per day or week
   b. _____ ounces wine per day or week
   c. _____ ounces beer per day or week
   If you have quit, when did you quit? _____
   Have you ever been counseled for alcohol or drug abuse? ___ yes ___ no
   Do you or have you in the past regularly used marijuana, cocaine, amphetamines or any other mind-altering drug?
   ___ yes ___ no

9. Do you drink coffee? ___ yes ___ no
   a. _____ cups per day (caffeinated)
   b. _____ cups per day (decaffeinated)
   Do you drink cola? ___ yes ___ no
   c. _____ ounces per day
   Do you drink tea? ___ yes ___ no
   d. _____ cups per day

10. Do you have a regular exercise program? ___ yes ___ no
    If yes, please describe: _____
    Number of days per week _____

11. How much sleep do you get at night? ___ hours
    Do you snore heavily? ___ yes ___ no

12. Number of meals eaten on an average day_____
    Number of glasses of water consumed in an average day _____
    Rank the content of fat of your diet ___ high ___ medium ___ low
    Rank the salt content of your diet ___ high ___ medium ___ low
    List your most common snack foods_____

13. Do you wear seat belts when in the car? ___ always ___ sometimes ___ never

14. Do you participate in any dangerous hobbies or activities? ___ yes ___ no
    Specify_____

15. Do you have smoke alarms in your home? ___ yes ___ no

16. Occupational history
    Please list all jobs you have held in adult life:

Jobs	Years
_____	_____
_____	_____
_____	_____
_____	_____

Have you had any exposure to known toxins, cancer-causing substances (carcinogens), or known hazardous materials? ___ yes
___ no
If yes, list substance and when exposed: _____

Table 9-10. Drug interactions

Interacting drugs	Adverse effects (probable mechanism)	Comments and recommendations
Acetaminophen, with		
Alcohol	Severe hepatotoxicity with therapeutic doses of acetaminophen in chronic alcoholics (mechanism not established)	Incidence unknown; warn patients
Anticoagulants, oral	Increased anticoagulant effect (mechanism not established)	Inconsistent effect; monitor prothrombin time
Benzodiazepines	Possible diazepam toxicity (mechanism not established)	Monitor clinical status
Beta-adrenergic blockers	Decreased acetaminophen clearance with propranolol (decreased metabolism)	Clinical significance not established
Alcohol, with		
Bromocriptine	Possible increased bromocriptine toxicity (mechanism not established)	Clinical evidence limited; warn patients
Cycloserine	Increased alcohol effect or convulsions (mechanism not established)	Avoid concurrent use; warn patients
Heparin	Increased bleeding (additive)	Avoid large amounts of alcohol
Hypoglycemics	Decreased hypoglycemic effect with chronic abuse (increased metabolism)	Avoid large amounts of alcohol
Sulfonylurea	Increased or prolonged hypoglycemic effect with acute ingestion of alcohol, especially in fasting patients (suppression of gluconeogenesis)	
Methotrexate	Increased hepatotoxicity in chronic alcoholics (mechanism not established)	Monitor hepatic function
Caffeine, with		
Alcohol	Caffeine may further decrease reaction time (synergism or antagonism)	Variable response
Contraceptives, oral	Possible caffeine toxicity (decreased metabolism)	Possibly significant with large doses of caffeine, especially with prolonged use
Iron, oral	Decreased iron effect (decreased absorption)	Give at least 2 hours apart
Theophyllines	Increased toxicity of both drugs in patients with liver disease (decreased metabolism)	Monitor methylxanthine as well as theophylline concentration in patients with liver disease
Verapamil	Possible caffeine toxicity (decreased metabolism)	Monitor cardiovascular status; based on studies in healthy men
Vitamin C, with		
Anticoagulants	Decreased anticoagulant effect (mechanism not established)	Occurs only occasionally; monitor prothrombin time
Estrogens	Increased serum concentration and possible increased toxicity of estrogens	Decrease vitamin C to 100 mg/day

From Rizack MD, Hillman CD: *Handbook of adverse drug interactions,* New York, 1991, The Medical Letter.

Vaccinations

Previous adult vaccinations should be listed. If persons are unaware of the previous vaccination history, practitioners are encouraged to seek previous medical records. Routine vaccinations to be listed should include the following:

- Tetanus and diphtheria
- Pneumococcal
- Influenza
- Hepatitis B
- Measles
- Mumps
- Rubella

Other vaccinations may be recorded if such are appropriate for the person's risk. An example is rabies vaccination in a veterinarian or animal handler. Please see also Chapter 57, Infectious Diseases and Immunizations. In reviewing vaccination history, the time is ideal for updating the person's vaccination status. Working knowledge of side effects and indications for the given vaccination are important for the practitioner to reassure the patient about the need for and the potential side effects of the procedure being performed. Knowing the mortality and morbidity figures outlined earlier in the chapter will help the practitioner to educate the patient about the need for a given vaccination.

Family medical history

Although family medical history is not a modifiable risk factor, the condition itself may be modifiable. In addition, these data may lead to counseling on future generations and genetic counseling for the patient or family members.

Assessment of this information is important to identify those conditions for which a person is at high risk so that other modifiable risk factors for that same condition can be addressed and improved upon. Most conditions are more strongly related to first-degree relatives. First-degree relatives include parents, siblings, and offspring. All important medical disorders or diseases of first-degree relatives should be outlined. Some of the more important disorders conveying higher risk to the individual are family history of the following:

- Cancer of the breast, colon, prostate, uterus, and ovaries
- Premature coronary artery disease
- Autosomal dominant disorders such as family hypercholesterolemia, Marfan's syndrome, polycystic kidney disease, Huntington's chorea, and neurofibromatosis
- Autosomal recessive disorders such as deafness, Wilson's disease, and hemochromatosis
- Inherited disorders specific for certain ethnic groups such as sickle cell disease or hemoglobinopathies[4] (see Chapters 38-40). Health conditions existent in a deceased parent that were not related to the specific cause of death are often overlooked by patients and should be carefully reviewed. Autopsy reports and medical records of deceased first-degree relatives may be helpful for the patient to outline a clear picture of his or her own family medical risk profile. Review of family medical history also presents an opportunity to counsel patients about appropriate screening and testing of their siblings, children, or parents for risk factors or diseases of importance uncovered by the interview.

Social history

The social history provides much information to the preventive practitioner for counseling and modification of risk factors. This portion of the questionnaire serves as a basis for areas of prevention often overlooked in the traditional physician-patient encounter. Therefore careful review of each facet of the social history with the questions in the questionnaire serving as a basis should be undertaken. These should include at least the following:

Tobacco. All tobacco use in the person's lifetime and particularly that used currently should be recorded and discussed. Smoking cessation options should be understood by the practitioner and referral for any cessation interventions should be available. Having patient education materials available that can be brought out at this point in the interview often serves as an opportunity to motivate a person to take active steps to modify his or her tobacco habit (see Chapter 16 Resources). Often persons have stopped smoking—sometimes even very recently—and will record that they do not smoke and sometimes even that they have not smoked in the past. They often feel guilt about this habit. Empathy from the physician that this is a difficult habit to break can serve to enhance the ability of the physician to motivate the patient. Use of other tobacco products such as chewing tobacco are ignored in the standard medical interview and should be surveyed in the preventive interview. One pouch of pipe tobacco contains 1 or 1½ oz. of tobacco.

Alcohol and illicit drugs. As with tobacco, alcohol consumption may be difficult to quantify as persons often minimize or underestimate their usage. Using the questionnaire as a basis for further discussion will help the practitioner to quantify alcohol usage and determine the degree of dependency that may be present for a given individual. This discussion also serves to outline the medical conditions associated with alcohol abuse. Many patients know of alcohol-related liver disease but are unaware of alcohol's effects on the heart, blood pressure, and bone marrow. Persons will often classify themselves as "moderate" drinkers of alcohol. Working with them to define what is meant by "moderation" serves as a foundation to establish whether alcohol is in fact a problem. Other questions may be added to the questionnaire under the heading Alcohol Use:

1. Have you ever had "blackouts" or been unable to recall events after a drinking episode?
2. Do you have a family history of alcoholism?
3. Have you ever lost work days because of alcohol consumption?
4. Do you drink one or two drinks even though you "shouldn't"?
5. Have you been unable to stop drinking for a period of one month or more?
6. Have you ever been to an Alcoholics Anonymous meeting?
7. Have you ever been in a fight while under the influence of alcohol?
8. Do you drink in the morning?
9. Have you ever had the shakes, DT's (delirium tremens), or hallucinations after drinking?

(For further discussion of assessing alcohol usage, see Chapter 15, Drug Dependence and Substance Abuse)

As with alcohol, use of illicit drugs is not often easily volunteered by patients. The patient must feel that the information discussed is confidential and will not be revealed even to family members who may be present with the patient at the time of the interview. A judgmental attitude must never be taken. Questions specifically about use of marijuana, cocaine, amphetamines, heroine, and other drugs should be asked even if the patient has listed "no" to those same questions on the questionnaire. This presents an opportunity also for the practitioner to review the health effects of any substances used by the patient and to discuss any fears the patient has about long-term health effects from previous usage. A working knowledge of this kind of information is important for the practitioner so that these questions may be encouraged and discussed freely.

Caffeine. Caffeine may or may not be associated with medical disease. Many studies have been conducted to evaluate the causal relationship of caffeine and a variety of medical diseases. The substance present in many foods and beverages does not appear to contribute in a significant way to the major causes of mortality but can cause symptoms that may be bothersome to the patient such as tremor, insomnia, and withdrawal headache. Quantifying caffeine consumption often unveils a caffeine dependency. See Table 26-7 for caffeine content of beverages and foods.

A caffeine table in the office can assist the practitioner in educating the patient about the relative caffeine content of the foods and beverages he or she consumes. This also serves as an opportunity to modify caffeine intake by suggesting other beverages or substitutes that have less caffeine content. Persons should be counseled to decrease caffeine intake gradually to avoid the symptoms of caffeine withdrawal. A common occurrence of caffeine withdrawal is the office worker who consumes coffee freely available during the work week on the job but consumes less on weekends. These persons frequently will encounter headache and caffeine withdrawal symptoms in the afternoon on Saturdays or Sundays. Demonstrating to patients the presence of these caffeine withdrawal symptoms can motivate them to decrease caffeine intake.

Exercise. Studies have shown that physical activity, recreational or occupational, is associated with decreased risk for coronary artery disease, colon cancer, stroke, and hypertension.[5] Exercise is also useful in the management of a number of diseases including diabetes, depression, and obesity (see Chapter 18).[5] Blair et al., in a study of 10,224 men and 3120 women, provided evidence that physical fitness is associated with lower cardiovascular disease, cancer, and all-cause mortality.[1] An important aspect of the preventive history therefore is an assessment of the patient's exercise level and counseling and encouragement for the patient to attain an optimal level of exercise. Ideally, if the patient is not engaged in a physically demanding job, he or she should be exercising at least 3 or 4 times per week for 30 to 40 minutes of aerobic activity. Heart rate during the aerobic period should be kept at a rate of 70% to 80% predicted maximum for that person's age. Target heart rate can be calculated for an individual as 220 minus the person's age and that number multiplied by .7 or .8 for **most** well people (see Chapter 19).

For the healthy individual, a simple guide to appropriate exercise level is that while exercising the person should be able to carry on a conversation, but because of some shortness of breath, has to work at maintaining that conversation. Inability to converse while exercising represents generally an excessive level of exercise. Ideally, exercise should be enjoyable and convenient so as to enhance long-term compliance. A social component to the exercise is often helpful in providing enjoyment and in ensuring long-

term compliance. Some persons should be encouraged therefore to participate in exercise with a spouse, friend, neighbor, or colleague whom he or she enjoys spending time with. Others enjoy this period as time alone. In each patient there is a key that assists in turning him or her on to a program. Mutual encouragement of persons participating in an exercise program often leads to that exercise becoming a habit. Care should be given in the selection of a specific exercise to any physical limitations of the patient. Exercise ideally should not aggravate pre-existing conditions such as low back pain, arthritis, or knee or ankle problems. A variety of activities can be recommended to the patient. When reviewing exercise, leisure activity should not be discouraged but only added to, so as to provide appropriate aerobic conditioning. Seasonal variation in exercise is to be encouraged as well. An assessment of the patient's previous exercise habits often gives clues to the kind of exercise to recommend to that person. A chart listing various exercises is often helpful to the practitioner in this portion of the interview. For further information please see Chapter 19, A Program for Fitness.

Sleep. Quantity and quality of sleep are important to assess. Chapter 17 outlines sleep patterns and disorders and Chapter 11 addresses the sleep problems of jet lag. Level of snoring is often helpful in uncovering undiagnosed sleep apnea. Use of sleep aids such as over-the-counter medications, prescription medications, or alcohol should be assessed because this information may not be volunteered.

Diet. Aspects of appropriate dietary assessment are discussed in detail in Part 5, Clinical Nutrition in Disease Prevention. A short list of questions on the preventive medicine questionnaire can lead to more detailed discussion in the interview. These questions should include number of daily meals, fat content, salt content, balance, and consumption of snack foods. This information along with previous questions of caffeine intake, alcohol consumption, and vitamin usage will help to provide an overview of the patient's nutrition level. This also provides an opportunity for counseling and intervention.

Safety. An assessment of safety habits in all people should include use of seat belts. Persons may admit to using seat belts but when questioned further, they may confine that use to trips or long distances or to certain automobiles. Discussing this as part of the medical interview helps to promote more general use of seat belts. Inquiries should also be made into high-risk recreational activities such as biking, motorcycling, and other sports. Appropriate counseling should be given for use of helmets, eye protection, hearing protection, and gloves. Questions about home safety are reviewed in Chapter 64, Safety in the Home and Automobile. A question about smoke alarms leads into a discussion of fire safety in the home and implementation of a plan if a fire occurs.

Table 9-11. Abbreviated list of sentinel health events (occupational)

Condition	Industry/occupation	Agent
Pulmonary tuberculosis	Physicians, medical personnel	*Mycobacterium tuberculosis*
Plague, tularemia, anthrax, rabies, and other infections	Farmers, ranchers, hunters, veterinarians, laboratory workers	Various infectious agents
Rubella	Medical personnel, intensive care personnel	Rubella virus
Hepatitis A, B, and non-A, non-B	Day care center staff, orphanage staff, medical personnel	Hepatitis A virus, hepatitis B virus
Ornithosis	Bird breeders, pet shop staff, poultry producers, veterinarians, zoo employees	*Chlamydia psittaci*
Malignant neoplasm of nasal cavities	Woodworkers, cabinet/furniture makers,	Hardwood dust
	Radium chemists and processors,	Radium
	Nickel smelting and refining	Nickel
Malignant neoplasm of larynx	Asbestos industries and utilizers	Asbestos
Malignant neoplasm of trachea, bronchus, and lung	Asbestos industries and utilizers	Asbestos
	Topside coke oven workers	Coke oven emissions
	Uranium and fluorspar miners	Radon daughters
	Smelters, processors, users	Chromates, nickel, arsenic
	Mustard gas formulators	Mustard gas
	Ion exchange resin makers, chemists	Bis (chloromethyl) ether
Mesothelioma	Asbestos industries and utilizers	Asbestos
Malignant neoplasm of bone	Radium chemists and processors	Radium
Malignant neoplasm of scrotum	Automatic lathe operators, metal workers	Mineral/cutting oils
	Coke oven workers, petroleum refiners	Soots and tars
Malignant neoplasm of bladder	Rubber and dye workers	Benzidine, naphthylamine, auramine, 4-nitrophenyl
Malignant neoplasm of kidney	Coke oven workers	Coke oven emissions
Lymphoid leukemia, acute	Radiologists, rubber industry	Ionizing radiation, unknown
Myeloid leukemia, acute	Occupations with exposure to benzene	Benzene
	Radiologists	Ionizing radiation
Erythroleukemia	Occupations with exposure to benzene	Benzene
Hemolytic anemia, nonautoimmune	Whitewashing and leather industry	Copper sulfate
	Electrolytic processes, smelting	Arsine
	Plastics industry	Trimellitic anhydride
Aplastic anemia	Explosives manufacture	TNT
	Radiologists, radium, chemists	Ionizing radiation
Agranulocytosis or neutropenia	Explosives and pesticide industries	Phosphorus
	Pesticides, pigments, pharmaceuticals	Inorganic arsenic
Toxic encephalitis	Battery, smelter, and foundry workers	Lead
Parkinson's disease (secondary)	Manganese processing, battery makers, welders	Manganese
Inflammatory and toxic neuropathy	Pesticides, pigments, pharmaceuticals	Arsenic and arsenic compounds
	Furniture refinishers, degreasing operations	Hexane
	Plastics, rayon industries	MBK, CS_2, other solvents
	Explosives industry	TNT
	Battery, smelter, and foundry workers	Lead
	Dentists, chloralkali plants, battery makers	Mercury
	Plastics industry, paper manufacturing	Acrylamide
	Microwave and radar technicians	Microwaves
	Radiologists	Ionizing radiation
	Blacksmiths, glass blowers, bakers	Infrared radiation
	Moth repellant formulators, fumigators	Naphthalene
Noise effects on inner ear	Many industries	Excessive noise
Raynaud's phenomenon (secondary)	Lumberjacks, chain saw operators, grinders	Whole body, segmental vibration
	Vinyl chloride polymerization industry	Vinyl chloride monomer

From Landrigan DL, Baker DB: Using occupational history to pinpoint the diagnosis, *Geriatrics:* 46(6):63-64, 1991.

Table 9-11, cont'd. Abbreviated list of sentinel health events (occupational).

Condition	Industry/occupation	Agent
Extrinsic asthma	Jewelry, alloy, and catalyst makers	Platinum
	Polyurethane, adhesive, paint workers	Isocyanates
	Plastic, dye, insecticide makers	Phthalic anhydride
	Foam workers, latex makers, biologists	Formaldehyde
	Bakers	Flour
	Woodworkers, furniture makers	Red cedar and other wood dust
Coalworkers' pneumoconiosis	Coal miners	Coal dust
Asbestosis	Asbestos industries and utilizers	Asbestos
Silicosis	Quarrymen, sandblasters, silica processors, mining, ceramic industries, and foundries	Silica
Talcosis	Talc processors	Talc
Chronic beryllium disease	Beryllium alloy workers, ceramic workers	Beryllium
Byssinosis	Cotton industry workers	Cotton, flax, hemp, and cotton-synthetic dusts
Acute bronchitis, pneumonitis, and pulmonary edema caused by fumes and vapors	Alkali and bleach industries	Chlorine
	Silo fillers, arc welders	Nitrogen oxides
	Paper, refrigeration, oil industries	Sulfur dioxide
	Plastics industry	Trimellitic anhydride
Toxic hepatitis	Solvent utilizers, dry cleaners, plastics industry	Carbon tetrachloride, chloroform, trichloroethylene
	Explosives and dye industries	Phosphorus, TNT
	Fumigators, fire extinguisher formulators	Ethylene dibromide
Acute or chronic renal failure	Battery makers, plumbers, solderers	Inorganic lead
	Electrolytic processes, smelting	Arsine
	Battery makers, jewelers, dentists	Inorganic mercury
	Fire extinguisher makers	Carbon tetrachloride
	Antifreeze manufacture	Ethylene glycol
Infertility, male	Formulators and applicators	Dibromochloropropane
Contact and allergic dermatitis	Leather tanning, poultry dressing plants, fish packing, adhesives, and sealant industry, boat building and repair	Irritants (e.g., cutting oils, solvents, acids, alkalis, allergens)

Occupational history

As noted earlier in this chapter, discussion of occupation often serves to establish rapport and comfort with the patient and to develop openness. Knowing the person's job title and company name are often not enough to know what the person actually does on the job and the health risks associated with the job. The patient should be asked to describe what he or she does on a daily basis and what safety precautions and protective equipment are used. Many substances encountered in the workplace have significant health effects. A partial list of offending agents is outlined in Table 9-11.

The occupational interview is an ideal time to discuss often neglected personal safety issues such as use of ear plugs, respirators, eye protection, and gloves. Listing all previous jobs also serves to outline potential health issues later in life. Frequently occupational disease has a long lag period for development of a related disease. Please see Chapter 62 for more detailed discussion of these issues. The occupational history is also an opportune time to ask

about stress. Questions such as "How is your job going?", "Have you noticed any increased pressure or stress on the job?", "Do you take regular vacations?", and "Do you use all of your allotted vacation time?" can help to assess the patient's stress level (see Chapter 12).

REVIEW OF MEDICAL SYSTEMS

Review of medical systems and risk factor profiles are tools used to determine a person's likelihood for common and important medical conditions.[3,8] These may be constructed and modified depending on the population served by the practitioner and the important health issues in that given population. Questions in the review of systems can be grouped by organ system or in a risk factor profile type format. The list can be simple or elaborate depending on multiple factors such as time allotted for the evaluation, educational level of the patient, and method of review of the questionnaire. The review of systems in Table 9-12 is designed for a comprehensive evaluation.

Areas can be expanded to provide emphasis. For exam-

Table 9-12. Review of medical systems

Yes	No	General
—	—	Do you have excess fatigue?
—	—	Has your weight changed in the past year?
		If so, how much? __ pounds (Circle: Loss or Gain)
		What has been your normal weight during the past few years? __ pounds
—	—	Have you had problems with dry skin, rash, eczema, or itching?
—	—	Have you had problems with psoriasis, skin cancer, or other skin conditions?
—	—	Have you had skin lesions that have changed in size, shape, color, or contour?
—	—	Are you concerned about any skin lesions that you think could be skin cancer?
—	—	Do you use deodorant soaps?

		Head and neck
—	—	Do you have frequent or periodic headaches?
—	—	Have you had dizziness or loss of consciousness (passing out)?
—	—	Have you had problems with memory?
—	—	Have you had seizures or convulsions?
—	—	Have you had problems with loss of vision, double vision, blurred vision, or seeing halos around lights?
—	—	Have you had cataracts or other eye disease?
		When was your last eye examination? _____
—	—	Have you had problems hearing or been told by others that you appear to have hearing loss?
—	—	Have you had ringing in the ears?
—	—	Have you had problems with sense of smell, nose bleeds, or breathing through the nose?
—	—	Have you had recurrent sinus infections or congestion?
—	—	Have you had problems with the teeth, gums, or throat?
—	—	Have you had problems with bad breath (halitosis)?
		Do you floss the teeth regularly?
		Date of last dental examination _____
—	—	Have you had goiter (increased size of the thyroid) or previous thyroid disease?
—	—	Have you had problems with swallowing or neck pain?
—	—	Have you had previous x-ray treatments (radiation) to the neck?
—	—	Have you had frequent hoarseness or a change in the character of your voice?

		Cardiopulmonary
—	—	Do you notice chest pain, ache, pressure, discomfort, or tightness?
		If so, how long does it last? _____ Is it caused by exertion? _____ by emotion? _____
—	—	Do you have discomfort in the arms, neck, or back?
—	—	Do you notice irregular or rapid heart beating?
—	—	Do you have shortness of breath on exertion, at night, or at rest?
—	—	Do you notice swelling of the feet, ankles, or hands?
—	—	Do you have a chronic cough?
—	—	Do you have hay fever or asthma?

		Gastrointestinal
—	—	Any trouble swallowing?
—	—	Are you bothered with heartburn?
—	—	Do you have abdominal pain?
—	—	Have you had black stools?
—	—	Have you had a change in bowel movements?
—	—	Have you passed blood with one or more bowel movements?
—	—	Have you had polyps in the colon or rectum?
—	—	Have you had a change in your bowel movements, frequent constipation, or intolerance to certain foods?

		Musculoskeletal
—	—	Have you had back pain?
		If so, does it go into the buttock, thigh, calf, or foot?
		(Circle: Right or Left)

Continued.

Table 9-12, cont'd. Review of medical systems.

Yes	No	General
—	—	Have you had joint pain, redness, or swelling?
—	—	Have you had pain in the legs when walking?
—	—	If so, does it improve quickly with rest?
—	—	Do you have tremor or shaking of the hands?
		Genitourinary—Men
—	—	Do you urinate at night?
		If so, number of times each night —
—	—	Have you had a kidney, bladder, or prostate infection in the past year?
—	—	Do you have problems emptying the bladder completely?
—	—	Do you have normal sexual drive (libido), erections, and ability to have normal sexual intercourse?
		Females
—	—	Do you have problems with control of urination?
—	—	Do you urinate at night?
		If so, number of times each night _____
—	—	Have you had bladder or urinary tract infections in the past year?
—	—	Have you noted blood in the urine?
—	—	Have you had discharge from the vagina?
—	—	Do you have discomfort with intercourse?
—	—	Have you had hot flashes, sweating at night, or dryness of the vagina?
		Age at time of first menstrual period _____
		Date of last menstrual period _____
		Number of pregnancies _____
		Number of births _____
—	—	Have you had vaginal spotting or bleeding at times other than your menstrual period?
—	—	Have your menstrual periods changed in frequency, regularity, or amount?
—	—	Do you have menstrual tension, pain, or other symptoms at around the time of your menstrual periods?
—	—	Have you experienced any recent breast tenderness, lumps, or nipple discharge?
		Mental Health
—	—	Is stress a major problem for you?
—	—	Do you feel depressed?
—	—	Do you desire stress or other counseling?
—	—	Do you often panic when stressed?
—	—	Do you have problems with appetite?
—	—	Do you cry frequently or feel "blue"?
—	—	Do you have problems with relationships?
—	—	Are you satisfied with your life?

ple, if safety issues are to be stressed, then questions pertaining to use of air bags, anti-lock brakes, firearms in the home, and posting of emergency phone numbers in the home may be added to the questionnaire. In another situation these may be left for verbal discussion by the physician or practitioner with the patient. Likewise, more intimate questions such as those related to sexually transmitted disease or to HIV risk factors may be listed in the questionnaire or instead left to personal discussion in the office. This information might include questions about homosexuality, multiple sexual partners, intravenous drug usage, and other sexually transmitted diseases. Similarly, questions pertinent to sexual function may or may not be listed in the questionnaire. Those questions listed in Table 9-12 related to male sexual dysfunction may at the practitioner's discretion be eliminated from the written questionnaire and asked instead in person. The art of discussing these issues in a nonthreatening and nonjudgmental fashion, making the patient feel comfortable and open, takes practice and consideration by the practitioner of his or her own individual biases and prejudices.

Questions to uncover problems of depression, anxiety, and stress are not as easily accomplished in a written questionnaire format. These issues may also often be overlooked by the practitioner. A set of questions that can be included as a framework are indicated at the end of Table 9-12. These may be expanded or modified depending on the practice setting. These questions serve as a take-off point for discussion of issues of concern to a patient that relate to his or her "mental health." The outlets an individual has to discuss stress and issues of personal concern should be ascertained. Many individuals have no close friend or confidant to discuss these problems. Providing a strategy for the individual to identify the appropriate person should be undertaken. Family issues such as problems with children, spouse, or parents often weigh heavily on a person's mind, and that individual often has a poorly constructed framework for dealing with those issues. The physician again can help to suggest resources in the community that may be helpful in these situations (see Chapter 12).

PHYSICAL EXAMINATION

The preventive physical examination includes the information contained in the general, routine, and often used medical physical examination, but with attention to detail in areas that may be overlooked by the "curative" practitioner. Attention to findings that portend increased risk for certain condition or disease are particularly emphasized in the preventive examination. The usual sequence of inspection, palpation, percussion, and auscultation should be followed where applicable. (A simple form of recording findings is contained in Table 9-13). Components of the examination include the following:

Vital signs

Height, weight, pulse, and blood pressure should be recorded. Blood pressure should be obtained in both arms and, if elevated, repeated with multiple measurements. Explanation of normal pulse and blood pressure should be discussed. Diagnosis of high blood pressure parameters should be given, particularly if screening blood pressures are elevated. Modifiable contributors to high blood pressure should also be reviewed in this situation.

General appearance

This aspect of the examination should assess intellectual status, emotional status, physical conditioning, and motivation. The patient should be observed throughout his or her time in the office both interacting with ancillary personnel and during the history and physical examination. "Body language" can be assessed. Does the patient fidget? Is the patient hostile or angry? Are fists clenched and fingernails bitten? Is the brow furrowed? Are answers to questions long and extensive or short and one word? Is there a dorsal stoop suggesting depression or poor posture? Does the patient move into the examination room easily and up and out of a chair and onto the examination table with normal effort or are distress or other abnormalities present? Is the person well groomed? Is recall appropriate? All of these questions and others can be assessed easily by observing the patient carefully.

Skin

The preventive medicine physician should have a working knowledge of skin cancers and their recognition. The entire skin should be examined. Suspicious skin lesions should be measured and fully examined with a hand lens. Precancerous and suspicious lesions should be removed and/or evaluated appropriately. During the skin examination, sun exposure and sun screens can be discussed. Skin typing and risk for development of melanomas are reviewed in Chapter 49, Skin Cancer and Protection of the Skin. Skin typing helps to identify those persons at high risk for skin cancer generally and for malignant melanomas specifically. Particular attention during the skin examination should be given to conditions that may be markers for systemic disease such as cafe au lait spots, neurofibromatosis, and acanthosis nigricans. Alterations of pigmentation should be noted. Unexplained bruises should alert the physician to possibility of physical abuse. Areas of moniliasis, especially of the groin (jock itch) may be continually perpetuated by the use of "effective" bacteriostatic or bacteriocidal "deodorant" soaps.

Head

Signs of head trauma, hair pattern, and symmetry should be noted.

Eyes

Pupils, conjunctivae, cornea, sclera, extraocular muscle movements, lens, and fundi should be examined. Ideally the pupils should be dilated for a full view of the optic fundi. The physician should begin with a +3 or +4 diopter level on the ophthalmoscope, progressively focus through the cornea and lens and finally onto the optic fundus.

Ears

Hearing loss is common in adults and often overlooked in a general physical examination. Hearing screening in the office with counseling for hearing protection should be undertaken.

Nose

Nasal mucosa and patency should be evaluated. Perforation should alert the physician to cocaine abuse or excessive picking of the nose. Nasal polyps and nasal obstruction are frequently overlooked as reversible conditions that, if corrected, can improve quality of life by improving sense of taste or smell.

Mouth, pharynx, and throat

Dentures should be removed for evaluation of the mouth. Condition of the teeth, mucosa, tongue, gums, and pharynx should be noted. Suspicious lesions should be referred for appropriate treatment and evaluation. Vocal

Table 9-13. Physical examination

Name_____

Height _____ Weight _____ Temperature _____ Pulse _____ Blood Pressure Right _____ Left _____ General Appearance_____

✔ **If normal**

If abnormal — write finding

Skin _____

Scalp/Skull_____

Nails_____

Eyes

Lids _____

Conjunctivae_____

Pupils_____

Extraocular muscles _____

Fundi_____

Cornea_____

Ear, nose, throat

Ext. Ear_____

Tympanic membrane _____

Hearing_____

Septum_____

Teeth_____

Gums _____

Tongue_____

Throat_____

Tonsils _____

Trachea_____

Neck_____

Thyroid _____

Lymph nodes

Cervical_____

Axillary_____

Inguinal _____ Other_____

Chest and lungs

Expansion_____

Auscultation _____

Breasts

Skin_____

Nipples _____

Masses_____

Heart

Rhythm _____

Insp/palp._____

Sounds_____

Murmur/extra sounds _____

Blood vessels

Peripheral pulses _____

Bruits_____

Carotids_____

Aorta _____ Other _____

Varicosities/edema_____

Abdomen

Scars _____

Organs_____

Masses_____

Tenderness_____

Hernia _____

Spine

Mobility/alignment _____

Tenderness_____

Extremities

Joints _____

Deformity_____

Neurologic_____

Gait _____

Coord._____

Reflexes_____

Sensory_____

Motor _____

Anus/rectum_____

External _____

Internal_____

Male

Genitalia _____

   Penis_____

   Scrotum_____

   Testes_____

Prostate _____

Female

Pelvis

   External _____

   Vagina_____

   Cervix_____

   Uterus_____

   Adnexa _____

cords may be visualized through indirect laryngoscopy. This technique can be mastered usually with practice. Smokers are often unaware of their "smoker's voice." Examination of the vocal cords and discussion of smoker's voice often can serve as a motivating factor for smokers to consider smoking cessation.

Lymph nodes

Major lymph node groups should be palpated. This includes those in the neck, axillae, and groin areas.

Thyroid gland

Position, regularity, and size of the thyroid should be noted using either the front or the back examination technique. Abnormalities may be further investigated by transillumination or auscultation.

Thorax

Structural abnormalities of the thorax such as kyphoscoliosis or pectus excavatum should be noted. The character of breath sounds should be described along with any abnormalities such as wheezing, rhonchi, or rales. If abnormalities occur, the patient should be re-examined after coughing to assess the true significance of the abnormality. Intercostal space and costochondral junction should be carefully palpated in patients with obscure chest pain.

Heart

The left border of cardiac dullness should be percussed either with the two-hand method or the two fingers (index and middle) on one hand method. Regularity of heart rhythm, heart sounds, murmurs, or abnormal or extra sounds should be noted. The patient should be examined in the sitting and supine position and if murmurs are present, maneuvers should be undertaken in an attempt to elicit the specific cause of the murmur. Most "innocent" murmurs are early systolic, soft, short, and transient, and exhibit little radiation. A paradoxically split-second sound may indicate left bundle branch block or left ventricular dysfunction. A widely split fixed second sound may indicate an atrial septal defect. The diastolic murmur of mitral stenosis is often heard best in the left lateral position with the bell portion of the stethoscope. Pericardial sounds are often heard best with the patient sitting and leaning forward in full expiration.

Peripheral circulation

The neck should be examined for jugular venous waves and the carotid arteries auscultated for presence of significant bruits. Care should be taken not to compress the carotid artery with the stethoscope so as to create a false carotid bruit. The abdomen should be auscultated for bruits, which may emanate from any of the abdominal vessels. Peripheral pulses in the extremities should be evaluated and recorded.

Abdomen

Symmetry, tenderness, organ enlargement, and any irregularity should be noted. Abdominal muscle relaxation may be attained by having the patient flex the knees.

Male genitalia

Testicles should be palpated in all males. Those men of high risk for testicular cancer should be instructed about self-examination. Examination of the inguinal area for hernias should also be undertaken. Examination of the spermatic cord may reveal an abnormality such as a varicocele or other fluid collections. Transillumination will help to distinguish fluid filled lesions from other more significant abnormalities. A varicocele is usually on the left side, prominent in the standing position, and less prominent in the supine position. The prostate is examined via the rectum. The rectal examination may be done either in the left lateral position or in the knee chest position.

Female genitalia

The bladder should be emptied before the pelvic examination. External genitalia inspection should include Bartholin's glands, Skene's glands, rectocele, and cystocele. The speculum examination should include the vagina and cervix. A Pap smear should be obtained of the cervix, the endocervix, and any suspicious areas. Palpation should ensue of the uterus and adnexa, and of the rectum and vagina by bimanual examination.

Rectal examination

This should include evaluation for pilonidal cyst, hemorrhoids, fissures, fistulas, and other abnormalities.

Extremities and musculoskeletal

The examiner should note asymmetry of limbs, swelling or decreased range of motion of joints, spinal curvature, muscle bulk, and flexibility. This portion of the examination provides an opportunity to discuss appropriate exercise choice.

Neurologic examination

This includes assessment of affect, memory, deep tendon reflexes, sensation, coordination, and motor function.

SUMMARY

The framework of a preventive history and physical examination has been presented. Following the accumulation of this data, a problem list can be assembled that includes medical conditions needing treatment and also significant risk factors and diseases the patient is most likely to encounter in his or her lifetime. This can then lead to a plan for (1) preventive habits to attend to; (2) changes in lifestyle to be made; (3) a screening protocol to be undertaken; and (4) a check list to record preventive interventions. The use of the preventive history and physical examination in the office setting should be based on individual style, specific aspects of the population served by the practitioner, the personality of the individual practitioner, the availability of office ancillary personnel, and the wishes and needs of the individual practitioner and patient. Incorporating preventive practices at the outset of setting up a practice is the ideal situation, but these principles can be incorporated into any existing practice.

REFERENCES

1. Blair SN et al: Physical fitness and all-cause mortality, a prospective study of healthy men and women, *JAMA* 262(17):2395-2401, 1989.
2. Boring CC, Squires TS, Tong T: Cancer statistics, 1992, *CA Cancer J Clin* 42:19-38, 1992.
3. Canadian Task Force on the Periodic Health Examination: The periodic health examination 1 and 2 (1984 update), *Can Med Assoc J* 130:1276-1285, 1984.
4. Goldstein JL, Brown MS. Genetic aspects of disease. In Wilson JD et al, editors, *Harrison's principles of internal medicine,* ed 12, New York, 1991, Mc-Graw Hill.
5. Koplan JP, Caspersen CJ, Powell EK: Physical activity, physical fitness, and health: time to act, *JAMA* 262(17):2437, 1989 (editorial).
6. Rizack MA, Hillman CD: *Handbook of adverse drug interactions,* New York, 1991, The Medical Letter.
7. *Monthly vital statistics report,* National Center for Health Statistics, Centers for Disease Control, U.S. Department of Health and Human Services, 40(8):(suppl 2), 1992.
8. U.S. Preventive Services Task Force. *Guide to clinical preventive services: an assessment of the effectiveness of 169 interventions,* Baltimore, 1989, Williams and Wilkens.
9. *Webster's third new international dictionary,* Springfield, Mass, 1976, GC Merrian.

RESOURCES

Health statistics

National Center for Health Statistics, U.S. Department of Health and Human Services, Public Health Service, Centers for Disease Control, Hyattsville, Maryland 20782.
Provides comprehensive monthly and yearly mortality and morbidity statistical information.

CA Cancer Journal for Clinicians, American Cancer Society.
Monthly journal free to clinicians available through local offices of the American Cancer Society. Each year publishes concise cancer and mortality statistics.

Exercise

Royal Canadian Air Force Exercise Plans for Physical Fitness, New York, 1962, Simon and Schuster. 80 pages.
The Royal Canadian Air Force fitness plan for men and women devised by a team of doctors, physical education specialists, scientists, and artists. Five basic exercises for men and 10 for women are designed to provide everyone, regardless of age or physical conditioning, with the opportunity to achieve and maintain physical fitness.

Anderson B: *Stretching,* Shetter Publications, P.O. Box 279, Bolinas, CA, 94924.
Provides information and advice for appropriate preparation for exercise. Available in 10 languages.

Nutrition and diet

Dietary Guidelines for Americans, ed 3, 1990. Prepared for the U.S. Departments of Agriculture and Health and Human Services by the Dietary Guidelines for Americans Committee.
This 27-page pamphlet provides guidelines for food selection and suggested weight.

Pennington JA: *Bowes and Church's Food Values of Portions Commonly Used,* ed 15, Philadelphia, 1989, JB Lippincott.
This 328-page book outlines foods, recommended daily dietary requirements, estimated safe and adequate daily vitamin and mineral requirements, mean heights, weights, and recommended energy requirements.

Stress

Bensen H: *Beyond the Relaxation Response,* New York, 1984, The New York Times Book Co., Inc. 180 pages.
Dr. Herbert Bensen, a cardiologist, presents a simple self-healing meditation technique for reducing stress.

Eliot MS, Breo DL: *Is it worth dying for?* New York, 1984, Bantam. 248 pages.
Dr. Eliot, a cardiologist who suffered a heart attack himself, discusses stress assessment and management.

Drug interactions

Rizack MA, Hillman CD: *Handbook of adverse drug interactions,* New York, 1991, The Medical Letter. 388 pages.
Provides a comprehensive resource for adverse drug interactions including over-the-counter preparations and an index of brand names and corresponding chemical names.

Part III

BEHAVIORAL AND PSYCHOLOGIC INFLUENCES IN HEALTH AND DISEASE

Chapter 10

DEPRESSION AND SUICIDE: RECOGNITION AND EARLY POSITIVE INTERVENTION

Michael P. Bennetts

Depression

Depressive (affective) disorders are extremely common illnesses, probably affecting almost 10 million Americans at any one time. All ages, races, cultures and socioeconomic classes are affected.[100] Fortunately, these disorders also represent the most treatable of psychiatric conditions; 80% to 90% of those affected respond to currently available treatments. With such a high success rate, it is a tragedy that so few of the people afflicted with these conditions seek professional help (rate of failure to seek help is estimated to be as high as 65% to 75%) and thus suffer unnecessarily. Many who go to primary care physicians for a bewildering array of somatic complaints may not be recognized as having an underlying (masked) depression. They represent a therapeutic lost opportunity and absorb huge medical resources before finally being diagnosed and treated appropriately.

Too often depression is underrecognized, undertreated, or inappropriately treated (as high as 75% of outpatients and 60% of the hospitalized) by the health care system.[15] Everyone experiences transient sad ("blue," "low," "down") feelings, which usually accompany loss, perceived failure, unhappy incidents or events, emotional letdowns, or occupational and relationship difficulties. Grief is a special form of natural temporary reaction to the loss of a loved person, pet, or prized possession. With time, healing occurs. Despite these natural sad reactions, people continue to function occupationally and socially. Reassurance or displays of affection help considerably.

In contrast, people with true depressive disorder have persistent difficulties with affective symptoms and signs for weeks, months, or even years. Depressive disorders pervasively affect feelings, thoughts, and actions, *with increasing inability to function in all meaningful areas of life*. Life changes from vibrant color to shades of drab gray.

DIAGNOSIS

Depression, as a transient feeling or symptom, is a universal experience. As a syndromal mental illness, it is probably experienced by 30% of the population at some point during their lifetimes.[96]

Depression may be seen as a continuum ranging from a symptom of sadness or the blues through normal grief to reactive or neurotic depressions and finally to the full expression in the form of endogenous and psychotic syndromes. At one end of the spectrum is normal functioning and short-lasting symptoms; at the other end is total inability to function and prolonged duration.

The best screening technique for depression is a good psychiatric history and mental status examination. The physician must be alert to look for the signs of symptoms of depression, a discussion of which follows.

DSM-III-R criteria

Clinical depression is best epitomized in the DSM-III-R criteria[2] for major depression (see box on p. 164). These criteria can be remembered more easily using the helpful mnemonic: SIG E CAPS (see box on p. 164).

Even more dramatic is the melancholic (endogenous) subtype of depression, which is characterized by prominent vegetative changes or disturbances of biologic functions as represented by the presence of at least five of the symptoms listed in the box on p. 164.[2]

Signs and symptoms of depression

Mood may be described as depressed, sad, unhappy, discouraged, demoralized, irritable, nonspontaneous, or

Major depression—DSM III-R

The presence of a change from previous functioning for at least a 2-week period of at least five of the following symptoms (one of the symptoms representing either [1] depressed mood or [2] loss of interest or pleasure) present nearly everyday:

1. Depressed mood as indicated either by subjective account or observation by others
2. Markedly diminished interest or pleasure in all, or almost all, activities
3. Significant weight loss or weight gain when not dieting, or decrease or increase in appetite
4. Insomnia or hypersomnia
5. Psychomotor agitation or retardation (observable by others)
6. Fatigue or loss of energy
7. Feelings of worthlessness or excessive or inappropriate guilt
8. Diminished ability to think or concentrate, or indecisiveness (either by subjective account or as observed by others)
9. Recurrent thoughts of death (not just fear of dying) recurrent suicidal ideation without a specific plan, specific plan for committing suicide, or a suicide attempt

From American Psychiatric Association: *Diagnostic and statistical manual of mental disorders,* ed 3, Washington, DC, 1987, American Psychiatric Association.

SIG E CAPS (prescribe energy capsules)

S = Sleep disturbance
I = Interests decreased
G = Guilt excessive
E = Energy decreased
C = Concentration decreased
A = Appetite disturbed
P = Psychomotor retardation or agitation
S = Suicide: thoughts, plans, and actions

Melancholia

1. Loss of interest or pleasure (anhedonia) in all, or almost all, activities
2. Lack of reactivity to usually pleasurable stimuli (does not feel much better, even temporarily, when something good happens)
3. Depression regularly worse in the morning (positive diurnal variation of mood)
4. Early morning awakening (at least 2 hours before usual time of awakening)
5. Psychomotor retardation or agitation (not merely subjective complaints)
6. Significant anorexia or weight gain (e.g., more than 5% of body weight in 1 month)
7. No significant personality disturbance before the first major depressive episode
8. One or more previous major depressive episodes followed by complete, or nearly complete recovery
9. Previous good response to specific and adequate somatic antidepressant therapy, for example, tricyclics, electroconvulsive therapy (ECT), monoamine oxidase inhibitor (MAOI), lithium

empty. Diurnal variation of mood may be present, with patients feeling worse in the morning and slightly better later in the day.

Common warning signs are changes in appetite, sleep, and energy. Appetite is usually decreased with attendant weight loss. Food becomes tasteless, and there is little pleasure in eating. A minority have hyperphagia, with associated weight gain. Sleep usually shows middle, terminal (typical early morning awakening), or paninsomnia. Some show hypersomnia, sleeping 12 or more hours each day. Energy may be decreased substantially to the point of amotivation, apathy, and chronic fatigue. Others may procrastinate. Agitation shows itself in pacing, hand wringing, fidgeting, and nervous smoking. Psychomotor retardation may manifest by extremely slow movement and speech and delayed responses to questioning.

Anxiety is often associated with mood disorders (70% to 80%),[113] particularly in the agitated depressive subtype. Other anxious symptoms may include phobias, obsessions, and state-dependent panic attacks (20%).[113] Loss of interest occurs in hobbies, work, personal relationships, and sexual activity (decreased libido).

Cognitive difficulties include decreased attention span, difficulties with concentration, slowed thinking, poverty of content of thought, indecisiveness, inability to complete tasks, impaired abstract thinking, decreased memory, and disorientation, which may reach the point of an affective pseudodementia.

Negative thinking, generalizations, and global negative conclusions are hallmarks of depression. Guilt can become so excessive as to reach the level of a full delusion for only minor previous transgressions. There may be extreme self-blame or shame, helplessness, hopelessness, crying spells, loss of capacity for pleasure and poor insight and judgment due to feelings of personal worthlessness.

Obsessive negative rumination and hypochondriacal preoccupation with bodily functions are frequent, including multiple somatic complaints: cardiac (e.g., atypical angina), gastrointestinal (e.g., constipation), and genitourinary (e.g., impotence), and orthopedic (e.g., back pain).

Patients with depressive symptoms experience poorer physical functioning than patients with many chronic medical conditions, including hypertension, diabetes, arthritis, and gastrointestinal and lung disorders.[52] In other words, depressed patients are as severely disabled as are those with chronic medical conditions.[116]

Preoccupation with death, reuniting with loved ones after death, or thoughts of the survivors' responses to their deaths are common. Delusions may occur, which tend to have mood-congruent themes of guilt, poverty, nihilism, deserved persecution, and somatic disturbances. Because of a belief that nothing will change, no attempts are made to improve things, thus reinforcing the belief that the situation is hopeless.[25] Victims tend to blame themselves for everything bad. Ten percent to 25% of those depressed have psychotic features.

Depressed individuals tend to become dependent, passive, helpless, insecure, needy, rejection-sensitive and avoid interactions leading to withdrawal, loneliness, and alienation.[25] Accident-proneness, frequent job changes, marital discord, cynicism, loss of sense of humor, and all-or-nothing thinking may point to covert depression. Inappropriate self-medication with, for example, alcohol, can be a clue to the diagnosis.

DIFFERENTIAL DIAGNOSIS

Depressive disorders manifest in several different forms, perhaps best placed in perspective by the diagnostic cascade, which basically divides them into four diagnostic levels (see upper right box).

The big three depressive disorders are *major depression, dysthymic disorder,* and *bipolar depression.* With major depression as our benchmark, we will now explore the differentiating features of the other forms of depression. Subtyping into dichotomies such as endogenous/nonendogenous, situational/nonsituational, psychotic/nonpsychotic, and primary/secondary have been popular, useful descriptively and in treatment planning, but not validated as distinct clinical entities.[51]

Psychotic depression is major depression with delusions or hallucinations that are usually mood-congruent-guilt, nihilism, etc. Episodes are more disabling and slower to recover and respond only when an antipsychotic is added to antidepressant or electroconvulsive therapy (ECT).

Dysthymia (Research Diagnostic Criteria [RDC]--chronic intermittent or chronic minor depression) is a chronic condition usually beginning early in life, in adolescence or adulthood, lasting at least 2 years (1 year for children and adolescents) with symptoms similar to those of major depression but not of sufficient severity to warrant a diagnosis. These individuals tend to say they have been depressed their whole lives and have a very negative view of their past, present, and future.

Double depression involves dysthymic patients who develop superimposed major depression (about 10% to 15%).[46]

Bipolar disorder depressed is very similar to major depression, but is characterized by a previous history of manic episodes. Bipolar II disorders show similar depressive episodes but a previous history of only hypomanic (less severe with reality contact maintained) episodes. The

---

Diagnostic cascade	
Diagnostic levels	*Depressive disorders*
Organic ↓	Organic affective disorder
	Secondary depressions—Medical illnesses drugs
Major/psychotic/ endogenous (Functional) ↓	Unipolar *major depression*
	Bipolar affective disorder, depressed
Minor/neurotic/ reactive ↓	*Dysthymic disorder* (old depressive neurosis)
	Cyclothymic disorder, depressed
	Adjustment disorder with depressed mood
Personality disorder (Reached by exclusion) (Longitudinal)	Chronic dysthymia
	Subaffective dysthymia
	Characterologic depression

---

vast majority of manics eventually become depressed at some point. Ten percent of unipolar depressions eventually proved to be bipolar in a 40-year follow-up study.[118]

Cyclothymic disorder is a much less severe form of bipolar disorder, with individuals showing depressive insecurity alternating with hyperactive aggressiveness.[25]

Seasonal affective disorder (SAD) is depression that comes with decreased daylight in the fall and winter and disappears as the day lengthens in spring and summer (or even is accompanied by hypomania). This condition is more common in latitudes further from the equator with very low winter sunshine (e.g., Alaska). (Reversed SAD is depression in summer and hypomania in winter). SAD tends to be associated with hypersomnia, hyperphagia, and psychomotor slowing and may represent a subtype of bipolar disorder. For further information, see Chapter 11.

Organic mood disorders are *secondary* to an organic cause, such as medical illness or drugs. The presence of depression should *always* lead the clinician to look for an organic etiologic agent. It may occur in the presence or aftermath of a serious illness.[17] Medical inpatients show depression in 20% to 32% of cases.[17]

MEDICAL ILLNESSES

Medical illnesses that may cause depression are legion.

1. *Neurologic diseases* such as multiple sclerosis, Parkinson's disease, partial complex seizure disorder, head trauma, cerebral tumors, cerebral vascular accident, dementing diseases, HIV encephalopathy, and sleep apnea may all be accompanied by or lead to depression.

2. More than 60% of hospitalized *cardiac* patients are

depressed. After a myocardial infarction, there is a high risk for depression for over 18 months.[33] Postcardiotomy patients are particularly at risk. The risk of death from cardiovascular disease is more than doubled in depressed outpatients.[87]

3. *Endocrine diseases,* such as hypothyroidism and hyperthyroidism, hyperparathyroidism, hyperadrenalism in the form of Cushing's disease, and adrenal insufficiency in Addison's disease, postpartum and menstrual depressions (late luteal phase dysphoric disorder).

4. *Infectious diseases* such as tertiary syphilis (GPI), multiple viral infections including influenza, AIDS, viral pneumonia, viral hepatitis, infectious mononucleosis, tuberculosis, or any other chronic infection.

5. *Nutritional disorders* such as various vitamin deficiencies, including B_{12} (pernicious anemia), C, folate, niacin, and thiamine deficiencies.

6. *Neoplastic diseases* such as cancer of the head of the pancreas, leukemia, disseminated carcinomatosis, or paraneoplastic limbic encephalopathy.

7. *Collagen diseases* such as rheumatoid arthritis and systemic lupus erythematosus (SLE).

8. *Liver disease.*

9. *Pharmacologic:* interactions leading to depression may be associated with any antihypertensive drug such as reserpine, alpha methyldopa, propranolol, hydralazine, thiazides, spironolactone, guanethidine, and clonidine; psychotropic drugs, such as phenothiazines, barbiturates, and benzodiazepines; alcohol and minor tranquilizers/sedatives (these are often initially taken to relieve distress, but eventually cause depression); amphetamine withdrawal, cocaine, narcotics, steroids, ACTH, contraceptives, insecticides, anticholinesterases, cimetidine, ranitidine, indomethacin; heavy metals such as thallium and mercury; chemotherapeutic agents such as cycloserine, vincristine, and vinblastine; amantadine, bromocriptine, carbamazepine, phenytoin, digitalis, disulfiram. (Approximately 200 specific drugs have been implicated as causes of depression, but only a few are regularly associated with it).[33] (Also see Chapter 14).

10. *Masked depressions* are depressions disguised as somatoform disorders such as hypochondriasis or Briquet's syndrome. Those affected are labeled as "hypochondriacs" or "crocks" and are often help-requesting rejectors covertly resisting efforts to help them.[25]

11. *Adjustment disorder with depressed mood* is a response to a clearly identifiable stress that would resolve as the stress diminishes. It is a maladaptive response with impairment in functioning or excessive and disproportionate intensity of symptoms. Patients with personality disorders or organic problems may be more vulnerable to developing these disorders.

12. *Situational or reactive depressions* tend to be associated with an overt precipitant and show more anger, self-pity, drug abuse, and suicidal behavior. The term remains popular despite lack of empirical validity. Despite the assumption that more of these conditions are psychologically than biologically caused, many respond to somatotherapy.[51]

13. *Chronic subaffective dysthymias* are subtle forms of depression with characterologic shift toward pessimistic, easily disappointed, anergic, avoidant, introverted, gloomy, passive, demanding, negativistic people who fear intimacy yet crave it.[25] There is equal debate that chronic, life-long, low-grade depressions are personality or character disorders or represent "subsyndromal" primary affective disorders[51] (see box on p. 165). Those with characterologic depressions tend to have lifelong problems with self-esteem, guilt, and poor interpersonal relationships.[51]

Forty percent of major depressions also have an Axis II (Personality Disorder) diagnosis, most commonly dependent, avoidant, narcissistic, or borderline personality disorders.[51] Unstable characterologic traits are the strongest predictor of poor social outcome.[51] Premorbid personality traits, such as introversion, may predispose to depression or affect the course of depression. Certain personality traits may represent attenuated forms of depression, and postmorbid personality changes may occur after depression.[51]

Secondary depression also refers to those following other psychiatric conditions such as alcoholism or schizophrenia. *Comorbid depression* exists alongside other psychiatric conditions and is often seen with alcoholism (33% to 59% of alcoholics have clinical depression), eating disorders (33% to 62% anorexics and bulimics are depressed), and anxiety (considerable overlap).[51] *Compound depression* (i.e., depression plus nonaffective psychiatric and/or medical condition) is common, with more difficult course, lower recovery rate, more suicidal ideation, and previous suicidal attempts.[49]

Grief, especially when unresolved, may be complicated and culminate in a major depressive syndrome. Acute grief may cause sadness, crying spells, rumination about involvement with the lost person, guilt, anger, denial, insomnia, and hypnogogic (as fall asleep) or hypnopompic (as wake up) hallucinations of the dead person.[25]

AGE-SPECIFIC FEATURES
Children

Childhood depression may be difficult to diagnose, particularly when depressive symptoms mix with hyperactivity, agitation, anxiety disorders, phobias, delinquency, school problems, or psychosomatic complaints.[100] Loss of a parental figure through death or divorce, child abuse, chronic illness or hospitalization, or having parents with psychiatric disorders lead to increased vulnerability. Children may respond to treatment or counseling of their parents in addition to their own individual and family therapy.

Adolescents

Adolescents tend to present with acting-out behavior, covering their depression by acting angry, negative, or aggressive; running away; truancy; school difficulties; delinquency; promiscuity; pregnancy; rejection sensitivity; poor peer relations; or poor hygiene.[100]

Geriatric

The elderly are particularly vulnerable to depression (10% to 65%).[100] They tend to present with cognitive deficits such as disorientation and memory loss, distractibility, and confusion to the point of an affective pseudodementia. Tragically, these affective pseudodementing symptoms can be misdiagnosed as Alzheimer's dementia, and the depression goes untreated.

Issues of aging, declining health, loneliness through loss of friends and family, and financial difficulties are factors predisposing to the development of depression. Only occasionally do the elderly admit to feelings of depression. Instead, they tend to focus more on multiple somatic symptoms, such as various aches, pains, fatigue, insomnia, or constipation, particularly in alexithymic (inability to express feelings in words) individuals (found particularly in men). Those tend to ascribe their symptoms to physical ailments and seek primary care rather than deal with the emotional issues.

Many physical illnesses tend to afflict older persons and are associated more commonly with depression, such as Parkinson's disease, cancer, arthritis, and Alzheimer's disease.[100] The elderly take many medications, which may cause drug interactions.

Treatment of depression in the elderly is often complicated by physical problems, which must be considered, particularly issues such as cardiotoxicity of antidepressants and altered pharmacokinetics in which medications are metabolized more slowly and thus require lower doses.

EPIDEMIOLOGY

It has been estimated that 23 million adult Americans are currently suffering from a major mental or behavioral disorder (excluding substance abuse, which probably doubles that number).[86] At some point in their lives, about 46 million persons will experience a major disorder, the most common of which are depression and anxiety.[86] More than 10% of the U.S. population (>30 million people) are vulnerable to depression.[25] Since 1910, each decade has brought with it an increased incidence of depression and the age at which that depression first appears has decreased in every generation since World War II (birth cohort effect).[25,34]

Depression is one of the most common problems seen by primary care physicians (30% of patients seen).[48] The prevalence of major depression in the general population is variously reported as 3% in a 6-month period, 5% to 8% for lifetime according to the National Institute of Mental Health Epidemiological Catchment Area (NIMH-ECA) Study. Other studies report 3% to 6%[25,103] in a 6-month period or 15% to 30% lifetime.[15] In addition, prevalence of dysthymia is 4.5% to 10.5%[33] (3.3% ECA lifetime: 4% women, 2% men). Up to 30% of the population may develop depression at some point in their lifetime.[96] Spontaneous remission occurs in up to 50%.[40] Fifty percent become chronic.[15]

Depression associated with mood/affective disorders affects about 8 million people in any 1-month period ECA[89] (major, bipolar, or dysthymic depressions). The estimated costs resulting from depression for 1980 were $16 billion (lost time from work representing $10 billion).[108] (Direct costs from inpatient and outpatient treatment of major depression alone were $2.1 billion.)[108]

The 6-month prevalence of depression associated with mood-affective disorders was 5.8% in 1982 (lifetime rate 8.3%) (i.e., 9.6 + 13.7 million people).[88] In that year only 33% of people with clinical depression received treatment, perhaps partly because of the misperception of depression as a personal weakness by 57% of the population.[86] Many are too ashamed or humiliated to ask for help. Physician attitude is extremely important: Acceptance of depression as a significant pathologic disorder helps, whereas discussing depression as "normal," "appropriate," or "insignificant" merely contributes to morbidity.

The incidence (new cases per year) of depression is 1/100 men, 3/100 women, and the prevalence is 2 to 3/100 men and 5 to 10/100 women.[46] The incidence of depression is greater among young, single, separated, or divorced women.[114] Separation or divorce causes 2.5 times more depression than marriage, although marital discord increases risk, too.[88] Women are depressed twice as frequently as men.[25] The NIMH-ECA study showed the lifetime risk for major depression in women to be 4.9% to 8.7% and 2.3% to 4.4% in men.[93] International rates vary from 4.7% to 25.8% in women and 1.2% to 12.3% in men.[9] In another paper by Kaplan et al.,[46] the figures given for men were 10% and for women 20%. Despite differences in studies, the relationship is constant. Differences in rate by sex are a result of underlying biologic causes,[34] not because of different treatment-seeking behavior. Men tend to forget depressive symptoms preferentially.

ETIOLOGY/RISK FACTORS
Biologic factors

Genetic factors. Depressive disorders tend to run in families, and gradually accumulating evidence implicates a genetic factor, particularly in recurrent depressive disorders. Further evidence of a genetic factor has been demonstrated in the field of bipolar disorders. If one twin is affected, the other identical twin has a 70% likelihood of developing the illness, whereas a nonidentical twin has a similar chance of developing the illness as other first-degree relatives, such as parents, siblings, or children of the proband. This incidence is about 15%, about twice as high as the general population. In second-degree relatives, the relative risk drops to about 7%. Adoption studies have shown much higher correlations between depressed adoptees (particularly bipolar depressives) and their biologic rather than their adoptive parents.

Genetic marker studies have supported linkage to chromosome 11 in one Amish family and X-linkage in several Middle Eastern families with bipolar disorder. Unipolar depression is more likely inherited polygenically.[25] The concordance rates for unipolar twin probands were 54% in monozygotic and 24% in dizygotic twins.[34] Prevalence of unipolar depression is 11% to 18% in relatives of patients (three times higher than controls—5% to 6%).[34]

Winokur et al. divided unipolar depressions on the basis of family history into sporadic depressive disorder with no ill family members, familial pure depressive disorder with family history of depression only, and depressive spectrum disorder with family history of alcoholism or antisocial behavior.[117]

Response of family members to biologic treatments tends to be similar (e.g., inherited patterns of metabolism of antidepressant medication). Early cholinergic REM induction may be a genetic vulnerability marker for depression.[34] Children of depressed parents may also learn maladaptive ways of handling life stressors because of the distorted family environment, thereby developing increased vulnerability to depression.

Biochemical factors. Biogenic neurotransmitters have been shown to regulate mood in the limbic system (e.g., norepinephrine and serotonin, which are closely linked to areas of the brain that control the drives of hunger, sex, and thirst). Improper balance of these neurotransmitters may be influential in the development of depressive symptoms.

Progressively more refined hypotheses of specific neurotransmitter abnormalities are available. Defective regulatory interactions among the most studied neurotransmitters—norepinephrine (NE $\downarrow$), dopamine (DA $\downarrow$), serotonin (5-Hydroxytryptamine-5HT $\downarrow$), acetylcholine (ACh $\uparrow$)—lead to depression.[3]

Norepinephrine is involved in the maintenance of arousal, alertness, and euphoria; and disturbances in its availability might lead to lack of energy and depressed mood.[100] Serotonin, an inhibitory neurotransmitter, when disturbed, may give rise to irritability, anxiety, and the sleep disturbances of depression.[100] Decreased serotonergic activity may increase vulnerability to depression. Its metabolite 5-hydroxyindoleacetic acid (5HIAA) is reduced in unipolar depression and may indicate patients prone to suicide.[3]

Acetylcholine hyperactivity/imbalance may account for withdrawal.[25] Increasing brain cholinergic activity induces shortened rapid eye movement (REM) latency. Depression may indicate a relative cholinergic over adrenergic predominance.[3] Physostigmine causes increased central cholinergic activity and rapidly induces depression or dramatically reduces mania. Thus cholinergic abnormalities may predispose one to develop depression.[3]

Hypothalamic-pituitary physiology is disturbed, causing alterations in releasing factors and, therefore, in the end organ hormonal secretions such as cortisol. Greater amounts are secreted and the diurnal variation is lost, which may partially explain the sleep disturbances associated with depression. Sleep may be phase advanced (turned ahead in the 24-hour cycle), leading to early REM onset and early morning awakening typical of depression. The suprachiasmatic nucleus of the hypothalamus functions as the biologic clock or pacemaker for circadian rhythms, such as sleep-wake cycle, REM sleep onset, cortisol secretion, and temperature control, which are phase advanced in depression.[3]

Biochemical imbalance may represent a genetic vulnerability triggered by prolonged stress, trauma, physical illness, or environmental conditions.[100] Changes in hormones, receptors, and calcium ion flux all occur. Receptor studies suggest decreased beta-adrenergic function or uncoupling between alpha 2-adrenergic receptors and adenylate cyclase in the postsynaptic cells in depression. Alpha adrenergic receptors may be challenged (e.g., by the alpha agonist clonidine) and reveal blunted growth hormone response in some depressed patients.[3]

Psychosocial factors

Any significant change, loss, or stress, such as divorce, death, unemployment, moving, promotion, financial problems, midlife crises, and sex role expectations, may trigger a depression. Premorbid personality, upbringing, and negative thinking style contribute to its development.

The loss may be of a person, attention from others, health, financial status, or control. It may be real or only threatened or imagined. A loss may be seen as devastating by a patient but only trivial to others.[25] Losses are worse when unexpected, related to ambivalently perceived objects, or occurring after previous losses in very dependent persons.

Retirement contributes to depression in older men who see their self-worth in terms of work and productivity.[100] The highest rates of depression among women are found among single, young, poor mothers of small children with little emotional or financial support.[100]

Marital strains or disputes and parenting stresses often contribute to depression. Depressed patients tend to function poorly as parents by withdrawing from or acting hostile to their children, who, in turn develop emotional problems themselves, including depression.

Patients in an environment with high levels of expressed emotion (i.e., the expression of criticism and hostility with overinvolvement of family members) are more likely to relapse.[104] Other issues that may contribute to depression include unexpressed anger, unresolved grief, all-or-nothing assumptions (e.g., "If I'm not liked/admired by everyone, I'm worthless"), negative self-fulfilling prophecies, and learned helplessness.[25]

SCREENING/ASSESSMENT

Clinicians must have an especially high index of suspicion for depressive symptoms and signs in those at risk for depression. Such persons may be characterized by:

- Recent loss (real or perceived)
- Previous history of depression
- Family history of depression (mania, suicide, alcoholism, psychiatric treatment)
- Eating, sleep or energy disorders
- Chronic illness or pain
- Adolescence
- Multiple unexplained somatic complaints
- Substance abuse

Screening in asymptomatic persons is not recommended by the U.S. Preventive Services Task Force[111,112] but should be focused on those with these risk factors.

The prevailing standard for the diagnosis of clinical depression is the opinion of an examining psychiatrist that a patient's symptoms meet DSM-III-R criteria.[2] In other words, a detailed psychiatric history and mental status examination is still the essential diagnostic assessment.[33] Most patients with depression, however, never get to see a psychiatrist. Most see nonpsychiatric physicians who often lack the skills and time to make the diagnosis, which is difficult to determine early in the illness.[83,96,47]

Questionnaires

Several validated screening questionnaires are available. Some are performed by the patients (subjective), whereas others are performed by the physician (objective). Subjective questionnaires include the following:

- *Beck Depression Inventory (BDI):* sensitivity 86%, specificity 82%, positive predictive value 30%.[13]
- *Zung Self-Rating Depression Scale (SDS):* most widely used screening tool; 82% with score > 55 have major depression by DSM-III-R criteria.[120,121] When physicians were alerted to positive Zung SDS scores, they detected depression in more patients (68% of 102) than when nonalerted (15% of 41).

Other self-administered questionnaires are the Center for Epidemiological Studies Depression Scale, The General Health Questionnaire, The Hopkins Symptom Checklist, the Mental Health Inventory, and The Hospital Anxiety and Depression Scale.[15]

Among the objective questionnaires is the Hamilton Psychiatric Rating Scale, which assesses depressive signs and symptoms. Other more complex psychologic tests helpful in diagnosis are the Minnesota Multiphasic Personality Inventory (MMPI) and the various projective tests, (e.g., the Rorschach and Thematic Apperception Tests [TAT].)

Biologic assessment tests

Dexamethasone suppression test (DST). This test is the most widely used and studied biologic test in psychiatry. One milligram of dexamethasone is given as a biologic challenge to the hypothalamic-pituitary-adrenal neuroendocrine system at 10 or 11 PM, and serum cortisols are taken at 4 PM and 11 PM the next day. Normal persons will suppress below 5 ng/ml. Biologically depressed individuals will show nonsuppression of cortisol secretion, as defined by a post-dexamethasone level of 5 ng or greater. This finding is found in about 50% of hospitalized major depressed patients and fewer (<40%) outpatients. Sensitivity is low and there are significant false-negative results. There are also many false-positive, which decreases the test's overall validity. A negative (suppressed) dexamethasone suppression test (DST) has little clinical significance. A positive (nonsuppressed) DST may make it easier for a patient to accept "chemical imbalance" and antidepressant medication. A persistently abnormal DST, or one that reverts to positive, is associated with high degree of relapse, rehospitalization, and possibly suicide.[3]

Urinary-free cortisol levels may be higher, particularly in psychotic depression and there may be a blunted ACTH (adrenocorticotropic hormone) response to CRH (corticotropin-releasing hormone).[3]

Thyroid releasing hormone (TRH) stimulation test. Five hundred micrograms of TRH is given to the patient intravenously and blood levels of thyroid stimulating hormone (TSH) are obtained at 15-, 30-, 45-, and 90-minute intervals. These levels are sometimes (about 25%) blunted in a group of unipolar patients (suggesting serotonin hyperactivity and/or noradrenergic hypoactivity) and elevated in bipolar depressed patients. This result may be a trait and not just a state marker. Subclinical hypothyroidism with increased basal TSH and antimicrosomal thyroid antibodies may be found in up to 20% of depressed patients.[3]

Sleep electroencephalogram (EEG) recordings. Major depressed patients characteristically show reduced REM latency below 90 minutes from the onset of sleep to the first REM phase and increased REM density in the first half of the night. They also show frequent awakenings, decreased total sleep, and decreased slow stage, or deep (stage 4) sleep. These changes in the REM architecture improve with subsequent biologic treatments. Antidepressants increase REM latency, phase delay REM onset, or completely eliminate REM sleep.[3] Short REM latency may be a predictor of relapse.[3]

These tests are generally not appropriate for routine screening because of poor sensitivity, significant numbers of false positive and false negative results, invasiveness, and high cost. An additional method of clarifying whether a major depression is present in the medically ill is to use a psychostimulant such as dextroamphetamine or methylphenidate as a challenge test.[17] Positive stimulant challenge tests may predict differential treatment response to adrenergic antidepressants such as imipramine.[3] Functional brain imaging techniques have been used to assess neuropathology of the depressive disorders.

EFFECTIVENESS OF EARLY DETECTION

Earlier detection and treatment alleviates symptoms sooner and speeds recovery,[100] reducing morbidity and duration.[88] The DART Program (Depression, Awareness, Recognition, and Treatment, since May 1988) is a major public health secondary prevention program sponsored by the National Institute of Mental Health to enhance professional (primary care and mental health specialists) and public awareness of depressive disorders as common serious illnesses requiring prompt diagnosis and treatment.[88] Seventy-four percent of patients with depression were seen in the general medical sector, 19% in the specialty mental health sector, and 10% in the human services sector. Twenty-one percent were not seen in any service setting.[88] Therefore, primary care has great potential value for recognizing and treating patients with depressive disorders who visit outpatient health facilities at least three times more often than average.[88]

Prospective studies of validated depression screening instruments suggest that they may help to increase physicians' awareness and detection of depression.[83,98,13]

Some are concerned about possible harmful false-positive labeling[13] and the stigma still associated with psychiatric referral. Greater acceptance of depression as a disorder than as a weakness may help public acceptance.[88]

Some authors favor general screening[83,47,98]; others do not (e.g., Canadian Task Force on the Periodic Health Examination).[13,14,15,32]

Better awareness, identification, and adequate follow-up are essential. Primary care physicians often do not provide adequate counseling, antidepressant medication, or psychiatric referral.[13,32] Complications can arise, such as suicide, recurrent episodes (50%), and iatrogenic morbidity due to unnecessary medical tests and treatment.[83,96]

COURSE AND PROGNOSIS

Depression is frequently (50% to 80%) recurrent or chronic. With age, episodes tend to become more frequent, severe, and complicated by residual symptoms. Because incomplete remissions tend to be followed by relapse, careful monitoring is extremely important. The highest rate of relapse is during the first few months after

recovery[51] (40% unipolars by 1 year). Unipolar depressives tend to average four to five lifetime recurrences, whereas bipolars tend to have ten. Those with primary unipolar depressions have a 90% rate of recovery, but those with secondary depressions have only a 23% rate.[51] Fifty percent to 60% of acute depressions remit spontaneously. There is a 43% recovery rate for dysthymics versus 75% for major depression. Dysthymia average duration is 5.5 years with a range from 2 to 20 years.[51]

Depressions lasting longer than 2 years are unlikely to spontaneously remit. Fifteen percent of depressives do not remit despite appropriate treatment. Chance of remission is low after 18 months of appropriate therapy.[25] Eighty percent relapse within 5 years of recovery, only 20% showing sustained recovery. The best predictor of relapse is the number of previous episodes (especially over three). Only 50% of recovered patients remained well more than 20 months.[50] In 15% (lifetime rate) depression is a fatal disease ending in death through suicide.

THERAPEUTIC INTERVENTIONS
Primary prevention

Unfortunately, there is insufficient epidemiologic data on which to base a "risk factor" intervention or primary prevention program.[88] Primary prevention basically involves helping individuals to feel good about themselves by enhancing self-esteem and teaching problem solving, stress management, and appropriate coping skills to decrease vulnerability to depression (see box on p. 171, top, for examples of programs).[86] Education offers the best hope for primary prevention. Far more resources, including financial and research, need to be devoted to psychoeducational approaches.

Secondary prevention

Depressive disorders respond well to treatment (secondary prevention)—some completely, others with some remaining morbidity—in a high proportion of cases. The type of treatment chosen depends on the particular presentation of the illness, its severity, whether it is a single or recurrent episode (treatments that were successful in the past are likely to be effective again), the patient's age and condition, request for a particular mode of therapy, and premorbid personality and coping style.

Treatment tends to be biologic at the organic and major depressive diagnostic levels with treatment of the underlying condition, removal of the offending medication, and/or biologic treatment of the underlying depression with antidepressant medications or ECT, as appropriate (see box on p. 171, bottom). The more minor and reactive levels of depression usually respond well to psychotherapeutic interventions and counseling. Unfortunately, many people avoid treatment, believing they should get better through their own efforts or simply live with depression until it

Primary prevention

Proactive positive intervention with:

Stressors	Environmental manipulation/modification
	Social support
	Work site stress programs
Response to stress	Relaxation techniques
	Biofeedback
	Time management skills
	Physical exercise
	Use of emotional outlets
Skills training/competence building around transitions	Parenting
	School entry
	Divorce
Healthy diet/nutrition	
Good judgment/choices	Marriage
	Career
	Retirement
Maternal support	Predelivery
	Postdelivery
Social health policies	Poverty
	Community breakdown
	Discrimination
Detection and referral	Depression
	Substance abuse

passes. (A 1986 Roper Poll reported that 78% of responders would avoid treatment, whereas only 12% would take antidepressant medication.) Many do not seek treatment because of feared effects on employment or perceived costs of treatment.[88] Depression is frequently treated inadequately and not enough use is made of MAOIs, lithium, and ECT in the United States.

Antidepressant medication. About 70% to 80% of depressed patients respond to antidepressants (versus 20% to 40% for placebo)[88,84] or augmentation strategies. ECT improves response to 80% to 85%. It is important to remember that 15% do not recover. Antidepressants tend to relieve neurovegetative symptoms most effectively. They

Biologic interventions

Tricyclic antidepressants
Heterocyclic antidepressants
Newer/third-generation antidepressants
MAOIs
Lithium
Anticonvulsants
ECT
Phototherapy
Sleep deprivation
Phase shifting

work by rebalancing neurotransmitter concentrations and receptor numbers (down regulation) and by altering calcium flux through membranes.[25]

Choice of a particular antidepressant, all of which are probably equally efficacious, depends on side effect profiles (which in turn depend on neurotransmitter and receptor profiles), previous responses or family members' responses, and physician's familiarity with this medication. (Table 10-1). Tricyclics are most effective in endogenous depression, with the strongest clinical predictor of good response being psychomotor retardation.[84]

Blood levels (12 hours after the last dose) can be helpful and tend to correlate with clinical response with nortriptyline (with therapeutic window between 50 and 150 ng/ml), imipramine, and desipramine.[109] Blood levels for other antidepressants are helpful in terms of compliance, rapid metabolism, and intolerance; but they do not correlate as well with clinical response.

Antidepressant side effects tend to occur early, and the patient often develops tolerance to them early. In other words, as long as the patient stays at the same dose, the side effect complained of will usually disappear within days. Exceptions to this general rule occur, such as dry mouth due to the anticholinergic effects of antidepressants. It is important to teach the patients to learn to tolerate side effects in the initial phases so that they can receive the eventual rewards.

Unfortunately, antidepressants take several weeks to become effective. Thus it is especially important to maintain frequent early contact between physician and patient to help patients through the initial phases when they may see the antidepressant as useless and merely causing more morbidity. Education and support by the physician leads to improved compliance and improved prognosis.

Antidepressants tend to improve appetite, weight, interests, pleasure, energy, psychomotor function, hopelessness, helplessness, and guilt, and to avert suicidal thoughts between 2 and 6 weeks after onset of therapy. Sleep pattern may improve first, during the first week (a hopeful sign). It is essential to treat adequately, i.e., sufficient time (up to 6 weeks) and in sufficient dosage before trying alternate strategy.

In a study involving 217 depressed patients, only 34% had received adequate antidepressant medication for at least four consecutive weeks, and only 3% received the highest therapeutic dose.[53] More than half of the patients in the National Institute of Mental Health (NIMH) Collaborative Program on the Psychobiology of Depression[53] had been treated with anxiolytics instead of antidepressants. Only 75% received any antidepressant, even after entry into tertiary care centers. Nearly 30% of inpatients received less than 100 mg of tricyclics (or their equivalent) per day.[54] After recovery, 47% of patients who relapsed had not been receiving an antidepressant in the month preceding the relapse.[55]

Table 10-1. Antidepressant drugs (presently available in U.S.)

Type	Drug	Usual therapeutic range (mg/day)	Side effects/comments*
Tricyclics			
Tertiary amines	Amitriptyline	75-300	S, ACh
	Imipramine	75-300	B
	Chlorimipramine	75-300	S, ACh
	Trimipramine	50-300	S
	Doxepin	50-300	S
Secondary amines	Nortriptyline	50-150	B, H
	Desipramine	75-300	B, H
	Protriptyline	15-60	A, ACh
Heterocyclics	Trazodone	150-600	S, O, H, C
	Maprotiline	75-250	
	Amoxapine	150-600	
Newer/third-generation	Fluoxetine	20-80	A, O, H, C
	Sertraline	50-200	O, H, C
	Bupropion	200-450	A, H, C
MAOIs	Phenelzine	45-90	
	Tranylcypromine	20-60	A, H
	Isocarboxazid	20-60	
Lithium		600-1800	

*S, Most sedating; A, most activating; ACh, most Anticholinergic; O, no anticholinergic; B, best blood levels; H, least hypotensive; C, least cardiotoxic.

MAOIs tend to have special effectiveness in atypical depressions characterized by marked anxiety, increased appetite, carbohydrate craving, hyperphagia, weight gain, excessive sleepiness (hypersomnolence), fatigue, self-pity, hypochondriacal, phobic and obsessive-compulsive features and reversed diurnal variation of mood (worse in evening).[21] Hysteroid dysphorics with histrionic personalities, emotional overreactivity, and extreme rejection sensitivity tend to respond to this group of drugs. They are particularly effective with melancholic depressions associated with panic attacks and should be given primary consideration over tricyclic antidepressants.[84] Although they sometimes cause hypotension, the elderly benefit from their use as well. The dangers associated with MAOIs have been exaggerated in the past and many people do very well on them. In the past they have been underused in American medicine, although this trend may be changing. Many patients can accept the dietary and medication restrictions fairly easily, thereby avoiding hypertensive crises. The most commonly used MAOI is phenelzine (Nardil), a hydrazine. Tranylcypromine (Parnate) is a nonhydrazine and is often activating.

Lithium revolutionized the treatment of manic depressive disorder, both acutely and prophylactically, by decreasing the frequency and severity of both manic and depressive episodes. Lithium has been analogized to insulin in the treatment of diabetics. This model helps in convincing patients and their families to comply with use of lithium. Lithium can be used to augment the effect of other antidepressant medications. More recently it has been discovered that various anticonvulsants help prevent relapses and also treat both depressions and manias, in particular, carbamazepine (Tegretol) and valproic acid (Depakene).

Stimulants, such as amphetamine, methylphenidate or pemoline, may be helpful in elderly, medically ill patients. Response is usually fairly rapid and sustained. Tolerance and dependence do not tend to occur.[25]

Maintenance of antidepressant treatment is extremely important after the acute episode. Many patients respond to the antidepressants initially and prematurely discontinue them. Within a few weeks thereafter they often relapse. When the drug is continued long enough, relapse of the underlying depression is prevented. It is wise to continue treatment at least for 3 to 4 months after resolution of multiple depressive symptoms and return to usual functioning to ensure that the episode has run its course. Length of time has been variously recommended from 4 to 12 months[85] before discontinuation by gradual taper. If discontinued too rapidly, there can be a brief period of discomfort with gastrointestinal (GI) complaints, listlessness, anxiety, and rapid eye movement (REM) rebound with nightmares.[57] Initially, maintenance was recommended at reduced (75 to 100 mg imipramine equivalence) dose, but increasing evidence suggests that it is better to use full acute therapeutic dosage, even for prevention. It is also very important to use maintenance antidepressants after a course of ECT.

Noncompliance is a frequent (probably 25% to 50% of patients)[84] occurrence, particularly in individuals who do not believe anything will help them or that they do not deserve to get better. Noncompliance can also occur when they feel threatened by or cannot handle the responsibility of becoming well, preferring their dependent depressive life-styles.[25]

Augmentation strategies to effect the antidepressant include adding lithium, cytomel(T_3), tryptophan, or stimulants in those patients failing on antidepressant alone. Psychotic depressives need the addition of an antipsychotic (75% response versus 41% amitriptyline alone or 19% perphenazine alone[107]) or ECT.

Between the 1930s and the 1950s, ECT was the only really effective biologic method to treat depression and was used extensively. With the development of antidepressants and their increasing use from the 1950s, ECT gradually became less popular. Nevertheless, it is still the most effective and most rapid known treatment for endogenous depression. Unfortunately, partly because of medicolegal issues, it has been relegated from a first line method of treatment to a treatment used only after more conservative approaches with various drugs have failed (i.e., in treatment resistant cases) or cannot be tolerated. It is extremely effective when appropriately prescribed in 80% to 90% of cases.[84] ECT may be life-saving in situations of high suicidal risk.

Experimental treatments. Pregnant women may prefer several experimental treatments herein described because they do not involve ingestion of medication and are (perceived as) safer.

Phototherapy exposure (particularly of seasonal affective disorder patients)[97] to bright (2500 to 10,000 lux) full-spectrum lights for various periods each day, often alleviates and, in certain cases, totally resolves these depressions. If a significant geographic factor is contributing to the depression, for example the Alaskan latitudes, a move toward the equator may be indicated to increase exposure to daily sunlight.

Sleep deprivation[81] is an effective technique to relieve depression temporarily. Unfortunately, it lasts only a day or two in most people, and the person may feel worse after recovery sleep. Depriving people of the latter part (partial sleep deprivation)[101] of their sleep may be more effective.

Phase shifting,[99] in which the time that people go to sleep is progressively advanced, can be helpful. This approach resets the biologic clock involved in controlling normal life rhythms, such as eating and sleeping cycles, which are disrupted during depressions.

Psychologic therapies. Psychologic therapies have been developed or modified specifically for the treatment of depression over the past 15 years, and their effectiveness has been supported through controlled studies.[105]

Psychotherapy is useful in persons who do not respond well to medication, persons who are intolerant to side effects, or those with medical contraindications to antidepressants.[105] Some prefer psychotherapy, wanting to avoid drugs. Psychotherapy may increase compliance and improve social and occupational functioning and coping capacity.

The physician-patient relationship is extremely important for treatment success. Empathy and establishing a trusting relationship in a supportive holding environment, characterized by positive expectation and the reversal of demoralization, may be the most important basis for all other therapies to work.

Insight-oriented therapies (psychodynamic, psychoanalytic) deal with internal conflicts, such as dependence/independence struggles or ambivalence about relationships, which are thought to cause the patient's disorder. Therapy is directed toward resolving these conflicts, many of which are rooted in early childhood from child-parent relationships. These conflicts are subsequently played out in transferential reactions in therapy. In the past, psychoanalysis typically took several years and required several treatments per week with goals of changing personality structure and not merely alleviating symptoms. Today, weekly short-term versions are increasingly used, such as those proposed by Malan[59] and Sifneos,[106] which tend to focus on a single dynamic issue.

Other short-term psychotherapies such as cognitive, behavioral, and interpersonal therapies tend to have standardized treatment manuals and explicit training procedures and seem to be supplanting or augmenting purely psychodynamic approaches. These approaches also have undergone the greatest empirical research.[105]

Cognitive/behavioral therapy is based on the premise that people's thoughts, attitudes, and views of the world and their experiences determine their emotions and subsequent behaviors. Because depressed people tend to think negatively about themselves, their environment (the world), and their futures (the negative cognitive triad), they expect to fail and make faulty conclusions (inferences) about the behaviors and thoughts of others. Treatment is devoted to correcting maladaptive beliefs and negative thought patterns/habits. Eventual acceptance of reality and logical thinking leads to enhanced functioning and improved self-esteem, thereby improving mood. The preventive aspect of the therapy is presumed to be the alteration of dysfunctional attitudes, such as associating self-worth with the approval of specific others or excessively high standards, dependency, or self-criticism.[104] Cognitive therapy lowers relapse and recurrence rates of unipolar nonpsychotic depressions.[104] At least 10 studies have demonstrated it to be as efficacious as antidepressant drugs in treating outpatient depression.[104]

Behavior therapy focuses on action and homework involving specific behaviors (e.g., positive activities and developing social skills) thereby giving patients a sense of accomplishment by setting realistic goals in stepwise fashion. Because depressed individuals give themselves too little self-reinforcement and too much self-punishment, behavioral strategies and techniques are designed to increase positive and decrease negative interactions and activities.[105]

Interpersonal therapy focuses on disturbed relationships rather than intrapsychic functions. These disturbed relationships cause depressive symptoms. By focusing on current interpersonal issues, patients are encouraged to become more aware of their patterns and develop better methods of relating and improved social functioning. Improved communication skills and the appropriate expression of suppressed emotions, including anger and grief, are encouraged.[105]

Combined treatments, blending psychotherapy and pharmacotherapy, may often be more effective than a single-treatment approach. Simply pushing pills on patients is often doomed to failure. The more arrows in their quivers (the more comfortable physicians feel with various approaches, both psychotherapeutic and pharmacotherapeutic), the better able physicians are to address and be effective with their patients' depressions. Controlled studies are accumulating as to the effectiveness of the psychotherapies, vis a vis controls, placebos, and antidepressant medications.[105]

Family involvement

Family and friends can be most helpful by encouraging the depressed person to seek appropriate treatment and by providing support and encouragement while the patient is depressed. They can help the patient feel worthwhile by maintaining the relationship with kindness, affection, respect, and caring.[100] Accepting that the person is suffering and in pain without being critical or disapproving is very supportive. Encouraging patients to pull themselves up by their bootstraps is not helpful. Helping the patient be busy and active breaks the cycle of withdrawal. It is important not to be impatient or to indicate that they believe depression is a sign of weakness. They also can be invaluable during times when suicide is a significant risk by providing containment and support.

Depressed individuals tend to marry similar souls (assortative mating) who also need treatment. Marital maladjustment is common, often leading to separation or divorce. Some depressed individuals even provoke their partners to leave, thereby avoiding having to wait passively for abandonment.[25] Marital therapy may be essential.

Not all people who are in a state of grief need formal intervention; they tend to respond to moral support and reassurance from family, friends, or religious support. Others are helped by physicians, psychiatrists, and other health professionals who review the historicity of the relationship with the departed person and use individual psychotherapy for persons who are overwhelmed. Self-help support groups, avoidance of alcohol and drug use, and specific antidepressants if grief gives way to major depression are indicated. Treatment-resistant cases should be referred to psychiatrists with special interest in the treatment of mood disorders or to tertiary care hospitals and universities.

Suicide

Suicide is defined as intentional, self-inflicted death. Suicidal behavior is an extreme expression of underlying psychopathology, not a diagnosis in itself.[22] Suicide exists as a spectrum from ideation-threat-plan-intent-attempt-completion.

EPIDEMIOLOGY

Suicide is the ultimate complication of depression in about 15% of cases. About 50,000 to 70,000 suicides occur annually[76]; 30% to 70% of these carried the diagnosis of major depression.[15,47,76] Identifiable depression may be causally related to 60% of suicides.[108]

In 1986, suicide was the eighth leading cause of death, affecting 30,904 Americans.[75,86] Because suicide is hard to prove, the true incidence probably is far greater. In fact, uniform operational criteria for declaring a death due to suicide have been developed only recently.[19] It is generally agreed that suicides are underreported. Suicide attempts occur in 1% of the population without lifetime mental disorder, 17% of dysthymics, 18% of those with major depressions, and 24% of those with bipolar disorders.[88]

Estimated suicide rate in the United States is 12.5:100,000 (0.01%) persons (in West Germany it is 36:100,000 and in Ireland 3:100,000, which may represent underreporting because of religious reasons).[86] In Canada the rate increased from 7.8 to 14.6 per 100,000 population from 1950 to 1986 and caused a loss of 122,908 potential life years (97,613 men and 25,295 women) in the 3700 suicides in 1986.[15] The tenth leading cause of death among adults in the United States, it is second only to homicide as the leading cause of death among young black men (see box below).[29]

Veterans Administration psychiatric patients in a large prospective study of 4800 patients had a suicide rate of 279:100,000 (12 times that of U.S. military veterans and 23 times the general civilian suicide rate).[82] Unfortunately, extensive efforts over the past three decades have not reduced the incidence of suicide in the United States.[37] Higher rates are consistently found in the West and South than in the Midwest and Northeast.[26]

Attempted suicides occur in an estimated 210,000 persons each year, causing 10,000 permanent disabilities, 155,500 physician visits, 259,200 hospital days, 630,000

Suicides in subpopulations: 1986[86]

Youth age 15-19	10.2/100,000
Men age 20-34	25.9/100,000
Men age >65	46/100,000
American Indians	14.1/100,000 (1985)

lost work days, and over $115 million in direct medical expenses.[95] Attempted suicides are often called parasuicides (nonfatal suicidal behaviors) by British authors.

American teenagers have the highest suicide rate in the world.[7] It has become the third leading cause of death in young persons (ages 15 to 24),[75] increasing dramatically in recent years.[11,18,30] It increases with each teenage year, peaking for youth at age 23.[102] Figures do vary; one author cites it as the fourth leading cause of years of potential life lost among teenagers.[20]

Suicide has tripled (i.e., increased by 300%) in the last 25 years. Drug abuse has been hypothesized as the main contributor to this increase.[79] Five thousand youths commit suicide and 500,000 to 1 million attempt it every year.[76,39] A particularly disturbing trend in adolescents are suicide clusters where several adolescents in the same community commit suicide in rapid copycat succession.[42]

People over 65 account for 25% of all suicides. High suicide rates for the elderly declined from 1950 to 1980, but then increased again.[26]

Female suicides peak at age 50 years, males at 75 years. Women attempt suicide three times more frequently than men, but men commit suicide three times more often than women. High-risk periods for women are premenstrual, postpartum, and seasonal.[44]

One percent to 2% of attempters do commit suicide each year, and a significant percentage (10% to 40%)[26] of eventual suicide victims have made previous attempts.[87] Two percent to 10% of attempters eventually commit suicide.[26] Six percent who attempt suicide leaving minimal provision for rescue complete suicide in the year after the attempt.[37]

RISK FACTORS

Although those at risk for suicide can be identified, those who will actually commit suicide cannot be identified. The fundamental problem with prediction is that suicide is a rare event.[37] The accuracy of a suicide prediction schedule for Veterans Administration neuropsychiatric patients was 0.20 (i.e., only 20% of patients predicted to commit suicide would actually do so).[58]

Similar risk factors appear to operate across the various life stages or phases, but their contributory weights differ.

Most people who engage in suicidal behavior suffer from mental illness.[79] Survivors of attempted suicide usually have adjustment or personality disorders.[79]

Psychiatric illness is the most important risk factor (70% to 98% of suicides; 90% suicide attempters).[29] The majority of suicides/attempters suffer from affective disorders (65% to 75%),[29] substance abuse (alcoholism 25%),[29] or schizophrenia[7,67] (depression rather than delusions increase the risk.)[24] Fifteen percent of those with depressive disorders and 20% of those with bipolar depression eventually commit suicide,[73] whereas 15% of alcoholics[73] and

2% to 13% of schizophrenics do so.[6,73] These patients are more likely to visit physicians than suicide prevention centers.[37] Three fourths of alcoholic suicides were committed by those suffering from concurrent depression.[73]

The risk of suicide is five to six times higher in psychotic depression.[25,94] Some suicides are covertly encouraged by hostile or depressed significant others who also may need to be treated to reduce suicidal risk.[25]

All suicide attempts or threats should be taken seriously, even though 85% to 95% of attempters do not commit suicide.[73] The apparent triviality of a suicide attempt may not be proportional to the seriousness of the risk and may be a rehearsal for a lethal attempt.[73] In a 40-year follow-up study of 225 recurrent unipolar depressives, all 15 who completed suicide had threatened suicide before.[31] It is important not to be afraid to ask patients about suicidal thoughts and behavior. There is a myth that direct questioning may give patients the idea of killing themselves. In fact, such questioning is the only way to identify those at risk for suicide. The typical suicide attempter wants something from others; in the truly presuicidal the wish to die relates to an internal state, such as hopelessness or unbearable pain, only.[73]

In a prospective study of 955 patients with major affective disorders, 25 suicides occurred in the first 4 years of follow-up; 13 (52%) occurred during the first year. Suicide appears to occur relatively early in the course of affective illness.[10] Predictors of these early suicides were severe hopelessness, near total anhedonia, severe anxiety, recent state-dependent panic attacks, depressive turmoil (rapid switching from depression to anxiety to anger), and moderate alcohol abuse. Suicides occurring after 1 year from presentation were associated with suicidal ideation, history of previous attempts, and suicidal intent (i.e., the more classically accepted predictors).[28]

Serious medical illnesses increase risk (5% of those with terminal illness kill themselves[91]). The risk increases from fourfold among cancer patients[63] to 66-fold among AIDS patients.[65] In comparison to the general population, patients in the hospital have a threefold higher risk of suicide (alcoholics, 70 times; epilepsy, 5 times; peptic ulceration, 5 times; dialysis, 10 to 50 times; and AIDS, 36 times).[69] Those who have had a family member commit suicide are nine times more likely than others to kill themselves.[15]

Biologic factors

Patients with low levels of 5-hydroxyindoleacetic acid (final breakdown product of serotonin) in the cerebral spinal fluid (CSF) are at high risk for suicide.[110] Impaired serotonergic activity may be a trait (i.e., the phenotypic expression of the genetic risk factor for suicide).[61] High levels of urinary 17-hydroxycorticosteroids are also at increased risk. Postmortem studies have revealed reduced

---

Psychobiologic model of suicide (combination leads to suicide)

Psychiatric disorder, particularly depression
Inherited biochemical predisposition for impulsivity and self-directed violence
Higher risk personality disorder, e.g., borderline or sociopathic type
Drug/alcohol abuse
Hopelessness
Stress
Being alone
Pain
Physical illness

Composite male high suicidal risk picture

Depressed	No friends
Elderly	No relatives
Physically ill	Hopeless
Disabled	Suicidal preoccupation
Unemployed	Specific plan
Alcoholic	Lethal means
Recently divorced	Suicide note
Living alone	Changed will
	Experience auditory hallucinations

Composite female high suicidal risk picture[23]

Depressed white (2:1 black)	Housewives
Midlife	Firearms
Divorced	Antidepressants
Widowed	Gifted with high IQs
Single, especially single parenthood	Gulf between endowments/achievement
Dropout activities/social networks	

Composite youth high suicidal risk picture[8,62]

Depressed	Parental divorce
Revenge-motivated	Family changes
Angry	Multiple moves
Aggressive	Family history of suicide
Impulsive	Conduct disorders
Accident prone	Substance abuse
History of injuries	Few life accomplishments
Romantic	Greater competition for education/jobs
Interpersonal problems	
Idealistic	Low self-esteem
Rigid	Humiliating life experience
Perfectionistic	Impending disciplinary crisis
Hopeless	Access to firearms

---

brain serotonergic activity in suicide victims.[60] These findings, although interesting, are not clinically useful.

Misdiagnosis and mistreatment of a depressed individual as primarily anxious, e.g., with benzodiazepines (central nervous system depressants) may worsen the illness.[79] Approximately 15% of suicides have a history of alcoholism, in whom the suicide rate is 10 times greater. Twenty-five percent to 30% of completers are reported to have been intoxicated at the time of their death[10] (see box[60] above).

Psychologic factors

Substantial risk exists with expressed suicidal intent, overt plan, or significant gesture.[79] Patients with the following traits are more likely to attempt suicide (see boxes at right):

- A history of previous suicide attempt (25% to 50% of completers). This characteristic is the best predictor of suicide.[61]
- Impulsivity (which has been associated with low levels of 5-hydroxyindoleacetic acid in CSF).
- Dependence, particularly in those who require constant reassurance and attention or who have unrealistic expectations, which are frequently unmet.
- Terminal illness, recent surgery, disfigurement (especially facial disfigurement).
- History of physical violence; violent temper; child, animal, or spouse abuse.
- Total hopelessness or overpowering feelings of loneliness or being "alone in the world." People with small social networks have a much greater risk of death than those with larger networks.[45] Suicide (egoistic) may occur when the individual has too few ties with the community.
- Family history of suicide.
- Marital status in increasing order of risk—single, widowed, divorced, separated,[69] especially with the attitude: "Without him/her, I am nothing." Marital history, living arrangements, recent life changes, stress, isolation, social, or occupational support should all be assessed.
- Recent bereavement.[7] The elderly widower may be particularly vulnerable to fantasies of reunion with his spouse, particularly around anniversaries.[79] The ratio for men/women is 4:1 in the 65 to 69 year age group and 12:1 in the over 85 group.[77]
- Intractable relationship problems, living alone, unemployed individuals, adolescents who have dropped out of school and geographic mobility. College students may have a lower risk with supportive milieu and mental health services available on campus.[8]
- Dentists, physicians, pharmacists, lawyers, musicians, police officers, and unskilled workers.[29]

- Blacks, especially black adolescents.
- Incarceration. Prison inmates in Canada had a suicidal rate of more than 60 per 100,000 in 1986 (four-fold greater risk than general population).[15]
- Dissolution of love relationship, starting or stopping psychotropic medication, drug intoxication, increased hopelessness, communication of suicidal intent and *sudden* improvement in previously depressed mood (perhaps partly related to resolution of conflict regarding suicide).
- Comorbid personality disorders (especially borderline and sociopathic).[44,61]
- Alienated or stigmatized groups such as homosexual adolescents. These groups attempt suicide three to seven times more often than heterosexuals.[113]
- Exposure to media coverage about suicide. During a newspaper strike in Detroit, suicides decreased. Rates increased particularly in adolescents after television shows involving peer deaths.[90] An association between exposure to media coverage of suicide and increased imitative youth suicide has been demonstrated.[36]
- Jewish suicides increased significantly under Nazi persecution in 1933-1945. The Catholic church no longer denies religious burial to suicides (Codex Juris Canonici).[90]

METHODS

A concrete suicidal plan, particularly if there has been rehearsal, is ominous. The most common method, firearms, is used by 60% of men and by over 33% of women. Drug overdose was preferred during the 1970s and today is the second most common means.[95] Amitriptyline is the most frequently used medication in suicide by overdose.[22] It ranks fifth among medical examiners' drug mentions after alcohol (in combination), heroin, cocaine, and codeine; secobarbital has dropped to thirteenth place.[73]

Alcohol intoxication is associated with 25% to 50% of all suicides,[7] and is especially common in suicides with firearms.[11] Men use potentially more lethal methods, such as firearms, hanging, jumping from heights, or drowning. Women tend to take drug overdoses, particularly psychotropic drugs mixed with alcohol or poisons or to slash their wrists.[29]

EFFECTIVENESS OF EARLY DETECTION

Because suicide is such a rare event, very large samples and lengthy follow-up are necessary for studies to demonstrate significant reduction in suicide rates. Suicide has been called "a permanent solution to a temporary problem" and if sufficient time is allowed to pass (people prevented from acting impulsively), people with suicidal ideation often judge their situations entirely differently, underscoring the importance of the time factor in suicide.

The physician can play a critical role identifying and treating the suicidal patient. Physicians commonly fail to inquire about suicidal ideation, only one in six being aware of suicidal ideation in their patients.[73] Seventy-five percent of patients who subsequently commit suicide see a physician (usually nonpsychiatrist) within 6 months of their death and 50% to 60% within 1 month of their death. Their complaints, mainly about somatic symptoms associated with depression, give the physician an opportunity to anticipate the possibility of suicide and refer the patient for psychiatric help. Even though two thirds communicate intent to commit suicide to friend, family, or physician, the communications are often difficult to interpret.[25] It is important to listen when a person talks about suicide, not to discount or deny it, and to realize that by talking about it or threatening to perform it, the patient may be crying for help.

Currently used suicidal intent scales lack sufficient sensitivity or specificity to be useful.[37] When the cutoff point on the Beck Hopelessness Scale is set to correctly identify 90% of suicides, it also yields 88% false-positive results.[5]

The single greatest contributor to suicide prevention is an early diagnosis of affective disorder, depressed.[73] Affective disordered patients who receive comprehensive psychiatric care have lower suicide rates than patients with other psychiatric illnesses.[43,64] Early diagnosis and adequate treatment of depression would also significantly decrease suicide.[56] It is important to remember that suicidal risk is coextensive with the depressive episode and, therefore, requires frequent reassessment.[73] Hence, the physician must be alert for signs and symptoms of occult depression to successfully administer prevention.

Only 12.1% of 313 teenaged students received medical care after suicide attempts.[113] Some patients who receive psychiatric consultation after attempted suicide find therapy to be of only limited benefit,[41] and over 40% choose not to remain in therapy.[68] Hospitalized suicide attempters who left prematurely attempted suicide more often subsequently than those who remained for psychiatric counseling.[38]

Although involuntary hospitalization can be of immediate benefit to those planning suicide, few reliable data are available regarding its long-term effectiveness.[119]

Although firearms are used in over half of all suicides[11,7,67,70] there is no direct evidence that removal of firearms can prevent suicide. On the other hand, places with reduced availability of firearms have lower suicide rates.[67] The more difficult it is to find the means with which to commit suicide (e.g., by restricting handgun availability or wrapping each pill in foil individually), the more likely a reduction in impulsive but not planned suicides.[61]

Elimination of domestic coal gas containing carbon monoxide led to a decrease in suicide in England.[12] Other methods, however, may be substituted after removal of an available suicide method (e.g., agricultural chemicals replacing undiluted vinegar in Surinam).[16]

Drugs prescribed by the physician are often used as a means of suicide, and in over 50% of suicides the drugs were prescribed by a physician within the preceding week or as a refillable prescription.[71] Therefore nonlethal quantities of prescription drugs should be prescribed, (e.g., less than 1500 to 2000 mg of standard tricyclic antidepressants at any one time). Because an overdose of 2 g of many antidepressants is potentially lethal, prescription amount should be limited and nonrefillable. Australian legislation to restrict the number of prescriptions for hypnotics may have been associated with a reduced rate of suicide, but the evidence was not conclusive.[35]

Early detection and treatment of substance abuse could potentially prevent suicide, but no conclusive proof is available.

CLINICAL INTERVENTION

The U.S. Preventive Services Task Force[111] does not recommend routine screening of asymptomatic adult persons for suicidal intent.[111] However, the American Academy of Pediatrics recommends questioning of all adolescents about suicidal thoughts during the routine medical history.[1]

Clinicians should assess risk factors for suicide and extent of preparatory actions (e.g., putting affairs in order, preparing will, giving prized possessions away, buying guns, refilling prescriptions, planning unexpected trip). They should specifically evaluate for depression, psychosis, intoxication, chronic alcohol abuse, recent loss, social support network and confidant, plans for the future, medical status, previous suicide attempts, appropriate demographic characteristics, history of recently starting or stopping psychotropics, orientation, suicidal ideas or wishes, intent to carry out these plans, feasibility, lethality, and allowing for the possibility of being saved (rescue plans) (see box below). There is some evidence that use of violent methods is predictive of future suicide.[10]

Patients with serious suicidal intent should be referred for psychiatric consultation or hospitalization. A policy of routine psychiatric consultation after attempted suicide reduces risk of suicide.[15] Hospitalization is mandatory for overt suicidal ideation complicated by injurious behavior, encephalopathy, substance abuse, or intoxication[79] (obtain toxicology screen). Clinicians should be particularly alert to signs of depression and alcohol and other substance abuse.

Previous attempters are less likely to seek help or share their feelings with others and more likely to react negatively to suicide prevention programs.[103]

The family should be contacted despite the patient's objections if suicidal risk is judged to be high[79] (i.e., confidentiality is breached in face of tissue damage/death). The closest available family member should be called to gain information and increase support. Patients and their families or friends should be made aware of available community resources, such as local community mental health centers. Significant others, including parents, should be counseled to remove potentially lethal prescription drugs and firearms from the home. Other family members may also be suicidal and merit assessment (see box below).[69]

Clinical diagnosis is the key to effective treatment, and the physician's office is the first line of defense and primary intervention center.[37] The physician's role in suicide prevention has been underemphasized (see box below).[8]

PREVENTION

Prevention is hard to detect because statistically nonsuicide is a nonevent.[73] There are three basic approaches to prevention:

1. Primary prevention. As for depression, help individuals to feel good about themselves by enhancing self-esteem and teaching problem solving, stress management, and appropriate coping skills so that

---

Why suicidal patients may be difficult to interview

Denial
Ambivalence
False improvement when removed from stress
Anger/hostility
Noncooperation
Distortions
Manipulativeness
Poor response to limit setting
Demandingness

Lethality = potential for causing death

High	*Low*
Precise plan	Vague plan
Next 24 to 72 hours	Rescue plans
Lethal method	
Available means	
Intent to die	
Poor impulse control	
No rescue plan	

Physicians' critical community leadership role

Educating the public
Continuing medical education
Restricting firearm availability
Guidelines for the media
Community clinics
Advocacy for insurance parity in mental health benefits
Political liaison with policymakers and civic leaders

they will not contemplate suicide as a solution.

2. Secondary prevention. Remove cause of distress driving them to suicide, psychiatric treatment of depression or other psychiatric illness.

3. Tertiary prevention. Physically restrain—hospitalization with suicide precautions; improved emergency treatment of overdose and self-inflicted gunshot wounds.

Because the primary contributor to suicide is affective disorder, suicide prevention is best accomplished through early and accurate diagnosis and effective treatment of depression and the prevention of further affective episodes (see box).[44]

High school curricula tend to be overinclusive and focus on stressful life events rather than mental illness. This approach is inappropriate based on current knowledge,[8] as 95% of those who commit suicide are psychiatrically ill at the time of death.[73] Short-term educational interventions are not effective for adolescent attempters, and exposure may stir up disturbing feelings without appropriate available treatment.[103] Focusing on mental state abnormalities (e.g., cognitive distortions) may be more helpful.[103]

Suicide hotlines and suicide prevention centers can provide valuable service in crisis intervention and triage, but this approach is not prevention in an epidemiologic sense.[37] The effectiveness of suicide hotlines in decreasing suicide rates is not conclusive,[15] although a small reduction among young white women was found in one study.[66] In the United States, over 200 centers offer variable educational, outreach, and supportive programs. Their availability has not been associated with reduction in the suicide rate. Only 2% of suicide victims have contacted a center before taking their lives.[37] Clients are more likely to be suicide attempters. According to the Canadian Task Force, there is only poor evidence supporting the effectiveness of crisis intervention in preventing suicide.[15] Thus crisis intervention seems to postpone rather than prevents suicide in the chronically suicidal.[37]

Hospitalization is indicated if risk is sufficient and there is good evidence that the person is suicidal. It is far better to err on the side of hospitalization than to allow the ultimate mistake. Overtly suicidal patients who refuse treatment should be hospitalized involuntarily, following state guidelines. Hospitalization itself does not solve the problem, as many patients commit suicide in the hospital. (In fact, hospitalized psychiatric patients have a suicide rate 30 times higher than the national average.[27]) In the first 24

to 48 hours, there should be strict precautions (from full restraints and constant 24-hour observation, even when going to the bathroom, to seclusion room with frequent checks every 15 minutes, to restrictions and close observation on the unit after removal of all harmful objects) (see box below).[27] The immediate post-discharge period also is characterized by particularly high rate.[10]

Suicidal patients are usually ambivalent about killing themselves. The impulse to kill oneself usually is brief and diminishes rapidly with treatment and a safe milieu. If every person thinking of suicide were hospitalized, they would fill every medical, surgical and psychiatric hospital bed.[22]

Outpatient treatment may be a valid alternative to hospitalization if there is suicidal ideation without a plan, no severe psychiatric disturbance, and low levels of anxiety and perturbation, supportive and responsible family members who will watch over the patient, and a willingness and commitment to outpatient treatment. Preventing suicide is a family concern and families need family therapy to understand, cope with, and monitor their own feelings evoked by self-destructive behavior in their loved one.[113]

Contracts against suicide are an effective preventive therapeutic strategy.[79] It is helpful to formulate a contract with the patient, verbally and in writing, to refrain from attempting suicide and to call the physician if resolve is weakening. Patients usually respect their agreement and do not break trust. Contact with the patient by telephone and in person should be made daily initially and frequently thereafter. It is important not to write prescriptions for lethal amounts of medication and to involve family in dispensing medication initially. Psychotherapy focus is on support and survival and, only later, on insight and exploration.

BIOLOGIC TREATMENTS

The risk of suicide decreases with appropriate optimal pharmacotherapy. Patients with major depression should be treated with antidepressant medication or ECT. Enhancing serotonergic brain function should reduce suicide risk, e.g., by antidepressants that inhibit serotonin reuptake (chlorimipramine, amitriptyline, imipramine and fluoxet-

---

Suicide prevention strategies

Hotlines
Crisis intervention centers
Media coverage: news, documentaries, movies
High school curricula
Individual treatment services

Hospital suicide prevention recommendations

Observe and document evidence of suicidal risk and behavior
Position patient on first floor; use unbreakable glass
Position patient near nurses' station
Remove sharp/dangerous objects
Avoid bathroom/room fixtures with opportunities for hanging
Reduce isolation
Provide supportive therapy
Prevent hoarding of medication
Examine suicide risk before issuing passes or discharge

ine), inhibit MAO (phenelzine), and increase serotonin turnover (lithium).[61]

Choice of antidepressants in the suicidal patient should be based on safety with risk of overdose. Newer antidepressants such as fluoxetine,[61] trazodone, and bupropion tend to be safer than tricyclic antidepressants. Psychotic symptoms merit antipsychotic medication. Severe agitation may require antipsychotics, IV benzodiazepines (such as lorazepam) or Amytal.

PSYCHOTHERAPY

It is important to establish a therapeutic alliance and to communicate hope to the patient. To relieve a sense of hopelessness, the patient should be encouraged to explore available options and alternative solutions and to focus on the temporary nature of suicidal feelings and intent. Psychotherapy helps to keep self-destructive dynamics in perspective. It is essential to involve family, friends, and significant others and to consider family therapy. Environmental manipulation by attending to worrisome matters that can be changed helps to reduce anxiety (e.g., contact with employer or significant other).

Continued reassessment is essential, particularly in the first phases of improvement from depression, when the patient develops sufficient energy to carry out a plan. Therapeutic home visits (i.e., leaving the hospital) with feedback from family, are important before final discharge. Abrupt cessation of physician contact may be interpreted by the patient as rejection.[73] Suicide completers are less likely to be in or stay in psychiatric treatment.[10]

Valente notes that suicidal risk decreases as adolescents learn to clarify problems, expand resources, use safer, more appropriate coping strategies, and rally significant others.[113] These same principles are applicable to other age groups as well in applied prevention.

No community has all the resources (especially experienced psychotherapists) to provide comprehensive care to all suicidal individuals,[37] and caring for these patients can be stressful, especially when one considers the medicolegal risks. (Hospitals and psychiatrists have been successfully sued, even though all safeguards to prevent suicide have been taken.) It is important to make careful diagnoses, treat appropriately, keep careful records, and obtain second opinions/consultations with difficult cases. (Interestingly, suicide prevention centers carry no liability insurance.)[37]

Many physicians who experience a patient suicide have many unresolved feelings and should be encouraged to discuss them with colleagues or supervisors. Suicide has been described as the ultimate hostility against the survivors. This sometimes includes the physician, giving rise to marked countertransference feelings, guilt, and grief. Physicians never know how many suicides they prevent and never forget the ones that are completed in spite of their best efforts. Psychiatrists need to limit the number of acutely suicidal patients they are treating, as these patients produce considerable emotional drain and stress.[29]

SUMMARY

Depressive disorders are common, serious conditions causing substantial morbidity and mortality and, therefore, merit early detection and prompt, effective treatment. Depression and suicide were presented from epidemiologic, risk factor, and diagnostic perspectives, underscoring the burden of suffering they cause as well as the availability and efficacy of preventive and treatment strategies. A biopsychosocial comprehensive approach is espoused during all phases, from screening and assessment through therapeutic interventions.

Acknowledgment

The author gratefully acknowledges Lillian Parmertor for her clerical support.

REFERENCES

1. American Academy of Pediatrics Committee on Adolescence: Suicide and suicide attempts in adolescents and young adults, *Pediatrics* 81:322-324, 1988.
2. American Psychiatric Association: *Diagnostic and statistical manual of mental disorders,* ed 3, revised. Washington, DC, 1987, American Psychiatric Association.
3. Ballenger JC: Biological aspects of depression: implications for clinical practice. In Frances AJ, Hales RE, editors: *Review of psychiatry,* vol 7, Washington, DC, 1988, American Psychiatric Press.
4. Barraclough B, Bunch J, Nelson B, et al: A hundred cases of suicide: clinical aspects, *Br J Psychiatry* 125:355-373, 1974.
5. Beck AT, Steer RA, Kovacs M: Hopelessness and eventual suicide: a ten-year prospective study of patients hospitalized with suicidal ideation, *Am J Psychiatry* 142:559-563, 1985.
6. Black DW, Winokur G, Warrack G: Suicide in schizophrenia: the Iowa Record Linkage Study, *J Clin Psychiatry* 46:14-17, 1985.
7. Blumenthal SJ: Suicide: a guide to risk factors, assessment, and treatment of suicidal patients, *Med Clin North Am* 72:937-971, 1988.
8. Blumenthal SJ: Youth suicide: the physician's role in suicide prevention, *JAMA* 264:3194-3196, 1990.
9. Boyd JH, Weissman MM: Epidemiology of affective disorders: reexamination and future direction, *Arch Gen Psychiatry* 38:1039-1046, 1981.
10. Brent DA, Kupfer DJ, Brochet EJ, et al: The assessment and treatment of patients at risk for suicide. In Frances AJ, Hales RE, editors: *Review of psychiatry,* vol 7, Washington, DC, 1988, American Psychiatric Press.
11. Brent DA, Perper JA, Allman CJ: Alcohol, firearms and suicide among youth: temporal trends in Allegheny County, Pennsylvania, 1960 to 1983, *JAMA* 257:3369-3372, 1987.
12. Brown JH: Suicide in Britain: more attempts, fewer deaths, lessons for public policy, *Arch Gen Psychiatry* 36:1119-1124, 1979.
13. Campbell TL: Controversies in family medicine: why screening for mental health problems is not worthwhile in family practice, *J Fam Pract* 25:184-187, 1987.
14. Canadian Task Force on the Periodic Health Examination: The periodic health examination, *Can Med Assoc J* 121:1194-254, 1979.
15. Canadian Task Force on the Periodic Health Examination: 1990 Update: 2. Early detection of depression and prevention of suicide,

Can Med Assoc J 142:1233-1238, 1990.

16. Caribbean Epidemiology Centre, PAHO: Paraquat poisoning in two Caribbean countries, *Carec Surveillance Report* 12:1-9, 1986.

17. Cassem EH: Depression secondary to medical illness. In Frances AJ, Hales RE, editors: *Review of psychiatry*, vol 7, Washington, DC, 1988, American Psychiatric Press.

18. Centers for Disease Control: *Youth suicide in the United States, 1970-1980*, Atlanta, 1986, Centers for Disease Control.

19. Centers for Disease Control: Operational criteria for determining suicide, *MMWR* 37:773-4, 779-80, 1988.

20. Centers for Disease Control: Years of potential life lost before age 65—United States, 1987, *MMWR* 38:27-29, 1989.

21. Davidson JT, Miller RD, Turnbull CD, et al: Atypical depression, *Arch Gen Psychiatry* 39:527-534, 1982.

22. Davidson L: Assessment and management of suicidal patients, *J Med Assoc Ga* 77:834-834, 1988.

23. Davidson L: Profiles of women at risk for committing suicide, *Clin Psychiatry News*, March 1991.

24. Drake RE, Gates C, Cotton PG, et al: Suicide among schizophrenics: who is at risk? *J Nerv Ment Dis* 172:613-617, 1984.

25. Dubovsky SL: Depression. In Dubovsky SL, editor: *Concise guide to clinical psychiatry*, Washington, DC, 1988, American Psychiatric Press.

26. Editorial: Prevention: the endpoint of suicidology, *Mayo Clin Proc* 65:115-118, 1990.

27. Farberow NL: Suicide prevention in the hospital, *Hosp Community Psychiatry* 32:99-104, 1981.

28. Fawcett J: Predictors of early suicide: identification and appropriate intervention, *J Clin Psychiatry* 49(Suppl 10):7-8, 1988.

29. Fawcett J, Shaughnessy R: The suicidal patient. In Flaherty JA, Channon RA, Davis JM, editors: *Psychiatry: diagnosis and therapy*, East Norwalk, Conn, 1988, Appleton & Lange.

30. Fingerhut LA, Kleinman JC: Suicide rates for young people, *JAMA* 259:356, 1988.

31. Fowler RC, Tsuang MT, Kronfol Z: Communication of suicidal intent and suicide in unipolar depression, *J Affective Disord* 1:219-225, 1979.

32. Frame PS: A critical review of adult health maintenance, Part 4, *J Fam Pract* 23:29-39, 1986.

33. Gaviria FM, Flaherty JA: Depression. In Flaherty JA, Shannon RA, Davis JM, editors: *Psychiatry: diagnosis and therapy*, East Norwalk, Conn, 1988, Appleton & Lange.

34. Goldin LR, Gershon ES: The genetic epidemiology of major depressive illness. In Frances AJ, Hales RE, editors: *Review of psychiatry*, vol 7, Washington, DC, 1988, American Psychiatric Press.

35. Goldney RD, Katsikitis M: Cohort analysis of suicide rates in Australia, *Arch Gen Psychiatry* 40:71-74, 1983.

36. Gould MS, Shaffer D: The impact of televised movies about suicide, *N Engl J Med* 318:707-708, 1988.

37. Greenberg SI: Suicide prevention update: thirty years later, *J Fla Med Assoc* 75:610-613, 1988.

38. Greer S, Bagley C: Effect of psychiatric intervention in attempted suicide: a controlled study, *Br Med J* 1:310-312, 1971.

39. Greydanus DE: Depression in adolescence: a perspective, *J Adolesc Health Care* 7:109S-120S, 1986.

40. Hankin JR, Locke BZ: The persistence of depressive symptomatology among prepaid group practice enrollees: an exploratory study, *Am J Public Health* 72:1000-1007, 1982.

41. Hengleveld MW, Kerkhof AJFM, van der Wal J: Evaluation of psychiatric consultations with suicide attempters, *Acta Psychiatr Scand* 77:283-289, 1988.

42. Idem. Cluster of suicides and suicide attempts—New Jersey, *JAMA* 259:2666-2668, 1988.

43. Jamison KR: Suicide and bipolar disorders, *Ann NY Acad Sci* 487:301-315, 1986.

44. Jamison KR: Suicide prevention in depressed women, *J Clin Psychiatry* 49 (Suppl 9):42-45, 1988.

45. Jones EN: American Association of Suicidology Presidential Address, 1988, *Suicide Life Threat Behav* 19:297-304, 1989.

46. Kaplan HI, Sadock BJ: Mood (affective) disorders. In Kaplan HI, Sadock BJ, editors: *Pocket handbook of clinical psychiatry*, Baltimore, 1990, Williams & Wilkins.

47. Kamerow DB: Controversies in family practice: is screening for mental health problems worthwhile? *J Fam Pract* 25:181-184, 1987.

48. Katon W: The epidemiology of depression in medical care, *Int J Psychiatry Med* 17:93-112, 1987.

49. Keitner GI, Ryan CE, Miller IW, et al: 12-month outcome of patients with major depression and comorbid psychiatric or medical illness (compound depression), *Am J Psychiatry* 148:345-350, 1991.

50. Keller MB: Chronic and recurrent affective disorders: incidence, course and influencing factors: proceedings of advances in biochemical psychopharmacology, *Adv Biochem Psychopharmacol* 40:111-120, 1985.

51. Keller MB: Diagnostic issues and clinical course of unipolar illness. In Frances AJ, Hales RE, editors: *Review of psychiatry*, vol 7, Washington, DC, 1988, American Psychiatric Press.

52. Keller MB: Depression: underrecognition and undertreatment by psychiatrists and other health care professionals, *Arch Intern Med* 150:946-948, 1990.

53. Keller MB, Klerman GL, Lavori PW, et al: Treatment received by depressed patients, *JAMA* 248:1848-1855, 1982.

54. Keller MB, Lavori PW, Klerman GI, et al: Low levels and lack of predictors of somatotherapy and psychotherapy received by depressed patients, *Arch Gen Psychiatry* 43:458-466, 1986.

55. Keller MB, Lavori PW, Lewis CE, et al: Predictors of relapse in major depressive disorder, *JAMA* 250:3299-3304, 1983.

56. Khuri R, Akiskal HS: Suicide prevention: the necessity of treating contributory psychiatric disorders, *Psychiatr Clin North Am* 6:193-207, 1983.

57. Lawrence JM: Reactions to withdrawal of antidepressants, antiparkinsonian drugs and lithium. *Psychosomatics* 11:869-877, 1985.

58. Mackinnon DR, Farberow NL: An assessment of the utility of suicide prediction, *Suicide Life Threat Behav* 6:86-91, 1976.

59. Malan DH: *The frontier of brief psychotherapy*, New York, 1976, Plenum.

60. Mann JJ, Stanley M: Postmortem monoamine oxidase enzyme kinetics in the frontal cortex of suicide victims and controls, *Acta Psychiatr Scand* 69:135-139, 1984.

61. Mann JJ, Stanley M: Afterword: suicide. In Frances AJ, Hales RE, editors: *Review of psychiatry*, vol 7, Washington, DC, 1988, American Psychiatric Press.

62. Maris R: The adolescent suicide problem, *Suicide Life Threat Behav* 15:91-109, 1985.

63. Marshall JR, Burnett W, Brasure J: On precipitating factors: cancer as a cause of suicide, *Suicide Life Threat Behav* 13:15-27, 1983.

64. Martin RL, Cloninger R, Guze SB, et al: Mortality in a follow-up of 500 psychiatric outpatients, *Arch Gen Psychiatry* 42:58-66, 1985.

65. Marzuk PM, Tierney H, Tardiff K, et al: Increased risk of suicide in persons with AIDS, *JAMA* 259:1333-1337, 1988.

66. Miller HL, Coombs DW, Leeper JD: An analysis of the effects of suicide prevention facilities on suicide rates in the United States, *Am J Public Health* 74:340-343, 1984.

67. Monk M: Epidemiology of suicide, *Epidemiol Rev* 9:51-69, 1987.

68. Morgan HG, Barton J, Pottle S, et al: Deliberate self-harm: a follow-up study of 279 patients, *Br J Psychiatry* 128:361-368, 1976.

69. Morgan HG, Vassilas CA, Owen JH: Managing suicide risk in the general ward, *Br J Hosp Med* 44:56-59, 1990.

70. Moscicki EK, Boyd JH: Epidemiologic trends in firearm suicides among adolescents, *Pediatrician* 12:52-62, 1985.

71. Murphy GE: The physician's responsibility for suicide. I. An error of omission, *Ann Intern Med* 82:301-314, 1975.

72. Murphy GE: The physician's responsibility for suicide. II. Errors of omission, *Ann Intern Med* 82:305-309, 1975.

73. Murphy GE: Prevention of suicide. In Frances AJ, Hales RE, editors: *Review of psychiatry,* vol 7, Washington, DC, 1988, American Psychiatric Press.

74. Reference deleted in galleys.

75. National Center for Health Statistics: Advance report of final mortality statistics, 1986, *Monthly Vital Statistics Report,* vol 37, no 6, Hyattsville, Md, 1988, Department of Health and Human Services.

76. National Institute of Mental Health. Depression: what we know, Washington, DC, Department of Health and Human Services. Publication No. DHHS (ADM) 85-1318, 1985.

77. Osgood NJ: Suicide in the elderly, *Postgrad Med* 72:123-130, 1982.

78. Reference deleted in galleys.

79. Pary R, Lippman S, Tobias CR: A preventive approach to the suicidal patient, *J Fam Pract* 26:185-189, 1988.

80. Reference deleted in galleys.

81. Pflug B, Tolle R: Disturbance of the 24-hour rhythm in endogenous depression and the treatment of endogenous depression by sleep deprivation, *Int Pharmacopsychiatry* 6:187-196, 1971.

82. Pokorny AD: Prediction of suicide in psychiatric patients: report of a prospective study, *Arch Gen Psychiatry* 40:249-257, 1983.

83. Prestidge BR, Lake CR: Prevalence and recognition of depression among primary care outpatients, *J Fam Pract* 25:67-72, 1987.

84. Prien RE: Somatic treatment of unipolar depression disorder. In Frances AJ, Hales RE, editors: *Review of psychiatry,* vol 7, Washington, DC, 1988, American Psychiatric Press.

85. Prien RF, Kupfer DJ: Continuation drug therapy for major depressive episodes: how long should it be maintained? *Am J Psychiatry* 143:18-23, 1986.

86. Public Health Service: US Department of Health and Human Services: *Promoting health/preventing disease. Year 2000 objectives for the nation; mental and behavioral disorders.* (Draft) PHS, 19-1–19-19, Philadelphia, 1989, WB Saunders.

87. Rabins PV, Harvic K, Koven S: High fatality rates of late-life depression associated with cardiovascular disease, *J Affect Disord* 9:165-167, 1985.

88. Regier DA, Hirschfeld RMA, Goodwin FK, et al: The NIMH depression awareness, recognition and treatment program: structure, aims and scientific basis, *Am J Psychiatry* 145:1351-1357, 1988.

89. Regier DA, Myers JK, Kramer M, et al: The NIMH Epidemiological Catchment Area Program: historical context, major objectives, and study population characteristics, *Arch Gen Psychiatry* 41:934-941, 1984.

90. Ringel E: Founder's perspectives—then and now, *Suicide Life Threat Behav* 18:13-19, 1988.

91. Robins E: Suicide. In Kaplan HI, Sadock BJ, editors: *Comprehensive textbook of psychiatry,* ed 4, Baltimore, 1985, Williams & Wilkins.

92. Reference deleted in galleys.

93. Robins LN, Helzer JE, Weissman MM, et al: Lifetime prevalence of specific psychiatric disorders in three sites, *Arch Gen Psychiatry* 41:949-958, 1984.

94. Roose SP, Glassman AH, Walsh BT, et al: Depression, delusions and suicide, *Am J Psychiatry* 140:1159-1162, 1983.

95. Rosenberg ML, Gelles RJ, Holinger PC, et al: Violence: homicide, assault and suicide. In Amler RW, Dull BH, editors: *Closing the gap: the burden of unnecessary illness,* New York, 1987, Oxford University Press.

96. Rosenthal MP, Goldfarb NI, Carlson BL, et al: Assessment of depression in a family practice center, *J Fam Pract* 25:143-149, 1987.

97. Rosenthal NE, Sack DA, Carpenter CJ, et al: Antidepressant effects of light in seasonal affective disorder, *Am J Psychiatry* 142:163-170, 1985.

98. Rucker L, Frye EB, Cygan RW: Feasibility and usefulness of depression screening in medical outpatients, *Arch Intern Med* 146:729-731, 1986.

99. Sack DA, Nurnberger J, Rosenthal NE, et al: The potentiation of antidepressant medications by phase advance of the sleep-wake cycle, *Am J Psychiatry* 142:606-608, 1985.

100. Sargent M: Depressive disorders: treatments bring new hope, DHHS Pub. No (ADM): 86-1491, 1986.

101. Schligen B, Tolle R: Partial sleep deprivation as therapy for depression, *Arch Gen Psychiatry* 37:267-271, 1980.

102. Shaffer D, Garland A, Gould M, et al: Preventing teenage suicide, *J Am Acad Child Adolesc Psychiatry* 27:675-687, 1988.

103. Shaffer D, Vieland V, Garland A, et al: Adolescent suicide attempters: response to suicide-prevention programs, *JAMA* 264:3151-3155, 1990.

104. Shaw BF: Cognitive-behavior therapies for major depression: current status with an emphasis on prophylaxis, Psychiatr J Univ Ott 14:403-408, 1989.

105. Shea MT, Elkin I, Hirschfeld RMA: Psychotherapeutic treatment of depression. In Frances AJ, Hales RE, editors: *Review of psychiatry,* vol 7, Washington, DC, 1988, American Psychiatric Press.

106. Sifneos PE: Short-term anxiety-provoking psychotherapy: its history, technique, outcome and instruction. In Budman S, editor: *Forms of brief therapy,* New York, 1981, Guilford Press.

107. Spiker DG, Perel JM, Hanin I, et al: The pharmacological treatment of delusional depression, Part II, *J Clin Psychopharmacol* 6:339-342, 1986.

108. Stoudemire A, Frank R, Hedemark N: The economic burden of depression, *Gen Hosp Psychiatry* 8:387-394, 1986.

109. Task Force on the use of laboratory tests in psychiatry: tricyclic antidepressants, blood level measurements and clinical outcome, *Am J Psychiatry* 142:155-162, 1985.

110. Traskman L, Asberg M, Berilsson L, et al: Monoamine metabolites in CSF and suicidal behavior, *Arch Gen Psychiatry* 38:631-636, 1981.

111. US Preventive Services Task Force: *Guide to clinical preventive services: screening for depression,* 173-175. Prepublication Copy, 1989.

112. US Preventive Services Task Force: *Guide to clinical preventive services: screening for suicidal intent,* 176-178, Prepublication, 1989.

113. Valente SM: Adolescent suicide: assessment and intervention, *J Child Adolesc Psychiatr Ment Health Nurs* 2:34-39, 1989.

114. Weissman MM: Advances in psychiatric epidemiology: rates and risks for depression, *Am J Public Health* 77:445-451, 1987.

115. Weissman MM, Merikangas KR, Boyd JH: Epidemiology of affective disorders. In Michaels R, Cavenar JO, Brodie HKH, et al, editors: *Psychiatry,* Philadelphia, 1986, JB Lippincott.

116. Wells KB, Stewart A, Hays RD, et al: The functioning and well-being of depressed patients: results from the Medical Outcomes Study, *JAMA* 262:914-919, 1989.

117. Winokur G, Behar D, Van Valkenburg C, et al: Is a familial definition of depression both feasible and valid? *J Nerv Ment Dis* 166:764-768, 1978.

118. Winokur G, Tsuang MT, Crowe RR: The Iowa 500: affective disorder in the relatives of manic and depressed patients, *Am J Psychiatry* 139:209-212, 1982.

119. Wise TN, Berlin R: Involuntary hospitalization: an issue for the consultation-liaison psychiatrist, *Gen Hosp Psychiatry* 9:40-44, 1987.

120. Zung WWK, King RE: Identification and treatment of masked depression in a general medical practice, *J Clin Psychiatry* 44:365-368, 1983.

121. Zung WWK, Magill M, Moore JT, et al: Recognition and treatment of depression in a family medicine practice, *J Clin Psychiatry* 4:3-6, 1983.

■ **RESOURCES** ■

The National Foundation for Depressive Illness, PO Box 2257, 245 7th Avenue, New York City, NY 10611, 1-800-248-4344.

Depression Awareness, Recognition and Treatment (DART) Program, The National Institute of Mental Health, 5600 Fishers Lane, Rockville, MD 20857.

The National Mental Health Association, 1021 Prince Street, Alexandria, VA 22314.

The National Depressive and Manic-Depressive Association, 53 W. Jackson Boulevard #618, Chicago IL 60654.

The National Alliance for the Mentally Ill, 2101 Wilson Boulevard, Suite 302, Arlington, WV 22201.

American Association of Suicidology, 2459 South Avenue, Denver, CO 80222.

Chapter 11

LIFE'S RHYTHMS

Enrico G. Camara

CHRONOPSYCHOLOGY

Human physical and mental processes vary greatly according to circadian (circa = around; dian = day) rhythms and other temporal cycles. *Chronopsychology* is the term used for the study of the effects of biologic rhythms on physical, cognitive, and emotional behavior.

A study of circadian rhythms requires frequent and regular sampling of different physiologic and biochemical variables over a 24-hour period. Such measurements indicate that most of these variables are not constant over the 24 hours but rather show a rhythmic change. Fig. 11-1 shows the normal circadian rhythms in a few variables. These rhythms persist even in environments where most external rhythmic cues are removed, indicating the existence of an internal body clock. Experiments in individuals studied in time-free environments show that our rhythms run in a cycle closer to 25 rather than 24 hours.[26]

In a normal environment, circadian rhythms are synchronized to a period of 24 hours by external rhythmic changes known as *zeitgebers*. In many animals and plants the alternation of light and dark synchronizes the internal clock to the 24-hour day. For humans, personal relationships and social demands or tasks (so-called social zeitgebers) are important in entraining our biologic rhythms.[13]

Circadian organization is an important phenomenon that serves to prime physiologic functions for imminent use and to switch off processes no longer required. Thus interdependent physiologic events and metabolic processes can be coordinated while incompatible processes are separated in time. This function has been termed *predictive homeostasis,* an organization of internal events attuned to environmental cues.[25] Thus a circadian system enables the body to prepare for waking—by increasing blood pressure, plasma adrenaline, and body temperature toward the end of the sleep period—and to prepare for sleep—by enabling us to "quiet down" in the evening.

Circadian rhythms not only help maintain physiologic functions but also allow incorporation of information about the environment. For example, our nocturnal inhibition of diuresis and micturition parallels our sleep-wake cycle, which parallels the environmental light-dark cycle. This incorporation helps us to not have our sleep disturbed by the need to urinate. Thus the anticipation of environmental events that have a regular 24-hour cycle enables animals to predict when regularly recurring daily events will occur and to initiate appropriate behavioral and physiologic responses sufficiently before the event to achieve an optimal response with a minimal time lag.

As mentioned earlier, human beings have a free-running period (rhythmicity in the absence of environmental cues) of approximately 25 hours in comparison with the earth day of 24 hours. If our circadian pacemakers were not reset, the timing of their endogenous rhythms would "lose" about 1 hour with respect to clock time each day. In subjects who are synchronized to a 24-hour day and then allowed to "free-run" in an environment free of time cues, sleep periods tend to get progressively later by about 1 hour each day.

The problem of Monday morning hangover (the "Monday morning blues") may be related to the tendency to free-run during the weekend. During weekends, one may go to bed progressively later and wake up later each day. On Monday morning, however, one has to wake up much earlier in relationship to subjective body time. Generally, by the end of the week the circadian system has had time to reentrain, and getting up earlier in the morning is easier.

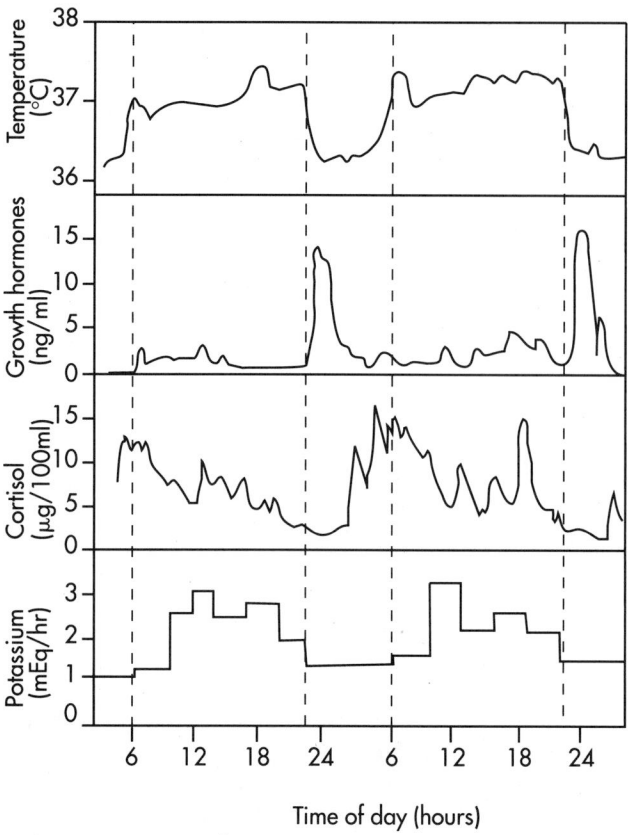

Fig. 11-1. Circadian rhythms in body temperature, plasma concentration of growth hormone and of plasma cortisol, and urinary excretion of potassium measured over 48 hours in a normal human subject.

OUR INTERNAL CLOCKS

That circadian rhythms are endogenous to the organism suggests the presence of identifiable anatomic correlates (i.e., "biologic clocks"). The suprachiasmatic nuclei of the hypothalamus (SNH) appears to be the chief coordinator of circadian rhythms.[31] Human beings have two major circadian pacemaking systems: body-temperature driving (X pacemaker) and rest-activity cycle driving (Y pacemaker); it is unclear if the SNH contains both or only one pacemaker (rest-activity).[26]

PHASE SHIFTING

A major conceptual advance in chronopsychology is the discovery that circadian systems can be phase-delayed (a transient lengthening of the cycle) or phase-advanced (a transient shortening of the cycle).[28] Phase resetting or shifting can occur with light pulses or with chemical agents such as methylxanthines, including theophylline and caffeine.[14] Light can induce a phase delay, a phase advance, or no phase shift at all, depending on when an animal is exposed to light in its subjective night or day. The largest phase delays occur in early subjective night, when a diurnal animal has just gone to sleep or a nocturnal ani-

mal has just woken up, and the largest phase advances occur in late subjective night. The circadian system is relatively unresponsive to light during the subjective day.

JET LAG

In humans the maximal phase delay and phase advance that can be obtained is approximately 2 hours.[26] Synchronization to the 24-hour period of the earth's rotation, however, allows in any one cycle a phase advance with respect to environmental time of only an additional half hour, while permitting a phase delay of 2.5 hours. Thus adaptation for most people is more rapid after westbound travel (requiring a phase delay) than after eastbound travel (requiring a phase advance). The experience of "jet lag" results when, in the process of readjustment, the endogenous circadian rhythms in sleep, alertness, gastrointestinal function, and mood are not synchronized with the new time zone, leading to the symptoms of malaise and fatigue.[3] Clearly these problems are in some way due to the slow adjustment to the new time zone of the internal clock and the dissociation between the clock and the new environment. Adjustment of the internal clock is brought about by zeitgebers in the new time zone and occurs after several days.

One can use various strategies to minimize the discomforts of jet lag.[23] For short stays adjustment cannot occur; however, it may be helpful to take a nap as soon as possible after the journey to make up for any loss of sleep. Scheduling meetings, when possible, to coincide with daytime in the old time zone is advisable. For longer stays, it is advisable to try to adjust circadian rhythms as rapidly as possible to the new time zone. One approach is to use the zeitgebers in the new time zone: scheduling sleep, activity, and meals in phase with the new local time; exposing oneself to social contacts; and exposing oneself to outdoors in the new time zone to achieve the natural light/dark cycle of the area. Others have advocated dietary measures to minimize jet lag.[16] High-protein breakfasts and lunches are recommended, as arousal is mediated by adrenergic mechanisms that are promoted by high-protein intake. High-carbohydrate suppers help stimulate sleep, which is mediated by serotonergic mechanisms promoted by high-carbohydrate diets.

The use of hypnotics or stimulants to prevent or treat jet lag has not been adequately investigated. Theoretically, one can use these agents at appropriate times in the new time zone. The administration of melatonin at a suitable time (i.e., just before bedtime on the new local time) has been reported to reduce the severity of symptoms of jet lag.[2] The mechanism by which the effect is produced is not known.

CIRCADIAN RHYTHMS AND MOOD DISORDERS

Circadian rhythmicity has many other implications for clinical and preventive medicine. Disorders of circadian timekeeping may underlie or be a result of a number of important diseases. This chapter focuses on circadian aspects of mood and cognitive disorders.

Affective disorders are those psychiatric disorders in which the primary disturbance is of affect or mood. They include states of depression, mania, and hypomania. Clinical depression is a large and heterogenous entity that may affect 10% of the female population and 5% of the male population.[12]

Disruption of biologic rhythms appears to be a major occurrence in patients with depression and related affective disorders. Affective disorders are episodic illnesses, (i.e., anyone who suffers one episode of depression or mania is likely to experience another). Periodicity characterizes the course of some manic-depressive patients.[15] Some patients regularly become depressed at the same time of year. General practitioners and outpatient and inpatient psychiatric services have reported depression associated with seasonal rhythms. Suicides appear to have a spring peak and a smaller peak in the fall.[33] There is circadian variation in the severity of depression; typically, depressed patients feel worse in the morning, whereas hypomanic patients feel worse in the evening.

The following observations in depressed patients point to a phase-advance of their circadian system[17]: the occurrence of early morning awakening, the consistently phase-advanced rhythm of rapid-eye-movement (REM) sleep, and the shifting to earlier times of body-temperature rhythms and a variety of neuroendocrine rhythms. Work at the National Institute of Mental Health (NIMH) has shown that in some manic-depressive patients, the phase of the rhythms of sleeping and waking and of body temperature were advanced during the patients' depressive periods and delayed during their hypomanic periods.[36]

Many antidepressant treatments alter the circadian rhythms of motor activity or neuroreceptor number; the mechanism of this action is unknown.[37] In animals a phase delay of these rhythms has been reported after chronic treatment with antidepressant drugs. Lithium salts, which are often effective in the treatment of depressive symptoms, have been reported to lengthen the period of the body-temperature rhythm markedly in healthy subjects, which results in a phase delay.[18] It has been proposed that antidepressant drugs act primarily to reverse the phase advance of circadian rhythms, which may be characteristic of depression.

SEASONAL AFFECTIVE DISORDER

A syndrome of annually recurring clinical depressions, which occurs in the late fall and winter within the temperate zone, was identified in the early 1980s and has been termed seasonal affective disorder (SAD).[30] Mean age of onset of this disorder is the early 20s. Women are affected at least four times more often than men. Onset of depressive symptoms is typically after the autumn equinox. The most difficult months are January and February, and spontaneous remissions typically occur after the spring equinox

during March and April. Common symptoms include sadness, anxiety, irritability, and decreased energy and libido. In addition, SAD is marked by prominent atypical vegetative changes that include fatigue, hypersomnia, increased appetite (especially for carbohydrates), and weight gain. It has been estimated that up to 10% to 15% of the population in the northern latitudes have SAD and that two to three times that number may have a subsyndromal form.[19] Light therapy of 2500 to 10000 lux intensity has been convincingly demonstrated to be clinically effective.[4]

The photoperiod is the interval between the first and last exposure to light each day. Because the duration of the photoperiod is the trigger to much seasonal behavior in the animal kingdom,[1] it was reasonable to propose that winter depression is a photoperiodic phenomenon, whose onset is triggered by the shortening of the photoperiod in autumn, and whose spontaneous recovery occurs due to the lengthening of the photoperiod in spring. In support of this hypothesis are the observations that winter depression peaks in December and that a trip to brighter climates results in a temporary loss of symptoms. The treatment of SAD with artificial light was designed on this basis, but it has since been shown that light therapy probably does not act through photoperiodic mechanisms.[7]

It has been proposed that the circadian rhythms of most patients with SAD are abnormally phase delayed.[21] This hypothesis predicts that these patients respond preferentially to morning light, which would provide a corrective phase advance. Consistent with this hypothesis, some investigators have shown that the onset of melatonin secretion occurs about 90 minutes later in these patients than in controls.[21] Other investigators, however, have not been able to replicate these findings.[7] Several studies demonstrate superior efficacy of morning light compared to evening light.[34] Other reports suggest that bright evening light can be effective for SAD patients, and the possibility of a second antidepressant "energizing" effect of light in addition to phase-shifting has been proposed.[32] At this point, the underlying etiology of SAD and the mechanism of action of light therapy is still unknown.

LIGHT THERAPY

There is broad agreement about the phase-shifting effects of light in humans: Morning light phase advances (shifts to an earlier time) the endogenous circadian pacemaker and its driven rhythms; evening light phase delays (shifts to a later time) the clock. Clinical applications of these effects are now being studied. Light therapy was effective in initial trials for patients with delayed sleep phase syndrome (DSPS) who have chronic inability to fall asleep and wake up at conventional clock time with consequent morning sleepiness and job-related difficulties.[29] Bright light during the night has been shown to improve substantially nighttime alertness and performance and may be useful for night shift workers.[6] In line with the phase advance hypothesis of nonseasonal depression, bright light appears to be effective for some of these patients, although they do not respond as well as do SAD patients.[20] Some patients with premenstrual depressive symptoms show evidence of phase-advanced circadian rhythms and respond to bright evening light.[27]

Light therapy is administered with bright fluorescent tubes of 2500 to 10,000 lux intensity in a box with a reflector and protected by a plastic diffusing screen. The antidepressant response usually occurs within 3 to 4 days of treatment, with a similar time course for relapse during withdrawal. Subjects are instructed to face the light apparatus, but not to look into it. Antidepressant response to 30 minutes of 10,000 lux light treatment has been high, with about 80% of subjects showing clinical remission within about 1 week of treatment, a rate comparable to most prior 2500 lux/2-hour studies.[35]

SHIFT WORK

Knowledge of circadian rhythms and their disruptions can also be helpful in public and occupational health, especially in the area of shift work. It is estimated that 25% of the working population rotates between day and night shifts.[9] Industries and service occupations that require night work abound and include nuclear power plant operators, factory workers, computer users, airline personnel, police, military personnel, doctors, nurses, and other health care professionals. Serious health consequences are becoming apparent in this population. Over 80% of shift workers have serious sleep disruption (insomnia at home and sleepiness at work), and there is evidence for increased levels of cardiovascular risk factors and gastrointestinal disorders among shift workers.[8] Sleepiness on the night shift is common and can cause accidents. Examples of night shift catastrophes include those at Three Mile Island, Chernobyl, and the Union Carbide plant in India.

Fatigue during night work is not unexpected, as people are expected to work at the lowest point of their circadian rhythms in mood, performance, adrenaline level, and deep body temperature. Fatigue also results from cumulative loss of sleep, as daytime sleep is being attempted when body temperature and the sympathetic nervous system are preparing the body for a new spell of activity. Every time a worker's shift changes, another change of routine occurs, with temporary mismatching between that routine and the internal clock. These workers also will be exposed to conflicting social zeitgebers because of pressure from family and friends to adjust to a "normal" existence. Most night workers revert to sleeping during conventional hours on days off. Thus the internal circadian rhythms of these workers rarely shift completely to match the work and sleep schedule of the night shift. Unlike jet lag, "shift lag" is a more permanent affliction. Although the problems of shift workers have been extensively documented, relatively few interventions have been developed based on circadian rhythm principles.

Certain people should avoid or be cautious about pursuing night work.[22] Epileptics are susceptible to seizures when fatigued and so cumulative sleep loss should be avoided. Asthmatics may have problems because bronchial sensitivity is greatest overnight, and allergic reactions to house dust and other allergens are at their peak. A person with diabetes should be advised against shift work in general because the insulin regimen will be difficult to judge accurately with irregular mealtimes. The elderly should also be aware that aging is associated with a decreased tolerance to shift work.

If one is required to perform shift work rotation, the sequence morning shift, evening shift, night shift is preferable to that of evening shift, morning shift, night shift[8] because the internal clock adjusts better to hours of work becoming later than earlier. This rationale also explains why adjustment to a westward-time zone is more rapid than to an eastward journey. Another general rule is that days off should be taken after night work so that any cumulative sleep loss can be made up before other shifts are worked.

When sleep/wake schedules are altered, performance falls to below normal. Performance tends to parallel changes in body temperature or plasma adrenaline (which are at a low at night). Decrements of performance at night of about 5% to 15% of the 24-hour mean are found in many types of tests.[24] Cumulative sleep loss also will produce further decrements in performance. Subjects who have lost sleep also are more likely to experience times when performance at a particular task is temporarily suspended while they appear to take a minisleep. Performance further deteriorates, with increasing time spent at repetitive tasks and those requiring vigilance suffering most.[5] This factor may be important when considering effects on workers who perform 12-hour shifts.

Short sleeps or naps can considerably ameliorate the performance decrements that can arise from a combination of prolonged hours, working during the circadian trough, and cumulative sleep loss. It is important to remember, however, that performance might be poorer immediately after waking from a nap, but this temporary decrement is usually over by about 12 minutes after waking.[10]

The model for an "ideal" night worker has been described by Minors and Waterhouse.[23] This worker will accept the changes in life-style that are involved and attempt to make use of the advantages it offers rather than be bothered by the disadvantages. This requires a dedication to work rather than conventional social life. The worker also should have a regular life-style with regard to times of sleep, mealtimes, and times for chores such as shopping and appointments. Such regularity will help to stabilize circadian rhythms to a 24-hour period.

Our knowledge of circadian rhythms and the effects of bright light may also be useful in helping the night-shift worker adapt. For a truly motivated person working in a supportive environment, adjustment can be accomplished by gradually delaying the sleep-wake (S-W) schedule by about 2 hours/day, starting several days before the first night shift. Using bright light (2500 to 10,000 lux) before bedtime, with the room dark during sleep, and exposing one's self only to dim light after waking will help the circadian rhythms to entrain to this schedule. Unfortunately, compliance to such an unusual sleep schedule is difficult.

Changing from the day to the night shift requires a typical shift worker to abruptly shift sleep time by about 12 hours after the first night of work. Eastman[11] has reported using bright light to facilitate such a shift. The easiest approach is to use bright light before sleep (to phase delay) and to apply the light later and later each day to gently "nudge" the oscillator along. Bedrooms need to be dark for sleeping and dim light exposure after awakening is assured through the use of dark welders' goggles whenever workers need to go outside during daylight hours. Such a technique can produce faster shifts than those expected from previously reported approaches. However, more research is needed to refine this method before it can be confidently and routinely recommended to shift workers.

It is ironic that the work schedules followed by members of the health professions (house officers, nurses, technical personnel, etc) are among the most disruptive for the circadian S-W cycle. It is time to address the problems of these disruptions, as medical personnel often handle life and death situations. In addition, the hospital environment needs to be redesigned to incorporate elements of normal temporal structure. Clearly, the goal should be to translate into good clinical practice the rapid strides made in understanding the pathophysiology of the circadian system.

REFERENCES

1. Arendt J: Role of the pineal gland and melatonin in seasonal reproductive function in mammals, *Oxf Rev Reprod Biol* 8:266-320, 1986.
2. Arendt J, Aldhous M, Marks V: Alleviation of jet lag by melatonin: preliminary results of controlled double blind trial, *Br Med J* 292:1170, 1986.
3. Arendt J, Marks V: Physiological changes underlying jet lag, *Br Med J* 284:144-146, 1982.
4. Blehar ML, Lewy AJ: Seasonal mood disorder: consensus and controversy, *Psychopharmacol Bull* 26:465-494, 1990.
5. Borland RG, et al: Performance overnight in shift workers operating a day-night schedule, *Aviat Space Environ Med* 57:241-249, 1986.
6. Campbell SS, Dawson D: Enhancement of nighttime alertness and performance with bright ambient light, *Physiol Behav* 48:317-320, 1990.
7. Checkley S: The relationship between biological rhythm and the affective disorders. In Arendt J, Minors DS, Waterhouse JM, editors: *Biological rhythms in clinical practice,* London, 1989, Boston: Wright.
8. Czeisler CA, Moore-Ede MC, Coleman RM: Rotating shift work schedules that disrupt sleep are improved by applying circadian principles, *Science* 217:460-463, 1982.
9. Danchik KM, Schoenborn CA, Elinson J Jr, editors: Basic data from wave 1 of the national survey of personal health practices and consequences: United States, 1979. Public Health Service: Hyattsville, MD, 1981. (DHHS publication no. (PHS) 81-1162).
10. Dinges DF et al: Performances after naps in sleep-conducive and alerting environments. In Johnson LC, et al, editors: *Biological rhythms, sleep and shiftwork,* Lancaster, 1981, MTP press.
11. Eastman CI: Squashing versus nudging circadian rhythms with artificial bright light: solutions for shift work? *Perspect Biol Med* 34:181-195, 1991.
12. *Economic Fact Book for Psychiatry.* Compiled by the Office of Economic Affairs, American Psychiatric Association, Washington, DC, 1987, American Psychiatric Press.
13. Ehlers CL, Frank E, Kupfer DJ: Social zeitgebers and biological rhythms, *Arch Gen Psychiatry* 45:948-952, 1988.
14. Ehret CF, Potter VR, Dobra KW: Chronotypic action of theophylline and of pentobarbital as circadian zeitgebers in the rat, *Science* 215:1407-1409, 1982.
15. Goodman FK, Jamison KA: The natural course of manic depressive illness. In Post RM, Ballenger JC, editors: *Neurobiology of mood disorders,* Baltimore, 1984, Wilkins & Wilkins.
16. Graeber RC, Sing HC, Cuthbert BN: The impact of transmeridian flight on deploying soldiers. In Johnson LC et al, eds: *Biological rhythms, sleep and shift work,* Lancaster, 1981, MTP Press.
17. Healy D: Rhythm and blues. Neurochemical, neuropharmacological and neuropsychological implications of a hypothesis of circadian rhythm dysfunction in the affective disorders, *Psychopharmacology* 93:271-295, 1987.
18. Johnson A, et al: Effect of lithium carbonate on circadian periodicity in humans, *Pharmakopsychiatr Neuropsychopharmakol* 12:423-425, 1979.
19. Kasper S, et al: Epidemiological findings of seasonal changes in mood and behaviour, *Arch Gen Psychiatry* 46:823-833, 1989.
20. Kripke DF, et al: Phototherapy for nonseasonal major depressive disorders. In Rosenthal NE, Blehar MC, editors: *Seasonal affective disorder and phototherapy,* NY, 1989, Guilford Press.
21. Lewy AJ, et al: Antidepressant and circadian phase-shifting effects of light, *Science* 235:352-354, 1987.
22. Minors DS, Scott AR, Waterhouse JM: Circadian arrythmia: shift-work, travel and health, *J Soc Occup Med* 36:39-44, 1986.
23. Minors DS, Waterhouse JM: Circadian rhythm in general practice and occupational health. In Arendt J, Minors DS, Waterhouse JM, editors: *Biological rhythms in clinical practice,* London, 1989, Boston: Wright.
24. Monk TH: The arousal model of time of day effects in human performance efficiency, *Chronobiologia* 9:49-54, 1982.
25. Moore-Ede MC: Physiology of the circadian timing system: predictive versus reactive homeostasis, *Am J Physiol* 250:R735-752, 1986.
26. Moore-Ede MC, Czeisler CA, Richardson GS: Circadian timekeeping in health and disease. Part 1. Basic properties of circadian pacemaker, *N Engl J Med* 309:469-476, 1983.
27. Perry BL, et al: Morning vs evening bright light treatment of late luteal phase dysphoric disorder, *Am J Psychiatry* 146:1215-1217, 1989.
28. Pittendrigh CS: Circadian rhythms and the circadian organization of living systems, *Cold Spring Harb Symp Quant Biol* 25:159-182, 1960.
29. Rosenthal NE, Joseph-Vanderpool JR, Levendosky AA: Phase shifting effects of bright morning light as treatment for delayed sleep phase syndrome, *Sleep* 13:354-361, 1990.
30. Rosenthal NE, et al: Seasonal affective disorder. A description of the syndrome and preliminary findings with light therapy, *Arch Gen Psychiatry* 41:72-80, 1984.
31. Rusak B, Zucker I: Neuronal regulation of circadian rhythms, *Physiol Rev* 59:449-526, 1979.
32. Sack R, et al: Morning vs evening light treatment for winter depression. Evidence that the therapeutic effects of light are mediated by circadian phase shifts, *Arch Gen Psychiatry* 47:343-351, 1990.
33. Souetre E, et al: Seasonality of suicides, *J Affect Disord* 13:215-225, 1987.

34. Terman M: On the question of mechanism in phototherapy for seasonal affective disorder: consideration of clinical efficacy and epidemiology, *J Biol Rhythms* 3:155-172, 1988.

35. Terman M, et al: Light therapy for seasonal affective disorder: a review of efficacy, Neuropsychopharmacology 2:1-33, 1989.

36. Wehr TA et al: Phase advance of the circadian sleep-wake cycle as an antidepressant, *Science* 206:710-713, 1979.

37. Wirz-Justice A: Circadian rhythms in mammalian neurotransmitter receptors, *Prog Neurobiol* 29:219-259, 1987.

RESOURCES

Society for Light Treatment and Biological Rhythms, P.O. Box 478, Wilsonville, OR 97070.

Association of Professional Sleep Societies, 1610 14th Street, N.W., Suite 300, Rochester, MN 55901.

Laboratory for Cicardian Medicine, Brigham and Women's Hospital, 221 Longwood Avenue, Boston, MA 02115.

Institute of Chronobiology, New York Hospital, 21 Bloomingdale Road, White Plains, NY 10605.

Chapter 12

STRESSES OF LIVING

Michael G. McKee

THE PROBLEM
Frequency, nature, and cost of stress problems

The pervasiveness of stress as a cause of illness[12,16] is summarized by Pelletier and Lutz[45] as follows: "Stress is widely recognized by health professionals, public policy makers, and corporate medical planners as a significant health factor. It is estimated that 60% to 90% of visits to health care professionals are for stress-related disorders." The effects of stress have been determined through research to be a significant contributor to many clinically defined illnesses, including hypertension, head and back pain, cardiovascular disease, immune disorders, gastrointestinal disorders, anxiety and depressive disorders, and eating disorders, as well as to injuries, violence, and suicide.[43,44]

Stress affects mental health as well as physical health according to *Healthy People 2000*,[56] a report of the U.S. Department of Health and Human Services: "The effects of stress are most commonly described as nervousness, tension, anger, irritation, depression, anxiety, and an inability to cope, as well as physical symptoms that include headache, muscle ache or tension, stomach ache or tension, and fatigue."[43] Addictions such as cigarettes and alcohol, and impaired performance as illustrated in lowered work productivity and higher absenteeism are also effected by stress.[35,50] Pelletier and Lutz[45] estimate that stress disorders cost business a minimum of $150 billion a year because of decreased productivity, absenteeism, and disability.

One study found that psychologic problems represented the most frequent health care requests.[23] The majority of adults in the United States report that they have emotional problems during a given year, yet fully 50% of them say that the problems they experience cannot be solved and one third feel helpless to make difficulties more tolerable. Although psychologic problems are the most frequent problems presented in health care settings, the majority of people still do not seek professional help. When they do reach out to a professional, physicians are frequently consulted.[56] However, the statement about stress may be masked, as in the presentation of stress-related symptoms without a description of the stress or with denial of the stress. Physicians are increasingly called on to learn how to decode the messages about stress and to recognize stress-related symptoms however they are presented, while they are also coping with all the pressures and demands of maintaining an ongoing practice. Almost none of these physicians will have received formal education in stress; Nathan's study reports that only one American medical school requires a course on stress.[38]

Because of these data, the *Healthy People 2000* report lists (among others) the following objectives to prevent and treat mental and behavioral disorders related to stress:

- Reduce to less than 35% the proportion of people age 18 and older who experienced adverse health effects from stress within the past year (baseline: 42.6% in 1985).
- Increase to at least 20% the proportion of people age 18 and older who seek help in coping with personal and emotional problems (baseline: 11.1% in 1985).
- Decrease to no more than 5% the proportion of people age 18 and older who report experiencing significant levels of stress, but who do not take steps to reduce or control their stress (baseline: 21% in 1985).
- Increase to at least 40% the proportion of work sites employing 50 or more people that provide programs to reduce employee stress (baseline: 26.6% in 1985).
- Establish mutual help clearinghouses in at least 25 states (baseline: 9 states in 1989).
- Increase to at least 50% the proportion of primary care providers who routinely review with patients their patients' cognitive, emotional, and behavioral

functioning and the resources available to deal with any problems that are identified (baseline data available in 1992).

- Increase to at least 75% the proportion of providers of primary care for children who include assessment of cognitive, emotional, and parent-child functioning, with appropriate counseling, referral, and follow-up, in their clinical practices (baseline data available in 1992).[56]

The *Healthy People 2000* report, issued in 1990,[56] may underestimate the stress problem. The 1991 study commissioned by Northwestern National Life Insurance Company, *Employee Burnout: Americas Newest Epidemic,*[39] found that 70% of workers said that job stress caused them frequent health problems and made them less productive. This finding was true across job levels nationwide, even though this study asked only about the effect of job stress, omitting any reference to the host of stressors encountered outside the job setting. Clearly, anything that reduces or prevents stress disorders helps the health of most Americans.

DEFINITION: WHAT STRESS IS
Stress reactions

Just defining stress is stressful. The term is used popularly in at least three major ways: (1) stressors, events that one experiences as stressful; (2) stress reactions, with particular emphasis on the physiologic responses detailed by Cannon[10] and Selye[51]; and (3) further consequences of stress reactions, with impairment of mental or physical functioning or performance. The common sense view of stress implies that stressful events lead rather inevitably to stress reactions and further consequences (i.e., that the relationship is linear); however, data suggest that the stress system is more complex than this. Much of stress is transactional, with perception and cognition playing major roles in the definition of an event as stressful. A given event becomes a stressor when it is perceived and defined as a threat, and except for a few universal stressors such as starvation or exposure to extreme cold, most stressors appear to exist in the eye of the beholder. Lazarus and Folkman[31] define psychologic stress as "a particular relationship between the person and the environment that is appraised by the person as taxing or exceeding his or her resources and endangering his or her well-being." Once an event is defined as stressful and reacted to as such, the result is not a linear sequence but a homeostatic network with reverberating feedback loops involving the central nervous system, the autonomic nervous system, the endocrine system, and the immune system.

Cannon[10] identified the *sympathoid-adrenal apparatus,* now conceptualized as the sympatho-adrenal-medullary axis, the response system needed for emergency reactions. An organism that does not face emergencies evidently does not need this mechanism. In the presence of emergencies, this network operates to maintain homeostasis. Multiple effects of the sympathetic stress reaction include increased cardiac output, increased stroke volume and systolic blood pressure, increased blood flow in skeletal muscles, increased muscle strength and muscle glycogenolysis, decreased blood flow to the skin, increased palmar sweating, slowed digestive processes, increased blood coagulation ability, release of sugar from the liver, and increased blood glucose concentration.[2]

The action of the sympathetic nervous system influences the physiology of emotion in many ways reflected in daily language. When people speak of "their hearts racing," "shaking with fear," "breaking out in a cold sweat," or "choking," they are describing sympathetic nervous system activity, which also includes tense muscles in the neck and upper back, bracing with the shoulders raised, an accelerated heart rate, dilated pupils, constricted throat, shallow respiration, cool hands, rigid pelvis and tight anus, inhibited extensor muscles and contracted flexors, and a locked diaphragm. These characteristics of excessive activity in the sympathetic nervous system, consistent with the name of the "fight-or-flight response," appear in similar form in animals and humans as a preparatory stage to running or fighting.

Selye[51] extended Cannon's concept of the "fight-or-flight response" to include two additional phases of stress response in an overall syndrome known as the *general adaptation syndrome*. The three stages in the syndrome are alarm, resistance, and exhaustion, with the first phase being similar to the fight-or-flight response, with marked emergency changes in endocrine and autonomic function.

Selye[51] focused on adrenocortical instead of sympathoadrenal-medullary changes and clearly conceptualized the stress response as leading to disease. During the second stage of the general adaptation syndrome, resistance, physiologic resources adapt in an effort to reestablish homeostasis. If the stress response continues, the stage of exhaustion follows, with premature aging caused by wear and tear. Selye's animal research clearly demonstrated that ulcers and hypertension, among other disorders, were produced by prolonged exposure to stressors in susceptible animals. The wear and tear process alone has been modified in explanations of psychosomatic disorders by Sternbach[52] to include the notion of response stereotype characterized by a particular idiosyncratic pattern of sympathetic response to stressful stimulation. It is as though the stress reaction were like a fingerprint, recognizable as such, but with clear-cut individual differences. When a person responds with a given pattern over and over and meets the second condition of a homeostatic weakness, a relative inability to return to resting level before another stressor is encountered, the given system (such as the gastrointestinal or cardiovascular system) is likely to suffer end organ damage secondary to chronic hyperarousal.

Asterita,[2] following the work of Wilson and Schneider,[60] describes four neurophysiologic pathways affected by stress in a way potentially contributing to disease. The first is the interneuronal stress response in which interference with normal functioning of neurotransmitter activity contributes to anxiety and depressive disorders. The second is the neurovascular stress response, which can contribute to hypertension and coronary artery disease, as well as lesser syndromes such as migraine headaches, primary Raynaud's disease, and severe menstrual cramps. The third is the neuromuscular stress response contributing to tension headaches, lower back pain, muscle spasms in various parts of the body, and fibrositis. The fourth is the neurohormonal stress response in which a variety of stress hormones are affected by chronic activation of the stress response, with elevated levels of adrenocorticotropic hormone (ACTH) and cortisol, epinephrine, and norepinephrine.

The stress disorders treated at the Cleveland Clinic fall into five main categories: psychophysiologic, emotional, interpersonal, performance problems, and bad habits related to stress. All are essentially disorders related to hyperarousal. Stress is a transaction that occurs when one perceives a threat in the environment based on a sensed mismatch of environmental demand and personal resources available to cope with it. One mobilizes in an emergency arousal because of this mismatch, with chronic overarousal contributing to these disorders.

Psychophysiologic. The more immediate physical symptoms of stress that lead to referrals to our applied psychophysiology and stress management program include gastrointestinal symptoms such as diarrhea, constipation, nausea, or vomiting; cardiovascular symptoms such as increased blood pressure or pounding or rapid heart rate; musculoskeletal symptoms such as tight and sore muscles; speech problems such as stuttering; respiratory symptoms such as shallow breathing or hyperventilation; peripheral vascular symptoms including cold hands and feet; dermatologic symptoms including itching, sweaty palms; and genitourinary problems such as urinary frequency or hesitancy. In reviewing referrals over the past several years to our program, we find that almost every department has referred patients thought to have symptoms primarily related to or secondarily exacerbated by stress. These problems include allergies; cardiologic problems such as changes in heart rhythm and coronary artery disease; dermatologic problems including alopecia and neurodermatitis; endocrinologic problems including diabetes; gastroenterologic problems including irritable bowel and ulcerative colitis; gynecologic problems such as infertility and severe menstrual cramps; hypertension; a variety of problems from internal medicine including particularly headaches; a range of autoimmune diseases; ophthalmologic problems including blepharospasm; otolaryngologic problems including stuttering and tinnitus; psychiatric problems such as anxiety disorders; pulmonary problems such as asthma; and pain problems from rheumatology. Surgical departments have referred patients for assistance in stress management before surgery and stress reduction during recovery.

Emotional. Emotional symptoms of stress that lead to referrals for stress management include various dimensions of fear and anger, such as panic and anxiety, irritability, hostility, and rage. Hyperarousal often causes motoric restlessness, hypervigilance, apprehensive expectation that something bad is about to happen, and autonomic overarousal in the sympathetic nervous system. One often feels pressured or harassed. With prolonged stress, self-esteem is usually lowered, with symptoms of depression including disturbed sleep and changes in eating patterns. Loss of initiative and interest in involvement with others, tearfulness, and feelings of being blue or sad also occur.

Interpersonal. In interpersonal disorders there is a disruption of social and family relationships, with tendencies to be either sad and withdrawn or irritable and difficult to get along with. Anger, as well as anxiety, is a common symptom of stress, and often the whole family is stressed by the anger, anxiety, depression of one stressed member.

Performance. Performance problems develop because prolonged stress tends to impair both mental and physical functioning, as does extreme acute stress. Increased difficulty focusing and concentrating, impairment of memory, a tendency toward increased confusion, such that one does less well on mental tasks are all characteristic. Physical symptoms include increased difficulty coordinating and loss of energy that reduces stamina. In general, the relationship between arousal and performance can be charted

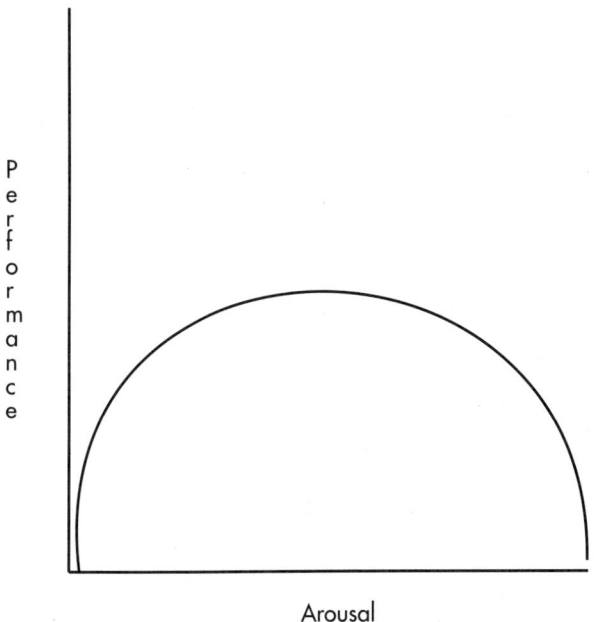

Fig. 12-1. Relationship between arousal and performance.

by an inverted U (∩), with too little arousal leading to low performance, and too high arousal leading to poor performance (Fig. 12-1). The acute stress response often initiates hyperarousal and the chronic stress hypoarousal.

Bad habits and addictive behaviors. Smoking, drinking alcohol, overusing caffeine, overusing tranquilizing medication, using street drugs, overeating, and sexual addictions are among the common habit problems that frequently develop in part as an effort to alleviate other stress symptoms. When one has symptoms in the other categories of stress reactions, the discomfort makes quick fixes very attractive, and addictions develop when one routinely turns to the quick fix for temporary respite from stress. The stress usually becomes greater as the problems contributing to the original stress responses are not dealt with, and as the habits themselves constitute additional problems.

Behavioral stress reactions of childhood. Sometimes children and teenagers don't come straight out and say they're unhappy. Instead they eat too much or too little, smoke dope every night or come home drunk, get pregnant, run away, drop out, or become a model adult with a waxen mask.

Behavior disorders are common stress reactions that usually constitute more stress in a vicious circle. Teachers, parents, and physicians are likely to encounter two major patterns: conduct disorder (known as behavior problem, antisocial disorder, aggressive personality, acting out, etc.) and anxiety/withdrawal disorder (known as personality disorder, overinhibited, neurotic, etc.).

Conduct disorder. Conduct disorder is characterized by behavior excesses (aggression, noncompliance, overactivity) and behavior deficits (in moral development, social skills, and learning abilities).[40] Children with conduct disorder may have failed to learn cultural norms of appropriate behavior or have learned less accepted norms (subculture). If adults can understand that these children generally are not trying to be bad but are trying to solve problems in a maladaptive way, they can be more patient. Conduct disorder seems to be common and may decrease with age. Most children have some behavior problems at times. The incidence is much more common in boys (ratios from 3:1 to 12:1), perhaps partly because school is a "feminine" environment.

Because conduct disorder is so annoying, it is noticed more often than anxiety or withdrawal. The basic behaviors are normal in children. Conduct disorder is determined when the behavior becomes maladaptive because it is excessively frequent, not age appropriate (e.g., temper tantrums are normal at age 3), excessive in quality (e.g., extreme physical aggression), inappropriate for setting (e.g., punching is okay in the boxing ring), or a combination of these. Without treatment, the prognosis is poor. Children do not outgrow conduct disorder, and more serious problems may develop as an adult.

Characteristics of these children elicit inappropriate responses from others, which in turn perpetuates acting out. Thus a vicious circle ensues. These children are difficult and frustrating to work with; in general they are not "likable" children.

Anxiety/withdrawal disorders. Anxiety disorders are characterized by behavioral deficits (too little interaction, little initiative, avoidant) and by behavioral excesses (fearful, nervous, tense). The child is self-conscious, seems to feel inferior, may appear sad or depressed, and is easily hurt. Anxiety/withdrawal disorder is probably as common as conduct disorder, but is less noticed. Because these children have less impact on others, they are likely to be ignored.

Anxiety/withdrawal disorder is diagnosed more in boys, although probably occurs more in girls, because it appears "abnormal" in boys. Again, basic behaviors are normal, but the child demonstrates an inability to play or work. The prognosis is probably poor, as this disorder is less studied. These children have great difficulty interacting with peers and adults. Their behavior may interfere with their ability to learn. They are generally more likable, but because they tend to be unresponsive, it is easy to "give up on them." Working with these children can be rewarding, as they often show dramatic improvement. It is easier to feel sympathetic toward them.

Burnout. One of the ironies of stress is that stress reactions themselves constitute a major source of stress, so that people in stress tend to spiral downward, often resulting in burnout.

Freudenberger[19] describes burnout as starting with an intense commitment to prove oneself, with the need to be of service leading to a denial and dismissal of one's own needs, followed by increased disengagement from others, and finally feelings of emptiness and depression. In the middle stages of burnout, one finds oneself fatigued and forgetful, working harder than ever, worrying more, sleeping badly, losing interest in sex, having vague physical complaints, increasingly cynical and isolated from others, and irritable and tense. Burnout tends to happen to the best and the brightest. If one does not care to begin with, the personal commitment, dedication, caring, and giving that ultimately lead to burnout is unlikely.

Individual, work group, and organization factors all contribute to burnout. The individual who is perfectionistic, who relates self-worth to achievement, who has difficulty saying no, and who tends to keep all feelings inside and to isolate oneself from others is at higher risk for burnout. So too is the worker whose workplace is characterized by excessive demands, competitiveness rather than cooperativeness, and punishment rather than reward. An organization that does not provide an opportunity for self-assessment and self-expression, and for stress reduction and problem-solving groups contributes to the development rather than the relief of burnout.

STRESSORS

This section reviews more common stressors in people's lives. Although stress is in the eye of the beholder, many people see through the same lenses. Some stressors seem to be primarily external (i.e., encountered), whereas others seem mainly internal (i.e., self-imposed).

External

Change. Many studies have documented that major life change is stressful for the average person. Holmes and Rahe[25] constructed a scale that assigns a value, which represents the amount of energy it takes to cope with any given change experienced during the past year. The most severe stressor on the scale is death of a spouse. Because both positive and negative events are stressful, getting married was set arbitrarily as the scale's mid-point. A life crisis can be defined as any change that requires one to modify important living patterns. Even going on a vacation temporarily disrupts normal patterns of living and in this sense constitutes a stressful demand. The more stress units one accumulates during a given year, the greater the likelihood of illness or injury in the next year.

What we often are unaware of is that we live in a time of major change. Toffler,[55] in *Future Shock,* describes the J curve of change, which characterizes much of life. He illustrates this with the speed of travel. If we asked how fast people could travel in a group in 6000 BC, the answer would be about 8 miles an hour in a camel caravan. By 1500 BC, 20 miles an hour in a horse-drawn chariot was possible. At the birth of Christ, it was still 20 miles an hour in a horse-drawn chariot. In 1800 one could travel 20 miles an hour in a horse-drawn chariot. It was 1880 before a steam locomotive could move at 100 miles an hour. But then the rate of change started to explode: Barely 50 years later a fighter plane would go 400 miles an hour; in the 1960s the SR-71 went 2000 miles an hour, and, a few years later a human being in space would go 18,000 miles an hour. For all of recorded history, very little had changed, and in a short period of time, the pace had exploded. The J curve also fits the explosion in the amount of available information and the pace of social change, such as the kind and amount of available street drugs. Although the world has always known horrors such as famine, pestilence, plague, war, and other forms of inhumanity, we have only recently lived with the accelerating pace of change that constitutes sort of a built-in daily dose of stress for most of us. Elkind[17] describes the "hurried child" who, like so many adults, feels there is no time for all that has to be done and feels the pressure of the "rat race."

For many of us, examining the changes that have occurred since our high school years is another way to illustrate the rate of change. Birth control pills, nuclear bombs, television, calculators, computers, fax machines, ballpoint pens, walkmen, cordless phones, car phones, jet planes,

polyester, street drugs (except in small amounts), high school sex (except for a few), step-families (in more than rare numbers), audiotape recorders, instantly developed pictures, long-playing records, compact discs, camcorders, VCRs, bypass surgery, health insurance, artificial organs, contact lenses, lasers, worldwide phone service, battery-powered watches, digital watches, satellites, space travel, microwave ovens, dishwashers, disposals, and self-cleaning ovens—none of these existed when I started high school! Toffler[55] would say that my mother, born in 1901, was born in the middle of history, that the world in which she was born is as different from the world of today as that world was from Julius Caesar's world.

The pace of change is so fast that it rips us apart from meaning. People are meaning makers and what threatens meaning threatens life itself, the rate of change perhaps being a significant contributor to a cruel statistic that has followed the J-curve—the incidence of childhood and adolescent suicide. Our coping mechanisms, both physiologic and psychologic, are surely tested by this exploding pace of change, these mechanisms having developed during all the centuries humankind lived on the horizontal part of the J and now needed as we climb the vertical.

It is ironic that even stress management programs constitute a source of stress in that they ask one to make major changes in patterns of thought and feeling and action. One of the reasons for failures in these programs is that people frequently have to undergo more stress before they achieve less, and this prospect is so threatening that they cannot change.

Work. A national survey, using a representative sample of people at all levels of the workplace hierarchy in different kinds of jobs in all geographic areas, found that 70% of people said that work stress alone resulted in frequent health problems and performance problems for them. One third said that they had seriously considered quitting their jobs in the previous year because of stress and another third said they expected to burn out in the near future. Forty-six percent found their jobs to be highly stressful.[39]

The most stressed employees were those who had too much work or too little control over their job. The combination of too much responsibility and too little authority appears almost to be a prescription for job stress. Erratic work schedules and too little work can also be stressful. Role ambiguity in which one is uncertain where responsibilities begin and end, is an additional source of job stress. A corporate culture in which loyalty is expected from the employee but not extended in return is also a significant source of stress. Uncertainty and insecurity in the workplace are an added source of stress, with rumors of takeovers increasing stress reactions and stress illnesses. Deadlines and the need to work fast are an additional stressor. Inadequate information, vague objectives, and inadequate or vague feedback about performance also increase stress

Table 12-1. Rotating, night shift, and 24-hour on-call workers' stress reactions

Physiologic[11]	Psychologic	Vocational and sociologic
Circadian rhythm disruption	Mood changes	Family responsibility and interactions disrupted
Insomnia	Absences	
Ulcers	Anger	Social interactions changed
Gastrointestinal disorders	Routine disruption	
	Confusion	Sexual patterns changed
	Compulsive eating and/or drinking	Community involvement altered
	Disruptions in planning	Performance decrement
	"Automatic pilot"	Greater job absences
		More injuries
		More tardiness
		Less job satisfaction and commitment

Table 12-2. Shift work and 24-hour emergency on-call stressors

Physiologic	Psychologic	Vocational and sociologic
Sleep interruption	Dealing with emergencies	Less interaction with peer group
Sleep deprivation	Dealing with emotionally upset people	Less interaction with family
Excessive fight-or-flight stress response	Apprehension: waiting for beeper to go off	"Living in different world—in a hardship post"
	Self-imposed pressure to "do it all" without complaint	Less time in office to do paper work

reactions among workers. Social isolation is stressful for most people.[29]

People and politics are always cited as major stressors in the workplace. Nonsupportive supervisors are a major source of stress cited by employees. The working environment, the physical conditions, and the ambiance are an additional source of job stress. Additionally, lack of opportunity for professional or personal advancement is stultifying and stressful.

American society is increasingly becoming an around-the-clock society, and stresses of shift work and on-call duty are a separate major category of job stress.[11] One analysis of the stressors, stress reactions, and stress moderators involved in shift and on-call work for personnel in an insurance company is presented in Tables 12-1 through 12-3.

Personal relationships. The great majority of people referred to us for stress-related disorders identify conflict with one or more family members as a major source of stress. Families appear to be more and more difficult to maintain.[8] Increasingly, both members in a marriage are on a career track, and increasingly children are growing up with both parents having demanding jobs in the work force.

The equation $I = 2^n - n - 1$ (with n equal to the number of family members and I representing the number of different groups that can interact) captures the number of different constellations of relationships within the family, including groups of various sizes. A marriage without children has only one relationship within the immediate family, and the adaptation required by marriage alone is a significant stressor. As the family grows to two children, there are 11 different constellations, child and child, parent and parent, four combinations of one parent and one child, two combinations of both parents and one child, two combinations of one parent and both children, and the whole family together; and just the complexity of the family becomes significantly stressful.

Most people have grown up with rules in their families that are unstated and often dysfunctional. Bringing different sets of rules into a family leads to clashes and/or repetition of past family problems. And increasingly, changing lives and changing times appear to be on a collision course. Families appear to be worse off economically than they were in the 1970s; the divorce rate has skyrocketed 700% since 1900. Families are responding to the economic crisis by working harder. Demographers project that half of all first marriages will end in divorce, and that about 60% of second marriages will end in divorce. Predictions are that 30% to 50% of all children born in the 1980s and 1990s will live in a stepfamily before they are 18.[15] Additionally, about 20% of children have only one parent, and 20% of children live in poverty. It is not that Americans seem to think that this is the way it should be. One study suggests that two thirds of Americans believe the family should sacrifice so that one parent can stay home to raise the children, but the trend continues the other way, with more than two thirds of all mothers in the work force and more than half of mothers of infants in the work force.

When you add a stepfamily to the equation, problems compound. Not only do the number of relationships go much higher, but every stepfamily is begun with a loss.[15] Step-parenthood does not seem to recreate the nuclear family, with studies suggesting that stepchildren are more like children in single parent families.

Although the constellation of the family and the per-

Table 12-3. Stress moderators

Physiologic	Psychologic	Vocational
Mastery of relaxation response	Positive attitude	Selection (e.g., "owl" or "lark"; spouse same shift)
Mastery of quieting reflex	Openness to discussing problems	Complete involvement in decision making about shift and on-call jobs
Good physical condition	Periodic opportunities to discuss stress	New performance evaluation criteria
	Sense of being one of elite group	Availability of exercise equipment
		Development of teams to cover office and on-call simultaneously
		Availability of space and training tapes to master control of physiologic reactivity
		If rotating shift, long duration and forward shift
		Job training to help develop attitude that beeper signals a challenge, not a threat
		Hardship pay
		Extra attention to communication to combat isolation

centage of women in the work force has changed greatly, the number of men who share the work at home has not increased as dramatically. If the ideal marriage for America now is sharing jointly in the workplace and at home, it hasn't happened; studies suggest that less than 25% of men help equally at home.

Americans seem confused about what they want in their families. The majority of adults think that those who have successful careers sacrifice too much family and personal life, but less than 25% prefer a marriage where, in the traditional style, the wife takes care of the home and children. Although they believe the traditional role for women wouldn't be personally satisfying, they tend to believe other families should pursue this life-style. The societal fabric that we have woven seems to be unraveling for American families. More and more men, and to a lesser extent women, tend to marry with a sense that if they don't like the marriage, if they are unhappy, they simply will divorce.

Difficult people. Difficult people come in all ages, all shapes, all sizes, and both sexes. They are angry and meek, blunt and indirect, too talkative and silent, blaming others and blaming themselves, hyperemotional and hyperrational. And on and on it goes. Difficult people exceed the normal boundaries. They have too much of this, too little of that. Davis et al.[13] described various agendas of people that can be very stressful for the physician. One of those agendas is that of a help-rejecting complainer who is always seeking assistance, but always finding it insufficient. Another is that of someone who presents as very fragile, as always seeking to be taken care of. Still another is the know-it-all stance, which makes it impossible for the physician to pass on any information.

Daily hassles. Daily hassles represent the other side of the stress picture, the opposite of enduring patterns or major life changes. Daily hassles are the small things that frustrate so many of us: the traffic light stuck on red, the driver who cuts in front of us or who goes too slowly in front of us, a child who isn't ready for school in the morning, the shoelace that breaks, the irritating phone call. When people's physiologic reactivity is monitored during the day, daily hassles tend to produce recurring fight-or-flight reactions.

Most of the people we see in consultation describe a day full of hassles, often secondary to their not having enough time for all of their activities. Interacting with children, spouses, and supervisors almost always produces some hassles in the course of the day, as does accomplishing all of the tasks, making the necessary purchases, running the necessary errands, and paying the bills.

Traumatic stresses. Traumatic stresses lead to posttraumatic stress disorder (PTSD). Children have been shown to be particularly vulnerable to PTSD.[46] According to DSM III-R[61] (the Diagnostic and Statistical Manual of the American Psychiatric Association),

> PTSD occurs when the individual has experienced an event that is outside the range of usual human experience and one that would be markedly distressing to almost anyone, e.g., serious threat to one's life or physical integrity; serious threat or harm to one's children, spouse or other close relatives or friends; sudden destruction of one's home or community; or seeing another person who has been, is being (or has recently been) seriously injured or killed as a result of an accident or physical violence.

Internal

Type A behavior. In 1973 Friedman and Rosenman's *Type A Behavior and Your Heart*[21] had a profound impact on the public. In 1984 Friedman and Ulmer published *Treating Type A Behavior and Your Heart,* reporting on a study indicating that type As who receive special counseling cut their heart attack rate by half, presumably as a result of changing their behavior patterns. Type A behavior was construed as having three main components: (1) anger and free-floating hostility; (2) time urgency and impatience, with a tendency to go at full speed; and (3) a high level of ambition and job involvement combined with insecurity.

Recent studies have indicated that there is no linear relationship between type A behavior and cardiovascular disease.[34] Indeed, there may be a nonlinear relationship, with younger Type As at risk and older Type As (older than 45), less likely to have severe coronary artery disease (CAD). The hypothesis is that those who survive the early years may represent a subsample of hardy people.

It is becoming increasingly clear that not all the ingredients of type A behavior carry the same risk for CAD. Indeed, rapid talk alone is one measure of speech that may not in itself predict increased risk for CAD. If the increased rate of speech is a function of enthusiasm and spontaneity, it may in fact represent less likelihood of developing CAD. The hostility and the anger appear to be the ingredients of type A that put one more at risk; if the rapid speech is a result of hostility and a sign of aggression, then it may in fact predict increased risk. Again, however, scores on a hostility scale on the Minnesota Multiphasic Personal Inventory (MMPI) predict CAD problems much more in a young group than in a post-50 group. The mechanisms behind the relationship between type A and CAD are not clear, but there are strong suggestions that one who is cynically mistrustful of the world and who is always on guard and hypervigilant has increased catecholamine and cortisol secretion associated with anger and increased testosterone secretion secondary to vigilance. When these individuals are subject to environmental challenges (when they are in environments that make type A demands), they may be hyperreactive on a frequent basis in a way that contributes to CAD.[48]

Co-dependency. Attention is being given increasingly to the impact on children of growing up in a family[8] with an addict, workaholic, alcoholic, or gambler or simply a dysfunctional family where there are inflexible roles, masked and indirect communication, lack of respect and support for individual differences, rigid rules, and insistence on perfection, where control and blame abound.[2] Growing up in a dysfunctional family often teaches one not to talk because the rule is that the family does not discuss the big problem. The problem remains the family secret even though everyone in the family and many people outside know the secret.[6] The corollary of "don't talk" is "don't feel" because if one can't talk about the extremely distressing feelings one experiences, it makes more sense simply to try not to feel, to suppress, and repress. The third rule in such families is "don't trust," because if one can't acknowledge and discuss feeling with the people upon whom one is dependent—parents, then it becomes difficult to trust them. Without this trust it is difficult to trust anyone.

Growing up in an environment that is out of control often causes one to try to compensate as an adult by controlling people and events because one cannot control one's own feelings. One may overfunction by taking on too many responsibilities because parents did not assume legitimate responsibility for the most important responsibility of all. Growing up under these conditions also causes low self-esteem secondary to a feeling that if one were really worthwhile, one's parents would not have the problems they have and certainly would engage in problem-solving activity at the very least. Thus as an adult, one may tend to become overly absorbed in other people's problems, to take care of other people, and to neglect oneself. A common pattern is to recapitulate the parents' marriage, by marrying an addict and developing the patterns of protecting the addict, covering up, losing control in a last ditch effort to establish control over the addict in the family, and being angry and out-of-control in many areas of life, both emotionally and behaviorally. The 12-step groups (based on the Alcoholics Anonymous program) are particularly effective in helping those who have grown up in dysfunctional families and who are co-dependent (see Resources).

Thought patterns. People tend to live by rules. Often the rules are hand-me-downs, coming from parents who got them from their parents, not rules consciously formulated to enhance functioning and reduce stress in current life. In fact, these rules often increase stress. Common rules that increase stress and often lead to perfectionistic striving and excessive work are "anything worth doing is worth doing well," and "anything worth starting is worth finishing." As Ellis and Harper[18] pointed out, stress does not go from action A to consequence C. Rather, it goes from A to B to C, B standing for what one believes about the situation. This philosophy is espoused eloquently by Epictetus who was born lame and a slave in ancient Greece, and who developed the philosophy of stoicism to give himself personal power and freedom from stress. Fundamental among his dicta were: "It is not events which disturb our lives, it is our judgment of events. . . . Never say that man's words make me angry; always say, I react with anger to that man's words."

The idea that one perceives and evaluates events is a powerful idea, enabling one to evaluate perception and thought patterns in any given instance, and to evaluate enduring rules that contribute to persistent patterns of perception, judgment, and thought, which can increase stress. People who tell themselves they must be perfect are subjecting themselves to standards that cannot be reached and thereby to chronic stress and frustration. The notion that one reacts to anger rather than someone else causing the anger is contrary to daily parlance in which "He really tics me off or she makes me furious" are examples of ways of talking that imply that somebody else has control over one's feelings and over stress.

Externalization of causality contributes to stress. So,

too, does permanence, in which factors that contribute to stressors are seen as never changing —*"It ·will always be that way."* A third stress-producing attitude is global attribution in which one focuses not on the effects of the immediate specific stress, but instead says *"Everything's going down the drain."* These factors have been shown to contribute to poor health in middle age, when they were evaluated at age 25 with the effects of mental and physical health controlled.

Thought patterns also enter into deciding whether a person will follow through with recommendations about enhancing health. Assessment of the possible risk and the cost of engaging in the preventive behavior will contribute significantly to a decision of whether or not to comply.

Life's stages

The importance of stressors and their impact on health is illustrated in the diagnostic system of the American Psychiatric Association,[1] which is based on five axes on which diagnoses are made, with axis IV being the severity of psychosocial stressors. The kinds of stressors considered include, along with those already discussed here, developmental such as phases of the life cycle (e.g., puberty, the transition to adult status, menopause, becoming 50, and physical illness or injury).

Infancy and childhood. Regarding family factors (for children and adolescents), the APA diagnostic manual states:

In addition to the above, for children and adolescents the following stressors may be considered: cold or distant relationship between parents; overtly hostile relationship between parents; physical or mental disturbance in family members; cold or distant parental behavior toward child; overtly hostile parental behavior toward child; parental intrusiveness; inconsistent parental control; insufficient social or cognitive stimulation; anomalous family situation, e.g., single parent, foster family; institutional rearing; loss of nuclear family members.[1]

Emotional, physical, and sexual abuse is more and more often uncovered in stressed children.

Karraker and Lake[29] note that, like the rest of us, infants are subject to stressors. They are subject to a variety of physiologic stressors in what William James has described as "the blooming, buzzing confusion" of the world in which they are born. Psychologically, separation is probably the major stressor starting around 7 or 8 months. Distressing interactions such as having a depressed mother are also significant stressors for infants. Events that infants experience as stressful may not, at first blush, seem stressful to adults, but they are categories of events that adults also find stressful: unpredictability, being out-of-control, uncertainty, and inconsistency with expectations and understandings.

Humphrey[26] has summarized sources of stress in children as including school conditions, home conditions, and self-concerns. School tends to be more stressful for boys than for girls. Test anxiety and subject anxiety are prevalent and manifest in increased muscle tension, difficulty concentrating, and restlessness. The one thing that seems to worry children most in school is pressure from teachers for competitiveness. At home, pressure to do things the parents' way is a major stressor as is lack of concern and lack of support. Self-imposed stressors are related to personal goals, self-esteem, values, social standards, ability, and personal characteristics (see box).

Adolescence. Each stage of life embodies certain tasks.[5,14] In adolescence these tasks center on establishing an identity—learning to answer "Who am I?" In their search, teenagers must learn to accept a new physical and

---

Childhood—illustrative case

A 10-year-old boy complained for the past year of almost chronic nausea and an urge to vomit, which made him almost phobic about places where a bathroom was not quickly available. His actual vomiting was infrequent. Medical examination did not reveal any basis for the nausea and vomiting. He was a bright, healthy, athletic, good-looking, and well-mannered boy. His parents were appropriately concerned and thought that perhaps he was putting too much stress on himself to do well in school and athletics. The boy's grandfather had been a famous athlete, and many people in the family said that this 10-year-old reminded them of him. He was an only child, and although his parents weren't obviously pushing him to emulate Grandfather, they certainly colluded in family discussions comparing the two. The 10-year-old seemed to have internalized the expectations that he would be an athletic superstar. When he was being monitored by biofeedback equipment, he showed a great deal of reactivity when discussing athletics. The parents were high achievers and clearly the expectations were that this 10-year-old would also do very well academically, and he had also internalized these expectations. He was bright and able to do well, but he had a great deal of anxious apprehension about examinations and reports. He resonated to the idea of "all this makes me sick," and "this makes me want to throw up." He was not, however, ready to abandon his high standards, and because he felt he had the talents to do very well, the therapeutic focus was more on convincing him that excessive arousal would interfere with performance and on reducing internal expectations to achievable ones. He was also bright enough to understand that he was afraid of failure, and that there was secondary gain when his nausea and vomiting kept him out of pressured situations. Once he was able to accept that he had alternatives—that he could choose not to compete—it was easier for him to relax and let go of his symptoms.

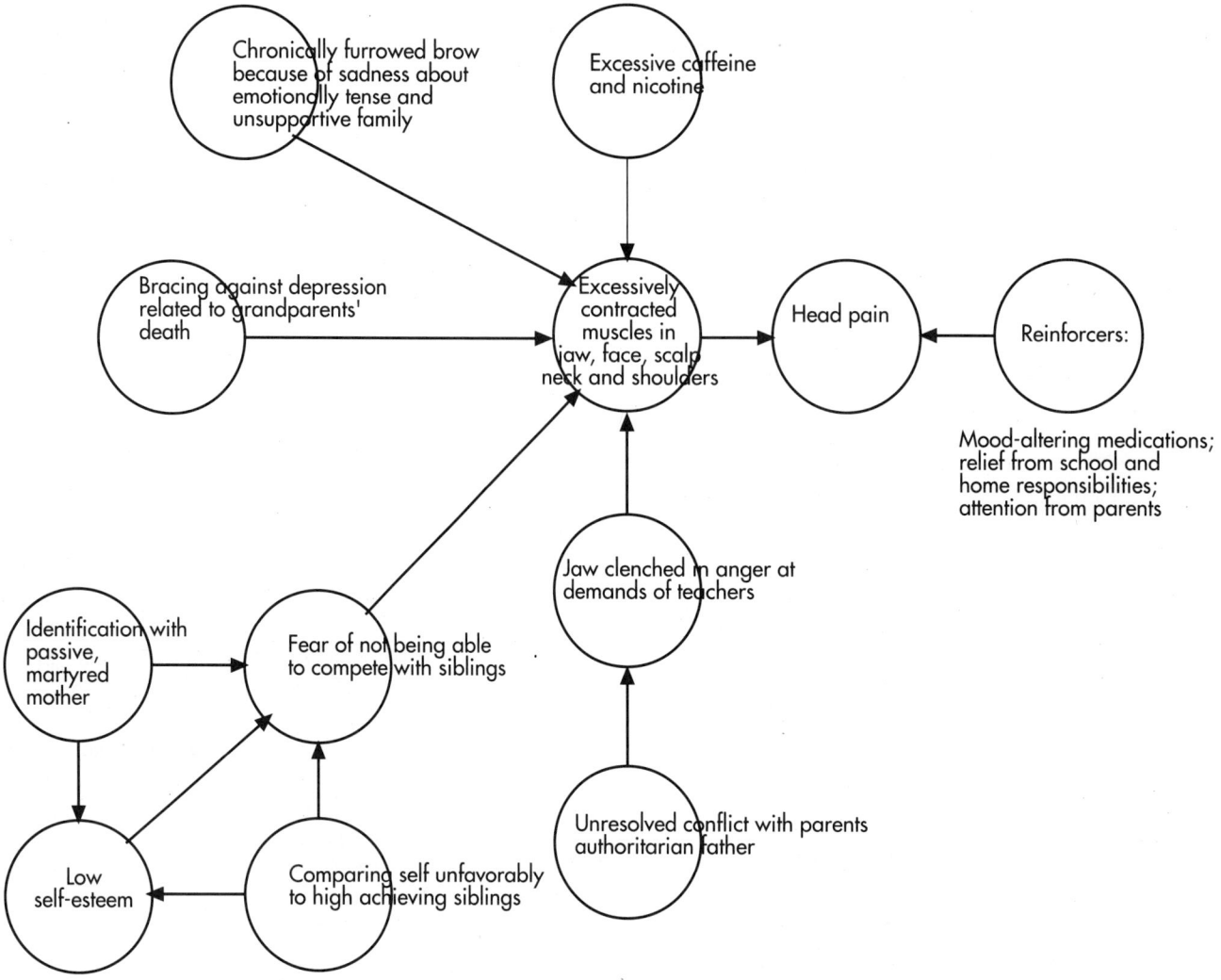

Fig. 12-2. Factors contributing to tension headaches in an adolescent.

sexual role, establish new friendships, strive toward emotional independence from their parents, and take steps towards economic independence. They must develop a greater capacity for abstract thinking, deal with social issues and personal values, develop socially responsible behavior, and start to prepare for marriage and family life. No wonder adolescence is often stressful.[41]

The responsibility a teenager should have depends on what he or she can handle. It is best to start with what is workable and build up to the adolescent's potential. A system for adding responsibilities one at a time should be established, so that when the teenager finally leaves home, it is just a small step—the additional responsibility of managing one's life outside the home. Rewards or privileges should be given for managing responsibilities well. Privileges are thus linked to responsibilities. When responsibilities are not paced appropriately, stress abounds.

Adolescence is a time of major change in physical and sexual characteristics. Sexual drives are very strong after

puberty and masturbation is almost universal. Venereal disease and pregnancy are high risks, and if teenagers are not capable of managing these risks, they clearly are not ready for sexual intercourse. Responsibility and personal values are primary considerations here. Counseling, listening, educating—not lecturing—may add reason to passion. What sexual behavior is appropriate depends on each person's rate of development, on values, and on ability to be responsible. What is inappropriate for one teenager may be appropriate for another. Sexual issues are almost always stressful for adolescents.

Teenagers often feel as if they were basic recruits in the Army, getting the worst jobs, having everything determined by authority figures, being harassed much of the time with punishment and little reward, yet told to respect their superiors. Often, they feel they lack identity—that they don't count. Often their response is anger (see box).

Diagramming the cause-and-effect chains contributing to symptoms can aid understanding and treatment plan-

---

Adolescence—illustrative case

This 15-year-old girl presented with recurrent, severe abdominal pain that had caused her to miss 45 days of school during the year. There was no demonstrable organic cause for her pain. She was a middle child, with sisters 2 years older and 2 years younger, a mother who was a homemaker, and a father in the clergy. She firmly and adamantly denied any stress in her life, as did her parents. Review of her development over the past year, however, suggested that the time she missed in school was putting her significantly behind her peers in dealing with major developmental tasks of adolescence, that she was failing to develop academically, to separate from family, to develop a peer group, to establish heterosexual relationships, and to develop an identity of independent competence.

Her psychosocial development had evidently proceeded normally until 2 years earlier, when they had moved from a small rural town to a major city. The move itself was probably stressful for her despite her denial, as it put her with a more socially advanced and sophisticated peer group and in more advanced classes. The coping methods that had worked up until age 13 in a small town no longer worked. Her main coping method had been to be a good girl, to be proper and correct, to work hard, to get good grades, and to be teacher's pet. Now those coping strategies weren't available to her because of her changed age and stage of life and because of the changed circumstances. Our impression was that she had adopted a pattern of somatization, rather than developing new and effective coping mechanisms. The worry, almost to the point of anguish, of her parents seemed to reinforce this pattern. She seemed well on the way to becoming the family invalid, while her older sister was socially popular and active and her younger sister was a successful student.

As a middle child, she had felt particular pressure to accommodate and to keep her feelings to herself, and she presented as quite repressive. Individual intervention was futile because she denied any stress, even when physiologic monitoring provided objective evidence of stress. Family therapy offered an opportunity to identify the pathologic patterns of reacting to stress and illness while they were being played out and was instrumental in initiating a turnaround. Progress was slow because she had to make up for much lost time in meeting developmental tasks.

---

ning. Fig. 12-2 diagrams factors contributing to tension headaches in an adolescent.

Early adulthood. After adolescence, young adults typically are oriented toward moving out of the house to develop families and careers of their own. In this stage there is the continued task of trying to define identity, followed by the task of becoming able to establish intimacy. Too often efforts are made for intimacy before personal identity is firmly established, so that the changing identity disrupts the intimacy patterns and impairs the relationship. Too often the demands of living up to expectations and rules of the family of origin, yet blending with another person in a marriage at the same time one is taking on responsibility for a career, becomes very stressful.[14] This situation is particularly stressful in an age of two-career families, which are difficult to maintain in their own right, but become more stressful when children are born. Children often constitute an overload on the family system, with marital happiness typically dropping after the birth of the first child and not recovering until the last child leaves home.

After marriage, developmental tasks include developing patterns of communication that are understandable to each partner, the patterns of family of origin often being quite divergent, and establishing shared expectations about how money is spent, about how tasks are accomplished, and about who is responsible for what. Establishing a satisfying sexual relationship is important as part of a pattern of communicating affection. Deciding which outside interests and friendships to pursue as a couple and which separately are major tasks. Patterns have to change to adapt to preg-

nancy, and after the birth of a child, tasks range from the pragmatic, such as childproofing the home, to practical future planning, such as anticipating educational costs, to establishing new patterns of communication to accommodate an additional family member.[14]

Moving into their 30s, adults become more independent, dropping away from mentors of the 20s, often working hard at consolidating careers, usually with very little personal time after all of life's responsibilities are attended to. Time pressure and feeling in a "rat race" are major stressors at this stage of life (see box).

Midlife transition. Many adults experience a midlife crisis near age 40.[5] This crisis occurs at a time when one perceives that one's life has reached the halfway point and is no longer going uphill, but is sliding downhill toward retirement, old age, and death. This perception leads many people to go through an agonizing appraisal of their personal and work lives. This philosophic crisis coincides with the reality that many parents are coping with adolescent children for the first time, often while simultaneously dealing with ill or dying parents. In addition, they may be coping with major job responsibilities that have accrued by midlife, along with facing the reality that one may not get the promotion or position that has been the dream for years. The demand for a great deal of work and multiple roles often overloads one's coping abilities.[42] Research suggests that the midlife crisis can be resolved in various ways, the most common being a reaffirmation of the path one is already on. Alternatively, one can choose to make a major change in family and/or work directions. If a posi-

---

Early adulthood—illustrative case

A 32-year-old, married female travel agent presented with nervousness and failure to become pregnant. She had married into a family in which all her husband's siblings had children and in which his parents emphasized the value of large families. The patient felt inferior and shamed and found it difficult to associate with her husband's family at their many large gatherings. When she didn't attend, however, her husband criticized her, so that she felt stressed whether she attended or stayed home. Her own family lived far away, had never been close, and was not supportive of her. Rather than developing emotional, intellectual, and physical intimacy with her husband, she was increasingly eliminating it, keeping her thoughts and feelings to herself, and, despite the desire to get pregnant, they were having sex very infrequently because of the chronic tension that existed between them. Involvement in a couples' self-help group together with couple's therapy and relaxation training for both of them was needed to reverse the negative spiral that had started in their marriage. Despite their problems, the couple had many strengths. They both had good jobs, were basically healthy, and had no financial problems. Thus the prognosis was more positive.

Midlife transition—illustrative case

A 42-year-old carpenter was brought to our service by his wife who said she discovered that he was having an affair and complained that he was drinking excessively and that his work and income were suffering. She was threatening divorce yet didn't really want it. He described common concerns of midlife, feelings that his youth was nearly over, and that his life was boring and dissatisfying. At the very time he was acting irresponsibly, there was increased demand on the couple to function responsibly, as each had aging mothers who were coping with widowhood and ill health, and their two children were in high school. He refused to acknowledge that he had any problems with stress and would not accept any treatment. Two years later his wife reported that indeed they had divorced and that his erratic and self-indulgent behavior had continued. She was expressing major symptoms of stress in every category.

---

tive resolution is not found, one may sink into despair.

Some theoretical work suggests that intimacy in relationships is more important for women than achievement and that women who have both achieved individuality and developed close relationships make midlife transitions more easily (see box).

Middle adulthood. Ideally, life settles down and improves and is less stressful during middle adulthood, with more time for marriage after children have left home. By this stage, peace has often been made with the conditions of the workplace. Middle adulthood is a time when men can develop more feminine sides of themselves, becoming kinder and gentler, and when women can develop a masculine side of themselves, becoming more assertive. In reality, however, middle adulthood may be the time when a couple discovers that they have very little in common once the children have left, and divorce follows. In addition even if one has made peace with the workplace, there may be a reduction in force, with a push for early retirement and/or with jobs abolished so that one is out of work at an age when it is difficult to find new employment. Increasingly, grown children come back to live at home, so that if there has been an improvement in the marriage after the children left, there is a subsequent disruption, with an adult returning home expecting the privileges of adulthood, but still stuck in an old childlike role of irresponsibility at home (see box).

Late adulthood and old age. As middle adulthood progresses into later adulthood, retirement from work often occurs. Most retired people are able to create new lives for themselves. Retirement is more stressful when a large part of one's identity has been the work identity, so that retirement brings a sense of emptiness and impotence. Retirement certainly results in major life changes, often financial changes, certainly social changes, and usually psychologic changes.[59] For many, the financial restrictions imposed by retirement pose stark reality stressors. For many, there is the sense of having been forced out of work, so that the reward for a lifetime of effort is being thrown out. For many, bridges haven't been built to a new way of life, so that there is a sense of uncertainty and dread as one looks ahead. For most, there is a sense that looking ahead to the next major milestone is to look ahead to illness and/or death.

Successful retirement usually requires preplanning several years before retirement. The process is like building a bridge from one stage of life to another, like outlining a new volume in one's autobiography before closing the present one. Many people don't plan; they just try to jump from one state to the next, sometimes falling short. They open a blank volume and wonder what to write. Those who do plan mainly focus on finances. This focus is essential but often not sufficient. Successful retired people tend to be busy, so it is wise to start planning and practicing the different ways in which you will be busy when you leave your job behind.

A couple needs to plan new patterns of relating. Many wives complain their husbands now want to manage them instead of the work force. The trick is to retire to something, as well as from something, to have a bridge to the

Middle adulthood—illustrative case

A patient presenting with the seemingly simple stress symptoms of a tension headache illustrates how such symptoms can reflect stressors in almost every area of life. The patient was a 51-year-old woman, married to a 60-year-old man. Her father had died 5 years earlier, and her 83-year-old mother was chronically ill. She was the parent of two children, a 22-year-old unmarried son and a 24-year-old daughter (herself a mother of a 1-year-old and a 3-year-old and currently going through a divorce). The patient was employed as an administrative assistant at a large corporation. She was taking anxiolytics and analgesics in an effort to relieve her head pain but was experiencing more side effects, including gastrointestinal upset and sleepiness, than therapeutic effect.

The following stressors were identified during the course of self-regulation training and psychotherapy as contributors to her headache:

- Too much work at the office
- Perfectionistic demands on herself at work
- A supervisor who was unclear in his expectations, selfish with compliments, and generous with criticism
- Deadlines and erratic pace of work
- A husband who
  - Teased by poking her in the ribs in a way that hurt rather than entertained
  - Teased by joking about her weight in a way that hurt rather than entertained
  - Had changed jobs 11 times in 10 years and who had been unemployed for 2 of those years, with resultant financial hardship
  - Was now retired without a pension and resultant financial hardship
  - Devoted a lot of his energy to bossing his wife when she was at home
  - A son who had graduated from college and come back home to live and who wanted the privileges of adulthood without the responsibilities

- A husband and son who were both deficient in communicating about feelings and who in general didn't talk much
- A daughter who frequently asked mother for help in child care on evenings and weekends as daughter was trying to develop a new social life of her own while going through divorce
- A son-in-law who appealed to mother to try to intervene to stop the divorce
- Grandchildren who were anxious, one acting out, the other clinging, secondary to the tension of divorce
- Regrets stirred up by daughter's divorce—regrets that despite the stress of divorce she herself hadn't left her husband when her children were little
- Pent up grief that had never been expressed at the time of her father's death because she had been the strong one, taking care of all of the practical details and taking care of emotional needs of other family members when her father died
- The need to hire nursing help for her mother; regular visits to her mother that placed further demands on evening and weekend time; coping with a mother who was guilt-inducing and manipulative, fearful of being abandoned
- A husband who drank too much and whose moodiness was in part secondary to alcohol; a pattern in herself of co-dependency, in which she was denying of her husband's alcohol problems, enabling and hyperresponsible
- A dissatisfying sexual relationship with a husband who was generally impotent and who blamed his impotence on her weight making her unattractive to him

She was able to master self-regulation and rid herself of headaches only after she learned to become more assertive, to set clearer limits, to create time for herself rather than everyone else, and to identify and manage unlabeled and unexpressed feelings.

---

future. Many organizations that address issues of aging and retirement are listed under Resources. Use their help. The myths about retirement need to be faced: "the trip" and "the move" often fail to live up to expectation; hobbies frequently pale, free time doesn't equate to freedom. Some people retire by choice, some are forced into retirement before their time, others struggle for years in the workplace just waiting to retire. Choice is always easier than force and planning is always better than chance. Richard Wilbur wrote:

"I read how Quixote in his random ride came to a crossing once, and lest he lose the purity of chance, would not decide whither to fair, but wished his horse to choose for glory lay wherever he might turn. His head was light with pride, his horse's shoes were heavy, and he headed for the barn."

Late adulthood and old age. Prolonged illness, institutionalization in a nursing home, becoming a burden to one's children, are fears that constitute major stressors for many older adults (see box).

Death and dying. Death of a family member is a major stressor whenever it occurs. On the life crisis scale, the most stressful item is death of a spouse. This event is more likely to be faced in late adulthood than in other times of life, with women four times as likely as men to have a spouse die.[9] The stages of reaction to death have been described as denial, bargaining, anger, sadness and loss, and finally acceptance. Developing a new life at this stage parallels developing a life back in young adulthood, leaving home, but without all the excitement of looking forward to a new life. The majority of persons over age 65 have grandchildren as well as children. Often the grandchildren

---

Late adulthood and old age—illustrative case

A 72-year-old woman presented with chronic tinnitus and episodic dizziness. The impression was that symptoms were in part secondary to hearing loss, but that they were in part functional. She felt that all of her significant friends were ill or dead. She wanted to focus on her children, but two had moved far away and the one who lived nearby was emotionally abusive. His wife had divorced him because of this behavior and he had turned much of his wrath on his mother. Her focus on her symptoms seemed both a way of trying to avoid this reality and a way of forcing someone to identify the stress in her life. While she was extremely reluctant to admit the reality, once she was able to do so and enter into supportive therapy, symptoms abated.

---

offer an extremely satisfying relationship and can help rebuild the will to live after a spouse's death. Group support can be particularly helpful during the grieving period,[51] more so at a time when families are less available for help.

STRESSORS FOR PHYSICIANS

Physicians, with high rates of drug and alcohol problems, depression, and suicide[33] are perhaps more aware than most of the multitude and magnitude of life stressors, which can be subsumed under the following general categories:

1. *Environmental:* These include major life changes and daily hassles along with the typically stressful environment of hospitals.
2. *Educational:* Like other professional fields, medicine requires continuous accumulation of new knowledge.
3. *Economic:* Health care is facing major economic pressures, with threats of more and more cutbacks in reimbursement.
4. *Biologic:* Exposure to many illnesses; easy availability of drugs; and sleep interruptions are all major stressors for physicians.
5. *Spiritual:* Whereas some people have spiritual beliefs that are strengthened by constant exposure to illness and death, others become alienated and lose faith.
6. *Social:* Physicians are expected to maintain a particularly controlled demeanor and propriety in social life.
7. *Psychologic:* Major psychologic stressors include perfectionistic demands on self that cannot be met.
8. *Familial:* Physicians are not immune from divorce. Work demands make it difficult to maintain healthy family relationships, with family members at risk for resenting that "patients always come first."
9. *Legal:* Physicians are increasingly subject to suit and to legal constraints that seem like straitjackets.
10. *Sociologic:* The once highly honored physician is now often suspected of being a money grabber who doesn't really care.
11. *Political:* Physicians, who once eschewed political involvement as nonprofessional, increasingly find they must protect their profession through political activities.
12. *Vocational:* Vocational stressors include too much work; patients and families who may be in bad moods/depressed, anxious, and angry because of illness; and frequent phone calls and interruptions.[36]

ASSESSING STRESS

If you suspect that stress is an important issue for one of your patients, you might ask the following:

- How do I know how stressed this person is? What are his/her symptoms?
- What are the causes of the symptoms?
- What can I do to help keep the person physically and mentally healthy?

Self-assessment

Asking a patient to complete the forms on stress symptoms and sources of stress is an effective way to establish effective communication (see Tables 12-4 and 12-5). Because everyone is under stress, people generally respond positively to a request to identify which stressors are in their life and which stress reactions bother them, realizing that everyone is going to have some of each.

Psychologic tests

In assessing stress, we use formal instruments such as the Minnesota Multiphasic Personality Inventory (MMPI),[57] which measures psychologic pathology along various dimensions and the California Psychological Inventory (CPI),[57] which presents a picture of coping skills and strengths and/or their absence. Computerized self-assessment questionnaires can be taken on-line at the office, making assessment of stress a routine part of examinations.

The simplest self-report methods are visual analog scales and ratings of magnitude. You can construct such a scale by simply drawing a line from 1 to 10 (Fig 12-3), to make a self-anchoring scale, in which one end is defined as no stress and the other end is defined as the worst stress imaginable. The person then assesses where he or she falls on the scale according to his or her own definitions of no stress and the worst stress.

Table 12-4. Sources of stress

Rate the following in terms of how much stress they cause you.

Work	Very much				Very little
Too much work	1	2	3	4	5
Too little authority	1	2	3	4	5
Politics	1	2	3	4	5
Difficult customers	1	2	3	4	5
Difficult supervisors	1	2	3	4	5
Difficult co-workers	1	2	3	4	5
Lack of clarity in job description	1	2	3	4	5
Lack of feedback	1	2	3	4	5
Excessive need for approval	1	2	3	4	5
Perfectionistic tendencies/unrealistic idealism	1	2	3	4	5
Too frequent interruptions	1	2	3	4	5
Juggling job and family demands	1	2	3	4	5
Crises and emergencies	1	2	3	4	5
Job instability and fear of unemployment	1	2	3	4	5
Too much responsibility, especially for people	1	2	3	4	5
Ongoing contact with "stress carriers" (alcoholics, anxious indecisive people, etc.)	1	2	3	4	5
Sexual harassment	1	2	3	4	5
Erratic work schedule and take-home work	1	2	3	4	5
Disparity between what I have to do on the job and what I would like to accomplish	1	2	3	4	5
Ambiguity of work tasks, territory, and role	1	2	3	4	5
Expecting too much of myself	1	2	3	4	5

Personal	Very much				Very little
Financial problems	1	2	3	4	5
Sexual problems	1	2	3	4	5
Marital or significant other problems	1	2	3	4	5
Problems with parents	1	2	3	4	5
Problems with children	1	2	3	4	5
Problems with other relations	1	2	3	4	5
Chronic illness in family member	1	2	3	4	5
Trouble speaking up for myself	1	2	3	4	5
Poor time management	1	2	3	4	5
Loneliness	1	2	3	4	5
Lack of confidence	1	2	3	4	5
Feeling of powerlessness	1	2	3	4	5
Effects of childhood abuse	1	2	3	4	5
Death of someone close	1	2	3	4	5
Divorce or separation	1	2	3	4	5
Spiritual alienation	1	2	3	4	5
Change in job	1	2	3	4	5
Change in residence	1	2	3	4	5
Health problems	1	2	3	4	5
Poor exercise and diet habits	1	2	3	4	5
Smoking	1	2	3	4	5
Drinking too much	1	2	3	4	5
Type A personality	1	2	3	4	5
Other _____	1	2	3	4	5

Table 12-5. Symptoms of stress

Rate how much you experience symptoms.

	Very much				Very little
Physical symptoms (e.g., headaches, GI upset, hypertension)	1	2	3	4	5
Deterioration in work performance (difficulty concentrating, increased errors, decreased efficiency)	1	2	3	4	5
Unhealthy habits (e.g., smoking, alcohol and substance abuse, overeating)	1	2	3	4	5
Deterioration in interpersonal relationships (e.g., increased conflict, decreased satisfaction, social withdrawal)	1	2	3	4	5
Subjective distress that interferes with well-being (e.g., tension, pressure, anxiety, depression)	1	2	3	4	5
Attitude change (e.g., decreased motivation, cynicism)	1	2	3	4	5
Fatigue, chronic tiredness	1	2	3	4	5
Insomnia (difficulty falling asleep and/or awakening frequently or early)	1	2	3	4	5
Anger and irritability	1	2	3	4	5
Other (list) _____	1	2	3	4	5

Little/no stress   Moderate stress   Extreme stress
1 2 3   4 5 6 7   8 9 10

Fig. 12-3. Self-assessment scale.

Name _____

HA = X   T = O

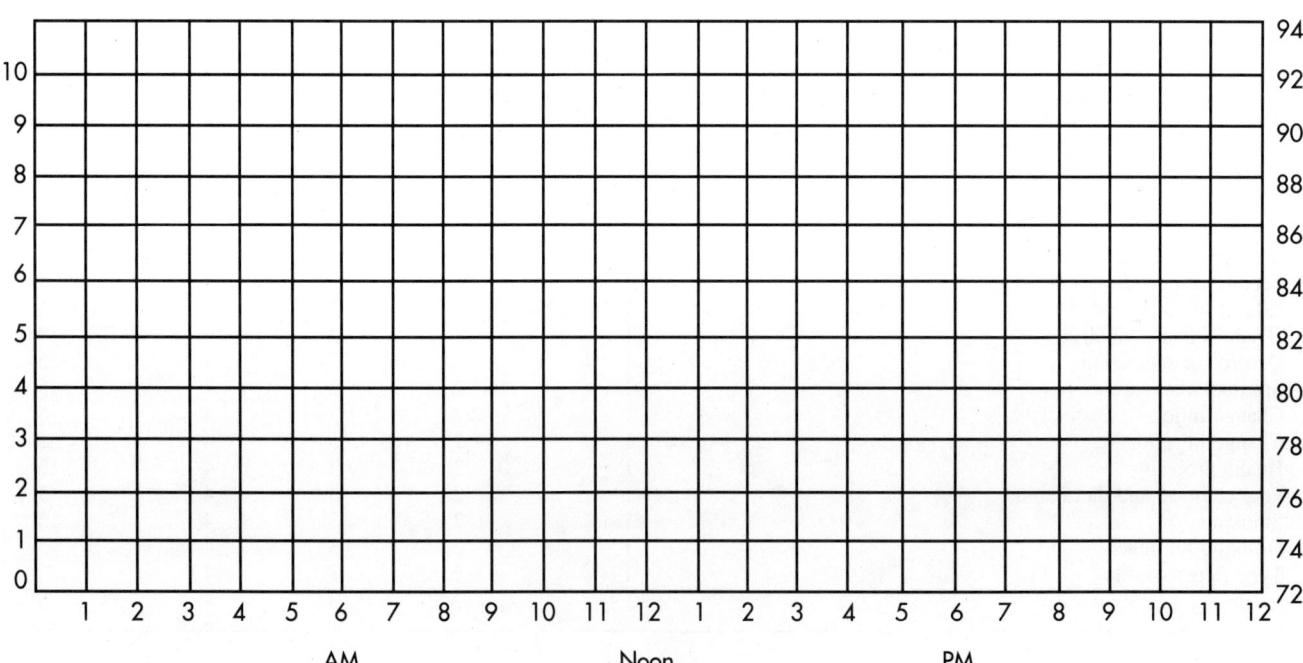

Fig. 12-4. Sample log.

Psychophysiologic profiling

Because stress is a psychophysiologic response, physiologic assessment is also important. The clinician will be alert to many of the physiologic changes simply by interviewing the patient and/or performing a physical examination. We use biofeedback equipment[49] in which muscle contraction levels in the jaw, face, and scalp, digital peripheral temperature, galvanic skin response, and heart rate are recorded at a baseline condition, under an imposed stressor (often Serial 7s, i.e., counting backwards from 100 by sevens under time pressure), during recovery and during a time of imagery of a recent significant stressor, and during self-relaxation and during assisted relaxation. The goal is to identify people who have excessively high resting levels of physiologic reactivity, excessively high levels of reactivity to imposed stressors and/or excessively slow or incomplete recovery from stressors, and/or inability to induce relaxation on one's own or when guided.

Diaries or logs can be used to monitor any particular symptom over time. Figs. 12-4 and 12-5 illustrate two headache logs in which severity of the headache can be recorded hourly or four times a day at breakfast, midmorning, noon, and later in the afternoon. Digital peripheral temperature is also monitored and recorded through an inexpensive hand-held thermometer to chart the correlation of vascular reactivity and headache experience. This chart can be modified for other symptoms.

Family report

Typically, one recognizes times of stress because:

- The body develops various symptoms including aches and pains
- The mind sends apprehensive thoughts and feelings of being pressured and harassed
- Habits tell you, as bad habits escalate to try to reduce stress
- Performance declines noticeably

If one doesn't hear any of the earlier messages, one's family usually can give messages, too. As the physician, if the patient is not listening to any of the other symptoms of stress is and not reporting them, it is useful to interview key family members. Spouses of type A personalities are always acutely aware of the type A behavior with which they live, even though the type A person may deny it. Anyone living with someone else who is irritable and/or withdrawn because of stress will be able to report the situation clearly. Often, it is a family member who sees the relationship between excessive drinking and stress, between school or work worries and physical symptoms. Asking a relevant family member to fill out the forms in this section, as they relate to the designated patient, can provide important information.

Name _____

Date _____

Headache rating (0-10)	Medication usage (type and milligram)	Comments and associated activity
5 AM		
6:00		
7.00		
8:00		
9:00		
10:00		
11:00		
Noon		
1 PM		
2:00		
3:00		
4:00		
5:00		
6:00		
7:00		
8:00		
9:00		
10:00		
11:00		
Midnight		
After		

Fig. 12-5. Sample log.

Interview and observation

Healthy People 2000[56] states:

Primary health care providers are urged to be alert to signs of mental and emotional disorders in their patients, giving particular attention to those going through major life transitions such as a recent divorce, separation, bereavement, unemployment, or serious medical illness. Co-morbidity of emotional disorders and alcohol and other drug use should also be considered.[7]

Normalizing stress is a key technique to obtain information from people who feel stigmatized by reporting stress or who feel that being stressed is a sign of personal weakness. Saying, "I know we are all under a lot of stress in the world we live in today, tell me about yours" can be a good starting point. Acknowledging that stress happens to people who care and who try is another way to offset possible feelings of stigma. Once the door is opened, using forms like those presented here can constitute a guided interview. Patients will communicate a great deal about themselves in nonverbal ways, too. The anxious patient will have motoric restlessness, autonomic hyperarousal, and vigilant scanning behavior as well as apprehensive expectations. Posture, movement, intonation, inflection, volume, eye contact, expression, and grooming all make

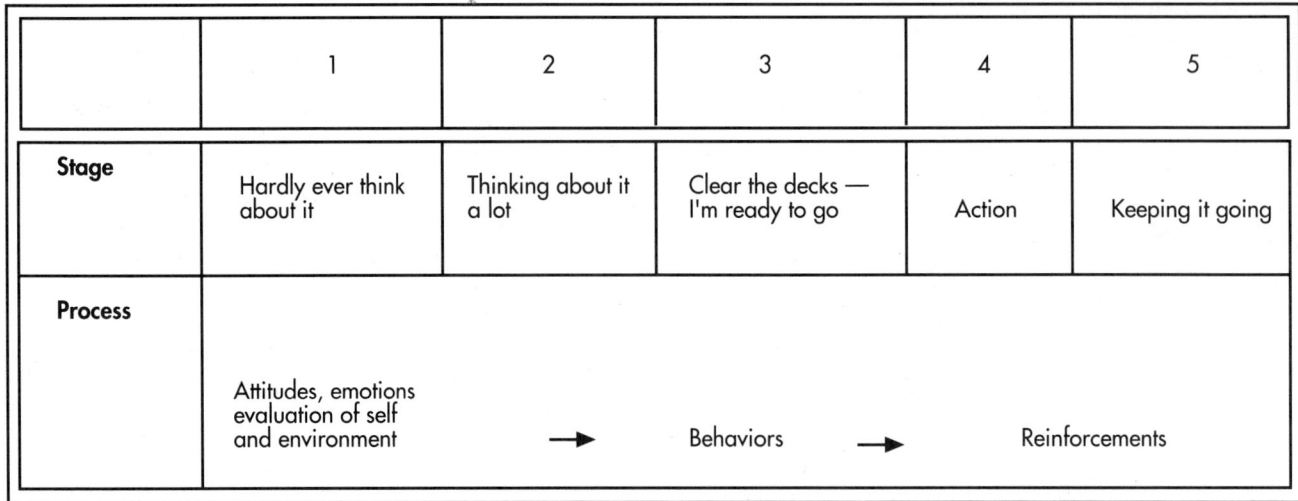

Fig. 12-6. Process and stages of change.

powerful statements about one's self-esteem and about how effectively one is coping with the multiple pressures in life.

MANAGING STRESS

Healthy People 2000[56] states:

Most adult Americans report having a great deal of stress in their lives. More than a fourth of those who acknowledge a great deal of stress say they do not consciously take steps to control or reduce it. Among those who do take steps, emotional denial, physical exercise, and stress avoidance are the most popular measures.[53] Yet the stress management literature describes an array of formal interventions, including relaxation, biofeedback, meditation, desensitization, development of coping responses, assertiveness training, imagery, diet, exercise, and weight control. A service industry is evolving, although the efficacy of most of the techniques has not yet been rigorously evaluated using physiologic measures, appropriate control groups, and random assignment procedures.

Everything we know about managing stress is stated in the Serenity Prayer: "God grant me the serenity to accept what I cannot change, the courage to change what I can, and the wisdom to know the difference." Acquiring the wisdom to know the difference and the skills to effect change or embrace serenity are the goals of the preventive and treatment modalities presented here. Programs to help people manage stress better often fail because they are targeted at people who are ready for action; most people, in fact, are not ready. Research by Prochaska et al.[47] indicates that many people who need to change are at earlier stages in the change process (Fig. 12-6), thus advice on how to act differently fails because thoughts and feelings haven't yet changed enough to enable action. In addition, reinforcements must be built in to maintain healthy habits.

Relaxation and meditation

An effective way[4] to induce deep relaxation and to master the skill is to practice in a quiet place where one won't be disturbed, find a comfortable sitting position, narrow attention as by counting to three slowly over and over, saying the number 1 to oneself each time one exhales, repeating a quieting phrase to oneself or using calming imagery such as a beach, and do this in a passive way by allowing the focus (not forcing it) and letting competing thoughts just drift through. The positions in meditation aren't always naturally comfortable, but in other ways meditation is a variety of relaxation. Practicing on a daily basis reduces susceptibility to stress-related disorders and enables mastery of briefer relaxation techniques to use throughout the day. For many people, going into daily life is like going into battle. It is necessary to be well conditioned and to have specific tactics to cope. A 15-minute period of deep relaxation each day is part of getting generally conditioned and developing a skill that can be used in response to stressors during the day. Meditative relaxation is a passive form of relaxation, which has various scripts.

A more active form of relaxation, which is particularly good for restless people and those with muscle aches and pains, is progressive muscle relaxation[27] in which the major muscle groups of the body are first tensed and then relaxed. The process progresses through all the muscle groups.

We tell people going through biofeedback training that any one of several strategies may be helpful in enhancing relaxation. They are encouraged to experiment both during the session and throughout the day to find which methods bring about the most relaxed sensations. An important concept that operates throughout all biofeedback techniques involves narrowing of the mind's activity to a sin-

Table 12-6. Modified progressive relaxation

Muscle area	Tensing instructions	Tension location
Hands	Clench and relax—right then left—then both fists	The back of your hands and your wrists
Upper arm	Bend elbows and fingers of both hands to your shoulders and tense the biceps	The biceps muscles
Lower arm	Hold both arms straight out—stretch—relax	The upper portion of the forearm
Forehead	Wrinkle the forehead and lift the eyebrow upward—relax	The entire forehead area
Eyes	Close the eyes tightly—relax	The eyelids
Jaws	Clench jaws—relax	The jaws and chin area
Tongue	Bring your tongue upward and press it against the roof of your mouth—feel tension—relax	The area in and around the tongue
Mouth	Press your lips tightly together, feel tension—relax	The region around the mouth
Neck	Press your head backward. Roll to the right and back; roll to the left and back, straighten—relax	The muscles in the back of the neck and at the base of the scalp, right and left side of neck
Neck and jaws	Bend the head forward. Press the chin against the chest, straighten—relax	The muscles in the front of the neck and around the jaws
Shoulders	Bring the shoulders up toward ears, shrug, and move around—relax	The muscles of the shoulders and the lower part of the neck
Chest	Take a deep breath slowly—hold it for 5 seconds—exhale slowly—relax	The entire abdominal region
Abdomen	Tighten stomach muscles, make the abdomen muscles hard—relax	The entire abdominal region
Back	Pull shoulders back—arch back from chair—relax	Lower back
Thighs	Press heels down hard, flex thighs—relax	The muscles in the lower part of the thighs
Legs	Hold both legs straight out, point your toes away from your face—relax	The muscles of the calf
Legs	Hold both legs straight out, point your toes toward your face—relax	The muscle below the kneecap

These exercises are designed for a sitting position and each one can be repeated once or twice. You may want to relax only certain muscle groups, you need not go through the entire list each time. The important thing is to remember to RELAX!

gle focus. One trainee mentioned that this is like "learning not to think." During the time of relaxation the idea is to increasingly close out the "mind chatter" and to cultivate awareness of your own subtle body rhythms. Listed are a number of helpful techniques to enhance the effectiveness of biofeedback training.

1. Concentrate on a very relaxing scene—maybe at the beach or in the mountains. Allow this scene to unfold and become vivid. Picture being in the scene, lying on the beach or sitting in the mountains.
2. Focus attention on hands and arms. Let them get very heavy. Let the feet and legs get heavy. Then picture each part of the body; see the muscles going loose and limp and feel heaviness develop.
3. Each time you breathe out, say the number 1 to yourself. Keep repeating this each time you breathe out, letting your breathing become slow and steady.
4. When other thoughts come to you, simply say to yourself, "I don't have to think about that now," and let the thoughts float in one side and out the other.
5. Concentrate on a single word or phrase like "peaceful" or "I feel quite quiet." Silently repeat it.

6. Simply stare at one spot. Passively let all your attention focus there. Let yourself go into a quiet and peaceful state of passive concentration.
7. As you become aware of the thoughts that constantly go through your mind, move the focus from those thoughts downward from your head so that you become aware of more subtle natural body rhythms such as breathing and heartbeat. Gradually let awareness of these rhythms replace the tension-producing chatter of the mind.
8. Focus attention on breathing. Breathe calmly and regularly. A deep breath that expands the diaphragm can be particularly useful in beginning a relaxation session.

We challenge patients to at least change one thing in their lives to be less stressed. We also want patients to be able to do a brief relaxation exercise such as the Quieting Reflex[54] in which, 10 times a day, they scan their mind and body, registering mood and tension, then tell themselves to let go, take a deep breath and let a wave of calm descend as they breathe out (Table 12-6).

Breathing

When one is stressed, subtle and chronic hyperventilation often is manifested by breathing that is mainly thoracic, the diaphragm is not used much and an odd effortless sighing occurs frequently. This breathing is described as a significant upward and forward motion in the upper sternum, with minimal expansion laterally.[20]

Subtle hyperventilation is such a common component in the stress response that learning to breathe normally and diaphragmatically can be an important stress reducer. We ask patients to put either a book or their hands over their belly while reclining in a lounge chair or lying on the floor and tell them that when they are breathing diaphragmatically the book or their hands will go up when they breathe in and go down when they breathe out. The diaphragm expands the air space by pushing down against the contents of the belly, forcing them up during inhalation.[20] With properly relaxed breathing, the shoulders and chest can be relaxed and still.

Chest breathing is appropriate during exercise but when present on a chronic basis, the effect is as if the patient were running a race while actually sitting still. That kind of chronic hyperventilation often leads to feelings of stress and anxiety. Diaphragmatic breathing is like a secret weapon for stress management because it can be used any time—sitting in a classroom, teaching a class, talking on the telephone, or driving a car. It can be used when someone is yelling at you, when someone is quizzing you, or when someone is pressuring you. It can be used without anyone else knowing that you are practicing stress management. It is thus an invaluable part of the armamentarium for managing stress.

Biofeedback

Biofeedback therapies are particularly appropriate for disorders of excessive arousal.[49] Biofeedback therapies for stress-related disorders generally teach lowered arousal. The biofeedback instruments that are used monitor physiologic functioning related to arousal, the most common measures being muscle tightness, sweating, and reduced blood flow to the periphery, all symptoms of increased arousal. Other forms of biofeedback instruments include those that give information on breathing rate and pattern, blood pressure, heart rate, and brain wave activity.

Biofeedback therapy always involves a therapist who conducts an initial assessment, develops a treatment protocol, and coaches the patient on how to acquire the skills needed for self-regulation. The Biofeedback Certification Institute of America has certified more than 1800 people in diverse fields, including many nurses, and certifies training courses as providing effective entry level training. The instruments provide feedback necessary for learning a skill. To learn any skill, one must have the required ability and motivation, must be rewarded for a correct response, and must have feedback about the results of efforts. Because most people do not have built-in feedback mechanisms to identify small changes in arousal level, the instruments provide the same effect one gets by looking in a mirror when trying to develop a special facial expression. They also guide and reinforce learning and help in self-awareness by indicating arousal associated with various aspects of one's life. This awareness is achieved when one realizes that reactivity peaks when discussing areas such as work or personal relationships.

Thoughts: changing threats to challenges

Stress develops when something in the environment is perceived as a threat, which one is unable to meet successfully because of limited capacity. Changing the perception of a threat to a challenge can be accomplished if one diminishes the size of the demand and increases a sense of personal competence. Many people live by rules such as "anything worth starting is worth finishing," which almost automatically creates stress. Because many of the rules we live by were built in when we were children, we often don't articulate them. Identifying the rules by which we live, the rules that constitute straitjackets, can be a major step in changing them.[18] It is important to write down reformulations. Various self-help books have multitudes of exercises to help accomplish this goal.

Stress inoculation

Stress inoculation[37] combines relaxation with developing more effective coping statements. For example, when facing a tough examination, one would learn to say ahead of time "I know I can handle this. I've been through tough examinations before. I'm preparing for it well." As the examination time approached, one would learn to say: "I am getting nervous, but some nervousness can be helpful to me. I can take the edge off excessive nervousness as I'm learning how to relax myself." In the examination, one would say: "I'm getting more anxious. I can focus on it and it won't overwhelm me. I can use my relaxation strategies and my focusing strategies and they will help." After the examination one could say: "I'm getting better at this. I'm not perfect, but these techniques are helpful and I'll keep practicing them."

Because many daily hassles fall into categories, such as traffic problems, irritating people, and difficult phone calls, stress inoculation strategies can be used to reduce the reactivity. The first steps are to use appropriate cognitive formulations, to take responsibility for one's own reactivity rather than blaming the situation, and to acknowledge that one's reactivity can be changed. The next step is to sit quietly, get relaxed, and visualize the scene approaching, reminding oneself that the situation can be handled. Finally, one can imagine oneself in the situation saying things such as "I knew I'd react to it, that's okay; I can reduce my reactivity," while doing the things that will help, such as slow breathing and saying "No point in creating another problem; this is bad enough without getting stressed out about it." Visualization should continue until the situation has passed. One should always congratulate oneself for learning how to handle the situation better by saying things such as "It's not perfect, but I'm doing better."

Assertiveness

How one deals with the agendas of difficult people depends on whether one interacts regularly with that person or whether it is a one-time encounter. If it is a repetitive interaction with someone who counts in one's life, it is helpful to learn to be assertive enough to discuss perceptions with the other person and try to work toward change.

If it is a one-time interaction, one might try stating the other person's agenda in the strongest terms, with some possibility they may back off from it. For example, "I gather there is no information that would make a difference to you in understanding this problem." This latter kind of response represents active listening to the fullest degree, listening for feelings, listening for underlying agendas, and repeating them back to the person. This technique represents empathy, which is a desirable listening characteristic. If it is joined with other characteristics of good personal interaction, such as warmth and genuineness, chances of effective communication are enhanced. A great risk in dealing with a difficult person is to react by also becoming difficult (i.e., by becoming angry, by attacking, or by retreating into silence or helplessness). In dealing with difficult people, one must work constantly to enhance self-awareness, to know when one is starting to get upset, to have an early warning system, and to recognize one's own danger signals.

When deciding to relate assertively to a difficult person, it is important to understand one's own rights. Davis et al.,[13] in the *Relaxation and Stress Reduction Workbook,* list legitimate human rights as including the right to make mistakes, the right to protest unfair treatment or criticism, the right to interrupt to ask for clarification, the right to negotiate for change, the right to say no, and the right not to take responsibility for someone else's problems. Assertive behavior is characterized by respecting self and others, and speaking up for oneself while letting others speak up for themselves. Passive behavior allows one to be pushed around and bulldozed. This outcome is particularly likely in relation to an aggressive person who fights, accuses, threatens, or intimidates.

In ongoing interactions with another person who has been difficult, the LADDER script described by Davis, et al.[13] provides an assertive approach (see box).

Assertive behavior interacts with one's beliefs and feelings. Which persons are difficult depends on both persons—one's beliefs, biases, patience, and mood at the moment. One has the power to make everyone easy. "There is nothing good or bad but thinking makes it so."

The LADDER script

"**L**ook at your rights.

Arrange a good time and place for discussion of the problem.

Define the problem as specifically as possible.

Describe your feelings in order to help the other person understand you.

Express your requests simply and explicitly.

Reinforce the other person's cooperation by having something to offer in return."

"The mind can make a heaven of hell, a hell of heaven." "Never say that person's words make me angry; always say I react with anger to that person's words." Realistically, that kind of serene stance is an ideal to which we may all aspire, but which none of us reach.

Time management

People in all age groups increasingly report that they feel they are in a "rat race," that they have no time, that a great stress in their life is the pressure of trying to get everything done in insufficient time. Standard time management strategies require record keeping of how time is actually spent to identify time wasters and exclude them from your repertoire. Time management strategies include categorizing goals into those most desired, those that can be delayed, and those that could be put off forever without making much of a difference. The goals can then be separated into 1-month, 1-year, and lifetime goals, with specific plans developed for at least one goal in each category.[30]

Special ways for parents to help stressed children, teens, and themselves

Parents can be effective "change agents," particularly by using positive reinforcement. They can improve a child's behavior regardless of the cause of the problem; they can decrease undesirable behaviors while at the same time increasing desired behaviors. Undesired behaviors must not just be decreased; they must be replaced with alternative positive behaviors. Positive reinforcement is anything that increases the likelihood that a behavior will occur again. The best reinforcers are "naturally occurring." Other examples are verbal and written praise, nods, smiles, stickers, and stars.

Punishment is generally less effective than positive reinforcement because it does not teach the child what do. Physical punishment teaches wrong behavior (how to hit; that physical aggression is an acceptable way to solve problems). Punishment is most effective if administered immediately, with an explanation of what is wrong, why it is wrong, and what could be done instead.

Time out to remove the child from the reinforcing situation is most effective when it is done calmly and the child is told why he or she is in time out and what must happen to leave. Time out should be kept short (a timer may be used) and contingent on better behavior. The time out area must be boring and not fun.

Give clear messages of what is expected. Repeat frequently. When possible, post a list of expectations.

Remember, the goal is to increase desirable behaviors and decrease undesirable behaviors. The following techniques can be useful for rule-breaking children:

1. Use systematic attention. Attention, whether to good or bad behavior, is reinforcing. Therefore, reinforce desirable behavior by attending to it; decrease undesirable behavior by ignoring it.
2. Use soft reprimands. Friends and siblings can reinforce acting out behavior. Do not call attention to misbehavior by yelling. Speaking softly also keeps the parent calmer and better able to cope.
3. Use "I messages." This lets the child know the impact of his/her behavior on others. It encourages more development (e.g., "When you do _____, I feel _____, and _____ may happen.").
4. Allow appropriate expression of negative emotions. It is okay to feel angry, sad, disappointed, etc. Children need to express appropriately.
5. Look for positives. Find strengths and likable qualities in children. Build on these qualities.
6. Change expectations. Don't ask too much of a child. Reevaluate and adjust goals.

Specific techniques with anxious/withdrawn children

Anxious and withdrawn children respond to physical closeness and touch. The presence of a calm adult may give the anxious child more courage. Be calm, self-assuring, and warm with these children. Speak quietly, offer unsolicited explanations of what might happen, how something might feel, etc. Gradually increase demands.

When dealing with children at risk, remember that behavior is what counts, that rewarded behavior is repeated, that rewards are internalized so they don't need to be given forever, and that nothing will work well without love and intimacy, warmth, genuineness, and empathy. Low self-esteem underlies almost all undesirable behavior.

It is important to help children and teens feel understood, even when their behaviors or opinions seem strange, silly, or thoughtless. Listen and say something supportive. Discussing, listening, empathizing, negotiating, and compromising are all preferable to ignoring, threatening, retaliating, giving false reassurance, becoming defensive, or setting unenforceable limits.

Helping teens

Too often, families jump headlong from concern to solution. This approach is like a physician ordering surgery when the patient merely complains of a pain. What's missing is diagnosis, considering different solutions, a joint agreement to try out one solution, and an alternate plan. Remember to go one step at a time. Impulsive problem solving helps prove the diction: "The problem is not the problem, the solution is." Solutions that make the original problem worse and/or add another problem only increase stress.

The parental attitude "do as I say, not as I do" is one of the major stressors for teens. Adults often act is if their teenagers could hear their every lecture, yet not see what they do. A second parental stressor is talking without listening. The most essential ingredient of effective communication with teenagers is listening to their feelings and communicating understanding. Another stressor is disciplining through power, which parents lose as teenagers grow up. Adults have to learn ways of persuading, negotiating, and compromising if they are to remain effective yet loving parents. They must learn to set limits that they can enforce. Consult your teenager. Discuss values and behavior, responsibilities and privileges, and rewards and punishments.

If parents don't like their teenager's friends, it is appropriate to ask why the teenager has chosen those friends. If the friends are in trouble, it may indicate that the teenager is in trouble, too, with a need for some appropriate intervention. If their teenager is not in trouble, objections to the friends may simply reflect rules and rigidities, and flexibility may be indicated.

Just as parents should not rule their teenagers by raw power, teenagers should not be allowed to tyrannize the house. Phone use, TV, and stereos are all privileges to be used responsibly. Parents need to set a good example and negotiate a system fair to the whole family.

The two kinds of discipline—discipline imposed from outside and self-discipline—are often negatively related: the more external the discipline, the less inner discipline is developed. Frequently, teenagers raised under extremely tight controls tend to run wild after leaving home because they have not had opportunities to develop self-discipline. Self-discipline is best taught by example. One of the best ways to give teenagers some discipline is to swallow a good dose of it first. Rule by reason is preferable to rule by fear, and rule by negotiation is preferable to rule by mandate.

One must also negotiate consistency in discipline with one's spouse—compromise. Get advice from an objective outside authority. Once a system is chosen, evaluate it. If it doesn't work, figure out why and change it. If a spouse's ideas don't work, avoid blame, and don't fight about it in front of your teenager. As parents, it's important to be consistent and present a united picture to the teenager.

One of the principles in developing good communication is to listen. It's important to accept what the other person says, even if one doesn't agree with it. By rephrasing what the other person says, one ensures understanding. Encourage talk by nods or in other ways to indicate that listening is taking place. If feelings are involved, label them. Empathize with the teenager's feelings. Give the gift of understanding. Avoid judging feelings. Feel free to state personal feelings and ideas but take full responsibility for them and don't try to impose them on the teenager.

Professionals can help teenagers manage stress and stress reactions. They can help them develop more appropriate expectations of themselves and the world, teach them ways to relax, help them feel good about themselves, and increase their self-esteem. Professionals can help families improve communication, manage anger, solve problems, resolve conflicts, influence behavior by reward, drop destructive patterns, and strengthen healthy habits.

Self-help groups. Social support protects one in stressful situations. Loving and caring friends and family help reduce stress reactivity. Self-help groups offer social support and acceptance along with a shared focus on a particular problem area. The *Healthy People 2000*[56] report states:

> During the past decade, autonomous mutual help groups have gained increasing recognition as complementary to clinical practice. Often referred to as self-help organizations, their members include people who share or have shared specific physical, mental, or emotional problems. These groups make significant contributions to positive outcomes for persons affected by mental and behavioral disorders, including the family members and formal and informal care givers of individuals with chronic conditions. An estimated 10 to 15 million people are members of mutual help groups in the United States, with 1.9 million adults turning to nonprofessional mutual help resources for personal or emotional problems in the course of a year.[32]

To locate a group that fits your need, national self-help clearinghouses can point the way (see Resources).

Psychotherapy

The goal of psychotherapy is to identify patterns of thought, feeling, and action so as to discover which of them are healthy and which are unhealthy. Then strategies are aimed at reducing the latter and strengthening the former. There are many psychotherapies and many psychotherapists. It is important to be able to establish rapport with the therapist and believe in the particular therapy approach. Ask about the therapist's experience with specific problems and about data on clinical and cost effectiveness for the kind of therapy being offered. Local mental health associations can provide information about available psychotherapists.

Psychopharmacology

The *Healthy People 2000*[56] report states:

> Psychopharmacologic interventions have proven to be highly effective in the treatment of mental disorders and are in wide-spread use. Psychotherapeutic agents accounted for one quarter of all outpatient prescriptions in 1984. There is growing evidence, however, that the effectiveness of pharmacologic interventions is enhanced by psychosocial interventions that are specifically designed and empirically tested.[24]

Various medications, as discussed in other chapters in this text, can be demonstrably helpful in managing stress symptoms.

Exercise and diet

Exercise and diet are important for conditioning one to respond to stress in a healthier manner. These approaches are reviewed at length in other chapters.

SUMMARY

Many strategies work to relieve stress. Although stress is unavoidable, it can be managed. Look over this list for ideas of ways to reduce stress. Try them out one at time, practice them often until they are learned.

- Exercise. Try physical activity to release tension—whether by walking, housework, or some sport. Walk as much as possible.
- Talk. Bottling up feelings increases stress. Talk over problems with a friend, family member, or counselor. Keep building channels to give and to receive support.
- Accept what can't be changed. Don't waste energy fighting something that can't be changed.
- Limit "worry time." If you worry too much, try to take control of it. Allow a limited time to worry every day and don't allow worry at any other time.
- Give in now and then. Work out conflicts with others so that no one suffers. Know when to back down a little.
- Don't try to "climb a mountain" when you're tired. Be aware of peak energy times and try to use them to maximum advantage. Tackle harder tasks at these times.
- Listen to your body. Be aware of your stress signals—sweaty hands, sore eyes, overeating, stiff neck, tiredness, rapid heart beat, headaches, etc. Stop and take a break by deep breathing, stretching, walking, or some other activity.
- Laugh! Have fun. Laughter is a great stress reliever. Look for ways to have fun and laugh. Look for humor in stressful situations.
- Avoid too many changes. Try to spread out the major changes in life such as changing jobs, getting married, taking a big loan, etc.
- Learn to say "NO!" Practice ways of saying "NO" or dealing with unreasonable requests to avoid feeling hassled or overloaded.
- It's okay to do nothing sometimes. Find a quiet place to unwind—even if it's just a comfortable chair.

Ways to ease stress

Eat and drink sensibly. (For healthy food and drink guidelines, see Chapter 22.

Assert yourself. You do not have to meet others' expectations or demands. It's okay to say "no." Remember being assertive allows you to stand up for your rights and beliefs while respecting those of others.

Stop smoking or other bad habits. Aside from the obvious health risks of cigarettes, nicotine acts as a stimulant and brings on more stress symptoms. Sometimes less can be more. Give yourself the gift of dropping unhealthy habits.

Exercise regularly. Choose noncompetitive exercise with reasonable goals. Aerobic exercise has been shown to release endorphins, a natural substance that helps you feel better and maintain a positive, upbeat attitude. (For specific guidelines, see Chapter 18.)

Study and practice relaxation techniques. Relax every day choosing from a variety of different techniques. Combining opposites—a time for deep relaxation and a time for aerobic exercise—is a sure fire way to inoculate your body from the effects of stress.

Take responsibility. Control what you can and leave behind what you cannot. When in doubt, think of the serenity prayer: *"Grant me the serenity to accept the things I cannot change, the courage to change the things I can and the wisdom to know the difference."*

Reduce stressors. Many people find life synonymous with too many demands and too little time. For the most part, these demands are ones we have chosen. Effective time-management skills involve delegating where appropriate, setting priorities (e.g., Does your house really have to be spotless?), pacing yourself, and taking time out for yourself.

Examine your values and live by them. The more your actions are in accordance with your beliefs, the better you will feel, no matter how busy your life is. Use this value when choosing your activities.

Set realistic goals and expectations. It's okay and healthy to realize you cannot be 100% successful at all things at once.

Sell yourself to yourself. When you are feeling overwhelmed, remind yourself of what you do well. Have a healthy sense of self-esteem.

- Plan ahead and plan to wait. Whenever possible, try to think ahead and avoid stress. For example, prepare for morning the night before. Don't rely on memory for addresses, directions, or appointments. Write them down. Be prepared to wait. Bring along a book or magazine.
- Take control of yourself even if you can't control the situation. When faced with stressful situations that you cannot control, work on your response to that situation. For example, when sitting in a traffic jam, try using a relaxation technique.
- Unwind after a stressful time. Reward yourself after stressful activities with something relaxing—a book, a TV show, lunch with a friend, or a leisurely bath.
- Break down large tasks into small parts. Decide which tasks are most important and do those first.
- Get enough sleep.
- Stop negative thinking before it overwhelms you. Be aware of overly negative thoughts. Substitute reasonable and positive thoughts.
- Make physical contact with loved ones. Hold hands, stroke a pet, or hug.
- Set realistic goals. Remember that the "success formulas" that work for others won't necessarily work for you.
- Notice your breathing. Try to take some slow deep breaths when feeling stressed.
- Think of stress as something to work on. Try to change the words used to think about sources of stress. Words, even in thoughts, affect attitudes and actions. Instead of thinking of the source of stress as a "problem," try thinking of it as a "project."

- Be positive. Try to look for and concentrate on the positive. Don't dwell on the negative.
- Learn from mistakes. When failures occur, be sure to remember past successes. Work out how to handle the situation better in the future.
- Choose words carefully. When speaking with someone else, be careful how you express yourself.
- Try delaying reactions to stressful situations or comments. For example, count to 10 before reacting.
- Learn a relaxation skill such as meditation or deep muscle relaxation.
- Imagine how you want things to be. Think about how you could handle expected stressful situations effectively. Picture yourself being successful.

We usually hand out the preceding suggestions adapted from materials of the Ohio Department of Mental Health, Pawtucket Heart Health Program, and Ohio Department of Health assembled by Hypertension Control and Cardiovascular Disease Prevention Program, Division of Chronic Diseases, Ohio Department of Health. We also hand out the summary represented in the acronym: Ease Stress (see box above).

The research describing the relationship between life stress and disease can be summarized briefly. The results are equivocal and contradictory but overall strongly suggest that stress is one of the factors in the cause-and-effect chain in the etiology of many diseases. The research is nomothetic; it looks for statistical relationships that hold across groups in which general principles of relationship exist. Clinical work is idiographic. It deals with individuals, and the challenge to the clinician is to define the way in which stress is relevant for each patient.

Excessive stress impairs mental health as well as physical health, reduces effectiveness at many tasks, and often contributes to bad habits that are intended to relieve tension. Assessing stress reactions and stressors can help the physician help patients change both themselves and their environments to reduce the negative effects of stress. In time this approach will contribute to improving the health, happiness, and effectiveness of the population and reduce mental health costs.

REFERENCES

1. American Psychiatric Association: *Diagnostic and statistical manual of mental disorders,* ed 3, Washington DC, 1987, APA.
2. Asterita ME: *The physiology of stress: with special reference to the neuroendocrine system,* New York, 1985, Human Sciences Press.
3. Beattie M: Co-dependent no more: how to stop controlling others and start caring for yourself, San Francisco, 1987, Harper & Row.
4. Benson H: The relaxation response, New York, 1976, Avon Books.
5. Berger KS: The developing person through the life span, New York, 1983, Worth Publishers.
6. Black C: *It will never happen to me,* Colorado, 1980, Medical Administration.
7. Blumenthal SJ: Suicide: a guide to risk factors, assessment and treatment of suicidal patients, *Med Clin North Am* 72:937-971, 1988.
8. Bradshaw J: *Bradshaw on: the family,* Dearfield Beach, Fla, 1988, Health Communications, Inc.
9. Caine L: *Being a widow,* New York, 1988, Penguin Books.
10. Cannon WB: *Bodily changes in pain, hunger, fear and rage,* ed 2, Boston, 1953, CT Branford Co.
11. Coleman RM: *Wide awake at 3 a.m. By choice or by chance,* New York, 1986 WH Freeman & Co.
12. Cummings N, Vanderbos G: The 20 year Kaiser-Permanente experience with psychotherapy and medical utilization, *Health Care Policy Q* 1(2), 1981.
13. Davis M, Eshelman ER, McKay M: *The relaxation and stress reduction workbook,* ed 3, Oakland, Calif, 1988, New Harbinger Publications.
14. Duvall EM: *Family development,* ed 4, New York, 1971 JB Lippincott.
15. Einstein E: *The step-family: living, loving and learning.* Boston, 1985, Shambhala.
16. Elite A: Stress management program. AFP Background Paper. San Francisco, California Department of Mental Health, July, 1986.
17. Elkind D: *The hurried child: growing up too fast too soon,* Reading, Mass, 1981, Addison-Wesley Publishing.
18. Ellis A, Harper RA: A new guide to rational living, North Hollywood, 1975, Wilshire Books.
19. Freudenberger H: *Burnout: How to beat the high cost of success,* New York, 1981, Bantam Books.
20. Fried R: *The hyperventilation syndrome: research and clinical treatment,* Baltimore, 1987, Johns Hopkins University Press.
21. Friedman M, Rosenman R: *Type "A" behavior and your heart,* New York, 1974, Alfred Knopf.
22. Friedman M, Ulmer D: *Treating Type "A" behavior and your heart.* New York, 1984, Alfred A. Knopf.
23. Good MD, et al: Patient requests in primary health care settings: development and validation of a research instrument, *J Behav Med* 6:151-168, 1983.
24. Hogarty GE: Social work research on severe mental illness: charting a future. Paper prepared for the NIMH Task Force on Social Work Research, Workshop on Social Work Research and Community-Based Mental Health Services, Bethesda, Md, 1989.
25. Holmes TH, Rahe RH: The social readjustment rating scale, *J Psychosom Res* 11:213-218, 1967.
26. Humphrey JH: *Stress in childhood,* New York, 1984, AMS Press.
27. Jacobson E: *You must relax,* New York, 1957, McGraw-Hill.
28. Karasek R, Theoreil T: *Healthy work: stress, productivity, and the reconstruction of working life,* New York, 1990, Basic Books.
29. Karraker KA, Lake M: *Normative stress and coping processes in lifespan developmental psychology: perspectives on stress and coping,* Hillsdale, NJ, 1991, Lawrence Erlbaum.
30. Lakein A: How to get control of your life and your time, New York 1973, Signet Books.
31. Lazarus RS, Folkman S: *Stress, appraisal and coping,* New York, 1991, Springer.
32. Louis Harris Associates Inc: A Study of the Sources, Correlates and Manifestations of Perceived and Experienced Stress in the United States. DHHS Contact No. 282-85-0063. Report submitted to the Office of Disease Prevention and Health Promotion, Department of Health and Human Services, 1985.
33. Maslach F: *Burnout—the cost of caring,* New York, 1986, Prentice-Hall.
34. Matthews KA, Weiss SM, Detre T, et al: *Handbook of stress, reactivity and cardiovascular disease,* New York, 1986, John Wiley and Sons.
35. McLeroy K, Green L, Mullen K, et al: Assessing the effects of health promotion in work sites: a review of the stress management evaluation, *Edu Q* 11(4):379-401, 1984.
36. McKee MG: Mixed messages and missed messages: communications gone awry. In Eisenberg MG, Falconer J, Sutkin LC, editors: *Communications in a health care setting,* Springfield, Ill, 1980, Charles C. Thomas.
37. Meichenbaum D: A self-instructional approach to stress-management: a proposal for stress-inoculation training. In Sarason I, Spielberger CD, editors: *Stress and anxiety,* vol 2, New York, 1975, John Wiley.
38. Nathan R: Effects of a stress management course on grades and health of the first year medical student. *J Med Edu* 62:514-517, 1987.
39. Northwestern National Life Insurance Co: *Employee burnout: America's newest epidemic,* 1991.
40. Offord DR: Conduct disorder: risk factors and prevention. In Shaffer D, et al, editors: *Prevention of mental disorders, alcohol and other drug use in children and adolescents,* Rockville, Md, 1989, US Department of Health and Human Services.
41. Paine RW: *We never had any trouble before,* New York, 1975, Stin and Dade.
42. Palmer S: *Role stress,* Englewood Cliffs, NJ, 1981, Prentice-Hall.
43. Pelletier K: *Mind as healer, mind as slayer,* New York, 1977, Dell Publishing.
44. Pelletier K, Herzing D: Psychoneuroimmunology: toward a mind and body model—a critical review. Advances, *J Advance Health* 5(1):27-56, 1988.
45. Pelletier KB, Lutz RW: Healthy people—healthy business: a critical review of stress management programs in the workplace. In Weiss SM, Fielding JE, Baum A, editors: *Perspectives in behavioral medicine: health at work,* Hillsdale NJ, 1991, Lawrence Erlbaum Associates.
46. Peterson C, Prout MF, Schwarz RA: *Post-traumatic stress disorder: a clinician's guide,* New York, 1991, Plenum Press.
47. Prochaska JO, Velicer WF, DiClemente CC, et al: Measuring process of change: application for the cessation of smoking, *J Consult Clinic Psychol* 56:520-528, 1988.
48. Roskies E: *Stress management for the healthy Type A,* New York, 1987, The Guilford Press.
49. Schwartz M, et al: *Biofeedback: a practitioner's guide,* New York, 1987, Guilford Press.

50. Seamonds B: Extension of research into stress factors and their effect on illness absenteeism, *J Occup Med* 25(1):821-822, 1983.
51. Selye H: *Stress in health and disease,* Boston, 1976, Butterworths.
52. Sternbach RA: *Principles of psychology. An introductory text and readings,* New York, 1966, Academic Press.
53. Strauss J, et al: The course of psychiatric disorder. III. Longitudinal principles, *Am J Psychiatry* 143:289-296, 1985.
54. Stroebel CF: *QR the quieting reflex,* New York, 1982, GP Putnam's Sons.
55. Toffler A: *Future shock,* New York, 1970, Random House.
56. US Department of Health and Human Services Public Health Service: *Healthy people 2000: national health promotion and disease prevention objectives,* Washington DC, 1990, US Government Printing Office.
57. Webb JT, McNamara KM, Rodgers DA: *Configural interpretations of the MMPI and CPI,* Columbus, Ohio, 1981, Ohio Psychological Publishing.
58. Wilbur R: *Poems of Richard Wilbur,* New York, 1963, Harcourt Brace Jovanovich.
59. Willing JZ: *The reality of retirement: the inner experience of becoming a retired person,* New York, 1981, William Morrow.
60. Wilson ES, Schneider C: The neurophysiologic pathways of disstress, *Stress/Pain Management Newsletter,* May-June 1981.

■ RESOURCES ■

Alcoholics Anonymous AA World Services, PO Box 459, Grand Central Station, New York, NY 10017.

American Association of Suicidology, 2459 S. Ash, Denver CO 80222.

American Psychiatric Association, 1700 18th Street, NW, Washington, DC 20009.

American Psychological Association, 750 First Street, NE, Washington, DC 20002-4242.

Association for Applied Psychophysiology and Biofeedback, 10200 West 44th Avenue, Suite 304, Wheatridge, CO 80033.

Association of Retired Persons, Widowed Persons Service, 1909 K Street, NW, Washington, DC 20049.

Battered Women Self-Help, Victims Services Agency, Two Lafayette Street, New York, NY 10007.

Children of Aging Parents (CAP), 2761 Trenton Road, Levittown, PA 19056.

Displaced Homemakers Network, 1411 K St, NW, Suite 930, Washington, DC 20005.

Emotions Anonymous, PO Box 4245, St Paul, MN 55104.

Growing Through Grief, PO Box 269, Arnold, MD 21012.

The League of Women Voters, 1730 M St, NW, Washington, DC 20036.

The National Council on Aging (NCOA), 600 Maryland Avenue, SW, West Wing 100, Washington, DC 20024.

National Council of Senior Citizens, 925 15th St, NW, Washington, DC 20005.

National Institute on Aging (NIA), 10000 Rockville Pike, Building 31, Room 5C35, Bethesda, MD 20205.

National Self-Help Clearinghouse, City University of New York Graduate Center, 22 W. 42nd Street, New York, NY 10036.

Older Women's League (OWL), 730 Eleventh Street, NW Suite 300, Washington, DC 20001.

Parents Without Partners, 8807 Colesville Road, Silver Springs, MD 20910.

Retired Senior Volunteer Program (RSVP), 806 Connecticut Avenue, NW Room M-1006, Washington, DC 20525.

Self-Help Clearinghouse, St. Clares-Riverside Medical Center, Denville, NJ 07834.

Self-Help Center, 1600 Dodge Avenue Suite S-122, Evanston, IL 60201.

Suicide Prevention Center, 184 Salem Street, Dayton, OH 45406.

Chapter 13

WOMEN'S ISSUES

Lilian Gonsalves
Gita Gidwani

"Frailty, thy name is woman." So wrote William Shakespeare at a time when he did not know about actuarial tables or the genetic advantages of the XX chromosomes. Over the last two decades an unprecedented expansion of knowledge and literature in the field of women's health has changed our beliefs and expectations about women's roles and identity in the context of work, family, and community. This chapter presents an overview of problems particular to women, especially depression, premenstrual syndrome, alcoholism, and violence, and addresses specific management and preventive strategies so that women can lead a fuller measure of health and a better quality of life.

CHANGING TIMES

Myths surrounding dysmenorrhea, menstruation, premenstrual syndrome, and menopause have always existed. Hippocrates suggested fumigation of external genitals by vapors of sweet wine, fennel seed, and root and rose oil. Chinese medicine recommended moxibustion, which involves a cone of wormwood on a slice of ginger placed on the abdomen, set aflame, and allowed to burn down to the skin. In 1865 Dr. Robert Battey in Georgia performed bilateral oophorectomy to cure dysmenorrhea, and in 1907 Polano claimed relief of dysmenorrhea by applying suction cups to the breasts.[30]

Victorians treated menstruation as an illness and believed that dysmenorrhea could be prevented or relieved by seclusion and rest with a minimum of needle work and piano playing and absolutely no singing. These traditional, negative attitudes towards menstruation, along with cultural taboos and religious beliefs involving isolation and ritual cleansing, exist in some cultures even today. It is not surprising then that in a random sample of 19-year-old Swedish women, 72% of whom reported dysmenorrhea,

only one fifth (21%) consulted a physician, although dysmenorrhea affected more than half of them quite severely, resulting in absenteeism from work or school.[6] Perhaps women accept dysmenorrhea as normal and do not believe that treatment is available. Studies of tracings of uterine contractions in both normal and dysmenorrheic women, the discovery of prostaglandins as a pathophysiologic explanation for the pain of dysmenorrhea, the relief of dysmenorrhea from oral contraceptives and nonsteroidal antiinflammatory drugs have all helped negate the psychogenic origin of dysmenorrhea.[3,19]

Premenstrual syndrome is no longer thought of as "a virgin's disease because in ancient time any woman who was married was usually pregnant."[22] Romans in the second century believed that "the menses are about to appear when a woman feels uneasy walking." Neither are menopausal women "peevish, irritable, morose and depressed."[61] Nor is it "a woman's last traumatic experience as a sexual being and an incurable narcissistic wound."[22] Exponential work in the field of reproductive neuroendocrinology has put such myths to rest.

Women today enjoy reproductive freedom because of landmark events that have taken place in the field of contraception and sterilization. Margaret Higgens Sanger (1883-1966), a nurse and daughter of a stonecutter father and tubercular mother (of Corning, New York,) observed women in the poorer sections of New York City who by the age of 35 were exhausted from repeated pregnancies or dead from self-induced abortions. Sanger undertook a study of contraception in Scotland[82] and later founded the International Planned Parenthood Federation in 1952. Her prime objective was liberation of women from "sexual servitude." Joined in her endeavors by a prominent gynecologist, Robert Latou Dickinson, Sanger encouraged research that led to the introduction of the birth control pill. This breakthrough was followed by sterilization by tubal ligation in 1970 and the advent of the laparoscope shortly thereafter. The easy availability of laparoscopic tubal ligation has made sterilization a safe and popular method of contraception for many women in the last two decades. All of these scientific developments have enabled women to be more autonomous and in control of their lives.

CHANGING ROLES

Freud, in 1933, stated "a man of about 30 strikes us as a youthful, somewhat unformed individual whom we expect to make powerful use of the possibilities for development opened up to him by analysis. A woman of the same age, however, often frightens us by her psychical rigidity and unchangeability."[27] Freud also formulated the feminine personality triad of "passivity, masochism, and narcissism" and proposed that the female superego is weak. Gilligan[31] criticized this approach as deriving from a male model and perspective and reflecting primarily male development. Important evidence is also emerging from other areas of the psychologic field. Baker and Miller[7] at the Wellesley College's Stone Center for Development Services and Studies have written that women have been socialized to view their relationships with others as central to their lives. Caring and providing support therefore is a woman's particular province and it is not surprising that women suffer more than men from the "contagion of stress." Women's lives are affected by the roles they take on (i.e., wife, mother, worker, caretaker). Whereas past generations of women organized their lives primarily to meet family-related objectives, some combination of work and family is a life-style preference for most American women today. Less than 12% of families today are "typical" (i.e., the father is the wage earner and mother is home with several children).[54] In 50% of marriages, both partners are employed, and 70% of married women with children under the age of 18 are in the work force.[49] By the year 2000 half of the women in the work force will be between the ages of 35 to 54, a shift from 1986 when the majority were between 25 and 44.[86]

Employment

Employment is associated with improved mental health when husbands help with child care. Mothers who have no difficulty arranging child care and who have husbands who share child care have very low depression levels.[71] Women who have the most complete role configuration as wife, parent, or worker experience fewer depressive symptoms than those who do not participate in marriage, parenthood, and employment.[48] Those women who have less education, low income, low socioeconomic status and who are unemployed are at a high risk for depression.[70]

Marital status

Marital status is another important role to consider. Weissman[87] reported in an Epidemiologic Catchment Area

(ECA) study that marriage conferred a greater protective advantage on men than on women, suggesting that psychologic symptoms in women are not intrinsic to femaleness, but to the conditions of subordination that characterize traditional female roles. Unhappily married women experience more depressive symptoms than either happily married or unmarried women. Women are three times as likely as men to be depressed in unhappy marriages. The number of women with young children who experience high levels of stress and depression is highest in single mothers with young children at home.[14] Along with child rearing, many women are also responsible for aging parents, the so-called "sandwich generation." This stress is also likely to increase the risk of depression.

Juggling multiple roles can be irritating, frustrating, and distressing; when these demands exceed a woman's resources for managing them, stress and strain result. Consequences of role strain include strained personal relationships, declining physical health, anger and hostility, dissatisfaction, anxiety, alcoholism, and depression.

Managing multiple roles

It is clear that role stress and strain are decreased if a woman's spouse approves and supports her choices and the woman is satisfied with her job, has no financial problems, and creates time for family activities. Dissatisfaction with child care, lack of a support network, and a poor coping style increase strain.

Paying attention to one's feelings and needs, regular exercise, relaxation techniques, and biofeedback are some ways of preventing stress. Others include provision of affordable, professional day care and child care facilities, foster grandparents, maternity and paternity leave policies, modification of men's career patterns, and better attention to the mental health needs of boys so that they can be prepared to anticipate more marital and domestic responsibilities.

WOMEN AND DEPRESSION

Women's risk for depression exceeds that of men by 2:1. This finding is consistent in the literature, occurs throughout many different countries and ethnic groups, and persists when income level, education, and occupation are controlled.[60] The incidence of bipolar illness, however, is equally reported in men and women.[87]

Why the gender difference in depression? It has been suggested that female gender role socialization produces maladaptive coping styles that increase the risk of developing depression. Women have been socialized to be passive, submissive and dependent and, therefore, have less perceived life control than men. This "learned helplessness training" predisposes women to depression.[77] As Guttentag and Salisan[34] have concluded, "Stress and powerlessness apparently are the deadly combination." In response to dysphoria, men tend to be more "instrumental" and engage in physical activities to distract them from their mood; women tend to be expressive and ruminative about the causes of their mood.[10] Help-seeking is not as threatening to the feminine image, and we know that women do report symptoms more readily and are more likely to seek help. Reproductive events, family and work roles, victimization, personality variables, social factors, and poverty are other factors associated with depression in women.[53]

Depression and reproductive factors

The extensive association of mood disorders around the time of reproductive endocrine change in some women cannot be ignored. A disproportionate occurrence of suicide attempts and psychiatric admission, occurring during the paramenstruum, postpartum, and menopause have been noted in the literature. Premenstrual syndrome (PMS), postpartum affective illness, and depression at midlife are discussed here.

Premenstrual syndrome. As a result of increased awareness of the phenomenon of PMS, women with menstrual cycle-linked cognitive, affective, and physical symptoms continue to seek help in ever-rising numbers. PMS, however, is not a new entity. Aristotle once said: "A menstruous woman would dull a mirror with a look and the next person to look into it would be bewitched." The first scientific paper about PMS was written by Frank,[25] an American gynecologist, in 1931, who summarized 15 cases of women with premenstrual symptoms. PMS research efforts have been ongoing since then, but past research has been compromised by serious methodologic problems, including unsophisticated methods of patient selection, no agreed upon definition of the syndrome, mainly open uncontrolled studies as opposed to double-blind placebo-controlled trials, and retrospective rating of symptoms, which tends to overestimate the prevalence of PMS.[1,24,32]

DSM III-R has tried to address these methodologic research problems by defining late luteal phase dysphoric disorder (LLPDD)[5] (see box at right). A diagnosis of LLPDD is made when at least five of the following symptoms occur in the last week of the luteal phase and remit within a few days of the onset of menses: affective lability, marked anger/irritability, tension, decreased interest in usual activities, fatigue, change in appetite, sleep problems, or physical symptoms such as bloating. These symptoms must interfere with work, social activities, or relationships and must be confirmed prospectively by daily self-rating during at least two symptomatic cycles. DSM III-R further advised that the disturbance is not merely an exacerbation of another psychiatric disorder such as major depression, dysthymia, or panic.

Etiologies. Numerous etiologies and explanatory models have been postulated to account for the constellation of premenstrual symptoms. Rubinow and Schmidt[73] recently discussed four models for understanding the development and expression of symptoms in PMS:

1. Biochemical or endocrine (i.e., decreased progesterone, elevated estrogen, elevated estrogen progesterone ratio, elevated prolactin).
2. Symptom exaggeration of special sensitivity model in PMS, which may represent an abnormal mood, behavioral, and somatic response to normal menstrual physiology.
3. PMS as a variant of affective disorder (i.e., it represents an entrainment of mood and behavioral changes with the menstrual cycle). Some evidence suggests that the occurrence of repetitive episodes in premenstrual depression may influence the develop-

---

Diagnostic criteria for LLPDD disorder (DSM III-R)

A. In most menstrual cycles during the past year, symptoms in B occurred during the last week of the luteal phase and remitted within a few days after onset of the follicular phase. In menstruating females, these phases correspond to the week before, and a few days after, the onset of menses. (In non-menstruating females who have had a hysterectomy, the time of luteal and follicular phases may require measurement of circulating reproductive hormones.)

B. At least five of the following symptoms have been present for most of the time during each symptomatic late luteal phase, at least one of the symptoms being either (1), (2), (3), or (4):
    (1) marked affective lability (e.g., feeling suddenly sad, tearful, irritable, or angry)
    (2) persistent and marked anger or irritability
    (3) marked anxiety, tension, feelings of being "keyed up" or "on edge"
    (4) markedly depressed mood, feelings of hopelessness, or self-deprecating thoughts
    (5) decreased interest in usual activities (e.g., work, friends, hobbies)
    (6) easy fatigability or marked lack of energy
    (7) subjective sense of difficulty in concentrating
    (8) marked change in appetite, overeating, or specific food cravings
    (9) hypersomnia or insomnia
    (10) other physical symptoms, such as breast tenderness or swelling, headaches, joint or muscle pain, a sensation of "bloating," weight gain

C. The disturbance seriously interferes with work or with usual social activities or relationships with others.

D. The disturbance is not merely an exacerbation of the symptoms of another disorder, such as major depression, panic disorder, dysthymia, or a personality disorder (although it may be superimposed on any of these disorders).

E. Criteria A, B, C, and D are confirmed by prospective daily self-ratings during at least two symptomatic cycles. (The diagnosis may be made provisionally prior to this confirmation.)

Modified from Diagnostic and Statistical Manual of Mental Disorders, ed 3, Appendix A, American Psychiatric Association.

ment of later major depression via a sensitization or kindling phenomenon.

4. PMS as a disorder of state regulation (i.e., it is characterized by a menstrual cycle-linked transition into a particular experiential state, which is usually characterized by dysphoria or irritability).

Schmidt et al.[76] lent support for this model in their study comparing the report of daily life events by women with prospectively confirmed PMS and asymptomatic control subjects. They found that PMS patients reported significantly more negative life events than the control group during the late luteal phase. In addition, PMS patients showed more distress with this event when it occurred premenstrually rather than postmenstrually.[76]

Co-morbidity of PMS and depression is common. Endicott and Halbreich[23] noted that 65% of women with major depressive disorder show signs of premenstrual exacerbation, including increased severity of symptoms, depersonalization, suicidal impulses, and the appearance of physical symptoms such as headache, gastrointestinal distress, and joint or muscle pain. Further, several studies have reported a good therapeutic response of PMS symptoms to antidepressant medications. Other evidence suggests that PMS responds to sleep deprivation, as has been noted in the past with regard to depression.[66] In addition, decreased premenstrual platelet serotonin uptake may occur in patients with PMS, as well as in those with depression.[85]

Fatigue is a common symptom in women seeking treatment for PMS.[75] Endicott et al.[24] noted that 95% of women who sought treatment for PMS reported depression, sleep and appetite changes, and *fatigue* compared with 51% of women who reported premenstrual distress but did not seek treatment. The relationship of PMS to glucose metabolism has also been studied, as symptoms associated with PMS such as fatigue, carbohydrate craving, and increased appetite are also symptoms of hypoglycemia. De Pirro et al.[21] noted a twofold increase in insulin binding to monocytes in the follicular phase as compared with the luteal phase, implying that changes in glucose tolerance may be related to the menstrual cycle. Denicoff et al.[20] however, found no significant difference in the frequency of hypoglycemia between follicular and luteal phases in 11 women who were administered two glucose tolerance tests during different phases of this cycle.

Clinical approach. The first step in making the diagnosis of LLPDD is to take a good history. It is important to gather information about the timing of symptoms relative to the menstrual cycle, and to have patients record symptoms prospectively for two to three consecutive cycles. A basal body temperature chart is helpful in correlating symptoms with the luteal phase. Patients with PMS show a discrete rise in the number and intensity of symptoms in the weeks after ovulation. A history of recurrent pelvic inflammatory disease, irregular painful menstrual cycles—

especially those associated with ovulation—menorrhagia, the use of an IUD, infertility, dyspareunia, cyclic or lower abdominal pain, cramping, and dysmenorrhea must be elicited (see box below). It is important to distinguish secondary dysmenorrhea, which is usually caused by an abnormality in the uterus or an abnormality in the pelvis and is not a symptom of PMS. The well-known causes of secondary dysmenorrhea (i.e., endometriosis [see box below], pelvic inflammatory disease, adenomyosis, uterine myomas, uterine polyps, congenital malformations of the mullerian system, cervical strictures of stenosis, and ovarian cysts) can all be found in these patients. If a careful history is not elicited, these symptoms will be missed and the patient not given a good gynecologic workup.

After obtaining a history, underlying medical and gynecologic diseases must be ruled out. For example, systemic lupus erythematosus, anemia, hypokalemia, and meningiomas can also present with fatigue, headaches, or joint pains. A general, physical, and pelvic examination must be performed to rule out medical causes and gynecologic pathology.

Routine laboratory studies, including complete blood count, electrolytes, kidney and liver profiles, thyroid function studies, estrogen, progesterone, and dehydroepiandrosterone sulfate (DHEAS), are useful in ruling out medical conditions and also in reassuring patients that hormone levels are not out of balance (see box on p. 221). Testosterone or other androgen-measuring hormone levels are useful in patients with symptoms of hirsutism and who complain of acne and severe bloating before their periods. Estrogen measurement, as well as determination of follicular stimulating hormone (FSH) function, is recommended

---

Differential diagnosis in the PMS patient

Pelvic inflammatory disease
Menorrhagia
Irregular, painful cycles, especially if associated with ovulation
Infertility
Primary or secondary dysmenorrhea
Dyspareunia
Use of IUD or oral contraceptives

Causes of secondary dysmenorrhea

Endometriosis
Pelvic inflammatory disease
Adenomyosis
Uterine myomas
Uterine polyps
Cervical stricture/stenosis
Ovarian cysts
Congenital malformation of the mullerian system

Condition	Helpful Tests
For all patients with PMS	CBC, electrolytes, kidney and liver profiles, thyroid function studies, psychologic tests
If perimenopausal symptoms present	Estrogen and FSH levels
For hirsutism, premenstrual acne, or bloating	Testosterone, DHEAS levels
If fibroids, polyps, endometriosis, or pelvic inflammatory disease suspected	Sedimentation rate, culture of the cervix, hysterosalpingography, pelvic sonogram, diagnostic laparoscopy, hysteroscopy, D&C

for patients whose symptoms are suggestive of imminent menopause as such patients benefit from low-dose estrogen. A pelvic sonogram, sedimentation rate, culture of the cervix, hysterosalpingography, diagnostic laparoscopy, hysteroscopy, and dilatation and curettage (D&C) are indicated if local conditions such as fibroids, polyps, or endometriosis are suspected. Psychologic tests, such as the Minnesota Multiphasic Personality Inventory (MMPI)[40] or Beck Depression Inventory,[11] administered a week before and a week after menses often lend objective evidence to the subjective reporting of symptoms.

Psychosocial issues must be evaluated, as the literature reports that women seeking treatment for PMS have a high lifetime history of affective and anxiety disorders. Keye et al.,[50] in a controlled study, noticed that women with premenstrual symptoms had higher scores on the MMPI than control subjects and were more likely to have thought of or attempted suicide. Harrison et al.,[39] in another controlled study, found that women seeking treatment for PMS had a higher lifetime history of depression, suicide attempts, panic disorder, and substance abuse; however, if those women with a primary psychiatric diagnosis were excluded, the incidence of these factors did not differ significantly between the PMS population and a control group. Psychiatric evaluation, therefore, should include a review of symptoms, with particular attention to vegetative symptoms of depression, bulimia, seasonal variation of depression, and alcohol and drug use. Early victimization and trauma also need to be explored, as does a family history of affective disorder and alcoholism.

Often it is necessary to assess spouse and family members to determine if interpersonal and situational stressors play a role. It is important to ask the question, "What brings you to treatment now?" Common responses in our clinic include increased awareness of PMS, worsening of symptoms despite seeing several physicians, being told that symptoms are "in your head," or being appropriately referred by a sensitive health care worker.

Experience at the Cleveland Clinic. The Premenstrual Syndrome Clinic of the Cleveland Clinic Foundation is conducted weekly in conjunction with the Departments of Gynecology, Nutrition, and Psychiatry. Patients presenting to the PMS Clinic prospectively rate and record the symp-

toms and basal body temperatures for two or three menstrual cycles and complete a standardized questionnaire pertaining to their medical history and an MMPI 1 week before and 1 week after a period. They are tested for thyroid dysfunction routinely; and estrogen, progesterone, FSH, and DHEAS levels are drawn on as needed. The patient is examined by a gynecologist, who takes a medical history and performs a pelvic examination, a psychiatrist who administers a semistructured interview, and a nutritionist who assesses whether dietary factors may be contributing to symptoms. The diagnosis of PMS is made through a team decision by examining symptom cards, correlating symptoms with basal body temperature graphs to confirm that the symptoms occur during the premenstruum, excluding a primary psychiatric diagnosis, and ruling out medical or gynecologic pathology that could account for symptoms.

We recently reviewed a series of 123 patients seen from November of 1987 to November of 1989. Of these women, 37.4% (n = 46) were diagnosed with PMS, 52.8% (n = 65) were given a psychiatric diagnosis, and 9.8% (n = 12) were believed to have a primary medical or gynecologic diagnosis.

Of those with a psychiatric diagnosis (Table 13-1), the most common diagnoses were major depression (32.3%) (n = 21) and adjustment disorder with depressed mood (29.3%) (n = 19). Other diagnoses were dysthymia (n = 7), marital discord (n = 6), alcohol abuse (n = 4), somatoform pain disorder (n = 3), personality disorder (n = 3), generalized anxiety disorder (n = 1), and grief reaction (n = 1). Of those with medical or gynecologic pathology (n = 12), the most common diagnoses were menopause (41.7%) (n = 5) and endometriosis (33.3%) (n = 4). One patient had irregular menses, one patient had a seizure disorder, and another had an ovarian cyst. These findings suggest that associated gynecologic and psychiatric disorders are often misdiagnosed as PMS, emphasizing again the need for a careful multidisciplinary evaluation.

Of the patients presenting with PMS (n = 46), the age range was from 26 to 44, with an average age of 35.2. The sample was predominantly physician referred, white, married or divorced (19.6% were single), and highly educated (only 6.5% had not completed high school). It is unclear

Table 13-1. Medical/gynecologic problems and psychiatric diagnoses

Problem	n	%	Diagnoses	n	%
Menopause	5	41.7	Major depression	21	32.3
Endometriosis	4	33.3	Adjustment disorder	19	29.3
Irregular menses	1	8.3	Dysthymia	7	10.8
Seizure disorder	1	8.3	Marital discord	6	9.2
Ovarian cyst	1	8.3	Alcohol abuse	4	6.2
			Somatoform pain disorder	3	4.6
			Personality disorder	3	4.6
			Generalized anxiety disorder	1	1.5
			Grief reaction	1	1.5

whether these features are characteristic of PMS patients in general or rather reflect sample bias, as we studied only patients seen at the Cleveland Cleveland Foundation rather than a sample from the general population.

History of physical or sexual abuse has been linked to the development of psychiatric morbidity, particularly depressive illness and pain disorders. In the course of conducting a weekly clinic, we noted that a significant percentage of these patients reported a history of physical or sexual abuse during childhood. Therefore, we decided to review this data in a systematic manner to examine whether patients with LLPDD had a higher than expected reporting of past abuse.

Only two studies to date have examined a history of past abuse among women presenting with PMS. Friedman et al.[29] examined the connection between premenstrual mood symptoms and sexual abuse in a sample of 45 psychiatric inpatients and postulated that sexual abuse predisposed to cyclic hormonal changes and PMS. Paddison et al.[64] reported that 40% of 174 women presenting with premenstrual complaints had a history of sexual abuse. Of those with LLPDD per DSM III-R criteria (n = 37), the rate of sexual abuse was 38%. The authors further noted that this rate did not differ significantly between high and low socioeconomic status.[64]

In our series, 17.3% of the patients presenting with premenstrual syndrome reported a history of abuse; this percentage was approximately the same as among those presenting with medical or gynecologic pathology (16.7% reported abuse) and was half the percentage of abuse reported by those with a psychiatric diagnosis (33.8% report abuse). We concluded from our review that patients with prospectively confirmed PMS did not have a higher rate of childhood abuse than a control group, whose symptoms were explained by medical or gynecologic pathology. By contrast, childhood abuse was twice as likely among patients reporting PMS who had an underlying primary psychiatric diagnosis. These findings parallel those of Harrison et al.[39] who found that PMS patients were similar to a control group along many parameters if patients with a primary psychiatric diagnosis were excluded from the group

studied. Our results differ from the results of a recent study by Paddison et al.[64] and underscore the need for careful psychiatric assessment of patients presenting with premenstrual complaints. Of our group, 52.8% had a psychiatric diagnosis other than LLPDD. One might wonder if attributing symptoms to PMS might be easier for certain patients than acknowledging other difficulties and psychiatric issues.

Treatment. Treatment strategies need to be individualized, as no replicated double-blind crossover placebo-controlled study confirms that any one treatment is preferable for any particular subgroup of women. The process of treatment begins in the evaluation itself. Gathering information in a systematic manner and having patients prospectively rate the symptoms over time gives them a sense of control.

Dietary interventions can be quite useful in the initial treatment of PMS. Decreased salt intake can help lessen swelling during the premenstruum, and decreased intake of methylxanthene (e.g., caffeine-containing foods) can partially alleviate irritability and anxiety.[32] Vitamin B_6 is commonly recommended for PMS patients for two reasons.[2] It is believed that vitamin B_6 reduces blood estrogen, increases progesterone, and thus improves symptoms; it also appears that vitamin B_6 suppresses aldosterone, producing diuresis and clinical improvement. Recommended doses are in the range of 100 to 300 mg/day, though caution is recommended, as high doses of pyridoxine have been associated with a sensory neuropathy.[74] Nicotine should be curtailed during the premenstruum, as it also contributes to anxiety and irritability.

Hormonal treatments also have been used to treat PMS symptoms with inconsistent results. Progesterone, either orally or as suppositories, is sometimes recommended during the late luteal phase. Double-blind studies of the efficacy of progesterone for premenstrual symptoms have been negative.[26] Oral contraceptives are sometimes useful in alleviating PMS symptoms. Because some authors believe that prostaglandins trigger many of the symptoms of PMS, prostaglandin synthetase inhibitors, such as naproxen and mefenamic acid, have been used to treat

PMS.[15] Some evidence suggests that these drugs improve fatigue, headache, and general premenstrual aches, as well as dysmenorrhea during the menstrual phase. Gonadotropin releasing hormone (GnRH) agonists are a relatively new modality for control of severe premenstrual symptoms.[57]

A number of psychotropic medications have been used to treat PMS. Rickels et al.[68] studied the anxiolytic buspirone under double-blind, placebo-controlled conditions. The symptoms of PMS dropped to 30% of baseline for patients who took buspirone during the last 12 days of their menstrual cycle and to 68% of baseline for the group treated with placebo. Harrison et al.[37] documented a decline in PMS symptoms to 20% of the pretreatment levels in 8 of 11 women treated with nortriptyline. Stone et al.[83] reported that eight of nine patients taking fluoxetine described a 50% improvement in their symptoms, as compared with one of six patients taking a placebo. In a randomized placebo-controlled, double-blind, crossover study with alprazolam for premenstrual dysphoria, 70% of the patients rated alprazolam as superior to placebo.[38] Recent studies of melatonin inhibitors have demonstrated positive effects with light therapy and atenolol[65] (see box below).

Psychosocial stressors can affect the PMS patient, and psychotherapeutic interventions are indicated for many PMS patients. Women have been socialized to be passive and submissive, with much learned helplessness in their lives. Underlying issues of passivity and control need to be explored so that women can be more autonomous and in charge of their lives all month long. In our experience, women have often presented because of marital problems or after a breakup in a relationship. Marital therapy or psychotherapy to work through issues of poor communication, hostility, control, passivity, and abuse in such cases is necessary to reduce stress and premenstrual dysphoria and to prevent a feeling of "my hormones take me over."

Prevention. Providing treatment in a caring and competent manner by sensitive physicians can benefit many women suffering from this otherwise disabling condition. More research in the area of PMS is necessary, as is easy access to PMS clinics. Recognition of medical and psychologic aspects is essential, as patients presenting with premenstrual complaints may indeed have other gynecologic or psychiatric disorders. Chemical dependency, past

---

Treatment

Diet
Vitamin B$_6$
Diuretics
Hormones
Prostaglandin inhibitors
Psychopharmacologic agents
Melatonin inhibitors

---

history of abuse, and depression often coexist in this patient population and must not be overlooked.

To assess the outcome among patients treated at our PMS clinic, 55 women who had been diagnosed with LLPDD per DSM III-R criteria during a 3-year period were surveyed. Of the 69% (n = 38) who responded, 66% (n = 25) reported moderate to marked improvement in their premenstrual symptoms. These findings underscore the need for an individualized treatment program for the LLPDD patient, with special attention to target symptoms, previous gynecologic and psychiatric therapies, and expectations from treatment (unpublished data).

Postpartum affective illness. The symptomatology of depressive disorders in the puerperium is similar to depressive disorders at other times. However, it is important to recognize special features of postpartum affective illness in terms of etiology, phenomenology, and consequences and to differentiate postpartum blues or maternity blues from major postpartum depression. The former consists of emotional lability and tearfulness seen 3 to 10 days postpartum. It occurs in 30% to 60% of new mothers and is usually self-limited. In contrast, major postpartum depression begins around the twentieth postpartum day and increases gradually over the next 5 to 6 weeks. Symptoms include extreme fatigue, weight loss, slowed thinking, skin changes, and depressed mood. These women often ruminate about being failures at motherhood and question their personal worth and femininity. Suicide is a serious hazard and, therefore, timely intervention with antidepressant medications and support is necessary.

Occasionally postpartum depression may be seen in combination with psychotic features. Postpartum psychosis occurs in 1 to 2 per 1000 births. Symptoms occur around the third week. Patients may appear perplexed, confused, and psychotic and the symptoms are mercurial (i.e., rapidly changing). Past psychiatric history of bipolar or unipolar disorders or a family history of affective disorders is a predisposing genetic factor. Other risk factors include having a first baby, being unmarried, birth by cesarean section, and perinatal death. It is important to remember that after a severe postpartum episode, the risk of future affective episodes after delivery is as high as one in three, making prophylaxis and prevention essential.[36]

Sometimes major postpartum depressions become chronic and may last weeks to months. This type of depression affects 10% to 20% of women and is associated with the acute stress of caring for an infant by a woman who is alone and unsupported and has poor coping skills.

Given the morbidity and mortality of postpartum affective illnesses, it is important to ensure family and psychologic support before and after delivery. Regular prenatal care with appropriate referral to a psychiatrist is most beneficial in the early diagnosis and management of postpartum illnesses. Women requiring prophylactic lithium or antidepressants also need to be identified in a timely fashion. A follow-up visit 2 weeks postpartum with the obstetric office nurse also will aid in the early recognition of severe postpartum depressions. Self-help and support groups, beginning in the second or third trimester and continuing 6 months postpartum are helpful in educating parents, especially new mothers. Timing of meetings, convenient locations, and child care for multiparae encourage participation.

Depression at midlife. Women enter midlife in different psychosocial situations. Contrary to popular beliefs, most women go through menopause without major difficulty. There appears to be a downward trend in the peak age of onset of depressive disorders, with younger women being more prone to depression and suicide; however, there does not appear to be a significantly greater risk for major depression during menopause than at other times.[55] A history of previous psychiatric illness, including unipolar or bipolar disorders, substance abuse, anxiety, and family history of affective disorders or alcoholism, is a predisposing factor to depression in midlife.[8] Psychosocial stressors of midlife include the empty nest syndrome, widowhood, divorce, and death of parents. Other losses include cessation of menses, decreased attractiveness and youth, and medical illness.[59] Bart and Grossman[9] noted that the highest rate of depression occurred in housewives experiencing maternal role loss who had overprotective or overinvolved relationships with their children. Many menopausal women describe a newfound freedom and increased energy level and increased pleasure in sexual activities.[59]

Physiologic changes of menopause include hot flashes and night sweats. Anxiety, dizziness, headaches, and vague somatic and depressive symptoms may indicate a psychiatric disorder or medical illness. A careful history, mental status examination, and physical examination are required to appropriately treat this subgroup of women.

Suicide in women

As the topic of suicide has been dealt with extensively in Chapter 10, only key factors pertaining to suicide in women will be reviewed here.

Women *attempt* suicide more frequently than men.[17] Sexual abuse, which is more frequently experienced by younger women than men, has been associated with suicide attempts and completions. Nevertheless, young men continue to outnumber young women in completed suicide.

The use of violent and potentially more lethal methods has increased among young women.[44] Research on suicide in professional women, such as chemists, nurses, physicians, medical students, pharmacists, and psychologists,[72] suggests a higher risk for suicide than women in the general population; however, an elevated risk was not found for teachers or student nurses. Perhaps easy access to lethal methods in the professional groups studied may account for the higher rate, as those who are knowledgeable

about means they use are more likely to complete the act. Suicide has also been closely linked to alcoholism and drug addiction, and the most common lifetime diagnosis for alcoholic women is depression. The incidence of completed suicides is higher in female alcoholics as compared to nonalcoholic women, and in 20% to 37% of suicides reported by Colliver and Malin,[18] the victim was either drinking or had a history of alcohol abuse.

Preventive aspects of suicide require a concerted effort of all physicians and mental health workers who come in contact with depressed women. The elimination of alcohol by these women or from consumption by the offspring of alcoholics would be a primary preventive goal. Aggressive identification of individuals with high suicide risks—such as previous attempters, white elderly females with primary depression or alcohol abuse, those who communicate their suicidal intent, those with a family history for affective illness or suicide, those with interpersonal problems, and those with easy access to lethal means—is essential, as is effective treatment of underlying affective illness (see box below). Early psychiatric intervention and continuous outpatient contact with this group of patients, especially during high-risk periods, such as postpartum, premenstrual, and seasonal, are likely to have a preventive impact on suicide.[46] Stricter handgun control laws and prescribing hypnotics and antidepressants in limited amounts are other methods of preventing suicide.[79] Finally, public health programs, using face-to-face contact, or the telephone interview have been suggested to reduce the incidence of suicide.[62]

Prevention of depression in women

The diagnosis and treatment of depression have been covered in detail elsewhere in this section and, therefore, will not be repeated. In treating depressed women, the following points need to be kept in mind:

1. A careful mental status examination is necessary to determine the presence or absence of risk factors in the woman's history.
2. Therapists must be knowledgeable about the psychology of women and gender differences in the etiology of depression.
3. As discussed earlier in the chapter, action and mas-

Risk factors for suicide in women

Elderly, white, professional
Has a major affective disorder
Abuses alcohol
Attempted previously
Has easy access to lethal means
Communicates suicidal interest
Has a family history of affective illness or suicide
Encounters high-risk periods such as postpartum, premenstrual, and seasonal

tery approaches may be particularly needed by depressed women, as women are usually not taught a broad range of problem-solving and coping skills.

4. Exercise, running, and weight lifting have been found to improve self-concept in clinically depressed women.[63]

5. Substance abuse and depression often coexist.

6. Women are the exclusive consumers of oral contraceptives, which can increase depression in some women and also interact adversely with other medications.

7. Psychotropic medications have slow metabolism and longer clearance times in women. Although research on interaction between antidepressants and reproductive events is sparse, these factors are important to bear in mind when treating the depressed woman.[33]

8. Depressed women must be encouraged and taught to become effective consumers by education and psychotherapy services.

WOMEN AND ALCOHOLISM

Alcohol abuse and dependence affect 10 million people in the United States, 30% to 50% of whom are estimated to be women.[58] As compared with men, women are better able to conceal their drinking and are more reluctant to seek treatment. A significant number of women appear to be cross-addicted to substances such as tranquilizers, sedatives, and amphetamines and are more likely to have histories of suicide attempts, previous depression, and sexual abuse.[4,89] Until the early 1970s, most of the research on alcoholism had been performed on male subjects. Jones and Jones[47] were the first to report that, even with single doses of alcohol under standard conditions, nonalcoholic women obtained a much higher blood alcohol level than men. This difference is related to the body water content, which is 65% for men and 55% for women.

Because alcohol is distributed throughout the body, in proportion to the water content of the body tissues, alcohol tends to be more diluted in the body of men than in women. Frezza et al.[28] reported a sex-related difference in blood alcohol concentrations in 20 men and 23 women and concluded that increased bioavailability of ethanol resulting from decreased gastric oxidation of ethanol may contribute to a higher vulnerability of hepatic injury of women as compared with men who consume similar amounts of alcohol. This fact may explain why, although women start drinking and begin their pattern for alcohol abuse at a later age than men, they present for alcohol treatment at about the same age as men. This rapid development of alcoholism or telescoping of the disease has an important consideration when treating women.[13] Drinking practices in women vary with age, with younger women having the highest rates of alcohol-related problems and middle-aged women being heavier drinkers, especially women 50 years or older who were not employed and whose children have left home.

Chronic alcohol abuse exacts a greater physical toll on women than on men. Alcoholic women have death rates 50% to 100% higher than alcoholic men and die more frequently from suicides, cirrhosis of the liver, alcohol-related accidents, and cardiac disease.[43]

The effect of alcohol on menstruation and fertility and PMS has also been studied. It has been reported that 20% of women who seek medical care for PMS also abuse alcohol.[35] Belfer et al.[12] evaluated alcohol use relative to the menstrual cycle in 34 alcoholic women, 50% of whom related their drinking to the menstrual cycle and overwhelmingly to the premenstruum as a key time.[12] Price et al.,[67] in a controlled study of women alcoholics, noted that a significantly greater number of women alcoholics suffered from severe PMS than their non-alcoholic counterparts, suggesting that PMS may increase alcohol use in some women. In addition, menstrual disorders (e.g., irregular cycles, menorrhagia, dysmenorrhea) have been associated with chronic heavy drinking, can have adverse effects on fertility, and may lead to early menopause.[43]

Because the literature suggests that women seeking treatment for PMS are often abusers of alcohol, a retrospective follow-up of patients seen at our PMS clinic over a 2-year period was conducted to examine the incidence of alcoholism and alcohol abuse in PMS patients. A diagnosis of alcohol abuse or alcoholism was made by a structured review of the PMS patient population to extract information correlating to the Michigan Alcoholism Screening Test (MAST).[78] The PMS patient was contacted if the evaluation was suggestive of alcohol abuse or alcoholism but did not contain enough information to categorize the patient or family members. This patient telephone interview was also based on the areas covered in the MAST to determine if a history of alcohol abuse or alcoholism was present in the patient or the patient's family. Although only 3.1% of patients with prospectively confirmed PMS were alcoholic or abused alcohol, more than 33% of the PMS patients had family members with a positive history for alcoholism or alcohol abuse, a much higher finding compared with that reported in the general population.[52]

A special problem of concern to women is fetal alcohol syndrome and fetal alcohol effects. Fetal alcohol syndrome has a current estimated incidence of 1 to 2 per 1000 live births and that of fetal alcohol effects of 3 to 5 per 1000 live births.[16] The syndrome is characterized by growth retardation, facial malformation, mental retardation, and neurobehavioral effects such as poor coordination, irritability in infancy, and hyperactivity in childhood. It also costs nearly a third of a billion dollars a year and is among the leading known causes of mental retardation in the western world. Alcohol causes fetal damage by interfering with maternal nutrition and being directly toxic to fetal cellular growth and metabolism. The literature suggests that a fetus exposed to 89 ml or more of absolute alcohol (equivalent of about six drinks of hard liquor per day) faces a serious risk of fetal alcohol syndrome.[84]

Preventive aspects

Important considerations in the treatment of alcoholic women must include a high index of suspicion for depression and cross-addiction to sedative hypnotics. Treatment programs need to be tailored to women's needs. Most alcohol programs today are male oriented, in which women are uncomfortable. In addition, programs do not provide child care, nor do they allow adequate alternatives for mothers who need to enter treatment programs. According to a 1986 National Council on Alcoholism study, this lack of child care was cited as the number one unmet need of alcoholic women.[58] Employee-related rehabilitation programs are not available to women because of their employment status, and most women who enter alcohol treatment programs have serious financial problems, which severely limit their treatment options to mainly public facilities. Self-help groups such as Alcoholics Anonymous and Women For Sobriety are useful as are female alcoholism counselors who are, themselves, recovered alcoholics.[13]

In terms of prevention, alcohol is a leading preventable cause of birth defects, and good prenatal care for all women is a must. Prevention programs promoting abstinence during pregnancy through public and physician education need to develop further. Additionally, efforts should be directed at public policy issues regarding the availability and marketing of alcoholic beverages, especially when targeted at the woman consumer.

Public service announcements aired on television and radio are useful in increasing community awareness and are effective in disseminating warnings to the general public. The current health warning on alcoholic beverage labels is a healthy start. Physicians should routinely ask patients about alcohol intake, and pregnant women should be asked about their alcohol use and advised to abstain from alcohol during pregnancy. One study of alcohol abuse found that clinicians missed the diagnosis in three of four alcohol abusing obstetric patients.[80] Longitudinal studies of health consequences, factors contributing to mortality and health service costs, and biochemical markers of alcoholism are much needed. Physicians can contribute to these efforts by influencing public policy and by setting healthy examples in their own alcohol use. Alcoholic mothers are limited in their parenting abilities and their children are at high risk for abuse and neglect. Enlistment of child protection services should be used as a resource to provide for the treatment and support of affected mothers and children.

WOMEN AND VIOLENCE

Battery is the single most significant cause of injury to women in this country . . . no woman is obliged to accept a beating and suffer because of it.

C. Everett Koop, MD, former Surgeon General
of the United States

Epidemiologic studies suggest that sexual and physical assault has been experienced by 38% to 67% of adult women before age 18, 15% of college women, and approximately 20% of adult women.[51] Thirty-one percent of married women report violence in their relationship. One of the more disturbing facts is that the majority of violent incidents are perpetrated by close friends or family members. In one survey, 49% of child sexual assaults were by acquaintances and 50% to 57% of sexual assaults reported by college students were by partners. Alcoholism and drug abuse are significantly higher in women who have been victimized.[56,89] In an outpatient study of bulimic women the rate of victimization was roughly double that of the general population.[69] Higher rates of depression and psychiatric disorders are commonly found in victims of interpersonal violence and those who have a history of being sexually abused as children.[42,45,81]

The mental health impact of violence is significant and once victimized, a woman can never again feel quite as invulnerable. Psychiatric sequelae include posttraumatic stress disorder (PTSD), in which victims essentially suffer from combat neurosis. Symptoms include reexperiencing the trauma with recurrent dreams and flashbacks and making every effort to avoid reexperiencing the trauma. Amnesia about the situation, feeling detached, psychic numbing, and diminished interest are examples of these behaviors. Others may show an increased arousal such as hypervigilance, insomnia, increased autonomic reactivity, and outbursts of anger. Hopelessness, helplessness, negative self-esteem, high levels of self-criticism, self-defeating interpersonal strategies, and difficulty maintaining intimate relationships are core features of victimized adult women.

When working with battered women, it is important to remember that batterment is found in all walks of life, on all socioeconomic levels, and in all educational, racial, and age groups. An accurate history is best obtained when the woman is approached alone, in private, and in a supportive therapeutic climate. Questions should be asked directly regarding how she was injured and about the duration, frequency, and severity of injury. If the person is vague or evasive, it is best to begin with gentle probing and open-ended general questions, moving on later to more specific concerns.

Batterment is highly subjective to repetition and the clinician should be watchful of women who show up with abrasions or contusions to the head, face, back, and arms in the emergency room. Abused women tend to be high users of emergency room services. Other clues to abuse include vague somatic complaints, especially hyperventilation, headaches, chest, back and pelvic pain, multiple miscarriages or abortions, frequent use of minor tranquilizers, or sleep medications. Abused women are more likely to be beaten when pregnant. Alcohol is also an important component of the violent situation, but in most cases the primary diagnosis is violence.

Prevention

Prevention consists of practical advice such as legal services, shelters, welfare services, telephone hotlines, social service organizations, the National Organization for Women, and community mental health centers. The best deterrent for ongoing abuse is to arrest the perpetrator. A night in jail may lead to constructive introspection and improved behavior. Separating the perpetrator and the victim is always helpful. In case of family violence, the whole family needs counseling to resolve fear, anger, and shame so that the family can function again. Adult victim advocacy programs provide supportive feelings and increased awareness of strengths and weaknesses. It is important to convey to victims that the abuse is a crime and it is not their fault. Guilt, disloyalty to parents, a general sense of depression, helplessness, and poor self-image need to be dealt with in psychotherapy.

Prevention of violence is a goal endorsed by policy makers. National representative statistics on violence, victimization, new instruments for history taking, funding priorities for projects, and focused interventions by community agencies are needed to aid primary prevention. Protocols for routinely identifying, treating, and properly referring victims of abuse to hospital emergency rooms must be extended. Coordinated, comprehensive violence prevention programs to include advocacy, alcohol and drug detoxification, and individual, couple, and family therapy are much needed. Physicians can serve as leaders in coordinating such prevention programs and educating the public and professionals who work with victims. Attitudes and behaviors that promote violence are learned and should be challenged early by educating girls and boys in school.

Therapists working with victims must be educated to take a careful and thorough history and be clear on their own beliefs that nothing justifies a violent, abusive response. Victims of violence rarely voluntarily describe abuse because they tend to be blamed by health care providers. It is also extremely painful to go through the details of abuse, and revealing abuse has often led to reduced quality of care and hostility from professionals. Caring, sensitive, trained clinicians go a long way in reducing the aforementioned behaviors.

SUMMARY

The future of medicine lies in the prevention, rather than treatment, of depression, PMS, alcoholism, and violence, common problems afflicting increasingly larger numbers of women. The education of women must start during adolescence, and it is important for a young girl to develop a good sense of self and grow up feeling comfortable with her body. Adolescent girls should be encouraged to be knowledgeable about the prevention of sexually transmitted diseases, contraception, reproduction, stress management, and the hazards of substance use. Adolescent girls and boys must be educated not to condone attitudes and behaviors that promote violence against women. It is our hope that women in the twenty-first century will be educated consumers, more in control of their lives and work in partnership with physicians at various health centers so that they can lead fuller, healthier lives.

REFERENCES

1. Abplanalp JM: Psychologic components of the premenstrual syndrome: evaluating the research and choosing the treatment, *J Reprod Med* 28:517-524, 1983.
2. Abraham GE: Nutritional factors in the etiology of the premenstrual tension syndromes, *J Reprod Med* 28(7):446-464, 1983.
3. Akerlund M, Andersson KE, Ingemarsson I: Effects of terbutaline on myometrial activity, uterine blood flow and lower abdominal pain in women with primary dysmenorrhea, *Br J Obstet Gynecol* 83:673-678, 1976.
4. Alcoholics Anonymous. *AA surveys its membership: a demographic report,* About AA: A newsletter for professional men and women. New York, 1984, General Service Office.
5. American Psychiatric Association: *Diagnostic and statistical manual of mental disorders,* ed 3, revised. Washington, DC, 1987, American Psychiatric Association.
6. Andersch B, Milsom I: An epidemiologic study of young women with menorrhea, *Am J Obstet Gynecol* 144:655-660, 1982.
7. Baker Miller J: *Toward a new psychology of women,* ed 2, Boston, 1986, Beacon Press.
8. Ballinger CB: Psychiatric morbidity and the menopause survey of a gynaecological outpatient clinic, *Br J Psychiatry* 131:83-89, 1977.
9. Bart PB, Grossman M: Menopause. In Notman MT, Nadelson CC, editors: *The woman patient: medical and psychological interfaces,* New York, 1978, Plenum Press.
10. Bassoff ES, Glass GV: The relationship between sex roles and mental health: a meta-analysis of twenty-six studies, *The Counseling Psychologist* 10:105-112, 1982.
11. Beck AT, Rush J, Shaw B, et al: *Cognitive therapy of depression,* New York, 1979, Gifford Press.
12. Belfer ML, Shader RI, Caroll M: Alcoholism in women, *Arch Gen Psychiatry* 25:540-544, 1971.
13. Blume SB: Women and alcohol: a review, *JAMA* 256(11):1167-1169, 1986.
14. Brown C, Ni Bhrolchain MN, Harris TO: Social class and psychiatric disturbance among women in an urban population, *Sociology* 9:225-254, 1975.
15. Budoff PW: The use of prostaglandin inhibitors for the premenstrual syndrome, *J Reprod Med* 28:7, 1983.
16. Clarren SK, Smith DW: The fetal alcohol syndrome, *N Engl J Med* 298:1063-1067, 1978.
17. Clayton PJ: Suicide, *Psychiatr Clin North Am* 8:203-214, 1985.
18. Colliver JD, Malin H: State and national trends in alcohol related morbidity: 1975-1982, *Alcohol Health Res World* 10:60-64, 1986.
19. Dawood M, McGuire J, Demers L: *Premenstrual syndrome and dysmenorrhea,* Baltimore, 1985, Urban and Schwarzenberg.
20. Denicoff K, Hoban C, Grover G, et al: Glucose tolerance testing in women with premenstrual syndrome, *Am J Psychiatry* 147:4, 1990.
21. DePirro R, Fusco A, Bertali A: Insulin receptors during the menstrual cycle in normal women, *J Clin Endocrinol Metab* 47:1387-1389, 1978.
22. Deutsch H: The menopause, *Int J Psychoanal* 65(1):55-62, 1984.
23. Endicott J, Halbreich V: Clinical significance of premenstrual dysphoric changes, *J Clin Psychiatry* 49:2, 1988.
24. Endicott J, Halbreich U, Schacht S, et al: Affective disorder and premenstrual depression. In Osofsky JH, Blumenthal SJ, editors: *Premenstrual syndrome: current findings and future direction,* Washington DC, 1985, American Psychiatric Press.
25. Frank RT: The hormonal causes of premenstrual tension, *Arch Neurol Psychiatry* 26:1053, 1931.
26. Freeman E, Rickels K, Sandheimer S, et al: Ineffectiveness of pro-

gesterone suppository treatment for premenstrual syndrome, *JAMA* 264:349-353, 1990.

27. Freud S: Femininity. In Stachey J, editor: *New introductory features on psychoanalysis.* standard ed, vol 22, London, 1964, Hogarth Press.

28. Frezza M, diPadova C, Pozato G, et al: High blood alcohol levels in women: the role of decreased gastric alcohol dehydrogenase activity and first-pass metabolism, *N Engl J Med* 322:95-99, 1990.

29. Friedman R, Hurt S, Clarkin J, et al: Sexual histories and premenstrual affective syndrome in psychiatric inpatients, *Am J Psychiatry* 139:1454, 1982.

30. Gidwani G: Dysmenorrhea—myths and facts, *Cleve Clin Q* 5:367, 1983.

31. Gilligan C: In a different voice: women's conception of the self and morality, *Harvard Educ Rev* 47(4):481-517, 1977.

32. Gitlin MJ, Pasnau RO: Psychiatric syndromes linked to reproductive function in women: a review of current knowledge, *Am J Psychiatry* 146:11, 1989.

33. Greenblatt DJ, Abernethy DR, Locniskar A, et al: Age, sex and nitrazepam kinetics: relation to antipyrine disposition. *Clin Pharmacol Ther* 38:697-703, 1985.

34. Guttentag M, Salisan S: Women, men and mental health. In Carter LA, Scott AF, editors: *Women and men: changing roles, relationships and perceptions,* New York, 1976, Aspen Institute.

35. Halliday A, Bush B, Cleary P, et al: Alcohol abuse in women seeking gynecologic care, *Obstet Gynecol* 68(3):322-326, 1986.

36. Hamilton JA: Postpartum psychiatric syndromes, *Psychiatr Clin North Am* 12:1, 1989.

37. Harrison WM, Endicott J, Nee J: Treatment of premenstrual depression with nortriptyline: a pilot study, *J Clin Psychiatry* 50:4, 1989.

38. Harrison W, Endicott J, Nee J: Treatment of premenstrual dysphoria with alprazolam, *Arch Gen Psychiatry* 47:3, 1990.

39. Harrison WM, Endicott J, Nee J, et al: Characteristics of women seeking treatment for premenstrual syndrome, *Psychosomatics* 30:4, 1989.

40. Hathaway SR, McKinley JC: A multiphasic personality schedule: I. Construction of the schedule, *J Psychol* 10:249-254, 1940.

41. Reference deleted in galleys.

42. Hilberman E, Munson K: Sixty battered women, *Victimology: An International Journal* 2:460-470, 1977-1978.

43. Hill SY: Biological consequences of alcoholism and alcohol-related problems among women. In *Special population issues. National Institute on Alcohol Abuse and Alcoholism.* Alcohol and Health Monograph No. 4. DHHS Pub No. (ADM) 82-1193, Washington DC, pp 43-73, 1982.

44. Holden C: Youth suicide: new research focuses on a growing social problem, *Science* 233:839-841, 1986.

45. Jacobson A, Richardson BC: Assault experiences of 100 psychiatric inpatients: evidence of the need for routine inquiry, *Am J Psychiatry* 144:908-913, 1987.

46. Jamison KR: Suicide prevention in depressed women, *J Clin Psychology* 49(9) (suppl):42-45, 1988.

47. Jones BM, Jones MK: Women and alcohol: intoxication metabolism and the menstrual cycle. In Greenblatt M, Schuckit MA, editors: *Alcoholism problems in women and children,* New York, 1976, Grune & Stratton.

48. Kandel DB, Davies M, Ravels V: The stressfulness of daily social roles for women: marital, occupational and household roles, *J Health Soc Behav* 26:64-78, 1985.

49. Keane JG: Changing population patterns. In *World almanac and book of facts: 1986,* New York, 1985, World Almanac.

50. Keye WR, Hammond DC, Strong T: Medical and psychological characteristics of women presenting with premenstrual syndrome, *Obstet Gynecol* 68:5, 1986.

51. Koss MP: The women's mental health research agenda: violence against women, *Am Psychol* 45:374-380, 1990.

52. Kotz M, Gonsalves L, Zuti R, et al: Familial alcoholism and patients with premenstrual syndrome, *Alcohol Clin Exp Res* 13:1, 1989.

53. McGrath E, Keita GP, Strickland B, Russo NF: *Women and depression: risk factors and treatment issues,* Washington DC, 1990, American Psychological Association.

54. McLaughlin S, Melber B: *The changing life course of American women: lifestyle and attitude changes,* Seattle, 1986, Battelle Memorial Institute.

55. Meyers JK: Six month prevalence of psychiatric disorders in three communities, *Arch Gen Psychiatry* 41(10):959-967, 1984.

56. Murphy WD, Coleman E, Hoon E, et al: Sexual dysfunction and treatment in alcoholic women, *Sexuality and Disability* 3(4):240-255, 1980.

57. Muse KN, Cetel NS, Fulterman LA, et al: The premenstrual syndrome. Effects of "medical ovariectomy," *N Engl J Med* 311:1345-1348, 1984.

58. National Council on Alcoholism: *A federal response to a hidden epidemic: alcohol and other drug problems among women,* Washington, DC, 1987, Author.

59. Neugarten BL: Time, age and the life cycle, *Am J Psychiatry* 136(7):887-893, 1979.

60. Nolen-Hoeksema S: Sex differences in depression, Stanford, Calif, 1990, Stanford University Press.

61. Novak E: Menstruation and its disorders, New York, 1923, Appleton.

62. Oast SP, Zitrin A: A public health approach to suicide prevention, Am J Public Health 65:146-147, 1975.

63. Ossip-Klein DJ, Doyne EJ, Bowman ED, et al: Effects of running or weight lifting on self-concept in clinically depressed women, *J Consult Clin Psychol* 57:158-161, 1989.

64. Paddison PL, Gise LH, Lebovits A, et al: Sexual abuse and premenstrual syndrome: comparison between a lower and higher socioeconomic group, *Psychosomatics* 31:3, 1990.

65. Parry BL, Berga SL, Mostofi N, et al: Morning versus evening bright light treatment of late luteal phase dysphoric disorder, *Am J Psychiatry* 146:1215-1217, 1989.

66. Parry BL, Wehr TA: Therapeutic effect of sleep deprivation in patients with premenstrual syndrome, *Am J Psychiatry* 144:6, 808-810, 1987.

67. Price WA, DiMarzio LR, Eckert JI: Correlation between PMS and alcoholism among women, *Ohio Med* 3:201-202, 1987.

68. Rickels K, Freeman E, Sandheimer S: Buspirone in treatment of premenstrual syndrome (letter to editor), *Lancet* 1:777, 1989.

69. Root MP, Fallon P: The incidence of victimization experiences in a bulimic sample, *J Interpersonal Violence* 3:161-173, 1986.

70. Ross CE, Huber J: Hardship and depression, *J Health Soc Behav* 26:312-327, 1985.

71. Ross CE, Mirowsky J: Child care and emotional adjustment to wives' employment, *J Health Soc Behav* 29:127-138, 1988.

72. Roy A: Suicide in doctors. *Psychiatr Clin North Am* 8:377-387, 1985.

73. Rubinow DR, Schmidt PJ: Models for the development and expression of symptoms in premenstrual syndrome, *Psychiatr Clin North Am* 12:1, 1989.

74. Schaumburg H, Kaplan J, Windebank A, et al: Sensory neuropathy from pyridoxine abuse: a new megavitamin syndrome, *N Engl J Med* 309:445-448, 1983.

75. Schinfeld JS, Cronin L, Parks-Truscs: Presenting premenstrual symptoms: another look. Presented at the International Symposium on Premenstrual Tension and Dysmenorrhea, South Carolina, September, 1983.

76. Schmidt PJ, Grover GN, Rubinow DR: State dependent alterations in the perception of life events in menstrual-related mood disorders, *Am J Psychiatry* 147:2, 1990.

77. Seligman MEP: *Helplessness: on depression, development and death,* San Francisco, 1976, WH Freeman.

78. Selzer ML: The Michigan Alcoholism Screening Test: the quest for a new diagnostic instrument, *Am J Psychiatry* 127(12):89-94, 1971.
79. Sloan JH, Rivara FP, Reay DT, et al: Firearm regulations and rates of suicide, *N Engl J Med* 322(6):369-373, 1990.
80. Sokol RJ, Miller SI, Martier S: *Preventing fetal alcohol effects: a practical guide for OB-GYN physicians and nurses*, Rockville Md, 1981, National Institute on Alcohol Abuse and Alcoholism.
81. Sorenson SB, Golding JM: Depressive sequelae of recent criminal victimization, *J Traumatic Stress* 3(3):337-350, 1990.
82. Speert H: *Obstetrics and gynecology in America: a history*, Baltimore, 1980, American College of Obstetricians and Gynecologists.
83. Stone AB, Pearlstein TB, Brown WA: Fluoxetine in the treatment of premenstrual syndrome, *Psychopharmacol Bull* 26(3):3-35, 1990.
84. Streissguth AP, Herman CS, Smith DW: Intelligence, behavior and dysmorphogenesis in the fetal alcohol syndrome: a report on 20 patients, *J Pediatr* 92:363-367, 1978.
85. Taylor DT, Mathew J, Ho BT, et al: Serotonin levels and platelet uptake during premenstrual tension, *Neuropsychology* 21:16-18, 1984.
86. US Department of Health and Human Services: (Draft) Promoting health, preventing disease: Year 2000 objectives for the nation, 1989.
87. Weissman MM: Advances in psychiatric epidemiology: rates and risks for major depression, *Am J Public Health* 77:445-451, 1987.
88. Weissman MM, Meyers JK: Affective disorders in a United States community: the use of research diagnostic criteria in an epidemiological survey, *Arch Gen Psychiatry* 35:104-131, 1978.
89. Wilsnack SC, Wilsnack RW, Klassen AD: Epidemiological research on women's drinking 1978-1984. In *Women and alcohol: health related issues*, Publication (ADM) 86-1139, US Department of Health and Human Services, 1986.

RESOURCES

Women and depression

Depression after delivery, PO Box 1281, Morrisville, PA 19067, (215) 295-3994. For women experiencing postpartum depression.

National Foundation for Depressive Illness, Inc., PO Box 2257, New York, NY 10611, 1-800-248-4344.

Provides referrals to support groups.

The National Alliance for the Mentally Ill, 2101 Wilson Blvd, Suite 302, Arlington, VA 22201, (703) 524-7600.

Provides information, emotional support and advocacy through local and state affiliates for families.

National Depressive and Manic Depression Association, Merchandise Mart, PO Box 3395, Chicago, IL 60654, (312) 939-2442.

For depressed persons and their families.

American Association of Suicidology, 2459 South Ave Denver, CO 80222.

For those who have experienced the suicide of someone close.

Depression/Awareness, Recognition and Treatment (D/ART), National Institute of Mental Health, Room 15C-05, 5600 Fishers Lane, Rockville, MD 20857.

A federal government/private sector effort to inform primary health care providers, mental health specialists and the general public about the most up-to-date treatments for depressive illness.

Healthy Mother, Healthy Babies Coalition (or state chapters) 409 12th Street SW, Room 309, Washington DC 20024, (202) 638-5577.

Information and education to improve maternal/infant health.

PMS Access, PO Box 9326, Madison, WI 53715, 1-800-222-4PMS.

For information on PMS, PMS clinics, support groups.

American College of Obstetricians and Gynecologists (ACOG), 409 12th Street SW, Washington DC 20024-2188, 1-800-673-8444.

For educational pamphlets on subjects related to women's health.

Women and alcoholism

National Clearinghouse for Alcohol and Drug Information (NCADI), PO Box 2345, Rockville, MD 20852, 1-800-729-6686.

National Council on Alcoholism and Drug Dependence, Inc., 12 West 21st Street, 8th Floor, New York, NY, 10010, 1-800-NCA-CALL.

Materials on alcoholism, fetal alcohol syndrome.

The National Institute on Drug Abuse, Treatment referral hotline 1-800-662-4357.

For drug treatment facilities in local communities.

Self-Help Groups: AA, Al-Anon, Adult Children of Alcoholics, Narcotics Anonymous, Women for Sobriety.

Listings of meetings can be obtained from headquarter offices with telephone numbers in local directories.

Relapse Prevention Hotline, 1-800-RELAPSE.

Women and violence

National Coalition Against Domestic Violence (NCADV), PO Box 15127, Washington DC 20003-0127, 1-800-333-SAFE.

A national organization of shelters and support service for battered women and their children.

Parents United, PO Box 952, San Jose, CA 95108, (408) 280-5055.

For abused children and for adults who were abused as children.

Child Help - Child Abuse Hotline, 1-800-422-4453.

Clearinghouse on Child Abuse and Neglect Information, PO Box 1182, Washington DC 20013, (703) 821-2086.

National Organization for Women (NOW), 1000 16th Street NW, Room 700, Washington DC 20036, (202) 331-0066.

Legal Aid Societies. Numbers are listed in local phone directories.

Chapter 14

THE PSYCHIATRIC EFFECTS OF MEDICATIONS

Donald A. Malone, Jr.

Many medications now used in the practice of medicine are known to have psychiatric side effects.[1,7] These side effects can be due to toxicity from the drug, but often are seen within the normal dosage range. Some of the side effects reported are widely known and frequently seen. Others are less common and can be confused with functional psychiatric disorders. Because the treatment of these particular side effects (usually withdrawal of the offending agent) is often rapidly effective, it is important to recognize the side effects early to avoid misdiagnosis or unneeded medical workup.

Most reports of adverse reactions in the literature describe the medical rather than the psychiatric and psychologic effects of medications. More recently, however, these other effects have been described. It is now becoming clear that a number of nonpsychotropic drugs have psychiatric and psychologic effects. Psychiatric syndromes, including depression,[17] anxiety,[30] mania,[44] dissociation,[19] and cognitive impairment,[34] have been related to nonpsychotropic medications. Of course, psychotropic medications also have distinct behavioral effects. As is the case with sedatives, these effects can in fact be part of the therapeutic action of the drug. Illicit drugs are used because of their behavioral effects and thus are also commonly recognized. For example, cocaine and amphetamines can induce a euphoric mood during the acute stage of usage and severe depression or paranoia with chronic use.

The accompanying box lists drugs that are known to lead to depression in certain patients.[10,17] Other drugs have also been implicated, although much less commonly. Interestingly, patients who have attempted suicide tend to be taking more medications than other patients who die of natural causes.[33] This finding may reflect the fact that

Drugs that may induce depression
Antihypertensive agents
Beta-blockers
Clonidine
Methyldopa
Reserpine
Thiazide diuretics
Gastrointestinal agents
Cimetidine
Metoclopramide
Hormones
ACTH
Corticosteroids
Oral contraceptives
Testosterone derivatives
Sedatives
Barbiturates
Benzodiazepines
Ethanol
Stimulants
Amphetamines
Cocaine

medical illness predisposes to depression rather than a direct drug effect. Nevertheless, it serves notice that patients on medications must be monitored for potential psychiatric effects.

Manic symptoms can also occur secondary to pharmacologic agents.[29,44] The agents most frequently implicated in causing secondary mania are listed in the following box. Numerous other agents have been reported to induce mania less frequently. Most have been implicated in only one or two case reports and are reviewed elsewhere.[44]

Drugs that induce mania

Anabolic steroids
Antidepressants
Corticosteroids
Isoniazid
Levodopa
Stimulants and sympathomimetics
Thyroxine

Drugs inducing cognitive impairment

Antiarrhythmic agents
  Digitalis
  Disopyramide
  Lidocaine
  Quinidine
Anticholinergic agents
  Tricyclic antidepressants
  Antiparkinsonian agents
Antihypertensive agents
  Beta-blockers
  Clonidine
  Methyldopa
Cimetidine
Corticosteroids
Lithium
Narcotics
Nonsteroidal antiinflammatory agents
  Ibuprofen
  Indomethacin
  Sulindac
Phenytoin
Sedatives
  Barbiturates
  Benzodiazepines

Anxiety symptoms can also be brought about by certain pharmacologic agents. In fact, agents such as yohimbine and lactate have been used as inducers of anxiety for research purposes.[30] The most common agents implicated in the induction of anxiety are *stimulants*, including commonly prescribed medications, such as *antihistamines*, illicit drugs such as cocaine and amphetamines, and commonly used substances such as caffeine. When an anxiety state is noted, it is thus important to inquire about both prescribed and over-the-counter medications.

Pharmacologic agents have also been noted to induce dissociative states, including transient amnesias, fugue states, depersonalization, and explosive disorders.[19] Agents implicated in the induction of dissociative states include *alcohol, sedatives, anticholinergic agents, beta-blockers, hallucinogens,* and *general anesthetics.* Differentiation of these drug-induced states from functional dissociative disorders can be difficult, and the removal of a possible offending pharmacologic agent can be diagnostic.

Cognitive impairment is another potential side effect of certain medications.[34] This impairment can present as either delirium or dementia and can be either acute or insidious in onset. This effect becomes particularly important in the elderly population, as they may already have some underlying cognitive impairment and are also more likely to be on various medications. The box above, right, summarizes the drugs most likely to induce cognitive impairment.

Other side effects that can mimic psychiatric disorders include hallucinations, delusions, nightmares, hyperactivity, amnesia, and catatonia.[1] Thus when a physician is treating a patient who is suffering from any type of psychiatric syndrome, the possibility that it is drug-induced must always be considered.

It can sometimes be difficult to determine whether psychiatric symptoms are due to medications, underlying disease, or a new psychiatric disorder. For example, a patient with multiple sclerosis may begin to experience some difficulty with memory and depression. The differential diagnosis would include the following: (1) cognitive dysfunction secondary to progression of multiple sclerosis, which has brought about a depressed mood; (2) an organic depression and cognitive impairment secondary to the corticosteroids the patient has been receiving for disease; and (3) a major depressive episode with subsequent difficulty

in attention and concentration, which has brought about a perceived impairment of memory. These three etiologies all have potentially effective, but different treatment options. The patient with worsening multiple sclerosis may require more intensive treatment. The patient with side effects from corticosteroids may require dose reduction, and the patient with major depression would be effectively treated with an antidepressant medication. Thus the consideration of drug-induced psychiatric effects in the differential diagnosis is essential to appropriate diagnosis and treatment.

That psychiatric effects can occur secondary to medications is relevant to preventive medicine in a number of ways. Reviewing potential side effects with the patient being placed on medication can enhance compliance. A patient who begins to suffer from a psychiatric side effect will be more likely to bring it to the physician's attention and have it effectively addressed. This communication can enhance a physician-patient relationship and, therefore, enhance compliance. If patients begin to suffer from unexpected side effects, it can strain the physician-patient relationship and present difficulties with medication compliance in the future. Patients may also attribute the psychiatric side effects to "emotional problems" and not complain to the physician. Thus the physician would remain unaware of potentially dangerous side effects.

The second issue relevant to preventive medicine is the importance of the quick recognition of psychiatric side effects. Telling the patient that these effects are due to a medication and not to a primary psychiatric disorder is often relieving. Thus compliance with regard to future medication will be enhanced. Quick recognition can also prevent worsening of these particular effects and possible dangerous consequences. For example, if a patient placed on a *beta-blocker* for hypertension becomes depressed, continuing this medication can lead to worsening of the depression. Severe depression can lead to suicidal ideation and potential death. Early discontinuation of the beta-blocker would prevent this potentially dangerous scenario.

Finally, the physician may choose different medications based on their potential psychiatric side effects. For example, if a patient has a long history of recurrent major depression, it would be wise to avoid the use of beta-blockers for the treatment of hypertension. Many other antihypertensive options do not carry the potential of inducing a recurrence of depression. Consequently, basing the treatment regimen on the patient's premorbid psychiatric state can effectively prevent potentially serious consequences and will also enhance compliance in patients.

The ability to predict and quickly recognize psychiatric side effects of medications can improve compliance, prevent psychiatric problems, and enhance treatment effectiveness. Because patients often find it difficult to discuss psychiatric symptoms with their physician, bringing up the possibility of their occurrence early in the course of treatment can enhance communication and compliance. The potential consequences of allowing these symptoms to go untreated can be severe.

DRUG-INDUCED PSYCHIATRIC EFFECTS
Antibiotics and antiviral agents

Antibiotic, antiviral, and antifungal agents have been associated with a number of psychiatric effects, including delirium, confusion, hallucinations, agitation, and mania[1]; however, none of the side effects are common. Most reports deal with individual case reports, which at times can also contain other factors that could have caused the side effect. Nevertheless, it is worthwhile to consider these agents as potential etiologic factors when psychiatric symptoms are encountered without known cause.

A number of case reports have documented various *cephalosporin* compounds as causing confusion or hallucinations. Altes et al.[2] reported a case of delirium in a patient with the acquired immune deficiency syndrome (AIDS), which was felt to be caused by ciprofloxacin. The delirium included symptoms of visual hallucinations. These symptoms immediately resolved when ciprofloxacin was discontinued. Patients with AIDS may be more sensitive to the adverse effects of medications, including antimicrobial agents.

Ceftazidime has also been associated with psychiatric effects and has been reported to cause both auditory and visual hallucinations.[3] This case, however, was somewhat

complicated by the presence of mild hypoxia. The psychiatric side effects of *cephalosporins* may be more common in the medically compromised patient and in the elderly. Patients with renal impairment are also more susceptible to toxic side effects if the dose has not been reduced appropriately.

Gentamycin and tobramycin have been reported to cause both disorientation and hallucinations.[9] It was once thought that patients who experienced acute confusional states as a result of gentamycin treatment probably had predisposing personality factors. Currently, this theory is no longer popular; in fact, patients with no prior psychiatric history can experience the same side effects. As with patients with renal impairment, it is important to remain vigilant about dosing.

As is the case with antibacterial agents, antiviral agents are not commonly associated with psychiatric side effects. Acyclovir has been associated with hallucinations, confusion, and on one occasion a psychotic depression.[43] Zidovudine also has been associated with hallucinations on rare occasion. *Antituberculous agents*, isoniazid in particular, have been reported to cause psychiatric symptoms including psychosis and depression.[5]

Most psychiatric effects secondary to antiinfectious agents are easily treated by switching to an agent of another class. However, this approach is not always possible. For example, the agent being used may be the only effective drug in a particular case. In these cases, the options become limited to decreasing the dose or treating the psychiatric side effects symptomatically. It may be possible to diminish the severity of the psychiatric symptoms by using *antidepressant*, *antianxiety*, or *antipsychotic agents* as appropriate.

Anticonvulsants

A number of neuropsychiatric effects have been attributed to anticonvulsant medications. Psychiatric symptoms that have been described include agitation, cognitive impairment, depression, psychosis, and mania.[1,39] Anticonvulsant agents that have been implicated include phenobarbital, phenytoin, ethosuximide, valproate, and carbamazepine. The medications with the most potential for psychiatric side effects appear to be phenobarbital and phenytoin. Cognitive impairment is clearly the most common of the reported effects. Actual behavioral changes on these medications appear to be uncommon. The barbiturates may lead to irritability, aggression, and hyperactivity, particularly in younger patients. In addition, ethosuximide has been reported to cause a number of cases of psychotic behavior.

Although cognitive dysfunction as a result of anticonvulsant treatment is of significant concern, it has been difficult to study because cognitive dysfunction can occur as a consequence of epilepsy itself.[45,47] Factors unrelated to medication may influence cognition, including patient age, frequency of seizures, and type of epilepsy. When cognitive dysfunction is apparent, however, alteration of the medication regimen may be the most important factor that a physician can control.

Different anticonvulsant medications may have very distinct effects on cognition. Phenobarbital seems to impair memory and concentration to a greater degree than the other anticonvulsants.[45] Phenytoin may have more effect on attention, problem solving ability, and visual motor tasks. Although carbamazepine seems to have some effect on tracking tasks, for the most part it is relatively free of significant cognitive impairment. Valproate, although not widely studied, in general seems to cause relatively minimal cognitive dysfunction. Therefore, if cognitive dysfunction becomes a problem in the treatment of the epileptic patient, it is reasonable to change to another anticonvulsant, particularly if a patient can be changed from phenobarbital or phenytoin to either carbamazepine or valproate.

Another important issue is the effect of polytherapy. The Collaborative Group for Epidemiology of Epilepsy has found that polytherapy significantly increases the adverse toxic effects of anticonvulsant medications.[13] Minimization of cognitive dysfunction can be achieved by changing to monotherapy, although this option is not always achievable because the control of epileptic seizures must also be considered.

In summary, anticonvulsant medications can cause neuropsychiatric side effects. Patients on these medications should be assessed for these side effects, particularly cognitive dysfunction. If cognitive dysfunction becomes a problem, the physician should consider either changing to an anticonvulsant with fewer cognitive effects or changing to monotherapy if possible.

Antidepressants and anticholinergic agents

A number of neuropsychiatric complications can occur with the use of antidepressant medications and anticholinergic agents. Many of the effects of antidepressants are often, but not always, secondary to their anticholinergic properties. Anticholinergic medications can result in cognitive impairment, which tends to occur most commonly in the elderly or medically compromised patient.[4]

Tricyclic antidepressants are those most commonly associated with neuropsychiatric symptoms. These can include cognitive impairment, mania, delirium, hallucinations, and paranoia.[41] The cognitive impairment secondary to antidepressants is directly related to the degree of anticholinergic properties of the particular medication. For example, amitriptyline is significantly more anticholinergic than its derivative nortriptyline. Therefore, amitriptyline is much more likely to impair cognitive abilities. If cognitive impairment becomes a problem, one can switch to a less anticholinergic antidepressant. In addition, it is reasonable to use antidepressants that have lower anticholinergic effects in the elderly patient.

Mania can occur with any of the antidepressant compounds. Most often it occurs early in the course of treatment, but it can occur at any time. The first symptoms of potential mania include mild euphoria, insomnia, and increased energy. If these symptoms are noted early on, the medication can be discontinued and a problem with mania often can be averted.

Agitation and increased anxiety can be side effects, particularly early on in treatment with an antidepressant. Antidepressants that have less sedative properties tend to cause problems more frequently. For example, fluoxetine or desipramine would be more likely to cause these symptoms than would amitriptyline or doxepin. Therefore, a patient who is anxious in addition to being depressed would respond better with a more sedating antidepressant. Panic attacks can also be exacerbated by any of these medications.

As noted earlier, *anticholinergic agents* can lead to cognitive impairment.[20] This common feature of anticholinergic toxicity can also be present in a more subtle form at nontoxic doses. One needs only to recall the classic description of belladonna toxicity "mad as a hatter" to note that anticholinergic toxicity can lead not only to cognitive impairment, but also to delirium and psychosis. Elderly and neurologically impaired individuals are more sensitive to the neuropsychiatric side effects of anticholinergic agents. When choosing agents for the treatment of depression in these populations, therefore, it would be most reasonable to consider agents that have minimal anticholinergic properties. These antidepressants would include trazodone, fluoxetine, bupropion, desipramine, and nortriptyline. The best treatment option in dealing with anticholinergic cognitive impairment is to discontinue or decrease the dose. *Cholinergic agonists* have been used but can cause problems with cardiac rhythm.

Antihypertensive agents and antiarrhythmics

Antihypertensive agents have long been associated with causing depression; however, they can also induce a number of other psychiatric symptoms.[36] Symptoms include insomnia, hallucinations, paranoia, cognitive impairment, and nightmares. With the possible exception of depression, however, these side effects tend to be uncommon.

Methyldopa is the antihypertensive agent most commonly associated with depression. Studies have noted depression to occur in at least 5% of patients treated, which may be secondary to central catecholamine- and serotonin-depleting actions of the medication. The most appropriate treatment is to change antihypertensive agents. Antidepressant medications may be beneficial if discontinuation alone does not resolve the symptoms. In addition to depression, methyldopa can commonly induce insomnia and nightmares. Acute confusional states have also been described, although much less often.

Clonidine is another centrally active antidepressant agent that can induce psychiatric symptoms. Depression has been reported to occur secondary to clonidine, but at a much lower incidence than methyldopa. The overall incidence of depression seems to be approximately 1.5%.[36] Sleep disturbance, anxiety, nervousness, and mild paranoia have been noted to occur, although at a fairly low rate.

Guanethidine and other adrenergic neuron blockers tend to be an infrequent cause of psychiatric symptomatology. Depression has been reported in a number of patients, but seems to be uncommon. Restlessness, insomnia, and paranoia have been reported rarely.

Beta-blocking agents, most commonly propranolol, have been associated with psychiatric side effects. Depression appears to occur relatively infrequently, but can become severe. The more lipophilic beta-blockers, such as propranolol, were once thought more likely to induce depression, but this theory has never been proven. Hallucinations, paranoia, insomnia, and nightmares can also occur with beta-blocking agents. All of the neuropsychiatric effects described with beta-blocking agents seem to be more common in the elderly, including cognitive impairment.[40] Studies have demonstrated that memory performance scores are consistently lower with beta-blocking agents than with placebo or other forms of antihypertensive agents. In summary, antihypertensive agents should be considered as potential etiologies when psychiatric symptoms, particularly depression or cognitive impairment, occur.

A number of neuropsychiatric side effects have been reported with *antiarrhthmic agents*.[1] Digoxin can produce symptoms of euphoria, confusion, amnesia, psychosis, and depression, particularly in high doses or in the elderly. However, cognitive dysfunction, depression, and emotional lability have also been reported at therapeutic serum concentrations.[16] Quinidine has been associated with confusion, agitation, and psychosis, which tend to be dose-related. They are frequently seen as results of quinidine toxicity, but have also been reported in therapeutic doses.[14] Procainamide and procaine derivatives in general have been noted to induce psychosis, agitation, depression, and anxiety. Again, these side effects are commonly dose related, but can occur at normal serum levels. They can usually be treated rather easily with a change to another antiarrhythmic agent.

Antineoplastic agents

A number of antineoplastic agents may cause neuropsychiatric side effects.[25,37] Most common are delirium, lethargy, affective symptoms, and psychosis. In many cases, these effects are dose related. The accompanying box outlines a number of chemotherapeutic agents and their associated neuropsychiatric symptoms. A complete discussion of the neuropsychiatric effects of the various chemotherapeutic agents is beyond the scope of this chapter. How-

---

Neuropsychiatric effects of chemotherapeutic agents[25,37]

Agent	Symptoms
Aminoglutethiamidine	Lethargy
L-Asparaginase	Delirium, EEG changes
5-Azacytadine	Delirium, depression
Corticosteroids	Agitation, depression, mania, psychosis
Cyclosporine	Hallucinations, mania
Cytosine arabinoside	Delirium
5-Fluorouracil	Delirium
Interferon	Delirium, paranoia
Methotrexate	Delirium, lethargy
Procarbazine	Delirium, mania
Vinblastine	Lethargy, depression
Vincristine	Dysphoria, hallucinations

---

ever, a few of the characteristics of certain agents are discussed.

Aminoglutethimide can cause a flulike syndrome, probably because of its relationship to glutethimide, a sedating agent. These symptoms tend to lessen after the first month of treatment and can be helped by adjusting the medication dose. L-Asparaginase has been documented to cause electroencephalographic (EEG) changes.[35] Thus its potential for causing delirium is not surprising. This delirium usually will resolve fairly rapidly and is not dose related. Another type of delirium can occur with the medication and can be longer lasting and related to a lack of asparagine.

Prednisone, dexamethasone, and other corticosteroids tend to cause their side effects in a dose-related manner. Manic or psychotic symptoms should be treated with haloperidol or other neuroleptic agents. It may be possible to prevent these side effects by pretreating with lithium. The symptoms that occur may continue for several weeks, even after the agent has been discontinued.

Cyclosporine-induced changes tend to be uncommon, but when they occur can be rather dramatic.[49] Reported cases tend to be of slow onset and may actually occur during the period of tapering the medication. 5-Fluorouracil appears to cause its side effect of delirium more commonly in the elderly. Interferon-induced encephalopathy may result in EEG changes and associated symptoms. The onset of these symptoms tends to be fairly rapid and may take several weeks to resolve.

Methotrexate causes greater symptoms when given at high doses intravenously. Sensorimotor signs can also occur and signal a need to discontinue treatment. Vincristine causes dysphoria and hallucinations in a dose-dependent manner.[24] This characteristic is present with a number of the chemotherapeutic agents and can often be treated by a small decrease in dose. Procarbazine, a weak inhibitor of monoamine oxidase, has been reported to cause psychosis and mania.

Antiparkinsonian agents

Psychiatric side effects can occur with a number of different medications used in the treatment of Parkinson's disease. For the most part, these medications can be grouped into two separate categories: *anticholinergic agents and dopamine agonists*. Anticholinergic agents have been discussed earlier in this chapter. As noted, they can lead to confusion, delirium, hallucinations, agitation, and bizarre behavior. That these symptoms occur much more frequently in the elderly is significant because most people with Parkinson's disease fall into this age range. The only effective treatment for dealing with these side effects is to reduce the dose of or eliminate the offending agent.

Dopamine agonists used in the treatment of Parkinson's disease include L-dopa, amantadine, and bromocriptine. Each of these agents, as well as other dopamine agonists, can induce psychiatric side effects.[27] The most significant of these side effects is psychosis.[46] When psychosis occurs early in the course of treatment, it is usually correlated with a history of a prior psychiatric illness. Long-standing treatment can also lead to psychotic symptomatology. Most of the psychotic symptoms that occur during treatment are paranoid thoughts, which often occur without a coexistent delirium or confusional state. Hallucinations tend to be visual and are mostly nocturnal, nonthreatening, and recurrent. Approximately one half of patients on L-dopa for over 2 years will develop this type of phenomenon. It tends to remit quickly when the medication is discontinued.[46] Interestingly, hallucinations as a symptom appear to correlate with the existence of nocturnal myoclonic activity.

Other psychiatric symptoms reported with dopamine agonists include vivid dreams, night terrors, depression, and mania.[38] These symptoms usually resolve rapidly upon discontinuation of the medication. With vivid dreams and night terrors, however, reassurance is often sufficient to allow continuation of treatment.

Hormonal agents

Oral contraceptives have been noted to cause psychiatric effects in patients without preexisting psychiatric illness.[18] Most patients who take these agents, however, will experience no change in mood. Some women will note an increased activity level, as well as an elevation of mood while on oral contraceptives. Several proposed mechanisms have been suggested, including monoamine oxidase inhibition, increased serotonin levels, direct effect on central nervous system (CNS) hormone receptors, and psychologic factors associated with the decreased likelihood of pregnancy. On the other hand, several reports of depression while taking oral contraceptives have been noted. The etiology of this side effect is not clear, but the symptomatology can be severe. Discontinuation of the hormonal agent results in eventual normalization of mood, but may take several weeks to occur. On occasion, a full affective disorder can be initiated by hormonal agents and requires antidepressant or antimanic treatment for its resolution.

Interestingly, hormonal agents, including estrogen and androgens, have been used to treat affective disorders, including depression.[26] However, data regarding whether this mode of treatment is effective is neither consistent nor convincing. What is clear, however, are that hormonal agents do affect mood and behavior differently in various women.

Anabolic steroids have also been noted to affect mood and behavior. This side effect will be more fully discussed in Chapter 21.

Narcotics and other analgesics

Narcotics have been associated with a wide variety of neuropsychiatric effects, including nightmares, agitation, euphoria, dysphoria, depression, paranoia, and hallucinations.[1] These side effects occur most commonly at higher dose levels or with patients who have more difficulty metabolizing the medications. For example, the elderly are much more prone to have cognitive impairment resulting from narcotic use than other patient populations. Meperidine, in particular, has been noted to cause symptoms of delirium.[15] CNS effects, in addition to delirium, include nervousness, tremors, myoclonus, and seizures. These effects have been attributed to the active metabolite of meperidine, normeperidine. This metabolite can accumulate over time because of its long half-life. Therefore, reversal of symptoms upon discontinuation of meperidine occurs gradually.

Most of the neuropsychiatric side effects described here tend to remit quickly after discontinuation of narcotics. If chronic narcotic use exists, however, the narcotic agents must be tapered gradually to avert withdrawal symptoms. If withdrawal symptoms are not an issue, other noncardiac analgesics can be substituted for the treatment of pain.

Narcotic analgesics are not the only analgesic agents to induce neuropsychiatric effects. Nonsteroidal antiinflammatory drugs have been noted to induce side effects such as depression, confusion, paranoia, hallucinations, and anxiety. These effects are usually minor and easily treated with a dose reduction or discontinuation of the agent. Severe symptoms, including psychosis, however, have been reported and require prompt treatment with neuroleptic medications in addition to discontinuing the agent.[21]

Respiratory agents and stimulants

Several alpha- and beta-adrenergic stimulants are used in the treatment of respiratory disease. Characteristic agents include ephedrine and phenylpropanolamine. These substances act in ways similar to that of amphetamines and cocaine. These two agents are not discussed in this section, but are referred to in Chapter 54. The most common neuropsychiatric side effects from these substances are agitation and anxiety.[22] Both the alpha-adrenergic stimulants, which are used as decongestants, and the beta-adrenergic stimulants, which are used as bronchodilators, can cause these symptoms. More serious effects have been documented. For example, phenylpropanolamine has been reported to induce acute mania, paranoia, and organic hallucinosis.[31] Discontinuation of the agent usually results in rapid reversal of symptomatology. The beta-adrenergic drug, albuterol, has also been reported to induce psychosis on rare occasion. The major side effect of beta-adrenergic agents, however, is anxiety, which is likely produced by direct central stimulation of beta-receptors. Methylxanthine derivatives may also cause symptoms of anxiety. These derivatives include caffeine and theophylline. Both anxiety and depression have been associated with long-term, high-dose caffeine ingestion.[12] It is possible, however, that depression predates heavy caffeine use and that coffee is used in an attempt to self-medicate depressive symptoms. Patients with panic attacks tend to use caffeine less frequently. It is clear, however, that any use of caffeine may greatly exacerbate their symptoms.

In summary, mild stimulants such as caffeine and those agents used as decongestants and bronchodilators cause relatively mild psychiatric effects. Anxiety is most common; however, more serious symptoms such as psychosis may occur. Discontinuation of the medication is the treatment of choice in most cases. Cases of prolonged symptoms after discontinuation have been noted only rarely.[23]

Sedatives

Barbiturate and benzodiazepine compounds have been noted to cause several different neuropsychiatric symptoms, including cognitive impairment, depression, hallucinations, nightmares, and paradoxical excitement or agitation.[1] In general, these side effects tend to be of minimal clinical significance, but they can be rather severe, particularly in the elderly patient. In patients with preexisting cognitive dysfunction, further cognitive impairment as a result of these agents is quite common. Paradoxical excitement or disinhibition is not very common but can be seen in the organically impaired individual. Chronic use of these substances can result in depressive symptoms,[32] which can occur insidiously over the course of treatment and usually respond to discontinuation of the agent. If symptoms do not remit upon discontinuation, however, antidepressant treatment may be indicated. Psychotic symptoms, particularly in patients with normal cognitive abilities, are rare, but have been reported.[50] Psychiatric symptoms may also manifest themselves during withdrawal from these compounds. These symptoms will be discussed in Chapter 15.

ISSUES IN SPECIAL PATIENT POPULATIONS

Psychiatric side effects of commonly used medications are uncommon in most patients. When they do occur, their overall impact is usually minimal. At higher dosage levels or in patients with a predisposition to these various effects, however, they can present a major problem, particularly in elderly and psychiatrically ill patients.

Geriatric patients are more sensitive to the side effects of medications for a number of reasons. Age-related changes in hepatic metabolism and renal clearance are two significant factors. In addition, the elderly are at much higher risk for cognitive impairment. Medications are much more likely to cause confusion or delirium in a patient who is cognitively impaired before using the drug. Thus sedatives, narcotics, beta-blockers, and other medications must be used with caution in this population. Periodic screening of gross cognitive function is important because moderate to severe cognitive dysfunction may go unnoticed if direct questioning of memory and orientation is not performed.

The psychiatric patient may have a number of symptoms that could be exacerbated by certain medications. For example, the patient with panic disorder will likely experience an increase in symptoms on medications such as theophylline, ephedrine, or albuterol. The patient who is prone to depressive symptoms should be carefully monitored when placed on medications such as beta-blockers or benzodiazepines. If severe psychiatric symptoms are present premorbidly or appear during the course of treatment, referral to a psychiatrist should be considered. Discontinuing the offending agent usually is recommended. In some cases, however, these medications are necessary and control of the symptoms may be achieved by additional medications or psychiatric therapies.

BEHAVIORAL TERATOLOGY

Behavioral teratology is a field of study that focuses on the adverse effects of teratogens on the functional development of the CNS and ultimately on behavior. The focus of teratology has long been on the more obvious structural effects of teratogens on the fetus. For example, the thalidomide effects were immediately obvious to the physician and others. If the effect of thalidomide had not been so dramatic, but had affected only behavior, it may well have gone unrecognized. These behavioral effects may not show up for a number of years and by that time the connection to the potential teratogen may not be realized. Thus not until the early 1970s was it understood that the same circumstances that can impair structural development in the fetus can also lead to functional impairment of the CNS.[8]

Behavioral teratology follows the principles and concepts of toxicology in general.[28] The result of behavioral teratogenicity is a delayed behavioral maturation along with impaired or abnormal behavior. In addition, the period during which the organism is susceptible to behavior teratogens is identical to the period of CNS development in the fetus. Time and duration of exposure of the agent are also significant. Despite these similarities to toxicology in general, it is much more difficult to recognize and accurately quantify the behavioral effects of agents.

The study of behavioral teratology also has a significant impact on the introduction of new substances into the marketplace. How intensely do we need to screen new agents for behavioral teratogenicity before their release? The answer is not entirely clear. For instance, barbiturates, phenytoin, and primidone have all been found to result in both physical and psychologic teratogenic effects. The psychologic components of these teratologic syndromes, however, may have not been recognized if not for the physical components. How many purely behavioral teratogens exist thus becomes difficult to determine.

The implications for behavioral teratogens in the study of preventive medicine are numerous. The prevention of all behavioral abnormalities that occur as a result of teratogenicity would be the ultimate goal, albeit difficult to achieve. At present, the physician must be aware of a number of known behavioral teratogens.

Known behavioral teratogens

The majority of research in behavioral teratology has been performed in animals. Little is known about possible effects in human populations. It is also not clear how applicable animal research is to human population with respect to behavioral teratogenic effects. The box below lists those compounds reported and confirmed as behavioral teratogens.

Although most studies are performed in animal populations, several known behavioral teratogens exist in humans, the best known of which is ethanol. Fetal alcohol syndrome has been described for a number of years in human populations and is most likely a major cause of cognitive impairment secondary to a teratogenic etiology.[11] When the fetal alcohol syndrome is fully expressed, it is fairly easily recognized. What is not known, however, is the frequency to which the syndrome is only partially expressed. A large number of children may be affected with more subtle behavioral or cognitive abnormalities than is presently known.

The problem of identifying and categorizing the behavioral effects of teratogens is enormous. In humans it would require following large numbers of exposed children as they develop through various stages of cognitive and emotional functioning. The difficulty involved in this type of research is obvious. Through careful observation of patients, it is hoped that some of these teratogens can be identified.

The actual teratologic effects of the substances listed earlier are discussed elsewhere.[6] Ethanol is used here as an example of potential neurobehavioral teratogenicity. Fetal alcohol syndrome can result in craniofacial abnormalities, growth deficiency, cardiac murmurs or septal defects, urogenital abnormalities, and skeletal and muscular deformities. CNS abnormalities are also a significant part of the syndrome.[42] These deficiencies can be manifested by mild to moderate retardation, microcephaly, irritability in infancy, hypotonia, poor coordination, and possible hyperactivity in childhood. Currently, it is not clear how much ethanol intake by the mother would be sufficient to cause the fetal alcohol syndrome. It is also unclear whether low doses of ethanol, which would be insufficient to cause the fetal alcohol syndrome, could cause more subtle abnormalities in behavior and cognition. What is certain is this field of study is in its infancy and further research is needed.

SUMMARY

A wide variety of medications can produce psychiatric effects. Whenever a clinician notices a change in behavior in a patient placed on a new medication, the medication must be suspected as a cause. Often it is difficult to tell whether the behavioral changes are due to progression of an underlying disease, a new psychiatric condition, or a medication side effect. The clinician must consider underlying emotional or psychiatric symptoms when prescribing new medications to patients. One can avoid exacerbation of certain psychiatric symptoms if care is taken when choosing a medication regimen. Psychiatric side effects of medications are not well studied. Therefore, it is up to the clinician in most cases to monitor for "behavioral side effects," as each patient's response to various medications can be idiosyncratic. Finally, the field of behavioral teratology is fairly new and difficult to document, but should always remain in the back of a clinician's mind.

REFERENCES

1. Abramowicz M, editor: Drugs that cause psychiatric symptoms, *Med Lett Drugs Ther* 31(808):114-118, 1989.
2. Altes J, Gasco J, DeAntonio J, et al: Ciprofloxacin and delirium, *Ann Intern Med* 110(2):170-171, 1989.
3. Al-Zehawi MF, Sprott MS, Hendrick DJ: Hallucinations in association with ceftazidime, *Br Med J* 297:858, 1988.
4. Baldessarini RJ, Cole JO: Chemotherapy. In Nichol AM, editor: *The new Harvard guide to psychiatry,* Cambridge, Mass, 1988, Harvard University Press.
5. Ball R, Rosser R: Psychosis and anti-tuberculosis therapy, *Lancet* 2:105, 1989.
6. Briggs GG, Bodendorfer TW, Freeman RK, et al: *Drugs in pregnancy and lactation: a reference guide to fetal and neonatal risk,* Baltimore, 1983, Williams & Wilkins.

Known behavioral teratogens in humans

Alcohol
Antimitotics
Antioxidants
Antipsychotics
Barbiturates
Lead
Methylmercury narcotics
Benatone and other anticonvulsants, stimulants, and vitamin A

7. Bullinger M: Psychotropic effects of non-psychotropic drugs, *Adv Drug React Ac Pois Rev* 6(3):141-167, 1987.

8. Butcher RE: A historical perspective on behavioural teratology, *Neurobehav Toxicol Teratol* 7:537-540, 1985.

9. Byrd GJ: Acute organic brain syndrome associated with gentamicin therapy, *JAMA* 238(1):53-54, 1977.

10. Cassem NH: Depression. In *Massachusetts General Hospital handbook of general hospital psychiatry,* ed 2, Littleton, Mass, 1987, PSG Publishing Co.

11. Clarren SK, Smith DW: The fetal alcohol syndrome, *N Engl J Med* 298(19):1063-1067, 1978.

12. Clementz GL, Dailey JW: Psychotropic effects of caffeine, *Am Fam Physician* 37(5):167-172, 1988.

13. Collaborative Group for Epidemiology of Epilepsy: Adverse reactions to anti-epileptic drugs: a multicenter survey of clinical practice. *Epilepsia* 27:323-330, 1986.

14. Delev D, Schmedding E: Acute psychosis as idiosyncratic reaction to quinidine: report of two cases, *Br Med J* 294:1001-1002, 1987.

15. Eisendrath SJ, Goldman B, Douglas J, et al: Meperidine-induced delirium, *Am J Psychiatry* 144:1062-1065, 1987.

16. Eisendrath SJ, Sweeney MA: Toxic neuropsychiatric effects of digoxin at therapeutic serum concentrations, *Am J Psychiatry* 144(4):506-507, 1987.

17. Gangat AE, Simpson MA, Naidoo LR: Medication as a potential cause of depression, *South African Med J* 70:224-226, 1986.

18. Glick ID, Bennett SE: Psychiatric complications of progesterone and oral contraceptives, *J Clin Psychopharmacol* 1(6):350-367, 1981.

19. Good MI: Substance-induced dissociative disorders and psychiatric nosology, *J Clin Psychopharmacol* 9(2):88-93, 1989.

20. Greenblatt DJ, Shader RI: Anticholinergics, *N Engl J Med* 288(23):1215-1219, 173.

21. Griffith JD, Smith CH, Smith RC: Paranoid psychosis in a patient receiving ibuprofen, a prostaglandin synthesis inhibitor: case report, *J Clin Psychiatry* 43(12):499-500, 1982.

22. Hall RCW, Beresford TP, Stickney SK, et al: Psychiatric reactions produced by respiratory drugs. *Psychosomatics* 26(7):605-616, 1985.

23. Hays DP, Johnson BF, Perry R: Prolonged hallucinations following a modest overdose of tripelennamine, *Clin Toxicol* 16(3):331-333, 1980.

24. Holland JF, Scharlau C, Gailani S, et al: Vincristine treatment of advanced cancer: a cooperative study of 392 cases, *Cancer Res* 33:1258-1264, 1973.

25. Kaplan RS, Wiernik PH: Neurotoxicity of antineoplastic drugs, *Semin Oncol* 9:103-130, 1982.

26. Klaiber EL, Broverman DM, Vogel W, et al: Estrogen therapy for severe persistent depressions in women, *Am J Psychiatry* 36:550-554, 1979.

27. Klawans HL: Psychiatric side effects during the treatment of Parkinson's disease, *J Neural Transm Suppl* 27:117-122, 1988.

28. Koëter HBWN: Behavioural teratology of exogenous substances: regulation aspects, *Prog Brain Res* 73:59-67, 1988.

29. Krauthammer C, Klerman GL: Secondary mania, *Arch Gen Psychiatry* 35:1333-1339, 1978.

30. Lader M, Bruce M: States of anxiety and their induction by drugs, *Br J Clin Pharmacol* 22:251-261, 1986.

31. Lake CR, Masson EB, Quirk RS: Psychiatric side effects attributed to phenylpropanolamine, *Pharmacopsychiatry* 21:171-181, 1988.

32. Lydiard RB, Laraia MT, Ballenger JC, et al: Emergence of depressive symptoms in patients receiving alprazolam for panic disorder, *Am J Psychiatry* 144(5):664-665, 1987.

33. Maris RW: *Pathways to suicide: a survey of self-destructive behaviors,* Baltimore, 1981, Johns Hopkins University Press.

34. Morrison RL, Katz IR: Drug-related cognitive impairment: current progress and recurrent problems, *Annu Rev Gerontol Geriatr* 9:232-279, 1989.

35. Moure JMB, Whitecare JP, Bodey GP: Electroencephalogram changes secondary to asparaginase, *Arch Neurol* 23:365-368, 1970.

36. Paykel ES, Fleminger R, Watson JP: Psychiatric side effects of antihypertensive drugs other than reserpine, *J Clin Psychopharmacol* 2(1):14-39, 1982.

37. Peterson LG, Popkin MK: Neuropsychiatric effects of chemotherapeutic agents for cancer, *Psychosomatics* 21:141-153, 1980.

38. Rego MD, Giller EL: Mania secondary to amantadine treatment of neuroleptic-induced hyperprolactinemia, *J Clin Psychiatry* 50(4):143-144, 1989.

39. Reynolds EH, Trimble MR: Adverse neuropsychiatric effects of anticonvulsant drugs, *Drugs* 29:570-581, 1985.

40. Richardson PJ, Wyke MA: Memory function—effects of different antihypertensive drugs, *Drugs* 35(Suppl 5):80-85, 1988.

41. Schoonover SC: Depression. In Bassuk EL, Schoonover SC, Gelenberg AJ, editors: *The practitioner's guide to psychoactive drugs,* ed 2, New York, 1983, Plenum Publishing Co.

42. Shaywitz BA: Fetal alcohol syndrome: an ancient problem rediscovered, *Drug Ther* 8:95-108, 1978.

43. Sirota P, Stoler M, Meshulam B: Major depression with psychotic features associated with acyclovir therapy, *Drug Intell Clin Pharm* 22:306-308, 1988.

44. Sultzer DL, Cummings JL: Drug-induced mania, causative agents, clinical characteristics and management. A retrospective analysis of the literature, *Med Toxicol Adverse Drug Exp* 4(2):127-143, 1989.

45. Trimble MR: Anticonvulsant drugs and cognitive function: a review of the literature, *Epilepsia* 28(suppl 3):537-545, 1987.

46. Turner TH, Cookson JC, Wass JAH, et al: Psychotic reactions during treatment of pituitary tumors with dopamine agonists, *Br Med J* 289:1101-1103, 1984.

47. Vining EPG: Cognitive dysfunction associated with antiepileptic drug therapy, *Epilepsia* 28(suppl 2):518-522, 1987.

48. Vorhees CV, Butcher RE: Behavioural tertogenicity. In Snell K, editor: *Developmental toxicology,* London, 1982, Croom Helm.

49. Wamboldt FW, Weiler SJ, Kalin NH: Cyclosporin-associated mania, *Biol Psychiatry* 19(7):1161-1162, 1984.

50. White MC, Silverman JJ, Harbison JW: Psychosis associated with clonazepam therapy for blepharospasm, *J Nerv Ment Dis* 170(2):117-119, 1982.

━━━━━━ **RESOURCES** ━━━━━━

The helpful resources are all included in the reference list. The *Physician's Desk Reference* also includes psychiatric effects of medications in their section on Adverse Reactions.

Chapter 15

DRUG DEPENDENCE AND SUBSTANCE ABUSE

Gregory B. Collins
Kirste Carlson
Teresa Conroy
Ora Frankel
David Golden
Howard Moliff

Substance abuse and dependency are large-scale public health problems that cause morbidity and mortality and are seen in nearly every type of medical practice. Abuse of alcohol and drugs affects nearly every American family in some way, as the lifetime expected prevalence rate of substance abuse is 17%.[46]

A recent government estimate of the cost of these disorders to our society exceeded $80 billion annually, and the human cost in suffering and wastage of lives is beyond measure. Because alcoholics and drug abusers use medical services excessively in proportion to their numbers, they are overrepresented in hospitals and clinics, where the medical, surgical, and psychologic sequelae of their disorders are treated. Although the physician is generally called on to diagnose and treat only the medical consequences of substance abuse, the physician also needs to recognize the opportunity to intervene in the underlying, often hidden, self-destructive, relentless, and perhaps fatal addictive process.

Prevention in the field of substance abuse is, in many ways, similar to prevention in other fields of medicine, with primary, secondary, and tertiary levels of activity. At the level of primary prevention of substance abuse, physicians carefully monitor the prescriptions they write, so as to limit availability and lessen the risk of dependence and abuse. Physician counseling of offspring of alcoholics to avoid drinking limits exposure in a high-risk population,

as susceptibility to alcoholism may be genetically influenced. These primary prevention efforts, although helpful, are modest compared to the involvement of physicians in secondary and tertiary levels of prevention of substance abuse.

Secondary level prevention occurs with the early identification and diagnosis of cases, so that treatment can begin at the earliest possible stage. Although substance abuse was long a neglected subject in medical training, physicians are now being taught in medical schools to recognize the signs and symptoms of substance abuse and are now well educated in the "disease model" of alcoholism and other addictions. This model emphasizes the primary, addictive nature of these illnesses, as well as the central theme of abstinence from mood-altering chemicals in recovery.

Tertiary prevention occurs through the involvement of physicians in the treatment and rehabilitation of alcoholics and other drug dependents. Here, too, the role of physicians has been expanding, from the narrow services of detoxification and organ restoration to the broader phases of psychologic, social, and even spiritual recovery. Physicians can and should play a major and decisive role in the rehabilitative process, as chemical dependency is a disease of the "mind, body, and spirit." Interested, committed physicians can combine elements of the art and science of medicine to relieve the suffering of not only these afflicted people, but also their aggrieved family members. Often the "turnarounds" are miraculous, and hope should never be abandoned.

COCAINE

Until recently, the popular myth was that cocaine was a nonaddictive substance that involved low risk to the user. However, with the deaths of sports figures Don Rogers and Len Bias and entertainers such as John Belushi, there is a growing appreciation that cocaine is both highly addictive and dangerous. Unfortunately, heightened public awareness of these dangers has not resulted in dramatic decreases in cocaine use, which is presently a virtual worldwide epidemic. The cocaine production and distribution industry is now rated as one of the largest industries in the world, and cocaine agriculture has become a mainstay in the economic vitality of producing countries. With the use of cocaine now widespread, primary care physicians must learn to recognize, diagnose, and manage its medical and psychiatric complications.[10]

The perception that cocaine was safe, had mood-elevating properties, and carried a high price tag (about $100.00 per gram, enough for an evening of recreational use) initially earned for cocaine the reputation of a drug associated with glamour, status, power, affluence, and sex appeal. This initial mystique of cocaine as a "jet set drug" has since abated, and today cocaine is used by individuals in every stratum of society. It has become more popular than heroin in the inner city. According to U.S. government figures,[43] the rate of cocaine-related emergencies and deaths tripled between 1976 and 1981. In 1983, a *Time* poll[1] reported that 4 to 5 million Americans used it at least once a month, and that 200,000 to 1 million were dependent. It also reported that, despite the cost, more blue-collar workers than professionals use cocaine. Cocaine "hotlines" indicate that approximately half the users are women. Younger people are increasingly involved, and cocaine is relatively commonplace in colleges and high schools.

Pharmacology

Pharmacologically, cocaine is an alkaloid, similar to atropine and belladonna; it is a potent vasoconstrictor and nerve-conduction blocker when administered locally. Recreational users generally begin by "snorting" cocaine. Taken intranasally, the drug is rapidly absorbed through mucous membranes. Heavy users and addicts adopt more efficient methods, such as crack smoking, freebase smoking, or intravenous (IV) administration. These methods allow the cocaine to reach the brain very rapidly, with the attainment of a nearly instantaneous "high."

Cocaine stimulates the central nervous system (CNS) "from above downward," affecting cognitive and mood centers first. Small amounts of the drug produce talkative-ness, elation, euphoria, motor restlessness, diminished fatigue and depression, and a sense of increased mental, physical, and sexual ability. However, severely depressed individuals do not experience mood elevation.[42] Depending on the individual's predisposition, other effects can include extreme hyperactivity, grandiose or paranoid delusions, and violence. The period of intense pleasure—30 to 60 minutes—is followed by depression and profound dysphoria; thus users want to repeat the experience to relieve "let-down" depression. At higher doses, users may become anxious and suspicious. They may resort to simultaneous use of IV opiates ("speedballing") to reduce the dysphoric effect. In the let-down phase, marked depression is common, with crying and suicidal thoughts. Some users may acutely experience seizures, respiratory arrest, or sudden death.

Cocaine potentiates sympathetic neurons with both excitatory and inhibiting functions. The drug probably prevents reuptake of catecholamines in the neuronal synapse and sensitizes neurons to sympathomimetic amines. Taken short term, cocaine acts as a powerful, pleasurable stimulant; but chronic cocaine use results in insomnia, diminished appetite, preoccupation with the drug, depression, and even delusions.

Role of the physician

The role of the physician should include making the diagnosis of cocaine abuse or dependency; treatment of acute, cocaine-related medical complications; and prevention of further abuse with education and treatment. Identifying cocaine-related problems depends to a large extent on physician awareness of the nonspecific signs and symptoms. A patient may come in to seek help for depression, insomnia, anxiety, or respiratory problems or perhaps because of a fall, a burn, or an accident. An employer may have made the appointment because of the worker's decreased efficiency on the job or recent poor attendance record. Often cocaine users stay up at night because of the stimulant properties of the drug, with resultant sleepiness at work or absenteeism the next day. Bringing up the subject should not be difficult. The physician might simply say, "I see a lot of drug use these days, so naturally I have to ask you about it." First inquire about alcohol and marijuana, which is what most cocaine users begin using. Once into the discussion, you might say, "Cocaine use is also common these days. Have you tried it?" If the answer is affirmative, ask "What kind of reaction did you get from it?" "When did you use it last?" "How much have you been using?" "Are you ever absent from work or school because of it?" "Has anyone in your family ever complained about your using it?" "How much do you spend on it?" "Is it getting out of control?" Positive answers from the patient or family members will usually indicate progressive, addictive use of the drug.

Diagnosis

Psychiatric and physical findings vary widely among individuals and also depend on the extent of cocaine use. Early psychologic/behavioral symptoms include anxiety, depression, excitability, garrulousness, hyperactivity, insomnia, motor restlessness, psychosomatic "aches and pains," relationship and job difficulties, and financial problems. Later, more profound psychiatric disturbance is evident, including auditory, olfactory, and visual hallucinations; delusions of parasites under the skin (Magnan's sign)[35]; fear of police; paranoid thoughts, possibly leading to violence; and suicidal ideation.

On physical examination, some patients may appear normal, whereas others may have conspicuous markers of drug abuse. The nasal mucosa may be atrophic or hemorrhagic. The nasal septum may be perforated because of vasoconstriction and necrosis from diminished blood supply. Rebound vasodilation may cause rhinorrhea and conjunctival and scleral injection. Pupils may be dilated but reactive. Voice coarseness may reflect chronic irritation from freebase or crack smoking. Needle tracks may be evident over venous injection sites. Cardiovascular signs and symptoms include mild hypertension, tachycardia, and other arrhythmias. Additional physical findings may include severe burns from explosions of volatile ether used in the freebasing distillation process, hyperpyrexia from the CNS effects, trauma from motor vehicle accidents, or attempted suicide or homicide. Some cocaine addicts become malnourished, with concomitant evidence of thiamine and vitamins B_6, A, and C deficiencies. Often, young cocaine abusers complain of chest pain after use of the drug. An electrocardiogram (ECG) may show indications of myocardial ischemia, premature ventricular contractions, or myocardial infarction. A chest film will show an occasional pneumothorax, pneumomediastinum, or pulmonary edema.

The patient should be examined for infection sites, especially skin abscesses and tissue cellulitis. Because addicts who take drugs IV may have subacute bacterial endocarditis, the presence of heart murmurs, indicating valvular vegetations, should be investigated. Possible complications from nonsterile drugs, syringes, and needles include AIDS, septic pulmonary emboli, pneumonia, brain abscesses, ophthalmic infections, and pulmonary granulomas. Users are also at risk for hepatitis; jaundice and laboratory evidence of hepatocellular dysfunction should be sought. In cases of central cardiorespiratory collapse, convulsions and coma occur. Unfortunately, sudden or unexplained death in a young person may well be the initial manifestation of cocaine abuse. Laboratory tests will establish a diagnosis. Urine toxicology will reveal the presence of cocaine breakdown products, benzoylecgonine and ecgonine methyl ester if ingestion has occurred within 48 to 72 hours. Toxicologic screens may also reveal the presence of other drugs, especially "downers" such as benzodiazepines, opiates, meperidine, or methaqualone, in addition to alcohol and marijuana.

Addiction to cocaine can develop rapidly, sometimes with only a few days of repeated use. The appearance of psychologic dependency predominates, as withdrawal produces no physical signs. Once addicted, users quickly progress to higher doses, purer drug, and more potent routes of administration. The initial "snorting" (intranasal use) of street cocaine gives way to freebasing or to IV use of purified or basified cocaine sulfate, with enhanced and more rapid CNS effects. Addiction can be profoundly disabling. Users may find themselves totally preoccupied with the drug and its effects. Even though they may try to stop, the compulsion to resume may be overwhelming. Addicts have been known to use millions of dollars worth of cocaine in a short time. Stories of $50,000 spent in 6 weeks are not unusual. With this degree of addiction, financial resources are quickly exhausted, and addicts must resort to selling the drug, to theft, or to prostitution.

Chronic cocaine use, especially if the drug is taken IV, may result in a psychosis indistinguishable from paranoid schizophrenia, with delusions that may be vague or fall into patterns. Auditory, visual, and olfactory hallucinations may occur in patients with a clear sensorium. Cocaine psychosis often is manifested by "bull horrors" (i.e., paranoid fear of the police) or "cocaine bugs" (Magnan's sign),[35] delusions of parasites under the skin that lead to itching, followed by compulsive scratching. Violence stemming from paranoid delusions is common. Behavior may eventually regress to stereotyped actions with endless concern for minute details. Hallucinations usually stop when cocaine is discontinued, but the paranoid delusions may persist.

In a series of cocaine-related deaths reported in Dade County, Florida, all routes of administration of the drug were implicated, including the intranasal route. Most deaths involved rapid onset of coma, sometimes with convulsions, progressing to respiratory suppression. In some users, death was the result of rapid cardiovascular collapse. Blood levels of cocaine varied widely. The lowest levels occurred in IV users, suggesting that even modest levels achieved by this route can be lethal. In 15 of the 68 subjects in the study, death resulted from trauma, including suicide, homicide, and vehicular accident.[58]

Treatment

Treatment for simple cocaine intoxication initially involves constant observation in a nonstimulating environment. Responsible family members can observe the intoxicated individual in an available examining room in the office or emergency room. The intoxication should dissipate relatively quickly and spontaneously. Obtaining a urine toxicology screen to check for the presence of additional drugs is recommended. For severe toxic overdose and coma, one should initiate basic supportive management, stabilizing the airway and circulatory system. Standard treatment consists of 100 ml of 50% dextrose and water and the opioid antagonist naloxone hydrochloride. For cocaine-induced central cardiovascular overstimulation (arrhythmias, hypertension, tachycardia), propranolol hydrochloride should be administered intravenously, with the patient continuously monitored.[44] A hypertensive crisis that does not respond to this regimen should be treated with an IV short-acting antihypertensive agent such as nitroprusside or the alpha-antagonist phentolamine. Agitation, seizures, or status epilepticus should be treated with IV diazepam. A short-acting barbiturate such as secobarbital or amobarbital can be given for sedation.[22] For toxic psychoses and severe paranoid reactions, haloperidol in 5 to 10 mg increments should be administered. For severe hyperthermia, continuous core temperature monitoring is critical. Treatment for cocaine-induced hyperthermia (core temperature above 40.5° C [105° F]) consists of an ice bath and monitoring of vital signs until the core temperature falls below 30° C (102° F).[23]

Withdrawal is generally characterized by irritability, depression, suicidal ideation, and a strong desire for the drug. It is best managed conservatively without replacement medications, although, we have enjoyed good success with 5 to 7 days of propranolol (Inderal) 10 mg tid and imipramine (Tofranil) 25 mg tid. Because there is no exact substitute medication for detoxification, the "cold turkey" approach is often used. Withdrawal symptoms and agitation usually abate within 4 to 5 days. Hospitalization is usually indicated in moderate to severe cases. Initial therapy for cocaine addiction involves detoxification and drug counseling in inpatient or outpatient drug and alcohol rehabilitation centers. Emphasis is on abstinence, not only from cocaine, but from all mood altering substances. The patient is strongly counseled to avoid situations and friends that put him/her in contact with the drug. Active participation in self-help support groups such as Cocaine Anonymous (CA), Narcotics Anonymous (NA), or Alcoholics Anonymous (AA) is encouraged. Outpatient professional counseling and supervision, including random urine monitoring, will improve the outcome. With reasonable compliance, the prognosis is good.

OTHER STIMULANTS

Among the other stimulants, amphetamine is the prototype drug. Although it was first synthesized in 1887 by Edeleano, its properties were not researched until 1920. In 1932, amphetamine was introduced as an over-the-counter inhaler (Benzedrine) for head colds, nasal congestion, and asthma. It was soon found to increase alertness and confidence, while decreasing fatigue and appetite. During World War II, amphetamine was used in Germany, Great Britain, Japan, and the United States to increase energy in combat troops.[34] In 1938, the Food and Drug Administra-

tion classified amphetamines as prescription drugs, although this rule was not strictly enforced until 1951, when it was passed as a federal law. Nevertheless, widespread use continued because physicians prescribed amphetamines quite freely. By the early 1950s, with attempts to limit the legal manufacture and sale of the drug, many clandestine laboratories appeared. Amphetamine abuse reached epidemic proportions in the late 1960s, with 50% of all manufactured amphetamines being diverted to illegal street sales. In the early 1970s, 14% of all psychoactive drugs prescribed by physicians were amphetamines. With the Controlled Substance Act of 1970, which imposed strict quotas on the manufacture of certain drugs and severe penalties for violation, the supply of amphetamines decreased.[34] In addition, about that time, knowledge of the potential dangers of drug abuse became widespread, contributing to a decrease in amphetamine abuse. Today, amphetamines are still abused by sophisticated addicts, but the newer amphetamine-like drugs, such as "Ice" (crystal methamphetamine) are more fashionable among stimulant abusers.

Medical uses of amphetamine compounds are basically limited to the treatment of narcolepsy and attention deficit disorders in children. Amphetamines are also sometimes useful in the treatment of certain types of depression, particularly in older patients with medical illnesses, and are the only effective medications in certain atypical depressions.[45] In other cases, it is quite useful as an adjunct to tricyclic antidepressant therapy.[27] Although amphetamine is still being prescribed for weight loss, many doubts have been raised about its long-term efficacy and safety in such treatments.[26] The anorectic effect of amphetamines is not long-lasting, and the risk of abuse or addiction exceeds the short-term benefit of weight loss.

Role of the physician

Patients who choose to obtain drugs from physicians rather than on the street are marked by their ability to simulate a straight, honest, and often helpless impression. Many patients, especially those who are experienced and skillful in obtaining the desired drug, are sufficiently cautious not to overdo the frequency of their visits and may be able to obtain prescriptions for a considerable period.[16] In general, any requests for amphetamines or "diet pills" should arouse suspicion. Patients may use many ploys to manipulate physicians to obtain stimulants, but they all lead to the same conclusion: The patient prescribes the drug he or she chooses through you. Typical ploys include "I'm allergic to . . ." (the patient shifts away from your suggestion and instead suggests their favorite drug); "My former doctor always gave me _____ for my weight problem;" or "My neighbor takes _____ for her weight problem." Such statements always pressure the physician to conform to the patient's expectation by prescribing controlled drugs. Although the physician may be tempted to offer small amounts, thinking that the situation is under control, it should be remembered that drug-abusing patients typically manipulate numerous physicians and pharmacies at the same time, so that even small amounts may be maintaining an addictive process.

Drug abusers may resort to more extreme methods to obtain controlled drugs, such as stealing prescription pads from the physician's office, altering prescriptions to get larger numbers of medications, or "misplacing" medications so that numerous refills are required. The physician should bear in mind that drug-dependent patients do not fit any stereotype. They come from all walks of life and may take great pains to appear conventional, appropriate, and disarming in the physician's office.

In many instances, the physician is alerted to the possibility of amphetamine abuse by the appearance of the patient or by members of the patient's family. One should note signs of social, economic, and emotional deterioration including job demotions, job loss, deteriorated physical condition, or unkempt appearance. Family members may describe the patient as having become unreliable, irritable, and unstable.[16] In spite of the physical signs and symptoms of autonomic arousal that may alert the physician to the presence of this class of drugs, the only truly definitive means of diagnosing acute ingestion is through a urine toxicology screen such as with the enzyme-multiplied immunoassay test (EMIT) assay. Corroborating information from cooperative pharmacies or family members may confirm a chronic abuse pattern and indicate addiction.

In the presence of good evidence, the physician may directly confront the patient. It is not unusual for the patient to deny drug abuse or dependence. Nonetheless, the physician must candidly express suspicion and evidence about the patient's drug misuse and show concern for the patient's well-being. The physician may feel angry at having been manipulated and may express this anger by refusing to see the patient again. Ideally, though, the patient should be told that despite these manipulations, the physician recognizes the signs and symptoms of drug dependency and is prepared to help.[16]

The physician should remember that the only presently acceptable indications for the use of amphetamines and their analogs are narcolepsy, childhood attention deficit disorder, and certain treatment-resistant depressions. Because these disorders are relatively uncommon, amphetamines should be used only rarely in medical practice. We do not recommend their use in weight control because the risk of addiction or drug diversion is relatively high. Patients seeking help for weight control should be given dietary guidelines, exercise regimens, and referral to obesity self-help groups such as Overeaters Anonymous or Weight Watchers. Involvement with these programs entail minimal risk for the patient or physician and produce far better, more long-lasting results than stimulant-induced weight loss.

Physicians are advised to formulate a "policy" that does not allow the prescription of stimulants for weight control. When put under pressure by demanding patients, the physician can take refuge in citing this policy. Regrettably, if the physician becomes known as being sympathetic to pleas for stimulant drugs, word will get around quickly, and the physician's office will become a magnet for all types of drug seekers, including many with criminal intent. In some cases, the physician's office becomes an armed fortress and is little more than a legalized drug distribution center for addicts. Generally, investigation and possible license suspension by the state medical board follows shortly thereafter. To avoid this negative chain of events, the physician is best advised to exercise caution and simply not prescribe amphetamines or other stimulants in clinical practice. In cases of suspicion that a patient is dependent on stimulant drugs, prompt referral for evaluation in a specialized chemical dependency treatment center is advisable. These centers, such as that found at the Cleveland Clinic Foundation, generally have success records in excess of 50%.[11,12]

Diagnosis

The acute effects of intoxication usually begin within 20 to 60 minutes after oral ingestion and immediately after IV administration of amphetamines. In high doses, they can produce euphoria or a "rush" (a burst of energy accompanied by a physical sensation in the head and neck). Other symptoms of the amphetamines' sympathomimetic effects during intoxication include increased confidence, elation, grandiosity, hyperarousal, hypervigilance, irritability, aggressiveness, hostility, hyperactivity, loquacity, emotional lability, anorexia, anxiety, panic, resistance to fatigue, decreased need for sleep, and impaired judgment. Amphetamines can also cause abdominal pain that can mimic an acute abdomen and may cause chest pain. Clinical signs of amphetamine use include dilated but reactive pupils, tachycardia, elevated temperature, elevated blood pressure, dry mouth, flushed skin, perspiration, chills, nausea, vomiting, psychomotor excitement, tremulousness, hyperactive reflexes, and (with prolonged use) repetitious compulsiveness behavior and body movements, such as bruxism, biting, and facial grimacing.

With chronic use of amphetamines, many medical and psychiatric complications can arise.[11] Malnutrition is common, especially after prolonged intravenous use with large doses. Hypertension may be exacerbated. Needle marks, as well as cutaneous abscesses, excoriations, and necrotizing angiitis, may be evident in intravenous users.[35] Evidence of infections such as sepsis and endocarditis are common with intravenous addicts. Death from amphetamine overdosage is associated with hyperthermia leading to hyperpyrexia, cardiovascular shock, and convulsions.[19,26]

Prolonged high-dose amphetamine use can result in a delusional state characterized by paranoid ideations which strongly resemble paranoid schizophrenia or bipolar mania.[25,26] The drug-induced state may be characterized by restlessness, irritability, and heightened perceptual sensitivity. Delusions of persecution or bizarre visual and auditory hallucinations may develop. Tactile hallucinations are distinct features in advanced cases and may range from vague skin discomfort to delusions and hallucinations of "bugs" crawling under the skin, much like Magnan's sign, or the "cocaine bugs" seen with cocaine use.[24] Disorientation and memory impairment, however, are not part of the syndrome. Amphetamine psychosis is frequently dose-related, is often associated with sleep deprivation, and generally resolves as amphetamines are excreted. Acute psychotic symptoms usually disappear within days or (at most) weeks after the drug is withdrawn; but fixed delusions and the tendency towards suspiciousness, misinterpretation, and mild paranoia may persist for months after the overt psychosis has ceased. Amphetamines can also precipitate latent psychotic reactions, which do not subside when the drug use ends.[53]

After prolonged heavy use of amphetamines, a withdrawal syndrome may occur. Often referred to as "crashing," this phenomenon is characterized by depressed mood, fatigue, disturbed sleep, and increased dreaming. Amphetamines suppress rapid eye movement (REM) sleep and cause a rebound increase in REM sleep after the drug is withdrawn.[24] Beginning within 24 hours after the last dose, the patient may sleep for increasing periods, up to 18 to 20 hours per day for the next 72 hours. Other symptoms include irritability, impulsivity, insatiable hunger, headaches, profuse sweating, muscle cramps, and stomach cramps. The depression generally peaks 48 to 72 hours after the last dose and persists for several weeks. Suicidal ideation occasionally occurs during this period. If depression persists longer, an underlying disorder should be considered and tricyclic antidepressant therapy instituted.

The epidemiology of amphetamine abuse often prompts individuals to try to facilitate their physical and intellectual performance through the use of stimulants. Examples include a diverse group of students, housewives, businessmen, professional athletes, and others who share involvement in episodic high-stress situations requiring increased energy, confidence, and concentration. Other patterns of misuse can be seen in patients with chronic depression or feelings of inadequacy who may be medicating themselves. "Recreational" drug users constitute another group of amphetamine abusers. Amphetamine dependence is characterized by a progression of drug use resulting in impairment of the user's health, social functioning, and occupational performance. Polydrug use is not uncommon among amphetamine abusers; frequently seen are combinations of amphetamines with a sedative-hypnotic or alcohol. Sometimes the problem associated with the secondary drug may bring the patient to the physician's attention and may mask the amphetamine abuse. Detecting coexistent drug dependency on barbiturates is especially important because, in the event of withdrawal, treatment must be initiated promptly to avoid serious complications such as convulsions.

Treatment

Treatment for patients presenting in an acutely intoxicated, agitated, or delusional state from amphetamines requires inpatient supervision. These patients should be placed in a quiet room and given reassurance. Intramuscular haloperidol (2 to 5 mg three times a day for 1 day, and as needed thereafter) should be started, if necessary, for control of agitation. Diazepam (10 to 20 mg orally or intramuscularly) may be substituted. Diazepam may also be the drug of choice if the patient has had seizures in the past. Later, if episodes of depression become notable during the withdrawal period, a tricyclic antidepressant may be added. It is also vitally important to establish a therapeutic relationship with the patient, explaining that episodes of depression, apathy, and lack of initiative may occur over the next 2 to 4 months and that this may tempt the patient to resume amphetamine use.

After the acute crisis has been resolved, the next step involves establishing follow-up care. Both outpatient and inpatient treatment options are available, depending on the individual patient's needs. Outpatient groups such as NA and AA can be a vital means of providing support for abstinence. Drug treatment centers are excellent for patients who need a more structured program. Inpatient treatment centers and residential homes are appropriate for those who are deeply immersed in the drug subculture (those with heavy drug use for many years, or those with criminal activity) and provide long-term resocialization treatment. After detoxification and acute rehabilitation therapy are completed, urine should be collected weekly for toxicology screens under supervision to check for the presence of any drugs. A contract should be established stating that if the patient is unable to remain abstinent as demonstrated through a positive urine sample, the patient will enroll in a more structured drug treatment center. The patient should be encouraged to overcome secrecy by confiding in doctors, pharmacists, and trusted family members and friends to establish a support system for recovery.

ALCOHOL

The primary care physician often plays a pivotal role in the course of the alcoholic's illness. Although the physician is in a unique position to help, he or she can also worsen the problem through benign neglect or mismanagement. To be effective, the physician must clearly understand the disease of alcoholism and the physician's front line role in treatment. Effective physician intervention involves the art and science of medical practice by combining common sense psychotherapy and physical restoration. Involvement concerns diagnosis, confrontation, detoxification, and follow-up. Competent intervention in these four areas may mean the difference between life and death.[9]

Role of the physician

The prospect of confronting an evasive, resistant, denying alcoholic is distressing for any physician. Experience has identified three basic steps in effective confrontation: (1) mutual recognition of worsening progression, (2) self-diagnosis, and (3) offering hope through treatment. An hour should be designated to interview the alcoholic with the spouse present. If both are denying, mature children should be included. Obtaining a good drinking history is the initial step. The physician should state concern about the possibility that the presenting complaint is related to a drinking problem and indicate that more discussion is indicated. Starting with the patient's first drinking, the physician should develop a chronologic history of the drinking to the present time. Alcohol problems in high school or college or heavy drinking in military service with serious consequences should be noted. Alcohol effects on the marriage, such as complaints from spouse, arguing and fighting, physical abuse, and alcohol-related divorce should also be identified. A good marital history should be obtained, listing all marriages and significant relationships and the reasons for breakups, separations, or divorces.

Absenteeism from work, including arriving late, leaving early, long lunch hours, declining performance, warnings on the job, or loss of job, should be explored. Alcohol-related health problems, hospitalizations, injuries, auto accidents, or surgery should be identified. Legal complications, such as arrests, convictions, charges of drunk driving, public intoxication, drunk and disorderly conduct, assault and battery, or alcohol-related felonies should also be described. Financial concerns should be explored. Is the spouse complaining about too much money being spent for drinking? Are bills unpaid or wages garnisheed? Has the patient ever had psychiatric difficulty involving alcohol or drugs in any way? Did he or she use psychotropic drugs, and if so, what type, how long, how many, and from whom? Is there dual dependency, (i.e., on psychotropic drugs as well as alcohol)? Remember that most drug-dependent persons obtain their medications from physicians, so that the patient's assurance that "I only take drugs when prescribed by a doctor" does not eliminate the possibility of medication dependency.

The pattern of drinking and drug use in the last year or two should be emphasized. Generally worsening progression is evident in the form of deterioration of functioning or health or in the form of more and more frequent episodes of intoxication. The physician should express that the situation is getting worse as time passes and should emphasize the need for immediate treatment to avoid further deterioration.

Fostering self-diagnosis is accomplished by recognizing that alcoholism is a stigmatized diagnosis, and that all the patient's defenses are usually geared toward avoiding the label of alcoholic being made by the physician. Thus it is often helpful to allow the patient the dignity of self-diag-

nosis. This step can be made easier with the help of a prepared alcoholism questionnaire, such as those available from AA or the Michigan Alcoholism Screening Test (MAST).[51] These tests help the patient perceive that his or her patterns and problems are those of an alcoholic. Often it is helpful to ask the hypothetical question, "If I asked if you were an alcoholic what would you say?" This question clearly gives the patient a chance for self-diagnosis and introduces the threatening word "alcoholic" nonjudgmentally. Usually after such a careful recitation of the many alcohol problems the patient has, the patient will concede to being an alcoholic or "becoming one."

Generally the term "alcoholic denial" suggests the patient's refusal to admit to any problem with drinking. More often, however, the patient refuses to acknowledge loss of control over drinking, thus denying the need for help. This aspect of denial often takes the form of promises to "cut down" or "do better" or in assertions that the patient wants to "go it alone." Because the patient has been struggling alone for years without success, however, there is little reason to suspect that the patient will do better now without outside help.

Diagnosis

Diagnosis of any medical condition, including alcoholism, is predicated on understanding and recognizing the disorder. Ethyl alcohol is an addictive drug, and it is now generally accepted that alcoholism is a disease of addiction and that the alcoholic has lost control over alcohol and other mood-altering chemicals.[29] Bearing in mind that the alcoholic has an addiction may help the physician to better understand the alcoholic's behavior, relapses, mood swings, and physical complications.

Addiction to alcohol can only be diagnosed by observing the consequences or symptoms of this process. Usually symptoms are reflected in deterioration of marital, occupational, emotional, spiritual, legal, financial, or physical well-being.[48] If drinking repeatedly causes problems in any one of these areas, the diagnosis of alcoholism can be made, even though the patient may believe he or she can stop drinking or can control alcohol use. Current thinking suggests that alcoholism is the result of complex genetic, environmental, psychologic, physical, and social factors.[37] Because of these complexities, most professionals pay little attention to how the alcoholic came to be addicted. Looking for underlying problems or causes before stable sobriety has been achieved is generally fruitless and may be detrimental. It is better to direct treatment at completely eliminating the use of alcohol and other psychoactive substances, while recognizing that the patient is suffering from a sick compulsion to return to alcohol or drug use.

Alcoholism is a great masquerader, disguising itself as a medical or psychiatric complaint. Patients rarely seek treatment for alcoholism. They are usually in the physician's office for one or more alcohol-related disorders, such as hypertension, seizures, gastritis, ulcers, tuberculosis, accidents, trauma, burns, pancreatitis, hepatitis, heart disease, anxiety, depression, personality disorder, or paranoid ideation. The spouse or another family member may also be symptomatic because of the alcoholic's drinking. The role of the physician is to "see through" these symptoms and to diagnose the drinking problem. If alcohol, drugs, or both have anything to do with the problem, the chemical abuse should be investigated further. Problems often arise because physicians tend to recognize only late-stage physical complications and withdrawal symptoms as indicative of alcoholism. Instead they should cultivate the skill of diagnosing alcoholism at a much earlier point in its progressive disability, when manifestations are subtle. The earliest signs of alcoholism generally are adverse effects on marriage and job, which often antedate by many years any detectable physical consequences. It is thus a good idea to ask, "Did this problem have anything to do with your drinking?" or "Had you been drinking when the problem occurred?"

Treatment and detoxification

The physician should offer hope through treatment by emphasizing that the downward spiral can be interrupted and that the patient and family do not have to continue to suffer. Patients invariably do better in specialized programs in hospitals and in Alcoholics Anonymous. The physician should be familiar with the treatment facilities in the area and be able to recommend those appropriate for the patient. Inpatient admission, especially in a specialized rehabilitation program, will greatly enhance outcome. Outpatient treatment should be considered only for stable, detoxified alcoholics who are in no medical danger. Modern, comprehensive-care treatment centers for chemical dependency are available in most parts of the country and have relatively high success rates (50% and greater in some centers).[12,41] The physician should be optimistic, hopeful, and firm.

Currently, minor tranquilizers such as chlordiazepoxide are finding favor for short-term detoxification because of their efficacy, safety, and ease of administration. A reasonable regimen for a tremulous, diaphoretic, middle-aged man, would be chlordiazepoxide, 50 mg orally four times a day, or diazepam, 20 mg orally three times a day. Dosages are then generally tapered to zero in 3 to 5 days. Doses must be individualized; some patients require higher doses and some need no medication at all. Multivitamins and thiamine are always indicated for older, more debilitated alcoholics. Thiamine should always be administered before giving intravenous glucose or any other carbohydrate to avoid inducing Wernicke's encephalopathy. Anticonvulsants have been shown by some investigators to prevent withdrawal seizures,[47] but in practice they should seldom be used unless a history of seizures is present. Intravenous fluid replacement is advisable if fluid loss has been substantial from diaphoresis, vomiting, or diarrhea.

Most alcoholics respond to reassurance, good nursing care, and moderate amounts of medication. Alcoholic detoxification is seldom a difficult management problem if the medication regimen is planned correctly and if other medical complications are ruled out.

During hospitalization, the patient must lay the groundwork for follow-up with the supervising physician and with AA. The role of AA in successful recovery cannot be overstated. As a rule, the patient must go to AA to maintain sobriety, and the physician should strongly endorse this organization and the facilitation of the patient's participation in it. The physician should not offer a treatment alternative to AA, although aftercare counseling and supervision in professional settings are strongly advisable. Knowledgeable physicians develop familiarity with local AA groups and cultivate friendships among them. The patient (with assistance, if needed) should call AA for help while in the hospital. AA representatives will either visit the alcoholic there or provide aftercare after discharge. The physician's role in aftercare is to inquire about abstinence and participation in the AA program and in professional counseling.

Continued sobriety usually hinges on regular and frequent attendance at self-help support group meetings (AA, for example) and at counseling sessions. The physician should not ignore this phase of treatment; it should be viewed as a diabetic patient's need to take insulin. Active participation in self-help and professional aftercare is far preferable to other treatment modalities, including disulfiram therapy. The use of disulfiram should be considered as adjunctive treatment only in selected cases and should be regarded as a treatment of only moderate effectiveness,[2,33] even when used in conjunction with AA.

After detoxification, psychoactive drugs should be avoided, especially sedatives, analgesics, and minor tranquilizers. Such medications, even when taken under the supervision of a well-meaning physician, are poorly tolerated by alcoholics; they carry significant risk for medication dependency or precipitating a relapse to drinking.

The physician should maintain close contact with both patient and spouse for at least 1 to 2 years. Follow-up visits may be scheduled to conform to a pattern of weekly, then biweekly, then monthly office visits, generally with the spouse included (or contacted by telephone) for verification of performance and compliance.

BENZODIAZEPINES AND SEDATIVE-HYPNOTICS
Benzodiazepines

The benzodiazepines are some of the most commonly prescribed and abused drugs in use today. In the mid-1970s diazepam (Valium) led *all* other drugs in number of prescriptions written.[18] A 1979 survey estimated that 3 million people (1.6% of Americans) had used benzodiazepines daily for a year or more.[36] The National Household Survey of 1985 reported 7.1% of responding households using some prescription tranquilizers the previous year.[14] In 1990 the American Psychiatric Association found that 1.65% of the U.S. population had used benzodiazepines for a year or more.[55] In spite of continued warnings about the danger of these drugs and their potential to create addiction and devastating side effects, the public continues to demand these medications, and some doctors continue to prescribe them liberally, perhaps excessively. Triazolam (Halcion) recently made the cover of *Newsweek* (August 19, 1991) because of mounting reports the drug may be less safe than its makers claim.[13] It is also sobering to note that benzodiazepines are the prescription drugs most often used in suicide attempts.[38] The issue for physician and patient alike is clearly safe and responsible use of this class of medications.

Benzodiazepines have largely replaced barbiturates, meprobamate, methyprylon, and methaqualone for the treatment of anxiety and sleep disorders because they are thought to be safer and less addicting. Included in the class of benzodiazepines are the "sleepers" such as triazolam (Halcion), oxazepam (Serax), and temazepam (Razepam or Restoril) and the "minor tranquilizers" such as lorazepam (Alzapam or Ativan), alprazolam (Xanax), chlordiazepoxide (Librium), diazepam (Valium), halazepam (Paxipam), clorazepate (Tranxene), prazepam (Centrax), clonazepam (Klonopin) and flurazepam (Dalmane, Durapam).

All of these drugs have the potential to produce tolerance, physical and psychologic dependence, and addiction in patients. Their mood-altering effects on the CNS are more or less similar to those of alcohol. In our clinical experience, many patients who become addicted to benzodiazepines have a history (perhaps unknown to the prescriber) of alcoholism. To complicate matters, the symptoms for which the benzodiazepines are often (perhaps inappropriately) prescribed may be consequences of alcoholism (including alcohol withdrawal) or alcohol abuse. These symptoms include excessive anxiety, insomnia, depression, relationship or job stress, and seizures.

Pharmacology. Pharmacologically all benzodiazepines are similar, although they do exhibit differences in potency as well as in duration of their effects. In action they all modulate anxiety through generalized CNS depression. They are appropriately prescribed for treatment of anxiety disorders (those *not* related to alcohol or other drug problems), insomnia (temporary and situational), and for control of seizures and muscle spasms.

Within the CNS, the sites of action of benzodiazepines are the gamma-aminobutyric acid (GABA) receptors in the brain. GABA is a neurotransmitter that inhibits neuronal excitability by binding to the neuron at a chloride channel and increasing the movement of chloride across its membrane. Benzodiazepine molecules enhance the action of GABA molecules by binding to them at the receptor site and increasing the frequency of channel openings. Barbiturates, on the other hand, increase the time a channel stays open.[5]

Sedative-hypnotics

Because of their extremely high potential for abuse and addiction, the drugs classified as sedative hypnotics are passing out of usage, particularly with outpatients. However, these medications, primarily phenobarbital, are appropriately used in control of grand mal seizures, for anesthesia, and for some insomnias. In most cases, they have been replaced by benzodiazepines. Included in this group are the short-acting barbiturates—amobarbital, methohexital, pentobarbital and secobarbital—and the long-acting barbiturates—barbital and phenobarbital—as well as the non-barbiturates—ethchlorvynol, glutethimide, meprobamate (immortalized by the Rolling Stones as "mother's little helpers"), methyprylon and methaqualone (this drug was withdrawn from the legal market in 1984). Many of these drugs are still in demand on the "street" drug market, and physicians may fall prey to cons if they prescribe them without extensive clinical data and knowledge of the patient.

Role of the physician

The role of the physician in treatment of benzodiazepine and sedative-hypnotic abuse and addiction begins with a careful and in-depth assessment of the patient's physical and psychologic functioning. Often the symptoms for which these drugs are prescribed are superficially identical to those for which the addicted patient complains once he or she is in withdrawal and/or seeking to obtain more drugs. This picture is complicated further because minimization and denial of drug or alcohol use and consequences are hallmarks of addiction. Therefore, the prudent physician will interview not only the patient but also (with permission) his or her significant others before making a diagnosis and offering a prescription for addictive drugs.

Diagnosis

Any patient who abuses these drugs or who takes them for longer than a few months is at risk for developing physical dependence and/or addiction. Signs of abuse include concurrent use of greater than four alcoholic drinks per week, concurrent use of any illicit drugs, taking more than the prescribed dose on a regular basis, or continued use of or desire for the drug in spite of poor therapeutic response. In addition addicted patients also show negative behavioral changes, including marital or relationship difficulties, job trouble or job loss, withdrawal from previous activities or friends, preoccupation with the drug, poor impulse control, driving under the influence, refusal or inability to stop using the drug in spite of requests from loved ones or health professionals, and other indicators of impaired judgment. The addicted patient will often obtain drugs from more than one doctor, alter prescriptions to increase the dose or number of pills, or even forge prescriptions to maintain or augment the supply of medication.

Signs and symptoms of intoxication. Intoxication from benzodiazepines and sedative-hypnotics resembles alcohol intoxication. Common manifestations include sedation, slurred speech, nystagmus, ataxia, and inappropriate affect. As with alcohol, individuals may react idiosyncratically with violence toward self or others. Particular care to avoid intoxication should be taken in prescribing these drugs to older persons and to individuals with decreased hepatic or renal capacity.

Signs and symptoms of withdrawal. Clinicians may observe a wide variety of signs and symptoms of withdrawal from benzodiazepines and other sedative hypnotics. In general, they represent a rebound of the symptoms the drug was originally taken to suppress. Primary among these signs and symptoms are anxiety and generalized CNS hyperexcitability culminating in a grand mal seizure or status epilepticus if untreated.

Common manifestations of withdrawal from benzodiazepines include anxiety and agitation, hyperactivity, insomnia, depression, perceptual abnormalities, headache, tinnitus, formication, pruritus, generalized gastrointestinal distress, palpitations or chest pain, flushing, incontinence, decreased libido, and urinary urgency or frequency.

Barbiturate and other sedative-hypnotic withdrawal is far more likely to result in seizure or psychosis, but early signs include muscle weakness, anxiety, and abdominal distress.[42]

The onset of withdrawal symptoms depends on the length of the drug's action. Withdrawal from short-acting benzodiazepines such as triazolam (Halcion) can occur within a few hours of the last dose. For the longer acting compounds, such as chlordiazepoxide or diazepam, withdrawal can be delayed by up to a week.

Intervention and treatment

Detoxification from barbiturates is generally best accomplished on an inpatient basis, as close nursing supervision is required to detect surreptitious self-medicating and to monitor the often high doses of barbiturates required in detoxification. Often barbiturate addicts have high tolerance and consume large amounts of medications—1000 to 1500 mg of pentobarbital (Nembutal) equivalent per day. The physician can establish the degree of tolerance (and the starting dosage of pentobarbital) by a "tolerance test" in which 200 mg of pentobarbital is given orally to a detoxifying patient. If there is no subsequent sleepiness, lethargy, or slurred speech within 2 to 3 hours, then tolerance is assumed, and 200 mg can be given three or four times a day under close observation to detect somnolence or respi-

ratory suppression. Medication is stopped if these occur. If this dose is inadequate to control withdrawal, 300 to 400 mg four times a day can be given, under close supervision, in extreme cases. Once the patient is stable and comfortable, gradual reduction of 10% to 15% of medication per day can be affected as long as the patient can tolerate the reduction. On the other hand, if the "test dose" produces somnolence or slurred speech, low doses of pentobarbital (e.g., 100 mg orally four times a day) may be initiated, then titrated gradually downward to zero.

For benzodiazepine withdrawal, we prefer to switch to longer-acting forms like chlordiazepoxide (Librium) or diazepam (Valium) for safety and for maintenance of effect. For severe benzodiazepine addicts, large doses may be required to control symptoms, which may include seizures. Up to 100 to 120 mg of diazepam or its equivalent may be needed daily in divided doses in severe cases. Once stable, tapering down can begin, but often progress is slow due to high levels of anxious distress as medications are lowered. In most cases, reductions of 10% every few days will produce good results, but in extreme cases, several months of gradual tapering may be required.

TOBACCO

"Nicotine is the deadliest drug used in the world. Cigarette smoking has caused more suffering and death to Americans than World War I, World War II, the Vietnam War, AIDS, heroin addiction, cocaine addiction, and terrorist attacks combined."[8] In the recovery community, tobacco use has somehow been viewed as a secondary addiction, taking a place far behind alcohol and drug abuse. Yet this addiction is a deadly threat to this community. In the United States, approximately 30% of the general population smoke; in the recovering population 80% smoke.[20] Keeping this statistic in mind when treating inpatients for drug and alcohol abuse, a decision has to be made as to how tobacco abuse is addressed.

Former Surgeon General C. Everett Koop has underscored tobacco addiction as being in the same league as other drugs such as cocaine and heroin. Many alcohol and drug rehabilitation units have taken a no-smoking stand, encouraging their patients to refrain from tobacco use as part of their recovery. This approach has met with limited success. For example, for a no-smoking policy to work, it is evident that staff members need to be smoke-free, yet many counselors and nurses smoke. Labor laws prevent discharging from employment for this reason, so sanctions against smoking staff members don't seem to work. In addition, many patients would lose their jobs if they did not complete treatment, so asking them to leave for smoking would have dire consequences.[57]

In the Cleveland Clinic Alcohol and Drug Rehabilitation Unit, the "smoke-free hospital" policy is enforced. Smoking breaks are provided to patients several times a day outside the hospital. Patients are encouraged to consider abstinence from tobacco as a part of their recovery but the decision is left to the patient.

For those who choose to try to stop tobacco use, several aids are provided. Nicorette gum is a nicotine-based product that provides its user with enough of this drug to help control cravings for tobacco. Nicotine transdermal patches provide the drug in a steady dosage with a convenient route of administration. Clonidine patches help control withdrawal symptoms. Support groups, such as Smoke-Enders and Smokers Anonymous, are also offered.

Treatment

As with all addictions, abstinence from nicotine leads to withdrawal symptoms. These symptoms include difficulty concentrating, increased appetite or hunger, cravings, gastrointestinal disturbances, stress intolerance, restlessness, nervousness, drowsiness, fatigue, depression, irritability, impatience, anxiety, headache, and tension.[15] Although nicotine replacement, using Nicorette gum, helps diminish the intensity of withdrawal experienced, this product has its own difficulties. Patients need adequate instruction and sufficient dosage to control cravings. Contraindications include cardiac disease, hypertension, peptic ulcer disease, pregnancy, and insulin-dependent diabetes mellitus. When using clonidine, the transdermal form is the preferred mode of administration. It has been documented to be useful in the treatment of opiate and alcohol withdrawal. Side effects from clonidine, which may limit its usefulness, are postural hypotension, light-headedness, dizziness, dry mouth, tiredness, and lethargy.[50]

Group support is also encouraged. Smokers Anonymous meetings are modeled after AA meetings and follow a similar 12-step approach to recovery. Other support groups are available through organizations such as the American Lung Association and the American Cancer Society.

Relapsing, as with other forms of addiction, is a fact of life. It is estimated that 80% of smokers fail to quit on the first attempt.[51] Even after several attempts at stopping the success rate is somewhere around 50%. Encouragement to stop is always offered and supported, and if relapse occurs, the patient is prodded to quit smoking again. Undoubtedly the best treatment is "prevention," that is, never starting to smoke in the first place. Prevention of smoking is now receiving serious national attention as a public health goal. It is hoped that the widespread morbidity and mortality of this addiction will eventually be reduced by these growing prevention efforts. See Chapter 16, Smoking Cessation, for further information.

MARIJUANA

Since the increase in popularity and use of marijuana in the early 1960s, volumes of research have been published to try to establish and classify the social and medical implications of this drug for modern society. Much of this work has been formerly clouded with emotion and prejudice, making objectivity a difficult task for practitioners treating patients who abuse this substance. Today, however more definite evidence points to acute and chronic sequelae from marijuana abuse as the consequences of long-term abuse of high-potency strains of marijuana have come to light.

Although the use of marijuana has declined over the last decade, it is still the most commonly used illicit substance in the United States. It is estimated that 10 to 12 million people use cannabis on a regular basis, down from a peak of 20 million users in the late 1970s.[7] It is also estimated that up to 40 million people have tried cannabis in the United States at least one time.[28] Occasional use of cannabis is far more common than daily use. Peer and sibling influence appears to be the strongest predictor of the initiation of cannabis use.[28] Children with parents actively using cannabis are far more likely to initiate and continue its use. Some evidence suggests that children from homes where alcohol is consumed regularly are more likely to begin experimentation with cannabis.

Pharmacology

Marijuana consists of the leaves, flowers, stems, and seeds of the plant *cannabis sativa*. This fibrous plant grows wild throughout most tropical regions of the world and has been used medicinally and recreationally for thousands of years. It was banned in the United States by the 1937 Marijuana Tax Act, as marijuana became recognized as a drug of abuse, used mainly by counterculture groups of musicians and intellectuals. Marijuana again became popular with the rebellious youth of the 1960s generation, continuing in popularity throughout the 1970s and 1980s. Only recently has a slight decrease in numbers of marijuana users been observed.

The term "cannabis" is used to describe the bioactive substances of the marijuana plant.[7] The most common method of using cannabis is to smoke or to ingest the dried plant parts. Other preparations of cannabis can be obtained by collecting the resin from the flowering tops of the plant, commonly referred to as "hash" or "hashish." Plant material can also be processed into a dark concentrated liquid called hash oil. In recent years more marijuana has been grown domestically by growers who develop potent, seedless strains called sensimilla, often doubling the percentage of bioactive substance within the plant.

Delta-9-tetrahydrocannabinol (*d*-9-THC) is the substance responsible for the mood-altering euphoria associated with cannabis use. Of the common methods of using cannabis, smoking maximizes the amount of bioactive substance absorbed to approximately 10% to 50%, compared to 1% to 10% when ingested.[7] *d*-9-THC has a high lipid solubility and is quickly absorbed into fatty tissue, resulting in a slow elimination time, up to 4 to 10 weeks in heavy cannabis users.[7] This slow elimination time becomes important in the treatment of cannabis abusers because measurable levels of marijuana metabolites can be obtained in urine samples long after the mood-altering effects have passed. These effects in humans usually last for only 3 to 5 hours when cannabis is smoked. The liver is responsible for almost complete metabolism of d-9-THC, with less than 1% of the unmetabolized d-9-THC present in urine.[7]

Diagnosis and effects of abuse

Due to a low level of toxicity, marijuana poses few acute medical problems. Emergency room visits are rare for exclusive use of cannabis, and a lethal dose of cannabis has yet to be determined in humans. The physician will be more likely to encounter medical complications associated with long-term chronic abuse of cannabis, rather than acute medical crises.

The CNS is the most affected system in cannabis intoxication, with the majority of users experiencing a change in mood, described as a feeling of well-being or euphoria.[7] There is also a decrease in attention span, short-term memory, and in the ability to perform memory-dependent tasks. Most users also experience an increase in appetite and lethargy. Simple reaction time appears to be unchanged, but complex reactions, in which information must be quickly processed by the brain, are impaired.[7] This effect may have serious consequences in the operation of automobiles or other equipment, during which information must be processed before a proper reaction is made. Learning is clearly made more difficult while intoxicated with cannabis due to decreases in attention span and short-term memory and due to increases in lethargy. Chronic use of cannabis among adolescents is said to produce an amotivational syndrome, but current research is controversial, with some studies noting this syndrome to be a psychologic variant that predisposes the person to cannabis use, along with chronic abuse of other substances.[7]

Cannabis has an extremely dysphoric effect on some users, causing an increase in anxiety, severe panic reactions, hallucinations, and confused thinking.[56] It has been shown to be detrimental in the treatment and maintenance of patients suffering from schizophrenia. Patients relapsing on cannabis have become psychotic, even after responding well to therapy.[56] It is critical for physicians treating schizophrenic patients to have knowledge of current and past potential for cannabis abuse.

The most medically significant effects of cannabis appear to be on lung tissue. Cannabis smoke is usually drawn deeply into the lungs and is held for the longest possible time to potentiate the absorption of cannabinoids into the bloodstream. By weight, cannabis contains approximately 10 times the respiratory irritants and has more carcinogens than tobacco. Evidence shows that chronic cannabis smokers face similar risks of developing lung cancer as tobacco smokers.[7]

Effects of cannabis on the cardiovascular system are usually minimal, but can be detrimental to persons with known arteriosclerotic heart disease. After the use of cannabis, most people experience mild tachycardia and orthostatic hypotension. People with known angina have reduced exercise tolerance before experiencing symptoms of chest pain.[7] Patients with known heart disease should avoid the use of cannabis.

Effects on the endocrine system are controversial. Serum testosterone levels and sperm production are slightly decreased, with little evidence of increases in infertility.[28] Some research has shown inhibition of ovulation, with more anovulatory menstrual cycles in women who are heavy marijuana users. The levels of luteinizing hormones are also slightly decreased with heavy marijuana use.[28] The physician should advise all women planning pregnancy to avoid the use of cannabis products.

Therapeutic uses

The therapeutic potential of cannabis has been controversial for years. Recent research has shown antiemetic effects of cannabis products in patients suffering chronic nausea from chemotherapy treatments. Although therapeutic effects are measurable with the use of THC, adverse effects are also frequently reported.[28] In light of the frequency of adverse reactions, other pharmacologic treatments are more effective at the present time. Cannabis has also been shown to lower intraocular pressure, with possible therapeutic effects in treating glaucoma. Studies have shown 30% to 50% decreases in intraocular pressure in patients with ocular hypertension.[28] However, more research is needed in this area to understand better the long-term benefits of cannabis in the treatment of glaucoma.

Treatment

Although marijuana does not show the severe physical withdrawal or acute medical problems associated with other substances of abuse, such as alcohol, opiates, and cocaine, signs of addiction are common in heavy cannabis abusers. The American Medical Association defines the characteristics of marijuana addiction as a preoccupation and compulsivity with the drug and potential for relapse.[39] The person compulsively using cannabis will show a preoccupation with all aspects of this drug. Obtaining and using cannabis will become the driving forces in the daily life of the addicted person, who will often risk loss of employment or relationships to use it.[39]

When cannabis addiction is severe, or when additional substances are also being abused, inpatient treatment is best recommended to disrupt the cycle of addiction and to confront denial and rationalization. This approach will also allow time for full medical and psychologic examination.[39] After inpatient treatment, the addicted person should be followed closely, with individual counseling and a 12-step program of recovery through AA and/or NA. Compliance with the program increases with random urine toxicology screens. Less severe cannabis addiction may be treated with outpatient treatment that should include strong group therapy, as well as individual counseling. Again, the 12-step programs of NA and AA provide the most essential and most accessible support system for the recovering addict.

HALLUCINOGENICS

Although the popularity of the hallucinogenic and psychedelic drugs has decreased in recent years, emergency room and law enforcement records indicate these substances are still available and are being used throughout the United States. Although many substances when ingested have the potential to cause perceptual distortions or hallucinations, this discussion will focus on the more common recreational drugs used to produce a mind-altering, hallucinogenic experience or effect. Phencyclidine (PCP) and lysergic acid diethylamine (LSD) are the most common hallucinogens found on the illicit market today. Other substances, such as mescaline, psilocybin, and the amphetamine derivatives, MDA, MDMA, and STP will be discussed in lesser detail because they are psychoactively very similar to LSD.

Although tolerance occurs quickly with most hallucinogenic substances, withdrawal symptoms have not been observed.[32] Because of the sensory distortion and intensity of the intoxication, these drugs are rarely used on a continuous, daily basis. More often it is the episodic experimentation by novice users who do not understand or expect the drastic mood-altering effect that comes to the attention of the physicians. Education on the unpredictable effects of the hallucinogenic drugs is probably the best method of reducing the incidence of experimentation with these substances.

Phencyclidine

PCP was developed and used as an anesthetic agent, but was discontinued for human use because of the high incidence of adverse postanesthetic reactions. These reactions included hallucinations, agitation, violence, and prolonged depression of consciousness.[3] These same symptoms pushed PCP into the illicit market as a recreational drug. PCP is most commonly referred to as "angel dust" or "hog" and may be sold erroneously as THC or LSD. It became popular in the 1960s, reaching a peak in the late 1970s, and gradually decreasing in popularity to a relatively stable level throughout the 1980s, with 5% of high school students and young adults reporting use of PCP.[6]

The most common method of using PCP is smoking, usually by mixing the powdered drug with tobacco or marijuana and rolling it into a cigarette. PCP can also be injected intravenously, ingested orally, or taken intranasally.

The effects of the drug can usually be recognized within a few minutes after administration and can last from 12 to 15 hours, depending on dose. The most common effects are feelings of euphoria and distortions of reality percep-

tion, time, space, and body image.[6] Arms and legs may appear longer or shorter; physical environments may seem larger or smaller than they actually are. These effects can produce extreme fear and panic in the user, causing bizarre behavioral changes, agitation, and violence.

Medical complications may include hypertension, hyperthermia, seizures, rhabdomyolysis, acute renal failure, apnea, cardiac arrest, and trauma. Medical management of PCP intoxication is mostly supportive, with symptomatic treatment of specific complications. Tranquilizing agents such as benzodiazepines and haloperidol may be used with the extremely agitated patient, and physical restraints are indicated with the combative patient.[3,6] Symptoms usually diminish within a few hours with supportive treatment, but can last days or weeks.[3] PCP can accumulate in adipose tissue with delayed release, causing a "flashback" or a recurrence of symptoms, making PCP an unpredictable and dangerous substance for recreational use.

Lysergic acid diethylamine

LSD was first synthesized in the laboratory in 1938, but it was not until the mid-1960s that it became a recreational drug. The rise in popularity followed the experimental use and publication by three Harvard professors: T. Leary, R. Alpert, and R. Metzner.[54] LSD peaked in popularity in the late 1970s, declining throughout the early 1980s, with an estimated 6% of high school students and young adults now reporting experimentation with this drug.[6]

The most common method of administering LSD is ingestion of the substance. The usual methods of oral administration are in small pills (microdots) or liquid LSD, often dropped on small pieces of blotter paper and sugar cubes. LSD can also be added to gelatin with the street name of "window pane." Other routes of administration include snorting, IV and subcutaneous injection, smoking, and conjunctival instillation of liquid LSD.[32] LSD is quickly absorbed from the gastrointestinal tract, with effects perceived within 30 minutes or less. The user may first feel a sense of being more alert and connected with the environment, followed by time distortion, visual illusions, and sound misperception. There may be a feeling of euphoria and peace, often described as a mystical or religious experience. Physiologic changes include tachycardia, hypertension, nausea, dilated pupils, and tremors.[32]

The experience may last from 6 to 18 hours, depending on dose. The extended duration of the intoxication along with the sensory distortions may become very frightening and anxiety provoking in individuals not expecting this experience or reaction. Fear and anxiety, combined with the intense high, can trigger a "bad trip," characterized by panic and feelings of breaking with reality. Long-term LSD psychosis has been disputed by many professionals, but similarities to schizophrenia have been observed.[32] Flashbacks are another controversial aspect of the LSD experience. It is unclear why some individuals experience flashbacks, but predisposing personality characteristics may be an important factor. Although withdrawal symptoms have not been observed with LSD, tolerance can develop quickly.[32]

Psilocybin, mescaline, and other substances

Psilocybin and mescaline are two naturally occurring substances with hallucinogenic effects when ingested. Psilocybin is a species of mushroom that grows wild in many regions of the world. Often these mushrooms are ingested whole or are boiled in tea. The intoxication is very similar to that of LSD, and the duration of the effects may be slightly shorter, but management of symptoms would be the same as for LSD. Mescaline is a substance derived from the peyote cactus, often introduced into the body by ingestion of cactus buds, or "buttons." Mescaline intoxication is similar to LSD, with adverse reactions much the same. Psilocybin and mescaline both have potential for causing "bad trips," best treated by supportive measures.

Throughout the 1980s, other substances with hallucinogenic effects have appeared on the illicit market. These mostly synthetic drugs are produced in clandestine laboratories. The most common synthetic drugs are the amphetamine derivatives, MDA and MDMA or "ecstasy." These substances produce a sympathomimetic response, visual illusions, and sound distortions, much the same as LSD, but with far more serious toxic effects. Overdose of these substances can produce lasting psychosis, anxiety, and panic. Physiologic symptoms may include tachycardia, hypertension, hyperthermia, and possible death.[27] Toxic doses of these drugs have not been determined because little human research has been performed. Residual symptoms may persist for much longer periods with the amphetamine derivatives than with other hallucinogens.

OPIATES

Opiates refer to a class of powerful analgesics derived from the poppy plant, *Papaver somniferum,* which contains over 20 alkaloids, including morphine and codeine. Altering the structure of morphine results in many synthetic opioids: heroin, hydrocodone, hydromorphone, and thebaine. The major medical uses of opiates are for the relief of pain, treatment of diarrhea, and the suppression of cough. Opioids are opium-like drugs that occur naturally or are synthetically produced and are used for analgesia and anesthesia.

Pharmacology

Opiates can be classified into three groups according to their functions: morphinelike agonists, mixed agonist-antagonists, and pure antagonists. Agonists such as morphine, heroine, codeine, and methadone produce their principal pharmacologic effects on the CNS and gastrointestinal tract by activation at the opioid receptor site on neurons throughout the brain and body. These agonist drugs typically have the strongest effects in producing an-

algesia and euphoria and have the highest addictive potential among opiates. Mixed agonists-antagonists have properties similar to opiates and also have the ability to block the effects of the drug at the opioid receptor sites. Butorphanol (Stadol), pentazocine (Talwin), and buprenorphine (Buprenex) are representatives of the agonist-antagonist class of opiates. Antagonists, such as naloxone and naltrexone, block the effects of opioids at the opioid receptor site and have no potential for abuse. Naloxone (Narcan) produces rapid withdrawal symptoms in opioid-dependent addicts. It is also the drug of choice to treat respiratory distress after acute opioid intoxication or overdose. Naltrexone (Trexan) has been found useful in the treatment of chronic opioid abusers. It may be taken orally and is effective in blocking the euphoric state from illicit opioid use[31] (see box on p. 253).

Diagnosis and effects

Psychologically, opioids usually cause a pleasant euphoria. Occasionally, and especially with the first use, some individuals experience a dysphoria, consisting of anxiety and fear, lethargy, apathy, sedation, mental clouding, lack of concern, inability to concentrate, nausea, and vomiting.[30] Frequent users describe either a euphoric state marked by feelings of peacefulness and increased energy, or a feeling of sedation with a dreamlike quality. Chronic opioid abusers may switch to IV use in an attempt to reexperience the original euphoric state.

Clinicians use several criteria to diagnose an addiction to opiates: a preoccupation with the acquisition of the drug, compulsive use in spite of adverse consequences, an inability to reduce the amount of use consistently to avoid adverse consequences, and a pattern of relapse after a period of abstinence.[4] Tolerance to opioids may develop at different rates among users. Dose, frequency of administration, and particular physiologic and psychologic responses are the influencing factors. If a pattern of repeated administration occurs, the clinician may find that a phenomenal increase in dose may be needed to prevent discomfort or to induce the euphoric state. Physiologically, tolerance appears to be due to both the induction of drug-metabolizing enzymes in the liver and the adaption of neurons in the brain to the presence of the drug.[30] Clinicians must also be aware of the phenomenon of cross-tolerance with opioid addiction; that is, as a patient develops a tolerance to one particular opioid he or she will have the same level of tolerance for all other natural or synthetically manufactured opioids. Cross-tolerance to other drugs, namely barbiturates and benzodiazepines and/or alcohol, does not occur with opiates.

Dependence is a physiologic phenomenon in which an individual does not function properly without the drug of choice. When the drug is withheld or unavailable, a series of withdrawal symptoms occur. Withdrawal from opioids is rarely life threatening, although the user is extremely

---

Classification of opioid analgesics by their ability to produce analgesia (agonists) or block the actions of morphine (antagonists)

Pure agonists	*Mixed agonist-antagonists*	*Pure antagonists*
Morphine	Nalbuphine (Nubain)	Naloxone (Narcan)
Codeine	Butorphanol (Stadol)	Naltrexone (Trexan)
Heroin	Pentazocine (Talwin)	
Meperidine (Demerol)	Buprenorphine (Buprenex)	
Methadone (Dolophine)		
Oxymorphone (Numorphan)		
Hydromorphone (Dilaudid)		
Fentanyl (Sublimaze)		

---

uncomfortable, anxious, and drug-seeking. Symptoms of withdrawal from opioids are restlessness, craving for the drug, sweating, extreme anxiety, fever, chills, violent retching and vomiting, increased respiratory rate (panting), cramping, insomnia, explosive diarrhea, and unbearable aches and pains. The magnitude of these withdrawal symptoms depends on the dose, frequency of drug administration, and the strength of the opiate used.[28]

Abusers of opioids fall into three categories. The first category is the nonmedical or "street" user of opioids, estimated to be well over 500,000 in number in the United States. Use includes multiple daily IV injections of various opioids. If intermittent IV abuse is considered, then the number of abusers may be well over 2 million.[31] The most often abused drug in this category is heroin, and because it is illegal, procurement and use often lead to criminal activities. A heroin addict may use over $500 worth of heroin in a day. Those most likely to use heroin are males living in urban settings. An antisocial disorder often predates heroin use, but if not, such a disorder frequently develops because of the pharmacologic effects of heroin addiction combined with the high cost of obtaining it.[4]

Drug dependence may also occur in the context of medical treatment for acute or chronic illnesses where pain control is a factor. According to Ford et al.,[21] the National Institute of Drug Abuse estimates that a total of 4 to 6.5 million Americans report recent use of opioid analgesics.[21] Often, this type of opioid-dependent patient will try to obtain prescriptions from more than one physician and will also be resistant to any other methods of pain control. As the dependence develops, patients may become involved in criminal activities, such as altering prescriptions and purchasing street supplies of drugs. In our experience, a significant number of these patients also abuse benzodiazepines and alcohol.

The third category of opioid abusers are found in methadone maintenance programs where heroin abusers are the primary population seeking treatment. Dole and Nyswander,[17] in studies done in the mid-1960s, found that methadone would block the effects of heroin and thus negate the euphoric properties of heroin use.[17] The goal of maintenance therapy is to give the abuser enough methadone to prevent the opioid withdrawal syndrome and also to block the euphoria produced by further opioid abuse. Studies have shown that as the overall health status of users improves, a decrease of criminal activities is seen, and the controlled addict may often be employed for the first time in many years.[52]

Treatment

Opiate detoxification is usually accomplished by discontinuing the abused drug (agonist) and substituting a noneuphoric drug. Typically, this substitute is a mixed agonist-antagonist, such as methadone or buprenophine. The substitute is then tapered down to a maintenance level (methadone), or is discontinued altogether. For cases of street opiate (heroin) use, usually 40 mg of methadone in divided doses will suffice to start. For recently acquired addictions or for those on milder opiates (codeine, propoxyphene), 20 to 30 mg of methadone in divided doses will often be adequate. Clonidine 0.1 mg by mouth can be used two to three times a day for milder addictions, perhaps with as needed supplementation of 100 mg of oral propoxyphene every 6 hours to reduce craving if this is a problem. Hypotension may occur with both methadone and clonidine detoxification and should lead to withholding doses or to changing the detoxification regimen. Addicts tolerant to daily large doses of high-grade pharmaceutical opiates may need 80 to 100 mg per day or more of methadone, usually given in four divided doses, with respirations closely monitored. Smaller "test doses" of 10 to 15 mg orally are usually given first to assure that the patient is telling the truth and is not exaggerating drug use, as sudden administration of high doses to a nontolerant person could be fatal. Naloxone (Narcan) injections of 1 mg are kept handy, just in case. Somnolence is the best indicator of overtitration and signals that medication should be held back. Once the patient is stabilized on the detoxification dosage, the medication can be tapered down in 5 to 20 days (or more), depending on severity.

SUMMARY

The physician plays a key role in the course of the addictive process with alcohol or drugs. Prevention at the primary level can be addressed by early counseling of those with strong family histories of alcoholism or drug dependency. Because research suggests a genetic predisposition to these disorders,[49] those at risk should be advised of their risks and should be encouraged to avoid alcohol and drugs. It is worth noting that offspring of alcoholics are *less* affected by alcohol than those with a negative family history and are, in a sense, more protected from the noxious and negative effects of alcohol. In turn, they may drink more without much consequence—for a while.

Early identification of "problem drinking," often seen in the teens or early twenties, can lead to "secondary prevention" counseling to interrupt the progressive cycle of the disorder at an early stage. To be effective, "tertiary prevention," the treatment of identifiable cases, requires proper physician attitudes and behaviors: a blend of compassion, firmness, vigilance, and optimism. The wise and experienced physician will cultivate the view that "it's never too late" to help an alcoholic or addict to recovery, and persistent use of the medical and psychologic tools available will save lives and relieve useless suffering.

Acknowledgments

With permission of Postgraduate Medicine, Gregory B. Collins, MD, author; Diagnosis, Gregory B. Collins, MD, author; Internal Medicine for the Specialist, Gregory B. Collins, MD and Ora Frankel, MD, authors; and Collins GB: The treatment of alcoholism: The role of the primary care physician. *Postgrad Med* 69:145-149, 1981.

REFERENCES

1. Andersen K: Crashing on cocaine, *Time*, 121(15):22-31, 1983.
2. Baekeland F, Lundwall L, Kissin B, et al: Correlates of outcome in disulfiram treatment of alcoholism, *J Nerv Ment Dis* 153:1-9, 1971.
3. Baldridge EB, Bessen HA: Phencyclidine, *Emerg Med Clin North Am* 8(3):541-550, 1990.
4. Belkin BM, Gold MS: Opioids. In Miller N, editor: *Comprehensive handbook of drug and alcohol addiction,* New York, 1991, Marcel Dekker.
5. Brier A, Paul SM: The GABA_A/Benzodiazepine receptor: implications for the molecular basis of anxiety, *J Psychiatry Residents* 24(2):91-104, 1990.
6. Carroll ME: PCP and hallucinogens, *Adv Alcohol Subst Abuse* 9(1-2):167-190, 1990.
7. Clark RF, Curry SC, Selorn BS: Marijuana, *Emerg Med Clin North Am* 8(3):527-539, 1990.
8. Cocores J: Nicotine. In Miller N, editor: *Comprehensive handbook of drug and alcohol addiction,* New York, 1991, Marcel Dekker.
9. Collins GB: The treatment of alcoholism: the role of the primary care physician, *Postgrad Med* 69(1):145-149, 1981.
10. Collins GB: Clues to cocaine dependency, *Diagnosis* 7(1):57-65, 1985.
11. Collins, Gregory B, Frankel O: Recognition and management of amphetamine abusers, *Internal Medicine for the Specialist* 8(3):135-146, 1987.
12. Collins GB, Janesz JW, Byerly-Thrope J, et al: The Cleveland Clinic Alcohol Rehabilitation Program: a treatment outcome study, *Cleve Clin Q* 52:245-251, 1985.
13. Cowley G, Springen K, Iarovici D: Sweet dreams or nightmares?! *Newsweek* 118(8):44-57, 1991.
14. Department of Health and Human Services: *National household survey on drug abuse: main findings,* Rockville, Md, 1985, DHHS Publication No. (ADM) 88-1586, 1988.
15. Department of Health Education and Human Services: *The health consequences of smoking—nicotine addiction: a report of the Surgeon General,* Washington, DC, US, 1988.
16. Detzer E, Miller B, Carlin AS: Identifying and treating the drug-misusing patient. *Am Fam Physician* 16(3):181-186, 1977.
17. Dole VP, Nyswander ME: The use of methadone for narcotic blockade, *Br J Addict* 63:55-57, 1968.
18. DuPont RL, editor: Abuse of benzodiazepines: the problems and the solutions. A report of the Committee of the Institute for Behavior and Health, Inc, *Am J Drug Alcohol Abuse* 14(Suppl 1):1-69, 1989.
19. Elinwood EH: Treatment of reactions to amphetamine-type stimulants, *Curr Psychiatr Ther* 15:163-169, 1975.
20. Emert V: Nic-addiction: treatment Field's smoking gun, *Prof Counselor* 2:44-48, 1988.
21. Ford M, Hoffman RS, Goldfrank LR: Opioids and designer drugs, *Emerg Med Clin North Am* 8:495-511, 1990.
22. Gay GR: Clinical management of acute and chronic cocaine poisoning, *Ann Emerg Med* 11:562-572, 1982.
23. Goldfrank L, Lewin N, Weisman R: Cocaine, *Hosp Physician* 17(5):26-45, 1981.
24. Gossop MR, Bradley BP, Brewis RK: Amphetamine withdrawal and sleep disturbance, *Drug Alcohol Depend* 10:177-183, 1982.
25. Griffith JD, Cavanaugh J, Held J, et al: Dextroamphetamine: evaluation of psychomimetic properties in man, *Arch Gen Psychiatry* 26:97-100, 1972.
26. Grinspoon L, Bakalar JB: Drug dependence: non-narcotic agents. In Kaplan HI, Sadock BJ, editors: *Comprehensive textbook of psychiatry/IV,* Baltimore, 1985, Williams & Wilkins.
27. Hayner GN, McKinney H: MDMA: the dark side of ecstasy, *J Psychoactive Drugs* 18(4):341-347, 1986.
28. Hollister LE: Cannabis, *Acta Psychiatr Scand Suppl* 345:108-118, 1988.
29. Jellinek EM: *The disease concept of alcoholism,* New Haven, Conn, 1960, College and University Press.
30. Julien R: A primer of drug action, ed 5, New York, 1988, WH Freeman and Co.
31. Kreek MJ: Tolerance and dependence: implications for the pharmacological treatment of addiction, In SO NIDA-Res-Monogr 76:53-62, 1987.
32. Kulig K: LSD, *Emerg Med Clin North Am* 8(3):551-559, 1990.
33. Kwentus J, Major LF: Disulfiram in the treatment of alcoholism: a review, *J Stud Alcohol* 40:428-446, 1979.
34. Lake CR, Quirk RS: CNS stimulants and the look-alike drugs, *Psychiatr Clin North Am* 7:689-701, 1984.
35. Magnan V, Saury: Trois cas de cocainisme chronique, *Comptes Rendus des Seances et Memoires de la Societe de Biologie,* Paris, 1889, Series 9, vol 1.
36. Mellinger GD, Balter MB: Prevalence of patterns of use of psychotherapeutic drugs: Results from a 1979 national survey of American adults. In Tognoni G, Bellantuono C, Lader M, editors: *Epidemiological impact of psychotropic drugs,* Amsterdam, 1981, Elsevier.
37. Milam JR: *The emergent comprehensive concept of alcoholism,* Kirkland, Wash, 1974, Alcoholism Center Associates.
38. Miller NS, Gold MS: Identification and treatment of benzodiazepine abuse, *Am Fam Physician* 40(4):175-183, 1989.
39. Miller NS, Gold MS, Pottash AC: A 12-step treatment approach for marijuana (Cannabis) dependence, *J Subst Abuse Treat* 6(4):241-250, 1989.
40. Morgan W: Abuse liability of barbiturates and other sedative hypnotics, *Adv Alcohol Subst Abuse* 9(1-2):67-82, 1990.

41. Noble EP: Third special report to the US Congress on alcohol and health. Rockville, Md, Alcohol, Drug Abuse, and Mental Health Administration, (HEW Publ No (ADM) 78-569), 1978.

42. Post RM, Kotin J, Goodwin FK: Effects of cocaine on depressed patients, *Am J Psychiatry* vol 131(5):511-517, 1974.

43. Public Health Service: *Drug abuse warning network,* 1976-1981 data [tape-SRVCD 48], Washington DC, 1981, National Institute on Drug Abuse.

44. Rappolt RT Sr, Gay G, Inaba DS: Propranolol: a specific antagonist to cocaine, *Clin Toxicol* 10(3):265-271, 1977.

45. Raskin DE: Amphet Use. Letter to the Editor, *J Clin Pharmacol* 3(4):262, 1983.

46. Robins LN, Helzer JE, Weissman MM, et al: Lifetime prevalence of specific psychiatric disorders in three sites, *Arch Gen Psychiatry* 41:949-958, 1984.

47. Sampliner R, Iber FL: Diphenylhydantoin control of alcohol withdrawal seizures: results of a controlled study, *JAMA* 230:757-762, 1976.

48. Schuckit MA: The disease alcoholism, *Postgrad Med* 64(6):78-84, 1978.

49. Schuckit MA: Genetics and the risk for alcoholism, *JAMA* 254:2614-2617, 1985.

50. Sees KL: Cigarette smoking, nicotine dependence and treatment, *West J Med* 152(5):578-584, 1990.

51. Selzer ML: The Michigan Alcoholism Screening Test: the quest for a new diagnostic instrument, *Am J Psychiatry* 12:1653-1658, 1971.

52. Senay E: Methadone maintenance treatment, *Int J Addict* 20(6-7):803-821, 1985.

53. Slaby AE, Martin SD: Drug and alcohol emergencies. In Miller N, editor: *Comprehensive handbook of drug and alcohol addiction,* New York, 1991, Marcel Dekker.

54. Smith DE, Seymour RB: Dreams become nightmares: adverse reactions to LSD, *J Psychoactive Drugs* 17(4):297-303, 1985.

55. The APA Task Force Report on Benzodiazepine Dependence, Toxicity and Abuse: Editorial, *Am J Psychiatry* 158(2):151-152, 1991.

56. Tunving K: Psychiatric effects of cannabis use, *Acta Psychiatr Scand Suppl* 72(3):209-217, 1985.

57. Twerski A: Nicotine in chemical dependency units, *Prof Counselor* 4(4):14, 1990.

58. Wetli CV, Wright RK: Death caused by recreational cocaine use, *JAMA* 241:2519, 1979.

RESOURCES

For patients and their families

Alcoholics Anonymous (AA), General Services Office, Box 459 Grand Central Station, New York, NY 10163.

Al-Anon Family Group Headquarters, Inc, PO Box 862, Midtown Station, New York, NY 10018-0862.

Cocaine Anonymous (CA), 3740 Overland Avenue, Suite G, Culver City, CA 90034.

Narcotics Anonymous (NA), PO Box 9999, Van Nuys, CA 91409.

Overeaters Anonymous (OA), 2190 190th Street, Torrence, CA 90504.

The preceding groups are usually listed in local phone directories, and most municipalities and counties have local Alcohol and Drug Boards who provide confidential services or referrals:

For the physician

1. American Society of Addiction Medicine (ASAM), 5225 Wisconsin Avenue, NW, Suite 409, Washington, DC 20016.

2. Cleveland Clinic Alcohol and Drug Recovery Center, 9500 Euclid Avenue, P-47, Cleveland, OH 44195.

3. Michigan Alcoholism Screening Test, (see Selzer ML: The Michigan Alcoholism Screening Test: the quest for a new diagnostic instrument, *Am J Psychiatry,* 12:1653-1658, 1971)

4. National Clearinghouse for Alcohol and Drug Information (NCADI), PO Box 2345, Rockville, MD 20852.

Chapter 16

SMOKING AND SMOKING CESSATION

Garland Y. (Gary) DeNelsky
Thomas L. Plesec

HEALTH EFFECTS OF SMOKING

Smoking has clearly been established as the chief preventable cause of morbidity and mortality in our society.[39] Beginning with the first (1964) *Surgeon's General Report,* which concluded that cigarette smoking causes lung and laryngeal cancer and chronic bronchitis, subsequent reports have determined that smoking causes coronary heart disease, atherosclerotic peripheral vascular disease, oral cancer, esophageal cancer, chronic obstructive pulmonary disease, intrauterine growth retardation, and low-birth-weight babies.[118] Smoking is now considered to be a probable cause of unsuccessful pregnancies, increased infant mortality, and peptic ulcer disease, a contributing factor for cancer of the bladder, pancreas, and kidney; and associated with cancer of the stomach.[118] Smoking has recently been established as a significant risk factor for stroke.[109] New associations between smoking and adverse health changes continue to be made (e.g., cataracts).[119] In addition, smokers seem to have a more negative attitude toward healthy behaviors, an attitude that can add to their already greater risk for diseases such as coronary heart disease.[8]

Put another way, smoking is responsible for approximately 390,000 excess deaths each year in the United States, or about one sixth of all deaths.[39] More recent estimates that include several additional heart disease categories place this figure at 434,000 smoking-attributable deaths,[106] or one in every five deaths in 1988—1200 Americans each day.[7,77,112,119] Smoking is responsible for an estimated 30% of all cancer deaths, including 87% of lung cancer deaths.[118] It causes about 30% of all cardiovascular deaths, and about 80% of all deaths from chronic obstructive pulmonary disease.[39] In 1984, 3.6 million years of potential life were lost through smoking in the United States[105]; in 1988, an estimated 6 million years of potential life were lost.[106] Whatever statistics are used, and from whatever perspective they are viewed, the loss of health and life due to smoking is indeed staggering. Louis W. Sullivan, Secretary of Health and Human Services, extended a dire warning: "Unless we act, we face a frightening possibility . . . at least 5 million American children who are alive today will die of smoking-related diseases. This is a catastrophe that policy makers, physicians, and community leaders must prevent."[111]

Nearly as dramatic as the losses due to smoking are the gains to be derived from quitting smoking. The 1990 *Surgeon General's Report,* which reviewed the health benefits of smoking cessation, concluded that smoking cessation has major, immediate health benefits for people of all ages, even those with smoking-related disease.[119] Stopping smoking decreases the risk of cardiovascular disease, lung cancer, other cancers, stroke, and chronic lung disease; after 10 to 15 years of abstinence, risk of dying from any smoking-related disease is nearly as low as that of persons who have never smoked.[119] Women who stop (not simply reduce) their smoking before pregnancy, or as late as the first 3 to 4 months of pregnancy, reduce the risk of having a baby of low birth weight to that of women who never smoked.[119]

The 1990 *Report of the Surgeon General on The Health Benefits of Smoking Cessation* documents advantages of ending tobacco use.[119] Previous reports identified causal links between smoking and cancers of the lung, larynx, esophagus, urinary bladder, and oral cavity. Further findings detailed connections between smoking and heart disease, stroke, peripheral artery occlusive disease, chronic obstructive pulmonary disease, and intrauterine growth retardation. More current evidence indicates benefits for ending smoking for persons of all ages, for those with existing diseases, for the fetus, and for infants and children. The 1990 report depicts how the risks of most smoking-related diseases decrease after cessation and with increasing duration of abstinence.[119]

Table 16-1 illustrates the overall mortality ratios among current and former smokers compared to those who never smoked. Because many smokers quit after a disease linked with smoking is identified, abstinence between 1 and 3 years seems to be associated with an increase in the mortality rate (in comparison with those who continue to smoke). When preexisting diseases are accounted for in the findings, it becomes evident that quitting smoking consistently and substantially extends the former smoker's length of life.[119]

Over the past 5 years, health concerns of another type have surfaced involving smoking. These latest fears involve the effects of smoke on the *passive smoker,* the person who breathes the smoke of another. It has been estimated that approximately 46,000 nonsmokers die from exposure to cigarette smoke each year,[127] with slightly more women than men perishing. Approximately three fourths of these deaths are from heart disease; most of the remaining are from cancer, primarily lung cancer.[127] Childhood smoke exposure has been demonstrated to impair physical and mental development.[103] The concern over involuntary smoking—the damage done to nonsmokers by the smoke of others—has led to a rapid growth of laws throughout the nation at the state and local levels that restrict or prohibit smoking. "Smoking can no longer be viewed simply as an issue of free choice by responsible adults. Rather, smoking is increasingly viewed as a public health hazard with the potential to injure innocent nonsmokers who are exposed to environmental tobacco smoke."[39]

It is not possible to place a dollar value on the lost lives, suffering, and diminished health engendered by smoking. But dollar estimates have been generated of the costs our society has to bear. It has been estimated that the costs of increased health care and insurance, and lost productivity, total $52 billion annually.[111] This cost could be viewed as a "hidden tax" of approximately $221 per person for each U.S. citizen.[111] The costs of the health outcomes of smoking have been calculated to be more than double the costs of cigarettes and other tobacco-related products, making the health effects of smoking "an industry larger than the cigarette business itself."[103] Smoking is not only the most preventable cause of death in the United States, but it is extremely expensive to the entire culture.

Based on the costs in terms of mortality, morbidity, needless suffering, and financial losses, it is hardly surprising that over 57,000 studies from dozens of countries have explored the phenomenon of smoking.[118] It is equally

Table 16-1. Overall mortality ratios among current and former smokers, relative to never smokers, by sex and duration of abstinence at date of enrollment, ACS CPS-II*

| | | Former smokers | | | | | |
| | | Duration of abstinence at enrollment (yr) | | | | | |
	Current smokers	<1	1-2	3-5	6-10	11-15	≥16
Men							
1-20 cig/day	2.22	2.49	2.38	2.03	1.63	1.38	1.06
≥21 cig/day	2.43	2.77	2.64	2.25	2.04	1.77	1.27
Women							
1-19 cig/day	1.60	1.58	1.96	1.41	1.14	1.10	1.01
≥20 cig/day	2.10	3.391	2.58	2.03	1.60	1.38	1.15

| | | Former smokers excluding those with cancer, heart disease, or stroke and those "sick" at interview | | | | | |
| | | Duration of abstinence at enrollment (yr) | | | | | |
	Current smokers	<1	1-2	3-5	6-10	11-15	≥16
Men							
1-20 cig/day	2.34	2.06	2.05	1.89	1.48	1.29	1.01
≥21 cig/day	2.73	1.85	2.15	1.90	1.77	1.65	1.19
Women							
1-19 cig/day	1.82	0.76	1.26	1.42	1.01	1.09	1.00
≥20 cig/day	2.46	3.33	2.15	1.44	1.46	1.18	0.95

From American Cancer Society unpublished tabulations.
*Mortality ratios are relative to those of never smokers. ACS CPS=American Cancer Society Cancer Prevention Study II.

understandable why so much effort has been directed toward smoking cessation, and recently, to prevention of smoking initiation. This chapter reviews some of the highlights in these areas.

THE EPIDEMIOLOGY OF SMOKING

Although tobacco use has been a part of the American culture for over four centuries, cigarette use is a relatively recent phenomenon.[102] The first automated cigarette machine appeared in 1881; before that, cigarettes had to be rolled by hand. But widespread adoption of cigarettes awaited the introduction of the first blended cigarette (Camels); compared to their counterparts, they were easily inhaled, thereby exposing the lungs and other organs to the many toxic and carcinogenic constituents in tobacco smoke.[102]

Smoking patterns for men and women have differed since cigarette use became widespread. During the first 50 years of this century, smoking was practiced principally by men, with more than half of the adult male population smoking by 1955.[55] In contrast, smoking rates for women remained at low levels during the early decades of the century and began rising with the gradual disappearance of the social restrictions that previously limited smoking by women. In 1964, the date of the first Surgeon General's report on smoking's health effects, men's rate of smoking had already begun to decline, whereas women's rate was still increasing.[37] Between 1965 and 1970, when many measures were undertaken to inform the public of the health hazards of smoking, men's smoking rate declined by nearly one fifth (from 52% to 42%), whereas women's rate increased slightly (from 32% to 33%).[102] From 1974 to 1985, smoking prevalence declined for both sexes, with the rate for men declining by about 1% per year, and the rate for women falling about one third as much.[37] By 1990, an estimated 28% of the adult population was smoking (30% of men, 26% of women).[39]

Paralleling these changes in smoking behaviors were the changes in mortality rates of smoking-related diseases, especially for women. Between 1965 and 1986, lung cancer death rates increased twofold to fourfold among older male smokers and fourfold to sevenfold among older female smokers.[118] Lung cancer replaced breast cancer as the number one cause of cancer death among women.[118] Death rates for older women smokers also increased markedly for chronic obstructive pulmonary disease.[122] Overall, there was a large increase in smoking-related deaths among American women between 1965 and 1985.

Factors in addition to gender are associated with differential smoking rates. A consistently higher percentage of blacks than whites have smoked through the past two decades; by the mid-1980s, approximately 6% more blacks than whites were still smoking.[37] However, the rate of smoking for blacks was declining slightly faster than that for whites.[37]

The most powerful predictor of smoking status is neither gender nor race, but educational level. In 1987, 44% of high school graduates (who did not proceed beyond high school) smoked, whereas only 16% of college graduates smoked.[85] From 1974 to 1985, smoking prevalence declined 4.8 times faster among college graduates than among people with less than a high school education.[85]

The National Health Interview Survey–Health Promotion and Disease Prevention–collected self-reported information about cigarette smoking in the United States. Data from that survey reprinted in the May 1992 issue of *Morbidity and Mortality Weekly Report* (MMWR) indicate that in 1990, an estimated 89.9 million (50.1%) American adults had ever smoked ("ever smokers") and 45.8 million (25.5%) were current smokers.[10] Approximately 44.1 million (49.1% of all smokers) were former smokers in 1990. Current smokers were estimated to be made up of 24.2 million (28.4%) men and 21.6 million (22.8%) women (Table 16-2).

Table 16-3 provides trends in the quit ratio by age and education for the United States from 1965 to 1987 for adults ages 20 and older.

In 1990 an estimated 24.2 million (28.4%) men and 21.6 million (22.8%) women were current smokers. From 1987 to 1990, overall prevalence declined an average of 1.1% annually.[10] The apparently accelerated decline in smoking has been attributed to a decrease in the social acceptability of smoking, the increased cost of cigarettes, and an increased awareness of the health consequences of active and passive smoking.[10] Published differences between the smoking quit rates of men and women (47.7% vs 40.1%, respectively) shrink when all forms of tobacco use are assessed (42.1% vs 39.9%). Former male cigarette smokers tend to use other tobacco products (cigars, pipes, snuff, chewing tobacco) more than do former female cigarette smokers.[119]

Smoking initiation

People learn to smoke early, or they do not learn at all. Ninety percent of all smokers start by age 19.[64] The rate at which young people take up smoking has declined significantly in the last two decades,[37] but this decrease is due entirely to the decrease in smoking behavior of young men. From 1974 to 1985, the percentage of young male smokers (between ages 20 and 24) declined from 45% to 33%, whereas the corresponding percentage for young women remained unchanged (34%).[37] The optimism this apparent reduction in smoking among men creates is tempered by information indicating an upsurge in the use of smokeless tobacco in young men.[108,109,123]

Children whose parents smoke are much more likely to become smokers themselves, with at least a fivefold increase in the likelihood of a teenager smoking if one or both parents smoke and an older sibling smokes.[49] It has been estimated that approximately 15% of teenagers currently smoke.[126] Those teenagers who do smoke tend to have a sense of invulnerability, distorted beliefs regarding

Table 16-2. Percentage of men and women who smoke cigarettes, by age group, race, Hispanic origin, and education United States, National Health Interview Survey, 1990*

Category	Men %	Men (95% CI†)	Women %	Women (95% CI)	Total %	Total (95% CI)
Age (yr)						
18-24	26.6	(24.3-28.9)	22.5	(20.6- 24.4)	24.5	(23.0-26.0)
25-44	32.9	(31.7-34.1)	26.6	(25.6- 27.6)	29.7	(28.9-30.5)
45-64	29.3	(27.8-30.8)	24.8	(23.5- 26.1)	27.0	(26.0-28.0)
65-74	18.3	(16.2-20.5)	15.6	(14.2- 17.0)	16.8	(15.5-18.1)
≥75	7.6	(5.8-9.4)	5.8	(4.7-6.9)	6.5	(5.6- 7.5)
Race‡						
White	27.9	(27.1-28.9)	23.5	(22.7- 24.2)	25.6	(25.0-26.2)
Black	32.6	(30.2-34.8)	21.2	(19.6- 22.8)	26.2	(24.8-27.6)
Asian/Pacific Islander	24.8	(20.4-29.2)	6.2	(4.1- 8.3)	16.4	(13.5-19.3)
American Indian/Alaskan Native	40.1	(29.4- 50.8)	36.2	(24.4-48.0)	38.1	(28.3-47.9)
Hispanic origin						
Hispanic	30.9	(27.8-34.0)	16.3	(14.1- 18.5)	23.0	(21.1-24.9)
Non-Hispanic	28.2	(27.4-29.1)	23.4	(22.7- 24.1)	25.7	(25.1-26.3)
Education (yr)						
<12	37.3	(35.4-39.2)	27.1	(25.7- 28.5)	31.8	(30.6-33.0)
12	33.5	(32.1-34.9)	26.5	(25.5- 27.5)	29.6	(28.7-30.5)
13-15	26.2	(24.5-27.9)	20.2	(19.0- 21.4)	23.0	(22.0-24.0)
≥16	14.5	(13.3-15.7)	12.3	(11.2- 13.4)	13.5	(12.7-14.3)
TOTAL	28.4	(27.6-29.2)	22.8	(22.1- 23.5)	25.5	(25.0-26.1)

*Sample size = 40,666; excludes 438 respondents with unknown smoking status.
†Confidence interval.
‡Excludes unknown, multiple, and other races.

Table 16-3. Trends in quit ratio (%) (percentage of ever cigarette smokers who are former cigarette smokers), by age and by education, NHISs, United States, 1965-1987, adults aged 20 and older

Year	Overall pop.	Age (years) 20-24	25-44	45-64	≥65	Less than high school graduate	High school graduate	Some college	College graduate
1965*	29.6	17.8	23.6	30.9	48.7	—	—	—	—
1966	29.5	17.0	23.4	30.9	50.5	33.3	28.0	28.7	39.7
1970	35.3	20.8	29.8	36.1	56.9	38.1	33.6	34.9	48.2
1974	36.3	20.9	29.3	39.7	57.8	38.0	35.2	36.6	47.9
1976	37.1	22.0	29.4	40.4	59.6	39.5	35.0	37.2	46.1
1977	36.8	22.9	29.6	39.5	58.7	38.3	34.0	36.8	48.6
1978	38.5	22.8	31.9	40.1	62.4	38.7	36.3	41.0	49.7
1979	39.0	22.6	31.8	42.4	61.7	40.8	36.7	37.5	50.6
1980	39.0	22.2	33.0	40.9	61.0	39.4	36.5	40.6	48.7
1983	41.8	21.4	34.3	46.4	64.7	42.1	38.7	41.2	54.9
1985	45.0	26.0	38.2	49.7	68.0	41.3	40.5	46.0	61.1
1987	44.8	23.8	37.2	49.2	79.2	44.3	41.1	45.5	59.1
Trend information									
(1965-87) Change† yr	0.68	0.26	0.61	0.84	0.86	0.44	0.55	0.74	0.88
Standard error (±)	0.04	0.06	0.05	0.06	0.06	0.05	0.05	0.08	0.13
R^2‡	0.96	0.64	0.93	0.95	0.96	0.88	0.92	0.90	0.83

Note: The data stratified by education are age adjusted to the 1985 population. NHIS=National Health Interview Survey.
*For 1965, data stratified by education were unavailable.
†In percentage points.
‡R^2 statistic is a measure of the strength of the linear relationship. R^2 values may range from 0.0 (no linear trend) to 1.0 (a perfect positive or negative linear relationship).

the health problems associated with smoking, and thrill-seeking attitudes that seem linked to risks of developing other problem behaviors (e.g., drug use).[103]

Smoking cessation

During that past two decades, an increasingly large percentage of smokers have quit. By 1987, more than 38 million Americans had quit, nearly half of all the living adults who ever smoked.[119] Benefits of quitting have been found for persons of all ages, even for those with preexisting disease.[119] The ratio of smokers who have quit to those who have ever smoked (quit ratio) rose from 29.6% in 1965 to 44.8% in 1987.[119] This increasing quit ratio included men and women, blacks and whites, and all educational and age subgroups; however, the quit ratios have not increased equally for all of these subgroups.[119] Between 1974 and 1985, the quit ratios increased more for black men than for white men or black women[37] and more for those with a college degree than for those with lesser education.[85] Overall smoking prevalence decreased 4.8 times faster among college graduates than among people will less than a high school diploma.[85]

Future trends in smoking

If the current trends continue, sometime during the middle 1990s more women will be smoking than men.[37] It has been estimated that by the year 2000, 20% of men and 23% of women will still be smoking.[86] At that time, a slightly higher proportion of blacks than whites will be smoking. But educational factors are expected to be much more significant in predicting who is smoking than either gender or race.[86]

AN OVERVIEW OF SMOKING AND QUITTING
The behavior of smoking

Smoking is a complex behavior. Quitting is a complex process. It is thus useful to review some of the more salient characteristics of both smoking and quitting before discussing actual methods of intervention.

Smoking is first of all an *addiction*. This observation is in contrast to earlier views that described tobacco use as "habituating."[121] The 1988 Report of the Surgeon General, probably the most exhaustive review of the addictive nature of smoking, concluded in its over 600 pages that:

1. Cigarettes and other forms of tobacco are addicting.
2. Nicotine is the drug in tobacco that causes addiction.
3. The pharmacologic and behavioral processes that determine tobacco addiction are similar to those that determine addiction to drugs such as heroin and cocaine.[121]

To a large degree, this report scientifically validated what many smokers had long suspected, especially after they attempted to quit. Nicotine, the addicting substance in tobacco, is a psychoactive drug that produces transient al-terations in mood, which are sufficiently rewarding to maintain self-administration.[121] Primary criteria for drug dependence—highly controlled or compulsive use, psychoactive effects, and drug-reinforced behavior—are all present with nicotine.[121] People get hooked and have considerable difficulty quitting, despite life-threatening reasons for doing so. It has been noted that "the inability to regulate behavior, despite contrary desires or significant deleterious consequences, is the core of addiction,"[103] a cardinal component of smoking behavior.

In addition, nicotine meets many other of the commonly accepted criteria for drug addiction including alteration of brain wave function, and development of withdrawal effects.[28] Nicotine also has direct mood-altering effects; substantial research (and much clinical evidence) indicates that nicotine reduces or "dampens" unpleasant emotional states and may directly stimulate "pleasure centers" in the brain.[89] Nicotine may also enhance performance, especially on monotonous tasks.[89]

Inhaling cigarette smoke is an extremely rapid and efficient means of delivering nicotine to the brain. Within 7 seconds of puffing, a quarter of the nicotine in inhaled smoke crosses the blood-brain barrier.[89] This rapid reinforcement of smoking behavior is undoubtedly a major element in why nicotine is so powerful in controlling behavior. Given all these factors, it is perhaps not so surprising that 85% of teenagers who smoke two or more cigarettes completely will become regular smokers.[75]

Multiplying these powerful, addictive properties of nicotine is the sheer frequency with which it is used. Assuming a smoker takes about 10 puffs per cigarette (a frequently cited number), a pack per day smoker will obtain approximately 73,000 nicotine "hits" each year. In less than 15 years—by the time an average smoker who began midway through the teenage years is around 30 years old—a pack per day smoker will have experienced over a million such nicotine "hits." No other addiction is so overly practiced.

Conditioning plays a major role in smoking as well. When a specific behavior (e.g., smoking) occurs in a particular situation (e.g., while driving an automobile) an association (or "linkage") is formed between the two. Gradually the association is strengthened to the point where the presence of the stimulus (driving) is sufficient to elicit the behavior (smoking). Smoking behavior becomes conditioned in this fashion to many situations: arising in the morning, having a cup of coffee, taking a "break," finishing a task, talking on the telephone, etc. Smoking can also become conditioned to emotional states, both negative (e.g., boredom, anger) and positive (e.g., excitement, joy). Smoking can even become linked to certain people in a smoker's life (e.g., ones "smoking buddies"). Pharmacologic and psychologic factors are closely linked in a conditioning process in which smoking becomes associated with multiple cues.[121]

Smoking thus becomes supported by a powerful addictive substance (nicotine) and associated with many environmental linkages or cues. Moreover, it appears that smokers develop a number of "psychologic meanings" of smoking. The authors have interviewed hundreds of smokers in their smoking cessation program at the Cleveland Clinic. When asked what special meanings smoking has to them, a number of common answers have emerged from these individuals. The accompanying box summarizes the more common categories of responses, which are smokers' attributions of what they feel smoking does for them.

Perhaps the most common "meaning" of smoking is an "old friend" (see box below). Persons who have gone through rough times in their lives point to their cigarettes as companions who have stayed by their side no matter what. "To me, quitting smoking is like losing my best friend," is a frequently heard statement in smoking cessation groups. Nearly as frequently heard is the comment that smoking is a special means of handling stress, especially intense, prolonged, or unanticipated stress. Some say it allows them to tolerate emotional upset and continue functioning, perhaps by "muffling" (buffering) their emotions, a property of nicotine described earlier. Some see smoking as a means of "buying time," especially in situations requiring difficult decisions. Others perceive smoking as an expander of their abilities (e.g., "The computer won't turn on if I don't have a cigarette in my hand!"). Smoking is used by some as a means of rewarding themselves after an accomplishment (e.g., by a student after finishing a chapter or a set of problems). Closely related is the feeling that smoking provides the basis for taking a true relaxation break. There are other "psychologic meanings" of smoking in addition to those in the box. All are attributions made by smokers, and while they may have little if any factual basis, they seem to have a powerful impact on the smoker, especially when the smoker contemplates quitting.

In essence the smoker anticipates a loss of emotional control, coping skills, and pleasures after quitting. Smoking thus becomes deeply embedded in a person's life, based on the powerfully addicting properties of nicotine; the sheer frequency with which smoking is repeated; the many

---

Some common psychologic meanings of smoking

1. An "old friend" or companion who is always there
2. A special means of handling stress, especially severe stress
3. A means of muffling anger (and other unpleasant emotions)
4. A way of "buying time"
5. An expander of one's abilities (e.g., writing, problem solving, handling difficult or ambiguous situations)
6. A means of rewarding oneself after an accomplishment

---

associations that come to exist between smoking and situations, emotions, and persons in the smoker's life; and the special attributions (psychologic meanings) that smokers make to smoking. No wonder that permanently stopping smoking becomes a real challenge to the would-be quitter. Yet despite the challenging nature of the task, by 1987 over 38 million Americans had successfully overcome their cigarette addictions.[119] Millions more have quit since then. How did they do it?

The process of quitting smoking

In theory, quitting smoking is relatively simple. The person quits, goes through withdrawal from nicotine, and gradually weakens and breaks the many associations through the process of extinction (e.g., has many cups of coffee without smoking so that eventually the stimuli associated with drinking coffee no longer are associated with the thought of smoking). Over time, as the person deals with a variety of life situations and stressors, the realization gradually emerges that the "psychologic meanings" of smoking were in fact myths. For example, a clearer perspective often develops about smoking as a "friend" when its departure results in the ex-smoker feeling healthier, less stressed, and more vigorous.

In actuality, quitting smoking is considerably more complicated. Although smoking cessation may appear to be a discrete event—one day a person smokes, the next day that person quits—in reality, there is a *process* involved. That process has been described in detail by Prochaska and DiClemente and their associates in a series of articles over the last decade.[27,91] According to their research, individuals in the "precontemplation stage" do not even consider the possibility of quitting. Those in the "contemplation" stage think about quitting, but make no active efforts to do so. When people move into the "action" stage they actually attempt quitting, if only for a few hours or days. Some move directly into the "maintenance" stage, which is of course the ultimate goal. Others go from maintenance to the "relapse" stage by beginning smoking again. Typically, these individuals cycle back to the contemplation stage, then to the action stage, etc.[91]

Indications that many people are in the contemplation stage is provided by findings that 90% of smokers attest that they know smoking is hazardous and express a desire to quit if they could find a way.[96] Sixty percent of smokers have been in the action stage at some point by trying to quit.[96] And perhaps most encouraging of all, by 1987 more than 38 million Americans had quit smoking cigarettes, nearly half of all living adults who ever smoked.[119] However powerfully addictive and overpracticed smoking is, tens of millions of people have already quit, more millions are trying, and most of the rest of those presently smoking are thinking about quitting.

For many, quitting smoking is a "try and try again" matter in which many attempts are made using a variety of methods before complete abstinence is achieved. Approximately 69% of former smokers use one method (usually a "cold turkey" approach) to end their smoking addiction, 27% use two to four methods, and 4% use five or more methods.[124] Persistence, both in terms of the quantity of quit attempts and the search for an effective method of quitting, seems to be a fundamental characteristic of successfully quitting.

The type of motivation individuals have seems to play an important role in how successful they will be in quitting. It has been found that those with higher levels of *intrinsic* motivation—where the rewards are internal to the individual—are more likely to succeed that those whose motivation is primarily extrinsic, based on some reward system outside themselves.[21] Although extrinsic motivators can produce immediate gains, they are often detrimental to long-term outcome by undermining intrinsic motivation.[22] Thus if people quit for their own health or self-preservation, they are more likely to succeed than if they quit primarily because others wish them to do so, or they receive some type of monetary reward for quitting. These "internal reinforcers" not only appear more likely to promote successful smoking cessation,[22] they also seem to help produce an enhanced sense of self-esteem and well-being.[88]

The only realistic goal for quitting is complete quitting. Cutting down the amount of smoking may be useful in preparation for quitting, but it is not a realistic long-term goal. "Controlled smoking"—whereby persons learn to smoke fewer cigarettes, or cigarettes with lower tar and nicotine content, or change their pattern of inhaling—may seem appealing to some smokers, but is not a realistic treatment goal.[121] Given the absence of convincing data on the long-term health effects of controlled smoking, "complete abstinence remains the most desirable alternative."[68]

When individuals actually quit smoking, most (but not all) experience some type of withdrawal syndrome.[80,121] Many different symptoms have been reported to comprise this syndrome, including craving for tobacco, irritability or anger, anxiety and tension, restlessness, impatience, depression, problems with concentration, drowsiness or fatigue, sleep disturbances, and increased hunger or appetite. Although individuals differ, most withdrawal symptoms appear within the first 24 hours after quitting, "peak" within the first few days of abstinence, and then gradually decline during the next week or two.[121] In the Cleveland Clinic's Smoking Cessation Program, the writers counsel their patients that withdrawal symptoms usually "peak" within 1 to 3 days after quitting, and then gradually decline to baseline levels between 10 and 14 days after quitting. This estimate is based on the findings that the withdrawal syndrome has a rapid onset and generally declines within 2 weeks.[16] It is indeed the rare patient that reports any purely physiologic withdrawal symptoms (other than now and then craving for tobacco, increased appetite, and occasionally, irritability) beyond 2 weeks of total absti-

nence. Patients who have a cigarette or two along the way, however, may report withdrawal symptoms for a considerably extended period of time, perhaps due to the lack of clearance of nicotine from their systems. In addition, individuals who use some form of nicotine replacement therapy (described below) tend to postpone or considerably modify their course of withdrawal. Table 16-4, which is adapted from materials from the National Cancer Institute, describes some common withdrawal symptoms, their suspected causes, their average duration, and suggested ways of obtaining relief from them.

As ex-smokers pass through withdrawal and beyond, they gradually weaken the many associations (linkages) between situations, emotions, and people and smoking. This process occurs through the mechanism of extinction.[121] Somewhat paradoxically, many of the strongest linkages are the most quickly eliminated because they are experienced so frequently in the person's life and, therefore, are more readily extinguished. Other, less frequently experienced linkages (e.g., weddings, reunions, unusual stressors) take much longer to extinguish because they are exposed more slowly to the extinction process. Some particularly strong and/or rarely experienced linkages may continue to elicit brief desires to smoke many months, even years, after quitting. People sometimes mistake these conditioned cravings for physiologic withdrawal symptoms.

As individuals progress through the quitting phase, they gradually seem to come to realize that their "psychologic meanings" of smoking were not as powerful as they had previously estimated. They learn they can live without their "old friend," that smoking was not a necessary or healthy tool for handling stress, that their abilities remained intact even when their cigarettes were gone, that they could learn new ways of handling their strong emotions, etc. In short, they come to realize that the "psychologic meanings" they attributed to their smoking were in fact *myths*. Gradually as this reality emerges, people really begin to feel more confident in themselves and more determined to remain smoke-free.

Another aspect of quitting that is remarkably underreported, even though clinicians working in the field of smoking cessation see it regularly, is that people who quit smoking report feeling better about themselves. Ex-smokers and nonsmokers have higher self-esteem than those who remain smokers.[88] The psychologic benefits of quitting deserve more attention and publicity.

Even after people successfully complete the steps necessary to quit smoking (i.e., survive the withdrawal period, break or weaken nearly all of their associations, and come to realize that their psychologic meanings of smoking were myths, not realities), they are not completely out of danger. *Maintenance* of nonsmoking after cessation remains a major problem in the treatment of cigarette smoking.[100] Maintenance will be described in greater detail later in the chapter.

Table 16-4. Withdrawal symptoms

Quitting smoking brings about a variety of symptoms associated with physical and psychologic withdrawal. Most symptoms decrease sharply during the first few days of cessation, followed by a continued, but slower rate in decline in the second and third week of abstinence. For some people, coping with withdrawal symptoms is like "riding a rollercoaster"—there may be sharp turns, slow climbs, and unexpected plunges. Most symptoms pass within 2 to 4 weeks after quitting.

Symptom	Cause	Average duration	Relief
Irritability	Body's craving for nicotine	2 to 4 weeks	Walks, hot baths, relaxation techniques, nicotine gum
Fatigue	Nicotine is a stimulant	2 to 4 weeks	Take naps; do not push yourself; nicotine gum
Insomnia	Nicotine affects brain wave function, influences sleep patterns; coughing and dreams about smoking are common	1 week	Avoid caffeine after 6 PM; relaxation techniques
Cough, dry throat, nasal drip	Body getting rid of mucus, which has blocked airways and restricted breathing	a few days	Drink plenty of fluids; try cough drops
Dizziness	Body is getting extra oxygen	1 or 2 days	Take extra caution; change positions slowly
Lack of concentration	Body needs time to adjust to not having constant stimulation from nicotine	a few weeks	Plan workload accordingly; avoid additional stress during first few weeks
Tightness in the chest	Probably due to tension created by body's need for nicotine; may be caused by sore muscles from coughing	a few days	Relaxation techniques, especially deep breathing; nicotine gum may help
Constipation, gas, stomach pain	Intestinal movement decreases for a brief period	1 or 2 weeks	Drink plenty of fluids; add fruits, vegetables and whole-grain cereals
Hunger	Craving for cigarette can be confused with hunger pang; oral craving, desire for something in the mouth	Up to several weeks	Drink water or low-calorie liquids; be prepared with low-calorie snacks
Craving for a cigarette	Withdrawal from nicotine, a strongly addictive drug	Most frequent first 2 or 3 days; can happen occasionally for months or years	Wait out the urge; urges last only a few minutes; distract yourself; exercise; go for a walk around the block

Adapted from materials from the National Cancer Institute.

METHODS OF SMOKING CESSATION

With a behavior as ubiquitous and tenacious as smoking, it is hardly surprising that a substantial number of different approaches to smoking cessation have emerged. This section reviews several of the leading methods and attempts to evaluate their efficacy. Because there are few randomized controlled trials of any of the methods, and other major methodologic weaknesses abound in the studies in this area, it is difficult to make direct comparisons of the efficacy of the methods and techniques used in smoking cessation.

Quitting on one's own

According to the 1985 Health Interview Survey, approximately 90% of former smokers report that they quit smoking without formal treatment programs or smoking cessation devices.[121] Another survey found that 85% of ex-smokers quit on their own.[38] A similar process can and does occur with other addictions; for example, it has been estimated (based on estimates derived from 10 studies) that approximately 30% of opioid-dependent persons spontaneously remit.[1] Of course, it is possible that "self-quitters" have talked with others, read self-help materials, and listened to media discussions of quitting, which helped their efforts along the way. It is also possible that for many "self-quitters," urgings to quit from their physicians or other health care professionals have played an important role. It should be kept in mind, however, that whatever accounts for "self-quitters" enabling themselves to quit—and we are not precisely certain as to what these processes may be—it has a more dramatic impact on reducing the number of smokers than all the smoking cessation methods and programs combined. In terms of sheer success, persons who quit on their own are more likely to be successful than those who seek help in quitting.[38] More will be said about quitting on one's own when physician interventions are discussed.

Education

Approximately a quarter century ago, when the multiple dangers of smoking were becoming very well known to the public, it was hoped that educating people about the dangers of smoking and the health benefits of quitting would be sufficient to motivate people to quit smoking.[110] Although education certainly plays an important role in motivating smokers to consider quitting, it is unclear how significant a role it plays in actual cessation. It has been speculated that gaining knowledge about smoking is a *necessary,* but not *sufficient,* variable in the smoking cessation process.[66] When comparisons are made between groups of individuals who have attempted quitting with groups who have not, lower levels of knowledge of the health consequences of smoking specifically predict those individuals who have not attempted cessation.[66] Knowledge acquisition is believed to be the first major step for behavior change in general and smoking cessation in particular.[33]

The type of educational information is also important. A review of methods that used fear-arousing education found that fear facilitates persuasion, fortifies the intention to quit smoking, and may even cause reductions in smoking; but it does not by itself lead to quitting.[97] Focusing on the positive reasons for quitting, such as better health, more attractive appearance, financial savings, and better self-image, may be stronger motivators for quitting.[110]

Evidence suggests that extensive educational campaigns have been successful in changing the public's attitudes about smoking. In a study of ex-smokers, the most common reason that precipitated smoking cessation was a general concern about health.[7]

For the past 25 years, there have been massive and continuing efforts to inform the public about the hazards of smoking and the benefits of quitting. The annual report of the Surgeon General, prepared by the Office on Smoking and Health, has been a leader in this effort.[96] The Office on Smoking and Health, the primary governmental agency concerned with the problems of smoking and its effects on health, also publishes the *Bibliography on Smoking and Health,* summarizing the world literature on smoking. Several other governmental agencies, including the National Cancer Institute, the National Heart, Lung and Blood Institute, the Centers for Disease Control, the National Institute on Drug Abuse, and the National Institute of Child Health and Human Development, are also quite involved in informing the public about the dangers of smoking, publishing information about smoking cessation, and sponsoring smoking- related research projects.[96] The Resources Section of this chapter provides detailed information about various sources of educational information.

In addition to the many formal programs designed to educate the public about smoking, there are many other less organized means of informing the public. Newspaper stories appear regularly documenting the hazards of smoking and the benefits of quitting. Magazines frequently carry articles and features on the subject. It needs to be kept in mind, however, that there are powerful forces working in the opposite direction. U.S. cigarette manufacturers spent $3.27 billion on cigarette advertising and promotion in 1988, the equivalent of $100 per second.[40] These advertisements and other promotional efforts portray smoking as glamorous, sexy, liberated, masculine, a mark of success, etc. Considering the magnitude of the campaign to promote cigarettes, antismoking educational efforts have helped provide an important counterbalance in the efforts to limit the influence of the tobacco industry's lures to smoke.

Despite all the educational efforts, however, there remains a surprising lack of information in certain areas regarding the dangers of smoking. A survey completed in the mid-1980s found that half of those surveyed did not know that smoking causes most cases of lung cancer, and half did not identify smoking as a cause of heart attacks.[125] The 1990 Surgeon General's Report reported that 30% to 40% of smokers surveyed in 1987 did not believe that smoking increases the risks of developing lung cancer, cancer of the mouth and throat, heart disease, emphysema, and chronic bronchitis or that smoking cessation decreases the risks from these diseases.[119] Overall, smokers know less about specific health consequences of smoking than nonsmokers.[124]

Continuing educational efforts are clearly crucial in the overall campaign for smoking cessation. For many persons, these efforts have probably been the decisive factor in quitting, especially for those who have quit on their own. Although these educational efforts may have been insufficient for others, they may have helped set the groundwork so that other approaches could be effective in helping achieve cessation.

Pharmacologic

Pharmacologic approaches to smoking cessation are not new. Among the earliest were smoking deterrents—substances designed to make smoking unpleasant. Included were such substances as silver nitrate, copper sulfate, or potassium permanganate, typically delivered via astringent mouthwashes or a gum. When these substances come in contact with the sulfides in tobacco smoke, the result is extremely distasteful. Vegetable-base products have also been used. The efficacy of all of these deterrents is quite doubtful[97]; they have never been validated scientifically.[121]

Next came products designed to substitute for nicotine, the highly addictive substance in cigarette smoke. Over 50 years ago, promising reports emerged that lobeline sulphate was an effective substitute for nicotine. Although short-term results were promising, long-term results were disappointing.[110] Lobeline turned out to be no more effective than a placebo, probably because it cannot mimic the full range of pharmacologic effects of nicotine.[97] Since 1980, few clinics have dispensed lobeline.[96]

A variety of drugs, many of them psychoactive, have also been studied to determine if they could ease the withdrawal effects of nicotine. Drugs studied include amphetamine, benzedrine sulphate, methylphenidate, fenfluramine, diazepam, phenobarbital, hydroxyzine, and meprobamate.[110] The results have been disappointing; none of these drugs has been found useful.[110]

Clonidine has also been studied as a possible aid to cessation. Useful in the treatment of hypertension, clonidine has been reported to diminish the symptoms of withdrawal of both alcohol and opiates.[45] One study did find that clonidine improved the 6-month cessation rate, but only for women.[45] Because the effect was relatively weak — only 27% of the clonidine-treated patients were still abstinent at 6 months — and because of the potentially hazardous side effects when clonidine is abruptly stopped, a clear recommendation for using clonidine cannot be made.[121]

Some experimental work has involved agents that block the rewarding pharmacologic effects of nicotine, similar to the use of naltrexone to block the reinforcing effects of opiates. Some preliminary data suggest that mecamylamine could be used as an antagonist to block the nicotine-mediated reinforcing effects of cigarette smoking.[121] Because mecamylamine blocks the effects of nicotine, however, it should precipitate withdrawal and, therefore, would not be indicated for acute cessation.[121] In addition, this drug also has some significant side effects, including ganglionic blocking and antihypertensive effects.[121]

Nicotine replacement therapy. The search to find chemicals that substitute for nicotine, block its use, neutralize its withdrawal effects, or block its reinforcing effects has been largely fruitless. During the 1980s, a new pharmacologic approach emerged: nicotine replacement therapy. The basic concept of this therapy is to provide an alternative delivery system for the nicotine that the smoker ordinarily obtains from smoking, thus permitting the smoker to quit smoking while remaining addicted to nicotine. While nicotine itself is of course a dangerous substance, the smoker would not be exposed to the many other poisonous products in tobacco smoke. This approach would permit smokers to quit smoking first and work on their addiction to nicotine later. It is also presumed that nicotine would be consumed in a more gradual fashion, avoiding the pleasurable nicotine "hit" that smokers feel a few seconds after they have inhaled tobacco smoke, which provides immediate reinforcement of the smoking behavior.

Nicotine polacrilex chewing gum. The first form of nicotine replacement approved by the Food and Drug Administration (FDA) was nicotine polacrilex chewing gum (Nicorette). A nicotine delivery system in which the nicotine is incorporated into an ion exchange resin base, the gum permits release of nicotine in the presence of saliva when the gum is chewed.[121] Between 20 and 30 minutes

of chewing can result in the release of approximately 90% of the nicotine.[35] Usually, when the gum is chewed, nicotine plasma levels rise slowly, peaking in about 20 to 30 minutes; the peak levels are usually below what the smoker had derived from smoking.[121] A number of studies, however, demonstrated that the gum produces nicotine levels sufficient to prevent withdrawal symptoms.[96]

Because of the widespread interest in nicotine chewing gum, a sizable research literature has developed, which Schwartz[96] has reviewed and summarized. About one third of patients were still using the gum 6 months or longer. A marked difference was noted in the median quit rates at 6 and 12 months: 23% were abstinent at 6 months, but only 11% at 1 year. These results are further inflated because many of those not smoking at follow-up were still using the gum, and hence still in treatment. According to Schwartz, "In my opinion, as long as the patient is using the gum, he or she is still in treatment, and follow-ups should be conducted posttreatment. It is the standard in smoking cessation evaluation to conduct follow-ups after treatment has ended."[96]

Nicotine chewing gum fared significantly better when it was used as part of another treatment, especially behavioral treatment.[90] When no more than advice, warnings, or booklets were given with the nicotine chewing gum, it produced low success rates,[80] sometimes lower than those provided by placebo gum.[96] This finding has led some to conclude that nicotine polacrilex gum alone in the physician setting is no more effective than placebo.[121] One recent study, however, found that especially for persons highly dependent on nicotine, the stronger (4 mg) gum was more effective than the weaker (2 mg) gum when used in combination with group counseling.[115] In addition, some studies suggest that nicotine gum may be helpful in limiting postcessation weight gain, a problem that can undermine efforts at quitting (especially for women).[51,65] It appears, however, that its use delays rather than prevents weight gain.[51] Its efficacy appears greatest when prescribed for those who are highly motivated and highly nicotine dependent, but it is not indicated for light to moderate smokers with a low degree of nicotine dependence.

An important, if not overriding, methodologic issue in virtually all of the studies that evaluate nicotine gum is the discontinuation of the gum itself. As Schwartz noted in his comprehensive review of the smoking cessation research literature, virtually all of the studies that evaluate nicotine replacement gum do not ascertain if the subjects remained abstinent *after* discontinuing the gum. "Results should be shown separately for subjects free of the gum and for those still using the gum. This is the only way to assess how effective Nicorette is in helping people to stop smoking and wean themselves of its addictive chemical, nicotine, on a long-term basis."[96]

Further complicating the issue of the effectiveness of nicotine replacement gum may be incorrect recommendations from physicians regarding use of the gum. In a recent survey, nearly 40% of internists would suggest gum to help patients cut down on smoking, and one fifth of those sampled incorrectly thought that patients should be advised to "swallow the juices from the gum so that the nicotine can be absorbed from the stomach."[19] Nicotine is actually poorly absorbed from the stomach due to the acidity of gastric fluid; the nicotine in nicotine gum is in fact absorbed by the mucous membranes of the mouth.[121]

Another complicating factor with nicotine replacement gum, which can stifle its acceptance by patients and hence its potential benefits, is adverse side effects. Common side effects include hiccoughs, nausea, and vomiting[110]; other reported side effects include excess salivation, insomnia, dizziness, irritability, headache, nonspecific gastrointestinal distress, eructation, jaw muscle ache, and anorexia.[96] It is also often considered unesthetic, irritates the mucosa, and is contraindicated for smokers wearing dentures or suffering from gastric ulcers and other dyspeptic syndromes.[5] Many heavily addicted smokers who might benefit from using nicotine replacement gum in conjunction with a smoking cessation program refuse to consider using the gum because they have previously experienced one or more of its side effects or because they simply find it difficult or distasteful to chew.

Despite all of the limitations with nicotine gum—its lack of effectiveness unless combined with some type of effective smoking cessation program, its side effects, and its contraindications (including women who are or may become pregnant)—until recently it was the only pharmacologic aid to smoking cessation that held any real promise. Perhaps that is why a recent survey found that about half of internists prescribe it "sometimes" and a quarter prescribe it "often."[19]

Transdermal nicotine systems. In December, 1991, a new pharmacologic aid, transdermal nicotine systems, became available in the United States. These systems use rate control membrane technology to deliver nicotine for 24 hours. Manufacturers of these patches provide three doses of transdermal nicotine, estimated to produce high (approximately 21 mg), medium (14 mg), or low (7 mg) levels of nicotine over 24 hours.[117] The recommended therapeutic program is for the person to stop smoking and simultaneously begin wearing the highest dose patch for 6 weeks. After 6 weeks, the patient switches to the medium-strength patch for 2 weeks, and then concludes with the low-strength patch for the final 2 weeks. Most of the patches are to be worn continuously.

The transdermal nicotine patch has several advantages over nicotine replacement gum. It does not have to be chewed correctly.[39] Because it is delivered directly through the skin, issues of unpleasant taste, gastrointestinal distress, or mandibular fatigue are eliminated. Because it needs to be "taken" only once per day, achieving the proper dosage appears to be simpler. Taken as prescribed, it automatically tapers the amount of nicotine delivered in

a manner designed to minimize unpleasant withdrawal effects. Nevertheless, it is not without some adverse effects. About half of the patients in a large multicentered trial reported transient itching or burning at skin sites, with 14% having definite or severe erythema noted at skin sites at least once during the trials.[117]

As with nicotine replacement gum, the nicotine patch is *not* to be used in conjunction with smoking, even smoking at a reduced level. Adding transdermal nicotine to the nicotine obtained from smoking exposes the patient to a potentially toxic acute nicotine overdose. Symptoms of such an experience—sometimes referred to as nicotine intoxication—can include nausea, vomiting, abdominal pain, diarrhea, headaches, sweating, and pallor.[121] Despite some anecdotal (newspaper) reports of heart attacks precipitated by the simultaneous use of transdermal nicotine and smoking, a clear connection has not been established. Yet nicotine poisoning through other means (e.g., ingestion of tobacco or of nicotine-containing pesticides) has resulted in severe reactions including convulsions, hypotension, coma, and death, with death usually caused by paralysis of respiratory muscles and/or central respiratory failure.[121]

In a large 9-center study of transdermal nicotine, over 900 patients were studied.[117] The transdermal nicotine was combined with group support systems in outpatient smoking cessation clinics. The transdermal nicotine system produced higher cessation rates than placebo at 6 weeks. Six-month cessation rates were significantly higher than placebo for those using the 21 mg patch, but the difference between the 14 mg patch and placebo approached but did not achieve statistical significance. At the end of 24 weeks, 26% of the 21 mg transdermal nicotine patients were not smoking, 18% of the 14 mg patients were not smoking, and 12% of the placebo patients were not smoking.[117] These rates, while respectable, certainly do not represent a breakthrough in smoking cessation. It was also noted that significant relapse occurred during the periods of down-titration of the transdermal nicotine and once the drug was discontinued completely.

Patients in this study reported significantly reduced withdrawal symptoms and nicotine craving while on the nicotine patch. Transdermal nicotine was well tolerated systemically and topically, and no serious systemic adverse events occurred.[117] The authors concluded that "transdermal nicotine systems show considerable promise as an aid to smoking cessation."[117]

Other, less extensive studies, have also concluded that transdermal nicotine delivery has some promise. One study, which used "low-intervention therapy" together with the nicotine patch found that either 24-hour transdermal nicotine delivery, or nicotine delivery during waking hours only, significantly enhanced cessation rates at 6 months.[23] Another study, which used the nicotine patch alone, found that the relatively high cessation rate while their subjects were on the transdermal nicotine shrank markedly when the patches were discontinued (17% cessation at 1 year).[113] The authors noted that this rate is lower than when nicotine chewing gum is combined with behavioral therapy.[113] As will be discussed later, this rate is also significantly lower than when behavioral therapy is used alone. One study in Germany that did combine transdermal nicotine with behavioral therapy recorded a 1-year cessation rate of 35% abstinence.[5] The authors of that study, after reviewing the relevant research by themselves and others where the nicotine patch was used without simultaneous psychologic or behavioral therapy, concluded the following: "A simultaneous behavioral smoking-cessation program is thus an essential precondition for successful application of the nicotine patch."[5] Other researchers in Europe using transdermal nicotine alone (i.e., without a smoking cessation program) achieved a 1-year abstinence rate of 12.5%.[29]

Although the transdermal nicotine system was designed as an alternative nicotine delivery system for use in smoking cessation, some have argued for its use in other applications. It has been argued that this new nicotine delivery system should be considered a potential long-term alternative to tobacco, which could make the virtual elimination of tobacco a realistic future target.[92] Another investigator found that transdermally administered nicotine reduced cigarette consumption in psychiatric patients who were not trying to stop smoking.[56] The authors suggest that the patch could be a useful adjunct in treating nicotine-addicted psychiatric patients in a nonsmoking environment.[56]

Delivering nicotine through a transdermal system appears to be a promising adjunct to smoking cessation programs. Like its predecessor, nicotine chewing gum, research thus far suggests it is rather weak when used alone, producing low long-term cessation rates that are barely higher than or no different from placebo. But as with nicotine chewing gum, transdermal nicotine shows considerably more promise when used in organized cessation programs, especially those that are behaviorally oriented. The types of patients most likely to benefit from the transdermal nicotine delivery system are yet to be identified. Several studies have concluded that the nicotine gum works best with subjects highly dependent on nicotine[96]; it is too soon to conclude if the same pattern will hold for the transdermal patch. Regardless of their relative merits, however, transdermal nicotine delivery systems are being heavily marketed. On that basis alone, they are likely to become an important element of the smoking cessation effort among physicians.

In summary, the exact mechanisms underlying nicotine addiction are not fully known. Similarly, the reasons for individual differences in initiation, withdrawal, relapse, and the reinforcing effect of tobacco use are not fully understood. A review of the literature on the psychopharmacology of smoking cessation by Nunn-Thompson and Si-

mon[80] provides a useful perspective on pharmacologic interventions. They classified drugs used in smoking cessation as nicotine replacements, nicotine antagonists, agents for lessening the symptoms of withdrawal, and smoking deterrents. They concluded that none of the drugs is completely effective, and that successful drug use for smoking cessation involves consideration of the psychologic as well as the physiologic aspects of nicotine addiction.[80] Although pharmacologic agents may help, they will probably never provide a complete answer to the challenge of smoking cessation.

Behavioral methods: aversive procedures

As behavior therapy has produced some of psychology's most important therapeutic advancements during the 1970s and 1980s, its techniques have been applied to the challenging area of smoking cessation. For purposes of discussion, behavioral methods may be divided into aversive procedures and self-management procedures.

Aversive procedures attempt to effect cessation by either pairing smoking with a noxious stimulus or exaggerating some aspect of smoking to the point where it becomes noxious to the smoker.

One of the earliest aversive procedures, termed *warm, smoky air,* involves blowing warm, stale smoke in subjects' faces while they smoke. This technique produced only limited success, and even those findings were criticized for invalid methodology.[96]

Another early method that did not achieve a permanent place in smoking cessation work was electroshock paired with smoking. It proved to be relatively ineffective when used alone.[71] Sensory deprivation, in which a person remains in bed with limited stimulation and hears periodic messages about the dangers of smoking, did not really generate much study, either.[110]

A much more popular and effective technique is rapid smoking. This technique requires the subject to inhale smoke from a cigarette every 6 seconds for the duration of the cigarette or until nauseated.[110] This method, as well as several similar methods, have some inherent dangers for patients with coronary artery disease including hypoxemia, increases in heart rate and blood pressure, and possible nicotine poisoning.[110] After carefully studying this issue, Hall et al.[52] concluded that rapid smoking was safe for healthy subjects, for patients with mild to moderate cardiopulmonary disease, and for those who have had previous, uncomplicated heart attacks.

As with many individual smoking cessation methods, rapid smoking has frequently been combined with one or more additional techniques. Indeed, as will be discussed later, multicomponent programs often produce superior results to those programs that rely on a single technique or procedure. Schwartz[96] found that rapid smoking had a median 1-year abstinence rate of 21% when used alone and 30% when combined with other procedures.[96]

Another aversive technique is satiation, which requires subjects to increase the number of cigarettes smoked instead of the rate of smoking. Where satiation has been used alone, the median quit rate 1 year later was 34.5%; however, more recent studies of this technique have been less encouraging, suggesting that satiation is less effective than rapid smoking.[96]

Another technique is smoke-holding, a variation of satiation. With this technique, subjects draw smoke directly into their mouths and hold it for 30 seconds while breathing normally through their noses and concentrating on the unpleasant sensations of the smoke, until feelings of nausea cause loss of desire to smoke.[116] This technique is safer than some of the other aversion techniques; unfortunately, insufficient data do not permit accurate evaluation.[96]

Covert sensitization is still another aversive technique. It is intended to produce avoidance behavior through the use of the subject's imagination. As described by Cautela,[9] the subject is asked to imagine receiving noxious stimulation while thinking of smoking; the subject can also imagine positive consequences when thinking of not smoking. Covert sensitization has been described as more likely to lead to reductions in smoking rather than quitting.[110] It has also been noted that quit rates are low when covert sensitization is used alone; when combined with other procedures, it adds little to their effectiveness; however, it may be useful as a maintenance technique.[96]

Overall, aversive techniques have produced a wide range of success rates. In the right combination they have some promise. They are probably not as widely used as they deserve to be due to public reluctance to go through unpleasant experiences to end smoking.

Behavioral methods: self-management procedures

One of the most basic techniques in behavior therapy is self-monitoring—recording the frequency of a behavior to establish a baseline. Not surprisingly, when a behavior is systematically recorded supposedly to establish a baseline (e.g., keeping a record of all foods eaten) the very act of recording can alter the behavior in question, even before the change is intended. This effect has certainly been found true in recording smoking behavior; recording smoking frequency and behavior is a "reactive" data gathering technique (producing its own behavior changes), causing changes in both smoking frequency and duration.[96]

Self-monitoring typically takes the form of a "smoking diary" (Table 16-5). For example, in the Cleveland Clinic's Smoking Cessation Program, the subject records each cigarette smoked, when it was smoked, where it was smoked, what (if any) people were present, and the prevailing emotion or mood the subject felt at the time. Later, the subjects are instructed to review their diaries to determine if their smoking follows any patterns or contains

Table 16-5. Smoking diary (sample)

No.	Time	Situation	People	Mood
1	7:10 AM	Breakfast	Alone	Tired
2	7:30	Car	Friend	Okay
3	7:50	Work	Alone	Rushed
4	9:00	Phone	Alone	Hassled
5	10:00	Break	Co-workers	Relaxed
6	10:45	Work	Client	Angry
7	11:30	Work	Alone	Hungry
8	12:00 PM	Lunch	Co-workers	Relaxed
9	1:15	Break	Co-workers	Relaxed
10	2:30	Phone	Alone	Anxious
11	5:00	Drive home	Friend	Okay
12	7:00	Supper	Friend	Calm
13	8:00	Bar	Friends	Happy
14	8:30	Bar	Alone	Lonely
15	9:00	Driving home	Alone	Drowsy
16	10:00	Watching TV	Alone	Okay
17	10:30	Watching TV	Alone	Bored
18	11:00	Bed	Alone	Tired

linkages of which they were previously unaware. This type of continuous recording results in the most positive control over smoking behavior.[96]

Self-monitoring is rarely used alone as a cessation technique, but instead is combined with other methods. One review of nearly a dozen smoking cessation studies where self-monitoring was combined with other techniques found a mean quit rate of 26% at the end of treatment and 13% at follow-up.[74]

Self-monitoring is often not a pleasant task for the subjects. While it can reduce smoking, it can also increase dropout rates in those smoking programs in which it is required.[43] Encouraging subjects to use it but not requiring them to do so, especially for a long time, may reduce the dropout rate.

Nicotine fading is another self-management technique. The basic idea is for the smoker to gradually decrease the amount of nicotine introduced into the body. One traditional approach is to simply reduce the number of cigarettes smoked each day rather than quitting "cold turkey." The evidence for gradual withdrawal of cigarettes is not very positive; as cigarettes are reduced, each cigarette can become more reinforcing.[96] This technique may have some value, however, in getting subjects down to a level at which quitting "cold turkey" is more achievable.

Nicotine fading, as the term tends to be used currently, typically refers to a reduction in nicotine but not in the number of cigarettes smoked. This reduction may be achieved through commercially available filters that become progressively stronger, or by "brand fading," changing brands to one increasingly weaker in nicotine. It should be remembered, however, that smokers often modify their smoking behavior when smoking low-nicotine cigarettes to maximize their nicotine intake.[4] Thus nicotine fading by changing brands is more of an ideal than a reality. Evaluation of nicotine fading has produced variable results; a comprehensive review of the outcome studies in this area reveal 1-year abstinence rates of between 7% and 46%, with a median rate of 25%.[96]

Stimulus control techniques are based on the finding that a wide variety of environmental stimuli (cues) are associated with and tend to trigger smoking. A gradual reduction in smoking is achieved by having subjects limit the situations in which they smoke. One variant of this technique is based solely on some type of cuing device (e.g., a timer); smoking is to occur only when the timer signals, with smoking gradually spread out as the time interval increases. More commonly, subjects are instructed to not smoke in certain situations that elicit smoking (e.g., while driving, telephoning, within 20 minutes of ending a meal, etc.). This process may be progressive, beginning with weaker linkages and building up to stronger ones.

The evidence does not support stimulus control as an effective means of achieving cessation,[121] but it does appear to help smokers reduce their smoking.[96] When used in multicomponent cessation programs (described later) it may be of some value, although its precise contribution is difficult to ascertain.[121]

Another self-management technique is contingency management or contingency contracting. The basic concept here is to reward subjects for not smoking, or conversely, to punish them for returning to smoking. One variation of this technique is to have subjects pledge to donate money to a disliked organization or individual for every cigarette smoked.[114] Another variation is to return money initially deposited by subjects if they complete the program, or if they do not smoke. Although some of the early studies in this area yielded promising results, more recent studies suggest that contingency management tends to lose its effectiveness once the treatment is over, or until the deposit is returned; nevertheless, 1-year abstinence rates in 13 contingency contracting trials ranged from 14% to 38%, with a median of 27%.[96]

Coping skills training

When smokers quit smoking, they are in all likelihood bound to have some recurring desires to smoke. As the period of abstinence becomes greater, these desires become less frequent and less intense. Coping skills training is intended to give the ex-smoker some skills with which to deal with the desires to smoke.

As described by Shiffman,[99] who emphasizes the use of coping skills in relapse prevention, coping skills may be behavioral or cognitive. Behavioral coping responses include eating or drinking, escape, relaxation, physical activity, and delay. Cognitive coping responses include reminding yourself of the health benefits of quitting, or the health dangers of smoking; distracting yourself mentally

from the desire to smoke; reminding yourself of how others will react to your resumption of smoking; reminding yourself of your reasons for quitting, etc. In the Cleveland Clinic's Smoking Cessation Program, considerable anecdotal evidence has suggested that recalling what is presented as the basic rule (that is repeatedly drummed into the minds of all participants)—"smoking is not an option in my life"—can be a useful cognitive coping response.

Coping skills training appears to be effective in enhancing short-term outcome, especially when combined with an aversive smoking procedure.[96] In studies of maintenance of abstinence, however, coping skills procedures results produce mixed results, with a number of negative results emerging[44] that could be more a function of compliance than weakness of the skills themselves. Coping skills training may be most effective for certain smokers who are less nicotine dependent or who rely more on smoking to cope with emotional stressors.[121]

A number of other behavioral techniques should be mentioned, although they have played a lesser role in cessation efforts. Relaxation training, while an apparently useful component of some programs, has demonstrated little efficacy as a cessation technique when used alone.[114] Systematic desensitization, which attempts to desensitize cues associated with smoking by pairing them with relaxation responses, has produced disappointing results.[96] Social support systems, such as development of a "buddy system" among group members and public announcements of those subjects successful at quitting, have enhanced abstinence rates in a behaviorally oriented program.[54] Involving spouses in a smoking cessation program provided no clear improvement in abstinence rates[121]; however, increasing the ratio of positive/negative behaviors of spouses toward their ex-smoking partners does have a favorable effect on abstinence.[13]

It is not surprising that behavioral methods have earned a respectable place in the smoking cessation field. Behavioral and psychologic factors in smoking are highly important; it is logical that techniques targeted at these aspects of smoking are likely to be beneficial. Self-management procedures that patients can learn and use much later on make a great deal of sense, as they encourage reliance on self rather than others; they can be particularly effective during the important maintenance phase of cessation.[96]

Hypnosis

Hypnosis seems to evoke a great deal of public interest. Advertisements for its use and claims of its success may be found in most newspapers, especially those in larger metropolitan areas. Its appeal probably lies in its promise of a rapid therapy requiring little personal effort and possessing almost magical qualities.

Hypnosis can take many forms: single or multiple sessions, individual or group settings. It can also use a variety of approaches: hypnotherapy, as an adjunct to verbal psychotherapy; hypnoaversion, which attempts to hypnotically induce an aversion to smoking; and self-hypnosis, used as an adjunct to supplement hypnotic treatment.[104] Many behavioral adjuncts are used with hypnosis including imagery, suggestions, self-relaxation, aversive methods, positive and negative reinforcement, substitute behavior, inconvenience ploys, and counseling.[96]

Spiegel[107] popularized the use of a single hypnotic session for the treatment of smoking. His hypnotherapy includes teaching the person self-hypnosis, which uses three standard suggestions: (1) Smoking is a poison to your body, (2) you need your body to live, and (3) you owe your body this respect and protection (of not smoking).[107] He reported a 1-year abstinence rate of 20% based on his single-session hypnosis. Others have obtained similar results with this technique.[79]

Success rates of multiple individual sessions have also been studied, although there have been few reports in this area since 1977. Schwartz,[96] who studied this topic comprehensively, concluded that multiple sessions appear to improve quit rates.

Group hypnosis has also been studied. One recent study reported just under 19% abstinence at 6 months.[79] In general, most group hypnosis is single session. The studies reviewed by Schwartz[96] yielded median percentage abstinence rates in the mid-30s, 6 months later.

The published literature on hypnosis is difficult to evaluate. In 1980, Holroyd[58] conducted a review of the hypnosis literature. She concluded "it seems clear from a review of the recent literature that hypnosis treatment for smoking is most effective when there are several hours of treatment, when an intense interpersonal interaction is part of treatment, when suggestions in the trance are designed to capitalize on the specific motivations of the individual patients, and when there is adjunctive counseling or follow-up telephone contact."

Schwartz comments that it is difficult to assess the true effect of hypnosis as a treatment for smoking, as most of the studies reported were weak in follow-up methodology.[96] A concluding comment by him is perhaps the best available summary on this issue:

> From my review of over 50 reports, comments, and critiques of the use of hypnosis to control smoking, I conclude that hypnosis produces only modest results when used alone, but when combined with other methods, the success rates are enhanced. The skill and experience of the therapist are very important. A single treatment of hypnosis seems most cost-effective, but multiple sessions appear to improve quit rates. As with any method, counseling and follow-up support are needed to maintain abstinence.[96]

It seems glaringly apparent that many of the claims of success made by hypnosis programs advertised in the telephone yellow pages and the daily newspapers are simply not supported by the facts. Despite this discrepancy, however, hypnosis seems to have a role to play in the field of smoking cessation. Perhaps the most important consideration is to keep people's expectations realistic. If people are looking for a "magic bullet" that will effortlessly make smoking vanish as though it never existed, hypnosis is not the answer. But it may prove to be a useful part of the process of quitting for motivated subjects who do not place all their hopes on this (or any other single) technique.

Acupuncture

Acupuncture, based on the Chinese science of presumed connections in the body, uses needles or staplelike attachments to treat the smoker, usually in the nose or ear, but sometimes in other parts of the body.[96] Acupuncture has been gaining in popularity among the public in the past decade despite the fact that its validation has been weak.[121] It claims to be able to reduce or eliminate withdrawal symptoms. After comprehensively reviewing the studies in this area, Schwartz concluded: "There is no evidence from this review than acupuncture may relieve withdrawal symptoms. Despite increasing popular interest in acupuncture as a treatment technique, it has not been demonstrated that acupuncture is able to promote smoking cessation."[96] Schwartz adds, however, that acupuncture may act as a placebo procedure to help the smoker to handle the addictive component of smoking. If this theory is true, the psychologic and social aspects of smoking remain to be dealt with,[96] suggesting that acupuncture may have something to contribute to multicomponent programs.

Multicomponent programs

It is abundantly clear that smoking is a complex behavior and quitting is an involved process. Thus it is understandable why treatment approaches involving a single method are likely to be less effective than multicomponent approaches that use several methods.[67]

In 1982 Lando[68] reported that combinations of treatments generally outperform any single constituent of treatment. The problem has been knowing *what* treatments to combine to obtain maximum benefit. Many multicomponent treatments are based on clinical intuition or on the effectiveness of a treatment when used by itself; few are based on an explicit theory of smoking cessation, addictive behavior, or behavioral change.[121] Thus even though multicomponent treatments are often effective, the reasons for their strengths are unclear.

Multicomponent programs using a variety of behavioral techniques have been studied most (including techniques such as aversive smoking, skills training, group support, and self-reward).[121] Some programs have achieved biochemically validated long-term cessation rates in the range of 30% to 40%.[30] It has been speculated that adding pharmacologic adjuncts (such as nicotine chewing gum) might make these cessation rates even higher,[30] especially for highly addicted smokers who have been unable to achieve even short-term abstinence despite repeated attempts.[121]

Although adding more components to smoking cessation programs increases their effectiveness, inclusion of too many procedures may overwhelm subjects and thereby reduce adherence to treatment. A point of diminishing returns may be reached by simply adding additional components to an already complex intervention.[121]

Self-help methods

As noted earlier, the overwhelming majority of ex-smokers quit smoking on their own, without the aid of any cessation program. Cessation programs do appear to be treating heavy smokers, the group at highest risk for morbidity and mortality.[38] In 1986, approximately 14.4 million of the 17 million smokers who attempted to quit smoking did so on their own.[38] One study found that those who attempted to quit on their own were nearly twice as successful as those who participated in a smoking cessation program, probably because self-quitters are not as strongly addicted.[38] Some estimates have been made of the percentages of those quitting on their own who turn to various types of self-help devices.[124]

A variety of self-help guides and books are available to help smokers who wish to quit on their own. Some of these are available free or at nominal cost through the resources described in the Resource Section of this chapter. Others may be purchased in bookstores or obtained through the mail. Some are built around a single concept or idea; others are considerably more complex. Schwartz[96] provides a fine summary of some of the more popular ones. It is difficult to assess their usefulness in helping people quit, but the fact that they are fairly widely used suggests they are at least of some value to some people.

In addition to written guides and books, a variety of aids are commercially available to assist in the smoking cessation process. These aids include filters that progressively reduce levels of tar, nicotine, and carbon monoxide; tablets or chewing gums that contain substances designed to create an unpleasant taste while smoking; vaporizers that look like a cigarette and release a substance that simulates the taste of a cigarette; a special "tobacco" that burns like a regular cigarette but contains no tobacco or nicotine; cigarette dispensers that unlatch a cigarette at predetermined intervals; and cigarette holding devices that discourage smoking by delivering a health risk message. The effectiveness of any or all of these aids is questionable. In 1982, an FDA panel of experts found that 43 of 45 active ingredients used in smoking deterrents were neither safe nor effective. Lobeline and silver acetate were still under study.[96]

THE ROLE OF THE PHYSICIAN IN SMOKING CESSATION

Physicians and other health care providers are in a unique spot. When their patients visit them, even for routine care, these patients are concerned about their health and, therefore, more likely to be receptive to suggestions that will improve or maintain it.[73] The physician's advice to quit smoking has been described as the most effective means of motivating smokers to make an attempt at quitting.[39] Physicians are thus in a powerful position to influence their patients to stop smoking. They are among the most respected professionals, and they have frequent contact with smokers (70% of smokers see a physician at least once a year).[39]

The enormity of cigarette-related morbidity and mortality and the clear potential for recovery from (or improvement of) many smoking-related problems provide powerful reasons for physicians to take an active role in altering their patients' smoking behavior.[109] The same symptoms that appear to increase a smoker's motivation to quit also bring the smoker to seek medical care, providing the physician with an excellent opportunity to encounter smokers at times when they are most motivated to quit.[109]

At the Cleveland Clinic Foundation patients are frequently reminded that persistence is a pivotal ingredient in successfully quitting, and that failure does not occur until one stops trying. In fact the successful quitter has generally failed on one or more previous quit attempts.[82] Similarly, the physician's advice to quit is not considered to have failed when it does not convince a smoker to quit; physician "failure" only occurs when the physician stops trying to get patients to quit. One study suggested that only 14% of physicians were optimistic about their ability to help patients quit, suggesting that motivational factors may play a key role in physician's involvement in the cessation process.[31]

To have an impact, the physician must of course communicate with the patient about smoking. Estimates vary as to how often this communication actually happens. One recent survey of internists, internal medicine residents, and family practice residents reported that 85% of these physicians at least brought up the subject of smoking with their smoking patients.[61] Other previous surveys of physicians reveal much smaller percentages advising their patients to stop; for example, ranges of between 10% and 44% have been reported.[39] More physicians in some subspecialties than others are likely to counsel their smoking patients to quit[128]; these differences appear to reflect training and subspecialty-specific priorities for counseling.

In one study that surveyed patients as to whether their physicians had told them to stop smoking, 41% replied affirmatively, with patients receiving this advice more frequently from nonsmoking than smoking physicians.[17] In another, 48.8% reported that their physicians had advised them to smoke less or stop smoking, with a tendency for this advice to be given more recently (in 1989 to 1990) than earlier (1979 to 1980).[42] It is possible of course that larger percentages of patients than these were actually advised about their smoking, but they either forgot or denied the messages. One survey reported that the majority of physicians (85%) stated that they brought up the subject of smoking with their patients; however, 34% never gave their patients self-help materials, 83% never used a quit date contract, and 73% never made appointments primarily for the purpose of discussing smoking.[61]

A number of surveys of physicians reveal that between 8 and 9 out of 10 believe it is their duty to help their patients stop smoking.[96] Smokers actually expect health care professionals to help them stop smoking.[62] Thus there seem to be a difference between what physicians feel is appropriate practice in this area and what they, and especially their patients, report they actually do.

Advising patients to quit smoking takes only a few minutes of physician time. Although this advice alone cannot be expected to produce large cessation rates, evidence suggests that it does have an impact. Presumably, physicians' lack of enthusiasm about attempting to intervene in their patients' smoking behavior may be largely based on unrealistic expectations of what their success rates should be. Simple but firm advice to quit smoking by the physician could double the rates reported for spontaneous cessation in this country.[50] Physicians tend to overestimate their patients' awareness of the hazards of smoking and underestimate their own influence in helping their patients to quit.

Schwartz[96] surveyed 12 studies of physician advice or counseling over a 16-year period and found that the median quit rate was 6% with a range of between 3% and 13% percent. (Higher rates have been reported for specific populations.[50]) If this success ratio were extended to all 50 million current smokers, 70% of whom see a physician at least once a year, over 2 million smokers would quit each year. When dentists and physicians are combined, just a 5% abstinence rate would result in more than 3.5 million people being cured of tobacco dependence annually, a yield 17 times greater than the results of saying nothing.[95] This approach would far and away be the most impressive smoking cessation program in history!

Specific physician interventions

Because quitting smoking is a process, and because smokers are at various stages in this process, how can physicians maximize their impact to help people quit? First, and perhaps of primary importance, all patients must be screened for smoking status.[39,59] To screen patients routinely and systematically, it has been proposed that smoking status (current smoker, former smoker, never smoked) become a new *vital sign,* along with blood pressure, pulse, temperature, and respiratory rate.[36,39] According to Fiore,[36] "this small but fundamental change in clinical practice will begin to address a current weakness in the way we practice medicine—the failure to universally assess, document, and intervene with patients who smoke."

A number of authors have proposed specific plans for physicians to follow to help their patients quit smoking.*

*References 11, 24, 36, 39, 50, 72, 73, 78, 96, 109.

There is a great deal of similarity and overlap among these plans. The following plan most closely approximates those proposed by Gritz[50] and by Stokes and Rigotti.[109]

Step 1: Assess smoking status/initiate discussion of smoking. It is important to assess smoking status with every patient. Even if a patient has quit or never began smoking it is good practice to confirm nonsmoking status on a regular basis. With patients who do smoke, it is imperative that smoking status be included in every contact. Chart reminders of those identified as smokers have been demonstrated to be an effective strategy for helping physicians consistently address the smoking issue at clinical appointments with patients who smoke.[12,72] Considering smoking a vital sign, as noted earlier, ensures that this topic will be covered at each patient visit.

If the patient is smoking, providing risk-benefit information is important; this information should be personalized and integrated with the patient's medical condition.[50] Discussion of environmental tobacco smoke and the documented effects of passive smoking on the health of others in the family can also be mentioned.[120,127]

Step 2: Assess patient's readiness for smoking cessation. Smoking patients vary a great deal in their attitudes toward smoking cessation. Some are not even thinking about quitting (precontemplators), some are thinking seriously about quitting but not ready to try (contemplators), and some are ready for action (action stage). Therefore, the messages that doctors convey need to be individualized according to the patient's stage of readiness.[78] If the patient is clearly in the "precontemplation" stage—not even thinking of quitting in the next 6 months—much more information about the risks of smoking and the benefits of quitting may need to be presented. Because smokers seem to have significantly more health worries and concerns than nonsmokers,[88] and because knowledge of the dangers of smoking has been described as necessary, but not sufficient to produce smoking cessation,[66] precontemplators may lack the necessary motivation to move further along in the quitting process. In this case, physicians will need to focus on trying to increase the patient's motivation to quit. Providing the patient with intrinsic motivators (e.g., reasons related to the patient's sense of self-preservation and self-esteem) seem to be superior to extrinsic motivators (e.g., social pressure) in bolstering successful attempts at quitting.[21]

If the patient is in the contemplation stage, less effort may need to be directed toward emphasizing the health issues and more toward underscoring the importance of trying to quit *now.* Such a patient needs to be encouraged to commit to a specific date for quitting. If the patient is in the action stage—actively attempting to quit—the emphasis needs to be on optimistically conveying the message, "keep at it until you get it right!", at the same time underscoring the need to learn from past efforts.[73]

Part of this smoking assessment needs to cover the issue of self-efficacy—how confident patients are about their ability to quit. Confidence will vary enormously among patients, but virtually all have some doubts. For the patient extremely low in self-efficacy, additional encouragement may be helpful. For example, encouraging patients to keep records of smoking behavior (self-monitoring), and recommending that they disrupt their normal smoking pattern in a variety of ways (e.g., not smoking in certain situations, smoking a less-favored brand, reducing their amount of smoking) can help develop a partial sense of control, leading to enhanced self-efficacy.[63] In addition, some of these patients may benefit from a more formalized smoking cessation program.

Step 3: Advise the patient to stop smoking. Brief but firm advice needs to be given at each and every contact with the patient. It may be framed quite simply: "I want you to stop smoking!"[59] The patient in fact may be in the precontemplation stage and not ready to take action on this recommendation. But hearing this message, repeated as often as necessary, may be crucial in helping the patient begin seriously thinking about quitting. For those patients in the contemplation stage, this recommendation may be sufficient to propel them into action.

Step 4: Set a date for quitting. Setting a specific date for quitting is clearly the most universally agreed-on component of the physician's intervention and the most important for maximizing cessation rates.[50] Encouraging the patient to select and commit to a quitting date within 4 weeks is preferable.[109] The patient may taper down the quantity of smoking before that date but should stop completely when that date arrives. Signing a written contract acknowledging the specific commitment to quit and the date of quitting can be helpful.[50] Specific forms are available for helping draft the contract.[47,81] The date itself should be during a time when the patient anticipates no unusual stress; however, once the date is selected, the patient should be strongly encouraged to adhere to it regardless of what develops in his or her life. If possible, involvement of family members or significant others in the patient's life to provide ongoing positive support can facilitate quitting and maintenance efforts.[42] The physician should keep a written record of the patient's commitment as a reminder to follow the patient's progress. Part VI of the Resources Section contains sample contracts that provide a tangible commitment by patients to a specific quit date to end their tobacco addiction.

For those remaining in the precontemplation stage, setting a date may not be immediately attainable. These individuals should be encouraged to *commit to a date when they will be ready to commit to quitting*. They need to be systematically followed by the physician in the same manner as those who have committed to quitting.

Step 5: Discuss/suggest specific treatment strategies. As noted earlier in this chapter, between 85% and 90% of all smokers quit on their own, without the aid of a formal smoking cessation program. For this reason, most smokers should at least try to quit on their own. As discussed earlier, quitting typically involves withstanding some withdrawal symptoms, which are usually short-lived; breaking the many associations between smoking and situations, emotions, and persons in the person's life; and gradually coming to realize that many of the special "psychologic meanings" people attributed to smoking were really myths. For the really heavily addicted smoker, especially the one who is not able to reduce his or her smoking to a pack per day or less by the day of quitting, use of a pharmacologic aid may be helpful. As noted earlier, however, there is little evidence that pharmacologic aids are of much greater benefit than simply advising patients to quit unless they are used as part of a behaviorally oriented smoking cessation program.[68,96]

The DeNelsky-Plesec Smoking Cessation Checklist[26] is provided in the Resources Section of this chapter. The physician may find it useful to give this checklist to patients to assist them in their quitting efforts. It provides information on preparing to quit, actual quitting, and maintenance. Sources of other self-help materials are also listed in the Resources Section.

Some smokers can benefit from a formal smoking cessation program. Individuals who have tried repeatedly on their own without successfully quitting or maintaining their quitting are most likely to benefit from such a program. As described earlier, multimodal programs that offer a variety of techniques are more likely to be successful than those that rely on a single technique. Collaboration between a physician and a formal smoking program has been suggested to be a more effective approach than if the two work separately.[94] The Resources Section of this chapter provides information for locating some smoking cessation programs.

Step 6: Offer follow-up. Follow-up visits to the physician or calls from nurses or other appropriate health care personnel can enhance the effectiveness of the physician's advice. Nurse-assisted smoking counseling in medical settings has been demonstrated not only to be more effective than physician-only advice, but also to minimize demands on physicians.[57] Calling the patient on the quit day may be especially helpful.[109] This call demonstrates to the patient that the physician is extremely serious about smoking and genuinely desires that the patient quit. Because many persons have considerable apprehension about quitting, reassurance from the physician or his or her nurse may be especially welcome at this time. A simple statistic such as "over 40 million smokers have quit, I know you can, too," may be quite encouraging.

If the patient is unable to quit or maintain abstinence, the physician should maintain a nonjudgmental attitude. The patient should be encouraged to learn from the experience, pick a new quit date, obtain whatever additional assistance may be helpful, and get it right the next time.[73] Persistence on the part of the physician is paramount. A recent analysis of 39 controlled smoking cessation trials by Kottke et al.[67] led to the following conclusions: "Success was not associated with novel or unusual interventions. It was the product of personalized smoking cessation advice and assistance, repeated in different forms by several sources over the longest feasible period."

This persistence can pay off, both in lives saved and improved health. It can also be quite cost-effective. In a recent analysis of cost-effectiveness, it was concluded that physician counseling about smoking during routine office visits is at least as cost-effective as a number of accepted medical practices, such as the treatment of mild hypertension or hypercholesterolemia.[18]

SPECIAL ISSUES IN SMOKING CESSATION
Weight gain

People who work in the field of smoking cessation frequently hear concerns about weight gain. The fear of postcessation weight gain, more than the weight gain itself,[70] may discourage many smokers from trying to quit; and the fear or actual occurrence of weight gain may precipitate relapse among those who have already quit.[119] In a study of smokers and former smokers, 47% of current and 48% of former smokers agreed that smoking helps control weight.[119]

Indeed, evidence suggests that smoking does help some people control their weight and that quitting smoking often results in weight gain.[121] A variety of factors may contribute to postcessation weight gain, including increased food consumption, decreased metabolism, and an increased preference for sweet-tasting, high-caloric foods.[121]

For most people who quit, however, the amount of weight gain is considerably less than anticipated. In a recent Surgeon General's Report, which reviewed 15 studies involving 20,000 persons, four fifths of ex-smokers did gain weight, but the average weight gain 1 year later was only 5 pounds.[119] Less than 4% of those who quit gained more than 20 pounds.[119] It is quite possible of course that many of those who gained even minimal amounts of weight after quitting found themselves in a significantly greater struggle *not* to gain weight than before.

In terms of health implications, the approximately 5-pound average weight gain associated with quitting smoking is minimal. There is evidence that this small weight gain is offset by favorable changes in lipid profiles and in body fat distribution from quitting smoking.[119] Most people are probably more concerned about the cosmetic effects of weight gain than the health effects.

Recommending exercise and providing appropriate dietary advice are probably the two most important avenues to limiting weight gain. In addition to burning calories, exercise may at least temporarily increase basal metabolic rate, thereby compensating to some degree for the lowered

metabolic rate often associated with quitting.[119] Dietary advice includes using appropriate amounts of low-calorie, high-bulk foods in one's diet and avoiding or eliminating simple sugars wherever possible. Inasmuch as it has been shown that quitting smoking can and often does lead persons to make other behavioral changes that promote health and prevent disease,[119] recommendations to exercise more and eat in a healthier fashion may be regarded more positively than might otherwise be expected.

Preventing initiation of smoking

As any fireman will attest, preventing fires is much more desirable than extinguishing them. Analogously, preventing smoking from starting is superior to helping those already hooked to quit. Unfortunately, the prevention of smoking has lagged substantially behind smoking cessation. For example, from 1974 to 1985, adult smoking decreased by an average of 1.3 million smokers per year.[86] This decline was not mirrored in the smoking rates of new smokers, which declined at a much smaller rate. In 1985, for example, approximately 3000 new young persons who were to become regular smokers started smoking each day; this rate adds up to over 1 million new smokers each year.[86] The gains this country is making in smoking cessation are to a large degree being offset by young people initiating smoking.

To prevent a behavior, it is helpful to understand its origins. It is believed that starting smoking, like quitting smoking, is a process. This process has been well described by Flay.[41] During the "preparation" or "anticipation" stage a knowledge or attitudinal base is formed. Family attitudes and behavior are important here; indeed, parental smoking is second only to peer influences as a predictor of adolescent smoking.[103] After preparation comes "initiation," trying that first cigarette. If there are sufficient social reinforcements for this first smoking, the neophyte smoker is likely to progress toward "continued experimentation." This quite typically leads to "regular but infrequent smoking," and finally, as the physiologic gratifications (psychoactive/addictive effects) of nicotine take over, to "habitual" or "adult" smoking.[41]

Parental attitudes and behavior set the stage for smoking initiation; peer influences appear to be the most potent factors in precipitating actual smoking.[103] Over half of adolescents report smoking their first cigarette with a friend; only 13% do so by themselves.[103] Mass media also play a role here by portraying the smoker as sexy, outgoing, successful, liberated, etc.

Some adolescents are more at risk for initiating smoking than others. The risk is greatest between ages 12 and 16, higher for adolescents who know less about the health risks and addictiveness of smoking and also higher for children who are rebellious, unconventional, and risk-taking.[103]

The physician can play an important role in preventing

smoking. Because children identify their doctors as second only to their mothers as sources of what they learn about health, the physician occupies a unique place in helping inoculate children against pressures to smoke.[83] Casually but regularly mentioning the dangers of smoking and its addictiveness to children during regular checkups helps set the stage.[39] With adolescents, it is most beneficial to point out how smoking alters here-and-now physiologic processes (such as heart rate, blood pressure, skin temperature, physical stamina) or causes other immediate negative effects (bad breath, smelly clothing) rather than to emphasize eventual morbidity and mortality.[41,103] Suggesting ways to deal with the pressures to smoke can also be quite helpful.[39] For those adolescents in the process or becoming (or are already) addicted, it is critical to urge them to stop smoking as soon as possible.

Some of the more promising approaches toward preventing smoking initiation involve helping youngsters learn how to resist peer pressure to smoke. Originally developed by Evans and his colleagues, this technique has been called the social influences or social inoculation approach.[32,41] These psychosocial approaches aim to give youngsters information about smoking (with emphasis on the here-and-now negative consequences) and on smoking prevalence. (Most adolescent smokers overestimate the prevalence of smoking in their age group.) They also attempt to help the juvenile develop a variety of ways to decline offers to smoke, strive to reinforce current nonsmoking, and seek commitments for future nonsmoking.[41,103] These approaches have the most positive outcomes in preventing smoking initiation.[118]

An involved professional can do much at other levels to help prevent smoking initiation. Pushing for tobacco control laws (with strict enforcement) that really work to eliminate access to tobacco products of underage youngsters, outlawing vending machines, and eliminating advertisements that glorify the deadly tobacco products would be strong steps in the right direction.[15] So would dramatically increasing the tax on tobacco products, which has been shown to result in reduced smoking among young people.[118] It has been demonstrated, for example, that community education regarding tobacco sales to minors plus more aggressive law enforcement efforts can substantially reduce over-the-counter sales to minors.[34] Nevertheless, additional legislation and community support addressing judicial obstacles and vending machine sales are sorely needed.[34]

Smokeless tobacco

Although cigarette, cigar, and pipe smoking has been steadily declining in the limited states over the past 25 years, the prevalence of both snuff and chewing tobacco has increased substantially.[121] In 1986, it was estimated that over 8% of male adolescents between ages 17 and 19 were users of smokeless tobacco products.[121]

It has been clearly documented that smokeless tobacco products produce addictions to nicotine; indeed, with fine-ground nasal snuff, blood levels of nicotine rise almost as fast as those observed after cigarette smoking,[93] although the rate of nicotine absorption with the use of oral snuff and chewing tobacco is more gradual.[121]

In 1986, an entire Surgeon General's report was devoted to smokeless tobacco.[123] Major findings of this report included the following: (1) over 12 million people used some form of smokeless tobacco in 1985, (2) the use of smokeless tobacco can lead to nicotine addiction, and (3) the scientific evidence is strong that smokeless tobacco can cause cancer, especially oral cancer. The overriding conclusion of this report was that "the oral use of smokeless tobacco represents a significant health risk. It is not a safe substitute for smoking cigarettes. It can cause cancer and a number of noncancerous oral conditions and can lead to nicotine addiction and dependence."[123]

Methods of smokeless tobacco cessation seem to be borrowed directly from those developed for smoking cessation. It has been suggested that because of the similarities between smokeless tobacco and nicotine replacement gum, the latter might serve as a particularly useful treatment of the former[123]; however, no clear evidence of such a relationship has been presented. As the number of people who are addicted to smokeless tobacco increases, more effort may need to be directed toward developing specific methods of smokeless tobacco cessation.

The problem of maintenance

The issue of maintenance remains perhaps the largest enigma in the field of smoking cessation. As noted earlier, smoking is a complex phenomenon. It is a powerful addiction, is incredibly overpracticed, builds up many, many associations (linkages) in a person's life, and develops personal psychologic meanings for people. It is no wonder that when people quit smoking, it is surprisingly easy for relapse to occur.

In reviewing the smoking cessation literature, it becomes apparent that virtually any type of program or technique, no matter how limited or ill designed, produces some initial quitters. But invariably significant relapse occurs during the first 12 months, and even beyond. If as many as one in three smokers who entered a particular program has not relapsed 1 year later, the outcome is considered good.[96] Similar findings apply to those who quit on their own. Between 1979 and 1985, each year over 1.3 million smokers quit; however, 75% to 80% of these individuals resumed smoking within 6 months.[6]

Opinions differ regarding lapses (short "slips") and relapses (complete returns to smoking). Much of this distinction may be semantic; an initial slip has been found to be highly predictive of a subsequent relapse.[2,121]

Some research has focused on the differences between successes and recidivists. Persons less likely to relapse include those who smoked less, those with higher personal adjustment, those who were highly motivated and in the right frame of mind initially, those having environments more conducive to not smoking, those with a more negative perception of smoking, those with lower cravings to smoke, those confident of their ability to quit (self-efficacy), and those with lower stress levels in their lives.[96] Factors that lead to relapse may be different for women and men, but it seems premature to draw firm conclusions about these differences.[127]

Shiffman[98] found that most relapse situations can be classified into one of four categories: (1) social situations marked by alcohol consumption, good feelings, and the presence of smokers, (2) relaxation situations marked by feelings of "unwinding," often after a meal, (3) work pressure marked by tension and frustration, and (4) emotional upset situations marked by negative affect.[98]

Most relapse crises—situations where ex-smokers feel a strong desire to return to smoking—occur in the presence of negative emotional states.[99] But one third of the relapse crises were linked to positive mood states and were frequently precipitated by other smokers, eating, and alcohol. Ex-smokers who had some type of coping response, either something appropriate to do (behavioral) or something relevant to think (cognitive) were much more likely to survive their relapse crises.[99] Persons who had been drinking alcohol were less likely to use behavioral coping responses, and depression diminished the effectiveness of coping responses.[101] The situations that precipitated relapse crises could not be reliably predicted from one crisis to another.[100] Similarly, the coping skills that people find effective vary from one situation to another, with behavioral coping skills being more consistently helpful in different situations than cognitive coping skills.[100]

A number of strategies can enhance maintenance. Social support in the workplace and community; support from family, friends, and co-workers; nonsmoking buddies, and follow-up support can all be useful.[96] Physicians verbally rewarding smoking cessation can be extremely helpful.

The most systematic approaches toward dealing with the problems of maintenance are found in the literature on relapse prevention. This term was coined by Marlatt,[73] who characterized it as a collection of cognitive and behavioral strategies and life-style change procedures aimed at preventing relapse in addictive behaviors of all types. The relapse prevention model proposes that initial smoking following a period of abstinence is likely to occur in certain types of high-risk situations. It further proposes that those individuals who have specific strategies to cope with the high-risk situations develop increased confidence in their ability to remain abstinent. The relapse prevention approach is to teach individuals the appropriate strategies, both behavioral and cognitive, to cope with their tendencies to lapse.[73]

A core concept in the relapse prevention model is called the abstinence violation effect (AVE). A goal of absolute abstinence potentially leads to a strong AVE. It is hypothesized that when an individual who is strongly committed to abstinence "slips," smoking will be dissonant with the self-image of an abstainer. It is then predicted that this dissonance will be resolved by a return to smoking. A related mechanism by which the AVE is hypothesized to work involves self-attribution of weakness following a slip. The negative emotional states resulting from this self-attribution may lead to continued smoking, turning what might otherwise have been a slip or a lapse into a true relapse.[73]

Predictably, the relapse prevention model of Marlatt and Gordon[73] does not push for a goal of absolute abstinence in the smoker who has quit. This approach can be contrasted with abstinence-based models, such as the one underlying AA. A recent study found that a commitment to absolute abstinence resulted in a *diminished* likelihood of relapse in clients treated for addiction to alcohol, opiate, and nicotine.[53] That study also found that for those individuals who did slip, commitment to an absolute goal of abstinence resulted in fewer relapses.[53] These findings of course runs counter to the predictions made by the AVE model; but even if the AVE model turns out to be incorrect, relapse prevention, with its emphasis on coping skills, has much to offer. Failure to perform any coping response is the single best predictor of relapse in a tempting situation.[99] Some studies have found that women tend to benefit more from relapse prevention skills training and men more from an absolute abstinence model in helping prevent relapse.[20]

Smokers frequently report that they smoke to help manage stress. Those who do relapse often report that they do so because of increased stress in their lives. It has been clearly demonstrated, however, that for people who quit and remain continuously abstinent for 6 months, their perceived level of stress decreases the longer they remain abstinent.[14] Thus although quitting may at first seem rather stressful, and this perceived level of stress increase may sabotage initial efforts at quitting, the longer people go without smoking, the less stressful their lives seem to become.

In reviewing the research on maintenance, contradictory findings abound and large gaps still remain in our knowledge base. In view of the continued high recidivism within the first year of quitting smoking, further developing our knowledge base about this critical period would seem to be of the highest priority.

SUMMARY AND CONCLUSIONS

Smoking has been clearly established as the single largest preventable cause of disease and death in our nation. Surgeon General Antonia C. Novella stated that smoking represents the most extensively documented cause of disease ever investigated in the history of biomedical research.[119] Smoking is also a powerful addiction, making smoking cessation a real challenge for most smokers. Despite the widespread death, disease, and disability that cigarettes cause, advertisement and promotion of tobacco products continue strong. In 1988, for example, the tobacco industry spent $3.27 billion on tobacco promotion, the second highest amount spent for promoting any product that year.[40] These promotional efforts are especially dangerous for adolescents because advertisements present these patently dangerous products in a deceptive fashion that appeals to youth.[15] They also may help to recapture ex-smokers who have recently quit.[25]

Notwithstanding its highly addictive nature, the money spent to promote it, and the powerful tobacco interests that fight every step of the way to maintain smoking at a high level and thus preserve their profits, smoking is definitely on the decline in the United States. Since 1964, when the first Surgeon General's Report was issued, there has been nothing less than a behavioral revolution. Nearly half of all living adults who ever smoked have quit; between 1964 and 1985 approximately three quarters of a million smoking-related deaths were postponed or avoided as a result of decisions to quit smoking or not to start.[118] Each of those avoided or postponed deaths represented an average gain in life expectancy of two decades.[121] This achievement is preventive health care at its best.

Other related, far-reaching changes have also occurred. The nonsmoker who wishes to breathe clean, smoke-free area has a much easier time of it. All domestic flights within the United States are now smoke-free. Many municipalities outlaw or place major restrictions on smoking in public places. An increasing number of workplaces either severely limit smoking or ban it altogether. In addition, surveys indicate that a majority of the population back these and additional actions such as increasing the cigarette tax, prohibiting the sale of cigarettes to minors, and placing a ban on cigarette advertising.[118]

As noted earlier in this chapter, most smokers have quit without the aid of any formal smoking cessation program. Quitting is most definitely a process, and that process has been given an immense boost by physicians and other health care personnel who have quit smoking themselves and have urged their patients to do so as well. There are no precise statistics regarding how many lives have been saved by these actions. In all likelihood, however, involvements by physicians and other health care professionals in the smoking cessation process represent one of the most major preventive efforts ever in health care.

Nevertheless, much work remains. Not all physicians counsel their smoking patients to quit. Many "hard core" smokers remain who will require new, innovative means to stop smoking. Special efforts must be directed at those "special populations" (described earlier) who have a higher than average rate of smoking. Maintenance of cessation is difficult; we need to learn more about this problem and ways to solve it.

But perhaps the biggest problem of all involves our youth, who continue to become addicted at an alarming rate. Prevention programs have mostly delayed, not eliminated, the onset of smoking.[46,84] Although adults are quitting smoking in large numbers each year, 3000 youngsters become new smokers each day.[86] Children see their parents and older siblings smoking; they see advertisements and other promotional efforts that romanticize smoking, they observe how easily youngsters can purchase tobacco products, and they know little about what "addiction" means. Even if they learn somehow what addiction really means, they never see this word on a cigarette package or in a tobacco advertisement. What they do see in cigarette advertisements are cartoon characters, designed to appeal to children.[40,87] The prevention of cigarette smoking in children might well begin at the preschool level for children of smokers, as attitudes and inclinations toward smoking seem to form at that time.[84]

In the final analysis, it is not enough to help individual patients quit smoking, although it is imperative that these efforts continue and intensify. As with most other important issues in our society, substantial economic and political forces are involved that cannot be ignored if we are really serious about eradicating smoking.

At an individual level, physicians can help continue to raise the consciousness of persons of all ages as to the dangers of smoking by improving the reporting of tobacco use as a cause of death on death certificates.[39] They can also make sure no magazines in their waiting rooms contain tobacco advertisements; a recent listing of magazines with no tobacco advertising appeared in the *Journal of the American Medical Association*.[76] Creating a smoke-free environment in their offices and medical centers seems fundamental. This policy not only sets a positive, healthy example to smokers and potential smokers, but also implies that passive smoking is harmful to nonsmokers. A medical center has an compelling obligation to shield persons in its environs from such exposure.[69]

At the organizational level, physicians and other health care professionals can work to achieve complete bans of smoking in all hospitals and clinics. This strategy not only provides a healthier environment for patients, visitors, and employees; but also provides a consistent message to patients.[60]

At the community level, school-based programs can help ensure that children of all ages are educated properly and provided with community support regarding the dangers of smoking, as well as given assistance in resisting the influence of peers and profit-oriented tobacco companies.[3] Specific involvement by doctors in the educational process have been described.[39]

Much more remains to be achieved at all levels of government to combat the deadly scourge of tobacco. At the local and state levels, a great deal can be accomplished through specific legislative involvement. It has been asserted that more can be accomplished at these levels than at the national level, where lawmakers seem to be more dependent on the financial contributions of special interest groups.[39] Clean air ordinances and laws that prohibit or severely limit smoking in public places and business establishments can be quite effective. As noted earlier, increasing the taxes on tobacco products seems to discourage use, especially among young people. Passing laws with real teeth in them that prevent children from having access to tobacco products can have major impact. Working to severely limit or altogether ban tobacco advertising would be a really major step, but one that can occur only with strong, sustained involvement of the health care community.

In addition, the courts may play a decisive role in the future of the tobacco industry. If, as recommended, the tobacco industry faced the same stark choices as manufacturers of other products face regarding adequate disclosure of dangers and compensation of injured parties, the death knell could be rung for these deadly products.[48]

We have come a long way in the past 25 years; we still have a long way to go. When we eventually succeed in making this a smoke-free society, we will have taken a truly enormous step toward establishing a healthier population. We will have conquered the current major preventable source of disability and death. We will then be able to turn our full resources and energies toward treating those whose diseases cannot be prevented.

REFERENCES

1. Anglin MD, Brecht ML, Woodard JA: An empirical study of maturing out conditioned factors, *Int J Addict* 21(2):233-246, 1986.
2. Baer JS, et al: Prediction of smoking relapse: analyses of temptations and transgressions after initial cessation, *J Consult Clin Psychol* 57(5):623-627, 1989.
3. Becker SL, et al: Community programs to enhance in-school antitobacco efforts, *Prev Med* 18:220-228, 1989.
4. Benowitz NL, et al: Smokers of low yield cigarettes do not consume less nicotine, *N Engl J Med* 309(31):129-142, 1983.
5. Buchkremer G, Minneker E, Block M: Smoking-cessation treatment combining transdermal nicotine substitution, *Pharmacopsychiatry* 24(3):96-102, 1991.
6. Carmody TP: Preventing relapse in the treatment of nicotine addiction: current issues and future directions, *J Psychoactive Drugs* 22(2):211-238, 1990.
7. Carmody TP, et al: A prospective five-year follow-up of smokers who quit on their own, *Health Educ Res: Theory Practice* 1:101-109, 1986.
8. Castro FG, et al: Cigarette smokers do more than just smoke cigarettes, *Health Psychol* 8(1):107-129, 1989.
9. Cautela JR: Treatment of smoking by covert sensitization, *Psycholo Rep* 26:415-420, 1970.
10. Centers for Disease Control: Cigarette Smoking Among Adults-United States, 1990, *MMWR* 41(20):354-355, 361-362, 1992.
11. Christen AG, et al: How-to-do-it quit-smoking strategies for the dental office team: an eight-step program, *J Am Dent Assoc* 20S-27S, 1990.
12. Cohen SJ, et al: Counseling medical and dental patients about cigarette smoking: the impact of nicotine gum and chart reminders, *Am J Public Health* 77(3):313-316, 1987.
13. Cohen S, Lichtenstein E: Partner behaviors that support quitting smoking. *J Consult Clin Psychol* 58(3):304-309, 1990.
14. Cohen S, Lichtenstein E: Perceived stress, quitting smoking, and smoking relapse, *Health Psychol* 9(4):466-478, 1990.
15. Connolly D: Kids' concept of cigarette code, *JAMA* 266(22):3126, 1991.
16. Cummings KM, et al: Reports of smoking withdrawal symptoms over a 21 day period of abstinence, *Addict Behav* 10:373-381, 1985.
17. Cummings KM, et al: Physician advice to quit smoking: who gets it and who doesn't, *Am J Prevent Med* 3(2):69-75, 1987.
18. Cummings SR, Rubin SM, Oster G: The cost-effectiveness of counseling smokers to quit, *JAMA* 261(1):75-79, 1989.
19. Cummings SR: Internists and nicotine gum, *JAMA* 260(11):1565-1569, 1988.
20. Curry SJ, et al: A comparison of alternative theoretical approaches to smoking cessation and relapse, *Health Psychol* 7(6):545-556, 1988.
21. Curry S, Wagner EH, Grothaus LC: Intrinsic and extrinsic motivation for smoking cessation, *J Consult Clin Psychol* 58(3):310-316, 1990.
22. Curry S, Wagner EH, Grothaus LC: Intrinsic and extrinsic motivation with a self-help smoking cessation program, *J Consult Clin Psychol* 59(2):318-324, 1991.
23. Daughton DM, et al: Effect of transdermal nicotine delivery as an adjunct to low-intervention smoking cessation therapy. A randomized, placebo-controlled, double-blind study, *Arch Intern Med* 151(4):749-752, 1991.
24. DeNelsky GY: Smoking cessation: strategies that work, *Cleve Clin J Med* 57,(5):416-417, 1990.
25. DeNelsky GY: Effectively countering tobacco advertisements: a useful tool in smoking cessation programs. Paper delivered at the 8th World Conference on Tobacco or Health, Buenos Aires, Argentina, March 31, 1992.
26. DeNelsky GY, Plesec TL: A stop smoking checklist, *Addict Program Manage* 4(8):105, 1990.
27. DiClemente CC, et al: The process of smoking cessation: an analysis of precontemplation, contemplation and preparation stages of change, *J Consult Clin Psychol* 59(2):295-304, 1991.
28. Edwards DD: Nicotine: a drug of choice? *Sci News* 129:44-45, 1986.
29. Ehrsam RE, et al: Weaning of young smokers using a transdermal nicotine patch, *Schweiz Rundsch Med Prax* 80(7):145-150, 1991.
30. Epstein LH, et al: Smoking research: basic research, intervention, prevention and new trends, *Health Psychol* 8(6):705-721, 1989.
31. Eraker SA, et al: Smoking behavior, cessation techniques, and the health decision model, *Am J Med* 78:817-825, 1985.
32. Evans RI: Smoking in children: developing a social pathological strategy of deterrence, *Prev Med* 5:122-127, 1976.
33. Farguhar JW, Maccoby N, Solomon DS: Community applications of behavioral medicine. In Gentry WD, editor: *Handbook of behavioral medicine,* New York, 1984 Guilford Press.
34. Feighery E, Altman DG, Shaffer G: The effects of combining education and enforcement to reduce tobacco sales to minors, *JAMA* 266(22):3168-3171, 1991.
35. Ferno O, Litchtneckert S, Lundgren C: A substitute for tobacco smoking, *Psychopharmacologia* 31:201-204, 1973.
36. Fiore MC: The new vital sign: assessing and documenting smoking status, *JAMA* 266(22):3183-3184, 1991.
37. Fiore MC, et al: Trends in cigarette smoking in the United States: the changing influence of gender and race, *JAMA* 261(1):49-55, 1989.
38. Fiore MC, et al: Methods used to quit smoking in the United States, *JAMA* 263(20):2760-2765, 1990.
39. Fiore MC, et al: Cigarette smoking: the clinician's role in cessation, prevention, and public health, *Dis Mon* 1990.
40. Fischer PM, et al: Brand logo recognition by children aged 3 to 6 years, *JAMA* 266(22):3145-3148, 1991.
41. Flay BR: Adolescent smoking: onset and prevention, *Ann Behav Med* 7(2):9-13, 1985.

42. Frank E et al: Predictors of physicians' smoking cessation advice, *JAMA* 266(22):3139-3144, 1991.

43. Glasgow RE: Smoking. In Holroyd K, Creer T, editors: *Self-management of chronic disease and handbook of clinical interventions and research,* Academic Press, 1986, Orlando, Fla.

44. Glasgow RE, Lichtenstein E: Long-term effects of behavioral smoking cessation interventions, *Behav Ther* 18:297-324, 1987.

45. Glassman AH et al: Heavy smokers, smoking cessation, and clonidine, *JAMA* 259(19):2863-2866, 1988.

46. Glynn TJ: Essential elements of school-based smoking prevention programs, *J School Health* 59(5):181-188, 1989.

47. Glynn TJ, Manley MW: *How to help your patients stop smoking: a National Cancer Institute manual for physicians,* Smoking, Tobacco and Cancer Program, Division of Cancer Prevention and Control, National Cancer Institute, US Department of Health and Human Services, WM 176 G586h, 1989:02NLM.

48. Gostin LO, Brandt AM, Cleary PD: Tobacco liability and public health policy, *JAMA* 266(22):3178-3182, 1991.

49. Green DE: *Teenage smoking: immediate and long term patterns,* National Institute of Education, US Department of Health, Education and Welfare, Washington, DC, 1979.

50. Gritz ER: Cigarette smoking: the need for action by health professionals, *Cancer J Clin* 38(4):194-212, 1988.

51. Gross J, Stitzer ML, Maldonado J: Nicotine replacement: effects on postcessation weight gain, *J Consult Clin Psychol* 57(1):87-92, 1989.

52. Hall RG, et al: Two year efficacy and safety of rapid smoking therapy in patients with cardiac and pulmonary disease, *J Clin Consult Psychol* 52:574-581, 1984.

53. Hall SM, Havassy BE, Wasserman DA: Commitment to abstinence and acute stress in relapse to alcohol, opiates, and nicotine, *J Consult Clin Psychol* 58(2):175-181, 1990.

54. Hamilton SB, Bornstein PH: Broad-spectrum behavioral approaches to smoking cessation: effects of social support and paraprofessional training in the maintenance of treatment effects, *J Consult Clin Psychol* 47(3):598-600, 1979.

55. Hammond EC, Grafinkel L: Smoking habits of men and women, *MMWR* 34:404-407, 1987.

56. Hartman N, et al: Transdermal nicotine and smoking behavior in psychiatric patients, *Am J Psychiatry* 148(3):374-375, 1991.

57. Hollis JF et al: Nurse-assisted smoking cessation in medical settings: minimizing demands on physicians, *Prev Med* 20(4):497-507, 1991.

58. Holroyd J: Hypnosis treatment for smoking: an evaluative review, *Int J Clin Exp Hypn* 28(4):341-357, 1980.

59. Hughes TR, Kottle TE: Doctors helping smokers: real world factors, *Minn Med* 69:143-145, 1986.

60. Hurt RD, et al: The making of a smoke-free medical center, *JAMA* 261(1):85-97, 1989.

61. Jelly MJ, Prochazka AV: A survey of physicians' smoking counseling practices, *Am J Med Sc* 301(4):250-255, 1991.

62. Joseph AM, Byrd JC: Smoking cessation in practice, *Prim Care* 16(1):83-98, 1989.

63. Kararck TW, Lichtenstein E: Program adherence and coping strategies as predictors of success in a smoking treatment program, *Health Psychol* 7(6):557-574, 1988.

64. Kandel DB, Yamaguchi K: *Developmental patterns of the use of legal, illegal, and medically prescribed psychotropic drugs from adolescense to young adulthood,* NIDA Research Monograph 56, US Department of Health and Human Services, Public Health Service, National Institute on Drug Abuse, 1986, pp 193-235.

65. Klesges RC, DePue K, Audrain J: Metabolic effects of nicotine gum and cigarette smoking: potential implications for postcesation weight gain? *J Consult Clin Psychol* 59(5):749-752, 1991.

66. Klesges RC, et al: Knowledge and beliefs regarding the consequences of cigarette smoking and their relationships to smoking status in a biracial sample, *Health Psychol* 7(5):387-401, 1988.

67. Kottke TE, et al: Attributes of successful smoking cessation interventions in medical practice: a meta-analysis of 39 controlled trials, *JAMA* 259(19):2883-2889, 1988.

68. Lando HA: A factorial analysis of pregnation, aversion, and maintenance in the elements of smoking, *Addict Behav* 7(2):143-154, 1982.

69. Leibowitz S: Creating a smoke-free environment in a medical center: an overview, *Bull N Y Acad Med* 65(7):757-773, 1989.

70. Leischow SJ, Stitzer ML: Smoking cessation and weight gain, *Br J Addict* 86(5):577-581, 1991.

71. Levine BA: Effectiveness of contingent and non-contingent electric shock in reducing cigarette smoking, *Psychol Rep* 34:223-226, 1974.

72. Manley M, et al: Clinical interventions in tobacco control, *JAMA* 266(22):3172-3173, 1991.

73. Marlatt GA, Gordon JR, editors: *Relapse preventions: maintenance strategies in the treatment of addictive behaviors,* New York, 1985, Guilford Press.

74. McFall RM, Hammen CL: Motivation, structure, and self-monitoring: role of non-specific factors in cigarette smoking, *J Consult Clin Psychol* 37:80-86, 1975.

75. McKennel AC, Thomas RK: Adults' and adolescents' smoking habits and attitudes. Government Social Survey, HM Stationery Office, London: cited in Russel, MAH: The smoking habit and its classification, *Practitioner* 212:791-800, 1974.

76. Medical News & Perspectives: Magazines without tobacco advertising, *JAMA* 266(22):3099-3102, 1991.

77. National Center for Health Statistics: Advance report of final mortality statistics, 1988, *Mon Vital Stat Rep* 39(7):2, 1990.

78. Nett LM: The physician's role in smoking cessation. A present and future agenda, *Chest* 97(2):28S-32S, 1990.

79. Neufeld V, Lynn SJ: A single-session group self-hypnosis smoking cessation treatment: a brief communication, *Int J Clin Exp Hypn* 36(2):75-79, 1988.

80. Nunn-Thompson CL, Simon PA: Pharmacotherapy for smoking cessation, *Clin Pharm* 8(10):710-720, 1989.

81. Ockene JK: Women and smoking. Promoting cessation, *J Am Med Wom Assoc* 44(2):60-63, 1989.

82. Pederson LL, Lefcoe NM: A psychological and behavioral comparison of ex-smokers and smokers, *J Chron Dis* 29:431-434, 1976.

83. Perry CL, Griffen G, Murray DM: Assessing needs for youth health promotion, *Prev Med* 14:379-393, 1985.

84. Philips BU Jr, et al: Expectations of preschool children to protect themselves from cigarette smoke: results of a smoking prevention program for preschool children, *J Cancer Educ* 5(1):27-31, 1990.

85. Pierce JP, et al: Trends in cigarette smoking in the United States: educational differences are increasing, *JAMA* 261(1):56-60, 1989.

86. Pierce JP, et al: Trends in cigarette smoking in the United States: projections to the Year 2000, *JAMA* 261(1):61-65, 1989.

87. Pierce JP, et al: Does tobacco advertising target young people to start smoking? *JAMA* 266(22):3154-3158, 1991.

88. Plesec TL: *Psychological characteristics of smokers, ex-smokers, and nonsmokers,* unpublished doctoral dissertation, Kent State University, 1978, UMI No. DEW:891-10828.

89. Pomerleau OF, Pomerleau CS: Neuroregulators and the reinforcement of smoking: towards a biobehavioral explanation, *Neurosci Behav Rev* 8:503-513, 1984.

90. Prignot J: Pharmacological approach to smoking cessation, *Eur Respir J* 2(6):550-560, 1989.

91. Prochaska JO, DiClemente CC: Stages and processes of self-change of smoking: toward an integrative model of change, *J Consult Clin Psychol* 51(3):390-395, 1983.

92. Russell MA: The future of nicotine replacement, *Br J Addict* 86(5):653-658, 1991.

93. Russell MA, et al: Nicotine intake by snuff users, *Br Med J*

283(6299):814-817, 1981.

94. Russell MA, et al: District programme to reduce smoking: effect of clinic supported brief intervention by general practitioners, *Br Med J* 295(6608):1240-1244, 1987.

95. Sachs DP: Smoking cessation strategies: what works, what doesn't, *J Am Dent Assoc* Suppl:13S-19S, 1990.

96. Schwartz JL: *Review and evaluation of smoking cessation methods: the United States and Canada, 1978-1985,* US Department of Health and Human Services. Public Health Service, National Institutes of Health. NIH Publication No. 87-2940, 1987.

97. Schwartz JL, Rider G: *Review and evaluation of smoking control methods: the United States and Canada, 1969-1977,* Washington DC, Department of Health, Education and Welfare, 1978; DHEW Publication (CDC), 79-8369.

98. Shiffman S: A cluster-analytic typology of smoking relapse episodes, *Addict Behav* 11:295-307, 1986.

99. Shiffman S: Relapse following smoking cessation: a situational analysis, *J Consult Clin Psychol* 50(1):71-86, 1982.

100. Shiffman S: Trans-situational consistency in smoking relapse, *Health Psychol* 8(4):471-481, 1989.

101. Shiffman S, Read L, Jarvik ME: Smoking relapse situations: a preliminary typology, *Int J Addict* 20:311-318, 1985.

102. Shopland DR, Pechacek TF, Cullen JW: Toward a tobacco-free society, *Semin Oncol* 17(4):402-412, 1990.

103. Silvis GL, Perry CL: Understanding and deterring tobacco use among adolescents, *Pediatr Clin North Am* 34(2):363-379, 1987.

104. Simon MJ, Salzburg HC: Hypnosis and related behavioral approaches in the treatment of addictive behaviors. In Hersen M, Eisler RM, Miller PM, editors: *Progress in behavior modification,* vol 13, New York, 1982, Academic Press.

105. Smoking-attributable mortality and years of potential life lost: United States, 1984, *MMWR* 36(42):693-697, 1987.

106. Smoking-attributable mortality and years of potential life lost: United States, 1988, *MMWR* 40(4):62-63, 1991.

107. Spiegel H: A single treatment method to stop smoking using ancillary self-hypnosis, *Int J Clin Exp Hypn* 18(4):235-250, 1970.

108. Squier CA: The nature of smokeless tobacco and patterns of use, *Cancer J Clin* 38(4):226-229, 1988.

109. Stokes J III, Rigotti NA: The health consequences of cigarette smoking and the internist's role in smoking cessation, *Adv Intern Med* 33:431-460, 1988.

110. Stone S, Perimutter KJ: Methods for stopping cigarette smoking. Health and Public Policy Committee. American College of Physicians, *Ann Intern Med* 105:281-291, 1986.

111. Sullivan LW: Family physicians and a smoke-free society, *Am Fam Physician* 42(5):1453-1454, 1456, 1990.

112. Sullivan LW: Statement on the ASSIST Federal Smoking Control Project, Washington, DC, October 4, 1991. In Making smoking prevention a reality, *JAMA* 266(22):3188-3189, 1991.

113. Tennesen P, et al: A double-blind trial of a 16-hour transdermal nicotine patch in smoking cessation, *N Engl J Med* 325(5):311-315, 1991.

114. Tiffany ST, Martin EM, Baker TB: Treatments for cigarette smoking: an evaluation of the contributions of aversion and counseling procedures, *Behav Res Ther* 24(4):437-492, 1986.

115. Tonnesen P, et al: Effect of nicotine chewing gum in combination with group counseling on the cessation of smoking, *N Engl J Med* 318(1):15-18, 1988.

116. Tori CD: A smoking satiation procedure with reduced risk, *J Clin Psychol* 34:574-577, 1978.

117. Transdermal Nicotine Study Group: Transdermal nicotine for smoking cessation, *JAMA* 266(22):3133-3138, 1991.

118. US Department of Health and Human Services: *Reducing the health consequences of smoking: 25 years of progress. A report of the Surgeon General,* US Department of Health and Human Services, Public Health Service, Centers for Disease Control, Center for Chronic Disease Prevention and Health Promotion, Office on Smoking and

Health. DHHS Publication No. (CDC) 89-8411, 1989.

119. US Department of Health and Human Services: *The health benefits of smoking cessation. A report of the Surgeon General,* US Department of Health and Human Services, Public Health Service, Centers for Disease Control, Center for Chronic Disease Prevention and Health Promotion, Office on Smoking and Health. DHHS Publication No. (CDC) 90-8416, 1990.

120. US Department of Health and Human Services: *The health consequences of involuntary smoking. A report of the Surgeon General,* US Department of Health and Human Services, Public Health Service, Centers for Disease Control, DHHS Publication No. (CDC) 87-8398, 1986a.

121. US Department of Health and Human Services: *The health consequences of smoking: nicotine addiction. A report of the Surgeon General,* US Department of Health and Human Services, Public Health Service, Centers for Disease Control, Center for Health Promotion and Education, Office on Smoking and Health. DHHS Publication No. (CDC) 88-8406, 1988.

122. US Department of Health and Human Services: *The health consequences of smoking: chronic obstructive lung disease. A report of the Surgeon General,* US Department of Health and Human Services, Public Health Service, Office on Smoking and Health. DHHS (PHS) 84-50205, 1984.

123. US Department of Health and Human Services: *The health consequences of using smokeless tobacco. A report of the advisory committee to the Surgeon General,* US Department of Health and Human Services, Public Health Service, NIH Publication No. 86-2874, 1986.

124. Vital and Health Statistics: *Smoking and other tobacco use,* United States, 1989. Series 10: Data from the National Health Survey, No. 169, DHHS Publication No. (PHS) 89-1597.

125. Warner KE: Cigarette advertising and media coverage of smoking on health, *N Engl J Med* 312:384-388, 1985.

126. Warner KF: Consumption impacts of a change in the federal cigarette excise tax. In *Smoking behavioral and policy conference series: the cigarette excise tax,* Cambridge, Mass, 1985, Institute for the Study of Smoking Behavior and Policy.

127. Wells AJ: Deadly smoke, *Occup Health Saf* 58(10):20-22, 44, 69, 1989.

128. Wells KB, et al: The practices of general and subspecialty internists in counseling about smoking and exercise, *Am J Public Health* 76(8):1009-1013, 1986.

━━━━━━━━━ **RESOURCES** ━━━━━━━━━

General information: available from the Office on Smoking and Health

Public Information, Office on Smoking and Health, Center for Chronic Disease Prevention & Health Promotion, Centers for Disease Control, 5600 Fishers Lane, Park Building, Room 1-16, Rockville, MD 20857.

Publication form #099-3652 (prepared 9/91) lists materials available (order through address or phone number above):

1) English (some Spanish) publications on smoking and other tobacco problems directed toward smokers, nonsmokers, children's health issues, and smokers over 50.

2) English and Spanish posters and stickers available to the public.

3) Technical information: A listing of technical infor-

mation related to smoking. *Smoking and Health: A National Status Report* (1988) includes information on smoking cessation programs available in each state.

4) Surgeon General Reports and executive summaries of these reports (1980-1990).

5) Address and phone numbers of organizations with information on smoking and health:
   a) 10 Government agencies
   b) 15 Nongovernment agencies

Resources for health professionals

How To Help Your Patients Stop Smoking: A National Cancer Institute manual for physicians, by Thomas J. Glynn and Marc W. Manley. Smoking Tobacco and Cancer Program, Division of Cancer Prevention and Control, National Cancer Institute, US Department of Health and Human Services, Public Health Service, National Institute of Health, 1989, NIH publication;/89-3064/G, CA-WM176G568h 1989:02NLM. To obtain a copy, write or call: National Cancer Institute, Building 31, 4B-43, 9000 Rockville Pike, Bethesda, MD 20892, 1-800-4-CANCER.

Clinical Opportunities For Smoking Intervention: A Guide For the Busy Physician, NIH publication 86-2178. National Heart, Lung, and Blood Institute. (Address listed under National organizations).

The Physician's Guide: How to Help Your Hypertensive Patients Stop Smoking, NIH publication 83-1271. National Heart, Lung and Blood Institute. (Address listed under National organizations).

Women and Smoking: promoting cessation, *J Am Med Wom Assoc* 44(2):60-63, 1989. Provides a step-by-step approach (including a sample behavioral contract) for helping the (female) smoker end their habit.

Self-help material for patients who smoke

Clearing the Air NIH publication 87-1647. Available from the National Cancer Institute (free) in English and Spanish. National Cancer Institute, Office of Cancer Communications, Bldg. 31, Room 4B43, Bethesda, MD 20892, 1-800-4-CANCER.

Smoking, Tobacco and Health: A Fact Book and *Pregnant? That's Two Good Reasons to Quit Smoking.* Available from the Office on Smoking and Health, 5600 Fishers Lane, Park Bldg., Room 110, Rockville, MD 20857.

Self-Help Guides: Call 1-800-4-CANCER for free guides for helping patients quit, or write: Office of Cancer Communications, Building 31, Room 4B39, Bethesda, MD 20014.

Self-help materials are available from the local offices of the American Cancer Society, American Lung Association, and American Heart Association. (Check phone book for local number).

Stop Smoking Checklist, Source: G. DeNelsky, PhD and T. Plesec, PhD, The Cleveland Clinic Foundation, Cleveland, OH 44195.

National organizations

American Cancer Society, 1599 Clifton Road, NE, Atlanta, GA 30329.*

American Heart Association, National Center, 7320 Greenville Avenue, Dallas, TX 75231.*

American Lung Association, 1740 Broadway, New York, NY 10019-4274.*

National Heart, Lung and Blood Institute, Smoking Education Program, National Institute of Health, Bldg 31, Room 4A-18, Dept A-1, 9000 Rockville Pike Bethesda, MD 20892.

*Provide group smoking cessation programs. Check phone book for local chapters.

TOBACCO (SMOKING) CESSATION CONTRACT

Name: _____ Date: _____

Age: _____ Health Professional: _____

Sex: _____ M _____ F

1. Tobacco products (e.g., cigarettes) _____ and rate of current consumption (e.g., one pack per day) _____.

2. Quit date: "I will totally end my use of tobacco on (specific date within the next month) _____."

3. In preparation for my quitting I will eliminate my use of tobacco in the following three situations frequently linked with my tobacco consumption (e.g., talking on the phone, immediately after eating, when bored, etc.):
   1. _____
   2. _____
   3. _____

4. I will call this office the week after quitting and the following week to report on my progress to (health professional's name) _____ _____. If I experience significant problems during this period I will call (above mentioned person) to obtain advice on how to proceed with quitting.

5. I understand the importance of ending my tobacco addiction and know that my motivation and effort are principal components in successfully quitting. I am determined to abide by this contract and will end my tobacco dependence on the quit date I specified above.

Patient's Signature: _____

Health Professional's Signature: _____

Date: _____

Nonsmoking contract

I understand that smoking is the single greatest preventable threat to my health. I have been advised by my health professional to end my tobacco addiction and will quit smoking on _____.

(Date)

_____   _____

Patient's Signature   Professional's Signature

_____

Today's Date

DeNelsky-Plesec Stop Smoking Checklist

Preparing to Quit

- Make a personal pact with yourself to quit.
- Pick a date for quitting completely (my date is _____).
- Write down, on a card, the three most important reasons for quitting. Carry that card with you from now on. Look at it several times each day.
- Before quitting, eliminate smoking completely in two or three of your high risk situations.
- Reduce consumption to one pack per day or less.
- Change to a less desirable brand of cigarettes.
- Discard your lighter; use matches. Carry your cigarettes in a different place.
- Spend a little time each day picturing in your mind stressful events occurring in the future and you not smoking.

Actual Quitting: The First Two Weeks.

- Get rid of ALL cigarettes! Put away all smoking related objects such as ashtrays. Ask people you live with not to smoke in your presence for two weeks.
- Spend as much time as possible with nonsmoking people.
- Keep busy, especially on evenings and weekends.
- Avoid "high risk" situations (large parties, bars, etc.).
- Spend lots of time in places that prohibit or discourage smoking (e.g., theaters, libraries).
- Drink plenty of fluids.
- Don't substitute food or sugar based products for cigarettes. Use approved substitutions (e.g., ice water, high bulk/low calorie foods, sugarless gum, mouthwash, brushing teeth).
- Begin (or increase) a regular exercise program.
- When experiencing withdrawal effects:
  1. Remind yourself of why you are quitting (from your card).
  2. Remind yourself that whatever discomfort you are experiencing is only a tiny fraction of the probable discomfort associated with continued smoking (i.e. painful diseases, surgery, chemotherapy).
  3. Practice deep breathing or other relaxation techniques.
- Remind yourself that you can free yourself from this unhealthy, expensive, messy habit and become a nonsmoker.

Maintenance of Quitting: After Two Weeks

- Remind yourself that the desire to smoke is linked to a great many situations, people, and emotional states.
- When you do have a desire to smoke, remember that it only lasts a few seconds; distract yourself, and leave the situation if necessary.
- After each desire to smoke has passed, give yourself a "pat on the back"—you have just made progress in breaking your habit forever.
- Save the money you wasted on cigarettes in a "special fund" and buy yourself something nice.

Maintenance of Quitting: After Two Months

- Be particularly vigilant when unusual life events occur (e.g. weddings, holidays, vacations).
- Be particularly vigilant when stressful life events occur (e.g. relationship problems, financial or work problems).
- Remind yourself regularly that continuing to not smoke is probably the most important gift you can give yourself.
- Remind yourself regularly that not smoking is completely within your personal control.
- NEVER lull yourself into thinking you are out of danger and you can safely have a cigarette or two—you cannot!
- If, by chance, you do slip and have one or more cigarettes, do not conclude that "all is lost." Return to complete abstinence immediately and learn from your experience.
- If you have gained significant weight since quitting, now is the time to do something about it.
- Each time you see a cigarette advertisement, remind yourself of why you quit. Also remember that a powerful industry spends billions of dollars each year trying to get people like yourself "rehooked."

From DeNelsky G, Plesec T: Cleveland Clinic Foundation, Cleveland, Ohio.

Chapter 17

SLEEP PATTERNS AND SLEEP DISORDERS

Dudley S. Dinner

This chapter will review principles of normal sleep and preventive aspects of common sleep disorders. Sleep is often ignored in the standard medical history and physical examination and can be incorporated easily into a discussion of prevention with a patient.

Sleep refers to a behavioral state that differs from alert wakefulness by a readily reversible loss of reactivity to one's environment. This reversibility differentiates sleep from other altered states of consciousness, such as coma or anesthesia.

In 1953 regularly occurring periods of rapid eye movements and associated phenomena during sleep were first reported in a study of normal subjects.[1] A few years later the EEG during sleep and its relation to rapid eye movements, body movements, and dreaming were reported, and a new classification of the stages of sleep was described.[15] The definition of the various sleep stages requires the polygraphic recording of the electroencephalogram (EEG), electrooculogram (EOG), and electromyogram (EMG). During the waking state the EEG is characterized by a medium-voltage rhythm in the alpha frequency of 8 to 13 Hz (cycles per second); the EOG shows the presence of rapid eye movements; and the EMG is high in amplitude, reflecting the presence of good muscle tone.

Non-rapid eye movement (NREM) sleep is divided into four stages, 1 to 4. Stages 1 and 2 may be referred to as light sleep and stages 3 and 4 as deep sleep. The EEG during stage 1 shows a loss of the dominant alpha rhythm, with replacement by a slower frequency activity in the theta range, 4 to 7 Hz, of lower amplitude (Fig. 17-1). Stage 2 sleep is characterized by the presence of theta activity and delta activity (1 to 3 Hz) of low to medium voltage. The other EEG patterns that are recorded from the parasagittal regions specific to stage 2 sleep are sleep spindles and K complexes (Fig. 17-1). Stage 3 sleep is characterized by high-amplitude delta activity that occupies 20% to 50% of the EEG recording, and stage 4 by the presence of more than 50% of this high-amplitude delta activity.[39] Stage 3 and 4 are often combined (Fig. 17-1). We have no rapid eye movements during any of the stages of NREM sleep. Slow rolling eye movements, predominantly horizontal, occur in stage 1 NREM sleep and are not present in the other stages. The EMG activity generally decreases progressively as one passes through the various stages of NREM sleep, reflecting a general decrease in muscle tone.

Rapid eye movement (REM) sleep is characterized by an EEG consisting of a low-voltage, irregular theta and delta activity similar to that of stage 1 NREM sleep and is associated with bursts of rapid eye movements and a dramatic decrease in EMG activity (Fig. 17-1).

The normal night sleep consists of constant cycling between NREM and REM sleep (Fig. 17-2). There are four to six cycles in each sleep period, beginning with a period of NREM sleep. The duration of each cycle varies but is approximately 90 minutes. From 15 to 25 minutes is needed to initiate sleep, and we first pass through stage 1 sleep, go into stage 2 NREM for a variable amount of time, then go into deep sleep (stages 3 and 4 NREM). The first REM period occurs approximately 90 minutes after sleep onset and is of short duration, a few minutes. REM sleep then recurs at fairly regular intervals, approximately every 90 minutes throughout the night. There is usually an increase in the duration of the subsequent REM periods over the night. Deep sleep, stages 3 and 4 NREM, are dominant during the first third of the night sleep, and REM sleep is prominent in the last third.

In NREM sleep the arousal threshold appears to increase with the depth of sleep. There is a parasympathetic

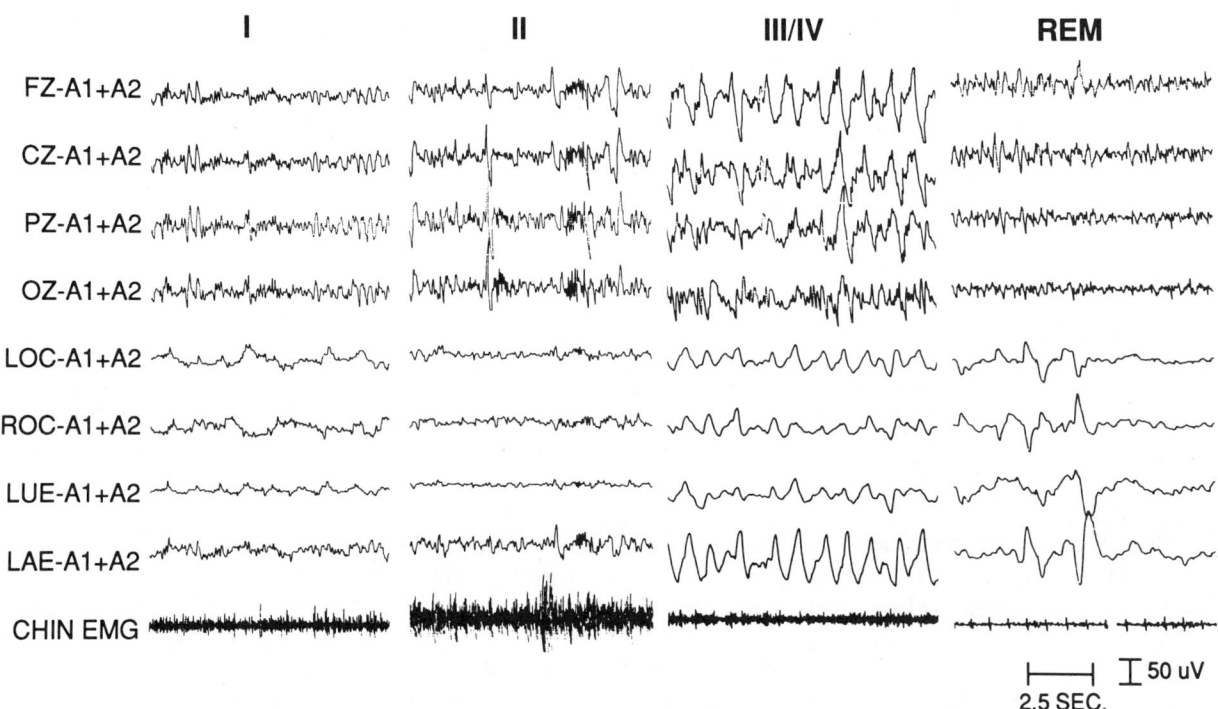

Fig. 17-1. The EEG, EOG, and EMG demonstrate the pattern of stages I, II, III/IV non REM and REM sleep. FZ, CZ, PZ, and OZ are the mid-frontal, vertex, mid-parietal and mid-occipital electrode locations. A1 and A2 are the left and right ear electrode positions. *LOC,* left outer canthus; *ROC,* right outer canthus; *LUE,* left under eye; *LAE,* left above eye electrode positions. (From Rechtschaffen A, Kales A, editors: *A manual of standardized terminology, techniques and scoring system for sleep stages of human subjects,* Los Angeles, Calif, 1968, UCLA Brain Information Service/Brain Research Institute.

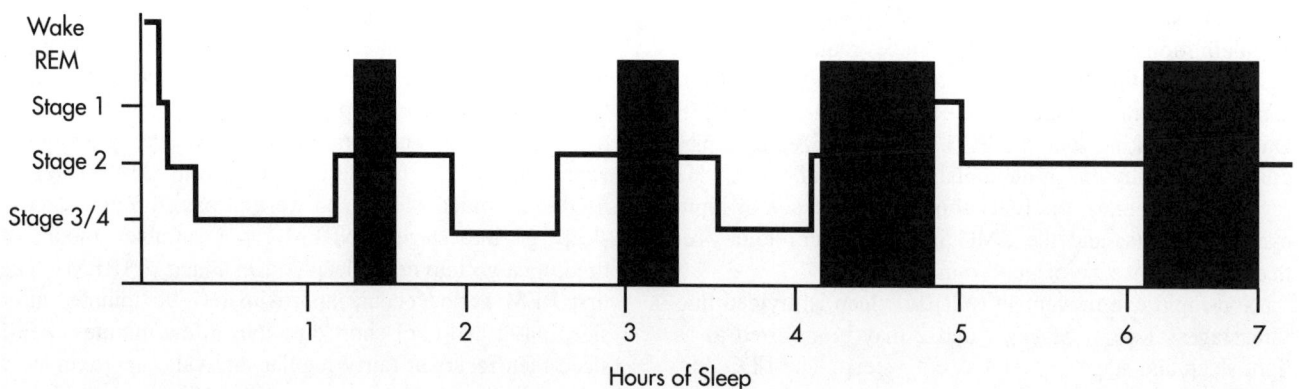

Fig. 17-2. Young adult sleep histogram.

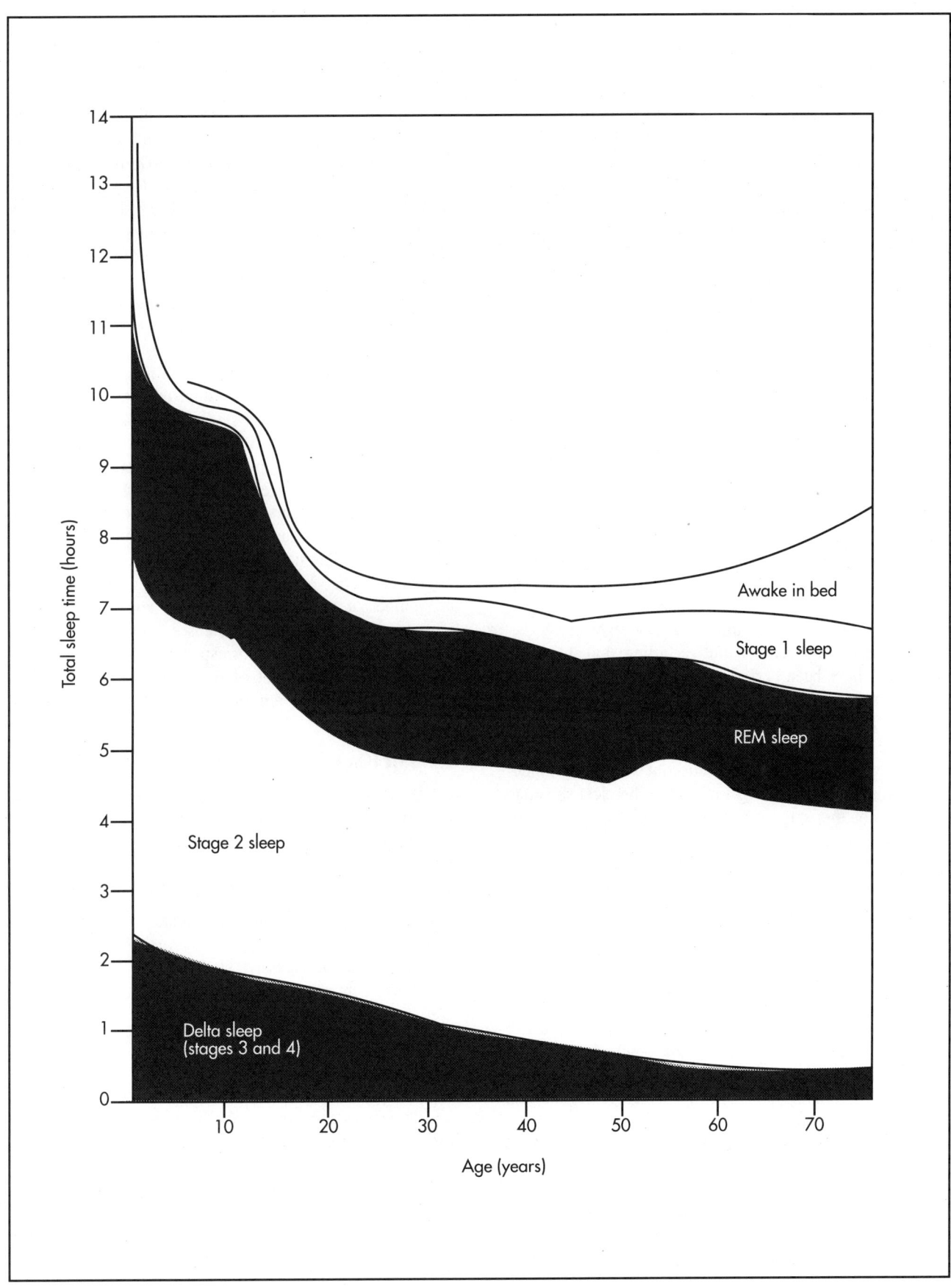

Fig. 17-3. Lifetime sleep patterns. (Modified from Williams RL, Karacan L, Hursen CJ: *Electroencephalography (EEG) of human sleep, clinical applications,* New York, 1974, John Wiley & Sons.)

predominance with a decrease in heart rate by approximately 10%. Blood pressure may also decrease. Respiration becomes slow and regular. Psychic activity is generally reduced, although hypnogogic hallucinations may occur during stage 1 NREM sleep. In REM sleep there is a dramatic decrease in muscle tone, which is punctuated intermittently by short bursts of rapid eye movements and other phasic movements (muscle twitches and jerks). There may be an increase in heart rate, systolic blood pressure, and respiratory rate, which may also become irregular. Penile erections in the male are characteristic of this state. Psychic activity in the form of vivid dreams is well recognized.

The physiologic role of sleep is as yet unknown. However, there appears to be a clear biologic need for both NREM and REM sleep. If a healthy person is selectively deprived of REM by systematic awakening when this appears in the night recording, a rebound in REM sleep occurs to levels higher than normal when undisturbed sleep is once again permitted. This increase in REM sleep occurs without affecting NREM sleep. Selective deprivation of NREM sleep produces a corresponding rebound in NREM during the recovery period. If subjects are deprived of all sleep, the recovery period is marked at first by an excess of NREM sleep, and the rebound in REM sleep is delayed until the second or third recovery night.

Many lesion and cellular unit recording studies in animal models have been performed to try to identify the centers concerned with NREM and REM sleep, and the waking state. The raphe nuclei in the brainstem tegmentum appear to be concerned with the production of NREM sleep. This region has a high concentration of serotonergic neurons, and serotonin is thought to be the chemical substrate important for this stage of sleep. The perilocus coeruleus and other cells in the dorsolateral tegmentum of the pons are thought to be important in the production of the manifestations of REM sleep. These regions project via a descending pathway to a nucleus in the medulla, the nucleus reticularis magno cellularis, which subsequently projects to the lower motor neurons in the spinal cord, producing an inhibitory effect and resultant dramatic hypotonia that is characteristic of the REM state. The ascending pathways from the pons are responsible for the bursts of rapid eye movements and dreams that are the other characteristic manifestations of REM sleep. In animals, electrical activity recorded from the pons, in the lateral geniculate and occipital region, ponto-geniculo-occipital activity, is the electrophysiologic hallmark of REM sleep in the animal model, occurring in association with the ascending manifestations of REM. The periodicity of REM, recurring throughout the night alternating with NREM sleep, is not understood. However, one hypothesis is the reciprocal interaction between the regions responsible for the production of NREM and REM sleep.

The amount of time we spend asleep in the 24-hour day and the proportion of the various stages vary with age (Fig. 17-3). The neonate sleeps for 15 to 16 hours each day, with approximately 50% in REM and 50% in NREM. At the age of 1 year the total sleep time has decreased to 12 to 13 hours, with approximately 30% in REM sleep. By the age of 2 to 3 years the total sleep time has decreased to 12 hours, with 25% in REM sleep. In young adults the total sleep time is 7 to 8 hours of sleep, with 20% to 25% in REM sleep. In young children there is also an abundance of deep sleep. Stages 3 and 4 NREM account for 30% to 40% of the total sleep time at the age of 2 to 3. This progressively decreases to the adult level of 20% to 25%.

In the young adult the average time in sleep stages as a percentage of total sleep time is approximately 5% in stage 1, 45% in stage 2, 25% in stages 3 and 4 NREM sleep, and 25% in REM sleep. There is no significant difference in the amount of sleep in males and females. The usual amount of sleep is between 7 and 8 hours. However, some people are long sleepers (over 9½ half hours per night), and some are short sleepers (less than 5½ hours per night). REM sleep predominates in the last third of sleep. As age progresses from young adulthood there is an increase in the number of nocturnal awakenings, and the amount of light sleep, NREM stage 1, increases from about 5% to as much as 15% in old age. Corresponding with this, there is a decrease in the amount of deep sleep, stages 3 and 4 NREM. However, the amount of REM sleep remains relatively constant.

CLASSIFICATION OF SLEEP DISORDERS

Diagnostic classification of sleep and arousal disorders was originally described by the Association of Sleep Disorder Centers.[2] Disorders were classified according to the two major presenting symptoms of insomnia and excessive daytime sleepiness. There were four major groups:

1. Disorders of initiating and maintaining sleep (insomnias)
2. Disorders of excessive sleepiness (hypersomnias)
3. Disorders related to specific sleep stages or arousals from sleep (parasomnias)
4. Disorders of sleep/wake schedule (circadian rhythm disorders)

Many conditions were listed as both insomnias and hypersomnias, as they may sometimes present either as an insomnia or with the chief complaint of excessive sleepiness. This classification did, however, provide a systematic approach to sleep disorders and allowed sleep specialists to communicate their experience easily.

Recently a new international classification of the sleep disorders has been established; see Table 17-1.[17]

The dyssomnias refer to the group of primary sleep dis-

Table 17-1. International classification of sleep disorders

I. Dyssomnias
  A. Intrinsic sleep disorders
    1. Psychophysiological insomnia
    2. Sleep state misperception
    3. Idiopathic insomnia
    4. Narcolepsy
    5. Recurrent hypersomnia
    6. Idiopathic hypersomnia
    7. Posttraumatic hypersomnia
    8. Obstructive sleep apnea syndrome
    9. Central sleep apnea syndrome
    10. Central alveolar hypoventilation syndrome
    11. Periodic limb movement disorder
    12. Restless legs syndrome
    13. Intrinsic sleep disorder (not otherwise specified)
  B. Extrinsic sleep disorders
    1. Inadequate sleep hygiene
    2. Environmental sleep disorder
    3. Altitude insomnia
    4. Adjustment sleep disorder
    5. Insufficient sleep syndrome
    6. Limit-setting sleep disorder
    7. Sleep onset association disorder
    8. Food allergy insomnia
    9. Nocturnal eating (drinking) syndrome
    10. Hypnotic-dependent sleep disorder
    11. Stimulant-dependent sleep disorder
    12. Alcohol-dependent sleep disorder
    13. Toxin-induced sleep disorder
    14. Extrinsic sleep disorder (not otherwise specified)
  C. Circadian rhythm sleep disorders
    1. Time zone change (jet lag) syndrome
    2. Shift work sleep disorder
    3. Irregular sleep-wake pattern
    4. Delayed sleep phase syndrome
    5. Advanced sleep phase syndrome
    6. Non–24-hour sleep-wake disorder
    7. Circadian rhythm sleep disorder (not otherwise specified)

II. Parasomnias
  A. Arousal disorders
    1. Confusional arousals
    2. Sleepwalking
    3. Sleep terrors
  B. Sleep-wake transition disorders
    1. Rhythmic movement disorder
    2. Sleep starts
    3. Sleep talking
    4. Nocturnal leg cramps
  C. Parasomnias usually associated with REM sleep
    1. Nightmares
    2. Sleep paralysis
    3. Impaired sleep-related penile erections
    4. Sleep-related painful erections
    5. REM sleep-related sinus arrest
    6. REM sleep behavior disorder
  D. Other parasomnias
    1. Sleep bruxism
    2. Sleep enuresis
    3. Sleep-related abnormal swallowing syndrome
    4. Nocturnal paroxysmal dystonia
    5. Sudden unexplained nocturnal death syndrome
    6. Primary snoring
    7. Infant sleep apnea
    8. Congenital central hypoventilation syndrome
    9. Sudden infant death syndrome
    10. Benign neonatal sleep myoclonus
    11. Other parasomnia (not otherwise specified)

III. Sleep disorders associated with medical/psychiatric disorders
  A. Associated with mental disorders
  B. Associated with neurological disorders
  C. Associated with other medical disorders

IV. Proposed sleep disorders

From Thorpy MJ: *The international classification of sleep disorders: diagnostic coding manual,* Rochester, Minn, 1990, American Sleep Disorders Association.

orders that may present either with a chief complaint of insomnia or excessive sleepiness. They are further subdivided according to whether the pathophysiologic factors responsible for their production are inside the body (intrinsic) or outside the body (extrinsic), or whether they are caused by disturbance in circadian rhythm. The second major subgroup of the primary sleep disorders is the parasomnias. The parasomnias are further subdivided based on pathophysiologic association.

PSYCHOPHYSIOLOGIC INSOMNIA

Psychophysiologic insomnia is a chronic insomnia caused by somatized tension and learned or acquired sleep-preventing associations. These patients are extremely concerned with the inability to sleep. This concern becomes a major pathogenetic factor in their insomnia. The more

concerned they become, the more they try to initiate sleep, and the more agitated and alert they become. They also associate many external factors with their insomnia. These patients often report that they sleep better away from home, such as in a hotel room or in the sleep laboratory.

Prevalence

This diagnosis constitutes approximately 15% of the patients with insomnia presenting to sleep disorder centers.[11] The condition usually starts in young adulthood and appears to be more frequent in females.

Clinical features

Patients frequently describe themselves as extremely light sleepers. They describe lying awake for a prolonged period of time, possibly hours, before falling asleep. During this time their minds usually are actively filled with various thoughts that are often inconsequential. They often describe having difficulty falling back to sleep if they awaken from sleep. In association with disturbed nocturnal sleep, they also describe fatigue and poor concentration during the daytime. However, they do not experience daytime sleepiness. Although there is no overt psychopathology, they may have an increase in associated stress-related symptomatology such as tension headache.

Complications

There are no specific medical or psychosocial effects other than the fact that many of these persons use hypnotics, usually benzodiazepines, on a chronic basis for sleep, or use alcohol to help initiate sleep.

Investigations

Polysomnography in these subjects demonstrates nonspecific findings of insomnia, with a prolonged sleep latency, increased wake time after sleep onset, increased number of awakenings, and a resultant decreased sleep efficiency. There also is an increase in light sleep (stage 1 NREM sleep) and a decrease in deep sleep (stages 3/4 NREM sleep). One may also find a reversed first-night effect in that the subjects often sleep better in the one night in the laboratory than they do at home.

Management

Treatment of these subjects consists of education in the principles of sleep hygiene, sleep restriction, and behavioral relaxation. Patients with psychophysiologic insomnia are often found to spend long hours in bed but report sleeping only a few hours. Sleep restriction consists of instructing these patients to decrease total time in bed. For example, if the subject complains of sleeping only 4 to 5 hours, he or she should restrict the total time in bed to 5½ to 6 hours. One should choose the desired waking time and then subtract the total bed time to define the time to go to bed.

A study found that, although sleep time initially did not increase, these subjects felt better during their waking hours and exhibited improved functioning after decreased total time in bed. Once the total sleep time improves, the time in bed can be increased by small increments.[45]

Behavioral management consists of relaxation techniques using biofeedback, meditation, self-hypnosis, and breathing techniques. Principles of sleep hygiene include a regular bedtime and a regular waking time.[26] The patient should have positive associations with the bedroom and go there only when ready to go to sleep. Working in bed should be avoided. The bedroom environment should be comfortable, and the bed should be comfortable. The room temperature should be comfortable, and the room should be dark. There should be no noises to disturb sleep. Eating

a large meal just before sleep should be avoided as this may cause a sleep disturbance. Conversely, a light snack before sleep may be beneficial. Caffeinated beverages in the evening can be detrimental because of their stimulant effect. Although alcohol may help initiate sleep, it is not recommended, as the resultant sleep may be fragmented, and a rebound insomnia phenomenon may occur.

SLEEP STATE MISPERCEPTION

This disorder is characterized by a complaint of insomnia without associated objective evidence of sleep disturbance on the polysomnogram.

Prevalence

This complaint represents less than 5% of patients presenting to sleep disorder centers with insomnia.[11] This condition appears to be more common in women and appears commonly in adulthood.

Clinical features

These patients usually present with chronic insomnia, complaining of difficulty initiating sleep, reduced quantity of sleep, excessive fatigue, and/or sleepiness during the daytime.

Investigations

Characteristic of the subjects with this diagnosis is that the polysomnogram shows no objective evidence of a sleep disturbance.[9] In marked contrast to their sleep architecture, these patients report in the morning questionnaire after the polysomnogram that their sleep during the test was extremely poor, they took a long time to initiate sleep, and they slept for a markedly short period of time.

Complications

There is no specific medical or psychologic effect. Similar to psychophysiologic insomnia, these subjects often use hypnotic medications on a chronic basis.

Management

These subjects are treated similarly to those with psychophysiologic insomnia.

NARCOLEPSY

Narcolepsy is characterized by excessive sleepiness and the REM-associated phenomena of cataplexy, sleep paralysis, and hypnogogic hallucinations. The term *narcolepsy* was introduced by Gelineau in 1880, who wrote "I propose to give the name narcolepsy to a rare, or at least at the present, little recognized malady characterized by an overwhelming desire for sleep which is sudden in occurrence, brief in duration and recurs at variable intervals".[21] The clinical tetrad was first defined in 1957 based on experience at the Mayo Clinic.[52]

Prevalence

Although initially thought to be a rare disorder, the prevalence was calculated to be 0.05% in the San Francisco Bay area[16] and 0.07% in the Los Angeles area.[14] The familial occurrence of narcolepsy is well described. In 1942 Krabbe and Magnussen found that 54 of 200 to 300 cases of narcolepsy came from 19 families. Yoss and Daly found a familial occurrence of narcolepsy in 10% of 400 cases.[52] Kessler, Guilleminault, and Dement[28] reported on the prevalence of narcolepsy among first-degree relatives of 50 narcoleptics. The prevalence of narcolepsy was 2.5%, a rate that was 60 times higher than in the general population. The results did not suggest a simple recessive or dominant mode of inheritance. Leckman and Gershon analyzed Kessler's data and concluded that they were compatible with a multifactorial mode of inheritance without dominance.[31a] Recent studies on the genetic basis of narcolepsy have centered on HLA antigen testing. Most studies have reported a very strong association between narcolepsy and the DR2 antigen, 84% to 100%, compared with the presence in normals of approximately 25% to 36%.[30]

Clinical features

The primary symptoms of the narcolepsy syndrome are excessive sleepiness with sleep attacks and cataplexy. The auxiliary symptoms are hypnogogic hallucinations, sleep paralysis, automatic behavior, and disturbed nocturnal sleep. The usual age of onset is 13 to 25 years; however, later onset is not rare and may be as late as 65 years. In a group of narcoleptics the incidence of manifestations is: sleep attacks, 100%; narcolepsy and cataplexy, 70%; hypnogogic hallucinations, 25%; sleep paralysis, 50%; and the full tetrad, 10%.[52]

Excessive sleepiness is the hallmark of the narcolepsy syndrome. An attack of irresistible sleep often occurs if the patient is in a relaxed situation, such as sitting and working at a desk, watching television, or reading. However, when excessive sleepiness is severe, he or she may fall asleep under unfavorable conditions, such as during work, conversation, or driving. The naps are characteristically of short duration, 30 seconds to as long as 15 or 20 minutes. On awakening from a nap these subjects characteristically feel refreshed.

Cataplexy consists of the sudden loss of muscle tone associated with an inability to move. The episodes may be partial, affecting only the eyelids and producing ptosis; affecting the face, causing sagging and an inability to continue speaking; or affecting the legs, producing a sensation of buckling at the knees without falling. Cataplexy may be complete, with significant involvement of all muscle groups, causing the person to fall to the ground. Cataplexy is usually provoked by emotion, laughter, anger, or excitement, particularly if the emotional event is sudden. Consciousness remains intact during the episode. The duration

is a few seconds to one or two minutes. The frequency of the episodes may vary from once or twice in a lifetime to many times per day. Cataplectic attacks may develop up to 10 years after the onset of the excessive sleepiness. A small percentage of subjects may experience the onset of the cataplexy before the excessive sleepiness, but in the majority of patients they start at the same time or within 5 years.

Sleep paralysis is characterized by the sudden inability to move at the onset of sleep or when awakening during the night or in the morning. It may occur in relation to night sleep or a narcoleptic sleep attack during the day. It usually terminates immediately if someone enters the room or addresses or touches the person. Consciousness during the attack is intact. However, there may be associated hypnogogic hallucinations, which represent the vivid imagery or dreams of REM sleep. The duration of these episodes varies from 1 to 10 minutes. The frequency may vary from a few episodes in the patient's lifetime to nightly.

Hypnogogic hallucinations consist of complex visual, auditory, or somatosensory hallucinations that occur in the period before falling asleep. They may also occur on awakening and are then called hypnopompic hallucinations. These often are accompanied by sleep paralysis. The duration may be from 1 to 15 minutes. The frequency also varies, as with the other REM-associated phenomena.

States of automatic behavior may occur if the patient continues his or her activity in spite of his or her drowsiness. The patient may fall asleep while walking and awaken in a different location without knowing how he or she got there.

Patients usually fall asleep extremely quickly at night, often within 10 to 15 seconds. However, disturbed nocturnal sleep is a common manifestation in this group of patients.

Pathophysiology

Cataplexy, hypnogogic hallucinations, and sleep paralysis are REM-associated clinical manifestations. Cataplexy is thought to be equivalent to the state of muscle hypotonia, which is a normal physiologic manifestation of the REM sleep state but that occurs inappropriately during the waking state, precipitated by emotional events. Sleep paralysis also represents the muscle hypotonia of the REM state, occurring during wakefulness at sleep onset or on awakening. The hypnogogic hallucinations represent the vivid imagery similar to the dream content of the REM state.

Investigations

The first EEG description of narcolepsy was made by Gibbs et al. However, no mention was made of REM sleep until the discovery of rapid eye movements in sleep[1] and the differentiation of sleep into NREM and REM sleep states.[15] The first polygraphic study of narcolepsy was published by Rechtschaffen, Dement et al.[40] in 1963. All of the nine patients studied demonstrated REM onset of sleep. In the evaluation of the patient with suspected narcolepsy, an all-night polysomnogram should be performed to assess the sleep architecture and disruption thereof and to exclude the presence of the sleep apnea syndrome and periodic limb movements as possible causes of the excessive sleepiness. Periodic leg movements appear to be increased in patients with narcolepsy. There have also been reports of an increased incidence of sleep apnea in these patients. This study may also demonstrate the onset of REM sleep within 10 to 15 minutes of sleep onset.[8] The polysomnogram is followed the next day by a multiple sleep latency test. The sleep latency (interval from the start of the recording to sleep onset) and the REM latency (interval from sleep onset to the onset of REM sleep) are measured in four or five 20-minute naps at 2-hour intervals over the day. The sleep latencies in patients with excessive sleepiness should have a mean of less than 5 minutes. In addition, in narcolepsy sleep-onset REM periods are present in at least two of the four or five naps experienced.

Complications

There are significant psychosocial effects of the excessive sleepiness in these patients. They may experience resultant difficulties in school, college, and career. They exhibit an increased risk of driving accidents as a result of the hypersomnolence or sleep attacks. Their sleepiness may also affect their social interaction.

Treatment

Management consists of counseling the patient and the family about the diagnosis. They should practice good sleep habits that consist of adequate nocturnal sleep and scheduled daytime naps. Medication is given independently for excessive sleepiness and cataplexy. For excessive sleepiness pemoline (Cylert) may be used, starting at the dosage of 18.75 or 37.5 mg daily and gradually titrating the dosage according to the clinical response. Methylphenidate (Ritalin) is an alternate stimulant medication, which can be started at a dosage of 5 mg daily and also titrated similarly to the pemoline. Amphetamines are also occasionally used in these patients. In the treatment of the cataplexy, protriptyline, starting at a dosage of 5 mg daily, or imipramine can be used. Viloxazine, a norepinephrinene uptake blocker is a newer compound that has been used for cataplexy in doses of 100 to 300 mg per day.[25] On occasion the nocturnal sleep disturbance in these patients needs to be addressed. Usually this can be improved by the use of benzodiazapines.

IDIOPATHIC HYPERSOMNIA

Idiopathic hypersomnia is a disorder of unknown etiology characterized by excessive daytime sleepiness and associated with prolonged nocturnal sleep and prolonged daytime naps of non-REM sleep.

Prevalence

Idiopathic hypersomnia is thought to account for 5% to 10% of patients presenting with excessive sleepiness to sleep disorder centers. The onset of the condition is in adolescence or early adulthood, affecting males and females equally.

Clinical features

Patients present with persistent, excessive sleepiness. They take naps that are prolonged (1 to 2 hours) compared with the short-duration naps that occur in narcolepsy.[24] They awaken from these naps unrefreshed in contrast to the refreshing quality of naps in narcolepsy. Nighttime sleep is described as normal or at times prolonged up to 10 to 12 hours.

Complications

Similar to narcolepsy, there may be significant psychosocial consequences as the result of the degree of excessive sleepiness that impairs daytime waking function.

Investigations

Polysomnography demonstrates normal sleep architecture, which may be prolonged.[25] The sleep latency may be reduced, such as in narcolepsy. The daytime multiple sleep latency test demonstrates short sleep latencies in each of the naps, with a mean of less than 5 minutes. However, no sleep-onset REM periods are present.

Treatment

Counseling of the patient and family about this diagnosis is necessary. These patients usually do not benefit from scheduled daytime naps. Stimulant medications may be used for management of hypersomnolence. However, these patients do not respond as well as narcoleptics to stimulants.

OBSTRUCTIVE SLEEP APNEA SYNDROME

Gastaut et al.[20] were the first to record multiple respiratory pauses during sleep in patients with the Pickwickian syndrome. Clinical sleep specialists then began studying respiration as a function of sleep. The first symposium on sleep-related respiratory problems was held in Italy in 1972, from which the concept of the sleep apnea syndromes arose.[32] One needs to be aware of certain definitions in relation to sleep apnea.

Apnea is defined as a cessation of airflow at the nose and mouth lasting at least 10 seconds.

Hypopnea is defined as a greater than 50% decrease of airflow at the nose and mouth lasting at least 10 seconds.

Apnea index is defined as the number of apneas per hours of sleep.

Hypopnea index is defined as the number of hypopneas per hour of sleep.

Central apnea is defined as a cessation of nasal and buccal air flow of 10 seconds or longer, accompanied by cessation of respiratory effort (Fig. 17-4).[32]

Obstructive apnea is defined as the cessation of airflow in spite of persistent respiratory effort (Fig. 17-5).[32]

Mixed apnea is defined as cessation of airflow associated with absent respiratory effort during the initial portion of the episode, followed by resumption of unsuccessful effort in the latter portion of the apnea episode (Fig. 17-6).[32]

A sleep apnea syndrome is diagnosed if apneas and hypopneas occur during NREM and REM sleep with a combined apnea and hypopnea index of greater than five episodes per sleep hour.

Prevalence

The obstructive sleep apnea (OSA) syndrome is the commonest cause of patients presenting to sleep disorder centers with excessive sleepiness, with a prevalence of 43% in a national cooperative study.[12] The prevalence in a young adult population has been estimated at between 1% and 10%.[31] The prevalence increases with age and it may affect 50% of males above the age of 60 years.[29]

The Stanford Sleep Disorder Center conducted studies of normal volunteers in 1972 and 1973 to establish normative data of apneas and hypopneas. The mean number of apneas was 6.70 (range 1 to 12) in the men and 2.1 (range 0 to 5) in women. In the subjects 40 to 60 years old, the males had a higher mean number of apneas than the females.[27] At the Cleveland Clinic from 1980 to 1981 we performed single-night studies of 82 normal subjects (38

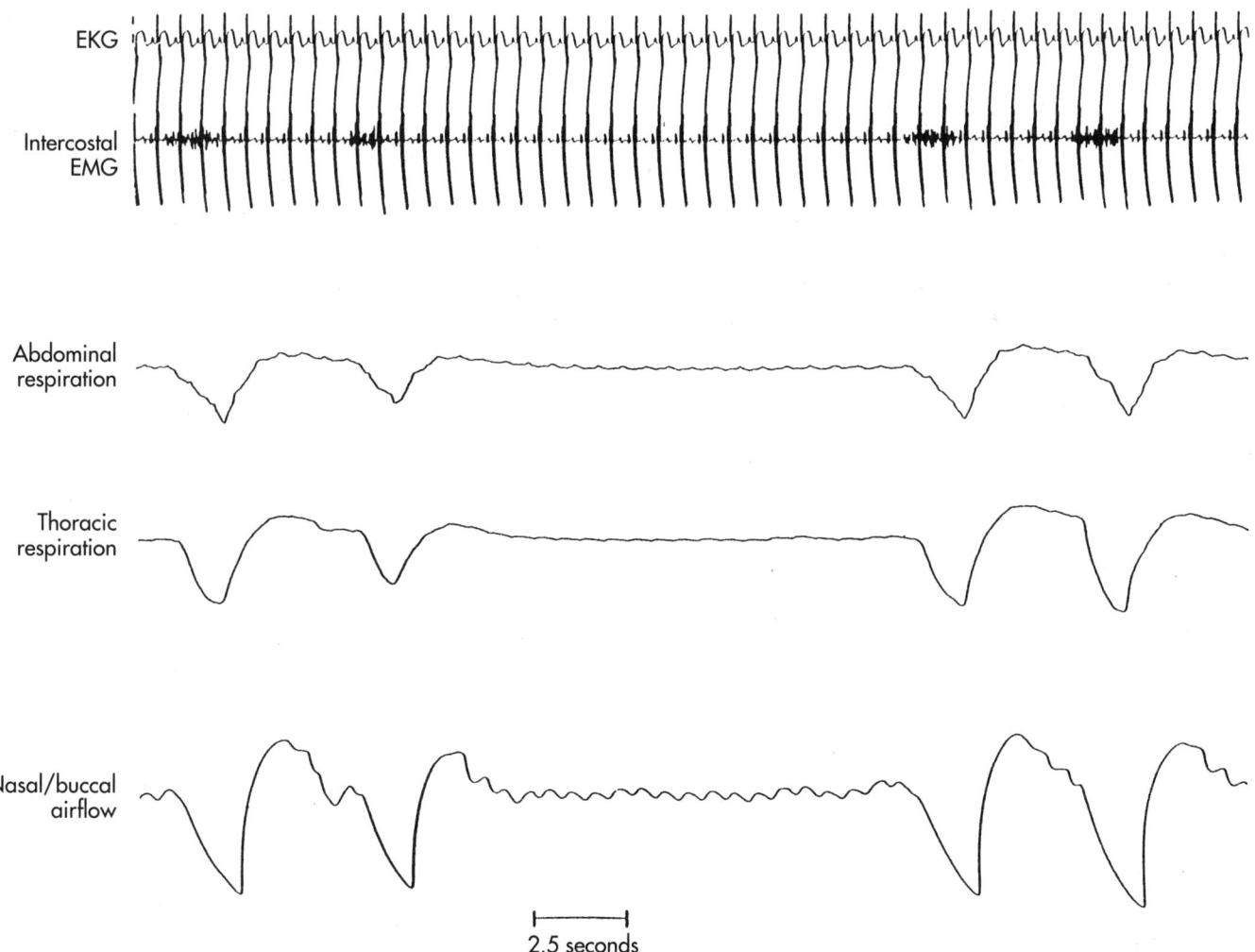

Fig. 17-4. Polysomnogram demonstrating episode of central sleep apnea. There is absent respiratory effort in association with absent airflow. (From Lugaresi E et al: *Sleep* 3:221-224, 1980.)

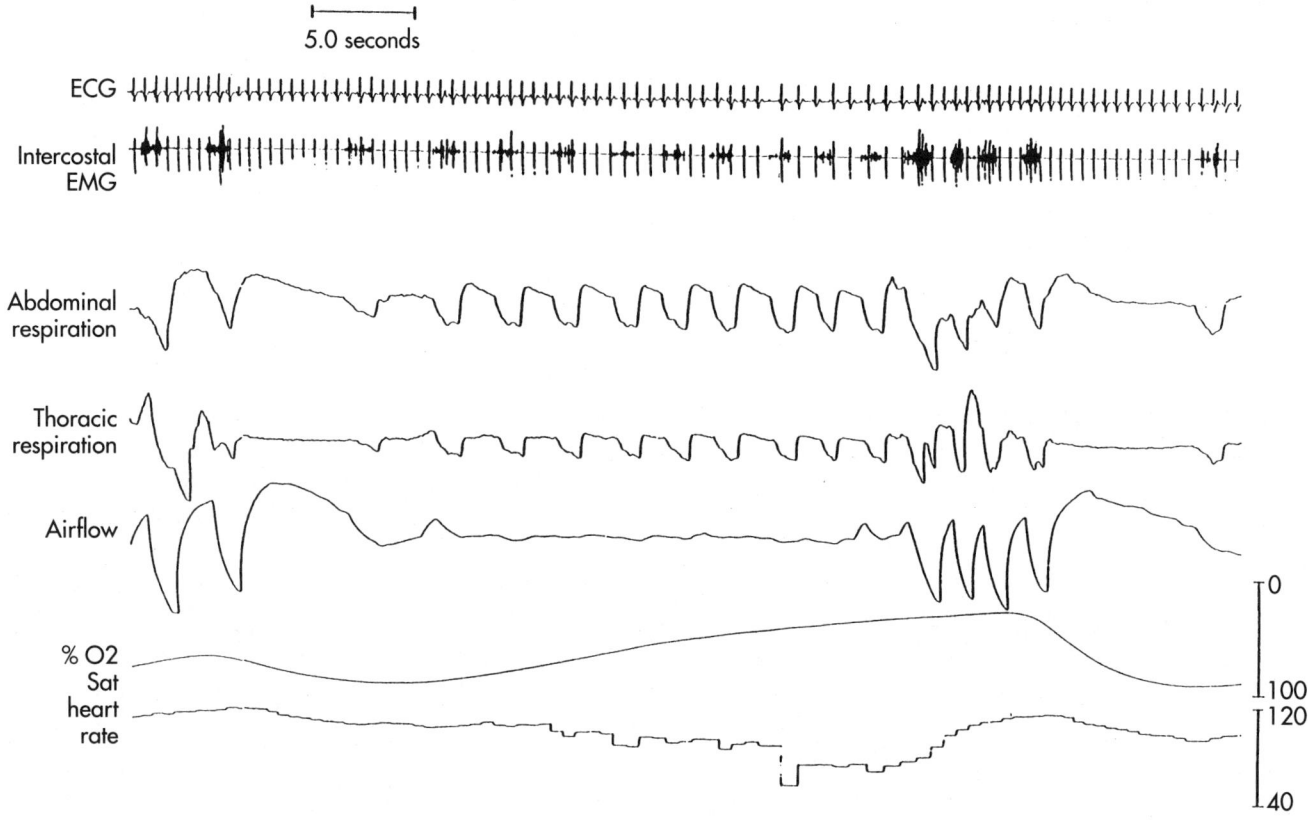

Fig. 17-5. Obstructive sleep apnea. In association with the apnea there is persistent respiratory effort demonstrated by the intercostal EMG and the monitors of abdominal and thoracic respiration. There is significant oxygen desaturation as the apnea progresses as well as bradycardia, and significant tachycardia as respiration restarts. (From Lugaresi E et al: *Sleep* 3:221–224, 1980.)

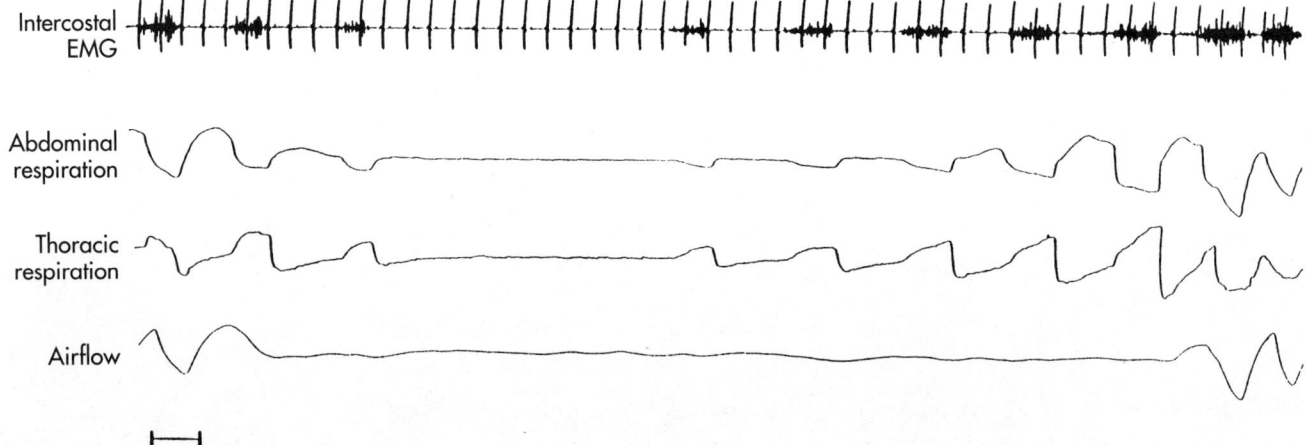

Fig. 17-6. Mixed sleep apnea. In association with the apnea there is absent respiratory effort in the initial portion of the apnea and then return of respiratory effort that is unsuccessful. (From Lugaresi E et al: *Sleep* 3:221-224, 1980.)

males and 44 females) between the ages of 20 and 65 without any sleep complaints. The mean apnea index was 0.62, and no subject had an apnea index of more than 4.5.

Pathophysiology

The site of the upper airway obstruction in OSA is in the pharynx. The pharynx is a collapsible tube that always remains open except during momentary closures during swallowing, regurgitation, and speech. The transmural pressure tending to cause the collapse of the pharynx is called the closing pressure (P Clos). Normally the pharyngeal musculature tends to keep the upper airway open; this pressure is called the muscular pressure (P Musc). The pressure in the pharynx, the luminal pressure (P Lumen), must be greater than the pressure outside the airway. Normally the airway resists closure. The subatmospheric pressure in the pharynx during inspiration tends to close the pharynx; this tendency is opposed by the contraction of the pharyngeal musculature. In addition, contraction of the genioglossus also exerts an outward pull opposing the large subatmospheric pressure in the pharynx. Two main factors influence the development of partial or complete upper airway obstruction during sleep, resulting in the development of episodes of obstructive apnea or hypopnea: (1) neuromuscular factors and (2) anatomic factors.

Neuromuscular factors

The medial pterygoid, tensor veli palatini, genioglossus, geniohyoid, and sternohyoid receive phasic activation during inspiration and must produce ventral movement of the soft palate, mandible, tongue, and hyoid bone, promoting a patent pharyngeal lumen. Similar contraction of the pharyngeal constrictors during inspiration stiffens the pharyngeal tube, also promoting its luminal patency. The current theory is that the decrease in the afferent activity to the pharyngeal muscles results in a decrease in the P Musc, causes pharyngeal narrowing with resultant hypopnea or apnea. As a result of the apnea or hypopnea, there is a drop in arterial Po_2, arousal with return of the pharyngeal musculature tone, and pharyngeal opening, allowing ventilation to occur. Besides being affected by sleep, the pharyngeal muscles are also affected by pharmacologic agents that tend to depress the reticular activating system, including anesthetics, hypnotics, and diazepam. The use of diazepam and alcohol has been shown to aggravate OSA.

Anatomic factors

The most common anatomic factor causing a decrease in the size of the pharyngeal lumen is fatty infiltration. Weight gain frequently produces a substantial increase in the severity of OSA, and weight loss may produce a significant improvement in the symptomatology of the OSA syndrome.[6a] Probably with weight gain or loss there is a gain or loss of fat in the pharynx or related structures such as the tongue, changing the size or configuration of the pharyngeal tube. Other anatomic abnormalities affecting the pharyngeal luminal size include retroposition of the mandible, an elongated soft palate, and enlarged tonsils.

The supraglottic resistance was shown to be increased in the awake state in patients with OSA. Narrowing of the pharyngeal lumen was demonstrated with computed tomography studies in awake OSA patients. Cephalometric studies have demonstrated certain abnormalities in OSA patients, including retroposition of the mandible, and have been used to make measurements to demonstrate a small pharyngeal airway.[41] The exact site of occlusion of the pharynx may vary, but there are two main areas of collapse: above the tongue, a narrowed oropharynx with posterior movement of the uvula and soft palate, and the base of tongue, respectively. Cineradiographic narrowing at these sites has been demonstrated, as has decreased EMG activity in the genioglossus during the obstructive apnea episodes.[27] This narrowing might also be accompanied by inward movement of the posterior and lateral walls of the pharynx. We have studied patients with OSA having undergone uvulopalatopharyngoplasty (UPP) with fiberoptic endoscopy and simultaneous EMG activity of the genioglossus and superior and middle pharyngeal constrictors, and have demonstrated the hypotonia during the apnea and return of EMG activity immediately before resumption of the airflow. Posterior movement of the tongue and hyoid bone allows the epiglottis to prolapse. The airway and the pressure at the margin of the epiglottis decrease, promoting further occlusion.

Clinical picture

Patients with OSA are frequently unaware of their nocturnal (sleep-related) symptoms and may deny their daytime (waking) symptoms. Thus it is beneficial to obtain a history from the bed partner or family members. One can divide the patient's symptomatology into sleep-related symptoms and waking symptoms.

Sleep-related symptomatology

Snoring is a major complaint of OSA patients. It frequently begins early in life and is present in childhood in 52% of cases and by the age of 21 years in 95%.[27] One may obtain the typical description of very loud snoring interrupted by quiet periods (caused by the apneas) followed by loud snorting as breathing restarts. Although 100% of patients with OSA snore, not all patients with snoring have the OSA syndrome. Thus other associated symptoms are necessary to make a clinical diagnosis.

Abnormal motor activity is frequently present in these patients. The bed partner will describe excessive movement and repetitive leg movements (nocturnal myoclonus) as well as thrashing movements as the patient struggles to resume breathing after the apneas. Sleepwalking has also been described in 10% of one OSA population group.[25]

Some patients awaken with the sensation of choking and may report that the airway feels closed and then feels as if it pops open. Some patients are awakened with a loud snort as they restart breathing after the apnea. Nocturnal enuresis was found in 5% and nocturia in 28% of 200 OSA patients.[25] The increased intraabdominal pressure associated with the increased respiratory effort during the obstructive apneas is thought to be the factor responsible for the nocturia. Increased intraabdominal pressure and associated awakening with occlusion may explain the nocturnal enuresis. Excessive nocturnal sweating is thought to be related to the excessive movement and activity that occur in these patients during sleep.

Daytime symptomatology

Excessive sleepiness is another characteristic manifestation of the OSA syndrome. However, it may not be present or apparent in the patient with mild OSA. The OSA syndrome is the commonest cause of excessive sleepiness in patients who present to sleep clinics.

Complaints of difficulty with cognitive ability are common in the OSA syndrome, particularly when the OSA is severe. These effects are secondary to the hypersomnolence.

Personality changes characterized by irritability and aggressiveness are not uncommon; they are reported by family members or friends.

Headache occurring on awakening in the morning is described usually as bifrontal or diffuse and lasts 1 to 2 hours. Patients usually awaken unrefreshed, have a sensation of mental fogginess, and may even demonstrate some confusion.

Physical findings

Obesity is a very commonly associated feature in patients with OSA. Two thirds of more than 1000 patients with OSA were 20% or more above ideal body weight.[25] The patients should be examined to identify specific anatomic factors that may contribute to the OSA, including a large tongue, elongated uvula and soft palate, prominent tonsilar tissue, and retrognathia. Mild to moderate systemic hypertension is common, especially in patients with severe OSA. Invasive studies of systemic arterial pressure during sleep have demonstrated transient increased levels occurring cyclically with each episode of apnea. When the apneas were repetitive, the systemic arterial pressure showed a step-wise increase over the night, to levels as high as 150 to 160 mm Hg diastolic. Pulmonary hypertension may also occur as an effect of OSA. Studies have shown a similar pattern of increase of the pulmonary arterial pressure with systolic pressures reaching 87 mm Hg and diastolic levels of 50 mm Hg.[27]

Complications

Both systemic hypertension and pulmonary hypertension may be complications of the OSA syndrome. Marked sinus dysrhythmia is characteristic of OSA. Holter ECG shows repetitive cycling of the sinus rhythm during sleep, associated with the apnea episodes. Marked sinus dysrhythmia with a fluctuation of greater than 50 beats per minute has been described in 78% to 100% of patients with OSA. Other significant cardiac dysrhythmias include sinus bradycardia of less than 30 beats per minute (9% to 10%), sinus arrest (9% to 11%), second-degree atrioventricular block (4% to 8%), and ventricular ectopy.[50] Anoxic seizures, generalized tonic clonic in nature, may occur but are extremely rare.

Investigations

Nocturnal polysomnography is the study necessary for the diagnosis and evaluation of the severity of OSA. Apneas and hypopneas occur during both NREM and REM sleep. There is a near absence of apneas during stages 3 and 4 NREM sleep. The apnea index is similar during NREM and REM sleep; however, the duration of apneas during REM sleep is significantly longer than in NREM.[18] One can define the severity of the OSA syndrome based on the apnea and hypopnea index. At the Cleveland Clinic we classify OSA as mild if the combined apnea and hypopnea index is between 5 and 20, moderate if the apnea and hypopnea index is between 20 and 50, and severe if the index is greater than 50.

Oxygen desaturation is an extremely significant consequence of the apneas and/or hypopneas. It is particularly severe in association with obstructive and mixed apneas rather than with central episodes. A drop in oxygen saturation of 5% or greater from the baseline value in association with an apnea or hypopnea is generally regarded as significant. In our laboratory we regard a drop in oxygen saturation to 85% or below as significant and express the amount of time spent at a level at or below an oxygen saturation of 85% as a percentage of the total sleep time. The greater this time, the more severe the degree of the OSA syndrome. The degree of cycling between bradycardia with the obstructive apneas, and tachycardia as breathing restarts, appears to increase with the severity and duration of the upper airway obstruction. The presence of sinus arrest or ventricular tachycardia in association with the apneas during sleep also indicates the severity of the OSA. The sleep architecture in relation to the OSA syndrome is disturbed with frequent arousals and awakenings after the respiratory abnormalities. A marked decrease of stages 3 and 4 NREM sleep occurs in severe OSA.[18]

Cephalometric x-rays are used to evaluate the soft tissues and skeletal structures important for OSA. Certain measurements can be taken to look for the size of the upper airway and to look for retrognathia.[41] Computed tomography of the neck has also been used to evaluate the size of the pharynx in patients with OSA.[41a,41b] Fluoroscopy of the upper airway during sleep has also been investigated to study the site of obstruction in OSA.[42,50] Fiberoptic endoscopy of the pharynx with the Meüller maneuver has been used to determine the site of collapse of the upper airway and has been used as a predictor for response to uvulopalatopharyngoplasty (UPP).[44a]

Treatment

1. Weight reduction. As the majority of patients with the OSA syndrome are overweight, a weight-reduction program is a component of the management program for these patients. Weight loss has been shown to significantly improve OSA in some patients.

2. Continuous positive airway pressure (CPAP). Nasal CPAP can be used in the majority of patients with the OSA syndrome.[48] It acts by producing a splint that keeps the upper airway patent. Approximately 15% to 20% of the patients who try CPAP do not comply with the use of this apparatus. The major reasons for noncompliance are the noise of the system, a sensation of claustrophobia, nasal congestion, dryness of the throat, and aesthetics. The level of CPAP necessary to maintain patency of the upper airway needs to be determined in the sleep laboratory through titration. The necessary pressure in the majority of subjects is between 7.5 and 12.5 cm H_2O.

3. Uvulopalatopharyngoplasty (UPP). This surgical procedure was introduced for the management of snoring. The procedure was first used for the management of obstructive sleep apnea at the Henry Ford Sleep Disorder Center.[19] This procedure involves the resection of the uvula, soft palate, any remaining tonsilar tissue, and redundant pharyngeal submucosal tissue in the posterior pharyngeal wall. The results of the surgery for obstructive sleep apnea are variable.[19] Approximately 50% of the patients have a greater than 50% reduction in the apnea index after surgery. The results of UPP in our center are similar in that approximately 50% of patients who underwent UPP had a greater than 30% reduction in apnea index, but only 50% demonstrated a dramatic reduction in apneas of greater than 90%.[51] As yet there is no single study that can predict with certainty that UPP will be successful for a particular individual. UPP is extremely effective for snoring; however, the patient may continue to have apnea in the absence of the usual snoring.

4. Tracheostomy. In the 1970s this was the treatment of choice in the surgical management of severe obstructive sleep apnea. However, today this procedure is rarely used.

5. Other surgery. If nasal obstruction is present because of a deviated septum or secondary to enlarged turbinates, this may need to be corrected. Tonsilar and adenoid enlargement are important causes of upper airway obstruction in children, but this is unusual in adult patients. Bony abnormalities such as micrognathia or retrognathia, may be important contributory factors for the upper airway obstruction and may need to be addressed.

Medications

Patients who have sleep apnea and associated hypoventilation while awake may respond to a trial of medrox-

yprogesterone acetate (60 mg per day).[49] However, this medication does not appear to be effective if there is no associated waking hypoventilation syndrome.[38,47] Protriptyline has been used in patients with mild sleep apnea with some benefit in doses of 10 mg bid.[7] The limiting factors on the use of this medication are usually the anticholinergic side effects (dry mouth, sexual impotence, constipation, and urinary retention).

CENTRAL SLEEP APNEA SYNDROME

The central sleep apnea syndrome is a disorder characterized by a cessation or decrease of airflow associated with decreased respiratory effort during sleep, usually associated with oxygen desaturation. This disorder was initially described by Guillemineault in 1973.[23a]

Prevalence

The exact prevalence of this condition is unknown. Central sleep apnea appears to increase in frequency with age. In young adults central apnea appears to be more common in men than in women. However, after menopause the occurrence is approximately equal.

Clinical features

The patients with the central sleep apnea syndrome usually present with insomnia, particularly an inability to maintain sleep. Awakenings may occur, and patients often experience a sensation of choking or gasping for air on awakening. These episodes, however, may also be completely asymptomatic and observed only by a bed partner. Because of the difficulty of maintaining sleep, patients experience daytime fatigue and excessive sleepiness. Snoring is not a prominent complaint.

Complications

Hemodynamic effects, such as systemic hypertension, pulmonary hypertension, and cardiac dysrhythmias, can occur but are much less prominent than in the OSA syndrome.

Treatment

1. Medications. Acetazolamide, a carbonic anhydrase inhibitor, has been used to treat central sleep apnea. When used over a 1- to 2-week period, this medication has been shown to reduce the number of central sleep apnea episodes. However, some such patients have been reported to develop obstructive apnea episodes. Theophylline and medroxyprogesterone acetate have also been used in the treatment of central sleep apnea.

2. Nasal CPAP. Nasal CPAP is also being used in the management of central sleep apnea. The general use of this form of treatment in central sleep apnea, however, needs further study. Administration of oxygen during sleep has also been shown to be of value in the treatment of central sleep apnea.

In the treatment of central sleep apnea, underlying

causes, such as nasal obstruction, congestive heart failure, and hypoxia, should be addressed.

PERIODIC LIMB MOVEMENT DISORDER

Periodic limb movement disorder is a condition characterized by repetitive, stereotyped limb movements that occur during sleep. Other terms have been used for this condition, including nocturnal myoclonus, periodic leg movements, and periodic movements in sleep. However, because these movements can affect both lower and upper limbs, the term periodic limb movements is preferred.

Prevalence

The prevalence of this condition is unknown. It is common in adults, increasing with age, and is thought to affect up to 34% of subjects over the age of 60 years. It is almost always present in patients with restless leg syndrome, is common in association with insomnia and narcolepsy, and is prominent in association with mild to moderate OSA but not with severe OSA. The prevalence of periodic limb movements in a group of subjects without any associated sleep complaints was 6%.[53] There appears to be no particular sex predominance.

Clinical features

Periodic movements are more common in the legs than in the arms. In the legs they typically consist of dorsiflexion of the big toe associated with flexion of the ankle, knee, and even hip. At times these movements may be bilateral. Although the patient is usually unaware of the repetitive limb movements, frequent arousals or even awakenings are associated with the movement. Usually the bed partner brings these episodes to the patient's attention. As the result of the repetitive limb movements, the patient may present either with a disturbance of maintenance of sleep with frequent awakenings or with excessive daytime sleepiness secondary to the sleep disturbance.

Investigations

The polysomnogram demonstrates the presence of repetitive limb movement during stages 1 and 2 NREM sleep predominantly (Fig. 17-7). There is a decrease in the amount of stages 3 and 4 REM sleep, and the movements are usually absent during REM sleep. The repetitive movements are usually monitored by electrodes over the tibialis anterior muscles and consist of repetitive bursts of EMG activity lasting 0.5 to 5 seconds. The interval between the repetitive movements is usually 20 to 40 seconds, with a range of 5 seconds to 120 seconds. The sleep architecture may demonstrate an arousal pattern associated with the leg movements consisting of a K complex or a complete awakening. One may construct a periodic limb movement (PLM) index, which is the number of episodes per hour of sleep. A PLM index of greater than 5 is abnormal.

Treatment

If periodic limb movements occur in association with another sleep disorder such as narcolepsy or OSA, the management must be directed at the primary disorder. Clonazepam has been used for treatment of periodic limb movements. It has been shown not to decrease the number of limb movements but rather to reduce the arousals associated with these. An alternate benzodiazepine, temazepam, with a shorter half-life than clonazepam has been used to avoid the side effect of daytime sedation. Other medications that have been used for periodic limb movements in association with restless leg syndrome include propoxyphene, baclofen, carbamazapine, and L-dopa.

RESTLESS LEGS SYNDROME

Restless legs syndrome is a condition characterized by an uncomfortable dysesthesia in the calves, usually in relation to sleep onset. The condition was first described by Ekbom in 1945.[54]

Prevalence

This is thought to be a common condition, with symptoms occurring in 5% to 15% of normal subjects.[53,55] Onset is usually in middle adulthood, and prevalence appears to increase with age. It is more common in females. Although usually occurring sporadically, restless legs syndrome appears to have a familial pattern as well.

Clinical features

The characteristic complaint is the uncomfortable crawling-like sensation in the calves, particularly at sleep onset, leading to an irresistible urge to get up and move around to relieve this discomfort, and the typical presentation of sleep onset insomnia. Although the symptoms typically occur at sleep onset, they also may occur at other times of the day, with prolonged sitting. It appears to be aggravated by pregnancy and associated with other conditions such as anemia and uremia. Virtually all patients with the restless legs syndrome demonstrate periodic limb movements during sleep.

Complications

The main effect of the restless legs syndrome is insomnia. Daytime fatigue and excessive sleepiness may be associated with this.

Treatment

Benzodiazepines, including clonazepam and nitrazapam, have been used in the treatment of the restless legs syndrome and associated periodic limb movement disorder. The benzodiazapines appear to reduce the number of arousals associated with the periodic limb movements rather than decrease the actual number of movements. Opioids have been used in the management of this condi-

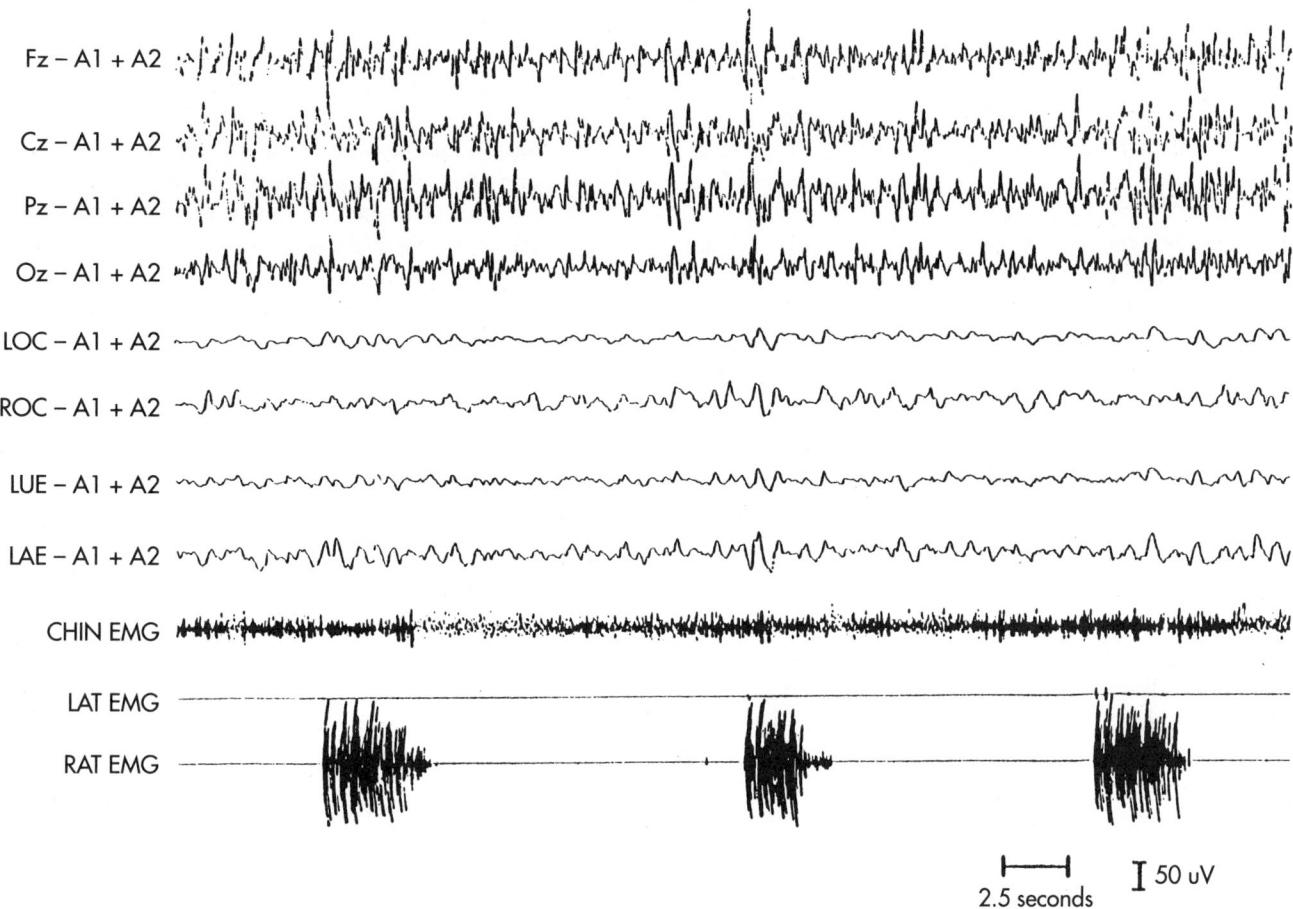

Fig. 17-7. Sleep-related myoclonus. *LAT,* left tibialis anterior; *RAT,* right tibialis anterior. The RAT EMG demonstrates repetitive leg movements.

tion and seem to be effective in suppressing the periodic movements as well as the symptoms of restless legs syndrome. Carbamazepine has been reported to have a therapeutic effect in the restless legs syndrome. Clonidine has also been reported as beneficial in the management of the restless legs syndrome. Baclofen, a GABA antagonist, has been reported to decrease the intensity of the periodic limb movements. Sinemet, consisting of L-dopa and a peripheral carboxylase inhibitor, has recently been shown to be effective in the management of the restless legs syndrome as well as of periodic limb movement disorder.

CIRCADIAN RHYTHM SLEEP DISORDERS

Most human behavior and physiologic processes have a temporal structure matching the 24-hour day-night schedule. The most apparent is our sleep-wake schedule.[13] Body temperature and the endocrine secretion of hormones also demonstrate this circadian rhythm. These circadian rhythms are generated internally. In the absence of environmental cues, these rhythms are said to "free-run." The periodicity of free-running rhythms is closer to 25 hours. It is thought that the circadian pacemaker exists in the hypothalamus in the suprachiasmatic nucleus. Destruction of

this nucleus in rodents has resulted in loss of circadian rhythmicity. Electrical and chemical stimulation of the suprachiasmatic nucleus can produce a phase shift of circadian rhythms. The biologic clock that drives body temperature internally synchronizes the sleep-wake cycle in a free-running environment. The circadian oscillator for temperature is fairly fixed at close to 25 hours; whereas that for sleep appears to be weaker, with a periodicity of between 25 and 60 hours. Recent studies have shown that temperature is a strong circadian influence on offset of sleep, with awakening occurring at the rising phase of the temperature cycle. REM sleep is also tied to the circadian rhythm of temperature; REM sleep appears just before the temperature nadir and continues on the rising phase of the circadian cycle in temperature. Environmental factors (Zeitgebers) influence the endogenous circadian rhythms. Psychosocial cues are often extremely important in the timing of sleep and wakefulness.

TIME ZONE CHANGE (JET LAG SYNDROME)

Jet travel and the resultant rapid changes in time zones are very frequent in today's world. This results in a disturbance in our sleep-wake schedule.

Prevalence

The exact prevalence of this condition is not known, but this is probably an extremely common condition. People over the age of 50 appear more likely to develop jet lag syndrome than young adults under the age of 30.

Clinical features

The main symptoms are disturbance of sleep and daytime fatigue. The severity of the jet lag syndrome is related to the direction of flight and the number of time zones crossed. Eastward flights shorten the day and require a phase advance, meaning the traveler's circadian rhythms have to decrease to less than 24 hours until they are in phase with local Zeitgebers. Westward flights lengthen the day and require a phase delay. It appears that subjects' rhythms readjust faster after westward flight than after eastward flights. Travelers adjust at a rate of about 1.5 hours per day after westward flights and at about 1 hour per day after eastward flights. As the result of the disturbance in sleep maintenance, individuals usually experience daytime fatigue. They may also encounter gastrointestinal distress, headaches, reduced cognitive skills, impaired motor coordination, muscle fatigue, and general malaise.

Management

The management of the jet lag syndrome may include gradual shift of the bedtime in the appropriate direction before travel. However, if the stay is to be short, one may want to maintain the usual "home" sleep-wake schedule. In the management of jet lag syndrome, one should follow certain procedures to enhance the phase resetting process (see box below). These include resetting one's watch to that of the destination at the onset of the trip. On arrival at one's destination one should adapt rapidly to the wake-activity schedule of the new destination. Before travel one may also try a gradual shift of one's bedtime in the appropriate direction for 2 to 3 nights before departure. However, if the stay in the new destination is to be short, 2 to 3 days only, one may consider maintaining the usual "home" sleep-wake schedule. One should also avoid activities that

---

may inhibit the phase resetting process such as taking prolonged naps or naps at inappropriate times, and excessive caffeine or alcohol. Short acting benzodiazepines may be used for the first few days after arriving in the new time zone to assist one in adjusting to the new sleep schedule. Short-acting benzodiazepines may be used for the first few days after arriving in the new time zone to help one to adjust to the new sleep-wake schedule.

SHIFTWORK SLEEP DISORDER
Circadian factors

The inability of the circadian system to adjust instantaneously to changes in routine that shiftwork schedules require is a major factor in this disorder. The realignment as measured by the temperature rhythm may take up to 14 days. During the process of realignment there may be sleep disruption, and the new time of wakefulness may be required during slower phases of psychologic functions normally occurring during sleep.

Sleep factors

Night workers get 5 to 7 hours less sleep per week than those working daytime shifts. This chronic sleep deprivation affects mood and performance ability.

Domestic "social" factors

Poor domestic adjustments may adversely affect the ability of the worker to cope with shift work. A common example is the childcare and household management tasks.

Prevalence

Approximately 20% of the U.S. workforce is involved in some form of shift work. Some people cope extremely well with a changing work shift, but others do poorly.

Clinical features

Those working a night shift may have difficulty in maintaining a normal amount of sleep during the daytime after the night shift, resulting in reduction in total sleep time. Individuals usually find the sleep unrefreshing. As a result of this chronic difficulty with maintenance of sleep and resultant sleep deprivation, excessive sleepiness and impaired cognitive ability may occur during the work shift.

Management

In the approach to the management of shift work, sleep should be sequentially delayed, shifting from days to evenings and then to nights. The duration of each shift should be more than 1 week. Short-acting benzodiazepines may be of benefit for one to two sleep periods after a shift change. Rapid rotation of shifts is becoming popular in Europe; for example, two morning shifts, two evening shifts, and two night shifts, followed by 2 days off.[36] Such a system allows the circadian system to maintain its diur-

---

> **Tips for prevention of jet lag**
>
> *Eastward flight (early morning arrival)*
>
> 1. Take a short (2 hour) nap immediately upon arrival
> 2. Remain awake for remainder of the day
> 3. On the first night, capitalize on sleep loss from day one
> 4. Take a short acting benzodiazepine hypnotic at bedtime for 2 to 3 nights (Triazolam 0.125 mg qhs or Temazepam 15 mg qhs)
>
> *Westward flight (afternoon arrival)*
>
> 1. Same as for eastward flight, but avoid nap

nal orientation and reduce the problems related to shift work.

DELAYED SLEEP-PHASE SYNDROME

This syndrome is characterized by the inability to fall asleep and awaken at conventional times. Sleep onset is often delayed to 3 or 4 AM. If the patient is allowed to sleep, such as on the weekend, the waking time may be 11 AM to noon. Attempts to advance the sleep onset fail, thus the patient usually presents with the chief complaint of sleep-onset insomnia. The pathophysiology of this condition is thought to be an inability to phase advance.

Prevalence

The prevalence of this condition is unknown, however, it represents a very small proportion of patients presenting to sleep disorder centers with insomnia. Subjects usually present during adolescence.

Management

The treatment is chronotherapy, which consists of systematically delaying the bedtime at 3-hour increments each day until the desired bedtime is reached. The patient is then required to adhere strictly to the new sleep-wake schedule. If he or she delays the bedtime and sleep onset time, there may be a relapse of the delayed sleep phase.

SLEEPWALKING

Sleepwalking is a complex behavior that usually occurs in the first third of sleep, arising from deep (stage 3/4) NREM sleep.[6]

Prevalence. Approximately 15% of children are thought to have walked at least once during sleep.[29] However, only 2.5% of children are habitual sleepwalkers. This condition is more common in children than in adolescents or adults. The most common age is between 4 and 8 years. There is a second peak between 10 and 15 years of age. The episodes of somnambulism usually occur within the first third of sleep. The individual frequently sits up, may perform repetitive movements, and then gets up and walks. He or she appears to be able to engage in complex behavior, walking through the home and negotiating furniture. The subject's eyes are usually open, with a blank expression. Episodes usually last less than 10 minutes. Patients usually have no recall of the episode. Younger individuals usually outgrow their sleepwalking during adolescence by the age of 15 years; however, later onset sleepwalkers have the behavior for a longer time. Psychologic factors may appear to exaggerate the sleepwalking.

Treatment. Sleepwalkers may be led back to bed. Parents of children who sleepwalk usually need reassurance that they will outgrow this during adolescence. Psychotherapy may be necessary in adults where underlying psychopathology is suspected. Benzodiazepines may be beneficial in suppressing these episodes by suppressing the as-sociated stages 3 and 4 NREM sleep. However, most individuals do not require medication.

REM SLEEP BEHAVIOR DISORDER

REM sleep behavior disorder is a clinical syndrome characterized by the occurrence of complex behavior in association with vivid dreams or nightmares.[43] The behavior originates from REM sleep associated with return of EMG tone, which is normally dramatically decreased during the REM state.

Prevalence

This syndrome is rare, affects mainly middle-aged or elderly individuals, but may begin at any age, and is more prominent in males than in females.

Clinical features

Two subgroups of patients present with REM behavior sleep disorder, an idiopathic group and a second group associated with neurologic disorders (Olivo-ponto-cerebellar degeneration, Guillain-Barré syndrome, subarachnoid hemorrhage).[33] Patients may present various complex behaviors, including talking, laughing, shouting, punching, and kicking as well as getting up out of bed. Frequently there is a history of the behaviors occurring in response to the dream content so that the patient appears to be acting out dreams.

Complications

The social effect of these episodes appears to be the most significant complication. However, the patient may injure himself or herself or the bed partner during the complex, often violent, behavior.

Treatment

This condition appears to be exquisitely sensitive to the benzodiazepine clonazepam, which is given at bedtime. An alternative medication is imipramine.

SLEEP-RELATED ENURESIS

Sleep-related enuresis is bedwetting occurring after the age when bladder control should have been achieved. Primary enuresis refers to the condition in which urinary continence was never achieved. Secondary enuresis refers to bedwetting that reappears after the child has been continent for over 6 months.

Prevalence

This appears to be related to age.[29] At the age of 5 years, 15% of boys and 10% of girls still have bedwetting at night. The prevalence drops to about 3% at the age of 12 years. In adults the prevalence is approximately 1%.

Clinical features

Anatomical abnormalities of the genitalia and urinary tract account for a small percentage of primary enuresis.

Secondary enuresis is thought to be often psychologic in origin. A psychologic factor such as a new sibling, parental separation, or divorce may be the precipitating factor. Other conditions may be responsible for secondary enuresis, including urinary tract infection, diabetes mellitus, diabetes insipidus, and nocturnal epilepsy. Nocturnal enuresis was also reported in a significant portion (36%) of patients with severe OSA. Nocturnal polysomnography has demonstrated that sleep-related enuresis is not related to a specific sleep state, such as arousal from slow-wave (stage 3-4) NREM sleep, as previously believed.[22]

Complications

Sleep-related enuresis has the effect of restricting the child's social activities, such as sleeping over at a friend's home or going away to camp. Psychologic effects of this condition are significant.

Treatment

It is essential to determine that there is no underlying secondary cause for bedwetting.[34] In older children and adults, psychologic factors may be important and need to be evaluated. In children, behavioral methods may be used.[23] Exercises to increase bladder capacity are recommended if the bladder capacity seems to be small.[46] Pharmacologic treatment may be tried, with imipramine in a dose of 1 to 2 mg/kg per day given at bedtime.[44] The mechanism of action of this medication is not clearly known, but it may be due to its anticholinergic effects. If underlying psychopathology is thought to be a factor in secondary enuresis, psychotherapy may be of value.

SNORING

Snoring is the sound occurring predominantly upon inspiration during sleep and results from the vibration of the soft tissue structures of the upper airway.

Prevalence

Habitual snorers are those who snore almost nightly. This is an extremely common phenomenon, occurring in about 19% of an unselected population.[32] Snoring is slightly more common in men (25%) than women (15%). The prevalence of snoring progressively increases with age, such that at the age of 41 to 64 years, 60% of males and 40% of females snore. Obesity is an important risk factor for the development of snoring. Among overweight men, 60% are habitual snorers, whereas in normal weight men, only 34% are habitual snorers in the age group of 30 to 59 years.[35]

Pathophysiology

Snoring is due to narrowing of the upper airway. It may occur continuously throughout sleep. When it occurs in association with OSA, it is interrupted by episodes of apnea resulting from complete occlusion of the upper airway.

Snoring is probably produced by vibration of the soft palate and uvula. Obesity causes narrowing of the upper airway and is an important contributory factor in the pathogenesis of snoring. Adenoid and tonsil enlargement, deviated nasal septum, turbinate hypertrophy, retrognathia, and micrognathia may be other anatomical factors that predispose to development of snoring. Benzodiazepines cause central nervous system depression and during sleep may aggravate the snoring. Alcohol may act in a similar way and increase the degree of hypotonia, aggravating snoring.

Clinical features

Snoring may be completely benign. However, transient decreases in arterial oxygen saturation may occur in association with snoring.[5] In addition, the pulmonary arterial pressure and systemic arterial pressure may increase in association with snoring. Snoring has been found to be an independent risk factor for the development of systemic hypertension. The risk for myocardial infarction and cerebral infarction also appears to be increased in snorers.

Management

Weight reduction is an important cornerstone of management of snoring in patients who are overweight. Sleep position may be important, as snoring may be predominant in the supine sleeping position. The use of a tennis ball sewn into a pocket in the back of a pajama top has been used to try to keep people off of the back while sleeping. Tongue-retaining devices may be used to prevent snoring when prolapse of the posterior genioglossus into the upper airway is an important contributing factor in patients who snore in the supine position. Surgery in the form of adenoidectomy, correction of a deviated nasal septum, or turbinectomy may be of value in patients in whom anatomic factors are important in pathogenesis of snoring. Uvulopalatopharyngoplasty was introduced for treatment of snoring before it was used in the management of OSA syndrome. Continuous positive airway pressure is another treatment modality that can be used in management of heavy snoring.

SUMMARY

We spend approximately one third of our lives asleep. Although sleep is essential and appears to have a restorative role, the precise function of sleep is still not known. The state of sleep can be defined electrophysiologically into the stages of non-REM and REM sleep. The raphe nuclei, thalamus, hypothalamus, and the nucleus of the solitary tract are the anatomical structures important in the genesis of non-REM sleep; the peri-locus coeruleus and other regions in the lateral pontine tegmentum and the nucleus reticularis magnocellularis in the medulla appear to be critical for the genesis of REM sleep. The initial classification of sleep disorders introduced in 1979 was based on the presenting complaint into those conditions presenting primarily with insomnia, those presenting with hypersomnia, the parasomnias and sleep-wake schedule disorders. In 1990 a new international classification of sleep disorders classified the conditions independent of their presenting complaint into the dyssomnias, which includes the primary sleep disorders, the parasomnias, and the sleep disorders associated with medical and psychiatric conditions.

This chapter has dealt with the major sleep disorders, dyssomnias, and parasomnias, which present to the clinician. Psychophysiologic insomnia is probably the most common condition that we see presenting with the chief complaint of insomnia. The OSA syndrome is the most common cause for patients presenting with the chief complaint of excessive daytime sleepiness. OSA together with narcolepsy accounts for approximately two thirds of the patients seen in sleep disorders clinics with daytime hypersomnolence. The definitive diagnosis of OSA syndrome and narcolepsy can be made on the basis of nocturnal polysomnography and the daytime multiple sleep latency test and is critical as both these conditions are amenable to specific treatments that are very different. Although the majority of the parasomnias are seen in childhood, one parasomnia recently described in adults' REM sleep behavior disorder is a condition that can be extremely gratifying to diagnose because of its exquisite responsiveness to treatment principally with clonazepam.

REFERENCES

1. Aserinsky E, Kleitman N: Regularly occurring periods of eye motility and concomitant phenomena during sleep, *Science* 118:273-274, 1953.
2. Association of Sleep Disorders Centers: Diagnostic classification of sleep and arousal disorders, *Sleep* 2:1-137, 1979.
3. Association of Professional Sleep Societies, APSS Guidelines Committee, Carskadon MA, chairperson: Guidelines for the multiple sleep latency test (MSLT): a standard measure of sleepiness, *Sleep* 9:519-524, 1986.
4. Baker TL et al: Comparative polysomnographic study of narcolepsy and idiopathic central nervous system hypersomnia, *Sleep* 9:232-242, 1986.
5. Block AJ et al: Sleep apnea, hypopnea and oxygen saturation in normal subjects: a strong male predominance, *N Engl J Med* 300:513-517, 1972.
6. Broughton RJ: Sleep disorders: disorders of arousal? *Science* 159:1070-1078, 1968.
6a. Browman CP, et al: Obstructive sleep apnea and body weight, *Chest* 85(3):435-438, 1984.
7. Brownell LG et al: Protriptyline in obstructive sleep apnea: a double blind trial, *N Engl J Med* 307:1037-1142, 1982.
8. Carskadon MA et al: Guidelines for the multiple sleep latency test (MSLT): a standard measure of sleepiness, *Sleep* 9:519-524, 1986.
9. Carskadon M et al: Self report versus sleep laboratory findings in 122 drug free subjects with the complaint of chronic insomnia, *Am J Psychiatry* 133:1382-1388, 1976.
10. Cartwright RD, Samelson CF: The effects of a non-surgical treatment for obstructive sleep apnea. The tongue retaining device, *JAMA* 248:705-709, 1982.
11. Coleman RM: Diagnosis, treatment and follow-up of about 8,000 sleep/wake disorder patients. In Guilleminault C, Lugaresi E, editors: *Sleep/wake disorders: natural history, epidemiology, and long-term evolution,* New York, 1983, Raven Press.
12. Coleman R et al: Sleep-wake disorders based upon a polysomnographic diagnosis—a national cooperative study, *JAMA* 247:997-1103, 1981.
13. Czeisler CA et al: Human sleep: its duration and organization depend on its circadian phase, *Science* 210:1264-1267, 1980.
14. Dement WC, Carskadon MA, Ley R: The prevalence of narcolepsy, *Sleep Res* 2:147, 1973.
15. Dement W, Kleitman N: The relation of eye movements during sleep to dream activity: an objective method for the study of dreaming, *J Exp Psychol* 53:399, 1957.
16. Dement WC et al: The prevalence of narcolepsy, *Sleep Res* 1:148, 1972.
17. Diagnostic Classification Steering Committee, Thorpy MJ, chairman: *International classification of sleep disorders: diagnostic and coding manual,* Rochester, Minn, 1990, American Sleep Disorders Association.
18. Dinner DS et al: Relationship of sleep apnea and sleep stages in obstructive sleep apnea, *Sleep Res* 19:224, 1989.
19. Fujita S et al: Surgical correction of anatomic abnormalities in obstructive sleep apnea syndrome: uvulopalatopharyngoplasty, *Otolaryngol Head Neck Surg* 89:923-934, 1981.
20. Gastaut H et al: Etude polygraphique des manifestations episodeques (hypiques et respiratoires) diurnes et nocturnes du syndrome de pickwick, *Rev Neurol* 112:573-579, 1965.
21. Gelineau J: De la narcolepsie, *Gaz Hop (Paris)* 53:626-628, 54:635-737, 1880.
22. Gillin JC et al: EEG sleep patterns in enuresis: a further analysis and comparison with normal controls, *Biol Psychiatry* 17:947-953, 1982.
23. Goel KM et al: Evaluation of nine different types of enuretic alarms, *Arch Dis Child* 59:748-753, 1984.
24. Guilleminault C, Faull KF: Sleepiness in non-narcoleptic, non-sleep apneic EDS patients: the idiopathic CNS hypersomnolence, *Sleep* 5:S175-181, 1982.
25. Guilleminault C et al: Viloxazine hydrochloride in narcolepsy: a preliminary report, *Sleep* 9:275-279, 1986.
26. Hauri P: *The sleep disorders,* ed 2, Kalamazoo, Mich, 1982, Scope Publications, Upjohn.
27. Hill MW, Guilleminault C, Simmons FB: Fiberoptic and EMG studies in hypersomnia-sleep apnea syndrome. In Guilleminault C, Dement W, editors: *Sleep apnea syndromes,* New York, 1978, Alan R Liss.
28. Kessler S, Guilleminault C, Dement WC: A family study of 50 REM narcoleptics, *Arch Neurol Scand* 50:503-512, 1974.
29. Klackbenberg G: Incidence of parasomnias in children in a general population. In Guilleminault C, editor: *Sleep and its disorders in children,* New York, 1987, Raven Press.
30. Kramer RE et al: HLA-DR2 and narcolepsy, *Arch Neurol* 44:853-855, 1987.
31. Lavie P: Sleep habits and sleep disturbances in industrial workers in Israel: main findings and some characteristics of workers complaining of excessive daytime sleepiness, *Sleep* 4:147-158, 1981.
31a. Leckman JF, Gershon ES: A genetic model of narcolepsy, *Br J Psychiatry* 128:276-279, 1976.
32. Lugaresi E et al: Some epidemiological data on snoring and cardiocirculatory disturbances, *Sleep* 3:221-224, 1980.
33. Mahowald MW, Schenck CH: REM sleep behavior disorder. In Kryger MH, Roth T, Dement WC, editors: *Principles and practice of sleep medicine,* Philadelphia, 1989, WB Saunders.
34. Mikkelsen EJ et al: Childhood enuresis. Sleep patterns and psychopathology, *Arch Gen Psychiatry* 37:1139-1144, 1980.
35. Mondini S et al: Snoring as a risk factor for cardiac and circulatory problems: an epidemiological study. In Guilleminault C, Lugaresi E, editors: *Sleep/wake disorders: natural history, epidemiology and long-term evolution,* New York, 1983, Raven Press.
36. Monk TH: Advantages and disadvantages of rapidly rotating shift schedules—a circadian viewpoint, *Hum Factors* 28:553-557, 1986.

37. National Institute of Mental Health, Consensus Development Conference: Drugs and insomnia, *JAMA* 251:2410-2414, 1984.

38. Rajagopal KR, Abbrecht PH, and Jabbari B: Effects of medroxyprogesterone acetate in obstructive sleep apnea, *Chest* 90(6):815-821, 1986.

39. Rechtschaffen A, Kales A, editors: *A manual of standardized terminology, techniques and scoring system for sleep stages of human subjects,* Los Angeles, 1968, UCLA Brain Information Service/Brain Research Institute.

40. Rechtschaffen A et al: Nocturnal sleep of narcoleptics, *Electroencephalogr Clin Neurophysiol* 15:599-609, 1963.

41. Riley R et al: Cephalometric analyses and flow volume loops in obstructive sleep apnea patients, *Sleep* 6:304-307, 1983.

41a. Suratt PM et al: Fluoroscopic and computed tomographic features of the pharyngeal airway in obstructive sleep apnea, *Am Rev Respir Dis* 127:487-492, 1983.

41b. Riley R, Powell N, Guilleminault C: Cephalometric roentgenograms and computerized tomographic scans in obstructive sleep apnea, *Sleep* 9:514-515, 1986.

42. Rojewski TE et al: Synchronous video recording of the pharyngeal airway in obstructive sleep apnea, *Am Rev Respir Dis* 127:487-492, 1983.

43. Schenck CH et al: Rapid eye movement sleep behavior disorder, *JAMA* 257:1786-1789, 1987.

44. Shaffer D, Costello AJ, Hill ID: Control of enuresis with imipramine, *Arch Dis Child* 43:665-671, 1968.

44a. Sher AE et al: Predictive valve of Müller's maneuver in selection of patients with UPPD, *Laryngoscope* 95:1483-1487, 1985.

45. Spielman AJ, Caruso LS, Glovinsky PB: A behavioral perspective on insomnia treatment, *Psychiatr Clin North Am* 10(4):541-553, 1987.

46. Starfield B, Mellits ED: Increase in functional bladder capacity and improvement in enuresis, *J Pediatr* 72:483, 1968.

47. Strohl KP et al: Progesterone administration and progressive sleep apneas, *JAMA* 245:1230-1232, 1980.

48. Sullivan CE et al: Reversal of obstructive sleep apnea by continuous positive airway pressure applied through the nares, *Lancet* 862-865, 1981.

49. Sutton JD Jr et al: Progesterone for the outpatient treatment of pickwickian syndrome, *Ann Intern Med* 83:476-479, 1975.

50. Walsh JK et al: Somnofluoroscopy: cineradiographic observation of obstructive sleep apnea, *Sleep* 8:294-297, 1985.

51. Wingkun EC et al: Polysomnography after oropharyngeal/nasal surgery for obstructive sleep apnea, *EEG Clin Neurophysiol* 1989.

52. Yoss RE, Daly DD: Criteria for the diagnosis of the narcoleptic syndrome, *Proc Staff Meet Mayo Clin* 32:320-328, 1957.

53. Bixler EO, Kales A, Vela-Bueno A, et al: Nocturnal myoclonus and nocturnal myoclonic activity in a normal population, *Research Commun Chem Pathol Pharmacol* 36: 129-140, 1982.

54. Ekbom KA: Restless legs, *Acta Med Scand Suppl* 158:1-123, 1945.

55. Ekbom KA: Restless legs syndrome, *Neurology* 10:868-873, 1960.

■ RESOURCES ■

American Sleep Disorders Association, 1610 14th Street NW, Suite 300, Rochester MN 55901-2200.

American Narcolepsy Association, P.O. Box 26230, San Francisco, CA, 94126-6230.

Part IV

PHYSICAL ACTIVITY AND FITNESS IN DISEASE PREVENTION

Chapter 18

PHYSICAL AND PSYCHOLOGIC BENEFITS OF A FITNESS PROGRAM IN HEALTH AND DISEASE

Donald T. Kirkendall

Habitual physical conditioning is known to be of benefit to the health of the population. Consistent physical training is common with coronary disease patients. However, there is increasing evidence that exercise is justified in a wide variety of clinical conditions, from cancer to HIV.

An adage suggests that exercise does not necessarily help one live longer, but helps one live "younger longer." Blair et al.[15] have suggested that consistent physical activity may influence longevity. They pointed out that all-cause mortality, independent of gender, was reduced with increasing levels of fitness (Fig. 18-1). Notice that the greatest reduction in death rate occurred between the sedentary group and those of low fitness. Further reductions in death rate were evident with increasing levels of fitness, but not to the degree seen between the two lowest categories. This indicates that even a moderate increase in physical activity benefits health.

To be convinced that physical activity is mandatory to good health, one must understand the adaptations that occur in consistent activity. The first section of this chapter deals with these adaptations. The second section discusses the application of exercise to a variety of clinical conditions. The medical and clinical aspects of these conditions are covered in other areas of this book. This section will point out the benefits of exercise in selected patient populations.

There are two issues involved with exercise. First, the application of exercise to selected disease states should be supervised and directed by some appropriate specialist and his or her associates (e.g., the cardiologist and exercise physiologist). The preventive medicine physician should support that effort. Other situations also lend themselves to primary care supervision. Second, exercise can serve as a supplement to other current therapeutic regimens, although in many cases (e.g., diabetes and hypertension) exercise has little effect on the underlying condition. In other illness (e.g., peripheral vascular disease and coronary disease), the proper use of exercise coupled with other therapies can favorably modify the disease itself. At the least, training typically increases the patient's functional reserve, permitting a greater range of daily living activities.

The pathophysiology and prevention of these conditions will be covered in other sections of this and/or other texts. In all cases, before placing a patient in an exercise program, the physician must conduct a complete history and physical, which usually includes a stress test. The exercise prescription principles outlined in Chapter 19 have broad application across numerous clinical populations but are based on these essential examinations. The key to understanding the use of exercise in selected patient populations is understanding the specific adaptations that occur after physical training and how these adaptations improve the status of a patient with selected clinical conditions.

ENERGY METABOLISM

Two types of adaptations will be discussed: long-duration, low-intensity (e.g., jogging) and short-duration, high-intensity exercises (e.g., weight training). Addition-

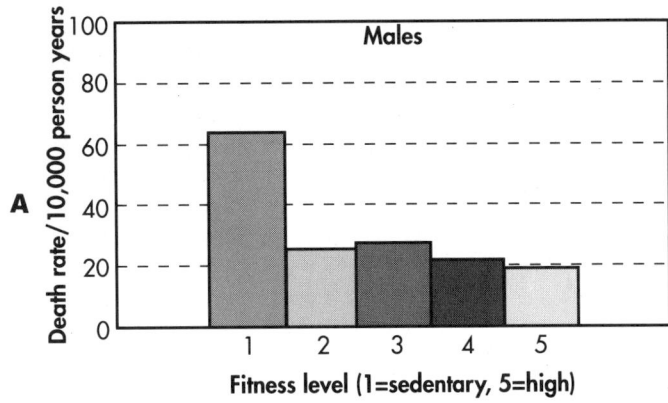

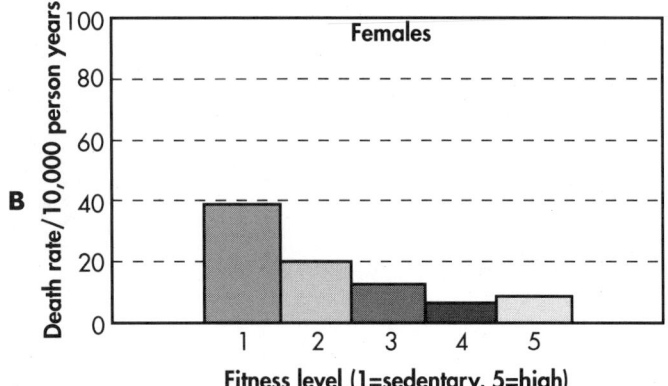

Fig. 18-1. Age-adjusted all-cause death rates by fitness level and gender. **A,** males; **B,** females.

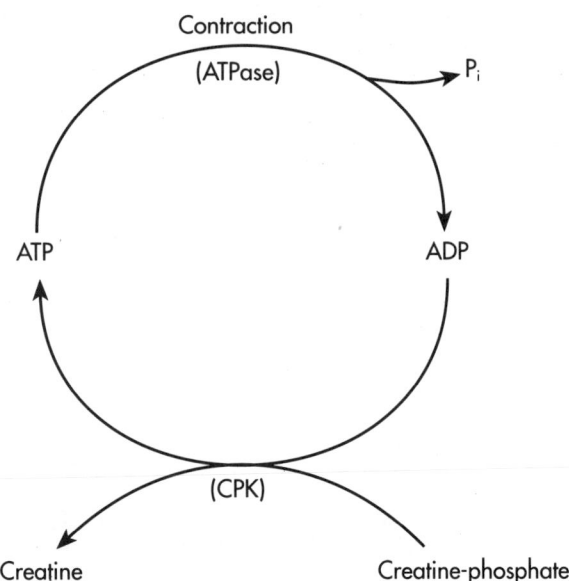

Fig. 18-2. Phosphagen replenishment of ATP.

ally, central adaptations (oxygen delivery systems) and peripheral adaptations (oxygen use systems) will be discussed. To understand the physiological modifications that follow such programs, we will take a brief look at the energy systems involved in each type of exercise. The reader is assumed to understand basic physiological function and the body's acute responses to physical exercise.

All our energy is derived from the sun. Energy is not created, but transferred. As a result, food contains energy transferred from the sun, which is then transferred to us, to be further transferred for use by individual cells. Although an array of compounds store energy for later use, the primary molecule is adenosine triphosphate (ATP). The high-energy phosphate bonds of the molecule are the site of stored energy. Enzymatic splitting of ATP to a diphosphate molecule (ADP) releases the energy for, in this discussion, muscular contraction. In muscle activity, ATP is required for myosin crossbridge movement and myosin-actin splitting for further contraction. Other uses of ATP during exercise include membrane transport and uptake of calcium into the sarcoplasmic reticulum. As the available supply of ATP is limited (total of about 3 oz in the whole body[112]) ATP must be constantly and rapidly replenished for the muscle to continue contracting. Two main meta-

bolic pathways continuously supply ATP. ATP may be produced from either anaerobic or aerobic mechanisms.

Anaerobic metabolism

Anaerobic metabolism occurs in two ways. The first and most rapid method is from a simple transfer of energy. Once an ATP molecule has been broken down and its energy used in muscular contraction, the energy-rich compound phosphocreatine (PC), with the aid of the enzyme creatine kinase, transfers its energy and phosphate (it too contains a high-energy bond) to the ATP molecule. The remainder is then free creatine. (Fig. 18-2). This system also has a limited capacity. However, it supplies energy at a fast rate (Table 18-1).

The second method of energy production involves the anaerobic degradation of glucose in the cytoplasm. The 6 carbon glucose molecule is eventually broken down into two three-carbon pyruvic acids. Along the way, two ATP molecules are used and four are produced with a net gain of two ATP molecules. During glycolysis, the electron carrier NAD is reduced. $NADH_2$ is oxidized, with the hydrogens being transferred to the pyruvic acid molecule, resulting in lactic acid (Fig. 18-3). This system is capable of producing energy at a reasonably high rate (Table 18-1), but its capacity is also limited. The declining pH from the production of lactic acid inhibits the rate-limiting enzyme PFK, slowing glycolysis. Thus a declining pH might be considered protection against the muscle proceeding toward irreversible damage from low pH.[113]

Aerobic metabolism

The aerobic metabolism of glucose proceeds in the mitochondria. In the presence of adequate oxygen and pyru-

Table 18-1. Characteristics of the three systems by which ATP is formed

System	Food or chemical fuel	O_2 required	Rate	Capacity	Maximal power (moles of ATP per minute)	Maximal capacity (total moles ATP available)
Anaerobic						
ATP-PC system	Phosphocreatine	No	Fastest	Few; limited	3.6	0.7
Lactic acid system	Glycogen (glucose)	No	Fast	Few; limited	1.6	1.2
Aerobic						
Oxygen system	Glycogen, fats, proteins	Yes	Slow	Many; unlimited	1.0	90.0

Modified from Fox EL et al: *Physiological basis of physical education and athletics,* ed 4, Dubuque, Iowa, 1988, William C. Brown.

vate deydrogenase complex, pyruvic acid is converted to acetyl coenzyme A (CoA). Through the Krebs cycle, CoA is re-worked to produce CO_2, electron carriers, and an ATP molecule. The electron carriers then proceed to the electron transport chain, where ATP and water are produced (Fig. 18-4). Fatty acids, once liberated from their glycerol backbone, are oxidized through beta oxidation. Numerous electron carriers and CoA are produced. The carriers go through the electron transport chain, and CoA passes into the Krebs cycle, with its accompanying electron carriers. Fatty acids are a huge reservoir of energy.

ENERGY METABOLISM AND EXERCISE

When a person exercises, increased energy is needed for the muscle contractions (among other things) needed for the activity. In the interaction of exercise and energy production, the nature of the activity determines the primary pathway for ATP production. The determinant is the performance time, or power output. The higher the power output (the less time taken to complete the activity), the greater is the reliance on the ATP-PC system and anaerobic glycolysis, with the resulting production of lactic acid. The lower the power output (and the more time taken to complete the task), the greater the energy production from aerobic metabolism (Fig. 18-5). Fig. 18-6 illustrates the interaction of the metabolic pathways described.

ADAPTATIONS TO TRAINING

The vast majority of clinical applications of exercise use aerobic training. Thus, this section will focus on aerobic training. Selected uses of resistance training will be discussed.

Physical training influences (1) the ability of the body to transport oxygen to the working muscles and (2) the working muscle's ability to use the delivered oxygen. These central and peripheral adaptations to training are the foundation of the clinical application of exercise.

In addition, selected principles influence the responses to training. For example, training programs need to *overload* the person. The training must be *progressive;* training volume or intensity must be increased systematically. Training is *specific.* Only those tissues that are stressed

will adapt. *Individual differences* affect training responses, and if training is interrupted, the adaptations *reverse,* unfortunately quickly.

CENTRAL ADAPTATIONS TO TRAINING
Adaptations seen at rest

Endurance training, be it of low or moderate intensity, results in well-defined adaptations. Central adaptations include changes in the circulatory, respiratory, and hematologic systems. Training studies typically show no change in resting cardiac output.[56] Cross-sectional and longitudinal studies of cardiac mass point to an enlargement of the heart, mainly in left ventricular mass. In endurance training, the left ventricular internal dimension increases and the mass increases out of proportion to the lean body mass, resulting in a true hypertrophy.[56,112] This functional change reverses with detraining.[56,112] An accompanying increase in plasma volume and total hemoglobin[102] is also reported. An increase in plasma volume will affect reporting of blood values. An increase in total content may be masked by the hemodilution, producing a "no change" result. A most notable case is with hemoglobin. Total hemoglobin may increase by nearly 25%, but plasma volume increases more, thus lowering hemoglobin concentration,[102] resulting in a pseudoanemia, which is occasionally seen, especially in females.

The most noted of training adaptations is a decrease in resting heart rate as a result of an increase in vagal tone and a decrease in sympathetic influence and intrinsic atrial rate.[138] With an increase in cardiac mass, a lower resting pulse rate, and no change in cardiac output, the stroke volume must rise.[56] This increase may be one of the most significant adaptations to training. Blood pressure at rest tends to decrease,[153,154] yet some[135] say the decrease in not enough to warrant the substitution of exercise for medical therapy.

The normal lung is generally not considered a limiting factor in exercise. Resting lung volumes are larger in trained people, mostly at the level of the inspiratory and expiratory reserve volumes.[85] Diffusion capacity of athletes is higher, probably because of a larger capillary-to-alveolus surface area. Maximum voluntary ventilation is

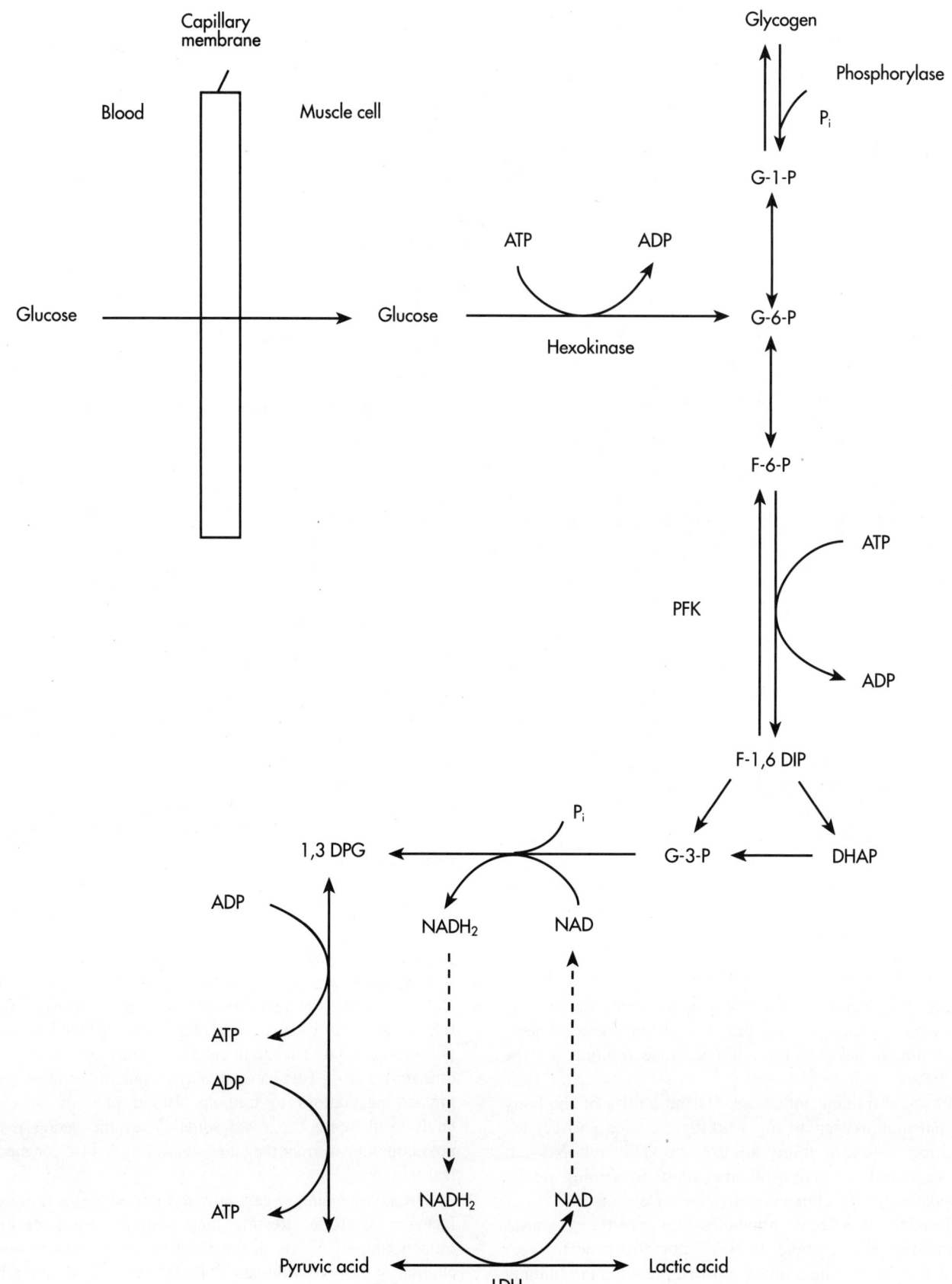

Fig. 18-3. Anaerobic glycolysis.

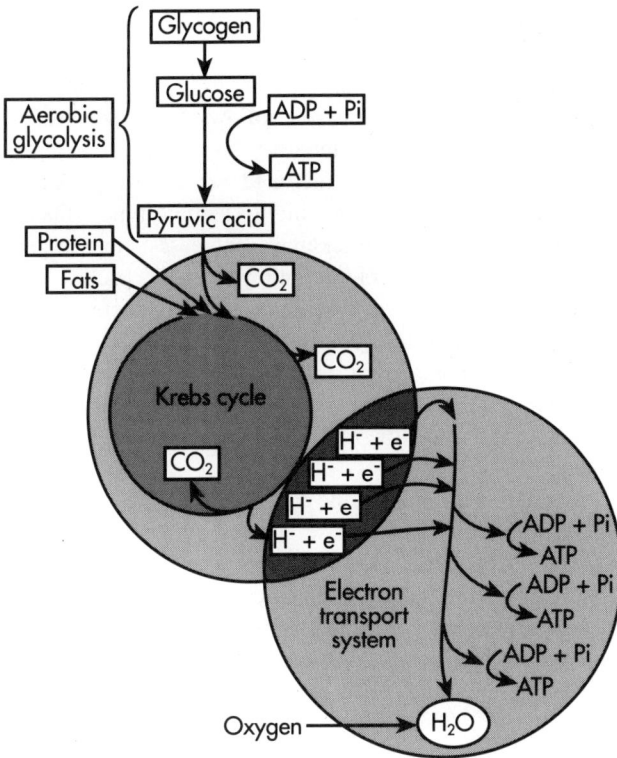

Fig. 18-4. The aerobic (oxygen) system.

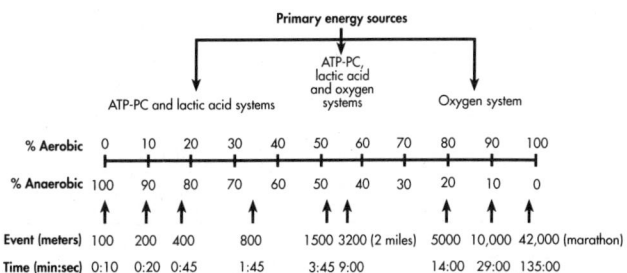

Fig. 18-5. The approximate percentage of contribution of aerobic and anaerobic energy sources in selected track events.

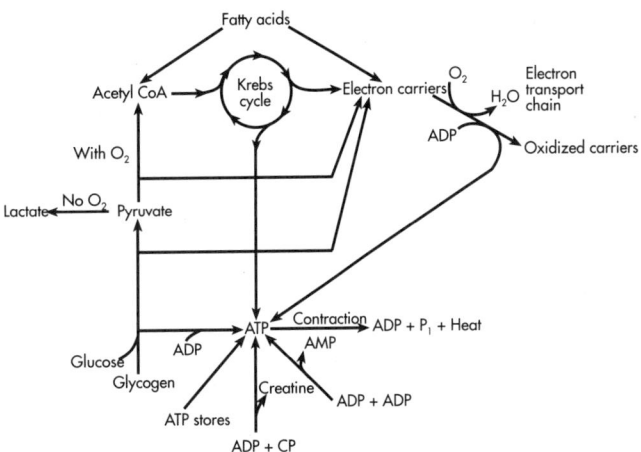

Fig. 18-6. Summary of ATP production.

increased, indicating a greater potential reserve.[56]

Other changes noticed at rest include a more favorable lipoprotein profile. Regardless of change in overall mass, training elevates HDL cholesterol while lowering total cholesterol and triglycerides,[152] yet wide variability requires that genetic factors be taken into account.[112] This opens the door to the use of training in the treatment of certain hyperlipidemias. Training, especially in concert with calorie restriction, can reduce the fat mass with little or no change in the fat-free mass.[128] This makes the use of exercise in concert with decreased calorie intake the method of choice for weight reduction. Connective tissue changes are seen as increases in trabecular bone thickness, resulting in an increase in bone density.[149] Cartilage is thickened, and ligaments and tendons are stronger, as are their attachments to bone.[155]

Responses to submaximal exercise

The adaptations discussed in this section are recorded during the performance of exercise at the identical power output. If a patient had a pretraining maximal power output of 200 watts and the submaximal power output used to record pretraining data was 100 watts, that power output was 50% of maximum. After training, assume that the patient improved work capacity to 300 watts. If the patient were to be cycled again at 100 watts (to record posttrain-

ing data), he or she would be working at 33% of maximum.

The most noticeable change is the reduction in heart rate (as discussed), making this figure usable in documenting training. A given power output before and after training requires the same amount of oxygen. As cardiac output and oxygen consumption are directly related, the cardiac output will be similar to pretraining cardiac output. Thus with a lower heart rate, the stroke volume will increase. Blood flow to the working muscles decreases[75,103] because of mechanisms discussed below.

Responses to maximal exercise

Training increases whole body maximal oxygen consumption and total power output by 5% to 25%,[1] depending on the initial level of fitness. Because of the direct relationship of cardiac output to oxygen consumption, cardiac output also increases to levels of 40+ L/min in world class athletes.[48,75] As the maximal heart rate may be unchanged or slightly lower this means that the stroke volume must have increased.[48,75] Relative blood flow in muscle is unchanged, but the total muscle mass recruited is in-

Table 18-2. Structural and functional characteristics of slow-twitch (Type I) and fast-twitch (Type II, A and B) muscle fibers

Characteristics	Fiber type		
	I	IIa	IIb
Neural aspects			
Motoneuron size	Small	Large	Large
Motoneuron recruitment threshold	Low	High	High
Motor nerve conduction velocity	Slow	Fast	Fast
Structural aspects			
Muscle fiber diameter	Small	Large	Large
Sarcoplasmic reticulum development	Less	More	More
Mitochondrial density	High	High	Low
Capillary density	High	Medium	Low
Myoglobin content	High	Medium	Low
Energy substrates			
Phosphocreatine stores	Low	High	High
Glycogen stores	Low	High	High
Triglyceride stores	High	Medium	Low
Enzymatic aspects			
Myosin-ATPase activity	Low	High	High
Glycolytic enzyme activity	Low	High	High
Oxidative enzyme activity	High	High	Low
Functional aspects			
Twitch (contraction) time	Slow	Fast	Fast
Relaxation time	Slow	Fast	Fast
Force production	Low	High	High
Energy efficiency, "economy"	High	Low	Low
Fatigue resistance	High	Low	Low
Elasticity	Low	High	High

creased, so the increased cardiac output is accommodated across a larger active area.[133]

PERIPHERAL ADAPTATIONS TO TRAINING
Changes seen at rest

Endurance training results in profound adaptation of the trained skeletal muscle. In light of the specificity principle, only those muscle fibers that are recruited will adapt. A fiber's characteristics are fixed by its motoneuron characteristics. Muscle fibers are classified by the speed of contraction as either slow contracting ("twitch") or fast twitch. The slow-twitch muscle (type I) is characterized by its low tension production, high aerobic capacity, and resistance to fatigue. Fast-twitch fibers (type II) are subdivided into two types. The pure fast-twitch fiber (type IIb) produces high tension, has a high glycolytic (thus a low aerobic) capacity, and fatigues quickly. There is also an intermediate fiber (type IIa). This fiber contracts quickly, has a better aerobic capacity than the IIb fiber, and is more resistant to fatigue like the type I fiber, making it a bit of a hybrid of both types. Table 18-2 summarizes some features of muscle fiber types.

Skeletal muscle is subservient to its motoneuron, and recruitment of the motoneuron follows the "size principle." As a result, in low-intensity submaximal exercise, the primary muscle fibers recruited are the small, slow-contracting, fatigue-resistant, highly aerobic type I fibers. As the intensity of the exercise increases, the larger, intermediate, faster contracting yet still aerobic and fatigue-resistant type IIa fibers are added to increase tension output. Finally, very-high-intensity exercises add the largest, fastest contracting, "strongest," and most fatigable anaerobic type IIb fibers[56,112] (Figure 18-7). The relative number of fast and slow muscle fibers is genetically determined.

In endurance training, the most recruited fibers are the type I, with some type IIa use. Thus the bulk of the adaptations will be found in these fibers that are recruited. A most noticeable change is the increase in myoglobin,[117] the oxygen-binding pigment of skeletal muscle, which would allow the muscle to "store" more oxygen. Glycogen stores are increased,[69,70] as are the number and size of mitochondria.[71,84] This leads to an increase in the aerobic enzymes of the Krebs cycle and electron transport chain[10,70,84] found in the mitochondria. In addition, fat stores increase in the muscle,[82,118] and fatty acids are more available from adipose tissue[17] and from mitochondrial enzymes of fat metabolism.[108]

In addition to the increase in intramuscular fuels of glycogen and fat, resting levels of ATP and phosphocreatine[51] are increased. Enzymes of glycolysis, although increased,[9,70,134] seem to be especially responsive to high-intensity training and even then do not change as much as aerobic enzymes, suggesting that our glycolytic capacity may be genetically determined.[56]

Training does not cause conversion of fiber type from type I to II or vice versa.[51,69] Training does result in a more aerobic profile of the intermediate IIa fiber, meaning it contracts slower and is more fatigue resistant.[112] Recruited muscle fibers are selectively hypertrophied. Endurance training increases the area of the type I and IIa fibers.[40,70] In addition, there appears to be an increased capillary bed that develops about the trained muscle, thus lowering the diffusion distance of oxygen.[2,3]

Changes seen during submaximal exercise

Cardiac output and oxygen consumption are directly related. A lack of change or a slight reduction in cardiac output should also reflect similar changes in oxygen consumption. Mechanical efficiency (skill) improvement may influence the reduction in oxygen consumption sometimes seen after training.[56] One of the most visible adaptations to training is a reduction in heart rate response to exercise performed at the same pretraining power output. There are many reasons for such a reduction. The cardiac hypertro-

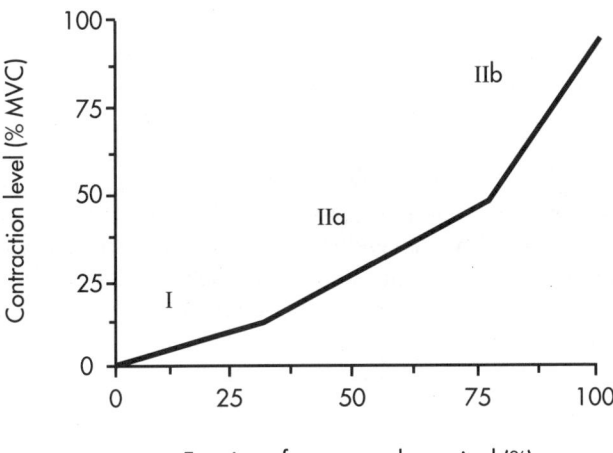

Fig. 18-7. Schematic demonstration of predicted orderly recruitment of motor units during voluntary activity as a function of contractile force. At lower forces, I units are recruited, and as force increases, IIa and IIb units are recruited. Adapted from Edgerton VR, et al: The matching of neuronal and muscular physiology. In Borer KT, Edington DW, and White TP, editors: *Frontiers of exercise biology,* Champaign, Ill, 1983, Human Kinetics Publishers.

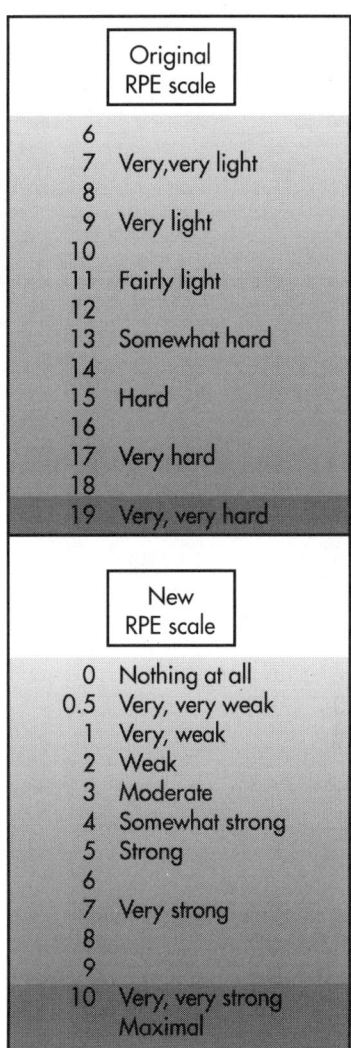

Fig. 18-8. Scales used for ratings of perceived exertion (RPE). Original scale (6-19) above and revised briefer scale (1-10) below. These scales are related to physiologic stress and can be used to establish exercise intensity for the purpose of training. From Borg GA: Psychological bases of perceived exertion, *Med Sci Sports Exerc* 14:377, 1982.

phy mentioned previously may result in a greater stroke volume. With little change in the cardiac output, a reduction in heart rate will follow. In addition, training results in reduced catecholamine production at identical power outputs (see previous discussion), thus reducing the sympathetic drive to the heart.[56]

After training, muscle blood flow (per kilogram of active muscle) decreases during submaximal exercise.[75,103] The increased activity of the muscle enzymes compensates by extracting more oxygen from the blood. With less blood passing through the active tissue bed and the cardiac output affected little, more blood is available to nonworking tissues. A main beneficiary is the skin, which leads to a greater ability to dissipate heat.[56]

Before training, the fuel of choice for the exercising muscle is carbohydrate. With training, there is a shift toward using fats as the primary fuel. This results in a decrease in the depletion of glycogen[97,133] and a decrease in the amount of lactic acid produced during work,[48,57] as well as an increase in the metabolism of lactic acid as a fuel by nonworking muscle fibers. The reasons for this are related to the changes in aerobic enzymes of the trained muscle noted previously. As the aerobic enzymes increase in their activity, the Krebs cycle is better able to compete for pyruvic acid. The power output needed to produce the same lactic acid level after training therefore is increased (an increase in the so-called "anerobic threshold", see reference 44). The shift from carbohydrate to fat as a fuel source also reduces the production of pyruvic acid (see Fig. 18-6) and is a reason for using exercise in weight control.

Changes seen at maximal exercise

Physical training generally improves a person's total work capacity. The percentage of improvement in maximal power output is related to the subject's pretraining fitness status; the lower the initial level of fitness in relation to age and gender, the greater the potential for improvement. Greater power output will probably require a larger active muscle mass to perform a given level of work. Thus, to supply the muscles (whose aerobic enzymes have been improved with training) with oxygen, a greater oxygen consumption is seen with concomitant increase in cardiac output. An interesting result is the lack of change, or even a small reduction, in maximum heart rate. Because there is little change in heart rate and improvement in car-

Table 18-3. Representative cross-sectional data comparing untrained vs endurance trained males

Variable	Untrained	Trained
Glycogen (mM/gm wet muscle)	85.0	120
ATP (mM/kg wet muscle)	3.8	4.8
Muscle enzymes		
PFK (mM/gm wet muscle)	50	50
SDH (mM/kg wet muscle)	5-10	15-20
Max VO2 (ml/kg/min)	30-40	60-80
Resting heart rate (bpm)	70	45
Resting stroke volume (ml/beat)	70	115
Maximal heart rate (bpm)	190	180
Blood volume (liters)	5.25	6.6
Hemoglobin (gm/100ml blood)	15.3	15
Left ventricle		
mass (gm)	210	300
cavity (mm)	43	55
wall thickness (mm)	10.4	10.55

From Fox EL, Bowers RG, Foss ML: Physiological basis of physical education and athletics, Dubuque, Iowa, 1988, WC Brown; and McArdle WD, Katch FI, Katch VL. Exercise physiology: energy, nutrition and human performance, Philadelphia, 1991, Lea & Febiger.

diac output and oxygen consumption, stroke volume must be increased.[49,133] More lactic acid is produced metabolically after training. This may be due to biochemical factors involved with glycolysis or perceptual factors whereby the person is more able to tolerate the declining muscle pH caused by the increase in lactic acid. Table 18-3 focuses on selected data to offer some perspective on the degree of change possible.

CORONARY HEART DISEASE

Coronary disease represents probably the widest area of application of systematic exercise training in clinical medicine. Cardiac rehabilitation programs have allowed the early placement of the postinfarction or postsurgery patient in the treatment mainstream not many years after absolute bed rest for extended periods was the norm. Although exercise is used in many circumstances, some situations still require caution (see the box on p. 315).

Rehabilitation programs are well documented.[128,143,172] Typically, soon after a coronary event, a phase I program of physical therapy and education begins. Phase II is usually in the early outpatient period, under some medical monitoring. Recently this phase has been performed in an out-of-hospital setting under medical monitoring. Activities are frequently of a light intensity and involve a variety of exercises. Phase III is a totally outpatient program still under medical guidance. Monitoring is minimal (exercise intensity monitored by either heart rate or perceived exertion, Fig. 18-8) and frequently is conducted at wellness centers, universities, YMCAs or YWCAs, and Jewish Community Centers. Activities include games and aerobic exercises and are closer to the exercise prescription guidelines of organizations like the American College of Sports Medicine. Occasionally a phase IV is included, which the patient conducts independently with only periodic checks with the physician. Time since the event or selected performance variables are the "graduation" criteria.

When one complies with the prescribed program, physical working capacity improves. The threshold for angina or ST segment depression occurs at a higher absolute power output (as high as +35%), which may lead to consideration of reductions in antianginal medications.[143] The improvement in work capacity is related to peripheral factors. If the oxygen consumption needed for any task is slightly reduced, then the cardiac output is also reduced, thus lowering the myocardial work requirement. The improvements in aerobic metabolism that influence the increase in the A-Vo2 difference will also reduce the heart rate, blood pressure, and muscle blood flow[34] during submaximal exercise, further reducing the myocardial demand.

All these benefits occur in lieu of changes at the cardiac level. There is little longitudinal evidence that exercise improves myocardial perfusion, be it measured by thallium 201 or angiography.[38,53,158] Anecdotal cross-sectional autopsy evidence suggests a larger coronary artery diameter in life-long runners.

Does cardiac rehabilitation stand up under scrutiny in the literature? Surprisingly, the four major studies of such programs showed improvements without statistical significance.[100,129,137,170] The reason for this lack of significance is related to "a high degree of non-adherence . . . a substantially lower than expected non-mortality rate in the usual care patients and inadequate sample size."[80]

In spite of all the apparent benefits of training, some patients do not improve with exercise. Those with significant myocardial damage or progression of the disease in spite of appropriate management may not realize any benefits. More data is needed on this set of coronary patients to understand their unique, and additional, limitations. The management of these individuals must be reconsidered separately.

Despite some statistical considerations as well as a lack of clear effects on the heart, the application of training in the postcoronary-event patient is one of the most widely practiced uses of exercise in the clinical community. Improvements in work capacity, psychological well-being, productivity, and other social and economic benefits, although sometimes difficult to document, are reasons to include training as a part of the therapeutic regimen.

PERIPHERAL VASCULAR DISEASE

Foley[55] first demonstrated that daily physical training (walking) was beneficial for patients with vascular disease. This contradicted the treatment at the time, which included reduction in walking intensity and smoking cessation in concert with medical or surgical management.[37] Patients

---

Contraindications to exercise training and conditions requiring special precautions

Absolute Contraindications
   Acute myocardial infarction
   Manifest circulatory insufficiency ("congestive heart failure")
   Rapidly increasing angina pectoris with effort
   Dissecting aneurysm
   Ventricular tachycardia at rest
   Severe aortic stenosis
   Active myocarditis
   Recent embolism, either systemic or pulmonary
   Thrombophlebitis
   Acute infectious disease
Relative contraindications
   Repetitive or frequent ventricular ectopic activity
   Uncontrolled or high-rate supraventricular dysrhythmia
   Ventricular aneurysm
   Moderate aortic stenosis
   Severe myocardial obstructive syndromes (subaortic stenosis)
   Untreated severe systemic or pulmonary hypertension
   Marked cardiac enlargement
   Severe anemia
   Uncontrolled metabolic disease (diabetes, thyrotoxicosis, or myxedema)
   Neuromuscular, musculoskeletal, or arthritic disorder that would prevent activity
   Overt psychoneurotic disturbance requiring therapy

Conditions requiring special consideration or precautions
   Controlled dysrhythmia
   Conduction disturbance
      Complete atrioventricular block
      Left bundle branch block
      Wolff-Parkinson-White syndrome
   Fixed-rate pacemaker
   Electrolyte disturbance
   Certain medication
      Digitalis
      Beta blockers and drugs of related action
   Angina pectoris and other manifestations of coronary insufficiency
   Cyanotic heart disease
   Intermittent or fixed right-to-left shunt
   Marked obesity
   Renal, hepatic, and other metabolic insufficiency

From American College of Sports Medicine: Guidelines for exercise testing and rehabilitation, ed 4, Philadelphia, 1991, Lea and Febiger.

---

feared the onset of ischemic pain. Once it was demonstrated that time (or distance) to the onset of pain could be increased, it was necessary to determine the best type of exercise and the mechanism responsible for the improvement.

An initial piece of information required before exercise training is the metabolic profile of the muscles distal to the disease. Typically the gastrocnemius is biopsied. Selected aerobic as well as anaerobic enzymes are elevated above normal in response to ischemia,[21] although Henriksson et al.[81] showed reductions in enzyme activity only in patients with occlusions in both legs. Smaller fibers (resulting to inactivity) yet similar capillary-to-fiber ratios were seen in the occluded leg. The latter finding suggests some degree of adaptation to the occlusive state.[81]

Many papers have addressed the aspect of training in PVD patients. The most common mode of training is walking. Training programs suggested in the literature* were typically 2 to 3 days per week, 30 to 60 minutes per day. In some cases basic calisthenics were performed (e.g., toes raises, stair climbing, leg raises, sit-stand, "squats"). In nearly every study, exercise to and beyond

*References 37, 41, 50, 52, 107, 144, 150.

the onset of pain was a requirement. The training programs varied from 2 to 11 months with patients who averaged 60+ years of age. Some of the referenced studies reported on subjects individually,[144] and others used large sample sizes of over 100.[50]

In the patients cited, those who *adhered* to the program (always an important requirement), including time (or distance) to the onset of pain and total distance walked, improved by up to 100% and more. This improvement was estimated by the use of blood flow measurement during exercise. Some studies showed no change in blood flow as a result of the training program,[41,107,150] but others did show an improvement.[52] Lactate production, indicative of anaerobic involvement, fell after training,[150] suggesting that the aerobic system had improved its ability to compete for pyruvic acid and to use the oxygen delivered. Sorlie[150] demonstrated this by showing that training elevated oxidative enzymes and the use of lipids as fuel, coupled with reduced lactate production. This increase in aerobic capacity might have occurred in the intermediate type IIa muscle fiber, which can show large increases in metabolic capacity in response to training. This possibility has yet to be demonstrated.

More efficient use of oxygen delivered to the working

muscles, in the absence of blood flow changes, allows time to pain to be increased as well as total walking distance. As seen in other clinical situations, exercise does little to the underlying disease, namely vascular narrowing. Rather, exercise allows the tissue distal to the lesion to raise its function in spite of its blood flow limitation.

The consistent requirement of walking to pain means that the exercise prescription needs to be modified to the patient's level of tolerance. It is unreasonable to expect a patient with PVD just entering a program to walk uninterrupted for 15 or more minutes. A patient should walk to pain, then rest before continuing until some time (say 10 to 15 minutes to start) or a distance requirement has been met. With training, that time or distance requirement will increase according to the mechanisms mentioned previously. Larsen[107] reported on one trained patient whose maximal walking distance was nearly 19 minutes, the rest were under 11 minutes. Total walking distances after training in the studies mentioned were typically less than 800 meters. Physician and patient expectations must be realistic.

HYPERTENSION

The role of exercise training in the treatment of hypertension remains controversial. Several studies have looked at the interaction of exercise with resting and exercise blood pressure responses. Many problems surround the interpretation of the literature. For example, was weight, body composition, diet, test location (laboratory vs. workplace vs. home) considered? What method was used for determining blood pressure and hypertensive classification and for determining improvement in aerobic power? Was the study cross-sectional or longitudinal and were control groups used? What methods were used to determine the mechanism of change, change in cardiac output and/or change in peripheral resistance? Because blood pressure is influenced by a multitude of factors, it is difficult to control all other factors and modify only one, like exercise, to get a reasonably definitive answer.

Two separate reviews in 1984 arrived at different conclusions. In Tipton's extensive review,[154] he said that "sufficient justification exists" to use physical training as supporting therapy for hypertensives. Given that the majority of studies indicate that systolic pressure can be reduced by 5 to 25 mm Hg, diastolic pressure can be lowered by 3 to 15 mm Hg, and in no study was training associated with elevation of resting pressure, exercise seems advisable for "hypertensive individuals regardless of age and individuals whose resting blood pressures are approximately 140/90 mm Hg." On the other hand, Seals and Hagberg[135] concluded from their review that the potential for approximately a 9 and 7 mm Hg reduction in resting systolic and diastolic blood pressure respectively was "inadequate for the recommendation of exercise conditioning as a replacement for pharmacological intervention."

Since 1984, several studies (reviewed in reference 155) on humans have examined the effect of chronic aerobic exercise on blood pressure. Four studies[22,47,101] have noted decreases in blood pressure and two[36,65] found no change. No study can be considered conclusive because of methodological concerns such as lack of control groups, lack of documentation about improvements in aerobic power, method of classifying subjects, or using normotensives only.

Gilders et al.[65] reported on a small sample (N = 8) of borderline or mild hypertensives who underwent 8 control weeks, 16 weeks of training, and 12 weeks of detraining. Cardiac output and peripheral resistance were monitored. They reported no changes in resting blood pressure throughout the study, indicating minimal influence of exercise on the subjects' resting blood pressure.

The American College of Sports Medicine has recently added resistance exercise to their position stand on exercise training (see Chapter 19). As such, the effects of weight training on blood pressure should be noted. Resistance training generally is considered to have little or no ability to improve aerobic power. Yet, in occupations with a moderate to high isometric component, the occurrence of hypertension has been reported to be quite low.[169] In addition to that epidemiologic data, controlled studies[77,88,169] on resistance training seem to suggest that resting blood pressure is lowered in normotensives[169] as well as borderline hypertensives.[77,88]

With aerobic exercise, systolic pressure rises to some steady level and diastolic pressure changes little with only slight changes in the mean arterial pressure.[56] During resistance exercise, both systolic and diastolic pressure rise, sometimes to dramatic levels. Macdougall (cited in reference 27) has reported transient intraarterial pressures as high as 450/310 during a bench press in weight lifters. Wiley et al.[169] used normotensives to study isometric handgrip training. With as little as four 2-minute contractions (3-minute rest between contractions) at 30% of maximal voluntary capacity (MVC), 3 days per week for 8 weeks, resting blood pressure declined by 12/15 mm Hg (systolic/diastolic respectively). With 50% of MVC for 45 seconds (1-minute rest) 5 days per week for 5 weeks, pressure declined 10/9 mm Hg. Detraining returned all subjects' pressure to prestudy levels.

Tipton has since updated his review.[155] The data reviewed look at a variety of mechanisms that might be involved in training-induced reductions in blood pressure, such as the sympathetic nervous system, metabolic implications, electrolyte/renal, calcium, kidney, other neural, and structural modifications in the cardiovascular system. The literature reflects Tipton's hypothesis favoring a reduction in the cardiac output after training. The more recent data have not changed his opinion regarding the use of exercise in the hypertensive. Tipton notes that the mode of exercise influenced outcome. In the spontaneously hy-

Table 18-4. Guide to grading disability (based on 40-year-old man)

Grade	Cause of dyspnea	FEV$_1$ (% pred)	Max Vo_2 (ml · min^{-1} · kg^{-1})	Exercise max V$_E$) (L · min^{-1})	Blood gases
1	Fast walking and stair climbing	>60	>25	Not limiting	Normal Pco_2, Sao_2
2	Walking at normal pace	<60	<25	>50	Normal Paco_2; Sao_2 above 90% at rest and with exercise
3	Slow walking	<40	<15	<50	Normal Paco_2; Sao_2 below 90% with exercise
4	Walking limited to less than one block	<40	<7	<30	Elevated Paco_2; Sao_2 below 90% at rest and with exercise

From Jones NL, et al. In Skinner JS, editor: *Exercise test and exercise prescription for special cases,* Philadelphia, 1987, Lea & Febiger.

pertensive rat, "marked reductions" in blood pressure were seen in rats trained by swimming, but most human studies neglect this type of activity.

The weight of evidence seems to imply that exercise, be it aerobic or resistance, does have a modest effect on resting blood pressure. The classification of the patient then influences the clinical decision to include an exercise program. According to Goldstein,[68] patients with a World Health Organization classification of stage 1 (mild, latent, or borderline with no signs of secondary organ involvement) demonstrate a mild reduction in hypertensive status when following a typical exercise prescription.[22] Other typical measures (e.g., diet, salt, weight control) are not to be ignored. Those with stage 2 hypertension (moderate or fixed hypertension with some secondary organ involvement) should first have their blood pressure under control. Then exercise should be used to support pharmacologic measures. Aerobic exercise is usually the choice, but some resistance or isometric exercise can be included. Exercise training in stage 3 hypertensives (advanced with signs/symptoms of secondary failure) "is absolutely contraindicated."[68] There is no evidence that aerobic training will lower blood pressure in the renal hypertensive patient.[155]

PULMONARY DISEASES
Chronic obstructive pulmonary diseases

Obstructive pulmonary diseases, whether chronic airflow obstruction, asthma, or chronic bronchitis, present a central limitation to the performance of exercise. Normally, the lungs offer little limitation to exercise. However, when ventilatory function is compromised, the physical working capacity and subsequent activities of daily living become difficult (see Chapter 55).

In some settings, disability is graded (Table 18-4), which offers some direction in assembling an individualized training program as patients work toward rehabilitation goals (see the box above, right). The following guidelines are based on the findings of Jones et al.[94] Patients with a grade I disability should perform daily exercise based on results of exercise testing and heart rate percent-

---

Objectives of rehabilitation exercise programs

Education of patients and relatives
  Disease process and management
  Improved compliance with therapy
  Practical advice regarding living with disability
Improvement in fitness and exercise performance
  Increased endurance
  Reduced respiratory muscle fatigue
  Increased strength
  Improved coordination and efficiency in everyday activities
Improved voluntary control of breathing pattern
  Increased tidal volume in exercise
  Reduced dyspnea in exercise and stressful situations
Increased flexibility
Improved confidence in physical abilities
Increased self responsibilities
Improved quality of life
  Increased physical and social activity
  Improved family relationships
  Increased sense of achievement through realistic goal setting and less reliance on others in work and at home

From Jones NL: Chronic obstructive respiratory disease. In Skinner JS, editor: *Exercise testing and exercise prescription for special cases,* Philadelphia, 1987, Lea and Febiger.

ages. Programs for these patients follow programs similar to those for coronary disease patients. The moderate dysfunction of the grade II patient forces a reduction of exercise intensity. An exercise heart rate at a moderate percentage (60% to 80%) of the ventilatory capacity (FEV$_1$ × 35) is used for monitoring the exercise intensity. Exercise may be performed more than once per day for shorter durations so that breathlessness does not limit the session. Grade III patients should work at an even lower percentage of capacity. This capacity might be so low that training adaptations may be minimal. Supplemental oxygen, training of individual muscle groups, and respiratory muscle train-

Table 18-5. Observed changes in selected variables after 5 months*

Group	n	$V_{O_2}max$	VC	FEV_1	FEF_{25-75}	GSI
Control	5 (3 males, 2 females)	−8	0	−5	−31	−10
Experimental	5 (3 males, 2 females)	+18	+9	+29	+26	+9

*Data represent percent change from baseline. VC, vital capacity; FEF_1, 1-second forced expiratory volume; FEF_{25-75}, forced expiratory flow; GSI, grip strength index.
From Keens T: Ventilatory muscle endurance training in normal subjects and patient with cystic fibrosis, *Am Rev Respir Dis* 116:853, 1977.

ing can be useful. The grade IV patient has the most severe limitation, and any exercise is limited by symptoms. Heart rate or perceived exertion (dyspnea) at the low intensities they can tolerate are reasonable indicators for controlling exercise intensity.

For patients who undertake an exercise program, the improvement in work capacity is unrelated to modification of the underlying disease. Rather, improvements are related to peripheral changes and increased tolerance to the changing blood gas admixture. A most important adaptation is related to an improvement in walking efficiency.[122] This is seen as improved posture and walking mechanics as well as reductions in unnecessary movements. This all results in a reduced oxygen requirement at submaximal power outputs, reducing the metabolic cost of breathing. The reduction in ventilation then raises the threshold needed to cause the onset of dyspnea.[119,162] The workload that results in the increase in blood lactic acid accumulation is raised in those who are able to train at such a moderate intensity.[161] Exercise tidal volume increases as a result of training, reducing the dead space/tidal volume ratio, improving gas exchange.[93] One of the blood adaptations, an increase in red cell mass, is seen in patients not receiving oxygen supplementation,[161,162] with the obvious improvement in oxygen carriage. Finally, ventilatory muscle training can result in small (but significant to the patient)[121] improvements in respiratory muscle capacity.[11] These adaptations obviously increase the daily activities they can accomplish (see Chapter 55).

Cystic fibrosis

Few cystic fibrosis patients exercise, despite the potential benefits. In spite of the lack of data documenting the benefits, the use of exercise for the cystic fibrosis patient is underprescribed,[90] especially when anecdotal reports suggest milder complications compared with nonexercising peers.[35,174]

Jankowski[90] suggests the following when training the cystic fibrosis patient. Training typically begins with the results of a clinical exercise test. The intensity of training usually begins at about 50% of capacity for about 1.5 to 3 months. Intensity is then gradually increased to about 75%. The cystic patient usually cannot exercise for long periods, so Jankowski typically breaks the time into three equal periods with rest between each. Starting with three 5-minute sessions at the desired intensity is advised. Increasing by 2 minutes each session every week will soon bring the patient up to the desired 1 hour of exercise (3 times 20 minutes). Frequency of training needs to be every other day, as the cystic fibrosis patient may take 48 hours to recover. The choices of exercise are the typical aerobic exercises of walking, jogging, cycling, and swimming. Special considerations (warm water, wetsuits, flotation devices) may be needed for swimming to protect the typically lean cystic patient from low water temperature.

Following such a program yields some predictable results. Table 18-5 displays some data regarding ventilatory and muscular performance data. In addition, respiratory muscle endurance has increase by 57%, with no change in aerobic power after only 4 weeks.[98] More controlled and longer training showed an increase in power output of 30%, a 15% increase in vital capacity, and a 17% increase in V_{O_2} max.[35] Summer camps are popular for cystic fibrosis patients. These serve as a good beginning to motivate the patient to continue the beneficial habit of exercise throughout the year.

DIABETES

Even before 1959, when Joslin[95] described the interaction of diet, exercise, and insulin, exercise served as a basic therapy for the patient with diabetes mellitus. Practical information for the diabetic is a result of the expanding knowledge base on the effects of physical training on metabolism.

Type I diabetes mellitus

Type I diabetes typically begins when physical activity is normally a part of everyday life. However, the fear of bringing on the hypoglycemic condition through exercise may force one to severely limit his or her activities. This inactivity may lead to other complications associated with a sedentary life, which may add other obstacles to an already difficult condition. However, if the diabetic knows about the disease, he or she can avoid risks that may come

Table 18-6. Exercise recommendations based on preexercise blood glucose levels (note that the exact levels may vary from patient to patient)

1. If blood glucose is:
Lower than 6 mmol/ liter→	Eat extra carbohydrates
*Between 6-16 mmol/ liter→	Exercise
*Higher than 16 mmol/ liter→	Postpone exercise session and check ketones in urine

2. If urinary ketones are:
*Negative→	Exercise
*Positive→	Inject insulin and postpone the exercise session until the urinary ketones have disappeared

3. Remember that the hypoglycemic response after an exercise session is still evident after 24 to 28 hr

*18 × mmol/liter = mg/dl
From Wallberg-Henriksson H: Exercise and diabetes mellitus, *Exerc Sport Sci Rev* 20:339, 1992.

Strategy to avoid hypo- or hyperglycemia in connection with exercise in type I diabetes mellitus

Food
   Eat a meal 1 to 2 hours before an exercise session
   Eat extra carbohydrates during exercise sessions that continue for more than 30 min (15 to 30 g carbohydrate every 30 min)
Insulin
   Inject insulin more than 1 hr before the exercise session
   Lower insulin dose before exercise session (to what level is individual and also depends on the type of exercise)
   When regular exercise is performed (> three times a week), the total insulin dosage will need to be lowered
Measuring blood glucose
   Measure blood glucose before, during, and after an exercise session
   Postpone the exercise session if the blood glucose is higher than 16 mmol liter and/or if ketone bodies are present in the urine

From Wallberg-Henriksson H: Exercise and diabetes mellitus, *Exerc Sport Sci Rev* 20:339, 1992.

---

with activity. There are many instances of professional athletes who have successfully competed while managing type I diabetes, notably tennis champion Don Budge.

In the normal person, increased glucose uptake by skeletal muscle during acute bouts of exercise is balanced by hepatic release of glucose. In addition, exercise typically results in a reduction in insulin as skeletal muscle increases its uptake of glucose. The type I diabetic receiving insulin may encounter hypoglycemia as the normal exercise-induced reduction in insulin fails to occur[167] as glucose is metabolized and blood sugar levels fall. The constant insulin level then prevents the liver from releasing sufficient glucose to supply the increased muscle uptake.[163,177] However, when ketosis is present, the opposite condition may occur,[164] and exercise should probably be delayed until ketosis disappears.[165] When exercises are of equal duration, higher intensity exercise results in a greater fall in blood glucose.[176] Excessive duration is also associated with hypoglycemia.[99] Increased glucose uptake and sensitivity to insulin seem to persist for up to 4 to 6 hours after exercise.[24]

Whether chronic exposure to the sequence of events just described will improve metabolic control is open to debate. Wallberg-Henriksson[165] suggests not, but does encourage exercise, intensive insulin therapy, and home blood glucose monitoring. Children with poor metabolic control showed the most improvement,[23,42] and those whose diabetic condition was well managed showed no changes.[89,106,132]

The lipid profile of the diabetic is usually improved with training, resulting in reductions in total cholesterol, triglycerides, and LDL-cholesterol,[39,79] with an increase in HDL-cholesterol.[166,175] In addition, insulin sensitivity (glucose uptake per unit of insulin) is improved by up to 20% with training,[166] but counter-regulatory hormones decrease.[59] These hormonal changes quickly disappear with a return to inactivity, and the insulin-resistant condition may worsen with bed rest.[165]

In a practical sense, the literature offers many suggestions (Table 18-6 and the box above). Individual differences may require alterations in these lists. Diabetes is a condition to which the standard exercise prescription can be applied, once appropriate medical clearance has been given. In addition, some physicians prefer to establish metabolic control first, then add exercise. Diet then is used to make adjustments (see Table 18-6), or possibly to alter the insulin dosage (see the box above). The box on p. 320 lists suggestions for avoiding exercise-related hypoglycemia.

A series of well-known conditions associated with type I diabetes deserve special mention. Patients with *diabetic retinopathy* are discouraged from participating in activities of very high intensity or activities that require a Valsalva maneuver.[165] This should not be interpreted to mean that exercise accelerates the progression of retinopathy.[12,72] Exercise related *albuminuria* is a common finding in diabetics and seems to be related to the degree of elevation in systolic pressure.[116] Thus activities that elevate systolic pressures above 180 to 200 mm Hg are to be avoided,[165]

Guidelines for avoiding hypoglycemia during and after exercise

1. Consume carbohydrates (15 to 30 g) for every 30 minutes of moderately intense exercise.
2. Consume a snack of slowly absorbed carbohydrate after prolonged exercise sessions.
3. Decrease the insulin dose
   a. Intermediate-acting insulin—decrease by 30% to 35% on the day of exercise.
   b. Intermediate- and short-acting insulin—omit dose of short-acting insulin that precedes exercise.
   c. Multiple doses of short-acting insulin—reduce the dose before exercise by 30% to 35% and supplement carbohydrates.
   d. Continuous subcutaneous infusion—eliminate mealtime bolus or increment that precedes or immediately follows exercise.
4. Avoid exercising muscle underlying injections of short-acting insulin for 1 hour.
5. Avoid late evening exercise.

From Vitug A, Schneider SH, Ruderman NB: Exercise and type I diabetes mellitus, *Exerc Sports Sci Rev* 16:285, 1988.

Long-term effects of regular exercise in type II diabetes mellitus: Possible positive effects

1. Improved blood glucose control
2. Increased peripheral insulin sensitivity
3. Improved blood lipid profile
4. Decreased hypertension
5. Contributing factors (together with diet) to weight reduction
6. Increased physical work capacity
7. Increased sense of well-being and quality of life

From Wallberg-Henriksson H: Exercise and diabetes mellitus, *Exerc Sports Sci Rev* 20:339, 1992.

---

with modes like walking or cycling to be encouraged. Patients with *autonomic neuropathy* are predisposed to postexertional hypotension and should be counseled to avoid exercises that result in rapid changes in body position, heart rate, or blood pressure, such as ball games and weight training.[165] These patients also seem to have problems with exercise in the heat that make them more likely to become dehydrated.[160] Patients with *peripheral neuropathy* need to pay particular attention to shoe selection and inspect their feet after each exercise session.[19] Cycling and swimming, because of the reduced stress on the feet, are the exercises of choice. In addition, the loss of sensation increases the risk of excessive stretching on muscles and connective tissues.[165] *Myocardial ischemia* is a common problem in the diabetic. Thus, before starting an exercise program, diabetics should have a thorough cardiovascular exam and stress test.[165]

Type II diabetes mellitus

Two types of type II diabetes exist. In the first type there is an impaired ability to secrete insulin, and the other type shows an impaired sensitivity to insulin.[165] Acute exercise decreases blood glucose well into the recovery period,[87,115] and this decrease appears to be related to exercise duration[126] and is most common in patients taking sulfonylureas or insulin.[165] After maximal, exhaustive exercise, a hyperglycemic condition can occur.[91]

Physical training (again following standard exercise prescription guidelines) has been shown to improve metabolic control, especially in younger diabetics.[16,104] However, minimal control is realized without weight loss.[105,142] Insulin sensitivity is improved,[104] most markedly in skeletal muscle tissue and adipose tissue[86] in patients with high insulin levels, while those patients with low insulin appear to show increased levels of insulin secretion.[104,165]

The association between obesity and type II diabetes clearly makes weight reduction a priority in any treatment plan.[83,173] Most people are aware that the most efficient method of weight loss is the combination of diet and exercise. This is true for the diabetic also. The preferred type of exercise is low-intensity, long-duration exercise. The higher the intensity, the greater is the reliance on carbohydrates for fuel. At lower intensities, a large fraction of the fuel can be derived from fats. Thus walking is an ideal activity.

The increased risk of coronary disease in diabetics[62,131] makes the improvement of lipid profiles a desired alteration. Female type II diabetics have shown such improvements[159] within a few months, but males have not shown any changes in up to 2 years.[142] Different training regimens and pretraining status may have accounted for the differences in these study results.[165]

In the care of the exercising type II diabetic, it is usually not necessary to increase carbohydrate intake unless the activity is extended. Patients under treatment with sulfonylureas may need some added carbohydrates before and during the activity.[165] The activity should be aerobic and chosen by the individual. The box above shows some potential benefits to the type II diabetic.

END STAGE RENAL DISEASE

Patients with end stage renal disease (ESRD) may experience multiple problems, which might include cardiovascular disease, muscular weakness, bone disease, metabolic and hormonal disorders, fatigue, and psychological problems. Many of these systemic problems can be influenced by exercise. As a result, the application of physical training has produced many favorable results.

Many patients with ESRD are limited in their ability to perform activities of daily living, much less a physical training program. The ability to perform exercise is limited by many factors, such as anemia, reduced hematocrit, cardiac function abnormalities, local muscular fatigue, elevated exercise lactic acid levels, and overall deconditioning.[124]

With the ESRD patient, the typical exercise prescription guidelines are followed. However, heart rate may not be the best indicator of exercise intensity; thus the perceived exertion scale (Fig. 18-8) is substituted. Usually the patient starts at a lower intensity and duration and gradually increases both. Training is typically performed on the off-dialysis days.[74]

Comprehensive studies of training in ESRD patients have been extensively reported.* Exercise and control groups of dialysis patients participated in a 12-month study.[66] Aerobic capacity improved by 21% and resting systolic pressure declined in the hypertensive patients from 155 to 124 mm Hg, which resulted in a corresponding modification or elimination of medications. Total cholesterol was unchanged, but the profile of fractions favored a reduction in their coronary risk factor. Depression was reduced, but other aspects of the psychological profile deteriorated. Hematocrit increased, as did hemoglobin.[66] After renal transplantation, training increased estimated maximal work capacity by nearly 30% after 6 weeks in a cardiac rehabilitation program.[151] There do not appear to be any reported training studies on continuous ambulatory peritoneal dialysis patients.

In other studies on ESRD patients, compliance has been a problem. For example, of 50 prestudy patients, only 14 completed a 12-week program.[136] Anxiety and hostility, by psychological inventory, were the primary predictors of noncompliance.

Although these studies focused on training on the nondialysis day, other investigators have studied the use of exercise during dialysis. Performing training at this time should positively affect compliance.[124] Training for 6 months at about 70% to 85% of capacity improved aerobic capacity by 26%.[125] A stationary cycle was placed in front of their dialysis chair, and the patient then pedaled from behind the cycle while seated in the chair. The patient began the program with 5 minutes of exercise, progressing to 30 minutes during treatments. A major improvement was the reduction in blood pressure in 75% of the hypertensive patients, with corresponding changes in medications. Lipids did not change and hematocrit rose slightly near the end of the program. Participation rates of those who enter such programs has been reported to be reasonable.[123] The later the exercise is performed during dialysis, the higher the heart rate, but the lower the blood pressure response, which further supports the use of perceived exertion as an intensity gauge.[124]

*References 25, 64, 66, 67, 76, 78.

OSTEOPOROSIS

Among the natural consequences of aging, the loss of bone density constitutes a major public health concern, especially in Western societies. The maintenance of bone health may reduce fractures, and the role of exercise in maintaining such health could be one of the most effective applications of exercise. The maintenance of bone health depends on the interaction of three variables, nutrition (calcium intake, vitamin D), functional stress (gravity and activity) and hormones (such as PTH, calcitonin, estrogen, growth hormone). Reducing any of these may result in a reduction in bone density. The influence of nutrition has been well documented. Elimination of gravity (space flight) results in rapid decrease in bone density. Bed rest and immobilization can also reduce bone density, but excess weight (obesity) can overload the bones and increase bone density. With aging and menopause come the reduction in estrogen and the resulting decrease in bone density. This problem is not limited to the aging female. Data suggest that in selected female subjects, training can disrupt the normal menstrual cycle. With the resulting loss of estrogen comes a reduction in bone density with a risk for stress fractures, most often documented in female runners during stressful training.[46,111] The estrogen problem is not as evident in males. Testosterone is converted to estrogen by extraglandular tissue, so a reasonable supply of estrogen continues throughout life. This section will focus on maintenance and improvement of bone health and is not directed to the heavily training young female.

Dense cortical and spongy trabecular bone have recently come under intense study. Bone mass is gained throughout adolescence. About 60% of the final bone mass is built up during the 2- to 3-year pubertal growth spurt, making nutrition in this period a critical factor.[149] A plateau is reached in about the third to fourth decade, followed by a progressive thinning or even disappearance of the trabecular aspects of the tissue.[114] The loss of mass during menopause proceeds at a rapid rate during the first 5 years (nearly 3.5% per year), followed by a small loss (<1% per year by the ninth year) in subsequent years.[60]

According to Wolff's law, bone will adapt to the recurring demands placed on it, as do most tissues. The load must be progressive. If one trains to jog 3 miles a day, the bone will adapt to some equilibrium by thickening trabecular bone. The number of years at this distance should not matter, as a new equilibrium has been reached.[149]

Part of the difficulty in interpreting the data is related to the site of measurement and the age of the subjects. Would walking or dancing be expected to increase bone density of the distal radius? Do premenopausal and postmenopausal women respond in the same manner? Is exercise beneficial for women already diagnosed as osteoporotic? Despite these unanswered questions, the research on this topic seems to support the use of exercise in the prevention and treatment of osteoporosis.

The specific type of exercise is critical when prescribing exercise. For example, a 6-month program of dancing resulted in no change in radial bone density,[168] while 9 months of running rewarded the subjects with an increased calcaneal density.[171] A series of long-term (3+ years) projects[145-147] studying elderly females (average, 81 years) showed that the activity (controlled calesthenics, rythmic exercise, walking) group and the calcium supplement group increased bone density of the radius by 2.3% and 1.6% respectively. The control group and combined calcium/exercise groups declined by 3.3 and .3% respectively. Specific loading of the arms of osteoporotic women resulted in nearly 4% gain in bone density over 5 months, while the controls lost nearly 2%, both at the radius.[7] Nine months of weight-bearing (walk/jog) and non–weight-bearing activities (rowing) resulted in a more than 5% increase in lumbar density, reaching more than 6% after an added year. These values returned nearly to baseline after 13 months of detraining.[43] In contrast, a walking program[28] showed a reduced bone mineral density of the spine roughly equivalent to the control group (5.6% vs. 4% respectively). As rowing loads the vertebra, the specific loading of the vertebra may be more important than the walking itself.[149] This is supported by the data that show fewer fractures in women who performed trunk extension exercises in comparison with women who performed trunk flexion exercises.[140] Therefore weight-bearing exercise, although beneficial, can be improved by supplementing specific sites (arms, lumbar vertebra) by incorporating some resistance exercise (weight lifting) and cross training, such as rowing.

The data support specific loading (weight lifting) to increase bone density and the (relative) lack of influence of aerobic exercise on bone density. It might be expected that the relationship of muscle strength and aerobic fitness to bone health has been explored.[149] This is especially interesting in light of the similar degrees of loss of strength and bone.[92] Because trunk extensor exercises improved lumbar bone density (as implied in reference 140 by fewer fractures), back extensor strength should correlate with bone density.[14] Even when an age adjustment is made, this correlation holds.[141] Site specificity is further supported by the relationship of grip strength to radial density.[14] Muscle strength was a better predictor of bone density than was age.[148] However, before one entirely accepts the site specificity hypothesis, one should remember that strength in remote muscle groups (e.g., forearm flexors) also predicts bone density in selected sites, such as the femoral neck or lumbar vertebra,[148] which may be explained by trunk stabilization during upper limb exercise.[149] With respect to aerobic fitness, a few studies find a significant relationship between oxygen consumption and bone density at selected sites.[29,127] However, the bulk of literature[13,14,43,120] found no such relationship. Thus aerobic fitness is not a very reliable indicator of bone density.[149]

The presented data shows that, although training can improve bone density, the degree of improvement is small, requires months or years, and shows the greatest percentage of improvement in sedentary people rather than in those already trained. According to Show-Hunter and Marcus[149] "it is difficult to conceive that a woman whose bone mass is in the 3rd percentile before exercise could ever achieve the 50th percentile for age from an exercise program, regardless of duration."

As a result of such considerations, exercise cannot be considered as a substitute for estrogen therapy. Should exercise, whether light intensity (walking, low-resistance, high repetition weight training), or higher intensity (more traditional weightlifting) be suggested in the older frail population? Low-intensity work has been suggested.[43] Types of activities include supervised rhythmic activities, supported (holding onto a chair) exercise, and low-intensity resistance training (sandbags, similar to what a physical therapist might use). These exercises need not be done to fatigue or exhaustion. The higher intensity work should be reserved for the younger people still laying down bone. However, training studies in nonagenarians[54] show that even this age group can tolerate weight training as well as show beneficial training effects.

HUMAN IMMUNODEFICIENCY VIRUS

Some believe that acute or chronic physical exercise can lead to suppression of the immune system. This might lead one to question the use of exercise in those with a challenged immune system.

Part of the problem with drawing conclusions about exercise and the immune system is the staggering number of parameters involved in immune status and their interactions (see Chapter 57 for a more detailed discussion of the immune system). Couple this with various exercise parameters, and conclusions are indeed difficult to determine. For example, do CD4, CD8, CD16 cell lines increase or decrease after different types of exercise? Is there a difference if the exercise is exhaustive or submaximal; if the exercise is high intensity and short duration vs. low intensity and long duration?

A change in immune function has obvious implications in individuals infected with human immunodeficiency virus-1 (HIV-1). Temoshak et al.[152] have suggested that exercise training is associated with improved immune status and increased survival time. Training resulted in small increases in CD4+ and less severe reductions in CD56 cells in HIV-1–positive men asymptomatic for AIDS-related complex or AIDS.[109]

Rigsby et al.[130] attempted to determine the influence of moderate, chronic physical training on T-lymphocyte function in HIV-1–positive men. A total of 37 HIV-1–positive males (Walter Reed ratings 1 to 5) were assigned to either a counseling group or a training group. Training consisted of stationary cycling, weight training, and flexi-

---

Contraindications for exercise during pregnancy*

Absolute contraindications

Heart disease
Ruptured membranes
Premature labor
Multiple gestation
Bleeding
Placenta previa
Incompetent cervix
History of three or more spontaneous abortions
   or miscarriages

Relative contraindications

High blood pressure
Anemia or other blood disorders
Thyroid disease
Diabetes
Palpitations or irregular heart rhythms
Breech presentation in the last trimester
Excessive obesity
Extreme underweight
History of precipitous labor
History of intrauterine growth retardation
History of bleeding during pregnancy
Extremely sedentary lifestyle

---

*From American College of Obstetricians and Gynecologists: *Exercise during pregnancy and postnatal period (ACOG) home exercise programs,* Washington, DC, 1985, ACOG.

bility exercises that required 1 hour per day, three days per week for 10 to 12 weeks of training. Strength and endurance both improved in the training group, but weight and body composition remained unchanged. A small, but statistically insignificant, increase occured in CD4+, CD8+, ratio, leukocytes and lymphocytes. The authors concluded two things. First, improved physical fitness resulted in an increase in physical reserves for the patients. Second, training did not have a negative effect on immune complexes studied. More data on the effect of training on HIV-1–positive patients is required, but these initial results certainly suggest the need for further research.

PREGNANCY

Pregnancy poses a unique dilemma, the competition between the exercising muscle and the fetus for a limited blood volume. There are questions about the risks and benefits to the mother, the fetoplacental unit, and the newborn. In addition, the interaction of pregnancy and exercise involves such a complex set of variables that research studies may be difficult to design and outcomes may not be detectable.[33]

The most obvious benefit of exercise during pregnancy is the maintenance of the fitness of the mother.[6,18,31-33] Other possible outcomes include labor facilitation, quicker recovery from birthing, improved emotional well-being, and improved lifestyle habits.[1]

Generally, if a woman is training and becomes pregnant, she can continue the training for a period of time. However, pregnancy is not the time to begin a training program.[56]

The American College of Sports Medicine[1] offers many suggestions regarding exercise and pregnancy: The frequency of exercise should be the typical 3 to 5 days per week with a duration of 15 to 30 minutes. Intensity should be monitored by the perceived exertion scale (Fig. 18-8)

Indications for discontinuing exercise during pregnancy*

Pain or bleeding
Dizziness or faintness
Pubic pain
Palpitations
Back pain
Rapid heart rates
Shortness of breath
Difficulty in walking

---

*From American College of Obstetricians and Gynecologists: *Exercise during pregnancy and postnatal period (ACOG) home exercise programs,* Washington, DC, 1985, ACOG.

rather than by heart rate because the maternal heart rate is elevated during pregnancy. Activities of choice include walking or weight-supporting exercises such as cycling or water-based programs. Whether weight training should be advised is still unknown. Extremes of heat (especially during the first trimester because of fear that hyperthermia might affect neural closure), humidity, hypoxia, or exercise duration should be avoided. For the training female, exercise in the first trimester should follow routine exercise prescription, including the avoidance of excessive heat. During the time when the risks of exercise are low, (second trimester), exercise can continue until discomfort requires a reduction in exercise duration or intensity. Third-trimester exercise usually decreases according to fatigue.

Certain conditions require special consideration (see the box above). Signs and symptoms (see the box above) may also force cessation of an exercise program. Although musculoskeletal complaints are frequent in the pregnant female, some evidence suggests a reduction in musculoskeletal problems during training.[5,6,31,33]

Risks of exercise include the concern of hyperthermia mentioned previously. In addition, there have been reports of varied fetal heart rates (absent medical intervention or birth abnormalities) in untrained women after exhaustive exercise.[5,26] What has received even less attention is the application of exercise in pregnant women with either co-existing disease or diseases particular to pregnancy.[31,33] In the absence of sound data, clinical judgment influences the physician in such cases.

CANCER

Epidemiologic reports point out that lifetime activity, whether occupational or recreational, can lower one's risk of colon or breast cancers.[58,61,63,157] Controlled studies are difficult because of the many factors associated with cancer. Any statements about the use of exercise in the prevention of cancer come from implications found in the epidemiologic literature.

The American College of Sports Medicine[1] offers suggestions regarding some mechanics in the use of exercise in cancer patients.

Before a patient begins an exercise program, functional capacity should be assessed through an exercise test. A low initial level of fitness is not uncommon. In addition, patients whose disease has metastasized to bone may need to be tested on a cycle for weight support.

Exercise intensity begins low (40% to 65% of heart rate reserve) and progresses according to patient tolerance. The clinical status of the patient governs frequency. Treatment regimens may require a more flexible approach to training days. Patients may have poor blood counts, IV solutions, fatigue, nausea, or malaise from treatments, or any number of limitations that would require postponing a training session. Weight training has been suggested to counter the muscle wasting sometimes seen in cancer patients. Low-intensity, high-repetition training using any of the commercial machines (for safety) is suggested. Serum enzymes are frequently used to follow the course of patients, and weight training elevates serum enzymes. Thus weight training should be avoided for at least 36 hours before venipuncture.

EXERCISE AND EMOTIONAL WELL-BEING

Improvement in emotional health is widely believed to be a benefit of physical training. Anecdotal evidence can be easily found to support better mental health. Executives say their efficiency and decision-making capacity are greater during training (Matzen, personal communication). Greenberg suggests that regular physical training "improves self-esteem, being perceived more positively by others, feeling more alert, having a better attitude toward work, decreased feelings of anxiety and being better able to manage stress."[73]

Stress management is frequently mentioned as a prime reason to pursue an exercise program. Whether stress reduction is in response to some biochemical alteration, such as a release of endorphins, or a sympathetic hormonal adaptation to physical or psychological stress, has not been conclusively demonstrated.[45] Bahrke and Morgan[8] have suggested that stress relief is a response to a "time-out" from the stressful environment. The elegant work of Dienstbier et al.[45] supports such a conclusion. However, some also suggest that the threshold for stress hormone release is raised (as noted by Dienstbier et al.), suggesting that stress levels previously perceived as grave would no longer be perceived as threatening. The influence of exercise on a variety of mental health dimensions seems to suggest that both short-term and long-term emotional well-being can be improved by training.

SUMMARY

Following a review of energy metabolism and the effect of training, the role of a physical conditioning program in improving function and the psychologic benefits of such a program (quality of life) are reviewed in those diseases where it is known to be of benefit.

REFERENCES

1. American College of Sports Medicine: *Guidelines for exercise testing and rehabilitation,* ed 4, Philadelphia, 1991, Lea and Febiger.
2. Andersen P: Capillary density in skeletal muscle of man, *Acta Physiol Scand* 95:203, 1975.
3. Andersen P, Henriksson J: Capillary supply of the quadriceps femoris muscle of man: adaptative response to exercise, *J Physiol (Lond)* 270:677, 1977.
4. Aniansson A, et al: Impaired muscle function with aging, *Clin Orthop Rel Res* 191:193, 1984.
5. Artral RM, MD Posner: Fetal responses to maternal exercise. In: *Exercise in pregnancy,* ed 2, Baltimore, 1991, Williams and Wilkins.
6. Artral RM, Wiswell RA, and Drinkwater B, editors: *Exercise in pregnancy,* ed 2, Baltimore, 1991, Williams and Wilkins.
7. Ayalon J, et al: Dynamic bone loading exercises for postmenopausal women: effect on the density of the distal radius, *Arch Phys Med Rehabil* 68:280, 1987.
8. Bahrke MS, Morgan WP: Anxiety reduction following exercise and meditation, *Cognitive Ther Res* 2:323, 1978.
9. Baldwin KM, et al: Glycolytic capacity of red, white and intermediate muscle: adaptive response to exercise, *Med Sci Sports* 4:50, 1972.
10. Barnard RJ, Edgerton V, and Peter J: Effects of exercise on skeletal muscle. I. Biochemical and histological properties, *J Appl Physiol* 28:762, 1970.
11. Bellman MJ, Mittman C: Ventilatory muscle training improves exercise capacity in chronic obstructive pulmonary disease patients, *Am Rev Respir Dis* 121:273, 1980.
12. Bernbaum M, et al: Cardiovascular conditioning in individual with diabetic retinopathy, *Diabetes Care* 12:740, 1989.
13. Bevier WC, Stefanik ML, and Wood PD: Bone density, aerobic capacity and body composition of moderately overweight adults (abstract), *Med Sci Sports Exerc* 20:s60, 1988.
14. Bevier WC, et al: Relationship of body composition, muscle strength and aerobic capacity to bone mineral density in older men and women, *J Bone Min Res* 4:421, 1989.

15. Blair SN, et al: Physical fitness and all cause mortality: a prospective study of healthy men and women, *JAMA* 262:2395, 1989.

16. Bogardus C, et al: Effects of physical training and diet therapy on carbohydrate metabolism in patients with glucose intolerance and non-insulin dependent diabetes mellitus, *Diabetes* 33:311, 1984.

17. Borensztajn J, et al: Effects of exercise on lipoprotein lipase activity in rat heart and skeletal muscle, *Am J Physiol* 229:394, 1975.

18. Brenner I, et al: Controlled prospective study of aerobic conditioning effects on pregnancy outcome (abstract), *Med Sci Sports Exerc* 23:S169, 1991.

19. Broadstone VL, et al: Diabetic peripheral neuropathy. Part I: sensorymotor neuropathy, *Diabetes Educ* 13:30, 1987.

20. Buck C, Donner AP: Isometric occupational exercise and the incidence of hypertension, *J Occup Med* 27:370, 1985.

21. Bylund AC, et al: Enzyme activities in skeletal muscles from patients with peripheral arterial insufficiency, *Europ J Clin Invest* 64:425, 1976.

22. Cade R, et al: Effect of aerobic exercise training on patients with systemic arterial hypertension, *Am J Med* 77:785, 1984.

23. Campaigne BN, et al: Effects of a physical activity program on metabolic control and cardiovascular fitness in children with insulin dependent diabetes mellitus, *Diabetes Care* 7:57, 1984.

24. Campaigne BN, Wallberg-Henriksson H, and Gunnarsson R: Glucose and insulin responses in relation to insulin dose and caloric intake 12 h after acute physical exercise in men with IDDM, *Diabetes Care* 10:716, 1987.

25. Carney RM, et al: Psychological effects of exercise training in hemodialysis patients, *Nephron* 33:179, 1983.

26. Carpenter MW, et al: Fetal heart rate response to maternal exertion, *JAMA* 259:3006, 1988.

27. Carswell H: BP spikes to 450/310 seen during weightlifting, *Medical Tribune*. Sept 14, p 33, 1983.

28. Cavanagh DJ, Cann CE: Brisk walking does not stop bone loss in postmenopausal women, *Bone* 9:201, 1988.

29. Chow RK, et al: Physical fitness effect on bone mass in postmenopausal women, *Arch Phys Med Rehabil* 67:231, 1986.

30. Clapp JF: Oxygen consumption during treadmill exercise before, during and after pregnancy, *Am J Obstet Gynecol* 161:1458, 1989.

31. Clapp JF: Exercise in pregnancy—a brief clinical review, *Fet Med Rev* 2:89, 1990.

32. Clapp JF, Capeless EL: The $V_{O_{2max}}$ of recreational athletes before and after pregnancy, *Med Sci Sports Exerc* 23:1128, 1991.

33. Clapp JF, et al: Exercise in pregnancy, *Med Sci Sports Exerc* 24:S294, 1992.

34. Clausen JP, Trap-Jensen J: Effects of training on the distribution of cardiac output in patients with coronary heart disease, *Circulation* 42:611, 1970.

35. Clement M, Jankowski LW, and Beaudry P: Prone immersion physical therapy in three children with cystic fibrosis: a pilot study, *Nurs Res* 28:325, 1979.

36. Cleroux J, Peronnet F, and DeChamplain J: Effects of exercise training on plasma catecholamines and blood pressure in labile hypertensive subjects, *Europ J Appl Physiol* 56:550, 1983.

37. Clifford PC, et al: Intermittent claudication: is a supervised exercise class worthwhile? *Br Med J* June, 1503, 1980.

38. Conner JF: Effects of exercise on coronary collateralization angiographic studies of six patients in a supervised exercise program, *Med Sci Sport* 8:145, 1976.

39. Costill DL, et al: Training adaptations in skeletal muscle of juvenile diabetics, *Diabetes* 28:818, 1979.

40. Costill DL, et al: Skeletal muscle enzymes and fiber composition in male and female track athletes, *J Appl Physiol* 40:149, 1976.

41. Dahllof A, et al: Metabolic activity of skeletal muscle in patients with peripheral arterial insufficiency. Effect of physical training, *Europ J Clin Invest* 4:9, 1974.

42. Dahl-Jorgensen K, et al: The effect of exercise on diabetic control and hemoglobin A1 (HbA1) in children, *Acta Paediatr Scand (suppl)* 283:53, 1980.

43. Dalsky G, Stocke KS, Eshani AA: Weight bearing exercise training and lumbar bone mineral content in postmenopausal women, *Ann Intern Med* 108:824, 1988.

44. Davis JA, et al: Anaerobic threshold alterations caused by endurance training in middle aged men, *J Appl Physiol* 46:1039, 1979.

45. Dienstbier RA, et al: Exercise and stress tolerance. In Sachs MH, Sachs ML, editors: Psychology of running, Champaign, Ill, 1981, Human Kinetics.

46. Drinkwater BL, et al: Bone mineral content of amenorrheic and eumenorrheic athletes, *N Engl J Med* 311:277, 1984.

47. Duncan JJ, et al: The effects of aerobic exercise on plasma catecholamines and blood pressure in patients with mild hypertension, *JAMA* 254:2609, 1985.

48. Ekblom B, et al: Effects of training on circulatory response to exercise, *Acta Physiol Scand* 24:518, 1968.

49. Ekblom B, Hermansen L: Cardiac output in athletes, *J Appl Physiol* 25:619, 1968.

50. Ekroth R, et al: Physical training of patients with intermittent claudication: indications, methods and results, *Surgery* 84:640, 1978.

51. Eriksson B, Gollnick P, and Saltin B: Muscle metabolism and enzyme activity after training in boys 11-13 years old, *Acta Physiol Scand* 87:485, 1973.

52. Ericsson B, Haeger K, and Lindall SE: Effect of physical training in intermittent claudication, *Angiology* 21:188-192, 1970.

53. Ferguson RJ: Effect of exercise capacity, collateral circulation and progression of coronary disease, *Am J Cardiol* 34:764, 1974.

54. Fiatarone MA, et al: High intensity strength training in nonagenarians: effect on skeletal muscle, *JAMA* 263:3029, 1990.

55. Foley WT: Treatment of gangrene of the feet and legs by walking, *Circulation* 15:689, 1957.

56. Fox EL, Bowers RW, and Foss ML: *Physiological basis of physical education and athletics,* ed 4, Dubuque, Iowa, 1988, William C. Brown Publishing.

57. Fox EL, McKenzie D, and Cohen K: Specificity of training: metabolic and circulatory responses, *Med Sci Sports* 7:83, 1975.

58. Frish RE, et al: Lower prevalence of breast cancer and cancers of reproductive system among former college athletes compared to non-athletes, *Br J Cancer* 52:885, 1985.

59. Galbo H: *Hormonal and metabolic adaptations to exercise,* Stuttgart, 1983, Georg Thieme Verlag.

60. Gallagher JC, Goldgar D, and Moy D: Total bone calcium in normal women: effect of age and menstrual status, *J Bone Mineral Res* 2:491, 1987.

61. Garabrant DH, et al: Job activity and colon cancer risk, *Am J Epidemiol* 119:1005, 1984.

62. Garcia MJ, et al: Morbidity and mortality in diabetics in the Framingham population: sixteen year follow-up study, *Diabetes* 23:105, 1974.

63. Garfinkel L, Stellman SD: Mortality by relative weight and exercise, *Cancer* 62:1844, 1988.

64. Gavin JR, et al: Endurance training improves insulin sensitivity in uremia, *Clin Res* 40:393, 1982.

65. Gilders RM, Voner C, and Dudley GA: Endurance training and blood pressure in normotensive and hypertensive adults, *Med Sci Sports Exerc* 21:629, 1989.

66. Goldberg AP, et al: Exercise training reduces coronary risk and effectively rehabilitates dialysis patients, *Nephron* 42:311, 1986.

67. Goldberg AP, Geltman EM, and Hagberg JM: The therapeutic effects of exercise training for hemodialysis patients, *Kidney Int* (suppl 24):S303, 1983.

68. Goldstein D: Clinical applications for exercise, Phys Sportsmedicine 17(8):83, 1989.

69. Gollnick PD, et al: Effect of training on enzyme activity and fiber composition of human skeletal muscle, *J Appl Physiol* 34:107, 1973.

70. Gollnick PD, et al: Enzyme activity and fiber composition in skeletal muscle of trained and untrained men, *J Appl Physiol* 33:312, 1972.

71. Gollnick PD, King D: Effects of exercise and training on mitochondria of rat skeletal muscle, *Am J Physiol* 216:1502, 1969.

72. Graham C, Lasko-McCarthy P: Exercise options for persons with diabetic complications, *Diabetes Educator* 16:212, 1990.

73. Greenberg JS: Comprehensive stress management, ed 3, Dubuque, Iowa, 1990, William C. Brown Publishing.

74. Greene MC, et al: Effect of exercise on lipid metabolism and dietary intake in hemodialysis patients, *Proc Dialysis Transplant Forum* 9:80, 1979.

75. Grimby G, Haggendal E, and Saltin B: Local xenon clearance from the quadriceps muscle during exercise in man, *J Appl Physiol* 22:305, 1967.

76. Hagberg JM, et al: Exercise training improves hypertension in hemodialysis patients, *Am J Nephrol* 3:209, 1983.

77. Harris RA, Holly RG: Physiological responses to circuit weight training in borderline hypertensive subjects, *Med Sci Sports Exerc* 19:246, 1987.

78. Harter HR, Goldberg AP: Endurance exercise training: an effective therapeutic modality for hemodialysis patients, *Med Clin North Am* 69:159, 1978.

79. Haskell WL: Exercise induced changes in lipids and lipoprotein levels, *Postgrad Med* 13:23, 1984.

80. Haskell WL: Coronary heart disease. In Skinner JS, editor: Exercise testing and exercise prescription for special cases. Theoretical basis and clinical application. Philadelphia, 1987, Lea and Febiger.

81. Henrikson J, et al: Enzyme activities, fiber types and capillarization in calf muscle of patients with intermittent claudication, *Scand J Clin Lab Invest* 40:361, 1980.

82. Hoeppeler H, et al: The ultrastructure of the normal human skeletal muscle: a morphological analysis on untrained men, women and orienteers, *Pflugers Arch* 344:217, 1973.

83. Holbrook TL, Barrett-Connor E, and Wingard DL: The association of lifetime weight and weight control patterns with diabetes among men and women in an adult community, *Int J Obesity* 13:723, 1989.

84. Holloszy JO: Effects of exercise on mitochondrial oxygen uptake and respiratory enzyme activity in skeletal muscle, *J Biol Chem* 242:2278, 1967.

85. Holmgren A: Cardiovascular determinants of cardiovascular fitness, *Can Med Assoc J* 96:697, 1967.

86. Horton ES: Role and management of exercise in diabetes mellitus, *Diabetes Care* 11:201, 1988.

87. Hubinger A, Franzen A, Gries FA: Hormonal and metabolic response to physical exercise in hyperinsulinemic and non-hyperinsulinemic type 2 diabetes, *Diabetes Care* 4:57, 1987.

88. Hurley BF, et al: Resistive training can reduce coronary risk factors without altering Vo_{2max} or percent body fat, *Med Sci Sports Exerc* 20:150, 1988.

89. Huttunen NP, et al: Effect of a once a week training program on physical fitness and metabolic control in children with IDDM, *Diabetes Care* 12:737, 1989.

90. Jankowski LW: Cystic fibrosis. In Skinner JS, editor: *Exercise testing and exercise prescription for special cases*, Philadelphia, 1987, Lea and Febiger.

91. Jenkins AB, et al: Regulation of hepatic glucose output during moderate exercise in non-insulin dependent diabetes, *Metabolism* 37:966, 1988.

92. Johnson T: Age-related differences in isometric and dynamic strength and endurance, *Physiol Ther* 62:985, 1982.

93. Jones NL: Pulmonary gas exchange during exercise in patients with chronic airway obstruction, *Clin Sci* 31:39, 1966.

94. Jones NL: Chronic obstructive respiratory disease. In Skinner JS, editor: *Exercise testing and exercise prescription for special cases*. Philadelphia, 1987, Lea & Febiger.

95. Joslin EP, Root HF, and White P, editors: The treatment of diabetes mellitus, Philadelphia, 1959, Lea & Febiger.

96. Karlsson J, et al: Muscle lactate, ATP and CP levels during exercise after physical training in man, *J Appl Physiol* 33:199, 1972.

97. Karlsson J, Nordesjo L, and Saltin B: Muscle glycogen utilization during exercise after physical training, *Acta Physiol Scand* 90:210, 1974.

98. Keens T: Ventilatory muscle endurance training in normal subjects and patient with cystic fibrosis, *Am Rev Respir Dis* 116:853, 1977.

99. Kemmer FW, Berger M: Therapy and better quality of life: the dichotomous role of exercise in diabetes mellitus, *Diabetes Metab Rev* 2:53, 1986.

100. Kentala E: Physical fitness and feasibility of physical rehabilitation after myocardial infarction in men of working age, *Ann Clin Res* 9(suppl):1, 1972.

101. Kiyonaga A, et al: Blood pressure and hormonal responses to aerobic exercise, *Hypertension* 7:125, 1985.

102. Kjellberg S, Rudhe U, and Sjostrand T: Increase in the amount of hemoglobin and blood volume in connection with physical training, *Acta Physiol Scand* 19:146, 1949.

103. Klassen G, Andrew G, and Becklake M: Effect of training on total and regional blood flow and metabolism in paddlers, *J Appl Physiol* 28:397, 1970.

104. Krotkiewski M, et al: The effects of physical training on insulin secretion and effectiveness on glucose metabolism in obesity and type 2 (non-insulin dependent) diabetes mellitus, *Diabetologia* 28:881, 1985.

105. Lampman RM, et al: The influence of physical training on glucose tolerance, insulin sensitivity and lipid and lipoprotein concentrations in middle-aged hypertriglyceridaemic carbohydrate intolerant men, *Diabetologia* 30:380, 1987.

106. Landt KW, et al: Effects of exercise training on insulin sensitivity in adolescents with type I diabetes mellitus, *Diabetes Care* 8:461, 1985.

107. Larsen OA, Lassen NA: Effect of daily muscular exercise in patients with intermittent claudication, *Lancet* Nov 19, 1966, 1093, 1966.

108. Lesmes GR, et al: Metabolic responses of females to high intensity interval training of different frequencies, *Med Sci Sports* 10:229, 1978.

109. Lewicki RH, et al: Effect of physical exercise on some parameters of immunity in conditioned sportsmen, *Int J Sports Med* 8:309, 1987.

110. Macdougall D, Magel J, Andersen K: Pulmonary diffusing capacity and cardiac output in young trained Norwegian swimmers and untrained subjects, *Med Sci Sports* 1:131, 1969.

111. Marcus R, et al: Menstrual function and bone mass in elite women distance runners: endocrine metabolic features, *Ann Intern Med* 102:158, 1985.

112. McArdle WD, Katch FI, and Katch VL: *Exercise physiology: energy, nutrition and human performance,* ed 3, Philadelphia, 1992, Lea and Febiger.

113. MacLaren DP, et al: A review of metabolic and physiological factors in fatigue, *Exerc Sports Sci Rev* 17:29, 1989.

114. Meema HE, Meema S: Cortical bone mineral density versus cortical thickness in the diagnosis of osteoporosis: a roentgenological-densitometric study, *J Am Geriatr Soc* 17:120, 1969.

115. Minuk HL, et al: Glucoregulatory and metabolic response to exercise in obese non-insulin dependent diabetes, *Am J Physiol* 240:E458, 1981.

116. Mogensen CE: Reduced progression of diabetic nephropathy by controlling hypertension, *Pract Cardiol* 9:156,

117. Mole P, Oscai L, and Holloszy J: Adaptations of muscle to exercise: increase in levels of palmityl CoA synthetase, carnitine palm-

ityltransferases and palmityl CoA dehydrogenase and in the capacity to oxidize fatty acid, *J Clin Invest* 50:2323, 1971.

118. Morgan T, et al: Effects of long-term exercise on human muscle mitochondria. In Pernow B, Saltin B, editors: *Muscle metabolism during exercise,* New York, 1971, Plenum Press.

119. Neff TA, Petty TL: Long-term continuous oxygen therapy in chronic airway obstruction, *Ann Intern Med* 72:621, 1970.

120. Nelson ME, Meredith CN, and Dawson-Hughes B: Hormone and bone mineral status in endurance-trained and sedentary postmenopausal women, *J Clin Endocrinol* 66:927, 1988.

121. Nicholas JJ, et al: Evaluation of an exercise therapy program for patients with chronic obstructive pulmonary disease, *Am Rev Respir Dis* 102:1, 1970.

122. Paez PN et al: The physiologic basis of training patients with chronic airway obstruction. I. Effects of exercise training, *Am Rev Respir Dis* 95:944, 1967.

123. Painter PL: Participation in exercise training during hemodialysis: a multicenter trial program (abstract), *Med Sci Sports Exerc* 19:s19, 1987.

124. Painter PL: Exercise in end stage renal disease, *Exerc Sports Sci Rev* 16:305, 1988.

125. Painter PL, et al: Effects of exercise training during hemodialysis, *Nephron* 43:87, 1986.

126. Paternostro-Bayles M, Wing RR, and Robertson RJ: Effect of lifestyle activity of varying duration on glycemic control in type II diabetic women, *Diabetes Care* 12:34, 1989.

127. Pocock N, et al: Muscle strength, physical fitness and weight but not age predict femoral neck bone mass, *J Bone Mineral Res* 4:441, 1989.

128. Pollack ML, Wilmore JH, and Fox SM: *Exercise in health and disease* Philadelphia, 1984, WB Saunders.

129. Rechnitzer P: Relation of exercise to the recurrence rate of myocardial infarction in men: the Ontario exercise-heart collaborative study, *Am J Cardiol* 51:65, 1983.

130. Rigsby LW, et al: Effects of exercise training on men seropositive for the human immunodeficiency virus-1, *Med Sci Sports* 24:6, 1992.

131. Robertson WB, Strong JP: Atherosclerosis in persons with hypertension and diabetes mellitus, *Lab Invest* 18:538, 1968.

132. Rowland TW, et al: Glycemic control with physical training in insulin dependent diabetes mellitus, *Am J Dis Child* 139:307, 1985.

133. Saltin B: Physiological effects of physical training, *Med Sci Sports* 1:50, 1969.

134. Saubert C, et al: Anaerobic enzyme adaptations to sprint training in rats, *Pflugers Arch* 341:30, 1973.

135. Seals DR, Hagberg JM: The effect of exercise training on human hypertension; a review, *Med Sci Sports Exerc* 16:207, 1984.

136. Shalom R, et al: Feasibility and benefits of exercise training in patients on maintenance dialysis, *Kidney Int* 25:958, 1984.

137. Shaw L: Effects of a prescribed supervised exercise program on mortality and cardiovascular morbidity inpatients after myocardial infarction, *Am J Cardiol* 48:39, 1981.

138. Sigviardsson K, Svanfeldt E, and Kilbom A: Role of the adrenergic nervous system in the development of training induced bradycardia, *Acta Physiol Scand* 101:481, 1977.

139. Sim DN, Neill WA: Investigation of the physiological basis for increased exercise threshold for angina pectoris after physical conditioning, *J Clin Invest* 54:346, 1974.

140. Sinaki M, Mikkelsen BA: Postmenopausal spinal osteoporosis: flexion versus extension exercises, *Arch Phys Med Rehabil* 65:593, 1984.

141. Sinaki M, Offord K: Physical activity in postmenopausal women: effect on back muscle strength and bone mineral density of the spine, *Arch Phys Med Rehabil* 69:277, 1988.

142. Skarfors ET, et al: Physical training as treatment for type II (non-insulin dependent) diabetes in elderly men: a feasibility study over two years, *Diabetologia* 30:930, 1987.

143. Skinner JS: *Exercise testing and exercise prescription for special cases. Theoretical basis and clinical application,* Philadelphia, 1987, Lea and Febiger.

144. Skinner JS, Strandness E: Exercise and intermittent claudication. II. Effect of physical training, *Circulation* 36:23, 1967.

145. Smith EL, et al: Deterring bone loss by exercise intervention in premenopausal and postmenopausal women, *Calc Tiss Int* 44:312, 1989.

146. Smith EL, Redden W, and Smith PE: Physical activity and calcium modalities for bone mineral increase in aged women, *Med Sci Sports Exerc* 13:60, 1981.

147. Smith EL, et al: Bone involution decrease in exercising middle-aged women, *Calc Tiss Int* 36:S129, 1984.

148. Snow-Harter C, et al: Muscle strength as an indicator of bone mineral density in young women, *J Bone Mineral Res* 5:589, 1990.

149. Snow-Harter C, Marcus R: Exercise, bone mineral density and osteoporosis, *Exerc Sport Sci Rev* 19:351, 1991.

150. Sorlie D, Myhre K: Effect of physical training in intermittent claudication, *Scand J Clin Invest* 38:217, 1978.

151. Squires RW, et al: Early exercise testing and training after renal transplantation (abstract), *Med Sci Sports Exerc* 17:184, 1985.

152. Temoshak L, et al: Intensive psychoimmunologic study of men with AIDS (abstract), Proceedings, Third International Conference on AIDS, Washington, DC, 1987.

153. Thompson PD: Modest changes in high-density lipoprotein concentration with prolonged exercise training, *Circulation* 78:25, 1988.

154. Tipton CM: Exercise, training and hypertension, *Exerc Sport Sci Rev* 12:245,

155. Tipton CM: Exercise, training and hypertension: an update, *Exerc Sport Sci Rev* 19:447, 1991.

156. Tipton CM, et al: The influence of physical activity on ligaments and tendons, *Med Sci Sports* 7:165, 1975.

157. Vena JE, et al: Lifetime occupational exercise and colon cancer, *Am J Epidemiol* 122:457, 1985.

158. Verani M: Effects of exercise training on left ventricular performance and myocardial perfusion in patients with coronary artery disease, *Am J Cardiol* 47:797, 1981.

159. Verity LS, Ismail AH: Effects of exercise on cardiovascular disease risk in women with NIDDM, *Diabetes Res Clin Pract* 6:27, 1989.

160. Vitug A, Schneider SH, Ruderman NB: Exercise and type I diabetes mellitus, *Exerc Sports Sci Rev* 16:285, 1988.

161. Vyas MN, et al: Response to exercise in patients with chronic airway obstruction, *Am Rev Respir Dis* 103:401, 1971.

162. Vyas MN, et al: Response to exercise in patients with chronic airway obstruction. I. Effects of exercise training, *Am Rev Respir Dis* 103:390, 1971.

163. Wahren J, et al: Glucose metabolism during leg exercise in man, *J Clin Invest* 50:2715, 1971.

164. Wahren J, Hagenfeldt L, and Felig P: Splanchnic and leg exchange of glucose, amino acids and free fatty acids during exercise in diabetes mellitus, *J Clin Invest* 55:1303, 1975.

165. Wallberg-Henriksson H: Exercise and diabetes mellitus, *Exerc Sport Sci Rev* 20:339, 1992.

166. Wallberg-Henriksson H, et al: Increased peripheral insulin sensitivity and muscle mitochondrial enzymes but unchanged blood glucose control in type I after physical training, *Diabetes* 31:1044, 1982.

167. Wasserman DH, Abumrad NN: Physiological bases for the treatment of the physically active individual with diabetes, *Sports Med* 7:376, 1989.

168. White MK, et al: The effects of exercise on the bones of postmenopausal women, *Int Orthop* 7:209, 1984.

169. Wiley RL, et al: Isometric exercise training lowers resting blood pressure, *Med Sci Sports Exerc* 24:749, 1992.

170. Wilhelmsen L: A controlled trial of physical training after myocardial infarction: effects on risk factors, nonfatal reinfarction and death, *Prev Med* 4:491, 1975.

171. Williams JA, et al: The effect of long distance running on appendicular bone mineral content, *Med Sci Sports Exerc* 16:223, 1984.

172. Wilson PK, Fardy PS, and Froelicher VF: *Cardiac rehabilitation, adult fitness and exercise testing,* Philadelphia, 1981, Lea and Febiger.

173. Wing RR: Behavioral strategies for weight reduction in obese type II diabetic patients, *Diabetes Care* 12:139, 1989.

174. Wood R, Boat T, and Doershuk C: Cystic fibrosis, *Am Rev Respir Dis* 113:833, 1976.

175. Yki-Jarvinen H, et al: Site of insulin resistance in type I diabetes: insulin-mediated glucose disposal in vivo in relation to insulin binding and action in adipocytes in vitro, *J Clin Endocrinol Metab* 59:1183, 1984.

176. Zander E, et al: Muscular exercise in type I diabetics. 1. Different metabolic reactions during heavy muscular work in dependence on actual insulin availability, *Exp Clin Endocrinol* 82:78, 1985.

177. Zinman B, et al: Glucoregulation during moderate exercise in insulin treated diabetics, *J Clin Endocrinol Metab* 46:641, 1977.

RESOURCES

American College of Sports Medicine: *Guidelines for exercise testing and rehabilitation,* ed 4, Philadelphia, 1991, Lea and Febiger.

Blair SN, et al: Physical fitness and all cause mortality: a prospective study of healthy men and women, *JAMA* 262:2395, 1989.

Fox EL, Bowers RW, Foss ML: Physiological basis of physical education and athletics, ed 4, Dubuque, Iowa, 1988, Wm C. Brown Publishing.

Galbo H: *Hormonal and metabolic adaptations to exercise,* Stuttgart, 1983, Georg Thieme Verlag.

McArdle WD, Katch FI, and Katch VL: *Exercise physiology: energy, nutrition and human performance,* ed 3, Philadelphia, 1992, Lea and Febiger.

Pollack ML, Wilmore JH, and Fox SM: *Exercise in health and disease,* Philadelphia, 1984, WB Saunders.

Skinner JS: *Exercise testing and exercise prescription for special cases. Theoretical basis and clinical application,* Philadelphia, 1987, Lea and Febiger.

Wilson PK, Fardy PS, and Froelicher VF: *Cardiac rehabilitation, adult fitness and exercise testing,* Philadelphia, 1981, Lea and Febiger.

Chapter 19

A PROGRAM FOR FITNESS

Donald T. Kirkendall

P.O. Astrand[4] quoted Starling as saying, "The physiology of today is the medicine of tomorrow." Research into the physical and psychologic benefits of consistent physical exercise supports both the health- and fitness-related benefits of physical training. As such the physician of today must be well versed in not only the benefits of exercise, but also the details of prescribing exercise programs to their patients. *Because many patients have a great deal of knowledge about exercise, the physician is expected to be knowledgeable, an example to patients, and a motivator.* Exercise suggestions depend on the patient's health status, goals, interests, and available resources.

When the physician or the patient broaches the topic of an exercise program, the question in both minds is, "How much exercise is needed?" A more telling question lurking in the background is, "What is the least that can be done to realize a benefit?" This chapter is designed to describe the logic behind the "exercise prescription" as well as some of the expected benefits of compliance to such a program.

The exercise prescription is an interplay of four variables: frequency (days/week), intensity, time (minutes/session), and type (selection of exercise mode). The common acronym is FITT. A fifth variable often neglected but no less important, is rate of progression; the speed at which one advances in training. The most recent review of the topic[1] served as the basis for this summary.

Physical fitness is an "umbrella" term that encompasses such variables as cardiorespiratory endurance, muscular strength and endurance, agility, power, body composition, and flexibility. Improvements in the above will improve one's "physical fitness." The most commonly measured variable is the maximal aerobic capacity, the body's maximal rate of consuming oxygen (Vo_2max). Reduction in risk factors of selected diseases of lifestyle have been linked to improvement in Vo_2max.

Vo_2max will improve with increases in exercise fre-

quency, intensity, time, or various combinations. One can expect increases of 5% to 30%[1] when the principles of the exercise prescription are followed, with 15% being a very reasonable expectation.[1] Increases in Vo_2max above these are typically due to low level of initial fitness and poor motivation or technique that lead to artificially low initial values. In addition, people who have undergone weight loss will show greater gains because Vo_2max is a weight-corrected figure. Genetic predisposition must be considered, as there appears to be a limit for the adaptation to physical training.[34]

FREQUENCY

When sedentary individuals begin a training program, the assumption is that their exercise frequency is zero days/week. Will exercising 1 day/week improve their endurance? Currently, the data suggest that training less than 2 days/week (while following the criteria for intensity and duration) has little effect on improving Vo_2max.[15,21,47,58,61] Training for 3 to 5 days per week, however, does show improvements in endurance consistent with those previously mentioned. The improvements tend to plateau at this frequency.[21,47,51] Should the frequency be increased to 6 or 7 days/week, improvements in performance are seen, but not as a result of further increases in Vo_2max.[42,47] Training frequencies of 6 to 7 days/week invite hazards (overuse injuries) that can be avoided.

INTENSITY AND TIME

Training intensity and duration are inversely related; that is, the more intense the exercise, the less time that it can be maintained. In addition, the total amount of work appears to be important to fitness improvements. As a result, if the total amount of work remains constant, long-duration, low-intensity training will result in degrees of improvement similar to shorter-duration, higher-intensity training.[1] If that is the case, would not the shorter time investment be the more desirable? The answer is probably no, because higher-intensity programs are related to reduced compliance[16,41,48,55] as well as increased cardiovascular[60] (see Chapter 20) and orthopedic[48,51] risks (see Chapter 20). To minimize the risks to the patient, low-to-moderate intensity training programs of longer duration (20 to 60 minutes per session) are most commonly undertaken.

Training intensity

Probably the most difficult variable to determine is the intensity of training. This is because there is the perception in the mind of the average patient and physician that a highly sophisticated technical exercise test, such as a treadmill stress test, is required before an appropriate training intensity can be prescribed. Although the scientific literature uses expired gases to document training changes, using such equipment would most likely be considered excessive in prescribing an exercise program. Details on the various methods for determining intensity are outlined below.

The minimum training level necessary to achieve an improvement in Vo_2max is suggested to be 60% of Vo_2max, or 50% of the heart rate reserve (maximum heart rate minus resting heart rate).[31] Working at levels below this minimum may still improve endurance. Large improvements in endurance are seen when one exercises between roughly 60% and 85% Vo_2max, but improvements plateau somewhat at levels above 85% of Vo_2max. This sigmoid curve (Fig. 19-1) suggests that light intensities result in small improvements, but moderate intensity results in great changes for small increases in effort. High-intensity efforts should probably be left for competitive athletes, because the additional improvements are minimal. This figure is modified in Table 19-1 to summarize the primary methods of determining intensity of effort.

It is well known that maximum heart rate response to exercise is reduced as one ages (Table 19-2). Thus the use of a set minimum exercise heart rate would result in differ-

The Exercise Prescription

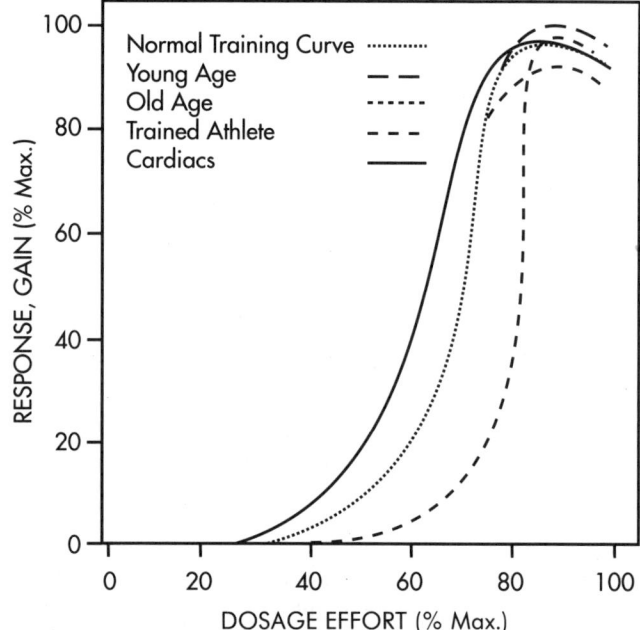

Fig. 19-1. Improvement anticipated from effort expended. A conceptual diagram illustrating training curves in various populations. Note that higher levels of fitness ("trained athlete") require higher exercise intensities. Also, note that age of onset of training affects the maximal physiologic gain. (From Wilson PK, Fardy PS, Froelicher VF: *Cardiac rehabilitation, adult fitness and exercise testing,* Philadelphia, 1981, Lea & Febiger.)

ing percentages of heart rate reserve for individuals of different ages. In addition, individuals taking beta adrenergic blocking agents would have a significantly lower exercising pulse rate,[62] *so a method that does not use heart rate might be better for such patients (see below).* Initial level of training also influences exercise intensity,[13,32,40,57] as a person with a low initial fitness level might realize improvements at 40% to 50% of Vo_2max. Those with higher initial fitness levels would require a higher training intensity.[58,61]

Table 19-1. Exercise intensity classification for 20 to 60 minutes of endurance exercise

Maximal HR	Maximal Vo_2 or HR reserve	Rating of perceived exertion (20-pt. scale)	Rating of perceived exertion (10-pt. scale)	Classification of intensity
<35%	<30%	<10	1	Very light
35-59%	30-49%	10-11	2	Light (fairly light)
60-79%	50-74%	12-13	3-4	Moderate (somewhat hard)
80-89%	75-84%	14-16	5	Heavy (hard)
>90%	>85%	>16	>6	Very heavy (very hard)

Modified from American College of Sports Medicine: The recommended quantity and quality of exercise for developing and maintaining cardiovascular and muscular fitness in healthy adults, *Med Sci Sports* 22:265, 1990.

Table 19-2. Estimated maximal heart rate response and confidence interval limits by age

Age	Estimated maximal heart rate	95% confidence limits
20	200	170-220
30	190	160-220
40	180	150-210
50	170	140-200
60	160	130-190
70	150	120-180

Modified from Wilson PK, Fardy PS, and Froelicher VF: *Cardiac rehabilitation, adult fitness and exercise testing,* Philadelphia, 1981, Lea & Febiger.

Determining the exercise intensity

As intensity is a key feature of the exercise prescription, accurate determination of this variable has garnered a great deal of attention, which has led to a variety of methods for its determination.

As a percentage of Vo₂max. If the gold standard of endurance is the maximum oxygen consumption, the training intensity also would be verified this way. To use Vo₂max this way requires expensive equipment that is probably not available to many practitioners. Computerized equipment that measures the volume of air breathed and fractions of expired air that are oxygen and carbon dioxide is required and may be available only in a cardiopulmonary laboratory. This method also requires the subject to wear a mouthpiece or face mask for gas collection purposes, which reduces patient comfort (Fig. 19-2). Once the Vo₂max has been established, the subject would have to exercise using the chosen type of activity and the same gas systems to determine the workload that would elicit the desired percentage of Vo₂max. The extra precision is gained at the expense of patient time, comfort, and effort, and technical requirements. Other methods, although only minimally less accurate, afford reasonable assurances of appropriate training intensity.

Percentage of maximal heart rate response. There are two ways to use maximal heart rate response. The first is to estimate maximal heart rate response based on the standard equation (220 minus age). This method is widely used in the popular press and commercial health clubs. One then needs only to multiply this figure by the desired training intensity (between 60% and 85%, but use a decimal such as .6 or .85) to determine a training heart rate. Obvious problems arise when the patient is on beta adrenergic blocking agents. A second way is to use the maximal heart rate determined from a maximal exercise test. This improves accuracy, as the age-related reduction in maximal heart rate has a variation of about ±15 beats (Table 19-2).[64] Therefore the maximal heart rate of 66% of a 50-

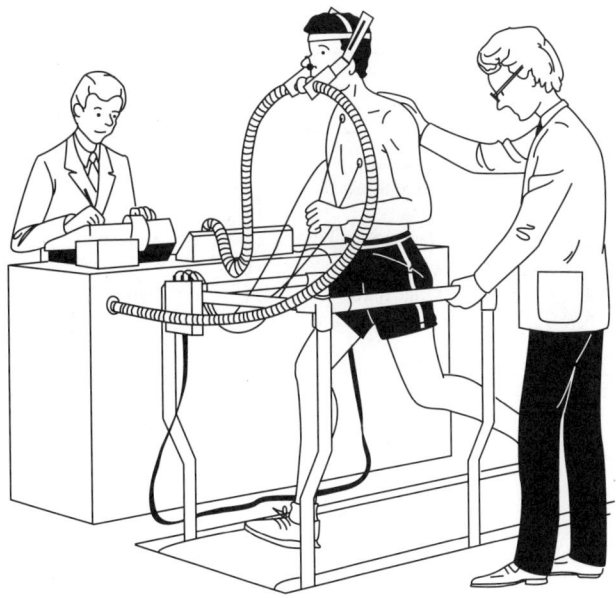

Fig. 19-2. Measuring aerobic capacity during an exercise tolerance test. (From Getchell LH, *Physical fitness: a way of life,* ed 3, New York, 1985, Macmillan.)

year-old patient would be between 155 and 185. Given this variability, a maximal heart rate determined from an exercise test is more desirable than an estimated heart rate, especially if the patient is on beta adrenergic blocking agents. In any case, using an estimated or known maximal heart rate gives a fairly conservative estimate of training intensity.

Percentage of heart rate reserve. The popular Karvonen[31] method narrows the training range by using a fraction of the heart rate reserve (HRmax minus HRrest) and adds it to the resting heart rate. The choice of an estimated or a known maximal heart rate should be influenced by the clinical condition of the patient. Training ranges are typically offered to the patient as a minimal and maximal desired training heart rate. The patient must then be instructed in the method and timing of taking a manual immediate postexercise pulse rate. Some patients may have access to commercial pulse rate meters, but acceptance of their universal accuracy is naive. Thus the patient needs to know *how* to take his or her own pulse rate. The timing is critical, as the exercise pulse rate declines rapidly in recovery, so the patient needs to start counting the pulse rate in the first seconds after exercise. Also to consider is the error one can make in taking a manual pulse rate. If the patient is taking a pulse for 6 seconds and he or she misses one beat, the patient made a 10 beat/minute error.

Rating of perceived exertion. A common and easily obtained figure during an exercise test is the rating of perceived exertion[15] (see Table 19-3). This scale uses a series of perceptual key words in response to the question, "How hard is the exercise?" The patient responds with a number

Table 19-3. Perceived exertion scales

10-point scale	Key word	20-point scale	Key word
0	Nothing at all	6	
0.5	Just noticeable	7	Very, very light
1	Very light	8	
2	Light	9	Very light
3	Moderate	10	
4	Somewhat hard	11	Fairly light
5	Hard	12	
6		13	Somewhat hard
7	Very hard	14	
8		15	Hard
9		16	
10	Very, very hard	17	Very hard
	Maximal	18	
		19	Very, very hard
		20	

From Borg GAV: Psychophysical basis of perceived exertion, *Med Sci Sports Exerc* 14:377, 1982.

Table 19-4. Hypothetical exercise test data from a 45-year-old male

Stage	Load (mph, % elevation)	Time (min)	HR	BP	RPE
A.					
Pretest			74	122/78	
I	3.5, 0%	0-2	112	136/80	2
II	3.5, 5%	3-4	135	150/76	3
III	3.5, 10%	5-6	154	168/74	5
IV	3.5, 15%	7-8	165	184/78	7
V	3.5, 17.5%	9-10	169	193/82	8
VI	3.5, 20%	11-12	172	204/80	10
B. 45-year-old male on a beta-adrenergic blocking agent					
Pretest			64	132/86	
I	3.5, 0%	0-2	82	138/84	1
II	3.5, 5%	3-4	106	144/88	2
III	3.5, 10%	5-6	117	154/84	3
IV	3.5, 15%	7-8	138	160/82	5
V	3.5, 17.5%	9-10	142	164/86	8
VI	3.5, 20%	11-12	147	170/84	10

Table 19-5. Training heart rates by various methods

Method	Resting HR	Maximal HR	60%	85%
A. For the normal male in Table 19-4, A				
% Estimated HRmax	n/a	175	105	149
% HRmax	n/a	172	103	146
% HR reserve	74	172	133	157
B. For the male on beta adrenergic blocking agents in Table 19-4, B				
% Estimated HRmax	n/a	175	105	149
% HRmax	n/a	147	88	125
% HR reserve	64	147	114	135

that corresponds to the appropriate key word. The training intensity typically relates to "moderate" to "hard" (or "heavy") intensities of exercise. The scale can be used two ways. First, the physician can see what heart rate corresponded to the above key words and use those heart rates as the training ranges. Second, simply abandon the use of heart rates altogether and just use the perceived exertion. (This may well be the method of choice for patients on beta adrenergic blockade.) Have the patient exercise to their interpretation of the key words "moderate" to "hard" (or "heavy"). This method is effective in confirming training intensity.[11,51]

An example. Consider Table 19-4, which details the results of two hypothetical exercise tests. Table 19-4, *A* is data from a normal individual and Table 19-4, *B* is from a person on a beta adrenergic blocking agent. Table 19-5 shows the differing methods of determining intensity. Notice that in the normal individual, the training range becomes narrowed by use of the percentage of heart rate reserve, suggesting that using an estimated HRmax gives a wider training range. In the case of the patient on the beta blocker, use of an estimated HRmax results in prescribing a training heart rate that exceeds the known maximal rate. Thus, when one is on medication that influences cardiac function, it is best to know the actual cardiac response. Any change in medication would necessitate reestablishing training ranges.

The decision to test. The previous discussion emphasizes that a known HRmax is more desirable than an estimated HRmax. Requiring an exercise test is based on the expectations for such a test. Generally there are two reasons for requesting an exercise test. First is to determine whether there are any underlying cardiovascular problems that might be uncovered by performing a stress test on an asymptomatic patient. The second is to determine a patient's functional capacity (level of fitness).[2]

Is the stress test sensitive (at finding the percentage of true positives) and specific (at finding true negatives) enough to make ordering one worthwhile? The stress test is generally thought to have a sensitivity of 66% to 75% and a specificity of up to 85% or above.[51,64] The likelihood of a patient having or not having coronary disease can be estimated from Fig. 19-3.[19] If, for example, based on history, physical, and risk factors, you estimate that a patient has about a 30% chance of having coronary disease, then assume that the stress test results indicate a negative test (<1 mm ST segment depression), enter the graph at the pretest likelihood (30%), move up to the dotted line, and determine that the posttest likelihood is less than 10%. If the test is positive by 2 to 2.49 mm ST segment depression, determine that the posttest likelihood is around 80%. In either case, more is known after the stress test than before.

In a survey of nearly 2000 cases over a 2-year period in

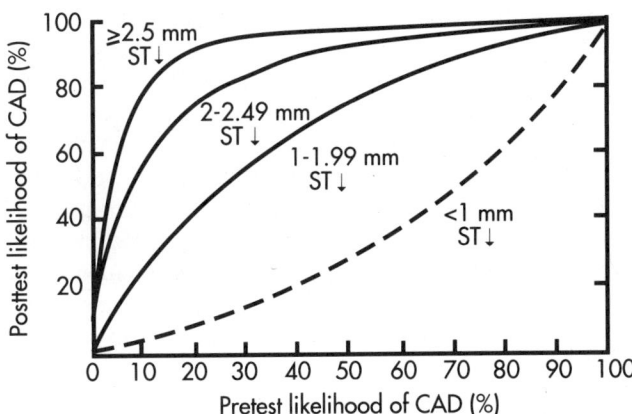

Fig. 19-3. Family of ST-segment depression curves (based on data derived from Diamond and Forrester) and likelihood of coronary artery disease (CAD). *ST*, ST-segment depression. (From Epstein SE: Implications of probability analysis on the strategy used for noninvasive detection of coronary artery disease, *Am J Cardiol* 46:491, 1980.)

patients over 40 years of age, only 25 males (1.3%) and 1 female (0.3%) were found to have coronary artery disease.[18] Age was the primary reason for ordering the test in this sample. Based on the clinical yield, the authors suggested that stress tests (for the detection of underlying coronary disease) be performed on males once while in their 40s, twice in their 50s, and every other year in their 60s. The recommendations for females were delayed by 1 decade, with a recommendation for a stress test on any patient with chest pain. Finally, they suggested that patients older than 40 who wish to undertake an exercise program should also have a stress test. This study is consistent with the American Heart Association guidelines with respect to the age criteria for a stress test. The American College of Sports Medicine[2] is more conservative and recommends 35 as the minimum age.

Another reason for considering an exercise test is to detect and evaluate dysrythmias. Clinically, a dysrythmia is most likely to occur immediately after exercise. Dysrythmias thought to be benign at rest may need to be observed under exercise stress.

The final decision about ordering a stress test is based on the expectations for the test. For asymptomatic individuals with minimal risk factors, the diagnostic yield (in terms of positive tests) will probably be minimal.[18] Yet the benefits of learning the posttest likelihood of coronary disease based on a negative test, obtaining a known maximal heart rate for prescribing intensity, and documenting a change in functional capacity (and thereby motivating the patient) might be reasons enough for ordering a stress test.

TYPE OF EXERCISE

The patient should enjoy the activity (or activities) chosen. If he or she does not, compliance is in question. As all patients have very busy schedules, the enjoyment factor weighs heavily on the decision to continue exercising. A period of time needs to be scheduled into the day, like any other appointment. Typically there are three times of the day to exercise: before the day begins, during the work day, and after the work day. Although each has advantages and disadvantages, few external factors limit exercise before the work day begins. This applies to exercise at home as well as when travelling. Although the choice of activities may be varied while at home, the opportunity to walk is available regardless of hotel facilities. In addition, some clinical common sense is needed when suggesting exercises. For example, low back pain or orthopedic problems of the legs would limit jogging or aggressive dance programs. Shoulder limitations might rule out swimming. Knee problems might not limit cycling or rowing, but would restrict jogging.

When all other factors are equal (frequency, intensity, duration), improvements in VO_2max are independent of the type of activity chosen.[1,38,49] However, this does not mean that patients are turned out on their own without further advice. The activity should be one that requires large muscle group(s) and is repetitive and rhythmic. The type of activity greatly influences the potential for developing an injury. Repetitive impact injuries (e.g., jogging, home-based or commercial dance) are related more to injuries[7,45,52,53] than non–weight-bearing activities (e.g., swimming, rowing, cycling, cross-country skiing). Beginners are especially prone to running injuries when exercising at 30 minutes/day, 3 days/week,[50] even more so in the elderly.[51]

Other thoughts to consider might be availability of facilities and expense. Although jogging is attractive because of its low expense (shoes and clothes) and availability (almost anywhere), the injury incidence is such that one should seriously consider other types of activity. Walking is an excellent choice, as it does not have the impact of running. Improvements can be realized if one understands that low-intensity exercise requires a longer time of activity. It is difficult to achieve the 60% to 85% training range while walking. Yet Fig. 19-1 demonstrates that even low-intensity exercise will improve aerobic capacity. Swimming is a reasonable alternative but obviously requires a pool. In addition, most exercise tests are performed on land, and cool water will lower the exercising pulse rate, so the patient should know this and not expect to achieve the pulse rate ranges seen when one exercises on land. Experience suggests that the target heart rate range should be lowered by 5 to 10 beats. However, no changes are needed if one is prescribing intensity based on perceived exertion.

Cycling, especially stationary cycling, is popular. The start-up expense can be high ($250 to $1000 or more for a good home cycle). Because there is no "breeze" when cycling indoors, sweat will drip through the chain mechanism and stain most floors or carpets. Suggest a towel under the cycle to protect the floor. If outdoor cycling is to be used, the individual must know that the cycling speeds needed to meet a target heart rate or perceived exertion can be substantial; neighborhood cycling is generally not a sufficient stimulus. The cyclist needs to find some area where interruptions (traffic, pedestrians, or traffic signals) are minimal and to use proper protective equipment. Mountain, or trail, cycling can be a very vigorous outing, provided that the skill, fitness, and equipment are appropriate for the terrain.

Rowing and cross-country ski machines give a good whole-body exercise (arms and legs). The patient should expect to pay $500 or more for a good machine. Commercial or home-based (television or videotape) dance programs are very popular but come with some of the lower extremity injury problems seen with running.[53] Weight training has little influence on Vo_2max.[1] However, circuit training (minimal rest between stations) has been shown to increase Vo_2max by up to 6%.[22,23,30,44] Games (e.g., tennis, badminton, soccer, basketball) offer a reasonable mode of exercise. However, the intermittent nature of games renders a training heart rate useless. The degree of effort depends on several other factors. There is a saying that notes the secondary importance of games in the development of fitness: "Get in shape to play the game, do not play the game to get in shape."

RATE OF PROGRESSION

A frequently omitted portion of the exercise prescription is the rate at which one progresses. The patient probably should not simply start at the rate of 3 days per week, 30 minutes per day, at an intensity of 75% heart rate reserve. The patient needs an initial period of adjustment to the activity; this implies a shorter time of exercise, lower intensity, and some reasonable frequency (2 to 3 days per week). The person then progresses to the guidelines of the exercise prescription. Typically, this means that the patient increases one of the three primary variables (frequency, intensity, or time), never two or all three simultaneously. Primary care physicians and orthopedists state that overuse problems can be directly related to the patient changing two or three training variables at the same time (some physicians extend training variables to include equipment, surface, environment, and more). For example, consider the person who was running 3 days/week, 30 minutes/day, at a particular intensity, then increases his or her frequency and duration, buys new shoes to run on trails in the mountains, and runs with friends who are better trained. Too many changes produce a high injury risk.

The rate of the increase is sometimes related to age.[2] For example, patients would increase one of the three variables every 2 weeks if they are in their 20s, and add 1 week for each decade. Patients in their 40s would increase their training roughly once a month and so on.

An example

Take the normal patient from Table 19-4, *A*. Assume for the moment that this person wants to exercise 4 days per week. He or she might start by exercising 3 days per week at a "light" to "moderate" intensity (note the heart rates that correspond to these perceptions), 10 to 15 minutes per day. After about a month, the patient might increase the frequency to 4 days per week while holding intensity and duration constant. After the next 4 weeks, the patient should increase the duration to 15 to 20 minutes/day while holding intensity and frequency constant. Four weeks later the patient should increase the duration to 20 to 25 minutes, then 4 weeks later increase the duration to 25 to 30 minutes per day. After 4 weeks at 4 days per week and 30 minutes per day at a "light" to "moderate" intensity, the patient should increase the intensity to the "moderate" to "hard" ("heavy") range (again, note the heart rates). This might appear to be a slow progression, but clinically the risk of injury is low. Besides, it took the person 20 or more years to obtain his or her pretraining fitness level, so the patient should not expect to gain a higher level of fitness in a very short time. Faster rates of progression are related to low compliance and injury risk.

MAINTENANCE OF FITNESS

To maintain a fitness level, the training must be regular[10,12,14,56]; thus patients should maintain their training at their comfortable frequency, intensity, and duration. Patients often question the effect of interruptions in their training regime. This has been investigated from two directions, reduction and cessation of training.

Reduction in training

Once a person has achieved some fitness level, will reductions affect fitness? Hickson et al. examined reductions in the training variables.[26-28] They found that if the intensity was constant, duration and frequency (training volume) could be reduced by up to two thirds without changes in Vo_2max (study duration was 15 weeks). If the volume was maintained, reductions in intensity of one third or two thirds resulted in reductions in Vo_2max (15-week study). Therefore the variable to be maintained is intensity.

Cessation of training

Patients also question the rate at which fitness is lost should training cease. Significant reductions in endurance capacity occur in as little as two weeks.[12,54] A 50% reduction in subjects' improvement has been shown to occur in 4 to 12 weeks of inactivity,[20,33,54] and a return to pretraining fitness levels has been reported to occur, in 10 weeks[20] to 8 months[35] of inactivity. Individuals with a long history of training seem to maintain their benefits for longer periods.[12]

MUSCULAR STRENGTH AND ENDURANCE

To emphasize one aspect of fitness such as endurance suggests that other aspects are of minimal importance. In

1990, the American College of Sports Medicine added a section on strength to its policy statements.[1]

Similar training variables are used when prescribing strength training. The type of exercise is limited typically to free weights (barbells) or some mechanical (machine) system. The skill required to adequately and safely perform free-weight exercises probably excludes free weights for most individuals. This then narrows the choice of activities to some machine-based system. Another choice is the type of contraction. Resistance exercise can be isometric (no joint movement), isotonic (controlled resistance, varying velocity of contraction), or isokinetic (controlled velocity of contraction, varying resistance). Strength improvements of 25% to 30% can be realized,[43] depending on the initial strength level. Caution should be used, however, because heavy resistance exercise can result in dramatic elevations in both systolic and diastolic blood pressure.[37,39]

Contractions can also be concentric (tension developed while the muscle is shortening) or eccentric (tension developed while the muscle is lengthening). Most resistance training encompasses both shortening and lengthening contractions. Many isokinetic machines have concentric as well as eccentric modes. Realize that the delayed soreness that is felt after exercise, be it from resistance or endurance modes, seems to be due to the eccentric component of the activity.[3]

The **frequency** of resistance training should be at least 2 days per week. In a comparison of 2 vs. 3 days per week, 2 days per week resulted in a 21% improvement in strength, and 3 days per week of resistance training showed a 28% improvement in strength.[9] Three quarters of the total improvement occurred in 2 days per week. This fraction of total improvement is consistent when compared with other studies of longer durations (number of sets multiplied by repetitions) and frequencies.[1,43]

The **intensity-time** relationship of resistance training greatly influences the degree of improvement seen. High-intensity, low-repetition training results in improvement in strength, and low-intensity, high-repetition training shows gains in local muscle endurance. Although each method will result in some degree of strength and local endurance,[43] a reasonable compromise is to perform sets of 8 to 12 repetitions to fatigue.[1,24,30] Time is further influenced by the selection of exercises. A minimum of 8 to 10 exercises that use the major muscle groups is suggested,[1] which practically works out to one complete circuit of most machine-based programs. Considering the shared use of such systems, this might take about an hour to complete. Programs of longer duration have poor compliance.[48]

The **rate of progression** varies from person to person. Rather than placing an age-related time limit (weeks) as in endurance training, resistance training progression is usually performance based. When the person can finish a set

of an exercise (12 repetitions) without experiencing failure, it is time to add resistance. For the machine user, that means adding a "plate," and for the free weight user, adding 5 to 10 pounds might be appropriate.

TRAINING EFFECTS ON BODY COMPOSITION

In its simplest model, the body is composed of two compartments, the fat compartment (fat mass, FM) and the fat-free compartment (fat free mass, FFM). Endurance programs are most effective at reducing FM and subsequently body mass, as endurance programs train the body to use fat as a fuel for the exercise.[51] Training studies on this topic typically show an average loss of 1.5 kg of mass. This loss of weight is usually achieved through a loss in percentage of weight as fat, with a maintenance of FFM. Nutritional intervention alone can result in greater reductions in mass, FM as well as FFM.[29,36,65] If exercise is added to the program, the loss of FFM is somewhat attenuated.[46,65] However, even during very low-calorie diets, the addition of exercise does not maintain the FFM,[36] *as these diets are "starvation diets" and cannot meet the full metabolic needs of the individual.*

Modifications to the exercise prescriptions are needed when weight loss is a primary goal. Longer duration and lower intensity programs are advisable; for example, a 3 day/week, 300 kcal expenditure-per-session program has been shown to be a reasonable threshold for reducing body mass and FM.[1,25,51] A program of 4 days per week at 200 kcal per session is also effective.[59] Less frequent participation and lower weekly volumes are not as effective in reducing FM or mass.

Table 19-6 can be used to estimate caloric expenditure for various activities. One can use 100 kcal per mile of walking/jogging or per .25 mile of swimming as a standard.

WARM-UP AND COOL-DOWN

The purpose of a warm-up is twofold. First, this period of gradual adjustment to the exercise intensity helps to elevate the body temperature to allow for the metabolic processes to operate at a more efficient level. Typically the person will perform some light calisthenics and stretching exercises. Most people will direct their efforts to the muscle groups to be used during the workout. However, this alone is probably reason enough to also direct the warm-up to muscle groups not used so that they, too, might be stressed to some degree. There is no standard time period for a warm-up. Warming up to the point of breaking into a sweat seems to be sufficient. It should be noted that, although flexibility is stressed during a warm-up, there are little hard data that suggest that flexibility is important in injury reduction. Also, performance does not seem to be consistently improved by warm-up. This does not mean we should not counsel about the importance of warm-up. The second reason for the warm-up is related to cardiovas-

Table 19-6. Energy cost of various activities*

Activity	Kilocalories† (kcal/min)	MET‡	Oxygen uptake (ml/kg·min⁻¹)
Archery	3.7-5	3-4	10.5-14
Backpacking	6-13.5	5-11	17.5-38.5
Badminton	5-11	4-9	14-31.5
Basketball			
Nongame	3.7-11	3-9	10.5-31.5
Game	8.5-15	7-12	24.5-42
Bed exercise (arm movement, supine or sitting)	1.1-2.5	1-2	3.5-7
Bicycling Recreation/transportation	3.7-10	3-8	10.5-28
Bowling	2.5-5	2-4	7-14
Canoeing (rowing and kayaking)	3.7-10	3-8	10.5-28
Calisthenics	3.7-10	3-8	10.5-28
Dancing			
Social and square	3.7-8.5	3-7	10.5-24.5
Aerobic	7.5-11	6-9	21-31.5
Fencing	7.5-12	6-10	21-35
Fishing			
Bank, boat, or ice	2.5-5	2-4	7-14
Stream, wading	6-7.5	5-6	17.5-21
Football (touch)	7.5-12	6-10	21-35
Golf			
Using power cart	2.5-3.7	2-3	7-10.5
Walking, carrying bag, or pulling cart	5-8.5	4-7	14-24.5
Handball	10-15	8-12	28-42
Hiking (cross-country)	3.7-8.5	3-7	10.5-24.5
Horseback riding	3.7-10	3-8	10.5-28
Horseshoe pitching	2.5-3.7	2-3	7-10.5
Hunting, walking			
Small game	3.7-8.5	3-7	10.5-24.5
Big game	3.7-17	3-14	10.5-49
Mountain climbing	6-12	5-10	17.5-35
Paddleball/racquet	10-15	3-12	28-42
Rope skipping	10-14	8-12	28-42

Running, 0% grade

Mph	Min/mile (min:sec)			
6.0	10:00	12.0	10.0	35
7.0	8:35	14.0	11.5	40.3
8.0	7:30	15.6	12.8	44.8
9.0	6:40	17.5	14.2	49.7
10.0	6:00	19.6	16.0	56

Activity	Kilocalories† (kcal/min)	MET‡	Oxygen uptake (ml/kg·min⁻¹)
Sailing	2.5-6	2-5	7-17.5
Scuba diving	6-12	5-10	17.5-35
Shuffleboard	2.5-3.7	2-3	7-10.5
Skating (ice or roller)	6-10	5-8	17.5-28
Skiing (snow)			
Downhill	6-10	5-8	17.5-28
Cross-country	7.5-15	6-12	21-42
Skiing (water)	6-8.5	5-7	17.5-24.5
Snow shoeing	8.5-17	7-14	24.5-49
Squash	10-15	8-12	28-42
Soccer	6-15	5-12	17.5-42
Softball	3.7-7.5	5-6	10.5-21
Stair-climbing	5-10	4-8	14-28
Swimming	5-10	4-8	14-28

*Energy cost values based on an individual of 154 pounds of body weight (70 kg).
†*Kcal,* a unit of measure based upon heat production. One Kcal equals approximately 200 ml of oxygen consumed.
‡*MET,* basal oxygen requirement of the body sitting quietly. One MET equals 3.5 ml/kg·min⁻¹ of oxygen consumed.
(Modified from Pollock ML, Wilmore JH, and Fox SM: *Health and fitness through physical activity,* New York, Churchill Livingstone, 1978.)

Table 19-6. Energy cost of various activities*—cont'd

Activity		Kilocalories† (kcal/min)	MET‡	Oxygen uptake (ml/kg·min^{-1})
Table tennis		3.7-6	3-5	10.5-17.5
Tennis		5-11	4-9	14-31.5
Volleyball		3.7-7.5	3-6	10.5-21
Walking, 0% grade				
Mph	**Min/Mile (min:sec)**			
2.0	30:00	2.5	2.0	7
3.0	20:00	3.7	3.0	10.5
4.0	15:00	5.5	4.6	16.1
Weight training, circuit		10	8.2	28

cular adjustment to the activity. Serious ECG abnormalities have been noted when exercise was begun without a warm-up period.[5] For that reason, a warm-up is always recommended.

A 5- to 10-minute period of light exercise/stretching after exercise is typically performed to assist in maintaining cardiac output and minimize the pooling of blood in the lower body that can occur after exercise. In addition, light exercise can also increase the rate of removal of lactic acid that may have accumulated during the activity. A shower after exercise should never be hot, as this can result in further peripheral pooling of blood. The period immediately after exercise seems to be the time when exercise dysrythmias are most likely. Thus a period of activity after the workout is needed to minimize this risk.

SUMMARY

Considering that reductions in functional capacity are related to inactivity and loss of FFM, the following recommendations can be made:

- Perform rhythmic activities that require the large, major muscle groups 3 days per week for 20 to 60 minutes per day at 60% to 85% of maximum heart rate reserve ("moderate" to "hard") while following a conservative rate of progression. *Suggest 4 to 5 days a week as a goal so that if 1 or 2 days are missed, the minimum of 3 days per week is still met.*
- Perform resistance activities 2 days per week at one set of 8 to 12 repetitions of 8 to 10 different lifts.
- Always include warm-up and cool-down activities.

REFERENCES

1. American College of Sports Medicine: The recommended quantity and quality of exercise for developing and maintaining cardiovascular and muscular fitness in healthy adults, *Med Sci Sports* 22:265, 1990.
2. American College of Sports Medicine: *Guidelines for exercise testing and prescription,* ed 4, Philadelphia, 1991, Lea & Febiger.
3. Armstrong RB: Mechanisms of exercise-induced delayed onset muscular soreness: a brief review, *Med Sci Sport Exerc* 16:529, 1984.
4. Astrand PO: Why exercise? *Med Sci Sports* 24:153, 1992.
5. Barnard RJ et al: Cardiovascular responses to sudden strenuous exercise—heart rate, blood pressure and ECG, *J Appl Physiol* 34:833, 1973.
6. Birk TJ, Birk CA: Use of ratings of perceived exertion for exercise prescription, *Sports Med* 4:1, 1987.
7. Blair SN, Kohl HW, Goodyear NN: Rates and risks for running and exercise injuries: studies in three populations, *Res Q Exerc Sports* 58:221, 1987.
8. Borg GAV: Pyschophysical basis of perceived exertion, *Med Sci Sports Exerc* 14:377, 1982.
9. Braith RW et al: Comparison of two vs three days per week of variable resistance training during 10 and 18 week programs, *Int J Sports Med* 10:450, 1989.
10. Brynteson P, Sinning WE: The effects of training frequencies on retention of cardiovascular fitness, *Med Sci Sports* 5:29, 1973.
11. Chow JR, Wilmore JH: The regulation of exercise intensity by ratings of perceived exertion, *J Cardiac Rehab* 4:382, 1984.
12. Coyle EF et al: Time course of loss of adaptation after stopping prolonged endurance training, *J Appl Physiol* 57:1857, 1984.
13. Crews TR, Roberts JA: Effects of interaction of frequency and intensity of training, *Res Q* 47:48, 1976.
14. Cureton TK, Phillips EE: Physical fitness changes in middle-aged men attributable to equal eight-week periods of training, non-training and retraining, *J Sports Med Phys Fitness* 4:1, 1964.
15. Davies CTM, Knibbs AV: The training stimulus, the effects of intensity, duration and frequency of effort on maximum aerobic power output, *Int Z Angew Physiol* 29:299, 1971.
16. Dishman RK, Sallis J, Orenstein D: The determinants of physical activity and exercise, *Public Health Reports* 100:158, 1985.
17. Dishman RK et al: Using perceived exertion to prescribe and monitor exercise training heart rate, *Int J Sports Med* 8:208, 1987.
18. Dunn RL, Matzen RN, VanderBurg-Medendorp S: Screening for the detection of coronary artery disease by using the exercise tolerance test in a preventive medicine population, *Am J Prev Med* 7:255, 1991.
19. Epstein SE: Implications of probability analysis on the strategy used for noninvasive detection of coronary artery disease, *Am J Cardiol* 46:491, 1980.
20. Fringer MN, Stull AG: Changes in cardiorespiratory parameters during periods of training and detraining in young female adults, *Med Sci Sports* 6:20, 1974.
21. Gettman LR et al: Physiological responses of men to 1, 3 and 5 day per week training programs, *Res Q* 47:638, 1976.
22. Gettman LR et al: The effect of circuit weight training on strength, cardiorespiratory function and body composition of adult men, *Med Sci Sports* 10:171, 1978.
23. Gettman LR et al: Physiological effects of circuit strength training and jogging, *Arch Phys Med Rehabil* 60:115, 1979.
24. Gettman LR, Ward P, Hagman RD: A comparison of combined running and weight training with circuit weight training, *Med Sci Sports*

Sports Exerc 14:229, 1982.

25. Gwinup G: Effect of exercise alone on the weight of obese women, *Arch Phys Med Rehab* 135:767, 1975.

26. Hickson RC, Rosenkoetter MA: Reduced training frequencies and maintenence of increased aerobic power, *Med Sci Sports Exerc* 13:13, 1981.

27. Hickson RC et al: Reduced training duration effects on aerobic power, endurance and cardiac growth, *J Appl Physiol* 53:225, 1982.

28. Hickson RC et al: Reduced training intensities and loss of aerobic power, endurance and cardiac growth, *J Appl Physiol* 58:492, 1985.

29. Hill JO et al: Effects of exercise and food restriction on body composition and metabolic rate in obese women, *Am J Clin Nutr* 46:622, 1987.

30. Hurley BF, Seals DR, Eshani AA: Effects of high intensity strength training on cardiovascular function, *Med Sci Sports Exerc* 16:483, 1984.

31. Karvonen M, Kentala K, Mustala O: The effects of training heart rate: a longitudinal study, *Ann Exp Biol Fenn* 35:307, 1957.

32. Kearney JT et al: Cardiorespiratory responses of sedentary college women as a function of training intensity, *J Appl Physiol* 41:822, 1976.

33. Kendrick ZB et al: Effects of training and detraining on cardiovascular efficiency, *Am Corr Ther J* 25:759, 1971.

34. Klissouras V, Pirnay F, Petit J: Adaptation to maximal effort: genetics and age, *J Appl Physiol* 35:288, 1973.

35. Knuttgen HG et al: Physical conditioning through interval training with young adults, *Med Sci Sports* 5:220, 1973.

36. Krotkiewski M et al: The effect of a very low calorie diet with and without chronic exercise on thyroid and sex hormones, plasma proteins, oxygen uptake, insulin C-peptide concentrations in obese women, *Int J Obesity* 5:287, 1981.

37. Lewis SF et al: Cardiovascular responses to exercise as functions of absolute and relative work load, *J Appl Physiol* 54:1314, 1983.

38. Lieber DC, Lieber RL, Adams WC: Effects of run training and swim training at similar absolute intensities of treadmill V$o_2$max, *Med Sci Sports Exerc* 21:655, 1989.

39. MacDougall JD et al: Arterial blood pressure response to heavy resistance training, *J Appl Physiol* 58:785, 1985.

40. Marigold EA: The effect of training at predetermined heart rate levels for sedentary college women, *Med Sci Sports* 6:14, 1974.

41. Martin JE, Dubbert PM: Adherence to exercise, *Exerc Sport Sci Rev* 13:137, 1985.

42. Martin WH, Montgomery J, Snell PG: Cardiovascular adaptations to intense swim training in sedentary middle-aged men and women, *Circulation* 75:323, 1987.

43. McDonagh MJN, Davies CTM: Adaptive response of mammalian skeletal muscle to exercise with high loads, *Europ J Appl Physiol* 52:139, 1984.

44. Messier JP, Dill M: Alterations in strength and maximal oxygen uptake consequent to Nautilus circuit weight training, *Res Q Exerc Sport* 56:345, 1985.

45. Oja P et al: Feasibility of an 18 months' physical training program for middle-aged men and its effect on physical fitness, *Am J Public Health* 64:459, 1975.

46. Pavlow KN et al: Effects of dieting and exercise on lean body mass, oxygen uptake and strength, *Med Sci Sports Exerc* 17:466, 1985.

47. Pollack ML: The quantification of endurance training programs, *Exerc Sport Sci Rev* 3:155, 1973.

48. Pollack ML: Prescribing exercise for fitness and adherence. In Dishman RK, editor: *Exercise adherence: its impact on public health,* Champaign, Ill, 1988, Human Kinetics Publishers.

49. Pollack ML et al: Effects of mode of training on cardiovascular function and body composition of middle-aged men, *Med Sci Sports* 7:139, 1975.

50. Pollack ML et al: Effects of frequency and duration of training on attrition and incidence of injury, *Med Sci Sports* 9:32, 1977.

51. Pollack ML, Wilmore JH: *Exercise in health and disease: evaluation and prescription for prevention and rehabilitation,* ed 2, Philadelphia, 1990, WB Saunders.

52. Powell KE et al: An epidemiological perspective of the causes of running injuries, *Phys Sportsmed* 14:100, 1986.

53. Richie DH, Kelso SF, Bellucci PA: Aerobic dance injuries: a retrospective study of instructors and participants, *Phys Sportsmed* 13:130, 1985.

54. Roskamm H: Optimal patterns of exercise for healthy adults, *Can Med Assoc J* 96:895, 1967.

55. Sallis JF et al: Predictors of adoption and maintenance of physical activity in a community sample, *Prev Med* 15:131, 1986.

56. Saltin B et al: Response to exercise after bed rest and after training, *Circulation* 38(suppl 7):1, 1968.

57. Saltin. B et al: Physical training in sedentary middle-aged and older men, *Scand J Clin Invest* 24:323, 1969.

58. Shephard RJ: Intensity, duration and frequency of exercise as determinants of the response to a training regime, *Int Z Angew Physiol* 26:272, 1969.

59. Sidney KH, Shephard RJ, Harrison J: Endurance training and body composition of the elderly, *Am J Clin Nutr* 30:326, 1977.

60. Siscovik DS et al: The incidence of primary cardiac arrest during vigorous exercise, *N Engl J Med* 311:874, 1984.

61. Wenger HA, Bell GJ: The interactions of intensity, frequency and duration of exercise training in altering cardiorespiratory fitness, *Sports Med* 3:346, 1986.

62. Wilmore JH, Ewy GA, Morton AR: The effect of beta-adrenergic blockade on submaximal and maximal exercise performance, *J Cardiac Rehab* 3:30, 1983.

63. Wilmore JH: Body composition in sport and exercise: directions for future research, *Med Sci Sports Exerc* 15:21, 1983.

64. Wilson PK, Fardy PS, Froelicher VF: *Cardiac rehabilitation, adult fitness and exercise testing,* Philadelphia, 1981, Lea & Febiger.

65. Zuti WB, Golding LA: Combining diet and exercise as weight reduction tools, *Phys Sportsmed* 4:49, 1976.

RESOURCES

American College of Sports Medicine, PO Box 1440, Indianapolis, IN 46206-1440.

American College of Sports Medicine: *Guidelines for exercise testing and prescription,* ed 4, Philadelphia, 1991, Lea & Febiger.

Dishman RK: *Exercise adherence: its impact on public health,* Champaign, Ill, 1988, Human Kinetics Publishers.

Pollack ML, Wilmore JH: *Exercise in health and disease: evaluation and prescription for prevention and rehabilitation,* ed 2, Philadelphia, 1990, WB Saunders.

Wilson PK, Fardy PS, Froelicher VF: *Cardiac rehabilitation, adult fitness and exercise testing,* Philadelphia, 1981, Lea & Febiger.

Chapter 20

EXAMINATION OF SCHOOL ATHLETES AND THEIR PREPARATION FOR COMPETITION

Andrew M. Tucker

The preparticipation physical examination for scholastic athletes is frequently considered with some contempt by participant and health care provider alike. The health care provider often must take time from a busy schedule to examine large numbers of adolescents, sometimes in a less-than-ideal setting. The athlete too dreads the endless lines, medical scrutiny, and potentially embarrassing situations. Many of us remember this, perhaps accepting it as a rite of passage or form of hazing mandatory to pursuing dreams of athletic glory.

Despite possible personal biases, the preparticipation evaluation deserves the best effort from those caring for our young athletes. Much has been written about the screening encounter, and although some aspects may be continuing sources of confusion and controversy, our present knowledge should enable us to conduct an examination that is effective and efficient. This chapter will review the many considerations for evaluation of our school athletes and their preparation for athletic competition.

THE CARE OF SCHOOL-AGE ATHLETES

A casual observer of U.S. society can plainly see that sports play a very prominent role, especially so at the junior high, high school, and collegiate levels. The number of participants has continued to rise with the proliferation of athletic opportunities for girls in the last 10 to 15 years. It is estimated that 5.8 million athletes participate in organized high school sports alone.[27] Millions more participate at the junior high and intercollegiate levels.

One obvious ramification of these imposing figures is the challenge to our health care system to evaluate the preparedness of millions of young athletes. This is basically accomplished through the preparticipation physical examination in private physician offices and mass screening evaluations. A review of the various state guidelines for scholastic preparticipation examinations indicates significant variability among specific requirements governing these evaluations.[10] Of the 45 states that responded, 35 require annual examinations. Six actually have no requirement regarding frequency of examination. Nine of the responding states have no official medical history and physical examination form. Of the 36 states with forms, nine did not include any medical history questions. Of those with medical history questions, the number of questions ranged from one to 200. A few of the states required specific lab testing, such as urinalysis, TB testing, and hemoglobin. Only three states provided examiners with a list of AMA-recommended contraindications for participation or recommendations for further evaluation. Although most states authorize only physicians to perform the evaluations, some states allow nurse practitioners or physician assistants to perform these examinations and three states do not specify who is authorized. It is clear that current knowledge needs to be applied by each state's athletic program regulatory bodies (usually high school associations) to encourage more uniform standards regarding the many aspects of preparticipation examinations.

Equally challenging for the health care system is providing medical coverage for the thousands of contests annually and caring for injury.

The National Athletic Training Association estimated the injury toll in high school sports alone to be approximately 1.3 million per year.[27] From 70% to 75% of all injuries were considered minor, with the athlete sidelined a week or less. One survey of injuries in 19 high school sports demonstrated an overall injury rate of 39 injuries per 100 participants.[12] Predictably football (81 injuries/100 participants) and wrestling (75/100 participants) demonstrated the highest injury rates. For female sports, comparable injury rates were seen for cross country, softball, gymnastics, and track and field (approximately 40 injuries/ 100 participants). Evaluation by a physician was required by 42% of all injuries. A more recent survey of high school sports injuries documented a total injury rate for collision sports (football, ice hockey, wrestling, and lacrosse) of 96.2/100 participants. Approximately 85% returned to activity in 7 days or less. The injury rates for boys' and girls' sports were similar if male collision sports were omitted, with boys sustaining a slightly higher rate.[35] Epidemiologic studies on injuries will differ depending on the definition of injury and the methods of recording and reporting; nonetheless, the implications for caring for the young athlete are obvious. Later we will see how information gained from the preparticipation evaluation can be used in an attempt to modify risk of injury.

Given the large number of participants, the incidence of death associated with participation must be regarded as very low. However, the few tragic events that occur have devastating effects in the local community, and often the shock waves are felt in distant regions. There are few data on the incidence of death associated with sports. Most attention is directed toward cardiac-related sudden death. Data have shown that those who die suddenly are more commonly male, have participated in a number of sports, and are likely to be of junior high or high school age at the time of death.[22] Most of these young athletes have demonstrable structural cardiovascular defects at time of autopsy.[22] In Maron's series, hypertrophic cardiomyopathy was the most common defect. In another review, hypertrophic cardiomyopathy and anomalous coronary arteries each accounted for approximately 20% of sudden cardiac death in those under age 30.[7] Unfortunately, sudden death is often the first manifestation of conditions such as hypertrophic cardiomyopathy.[21]

Collision sports such as football and ice hockey place the participant at increased risk of catastrophic injuries from head and neck trauma. Catastrophic football injuries are more common in high school players aged 16 to 18; the increased prevalence in this age group is attributed to such factors as lack of physical conditioning, inferior equipment or improperly fitted equipment, lack of knowledge of coaches, and unavailability of medical care.[6] There is evidence that football has become safer because

of equipment standards and rules modifications. In 1968, 36 deaths occurred in football, 20 caused by head injuries in high school. In 1990, no deaths occurred directly because of football for the first time since record keeping began in 1931.[24] The proper fitting of quality equipment, adequate supervision, use of proper coaching techniques, and continued modification of rules governing play will, we hope, continue to have a beneficial effect.

Environmental variables, such as ambient temperature and humidity, are often neglected in studies of mortality in athletes.[20]

We will see how the preparticipation examination could reduce cardiac-related mortality by identifying those at risk before they participate. However, there will always be a few who are at great risk who are entirely asymptomatic. Many coaches, parents, and administrators may gain a false sense of security from the preparticipation examination and overestimate its ability to ensure problem-free participation. The grim reality is that careful examinations by knowledgeable providers will not entirely prevent tragic outcomes on the playing fields. We hope preparticipation screening will minimize these tragedies.

GOALS OF PREPARTICIPATION SCREENING

There has been much discussion regarding the goals of the preparticipation examination. It seems reasonable to use the encounter as the adolescent's continuous medical care. Studies support this inclination. Goldberg et al. showed nearly 80% of the high school population used this encounter as their annual health assessment.[15] However, others have pointed out that this places an unnecessary and unfair burden on the preparticipation encounter.[13] Defining the goals of the examination helps define the appropriate content of the encounter.

The primary goal of the examination "should be the detection of athletes who would be at medical risk if they engaged in competition."[15] This includes the detection of underlying conditions that may increase the risk of sudden death (e.g., hypertrophic cardiomyopathy) as well as known or unknown medical conditions that might manifest or be worsened with participation (e.g., exercise-induced asthma). Another primary goal is the uncovering of physical deficiencies that might put the participant at increased risk for injury, such as an inadequately rehabilitated knee injury.[2] Poor flexibility (e.g., of the hamstrings or Achilles tendon) may be a risk factor for acute injuries (strains) and overuse conditions (tendinitis, patellofemoral syndrome) and can be the target of a specific stretching regimen. Identification of these deficiencies and proper rehabilitation of residual injury can decrease the risk of further injury.[1] At minimum, the preparticipation examination should meet these goals. Thus the content of the history and physical examination, as will be seen in a later section, can be focused or narrowed in scope to accomplish these goals.

There are many other potential goals. One may evaluate size and level of maturity of the younger athlete to make recommendations ensuring safe and satisfying participation.[4,8,19] The open epiphyseal plates in a skeletally immature athlete represent potential sites of injury. Exposing the skeletally immature athlete to collision sports against more mature counterparts may be an important risk factor for injury.[23] In addition, the immature athlete is usually at a competitive disadvantage in regard to speed, strength, and power, and thus may be more likely to fail in his or her efforts to make the team. This potentially negative psychological trauma can have lasting effects. Thoughtful counseling with the participant and parents may help avoid this situation.

Another potential goal is the assessment of fitness in an individual so that performance and participation can be maximized.[2,4,15] Evaluation of parameters such as flexibility, strength, and body composition can be the basis for appropriate training modifications. Exercise physiologists, athletic trainers, and physical therapists are often utilized to help make these determinations. Assessment of body composition and determination of appropriate weight are important, especially in sports where weight-loss techniques are frequently abused (e.g., wrestling, gymnastics).

The preparticipation encounter can serve as the athlete's entry into the local health care or sports medicine system.[23] The establishment of a relationship with a trusted physician can provide an important resource to the athlete regarding health-related issues.

Finally, the preparticipation examination serves to fulfill state and local legal and insurance requirements.[19] As mentioned, requirements vary from state to state and among school systems. The physician should know the state and local requirements where he or she practices.

The preparticipation evaluation is not intended to substitute for the young participant's continuous health care as provided by a family physician or pediatrician. The fact that it often does, emphasizes a gap in our country's health care delivery system. Participants and parents need to understand this important point. Unfortunately, the survey of the states' guidelines revealed only one state that included in its form a statement of the purpose and limitations of the preparticipation examination.[10] Until this figure increases, many athletes and parents will probably continue to misunderstand and misuse this annual evaluation.

COST EFFECTIVENESS OF PREPARTICIPATION SCREENING

Those who have been involved with large-scale preparticipation screening know that it is not a "high-yield" process, with low rates of disqualification and referral. The population being screened is generally very healthy, with few ongoing medical problems and even fewer conditions that will exclude the individual from participation. The cost effectiveness of preparticipation screening has been

questioned. One study performed a cost-benefit analysis of screening examinations for two groups of high school students in Houston and demonstrated a cost of $4537 for each disqualification.[28] The disqualification rate in that study was similar to other series that will be reviewed in the next section of this chapter. The authors made recommendations that could increase the cost effectiveness of the screening examination:

- Having subspecialty consultation available at the exams, thus minimizing expensive referrals
- Using the station exam method to screen large groups of athletes in a relatively short time
- Requiring physical examinations at only entry levels of competition (junior high, high school, college) with encounters scheduled in the intervening years to screen for new problems
- Avoiding unnecessary tests (urine, hemoglobin) that have been shown to be cost-ineffective screening methods

The first two points are very worthwhile considerations, although office-based examination by a primary care physician does have certain advantages over the mass screening method (see later discussion). The latter two points have gained growing acceptance by many sports medicine authorities.[19,23] Three states require a preparticipation examination every 3 years, and one state requires evaluation only upon entering middle or junior high school.[10]

Some have suggested that widening the scope of the screening examination would increase the cost effectiveness, because a number of non–sports-related diagnoses would be documented.[28] We discovered this approach is supported by the finding that the preparticipation examination is often the only encounter between the adolescent and the health care system,[15,28] and thus the screening encounter could help to plug a gap in our health care delivery system. However, if the primary goal of the preparticipation examination is to determine conditions that predispose to injury or death, it would be inappropriate to expand the screening examination so it can serve as the adolescent's annual primary care visit. Expanding the examination potentially decreases its efficiency and effectiveness.[13] The content of the examination is discussed in a later section.

While the number of disqualifications is predictably small, the identification of orthopedic and medical conditions that may interfere with activity is potentially more important. Diagnosing and rehabilitating an athlete's unstable shoulder or ankle before competition may prevent a serious and costly injury later. Indeed, a West Point study demonstrated that identification and rehabilitation of residual knee injuries decreased the rate of reinjury.[1] Likewise, athletes with conditions such as exercise-induced asthma or severe bee sting hypersensitivity can be identified and preventive measures taken, thereby potentially preventing an emergency room visit or hospitalization. There are

Table 20-1. Outcomes of recent preparticipation evaluations

Study	Method	Number	Temporary disqualification requiring evaluation	Eventual disqualification	No disqualification but "MD attention advised"
Risser et al., 1982	Station/individual	763	16	2	213
Tennant, 1981	Station	271	32	N/A	217
Goldberg et al., 1980	Station	701	104*	9	N/A
Linder et al., 1981	Station	1268	64	2	N/A
Thompson et al., 1982	Station	2670	31	N/A†	257‡
Hough and McKeag, 1982	N/A	989	10%	1.1%	N/A

*Includes 40 with proteinuria. None had positive workup.
†One found to have hypertrophic cardiomyopathy; one found to have severe mitral stenosis.
‡Includes 2+ or greater proteinuria on dipstick urinalysis.

many such examples of how the screening encounter can benefit the athlete, trainer, or team physician. Such benefits are difficult to prove in studies.

The preparticipation screening examination may not stand up to rigid cost-benefit analyses. However, we have discussed certain measures that can maximize its cost effectiveness. Again, one of the most important measures is to involve *interested* and *qualified* physicians in an adequate setting so that the young athletes may gain the most benefit.

OUTCOMES OF PREPARTICIPATION SCREENING

We have alluded to the low rates of disqualification resulting from preparticipation screening. Several recent studies allow evaluation of outcomes of preparticipation screening.* Nearly all of these screening examinations were conducted by the station method. The contents of the history forms and physical examination methods were not always available for comparison. Likewise, the numbers of referrals and actual disqualifications are not easily compared because of differing methods and study objectives. Nonetheless, review of the available data presents important information (see Table 20-1) for examining physicians.

The outcomes shown underscore the low rates of disqualification for the preparticipation examination. This should not be surprising. As previously mentioned, the population being screened is young and generally very healthy. Therefore the incidence of potential disqualifying conditions is low. In addition, a selection process may be at work, as children with significant health problems are usually prevented or discouraged from participating in organized sports at the elementary and junior high school level.

Not only is the incidence of disqualifying conditions low, but those very conditions being sought (e.g., hypertrophic cardiomyopathy) can be both asymptomatic and

*References 15, 17, 18, 28, 33, 34.

undetectable on routine physical examination. Thus false-negative examinations will occur.

One could speculate about an element of underreporting in this population. Adolescents intent on playing their desired sport(s) may withhold information if they perceive they could be jeopardizing their permission to play. Likewise, some students may unknowingly omit or withhold information because they might think it irrelevant or unimportant. These instances may be minimized by requiring the parent or guardian to review or complete the history form. Unfortunately, several states do not include a history form in the recommended preparticipation screening forms they provide to school systems or physicians.[10]

It is instructive to note that the outcome of the preparticipation examination can depend significantly on the examiners themselves. The type of specialists involved and their knowledge of sports medicine will affect the findings and rates of referral. As has been noted, the participating physicians "tended to be more sensitive to aspects of the exam that were related to their particular interest."[18] In another study, Thompson et al. reported that the high incidence of musculoskeletal findings was attributable to the large number of orthopedists involved.[34] One could predict that primary care physicians minimally exposed to sports medicine might fail to diagnose musculoskeletal problems. As previously mentioned, the presence or ready availability of certain specialists (most notably cardiologists and orthopedists) can potentially improve the sensitivity of the examinations and perhaps minimize referrals.

More important than disqualification or referral rates is the issue of prevention: Does the screening examination make sports participation safer for the participants? If the issue is cardiac-related sudden death, it has been estimated that of 200,000 potential athletes, 1000 are at risk because of a cardiac abnormality, and ultimately only one would die during participation from that cardiac abnormality.[9] Can the system prevent that one out of 200,000 cardiac deaths? Obviously this is a difficult question to answer. We have learned that injuries can be decreased if vulnerable joints are identified and rehabilitated.[1] This author be-

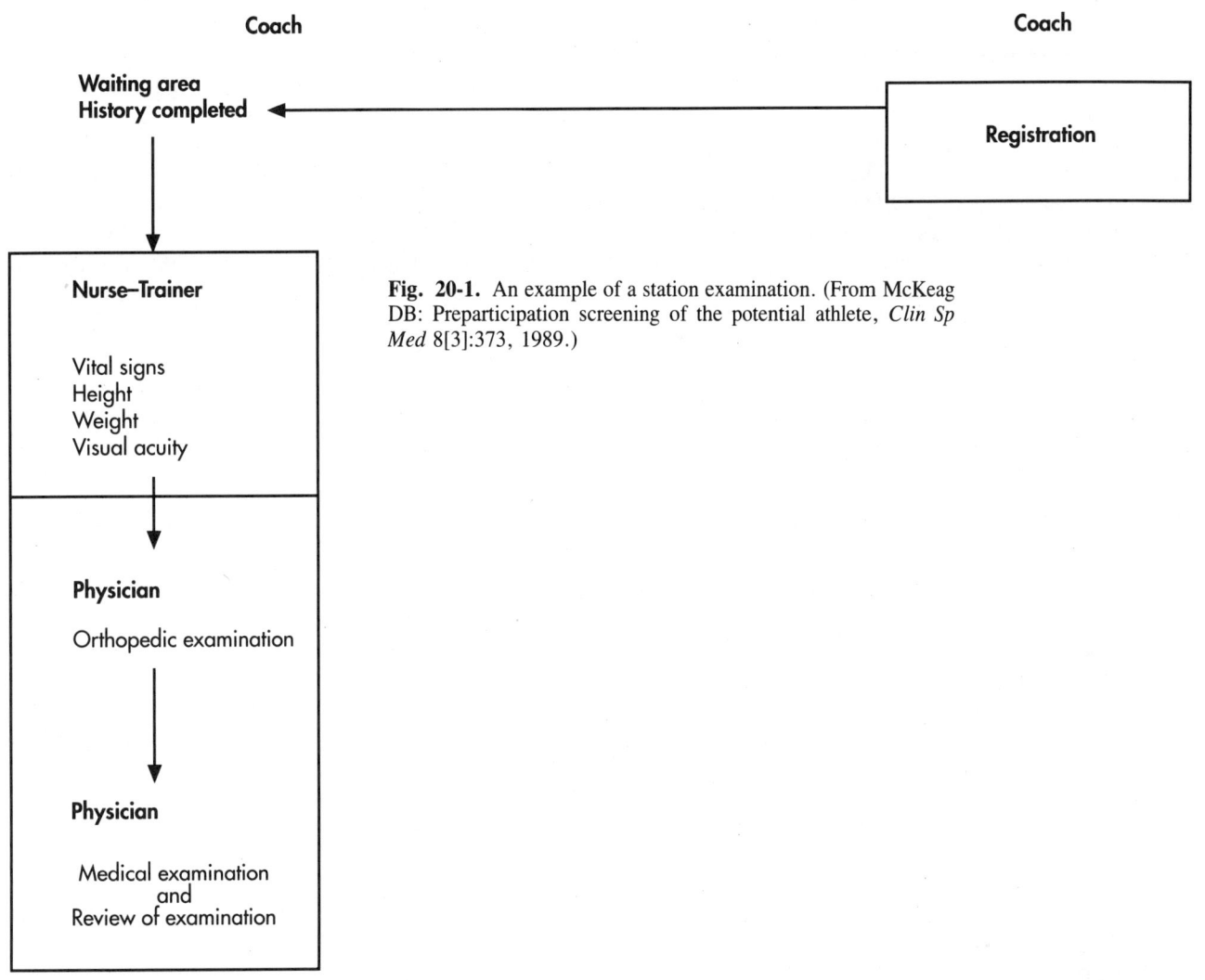

Fig. 20-1. An example of a station examination. (From McKeag DB: Preparticipation screening of the potential athlete, *Clin Sp Med* 8[3]:373, 1989.)

lieves that the preparticipation evaluation does make a difference for those who are participating. Involving *knowledgeable* people *who care* about the well-being of young athletes is an important way of maximizing the outcome of the preparticipation examination and ensuring the greatest chance for safe and enjoyable participation.

THE METHODOLOGY OF SCREENING

Preparticipation screening methods have varied in type, frequency, and timing. These will be reviewed here.

Examination method

Three basic types of screening have been used: office-based screening, multiple station mass screening, and the "line-up" examination. Examination in a primary care physician's office offers many advantages. It usually is the most comfortable and private setting, which encourages patient rapport. The discussion of the most private and sensitive issues, such as chemical abuse or issues of sexuality, is encouraged in this setting.[23] The availability of medical records enables the physician to follow up on old injuries or previously treated medical conditions, thus promoting continuity of care.[18] The private office evaluation obviates the organizational challenges presented by scheduling mass screening evaluations.[18]

The disadvantages of office-based examinations include decreased efficiency and cost effectiveness, as well as increased cost to the athlete.[23] Also, as physicians' knowledge and interest in sports medicine varies greatly, the examinations may lack consistency in findings and recommendations.[23]

The station exam is probably used to perform the bulk of screening examinations. The organization varies but usually involves a physician or physicians in conjunction with support personnel that may include nurses, trainers, therapists, coaches, or parents. An example of a typical station setup is given in Fig. 20-1. Additional stations may be used if other parameters are measured, such as body fat determination by skin calipers, flexibility, or muscle strength. These parameters are usually measured by physical therapists, trainers, or exercise physiologists.

The station examination has several advantages.[18] It is a standardized examination that offsets the physician variability in office examinations. Station examinations can be administered to large numbers of athletes over a relatively short time and thus are more efficient and cost effective than office examinations.[18] Often specialty consultation can be made available, thus potentially minimizing referrals. The mass station examination often is administered by physicians who have a genuine interest in sports medicine and thus may bring more knowledge that is pertinent to the examinations.

Other potential benefits include the fostering of cooperation among health professionals, the involvement of the coaching staff with the care of the athletes, and the development of a data base for research purposes.[18]

A potential disadvantage of the station examination is the relative lack of privacy, which lessens the opportunity to discuss personal issues. Often adequate planning will enable at least one private "station" to be available, where this sort of exchange can occur, thus combining the best of both the private and station examinations.[19]

The line-up examination was a common mode of examination in the past, probably because it was very time efficient. The patient must endure lack of privacy and potential embarrassment. The physician's examination accuracy is invariably compromised. Many sports medicine authorities have condemned this type of examination.

Examination frequency

The screening examination is often required annually. The survey of state examination requirements[10] reported that more than three fourths require annual evaluations for sports participation. Some schools engage in screening evaluations before each new sport season. Many authorities now recommend a screening physical examination at the beginning of a new level of competition (e.g., junior high, high school, college) with intercurrent interviews at the start of each new sport season to screen for new problems or evaluate rehabilitation of old injuries.[19,23] This approach makes judicious use of the time of the athlete and health care provider without compromising quality of care.

Examination timing

Preparticipation evaluations must allow sufficient lead time to allow for adequate rehabilitation/treatment of injuries or deficiencies, or further investigation of new findings. However, the evaluation should not take place so long before a season or school year that the development of new problems might become a significant factor. Scheduling the evaluation 4 to 6 weeks before a season seems to satisfy both considerations.[19,23]

PREPARTICIPATION HISTORY

The medical history is the cornerstone of diagnosis, and its role in preparticipation examinations is no less impor-

tant. Many authors have emphasized the need for an effective screening history.[11,15,19,23,30] Studies have proved the effectiveness of the history as a screening tool. In one survey the history was positive in seven of nine students disqualified from activity and in 74% of the students requiring further evaluation.[15] The history is generally regarded as the most sensitive and specific part of this screening evaluation.

Adherence to the specific goals of the screening encounter allows effective history-taking with relatively few questions. Many authors recommend a history form with fewer than a dozen questions.[4,8,11,30,34]

The history should focus primarily on the cardiovascular, musculoskeletal, and neurologic systems as well as adequately cover questions of general health.[11] As we will see, these systems have the most relevance to safe participation by the young athlete. There is no single "correct" form. An example of the form the Cleveland Clinic Foundation uses in preparticipation evaluations is given in Fig. 20-2. In addition to covering the necessary areas, the forms should be brief, easy to read, and understandable by the athletes/parents, and should allow adequate space for elaboration of positive findings.

Although sudden cardiac death is relatively rare, it attracts widespread attention from parents, coaches, and administrators. Therefore a primary goal of the examination is detection of cardiac abnormalities that may place the athlete at an increased risk through participation. The more common causes of sudden cardiac death in patients under 35 years of age are listed in the box below. Although coronary artery disease is the common cause of death in those older than 35, structural abnormalities are the most common causes of sudden cardiac death in this younger population. Although sudden death is often the initial presentation of such cardiac problems, prodromal symptoms can at times identify the at-risk individual. The examiner should specifically ask the prospective participant about a history of syncope/near syncope with exercise, a family history of atraumatic sudden death and/or premature atherosclerosis, and a personal history of seizures.[5] The presence of syncope may indicate a malignant dysrhythmia associated with hypertrophic cardiomyopathy or anomalous coronary circulation. A history of atraumatic sudden death in a

---

> **Common causes of sudden death in young athletes**
>
> Hypertrophic obstructive cardiomyopathy
> Idiopathic concentric left ventricular hypertrophy
> Atherosclerosis
> Aberrant origin of the left coronary artery
> Hypoplastic coronary arteries
> Ruptured aorta

From Strong WB, Steed D: Cardiovascular evaluation of the young athlete, *Pediatr Clin North Am* 29(6):1325, 1982.

Date of Exam_____/_____/_____   Cleveland Clinic Foundation   **A   B   C**
School Official _____   **PREPARTICIPATION**   **Contact:** Coach ☐
Exam Doctor _____   **SPORTS EXAM**   School Nurse ☐
                                                                       Family Doctor ☐
                                                                       Family Dentist ☐

THIS IS NOT A SUBSTITUTE FOR A REGULAR PHYSICAL EXAM PERFORMED BY YOUR FAMILY DOCTOR

Name _____   Grade _____ Age _____ Birthdate _____/_____/____
School _____   Sport _____ Sex _____
Parents _____   Address _____ Phone _____
Family Doctor _____   Address _____ Phone _____

HISTORY: Answer **No** or **Yes** with details and dates. Use reverse side if necessary.

I.   Have you ever sustained **an injury** which prevented you from playing sports for **more than one day
     and** have you had any injuries **such as** (circle): skull fracture - **brain surgery**
     concussion - knocked out, **neck pain**/injury - arm/finger **numbness**, **back pain**/injury - leg/toe
     numbness, heatstroke/fainting - exhaustion, broken bone - **fracture**, joint **dislocation** - out of place,
     deep bruise - muscle pull, ligament **sprains**, tender kneecap/shin, **trick knee** - catching/locking,
     _____
     _____

II. Do you have a history of **and/or** take medicine (specify) for any medical problems **such as** (circle):
     asthma - allergy - wheezing - short of breath, heart **murmur**/palpitation - rheumatic fever - **high blood
     high blood pressure**, diabetes - high/low **sugar**, fainting - **seizure**, yellow jaundice - **hepatitis**,
     severe influenza/cold - **mononucleosis** - weakness, **anemia** - bruise easily - bleeding - sickle cell,
     loss of eyesight, hearing, testicle, kidney, etc., **hernia** - rupture - bulging, skin disease - boils - **rash**,
     or other?
     _____
     _____

III. Are you allergic to any medicine such as (circle) penicillin, iodine, novocaine or other?
     _____

IV. Any family history of medically unexplained or cardiac caused sudden death under age 50?
     _____

V.   L.M.P. _____

BP____/____ P_____ Ht_____ Wt_____ Gross vision: R____ L____, Pupils R____ L____ LAB: UA_____
EXAM:

1. Upper Extr: AC jts _____   4. Heart: _____
          Symm _____   5. Lungs: _____
          ROM _____   6. Skin: _____
2. Spine: Neck _____   7. Abdo: Spleen _____
          Fwd Bend _____   Liver _____
          Curve _____   8. GU: Hernia _____
3. Lower Extr: Gait _____   Testicles _____
          1-Hop _____   9. Dental _____
          Duck _____   10. Other _____
          Symm _____   _____
          ROM _____   _____

IMPRESSION:

☐ Satisfactory Exam
☐ Recommend further evaluation/rehabilitation regarding: _____

Contact your: School Nurse — Coach — Family Doctor — Family Dentist
_____

CLEARANCE:

A — Cleared for: Collision — Contact — Noncontact sports
B — Cleared for: Collision — Contact — Noncontact sports after completing eval/rehab
C — NOT cleared for: Collision — Contact — Noncontact sports due to: _____
                          _____

Fig. 20-2. The preparticipation form used at the Cleveland Clinic Foundation.

young first- or second-degree relative can alert the examiner to the possibility of a family history of hypertrophic cardiomyopathy or Marfan's syndrome. Seizures and sudden death have been associated with a prolonged QT syndrome.[5] A family history of sudden death before age 50 may indicate premature atherosclerosis and would warrant screening the participant with a lipid profile. Elevated lipid levels alone, of course, would not be a contraindication to participation.[5] A positive response to these personal or family history questions necessitates very careful cardiac physical examination. Some would recommend a cardiologic consultation on the basis of a positive response to any of these questions, even if the physical examination proves negative.[5]

Some have found certain common complaints such as chest pain and easy fatigability to be nonspecific for screening purposes.[32] Chest pain as a symptom of serious cardiac disease in the young is thought to be unusual. The complaint is more worrisome if the pain is substernal, is associated with exertion, and requires stopping activity for relief.[32] Similar symptoms may be produced by exercise-induced asthma, hence close questioning and follow-up, both clinical and testing, are indicated (e.g., stress test with pre- and postpulmonary function testing). Mitral valve prolapse is not uncommon and can be associated with atypical chest pain, characteristically sharp and of short duration. Likewise, easy fatigability is thought to be an unreliable symptom for screening purposes. Often the young participant's perception of his or her fatigability does not correspond with objective measurements.[32]

The musculoskeletal history is an obviously important point. In one study, musculoskeletal findings represented two thirds of all identified risk factors.[34] In another study the most frequent positive response to the health history form was a history of a previous injury (about 27%).[18] The most common sports injuries are actually reinjuries of a previously damaged joint.[29] However, we have learned that proper rehabilitation of an injured joint has been found to decrease the risk of reinjury.[1] Inquiry into past injury can direct the physical examination to questionable areas so that previous injury can be rehabilitated before competition.

A history of concussion is significant for contact/collision sports.[11] A study of high school football players in Minnesota reported a fourfold increase in the risk of suffering a concussion if the player had a positive history of prior concussion.[14] A history of temporary paresis or paralysis may indicate cervical spine instability or cervical spinal stenosis. Young athletes frequently downplay neurologic symptoms, ascribing them to the common "stinger" or "burner," a brachial plexus stretch injury commonly experienced by those participating in collision sports, especially football. A positive response to any of these screening questions requires careful neurologic examination and possibly further diagnostic testing such as cervical spine radiographs or magnetic resonance imaging. Neurologic/neurosurgical consultation should be sought for histories of frequent (greater than three per season) or severe concussion, or transient paraplegia/quadriplegia.

Other information that is pertinent includes any history of prior heat-related illness. Research indicates that those who have suffered from a heat-related illness have an increased likelihood of experiencing a recurrence.[11] An individual with such a history deserves close monitoring during practices and competitions held during conditions of high heat and humidity.

Finally, a brief survey of chronic medical problems, previous surgeries, allergies to medications or insect stings, and tetanus immunization status is pertinent. The athlete should have an opportunity on the history form to indicate a desire to discuss any health-related issues. Athletes of this age, like their nonathletic counterparts, are facing important decisions about alcohol, drugs, smokeless tobacco, and issues of sexuality. As noted, the encounter in a private practitioner's office is ideally suited to accomplishing this goal of discussing any of these issues. However, these important issues also can be identified during mass screening examinations, with appropriate follow-up arranged.

Ideally, the prospective athlete and his or her parent should complete the history form before the preparticipation evaluation. At the time of the evaluation, a health care provider should review the history form with the athlete before the actual examination. A nurse or physician assistant is an ideal person to review the form with the athlete. Clarifying or elaborating on questionable areas before the actual physical examination can help the physician to focus the examination on these areas.

The importance of the history in the overall evaluation process cannot be overemphasized. Relatively few questions are needed to produce a history covering those few items that are most pertinent to safe participation by a scholastic athlete. The responses to those questions will go a long way in determining the fitness of an individual to participate in various sports.

PHYSICAL EXAMINATION

The content and extent of the physical examination is governed by the same principles that directed the history. The examination should be relatively brief and should focus on areas that are most pertinent to the safe participation of athletes; thus the emphasis is placed on the cardiopulmonary and musculoskeletal examinations. However, the examiner must be prepared to pursue other areas of the examination should the young athlete's medical history indicate. For example, a history of serious head injury necessitates a screening neurologic examination.

In addition, the examiner should be aware of the athlete's intended sport(s) when performing the physical examination. This allows the examiner to pay particular attention to parts of the examination that are most relevant to a given sport.[23] A prospective basketball player's knees and ankles need special attention, and a baseball player's throwing arm will require scrutiny. The ear and throat examination is of questionable benefit in most athletes but is extremely pertinent to a swimmer or diver.

The examination should begin with accurate measurements of height, weight, visual acuity, and blood pressure. Standard tables can be used to evaluate height and weight. Significant variations from the norm may warrant further investigation. The examiner should be aware of the possibility of steroid use in an extremely well-muscled athlete who has made rapid weight gains in a short time. Of course, judgments must be made carefully, as adolescent bodies are capable of rapid changes (author's personal experience). Significantly underweight athletes may arouse concern for malnutrition or eating disorders. Special attention should be paid to weight in those involved in sports in which weight control is especially important (e.g., wrestling, gymnastics).

Visual acuity is screened using the standard Snellen chart. Visual problems are often noted in screening examinations and are a frequent cause of referral. Eye protection is available for those with significant impairment, but thorough discussion of the risks of contact/collision sports with participant and parents is essential.

Blood pressure is determined with particular attention to the appropriate size cuff. Goldberg et al. found 10 cases of previously undetected hypertension in a group of 701 athletes.[15] The American Academy of Pediatrics places no restrictions on those with mild hypertension. Those with moderate to severe hypertension deserve consultation and possible individualized restriction.[3] Coarctation of the aorta can be easily ruled out at the time of the examination. Prolonged isometric activity (e.g., weightlifting) can produce significant elevations in blood pressure. This type of activity should be discouraged in those with a diagnosis of hypertension.[23]

The head and neck is often included in the examination, although most practitioners would probably agree that significant findings that bear on safe participation are rare. As noted previously, swimmers and divers are the athletes who deserve close examination of the ears, nose, and throat. Checking pupil equality in all athletes is also important. In cases of head injury, it is extremely beneficial to have prior documentation of unequal or equal pupils on screening examination. Aside from these two instances, otoscopic and ophthalmologic examinations are time consuming and usually of little utility.

The cardiopulmonary examination deserves special emphasis. As noted previously, sudden cardiac death in young athletes is associated with underlying structural cardiac abnormalities in most cases. The potential benefit of careful history taking was discussed in the last section of this chapter. Likewise, a subtle murmur may be the only

clue to an underlying cardiac abnormality that may place the individual at increased risk with participation. Of course, innocent murmurs are infinitely more common. The examiner needs to be able to distinguish the pathologic murmur from the benign. Consultation with a cardiologist is necessary in some cases and should be done without hesitation in cases of indecision.

It is important that the examiner have a quiet place to perform this part of the examination. Many examiners know the frustration of trying to auscultate in a noisy room or gymnasium.

The lungs are auscultated for pathologic sounds. If undiagnosed exercise-induced bronchospasm is suspected by history, the athlete may be exercised in an effort to bring out audible wheezing. A complaint of coughing during or after exercise should alert the examiner to this possible diagnosis.

The cardiovascular examination includes palpation of peripheral pulses to rule out coarctation of the aorta. The precordium is inspected and palpated for heaves and thrills. As noted, murmurs are a common finding in the adolescent age group. Innocent murmurs far outnumber pathologic murmurs. Table 20-2 reviews the common innocent murmurs heard in children and lists the differential diagnosis of murmurs in young athletes expanded on in the box below.

Careful evaluation of all heart sounds and murmurs is essential. Strong and Steed have concisely organized the process of evaluating murmurs.[32] If the first heart sound is easily heard, the murmur is not holosystolic, helping to rule out a ventricular septal defect or mitral insufficiency. If S_2 is of normal quality with normal splitting, tetralogy of Fallot, atrial septal defect, and pulmonary hypertension are unlikely. With no audible ejection click, aortic and pulmonary valvular stenosis are unlikely. If no continuous murmur is heard, patent ductus arteriosus is ruled out. An early diastolic decrescendo murmur is suggestive of aortic insufficiency. It is important to remember that the intensity

---

Differential diagnosis of murmurs in young athletes

Normal
Aortic stenosis
   (congenital or hypertrophic obstructive cardiomyopathy)
Pulmonary stenosis
Coarctation of the aorta
Atrial septal defect
Ventricular septal defect
Patent ductus arteriosus
Mitral insufficiency
   (rheumatic or prolapse)
Aortic insufficiency

From Strong WB, Steed D: Cardiovascular evaluation of the young athlete, *Pediatr Clin North Am* 29(6):1325, 1982.

Table 20-2. Common benign murmurs in children

Type	Characteristic	Etiology	Differential diagnosis	Notes
Pulmonary flow murmur	Grade 1/6 or 3/6 ejection murmur; left upper sternal border	Flow across normal pulmonic valve	ASD, valvular PS	Most common innocent murmur
Still's murmur	Grade 1/6 to 3/6 vibratory systolic murmur; halfway between lower sternal border and apex	Vibrations under aortic valve	Small VSD, subvalvular AS, mitral regurgitation	Very characteristic sound, sometimes musical
Venous hum	Grade 1/6 to 3/6 continuous murmur through the second sound; one or both upper sternal borders	Turbulent flow at confluence of veins; disappears when neck is turned or patient supine	PDA	Maneuvers mentioned make diagnosis easy
Carotid bruit	Grade 1/6 to 3/6 ejection murmur; in the neck	Turbulence in carotid blood flow; murmur fainter as approach upper sternal borders	Valvular stenosis	

Abbreviations: *ASD*, Atrial septal defect; *PS*, pulmonic valve stenosis; *VSD*, ventricular septal defect; *PDA*, patent ductus arteriosus.
From McKeag DB: Preparticipation screening of the potential athlete, *Clin Sport Med* 8(3):373, 1989.

of a murmur does not necessarily correlate with the extent of pathology.

Physical examination maneuvers may help distinguish the murmur of hypertrophic cardiomyopathy. Because the murmur will increase in intensity with decreases in ventricular filling, sitting upright or standing will increase the murmur; conversely, squatting will decrease the murmur intensity.

Certain rhythm disturbances are common in well-conditioned athletes and include premature atrial contractions, premature ventricular contractions, or, less commonly, paroxysmal supraventricular tachycardia and atrioventricular block. PACs and PVCs may be associated with caffeine, tobacco, alcohol, and medications (e.g., bronchodilators). It has been generally accepted that unifocal premature contractions that disappear with exercise are benign.[32] An exercise test may be necessary to prove that exertion suppresses the premature contractions. A diagnosis of myocarditis should be entertained in cases of frequent PVCs, bigeminy, or trigeminy.

Rhythm disturbances such as paroxysmal supraventricular tachycardia or Wolff-Parkinson-White syndrome do not necessarily preclude an athlete from competition. If symptoms are well controlled on medications, participation is often allowed by cardiologists. Likewise, if an accessory pathway's conduction is found to be too slow to predispose the ventricle to a malignant dysrhythmia, treatment may not be necessary. An exercise stress test is often used in these patients to evaluate the cardiovascular response to exercise.[32] Some centers are now using an echocardiogram in conjunction with an exercise stress test to better evaluate the athlete's cardiac response to exercise.

It should be noted that a number of electrocardiographic abnormalities are found in a higher percentage of the athletic population, including bradycardia, first-degree heart block, Wenckebach type of second-degree heart block, junctional rhythm, and ST and T wave abnormalities.[31]

If the history and/or physical examination is worrisome, ECG and chest radiograph is an appropriate next step in evaluation. If these studies are normal, a life-threatening defect is unlikely.[5] If doubt persists, consultation with a cardiologist familiar with the problems of active young people should be sought without hesitation. Other tests that may be indicated include an exercise stress test, echocardiography, Holter monitoring, and cardiac catheterization. As noted previously, some authorities recommend echocardiography before and after the exercise stress test to see whether activity brings out wall-motion abnormalities.

Abdominal examination should be accomplished to rule out hepatic or splenic enlargement. Infectious mononucleosis can be a common cause of splenomegaly in the adolescent population. Splenomegaly warrants disqualification for all but moderately strenuous (e.g., table tennis) or nonstrenuous noncontact sports (e.g., golf).[3]

The male genitourinary examination may detect an undescended testicle or testicular mass. Those with a testicular absence should be counseled regarding risks in contact or collision sports. Inguinal hernia may require further consultation to assess the risks of possible complication. Many surgeons are now recommending elective repair at the end of the competitive season rather than restriction from activity.

Pelvic examination in female athletes may be indicated if the history reveals abnormalities of the menstrual cycle.

Many recommend the use of Tanner staging to assess physical maturity, with subsequent counseling about injury risk for skeletally immature athletes in collision sports.

Table 20-3. Example of a screening musculoskeletal examination

Athletic activity (instructions)	Observations
1. Stand facing examiner	AC joints; general habitus
2. Look at ceiling, floor, over both shoulders, touch ears to shoulder	Cervical spine motion
3. Shrug shoulders (examiner resists)	Trapezius strength
4. Abduct shoulders 90 degrees (examiner resists at 90 degrees)	Deltoid strength
5. Full external rotation of arms	Shoulder motion
6. Flex and extend elbows	Elbow motion
7. Arms at sides, elbows at 90 degrees flexed; pronate and supinate wrists	Elbow and wrist motion
8. Spread fingers; make fist	Hand and finger motion and deformities
9. Tighten (contract) quadriceps; relax quadriceps	Symmetry and knee effusion, ankle effusion
10. "Duck walk" four steps (away from examiner)	Hip, knee, and ankle motion
11. Back to examiner	Shoulder symmetry; scoliosis
12. Knees straight, touch toes	Scoliosis, hip motion, hamstring tightness
13. Raise up on toes, heels	Calf symmetry, leg strength

From McKeag DB: Preparticipation screening of the potential athlete, *Clin Sport Med* 8(3):373, 1989.

Some evidence exists that matching skeletally immature athletes with their more mature counterparts is a major risk factor for injury.[23] Consideration also should be given to the psychologic effects of pitting the immature against the mature who have the competitive advantage, especially in collision/contact sports.[13] The effect of "not making the team" can be significant to the young fragile psyche. This author is not advocating disqualification from a sport on the basis of physical maturity. However, sensitive counseling about the physical and psychologic issues of maturity "mismatching" is recommended. Appropriate matching of individual and sport may maximize enjoyment of participation and reduce risk of injury.

A skin examination is most important for those involved in contact or collision sports. A number of dermatologic infections require deferred clearance, including herpes, impetigo, and louse or scabies infestation.

The importance of the musculoskeletal examination has been emphasized. In one study, musculoskeletal findings represented two thirds of all identified risk factors.[34] In another study the results of the health history form indicated the most frequent positive response was a history of a previous injury requiring treatment by a physician (about 27%).[18] Knee instability is perhaps the most common orthopedic condition resulting in disqualification. Goldberg's study showed five of the nine athletes disqualified had significant knee instability.[15] An additional 21 required further knee evaluation and rehabilitation before being allowed to participate. Ankle injuries are among the most common in sports and are often inadequately rehabilitated before the return to competition.

A screening musculoskeletal examination can be accomplished in a short time. An example of such an examination is given in Table 20-3. The emphasis is on documenting full range of motion and symmetrical strength about the major joints. In addition, further evaluation should be conducted of those joints that (1) have been previously injured, (2) are of particular importance for the sport(s) to be played by the individual, or (3) show an abnormality on the screening portion of the examination.

As previously noted, assessment of fitness may be a secondary goal of preparticipation evaluations. This could be accomplished at the time of the preparticipation encounter. Evaluation of variables such as flexibility, strength, and body composition may aid coaches and trainers in modification of athletes' training to optimize performance. These special evaluations are often impractical for an examiner performing office-based examinations. However, the involvement of athletic trainers, physical therapists, and exercise physiologists in a station approach permits efficient evaluation of these variables. This information may be used to maximize performance and possibly to reduce risk of injury. The relationship between ligamentous laxity and "tightness" to injury remains unclear. Some data suggest that injury rates are higher for "loose" knees and ankles.[25] Other data in a high school population found no difference in injury rates between "loose" and "tight" players.[16] Regardless, those athletes with poor flexibility are given stretching exercises, and those with ligamentous laxity are started on strengthening programs.

At the conclusion of the preparticipation examination, the physician decides the participant's eligibility status. Various authors have proposed similar classification schemes based on the findings of the history and physical examination. At the Cleveland Clinic Foundation, examiners have a choice of three categories of clearance:

Category A: complete clearance for participation in a designated sports classification (collision/contact/noncontact).

Category B: clearance pending notification of a responsible person (e.g., coach, family doctor, parent). This represents a scenario in which special treatment or equipment is required but activity is not limited.

Category C: clearance deferred until further evaluation, treatment, or rehabilitation is accomplished (e.g., evaluation of a questionable heart murmur).

When the young athlete's primary care physician performs the evaluation, communication to the parents regarding the category of clearance is usually hastened. However, private physicians must remember to communicate any restrictions to the athlete's coach and/or athletic trainer. Often, the examining physician is employed by or has a relationship with the respective school and is not the athlete's primary care physician. In this case, the examining physician should make a special effort to communicate any significant findings or restrictions in participation to the athlete's parents and primary care physician. At the Cleveland Clinic Foundation we give copies of our evaluation to the athlete, which are to be passed on to the athlete's parents and, if necessary, to the athlete's primary care physician. In this way, the problems of continuity of care inherent in this method of evaluation can be alleviated. Table 20-4 represents the classification of sports used by the American Academy of Pediatrics. The American Academy of Pediatrics policy statement on recommendations for participation is shown in Table 20-5.

USE OF LABORATORY TESTS AND PROCEDURES

Dipstick urinalysis and hemoglobin/hematocrit determination have often been included in the preparticipation examination. However, many authorities now are not recommending the inclusion of these as screening tests.[4,8,19,23]

Proteinuria is commonly seen during childhood and adolescents. One study of junior high and high school preparticipation examinations showed proteinuria was seen in 62% of all urinalyses, 17% if trace protein was excluded.[26] However, proteinuria has been shown to be a benign event in all but 0.8% of cases.[26]

In another study[15] 40 of 701 students had a positive dipstick test for urine protein. None of the 40 had a significant urologic abnormality upon consultation. The logistics of administering large-scale urine dipstick testing are considerable. The time and costs of needless consultation are also significant. It appears the dipstick test and resulting consultation can be eliminated without compromising the quality of care to the young athlete.

Positive urine dipstick testing for blood can also be very misleading because of contamination of specimens in female athletes during their menstrual periods.

Hemoglobin determination as a screening test is also of questionable benefit. Without a positive history, hemoglobin testing is not likely to detect an anemia that would adversely affect performance.[23] However, performance may be impaired when iron stores are depleted before any evi-

Table 20-4. Classification of sports

Contact/collision	Limited contact/impact	Noncontact		
		Strenuous	**Moderately strenuous**	**Nonstrenuous**
Boxing	Baseball	Aerobic dancing	Badminton	Archery
Field hockey	Basketball	Crew	Curling	Golf
Football	Bicycling	Fencing	Table tennis	Riflery
Ice hockey	Diving	Field		
Lacrosse	Field	Discus		
Martial arts	High jump	Javelin		
Rodeo	Pole vault	Shot put		
Soccer	Gymnastics	Running		
Wrestling	Horseback riding	Swimming		
	Skating	Tennis		
	Ice	Track		
	Roller	Weight lifting		
	Skiing			
	Cross-country			
	Downhill			
	Water			
	Softball			
	Squash, handball			
	Volleyball			

From AAP policy statement, recommendations for participation in competitive sports, *Pediatrics* 81(5):737, 1988.

Table 20-5. Recommendations for participation in competitive sports

		Limited contact impact	Non-contact		
	Contact collision		Strenuous	Moderately strenuous	Non-strenuous
Atlanto-axial instability	No	No	Yes*	Yes	Yes
*Swimming: no butterfly, breast stroke, or diving starts					
Acute illnesses	*	*	*	*	*
*Needs individual assessment (e.g., contagiousness to others, risk of worsening illness					
Cardiovascular					
Carditis	No	No	No	No	No
Hypertension					
Mild	Yes	Yes	Yes	Yes	Yes
Moderate	*	*	*	*	*
Severe	*	*	*	*	*
Congenital heart disease	†	†	†	†	†
*Needs individual assessment, see reference 2					
†Patients with mild forms can be allowed a full range of physical activities; patients with moderate or severe forms, or who are postoperative, should be evaluated by a cardiologist before athletic participation, see reference 2					
Eyes					
Absence or loss of function of one eye	*	*	*	*	*
Detached retina	†	†	†	†	†
*Availability of American Society for Testing and Materials (ASTM)-approved eye guards may allow competitor to participate in most sports, but this must be judged on an individual basis, see references 3, 4					
†Consult ophthalmologist					
Hernia					
Inguinal	Yes	Yes	Yes	Yes	Yes
Kidney					
Absence of one	No	Yes	Yes	Yes	Yes
Liver					
Enlarged	No	No	Yes	Yes	Yes
Musculoskeletal disorders	*	*	*	*	*
*Needs individual assessment					
Neurologic					
History of serious head or spine trauma, repeated concussions, or craniotomy	*	*	Yes	Yes	Yes
Convulsive disorder					
Well controlled	Yes	Yes	Yes	Yes	Yes
Poorly controlled	No	No	Yes†	Yes	Yes‡
*Needs individual assessment					
†No swimming or weight lifting					
‡No archery or riflery					
Ovary					
Absence of one	Yes	Yes	Yes	Yes	Yes

From AAP Policy Statement, *Pediatrics* 81(5):737, 1988.

Continued.

Table 20-5. Recommendations for participation in competitive sports—cont'd

	Contact collision	Limited contact impact	Non-contact		
			Strenuous	Moderately strenuous	Non-strenuous
Respiratory					
Pulmonary insufficiency	*	*	*	*	Yes
Asthma	Yes	Yes	Yes	Yes	Yes
*May be allowed to compete if oxygenation remains satisfactory during a graded stress test					
Sickle cell trait	Yes	Yes	Yes	Yes	Yes
Skin					
Boils, herpes, impetigo, scabies	*	*	Yes	Yes	Yes
*No gymnastics with mats, martial arts, wrestling, or contact sports until not contagious					
Spleen					
Enlarged	No	No	No	Yes	Yes
Testicle					
Absent or undescended	Yes*	Yes*	Yes*	Yes*	Yes*
*Certain sports may require protective cup, see reference 3					

dence of anemia is detected. More study in this area is needed.

Other diagnostic tests used frequently are related to evaluation of the cardiovascular system: chest x-ray, ECG, and echocardiography. None of these is recommended in the routine screening process. However, an examiner should not hesitate to use them if the history or physical examination warrants.

SUMMARY

Available information should allow standardization of the preparticipation evaluation of school-age athletes, whether the encounter takes place in a private office setting or as part of mass screening examinations. Many authorities now advocate a complete screening examination only for new levels of competition, with annual or seasonal limited encounters to update information.

The encounter should be accomplished in an efficient manner and focused on those items that pertain to safe sports participation. The history, which can be covered in a relatively few questions, is the most sensitive portion of the encounter. The physical examination focuses on the cardiovascular and musculoskeletal examinations, with flexibility to expand the evaluation depending on the participant's history. Laboratory testing is of questionable benefit in the screening setting.

The goal is safer and more enjoyable sports participation for millions of young athletes.

REFERENCES

1. Abbott HG, Kress JB: Preconditioning in the prevention of knee injuries, *Arch Phys Med Rehabil* 50:326, 1969.
2. Allman FL, McKeag DB: Prevention and emergency care of sports injuries, *Fam Pract Recert* 5(4):141, 1983.
3. American Academy of Pediatrics Policy Statement: Recommendations for participation in competitive sports, *Pediatrics* 81(5):737, 1988.
4. Blum RW: Preparticipation evaluation of the adolescent athlete, *Postgrad Med* 78(2):52, 1985.
5. Braden DS, Strong WB: Preparticipation screening for sudden cardiac death in high school and college athletes, *Phys Sportsmed* 16(10):128, 1988.
6. Brooks WH, Young AB: High school football injuries; prevention of injury to the central nervous system, *South Med J* 69(10):1258, 1976.
7. Chillag S et al: Sudden death: myocardial infarction in a runner with normal coronary arteries, *Phys Sportsmed* 18(3):89, 1990.
8. Dyment PG: Another look at the sports preparticipation examination of the adolescent athlete, *J Adolesc Health Care* 7:130s, 1986.
9. Epstein SE, Maron BJ: Sudden death and the competitive athlete: perspectives on preparticipation screening studies, *J Am Coll Cardiol* 7:220, 1986.
10. Feinstein RA, Soileau EJ, Daniel WA: A national survey of preparticipation physical examination requirements, *Phys Sportsmed* 16(5):51, 1988.
11. Fields KB, Delaney M: Focusing the preparticipation sports examination, *J Fam Pract* 30(3):304, 1990.
12. Garrick JG, Requa RK: Injuries in high school sports, *Pediatrics* 61(3):465, 1978.
13. Garrick JG, Smith NJ: Pre-participation sports assessment, *Pediatrics* 66(5):803, 1980.
14. Gerberich SG et al: Concussion incidences and severity in secondary school varsity football players, *Am J Public Health* 73(12):1370, 1983.
15. Goldberg B et al: Pre-participation sports assessment—an objective evaluation, *Pediatrics* 66(5):736, 1980.
16. Godshall RW: The predictability of athletic injuries: an eight year study, *J Sport Med* 3(1):50, 1975.
17. Hough DO, McKeag DM: Preparticipation examination results from Michigan State University (unpublished data), 1982.

18. Linder CW et al: Preparticipation health screening of young athletes, *Am J Sport Med* 9(3):187, 1981.

19. Lombardo JA: Pre-participation physical evaluation, *Prim Care* 11(1):3, 1984.

20. Luckstead EF: Sudden death in sports, *Pediatr Clin North Am* 29(6):1355, 1982.

21. Maron BJ et al: Sudden death in patients with hypertrophic cardio-myopathy: characterization of 26 patients with functional limitation, *Am J Cardiol* 41:803, 1978.

22. Maron BJ et al: Sudden death in young athletes, *Circulation* 62(2):218, 1980.

23. McKeag DB: Preparticipation screening of the potential athlete, *Clin Sport Med* 8(3):373, 1989.

24. National Operating Committee on the Standards for Athletic Equipment, *Football Protective Equipment Research Summary,* September 25, 1991.

25. Nicholas JA: Risk factors, sports medicine and the orthopedic system: an overview, *J Sport Med* 3(5):243, 1975.

26. Peggs JF, Reinhardt RW, O'Brien JM: Proteinuria in adolescent sports physical examinations, *J Fam Pract* 22(1):80, 1986.

27. Public Relations, *Athletic Training* 24(4):360, 1989.

28. Risser WL et al: A cost-benefit analysis of preparticipation sports examinations of adolescent athletes, *J School Health* 55(7):270, 1985.

29. Robey JM, Blyth CS, Mueller FO: Athletic injuries, application of epidemiologic methods, *JAMA* 217(2):184, 1971.

30. Runyan DL: The pre-participation examination of the young athlete, *Clin Pediatr* 22(10):674, 1983.

31. Salem DN, Isner JM: Cardiac screening for athletes, *Orthop Clin North Am* 11(4):687, 1980.

32. Strong WB, Steed D: Cardiovascular evaluation of the young athlete, *Pediatr Clin North Am* 29(6):1325, 1982.

33. Tennant FS, Sorenson K, Day CM: Benefits of preparticipation sports examination, *J Fam Pract* 13(2):287, 1981.

34. Thompson TR, Andrish JT, Bergfeld JA: A prospective study of preparticipation sports examinations of 2670 young athletes: method and results, *Clev Clin Q* 49(4):225, 1982.

35. Whieldon TJ, Cerny FJ: Incidence and severity of high school athletic injuries, *Athletic Training, JNATA* 25(4):344, 1990.

━━━━━━━━━━ **RESOURCES** ━━━━━━━━━━

High school preparticipation requirements

National Federation of State High School Association, 11724 Northwest Plaza Circle, P.O. Box 20626, Kansas City, MO 64195.

Injuries, epidemiology

National Athletic Trainers Association, Inc., 2952 Stemmons, Suite 200, Dallas, TX 75247.

National Collegiate Athletic Association, 6201 College Boulevard, Overland Park, KS 66211-2422.

Fatal/Catastrophic Injuries in Football, Fred Mueller, PhD, Director, Annual Survey of Football Injury Research, 205 Woollen Gym, University of North Carolina, Chapel Hill, NC 27599-8605.

Equipment testing

National Operating Committee on Standards for Athletic Equipment, 11724 Northwest Plaza Circle, P.O. Box 20626, Kansas City, MO 64195-0626.

Chapter 21

STEROIDS AND OTHER PERFORMANCE ENHANCERS

Robert J. Dimeff

OVERVIEW
History

For over 3000 years, athletes have used numerous agents and techniques to improve performance. Most of these agents have had little or no ergogenic effect. Many have been associated with serious short- and long-term adverse effects. It is often asked why an elite athlete would subject his or her body to the potential ill effects of these agents. More recently, the question has arisen as to why nonathletes would use these agents. To discuss treatment and prevention of abuse of these drugs, it is imperative to understand the rationale for their use.

Rationale

Numerous factors influence athletic performance. Cardiovascular fitness and muscular strength and conditioning are key to success in sports. Indeed, systematic exercise training over prolonged period is the most effective method for improving physical performance. Skills such as eye/hand coordination are another important component in determining performance. Many aspects of skill are inherited; however, they can be influenced by training. General nutrition for training and competition is another important component that influences athletic performance. General and athletic nutrition are discussed elsewhere in this text. Baseline psychologic makeup and acute psychologic changes also highly affect performance. The ability of an athlete to prepare mentally for competition is often the difference between athletic success and failure. Proper rest allows the body time to recover from the stresses of training and competition and also allows the athlete to be more alert and attentive and improves reaction time. The location of the event also influences athletic performance. These effects may range from simply a change in playing surface that causes excessive physical stress to competing in a hostile, foreign gymnasium. In addition to being a "visiting" athlete, the athletic preparation and prowess of the opponent also influences athletic performance. Genetic differences in size, strength, quickness, balance, coordination, muscle composition, and metabolic efficiency all also play a role in athletic performance. These differences are completely out of the athlete's control.

Ergogenic aids are the final factor that play a role in athletic performance. Performance-enhancing or ergogenic aids include any physical, mechanical, nutritional, psychologic, or pharmaceutical substance or treatment that either directly improves physiologic variables associated with exercise performance or removes subjective restraints that may limit physiologic capacity. These aids allow individuals to perform more work than they would otherwise be capable of performing. Ergogenic aids do not result in more than a 7% increase in work output. Nevertheless, at high training regimen, large increases in training effort are required to prompt small improvement in performance; thus a small increase in work output can make a large difference in results.[71]

A rationale for using ergogenic agents is the fame and fortune that accompany athletic success. The opportunity to obtain a college scholarship based on athleticism allows young people to advance their education and improve their sports skills. This opportunity can lead to further exposure, which may result in a professional athletic career, Olympic opportunities, or contacts for professional advancement outside sport. At the more elite levels, other important factors come into play, including securing a lucrative sports contract, working simply to make the team, or striving to succeed and win the gold medal. When taking all factors into account, it is easy to understand why an athlete may turn to ergogenic aids. Viewed in the context of a training program (which may emphasize proper rest, nutrition, strength and conditioning, and sport-specific training), ergogenic aids may simply be considered another part of the training regimen. Certainly this explanation does not justify the use of the agents; however, the rationale behind their use becomes apparent.

A growing number of nonathletes are beginning to use ergogenic aids for cosmetic purposes. This group tends to be adolescent and young adult men who are taking drugs to develop larger muscles, appear leaner, and look more attractive to members of the opposite sex.[42] These individuals tend to have low self-esteem and poor self-confidence and are using the drugs to compensate.

It is helpful to classify ergogenic aids according to their major effect:

1. Provide supplementary source of fuel
2. Increase metabolism and/or transport of fuel to increase the available energy
3. Remove waste products that may contribute to fatigue
4. Increase the quality and efficiency of work output
5. Improve efficiency of the nervous system input into the physiologic systems[71]

In general, the type of sport determines the type of ergogenic aid an athlete uses. Sports that require significant aerobic endurance, such as long-distance cycling, swimming, and running, lead to the use of agents that improve aerobic fitness. Sports that require strength and power, such as football, Olympic weightlifting, and sprinting, lead to the use of agents that improve muscular power.

Epidemiology

It is difficult to estimate the prevalence of ergogenic use because the recent establishment of strong laws and rules against their use have made athletes less willing to talk about the problem. Conservative estimates suggest that there are 1 to 2 million users of anabolic steroids in the United States. Although anabolic steroids are probably the most frequently used ergogenic agent, many other substances are also used. Again because of the stigma associated with use of ergogenic aids, it is extremely difficult to estimate how widespread these practices are.[42,188,341]

Economics

Over $100 million a year is spent illegally in the United States on ergogenic aids.[67,237] An even larger amount is spent on legal substances promoted as performance-enhancing aids. These agents are often sold by nutrition centers and mail order catalogs. Cost may be as little as $70 for a 6-week course of testosterone cypionate to $2000 for an 8-week course of growth hormone. The recent change of anabolic steroids and related compounds to schedule III substances has led to a significant increase in their black market price. The prohibitive cost may make it difficult for many individuals to afford these agents; however, the wealthier athlete will still not be daunted by the expense.

Ethics

There are numerous arguments for and against the use of ergogenic aids. One of the strongest arguments is that their use is a form of cheating and, therefore, is unethical. The spirit of competition is that the athlete with the best performance should win. By using performance-enhancing agents, this spirit of competition is violated. Additionally, an athlete who perceives that the opponent is using ergogenic aids, will be further tempted to use them to level the playing field. Those who will not use the agents are forced to compete at a perceived or real disadvantage that may require participation at a lower level, result in being cut from the team, or lead to retirement from competition.

THE AGENTS
Anabolic/androgenic steroids

Anabolic/androgenic steroids (AAS) have been used by athletes to improve performance for over three decades. Sports medicine specialists believe AAS are the most commonly abused ergogenic aids. Over 1 million users of AAS are estimated in the United States. Approximately 2% of students between the ages of 10 and 14 and 5% to 10% of high school students have used AAS. Approximately 5% of college athletes currently use AAS.[6,32,42,188,342] Because of recent legal and administrative changes associated with AAS it is difficult to estimate the percentage of Olympic and professional athletes currently using these agents.

Historical development. In 1931, researchers[209] injected an extract of human male urine into castrated male dogs and noted an increase in metabolic rate proportional to the dose administered. Kochakian and Murlin,[207] in 1935, discovered that injecting a similar extract caused a decrease in protein metabolism and an increase in lean body mass, with only a slight increase in metabolic rate. They were able to obtain similar results using testosterone, testosterone acetate, and androstenedione.[207a,207b]

In 1944, Kochakian[206] discovered a dichotomy between the anabolic and androgenic effects of androstene 3-alpha 17-beta diol. This discovery led to the belief that it may be possible to completely separate the anabolic effects from the androgenic effects. The anabolic effects are the increase in protein synthesis, which leads to an increase in lean body mass. The androgenic effects, or masculinizing effects, include male-pattern baldness, acne, deepening of the voice, increased libido, increased aggression, and other changes.[163,190,214,370]

In the 1950s, a variety of testosterone analogs apparently were being used by Russian weightlifters as reported by Ziegler.[350] In 1956, Ziegler and Ciba, working together, developed methandrostenolone (Dianabol), an oral anabolic steroid. Since then, numerous individuals have attempted unsuccessfully to alter the side chains of these agents to completely separate the anabolic and androgenic qualities. It has also become apparent that for a steroid to be active orally, it must be alkylated at the C-17-alpha position. This alkylization results in many of the adverse effects seen with usage of the oral anabolic steroids. Injectable anabolic steroids are usually esterified at the C-17-beta position.[140,351,368,370]

Physiology and biochemistry. AAS are analogs of testosterone. To understand their mechanism of action and their side effects, it is important to understand basic testosterone metabolism.

Leuteinizing hormone (LH) released from the anterior pituitary stimulates the interstitial cells of Leydig to produce testosterone. Follicle-stimulating hormone (FSH), also released from the anterior pituitary, may augment testosterone secretion by regulating the number of LH receptors on the Leydig cell plasma membrane. FSH and LH secretion are controlled by gonadotropin-releasing hormone (GnRH), which is produced in the hypothalmus. Testosterone production results in feedback inhibition at the hypothalamic and pituitary levels to control release of GnRH, FSH, and LH. Inhibin, released by the sperm-producing Sertoli cells, also results in feedback inhibition at the hypothalmic and pituitary levels.[140,351,368]

Testosterone is produced from cholesterol by a series of chemical reactions. The first four enzymes involved in this synthesis are present in both the adrenal and testes and result in the production of androstenedione. 17-Beta-hydroxy-steroid hydrogenase, present in the testes, converts androstenedione into testosterone. In the peripheral tissues, plasma testosterone is metabolized by several pathways. The two most important are aromatization to estradiol and irreversible reduction to dihydrotestosterone by 5-alpha-reductase.[351,368]

The main functions of testosterone and dihydrotestosterone are to (1) promote the development of male sex characteristics during embryogenesis, (2) initiate and maintain sperm production, (3) regulate FSH and LH secretion, and (4) promote secondary sex characteristics.

At the cellular level, testosterone may exert its effect by a variety of methods.[140,351,368] First, the binding of free testosterone to the membrane receptor may stimulate a series of reactions leading to the production of cyclic adenosine monophosphate (cAMP), which activates a series of catalytic reactions leading to the effects of testosterone. Second, testosterone may bind with the cell membrane receptor, leading to an increase in cytoplasmic calcium concentration, which then triggers the effects. Finally, the testosterone receptor complex itself may stimulate the cell at the nuclear level. Following transportation of the testosterone receptor complex or reduced testosterone to the nucleus, various chromosomes are stimulated, resulting in DNA replication and transcription. The messenger RNA is then translated into various proteins. Decreased production of membrane testosterone receptors and cytoplasmic receptors occurs as a result of this nuclear stimulation.

Because AAS are analogs of testosterone, it is postulated that they work by the same biochemical reactions*; that is, direct or indirect stimulation of protein synthesis. In muscle cells, this would result in an increase in production of the proteins responsible for muscle contraction (actin, myosin, troponin, tropomysin, and others) energy production, and storage. A permanent increase in intracellular calcium concentration may also occur as a result of AAS use. This inotropic effect could lead to an increase in force and speed of muscle contraction and an acceleration of enzymatic reactions required for aerobic and anaerobic performance.

The most important anabolic effect of AAS is really their anticatabolic effect.[44,109,351,370] After strenuous activity, natural glucocorticoids are released, which result in breakdown of tissue. By some uncertain mechanism—perhaps the inhibition of cortisol from entrance into muscle and liver tissue—AAS prevent this tissue breakdown. This allows the athlete using AAS to exercise more intensely and frequently, as they do not experience the same degree of muscle damage and soreness after strenuous training. Because they are not breaking down their tissue as much, AAS users retain more of their strength and conditioning gains.

Another effect of AAS is an increase in aggressive behavior. Natural androgens cause an increase in aggression.† Because all AAS have both anabolic and androgenic effects, the AAS user usually experiences an increase in aggression. During the training session, this increase in aggression or aggressive behavior may allow the athlete to do more work, resulting in further overload of the metabolic systems, and thus promoting further strength and conditioning adaptations.‡

Administration. AAS can be administered in various ways. These agents are divided into oral (C-17-alpha alkylated steroids) and injectable (C-17-beta esterified steroids) forms. The injectable agents may be water or oil based; water-based AAS have a more rapid onset, less duration, and more rapid excretion than oil-based AAS.[140,161,214,351,370]

A cycle refers to a period of time that an individual is taking AAS and may range from 2 to 16 weeks. This cycle is followed by a equal or longer rest or recovery period. The justification for this regimen, from the user's standpoint, is that it allows the body time to recover to baseline hormone levels.

---

*References 19, 140, 171, 179, 304, 305, 308, 331, 351, 370.
†References 13, 212, 242, 253, 260, 279, 284, 297.
‡References 109, 121, 163, 168, 214, 351, 367.

Stacking refers to the use of more than one AAS during a cycle. This technique may allow the receptors to be saturated at the lower dose of each drug, thus minimizing the potential side effects and maximizing the anabolic effect.[161,214,370] Pyramiding refers to starting a drug at a low dose, gradually increasing to a plateau, and then gradually decreasing until the drug is discontinued. The purported benefit of this method is that as AAS are administered and down regulation begins, a larger and larger dose is required to saturate the receptors. Finally, a plateau is reached whereby the drug has no further benefits despite the high dosage. At this time, the individual begins to taper the drug over the course of a few weeks to minimize sudden withdrawal effects.[161,214,370] Another method of cycling is the dosepack technique, whereby AAS are begun at a very high dose and gradually tapered over the course of a few weeks. This technique saturates a maximum number of receptors immediately, and the rapid decrease in dose may minimize side effects.[299]

The total dose of steroids that an athlete takes may easily exceed 100 times the therapeutic dose for a given drug. The athlete will experiment with various drugs in an attempt to achieve the desired effects. Because the response to each AAS drug varies among individuals and within the same individual, it is necessary for the athlete to alter dosage schedules.

Oral AAS remain in the body and can be detected by urine drug testing from 2 to 14 days after administration. Injectable AAS are usually detectable up to 4 weeks after administration. However, some injectable agents, particularly the oil-based AAS, can be detected more than 12 months after injection.[87,148,161,270] The AAS may certainly remain effective even though they are not detectable in the urine.

Beneficial effects. The purported benefits of AAS use in the athlete include (1) increased lean body (muscle) mass, (2) increased strength, (3) increased aerobic capacity, and (4) increased aggressive behavior.*

Most of the AAS research is technically flawed. Current research efforts are difficult for several reasons. First, it is unethical to administer megadoses of AAS in a double-blind, random protocol. Second, athletes invariably know when they are taking the AAS compared to the placebo. Finally, many athletic organizations now ban the use of these agents.

In a classic review of the literature in 1984, Haupt and Rovere[163] found that AAS use consistently results in an increase in strength, body size, and weight if the athlete trains intensively in weightlifting immediately before the start of AAS use and continues the intensive weight training during the AAS regimen, if the athlete consumes a high-protein diet (2.2 mg/kg/day), and if the changes in

strength are measured using a single repetition maximum lift for those resistance exercises with which the athlete trains. Their review did not demonstrate improvement in aerobic performance as measured by VO₂ max and running and swimming times. Some reports, however, have demonstrated increased aerobic capacity in AAS users.[185,200] While this debate continues, endurance athletes continue to use AAS as part of their training program.

As stated earlier, AAS cause an increase in aggression. Users often experience a state of euphoria and increased energy, which enhances their training efforts. Numerous studies have demonstrated that the placebo effect is very real and may account for 10% to 30% of the gains made by the athlete using AAS.[10]

Because of contradictory studies, for many years physicians stated publicly that AAS had no effect on improving athletic performance. The athletes who used these drugs in conjunction with their training programs knew otherwise. This discrepancy in beliefs led to a large credibility gap between physicians and athletes. Athletes view the medical community and medical research with significant skepticism. It is imperative that this gap be bridged if the sports medicine community and the athletic fraternity are to develop the mutual respect needed to decrease the use of these agents.

Adverse effects. AAS are associated with many adverse effects.* Most are mild, some are severe, and some are theoretical. Most of the side effects are hepatic, endocrine and reproductive, cardiovascular, and psychologic; but other organ systems also can be involved.

Liver abnormalities occur in users of oral preparations. In general, there is elevation of the enzymes gamma-glutamyl transpeptidase (GGTP), serum glutamic-oxaloacetic transaminase (SGOT), serum glutamate-pyruvate transaminase (SGPT), alkaline phosphatase, lactate dehydrogenase (LDH), and bilirubin. Intense training alone may elevate these enzymes; therefore, fractionation of alkaline phosphatase and LDH should be used to establish hepatocellular dysfunction. Cholestatic jaundice may develop in a very small percentage of users.

Severe hepatotoxicities include peliosis hepatis and hepatic tumors. Peliosis hepatis is a condition in which potentially life-threatening, blood-filled cysts develop in the liver. Fewer than 30 cases have been reported in the literature.[163,183,214] Nearly all patients were treated with AAS for medical conditions, used oral agents, and took the medications continuously for over 6 months. Some authors feel that peliosis hepatis may actually be a precancerous lesion that can become malignant with prolonged AAS exposure.

Thirty-eight cases of AAS-induced hepatic tumors have been reported in the literature; 30 were considered malig-

*References 8, 9, 30, 78, 121, 161, 163, 168, 169, 170, 185, 186, 187, 189, 199, 214, 276, 333, 336, 354, 369, 370.

*References 161, 163, 190, 214, 351, 370.

nant, 35 occurred in patients being treated for a variety of medical conditions. Only three of the malignant tumors were reported in healthy adult men using AAS to enhance athletic performance.[75,145,163,214,280] Nearly all the liver tumors occurred in individuals who were taking the orally active anabolic steroids. Regression of hepatocellular carcinoma after the discontinuation of AAS has been reported,* suggesting that these lesions may not be truly malignant. A recent change in nomenclature describes androgenic-associated hepatic tumors. These tumors appear to have androgen receptors and develop and grow in response to androgenic steroid administration. When the steroids are discontinued, the tumor regresses. Nonandrogenic-associated hepatocellular carcinoma, regardless of how well differentiated, is relentlessly progressive and malignant.

AAS are associated with numerous cardiovascular effects.† Reversible hypertension occurs, especially with the use of highly androgenic AAS such as testosterone, which may be related to fluid retention. There is an almost universal, reversible increase in low-density lipoprotein cholesterol (LDL-C) and decrease in high-density lipoprotein cholesterol (HDL-C) during AAS use. The long-term significance of these changes is uncertain.

It has recently been reported that concentric myocardial hypertrophy appears to occur only in weightlifters who use AAS.[55,343] This finding contradicts previous studies suggesting that all serious weightlifters develop a concentric hypertrophy. These previous studies may have been flawed by not addressing AAS use in the weightlifters.

Acute myocardial infarctions in athletes with normal coronary arteries who use AAS has been reported.[31,231,246,252] A few case reports of stroke, pulmonary embolus, and arterial thrombosis in steroid users have also been published.[116,120,126,216] These significant cardiovascular events are probably related to hypercoagulability rather than artherosclerotic changes.

The long-term cardiovascular effects of AAS are largely unknown. Recent evidence suggests that serious complications may occur and studies are currently underway to evaluate these risks.[68]

The endocrinologic effects of AAS use in the male include a decrease in natural FSH, LH and testosterone production, azospermia including abnormal sperm morphology and decreased counts, and testicular atrophy, all of which appear to be reversible.[2,180,204,239,241] Gynecomastia, due to the peripheral conversion of AAS to estrogen, is irreversible.[189,214,351,370] AAS users self-administer tamoxifen with some success to treat this condition; however, surgical intervention is often required.[123,161] Sebaceous gland activation and changes in normal skin bacterial flora cause an increase in acne.[202,203] Relative glu-

cose intolerance, priapism and alopecia may also occur.[57,189,214,370]

Vocal cord hypertrophy, which results in deepening of the voice; male pattern baldness; hirsutism; and cliteromegaly are irreversible changes due to AAS use in women. Breast tissue atrophy and menstrual abnormalities are common and are reversible. Female users also have significant acne and abnormalities in glucose tolerance.[161,189,214,370]

AAS use may decrease connective tissue strength; anecdotally, this is manifested as muscle tears and tendon ruptures.* The rate of increased muscle strength is greater than the rate of increased tendon strength in response to AAS use and resistance exercise. This results in rupture of the tendon before the development of muscle fatigue.

AAS use causes a transient decrease in concentration of serum immunoglobulins and killer cell function.[48] This may result in frequent minor infections and theoretically an increased risk of malignancy. Two cases of Wilms' tumor and one case of prostate cancer have been reported in athletes using AAS.[294,300,335,370] Five cases of leukemia have been reported in patients with aplastic anemia who were treated with AAS.[84,98,201,277,370]

Perhaps the most significant short- and possibly long-term adverse effects of AAS use are psychologic. Increased aggression, change in libido, anxiety, panic disorder, psychosis, depression, mania, and addiction have all been reported in steroid users.† Although the exact incidence of these findings is unknown, research is ongoing to further define the incidence. Approximately 7% of steroid users will experience depression after withdrawal from steroids, and up to 10% may experience hypomania or mania while taking steroids. The incidence of steroid dependence may be as high as 15%.[87]

Subjectively, users often complain of headaches, dizziness, nausea, anorexia, increased appetite, euphoria, muscle spasms, rash, scrotal pain, dysuria, and insomnia.[87,163] Due to possible needle contamination, there is an increased risk of hepatitis B and HIV infection, and cases have been reported.[315,326]

Young athletes may also experience premature closure of the growth plates with resultant short stature and are at increased risk for abnormal psychosexual maturation.[86,190,214]

Human chorionic gonadotropin

Physiology. Human chorionic gonadotropin (HCG) is a glycoprotein hormone secreted by the trophoblastic epithelium of the placenta and purified from the urine of pregnant women.[368] HCG consists of two noncovalently linked subunits. Its alpha subunit is nearly identical to the alpha subunit of FSH, LH, and thyroid stimulating hormone

---

*References 112, 143, 182, 184, 262, 317.
†References 1, 14, 58, 65, 124, 172, 189, 214, 220, 222, 229, 285, 344, 351, 355, 370.

*References 161, 189, 214, 218, 254, 372, 377.
†References 7, 39, 40, 41, 60, 87, 122, 163, 166, 168, 196, 214, 235, 275, 291, 292, 293, 339, 376.

(TSH). The beta subunit of HCG and LH are related, but at the carboxy-terminal of HCG there is an additional 30-amino acid sequence. Due to its structural resemblance to LH, HCG is able to stimulate Leydig cells to increase testosterone production.

HCG produced by the trophoblastic cells in pregnant women is responsible for maintaining the corpus luteum. Cancer patients may develop ectopic production of this hormone, and the presence of a detectable level in a man or nonpregnant woman is indicative of an underlying tumor. Trophoblastic neoplasms of the placenta such as hydatidiform mole and choriocarcinoma; germ cell tumors; adenocarcinoma of the ovary, pancreas, and stomach; hepatomas; and islet cell carcinomas may all produce ectopic HCG. Tumors of the breast, bladder, adrenal, mediastinum, gonads, melanocytes and GI tract also have been reported to produce HCG.[83,368,373]

Administration. HCG is available in vials of 5000 to 20,000 International Units (IU). Because of its LH-like effect, HCG is used to establish or restore fertility in men with a secondary hypogonadism. The dose of HCG required to maintain a normal testosterone level ranges from 1000 to 5000 IU per week. The dose required for the induction of spermatogenesis is higher, usually 2000 to 5000 IU of HCG three or more times a week. The dosage is adjusted until clinical parameters and serum testosterone levels indicate normal adult male development.[83,368,373]

The athlete uses HCG to increase natural testosterone production by the testes.[335,349a,351] The increased serum testosterone levels then have the same potential beneficial effects as exogenously administered testosterone. HCG may be used alone or in conjunction with AAS. When used alone, HCG will cause a rapid increase in serum testosterone level. When used in conjunction with AAS, HCG will prevent or reverse testicular atrophy. HCG also is used on withdrawal from an AAS cycle to "naturally" stimulate endogenous testosterone production. Most athletes use a therapeutic dose of HCG, 1000 to 5000 IU per week.

Beneficial effects. High doses of HCG may be used to induce ovulation in women with infertility due to chronic anovulation.[83,368,373] It is generally given in conjunction with human menopausal gonadotropin (HMG, Pergonal). HMG is obtained from the urine of postmenopausal women and contains 75 IU of FSH and LH per vial.

HCG can be used clinically to assess testicular function.[83,368] The ability of Leydig cells to produce testosterone in response to gonadotropin stimulation is assessed after administration of HCG; 2000 IU are given intramuscularly for 4 days and plasma testosterone levels are measured before the first dose and 24 hours after the fourth dose. Normal prepubertal boys respond with an increase in plasma testosterone of about 300 ng/%. Normal men respond with a larger increase in testosterone, the magnitude of which peaks early in puberty.

Adverse effects. Most of the adverse effects of HCG are due to the increased testosterone level.[349,351] Water retention, hypertension, change in mood and libido, headaches, gynecomastia, and morning sickness may result from HCG use.

Growth hormone and related compounds

Physiology. Growth hormone (GH), produced in the anterior pituitary gland, is a single-chain polypeptide composed of 191 amino acids.[83,368,373] Originally, GH was produced by chemical extraction from the pituitary glands of human cadavers. In 1985, the use of this compound was suspended after the several GH users developed Creutzfeldt-Jakob disease.[59] GH is now produced by means of recombinant DNA technology.

GH secretion is stimulated by GH-releasing factor and inhibited by somatostatin, both of which are released from the hypothalamus. Many factors influence this response. Sleep, resistance exercise training, hypoglycemia, glucagon, estrogen, vasopressin, numerous amino acids (arginine, lysine, ornithine), serotonin, norepinephrine, dopamine, and a variety of other drugs may cause an increase in growth hormone response.* Obesity, hypokalemia, thyroid abnormalities, exogenous glucocorticoid use, Cushing's disease, hyperglycemia, progesterone, phenothiazine administration, and depression may blunt the growth hormone response.[83,234,368,373]

The degree of GH release also varies with age, level of maturity, diet, sex, baseline cardiorespiratory fitness, and intensity and duration of exercise. Released in a pulsatile fashion, GH has its peak effect about 60 minutes after release, and the level returns to baseline in approximately 200 minutes.[83,155] In the well-trained athlete, the peak concentration is less and the level returns to baseline within 30 minutes.[79]

GH affects growth of every tissue and organ in the body. Somatic growth is mediated by somatomedins, protein-bound hormones that are produced in the liver and released in response to GH. Somatomedin levels peak 3 hours after a GH surge, and remain elevated for 9 to 24 hours.[33,83]

Human GH increases intracellular transportation of amino acids and production of messenger RNA, resulting in an increased rate of protein synthesis. GH conserves muscle glycogen and glucose during exercise by directly stimulating lipolysis and increasing the sensitivity of fat to catecholamines. Inhibition of glucose uptake and use by muscle cells also occurs. Increased mobilization of free fatty acids and decreased glucose intake will decrease body fat, improve body composition, and preserve muscle glycogen stores during endurance events.†

---

*References 70, 79, 83, 101, 102, 174, 196, 214, 234, 337, 348, 373.
†References 33, 79, 83, 111, 113, 115, 125, 192, 234, 303, 310.

Human GH enhances the synthesis of collagen required for growth and development of bones, cartilage, tendons, and ligaments. This effect may increase axial growth in young users who have open epiphyseal growth plates. Stimulation of collagen synthesis by use of GH may also promote the healing of soft tissue injuries.[33,83,234,303]

Beneficial effects. Four effects of GH are perceived as beneficial to the athlete: (1) increased amino acid uptake and protein synthesis in skeletal muscle, (2) increased lipolysis, (3) increased axial growth (height) in the skeletally immature, and (4) enhanced healing of musculoskeletal injuries.

Skeletal muscle hypertrophy may be either GH dependent or work dependent.[141] Animal studies have shown that muscle hypertrophy can occur with GH treatment alone; however, there is less strength per mass than with work-dependent muscle hypertrophy.[142] GH administration will increase lean body mass, volume, and strength in GH-deficient humans.[83,113,303,310,359] GH administration may increase muscle size, volume, and strength in athletes; however, no controlled studies have been conducted to support this hypothesis.[33,79,234,303,375] Anecdotally, illicit users of GH feel there is a true anabolic effect.

GH may be used by short or average height and weight athletes who are genetically gifted in an attempt to increase size. Medical research in this area is not possible because of obvious ethical considerations.

Musculoskeletal injuries probably heal quicker with GH use because of increased protein synthesis. This effect would certainly be of value for an injured athlete trying to participate in continued training and competition.

Medically, the drug is intended for use in individuals who are deficient in natural GH. Use of the medication in these individuals allows normal growth and prevents pituitary dwarfism.[33,83,303,368,373]

Adverse effects. Little is known about the side effects of GH use in the non-GH-deficient athlete. GH excess in the nonathlete may result in gigantism in children and acromegaly in adults.[33,83,368,373] Gigantism is due to increased linear bone growth and acromegaly is due to increased growth of all tissues. Excessive skeletal growth results in the characteristic features of acromegaly: increased skull size, prominent cheek bones, protruding jaw, frontal bossing, and large, broad hands and feet. Organomegaly of the heart, liver, kidney, spleen, colon, and salivary glands can occur. Cardiovascular disease including hypertension and cardiomyopathy are not uncommon; most patients with acromegaly die of cardiac failure. Although skeletal muscle hypertrophy occurs, it is generally myopathic and thus results in muscle weakness. Thick skin, hirsutism, fibroma musculosum, ecanthosis nigricans, hypersecretion of sebaceous glands, hyperhydrosis, peripheral neuropathy, colonic polyps, glucose intolerance, and diabetes mellitus may also occur.

No case reports or studies of adverse effects of GH use

in the athlete have been published. If the use of GH in this population increases, such reports may appear.

Administration. In the treatment of pituitary dwarfism, the usual dose of GH is 1 to 2 ml/week.[83,140,286,368,373] Athletes using this agent will use 1 to 2 ml/day. Current black market prices are about $250 for a 10 ml vial; an 8-week cycle of GH costs nearly $2000. Because of the expense, many users use this agent sparingly and only in conjunction with AAS.[299]

Humatrope (somatropin) (Eli Lilly, Indianapolis, Ind.) contains the correct 191-amino acid sequence of GH. Protropin (Somatren) (Genetech, South San Francisco, Calif.) is a 192-amino acid sequence.[286] Although Protropin is more readily available on the black market, it is thought inferior to Humatrope because of the additional amino acid. The extra amino acid may lead to antibody production to the exogenous GH, thereby rendering it ineffective. There is less chance of developing immunity to Humatrope.

With advancing recombinant DNA technology, the production of somatomedin C and other somatomedins will occur. Because of the specificity of somatomedins for skeletal muscle, this organ should be the only one affected. The result will be avoidance of most of the potential adverse effects of GH.

Stimulants

The athlete uses AAS, HCG, and GH to improve work output and efficiency. Stimulants are used to affect nervous system control. The central nervous system (CNS) coordinates muscle cell activity during exercise. Most people operate at a level of neural inhibition that prevents the expression of true strength capacity. In the early stages of strength training, neural facilitation reduces this inhibition and accounts for the rapid improvements of strength seen during the early phases of training.[117,210,261] Psychologic manipulation such as hypnosis, biofeedback, and placebo may also improve neural activity. The use of stimulants may also achieve this effect; they are also used as ergogenic aids because of their ability to mask, delay, or alter the perception of fatigue.[71,162,353]

Amphetamines

Historical development. Amphetamine is a sympathomimetic amine that mimics the actions of endogenous hormones such as epinephrine and norepinephrine. Amphetamines have been used for many years as an ergogenic aid and were first synthesized in 1887. In the 1930s, Piness et al.[289] established the pressor effects of amphetamine. In 1935, Prinzmetal and Bloomberg[295] treated narcolepsy with amphetamine, taking advantage of its central stimulant effect. The Germans demonstrated that time of running to exhaustion was increased with the use of intramuscular amphetamine, and actually may have used this drug during World War II to delay the onset of fatigue in military troops.[353] In the late 1940s, experimental research showed enhanced endurance in cycling and hand ergometry.[81,225]

Amphetamine abuse began to occur in the 1940s and became widespread in the United States in the 1960s. In 1969, over 13% of American college students had used amphetamines at least once. Research in the National Football League (NFL) between 1972 and 1975 revealed that approximately 70% of players used amphetamine at least sometimes during participation and over 50% used amphetamines regularly.[351] In 1985, 8% of college athletes had used amphetamines within the past year; 37% of this group used this agent to improve performance and 61% used it for recreational purposes.[6] However, the incidence of use by college athletes fell from 8% in 1985 to 3% in 1989.[6] The reasons for this decline are uncertain. It may be the result of current education and awareness programs, the status of amphetamine as a controlled substance, other variables, or a combination of these factors.

Biochemistry and physiology. In addition to the peripheral alpha and beta actions common to these indirectly acting sympathomimetic agents, amphetamine also has a powerful CNS stimulant effect. The purported action of amphetamines on the peripheral and central nervous systems includes (1) displacement of catecholamine causing direct release into the synaptic cleft, (2) action as a catecholamine agonist, (3) inhibition of catecholamine reuptake at the synaptic cleft resulting in increased bioavailability, and (4) inhibition of monaminoxidase resulting in decreased degradation and increased effective concentration.[140,225,351]

The most powerful CNS effect of amphetamine is the behavioral response. Clinically, this response is manifested as increased alertness, decreased sense of fatigue, and a delay in the point of fatigue during prolonged intense exercises. This effect is more marked when performance is reduced by fatigue or lack of sleep. Other central effects include elevation of mood, increased motor and speech activity, improved self-confidence, and decreased appetite.[71,162,225,351] The most prominent peripheral effects are elevation of systolic and diastolic blood pressure with reflex bradycardia and increased lipolysis.

Beneficial effects. Studies have shown that amphetamine use can enhance some skills that play a key role in athletic performance, including speed, power, endurance, concentration, and fine motor coordination.[52,81,329] Smith and Beecher[329] showed an improvement in performance in throwers, runners, and swimmers given amphetamine in doses of 14 mg/kg. Amphetamine does not prevent fatigue but rather masks the physiologic symptoms. Amphetamine restores the reaction time in weary athletes but does not appear to improve reaction time or diligence in well-rested athletes. Enhanced lipolysis, by sparing muscle glycogen stores, may improve aerobic endurance. Due to their psychologic effects, these agents may be ergogenic in strength and power sports.[71,162,225,353]

Adverse effects. Most of the adverse effects of amphetamine are related to the CNS action: anxiety, nervousness, agitation, anorexia, insomnia, paranoia, and hallucinations.[140,162,225,353] Palpitations and hypertension with subsequent cerebrovacular accident (CVA) and myocardial infarction (MI) may occur.

Sympathomimetic agents. Athletes use numerous other sympathomimetic amines.[162,225,353] Drugs such as ephedrine, phenylephrine, phenylpropanolamine, and pseudoephedrine are structurally similar to amphetamine. Beta-agonists such as albuterol, isoetharine, terbutaline, metaproterenol, and clenbuterol are also used for their potential ergogenic effects.

Biochemistry and physiology. The amphetamine lookalikes, such as phenlypropanolamine and ephedrine, are indirect sympathomimetic agents.[140,162,353] These drugs displace norepinephrine and other neurotransmitters from their storage sites causing CNS stimulation, but not to the degree of amphetamine. The central effects are similar to amphetamine and include increased alertness and decreased fatigue. These drugs also have a direct peripheral effect on the alpha- and beta-receptors causing increased blood pressure and heart rate, bronchodilation, and probable increased peripheral lipolysis.

Beneficial effects. Many endurance, strength, and power athletes use sympathomimetic agents by inhalation or orally to improve performance.[162,225,353] The beneficial effects of sympathomimetic agents are similar to amphetamine: improved speed, power, endurance, concentration, fine motor coordination, lipolysis, and reaction time, especially in fatigued athletes. Elevated mood and increased alertness also occur. Recent evidence suggests that inhaling albuterol before activity increases power.[16,325] Clenbuterol, a potent beta-adenergic agonist, may promote skeletal muscle development and improve lipolysis, making it an attractive supplement to both strength and endurance athletes.[374]

Adverse effects. Adverse effects of sympathomimetic amines and beta-agonists are similar to amphetamine: nervousness, irritability, anorexia, tachycardia, palpitations, confusion, paranoia, hallucination, CVA, and MI.[140,162,225,353] Beta-agonist use may result in tachycardia, hypertension, agitation, and tremor.[140,286]

Caffeine. Coffee is the major source of caffeine, the most widely consumed drug in North America. A methylxanthine, caffeine shares properties with other drugs in this group, which includes theophylline and theobromine.[140]

Beneficial effects. Caffeine affects athletic performance in three main ways.[162,225,353] First, it is a CNS stimulant; it improves neuromuscular activation to coordinate muscle activity, increases lipolysis as a result of catecholamine release, and increases mental alertness. Second, it is a direct adipocyte receptor stimulant, which increases lipolysis. Third, it directly stimulates the muscle cell to decrease glycogenolysis and increase free fatty acid metabolism.

Caffeine also increases GI secretions, resting blood pressure, heart rate, stroke volume, cardiac output, oxygen consumption, metabolic rate, and skeletal muscle contractility.[140]

Aerobic performance may be improved in caffeine users secondary to muscle glycogen sparing and increased fat mobilization and utilization.* Performance may also be improved by increased alertness, reduced perception of fatigue, shortened reaction time, and increased capacity for attention requiring tasks. No proven benefits of caffeine have been demonstrated for short-term, high-intensity work.[162,225,353]

Adverse effects. Nervousness, irritability, insomnia, tachycardia, hypertension, GI distress, xerostomia, tinnitus, myalgia, headache, and scotomata can occur with acute caffeine use. Peptic ulcer disease, delirium, seizure and coma, cardiac dysrhythmias, and ectopy are more severe effects.[140,162,225,353]

Ergogenic effects of caffeine do not seem to occur until the urine concentration is greater than 12 μg/ml. For this reason, the International Olympic Committee (IOC) bans athletes with urine caffeine concentrations over 12 μg/ml; the National Collegiate Athletic Association (NCAA) limits caffeine concentration to 15 μg/ml.[154,225,353] Two hours after the consumption of 2 cups of coffee, 48 ounces of Coca-Cola, or 1 vivarin tablet, the urine concentration of caffeine will be about 3 μg/ml.[154]

Cocaine. Cocaine is a CNS stimulant similar to amphetamine. This drug has been used for centuries as a mood-altering agent and stimulant. This dangerously addictive drug is used by athletes for social and recreational purposes rather than for ergogenic effects. Depending on the route of administration, the drug achieves peak effect within seconds to minutes and the effects last from minutes to hours.[140,162,226,353]

Beneficial effects. In theory, cocaine could have a beneficial effect by enhanced endurance and improved sense of mental prowess; however, objective observers note that athletic performance deteriorates with acute cocaine use.[340]

Adverse effects. Mild adverse effects of cocaine include insomnia, anorexia, delirium, confusion, and paranoia. Serious complications include psychosis, seizures, CVA, MI, cardiac dysrhythmia, and sudden death.†

Blood doping/erythropoietin/iron

The use of blood transfusion, erythropoietin, and iron supplementation may increase the oxygen-carrying capacity of the blood, increase buffering capacity for metabolic wastes, and decrease cardiac workload for a given aerobic performance. If these methods do improve energy delivery and waste removal, aerobic performance will improve. This is the basis and rationale for the use of these techniques by the athlete.

Physiology. During aerobic exercise there is a significant increase in blood flow to the exercising muscles. This increased blood flow delivers important nutrients and removes metabolic waste products. During prolonged exercise skeletal muscle uses glucose and fatty acid as energy sources; oxygen is required to fully metabolize these energy sources to obtain maximum adenosine triphosphate (ATP) production. Oxygen is delivered to the tissues primarily by binding to the hemoglobin in red blood cells; a small amount of oxygen is in dissolved form in the plasma. Red blood cells also transport numerous metabolic waste products from the tissues.[368,373]

Methods to increase oxygen delivery to the system would include increasing (1) the amount of oxygen dissolved in the plasma, (2) the amount of oxygen combined with hemoglobin, and (3) the total amount of hemoglobin.

Erythropoietin, a renal glycoprotein hormone released in response to a low hematocrit, directly stimulates red blood cells forming units in the bone marrow. This results in an increase in hematocrit and oxygen-carrying capacity, which may improve aerobic endurance. The increased hematocrit increases the buffering capacity of the blood for lactic acid and other metabolic wastes; this increase may result in a delay in the onset of fatigue associated with exercise. Also with the increased hematocrit, a smaller portion of the cardiac output is able to supply the same amount of oxygen to exercising muscles, leaving a larger component of the cardiac output to be diverted to the skin for heat dissipation. The improved heat transfer decreases the risk of dehydration; dehydration will definitely interfere with athletic performance.[103,191]

Erythropoietin has a serum half-life of approximately 4 hours, but there are prolonged effects because the life span of the resultant red blood cell is 120 days. Recombinant erythropoietin has been available since 1987 and from a physiologic and immunologic standpoint, it is identical to the natural human erythropoietin.[4,103,314]

Blood doping is another method to increase the total amount of hemoglobin. Heterologous blood doping involves the transfusion of donated packed red blood cells 1 to 7 days before competition. Autologous blood doping involves donating two or more units of blood at least 8 weeks before competition, and then reinfusing the thawed, resuspended blood 1 to 7 days before the event. After transfusion, the hematocrit stays elevated for approximately 7 days and then gradually decreases over the subsequent 3 to 4 months.[4,191]

Iron is required for the synthesis of hemoglobin and myoglobin and is an important component of the electron transport chain. It is believed that iron deficiency, with or

*References 20, 63, 108, 175, 228, 342, 360.
†References 49, 76, 140, 162, 226, 230, 353.

without anemia, will impair aerobic performance.* Certainly, anemic athletes have a decreased oxygen-carrying capacity. Iron deficiency without anemia may impair endurance training and performance by decreasing ATP production from the electron transport chain, which requires elemental iron as a cofactor. This impairment may be manifested clinically by complaints of fatigue, decreased performance, and increased running time. Laboratory investigations may reveal a decreased hemoglobin and hematocrit with a decreased mean corpuscular volume, decreased mean corpuscular hemoglobin, increased red blood cell distribution width, and a low ferritin level.

In the human, the ferrous form of dietary iron is more readily absorbed than the ferric form with the absorption taking place in the duodenum and proximal jejunum. Vitamin C promotes iron absorption, most likely secondary to maintaining the iron in the reduced ferrous form. Carbohydrates are also necessary for adequate iron absorption.[368]

Administration. The amount of erythropoietin required to increase the hematocrit is uncertain. About 75 U/kg of erythropoietin three times a week is required to maintain a hematocrit of 35% in anephric patients.[103,104,105,106,371] Athletes with a normal hematocrit will raise their hematocrit to about 50% using 20 to 40 U/kg three times a week for 6 weeks.[94] For a given individual, there appears to be a consistent dose-dependent increase in hematocrit in response to erythropoietin administration; however, the response varies among individuals.[103,191] After erythropoietin administration, the hematocrit begins to rise within 7 days and will continue to rise for 5 to 10 days after the last injection. The hematocrit remains increased for the life span of the red blood cell, which is approximately 120 days.

For blood doping to improve aerobic performance, about 900 to 1800 ml of autologous or 2000 ml of homologous blood are required.† Packed red blood cells are transfused with normal saline at a hematocrit of 50% 7 days before the event. The postinfusion hypervolemia leads to a shift in protein-free plasma from the intravascular to the interstitial compartments. The result is an eventual normovolemia with a greater hemoglobin concentration. The hematocrit remains constant for approximately 7 days after infusion and then gradually declines over the succeeding 100 days.

For autologous transfusion, two units of blood are removed at least 8 weeks before the event.[4,191] The donated blood is then frozen in glycerol to interrupt the aging process; this process actually allows storage for up to 10 years. During the 8 weeks after donation, the athlete continues to train and the hemoglobin will return to normal, prephlebotomy level. After thawing and resuspension in saline to a hematocrit of 50%, the blood is infused 1 to 7 days before competition.

The current United States Recommended Daily Allowance (RDA) for iron is 18 mg/day of elemental iron for menstruating women and boys and 10 mg/day for men. The average diet supplies about 5 to 6 mg of elemental iron per 1000 calories consumed. An athlete consuming less than 2000 calories a day may not be taking in enough iron. In addition to insufficient intake, heel strike hemolysis, GI and renal blood losses, menstruation, and possibly sweat loss may lead to iron deficiency. The diagnosis of iron deficiency with or without anemia is confirmed with a complete blood count, and more important, a ferritin level.[38,50,165,273]

Some normal athletes are found to be "anemic" during routine bloodwork.[50,273] As an adaptation to aerobic exercise training, there is an increase in intravascular volume with no change in the number of red blood cells, which results in a dilutional anemia. This condition, which requires no treatment, can be differentiated from true anemia by the absence of symptoms, normal red blood cell indices, and a normal ferritin level.

Administration of iron should be made only to individuals who are documented to be iron deficient.[38,50,165,273,306] The best sources of dietary iron are beef and pork products, which contain the ferrous form. Vegetable sources, such as spinach, broccoli, and peas, contain the ferric form, which is less readily absorbed. Supplementation with ferrous sulfate or gluconate may be used to treat iron deficiency. Supplementation should be continued until laboratory and clinical parameters return to normal.

Beneficial effects. Blood doping and erythropoietin use will improve endurance performance by increasing hematocrit.* There is an increased arterial-venous oxygen difference, increased maximum oxygen consumption (Mvo_2), increased endurance capacity, and improved carbon dioxide and waste removal from tissues. With a hematocrit over 50%, there is decreased heart rate, cardiac output, and lactate for exercise at a given intensity.

It is believed that the optimum hematocrit for improvement in athletic performance is about 55%. The total amount of erythropoietin required to achieve this level is uncertain.[94] About 900 to 1800 ml of autologous blood and 2000 ml of heterologous blood are needed for improvement in athletic performance.* Iron supplementation in a nondeficient athlete will result in no improvement in hematocrit or athletic performance.[38,271,306]

Adverse effects. Hyperviscosity is the most serious adverse effect of blood doping and erythropoietin use.[4,94,103,191,298] As the hematocrit approaches 60%,

---

*References 38, 54, 165, 272, 278, 313.

†References 21, 36, 43, 99, 100, 282, 301, 302, 312, 332, 363, 364, 365.

*References 4, 31, 36, 43, 99, 100, 191, 282, 301, 302, 312, 332, 363, 364, 365.

blood viscosity increases, which may lead to myocardial infarction, cerebrovascular accident, and peripheral artery thrombosis. Early symptoms of increased viscosity include headache, dizziness, vertigo, tinnitus, visual changes, angina, and intermittent claudication. Dehydration, which frequently occurs with exercise, will compound this syndrome by further increasing the hematocrit. Although parenterally administered erythropoietin lasts only 3 to 5 days, there are prolonged effects because the serum life of the red blood cell produced is 120 days. In addition because the response to erythropoietin is uncertain, there is a significant risk for hyperviscosity. For these reasons, individuals using these techniques must have their hematocrit levels monitored closely.

Blood doping itself carries all the potential complications of transfusion including venous thrombosis, phlebitis, sepsis, transfusion reaction, delayed red blood cell destruction, and disease transmission such as HIV and hepatitis B.*

Erythropoietin and blood doping are banned by the IOC, NCAA, and most other governing bodies. Unfortunately, no tests are currently available to accurately detect the use of these techniques. Athletes discovered to be using these techniques are banned from competition, have their achievements stricken from the records and their medals rescinded, and place their entire athletic careers in jeopardy.

The use of iron may lead to nausea, vomiting, abdominal pain, and distention, all of which may interfere with athletic performance. Potential toxic effects include bloody diarrhea, lethargy, restlessness, shock, acidosis, hepatic necrosis, and GI obstruction. Toxic effects are usually not seen unless large amount of iron are ingested.[368,373]

Protein and amino acid supplements

Biochemistry. (Refer to Part V, Clinical Nutrition in Disease Prevention.)

Dietary protein is broken down into amino acid building blocks, which are then used by the body for a variety of purposes. Amino acids are the precursors for protein and muscle synthesis, form enzymes and hormones to regulate cellular processes and reactions, maintain and repair body tissue, and form hemoglobin and antibodies. Through a series of enzymatic reactions (gluconeogenesis), amino acids may be converted into glucose and tricarboxcylic acid cycle (TCA) precursors to provide energy in the form of ATP. Used as an energy source, amino acids and proteins provide 4 Cal/gram.

Of the 21 amino acids present in the human body, histidine, leucine, isoleucine, valine, lysine, methionine, phenlylalanine, threonine, and tryptophan are essential or unable to be synthesized in vivo. Animal protein, milk, egg yolks, and soy are complete proteins in that they con-

tain all of the essential amino acids. Grains are low in lysine content and vegetables are low in methionine content.

Physiology. After absorption, dietary protein and amino acid supplements are used for a variety of body functions. The amino acids are used as protein precursors in muscle hypertrophy associated within strength training. During endurance training, the amino acids are used as TCA intermediates leading to increased oxidation of acetyl coenzyme A (CoA) and increased ATP production. Amino acids can be converted to glucose through gluconeogenesis and can be oxidized by the muscle to provide energy. The branched-chain amino acids (leucine, isoleucine, and valine) are most readily oxidized during aerobic exercise, but no studies have found improved performance with their use.*

Specific amino acids (arginine, ornithine, lysine, phenlyalanine, and methionine) have been shown to increase GH levels.[101,102,174,234,337] Supplementation with these specific amino acids may increase GH secretion and theoretically lead to the beneficial effects observed with GH use. No studies, however, have shown improvement in strength or body composition in athletes using large quantities of amino acid supplements.[101,102,174,257,337]

Administration. The current recommended daily allowance for protein is 0.8 g/kg/day. Most athletes eating a normal western diet consume at least 1.5 g/kg/day.† Athletes involved in heavy resistance exercises, such as weightlifting and body building, or long endurance training, may require over 2.2 g/kg/day of protein.‡ For practical purposes, protein should make up approximately 10% to 20% of the total daily calories.

The complete proteins—that is, animal, milk, egg, and soy—should be the protein foundation of a healthy athletic diet. Vegetarians may be deficient in lysine, methionine, and other amino acids and may require specific amino acid supplementation. After ingestion the rates of absorption of simple amino acids and protein are similar.

Beneficial effects. In an athlete who may be deficient in dietary protein calories, amino acid and protein supplements may be beneficial. Specifically, vegetarians may benefit from supplementation with lysine and methionine. The branched-chain amino acids, which can be used as an energy source in endurance activities, have not been shown to improve athletic performance. Arginine, ornithine, lysine, and other amino acid supplements, which have been shown to increase growth hormone release, have not shown an increase in strength or improvement in body fat in athletes.

To summarize, amino acid and protein supplementation does not improve athletic performance unless there is a dietary insufficiency.[38,46,88,167]

---

*References 4, 35, 37, 80, 149, 192, 288, 344.

*References 26, 128, 258, 319, 351, 353.
†References 38, 46, 88, 150, 167, 221.
‡References 38, 46, 51, 61, 215, 221, 236.

Adverse effects. Amino acids and protein supplements cause few side effects.[257,327,351] Dehydration, gout, hypocalcemia from urinary calcium losses, and renal and hepatic damage from excessive nitrogen load may result from amino acid supplementation. More important, excessive dietary protein may result in a carbohydrate deficiency, which has been proven to interfere with athletic performance.

Vitamins and minerals

Biochemistry and physiology. (Refer to Part V, Clinical Nutrition in Disease Prevention.)

Many vitamins and minerals are required for optimum nutrition, and many supplements are available. Vitamins are divided into fat soluble and water soluble, and their primary function is to act as cofactors and coenzymes for numerous cellular reactions. The fat soluble vitamins are A, D, E, and K. There are numerous water-soluble vitamins including the B vitamins, C, niacin, folate, biotin, and pantothenic acid.

Calcium, phosphorus, iodine, and iron are the most important minerals. Numerous trace minerals such as magnesium, zinc, copper, cobalt, selenium, manganese, nickel, chromium, fluoride, and silicon are essential for optimum biochemical and physiologic processes.

Vitamin and mineral deficiencies in the athlete consuming an adequate, well-balanced diet are extremely rare. However, the athlete who is amenorrheic or oligomenorrheic or who is avoiding dairy products may be calcium deficient.[46,90,91,191,296] Iron deficiency and anemia have been discussed previously in the section on blood doping/erythropoietin/iron.

Chromium picolinnate is a commonly used supplement. Chromium is an essential component of glucose tolerance factor that facilitates insulin action in sensitive tissues and is necessary for normal glucose tolerance.[368,373] A deficiency of chromium leads to reversible glucose intolerance, ataxia, and peripheral neuropathy.[29] The incidence of chromium deficiency in healthy patients, however, is extremely rare, and there is no evidence of improved performance in athletes who are not deficient and use a chromium supplement.[352]

Boron, zinc, magnesium, selenium, and other minerals are also promoted as ergogenic elements. As with vitamins, unless the athlete is deficient, there is no evidence that use of these supplements will improve athletic performance.[307,353,356,357]

Administration. Vitamins and minerals are available as oral preparations; some are available for parenteral administration. The body readily absorbs these substances based on need and bioavailability. Excesses are excreted in the stool and urine to maintain homeostatic balance.

Beneficial effects. In studies of trained athletes, the use of vitamin and mineral supplements has resulted in no significant change in hemoglobin and hematocrit, Mvo_2,

peak exercise speed, and lactate levels.* Unless the individual is deficient in a vitamin or mineral, there is no evidence to support improved athletic performance with supplementation. With a well-balanced diet, vitamin and mineral deficiencies are rare, with the exception of iron and calcium. For these reasons, the use of vitamin and mineral supplements should not be encouraged. Nevertheless, up to 80% of athletes use a multivitamin daily. Because of a variety of unhealthy dietary practices in the athlete, it is reasonable to suggest a one-a-day multivitamin and mineral supplement.[17,362]

Adverse effects. The use of a daily multivitamin has not been associated with serious deleterious effects. Megadosing of vitamins, however, may cause serious adverse effects.[351,368,373] Toxic levels of vitamin A result in acute hydrocephalus, pseudotumor cerebri, cirrhosis, bony resorption, hypercalcemia, and hypertriglyceridemia and may have teratogenic effects. Excessive vitamin D may lead to hypercalcemia, apathy, headache, anorexia, hypertension, nephrolithiasis, cardiac dysrhythmia, ectopic calcification, and bone pain. Toxic levels of vitamin E may cause generalized fatigue and weakness, headache, nausea, diarrhea, and hypercholesterolemia. Adverse effects of water-soluble vitamins are rare; however toxic doses of niacin cause urticaria, flushing, bronchospasm, hyperuricemia, hyperglycemia, hepatitis, and hypertension. Vitamin C intoxication may be manifested by nausea, vomiting, diarrhea, and vitamin B_{12} destruction. Toxic doses of pyridoxine may cause a sensory neuropathy. Other adverse effects of vitamins may also be noted.

Supplementation with large doses of minerals is unlikely to cause serious side effects. Excessive calcium supplementation may lead to hypercalcemia and many side effects similar to vitamin D intoxication. Iron toxicity has been previously discussed in the section on blood doping/erythropoietin/iron. Excessive intake on the trace minerals results in few side effects, and most will be unabsorbed or excreted unchanged in the urine.[368,373]

Miscellaneous

Sodium bicarbonate. The use of oral sodium bicarbonate before exercise may delay or prevent acidosis-induced muscle fatigue.† The bicarbonate acts as a proton sink, allowing for more rapid removal of the lactic acid produced during exercise. A regimen of 300 mg/kg of sodium bicarbonate taken 30 minutes before high-intensity, short-duration exercise has been found to decrease lactic acid levels and improve performance time.[361] It appears to be a more effective supplement in exercise that involves the lower extremities; no effect has been demonstrated in aerobic or upper extremity anaerobic activity. The side ef-

---

*References 15, 17, 46, 165, 271, 306, 351, 356, 357, 362.
†References 71, 130, 144, 173, 219, 251, 351, 361.

fects of acute sodium bicarbonate loading include significant GI distress, eructation, flatulence, and diarrhea; chronic bicarbonate use may result in electrolyte disturbances.

Phosphate. Phosphate loading theoretically increases concentration of 2,3-diphosphoglycerate (2,3-DPG) in red blood cells.[351] This increase results in a shift of the oxygen dissociation curve to the right, leading to increased oxygen unloading at the tissue level. The phosphate may also act as a proton sink, thereby buffering the lactic acid produced during exercise; 500 mg or more of sodium phosphate is consumed daily to achieve this effect. This regimen has been shown to possibly increase learning efficiency; however, no studies have confirmed improvement in high-intensity exercise performance.[47,93,178,211] Excessive phosphate administration may cause hyperphosphatemia.

Diuretics. Diuretics are used by athletes for a number of reasons.[351,353] Wrestlers, boxers, and jockeys may use diuretics to achieve rapid weight loss to make a specific weight class. Gymnasts and dancers use diuretics to improve body image. Diuretics are also used by athletes abusing a variety of banned substances to reduce urine concentration of the banned drugs. Dehydration associated with diuretic use results in a decrease in overall athletic performance. Serious electrolyte abnormalities associated with diuretic use may also lead to potentially life-threatening conditions. Diuretics are banned by the NCAA, IOC, and numerous other governing bodies because of the masking effect on urine drug testing and the unnatural weight loss associated with their use.

Alcohol. Alcohol is a CNS depressant and, as such, causes impairment of psychomotor skills and deleterious effects on athletic performance.[53,269,353] Accuracy, balance, steadiness, reaction time, complex and fine motor coordination, visual tracking, and information processing are adversely affected with acute alcohol use. Alcohol use may lead to a decrease in aerobic capacity; however, there is no change in muscle strength or endurance.[27,250] Athletic performance may be adversely affected by social use of alcohol the day before an event.[53] Symptoms of acute alcohol ingestion include euphoria, impaired judgment, nystagmus, cardiac dysrhythmia, coma, and death. Chronic alcohol use results in CNS, cardiac and GI deterioration. Used in low doses, alcohol may have an anxiolytic and antitremor effect and, therefore, is ergogenic in sports such as archery and riflery where a steady hand is required for optimum performance.[208] For this reason, alcohol use is banned by the NCAA and IOC in these events.

Beta-blockers. The use of beta-blockers by an athlete results in a decrease in aerobic and anaerobic endurance and power.[345,351] Bronchospasm, hypotension, bradycardia, atrioventricular block, sleep disturbance, impotence, and hypoglycemia may result from beta-blocker use.[140,286,368,373] However, anxiolysis, bradycardia, and the antitremor effects of beta-blockers are ergogenic in sports requiring steadiness such as archery and riflery.[213,351,353] Beta-blocker use by anxious musicians has also reportedly improved performance.[110] The IOC and NCAA ban the use of beta-blockers in those sports that require a steady hand.

Narcotics. Narcotics are used clinically for pain management and cough suppression and as an adjunct in the treatment of acute cardiogenic pulmonary edema. The use of narcotics by the athlete does not result in an ergogenic effect; however, it may allow the injured athlete to compete in spite of pain. In a 1989 survey,[6] nearly one third of college athletes admitted to use of narcotics within the previous year; 95% of these used the narcotics for control of pain associated with an injury. The use of narcotics may allow the injured athlete to compete through pain at the risk of masking medical or orthopedic problems. This practice could result in more serious long-term sequelae.[353]

Acute narcotic use causes sedation, clouding of sensorium, difficulty in mentation, euphoria, dysphoria, decreased visual acuity, nausea, vomiting, constipation, and other effects that could adversely affect athletic performance. Chronic narcotic use has not been shown to have adverse effects on athletic performance. Although short-term narcotic use for control of severe pain is unlikely to lead to narcotic dependence, tolerance does develop in the chronic user, leading to increased dosage and possible addiction. Narcotics are banned by the IOC and other governing bodies.[353]

RECOGNITION AND TREATMENT OF ABUSE
History

With most medical conditions, the history is the most important factor in identifying the pathology. Abuse of performance-enhancing agents is no exception. The interview should begin with general questions and lead to more specific ones. Because most athletes and potential users of ergogenic aids are young and healthy, they rarely seek medical attention.

The best opportunity for discussion of this topic is at the time of the preseason and postseason physical examinations. Because many of these physical examinations are in an open, group setting, however, there is little opportunity for confidential discussion. One method to circumvent this lack of privacy is to have a separate private station during the physical examination. This approach will give the athlete the opportunity to discuss not only the use of ergogenic substances but also other pertinent health issues such as drug and alcohol abuse, sexually transmitted disease, HIV, and many other health concerns. The private physician office is another location where preseason evaluations are performed; here, too, is an excellent opportunity to discuss these issues.

The interview may begin with general questions regarding the athlete's overall health status, general nutrition, and strength and conditioning programs. This approach easily leads into directly asking athletes if they are using any special techniques or supplements to improve their athletic performance. Specific questions can then be asked as guided by the patients' responses. If the physician is perceived as being honest, sincere, and concerned about the welfare of the athlete, it is usually easy to obtain accurate historical information. If the physician is perceived as uninterested, judgmental, or a threat, the history is unlikely to be fruitful. If the patient admits to using ergogenic techniques, determine how recently, how much, and how often they were used. Inquire about potential side effects and address any other concerns that the athlete expresses.[189]

Once a user has been identified, a systematic review of adverse effects should be made. A review of pertinent adverse effects may also assist in identifying an athlete who denies but is suspected of ergogenic use.[189,227]

Physical examination

The physical examination can be extremely helpful in identifying the user of ergogenic aids. A complete examination should be performed on all athletes before competition; during this evaluation specific abnormalities may be noted.

AAS users may have a sudden and dramatic increase in size, weight, and strength. Other findings on physical examination may include hypertension, tachycardia, scleral icterus, cardiac hypertrophy, tender or nontender hepatomegaly, gynecomastia, testicular atrophy, alopecia, acne, needle marks, and significant psychologic swings, ranging from major depression to mania and psychoses. Physical findings in the female may also include vocal cord hypertrophy with deepening of the voice, alopecia, cliteromegaly, and breast tissue atrophy.

Physical findings in users of HCG may include hypertension, water retention, gynecomastia, needle marks and psychologic changes in mood and libido. Decreased body fat and increased lean body mass and strength may be observed in users of GH; acromegalic features and other physical findings appear to be extremely rare.

Athletes using erythropoietin and blood doping will have few physical findings. Indications of blood donation or transfusion such as hematoma, phlebitis, and puncture wounds in the antecubital fossa may be the only physical findings. After blood donation, aerobic performance may decline secondary to the phlebotomy-induced anemia; this may be noted by a coach or other person close to the training athlete.

Athletes using stimulants such as amphetamine, caffeine, ephedrine, and phenylpropanolamine may be found to have tachycardia, hypertension, palpitations, anxiety, agitation, tremulousness, anorexia, and weight loss. Users

of amino acid and protein supplements, vitamin and mineral supplements, bicarbonate, and phosphate will have no obvious physical findings. Diuretic users may be found to have orthostatic hypotension and other findings consistent with dehydration.

Athletes using alcohol solely as an ergogenic aid will have few, if any, physical findings. Mood disturbance, sedation, and impairment of psychomotor skills may be present with acute alcohol use. Findings of chronic alcohol abuse are discussed elsewhere in this textbook (refer to Chapter 15). Beta-blocker use by athletes may be manifested by hypotension, bradycardia, and bronchospasm. Long-term side effects of beta-blockers are rarely seen in the athlete, as these medications are used only during the actual time of competition. Use of narcotics by the athlete may be difficult to detect; however, sedation, and dysphoria may be observed. If injectable narcotics are used, needle marks may be apparent.

Investigations

Routine laboratory investigations may uncover abnormalities suggestive of abuse of one or more of these techniques. Other testing may be required to fully evaluate the athlete. Additionally, a variety of tests may be helpful to confirm ergogenic use when it is suspected.[189,191,227] The use of AAS may cause elevation of SGOT, SGPT, alkaline phosphatase, LDH, and bilirubin. FSH, LH, and natural testosterone will decrease; however, if a testosterone preparation is being used, the testosterone level will increase significantly. Hypertriglyceridemia and hypercholesterolemia with an increase in LDL-C and a decrease in HDL-C will be present. A sperm count may be necessary to evaluate testicular function. Routine chest x-ray study and electrocardiagram (ECG) may reveal nonspecific signs of left ventricular hypertrophy.

Blood doping and erythropoietin use will result in an increase in hemoglobin and hematocrit if the athlete is tested within 2 to 3 months of using these techniques. Bicarbonate use may cause metabolic alkalosis and hyperkalemia. Phosphate loading may lead to hyperphosphatemia and hypocalcemia. The use of diuretics may cause hypokalemia, hypercholesterolemia, hypertriglyceridemia, and hyperuricemia. Use of alcohol as an ergogenic aid may result in an increase in SGPT, SGOT, and GGTP. The use of HCG, GH, stimulants, amino acids and protein supplements, vitamins and minerals, narcotics, and beta-blockers as ergogenic aids will result in no significant laboratory abnormalities.

Treatment

Once it is determined that an athlete is using an ergogenic aid, treatment should be initiated. It is important to treat any significant side effects and to be prepared for the development of withdrawal effects. After cessation of AAS and to a lesser extent, HCG and GH, the athlete must realize that a significant amount of body size and strength will be lost. In the case of AAS, major depression may be associated with withdrawal and this issue needs to be addressed and treated. Fluoxetine hydrochloride (Prozac) has been extremely successful in treating major depression associated with AAS withdrawal.[235] The treatment of athletes using blood doping or erythropoietin, which can cause hyperviscosity syndrome, may require phlebotomy, strict avoidance of dehydration, and close monitoring of the hematocrit. Potassium replacement may be necessary to treat hypokalemia associated with diuretic use. Bradycardia and cardiac dysrhythmia associated with beta-blocker use may require cardiac monitoring and treatment. The use and withdrawal of most of the other ergogenic aids generally require no other specific evaluation or treatment.

PREVENTION

As with other drugs of abuse, prevention is key in the war against the use of ergogenic substances. Many of the prevention programs are modeled after programs designed to prevent the abuse of drugs and alcohol.

The players

Prevention programs must be geared toward all individuals associated with athletics. Certainly, the athlete is the primary player in the game of prevention. Without adequate involvement of the athlete, it will be impossible to prevent the use of ergogenic aids. Athletes hold their coaches in high esteem. Because of the value placed on the coach's opinion by the athlete, it is extremely important that the coaching staff be involved in the prevention program.

The medical aspect of sport is another integral factor in preventing ergogenic substance use. Physicians, the nursing staff, physical therapists, and athletic trainers may all play a role. In particular, the athletic trainer in whom the athlete often maintains a high degree of confidence may be the most important health care provider for the athlete. In this capacity the athletic trainer is an important member of the prevention team.

Role models and peers are also involved in the overall program. Athletes who have succeeded at a high level of competition without the use of ergogenic substance can enlighten other athletes. The athlete who has been damaged physically, psychologically, and economically by the use of ergogenic aids may be used as an example of why these agents should be avoided. Other peers of the athlete can be helpful in pressuring the athlete to make the appropriate decision regarding the use of ergogenic aids.

Teachers and administrators from the elementary school to the professional and international levels should also be involved in this process. By virtue of their academic status, teachers provide the educational process by which prevention may begin and prosper. Through their policies and actions, administrators may help to foster and stabilize the development of overall prevention programs. By working together, teachers and administrators can promote an environment that condemns the use of ergogenic aids.

The family plays an important role in preventing the use of ergogenic aids. Parents, grandparents, siblings, and other family members must support the athlete regardless of the outcome of competition. Promotion of fair play during training and competition may more likely lead athletes to view the use of ergogenic aids as a form of cheating; therefore, they may be less likely to use these techniques. A family that equates winning with success, however, may inadvertently promote the use of ergogenic techniques as the athlete attempts to win at all costs. Unfortunately, this attitude is often held by all those involved with the athlete. Until the "win at all cost" philosophy changes, preventing the use of ergogenic techniques will be extremely difficult.

Education

General program. A proactive educational program geared toward the athlete and those having influence on the athlete is a significant deterrent to the use of ergogenic aids. This program can be introduced with other health topics such as illicit drug abuse and sex education. The programs must start at an elementary and junior high school level and should be continued through high school, college, and professional ranks. A variety of techniques may be used for this process. Speeches and seminars geared toward all groups are an effective means of education. The involvement of sports medicine specialists in the education of all involved in the care of the athlete is essential. The sports medicine specialist may be an orthopedic surgeon, primary care or other physician, physical therapist, athletic trainer, nutritionist, exercise physiologist, podiatrist, or psychologist.

The use of printed materials, such as posters, billboards, and brochures, can be an effective means to educate a large number of people. Motivational speakers, including both successful athletes or athletes who have been damaged by the use of ergogenic substances, may arouse an emotional response that may deter use. It is extremely important, regardless of the means of education, that educators provide accurate and honest information. Failure to do so will result in a loss of trust by the athletic population; it will be impossible to restore this faith. Athletes who are constantly pushing the limits and experimenting with a variety of techniques to gain the competitive edge will not be frightened by claims of flamboyant problems associated with the use of ergogenic aids.

All groups should be made aware of the potential risks and adverse effects associated with the use of these techniques. They must be educated to recognize the signs and symptoms of abuse, to identify the potential abuser, and to understand the rationale for use. Improvement in athletic performance is the most common reason for use of these techniques. Improvement in appearance and self-esteem, peer pressure, coaching and parental pressure, and possible financial reward are other reasons for abuse.

The adolescent athlete is at great risk for abuse of ergogenic techniques. The adolescent years are a time for establishing independence. Experimentation is part of this growth process; growth-enhancing, limit-testing behavior is ultimately positive and contributes to optimal competence. It is during this time that the use of illicit drugs is extremely common. The need to come to terms with one's self in relation to drugs of abuse becomes a major developmental task during this phase of maturation. This drug experimentation, which can be considered usual but not normal, may cross over and lead to experimentation with ergogenic techniques. The adolescent athlete is used to a high level of stimulation during competition and, therefore, may use ergogenic agents to fulfill this thrill-seeking drive. The adolescent athlete is often looked up to by many classmates. To maintain this reputation and "macho" image as a leader, the athlete may be the first to experiment with these techniques. Being with the "in crowd" is very important at this stage of development, and this need puts the athlete at an even greater risk for abuse of these agents.

There are many healthy, legal, and ethical means for improving athletic performance. Education regarding proper use of these techniques to maximize performance may deter the use of ergogenic aids.

Nutrition. Proper nutrition and hydration are essential during all phases of athletic performance. The main dietary goal is to supply adequate nutrition to optimize training. The metabolism of carbohydrates and fats during exercise provides most of the energy required for exercise. Numerous studies have shown* that a high-carbohydrate diet results in improvement in athletic performance and increased muscle glycogen stores.* Carbohydrate deficiency results in staleness, overtraining, and an inability to complete training workouts. Carbohydrates should make up 65% to 75% of the total calories consumed.

After completing an exercise session, the muscle glycogen stores depleted during the exercise must be replenished. A high-carbohydrate diet accomplishes this most efficiently.[22,62,64,177,287] Research has shown that 24 hours after exercise, there is no difference in the rate of muscle glycogen synthesis comparing the consumption of simple versus complex carbohydrates.[64,200] However, 24 to 48 hours after exercise, a complex carbohydrate diet results in higher muscle glycogen stores. Good sources of carbohydrate include breads, cereals, pastas, grain products, fruits and vegetables, dairy products, beans, and peas. Sugary foods, such as cakes, pies, cookies, and soft drinks are high in carbohydrate but contain few other nutrients.

During exercise, protein is a minor source of energy; gluconeogenesis from the catabolism of protein and amino acids provides only 5% to 10% of the energy during prolonged exercise.[38,46,88,167,221] The current U.S. RDA for protein is 0.8 g/kg/day. Most athletes eating a normal western diet consume at least 1.5 g/kg/day. Research has suggested athletes involved in prolonged endurance events and in heavy resistance exercises, such as weightlifting and body building, may require over 2.2 g/kg/day of protein. For this reason, these athletes may need an amino acid or protein supplement.

Fat is an important energy source for the athlete involved in prolonged low-intensity exercise.* With moderate or heavy intensity exercise of short duration, carbohydrate from muscle and liver glycogen is the main energy source. As the intensity of exercise decreases and the duration increases, however, a greater percentage of energy is derived from fat. Fat is not used until exercise lasts at least 20 minutes; after 3 hours of continuous exercise, over 50% of the energy is supplied in the form of free fatty acids. With improved endurance training, general cellular and physiologic adaptations result in improved fat use.[259,320,366] Fat should make up no more than 15% to 20% of the total calories in the diet of an athlete.

Water is the most critical nutrient for an athlete during training and competition. Sweat losses, which are affected by overall conditioning and acclimatization, can range from 1.5 to 3 L/hr. Two percent dehydration results in impairment of thermal regulation, 3% dehydration leads to reduction of muscle endurance; 4% dehydration results in a decrease in muscle strength and endurance, and dehydration of over 6% may lead to heat exhaustion and heat stroke.[167]

Because thirst is an inadequate indicator of fluid losses, it is important to maintain oral hydration during training.[38,46] Four to eight ounces of cool water should be consumed every 15 to 20 minutes during exercise; 5% to 8% carbohydrate liquids may also be used. Carbohydrate liquids, in addition to providing hydration, will help preserve muscle glycogen stores. The carbohydrate drinks are most beneficial when the duration of exercise is over 40 to 60 minutes.[118,157-159,256,324]

Preevent nutrition. The goals of the preevent meal are to ensure adequate carbohydrate, prevent dehydration, avoid GI irritation, and provide a relatively empty stomach and yet avoid hunger pangs.[38,46,167] The meal should be pleasant and satisfying and consumed 2 to 5 hours before competition. If the athlete cannot consume a solid meal, a liquid carbohydrate meal may be consumed up to 60 minutes before the event. It is recommended, however, that carbohydrate feedings be avoided 15 to 60 minutes before exercise, as this may cause an increase in serum insulin

*References 24, 38, 46, 62, 66, 72, 73, 146, 157, 159, 167, 264, 322, 324.

*References 11, 38, 107, 164, 240, 281.

level leading to hypoglycemia.[268,316] This hypoglycemia may decrease performance during high-intensity exercise, but it appears to have little deleterious effect on performance during moderate intensity exercise.[321] Carbohydrate ingested immediately before a high-intensity exercise may improve performance due to an increase in carbohydrate bioavailability.[56]

The preevent meal should have minimal bulk, low salt, and provide adequate fluid of at least 16 ounces. It is also important that the pregame meal be composed of foods that the athlete is used to eating. Experimentation with new foods on the day of the competition should be avoided.

Carbohydrate loading is a dietary technique that may improve performance in endurance events, such as cross country skiing, distance cycling, running, and swimming. This technique should be used only in well-trained athletes. It will improve endurance in exercise that lasts over 60 to 90 minutes by allowing muscle to store two to three times more glycogen than normal. The classic carbohydrate[23,24] loading regimen developed in the 1960s involved 3 days of intense exercise on an extremely low (less than 10%) carbohydrate diet to deplete muscle glycogen stores. Days four, five, and six are spent resting and consuming a high (over 80%) carbohydrate diet. The competition is then held on day seven with consumption of a normal high carbohydrate precompetition meal. This technique increases muscle glycogen stores up to three times baseline; however, it is extremely strenuous and may lead to injury, fatigue, and irritability. The modified carbohydrate regimen[323] involves a moderate (50%) carbohydrate diet on day one, two, and three and a high (over 80%) carbohydrate diet on days four, five, and six with a high-carbohydrate, precompetition meal. In association with this diet, exercise is tapered on days one through five with rest on day six. The modified technique results in an increase in muscle glycogen stores similar to the classic regimen; however, it is safer and less strenuous.[323]

Event nutrition. During sporting events that last less than 1 hour, water alone may be used. Four to 8 ounces of cool water should be consumed every 15 to 20 minutes to prevent dehydration. Increased volumes are required in hot, humid weather, especially in the unacclimatized, less-trained athlete. Carbohydrate should be consumed during competition of greater than 45 to 60 minutes duration. The carbohydrate will help maintain blood glucose and liver glycogen and spare muscle glycogen stores. The most effective carbohydrate supplements during exercise are the 5% to 8% carbohydrate solutions.[38,46,160,167,176] The glucose supplements are felt to be superior to fructose solutions, as the latter may cause a delay in gastric emptying and GI distress.[158,263,265] The minimal amount of carbohydrate needed for effectiveness is 22 g/hour; some experts recommend up to 250 g/hour.[46,72,157,160] Solid carbohydrate sources are also beneficial but obviously do not pro-

vide the necessary liquid to prevent dehydration. Compared to solids, liquid supplements provide both fluid and carbohydrate and have faster gastric emptying.

Postevent nutrition. The goals of postevent nutrition are to replace fluid losses and replenish glycogen stores.[38,46,167] The volume of fluid loss during competition can be calculated from the difference between preevent and postevent weights. Close monitoring of weight, especially early in the sport season, should be practiced to minimize dehydration and fluid imbalance. Assuming 16 ounces of fluid represents 1 pound of weight loss, a 10-pound weight loss would require replacing a total of 160 ounces. Half of this volume should be consumed within the first 8 hours and the remaining half within 24 hours to bring the weight to approximately the preevent level.

The rate of glycogen synthesis is highest immediately after exercise, and repletion of stores depends on the availability of carbohydrate from the diet.[22,62,64,177,287] Both simple and complex carbohydrates should be consumed immediately after the termination of activity; 100 g of carbohydrate within the first hour and 100 g every 2 to 4 hours thereafter is recommended. From a practical standpoint, it is difficult to eat solid, complex carbohydrate foods immediately after competition. For this reason, immediately and early after exercise, simple, liquid carbohydrates should be consumed with the addition of complex carbohydrates as soon as they can be tolerated.

To summarize, a well-balanced diet high in carbohydrate and low in fat that provides adequate fluid, vitamins, and minerals can be an extremely effective method of improving athletic performance. By educating the athlete and those associated with the athlete about proper nutrition, the use of ergogenic aids may be prevented and proven to the athlete to be unnecessary.

Equipment and training. Good coaching can tremendously impact athletic performance. A good coach knows all facets of athletic participation, including use of sport-specific skills and proper technique; adequate adjustment of training programs; repetition in practice; appropriate rest and rehabilitation from training, competition, and injury; and mental preparation for the sport. A coach who is well versed in these techniques can give this knowledge to the athlete to allow him or her to compete at peak form.

It is also extremely important that proper equipment be used for practice and competition. The athlete, coaches, and trainers need to ensure that all equipment is in proper working condition and of high quality. Equipment varies with the sport and may include items such as proper footwear, adequate pads and braces, protective eyewear, helmets, appropriate outerwear, jock straps and sport bras, balls, pucks, bats, sticks, and training equipment such as weights, sleds, and trampolines. Another important piece of equipment is the playing surface. The playing surface may be concrete, asphalt, cinder, clay, grass, Astroturf, wood, dirt, sand, rubber, mud, or other material. Irregularities in the playing surface may cause injury and should be repaired promptly. Those involved in athletics need to be aware of the risk factors associated with practice and competition on these surfaces and appropriately alter schedules. By maintaining high-quality athletic equipment and practice standards, an athlete will be better able to achieve excellence without the use of ergogenic aids.

Strength and conditioning. As an adjunct to proper training, overall fitness is essential to maximize success in sports (see Chapter 19). There are two basic aspects of fitness, anaerobic or muscle strengthening and aerobic or cardiovascular conditioning. Depending on the sport involved, the amount of training in either of these areas may be altered. It is here that a well-trained strength and conditioning coach can help the athlete improve performance without the use of ergogenic substances.

Cardiovascular conditioning. The goal of aerobic training is to provide sufficient cardiovascular overload to cause cardiac changes that improve efficiency.* Upon initiation of a cardiovascular training program, there is considerable potential for improvement; at higher levels of fitness, however, there is little room to improve cardiovascular performance. Beneficial physiologic changes depend primarily on the intensity of work overload.† A minimum threshold must be reached before aerobic improvements occur; although a variety of methods can be used to determine this threshold, all techniques use some percentage of maximum cardiovascular function.‡ Maximum cardiovascular function may be determined directly by a maximum cardiovascular test in which the athlete runs to exhaustion. Indirect determination of maximal heart rate can be made by using submaximal testing or standard formulas. The most commonly used formula is the equation 220 minus the age in years (see Chapter 19). The difference between the maximal heart rate and the resting heart rate (first morning pulse) is the heart rate reserve. To improve cardiovascular performance, exercise intensity must raise the heart rate into the training heart zone; the training heart zone is the sum of the resting heart rate and 60% to 85% of the heart rate reserve. Greater intensity of training results in greater improvement.§

The actual duration of exercise required for improvement is not well established; however, 20 to 30 minutes of continuous training is probably enough if it is performed at the proper intensity.‖ An athlete involved in long duration sports, such as marathon running, must train at a longer duration. The frequency of exercise is also important; three to five sessions per week yields the best results.** With any aerobic program, a recovery or rest period is needed to prevent breakdown. As overall cardiovascular conditioning improves, exercise intensity, duration, and

frequency must be increased to provide adequate stress for continued cardiovascular adaptation.

Three methods of aerobic training may be used. In interval training, repeated exercise bouts are interspersed with periods of rest or relief.[96,117,119,205,243] The intensity, duration, number of intervals, length and type of rest, and number of sets per session can all be modified depending on the goals. Interval training allows the athlete to train at extremely high intensity levels for a relatively long time by interspersing the intervals with relative rest periods.

Continuous training, the second method of aerobic training, involves steady paced exercise performed at moderate- to high-intensity for sustained duration.[96,117,243] The athlete will train at distances two to five times the actual race distance. This type of training is good for beginners. It can be performed with relative comfort and appears to produce the largest aerobic adaptation. This technique is also best suited for individuals involved in endurance sports.

Fartlek or speed play is a third method of aerobic training.[243] Training is based on how it feels at the time of the activity. If the athlete feels overworked, the intensity is decreased. If the athlete feels underworked, the intensity is increased. Fartlek is good for general conditioning during the off-season. Fatigue, nausea, and lethargy after exercise are signs of overuse and suggest that exercise should be decreased.

Muscular conditioning. The goal of muscular conditioning is to provide sufficient resistance to overload muscles, allowing them to achieve their maximum tension-developing or force output capacity through the entire range of motion.* The degree and method of strength training are determined by the sport and position of the athlete. The ultimate strength is determined by anatomic and physiologic factors within the muscle. With strength training, muscle fibers enlarge as an adaptation to the increase in workload; this result allows for an increased ability to exert force through a range of motion.†

Strength, defined as the maximum tension generated by a muscle group, depends on the size, shape, fiber type, architecture, and orientation of the muscle fibers.[117,210,243,347] The intensity of exercise is the resistance lifted per repetition and is the most important factor in determining strength improvements.[5,117,233,243]

A set refers to a group of repetitions and usually ranges from three to six per weightlifting session. The use of multiple sets induces faster and greater development in strength, power, and muscle endurance than use of a single set.[5,85,117,243] Repetition continuum refers to the number of lifts per set. Lifting less than seven repetitions per set is most effective for developing strength and power.[5,97,117,233,243] Lifting 7 to 20 repetitions per set re-

*References 5, 12, 77, 117, 119, 134, 223, 224, 243, 255, 325, 358.
†References 5, 25, 45, 117, 127, 197, 243, 319, 358.
‡References 3, 5, 82, 117, 138, 156, 243, 245, 249.
§References 5, 12, 45, 77, 117, 127, 197, 224, 243, 318, 358.
‖References 3, 5, 117, 119, 224, 243, 255, 318, 358.
**References 3, 5, 12, 77, 117, 119, 134, 224, 290, 358.

*References 5, 85, 97, 117, 210, 243.
†References 5, 89, 95, 117, 147, 210, 217, 238, 243, 247, 309, 338, 346.

sults in strength and power gains and also improves endurance. Lifting more than 20 repetitions per set trains the muscle primarily for endurance with little improvement in strength and power. The maximum voluntary contraction is a lift in which the athlete attempts to recruit as many muscle fibers as possible to develop the force. The last lift of a set should be a maximum lift to maximize strength training.[5,34,117,151,243] Frequency refers to the number of weightlifting sessions per week; the optimum number is three to four per week.* The rest period refers to the time between individual exercises, between sets, and between sessions. During a weightlifting session, the rest period between exercises determines the extent to which aerobic and anaerobic energy sources will be involved in the succeeding exercises.[117,243] For maximum strength and power training, 2 to 3 minutes between exercises is required. With low-intensity exercise, rest periods should be less than 30 seconds. Volume refers to the amount of work performed and is determined by the weight, repetition, and number of sets.

Overload is a key factor in any strength program. To effectively improve physiologic performance and efficiency, the muscle must be overloaded. A load of 60% to 80% of the muscle's force-generating capacity is usually sufficient to produce strength gains. By manipulating resistance, repetitions, rest intervals, number of sets, frequency, and type of activity, one may achieve these goals.†

Specificity is another key factor in strength training. The metabolic and physiologic responses to overload are specific. In general, strength training increases only the strength of the exercised muscle. The athlete must train the muscle similarly to its use during the sport, including flexibility, endurance, and strength.[5,117,243]

There are numerous methods of weight training. Isometric exercise refers to the contraction of a muscle at a constant length. This exercise requires training at several points through the range of motion and its use is limited in sports because of the specificity of joint angle and body position.‡

Isotonic exercise refers to lifting constant weight or "free weights" through a range of motion. For a given weight, faster rates of lifting generate better strength improvements.[135,136,193,194,330] Eccentric exercise (contraction with the muscle lengthening) is more effective than concentric exercise (muscle contraction with the muscle shortening) for developing strength.[28,181] The one drawback to using free weights is that the resistance can be no greater than the maximum strength at the weakest point in the range of motion.

Isokinetic exercise refers to resistance exercises performed at a constant speed. These exercises activate the largest number of muscle cells and overload muscles to al-

low them to achieve their maximum tension developing capacity at every point in the range of motion.* Use of faster speeds results in specific training at the angular velocity used in the exercise; this should mimic the activity of the sport in which the athlete is participating.

Circuit weight training is a general conditioning program that attempts to improve body composition, strength, endurance, and cardiovascular fitness.[117,133,135-137,198,243] This training requires rapid lifting of low to moderate resistance weights for 30 to 60 seconds. This causes an increase in the heart rate. There is a short rest period followed by another exercise, and this cycle is repeated for 15 to 30 minutes. Theoretically, circuit weight training improves not only muscle strength and endurance, but also cardiovascular conditioning.

It is obvious that there is more to strength training than simply lifting weights. Proper education by trained individuals is the most effective method for increasing muscle strength. Not only is the knowledge of using the weights important, but a number of other variables need to be considered. The choice of exercise should be specific for the sport so that the program mimics the angular speed and type of contraction used in the skill. The resistance and rest periods used during the exercise program must also be specific to the sport. The program needs to be changed to optimize strength and power gains and also to fight boredom. This cycle can be repeated daily, weekly, monthly, or yearly. The most effective means of producing increases in muscle strength, endurance, and size is through a structured exercise program.[117,243] By educating the athletic population about these techniques, the use of ergogenic aids will be decreased.

Psychologic techniques. Instruction on the psychologic aspect of training and competition can be extremely helpful.† Specialists trained as sports psychologists can make a tremendous difference in athletic performance. Optimum athletic performance requires optimum stimulation. If the level of stress is too low, performance declines; if the level of stress is too great, anxiety develops, which also interferes with performance. The level of stimulation required for optimum performance varies from athlete to athlete and from competition to competition within the same individual. This fluctuation may be altered with mental training. The ability to "psyche up" can be learned and will improve athletic performance in situations where stimulation is low. A variety of feedback techniques have been developed, which may work to relax the athlete in situations where the stimulation is too great. Techniques, such as biofeedback, rehearsal, imagery, and self-talk, may help the athlete establish the mental toughness required to succeed at a high level. With experience and proper psychologic instruction, the mental health of the athlete is sta-

*References 5, 34, 117, 139, 151, 243.
†References 5, 18, 34, 85, 97, 117, 139, 151, 233, 243.
‡References 5, 28, 117, 131, 152, 193, 243, 266.

*References 74, 133, 135, 136, 193, 330.
†References 114, 132, 232, 244, 248, 274, 283, 311, 328.

bilized and athletic performance is improved. Proper use of sports psychology may also deter the athlete from using ergogenic aids.

Genetics. As stated earlier, genetics play a key role in the development of an athlete. Despite proper nutrition, equipment, training, strength and conditioning, and psychologic training, most athletes will not be able to compete at professional or international levels due to genetic limitations. Parents, coaches, and the athletes themselves need to recognize and accept these genetic limitations. By setting realistic goals and using the previously mentioned training techniques, athletes will optimize their performance without the use of ergogenic aids.

Philosophy. The "win at all cost" attitude permeates society. The rationale of the "ends justifying the means" is used by athletes to justify their use of ergogenic aids. The best prepared athlete should be the one who wins the event. The use of ergogenic aids to make up for the difference in preparation is not fair. It is a method of cheating, and the old adage "cheaters never win" should be followed. Until society changes its philosophy of defining a winner, however, the use of ergogenic aids will thrive. A winner should be defined as the athlete who gives it his or her all in practice and competition regardless of the final outcome. Cheating, in sports and in life, is unethical and should not be tolerated.

Expense

For many athletes the expense involved in using ergogenic aids can be tremendous. Many of these techniques involve the use of expensive medical intervention. The cost of the agents themselves can be tremendous. The recent change in legislation resulting in AAS and related compounds being defined as schedule III drugs has caused a significant increase in price. With the new law, the penalties for transportation and distribution of AAS may result in a fine of up to $500,000 and a prison term of up to 15 years.[123] Before this legislation, AAS freely entered the country and were freely distributed by physicians and veterinarians. The result was easy access to relatively inexpensive drugs. Now that this source has been limited, users of these agents are turning to the black market where quality is often questioned and prices have significantly risen.

The effect of legislation to control to AAS, HCG, and GH has significantly increased the cost of these drugs, which has decreased availability to many potential users. The expense of the agents is a deterrent to the athlete. Finances are also a problem for the athletic governing bodies. The development of education, treatment, and testing programs can be extremely expensive. The money to pay for these programs must come from somewhere. For the professional leagues and IOC, financial backing is available. At the junior high and high school levels, and to a lesser extent at the college level, the financial burden is

great. Often the program must be sacrificed due to loss of support. Professionals at all levels who volunteer their time can assist in the development and maintenance of a program to fight the use of ergogenic aids.

Drug testing

Drug testing, extremely important in preventing the use of ergogenic aids, is controversial, with strong vocal proponents on both sides of the issue.[69,92,129] Before drug testing can be instituted, rules must be established to govern how the results are used. Prevention and treatment programs should be established to avoid inconsistencies in the treatment of any given athlete.

Those who demand drug testing do so for a variety of reasons. First, the athlete is a highly visible person in society and is often "looked up to" by the younger population and peers who may mimic their behavior. Use of ergogenic aids gives the sport a bad name. Second, the athlete may be experiencing significant side effects from using ergogenic aids. Drug testing may allow early detection of ergogenic users and subsequent referral for appropriate treatment. Third, the use of ergogenic aids is unethical and a form of cheating. It is not fair that one or more competitors use these substances to improve performance. Drug testing will detect some of the cheaters. The risk of potentially being tested may deter the use in other athletes. Urine drug testing will help to level the playing field, thereby allowing the best prepared athlete to win the competition.

Those who argue against drug testing also raise many issues. First, random urine drug testing is a violation of civil liberties; the athlete is forced to submit a urine specimen at a moment's notice. The athlete is singled out for testing while others in the academic or work environment have no such worry. Another issue is the concern about randomization of the testing. Who will be tested? When will they be tested? Will the test be unannounced? Will "just cause" testing be used? Third, many ergogenic drugs and techniques cannot be detected through testing at this time, and newer drugs and techniques are constantly being developed. Because the new techniques are often expensive, only the smart or rich athlete can use them; therefore, the testing will be biased. Fourth, as with any testing program, there may be false-positive and false-negative test results, all of which carry significant ramifications. A final argument against drug testing is that it is extremely expensive; tests for the detection of AAS alone approach $150 to $200 per test. Other expenses include the use of administrative, laboratory, and urine collection personnel. This amount is cost-prohibitive when dealing with a junior high or high school program. At the college level, selective testing must be performed because of the significant expense.

Although all drug testing programs have problems, there is no question that the risk of being tested may deter the use of ergogenic aids. With the institution of testing for ergogenic substance abuse at the collegiate and professional levels, it will be interesting to determine whether changes in drug use occur in the next decade.

Penalties

Although random drug testing is important in the prevention of the use of ergogenic aids, it will not be effective unless there are significant penalties. The penalties should be unbiased, consistent, and harsh and they should fit the crime. In a sport where millions of dollars can be riding on a result, there should be a significant financial penalty. The use of some of these agents carry significant legal ramifications. If the penalty is minimal, the effectiveness of prevention of the use of ergogenic aids through education and drug testing will also be minimal. The current NFL policy[267] requires a 4-week suspension for the first positive test for use of ergogenic agents. The second positive test results in suspension for the balance of the season without pay. Refusal or failure to supply a specimen for analysis is considered a positive test, and deliberate distortion of the urine sample results in a more severe penalty than use of the agents themselves. With the NFL substance abuse policy as a model—random, weekly drug testing during the preseason, the season, the postseason, and the off-season—the use of ergogenic substances in the NFL is thought to be decreasing. Other organizations are establishing similar programs.

REFERENCES

1. Alen M et al: Serum lipids in power athletes self-administering testosterone and anabolic steroids, *Int J Sports Med* 6:139-144, 1985.
2. Alen M et al: Androgenic-anabolic steroid effects on serum thyroid, pituitary and steroid hormones in athletes, *Am J Sports Med* 15:357-361, 1987.
3. *ACSM Guidelines for graded exercise testing and exercise prescription*, Philadelphia, 1980, Lea and Febiger.
4. American College of Sports Medicine Position Stand: Blood doping as an ergogenic aid, *Med Sci Sports Exerc* 19:540-543, 1987.
5. American College of Sports Medicine Position Stand: The recommended quantity and quality of exercise for developing and maintaining cardiorespiratory and muscular fitness in healthy adults, *Med Sci Sports Exerc* 22:265-274, 1990.
6. Anderson WA et al: A national survey of alcohol and drug use by college athletes, *Physician Sports Med* 19:91-104, 1991.
7. Annitto WJ, Layman WA: Anabolic steroids and acute schizophrenic episode, *J Clin Psychol* 41:143, 1980.
8. Ariel G: The effect of anabolic steroid (methandostenolone) upon selected physiologic parameters, *Athletic Train* 7:190-200, 1972.
9. Ariel G: The residual affect of an anabolic steroid upon isotonic muscular force, *J Sports Med Phys Fitness* 14:103-111, 1974.
10. Ariel G, Seville W: Anabolic steroids: the physiologic effects of placebos, *Med Sci Sports Exerc* 4:124-126, 1972.
11. Askew EW: Role of fat metabolism and exercise, *Clin Sports Med* 3:605-621, 1984.
12. Atomi Y et al: Effects of intensity and frequency of training on aerobic work capacity of young females, *J Sports Med* 18:3-9, 1978.
13. Bahrke MS et al: Psychological and behavioral effects of endogenous testosterone levels in anabolic/androgenic steroids among males, a review, *Sports Med* 10:303-37, 1990.

14. Baldo-Enzi et al: Lipid and apoprotein modification in body builders during and after self-administration of anabolic steroids, *Metabolism* 39:203-207, 1990.
15. Barnett DW, Conlee RK: The effects of commercial dietary supplementation on human performance, *Am J Clin Nutr* 40:586-590, 1985.
16. Bedi JF et al: Enhancement of exercise performance with inhaled albuterol, *Can J Sports Sci* 13:144-148, 1988.
17. Belko AZ: Vitamins and exercise—an update, *Med Sci Sports Exerc* 19:S191-S196, 1987.
18. Berger RA: Effect of varied weight training programs on strength, *Res Q* 33:168-181, 1962.
19. Bergink EW et al: Metabolism and receptor binding of nandrolone and testosterone under in vitro and in vivo conditions, *Acta Endocrinol* 110:31-37, 1985.
20. Berglund B, Hemmingsson P: The effects of caffeine ingestion on exercise performance at low and high altitudes in cross country skiers, *Int J Sports Med* 3:234-236, 1982.
21. Berglund B, Hemmingson P: Effect of reinfusion autologous blood on exercise performance in cross-country skiers, *Int J Sports Med* 8:231-233, 1987.
22. Bergstrom J, Hultman E: Muscle glycogen synthesis after exercise: an enhancing factor localized to the muscle cells in man, *Nature* 210:309-10, 1966.
23. Bergstrom J, Hultman E: A study of the glycogen metabolism during exercise in man, *Scand J Clin Lab Invest* 19:218-228, 1967.
24. Bergstrom J et al: Diet, muscle glycogen and physical performance, *Acta Physiol Scand* 7:140-150, 1967.
25. Blair SN et al: Improving physical fitness by exercise training programs, *South Med J* 73:1594-1596, 1980.
26. Blomstrand E et al: Administration of branched-chain amino acid during sustained exercise: effects on performance and on plasma concentration of some amino acid, *Eur J Appl Physiol Occup Physiol* 63:83-88, 1991.
27. Bond V: Effects of small and moderate doses of alcohol on submaximal cardio-respiratory functions, perceived exertion and endurance performance in abstainers and moderate drinkers, *J Sports Med* 23:221-8, 1983.
28. Bonde-Peterson F: Muscle training by static, concentric and eccentric contractions, *Acta Physiol Scand* 48:406-416, 1960.
29. Borel JS, Anderson RA: Chromium. In Frieden E, editor: *Biochemisty of the essential ultra-trace elements*, New York, 1984, Plenum Press.
30. Bowers RW, Reardon JP: Effects of methandostenolone (dianabol) on strength development and aerobic capacity, *Med Sci Sports Exerc* 4:54, 1972.
31. Bowman S: Anabolic steroids and infarction, *Br Med J* 300:750, 1990.
32. Boyea S et al: Ergogenic drug use among high school athletes: a three year sequential study, *Med Sci Sports Exerc* 22:S63, 1990.
33. Bradley CA, Sodeman TM: Human growth hormone, its use and abuse, *Clin Lab Med* 10:473-478, 1990.
34. Braith RW et al: Comparison of a two versus three days per week of variable resistance training during 10 and 18 week programs. *Int J Sports Med* 10:450-454, 1989.
35. Braude IA: Transfusion reactions from contaminated blood: the recognition and treatment, *N Engl J Med* 258:1289-1293, 1958.
36. Brien AJ, Simon TL: The effects of red blood cell infusion on 10-KM race time, *JAMA* 257:2761-2765, 1987.
37. Brittingham TE, Chaplin H: Febrile transfusion reactions caused by sensitivity to donor leukocytes and platelets, *JAMA* 165:819-25, 1957.
38. Brotherhood J: Nutrition and sports performance, *Sports Med* 1:350-389, 1984.
39. Brower KJ: Anabolic androgenic steroids in suicide, *Am J Psychol* 146:1075, 1989.

40. Brower KJ et al: Anabolic-androgenic steroid dependence, *J Clin Psychol* 50:31-33, 1989.

41. Brower KJ et al: Evidence for physical and psychological dependence on anabolic androgenic steroids in eight weight lifters, *Am J Psychol* 147:510-512, 1990.

42. Buckley WE et al: Estimated prevalence of anabolic steroid use among male high school seniors, *JAMA* 260:3441-3445, 1988.

43. Buick FJ et al: Effect of induced erythrocythemia on aerobic work capacity, *J Appl Physiol* 48:636-642, 1980.

44. Bullock G et al: The effects of catabolic and anabolic steroids on amino acid incorporation by skeletal muscle ribozomes, *Biochem J* 108:417-425, 1968.

45. Burke EJ, Franks BD: Changes in VO_2 max resulting from bicycling training at different intensities holding total mechanical work constant, *Res Qu* 46:31-37, 1975.

46. Burke LM, Read RSD: Sports nutrition approaching the 90's, *Sports Med* 8:80-100, 1989.

47. Cade R et al: Effects of phosphate loading on 2, 3-diphosphoglycerate and maximal oxygen uptake, *Med Sci Sports Exerc* 16:263-268, 1984.

48. Calabrese LH et al: The effects of anabolic steroids and strength training on the human immune response, *Med Sci Sports Exerc* 41:386-392, 1989.

49. Cantwell JD, Rose FD: Cocaine and cardiovascular events, *Physician and Sportsmedicine* 11:77-82, 1986.

50. Carlson DL, Mawdsley RH: Sports anemia: a review of the literature, *Am J Sports Med* 14:109-112, 1986.

51. Celejowa I, Homa M: Food intake, nitrogen and energy balance in Polish weightlifters during a training camp, *Nutr Metab* 12:259-274, 1970.

52. Chandler JV, Blair SN: The effect of amphetamines on selected physiological components related to athletic success, *Med Sci Sports Exerc* 12:65-69, 1980.

53. Clarke N: Social drinking in athletes, *Physician and Sportsmedicine,* 17:95-100, 1989.

54. Clement DB, Sawchuk LL: Iron status and sports performance, *Sports Med* 1:65-74, 1984.

55. Climstein M et al: The effects of anabolic steroids on left ventricular performance of elite power lifters and endurance athletes, *Med Sci Sports Exerc* 22:S64, 1990.

56. Coggan AR, Coyle EF: Effect of carbohydrate feedings during high-intensity exercise, *J Appl Physiol* 65:1703-1719, 1988.

57. Cohen JC, Hickman R: Insulin resistance and diminished glucose tolerance in power lifters ingesting anabolic steroids, *J Clin Endocrinol Metab* 64:960-963, 1987.

58. Cohen JC et al: Hypercholesterolemia in male power lifters using anabolic-androgenic steroids, *Physician and Sportsmedicine* 16:49, 1988.

59. Committee on Growth Hormone Use: Degenerative neurologic disease in patients formally treated with growth hormone, *J Pediatr* 108:10-12, 1985.

60. Conacher GN: Violent crime possibly associated with anabolic steroid use, *Am J Psychol* 146:679, 1989.

61. Consolazio CF et al: Protein metabolism during intensive physical training in the young adult, *Am J Clin Nutr* 28:29-35, 1975.

62. Costill DL, Miller JM: Nutrition for endurance sport: carbohydrate and fluid balance, *Inter J Sports Med* 1:2-14, 1980.

63. Costill DL et al: Effects of caffeine ingestion on metabolism and exercise performance, *Med Sci Sports Exerc* 10:155-158, 1978.

64. Costill DL et al: The role of dietary carbohydrates in muscle glycogen synthesis after strenuous exercise, *Am J Clin Nutr* 34:831-836, 1981.

65. Costill DL et al: Anabolic steroid use among athletes: changes in HDL-C levels, *Physician and Sportsmedicine* 12:113, 1984.

66. Costill DL et al: Effects of repeated days of intensified training on muscle glycogen and swimming performance, *Med Sci Sports Exerc* 20:249-254, 1988.

67. Cowart V: Some predict increased steroids use in sports despite drug testing, crackdown on suppliers, *JAMA* 257:3025, 1987.

68. Cowart VS: Study proposes to examine football players, power lifters for possible long-term sequelae from anabolic steroid use in 1970's competition, *JAMA* 257:3021, 1987.

69. Cowart VS: Drug testing programs face snags and legal challenges, *Physician and Sportsmedicine,* 16:165-173, 1988.

70. Cowart VS: Human growth hormone: the latest ergogenic aid? *Physician and Sportsmedicine* 16:175-190, 1988.

71. Coyle EF: Ergogenic aids, *Clin Sports Med* 3:731-742, 1984.

72. Coyle EF: Muscle glycogen utilisation during prolonged strenuous exercise when fed carbohydrates, *J Appl Physiol* 61:165-172, 1986.

73. Coyle EF, Coggan AR: Effectiveness of carbohydrate feeding in delaying fatigue during prolonged exercise, *Sports Med* 1:446-458, 1984.

74. Coyle EF et al: Specificity of power improvements through slow and fast isokinetic training, *J Appl Physiol* 51:1437-1442, 1981.

75. Creagh TM: Hepatic tumours induced by anabolic steroids in athlete, *J Clin Pathol* 41:441-443, 1988.

76. Cregler LI, Mark H: Medical complications of cocaine abuse, *N Engl J Med* 315:1495-1500, 1986.

77. Crews TR, Roberts JA: Effects of interaction of frequency and intensity of training, *Res Qu* 47:48-55, 1976.

78. Crist DM: Effects of anabolic andergenic steroids on neuromuscular power and body composition, *J Appl Physiol* 54:366-370, 1983.

79. Crist DM et al: Body composition response to exogenous GH during training in highly conditioned adults, *J Appl Physiol* 65:579-584, 1988.

80. Curran JW et al: Acquired immune-deficiency syndrome associated with transfusion, *N Engl J Med* 310:69-75, 1984.

81. Cuthbertson DP, Knox JA: The effects of analeptics on the fatigued subject, *J Physiol* 106:42-58, 1947.

82. Davies B et al: Maximum oxygen uptake utilizing different treadmill protocols, *Br J Sports Med* 18:74-79, 1984.

83. DeGroot LJ et al editors: Endocrinology, ed 2, Philadelphia, 1989, WB Saunders.

84. Delamore IW, Geary CG: Aplastic anaemia, acute myeloblastic leukaemia and oxymetholone, *Br Med J* 2:743-745, 1971.

85. Delorme DL: Restoration of muscle power by heavy resistance exercise, *J Bone Joint Surg* 27:645-667, 1945.

86. Dimeff RJ: Prevalance of drug use by pediatric athletes, *Dialogues Pediatr Urol* 15:2-4, 1992.

87. Dimeff RJ et al: Psychiatric effects of anabolic steroids, manuscript in preparation.

88. Dohm GL: Protein nutrition for the athlete, *Clin Sports Med* 3:595-605, 1984.

89. Dons B et al: The effect of weight-lifting exercise related to muscle fiber composition and muscle cross-sectional area in humans, *Eur J Appl Physiol* 40:95-106, 1979.

90. Drinkwater BL et al: Bone mineral content of amenorrheic and eumenorrheic athletes, *N Engl J Med* 311:277-281, 1984.

91. Drinkwater BL et al: Menstrual history as a determinant of current bone density in young athletes, *JAMA* 263:545-548, 1990.

92. Duda M: IOC rescinds ban on birth control drug, *Physician and Sportsmedicine* 16:175-179, 1988.

93. Duffy DJ, Conlee RK: Effects of phosphate loading on leg power and high intensity treadmill exercise, *Med Sci Sports Exerc* 18:674-677, 1986.

94. Dying to win: rEPO, blood doping, and athletics, a current issue session, American College of Sports Medicine National Meeting, Orlando, Fla, 1991.

95. Ebbeling CB, Clarkson PM: Exercise-induced muscle damage in adaptation, *Sports Med* 7:207-234, 1989.

96. Eddy DO: The effect of continuous and interval training in women and men, *Eur J Appl Physiol* 37:83-92, 1977.

97. Edstrom L, Grimby L: Effect of exercise on the motor unit, *Muscle Nerve* 9:104-126, 1986.

98. Ehrlich LR: Arsenic, oxymetholone, and leukemia, *Ann Int Med* 79:288, 1973.

99. Ekblom B et al: Responses to exercise after blood loss and reinfusion, *J Appl Physiol* 33:157-180, 1972.

100. Ekblom B et al: Central circulation during exercise after venesection and reinfusion of red blood cells, *J Appl Physiol* 40:379-383, 1976.

101. Elam RP: Morphological changes in adult males from resistance exercise and amino acid supplementation, *J Sports Med Phys Fitness* 28:35-40, 1988.

102. Elam RP et al: Effects of arginine and ornithine on strength, lean body mass and urinary hydroxyproline in adult males, *J Sports Med Phys Fitness*, 29:52-57, 1989.

103. Erslev AJ: Erythropoietin, *N Engl J Med*, 324:1339-1344, 1991.

104. Eschbach JW: Treatment of anemia of progressive renal failure with recombinant human erythropoietin, *N Engl J Med* 321:158-163, 1989.

105. Eschbach JW et al: Correction of anemia of end-stage renal disease with recombinant human erythropoietin: results of a combined phase I and II clinical trial, *N Engl J Med* 316:73-78, 1987.

106. Eschbach JW et al: Recombinant human erythropoietin in anemic patients with end-stage renal disease, results of a phase III multicenter clinical trial, *Ann Int Med* 111:992-1000, 1989.

107. Essen B et al: Utilization of blood-borne and intramuscular substrates during continuous and intermittent exercise in man, *J Physiol* 265:489-506, 1977.

108. Essig D et al: Effects of caffeine ingestion on utilization of muscle glycogen and lipid during leg ergometer cycling, *Int J Sports Med* 1:86-90, 1980.

109. Fahey TD, Brown CH: The effects of anabolic steroid on the strength, body composition, and endurance of college males when accompanied by a weight training program, *Med Sci Sports Exerc* 5:272-276, 1973.

110. Faigel HC: Effects of beta-blockade, *Clin Pediatr* 30:441-445, 1991.

111. Fain JN et al: Effect of growth hormone and dexamethasone on lipolysis and metabolism in isolated fat cells of other rat, *J Biol Chem* 240:3522-3529, 1965.

112. Farell GC et al: Androgen-induced hepatoma, *Lancet* 1:430-431, 1975.

113. Federspil G et al: Role of growth hormone in lipid mobilization stimulated by prolonged muscular exercise in the rat, *J Hormone Metab Res* 7:484-488, 1975.

114. Feigley DA: Psychological burnout in high-level athletes, *Physician and Sportsmedicine* 12:109-119, 1984.

115. Fenter WM et al: The role of growth hormone in the mobilization of fuel for muscular exercise, *Q J Exp Physiol Cognitive Med Sci* 50:406-16, 1965.

116. Ferenchick GS: Are androgenic steroids thrombogenic? *N Engl J Med* 322:476, 1990.

117. Fleck SJ, Kraemer WJ: *Designing resistance training programs,* Champagne, Ill, 1987, Human Kinetic Books.

118. Flynn MG et al: Influence of selected carbohydrate drinks on cycling performance and glycogen use, *Med Sci Sports Exerc* 19:37-40, 1987.

119. Fox EL: Frequency and duration of interval training programs and changes in aerobic power, *J Appl Physiol* 38:481-484, 1975.

120. Frankle MA et al: Anabolic androgenic steroids and a stroke in a athlete: case report, *Arch Phys Med Rehabil* 69:632-633, 1988.

121. Freed DLJ et al: Anabolic steroids in athletics: crossover double-blind trial in weightlifters, *Br Med J* 2:471-473, 1975.

122. Freinhar J, Alvarez W: Androgen-induced hypomania, *J Clin Psychol* 46:354-355, 1985.

123. Friedl KE, Yesalis CE: Self-treatment of gynecomastia in body builders who use anabolic steroids, *Physician and Sportsmedicine* 17:67-79, 1989.

124. Frohlich J et al: Lipid profile of body builders with and without self-administration of anabolic steroids, *Eur J Appl Physiol* 59:98-103, 1989.

125. Fryburg DA et al: Growth hormone acutely stimulates forearm muscle protein synthesis in normal adults, *Am J Physiol* 260:499-504, 1991.

126. Gaede JT, Montine TJ: Massive pulmonary embolus in anabolic steroid abuse, *JAMA* 267:2328-2329, 1992.

127. Gaesser GA, Rich RG: Effects of high and low-intensity exercise training on aerobic capacity and lipids, *Med Sci Sports Exerc* 16:269-274, 1984.

128. Galiano FJ et al: Physiological, endocrine and performance effects of adding branch chain amino acids to a 6 percent carbohydrate-electrolyte beverage during prolonged cycling, American College of Sports Medicine, National Meeting, Orlando, Fla, 1991.

129. Gall SL et al: Who tests which athletes for what drugs? *Physician and Sportsmedicine* 16:155-161, 1988.

130. Gao JP et al: Sodium bicarbonate ingestion improved performance in interval training, *Eur J Appl Physiol Occup Physiol* 58:171-174, 1988.

131. Gardner G: Specificity of strength changes of the exercised and nonexercised limb following isometric training, *Res Q* 34:98-101, 1963.

132. Gauron EF: The art of cognitive self-regulation, *Clin Sports Med* 5:91-101, 1986.

133. Gettman LR, Pollock ML: Circuit weight training: a critical review of its physiological benefits, *Physician and Sportsmedicine* 9:44-60, 1981.

134. Gettman LR et al: Physiological responses of men to one, three, and five day per week training programs, *Res Q* 47:638-646, 1976.

135. Gettman LR et al: The effect of circuit weight training on strength, cardiorespiratory function and body composition of adult men, *Med Sci Sports Exerc* 10:171-176, 1978.

136. Gettman LR et al: Physiological changes after 20 weeks of isotonic versus isokinetic circuit training, *J Sports Med Phys Fitness* 20:265-274, 1980.

137. Gettman LR et al: A comparison of combined running and weight training with circuit weight training, *Med Sci Sports Exerc* 14:229-234, 1982.

138. Gibson TM et al: An evaluation of a treadmill work test, *Br J Sports Med* 13:6-11, 1979.

139. Gillam GM: Effects of frequency of weight training on muscle strength enhancement, *J Sports Med* 21:432-436, 1981.

140. Gilman AG et al, editors: *Goodman and Gilman's the pharmacological basis of therapeutics,* ed 8, New York, 1990, Pergamon Press.

141. Goldberg AL: Work-induced growth of skeletal muscle in normal and hypophysectomized rats, *Am J Physiol* 213:1193-1198, 1967.

142. Goldberg AL, Goodman HN: Relationship between growth hormone and muscular work in determining muscle size, *J Physiol* 200:655-666, 1969.

143. Goldfarb S: Sex hormones and hepatic neoplasia, *Cancer Res* 36:2584-2588, 1976.

144. Goldfinch J et al: Induced metabolic alkylosis and its effect on 400 M racing time. *Eur J Appl Physiol* 57:45-48, 1988.

145. Goldman B: Liver carcinoma in an athlete taking anabolic steroids, *J Am Osteopath Assoc* 85:56, 1985.

146. Gollnick PD, Matoba H: Role of carbohydrate in exercise, *Clin Sports Med* 3:583-593, 1984.

147. Gonyea WJ et al: Exercise induced increased in muscle fiber number, *Eur J Appl Physiol* 55:137-143, 1986.

148. Gradeen CY et al: Urinary excretion of furazabol metabolite, *J Anal Toxicol* 14:120-123, 1990.

149. Grady GF, Chalmers TC: Risk of post-transfusion hepatitis, *N Engl J Med* 271:337, 1964.

150. Grandjean AC: Macronutrient intake of US athletes compared with

the general population and recommendations made for athletes, *Am J Clin Nutr* 49:1070-1076, 1989.

151. Graves JE: Effect of reduced training frequency on muscular strength, *Int J Sports Med* 9:316-319, 1988.

152. Graves JE et al: Specificity of limited range of motion variable resistance training, *Med Sci Sports Exerc* 21:84-89, 1989.

153. Grossi T: New laws effect steroids supply, not demand, *The Cleveland Plain Dealer,* 1D, May 10, 1992.

154. Guide to banned medications, *Sportsmediscope* 7:1-5, 1988.

155. Hall K: Effective intervenous administration of human growth hormone on sulfation factory activity in serum of hypopituitary subjects, *Acta. Endocrinol* 66:491-497, 1971.

156. Hammond HK, Froelicher VF: Exercise testing for cardiorespiratory fitness, *Sports Med* 1:234-239, 1984.

157. Hargreaves ML et al: Effect of carbohydrate feedings on muscle glycogen utilisation and exercise performance, *Med Sci Sports Exerc* 16:219-222, 1984.

158. Hargreaves M et al: Effect of fructose ingestion on muscle glycogen usage during exercise, *Med Sci Sports Exerc* 17:360-363, 1985.

159. Hargreaves ML et al: Effects of pre-exercise carbohydrate feedings on endurance cycling performance, *Med Sci Sports Exerc* 19:33-36, 1987.

160. Hasson SM, Barnes WS: Effect of carbohydrate ingestion on exercise of varying intensity and duration: practical implications, *Sports Med* 8:327-344, 1989.

161. Hatfield FC: *Anabolic steroids, what kind and how many,* Los Angeles, 1982, Fitness Systems.

162. Haupt HA: Drugs in athletics, *Clin Sports Med* 8:561-582, 1989.

163. Haupt HA, Rovere GD: Anabolic steroids: a review of the literature, *Am J Sports Med* 12:469-484, 1984.

164. Havel RJ et al: Travel rate and oxidation of different free fatty acids in man during exercise, *J Appl Physiol* 19:613-618, 1964.

165. Haymes EM: Nutritional concerns: needs for iron, *Med Sci Sports Exerc* 19:S197-S200, 1987.

166. Hays LR et al: Anabolic steroid dependence, *Am J Psychol* 147:122, 1990.

167. Hecker AL: Nutritional conditioning for athletic competition, *Clin Sports Med* 3:567-582, 1984.

168. Hervey GR: Are athletes wrong about anabolic steroids? *Br J Sports Med* 9:74-77, 1975.

169. Hervey GR et al: Effects of methandienone on the performance and body composition of men undergoing athletic training, *Clin Sci* 60:457-461, 1981.

170. Hickson RC, Kuroskwi TT: Anabolic steroids in training, *Clin Sports Med* 5:461-469, 1986.

171. Hickson RC et al: Skeletal muscle cytosol (3H)-methyl trienolone receptor binding and serum androgens: effects of hypertrophy and hormonal state, *J Steroid Biochem* 19:1705, 1983.

172. Hurley BF et al: High-density-lipoprotein cholesterol in body builders vs. power lifters—negative effects of androgen use, *JAMA* 252:507-513, 1984.

173. Inbar O et al: The effect of alkaline treatment on short term maximal exercise, *J Sports Sci* 1:95-104, 1983.

174. Isidori A et al: A study of growth hormone release in man after oral administration of amino acids, *Curr Med Res Opin* 7:475-481, 1981.

175. Ivy JL et al: Influence of caffeine and carbohydrate feedings on endurance performance, *Med Sci Sports Exerc* 11:6-11, 1979.

176. Ivy JL et al: Endurance improved by ingestion of a glucose polymer supplement, *Med Sci Sports Exerc* 15:466-471, 1983.

177. Ivy JL et al: Muscle glycogen synthesis after exercise, effect of time of carbohydrate ingestion, *J Appl Physiol* 64:1480-1485, 1988.

178. Jain SC et al: Effect of phosphate supplementation on oxygen delivery at high altitude, *Int J Biometeriol* 331:249, 1987.

179. James VH et al: Effect of an anabolic steroid (methandienone) on the metabolism of cortisol in the human, *J Endocrinol* 25:211-220, 1962.

180. Jarow JP, Lipshultz LI: Anabolic steroid-induced hypogonadotropic hypogonadism, *Am J Sports Med* 18:429-431, 1990.

181. Johnson BL et al: A comparison on concentric and eccentric muscle training, *Med Sci Sports Exerc* 8:35-38, 1976.

182. Johnson FL: Hepatoma associated with androgenic steroids, *Lancet* 1:1294-1295, 1975.

183. Johnson FL: The association of oral-anabolic steroids in life threatening disease, *Med Sci Sports Exerc* 7:284-286, 1975.

184. Johnson FL et al: Association of androgenic-anabolic steroid therapy with development of hepatocellular carcinoma, *Lancet* 2:1273-1276, 1972.

185. Johnson LC, O'Shea JP: Anabolic steroid: effects on strength development, *Science* 164:957-959, 1969.

186. Johnson LC et al: Anabolic steroid: effects on strength, body weight, oxygen uptake and spermatogenesis upon mature males, *Med Sci Sports Exerc* 4:43-45, 1972.

187. Johnson LC et al: Effect of anabolic steroid treatment on endurance, *Med Sci Sports Exerc* 7:287-289, 1975.

188. Johnson MD et al: Anabolic steroid use by male adolescents, Pediatrics 83:921-925, 1989.

189. Johnson MD: Anabolic steroid use in adolescent athletes, *Pediatr Clin North Am* 37:1111-1123, 1990.

190. Johnston CC, Longcope C: Premenopausal bone loss-a risk factor for osteoporosis, *N Engl J Med* 323:271-272, 1990.

191. Jones M, Pedoe DST: Blood doping—a literature review, *Br J Sports Med* 23:84-88, 1989.

192. Jorgensen JOL et al: Beneficial effects of growth hormone treatment in growth hormone-deficient adults, *Lancet* 1:1221-1225, 1989.

193. Kanehisa H, Miyashita M: Effect of isometric and isokinetic muscle training on static strength and dynamic power, *Eur J Appl Physiol* 50:365-371, 1983.

194. Kanehisa H, Miyashita M: Specificity of velocity in strength training, *Eur J Appl Physiol* 52:104-106, 1983.

195. Karagiorgos A et al: Growth hormone response to continuous and intermittent exercise, *Med Sci Sports Exerc* 11:302-307, 1979.

196. Kashkin KB, Kleber HD: Hooked on hormones? An anabolic steroid addiction hypothesis, *JAMA* 262:3166-3170, 1989.

197. Kearney JT et al: Cardiorespiratory responses of sedentary college women as a function of training intensity, *J Appl Physiol* 41:822-825, 1976.

198. Kelemen MH, Stewart KJ: Circuit weight training—a new direction for cardiac rehabilitation, *Sports Med* 2:385-388, 1985.

199. Keul J et al: Anabole hormone: schadigung leistungsfahigkeit und stoffwechses, *Med Klin* 71:497-503, 1976.

200. Kiens B et al: Benefit of dietary simple carbohydrates on the early post-exercise muscle glycogen repletion in male athletes, *Med Sci Sports Exerc* 22:S88, 1990.

201. King JB, Burns DG: Aplastic anaemia, oxymetholone and acute myeloid leukaemia, *South African Med J* 46:1622-1623, 1972.

202. Kiraly CL et al: Effect of androgenic and anabolic steroids on the sebaceous gland in power lifters, *Acta Derm Venereol* 67:36-40, 1987.

203. Kiraly CL et al: The effect of testosterone and anabolic steroids on the skin surface lipids and the population of a propionibacteria acnes in young post pubertal men, *Acta Derm Venereol* 68:21-26, 1988.

204. Knuth UA et al: Anabolic steroids and semen parameters in body builders, *Fertil Steril* 52:1041-1047, 1989.

205. Knuttgen HG et al: Physical conditioning through interval training with young male adults, *Med Sci Sports Exerc* 5:220-226, 1973.

206. Kochakian CD: Comparison of renotropic with androgenic activities of various steroids, *Am J Physiol* 142:315-325, 1944.

207. Kochakian CD, Murlin JR: The effect of male hormone on the pro-

tein and energy metabolism of castrate dogs, *J Nutr* 10:437-459, 1935.

207a. Kochakian CD: Testosterone, testosterone acetate, and the protein and energy metabolism of castrate dogs, *Endocrinology* 21:750-755, 1937.

207b. Kochakian CD, Murlin JR: The relationship of the synthetic male hormone, androstenedione, to the protein and energy metabolism of castrate dogs and the protein metabolism of a normal dog, *Am J Physiol* 117:642-657, 1936.

208. Koller WC, Biary N: Effect of alcohol on tremors: comparison with propanalol, *Neurology* 34:221-222, 1984.

209. Kopera H: The history of anabolic steroids and a review of clinical experiences with anabolic steroids, *Acta Endocrinol* 110:11-18, 1985.

210. Kraemer WJ et al: Physiological adaptations to resistance exercise-implication for athletic condition, *Sports Med* 6:246-256, 1988.

211. Kreider RB et al: Effects of phosphate loading on oxygen uptake, ventilatory anaerobic threshold, and run performance, *Med Sci Sports Exerc* 22:250-256, 1990.

212. Kreuz LE, Rose RM: Assessment of aggressive behavior and plasma testosterone in young criminal population, *Psychosom Med* 34:321-332, 1972.

213. Kruse P et al: Beta blockade use in precision sports: effect on pistol shooting performance, *J Appl Physiol* 6:417-420, 1986.

214. Lamb DR: Anabolic steroids in athletics. How well do they work and how dangerous are they? *Am J Sports Med* 12:31-39, 1984.

215. Laritcheva KA et al: Study of energy expenditure and protein needs of top weightlifters. In Parizkova J, Rogozkin VA, editors: *Nutrition, physical fitness and health,* Baltimore, Md, 1978, University Park Press.

216. Laroche GP: Steroid anabolic drugs and arterial complications in an athlete—a case history, *Angiology* 41:964-969, 1990.

217. Larsson L, Tesch PA: Motor unit density in extremely hypertrophied skeletal muscles in man, *Eur J Appl Physiol* 55:130-136, 1986.

218. Laseter JT, Russell JA: Anabolic steroid-induced tendon pathology: a review of the literature, *Med Sci Sports Exerc* 23:1-3, 1991.

219. Lavender G, Bird SR: Effect of sodium bicarbonate ingestion upon repeated sprints, *Br J Sports Med* 23:41-45, 1989.

220. Leeds EM, et al: Effects of exercise in anabolic steroids on total and lipoprotein cholesterol concentration and male and female rats, *Med Sci Sports Exerc* 18:663, 1986.

221. Lemon PWR: Protein and exercise: update 1987. *Med Sci Sports Exerc* 19:S179-S190, 1987.

222. Lenders JWM et al: Deleterious effects of anabolic steroids on serum lipoproteins, blood pressure, and liver function in amateur body builders, *Int J Sports Med* 9:19-23, 1988.

223. Lewis SF et al: Cardiovascular responses to exercise as functions of absolute and relative work loads, *J Appl Physiol* 54:1314-1323, 1983.

224. Liang MT et al: Aerobic training threshold, intensity, duration and frequency of exercise, *Scand J Sports Sci* 4:5-8, 1982.

225. Lombardo JA: Stimulants and athletic performance: amphetamines and caffeine, *Physician and Sportsmedicine* 14:128-140, 1986.

226. Lombardo JA: Stimulants and athletic performance: cocaine and nicotine, *Physician and Sportsmedicine* 14:85-90, 1986.

227. Lombardo JA et al: Recognizing anabolic steroid use, *Patient Care* 19:28-47, 1985.

228. Lopes JM et al: The effect of caffeine on skeletal muscle function before and after fatigue, *J Appl Physiol* 54:1303-1305, 1983.

229. Lorimer DA, Hart LL: Cardiac dysfunction in athletes receiving anabolic steroids, DICP, *Ann Pharmacotherapy* 24:1060-1061, 1990.

230. Lowenstein DH et al: Active neurological and psychiatric complications associated with cocaine abuse, *Am J Med* 83:841-846, 1987.

231. Luke JL et al: Sudden cardiac death during exercise in a weight lifter using anabolic androgenic steroids: pathological and toxiological findings, *J Forensic Sci* 35:144-147, 1990.

232. Lynch GP: Athletic injuries in the practicing sports psychologist: practical guidelines for assisting athletes, *Sports Psychol* 2:161-167, 1988.

233. MacDougall JD et al: Biochemical adaptation of human skeletal muscle to heavy resistance training and immobilization, *J Appl Physiol* 43:700-703, 1977.

234. Macintyre JG: Growth hormone in athletes, *Sports Med* 4:129-142, 1987.

235. Malone DA, Dimeff RJ: The use of fluoxetine in depression associated with anabolic steroid withdrawal: a case series, *J Clin Psychiatry* 53:130-132, 1992.

236. Marable NL et al: Urinary nitrogen excretion as influenced by a muscle-building exercise program and protein variation, *Nutr Reports Int* 19:795-804, 1979.

237. Marshall E: The drug of champions, *Science* 242:183-184, 1988.

238. Matoba H, Gollnick PD: Response of skeletal muscle to training, *Sports Med* 1:240-251, 1984.

239. Matsumoto AM: Effects of chronic testosterone administration in normal men: safey and efficacy of high dose testosterone and parallel dose-dependent supression of leutenizing hormone, follicle-stimulating hormone, and sperm production, *J Clin Endocrinol Metab* 70:282-287, 1990.

240. Maughan RJ et al: Fat and carbohydrate metabolism during low intensity exercise: effects of the availability of muscle glycogen, *Eur J Physiol* 37:7, 1978.

241. Mauss J et al: Effect of long-term testosterone oenanthate administration on male reproduction function: clinical evaluation, serum FSH, LH, testosterone, and seminal fluid analysis in normal men, *Acta Endocrinol* 78:373-384, 1975.

242. Mazur A, Lamb TA: Testosterone, status and mood in human males, *Horm Behav* 14:236-246, 1980.

243. McArdle WD, Katch FI, Katch VL: *Exercise physiology—energy, nutrition and human performance,* ed 2, Philadelphia, 1986, Lea and Febiger.

244. McCauley E: Sports psychology for the 1980's: some current developments, *Med Sci Sports Exerc* 19:S95-S97, 1987.

245. McConnel TR: Practical considerations in the testing of VO2 max in runners, *Sports Med* 5:57-68, 1988.

246. McDermott J: Steroids cited in teens' death, *Cleveland Plain Dealer,* 1989, pp 1a & 8a.

247. McDonagh MJN, Davies CTM: Adaptive response of mammalian skeletal muscle to exercise with high loads, *Eur J Appl Physiol* 52:139-155, 1984.

248. McKee MG: Burnout and the athlete, *Surgical Rounds for Orthopaedics* 1:23-28, 1990.

249. McMiken DF, Daniels JT: Aerobic requirements and maximum aerobic power in treadmill and track running, *Med Sci Sports Exerc* 8:14-17, 1976.

250. McNaughton L, Preece D: Alcohol and its effect on sprint and middle distance running, *Br J Sports Med* 14:481-482, 1982.

251. McNaughton L et al: Anaerobic work and power output during cycle ergometry exercise: effects of bicarbonate loading, *J Sports Sci* 9:151-160, 1991.

252. McNutt RA et al: Acute myocardial infarction in a 22-year-old world class weight lifter using anabolic steroids, *Am J Cardiol* 62:164, 1988.

253. Meyer-Bahlburg FL et al: Aggressiveness and testosterone measures in man, *Psychosom Med* 36:269-274, 1974.

254. Michna H, Stang-Voss C: The predisposition to tendon rupture after doping with anabolic steroids, International, *J Sports Med* 4:59, 1983.

255. Milesis CA et al: Effects of different durations of training on cardiorespiratory function, body composition and serum lipids, *Res Q* 47:716-725, 1976.

256. Millard-Stafford ML et al: Effect of glucose polymer diet supplement on responses to prolonged successive swimming, cycling and running, *Eur J Appl Physiol* 58:327-333, 1988.

257. Mitchell M, Dimeff RJ: Effects of arginine and lysine supplementation on body composition and strength in highly conditioned weight lifters, (Manuscript in preparation, 1992.)

258. Mitchell M et al: Effects of amino acid supplementation on metabolic responses to ultraendurance triathalon performance, American College of Sports Medicine, National Meeting, Orlando, Fla, 1991.

259. Mole PA et al: Adaptation of muscle to exercise. Increase in levels of palmityl CoA synthetase, carnitine, palmityltransferase, and palmityl CoA dehydrogenase and the capacity to oxide fatty acids, *J Clin Invest* 50:2323, 1971.

260. Monti PM et al: Testosterone in components of aggressive and sexual behavior in man, *Am J Psychol* 134:692-694, 1977.

261. Moritani T, DeVries HA: Neurofactors versus hypertrophy in the time course of muscle strength gain, *Am J Phys Med* 82:521-524, 1979.

262. Mulvihill JJ et al: Hepatic adenoma in Fanconi anemia treated with oxymetholone, *J Pediatr* 87:122-124, 1975.

263. Murray R: The effects of consuming carbohydrate-electrolyte beverages on gastric emptying and fluid absorption during and following exercise, *Sports Med* 4:322-351, 1987.

264. Murray R et al: The effect of fluid and carbohydrate feedings during intermittent cycling exercise, *Med Sci Sports Exerc* 19:597-604, 1987.

265. Murray R et al: The effect of glucose, fructose and sucrose ingestion during exercise, *Med Sci Sports Exerc* 21:275-282, 1989.

266. Myers CR: Effect of two isometric routines on strength, size and endurance in exercise and non-exercised arms, *Res Q* 38:430-440, 1967.

267. National Football League substance abuse policies, 1990.

268. Naveri H et al: Gastric emptying and serum insulin levels after intake of glucose-polymer solutions, *Eur J Appl Physiol* 58:661-665, 1989.

269. Nelson D: Effects of ethyl alcohol on performance of selected gross motor test, *Res Qu* 30:312-320, 1959.

270. Nerducci WA et al: Anabolic steroids—a review of the clinical toxicology and diagnostic screening, *Clin Toxicol* 28:287-310, 1990.

271. Newhouse IJ et al: The effect of prelatent/latent iron deficiency on physical work capacity, *Med Sci Sports Exerc* 21:263-268, 1989.

272. Nickerson HJ, Tripp AD: Iron deficiency in adolescent cross-country runners, *Physician and Sportsmedicine* 11:60-66, 1983.

273. Nickerson HJ et al: Causes of iron deficiency in adolescent athletes, *J Pediatr* 114:657-663, 1989.

274. Nideffer RM: Psychological preparation of the highly competitive athlete, *Physician and Sportsmedicine* 15:85-92, 1987.

275. O'Carroll R: Psychiatric effects of steroids, *Lancet* 1:1212, 1987.

276. O'Shea JP: The effects of an anabolic steroid on dynamic strength levels of weight lifters, *Nutr Reports Int* 4:363-370, 1971.

277. Obeid DA et al: Fanconi anemia oxymetholone hepatic tumors and chromosone aberrations associated with leukemic transition, *Cancer* 46:1401-1404, 1980.

278. Ohira Y et al: Work capacity, heart rate, and blood lactate responses to treatment, *Br J Hematol* 41:365-372, 1979.

279. Olweus D et al: Testosterone, aggression, physical and personality dimensions in normal adolescent males, *Psychosom Med* 42:253-269, 1980.

280. Overly WL et al: Androgens and hepatocellular carcinoma in an athlete, *Ann Int Med* 100:158-159, 1984.

281. Owens JL et al: Influence of moderate exercise on adipocyte metabolism and hormonal responsiveness, *J Appl Physiol* 43:425-430, 1977.

282. Pace N et al: Increase in hypoxic tolerance of normal men accompanying the polycythaemia induced by transfusion of erythrocytes, *Am J Physiol* 148:152-163, 1947.

283. Paivio A: Cognitive and motivational functions of imagery and human performance, *Can J Appl Sci* 10:22S-28S, 1985.

284. Perskey H et al: Relation of psychologic measures of aggression and hostility to testosterone productions in man, *Psychosom Med* 33:265-277, 1971.

285. Peterson GE, Fahey TD: HDL-C in five athletes using anabolic-androgenic steroids, *Physician and Sportsmedicine* 12:120, 1984.

286. *Physicians desk reference,* ed 46, Montvale, NJ, 1992, Medical Economics Data.

287. Piehl K: Time course for refilling of glycogen stores in human muscle fibres following exercise-induced glycogen depletion, *Acta Physiol Scand* 90:297-302, 1974.

288. Pineda AA et al: Delayed hemolytic transfusion reaction: an immunologic hazard of blood transfusion, *Transfusion* 18:1-7, 1978.

289. Piness G et al: Clinical observations on phenylaminoethanol sulphate, *JAMA* 94:790-791, 1930.

290. Pollock ML et al: Effects of frequency of training on working capacity, cardiovascular function and body composition of adult men, *Med Sci Sports Exerc* 1:70-74, 1969.

291. Pope HG, Katz DL: Body builders psychosis, *Lancet* 1:863, 1987.

292. Pope HG, Katz DL: Affective and psychotic symptoms associated with anabolic steroid use, *Am J Psychol* 145:47, 1988.

293. Pope HG, Katz DL: Homocide and near-homocide by anabolic steroid users, *J Clin Psychol* 51:28-31, 1990.

294. Prat J et al: Wilms' tumor in an adult associated with androgen abuse, *JAMA* 21:2322-2323, 1977.

295. Prinzmetal M, Bloomberg W: The use of benzedrine for the treatment of narcolepsy, *JAMA* 104:2051-2054, 1935.

296. Prior JC et al: Spinal bone loss in ovulatory disturbances, *N Engl J Med* 323:1221-1227, 1990.

297. Rada RT et al: Plasma testosterone in aggressive behavior, *Psychosomatics* 17:138-141, 1976.

298. Raine AEG: Hypertension, blood viscosity, and cardiovascular morbidity in renal failure: implications of erythropoietin therapy, *Lancet* 1:97-100, 1988.

299. RJ, anonymous; Personal correspondence, July, 1990.

300. Roberts JT, Essenhigh DM: Adenocarcinoma of prostate in 40-year-old body-builder, *Lancet* 2:742, 1986.

301. Robertson RJ et al: Effect of induced erythrocythemia on hypoxia tolerance during physical exercise, *J Appl Physiol* 53:490-495, 1982.

302. Robertson RJ et al: Hemoglobin concentration and aerobic work capacity in women following induced erythrocythemia, *J Appl Physiol* 57:568-575, 1984.

303. Rogol AD: Growth hormone: physiology, therapeutic use, and potential for abuse, *Exerc Sports Sci Rev* 17:353-377, 1989.

304. Rogozkin VA: Metabolic effects of anabolic steroids in skeletal muscle, *Med Sci Sports Exerc* 11:160-163, 1979.

305. Rogozkin VA, Feldkoren B: The effects of retabolil and training on activity of RNA-polymerase in skeletal muscles, *Med Sci Sports Exerc* 11:345-347, 1979.

306. Rowland TW: The effect of iron therapy on the exercise capacity of nonanemic iron-deficient adolescent runners, *Am J Dis Child* 142:165-169, 1988.

307. Ruddel H et al: Impact of magnesium supplementation on performance data in young swimmers, *Magnes Res* 3:103-107, 1990.

308. Saartok T et al: Relative binding affinity of anabolic androgenic steroids: comparison of the binding to the androgen receptors in skeletal muscle and in prostate as well as to sex hormone-binding globulin, *Endocrinology* 114:2100, 1984.

309. Salmons S, Heriksson J: The adaptive response of skeletal muscle to increased use, *Muscle Nerve* 4:94-105, 1981.

310. Salomon F et al: The effects of treatment with common human growth hormone on body composition and metabolism in adults with growth hormone deficiency, *N Engl J Med* 321:1797-1803, 1989.

311. Samples B: Mind over muscle: returning the injured athlete to play, *Physician and Sportsmedicine* 15:172-180, 1987.

312. Sawka MN et al: Erythrocyte reinfusion and maximal aerobic

power: an examination of modifying factors, *JAMA* 257:1496-1499, 1987.

313. Schoene RB et al: Iron repletion decreases maximal exercise lactate concentrations in female athletes with minimal iron deficiency anemia, *J Lab Clin Med* 102:306-312, 1983.

314. Schwartz AB et al: Erythropoietin for the anemia of chronic renal failure, *Am Fam Physician* 37:211-215, 1988.

315. Scott MJ, Scott MJ: HIV infection associated with injections of anabolic steroids, *JAMA* 262:207-208, 1989.

316. Seidman DS et al: The effect of glucose polymer beverage ingestion during prolonged outdoor exercise in the heat, *Med Sci Sports Exerc* 23:458-469, 1991.

317. Shapiro P et al: Multiple hepatic tumors in peliosis hepatis in Fanconi's anemia treated with androgen, *Am J Dis Child* 131:1104-1106, 1977.

318. Sharkey BJ: Intensity and duration of training in the development of cardiorespiratory endurance, *Med Sci Sports Exerc* 2:197-202, 1970.

319. Sharp R et al: Effects of a commercial amino acid supplement on adaptations to cycle ergometry training, American College of Sports Medicine, National Meeting, Orlando, Fla, 1991.

320. Shepherd RE et al: Effect of physical training on control mechanisms of lipolysis in rat fat cell ghosts, *J Appl Physiol* 42:884-888, 1977.

321. Sherman WM: Carbohydrate feedings one hour before exercise improves cycling performance, *Am J Clin Nutr* 54:866-870, 1991.

322. Sherman WM et al: The effect of exercise and diet manipulation on muscle glycogen and its subsequent utilization during performance, *Int J Sports Med* 2:114-118, 1981.

323. Sherman WM et al: The effect of exercise-diet manipulation on muscle glycogen and its subsequent utilisation during performance, *Int J Sports Med* 2:114-118, 1981.

324. Sherman WM et al: Effects of a 4H preexercise carbohydrate feeding on cycling performance, *Med Sci Sports Exerc* 21:598-604, 1989.

325. Signorile JF et al: Effects of acute inhalation of the bronchodilator, albuterol, on power output, *Med Sci Sports Exerc* 24:638-642, 1992.

326. Sklarek HM et al: Aids in a body builder using anabolic steroids, *N Engl J Med* 311:1701, 1984.

327. Slavin JL et al: Amino acid supplements: beneficial or risky? *Physician and Sportsmedicine* 16:221, 1988.

328. Smith AM et al: Emotional responses of athletes to injury, *Mayo Clin Proc* 65:38-50, 1990.

329. Smith GM, Beecher HG: Amphetamine sulphate in athletic performance, *JAMA* 170:542-547, 1959.

330. Smith MJ, Melton P: Isokinetic versus isotonic variable resistance training, *Am J Sports Med* 9:275-279, 1981.

331. Snochowski M et al: Androgen and glucocorticoid receptors in human skeletal muscle cytosol, *J Steroid Biochem* 14:765-771, 1981.

332. Spriet LL et al: Effect of graded erythrocythemia on cardiovascular and metabolic responses to exercise, *J Appl Physiol* 61:1942-1948, 1986.

333. Stamford BA, Moffatt R: Anabolic steroid: effectiveness as an ergogenic aid to experienced weight trainers, *J Sports Med* 14:191-197, 1974.

334. Stone HO et al: Effects of erythrocytes on blood viscosity, *Am J Physiol* 214:913-918, 1968.

335. Strauss RH et al: Side effects of anabolic steroid in weight-trained men, *Physician and Sportsmedicine* 11:86-99, 1983.

336. Tahmindjis AJ: The use of anabolic steroids by athletes to increase body weight and strength, *Med J Australia* 1:991-993, 1976.

337. Takahara J et al: Stimulatory effects of gamma-hydroxybutyric acid on growth hormone and prolactin release in humans, *J Clin Endocrinol Metab* 44:1014-1017, 1977.

338. Taylor NAS, Wilkinson JG: Exercise-induced skeletal muscle growth: hypertrophy or hyperplasia? *Sports Med* 3:190-200, 1986.

339. Tennant F et al: Anabolic steroid dependence with opioid-type features, *N Engl J Med* 319:578, 1988.

340. Tennant FS: Dealing with cocaine use by athletes, *Med Digest* 6:1-3, 1984.

341. Terney R, McClain LG: The use of anabolic steroids in high school students, *Am J Dis Child* 144:99-104, 1990.

342. Toner MM et al: Metabolic and cardiovascular responses to exercise with caffeine, *Ergonomics* 25:1175-1183, 1982.

343. Ullrich I et al: Cardiac hypertrophy in weightlifters: only in steroid users? *Med Sci Sports Exerc* 22:S64, 1990.

344. Urhausen A et al: One and two-dimensional echocardiography in body builders using anabolic steroids, *Eur J Appl Physiol* 58:633-640, 1989.

345. Van Baak MA: Beta adrenoceptor blockade and exercise, an update, *Sports Med* 4:209-225, 1988.

346. Van Linge B: The response of muscle to strenuous exercise, *J Bone Joint Surg* 44B:711-721, 1962.

347. Vander AJ et al: *Human physiology the mechanism of body functions*, ed 4, New York, 1985, McGraw-Hill.

348. Vanhelder WP et al: Growth hormone responses during intermittent weight lifting exercise in men, *Eur J Appl Physiol* 53:31-34, 1984.

349. Voy RO: IOC bans human chorionic gonadotropin, *Sportsmediscope* 7:11, 1988.

350. Wade N: Anabolic steroids: doctors denounce them, but athletes aren't listening, *Science* 176:1399-1403, 1972.

351. Wadler GI, Hainline B: *Drugs and the athlete*, Philadelphia, 1989, FA Davis.

352. Wagner JC: Use of chromium and cobalamide by athletes, *Clin Pharm* 8:832-834, 1989.

353. Wagner JC: Enhancement of athletic performance with drugs: an overview, *Sports Med* 12:250-265, 1991.

354. Ward P: The effect of an anabolic steroid on strength and lean body mass, *Med Sci Sports Exerc* 4:277-282, 1973.

355. Webb OL, et al: Severe depression of high-density lipoprotein cholesterol levels in weight lifters and body builders by self-administered exogenous testosterone and anabolic-androgenic steroids, *Metabolism* 33:971, 1984.

356. Weight LM et al: Vitamin and mineral status of trained athletes including the effects of supplementation, *Am J Clin Nutr* 47:186-191, 1988.

357. Weight LM et al: Vitamin and mineral supplementation: effect on the running performance of trained athletes, *Am J Clin Nutr* 47:192-195, 1988.

358. Wenger HA, Bell GJ: The interactions of intensity, frequency and duration of exercise training in altering cardiorespiratory fitness, *Sports Med* 3:346-356, 1986.

359. Whitehead HM et al: Growth hormone treatment in adults with growth hormone deficiency: effect on muscle fibre size and proportions, *Acta Paediatr Scand Suppl* 356:65-67, 1989.

360. Wilcox AR: The effects of caffeine and exercise on body weight, fat pad weight and fat cell size, *Med Sci Sports Exerc* 14:317-321, 1982.

361. Wilkes D et al: The effect of acute induced metabolic alkylosis on an 800 M racing time, *Med Sci Sports Exerc* 15:277-280, 1983.

362. Williams MH: Vitamin and mineral supplements to athletes: do they help? *Clin Sports Med* 3:623-637, 1984.

363. Williams MH et al: Effect of blood reinjection upon endurance capacity in heart rate, *Med Sci Sports Exerc* 5:181-186, 1973.

364. Williams MH et al: Effect of blood infusion upon endurance capacity and ratings of perceived exertion, *Med Sci Sports Exerc* 10:113-118, 1978.

365. Williams MH et al: The effect of erythrocythemia upon 5-mile treadmill run time, *Med Sci Sports Exerc* 13:169-175, 1981.

366. Williams RS, Bishop T: Enhanced receptor cyclase and coupling and augmented catecholamine-stimulated lipolysis in exercising rats, *Am J Physiol* 243:E345-E351, 1982.

367. Wilson JD, Griffin JE: The use and misuse of androgen, *Metabolism* 29:1278-1295, 1980.

368. Wilson JD et al, editor: *Harrison's principles of internal medicine,* ed 12, New York, 1991, McGraw-Hill.

369. Win-May M, Mya-Tu M: Effect of anabolic steroids on physical fitness, *J Sports Med Phys Fitness* 15:266-271, 1975.

370. Windsor RE, Dumitru D: Anabolic steroid use by athletes. How serious are the health hazards? *Postgrad Med* 84:37-49, 1988.

371. Winearls CG et al: Effect of human erythropoietin derived from recombinant DNA on anaemia of patients maintained by chronic haemodialysis, *Lancet* 2:1175-1178, 1986.

372. Wood TO et al: The effect of exercise in anabolic steroids on the mechanical properties of crimp morphology of the rat tendon, *Am J Sports Med* 16:153-158, 1988.

373. Wyngaarden JB et al, editors: *Cecil textbook of medicine,* ed 19, Philadelphia, 1992, WB Saunders.

374. Yang YT, McElligott MA: Multiple actions of beta adrenergic agonists on skeletal muscle and adipose tissue, *Biochem J* 261:1-10, 1989.

375. Yarasheski KE et al: Effects of growth hormone in resistance exercise on muscle growth in young men, *Am J Physiol* 262:e261-267, 1992.

376. Yates WR et al: Illicit anabolic steroid use: a controlled personality study, *Acta Psychiatr Scand* 81:548-550, 1990.

377. Yu-Yahiro JA et al: Morphologic and histologic abnormalities in female and male rats treated with anabolic steroids, *Am J Sports Med* 17:686-689, 1989.

■■■■ **RESOURCES** ■■■■

Drugs

Duchaine D: *The underground steroid handbook,* Venice, Calif, 1989, HLR Technical Books.

Newsom MM, editor: *Drug free,* Colorado Springs, 1989, USOC Drug Education Program.

Voy RO: *Drugs, sport and politics,* Champaign, Ill, 1991, Leisure Press.

Wadler GI, Hainline B: *Drugs and the athlete,* Philadelphia, 1989, FA Davis.

Williams MH: *Beyond training—how athletes enhance performance legally and illegally,* Champaign, Ill, 1989, Leisure Press.

Yesalis CE, editor: *Anabolic steroids in sport and exercise,* Champaign, Ill, 1993, Human Kinetics Publishers.

Drug testing information

USOC Drug Education Program, 1750 East Boulder Street, Colorado Springs, CO 80909.

NCAA Drug Education Program, 6201 College Blvd., Overland Park, KS 66211-2422.

Performance improvement

Berning J, Steen SN, editors: *Sports nutrition for the 90's: the health professionals handbook,* Gaithersburg, Md, 1991, Aspen Publications.

Clark N: *Nancy Clark's sports nutrition guidebook,* Champaign, Ill, 1990, Leisure Press.

Fleck SJ, Kraemer WJ: *Designing resistance training program,* Champaign, Ill, 1987, Human Kinetics Books.

Wells CL: *Women, sport and performance—a physiological prospective,* ed 2, Champaign, Ill, 1991, Human Kinetics Books.

American College of Sports Medicine position stands

Blood doping as an ergogenic aid, *Med Sci Sports Exerc* 19:540-543, 1987.

Recommendation quantity and quality of exercise for developing and maintaining cardiorespiratory and muscular fitness in healthy adults, *Med Sci Sports Exerc* 22:265-274, 1990.

The use of anabolic-androgenic steroids in sports, *Med Sci Sports Exerc* 19(5):534-539, 1987.

CLINICAL NUTRITION
IN DISEASE
PREVENTION

Part V

Chapter 22

NUTRITION GUIDELINES FOR DIET AND HEALTH

Susan M. Kleiner

Since the dawn of humanity, one of the most pressing problems has been satisfying hunger. Whatever was available and edible was eaten, regardless of nutritive value. As we extended horizons beyond familiar lands, familiar foods became scarce, and diets adapted to the changing environments.

Even though the nutritional value of foods was not always a consideration, certain foods have always been more desirable than others because of taste, odor, and texture, giving a sense of satisfaction when eaten. Depending on the local climate, geographic location, soil productivity, vegetation, and fauna, diets in different parts of the world became dramatically different. As late as the year 1900, physiologists assumed that food had little to do with health, because despite a great dietary diversity, health standards worldwide were similar.[9]

Because all humans had to eat, the scientific study of nutrition began early in human history. Questions about food, its contents, and its chemistry are ancient. Investigations by the people of the island of Chios into the uses of starch as both a food and an adhesive were reported by Pliny in the first century AD.[9]

By the first half of the twentieth century, the classical science of human nutrition was advancing rapidly. Scientists had unraveled the major questions concerning the energy-yielding nutrients: protein, fat, and carbohydrate. By 1940, with the exception of folic acid and vitamin B_{12}, all the known essential nutrients, amino acids, vitamins, fatty acids, carbohydrates, and inorganic elements had been identified, isolated, and characterized chemically, and their pathological roles in human deficiency diseases were being illustrated.

In 1943, Recommended Dietary Allowances (RDAs) were published for the first time by the Food and Nutrition Board of the National Academy of Sciences. The first edition was published to provide "standards to serve as a goal for good nutrition" and reflected the best scientific judgment of the time.[17] This judgment was based on the understanding of population needs and the prevention of deficiency diseases.

As the prevalence of nutritional deficiency diminished in the United States, diseases of nutritional excess and dietary imbalance came to the fore. At the end of World War II, nutrition research shifted focus from the role of diet in deficiency diseases to the role of diet in chronic diseases, such as coronary heart disease and cancer.[17] According to the National Center for Health Statistics, of the 10 leading causes of death in 1987, five—coronary heart disease and generalized atherosclerosis, stroke, some types of cancer, and diabetes—have been associated with dietary excesses or imbalances, and another three—cirrhosis of the liver, accidents, and suicides—are often the result of excessive alcohol intake. Together, these eight conditions account for as much as 70% of all U.S. deaths each year (Table 22-1).[25]

Dietary and nutrition advice can no longer be based solely on the prevention of the classical deficiency diseases. Laboratory and epidemiologic studies have given clear support for the link between diet and chronic disease, and several reports have been issued addressing the public health importance of dietary risk factors in chronic disease prevention. In addition to the influence that dietary risk factors pose on single chronic diseases, the complex role that these risk factors play in the entire spectrum of chronic diseases—atherosclerotic cardiovascular diseases, cancer, diabetes, obesity, osteoporosis, dental caries, and chronic liver and kidney diseases—may be greater than we yet realize.

Table 22-1. Estimated total deaths and percentage of total deaths for the 10 leading causes of death: United States, 1987

Rank	Cause of death	Number	Percent of total deaths
1*	Heart diseases	759,400	35.7
	(Coronary heart disease)	(511,700)	(24.1)
	(Other heart disease)	(247,700)	(11.6)
2*	Cancers	476,700	22.4
3*	Strokes	148,700	7.0
4**	Unintentional injuries	92,500	4.4
	(Motor vehicle)	(46,800)	(2.2)
	(All others)	(45,700)	(2.2)
5	Chronic obstructive lung diseases	78,000	3.7
6	Pneumonia and influenza	68,600	3.2
7*	Diabetes mellitus	37,800	1.8
8**	Suicide	29,600	1.4
9**	Chronic liver disease and cirrhosis	26,000	1.2
10*	Atherosclerosis	23,100	1.1
. . .	All causes	2,125,100	100.0

From National Center for Health Statistics 1988, USDHHS publication 88-50210, Washington, DC, 1988.
*Causes of death in which diet plays a part.
**Causes of death in which excessive alcohol consumption plays a part.

THE NUTRIENTS

The fundamental principles of human nutrition remain the same regardless of race, sex, or age. Carbohydrate, protein, fat, vitamins, minerals, and water are the six classes of nutrients found in foods. Nutrients are substances the body uses for the growth, maintenance, and repair of tissues. *Essential* nutrients are those that the body cannot manufacture in sufficient amounts to meet its needs, and so must be obtained from the diet.

The macromolecules carbohydrate, protein, and fat are the only energy-yielding or calorie-containing nutrients. When completely metabolized, a gram of carbohydrate provides approximately 4 calories, a gram of protein also provides approximately 4 calories, and a gram of fat provides approximately 9 calories. Alcohol, considered a drug rather than a nutrient because it does not support growth, is also energy-yielding, providing 7 calories per gram. The energy content of food therefore depends on the total amount of protein, carbohydrate, and fat it contains.[26] (Fat calories may actually yield more than 9 calories per gram. This will be discussed further in the section on obesity.)

Most foods are a mixture of the energy-yielding nutrients, although one nutrient may predominate over the other two. For instance, even though bread is popularly considered a carbohydrate food, and meat a protein food, both of these are actually mixtures of all three major nutrients. Bread is rich in carbohydrates but also contains some protein and traces of fat. Meats are protein-rich, but are also sources of fat.

Vitamins are fundamentally different from the macromolecular energy-yielding nutrients (see box). Vitamin molecules are much smaller in size and are required by the body in minute amounts compared with the body's re-

---

The 13 vitamins

Water-soluble vitamins	Fat-soluble vitamins
B vitamins	Vitamin A
Thiamin	Vitamin D
Riboflavin	Vitamin E
Niacin	Vitamin K
Vitamin B_6	
Vitamin B_{12}	
Folate	
Biotin	
Pantothenic acid	
Vitamin C	

---

quirements for protein, carbohydrate, and fat. By definition, vitamins are essential organic nutrients required by the body in small amounts. Vitamins may catalyze energy-yielding reactions, but vitamins alone do not yield energy.[26]

There are 13 different vitamins, separated into two classes: water-soluble (B vitamins and vitamin C) and fat-soluble (vitamins A, D, E, and K). Because of their organic nature, vitamins are destructible. Food handling and preparation techniques designed to reduce vitamin losses are important to preserve the nutritional quality of foods.

Minerals are small inorganic atoms or molecules, and only some of them are essential nutrients, required in small amounts (see box). Like vitamins, minerals do not yield energy, although some may be essential for energy production. Unlike vitamins, minerals are indestructible because of their elemental nature. Food handling and processing cannot destroy the mineral content of foods.

```
┌─────────────────────────────────────────────────┐
│  Minerals                                        │
│                                                  │
│  Major minerals              Trace minerals      │
│  Calcium                     Iron                 │
│  Phosphorus                  Iodine               │
│  Potassium                   Zinc                 │
│  Sodium                      Chromium             │
│  Chloride                    Selenium             │
│  Magnesium                   Flouride             │
│                              Molybdenum           │
│                              Copper               │
│                              Manganese            │
└─────────────────────────────────────────────────┘
```

Many minerals are nutrients, but all minerals are not essential nutrients. The functions of many of the minerals are still under investigation, and their roles in human physiology and metabolism are yet to be determined. The essential minerals are grouped into two classes based on the amount of the mineral found in the human body, and hence the amounts required in the diet. Therefore the major minerals are found in the greatest concentrations and are required in the greatest amounts, and the trace minerals are found in the smallest concentrations and are required in smaller amounts.[26]

Water is essential, and is the most important nutrient. We can live for weeks without food, but we can only live a few days without water. It provides a medium for almost all of the body's biochemical reactions, as well as participating in many metabolic reactions. Water provides for the transport of nutrients to cells and waste away from cells, and it is a major part of almost every body tissue.[26]

NUTRIENT RECOMMENDATIONS

A nutrient *requirement* is the amount of nutrient used or required by the body to maintain growth and health, and prevent signs or symptoms of deficiency disease. A nutrient *recommendation* is an estimation of the amount of a nutrient that should be present in the diet based on factors such as food preference and availability, destruction of nutrients caused by food handling and preparation, nutrient bioavailability, and caloric content of the diet. Nutrient recommendations therefore have many margins of safety built in and are always greater than nutrient requirements.

Many countries and world organizations have developed nutrient recommendations. In the United States, the Recommended Dietary Allowances, or RDAs, were first published by the National Research Council in 1943, during World War II. The RDAs were to serve as a guide for advising the military on nutrition problems related to national defense. Since then, the RDAs have come to serve many other purposes. They are frequently used for planning and evaluating food programs and menus for subgroups and populations, for establishing safe and adequate

nutrition standards for food assistance programs, for designing nutrition education programs, and for developing new products in industry.

The RDAs are based on population statistics and therefore were never intended to be used to evaluate individual diets. However, for lack of a better tool, the RDAs are presently used as a standard of comparison for individual food intakes averaged over a minimum of 3 days.[15]

The Recommended Dietary Allowances (RDAs) should not be confused with the U.S. Recommended Daily Allowances (USRDAs). The USRDAs were derived from the 1968 RDAs (seventh edition), to be used by the Food and Drug Administration (FDA) as standards for nutritional labeling, and they have never been updated.

Since 1943, the RDAs have been revised at regular intervals, and the tenth edition of the RDAs was published in 1989, 9 years after the ninth edition. The RDAs are a scientific consensus of recommended levels of essential nutrients needed by the majority of healthy Americans (97.5%) to achieve adequate nutritional status. Formulating this consensus is an extremely difficult task, and the latest edition was delayed 4 years as nutrition experts disagreed about the specific dietary recommendations for healthy Americans. Experts disagree because limited experimental data are available on which to base recommendations concerning nutritional requirements. Additional factors such as age, genetic make-up, diet history, and physiological/medical conditions also affect the nutritional requirements of individuals and can further confound the process of determining minimum and optimum recommendations.[15]

In addition to the 19 nutrients for which RDAs have been set, the RDA committee has set ranges of "Estimated Safe and Adequate Daily Dietary Intakes" for selected vitamins and minerals. These nutrients lack a sufficient quantity of research data on which to base absolute recommendations but are recognized as essential nutrients in the diet. Therefore the committee has provided ranges of recommended intakes.[15]

The tenth edition of the RDAs underwent some modest revisions, reflecting advances in scientific knowledge in the past 9 years or new interpretations of data by the scientific committee. The two most significant changes are a revision of the age groupings and the height and weight values for reference adults in each age-sex class. The age group of 19 to 22 years has been extended through age 24 for both sexes based on the estimated age of 25 years for the attainment of peak bone mass. The reference heights and weights now represent the actual median values for the U.S. population by age, based on data collected in the second National Health and Nutrition Examination Survey (NHANES II) instead of arbitrary ideal values used in previous editions (Tables 22-2 and 22-3).[14]

Many experts agree that the RDAs in their present format are incomplete. They do not reflect optimal levels of

Table 22-2. Food and nutrition board, National Academy of Sciences, National Research Council Recommended Dietary Allowances,* Revised 1989

Designed for the maintenance of good nutrition of practically all healthy people in the United States

Category	Age (years) or condition	Weight† (kg)	Weight† (lb)	Height† (cm)	Height† (in)	Protein (g)	Fat-soluble vitamins Vitamin A (µg RE)‡	Vitamin D (µg)§	Vitamin E (mg α-TE)‖	Vitamin K (µg)
Infants	0.0-0.5	6	13	60	24	13	375	7.5	3	5
	0.5-1.0	9	20	71	28	14	375	10	4	10
Children	1-3	13	29	90	35	16	400	10	6	15
	4-6	20	44	112	44	24	500	10	7	20
	7-10	28	62	132	52	28	700	10	7	30
Males	11-14	45	99	157	62	45	1000	10	10	45
	15-18	66	145	176	69	59	1000	10	10	65
	19-24	72	160	177	70	58	1000	10	10	70
	25-50	79	174	176	70	63	1000	5	10	80
	51+	77	170	173	68	63	1000	5	10	80
Females	11-14	46	101	157	62	46	800	10	8	45
	15-18	55	120	163	64	44	800	10	8	55
	19-24	58	128	164	65	46	800	10	8	60
	25-50	63	138	163	64	50	800	5	8	65
	51+	65	143	160	63	50	800	5	8	65
Pregnant						60	800	10	10	65
Lactating	1st 6 months					65	1300	10	12	65
	2nd 6 months					62	1200	10	11	65

From NAS/NRC Subcommittee on the 10th edition of the RDAs, Washington, DC, 1989, National Academy Press.

*The allowances, expressed as average daily intakes over time, are intended to provide for individual variations among most normal persons as they live in the United States under usual environmental stresses. Diets should be based on a variety of common foods to provide other nutrients for which human requirements have been less well defined. See text for detailed discussion of allowances and of nutrients not tabulated.

†Weights and heights of reference adults are actual medians for the U.S. population of the designated age, as reported by NHANES II. The median weights and heights of those under 19 years of age were taken from Hamill et al. (1979). The use of these figures does not imply that the height-to-weight ratios are ideal.

‡Retinol equivalents. 1 retinol equivalent = 1 µg retinol or 6 µg β-carotene. See text for calculation of vitamin A activity of diets as retinol equivalents.

§As cholecalciferol. 10 µg cholecalciferol = 400 IU of vitamin D.

‖α-Tocopherol equivalents. 1 mg d-α tocopherol = 1 α-TE. See text for variation in allowances and calculation of vitamin E activity of the diet as α-tocopherol equivalents.

¶1 NE (niacin equivalent) is equal to 1 mg of niacin or 60 mg of dietary tryptophan.

dietary intake. Rather, the RDAs are safe and adequate levels with margins of safety built into the recommendations to account for biological variability with the population. Key questions regarding the dietary needs of the elderly, and recommendations for intakes of nutrients such as vitamins A, E, and C, and fiber, linked with the prevention of chronic diseases, are not addressed by the RDAs. According to the RDA committee, much more research will be needed to establish such recommendations.[15]

Since the data on many of the minerals and vitamins now support dosages above the RDA for the treatment and prevention of certain diseases, it has become especially critical to be aware of the toxic potentials of these nutrients. When vitamins and minerals are consumed in pharmacologic doses rather than nutritional doses, they may act more like drugs than nutrients. The minimum toxic doses and safety indices for vitamins and minerals with RDA values are listed in Tables 22-4 and 22-5.

FUNCTIONS OF THE NUTRIENTS
Carbohydrates: Sugar, Starch, and Fiber

The nutrient class of carbohydrates is divided into two subclasses: simple carbohydrates and complex carbohydrates. The simple carbohydrates are all monosaccharide and disaccharide sugars. Complex carbohydrates are polysaccharides called starch, and some fibers.

The most familiar simple carbohydrate is the disaccharide sucrose, or table sugar. Other simple carbohydrates are the monosaccharides glucose, fructose (fruit sugar), and galactose (found only as part of lactose), and the disaccharides lactose (milk sugar) and maltose.[26]

As a carbohydrate, sugars yield 4 calories per gram. Other than providing energy, sugars add sweetness to foods, making them more appetizing. The major detrimental health effect from moderate sugar consumption is tooth decay. If dental hygiene is properly maintained, this

	Water-soluble vitamins						Minerals						
Vitamin C (mg)	Thiamin (mg)	Riboflavin (mg)	Niacin (mg NE)¶	Vitamin B$_6$ (mg)	Folate (µg)	Vitamin B$_{12}$ (µg)	Calcium (mg)	Phosphorus (mg)	Magnesium (mg)	Iron (mg)	Zinc (mg)	Iodine (µg)	Selenium (µg)
30	0.3	0.4	5	0.3	25	0.3	400	300	40	6	5	40	10
35	0.4	0.5	6	0.6	35	0.5	600	500	60	10	5	50	15
40	0.7	0.8	9	1.0	50	0.7	800	800	80	10	10	70	20
45	0.9	1.1	12	1.1	75	1.0	800	800	120	10	10	90	20
45	1.0	1.2	13	1.4	100	1.4	800	800	170	10	10	120	30
50	1.3	1.5	17	1.7	150	2.0	1200	1200	270	12	15	150	40
60	1.5	1.8	20	2.0	200	2.0	1200	1200	400	12	15	150	50
60	1.5	1.7	19	2.0	200	2.0	1200	1200	350	10	15	150	70
60	1.5	1.7	19	2.0	200	2.0	800	800	350	10	15	150	70
60	1.2	1.4	15	2.0	200	2.0	800	800	350	10	15	150	70
50	1.1	1.3	15	1.4	150	2.0	1200	1200	280	15	12	150	45
60	1.1	1.3	15	1.5	180	2.0	1200	1200	300	15	12	150	50
60	1.1	1.3	15	1.6	180	2.0	1200	1200	280	15	12	150	55
60	1.1	1.3	15	1.6	180	2.0	800	800	280	15	12	150	55
60	1.0	1.2	13	1.6	180	2.0	800	800	280	10	12	150	55
70	1.5	1.6	17	2.2	400	2.2	1200	1200	320	30	15	175	65
95	1.6	1.8	20	2.1	280	2.6	1200	1200	355	15	19	200	75
90	1.6	1.7	20	2.1	260	2.6	1200	1200	340	15	16	200	75

Table 22-3. Estimated safe and adequate daily dietary intakes of selected vitamins and minerals*

		Vitamins	
Category	Age (years)	Biotin (µg)	Pantothenic acid (mg)
Infants	0-0.5	10	2
	0.5-1	15	3
Children and adolescents	1-3	20	3
	4-6	25	3-4
	7-10	30	4-5
	11+	30-100	4-7
Adults		30-100	4-7

		Trace elements†				
Category	Age (years)	Copper (mg)	Manganese (mg)	Fluoride (mg)	Chromium (µg)	Molybdenum (µg)
Infants	0-0.5	0.4-0.6	0.3-0.6	0.1-0.5	10-40	15-30
	0.5-1	0.6-0.7	0.6-1.0	0.2-1.0	20-60	20-40
Children and adolescents	1-3	0.7-1.0	1.0-1.5	0.5-1.5	20-80	25-50
	4-6	1.0-1.5	1.5-2.0	1.0-2.5	30-120	30-75
	7-10	1.0-2.0	2.0-3.0	1.5-2.5	50-200	50-150
	11+	1.5-2.5	2.0-5.0	1.5-2.5	50-200	75-250
Adults		1.5-3.0	2.0-5.0	1.5-4.0	50-200	75-250

*Because there is less information on which to base allowances, these figures are not given in the main table of RDA and are provided here in the form of ranges of recommended intakes.

†Because the toxic levels for many trace elements may be only several times usual intakes, the upper levels for the trace elements given in this table should not be habitually exceeded.

From NAS/NRC Subcommittee on the tenth edition of the RDAs, Washington, DC, 1989, National Academy Press.

should represent little problem. Naturally sweet foods, such as fruits and fruit juices, are excellent sources of essential vitamins and minerals, are generally low in calories, and are high in fiber (especially whole fruits). However, if sugar is eaten in excess, such as in foods cooked, baked, or prepared with added sugar, it may cause detrimental health effects.

When consumed in excess, sugar may add too many calories to a diet, leading to obesity, and the possible chronic diseases for which obesity is a risk factor. Sweetened foods are also often high in fat, adding even more calories to the diet. Additionally, foods high in sugar are generally low in other nutrients such as vitamins and minerals. These "empty-calorie" foods in the diet can easily replace lower calorie but more nutrient-dense foods, such as fruits and vegetables. If this is a frequent dietary pattern, it can result in nutrient insufficiencies, or even nutrient deficiencies.

Complex carbohydrates, or starches, are highly recommended for a healthy diet. Also yielding 4 calories per gram, starchy foods are generally nutrient-dense, containing many vitamins, minerals, and fiber, in addition to carbohydrate. Diets high in complex carbohydrates are usually lower in fat, sugar, and calories, more nutrient dense, and higher in fiber. As will be discussed in further chapters, these results are exactly the recommendations by many health professionals and organizations for the dietary promotion of health and prevention of disease.

For protein to be utilized for its unique functions, adequate carbohydrate (and fat) must be available in the diet. This is referred to as the protein-sparing effect of carbohydrate. If consumption of carbohydrate and fat is inadequate to meet the body's caloric requirements, nitrogen will be stripped from protein molecules and excreted to use protein as energy. The protein then becomes unavailable as a source of nitrogen and amino acids.[26]

Table 22-4. Mineral safety index*

Mineral	Recommended adult intake†	Minimum toxic dose	Mineral safety index
Calcium	1200 mg	12,000 mg	10
Phosphorus	1200 mg	12,000 mg	10
Magnesium	400 mg	6000 mg	15
Iron	18 mg	100 mg	5.5
Zinc	15 mg	500 mg	33
Copper	3 mg	100 mg	33
		<3 mg‡	<1
Fluoride	4 mg	20 mg	5
		4 mg§	1
Iodine	0.15 μg	2 mg	13
Selenium	0.2 μg	1 mg	5

*From Hathcock JN: Quantitative evaluation of vitamin safety, *Pharm Times,* May, 1985.
†The RDA (except those for pregnancy and lactation) or the U.S. recommended daily allowance, whichever is higher.
‡For people with Wilson's disease.
§Level producing slight fluorosis of dental enamel.

Table 22-5. Vitamin safety index*

Vitamin	Recommended adult intake†	Minimum toxic dose	Vitamin safety index
Vitamin A	5000 IU	25,000 to 50,000 IU	5 to 10
Vitamin D	400 IU	50,000 IU	125
		1000 to 2000 IU‡	2.5 to 5
Vitamin E	30 IU	1200 IU	40
Vitamin C	60 mg	2000 to 5000 mg	33 to 83
		1000 mg§	17
Thiamin (B₁)	1.5 mg	300 mg	200
Riboflavin	1.7 mg	1000 mg	588
Niacin	20 mg	1000 mg	50
Pyridoxine (B₆)	2.2 mg	2000 mg	900
		200 mg‖	90
Folacin	0.4 mg	400 mg	1000
		15 mg¶	37
Biotin	0.3 mg	50 mg	167
Pantothenic acid	10 mg	10,000 mg	1000

*Adapted from Hathcock JN: Quantitative evaluation of vitamin safety, *Pharm Times,* May, 1985.
†The individual RDA (except those for pregnancy and lactation) or the U.S. recommended daily allowance, whichever is higher.
‡For infants and also for adults with certain infections or metabolic diseases; 50,000 IU for most adults.
§To produce slightly altered mineral excretion patterns.
‖For antagonism of some drugs; 2000 mg for most adults.
¶For antagonism of anticonvulsants in epileptics; 400 mg for most adults.

Foods high in starch include all kinds of breads, cereals, grains, noodles and pastas, dried beans and peas, potatoes, yams, corn, and peas.

Fiber is a general term for the relatively indigestible polysaccharides cellulose, hemicellulose, pectins, gums, and mucilages, as well as the nonpolysaccharide lignins, all found in plant products. The term *dietary fiber* represents the residue of plant food resistant to hydrolysis by human digestive enzymes.

The classifications for fiber are based primarily on their solubility in water. Water-insoluble fibers include lignin, cellulose, and the hemicelluloses. These fibers have been shown to accelerate intestinal transit and fecal weight, slow starch hydrolysis, and delay glucose absorption. Water-soluble fibers, including pectin and gums, delay intestinal transit, gastric emptying, and glucose absorption and decrease serum cholesterol concentration.[5]

Food sources of water-insoluble fibers include vegetables, wheat, and grains. Sources of water-soluble fibers include fruits, oats, barley, legumes, and psyllium.

Protein

Amino acids are the building blocks of proteins. There are 20 amino acids, but 9 are essential amino acids that must be consumed in the diet, along with enough nitrogen for synthesis of the other 11 amino acids, to support total protein synthesis (see box). All essential amino acids must be present in their required amounts to promote protein synthesis. If there is less of one amino acid than is necessary, fewer complete proteins will be manufactured. The body does not build partial proteins. The unavailable amino acid that limits protein production is called the *limiting amino acid*.[26]

Protein quality of food is determined by the array and amounts of essential amino acids present. A poor-quality or incomplete protein contains an imbalance of amino acids and causes protein production inefficiency in the body. The limiting amino acid in the food protein will cause the body to waste other amino acids during protein produc-

tion, because they cannot be utilized to make complete proteins without the correct amount of the limiting amino acid, and they cannot be stored.

A complete protein contains all the amino acids essential in human nutrition in amounts adequate for human use. A high-quality protein is an easily digestible complete protein. Egg protein has been determined by the Food and Agriculture Organization/World Health Organization (FAO/WHO) to be the highest quality protein and is used as a standard against which to measure the quality of other proteins. According to this standard of biological value, the quality of egg protein equals 100, followed by fish, beef, milk, rice, and corn, in order of biological value.[26]

Generally, protein derived from animal foods (beef, poultry, fish, pork, milk, eggs) is complete protein, and protein derived from plant foods (vegetables, grains, legumes) is incomplete. There are exceptions to this rule. Gelatin is an incomplete protein, and rice and potatoes are complete proteins, although the total amount of protein available per serving from rice or potatoes is small. Incomplete, poor-quality protein foods can be eaten together to complement the missing amino acids in each food, or a small amount of complete protein eaten with an incomplete source, thereby forming complete proteins.

In parts of the world where animal products are scarce, this has been a practice of good nutrition for centuries. In China, rice is eaten at virtually every meal. This complete protein is often eaten with tofu (soybean curd), an incomplete protein, forming a complementary, higher-biological-value, complete protein meal. In Mexico, corn tortillas are combined with beans and a little cheese or meat to create complete proteins.

Fats

Fatty acids are divided by structure into three categories, referring to their level of carbon bond saturation. Those chains with all carbon atoms bound to hydrogen atoms, and therefore all single C-C bonds, are said to be saturated. If the fatty acid chain contains one double bond, the fat is monounsaturated, and if there are two or more double bonds, the fat is polyunsaturated.

Saturated fats are the building blocks of serum cholesterol, and are known to be the major dietary source of increased serum cholesterol, a risk factor for cardiovascular disease (see Chapter 24). Saturated fats in food can be identified visibly because they are solid when refrigerated and remain semisolid at room temperature. They are found predominantly in animal foods, such as meats, lard, butter, and whole milk dairy products. They are also a major part of the fat in cocoa butter, coconut, and the tropical oils—palm, palm kernel, and coconut. Saturated fats should be limited in the diet.

Hydrogenated fats are vegetable oils (unsaturated) that have been processed to add hydrogens back to the fatty acid chains, thereby saturating them. Hydrogenated fats

Amino acids	
Essential	**Nonessential**
Histidine	Alanine
Isoleucine	Arginine
Leucine	Asparagine
Lysine	Aspartic acid
Methionine	Cysteine
Phenylalanine	Glutamic acid
Threonine	Glutamine
Tryptophan	Glycine
Valine	Proline
	Serine
	Tyrosine

are less prone to oxidation than vegetable oils and have the physical properties of animal fats. Hydrogenated fats are found in shortenings and margarines, and are commonly part of the manufacturers' recipes for crackers and baked goods, to help make products flaky and crispy and to extend shelf life. Hydrogenated fats should be limited in the diet.

At one time, monounsaturated fats were considered neutral in the diet. However, several population studies and laboratory investigations have demonstrated that monounsaturated fats in the diet are associated with decreased risk of cardiovascular disease. These fats are found predominantly in peanut oil, olive oil, and canola oil, and should be the major fat component in a health-promoting diet.

Within the category of polyunsaturated fatty acids, two families that differ structurally have been recognized as very important to health. The first, omega-6 fatty acids, have their endmost double bond six carbons from the methyl end of the chain. Humans cannot manufacture this fatty acid structure and so it must be consumed in the diet. Linoleic acid (18:2) is an essential omega-6 fatty acid, and it is found widely in vegetable oils and meats.

The second family of polyunsaturates important to health are the omega-3 fatty acids. Omega-3 fatty acids have their endmost double bond three carbons away from the methyl end of the chain. This polyunsaturate also cannot be manufactured in the human body to maintain health. Until recently, linolenic acid (18:3) was considered the only essential omega-3 fatty acid. Two other omega-3 fatty acids are now considered virtually essential: eicosapentaenoic acid (EPA; 20:5) and docosahexaenoic acid (DHA; 22:6). The chief jobs of these two fatty acids are maintenance of the retina and the cerebral cortex, and assistance in the prevention of atherosclerosis and cerebral stroke[26] (see Chapter 24.)

If linolenic acid is consumed in the diet, the body can manufacture EPA and DHA, but at a very slow rate. Because of the recent recognition of their importance in health, these two fatty acids are recommended for inclusion in the diet. The best dietary sources of linolenic acid are leafy vegetables and vegetable oils. The best sources of EPA and DHA are fish, especially cold water, fatty fish like salmon and mackerel, and seafoods.

The Water-soluble vitamins

Thiamin. The beginning of the new age in vitamin research began in Japan in 1887, when Takaki demonstrated that diet was an effective treatment for the disease beri-beri. By 1896, research by Eijkman and Grijns associated the feeding of polished rice with the production of symptoms of polyneuritis in pigeons and identified the properties of the dietary factor that cured these symptoms. In 1911, Funk produced a concentrated form of active anti-beri-beri factor (later identified as thiamin and niacin),

and called it "vitamine." In 1937, three different laboratories isolated the vitamin once known only as B_1 and now known as thiamin.

Thiamin pyrophosphate (TPP) is the coenzyme that plays a pivotal role in the enzyme-catalyzed reactions of carbohydrate metabolism. Involved in the decarboxylation of alpha-keto acids, it assists the decarboxylation of pyruvate to acetaldehyde and the oxidation of alpha-ketoglutarate to succinyl-CoA. TPP is essential to the formation or degradation of alpha-ketols.

In addition to its function in carbohydrate metabolism and biosynthesis of essential compounds that affect nervous system composition, thiamin appears to have a less well understood role in neurophysiology. TPP has been identified in the axonal membranes of nerves, and enzymes involved in its formation and cleavage are in nervous tissue. A subacute necrotizing encephalomyelopathy in patients with Leigh's syndrome results from the presence of an inhibitor of TPP-ATP phosphoryl transferase.[13]

Beri-beri is the disease resulting from thiamin deficiency in humans. Clinical signs involve the nervous and cardiovascular systems. In adults, symptoms observed are mental confusion, anorexia, muscle weakness, ataxia, peripheral paralysis, ophthalmoplegia, edema, muscle wasting, tachycardia, and an enlarged heart. In infants, symptoms appear rapidly and may be severe. Nervous system involvement includes peripheral neuropathy, Wernicke's encephalopathy, and the amnesic psychosis of Korsakoff syndrome.[26]

An excess of water-soluble vitamin generally results in the excretion of the excess as waste from the body. However, in almost every instance of these vitamins, there is an exception to this rule. Parenteral doses of thiamin greater than 400 mg cause nausea, anorexia, lethargy, solemness, mild ataxia, heaviness in the limbs, and a diminution of gut tone.

Thiamin deficiency was most commonly observed in the Far East, where milled, nonenriched rice was the mainstay of the diet. In Japan, where white rice was eaten with raw fish, the microbial thiaminases contained in the raw fish assisted with the hydrolysis of whatever thiamin was available in the meal, and rendered it biologically inactive. Tea may also contain some antithiamin factors. All of these practices placed the populations of this region at high risk for thiamin deficiency.

Chronic alcoholism is a common cause of thiamin deficiency for several reasons. The diet of an alcoholic may be nutritionally poor, placing the alcoholic at general nutritional risk. Second, alcohol impairs thiamin absorption and storage. It is critical that such patients be examined for the presence of thiamin and all B-vitamin deficiencies.

Thiamin requirements are linked with carbohydrate ingestion and are therefore highly variable. Other influencing factors include high levels of physical activity, pregnancy, lactation, fever, and hyperthyroidism. Therefore, the recommended dietary allowance (RDA) for thiamin is based on a ratio with calorie intake, at 0.5 mg/1000 calories, with a minimum intake of 1 g per day, for healthy adults.[15]

Individuals on low-calorie diets (less than 2000 calories/day) should ingest at least 1 g of thiamin per day. Individuals consuming higher calorie diets need to increase their thiamin intakes. Generally, as calorie intake increases, nutrient intake increases as well, so that there is no need to supplement the diet. However, if 1000 calories or more within the diet consistently come from nutrient-poor foods (e.g., sweets, fried foods), thiamin may be insufficient in the diet. Instead of supplementing the diet with thiamin, the patient should be counseled on methods to improve the nutrient density of the diet.

The food sources most abundant in thiamin include unrefined and enriched cereal grains, liver, heart, kidney, and lean cuts of pork.

Riboflavin. Riboflavin was identified and synthesized in 1935, and its coenzyme form, flavin adenine dinucleotide (FAD), was defined in 1954. From 70% to 90% of riboflavin in tissue is as FAD and flavin mononucleotide (FMN). In addition to its function as flavin nucleotides (FAD and FMN), riboflavin serves as prosthetic groups of flavoproteins, serves in the oxidative degradation of pyruvate, fatty acids, and amino acids, and functions in electron transport during hydrogen atom transfer.[12]

Pure riboflavin deficiency is virtually never observed in patients. More commonly, ariboflavinosis presents as part of multiple nutrient deficiencies. Primary riboflavin deficiency from an inadequate diet usually occurs as part of limited access to food or enforced food deprivation. Milk is an excellent source of riboflavin, and individuals with lactose intolerance may avoid milk, resulting in a diet that is insufficient in riboflavin as well as calcium.

Secondary riboflavin deficiency may occur from poor absorption in the small bowel, defective utilization from hormone imbalances, increased destruction from phototherapy for neonatal jaundice or from long-time use of barbiturates, and increased excretion in catabolic patients undergoing nitrogen loss or use of certain antibiotics and phenothiazine drugs. All of these conditions mandate an increased vitamin requirement.[12]

The RDA for riboflavin is also derived from an energy-intake ratio and is set at 0.6 mg/1000 kcal, with a daily minimum recommendation of 1.2 mg for healthy adults. Growth, pregnancy, lactation, and illness stimulate the utilization of riboflavin and thus increase daily requirements.[15] Good food sources of riboflavin include eggs, lean meats, milk, broccoli, and enriched breads and cereals.

Niacin. Unique among the investigations of the vitamins, knowledge of the bichemical function of niacin preceded the discovery of its nutritional significance. The vitamin niacin exists in two forms: nicotinic acid and nicoti-

namide. Nicotinic acid was first prepared chemically in 1867. In 1934, nicotinamide was isolated by Warburg and Christian from the coenzyme triphosphopyridine nucleotide (TPN), now known as nicotinamide adenine dinucleotide phosphate (NADP). In 1935, nicotinamide was also isolated by Von Euler from a conenzyme now known as nicotinamide adenine dinucleotide (NAD). Not until 1937 did Elvejhem demonstrate that nicotinic acid cures black tongue disease in dogs. This disease was observed to parallel the disease of pellagra in humans, and the correlation of human pellagra with deficiency of nicotinic acid quickly followed.[11]

Nicotinamide is the active form of the vitamin. The body can easily convert nicotinic acid to nicotinamide. Humans also have the ability to metabolize the amino acid tryptophan to an altered form of the vitamin, nicotic acid mononucleotide, which is a common intermediate in the conversion process of nicotinic acid to its coenzymes. Because of the tryptophan-niacin relation, units of available niacin are stated as niacin-tryptophan equivalents. The nicotinamide equivalents (NE) relationship is 60 mg tryptophan equals 1 mg niacin.[11]

The NAD and NADP-containing coenzymes are pyridine-linked dehydrogenases involved in oxidation-reduction reactions and in electron transfer, especially in the metabolism of glucose, fat, and alcohol. There are more than 200 of these enzymes. Nicotinamide is also an essential part of the tetra-aqua-di-nicotinato-chromium complex, or the glucose tolerance factor, known to be a critical element of glucose tolerance.[26]

The name for niacin deficiency disease, pellagra, originated in Italy, and means "rough skin." It has been associated with cultures that subsist chiefly on corn as the staple of their diet.[11] The typical symptoms of pellagra present as a combination of dermatitis, dementia, and diarrhea. The dermatitis is bilateral and symmetrical, and is found especially on skin exposed to the sun. Patients often have a painful flush and rash, itching, burning, and excessive sweating. Mental changes include fatigue, insomnia, and apathy, which may proceed into an encephalopathy characterized by confusion, disorientation, hallucination, loss of memory, and eventually frank organic psychoses. The mucosal lining of the gut may experience widespread inflammation, and this may be accompanied by vomiting and dysphagia. The oral cavity may show glossitis and stomatitis.[11]

Pharmacologic doses of nicotinic acid (10 times the RDA or more) have been used for the treatment of Hartnup disease, carcinoid syndrome, and atherosclerosis (see Chapter 24). Close supervision of patients is required because excesses of nicotinic acid (but not the amide) produce vascular dilation or flushing accompanied by a sensation of burning or stinging in the face and hands. Pruritus, nausea, vomiting, and diarrhea have been reported at the outset of therapy but often abate with continued treatment.

Additional negative side effects include abnormal glucose tolerance, hyperuricemia, peptic ulcer, hepatomegaly, jaundice, and increased serum transaminases. High chronic doses of nicotinic acid appear hepatotoxic.[11]

The recommended dietary allowance for niacin is based on energy metabolism and average tryptophan consumption. An RDA of 6.6 NE/1000 kcal and not less than 13 NE at caloric intakes of less than 2000 calories is recommended for all healthy adults. The RDA for niacin is adjusted for infants, children, and women during pregnancy and lactation.[15]

The best food sources of niacin are yeast, lean meats, liver, and poultry. Milk, canned salmon, and several leafy green vegetables contribute lesser, but considerable, amounts. Protein contributes a significant amount of niacin equivalents because of the tryptophan content.

Vitamin B_6. Vitamin B_6 is a family of compounds containing three forms: pyridoxine, pyridoxal, and pyridoxamine. Its coenzyme forms are pyridoxal phosphate (PLP) and pyridoxamine phosphate (PMP). All three forms of the vitamin can be converted to PLP. Even though vitamin B_6 was isolated and synthesized in 1938-1939, not until 1950 was a deficiency in humans demonstrated by antagonist induction.

Vitamin B_6 is intimately related to amino acid metabolism. PLP and PMP serve primarily as coenzymes in transamination reactions. PLP is also part of decarboxylation and racemization of α-amino acids, in other metabolic transformations of amino acids, and in the metabolism of lipids and nucleic acids. Glycogen phosphorylase depends on PLP as its essential coenzyme.

Similar to riboflavin, vitamin B_6 deficiency rarely occurs alone and is most commonly observed in people with limited diets and multiple B-vitamin deficiencies. Vague symptoms of vitamin B_6 deficiency are weakness, irritability, and insomnia. In frank vitamin B_6 deficiency, more clearly defined symptoms of growth failure, impaired motor function, and convulsions are observed.[14]

In addition to a vitamin-deficient diet as the cause of deficiency symptoms, several drugs are vitamin B_6 antagonists. Alcohol is the most commonly used vitamin B_6 antagonist. During alcohol metabolism, the production of acetaldehyde destroys PLP, and PLP is excreted. Isoniazid, an inhibitor of the growth of the tuberculosis bacterium, binds and inactivates vitamin B_6, as does penicillamine, used in the treatment of Wilson's disease.[26]

Symptoms of vitamin B_6 toxicity have been reported. Megadoses of 2 to 6 g/day of pyridoxine in the human, usually for treatment of carpal tunnel syndrome, preeclampsia edema, or premenstrual syndrome, have resulted in toxicities ranging from dependency to a peripheral neuropathy similar to that which occurs from vitamin B_6 deficiency.[14]

The RDA for vitamin B_6 is based on protein intake and has been set at 0.016 mg/g protein for healthy adults. Adjustments in the RDA are made for growth, pregnancy, and lactation. Using twice the RDA for protein for women and men, the upper boundary of acceptable protein intakes, the RDA was set at 2.0 mg/day for men (126 g protein/day) and 1.6 mg/day for women (100 g protein/day).[15] As protein intake increases, the requirement for B_6 increases. However, because most sources of protein are also good sources of vitamin B_6, maintaining a healthy ratio of vitamin B_6 and protein generally is not a problem.

Vitamin B_6 is widely distributed in animal and plant foods. Good sources of the vitamin are meats, poultry, fish, yeast, certain seeds, and bran. More limited sources are milk, eggs, and green leafy vegetables.

Vitamin B_{12}. Pernicious anemia, ultimately identified as the vitamin B_{12} deficiency disease, was first recognized in 1855, but the vitamin itself was not synthesized until 1972. The terms *vitamin B_{12}* and *cobalamin* refer to all members of a group of large cobalt-containing corrinoids that can be converted to methylcobalamin (methyl B_{12}) or 5-deoxyadenosylcobalamin (coenzyme B_{12}), the active vitamin B_{12} coenzymes. The pharmaceutical preparation of vitamin B_{12} is cyanocobalamin.[15]

Coenzyme B_{12} functions in reactions having a 1,2 shift in hydrogen from one carbon of the substrate molecule to the next, usually with a 2,1 shift of some other group such as hydroxyl, amino, alkyl, or carboxyl. For example, one such metabolic conversion is methylmalonate to succinate, a reaction present in the degradation pathways of certain amino acids and odd-chain fatty acids, which are involved integrally in both fat and carbohydrate metabolism. In vitamin B_{12} deficiency, the blockage of this reaction results in the characteristic increased urinary excretion of methylmalonic acid.

Methylcobalamin catalyzes the transmethylation from a folic acid cofactor to homocysteine to form methionine. This reaction releases the unmethylated folate cofactor for other functions related to nucleic acid synthesis. It is this B_{12}–folate interaction that may explain the similarities between vitamin B_{12} and folate deficiency signs.[7]

Vitamin B_{12} is also involved in the maintenance of the myelin sheath that protects nerve fibers and promotes their normal growth. In addition to these main functions, bone cell activity and metabolism seem to depend on the presence of vitamin B_{12}, possibly because of the interrelationship of B_{12} and folate and their joint influence on nucleic acid synthesis.[26]

The absorption of vitamin B_{12} occurs at receptor sites in the ileum, dependent on a highly specific binding glycoprotein (Castle's intrinsic factor), secreted by the stomach. Approximately 1% to 3% of the vitamin is also absorbed by simple diffusion. The vitamin is recycled through enterohepatic circulation from bile and other intestinal secretions.[15]

Vitamin B_{12} deficiency results in macrocytic, megaloblastic anemia, from the slow DNA synthesis of folate deficiency caused by insufficient methylcobalamin. Either vitamin B_{12} or folate will reverse these symptoms. However, folate cannot reverse the additional neurological symptoms of B_{12} deficiency because of demyelination of the spinal cord, brain, and optic and peripheral nerves. Neuropsychiatric manifestations of vitamin B_{12} deficiency are seen in the absence of anemia, if folate has reversed the hematologic symptoms.[26]

Because vitamin B_{12} is ubiquitous in animal foods, but virtually only animal foods, dietary deficiency of vitamin B_{12} is rare except in pure vegans. Vitamin B_{12} deficiency seen in the United States is more commonly due to poor absorption. Pernicious anemia is due to inadequate secretion of intrinsic factor, leading to diminished vitamin absorption.

The RDA for vitamin B_{12} is 2 μg daily for healthy adults. Additional allowances are made for growth, pregnancy, and lactation.[15] Toxic symptoms have not been identified from daily oral ingestion of up to 100 μg of vitamin B_{12}.

Vitamin B_{12} is found almost exclusively in products with animal origins, such as meat, poultry, fish, milk, cheese, and eggs. Pure vegans (vegetarians who limit their diets to vegetable products only) need to supplement their diets with vitamin B_{12}-fortified soy "milk" or meat replacements, vitamin B_{12}-enriched yeast, and bacterially-fermented products. Because of the ability of the body to recycle vitamin B_{12}, deficiency symptoms may not appear in vegans for many years if they were previously meat eaters or if their diets are slightly contaminated with bacteria that produce the vitamin.

Folate. The vitamin folate, first synthesized in 1945, is also known as folacin, folic acid, and pteroylglutamic acid (PGA). The coenzymes, tetrahydrofolic acid (THFA) and dihydrofolate (DHF), catalyze the transport of single carbon fragments from one compound to another in amino acid metabolism and nucleic acid synthesis.

Folate deficiency may occur from a state of decreased absorption or increased requirements, as well as a nutrient-poor diet. A diet containing a large percentage of calories from alcohol or other foods that are not nutrient-dense can result in folate deficiency symptoms. Because folate is critical to DNA synthesis, any conditions causing rapid cell multiplication may induce folate deficiency. Deficiency of the vitamin leads to impaired cell division and alterations of protein synthesis, and two of the first symptoms of folate deficiency are macrocytic, megaloblastic anemia, and GI tract deterioration.[26]

Drugs that have a structure similar to folate interact with folate at its enzyme binding site and block normal metabolic pathways. Drugs used to treat cancer, such as methotrexate, function in this manner. Aspirin also displaces folate from its carrier protein, increasing folate excretion. Folic acid and the anticonvulsant drug phenytoin inhibit uptake of each other at the gut cell membrane, and

megadoses of folate (100 or more times the RDA) should be avoided when phenytoin therapy is indicated.[7]

The RDA for folate is approximately 3 μg/kg body weight for adults and adolescents. The standard reference RDA is 200 μg for adult males and 180 mg for adult females. Additional adjustments are recommended for infants, children, and pregnant and lactating females[15] (see Chapter 23).

Toxic doses of folate have been sporadically reported, and excessive intakes of folate are not recommended. Megadosing of folacin is contraindicated in patients with nutrient-poor diets, because it may mask some of the symptoms of vitamin B_{12} deficiency.

Folate is found abundantly in vegetables, especially green leafy vegetables. Other foods, such as meats, milk, and milk products, are very poor sources of folate. Because of this limited distribution in foods other than vegetables, folate-deficiency anemia is probably the most common of all vitamin deficiencies, especially among the poor and pregnant women in the United States and other parts of the world.

Biotin. Biotin was synthesized in 1943, but its functions were not elucidated until the 1950s and 1960s. Biotin is a sulfur-containing vitamin that is synthesized in the lower gastrointestinal tract by microorganisms and some fungi.[15] Even though it is produced in the human gut, biotin is considered an essential vitamin because there is not enough research data to show that a sufficient amount of biotin is produced and absorbed by the gut to maintain health.

Most carboxylation reactions depend on a biotin-containing enzyme. Biotin is the prosthetic group on pyruvate carboxylase and acetyl CoA carboxylase, for instance, giving biotin an essential role in gluconeogenesis and fatty acid synthesis. The biotin enzymes propionyl-CoA carboxylase and 3-methylcrotonyl CoA carboxylase, are required for propionate metabolism and the catabolism of branched-chain amino acids.[15]

Because biotin is widespread in foods, a dietary biotin deficiency is rare. Patients fed artificial formulas of purified nutrients have, on occasion, experienced biotin deficiency when biotin was lacking in the formulation. Researchers can induce biotin deficiency by feeding subjects avidin, a glycoprotein found only in raw egg whites that binds biotin, making it biologically unavailable.[26] Humans who consume more than two dozen raw egg whites a day can induce biotin deficiency. Cooking the eggs denatures the protein and eliminates its binding potential. Signs of biotin deficiency include anorexia, nausea, vomiting, glossitis, pallor, mental depression, alopecia and a dry scaly dermatitis, and an increase in serum cholesterol and bile pigments.[10]

Because there is minimal research on biotin requirements, the RDA committee of the NRC has established a range of "estimated safe and adequate daily dietary intake" for biotin. According to this range 30 to 100 μg of biotin per day is recommended for healthy U.S. adults. There have been no reports of biotin toxicity.[15]

Biotin is widespread in foods, but its most abundant sources are liver, egg yolk, soy flour, cereals, and yeast.

Pantothenic acid. Pantothenic acid was first described as a compound in 1933, but the first identification of a biochemical function came in 1947. In 1948, the compound in tissues containing pantothenic acid was named *coenzyme A* (for acetylation coenzyme). As a component of coenzyme A, pantothenic acid is involved in fatty acid synthesis, fatty acid oxidation, the transformation of pyruvate to acetyl-CoA, and acetylation reactions. As an acyl carrier protein, pantothenic acid plays a role in fatty acid synthesis analogous to the role of CoA in fatty acid oxidation. It carries the acyl group from one enzyme to the next for the six steps needed to add each 2-carbon unit.

Frank dietary vitamin deficiencies have been observed in animals but not in humans. Deficiency symptoms have been produced in humans only by the administration of a pantothenic acid antagonist or by feeding a vitamin-deficient synthetic diet. In such experiments, subjects experienced fatigue and developed postural hypotension and rapid heart rate on exertion, gastric distress with anorexia and constipation, and a numbness and tingling of the hands and feet ("burning feet" syndrome).[15]

An "estimated safe and adequate daily dietary intake" range of 4 to 7 mg/day for healthy adults has been established by the RDA committee for pantothenic acid. An actual RDA value cannot be set because of lack of sufficient research data on human requirements.[15]

Pantothenic acid is widespread in foods, and typical diets generally provide adequate amounts of the vitamin. Meat, fish, poultry, whole grain cereals, and legumes are particularly good sources.

Vitamin C. Perhaps the earliest controlled human clinical trial was the investigation by James Lind of treatments for scurvy (conducted in 1742, published in 1752). In his "Treatise of the Scurvy," Lind recounts that of six different treatment methods given to six pairs of scorbutic sailors, the patients given lemon juice recovered.[8]

Some animals possess the ability to synthesize vitamin C; humans do not. Among the two active forms of the antioxidant vitamin C, L-ascorbic acid is the most prevalent. Its oxidized form, dehydroascorbic acid, is also present in the diet.

There is no clearcut definition for the functions of vitamin C, but it is categorically established that it is essential for the prevention and cure of scurvy. Vitamin C is a cofactor of hydroxylating enzymes involved in reactions requiring molecular oxygen. For instance, vitamin C is an active cosubstrate involved in the action of prolyl and lysyl hydroxylases (proline, lysine); in the conversion of proline (in a polypeptide chain) to hydroxyproline (collagen); in the hydroxylation of tryptophan to 5-hydroxy tryptophan

(to seratonin); and in the hydroxylation of 3,4-dihydroxyphenylethylamine (dopamine) to norepinephrine.[15]

As a protective reducing agent, vitamin C is involved in many other reactions involving many other compounds, such as tyrosine, folic acid, histamine, corticosteroids, neuroendocrine peptides, and bile acids. It can affect functions of leukocytes, macrophages, immune responses, wound healing, and allergic reactions.[15]

Because of its reducing properties, vitamin C alters ferric iron to its more absorbable form, ferrous ion. When consumed in conjunction with nonheme, ferric iron from plant foods, vitamin C enhances the absorption of iron. This may also be true for inorganic copper. These changes may have tremendous influences on iron and copper nutriture, especially in pure vegetarians.[8]

Vitamin C may play a significant role in several physiological systems that are essential to disease prevention, such as lipid metabolism and immune function. It is no wonder that in 1970, Linus Pauling speculated that megadoses of vitamin C could cure everything from cancer to the common cold. Even though there is more research data pertaining to this vitamin than any other, a tremendous amount is still unknown or not well understood. However, the latest research reports lend some support to the clinical use of vitamin C in the prevention and treatment of certain diseases (see Chapter 24). This therapy uses vitamin C as a drug, rather than in its role as a vitamin, because vitamins are needed in only minute amounts by the body.[8]

There are classically two early signs of vitamin C deficiency: scorbutic gums, a symmetrical condition where the gums around the teeth bleed easily but are not infected; and petechial hemorrhages. Additional early clinical signs are joint pain, follicular hyperkeratosis, and atherosclerotic plaques.[26]

Vitamin C nutriture varies seasonally, with higher plasma levels seen during the summer months and the lowest occurring at the end of the winter months. Marginal vitamin C deficiency has been observed in the elderly and in patients suffering from chronic or acute diseases. Cigarette smokers have lower concentrations of serum and leukocyte ascorbic acid. This is explained by both a lower dietary vitamin C intake and an increased metabolic turnover in smokers.[8]

In 1989, the RDA subcommittee recognized the multiple roles that vitamin C may play in chronic disease prevention. However, because there was a lack of substantial data to allow the subcommittee to make any recommendations based on its disease-preventing potential, and RDAs are based on a philosophy of prevention of deficiency diseases rather than prevention of chronic diseases, the 1989 RDA for vitamin C is set somewhere "between the amount necessary to prevent overt symptoms of scurvy (approximately 10 mg/day in adults) and the amount beyond which the bulk of vitamin C is not retained in the body, but rather is excreted as such in the urine (approximately 200 mg/day)."[15] The RDA for healthy adults is 60 mg daily. Regular cigarette smokers are recommended to ingest at least 100 mg daily. Adjustments of RDAs are made for growth, pregnancy, and lactation.[15]

The practice of megadosing with vitamin C is common, and it is not surprising that instances of vitamin C toxicity have been reported. Nausea, abdominal cramps, and diarrhea are often reported from intakes of 1 g or more. Ascorbic acid interferes with the anticoagulants warfarin and heparin. Megadoses of vitamin C obscure the results of urinary glucose monitoring tests. In susceptible individuals, large doses may cause hemolytic anemia, kidney stones, and gout.[26]

Individuals taking chronically large doses may adjust their metabolism of vitamin C by limiting absorption and destroying and excreting more of the vitamin than usual. If the megadoses are suddenly reduced to normal, scurvy may develop because of the increased metabolic turnover of the vitamin. One report of two cases of infantile "rebound scurvy" referred to babies born to mothers who had been consuming approximately 400 mg of ascorbic acid daily during gestation. On an otherwise adequate intake, the infants developed scurvy because they had adapted to the megadose amounts during gestation.[2]

The primary source of vitamin C in the diet of Americans is citrus fruits. Other foods, such as green and red peppers, collard greens, broccoli, brussel sprouts, cabbage, spinach, tomatoes, potatoes, cantaloupe, and strawberries are also excellent sources of vitamin C, providing 30 mg of vitamin C in a serving of less than 50 calories. Meat, fish, poultry, eggs, and dairy products contain much less ascorbic acid, and grains contain none.

Fat-soluble vitamins

Vitamin A. In 1915, two pairs of noted scientists identified a fat-soluble growth factor in foods; McCollum and Davis found it in butter and egg yolk, and Osborn and Mendel in cod liver oil and butter. They termed this factor *fat-soluble A,* and it was the first fat-soluble vitamin recognized.[21]

Vitamin A is now the umbrella term for a group of compounds collectively termed retinoids. Retinol, retinaldehyde, and retinoic acid are naturally occurring compounds with some vitamin A activity. There are also a number of synthetic analogs with or without vitamin A activity. In addition, carotenoid plant pigments can be converted to vitamin A by the liver and are considered vitamin A precursors, or provitamin A. The most active of the precursors is beta-carotene, which when metabolically split yields one molecule of retinol.

The primary unit of biologic activity for vitamin A is 1 µg of all-trans retinol. One retinol equivalent (RE) therefore equals 1 µg retinol, or 6 µg beta-carotene, or 12 µg other provitamin A. Using the system of international units (IU), 1 RE equals 3.33 IU vitamin activity from retinol, or 3.33 IU carotenoids, or 10 IU vitamin activity from beta-carotene.[26] The transport of vitamin A depends on retinol binding protein (RBP), and each form of vitamin A has its own binding proteins as well.[21]

Vitamin A is the most versatile of the fat-soluble vitamins. Its physiological functions can be considered from two perspectives: (1) those functions dependent specifically on vitamin A and (2) those functions that are negatively affected during vitamin A deficiency. In the first category are vision and the promotion of night vision, and the differentiation and growth of some types of cells. In the second category are food intake, amino acid metabolism, differentiation of mucus-secreting cells and other epithelial cells, the immune system, reproduction, and ultimately the structure and function of most cells and organs of the body.[21]

Avitaminosis A is a major nutritional problem among the poor. The prevalence of vitamin A deficiency increases with deteriorating economic status. In humid tropical areas, where refrigeration is virtually unavailable, 5% to 10% of toddlers may have demonstrable vitamin A deficiency. It is estimated that 250,000 preschool children go blind each year in Asia alone, primarily because of avitaminosis A.[23]

The symptoms of vitamin A deficiency are predominantly ocular and range in increasing severity from night blindness and conjunctival xerosis to corneal xerosis, ulceration, and sometimes liquefaction. These ocular manifestations are often collectively referred to as xeropthalmia. Other symptoms include anorexia, hyperkeratosis, increased susceptibility to infection, and metaplasia and keratinization of respiratory tract epithelial cells.[15]

Vitamin-A deficiency usually occurs from dietary vitamin A insufficiency, fat malabsorption, or protein deficiency (lack of RBP). Vitamin A deficiency is also associated with a lack of cow's milk during growth. Use of unfortified skim milk has caused problems. Males appear more vulnerable than females, and xeropthalmia is rare during pregnancy, although night blindness may be common.[21]

In addition to their vitamin functions, some retinoids are under investigation for their hypothesized ability to prevent, suppress, or retard some cancers of the skin, bladder, and breast. Some synthetic retinoids are already used as drugs for the treatment of some skin disorders and severe acne. Unrelated to their provitamin activity, carotenoids are under investigation for their potential anticancer capabilities related to their antioxidant properties. To date, there is insufficient data to recommend specific amounts of either retinoids for treatment purposes, or carotenoids for prevention. However, this is an area of intense experimentation with the potential for promising results. Studies suggest that a generous intake of carotenoid-rich foods may be of benefit in cancer prevention, and several synthetic retinoids may ultimately be a therapy of choice for specific cancers.

On the basis of body weight, the RDA for vitamin A is 1000 RE for men and 800 RE for women. The allowance is adjusted for growth, pregnancy, and lactation.[15]

Excessive intakes of preformed vitamin A are toxic. Manifestations include headache, vomiting, diplopia, alopecia, dryness of the mucus membranes, desquamation, bone abnormalities, and liver damage. Symptoms can occur with daily intakes through food and supplementation of 15,000 μg retinol (50,000 IU) in adults and 6000 mg retinol (20,000 IU) in children. Preformed vitamin A is teratogenic, and fetal abnormalities have been observed in women ingesting therapeutic doses (0.5 to 1.5 mg/kg) of 13-cis retinoic acid (isotretinoin) during the first trimester of pregnancy.[15]

Carotenoids are not known to be toxic because of their reduced absorption at high doses and limited conversion to vitamin A in the body. However, large doses taken chronically will color the adipose tissue stores, thereby coloring the skin yellow, especially the palms of the hands and the soles of the feet.[15]

The most significant sources of retinol are fortified milk, cheese, cream, butter, fortified margarine, eggs, and liver. The best sources of beta-carotene are spinach and other dark, leafy greens, broccoli, deep orange fruits, such as apricots and cantaloupe, and vegetables, such as squash, carrots, sweet potatoes, and pumpkin.

Vitamin D. Vitamin D deficiency disease, or rickets, was described in the mid-17th century. Even though the cause of rickets had not been identified, rickets was effectively cured by Huldchinsky in 1919, using ultraviolet rays from a mercury vapor lamp. By 1922, McCollum had identified a second fat-soluble factor in cod liver oil that was different from fat-soluble A, and in 1938, vitamin D was isolated. It was not until the early 1970s, however, that the fully metabolically active form, 1-25-OH-cholecalciferol, was identified and established as an active hormone.[3]

Vitamin D is different from all the other nutrients in that the body can synthesize it with the help of sunlight. In a sense, then, with adequate exposure to sunlight, vitamin D is not an essential nutrient. When synthesized in the body, vitamin D travels to a target tissue to promote its metabolic or physiologic function. In this way, it acts not as a vitamin, but as a hormone. Exposure to ultraviolet light catalyzes the synthesis of cholecalciferol (vitamin D) from 7-dehydrocholesterol (provitamin), in the skin. Cholecalciferol travels to the liver, where it is hydroxylated to 25-hydroxycholecalciferol. This intermediate compound then travels to the kidney and is hydroxylated a second time to 1,25-dihydroxycholecalciferol, the activated hormone of vitamin D.[3]

In most urban parts of the world, few people are exposed to enough sunlight year-round to produce adequate supplies of vitamin D without dietary supplementation. When adequate exposure to sunlight is not possible, dietary consumption of the organic compound is required. As such, vitamin D is an essential micronutrient, and in this manner, vitamin D does function as a vitamin.

Vitamin D is part of a cooperative group of other nutrients and compounds essential to healthy bone growth and maintenance. The main action of vitamin D is the promotion of normal bone mineralization by the elevation of the concentrations of plasma calcium and phosphorus to levels that allow normal bone mineralization. When plasma calcium is low, this action prevents tetany from hypocalcemia. Maintenance of mineral blood levels is accomplished by vitamin D through the enhancement of calcium and phosphorus absorption from the intestinal tract; mobilization of calcium from bone; and stimulation of renal reabsorption of calcium. Vitamin D may also function at the calcification sites of bone and may be involved in muscle strength.[26]

Hypovitaminosis D develops in three stages, reflecting depletion of vitamin D, accompanied by secondary hyperparathyroidism. Vitamin D deficiency disease is called rickets in children, and osteomalacia in adults.[3] Stage I in some infants involves an inability to maintain normal blood calcium levels, resulting clinically in generalized convulsions or attacks of tetany. No radiologic skeletal signs are apparent. Stage I represents a period of functional hypoparathyroidism.

Stage II presents with a secondary hyperparathyroidism stimulated by the hypocalcemia of the preceding stage, which corrects the blood calcium levels and lowers the blood phosphorus level. At this point, the skeletal changes associated with rickets begin to appear, and alkaline phosphatase levels in the blood increase.

Stage III is reached when the body's calcium reserves are exhausted. The skeleton is very demineralized, the parathyroid glands can no longer maintain a normal blood calcium level, and there are very marked clinical signs of rickets and osteomalacia.

Because a substantial portion of the U.S. population is not exposed to enough sunlight for adequate synthesis of vitamin D, an RDA has been established. The RDA for vitamin D for adults beyond 24 years of age is 5 μg (200 IU) daily. An allowance is established for growth, pregnancy, and lactation.[15]

Toxicity from excessive intakes of vitamin D have been reported, especially in children. Toxic effects include hypercalcemia and hypercalciuria. These conditions can lead to deposition of calcium in soft tissues and irreversible renal and cardiovascular damage. The consumption of as little as 45 μg (1800 IU) per day of cholecalciferol has been associated with toxic symptoms in young children.[15]

The best food sources of vitamin D in the U.S. are fortified milk products. Processed cow's milk provides 10 μg of cholecalciferol per quart and is the primary source of the vitamin in children. Eggs, butter, and fortified margarine are the solid food sources of vitamin D.

Vitamin E. The importance of vitamin E was established in 1922 when this fat-soluble factor was shown to prevent fetal death in animals fed a diet containing rancid lard. Not until 1968 was vitamin E recognized formally as an essential nutrient for humans. Since then, there have been many discoveries relating to nutritional and clinical aspects of vitamin E. With the advent of high-performance liquid chromatography (HPLC), the many isomers of the vitamin E family have been identified.[4]

Two groups of compounds have vitamin E biological activity. Most important are the tocopherols; second are the tocotrienols. The most active form of vitamin E, alpha-tocopherol, is also the most widely distributed in foods. Because there are so many different isomers, each with varying levels of activity, vitamin E activity is expressed as RRR-alpha-tocopherol equivalents (alpha-TEs). One alpha-TE is the activity of 1 mg of RRR-alpha-tocopherol.[15]

The chief function of vitamin E in the body is as an antioxidant. By its presence, it neutralizes free radicals, which could otherwise initiate the chain reaction, especially in membranes containing large amounts of highly unsaturated fatty acids. Through this antioxidant activity, vitamin E stabilizes cell membranes, regulates oxidation reactions, and protects polyunsaturated fatty acids, vitamin A, and vitamin C.[4,15]

Until recently, vitamin E deficiency in humans was observed only through experimental induction. It is now apparent that deficiency occurs in two classes of subjects: (1) premature, very low birth weight infants, and (2) patients unable to absorb fat normally. In adults, symptoms of hypovitaminosis may take years to develop. The primary signs of deficiency are hemolysis and possible anemia, reproductive failure, neuronal degeneration, and nutritional muscular dystrophy.[15]

Because of its close association with unsaturated fatty acids, it is not surprising that the dietary requirement for vitamin E is linked to consumption of polyunsatured fatty acids (PUFA). The vitamin E requirement increases when PUFA intake increases. A ratio (mg RRR-alpha-tocopherol to grams of PUFA) of 0.4 has been suggested when the primary PUFA in the diet is linoleic acid, as in most U.S. diets. Based on the customary diets of Americans, and body weight, the RDA subcommittee has established a dietary recommendation of 10 mg of alpha-TEs per day for adult men and 8 mg/day for women. An allowance for growth, pregnancy, and lactation has been established as well.[15]

Unlike the fat-soluble vitamins A and D, vitamin E is relatively nontoxic in excessive amounts. Possible GI disturbances have been reported in some individuals taking more than 600 mg/day. High doses may enhance the effects of anticoagulant drugs. Patients undergoing such treatment should avoid megadoses of vitamin E.[15,26]

Vitamin E is found widely in foods, and the richest sources in the U.S. food supply are vegetable oils and products made from them. Wheat germ and nuts are high in the vitamin, and fruits and vegetables supply appreciable amounts.

Vitamin K. Vitamin K was discovered serendipitously while Dam was studying cholesterol metabolism in chicks fed fat-free diets. Subcutaneous and intraperitoneal hemorrhages were observed in the chicks after a few days, and he named the fat-soluble factor absent from the diet and identified with these symptoms "vitamin K" for the "koagulation" vitamin.[20]

Vitamin K is the name for a group of compounds that all contain the 2-methyl-1,4-naphthoquinone moiety; these include phylloquinone, menaquinones, and menadione. Vitamin K-dependent compounds are responsible for the carboxylation reaction of prothrombin formation in the liver, and at least five other proteins involved in the regulation of blood clotting. Other K-dependent proteins are plasma serine protease and some gamma-carboxyglutamic acid proteins in plasma, bone, and kidney.[20]

Microbiologic flora of the normal gut synthesize the menaquinones in amounts that may supply a significant part of the requirement for vitamin K. Vitamin K is also widely distributed in foods. For these reasons, vitamin K deficiency is rare and usually occurs secondary to disease or drug therapy with K-antagonists. Anticoagulant drugs, such as 4-hydroxy coumarins, or warfarin, are vitamin-K antagonists, and patients undergoing any therapies involving these drugs should be closely monitored for vitamin K status. Patients chronically treated with broad-spectrum antibiotics or on long-term hyperalimentation and patients with chronic biliary obstruction or with lipid malabsorption syndromes are prone to vitamin K deficiency. Large amounts of vitamin E may also antagonize the action of vitamin K. Although vitamin K has other functions, the primary deficiency symptom is increased clotting time and resultant hemorrhage.[20]

According to the RDA subcommittee, a dietary intake of 1 μg/kg body weight should be sufficient to maintain normal blood clotting time in adults. The established RDA value for a 79 kg man is 80 μg/day, and for a 63 kg woman, it is 65 μg/day.[15]

There have been no toxic symptoms identified with excessive ingestion of vitamin K. However, large doses of parenterally administered menadione in newborns may cause hemolytic anemia, hyperbilirubinemia, and kernicterus.[15]

The most significant sources of vitamin K are bacterial synthesis in the gut; green, leafy vegetables, liver, cabbage-type vegetables, and milk.

The major minerals

The major minerals are those found in the body in amounts greater than 5 grams. They all function as great mediators of fluid balance and blood pressure, and individually influence such important factors as bone metabolism, enzyme function, and nerve impulse transmission.

Sodium. Sodium is the chief extracellular cation and is the principal regulator of extracellular fluid balance. Sodium is also essential for acid-base balance, the regulation of osmalarity, and nerve impulse transmission.[26]

Because of the kidney's ability to conserve sodium, deficiency is uncommon, even in individuals on very low sodium diets. Deficiency can occur, however, under extreme environmental conditions causing heavy and persistent sweating, or from trauma, chronic diarrhea, or renal disease.

Sodium recommendations are based on calculated estimates of requirements during growth, and for replacement of obligatory losses. The minimum average requirement of sodium for adults under normal conditions is no more than 5 mEq/day (115 mg sodium or 300 mg sodium chloride). The RDA subcommittee, in establishing a minimum allowance of sodium intake, has considered the wide variation of physical activity and environmental exposure of Americans, as well as the tendency for consumption of large amounts of sodium to bring on or exacerbate hypertension (see Chapter 24). The minimum sodium requirement for healthy adults established by the RDA subcommittee is 500 mg/day. The Food and Nutrition Board Committee of the National Research Council has recommended that daily intakes of sodium chloride be limited to 6 g (2.4 g of sodium) or less.[15]

The most significant sources of sodium are salt, soy sauce, commercially prepared processed foods and snack foods, and softened water. Moderate quantities are found in whole, unprocessed foods.

Chloride. Chloride is the chief anion in the extracellular fluid and, like sodium, is essential in maintaining fluid and electrolyte balance. It is also a principal component of hydrochloric acid, secreted in the stomach during digestion of protein.[26]

Dietary deficiency of chloride parallels sodium; it occurs only as a result of heavy, persistent sweating, chronic diarrhea or vomiting, trauma, or renal disease, resulting in hypochloremic metabolic alkalosis.

The minimum estimated requirement of chloride for healthy adults established by the RDA subcommittee is 750 mg/day. Dietary sources of chloride are almost exclusively from sodium chloride, with a smaller amount from potassium chloride and water.[15]

Potassium. In contrast to the sodium cation, the potassium cation is more concentrated inside, rather than outside, the cell. As the body's chief intracellular electrolyte, potassium plays a major role in the maintenance of normal fluid and acid-base balance, and is critical to nerve transmission and muscle contraction through its active participation in the sodium-potassium ion exchange pump. Potassium also plays a catalytic role in protein and carbohydrate metabolism.[26]

Potassium deficiency is unlikely, but possible. Diets void of fresh fruits and vegetables can result in potassium deficiency. Abnormal conditions, such as diabetic acidosis, dehydration, or potassium-depleting diuretics, can promote potassium deficient states. Large potassium losses may occur through prolonged vomiting, chronic diarrhea, or laxative abuse. Symptoms of potassium deficiency include weakness, anorexia, nausea, listlessness, apprehension, drowsiness, and irrational behavior. If hypokalemia is severe, potentially fatal cardiac dysrhythmias can occur.[15]

Potassium is less well conserved by the body than sodium. To maintain normal body stores and normal plasma and fluid concentrations, an intake of approximately 40 mEq/day has been estimated.[15] The minimum adult requirement recommended by the RDA committee is 1600 to 2000 mg (40 to 50 mEq) per day. Additionally, the NRC has recognized evidence of benefits of higher potassium intakes to hypertensive patients. Along these lines, the NRC Committee on Diet and Health recommends an increased intake of fruits and vegetables by adults to equal about 3500 mg (90 mEq) of potassium per day. The RDA committee does not recommend increases in potassium intakes during pregnancy or lactation, but recommendations considering childhood growth requirements are established.[15]

Incidences of hyperkalemia are predominantly associated with acute intoxication from enteral or parenteral supplements. Hyperkalemia can result in potentially fatal cardiac arrest.[15]

The richest sources of dietary potassium are unprocessed foods, especially fruits, many vegetables, legumes, and fresh meats.

Calcium. Calcium is the most abundant mineral in the body, and 99% of the body's calcium is stored in the skeleton. The other 1% is found in extracellular fluids, intracellular structures, and cell membranes, and plays critical roles in normal muscle contraction and relaxation, proper nerve functioning, blood clotting, blood pressure, and immune defenses.[26]

Blood calcium concentrations are maintained within a very narrow range that is tightly controlled by a system of hormones. 1,25-dihydroxycholecalciferol, parathyroid hormone, calcitonin, estrogen, testosterone, and possibly others control calcium absorption and excretion, as well as bone metabolism.[1]

In the face of inadequate dietary intake or absorption, blood calcium is maintained at the expense of bone. In children, this results in inadequate bone mineralization. In adults, mineral is withdrawn from bone, resulting in reduced bone mineral density and strength.

Intestinal calcium absorption is affected by several nutritional and physiological factors. During periods of increased requirements and/or low dietary intake, calcium absorption is enhanced. Vitamin D promotes calcium absorption through the production of calcium-binding protein. Dietary protein enhances calcium absorption when the protein intake range is between inadequate and adequate, but excess dietary protein may increase calcium excretion. Lactose may also facilitate calcium absorption.[15] Gastric acidity assists calcium absorption by maintaining calcium solubility, a possible partial explanation for impaired calcium absorption in the elderly.

Phytate, found in oatmeal and whole grains, and oxalate, found in rhubarb, spinach, and other vegetables, bind calcium (and other minerals such as iron and zinc) to prevent absorption. Certain fibers may also hinder calcium absorption. Foods high in these factors are not useful dietary calcium sources.

Calcium deficiency disease is known as rickets in the young, and osteomalacia in adults. Deficient calcium uptake threatens the integrity of bones; however, vitamin D deficiency is the most common cause of rickets and osteomalacia. Rickets results in soft bones and stunted growth in children.

Osteoporosis, a disease of bone loss in adults, particularly postmenopausal women, may be caused by several factors, including inadequate lifetime calcium availability and reduced estrogen production, but ultimately results in bone softening and loss of bone integrity, similar to osteomalacia. However, treatments for osteoporosis are not as straightforward and well-defined as for osteomalacia, a true deficiency disease.

Studies appear to agree that concurrent calcium intake in osteoporotic women does not correlate with bone mineral status, unless lifetime high-calcium food consumption patterns were established in childhood. Investigations into maintenance of bone mineral mass have found that those individuals with higher lifetime calcium intakes have greater bone mass as they age. The assumption has been made that those individuals who attain a higher peak bone mass can maintain a healthier level of bone density with age, even though bone loss still occurs.[1,15]

The 1989 RDA for optimal calcium intake for women is based on the attainment of peak bone mass at about 25 years. The RDA committee stresses the importance of meeting recommended allowances at all ages, but with special attention to intakes throughout childhood to age 25 years.[15]

An intake of 1200 mg is recommended for both sexes from ages 11 to 24; 800 mg is recommended for all adults. Allowances for pregnancy, lactation, and childhood growth are established.[15]

World health organizations generally recommend lower intakes of calcium. Calcium recommendations for Thai women are 400 mg/day, and evidence exists that various population groups do maintain normal calcium status at lower intakes than the RDA.[15] However, because there is a long period of time before changes in calcium status can be detected, and often the first sign of poor lifetime status is a bone fracture representing osteoporosis, the RDA subcommittee has chosen to maintain these relatively higher recommendations.

Recommended calcium intakes from the National Institutes of Health Consensus Development Conference on Osteoporosis were 1000 mg for premenopausal or estrogen-treated women, and 1500 mg for postmenopausal women who are not treated with estrogen.[18]

No adverse effects have been observed in healthy adults consuming up to 2500 mg of calcium daily; however, high intakes may induce constipation and increase the risk of urinary stone formation in males. High calcium intakes may inhibit absorption of zinc, iron, and other minerals. Excessive intakes can ultimately impair renal function.[15]

Calcium is significantly found almost exclusively in milk and milk products. Even though some greens appear to be good sources of calcium, the fibers and oxalates that bind the calcium render it biologically unavailable to humans. Therefore calcium is not always efficiently absorbed from green vegetables, whereas it is known to be efficiently absorbed from milk. Daily consumption of low-fat or nonfat milk products is essential for the adequate consumption of calcium.

Phosphorus. The second most abundant mineral in the body, 85% of phosphorus in the adult is found as calcium phosphate salts in bone. It is also present in soft tissues as a soluble phosphate ion; in lipids, proteins, carbohydrates, and nucleic acid in an ester or anhydride linkage; and in enzymes as a modulator of their activities. Phosphorus plays key roles in energy transfer through the active phosphate bonds of adenosine triphosphate (ATP), creatine phosphate, and similar compounds.[1,15]

Because phosphorus is efficiently absorbed and is found almost ubiquitously in foods, dietary deficiency usually does not occur. Deficiencies have been seen in premature infants fed exclusively cow's milk, and deficiency has been induced in patients receiving aluminum hydroxide as an antacid for prolonged periods. Aluminum hydroxide binds phosphorus, making it biologically unavailable. Symptoms of phosphorus deficiency include bone loss characterized by weakness, anorexia, malaise, and pain.[15]

The RDA for phosphorus is set at a 1-to-1 ratio with calcium. Recommendations are 800 mg for children 1 to 10 years, 1200 mg for ages 11 to 24, and 800 mg for adults beyond 24 years. A 1200 mg/day recommendation is given for pregnancy and lactation, and special consideration is given for infants.[15]

Excessive intakes of phosphorus in humans, at a calcium-phophorus ratio of less than 1-to-2, have resulted in lowered blood calcium levels.[15]

The greatest dietary sources of phosphorus are animal protein foods, such as meat, fish, poultry, milk, and milk products. Processed foods and soft drinks are also usually high in phophorus.

Magnesium. As part of the Mg-ATP complex, magnesium functions in hundreds of biosynthetic reactions. It is best known for its participation in protein synthesis, bone mineralization, enzyme action, muscular contraction, transmission of nerve impulses, and maintenance of teeth.[15]

Dietary intake of magnesium in the United States is generally below the RDA, although deficiency symptoms caused by dietary inadequacies have not been observed in healthy adults. Magnesium depletion has been reported in association with various disease states: gastrointestinal tract abnormalities, renal dysfunction, general malnutrition, alcoholism, and iatrogenic causes.[15,22]

The most prominent signs of magnesium deficiency include nausea, muscle weakness, irritability, mental derangement, myographic changes, and depressed pancreatic hormone secretion. In extreme cases, convulsions, hallucinations, dysphagia, tetany, and growth failure in children may occur.[26]

The RDA for adults is based on a value of 4.5 mg/kg, with a standard daily recommendation of 280 mg for women and 350 mg for men. Additional recommendations are given for pregnant and lactating women, and infants and children.[15]

Toxicity symptoms are unknown in healthy adults. Hypermagnesemia has occurred in individuals with impaired renal function consuming excessive doses of magnesium. Early toxicity symptoms include nausea, vomiting, and hypotension. More severe symptoms can include bradycardia, cutaneous vasodilation, electrocardiographic changes, hyporeflexia, central nervous system depression, respiratory depression, coma, and asystolic arrest.[15,26]

Foods with the highest concentrations of magnesium are unprocessed; removal of the germ and outer layers of cereal grains results in a greater than 80% loss of magnesium. The best dietary magnesium sources are nuts, legumes, whole grains, dark green vegetables, and seafoods.

The trace minerals

There are 13 trace minerals known to be essential for animals, but scientists have established human essentiality for only nine. Of these nine, iron, zinc, iodine, and selenium have been studied in enough detail to establish recommended dietary allowances. Safe and adequate daily dietary intake *ranges* have been recommended by the RDA committee for copper, manganese, fluoride, chromium, and molybdenum, because further research is necessary to make absolute recommendations. Arsenic, nickel, silicon, and boron are known to be essential to animals, but their essentiality in the human diet is now under investigation.

Iron. Every cell contains iron. Iron is a functional constituent of hemoglobin, myoglobin, and a number of oxidizing enzymes. Iron is essential for many of the oxidation-reduction reactions of the metabolic pathways to proceed. Storage forms of iron include ferritin, hemosiderin, and transferrin.[26]

The body's iron content is regulated mainly by the absorption capability of the intestinal mucosa. This capability changes depending on body iron stores, the amount of available iron in a meal, and the ionic state of the iron, as well as several other dietary factors that influence iron's bioavailability.[15]

Normally, approximately 10% to 15% of dietary iron is absorbed, although there is interindividual and intraindividual variation. If iron intake is low or requirements increase, the capacity of the intestinal mucosa to absorb iron increases. If iron status is good, then absorption may be more moderate. Unfortunately, if iron intake is significantly diminished long enough, intestinal absorptive capacity cannot overcome the potential for iron deficiency. In the same way, if iron intake is significantly high, mucosal absorption cannot protect against toxicity.[26]

There are three stages of impaired iron status. Iron stores are diminished in the first stage, referred to as iron depletion, and there is a decrease in plasma ferritin to below 12 μg/liter. No functional impairment is observed.[15]

The second stage is iron-deficient erythropoiesis. Hemoglobin levels are within normal reference ranges; however, red cell protoporphyrin levels are elevated, transferrin saturation is reduced to less than 16% in adults, and work capacity may be impaired.[15]

The final stage is iron deficiency anemia, when total blood hemoglobin levels are below normal. Severe iron deficiency anemia exhibits microcytosis with hypochromia.[15]

The RDA committee has recognized that iron deficiency may be observed primarily during four periods of life:

- 6 months to 4 years, because of low iron stores, low iron content of milk, and increased growth requirements
- Early adolescence, because of increased growth requirements
- Female reproductive years, because of menstrual losses
- During pregnancy, because of increased blood volume of mother, demands of fetus and placenta, and blood losses during childbirth[15]

The RDA for adults in the U.S. is based on the typical diet, with an estimated iron absorption of 10% to 15%. An intake of 10 mg/day is recommended for adult males, 15 mg/day for females aged 11 to 50, and 10 mg/day for women older than 50 years. Additional allowances are made for growth of infants and children, and for pregnant women.[15]

The most common instances of iron toxicity in otherwise healthy people in the U.S. occur in children who ingest the medicinal iron supplements formulated for adults. The lethal dose of ferrous sulfate for a 2-year-old child is approximately 3 g. The lethal dose for adults ranges from 200 to 250 mg/kg body weight. People with the genetic defect that causes idiopathic hemochromatosis are at risk for iron overload. Iron toxicity may result in tissue damage, especially to the liver, and infections resulting from the iron-rich environment.[15,26]

Meats, fish, and poultry rank the highest in iron per serving, providing about one third of the iron in the average American diet. Whole-grain or enriched breads and cereals also provide about one third of the nation's dietary iron. Legumes, dark greens, and some fruits such as peaches, prunes, and apricots are also rich in iron. Although it is an excellent source of many nutrients, milk is a poor source of iron.

All forms of iron are not absorbed equally well. Heme iron, found as part of hemoglobin and myoglobin, is the best absorbed form of iron, at a rate of about 23%. In meat, poultry, fish, and dairy products, 40% of the iron is heme iron; these are the only sources of dietary heme iron. The majority of iron in the diet is nonheme iron, which is the remaining 60% of iron from animal tissues, and fruit, vegetable, and grain sources. Nonheme iron is absorbed at a much lower rate of about 2% to 20%.[26]

The absorption of nonheme iron depends on dietary factors and iron stores. When iron stores are low, absorption of both heme and nonheme iron is enhanced. Certain dietary combinations can also enhance or inhibit nonheme iron absorption. When organic acids, especially ascorbic acid, and/or animal tissue from meat, fish, or poultry, (the MFP factor) are present in a meal, nonheme iron absorption is increased. Both factors present in a meal will influence absorption to the greatest extent.[26]

Factors that inhibit absorption are calcium phosphate, phytates, bran, polyphenols in tea, and antacids.

Zinc. Zinc is a cofactor for more than 70 enzymes that are essential to the healthy function of eyes, liver, kidneys, muscles, skin, bones, and male reproductive organs. Zinc functions in association with insulin, protein and nucleic acid synthesis, immune function, vitamin A transport, taste perception, wound healing, and fetal growth and development.[15,26]

Pockets of the U.S. population may experience marginal zinc status. Children, pregnant women, the elderly, and poor may be at greatest risk of marginal zinc status in the United States, although overt deficiency symptoms may not be apparent.[26]

General signs of dietary zinc deficiency include loss of appetite, growth retardation, skin changes, and immunological abnormalities. Severe zinc deficiency affects the function of nearly all systems. Pronounced zinc deficiency in men has resulted in hypogonadism and dwarfism.[15]

The RDA for zinc is set at 15 mg/day for adult men, and 12 mg/day for adult women, because of the lower body weight in women. Additional recommendations are established for growing infants and children, and pregnant and lactating females.[14]

Zinc toxicity occurs in two forms. Acute toxicity after the ingestion of 2 g or more of zinc sulfate results in gastrointestinal irritation and vomiting. More commonly,

moderately elevated zinc intakes are not easily detected and may have more subtle effects. Supplemental zinc intakes of 18.5 mg have resulted in impaired copper status. Higher intakes may cause more severely impaired copper status, further compromising biological function. Other results of excessive zinc supplementation include diminished immune function and suppressed levels of high-density lipoproteins.[15]

As with iron, the bioavailability of zinc varies depending on the food source, and the absorption of zinc varies with nutritional status. Small amounts of zinc are better absorbed than large amounts, and people in good zinc status absorb less zinc that those in a depleted state.

Americans consume approximately 70% of their dietary zinc from animal sources. Animal foods contain the most bioavailable form of zinc, with meat, liver, eggs, and seafoods (especially oysters) offering the greatest amounts of zinc. Whole grain products contain zinc, but in a less available form. Also, high concentrations of phytate and dietary fiber seem to impair zinc utilization.

Iodine. Essential in the diet in minute amounts, iodine plays a principal role in thyroxin and triiodothyronine synthesis. Dietary iodine is converted to iodide in the GI tract.[26]

Iodide deficiency is known as simple goiter, resulting in an enlarged thyroid gland, sluggishness, and weight gain. During pregnancy, goiter will have severe effects on fetal growth and development.[26]

Iodine deficiency disease can be treated by providing adequate iodine. The incidence of endemic goiter in the United States fell sharply with the introduction of iodized salt in 1924. Natural goitrogens found in cabbage and cassava have been implicated in the pathogenesis of goiter internationally but are not known to cause problems in the United States.[15]

The RDA for adult consumption of iodine is 150 μg/day. Additional allowances for growth of infants and children, and for pregnancy and lactation, have been established.[15]

Excessive iodine intakes can also lead to thyroid enlargement. Iodine intakes of Americans increased dramatically during the 1960s and 1970s, when consumption of salt increased, as well as consumption of iodates from dough conditioners and disinfectants used in the dairy industry. As salt intake has declined and the food industry has become more aware of the risk of overuse of iodine products, the problem has diminished. The average intake of iodine in the United States is now down to about 200 to 500 μg/day. The toxic levels thought to induce harm are over 2000 μg/day in adults.[15]

The natural availability of iodine in food varies geographically. Because seawater is naturally high in iodine, seafoods, water, and iodine-containing mist from the ocean that "seeds" the soil are important sources in coastal areas. Further inland, the iodine content of plant and animal products is more variable, depending on the growing and processing practices of farmers and food manufacturers. Iodized salt plays a major role as a vehicle for iodine consumption, providing 76 μg of iodine per gram of salt. Also, advances in the ability to transport food nationwide have diminished the potential for the development of endemic goiter.[15]

Selenium. The essentiality of selenium in the human diet was not established until 1979. Chinese scientists reported an association between low selenium status and Keshan disease, a cardiomyopathy that affects primarily young children and women of childbearing age. Selenium supplementation was pivotal in the prevention of the disease.[15]

Selenium is present at the active site of glutathione peroxidase, an enzyme that catalyzes the breakdown of hydroperoxides. Selenium has a close metabolic interrelationship with vitamin E, another antioxidant, although their functions are complementary rather than duplicative. Other functions for selenium are being investigated.[26]

Dietary selenium deficiency is uncommon in the United States. Patients on total parenteral nutrition may be at risk of selenium deficiency, and feeding solutions should be checked for selenium content. Deficiency symptoms include anemia and heart disease.[15,26]

Because the data for establishing requirements for selenium are still scant, the RDA for selenium has been set somewhat arbitrarily, particularly the extrapolated values for infants and children. The RDA is 70 μg/day for adult males and 55 μg/day for adult females. Additional allowances have been set for growth of infants and children, and for pregnancy and lactation.[15]

Selenium toxicity can result from intakes of approximately 5 mg/day from food, resulting in fingernail changes and hair loss. Higher supplemental intakes can result in nausea, abdominal pain, diarrhea, nail and hair changes, peripheral neuropathy, fatigue, and irritability.[15]

The selenium content of foods varies with the amount in the soils in which the food is grown. Seafoods, kidney, liver, and other meats are good sources of selenium. Grains and seeds can be good sources of selenium; however, the content is variable. Fruits and vegetables are generally poor selenium sources.

Copper. Much of what is known about the role of copper comes from animal research. Copper is part of several proteins and enzymes, is essential for the proper utilization of iron, and is involved in collagen synthesis, wound healing, and maintenence of the myelin sheath around nerve fibers.[26]

Copper deficiency is rare but has been observed in children with protein deficiency and iron-deficiency anemia. Excess zinc interferes with copper absorption and can cause deficiency. Symptoms of copper deficiency include anemia, bone changes, and disturbed growth and metabolism in children.[26]

The estimated safe and adequate dietary intake range for copper is 1.5 to 3.0 mg/day for adults, with allowance for growth in infants and children.[15]

Copper toxicity is extremely rare. Symptoms of toxicity include vomiting and diarrhea at intake of 10 to 15 mg. Larger amounts can be fatal.[26]

Organ meats, especially liver, are the richest sources of copper in the diet. Because the preceding are rarely recommended as part of a daily diet because of their high concentrations of cholesterol, seafoods, nuts, and seeds are considered the more healthful sources to include as a regular part of the daily diet. Although concentrations are highly variable depending on the plumbing and hardness, drinking water can be a significant source of copper in the diet.

Manganese. Manganese is a facilitator of many cellular processes. It is an activator of decarboxylases, hydrolases, kinases, and transferases. There are two manganese metalloenzymes: pyruvate carboxylase and superoxide dismutase.[15]

Manganese deficiency has been recorded in only one human fed a purified diet for a vitamin-K-deficiency study. Manganese was inadvertently omitted from the dietary formulation.[15]

The estimated safe and adequate range for dietary intake of manganese has been set at 2.5 to 5.0 mg/day for adults. Growth allowances for infants and children have been derived through extrapolation on the basis of body weight and expected food intake.[15]

Manganese toxicity has been observed to result from environmental contamination, such as with miners inhaling manganese dust. Symptoms of toxicity exhibit as nervous system disorders.[26]

Manganese is widely distributed in foods, but the richest sources are whole grains and cereals, followed by fruits and vegetables.

Fluoride. In fact, there is controversy over the actual essentiality of fluorine in human nutrition. However, because of its valuable effects on dental health, fluorine is clearly a beneficial element for humans.

Fluoride, a binary compound of the element fluorine, is found predominantly incorporated into the tissues of bones and teeth. Fluoride replaces the hydroxy portion of hydroxyapatite in bones and teeth. This makes teeth more resistant to decay. The role of fluoride in protection against osteoporosis is less clear. Theoretically, high fluoride intake in combination with adequate calcium and vitamin D should increase bone mass and reduce the incidence of fractures. However, definite evidence for this effect is lacking, and side effects to fluoride therapy may be severe. Research into this area is continuing.[26]

The only fluoride deficiency symptom identified is increased susceptibility to tooth decay. On the other hand, fluorosis, the disease of excess fluoride, exhibits a discoloration of teeth, nausea, diarrhea, chest pain, itching, and vomiting. Severe cases may affect bone health, kidney function, and possibly muscle and nerve function.[15,26]

The estimated safe and adequate range of intakes of fluoride for adults is 1.5 to 4.0 mg/day. This amount is reduced in children to avoid mottling of the teeth.[15]

The most significant dietary source of fluoride is drinking water, whether naturally or artificially fluoridated. Tea and seafood may also supply substantial amounts of fluoride to the diet.

Chromium. Chromium participates in carbohydrate and lipid metabolism. Working closely with insulin as part of a poorly understood complex, the glucose tolerance factor (GTF), chromium facilitates the uptake of glucose into cells and the release of energy. In a chromium deficient state, insulin action is impaired, and a diabetes-like condition results. Impaired glucose tolerance in malnourished children, in some mild diabetics, and in middle-aged subjects has improved with chromium supplementation.[15,26]

In animals, chromium deficiency raises serum cholesterol and low-density lipoprotein concentrations, and lowers high-density lipoprotein fractions. In adults, chromium deficiency has been associated with coronary artery disease.[26]

The range of estimated safe and adequate dietary intake of chromium for adults is 50 to 200 μg/day. Recommendations for infants and children are based on extrapolated data from expected food intakes.[15]

Chronic occupational exposure to chromium dust has been correlated with an increased incidence of bronchial cancer. Chromium toxicity is unknown as a nutritional disorder.[15]

The most significant dietary sources of chromium are meat, unrefined foods, fats, and vegetable oils.

Molybdenum. Required in minute amounts, molybdenum plays an essential role in human physiology as part of several metalloenzymes: aldehyde oxidase, xanthine oxidase, and sulfite oxidase.[15]

Human molybdenum deficiency has been induced only in a patient on total parenteral nutrition. Excesses of molybdenum intake have been observed only as a result of high environmental concentrations. Dietary intake of 10 to 15 mg/day may have caused high incidences of a goutlike syndrome.[15]

The range of safe and adequate dietary intake is estimated at 75 to 250 μg/day for adults and older children. The range for other age groups is derived through extrapolation on the basis of body weight.[15]

The molybdenum content of foods varies geographically. The foods that are the richest sources of molybdenum include milk, beans, breads, and cereals.

DIETARY GUIDES AND GUIDELINES

Diet guides and guidelines pick up where the RDAs leave off. The RDAs offer nutrient recommendations, but people eat *food* and can relate to, understand, and use rec-
ommendations only when given in a format that describes food. Dietary guides and guidelines are published by the U.S. government, by industry, and by health organizations. They are an excellent way of translating the science of nutritional requirements into practical information about food.

Food group plans help most with dietary adequacy, balance, and variety. The most popular and simple diet guides group foods into four food groups.

The Four Food Group Plan published by the National Dairy Council groups foods by similarity of origin and nutrient content. In fact, the Four Food Group Plan has been modified into a plan that consists of five groups: milk and milk products, breads and cereals, vegetables and fruits, meat and meat alternates, and miscellaneous[26] (see the box on p. 406).

One major assumption of the Four Food Group Plan is that as long as one consumes a variety of foods from all four major food groups, selects predominantly unprocessed foods, and consumes at least the minimum number of suggested servings, enough of all the essential nutrients will be consumed. This is not always a safe assumption; however, this food guide creates a good foundation for diet planning.

One of the drawbacks of the Four Food Group Plan is an inconsistency in fat and calorie values among the foods within the same group. For instance, milk, cheese, and ice cream are all grouped within milk and milk products, and servings are determined on the basis of calcium, riboflavin, protein, and vitamin B_{12} content, with no consideration for fat or calorie content. Therefore it may be very easy to overconsume fat and calories if one uses the Four Food Group Plan as the sole guide to diet planning. Another potential problem with this plan is that even if the rules are carefully followed, one can still fail to meet the day's needs for vitamin B_6, vitamin E, iron, magnesium, and zinc.

A second popular diet guide, the Exchange System, sorts foods and serving sizes by calories and proportions of carbohydrate, fat, and protein. The exchange system is based on six lists of foods: milk, vegetables, fruits, starches and breads, meat, and fat (see the box on p. 407 and Table 22-6). The meat and milk lists are subdivided into low-, medium-, and high-fat categories.[26]

Because foods are grouped by major nutrient content rather than outward similarities, some foods might not be where one might expect to find them. For example, potatoes are a starchy vegetable but are more similar to breads than to vegetables and are therefore grouped in the starch/bread list. Olives and bacon, which are very high in fat, are grouped as fats, rather than as vegetable and meat, as one might presume.

The term *exchange* is useful, because depending on the calorie and nutrient contents of the foods, certain foods can be "exchanged" for other foods within the selected diet

The four food group plan

Milk and milk products

Calcium, riboflavin, protein, vitamin B$_{12}$, (vitamin D and vitamin A, when fortified).

2 servings per day for adults.

3 servings per day for children.

4 servings per day for teenagers, pregnant/lactating women, women past menopause.

5 servings per day for pregnant/lactating teenagers.

Serving = 1 c milk or yogurt; ¼ c Parmesan cheese or process cheese spread; 2 c cottage cheese; 1½ c ice cream or ice milk; 2 oz process cheese food; 1⅓ oz cheese.
- Nonfat milk, buttermilk, low-fat milk, plain yogurt (lowest in kcalories).
- Whole milk, cheese, fruit-flavored yogurt, cottage cheese (moderate in kcalories).
- Custard, milk shakes, pudding, ice cream (highest in kcalories).

Breads and cereals

Riboflavin, thiamin, niacin, iron, protein, magnesium, folate, fiber.

4 servings per day.

Serving = 1 slice bread; ½ to ¾ c cooked cereals, rice, or pastas; 1 oz ready-to-eat cereals.
- Whole grains (wheat, oats, barley, millet, rye, bulgur) enriched breads, rolls, tortillas (lowest in kcalories).

- Rice, cereals, pastas (macaroni, spaghetti), bagels (moderate in kcalories).
- Pancakes, muffins, cornbread, biscuits, presweetened cereals (highest in kcalories).

Vegetables and fruits

Vitamin A, vitamin C, riboflavin, folate, iron, magnesium, low in fat, no cholesterol.

4 servings per day.

Serving = ½ c or typical portion (such as 1 medium apple, ½ grapefruit, or 1 wedge lettuce).
- Apricots, bean sprouts, broccoli, brussels sprouts, cabbage, cantaloupe, carrots, cauliflower, cucumbers, grapefruit, green beans, green peas, leafy greens (spinach, mustard, and collard greens), lettuce, mushrooms, oranges, orange juice, peaches, strawberries, tomatoes, winter squash (lowest in kcalories).

- Apples, bananas, canned fruit, corn, pears, potatoes (moderate in kcalories).
- Avocados, dried fruit, sweet potatoes (highest in kcalories).

Meat and meat alternates

Protein, phosphorus, vitamin B$_6$, vitamin B$_{12}$, zinc, magnesium, iron, niacin, thiamin.

2 servings per day for adults, children, teenagers.

3 servings per day for pregnant/lactating women/teenagers.

Serving = 2 to 3 oz lean, cooked meat, poultry, or fish; 1 oz meat, poultry, or fish = 1 egg, ½ to ¾ c legumes, 2 tbsp peanut butter, ¼ to ½ c nuts or seeds.

- Poultry, fish, lean meat (beef, lamb, pork), dried peas and beans, eggs (lowest in kcalories).
- Beef, lamb, pork, refried beans (moderate in kcalories).
- Hotdogs, luncheon meats, peanut butter, nuts (highest in kcalories).

Miscellaneous group

Sugar, fat (vitamin E), salt, alcohol, kcalories.

No serving sizes are provided because servings of these foods are not recommended. Concentrate on the four food groups that provide nutrients; the foods in the miscellaneous group will find their way into your diet as ingredients in prepared foods, or added at the table, or just as "extras." Note that some of the following items could be placed in more than one group or in a combination group. For example, potato chips are high in both salt and fat; doughnuts are high in both sugar and fat.

- Miscellaneous foods, not high in kcalories, include spices, herbs, coffee, tea, and diet soft drinks.
- Foods high in fat include margarine, salad dressing, oils, mayonnaise, cream, cream cheese, butter, gravy, and sauces (highest in kcalories).
- Foods high in salt include potato chips, corn chips, pretzels, pickles, olives, bouillon, prepared mustard, soy sauce, steak sauce, salt, and seasoned salt (highest in kcalories).
- Foods high in sugar include cake, pie, cookies, doughnuts, sweet rolls, candy, soft drinks, fruit drinks, jelly, syrup, gelatin desserts, sugar, and honey (highest in kcalories).
- Alcoholic beverages include wine, beer, and liquor (highest in kcalories).

Modified from Whitney EN, Hamilton EMN, Rolfes SR: *Understanding nutrition,* ed 5, St. Paul, Minn., 1990, West Publishing.

The exchange system

1. Starch/breads

1 slice bread is like:
¾ c ready-to-eat cereal.
⅓ c cooked beans.
½ c corn.
1 small (3 oz) potato.
(1 bread = 15 g carbohydrate, 3 g protein, trace of fat, and 80 kcal.)

2a. Meats (lean)

1 oz lean meat is like:
1 oz chicken meat without the skin.
1 oz any fish.
¼ c canned tuna.
1 oz low-fat cheese.*
(1 lean meat = 7 g protein, 3 g fat, and 55 kcal.)
(One 3-oz portion of meat (such as a hamburger patty) = 3 meat exchanges. One meat exchange = ⅓ of a 3-oz hamburger patty.)

2b. Meats (medium-fat)

1 oz medium-fat meat is like 1 oz lean meat in protein content, but has 5 g fat
(2 g more fat than lean meat).
Examples:
1 oz pork loin.
1 egg.
¼ cup creamed cottage cheese*
(1 medium-fat meat = 7 g protein, 5 g fat, and about 75 kcal.)

2c. Meats (high-fat)

1 oz high-fat meat is like 1 oz lean meat in protein content but is estimated to have an extra "1 fat"—that is, to have the 3 g fat of a lean meat and 5 g additional fat.
Examples:
1 oz country-style ham.
1 oz cheddar cheese.*
1 small hotdog (frankfurter).†
(1 high-fat meat = 7 g protein, 8 g fat, and 100 kcal.)

2d. Legumes

Legumes are an odd kind of plant food. They are like meats because they are rich in protein and iron, but many are lower in fat than meat. Besides, they contain a lot of starch. They can be treated as follows: 1 c legumes = 1 lean meat + 2 starch. (1 c legumes = 30 g carbohydrate, 13 g protein, 3+ g fat, and 215 kcal.) Legumes can also be considered similar to breads in being rich in complex carbohydrate, and the additional protein can be ignored. However, this treatment underestimates their kcalorie value, especially that of the higher-fat legumes such as peanuts.

Whatever you do with legumes on paper, however, use them often in cooking. You will learn many more reasons why they are an inexpensive, nutritious, high-quality, and health-promoting food.

2e. Peanut butter

Peanut butter is like a meat in terms of its protein content. It is estimated as:
1 tbsp peanut butter = 1 high-fat meat (1 tbsp peanut butter = 7 g protein, 8 g fat, and 100 kcal.)

3. Vegetables

½ c carrots is like:
½ c greens.
½ c brussels sprouts.
½ c beets.
(1 vegetable = 5 g carbohydrate, 2 g protein, and 25 kcal.)

4. Fruits

½ small banana is like:
1 small apple
½ grapefruit.
½ c orange juice.
(1 fruit = 15 g carbohydrate and 60 kcal.)

5. Milks

1 c nonfat milk is like:
1 c nonfat yogurt, plain.
1 c nonfat buttermilk.
½ c evaporated nonfat milk.
(1 milk = 12 g carbohydrate, 8 g protein, trace of fat, and 90 kcal.)

6. Fats

1 tsp butter is like:
1 tsp margarine.
1 tsp any oil.
1 tbsp salad dressing.
1 strip crisp bacon.
5 large olives.
10 whole Virginia peanuts.
(1 fat = 5 g fat and 45 kcal.)

Modified from Whitney EN, Hamilton EMN, Rolfes SR: *Understanding nutrition,* ed 5, St. Paul, Minn., 1990, West Publishing.
*Cheeses are grouped with milk in food group plans because of their calcium content but with meats in this system because, like meat, they contribute kcalories from protein and fat and have negligible carbohydrate content.
†The frankfurter counts as 1 high-fat meat exchange plus 1 fat exchange.

Table 22-6. The six exchange lists

List	Portion size	Carbohydrate (g)	Protein (g)	Fat (g)	Energy (kcal)
Starch/bread*	1 slice	15	3	Trace	80
Meat†	1 oz				
Lean		—	7	3	55
Medium-fat		—	7	5	75
High-fat		—	7	8	100
Vegetable‡	½ c	5	2	—	25
Fruit	1 portion	15	—	—	60
Milk	1 c				
Nonfat		12	8	Trace	90
Low-fat		12	8	5	120
Whole		12	8	8	150
Fat	1 tsp	—	—	5	45

From Whitney EN, Hamilton EMN, and Rolfes SR: *Understanding Nutrition,* ed 5, St Paul, Minn, 1990, West Publishing.
NOTE: This is the U.S. exchange system.
*This list includes starchy vegetables such as lima beans and corn, as well as cereal, bread, pasta, and other grain products.
†This list includes cheese and peanut butter as well as meat.
‡This list includes low-kcalorie vegetables only.

Table 22-7. Diet planning with the exchange system using the Four Food Group Pattern

Pattern from four food group plan	Selections made using the exchange system	Example	Energy cost (kcal)
Milk—2 c	Milk list—select 2 exchanges	2 c nonfat milk	180
Meat—2 servings (2 to 3 oz each)	Meat list—select 6 exchanges*	6 oz lean meat	330
Fruits and vegetables—4 servings	Fruit and vegetable lists—select 4 exchanges	2 vegetable exchanges;	50
		2 fruit exchanges	120
Grains (breads and cereals)—4 servings	Starch/bread list—select 4 exchanges	2 bread exchanges; 2 starchy vegetable exchanges	320
Total			1000

*In the Four Food Group Plan, one serving is 2 to 3 oz. In the exchange system, one exchange is 1 oz.
From Whitney EN, Hamilton EMN, and Rolfes SR: *Understanding Nutrition,* ed 5, St Paul, Minn, 1990, West Publishing.

guide pattern. For example, if an individual's diet pattern calls for nonfat milk from the milk group, and three fat exchanges are allowed from the fat group, then lowfat milk can still fit into this pattern because it is counted as one nonfat milk and one fat exchange. The exchange system is therefore helpful in assisting with calorie and fat balance, but because the amounts of vitamin and minerals may vary greatly among the foods within one exchange, the user must choose a variety of foods from all of the exchanges to achieve nutritional adequacy.

Numbers of servings are not suggested as part of the exchange system. Exchange servings must be computed in accordance with individual calorie and fat intake goals (Table 22-7). By combining the Four Food Group Plan as the basic pattern and the Exchange System as the list for choosing foods, one can design a diet that promotes both nutritional adequacy and balance.

The diet guides discussed above primarily emphasize

the prevention of nutritional deficiency. More recently, this focus has changed to chronic disease prevention and health promotion. Dietary guidelines for the general public have been published by government agencies and other health organizations to help guide the public into more healthful dietary choices. Limits on the dietary intake of calories, fat, cholesterol, sugar, salt, fiber, and alcohol have been suggested as part of a campaign to decrease the nation's risk of many chronic illnesses, including heart disease, cancer, diabetes, and liver disease (see the box on p. 409).

The final numbers of servings from the exchange lists therefore should conform with some predetermined amount of calories, fat, cholesterol, sugar, salt, fiber, and alcohol desired in the diet, and follow the basic Four Food Group Plan to achieve nutritional adequacy. Dietary guideline goals can assist with the determination of the amounts and types of fat, sugar, fiber, and alcohol (Tables 22-8 and 22-9).

Dietary guidelines for Americans

1. Eat a variety of foods
2. Maintain healthy weight
3. Choose a diet low in fat, saturated fat, and cholesterol
4. Choose a diet with plenty of vegetables, fruits, and grain products
5. Use sugars only in moderation
6. Use salt and sodium only in moderation
7. If you drink alcoholic beverages, do so in moderation

From *Dietary Guidelines for Americans*, ed 3, USDA, USDHHS, 1990.

Table 22-8. A sample diet plan

Exchange	Energy (kcal)*
7 starch/bread	560
6 medium-fat meat	450
2 vegetable	50
3 fruit	180
2 nonfat milk	180
4 fat	180
	1600

From Whitney EN, Hamilton EMN, and Rolfes SR: *Understanding Nutrition*, ed 5, St Paul, Minn, 1990, West Publishing.
*This diet derives about 20% of its kcalories from protein, about 30% from fat, and nearly 50% from carbohydrate.

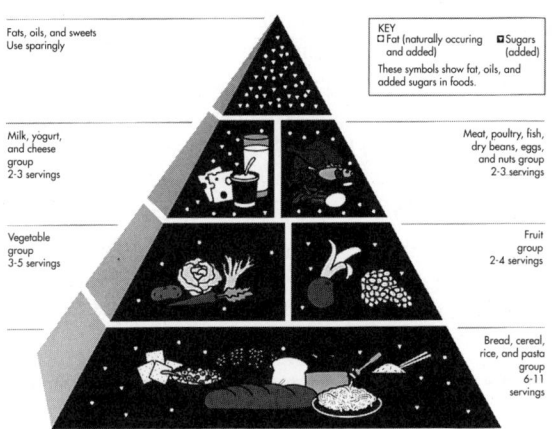

Food Guide Pyramid
A Guide to Daily Food Choices

Fig. 22-1. Food Guide Pyramid. From USDA/DHHS, US Department of Agriculture and US Department of Health and Human Services.

Table 22-9. Diet patterns for different energy intakes

	Energy level (kcal)*						
Exchange	1200	1500	1800	2000	2200	2600	3000
Starch/bread	4	6	8	9	11	13	15
Meat	5	5	5	6	6	7	8
Vegetable	3	3	4	5	5	6	6
Fruit	3	3	4	4	4	5	6
Milk	2	3	3	3	3	3	3
Fat	4	5	6	7	8	10	12

From Whitney EN, Hamilton EMN, and Rolfes SR: *Understanding Nutrition*, ed 5, St Paul, Minn, 1990, West Publishing.
*These patterns of exchanges supply about 30% of the kcalories as fat, in accordance with the view that a moderate fat intake is desirable.

The USDA has adopted a food pyramid to visually rank the kinds of food that Americans should eat daily for health promotion and disease prevention. The pyramid emphasizes the need to eat more fruits, vegetables, and grains, and less fat and sugar (Fig. 22-1).[26]

Breads and grains make up the foundation of the pyramid with 6 to 11 servings suggested daily. Vegetables (3 to 5 servings) and fruits (2 to 4 servings) share the next layer. The next highest level is the milk group and the protein foods group (2 to 3 servings each). The smallest top layer symbolizes fats, oils, and sweets, with instructions to "use sparingly."

REFERENCES

1. Avioli LV: Calcium and phosphorus. In Shils ME, Young VR, editors: *Modern nutrition in health and disease,* ed 7, Philadelphia, 1988, Lea & Febiger.
2. Cochrane WA: Symposium on nutrition. Overnutrition in prenatal and neonatal life: a problem? *Can Med Assoc J* 93:893, 1965.
3. DeLuca HF: Vitamin D and its metabolites. In Shils ME, Young VR, editors: *Modern nutrition in health and disease,* ed 7, Philadelphia, 1988, Lea & Febiger.
4. Farrell PM: Vitamin E. In Shils ME, Young VR, editors: *Modern nutrition in health and disease,* ed 7, Philadelphia, 1988, Lea & Febiger.
5. Gorman MA, Bowman C: Position of the American Dietetic Association: health implications of dietary fiber, *J Am Dietet Assoc* 88(2):216-221, 1988.
6. Hathcock JN: Quantitive evaluation of vitamin safety, *Pharm Times* 51:104-113, 1985.
7. Herbert VD, Colman N: Folic acid and vitamin B_{12}. In Shils ME, Young VR, editors: *Modern nutrition in health and disease,* ed 7, Philadelphia, 1988, Lea & Febiger.
8. Hornig DH, Moser U, Glatthaar BE: Ascorbic acid. In Shils ME, Young VR, editors: *Modern nutrition in health and disease,* ed 7, Philadelphia, 1988, Lea & Febiger.
9. McCollum EV: *A history of nutrition,* Boston, Mass, 1957, Houghton Mifflin.
10. McCormick DB: Biotin. In Shils ME, Young VR, editors: *Modern nutrition in health and disease,* ed 7, Philadelphia, 1988, Lea & Febiger.
11. McCormick DB: Niacin. In Shils ME, Young VR, editors: *Modern nutrition in health and disease,* ed 7, Philadelphia, 1988, Lea & Febiger.
12. McCormick DB: Riboflavin. In Shils ME, Young VR, editors: *Modern nutrition in health and disease,* ed 7, Philadelphia, 1988, Lea & Febiger.

13. McCormick DB: Thiamin. In Shils ME, Young VR, editors: *Modern nutrition in health and disease,* ed 7, Philadelphia, 1988, Lea & Febiger.
14. McCormick DB: Vitamin B$_6$. In Shils ME, Young VR, editors: *Modern nutrition in health and disease,* ed 7, Philadelphia, 1988, Lea & Febiger.
15. NAS/NRC Subcommittee on the Tenth Edition of the RDAs: *Recommended dietary allowances,* ed 10, Washington, DC, 1989, National Academy Press.
16. National Academy of Science, National Research Council, Food and Nutrition Board: *Diet and health. Implications for reducing chronic disease risk,* Washington, DC, 1989, National Academy Press.
17. National Academy of Science, National Research Council, Food and Nutrition Board: *Recommended dietary allowances,* ed 10, Washington, DC, 1989, National Academy Press.
18. National Institutes of Health: Osteoporosis, consensus development conference statement, 5(3), 1984.
19. Reference deleted in proofs.
20. Oldon RE: Vitamin K. In Shils ME, Young VR, editors: *Modern nutrition in health and disease,* ed 7, Philadelphia, 1988, Lea & Febiger.
21. Olson JA: Vitamin A, retinoids, and carotenoids. In Shils ME, Young VR, editors: *Modern nutrition in health and disease,* ed 7, Philadelphia, 1988, Lea & Febiger.
22. Shils ME: Magnesium. In Shils ME, Young VR, editors: *Modern nutrition in health and disease,* ed 7, Philadelphia, 1988, Lea & Febiger.
23. Sommer A: *Nutritional blindness.* Oxford, 1982, Oxford University Press.
24. USDA/DHHS Human Nutrition Information Service: *Food guide pyramid,* Hyattsville, Maryland.
25. US Department of Health and Human Services, Public Health Service: *The Surgeon General's report on nutrition and health,* Washington, DC, 1988, DHHS (PHS) Publication No. 88-50210.
26. Whitney EN, Hamilton EMN, and Rolfes SR: *Understanding Nutrition,* ed 5, St Paul, Minn, 1990, West Publishing.

RESOURCES

American Dietetic Association, 216 W. Jackson Blvd., Chicago, IL 60606.

The American College of Nutrition, 722 Robert E. Lee Drive, Wilmington, NC 28412.

Executive Health's Good Health Report, newsletter, P.O. Box 8880, Chapel Hill, NC 27515.

Food & Nutrition News, newsletter, National Livestock and Meat Board, 444 N Michigan Ave., Chicago, IL 60611.

Guide to Good Eating. The Four Food Groups, ed 5, 1989. National Dairy Council, Rosemont, IL 60018-4233.

NAS/NRC Subcommittee on the Tenth Edition of the RDAs: *Recommended dietary allowances,* ed 10, Washington, DC, 1989, National Academy Press.

National Center for Nutrition and Dietetics, toll-free consumer nutrition hotline, (800) 366-1655.

Nutrition & the M.D., newsletter, PM, Inc, 14545 Friar, #209, Van Nuys, CA 91411.

Nutrition and your health: dietary guidelines for Americans, ed 3, USDA, USDHHS, 1990.

Shils ME, Young VR, editors: *Modern nutrition in health and disease,* ed 7, Philadelphia, 1988, Lea & Febiger.

USDA Human Nutrition Information Service, 6505 Belcrest Rd. Hyattsville, MD 20782.

Chapter 23

SPECIAL NUTRITIONAL NEEDS THROUGH THE LIFE CYCLE

Susan M. Kleiner
Karen-Rae Friedman-Kester

Human growth, development, and health maintenance require attention to diet and nutrition. Although the nutrients that are needed remain the same throughout the life cycle, the amounts that are needed change, depending on the life stage. Health maintenance and disease prevention are the primary goals throughout life, but each stage of the life cycle presents a distinct set of nutritional priorities. As we age, disease management may impact significantly on nutritional requirements and dietary planning.

MATERNAL AND INFANT NUTRITION

The factors most closely associated with maternal health and birth risk and outcome are genetic, environmental, behavioral, and nutritional. Although the exact contribution of nutrition cannot be distinguished from the other factors, it is clear that an inadequate diet during pregnancy increases the probability of a low birth weight infant, who then has an increased risk of morbidity and mortality.[44]

The infant mortality rate (the number of deaths of infants below 1 year of age per 1000 live births) in the United States in 1985 was 10.6[29]; it was only marginally better in 1986, at 10.4.[44] Although rates among countries are not strictly comparable because of differences in definitions, the rates in several industrialized countries are considerably lower than in the United States. In 1983 the infant mortality rate in Finland was 6.5, and in the same year it was 6.6 in Japan.[44]

Among the subgroups in the United States black Americans have the highest rate of infant mortality: twice the rate of white Americans. In 1985 the rate of infant mortality was 18.2 among black, compared to 9.3 among white, Americans.[44]

Low birth weight (LBW), defined as less than 2500 g, or 5.5 lb, is the single most important factor contributing to the U.S. infant mortality rate. In 1985 LBW babies accounted for 6.8% of all births in the United States, 67% of all infant deaths during the first month of life, and 60% of all infant deaths.[44]

Medical, social, behavioral, and dietary factors are associated with an increased risk of LBW. Maternal characteristics associated with risk of LBW include many previous pregnancies, previous LBW delivery, anemia, hypertensive disorders of pregnancy, chronic illness, low prepregnancy weight, short stature, low gestational weight gain, and low caloric intake during pregnancy. Low socioeconomic status, low educational level, minority race, single marital status, adolescence, inadequate prenatal care, and use of drugs, alcohol, or cigarettes have also been identified as LBW risk factors.[44,45]

Dietary risk factors include an inadequate intake of calories or essential nutrients, such as protein, vitamins, and minerals. The greater the number of risk factors, the greater the risk to mother and child.[44]

Since the 1940s it has been well documented that the mother's nutritional state before and at the time of conception and the adequacy of her diet during pregnancy influence the well-being of the infant.[44] The diet of a lactating mother continues to influence her child's health for as long as she nurses the child. The nutritional adequacy of the diets of all pregnant women should be assessed. Women should be educated regarding the importance of diet and pregnancy outcome and encouraged to follow healthy dietary guidelines for pregnancy. Dietary counseling should be available to those women who need extra support.

Clearly, those women at greater risk, such as adolescents, should be counseled and monitored regularly for the nutritional adequacy of their diets.

Nutrient requirements and dietary allowances of adult and adolescent pregnancy

While a woman is pregnant, she must consume the basic nutrient requirements to maintain her own body tissues and functions. Nutrients must also be supplied for the growth of new tissue of the placenta and fetus and of the reproductive tissues that support pregnancy and prepare for lactation. Approximately one third of the total weight gain during pregnancy is accounted for by increases in blood volume and total body water. These tissue increases have a high requirement for protein, minerals, and electrolytes. Metabolic demands are increased by the formation and maintenance of new tissue and the increased energy demands of movement. As part of pregnancy and preparation for lactation, additional fat and protein are stored in the woman's body. The increase in nutrient demands during pregnancy versus the nonpregnant state is not equal for all nutrients but is specific to each nutrient in relation to its functions and to the timing of each of the growth phases for which it is essential.[4]

Energy. The World Health Organization and the Committee for Recommended Dietary Allowances (RDA) of the National Research Council have estimated energy allowances for pregnancy on the basis of the total estimated energy cost of pregnancy. For a full-term pregnancy, during which the mother has gained 12.5 kg (27.5 lb) and has given birth to a 3.3 kg (7.3 lb) baby, total energy cost has been estimated to be 80,000 kcal. To establish a daily energy cost of pregnancy, the gross energy cost (80,000 kcal) is divided by the approximate duration of pregnancy (250 days after the first month), yielding a rounded average value of 300 kcal/day for the entire pregnancy.[33]

A greater energy allowance is provided for the adolescent than the adult woman (see RDA table, Chapter 22). The pregnant adolescent must meet her own energy requirements for growth, as well as her gestational growth requirements. A woman who is underweight before pregnancy or who has high physical activity demands should also consume a greater number of calories.

Food restriction and weight reduction diets are absolutely not recommended during pregnancy. The incidence of LBW infants is higher among women whose weight gain is low. Adequate use of nitrogen may be imperiled if caloric intake falls below 36 kcal/kg of pregnant weight, since adequate energy is required for the sparing of protein and efficient use of nitrogen.[35]

Protein. Additional protein is required during pregnancy to support the growth needs of the mother and the fetus. The exact magnitude of the required increase in dietary protein remains uncertain, since different methods of estimation yield different results. Epidemiologic studies of the diets of pregnant women in developed countries indicate that their self-selected diets are generally somewhat higher in protein than the theoretical requirements.[32]

It is generally assumed that dietary protein is converted to fetal, placental, and maternal tissue at 70% efficiency. An additional allowance of reference protein needed to support the deposition of new tissue is calculated to be 1.3, 6.1, and 10.7 g/day during the first, second, and third trimesters of pregnancy, respectively. A maintenance requirement is also associated with the added lean tissue. To allow for this, as well as the uncertainty about the rate of tissue deposition, the RDA subcommittee recommends 10 g of protein per day, in addition to the mother's pregravid allowance, throughout pregnancy.[32]

This recommendation is based on an adequate energy intake. Adolescent and pregravid underweight women should be strongly encouraged to consume adequate calories in order to spare their use of protein for nitrogen, rather than energy needs.

Vitamins

Folate. The functions of folate in DNA synthesis and in erythrocyte maturation are particularly important during pregnancy, and folate is the only nutrient for which the RDA during pregnancy is twice the nonpregnancy allowance. Pregnancy increases the incidence of folate deficiency among populations with low or marginal intakes of the vitamin.[32]

The most controversial subject related to dietary folate and pregnancy outcome is the cause of neural tube defects. Early investigations observed the possibility that folic acid might be involved in the causation of neural tube defects.[19] Two intervention studies followed, in which vitamin supplementation around the time of conception was given to women who had had a pregnancy with a neural tube defect.[43,25] These studies suggested that folic acid or other vitamin supplementation might reduce the risk of a recurrence, but both studies were fraught with design problems.

In 1991 the report of a randomized double-blind prevention trial to determine whether supplementation with folic acid or a mixture of seven other vitamins (A, D, B_1, B_2, B_6, C, nicotinamide) around the time of conception can prevent neural tube defects was published. The study used a factorial design, was conducted at 33 centers in seven countries, and followed 1817 women at high risk of having a pregnancy with a neural tube defect, because of a previous affected pregnancy. The women were randomized into four groups: folic acid, other vitamins, both, or neither. Folate supplement capsules contained 4 mg folic acid, and multivitamin capsules contained 4000 IU vitamin A, 400 IU vitamin D, 1.5 mg B_1, 1.5 mg B_2, 1.0 mg B_6, 40 mg C, and 15 mg nicotinamide. Matched placebo capsules were used for the nonsupplemented group. Supplementation was given until 12 weeks of pregnancy.[28]

In 1195 women with completed pregnancies the fetus or

infant was known to have or not have a neural tube defect. Twenty-seven of these had a known neural tube defect, 6 in the folic acid groups and 21 in the two other groups, a 72% protective effect (relative risk 0.28, 95% confidence interval 0.12 to 0.71). The other vitamins showed no significant protective effect, and no detectable adverse effects were noted in the supplemented groups.[28]

The authors suggest that their results pertain particularly to women at high risk of neural tube defects. However, they also suggest that there is no reason to believe if folic acid causes the defect, that the preventive effect of folic acid supplementation is restricted to this group.

Several unanswered questions are raised in this study. There was no difference between the initial folate nutriture of the women with poor versus good pregnancy outcomes. Studies of women in the United Kingdom, where one of the highest rates of neural tube defects exists, do not indicate that they are unusually deficient in folic acid. And finally, although the study may have established a basis for folic acid supplementation of women who have had a previously affected pregnancy, the supplement dosage has not been determined.[28]

The RDA for pregnant women is set at 400 μg/day on the basis of a 50% food folate absorption. The RDA subcommittee states, "This level can be met by a well-selected diet without food fortification or oral supplementation."[32]

All women do not consume a well-selected diet. Foods high in folacin include liver, dark-green leafy vegetables, dry beans, peanuts, wheat germ, and whole grains. In the face of a limited dietary supply of folate, supplementation for women planning a pregnancy and during the first trimester may be an appropriate prophylactic measure. Supplements in the recommended dose of 200 to 400 μg/day have been suggested by the Committee on Nutrition of the American College of Obstetricians and Gynecologists[4]; supplements of 400 μg/day are advocated by the 1980 RDA subcommittee.[31] Supplementation is clearly justified in instances of low intake or for women who have unusually high requirements, such as those carrying twins and pregnant adolescents. Women with a history of long-term use of oral contraceptive agents should receive careful assessment of folic acid status.[46]

Excessive intakes of folic acid inhibit uptake of the anticonvulsant drug phenytoin at the gut cell membrane and possibly at the brain membrane. In laboratory animals large folic acid doses may produce kidney damage and hypertrophy. Toxic effects have not been reported in women given 10 mg/day of folic acid continuously for 4 months.[32]

Folate status may be assessed by dietary analysis (see Chapter 25) and measurements of serum and erythrocyte folate levels. Evidence of defective DNA synthesis is seen as hypersegmentation of cells and abnormality in the sensitive deoxyuridine (dU) suppression test. Overtly megalo-blastic bone marrow and macrocytic anemia are late consequences of folate deficiency.[32]

Vitamin B$_{12}$. Megaloblastic anemia during pregnancy is most often due to folacin deficiency, but deficiency of vitamin B$_{12}$ must be ruled out. Both vitamins are required for cell division.

There is generally little concern about meeting the recommendations for dietary B$_{12}$, as long as the diet contains animal products. Maternal body stores are normally sufficient to meet the needs of pregnancy. The RDA subcommittee recommends a slight increment of 0.2 μg/day of B$_{12}$ above the pregravid allowance, for an RDA of 2.2 μg/day.[32] Strict vegans, who consume no animal products, will be unable to meet the RDA, and their diets should be supplemented.

Vitamin B$_6$. The need for vitamin B$_6$ increases with the increased requirement for protein during pregnancy. The RDA for vitamin B$_6$ increases by 0.6 mg/day for pregnant versus nonpregnant women, for an RDA of 2.2 mg/day. The requirement for pregnant adolescents is increased to meet their own growth demands, as well as that of the growing fetal and maternal tissues. Some studies have indicated a possible link between maternal nausea and vomiting, and vitamin B$_6$ status. However, a clear connection remains to be observed, and additional research is necessary before any conclusions may be drawn.[4,46] Another area of investigation is that many biochemical parameters associated with vitamin B$_6$ metabolism are altered with the use of oral contraceptives. Special attention may be needed by women who have used oral contraceptives for an extended period without sufficient time for normalization of B$_6$ metabolism before conception.[4]

Vitamin A. Vitamin A and carotene cross the placenta. Although some subgroups of society do not consume adequate vitamin A, there is no increased RDA for pregnant women. Women who eat an adequate diet do not require any vitamin A supplementation.

The recent concern with vitamin A in the United States is more a matter of toxicity than of deficiency. Vitamin A and its analogs are teratogens. The introduction of isotretinoin (Accutane), a vitamin A analog, for the treatment of cystic acne, has been associated with many cases of birth defects and spontaneous abortions.[46] Extreme caution should be used in recommending this drug to a woman during her reproductive years.

Other vitamins. Small increases in the RDAs for pregnancy are suggested for vitamins D, E, C, thiamin, riboflavin, and niacin (see RDA table in Chapter 22). Pregnant adolescents may require greater increments, especially of the B vitamins, to meet growth requirements. Little is known about the dietary requirements for vitamin K, biotin, and pantothenic acid, especially during pregnancy. No increases in the RDA for vitamin K, or for the estimated safe and adequate daily dietary intake range for biotin or pantothenic acid are suggested for pregnant women.

Megadosing of vitamins during pregnancy should be strongly discouraged. Several vitamins, including water soluble vitamins, can cause toxic effects on the developing fetus. In large doses the vitamins have pharmacologic effects that can be detrimental to the growing tissues. For instance cases of "conditioned infantile scurvy" have been reported in the infants of women who supplemented their vitamin C intake during pregnancy at a level of approximately 400 mg daily. The infants appear to have been born conditioned to a larger vitamin C requirement than normal. When these greater requirements were not met, the infants developed the classic signs of scurvy.[7]

Minerals

Calcium and phosphorus. The calcium recommendation during pregnancy is increased 50% above the nonpregnant RDA, to 1200 mg/day.[32] The fetus acquires its calcium during the last trimester of pregnancy, when skeletal growth is maximal and teeth are being formed. Additional calcium is stored in the maternal skeleton as a reserve for lactation.[46]

Although the absolute amount of calcium required for successful pregnancy outcome is significantly smaller than the RDA increase and calcium is not used by the fetus until the third trimester, studies suggest that maternal retention begins early in pregnancy for later use by the fetus.[4] Also, balance studies suggest that if maternal intake of calcium is low, then stores of calcium will be depleted to meet fetal needs. These two factors support an increased calcium recommendation. This increase is even more critical in cases of frequent pregnancies and consistently low calcium intakes.

The calcium absorption rate has been reported to increase during adolescent pregnancy.[32] Although the RDA subcommittee does not recommend an additional increment in calcium allowance for pregnant adolescents, it is possible that they may have greater calcium requirements. The RDA for women less than 24 years old is 1200 mg/day.[32] It may be prudent to increase the calcium recommendation for adolescents to cover the needs of increasing maternal bone mass, as well as gestational requirements.

Clearly it is essential that dietary calcium nutrition be assessed in all women, since few women consume even 800 mg of calcium on a daily basis.[32] Dietary supplementation should be considered for those women unable to meet their needs through diet.

Phosphorus is an essential component of bone mineral. It occurs in the bone mass at a ratio with calcium of one part phosphorus to two parts calcium. Calcium-phosphorus balance relates to maintenance of normal neuromuscular action. The pregnancy RDA for phosphorus is 1200 mg/day, set to provide a calcium-phosphorus ratio of 1.[32]

Dietary phosphorus can affect the metabolism of, and requirement for, calcium. A high dietary phosphorus intake increases fractional reabsorption of calcium and causes urinary calcium to decrease. The U.S. diet is generally high in phosphorus, because of its wide availability in meats, processed foods, and soft drinks. Animal studies have indicated that excessive phosphorus intake led to secondary hyperparathyroidism, resulting in loss of calcium from the skeleton. This has not been shown in humans when adequate levels of dietary calcium are consumed.[32]

Magnesium. The pregnancy RDA for magnesium, 320 mg/day, is slightly increased over the nonpregnant allowance (280 mg/day). However, this value is based solely on the amount of magnesium accumulated by the mother and fetus during pregnancy.[32] There is an incomplete understanding of the role of magnesium during pregnancy.[46]

Dietary surveys indicate that magnesium intakes of some segments of the population are lower than current recommendations. However, biochemical measures are not yet available to measure magnesium status equivocally. Therefore there is no unequivocal evidence that magnesium deficiency is a problem among healthy Americans.[32]

Less magnesium is available in the U.S. diet today. Generally good food sources include green vegetables, nuts, seeds, dried beans, whole grains, and meats. The decline in magnesium availability is due to the decreased use and refinement of grains and flour.[30] The magnesium nutriture of pregnant women should be assessed. Women should be encouraged to consume plenty of whole grains, as well as the other foods indicated. If magnesium intake is inadequate, supplementation should be considered.

Iron. The pregnancy RDA for iron (30 mg/day) is double the nonpregnant allowance (15 mg/day). During pregnancy iron is used to replace the usual basal losses, to allow expansion of the red cell mass, to provide iron to the fetus and placenta, and to replace blood loss during delivery.[32]

The fetus accumulates most of its iron during the last trimester. At this time the fetus acts as a true parasite and draws on mother's iron in spite of her own nutritional status. Therefore maternal iron deficiency does not usually cause an infant to be born anemic.[46] Iron deficiency anemia can place the mother at risk and should be prevented.

Maternal iron status should be monitored regularly, and biochemical values compared to reference standards for pregnant women. The increased iron requirement for pregnancy can rarely be met by the normal U.S. diet. Daily iron supplementation is usually recommended throughout the course of pregnancy.[32]

Sodium. Increased fluid retention is normal during pregnancy. Restriction of dietary sodium has been common in pregnant women in the past to control edema, but moderate edema is normal during pregnancy and should not be treated with diuretics and low-sodium diets. Sodium restriction stresses the renin-angiotensin-aldosterone mechanism in order to maintain homeostasis.[4] Neonatal hyponatremia has been observed in the newborns of women who have unduly restricted their sodium intake before delivery.[46] Certainly a moderation of the usually high sodium intake representative of the normal American diet may be prudent, but no less than 2 to 3 g of sodium (5 to 7.5 g or 1 to 1.5 teaspoons of salt) should be consumed daily.[46]

Other minerals. The present state of knowledge of many of the trace minerals makes it clear that they are integrally involved in growth, health maintenance, and reproduction, but we do not yet have enough data to set recommended allowances for many of these nutrients during pregnancy. There is a small incremental pregnancy RDA for zinc, iodine, and selenium. Estimated safe and adequate daily dietary intake ranges have been suggested by the RDA subcommittee for copper, manganese, fluoride, chromium, and molybdenum (see RDA table in Chapter 22).

It is important to assess the diets of pregnant women not only for consumption of foods from all food groups but also for variety of types of foods within each category. Consumption of whole grains, beans, green and yellow vegetables, and a variety of fruits will help ensure an adequate intake of trace minerals. Since toxic levels of many of the trace elements may not be much higher than usual intakes, pregnant women should not take supplements that would greatly exceed the upper limits recommended.[46]

Practical tips for increasing dietary nutrients

Even if a woman's pregravid diet has been healthy, increases in certain specific foods are required during pregnancy. In order to meet the necessary minimum caloric and nutrient needs easy food combinations to add to the diet are 8 oz skim milk, 1 whole wheat bagel, and two fruits; or 1 cup lowfat yogurt, 1 baked potato, and 1 fruit. Other combinations can be designed by using Table 23-1.

Table 23-1. Food guide for pregnant and lactating women

Food groups	Recommended daily intake (number of servings)	Serving content
Milk and milk products —Calcium, riboflavin protein, B_{12}, and D and A when fortified	4 a day for women 5 a day for adolescents Low-fat products	1 C milk/yogurt 2 C cottage cheese 1⅓ oz cheese
Breads and cereals —Riboflavin, thiamin, niacin, iron, protein, magnesium, folate, fiber	6-11 a day whole grain or enriched	1 slice bread ½ C cooked cereal, rice, or pastas 1 oz ready-to-eat cereal
Vegetables —Vitamin A, folic acid, riboflavin, iron, magnesium, fiber	3-5 a day green and yellow starchy and all others	½ C cooked or chopped raw 1 C leafy raw
Fruits —Vitamin C, vitamin A fiber	2-4 a day citrus, melons, berries, all others	1 whole; ½ C juice ¼ melon ½ grapefruit ½ C cooked/canned ¼ C dried
Meat and meat alternates —Protein, phosphorus, vitamin B_6, B_{12}, zinc, magnesium, iron, niacin, thiamin	3 a day lean meat, poultry, fish, shellfish, and vegetable protein sources	2-3 oz lean cooked 2 eggs; 4 egg whites 1 C cooked dried beans or peas 2 tbsp peanut butter
Fats —Vitamin A, vitamin E	3-6 a day Unsaturated vegetable oils salad dressings, spreads, nuts; as needed for calories	1 tsp spreads 1 tsp vegetable oils 1 tbsp salad dressing 1 oz nuts
Sweets —Energy	Consume in moderation as needed for calories	
Alcohol —Energy	Not recommended	
Water	8 or more glasses/day 2-3 L during lactation	

Modified from National Research Council: *Diet and health, implications for reducing chronic risk,* Washington, DC, 1989, National Academy Press.

Safe food practices for pregnant women

Alcohol. The adverse effects of excessive alcohol consumption on fetal development have been well documented. The fetal alcohol syndrome (FAS) is manifested by specific anomalies of the eyes, nose, heart, and central nervous system, accompanied by growth retardation, small head circumference, and mental retardation. FAS babies have a high rate of infant mortality. The children who survive are generally permanently disabled.[46]

It is now recognized that moderate alcohol drinking during pregnancy may cause offspring to have "fetal alcohol effects." These infants show more subtle features of FAS, and women experience higher rates of spontaneous abortion, abruptio placentae, and low birth weight delivery.[46]

Light drinking has also been associated with poor pregnancy outcome, particularly birth of LBW infants. In a large prospective study of 31,604 pregnancies the percentage of newborns below the 10th percentile of weight for gestational age increased sharply with increasing alcohol intake. After adjustment for other risks a reduction in mean birth weight was seen in drinkers compared with nondrinkers. In this cohort only women consuming less than one drink each day avoided a clinically significant increased risk for producing a growth-retarded infant.[27]

Because a safe level of alcohol intake has not been established, and consumption of empty calories from alcohol may replace intake of important nutrient-dense calories from other foods, the Surgeon General recommends that pregnant women avoid alcohol entirely.[45]

Caffeine. Caffeine crosses the placenta and reaches the fetus. In large doses it has been shown to be teratogenic in animal studies, but there is no clear epidemiologic evidence of similar effects in humans. Results of studies of humans and the effect of caffeine consumption on birth defects have been equivocal. Although the data do not provide significant evidence that caffeine affects pregnancy outcome, the Food and Drug Administration advises pregnant women to eliminate or limit consumption of caffeine-containing products as a precautionary measure.[44]

Artificial and nonnutritive sweeteners. These products are generally contraindicated during pregnancy. Because saccharin has been shown to be carcinogenic in rats, its use during pregnancy is not advisable. Studies of aspartame (Nutrasweet) have not shown evidence of risk to human fetuses, and aspartame does not readily cross the placental barrier. However studies have not thoroughly considered the potential effects of very high intakes of aspartame. This potential exists because of its availability in a multitude of food products, ranging from soft drinks to yogurt. Because limited data are available, it is prudent that use of aspartame be limited during pregnancy.[46]

Acesulfame K (Sunette or Sweet One), was approved by the FDA in 1988 as a sugar substitute in packet or tablet form and in a variety of food products. The Center for Science in the Public Interest claims that this additive is inadequately tested and should be avoided. A safety ruling by the FDA is pending.[20]

During pregnancy the safest recommendation for sweetening foods and beverages is the use of sugar or other natural sweeteners such as honey or molasses. Because these sweeteners offer little other than pure carbohydrate calories, their use should be moderated so as not to substitute for other important nutrient-dense calories in the diet. However, used moderately, these natural sweeteners add very few calories and much variety to the pregnant woman's diet:

1 tsp sugar, white granulated	= 15 cal
1 tsp honey	= 21 cal
1 tsp molasses, light	= 17 cal
1 tsp maple syrup	= 17 cal

Other issues

Vegetarian food patterns. Many levels of animal food consumption are labeled as "vegetarian." If the food plan excludes only red meat, all meats and poultry, or all meats, poultry, and fish, ample primary protein and other nutrients may still be obtained from dairy foods and eggs (lactoovovegetarian). Emphasis should be placed on the use of low-fat dairy products, egg whites, and vegetable protein sources, such as dried beans and peas combined with grains or dairy foods. Iron nutriture should be stressed, especially if the woman also restricts eggs in her diet (lactovegetarian).

Vegans, or strict vegetarians who include no animal products in their diets, can still consume adequate protein for successful pregnancy outcome, but careful menu planning is required. Proteins must be complemented to obtain an adequate amount of essential amino acids, and the number of protein servings for meat and meat alternates group should be closely followed (see box).

Because dairy products are not included in the vegan diet pattern, calcium and vitamin B_{12} may have to be supplemented by fortified products, nutritional yeasts, or vitamin-mineral supplements. The high fiber and phytate content of this diet may cause a decrease in the bioavailability of calcium and other minerals. Iron and zinc supplementation may also be indicated.

The greatest problem with a vegan diet during pregnancy is the volume of food that must be consumed during periods when a mother may not be able to consume much food. The high fiber content of the diet also poses some inhibition to consumption of adequate amounts of food to meet total daily requirements.

A vegan woman must take special care in planning a well-balanced diet complete with complementary protein sources and any fortified or supplemental foods required. She must consume enough food to meet the daily requirements of pregnancy. By following these recommendations a vegan woman can achieve a successful pregnancy.

Vegetable sources of critical nutrients

Certain nutrients usually obtained from animal foods may be in short supply in a vegetarian diet. Alternative sources of these nutrients are listed here. Vegans, who eat no animal foods, can use only the vegetable sources listed. Part-time vegetarians and those who eat fish are at less risk of nutrient deficiencies.

Nutrient	Sources
Protein	Legumes combined with grains, nuts or seeds, or any plant food combined with eggs or dairy products
Calcium	Dairy products, dark leafy greens, fortified soy milk, legumes, peanuts, almonds, and seeds
Iron	Legumes, dark leafy greens, torula yeast, dried fruits, whole and enriched grains, cooking in cast-iron pots, food that contains vitamin C (citrus fruits, peppers, tomatoes) with any iron-rich food
Vitamin B_{12}	Dairy products, eggs, nutritional yeast, foods fortified with B_{12}, fermented soy products, supplements
Riboflavin	Dairy products, eggs, whole and enriched grains (if eaten daily), brewer's yeast, dark leafy greens, legumes
Vitamin D	Fortified milk, fortified soy milk, exposure of skin to sunshine

Food contaminants. A number of contaminants are found in foods, as a result of both natural phenomena and human pollution or neglect. Most heavy metals are known to be embryotoxic.[46]

To prevent the possibility of contaminating food with lead, fruit juice and acidic foods should be stored in glass or plastic containers. The use of leaded crystal or ceramic food containers, especially imported or handcrafted ceramics, should be avoided. Tap water from older homes, which may have lead pipes and faucets, should be tested for lead content.[20]

Large predatory fish have a greater potential to contain high levels of mercury. Pregnant women should therefore avoid eating swordfish, shark, or marlin. Tuna intake should be limited to ½ lb/wk.

Foods contaminated with pesticides and polychlorinated biphenyls (PCBs) should also be avoided.[46] Fish from the Great Lakes and the Hudson River and freshwater fish from other inland waterways, especially those caught by recreational fishing, may be contaminated with PCBs. Fish likely to contain high levels of PCBs include freshwater carp, wild catfish, lake trout, whitefish, bluefish, mackerel, and striped bass. Because pesticides and PCBs accumulate in fat, low-fat fish and meats, when trimmed, have lower levels of contamination.[20]

Bacterial contamination and raw foods. Perhaps bacterial contamination of foods is the most common form of contamination. While traveling in foreign countries pregnant women should avoid buying foods from street vendors and should eat only cooked foods, including fruits and vegetables. All foods should be eaten while still hot. Only boiled or bottled water should be used, including water used to make ice cubes.[21]

Soft cheese such as Mexican-style cheese, Brie, and Camembert, although not raw, may be contaminated with *Listeria*. Pregnant women should avoid eating these cheeses.[20]

Raw or unpasteurized milk and raw or undercooked shellfish, fish, eggs, poultry, or meat should never be consumed by pregnant women. Meat and fish should be cooked thoroughly to kill bacteria and parasites. Partially cooked hamburgers, rare roast beef, and dishes made with raw or lightly cooked eggs, such as homemade eggnog, ice cream, and Caesar salad dressing, may increase the risk of bacterial infection. Care should be taken with foods that are nibbled, such as raw cookie dough or pancake batter containing raw eggs.[20]

Nutritional needs of the lactating woman

Lactating women have greater nutritional requirements than nonlactating women and, in many cases, than pregnant women (see RDA table in Chapter 22). The energy and protein requirements for lactation are greater than during pregnancy. The RDA subcommittee recommends an increase of 500 kcal/day throughout lactation. Assuming that weight gain during pregnancy was appropriate, this recommendation may permit readjustment of maternal body fat stores on termination of breast-feeding. If maternal weight gain was subnormal or if weight during lactation falls below the standard for height and age, the RDA for increased energy intake is raised to 650 kcal/day during the first 6 months.[32] Dietary energy restriction is contraindicated during lactation, as sufficient energy is required for satisfactory milk production.

The average protein requirement for lactation is estimated from milk composition and the mean volume of milk produced, adjusted for 70% efficiency in the conversion of dietary protein to milk protein. The RDA increment for lactating women is 15 g/day during the first 6 months (total RDA is 65 g/day) and 12 g/day thereafter (total RDA is 62 g/day).[32]

The fat soluble and water soluble vitamins in human milk can be altered by maternal deficiencies or excessive intakes. Care should be taken to assess the diets of lactating women to account for any dietary anomalies. It is common for lactating women to continue with prenatal vitamin-mineral supplementation throughout lactation; however, this is no substitute for a well-balanced diet.

The macromineral content of breast milk is not influenced by maternal intake. Calcium and phosphorus content of breast milk are maintained despite poor dietary intake by maternal bone demineralization. Therefore it is essential that the mother's diet contain adequate calcium and phosphorus to prevent bone demineralization.[46]

The micromineral content of human milk may be slightly influenced by maternal intake. To protect the mother's reserves, her diet should be adjusted to provide the minerals lost in milk.[4]

Approximately 87% of the volume of breast milk is water. A generous fluid intake, close to 3 L/day, is essential to prevent dehyration. An easy recommendation for a woman to follow is that she drink fluids every time she is breast-feeding her infant.[4]

The diet during pregnancy is an excellent basis for diet during lactation. The 200 calories added since pregnancy should be provided by foods that meet the higher needs for vitamin A, vitamin C, niacin, riboflavin, and zinc. Milk is an excellent source of several of these nutrients, as well as protein and calcium. Citrus fruits and green leafy and yellow vegetables should be consumed in amounts slightly higher than during pregnancy.

The contamination of human milk through maternal food consumption or exposure of the mother to the environment is a risk that continues to be studied. It is clear that human milk is a variable source of contaminants, but it is difficult to define a "safe" level of exposure to these compounds. However very few cases of illness caused by transmission of environmental chemicals through breast milk have appeared.[46] In order to minimize exposure breast-feeding mothers should follow the suggestions listed in the section, Safe Food Practices During Pregnancy.

Infants may react to a food in the mother's diet. Reactions range from colic to other allergic symptoms. If these symptoms develop in a breast-feeding infant and can be reasonably attributed to food sensitivity, then maternal dietary elimination trials may be considered. Foods most frequently associated with allergic reactions in childhood, such as cow's milk and soy products, are naturally suspect.

Alcohol and caffeine are passed from the mother's bloodstream into breast milk. Excessive alcohol intake by nursing mothers may result in pseudo Cushing's syndrome in the infant.[46] Lesser alcohol intakes have been shown to impair infant muscle coordination and reduce the volume of breast milk consumption. Alcohol consumption should be avoided before nursing and limited during lactation.

Caffeine can accumulate in the infant over time. Wakeful, hyperactive infants sometimes are victims of caffeine stimulation. A mother who drinks six to eight caffeine-containing beverages per day may induce a case of "coffee nerves" in her infant.[46] Caffeine consumption should be avoided before nursing and limited during lactation.

Nutritional needs and dietary requirements of infants

Breast-fed infants. Breast milk, provided that the mother is healthy and well nourished, is more nutritious than infant formula for most babies. But formula feeding, appropriately conducted, is a highly acceptable substitute.

Breast milk is more easily digested by the baby, and less likely to cause allergies and stomach upsets. It contains the ideal biochemical/nutritional composition to meet the infant's needs. The protective effects of breast milk against a range of infections, particularly diarrheal disease, are attributed both to its cleanness and inaccessibility to contaminants and to its content of maternal humoral "host resistance factors." These immune factors include secretory immunoglobulin A (IgA), lactoferrin, lysozyme, and the bifidus factor, and as many white cells, notably macrophages and lymphohyctyes, as are present in the blood.[21]

Breast-feeding promotes a special maternal-infant bonding that is only partially duplicated during bottle feeding. The skin-to-skin contact, as well as the maternal hormonal responses to breast-feeding, trigger a unique set of factors that promote an intense attachment between the mother and infant.[46,21]

Colostrum, or first milk, is a yellowish liquid that is higher in protein, minerals, vitamin A, and antibodies and lower in fat and sugar than true milk. It is easier for the newborn to digest and use than true milk, which "comes in" in a few days. In addition to its important nutritional and immunologic functions, colostrum has an important laxative effect on the newborn, helping to clean out any meconium collected in the infant's bowels.[14]

True breast milk is produced 2 to 3 days after delivery. Newborns should nurse from both breasts at each feeding for at least 10 minutes at each breast. A newborn baby may nurse 8 to 12 times in 24 hours.

A new mother can assess whether an infant is getting enough milk by observing the following:

1. Six to eight wet diapers per day
2. One or more bowel movements per day
3. Consistent weight gain
4. Apparent infant satisfaction between feedings

Bottle-fed infants. Even though breast milk has some characteristics that cannot be duplicated by even the most sophisticated formula, formula feeding, when appropriately conducted, is a highly acceptable substitute. Mothers who are anxious about breast-feeding, those who cannot be with their infant because of demands outside the home (and cannot or wish not to express breast milk), or those who are physically or mentally handicapped and cannot breast-feed should feel confident that formula feeding will meet their infant's nutritional needs. Maternal-infant bonding can also occur with bottle feeding.

Whether formula fed or breast-fed, a newborn will depend on milk as the sole source of nutrition for the first 4 to 6 months of life. It must therefore be absolutely appropriate for the infant's nutritional needs. Breast milk, commercial formulas (both cow's milk and soy based), and evaporated milk formula all adequately fill these specifications. Other formulas, such as the hypoallergenic formulas and the premature infant formulas, are more highly specialized to provide for the specialized needs of the infants.[40]

A classification system has been suggested to characterize the most important properties of the range of available formulas[6]:

- Starting formulas: intended to fulfill all the nutritional requirements for the healthy infant through the first 6 months of life. These can be used to supplement other foods up to 1 year. Starting formulas may also be called complete formulas. (Examples are SMA, Nursoy, Wyeth Laboratories, Inc., Philadelphia, Pennsylvania; Similac, Ross Laboratories, Columbus, Ohio; Enfamil, ProSobee, Mead Johnson Laboratories, Evansville, Indiana.)
- Adapted formulas: composition is closer to human milk than that of starting formulas; also termed humanized formulas.
- Follow-up formulas: used after 6 months and only as part of a mixed feeding regimen. (Examples are Carnation Follow-Up Formula, Carnation Nutritional Products; whole cow's milk; and evaporated milk.)
- Medical formulas: for special dietary use in specific disorders; also called therapeutic formulas. (Example: Alimentum, Ross Laboratories, Columbus, Ohio.)

The American Academy of Pediatrics (AAP) Committee on Nutrition and the European Society of Paediatric Gastroenterology and Nutrition (ESPGAN) set standards for the composition of infant formulas. Both recommendations contain minimum levels for most components necessary to meet the individual infant's requirements. Maximum levels are also set to prevent toxic doses of excessive nutrients.[6]

There may be slight differences between starting infant formulas on the market, but most times these differences lack nutritional significance and are purely for promotional effect. It is important than any formula used at any time correspond to the AAP and ESPGAN standards and guidelines.

Modern formula feeding is convenient and safe, as long as several factors are observed. It is important not to become casual about the mechanics of formula preparation. The water supply must be clean and safe, the nursing equipment sanitary and comfortable, and the formula prepared precisely according to directions. Expiration dates should be checked and observed on all types of formulas.

Commercial formulas are of four types:
- Powder: least expensive, convenient for supplementing breast-feeding. Mix desired amount with water; able to make one bottle at a time; powder stays fresh for 1 month after opening.
- Concentrated liquid: more convenient and more expensive than powder. Mix equal amounts of formula with water; the open refrigerated can stays fresh for 48 hours.
- Ready-to-pour: more convenient and more expensive than preceding types. Pour into bottles and feed; the open refrigerated can stays fresh for 48 hours.
- Nursette: most convenient and most expensive; a 4 oz formula-filled bottle. Take off cap and put on nipple.

The standards for energy content and nutrient composition of infant formulas are based on the average energy content and distribution of nutrients in mature human milk, taking into account the variations in infant requirements. Whole cow's milk and diluted cow's milk do not meet these standards. The type and amount of protein, fat, carbohydrate, and micronutrient contents of cow's milk are not balanced compared with the set standards. Infants also have a difficult time digesting and absorbing the fat from cow's milk. Cow's milk is therefore excluded as an acceptable starting formula (Table 23-2).

Table 23-2. Major characteristics of human milk and cow's milk

Characteristic (g/100 ml)	Human milk	Cow's milk
Energy (kcal/100 ml)	70	67
Protein	0.9	3.5
Whey/casein ratio	80:20	20:80
Casein	0.2	2.7
Whey	0.7	0.6
α-Lactalbumin	0.26	0.11
Lactoferrin	0.17	Trace
β-Lactalbumin	None	0.36
Lysozyme	0.05	Trace
Serum albumin	0.05	0.04
IgA	0.10	0.003
Nonprotein nitrogen	0.5	0.03
Carbohydrate	7.0	5.0
Carbohydrate source	Lactose	Lactose
Fat	2.7-4.5	3.5
Linoleic acid (%)	10-15	4
Calcium (mg/L)	340	1200
Phosphorus (mg/L)	150	955
Ca/P ratio	2.3	1.3
Iron (mg/L)	1	0.5
Sodium (mEq/L)	7	25
Potassium (mEq/L)	14	35
Renal solute load	80	220
Oral solute load	250	263

Adapted from Brostrom K: Human milk and infant formulas. In Suskind RM, editor: *Textbook of pediatric nutrition*, New York, 1981, Raven Press.

Some infants may be intolerant to certain formula preparations. They may be sensitive to the cow's milk protein or to lactose in the formula. There are many other potential problems, as well. Possible symptoms of sensitivity include eczema, hives, respiratory congestion, wheezing, gassiness, vomiting, diarrhea, and bloody stools. Many therapeutic formulas meet the specialized needs of these children. If an infant displays any of these characteristics, consultation with a pediatric medical specialist or dietitian is recommended.

Supplementing milk feedings. During his or her first year an infant passes through three fairly distinctive feeding patterns. Milk feeding is the sole nutritional source from 0 to 6 months of age. From 4 to 6 months of age, the child passes through a transitional period, in which he or she begins eating solid foods. This period lasts through 12 months. From about 8 months on a baby takes on much more adultlike feeding characteristics. These ages are not exact, but represent developmental stages that should occur at approximately the times indicated during the first year of life.[40]

Physiologically the full-term infant's nutritional needs can virtually be met by breast milk or a proper formula. Pancreatic amylase production may be inadequate for complete digestion of starch until 4 to 5 months. Early feeding of solid foods may result in allergy caused by absorption of unaltered protein by an immature gastrointestinal wall.[4]

Developmentally the disappearance of the primitive extrusion reflex is an essential preliminary to the willing acceptance of spoon feeding. A child must be able to sit upright and have complete head control in order to accept food and swallow properly.

There are a few reasons to supplement the diet of a breast- or formula-fed infant at certain points during the first year. Factors that influence this decision include birth weight and degree of maturity, type of milk or formula, use of iron-fortified cereal or formula, presence of fluorine in water and amount consumed by the infant plain or in formula, exposure to sunshine, and inclusion of juices containing ascorbic acid. If the recommended allowances (see RDA tables in Chapter 22) are met by the foods consumed, supplements are unnecessary.[4]

Nutrients that may require supplementation during the first year include vitamins C and D, fluoride, and iron. If necessary supplementation regimens may include vitamin D (400 IU), vitamin C (35 mg or 3 oz orange juice), fluoride (0.25 mg), and iron (5 to 10 mg at 4 months of age).[40]

Moving to solid foods. Solid foods must be introduced in a careful and regimented manner. To identify possible food intolerances and sensitivities new foods should be introduced one at a time, for 3 or 4 days at a time. If no abnormal symptoms occur, another new food may be introduced (see box).

First foods introduced are usually cereals. Iron-fortified infant rice cereal is a good selection, as it supplies iron and provides a smooth, semiliquid texture that is helpful in a first food. Cereal should be followed first by vegetables and then by fruits that are mashed or chopped. These provide vitamins A and C and a lumpier texture that encourages the development of chewing and tongue control. When vegetables are introduced before fruits, the baby does not develop a taste preference for sweets before developing a taste for vegetables.[40]

Finger foods, such as breads and cereals, can be added at about the same time as fruits and vegetables. These encourage finger dexterity and hand-mouth coordination, as well as supplementing the B vitamins and iron.[40]

Table foods for babies

6-8 months old

Mashed bananas or small slices
Applesauce
Cooked cereals
Cheerios
Toast, lightly buttered and cut
Graham cracker
Arrowroot cookies
Mashed potato
Soft cooked vegetables, mashed
Cottage cheese
Yogurt
Pudding
Vanilla ice cream
Chicken liver and other tender meats mashed or chopped

9 months-1 year

Apples, peeled and cut
Orange sections, peeled and membranes removed
Egg, boiled or scrambled
Cheeses, soft
Soft custards
Carrots and other vegetables, cooked soft
Egg noodles
Rice
Toast
Bagel
Tender meats: lamb, veal, some beef
Wieners, cut in cubes, not round slices
Spaghetti with meat sauce
Fish, without bones
Large cut meatballs

Dietary guidelines for infants. The dietary guidelines for adults have emphasized prevention of disease processes. Prevention is not the aim of the dietary guidelines for infants. Guidelines for infants less than 2 years of age emphasize appropriate growth rather than prevention and include the following four recommendations, which are consistent with the American Academy of Pediatrics and the American Dietetic Association recommendations.[17]

GUIDELINES FOR CHILDREN

Like the infant recommendations, the dietary guidelines for children over 2 years of age also differ from the adult guidelines. These recommendations are designed to promote adequate growth and prevent disease.

DIETARY RECOMMENDATIONS FOR CHILDREN ABOVE 2 YEARS OF AGE[3]

1. Diet should be nutritionally adequate, consisting of a variety of foods.
2. Caloric intake should be based on growth rate, activity level, and content of deposits of subcutaneous fat so as to maintain desirable body weight.
3. Total fat intake should be approximately 30% of calories, with 10% or less from saturated fat, about 10% from monounsaturated fat, and less than 10% from polyunsaturated fat. The emphasis should be on reducing total fat and saturated fat rather than increasing polyunsaturated fat.
4. Daily cholesterol intake should be approximately 100 mg cholesterol per 1000 calories, not to exceed 300 mg. This allows for differences in caloric intake in various age groups.
5. Protein intake should be about 15% of calories, derived from varied sources.
6. Carbohydrate calories should be derived primarily from complex carbohydrate sources to provide necessary vitamins and minerals. Thus, the total percentage of calories from carbohydrates would be about 55%.
7. Excessive salt intake may be associated with hypertension in susceptible persons. On the whole, the American diet contains excessive amounts of salt. Therefore a limitation on most highly salted processed foods and sodium containing condiments and the elimination of added salt at the table are recommended.

CHILDHOOD BEHAVIOR AND ALLERGIES
Hyperkinesis and the elimination diet

The relationship of food allergies to behavior has been correlated by anecdotal reports since the 1920s.[41] Because the relationship was anecdotal it was often discounted by the medical profession. Hyperkinesis is considered a learning disability affecting school age children. Estimates of the prevalence of this disorder vary, but evidence indicates that it may be 4% to 5% of all school age children.[34] A problem in discussing hyperkinesis is the difference of

opinion as to whether the disorder exists, or is simply a convenient label for rambunctious kids.[13]

Some authorities believe that hyperactivity is a discrete entity; others believe that it is a group of attention problems not represented by a single syndrome. More recent suggestions indicate the condition actually comprises numerous individual disorders with a similar manifestation. Furthermore, incidence varies dramatically in different countries and the criteria used for diagnosis of hyperactivity are extremely subjective and cannot be correlated in 80% of cases.[9] For example, the diagnosed incidence in North America is 20 to 40 times greater than in England.[13]

A learning disability is a disorder that causes a student difficulty in learning; it is thought to be related to a central nervous system dysfunction.[5,37] Whereas some studies have examined the central nervous system for answers, others have considered genetic predisposition, environmental toxins, and psychosocial family interaction.[37,39] One suggestion has implicated an allergen affecting the central nervous system, causing swelling in the neural connections affecting aggression.[39] The avenue for allergen exposure has been hypothesized to be food.

Another controversy linking diet to hyperkinesis began in the early 1970s. At that time Dr. Ben Feingold reported to the American Medical Association that food additives were responsible for 40% to 50% of the hyperactivity in children in his practice.[15] Numerous studies were conducted to prove or disprove his theory. These studies included atomic mineral analysis of hair to examination of vitamin metabolism and carbohydrate metabolism. Findings ranged from high mineral levels of cadmium, lead, and manganese and low levels of cobalt to inappropriate metabolism of the B vitamins. Additional studies indicated hypoglycemia or food additives as the primary culprits.[26,22,17,38,23]

Dietary guidelines for infants

The goal of the infant diet is to provide the nutrients and calories needed for the achievement of maximum growth potential.
1. Underfeeding and overfeeding can be avoided by responding to the infant's hunger signals, rather than an adult time schedule.
2. Solid foods should be introduced slowly and individually, with the goal of ultimately providing a variety of foods.
3. Sweet and salty foods should be offered in moderation and should not replace important nutrient-dense foods in the diet.
4. Whole fat dairy products should be used at least until the age of 2 years, unless otherwise cautioned by a pediatric specialist.

Until Feingold announced his theory, the prevailing belief was the disorder resulted from an injury to the diencephalon, leading to increased sensitivity of the central nervous system to stimuli. Treatment most often was administration of amphetamines.[13,9,39,15]

The alternative to amphetamine use has been diet modification. The diet most often recommended by advocates of the diet-induced hyperkinesis theory is the Feingold Kaiser Permanente (K-P) diet. This diet is free of all artificial colors and flavorings and relatively low in simple sugars.[15] The effectiveness of this treatment has caused great debate.[13]

The scientific studies that reject the diet/behavior hypothesis have drawn conclusions such as "Diet may play a role in a small subgroup of hyperactive children" and "Diet cross over studies have demonstrated a limited positive association between diet and hyperactivity."[13,26] In one study rejecting the diet/behavior elimination hypothesis, results showed that diet made a significant difference in 5% of the children and this difference was attributed to potential food allergies.[22]

Proponents of the K-P diet cite objections to the methodology of the studies used to disprove the K-P diet. These objections include the following:

- Challenge doses were only 2% to 8% of the amount of additive commonly consumed by children whereas other additive studies on food safety use test doses 10 to 100 times average consumption levels.[27,38]

- Many of the challenge studies on humans were not totally controlled and therefore the animal studies that have been ignored and were totally diet controlled should be considered; these studies indicate that hyperactivity increased 63% and avoidance learning decreased 28% with exposure to additives.[38]

Furthermore, the work of W. Crook, C. K. Connors, J. Egger, B. Kaplan, and other physicians has indicated that hyperactive behavior may have multicausitive agents such as food, vitamin deficiencies, environmental toxins, extensive antibiotic use, and individual food allergies such as those to corn, milk, or citrus.[10]

Other studies examined yellow food coloring (tartrazine) and found that its ingestion increased out-of-seat behavior and off task behavior, as well as other clinical manifestations.[8] Studies on caffeine ingestion from soda pop and chocolate indicate that they can also cause restlessness.[30]

In conclusion, although all of the evidence as to the causes of hyperactivity is not in, when diet and/or environment is implicated, the use of an elimination diet (Table 23-3) and other environmental manipulation may be indicated before beginning medication.

Lactose intolerance

Lactose intolerance, or the inability to digest milk sugar, is not a defect, but rather a natural often expected progression caused by a decline in the ability of the brush border of the small intestine to produce lactase.[42] This recessive homogenous trait is called milk malabsorption and affects the majority of the non-Caucasian world.[30]

The incidence among different ethnic groups varies (see box). The heterogenous trait (Ll) or homogenous trait (LL) that allows lactose digestion beyond weaning is most often seen in people of Northern European origin.[30] Lactose malabsorption is not usually seen in toddlers but often manifests itself at 5 or 6 years of age.[2] Reports that aging can reduce lactase activity have not been confirmed. The effect may be due to malnutrition, disease state, or drug interaction.[2] Symptoms of malabsorption include gastric upset, bloating, gas, diarrhea, and in some cases nausea and vomiting.[8,33]

Secondary lactose deficiency can result from medication, some intestinal disease processes, and malnutrition.[44,2] Lactose intolerance is an issue in the United States because dairy products are an integral part of the

Table 23-3. Elimination diet

	Allowed	Not allowed
Vegetables	All but those specifically prohibited	Corn
Fruit	All but citrus (oranges, grapefruit, tomato, etc.)	Citrus
Meat	Any unprocessed meat, poultry, or fish	Hot dogs, sausage, luncheon meat, and bacon
Grain	Oats, rice, barley, and the grain alternatives amaranth, quinoa, and buckwheat	Wheat, corn
Dairy	Soy or rice substitute	Milk, cheese
Miscellaneous		Sugar, yeast, food coloring, food additives, chocolate, soda pop, fruit drink, artificial colors

Remind patients to read processed food labels carefully for hidden ingredients. Symptoms may be related to cumulative foods so with elimination of all disallowed foods on the diet, symptoms should disappear after a few days. Then add one type of food each 3 days; if symptoms reappear, eliminate that food to determine whether the symptom disappears.

Modified from Crook W: *Help for the hyperactive child*, Jackson, TN, 1991, Professional Books.

American diet and 75% of all the calcium (a key nutrient in the growth of bone and the prevention of osteoporosis) and 20% of vitamin B_{12} are ingested in dairy products.[2] Therefore substitutes for milk in recipes and for daily calcium are essential.

Nondairy high-calcium food substitutes are available (Table 23-4), as are calcium fortified orange juice and calcium substitutes (see the bioavaliability information in Chapter 22). Non-milk-containing commercial products, predigested lactose products, and lactase containing tablets are readily available in drug stores, grocery stores, and health food stores.

Drinking milk is not essential as long as the nutrients usually provided by the milk are supplied via other foods. The emphasis on milk drinking is due to the convenience with which it supplies nutrients. As long as other sources of protein, calcium, and vitamin B_{12} are found, health is not dependent on ability to digest milk.

NUTRITION AND ADOLESCENCE

One of the hallmarks of the adolescent diet in the United States is its fast food and convenience food content. The result is a diet high in fat and sodium. Since eating food is an important social phenomenon during these years, it is important to teach teens how to select healthy foods within their own socially acceptable food environments.

For instance most fast food establishments now offer lower-fat selections. Choosing a salad, chili, or baked potato stuffed with vegetables allows an adolescent to eat with friends and maintain a lean menu. Fried foods should always be avoided because of their high fat content. Broiled chicken sandwiches are much lower in fat. Select-

ing only one regular sized sandwich, rather than the double- or triple-sized fare, also decreases the amount of fat and sodium in a meal.

All adolescents should be encouraged to consume low-fat dairy products. Low-fat frozen yogurts are now offered as alternatives to ice cream at nearly all dessert establishments.

Vending machine foods become popular at this age. Healthier selections include peanuts, popcorn, fig bars, cheese and crackers, peanut butter and crackers, dried fruits, candied popcorn (Cracker Jack) and pretzels. Fresh fruit, fruit juices, and milk are always preferable to soda pop.

Candy is a favorite food at this time. Those types that are lower in fat are also lower in calories. Such candies as licorice, jelly beans, hard candy, and peppermint patties meet many of the flavor requirements, without much of the fat and calories.

NUTRITION AND AGING

"Getting older is good, but getting old isn't so good," said one 99-year-old patient.[47] The real problem for the practitioner is determining when a patient has left middle age and entered the "golden years." One definition that

---

Incidence of lactose intolerance in adults

Ethnic group	Percentage intolerant
African blacks	97-100
Dravidian Indians (India)	95-100
Orientals	90-100
North American Indians	80-90
Central/South American Indians	80-90
Mexican Americans	70-80
North American blacks	70-75
Mediterraneans	60-90
Jews	60-80
Central and Northern Indians (India)	25-65
Middle Europeans	10-20
North American caucasians	7-15
Northwestern Indians (India/Pakistan)	3-15
Northern Europeans	1-5

Skinner-Martens S, Martens RA: *The milk sugar dilemma: living with lactose intolerance,* ed 2, East Lansing, MI, 1987, Medi-ed Press.

Table 23-4. Alternate sources of calcium for lactose restricted diets

Food	Amount	Calcium (mg)
Collards, cooked	½ c	74
Soy milk	1 c	10
Mackerel, canned including bones	3 oz	205
Dandelion greens, cooked	½ c	73
Turnip greens, cooked	½ c	99
Mustard greens, cooked	½ c	52
Kale, cooked	½ c	89
Tortillas, corn	2-6 inch	84
Molasses, blackstrap	1 Tbsp	137
Orange	1 medium	56
Salmon, canned including bones	3 oz	181
Sardines, canned including bones	2 medium	92
Boston baked beans	½ c	155
Herring, cooked	3 oz	63
Soybeans, cooked	½ c	87
Broccoli, cooked	½ c	89
Artichoke, cooked	1 medium	47
White beans, cooked	½ c	80
Kidney beans, cooked	½ c	25
Almonds, dried	1 oz	75
Tofu (soy bean curd), firm	½ c	130

Hodgkins MS, editor: *Diet manual,* ed 7, Seventh Day Adventists Diet Assoc, Loma Linda, CA, 1991

Table 23-5. Nutritional problems caused by compensation of patients for problems with aging

Primary problem	Secondary problem	Intervention
Incontinence	May lead to reduction in fluid consumed to reduce bathroom accidents, possibly causing constipation and dehydration	Patient should consume eight 8-oz glasses of fluid per day
Poorly fitted dentures or problems with chewing from loosened teeth; reduction in swallowing caused by decreased saliva production	Reduced intake of fresh fruits and vegetables, leading to constipation, and reduced vitamin and mineral intake	Fix teeth; eat canned and cooked vegetables
Malabsorption, gas, heartburn, swallowing of air while eating, or medication interaction	Reduced choices of food; may prevent patient from eating; embarrassment may cause patients to avoid social interactions that require eating or to change eating habits that prevents adequate nutrition	Check for medication interaction
Obsessive concern about cholesterol	Reduced intake of iron caused by lack of animal products in diet	Suggest prunes, lima beans, and iron fortified cereals

works well for the practitioner, if not for the age conscious patient, is based on the concept of technical life span.[48] The technical life span (TLS) of a human is based on when organs are worn out through old age. It has been defined as 120 years.

The first 60 years are easily distinguished by time segments of infancy, childhood, teenage years, young adult, and middle age; the second 60 years have been classified into three segments of time: aging (60 to 80 years old), elderly (80 to 100 years old), and aged (100 to 120 years old).[48]

Changes occur during these years in coordination and reaction time and in organ and metabolic function that affect all systems of the body, including the cardiovascular system, the pulmonary system, and the digestive system.[1]

Alteration in eating habits to compensate for changes may be innocuous or may lead to serious complications. Included in Table 23-5 are some examples of specific common problems and their consequences.

Currently the percentage of the population over 65 is calculated at 10% but it is estimated that it will increase to 20% by the year 2030.[1] Many older people have no serious medical problems and often do not consider themselves old, as they lead active lives. This attitude can lead to a tendency to ignore small problems until they become major.

Other persons in this age group have significant impairments or problems in daily living. They may still live independently with some help from family or neighbors. Grocery shopping and meal preparation are often key issues.

Determining whether older patients are eating properly requires the practitioner to consider issues such as ability to regularly shop for food, financial means to buy food, and the ability to prepare meals.

It is assumed that the healthy aging person has no special needs; however, the aged individual does have some changes that affect nutritional requirements. These changes include a reduction in lean body mass, which occurs with aging. The amount of lean body mass is directly correlated with basal caloric requirements.[34] The result is a decrease in the number of calories needed per day. The only option available to prevent lean body mass loss is exercise that promotes strength training. If basal metabolic needs drop, the patient must obtain nutrients from fewer calories or the result will be excessive weight gain.

Other changes affecting nutritional requirements are associated with vitamins and minerals such as vitamin D and calcium. The major source of vitamin D is exposure to the sun; in most older individuals the ability of the skin to convert the precursor to vitamin D is reduced, as is exposure to the sun, especially for people living in the north.[16] This leads to problems with calcium absorption and retention (see Chapter 22). Therefore, calcium supplementation for nonmilk drinkers is essential. Table 23-4 lists nondairy sources of calcium.

Another change that occurs is a decrease in hemoglobin, especially in men, as testosterone levels fall. Hemoglobin levels for diagnostic determination of anemia for older men should therefore be similar to women's levels so as to avoid men being falsely labeled as anemic and thereby supplemented unnecessarily. The intake of iron-containing foods may be poor and iron supplementation leads to constipation.

Vitamin A is also an issue, but for the opposite reason. Vitamin A is known to have toxic effects in large doses (see Chapter 22) and older individuals do not clear the retinol esters as fast as younger people. This may lead to potential complications such as toxicity.[24]

The vitamin B complexes may be depleted in the elderly, secondary to atrophic gastritis or reduced stomach acid secretions. Supplementation may be needed.[25]

The current recommended dietary allowances for aging adults lump all people 51 years and older together. Therefore little specific information is available on needs of the aging population. The current RDA for protein for healthy older Americans is 0.75 g/kg of body weight.[32] Although some research finds this amount inadequate, other national standards are not available.[33] Other recommendations include consuming a minimum of eight 8 oz glasses of fluid per day and obtaining adequate fiber through the consumption of fruits, vegetables, legumes, and whole grain cereals.[32]

Current research focuses on prevention of aging. Some research has considered aging as a result of a toxic side effect of normal metabolism.[11] Others have considered gene control as the cornerstone of the aging process.[12]

What has been established is that aging is related to metabolic rate, or the rate at which oxygen is used to perform life processes. This rate is correlated to free oxygen radical production and aging as well as presence of free oxygen radicals and other disease processes (see Chapter 24).[11]

It has not been determined which is the cause and which is the effect in the relation of increased free radicals to aging.[36] The use of antioxidants may act as a regulatory gene change to alter longevity or simply remove potentially damaging free oxygen radicals from the circulation.[11,37] These antioxidants include enzymes such as superoxidase dismutase (SOD) and glutathione peroxidase as well as vitamins such as α-tocopherol, carotenoids, and ascorbic acid.[11,36] None of these antioxidants is 100% effective, as free radical damage is found in even young, healthy organisms, but the efficiency of the body to correct for free radical damage may diminish with age.[36]

Although research into ingestable antioxidants appears promising, advocating megadoses of potentially toxic vitamins (see Chapter 22) is premature and potentially harmful.

REFERENCES

1. Albanese AA, Wein EH: Nutritional problems of the elderly, *Aging* 311-312, 1980.
2. The American Dietetic Association: *Handbook of clinical dietetics*, New Haven, CT, 1981, Yale University Press.
3. American Heart Association: *Circulation* 67:1411A, 1983.
4. Beal VA: *Nutrition in the life span*, New York, 1980, John Wiley and Sons.
5. Biehler RF, Snowman J: *Psychology applied to teaching*, Boston, 1986, Houghtin-Mifflin.
6. Brostrom K: Human milk and infant formulas: nutritional and immunological characteristics. In Suskind RM, editor: *Textbook of pediatric nutrition*, New York, 1981, Raven Press.
7. Cochrane WA: Symposium on nutrition. Overnutrition in prenatal and neonatal life: a problem? *Can Med Assoc J* 93:89, 1965.
8. Collins-Williams C: Clinical spectrum of adverse reactions to tartrazine, *J Asthma* 22(3):139-143, 1985.
9. Connors CK, Wells KC: *Hyperkinetic children: a neuropsycosocial approach*, Beverly Hills, CA, 1986, Sage Publishing.
10. Crook W: *Help for the hyperactive child*, Jackson, TN, 1991, Professional Books.
11. Cutler R: Antioxidants and aging, *Am J Clin Nutr* 53:373s-379s, 1991.
12. Cutler RG: Longevity is determined by specific genes: testing the hypothesis. In Adelman R, Roth G, editors: *Testing the theories of aging*, Boca Raton FL, 1982, CRC Press.
13. Dworkin PH: *Learning and behavior problems of schoolchildren*, Philadelphia, 1985, WB Saunders.
14. Eiger MS, Olds SW: *The complete book of breastfeeding*, New York, 1981, Bantam Books.
15. Feingold B: *Why your child is hyperactive*, New York, NY, 1974, Random House.
16. Fielding JE, Frier HI: *Nutrition research: future directions and applications*, New York, 1991, Raven Press.
17. Hamilton EMN, Whitney EN, Sizer FS: *Nutrition concepts and controversies*, St Paul, MN, 1979, West Publishing.
18. Heath MK, editor: *Diet manual including a vegetarian meal plan*, ed 6, Loma Linda, CA, 1982, Seventh Day Adventist Dietetic Association.
19. Hibbard ED, Smithells RW: Folic acid metabolism and human embryopathy, *Lancet* 1:1254, 1965.
20. Jacobson MF, Lefferts LY, Garland AW: *Safe food: eating wisely in a risky world*, Los Angeles, 1991, Center for Science in the Public Interest and Living Planet Press.
21. Jelliffe DB, Jelliffe EFP: Current concepts in nutrition. "Breast is best": modern meanings, *N Engl J Med* 297:912-915, 1977.
22. Johnson C: *The diagnosis of learning disabilities*, Boulder, CO, 1981, Pruett Publishing.
23. Kavale KA, Forness SR: Hyperactivity and diet treatment: a meta-analysis of the Feingold hypothesis, *J Learn Disabil* 16(6):324-330, 1983.
24. Krasinski SD et al: Relationship of vitamin A and E intake to fasting plasma retinol, retinol binding protein, retinyl ester carotene, alpha tocopheral and cholesterol among elderly people and young adults: increased plasma retinyl esters among vitamin A supplement users, *Am J Clin Nutr* 49:112-120, 1989.
25. Laurence KM et al: Double-blind randomised controlled trial of folate treatment before conception to prevent recurrence of neural-tube defects, *Br Med J* 282:1509-1511, 1981.
26. Mattes JA: The Feingold diet: a current reappraisal, *J Learn Disabil* 16(6):319-323, 1983.
27. Mill JL et al: Maternal alcohol consumption and birth weight: how much drinking during pregnancy is safe? *JAMA* 252:1875-1879, 1984.
28. MRC Vitamin Study Research Group: Prevention of neural tube defects: results of the Medical Research Council Vitamin Study, *Lancet* 338:131-137, 1991.
29. National Center for Health Statistics: Advance report of final mortality statistics, 1985, *Monthly Vital Statistics Report* 36:1-44, 1987.
30. National Research Council: *Diet and health: implications for reducing chronic risk*, Washington, DC, 1989, National Academy Press.
31. National Research Council: *Recommended dietary allowances*, ed 9, Washington, DC, 1980, National Academy Press.
32. National Research Council: *Recommended dietary allowances*, ed 10, Washington, DC, 1989, National Academy Press.
33. Newcomer AD, McGill DB: Clinical consequences of lactase deficiency, *Clin Nutr* 3(2):53-54, 1984.
34. O'Brien S, Obrzut JE: Attention deficit disorder with hyperactivity: a review and implications for the classroom, *J Special Educ* 20(3):281-297, 1986.
35. Oldham H, Sheft BB: Effect of caloric intake on nitrogen utilization during pregnancy, *J Am Diet Assoc* 27:847-854, 1951.
36. Pacifici RE, Davies JA: Protein lipid and DNA repair systems in oxidative stress: the free radical theory of aging revisited, *Gerontology* 37:166-180, 1991.
37. Prinz RJ, Roberts WA, Hantman E: Dietary correlates of hyperactive behavior in children, *J Consult Clin Psychol* 48(6):760-769, 1980.

38. Rimland B: The Feingold diet: an assessment of the reviews by Mattes, by Kavale and Forness and others, *J Learn Disabil* 16(6):331-333, 1983.

39. Ross DM, Ross SA: *Hyperactivity: research theory and action,* New York, NY, John Wiley and Sons, 1976.

40. Satter E: *Child of mine: feeding with love and good sense,* Palo Alto, CA, 1983, Bull Publishing.

41. Shannon WR: Neuropathic manifestations in infants and children as a result of anaphylactic reactions to foods contained in their dietary, *Am J Dis Child* 24:89, 1922.

42. Skinner-Martens S, Martens RA: *The milk sugar dilemma: living with lactose intolerance,* ed 2, East Lansing, MI, 1987, Medi-Ed Press.

43. Smithells RW et al: Possible prevention of neural-tube defects by periconceptional vitamin supplementation, *Lancet* 1:339-340, 1980.

44. The Surgeon General's Report on Nutrition and Health: U.S. Department of Health and Human Services, Public Health Service, DHHS (PHS) Publication No. 88-50210, Washington, DC, 1988.

45. Williams SR: Nutrition for high-risk populations. In Williams ST, Worthington-Roberts BS, editors: *Nutrition throughout the lifecycle,* St. Louis, 1988, Times Mirror/Mosby Publishing.

46. Worthington-Roberts BS: Maternal nutrition and the course and outcome of pregnancy, In Williams ST, Worthington-Roberts BS, editors: *Nutrition throughout the lifecycle,* St. Louis, 1988, Mosby-Year Book.

47. Young S: Personal communication.

48. Watkins DM: Goal: "Rectangularize" survival; objective: change behavior. In *Clinics in Geriatric Medicine* 3(2):237-252, 1987.

RESOURCES

(See also Resources for Chapter 26)

Administration on Aging, Office of Human Development Services, U.S. Department of Health and Human Services, 330 Independence Avenue SW, Washington, DC 20201.

American Academy of Pediatrics, 141 Northwest Point Blvd., P.O. Box 927, Elk Grove Village, IL.

Area Agencies on Aging, 1828 L Street SW, Suite 400, Washington, DC 20036. (See your phone book for the agency near you.)

Beech-Nut Nutrition, Info. Line, (800) 523-6633.

Carnation Good Start Product Line, (800) 782-7766, Ext. 565.

Center for Science in the Public Interest, 1875 Connecticut Ave, Suite 300, Washington, DC 20009-5728.

Duke University Medical Center, Dr. C. Keith Connors, Professor of Medical Psychology, Durham, NC 27710.

Gerber Products Co., Breast Feeding Info. Line, (800) 421-4221.

Johnson & Johnson Consumer Products, Inc., Product Info. Line, (800) 526-3967.

Antism Research Institute, 4182 Adams Avenue, San Diego, CA 92129. Send a self-addressed, stamped envelope.

La Leche League, 9616 Minneapolis Avenue, Box 1209, Franklin Park, IL 60131-8209.

Mothers' Home Business Network, P.O. Box 423, East Meadow, NY 11554.

Children's PKU Network, 10525 Vista Sorrento Pkwy., No. 204, San Diego, CA, 92121.

Nursing Mothers Council, Inc., Liaison Officer, P.O. Box 50063, Palo Alto, CA 94303.

Playtex Family Products Corp., Product Info. Line, (800) 222-0453.

Chapter 24

NUTRITION, DISEASE, AND PREVENTION

Susan M. Kleiner
Karen-Rae Friedman-Kester

As we approach the twenty-first century, the numerous deaths caused by infectious disease and nutrient deficiencies have been superseded by chronic diseases. More than 1.25 million heart attacks occur each year in the United States, and more than 500,000 people die as a result. More than 475,000 Americans died of cancer in 1987. During the same period, there were more than 900,000 new cases. More than 60 million Americans may have blood cholesterol levels that are too high. Approximately 2 million Americans suffer from stroke-related disabilities. About 58 million Americans have high blood pressure. Approximately 11 million Americans have diabetes, and approximately 34 million adults are obese.[78]

In 1985, illness and deaths of coronary heart disease cost Americans an estimated $49 billion in direct health care costs and lost productivity. The costs of cancer for 1985 were estimated at $72 billion.[78]

Many of the current leading causes of death in the United States have been linked to diet. In fact, according to the U.S. Surgeon General, 5 of the 10 leading causes of death have been associated with dietary intake and an additional 3 have been linked to excessive alcohol consumption.[78] Other illnesses that are not among the 10 most common causes of death add an even higher toll to the nation's public health, such as obesity, dental caries, gastrointestinal diseases, and osteoporosis.

As research increases our understanding of the causes of many of these chronic diseases, the dietary recommendations for the prevention of individual conditions have converged.[78] In fact, except for very minor alterations, there is just one diet to promote the prevention of dietary-related chronic disease and obesity. The following sections discuss the rationale behind the dietary recommendations for the prevention of each disease.

OBESITY

Obesity is a disorder, or group of disorders, that afflicts 20% to 40% of adults in the United States,[23] and 27% of children aged 12 to 17 years.[28] It is responsible for increasing the risks of developing diabetes, hypertension, cardiovascular diseases, diseases of the digestive system, and some cancers. In children, obesity is linked to hypertension, psychosocial dysfunction, respiratory disease, diabetes, and some orthopedic disorders.[26]

Obesity is more prevalent among women than men, among blacks than among whites,[8] and among black women than white women.[20] In women, poverty and race are independent predictors of overweight; educational and socioeconomic levels are inversely related to weight.

This disorder, which has an overwhelming impact on the public health of the nation, has historically received only marginal attention from the medical community. Its causes and cures have been oversimplified. Overfat patients who have been unable to lose their extra weight have been labeled sloppy, lazy, and noncompliant. During the past few years, physicians and other health care professionals have begun to recognize the complex nature of obesity as a disease, and its treatment has spawned the education of experts in the subspecialty.

To formulate a program of prevention, obesity must be defined, and its causes must be considered. *Obesity* is generally defined as an excessive accumulation of fat. According to body composition assessments of Americans, normal-weight body fat percentages are 15% to 20% for men and 22% to 25% for women.[87] These are generous ranges, and body fat percentages greater than these are considered obese.

Although obese individuals clearly are overfat, they may also have increased amounts of lean tissue, which may account for 23% to 29% of their overweight.[87] However, when expressed in percentages, lean tissue decreases in relation to fat. A 70-kg nonobese man may have 20% fat and 80% lean tissue. When that man increases his weight by 50% (35 kg) to 105 kg, his percentage of body fat increases to 38.4%, and his lean mass decreases to 61.6% in comparison.

Measurement

The measurement of percentage of body fat is most effectively done in the clinical setting by using skinfold calipers to measure fatfolds. This is a technique-sensitive measure that must be performed by a trained and experienced individual; otherwise, it will be inaccurate and unreliable. Although skinfold measures are not always precise, when made by a trained technician, the measurements are reliable and can track changes in body composition.

The body-mass index (BMI) derived from weight and height (weight [kg]/height [m]^2) is frequently used as an indirect correlate of obesity and is a practical measure in the clinical setting. Overweight is defined as a BMI of 25 to 30; obesity is defined as a BMI above 30.[8]

The pattern of regional distribution of body fat may be as significant a morbidity cofactor as the fatness itself, particularly in women. Android or central obesity, the predominant distribution of fat in the central abdominal area, is most associated with male pattern obesity. Gynoid or peripheral obesity is typically associated with the female pattern of fat distribution in the lower extremities around the hip or femoral region and to some extent in the arms.[30]

Although typically seen in their corresponding sex, either pattern may occur in males and females. The gynoid pattern of fat distribution is more benign than the android pattern. In women, risk for impaired carbohydrate metabolism, and presumably diabetes, is correlated with android obesity, and not obesity per se.[30] In men, moderate central obesity increases the risk for hypertension[30] and elevated plasma lipid and lipoprotein levels.[6]

Causes

Genetics and environment. Obesity is both a genetic and an environmental disorder. Whether each or both is operative in producing the condition of excess weight and to what degree are case-dependent. Studies assessing the relative importance of genetics versus environment have been conducted on samples of identical and fraternal twins.

The effects of genetics and environment on the BMI of

identical and fraternal twins, reared apart or reared together, were studied with statistical analyses.[77] According to the results, genetics explained 70% of the variance for men and 66% of the variance for women, making an overwhelming contribution to the ultimate BMI of the twin pairs who were reared apart. Of the potential environmental influences, only those unique to the individual and not those shared by family (common-household) members were important, contributing about 30% of the variance. Sharing the same childhood environment did not contribute to the similarity of the BMI of twins later in life. The authors conclude that genetic influences on BMI are substantial, whereas childhood environment has little or no influence.

A landmark study was conducted by Bouchard and associates to evaluate the response to long-term overfeeding in identical twins.[6] This intervention method could determine whether there are differences in the responses of different persons to long-term overfeeding and assess the possibility that genotypes are involved in such differences.

Twelve pairs of young adult male identical twins were overfed 1000 kcal per day, 6 days per week, for a total of 84 days during a 100-day period. Each man consumed an excess of 84,000 kcal above his previously determined caloric requirements.

Overfeeding resulted in highly variable individual changes in body composition and topography of fat deposition. The mean weight gain was 8.1 kg, but the range was 4.3 to 13.3 kg. On average, about 29,000 kcal did not appear as weight gain when constants were used to convert tissue gains into energy equivalents, and the authors presumed that this energy was dissipated in some way. One third of the weight gained by the group as a whole was in the form of fat-free mass. The man who gained the most weight had no evidence of energy dissipation by any mechanism, whereas in the man who gained the least weight only about 40% of the extra calories were deposited as body tissues.

Genetic factors explained the intrapair similarity in the adaptation to long-term overfeeding and the variations in weight gain and fat distribution between the pairs of twins. Within pairs, similarities of response to overfeeding were remarkably significant ($p < 0.05$) with respect to body weight, percentage of fat, fat mass, and estimated subcutaneous fat, with about three times more variance between pairs than within pairs (r = 0.5). When statistical adjustments were made to account for gains in fat mass, the within-pair similarity for changes in regional fat distribution and amount of abdominal visceral fat became particularly evident ($p < 0.01$). There was six times the variance among pairs as within pairs (r = 0.7). Genetic factors may govern the tendency to store energy as either fat or lean tissue and the various determinants of the resting expenditure of energy.

It is clear that genetics plays a role in the expression of

obesity. However, genetics can only predispose an individual to a trait or condition. The environment influences the expression of the trait.

The two significant environmental factors that impact body weight are energy expenditure and energy consumption (thyroid function is not considered here, as it is not related to the nutrition discussion). The largest and least variable portion of daily energy expenditure is resting metabolism. The rate of energy expenditure from resting metabolism is dependent on age, sex, body size, and lean body mass. Other normal contributors are more variable; these include physical activity and thermic effect of food.

Energy expenditure. Energy expenditure plays an important role not only in the development of obesity but also in the ability to maintain weight loss. In a study examining the southwestern Indian population, it was found that even after adjusting for other energy expenditure–influencing factors, the risk of gaining weight in a 2-year follow-up period was significantly higher among individuals with low 24-hour energy expenditures than individuals with high 24-hour energy expenditures.[67] After 4 years, individuals with the slowest resting metabolism gained an average of 2.75 kg per year. The middle and highest tertile groups averaged a gain of 0.23 kg and a loss of 0.07 kg per year. The data suggest that low resting metabolic rate and 24-hour energy expenditure are significant predictors of gains in body weight.

Weight control is highly affected by physical activity. Although weight loss is possible without exercise, weight maintenance is much more difficult without it.[12] Regular physical activity appears to affect both physiologic and psychologic states. Physiologically, it may affect metabolic rate by increasing lean body mass. Appetite is also affected. Psychologically, it increases the feeling of well-being and decreases depression[19] (see Chapter 18).

Dietary fat. It has been a long held belief that "a calorie is a calorie" regardless of its macronutrient source. However, this concept of energy balance for weight control is changing. The theory suggests that on isocaloric diets, individuals consuming high-fat foods will have higher amounts of body fat than individuals consuming high-carbohydrate diets.

Several studies have indicated that there is a positive relationship between dietary fat and body fat, but an inverse relationship between carbohydrate intake and body fat. Total calories were not related to body weight or body fat in most studies.[16] Some studies further indicate that the relationship is specifically associated with saturated fat, rather than polyunsaturated fat, intake.

The actual caloric content of a gram of fat has been questioned. According to the traditional Atwater values, a gram of fat contains 9 calories, a gram of protein contains 4 calories, and a gram of carbohydrate contains 4 calories. Several studies offer differing values, but the basic conclusion is that when digested and metabolized, fat may offer more calories per gram, or carbohydrate may offer fewer calories per gram, than previously suspected. Also, the energy costs of converting and storing adipose tissue from dietary carbohydrate are three times higher than those of dietary fat.[16]

Other explanations why calories from fat appear more obesity-promoting than calories from carbohydrate include the following: (1) higher-fat foods may be perceived as more palatable and be preferred to carbohydrate foods; (2) a higher caloric intake results with a higher-fat diet; (3) little dietary carbohydrate is used for adipose tissue synthesis under normal feeding conditions; (4) fat oxidation is not directly regulated by fat intake.[16]

Since dietary fat appears to turn into body fat more readily than dietary carbohydrate, altering dietary compo-

Table 24-1. Convergence of Recommendations*

Change diet ⇨	Reduce fats	Control calories	Increase starch† and fiber	Reduce sodium	Control alcohol
Reduce risk ⇩					
Heart Disease	✓	✓		✓	
Cancer	✓	✓	✓		✓
Stroke	✓	✓		✓	✓
Diabetes	✓	✓	✓		
Gastrointestinal Diseases‡	✓	✓	✓		✓

From U.S. Department of Health and Human Services: Surgeon General's Report on Nutrition and Health, DHHS Publication No. 88-50210, Washington, DC, 1988, U.S. Government Printing Office.
*To reduce the risk of diseases or their complications.
†Starch refers to complex carbohydrates provided by fruits, vegetables, and whole grain products.
‡Primarily gallbladder disease (fat and energy), diverticular disease (fiber), and cirrhosis (alcohol).

sition to one higher in carbohydrate and lower in fat may be an effective approach to prevent development of obesity. This guideline is consistent with the dietary guidelines suggested for the prevention of chronic diseases associated with diet (Table 24-1).

Dietary carbohydrate and fiber

In addition to a high-carbohydrate diet, a diet high in fiber has been shown to have beneficial effects in weight loss and weight management. The exact mechanisms for this effect are still unknown; proposed theories include the following: (1) fiber in food acts as a caloric dilution element by decreasing intestinal transit time, thereby decreasing absorption; and (2) fiber can decrease gastric emptying, which may in turn reduce hunger and prolong satiety.

In an investigation of five breakfast cereals with differing fiber levels, a negative association was found between fiber content of the cereal and caloric intake.[46] When high-fiber cereals were eaten at breakfast, food intake at lunch was decreased, reducing daily caloric consumption.

Other studies have used fiber supplements to design a high-fiber diet. The use of fiber supplements for weight loss is not recommended, since large doses of fiber may interfere with mineral absorption and nutriture (see Chapter 22). The use of fiber supplements also does not promote the consumption of a low-fat, high-carbohydrate diet. Certain individuals may continue to consume a high-fat diet while using fiber supplements.

Further research needs to be done in this area, but it is prudent to recommend that a healthy weight-loss diet include high-fiber foods such as whole-grain breads and cereals, fruits, and vegetables. The goal of including 20 to 35 g of fiber in the diet daily is recommended by the National Cancer Institute[60]: a serving of food is considered high in fiber if it contains 3 g of fiber (see Chapter 26).

Weight maintenance

The dieting-rebound cycle (yo-yo dieting or weight cycling) is a trap that many overweight, as well as normal weight, individuals fall into. However, the obese are particularly prone to this phenomenon, and it may have independent effects on obesity.[30] This loss-regain cycle may enhance metabolic adaptations to fasting and refeeding such that it becomes increasingly more difficult for people to lose weight, and increasingly easy to regain. As weight is continually lost, more lean tissue is lost. As weight is regained, more adipose tissue replaces lean tissue, thus dramatically altering body composition, and therefore metabolic rate. The reduced amount of metabolically active tissue plunges the dieter into a chronic cycle of weight gain.[15]

Dr. John Foreyt, director of the Diet Modification Clinic at Baylor College of Medicine, has listed the following predictors of success and failure for long-term weight maintenance[22]:

Predictors of success

1. Regular physical activity
2. Social support (positive support from family, friends, colleagues)
3. Internal motivation ("I will get in control of my life")
4. Focus on positive changes (feeling good, having more energy, getting healthy, etc.)

Predictors of failure

1. Negative feelings
2. Social situations (pressure to eat, irregular eating patterns)
3. Testing oneself (tempting fate)

Foreyt recommends a team approach to weight loss treatment and management, including a dietitian to help increase the chances that clients will maintain weight losses. Longer treatments are related to better initial weight losses and improved maintenance. Programs of at least 6 months in length, followed by access to a long-term support group for maintenance, are the most successful.[22]

Patients and caregivers should set reasonable weight loss goals. Rigid dieting, weight cycling, and excessive preoccupation with weight can be as harmful as overweight. For some individuals, focusing on medical risks of overweight, and the health benefits of weight loss, may be more helpful than emphasizing weight loss itself. Even small reductions in weight can positively affect health parameters such as blood glucose level, blood pressure, and serum triglyceride and lipoprotein levels. Reasonable weight loss goals may be reached within small increments of time, and changes in health parameters can reinforce positive behavior changes.

Gradual changes in dietary patterns and physical activity seem to promote weight maintenance better than quick, drastic changes.[75] Dietary fat should slowly be replaced with complex carbohydrates, so that the dieter does not become overwhelmed with feelings of hunger and deprivation.

Reducing fat intake is one of the most important factors to weight loss and maintaining that loss. It is also important for reducing risk factors for chronic diseases such as high blood cholesterol level and certain types of cancer. Diets should contain no more than 30% of calories from fat, and no more that 10% of calories from saturated fat.

To lose weight on a low-fat, high-carbohydrate diet with little or no restriction in total caloric intake, a total fat intake of 20% to 25% of total calories or less should be maintained. Table 24-2 translates this recommendation into actual daily fat gram intakes for various caloric needs. (See Chapter 26 for information on figuring target fat rates and for specific healthy diet plan information.)

The majority of individuals who try to lose weight regain it after treatment.[22] It is essential that patients trying to lose weight be counseled in behavioral principles and coping skills. Weight loss and management strategies should be developed by a multidisciplinary approach, including medical, nutritional, social, and psychologic specialties. In this way, the weight loss plan actually becomes the patient's new life-style plan, thereby supporting the ultimate achievement of permanent weight loss.

Obesity must be viewed as a chronic disease, rather than a behavioral abnormality. Once it is viewed as a condition to be controlled, the goals of treatment and the criteria defining success will change their emphasis to positive alterations in health parameters, such as decreases in blood glucose and serum cholesterol levels and blood pressure. Long-term weight maintenance may be sufficient to decrease morbidity.

No studies have quantified the cost-effectiveness of weight reduction in management of diabetes, hypertension, and hypercholesterolemia. However, weight reduction is widely supported as an important step in effective management of these major chronic diseases.[26]

DIABETES MELLITUS

Diabetes mellitus is the seventh leading cause of death in the United States.[78] It is associated with high blood glucose levels and a deficiency in or resistance to insulin leading to inappropriate carbohydrate metabolism. At one time diabetes was defined as juvenile onset or adult onset; it has more recently been defined as insulin-dependent diabetes mellitus (type I [IDDM]) and non-insulin-dependent diabetes mellitus (type II [NIDDM]).[18] The difference is associated with the medicinal treatment of this disorder (insulin vs. hypoglycemic agents). All diabetics, whether type I or type II, are encouraged to follow a diabetic diet (see General Recommendations). The number of Americans suffering from diabetes is approximately 11 million people.[78] The complications of diabetes include ketosis, coma, hypertriglyceridemia, coronary artery disease, stroke, retinopathy, peripheral vascular disease, and impaired renal function.[42]

Type I diabetes is prevalent in 5% of all diabetics and is associated with a loss of function of the islets of Langerhans in the pancreas and thus the reduced or complete stoppage of insulin production.[17] Insulin is necessary to transport circulating glucose into the cell from the bloodstream. There has been some suggestion that type I diabetes is linked to the immune system. Its prevalence is significantly higher among whites than blacks, and siblings of type I diabetics are at increased risk.[18]

Type II diabetes has been associated with obesity. In fact, 80% of type II diabetics are obese.[34] The pancreas produces insulin but does not produce enough insulin or may produce insulin that is biologically less active.[7] Obese patients with type II diabetes often become asymptomatic and have normal glucose tolerance test results after weight loss. The number of type II diabetics has been known to rise in times of plenty and drop during times of food rationing or reduced food availability.[7] (See Chapter 55 for a

Table 24-2. Fat grams in a diet of 20% to 25% of calories as fat

Calories/day	Grams of fat/day
1200	27-33
1400	31-39
1600	36-44
1800	40-50
2000	44-56
2200	49-61
2400	53-67

more extensive discussion of causes of endocrine disorders.)

One method that can be used to assess patients at risk for type II diabetes is high waist/hip ratio. The *waist/hip ratio* (W:H) is determined by measuring the circumferences of the waist and hip and computing the ratio. The android distribution of fat is associated with the risk for diabetes. Normally, in women, the waist is smaller than the hip, and thus a normal W:H ratio is less than 1. In the android pattern of fat distribution, the waist measurement increases, while the hip measurement may remain stable or only slightly enlarged.[30]

There is also a correlation of higher incidence of diabetes within families and among identical twins, suggesting a genetic link.[17,18] Other factors that have been correlated with higher incidence of the disease include lower socioeconomic status, less schooling, and unemployment. Nonwhites also have a significantly higher incidence of type II diabetes than whites. This may be both genetic and associated with socioeconomic status.[18]

Means of prevention of type I diabetes are not yet known; onset of type II diabetes can be prevented or postponed through maintaining ideal body weight in terms of percentage of body fat or dieting to achieve it. Therefore, the approach to treatment of diabetes relies heavily on diet and exercise. (See Chapter 18 for more discussion of exercise.) Blood sugar level should be monitored before, during, and after exercise. A regular and consistent exercise program is a key to preventing blood sugar level swings.[11] It should be noted that although exercise and diet are used to control diabetes, no clear evidence indicates that lack of exercise, high refined sugar intake, or increased calorie intake (except in obesity) is linked to the development of diabetes.[18] Current guidelines for controlling diabetes include the following protein, fiber, carbohydrate, and fat intake recommendations:

That protein be limited to the recommended dietary allowance (RDA) for protein of 0.8 g/kg of body weight.[85] (Therefore, a patient who weighs 150 lb, or 68.18 kg, has a protein need of 54.55 g.)

That fat consumption be limited. (See the obesity chart for examples of grams of fat in a 20% to 25% fat diet.)

That the majority of foods be selected from those high in fiber or complex carbohydrates.

Changing lifelong eating patterns is extremely difficult, especially when one must coordinate eating with times of increased physical activity. Therefore, it is highly recommended that the caloric level and diet pattern designed for a patient be planned with the expertise of a dietitian who will teach the patient the diet and provide information on foods that contain hidden sugars and fats. If these recommendations are followed, the risk of complication to diabetes is greatly reduced.

HYPERTENSION

Hypertension is a disease, or it can be a symptom of another disease. Both environment and genetics play a significant role in hypertension as a primary disease.[69] Approximately 70% of the adult population in the United States have a chronically increased arterial pressure.[24] Of hypertensive patients 10% have secondary hypertension, indicating that the cause is another pathologic process, such as kidney disease. Concern about hypertension is raised by its epidemiologic link to atherosclerosis as well as aneurysms.[32] Maintaining ideal body weight can help reduce the blood pressure of many hypertensive patients.[30] (See the discussion of obesity.)

Until recently, sodium was assumed to be the primary dietary cause of hypertension. Although clinicians continue to recommend moderate sodium intake (approximately 3 to 4 g, or 6 g of table salt, per day[18]), it is now known that only one tenth of individuals in the general population and one third to one half of patients with diagnosed hypertension are sodium sensitive. Reducing sodium in a non–sodium-sensitive patient does not alter blood pressure.[53]

To determine whether a patient is sodium sensitive, a 2-g sodium diet, generally referred to as a "no added salt" diet, should be implemented for 1 month. The patient should be referred to a registered dietitian for nutrition education and monitoring. If there is no blood pressure response, and the patient has complied with the diet recommendation, the patient is likely a nonresponder to sodium restriction.

When sodium restriction is indicated the patient must be taught that sodium exists in other forms than sodium chloride (table salt). This includes preservatives and other additives, such as sodium benzoate, sodium phosphate, hydrolyzed vegetable protein, whey solids, monosodium glutamate (MSG), and many processed foods, such as ketchup, tomato sauce, soy sauce, and canned soup. The patient should also be aware that many medications, such as antacids, laxatives, and sleeping aids, may contain sodium. Another source of sodium is conditioners used to soften hard water.

If the patient needs a specific low-sodium diet to make life-style changes, a registered dietitian is best equipped to teach the new diet. Salt substitutes can be purchased at most grocery stores; however, they have a strong metallic taste and are not palatable to many patients. The use of salt substitutes by patients should be overseen by the physician, as they substitute potassium, which may be contraindicated, for sodium.

In the search to find another cause of primary hypertension, calcium has received a fair amount of attention. Although many epidemiologic studies have found that low consumption of calcium led to hypertension,[39] others have not supported this finding.[71] Better evidence can be found through using high-calcium diets (1 to 1.5 g/day for at least 6 weeks) to lower blood pressure.[35,39]

Although this research is promising, not all patients respond to increased calcium in the diet and it is the physician's role to determine whether the patient is likely to benefit from increased calcium intake, as excessive calcium may also contribute to some hypertension.[69] Therefore, the current recommendation is to meet the RDA for calcium for all patients as it is protective against osteoporosis and possibly hypertension.

RENAL DISEASE

Although diet modification is a significant portion of treatment for renal disease, at this time no diet modification is recommended for prevention of renal disease. However, diabetic patients who have an increased risk for renal disease can prevent such complications by following a diabetic diet. A diabetic diet and good blood sugar level control can reduce side effects of renal impairment.[42]

CORONARY HEART DISEASE

Although more than 500,000 Americans die of heart disease each year,[78] there has been a progressive improvement in the prevalence of the disease. Overall mortality from heart disease has declined 40% in the past 20 years, or about 3% per year.[27] This decline is probably linked in part to favorable changes in cardiovascular risk factors such as dyslipidemia, hypertension, and glucose intolerance, as well as life-style changes such as dietary modifications, increased exercise, and decreased cigarette smoking.[72]

Treatment of hyperlipidemia to prevent coronary heart disease (CHD) has been advocated by the National Heart, Lung and Blood Institute through the development of the National Cholesterol Education Program (NCEP).[57] The NCEP provides guidelines for the screening and treatment of plasma cholesterol levels in adults (Table 24-3).

Dietary therapy is the mainstay of treatment and prevention. According to the NCEP treatment paradigm, all patients should receive general dietary and risk-factor education. Borderline-high-risk and high-risk individuals should be provided with diet instruction.[57] The step-one diet should be followed for 3 months[58] (Table 24-4). If the

Table 24-3. Recommendations of the adult treatment panel of the national cholesterol education program for classification of patients*

Classification based on T-Chol*	Classification based on LDL* cholesterol
Desirable blood cholesterol: <200 mg/dl (<5.17 mmol/L)	Desirable LDL cholesterol: <130 mg/dl (<3.36 mmol/L)
Borderline high blood cholesterol: 200-239 mg/dL (5.17-6.18 mmol/L)	Borderline-high-risk LDL cholesterol: 130-159 mg/dl (3.36-4.11 mmol/L)
High blood cholesterol: ≥240 mg/dl (≥6.21 mmol/L)	High-risk LDL cholesterol: ≥160 mg/dl (≥4.13 mmol/L)

From National Cholesterol Education Program: *Report of the expert panel on detection, evaluation and treatment of high blood cholesterol in adults,* Bethesda, Md, 1988, NIH publication no 88-2925, National Institutes of Health.

*LDL, low density lipoprotein; T-chol, total cholesterol. To convert mmol/L to mg/dl, multiply mmol/L by 38.86.

Table 24-4. Dietary therapy for high blood cholesterol level

Nutrient	Recommended intake	
	Step-one diet	Step-two diet
Total fat	<30% total kcal*	<30% total kcal
Saturated fat	<10% total kcal	<7% total kcal
Polyunsaturated fat	≤10% total kcal	≤10% total kcal
Monounsaturated fat	10-15% total kcal	10-15% total kcal
Carbohydrates	50-60% total kcal	50-60% total kcal
Protein	10-20% total kcal	10-20% total kcal
Cholesterol	<300 mg/day	<200 mg/day
Total calories	Maintain IBW*	Maintain IBW*

From National Cholesterol Education Program: *Report of the expert panel on detection, evaluation and treatment of high blood cholesterol in adults,* Bethesda, Md, 1988, NIH publication no 88-2925, National Institutes of Health.

*kcal, calories; IBW, ideal body weight.

cholesterol goal is not achieved, referral to a registered dietitian with a retrial of the step-one diet or a move to the step-two diet should be recommended. Drug treatment should be considered only after a minimum of 6 months of dietary intervention.

The NCEP treatment panel estimates that dietary changes can improve lipid levels by 10%. In fact, the observed reductions in total serum cholesterol levels produced by dietary interventions published in the Lipid Research Clinics Trial[47] and MRFIT[80] were 4.9% and 5%, respectively. Others have estimated that a lifelong program of dietary modification would result in a 6.7% decline in total serum cholesterol levels.[79] Although this reduction may seem small, every 1% decrease in blood cholesterol level leads to a 2% reduction in CHD risk. In addition, even a 5% reduction in lipid levels can be enough to allow many patients to prevent or markedly reduce the use of medications, thereby improving their quality of life.[59]

Improvements in quantity and quality of life are the goals of lipid treatment and intervention. According to computer-generated model estimates of life expectancy and morbidity, among low-risk individuals the average increased life expectancy associated with dietary intervention alone is usually small, ranging from 0.08 year for 65-year-old men with a baseline serum cholesterol level of 5.7 mmol/L (221.5 mg/dl) to 0.32 year for 35-year-old men with a baseline serum cholesterol level of 7.8 mmol/L (303.1 mg/dl).[31] However, among the same individuals with combined diet and drug intervention, the additional years of life free of symptomatic coronary heart disease were approximately twofold greater than the forecasted changes in life expectancy. The maximum benefit was forecasted among younger women and men (35 years old);

older men and women received less benefit. The benefits of dietary intervention alone were again small, with a maximum delay of 0.75 year predicted for 35-year-old men with cholesterol levels of 7.8 mmol/L.

The authors state that more intensive dietary intervention than that used in the Lipid Clinics Trial and the MRFIT could further reduce serum cholesterol, and therefore extend both the years of freedom from disease and life expectancy. The model suggests that high levels of serum cholesterol should be aggressively treated early with diet and medication. There is decreasing benefit when intervention is initiated later in life.[31]

The nutrition recommendations of the NCEP are designed to encourage the development of healthy eating patterns in all adults and to assist individuals to lower blood cholesterol to desirable levels. They are essentially the same as those recommended by the American Heart Association and the National Research Council.

The panel recommends the following pattern of nutrient intake for all Americans[57]:

1. Less than 10% of total calories from saturated fatty acids.
2. An average of 30% of total calories or less from all fat.
3. Dietary energy (calories) levels needed to reach or maintain a desirable body weight.
4. Less than 300 mg/day of cholesterol.

In addition to these recommendations, The American Heart Association has added the following prudent diet strategies to reduce hyperlipidemia (especially hypercholesterolemia) and hypertension[37]:

1. Cholesterol intake should be less than 100 mg/1000 kcal, not to exceed 300 mg/day.
2. Protein should contribute approximately 15% of calories.
3. Carbohydrate should contribute 50% to 55% or more of calories, with an emphasis on complex carbohydrates.
4. The sodium intake should be reduced to 1 g/1000 kcal, not to exceed 3 g/day.
5. If alcoholic beverages are consumed, intake should be limited to 15% of total calories, not to exceed 50 ml of ethanol/day.
6. A variety of foods is recommended.

Recommendations regarding specific dietary fats have become more concrete as longitudinal diet studies are completed. These recommendations are reflected in the step-one and step-two diets of the NCEP.

Information from the Seven Countries Study[4] indicated that monounsaturated fatty acids may be protective against CHD. Although study subjects on the isle of Crete ate a diet that contained 40% of its calories in fat, they had a very low incidence of CHD. It was speculated that the high concentration of the monounsaturated fatty acid (MUFA) oleic acid derived from olive oil might be protective.

The typical American diet contains 37% of calories from fat, 14% of which are from MUFA, 13% from saturated fat (SFA), and 7% from polyunsaturated fat (PUFA). The subjects on Crete ate a diet of 26% of calories from MUFA, 8% of calories from SFA, and 3% of calories from PUFA.

Fifteen-year follow-up data from the study indicate that relationships between death rates and dietary factors were positive for SFA and negative for MUFA. Death rates were negatively related to the ratio of MUFA to SFA.[41]

These data have led to laboratory tests of the effect of diets high in MUFA, versus PUFA and SFA. From all of the research on dietary fats and lipid levels, some general conclusions can be drawn[44]:

1. A diet low in SFA is effective in lowering elevated plasma levels of total and LDL cholesterol.
2. Partially replacing the calories from SFA with carbohydrate calories can lead to reductions in plasma total cholesterol, LDL cholesterol, and high density lipoprotein (HDL) cholesterol levels and may cause slight (not statistically significant) elevation in triglyceride levels.
3. Partially replacing the calories from SFA with omega-6 (Ω_6) fatty acids (general polyunsaturated) leads to a decrease in both LDL cholesterol and HDL cholesterol levels.
4. Partially replacing the calories from SFA with MUFA leads to a decrease in plasma total cholesterol and LDL cholesterol levels at least as great as

that produced by diets that either are low in total fat or that partially replace SFA with Ω_6 fatty acids. Using MUFA does not significantly change HDL cholesterol or triglyceride levels.

The positive effect of Ω_3 fatty acids from fish oil (principally eicosapentenaeoic acid [EPA] and docosahexaenoic acid [DHA]) on CHD risk has been documented by epidemiologic and laboratory studies.[33] Consumption of large amounts of fish oil (90 to 120 g/day) markedly lowers plasma triglyceride levels by inhibiting very low density lipoprotein (VLDL) production. Smaller quantities (8 g/day) also show an effect on triglyceride levels.

Fish oils have little effect on total cholesterol levels, but HDL cholesterol level may be increased by 5% to 10% when fish oil is consumed. The mechanisms responsible for these effects are unknown. Ω_3 fatty acids are antithrombotic, they reduce platelet aggregation (and blood clots), and they are also anti-inflammatory.[44]

The amount of Ω_3 fatty acids required for effective management of plasma lipids is not known, but it is prudent to recommend that Americans increase their consumption of fish, since it has been shown to affect CHD risk beneficially. Substituting fish for other foods high in SFA is an effective way to reduce SFA and total fat in the diet. All types of fish are recommended, but those highest in Ω_3 fatty acids are the oilier fish, such as mackerel, salmon, albacore tuna, sablefish, halibut, shark, snapper, and trout. Seafoods that are generally high in Ω_3 fats include mussels, oysters, and squid.

Fish oil supplements are not recommended. Questions regarding safety, proper dosages, duration of treatment, and side effects of long-term ingestion make their use inadvisable. In addition, when taken in the recommended doses by the manufacturers, supplements contain very small amounts of Ω_3 fatty acids.[44] These amounts can easily be obtained by adding two to three fish meals to the diet each week.

In addition to recommendations regarding fats, cholesterol, and calories, several other dietary factors have recently been recognized in relation to the prevention of CHD. Dietary fiber should be part of an overall healthy diet. Studies suggest that dietary fiber reduces not only fasting lipoproteins but postprandial lipoproteins, as well.[1,68] More specifically, diets high in water-soluble fibers from oats and dried beans significantly lower serum cholesterol concentrations[2,3] (see Chapters 22 and 26). The Sports and Cardiovascular Nutritionists Practice Group of the American Dietetic Association recommends a daily intake of 15 to 25 g of water-soluble fibers for prevention and treatment of CHD.[44]

The newest dietary research has linked antioxidant vitamins with CHD risk.[45] Epidemiologic data indicate interesting relationships among vitamin E, β-carotene, vitamin C, and heart disease risk factors. β-Carotene and vitamin

C have been found in lesser amounts in smokers. There is more oxidized vitamin E in the lungs of smokers. An inverse relationship has been documented between vitamin C status and blood pressure in normotensive individuals. A direct relationship has been documented between HDL cholesterol and plasma vitamin C levels.

Although promising, these data are quite preliminary, and it is too soon to make recommendations regarding specific doses of these vitamins. However, a diet high in fruits and vegetables will provide generous amounts of all vitamins, including vitamins C, E, and β-carotene. (See the dietary guidelines in Chapter 22 and the discussion of coffee and caffeine in Chapter 26.)

A diet for the prevention of heart disease for the general healthy population follows the basic dietary guidelines of the USDA and NIH (see Chapter 22). The step-one and step-two diets have been developed for the treatment of hyperlipidemia but can be followed by individuals that are highly motivated to decrease their chronic-disease risks.

CANCER

Cancer is not one disease but a group of diseases that can affect any organ or tissue in the body. The development of cancer is a multistep process that can take decades or appear to be a matter of weeks or months.[82] Life-style, including diet, has been indicated as one factor that can affect patient risk of these diseases. The risk due to diet may be increased by excessive intake or carcinogenic content of certain foods. Some foods may lower risk by "protecting" against specific cancers.[13]

The dietary guidelines to lower cancer risk are similar to those for other disease states although the rationales for the recommendations may differ.

These basic recommendations[70] include the following:

- Reducing fat consumption to no more than 30% of total calories. This includes all fats, saturated and unsaturated.
- Increasing the amount of fiber and whole grain cereals in the diet.
- Increasing the consumption of fruit and vegetables.
- Reducing the amount of alcohol consumed to a moderate level.
- Reducing the consumption of cured and smoked meats.
- Reducing the consumption of charcoal broiled foods.

The rationale for these guidelines includes direct associations that have been discovered between fat consumption and numerous cancers, including intestinal and colorectal cancer[38] and breast and prostate cancer.[43,49,64] Increased animal protein intake has also been examined as a culprit for increased cancer risk, specifically risk of breast, endometrium, prostate, colorectum, pancreas, and kidney cancers. Although a correlation exists, a stronger correlation has been demonstrated with the fat component of the ani-

mal product rather than the protein component. By-products of bile acids used to digest fat may be the cause.[13]

The recommendation to increase intake of whole grain foods as well as fruits and vegetables is based on the protective role against cancer that fiber appears to provide to the large bowel. This may be due to decreased transit time or influences on the fecal flora of the large intestine.[13] Epidemiologically, societies that consume a high-fiber diet have a lower incidence of bowel cancer than those that consume lower-fiber diets.[50,51] Some studies have not directly correlated fiber with incidence, and in 1982 the Committee on Diet Nutrition and Cancer stated that there is no conclusive evidence that dietary fiber provides a protective mechanism against cancer.[13] Yet the American Institute for Cancer Research interprets the committee's recommendations through their professional reference guide as a need to increase intake of whole grain foods, fruits, and vegetables.[70]

Other components of fruits and vegetables besides their fiber content have also been examined for protective roles against cancer and have shown promising results. These include vitamin A, retinoids, carotenoids, vitamin C, and calcium.

The original studies on vitamin A included the retinoids and carotenoids because of their precursor relationship to vitamin A.[50] More recent studies have examined the possible independent role of carotenoids as antioxidants in protecting against cancers.[88] Cancers studied included lung, larynx, bladder, esophagus, stomach, colon, and prostate.[9,13,29,40,54,55,73,86]

Study results have shown evidence of a protective effect and recommended eating foods rich in vitamin A and its precursors; however, the National Research Council cautions against using vitamin supplements because of the toxic nature of vitamin A.[13] Addition of a variety of fruits and vegetables to the daily diet is recommended.

Studies of vitamin C or ascorbic acid have also indicated a protective mechanism against some cancers, specifically esophageal,[55] laryngeal,[29] and gastric cancer.[14] One mechanism for the protective nature of vitamin C may be its inhibition of nitrosamines.[56] The correlation of nitrosamines with cancer, especially liver cancer, is the reason for the restrictions on intake of cured and smoked meats as well as charcoal broiled meats, which contain large amounts of nitrosamines.[13,83] Again inclusion of fruits in the diet rather than supplementation is recommended.

Studies of the protective role of calcium in patients predisposed to colorectal cancer have also shown promising results; additional intake of calcium beyond the current RDA or no more than 1.5 times the RDA is needed.[48,76] Supplementation beyond the RDA is not currently recommended, although many people need supplements to reach the current RDA.

Numerous other vitamins and minerals are being studied for a causative or preventive role in cancer. The mechanisms vary from prevention of carcinogen formation to increased detoxification to control of cell replication, differentiation, expression of malignancy, or cell communication.[83] At this time, these roles are not understood and no nutritional recommendation can be made.[13,52]

The use of specific foods to prevent cancer, such as broccoli and other cruciferous vegetables (cauliflower, cabbage, brussels sprouts), has also received attention in the research community. Although a relationship exists between consumption of these foods and reduced risk of developing cancer the mechanism is unclear. Therefore, eating a variety of fruits and vegetables including the crucifers is recommended.[66,89]

The recognition that alcohol plays a role in cancer was understood as early as the 1930s when one study in France identified 95% of esophageal cancer patients as alcohol abusers.[65] Other studies have identified a correlation of hepatomas, as well as tongue, hypopharynx, larynx, and colorectal cancers, with excessive alcohol use, including excessive beer drinking.[13] Therefore, alcohol should be consumed in moderation, if at all.

AIDS

Acquired immunodeficiency syndrome (AIDS) has no nutritional cure; nor can it be prevented through nutritional means. The reason for its inclusion in this chapter is that the side effects and progress of the disease have been curtailed to some degree through careful nutrition intervention. Furthermore, the major review on nutrition and human immunodeficiency virus (HIV) infected patients commissioned by the FDA states that HIV-infected patients at risk for malnutrition require nutrition intervention.[63]

The incidence of malnutrition in patients with AIDS has been as high as 96% of all patients.[25] The problem is partially the result of difficulty of food intake, but malnutrition is also caused by foodborne infections, such as severe gastroenteritis, diarrhea, and dehydration. These infections can be prevented through careful food handling and choice of foods (see recommendations). Diarrhea may also result from diets that are too high in fiber or from lactose intolerance. Excessive caffeine intake can also increase diarrhea. Restriction of foods high in fiber or containing caffeine or lactose may help prevent malnutrition.[74]

Uninfected relations will not contract AIDS as a result of eating with or sharing the same eating utensils as someone who has AIDS. The purpose of these guidelines is to prevent the AIDS patient from becoming infected with an opportunistic infection. Recommendations for safe food handling[36] are as follows:

Do not share drinks or eating utensils during the meal with another person.

Wash hands and utensils with hot soapy water before preparing food.

Do not use wooden utensils or cutting boards. Use plastic and wash it in hot soapy water.

Do not use the same cutting board for raw meats and poultry as for other raw or cooked foods such as salads.

Use dish towels or rags that are freshly laundered. Use them once and relaunder.

Cook foods until well done (165° F to 212° F); this applies to meat, poultry, fish, and eggs

Do not save leftovers more than 3 days.

Thaw frozen food in the refrigerator, not in the pantry.

Avoid cracked eggs or foods with raw eggs such as homemade mayonnaise, egg nog, caesar salad dressing, or hollandaise sauce.

Use only pasteurized milk products.

Avoid sushi and other raw fish, poultry, or meat.

Wash, then peel all fruits and vegetables; avoid fruits and vegetables that have any mold on them.

Avoid foods when uncertain of their freshness.

Avoid foods from any source that may not be safe. This includes food carts or buffets where food is kept warm and bacteria can grow.

If traveling, be aware that many foods that do not cause problems for the general public can cause AIDS patients problems. This includes water, ice cubes, and any other product that may be handled in a local tradition yet not cooked thoroughly.

Consume foods that were cooked recently rather than chilled and rewarmed.

Patients with AIDS are often willing to try any therapy offered to them, including fad diets and magic elixirs. The use of megavitamins and/or minerals to boost immune function has not proved successful and may create vitamin and mineral toxicities.[21] No scientific evidence supports the use of any fad diet to promote wellness or remission in AIDS patients.

Therefore, consumption of a nutritionally sound diet high in protein and calories with adequate fluid is the best option for patients with AIDS. If any sign of diet intolerance or malnutrition occurs, referral to a registered dietitian with AIDS experience is a must.

Recommendations for nutrition monitoring of AIDS patients are as follows:

Conduct or refer patient for a complete nutritional evaluation.

Monitor patient weight.

Recommend a high-calorie, high-protein diet.

Recommend a nutritional consultation with a registered dietitian at the first sign of anorexia, nausea, weight loss, dehydration, diarrhea, or malnutrition.

If patient intake is poor, consider dietary supplements such as calorie boosters and multivitamins.

IMMUNE SYSTEM

The immune system is highly responsive to the nutritional status of the patient. Whether a patient has cancer,

AIDS, or a suppressed immune system caused by primary malnutrition, apart from consuming a diet that includes appropriate calories, protein, and nutrients, there is no magic formula for boosting the immune system. However, research is continuing.

In animal studies vitamin E and vitamin A have been shown to increase immune function. In human studies β-carotene increased T cells in young men and vitamin C ingestion improved immune response.[5] All three nutrients have produced reduction in tumor growth, but further research is needed to support advocating vitamin supplementation beyond consuming appropriate foods.

Appropriate foods include those specified in the cancer guidelines: addition of whole grains and a variety of fruits and vegetables and reduction in excessive fats. As discussed, this has been shown to reduce the risk of some diseases. Equally important is intake of adequate nutrients to maintain a strong immune system when a disease process is present. Therefore, the patient who has a suppressed immune system needs to receive a healthy diet but should not limit foods if at risk for weight loss or malnutrition as this can further reduce the efficiency of the immune system.[10] The use of nutritional support to prevent malnutrition may be appropriate.

OSTEOPOROSIS

The growth of the skeleton requires a positive calcium balance. Although adult stature is reached in the teen years, the skeleton continues to accumulate mass until age 30 to 35. During the fifth decade of life, bone mass begins to decline slowly in both sexes, but the rate of loss accelerates greatly about the time of menopause in women and remains high for several years. Bone loss accelerates much later in men, by a decade or more. This loss results in gradually diminishing bone strength and increased risk of fractures.[62]

Menopause-related bone loss is due for the most part to estrogen deficiency and cannot be prevented by high-calcium intake (see Chapters 18 and 30). Age-related involutional loss continues at a slower rate thereafter; some of the loss is calcium-related. Peak bone mass appears to be related to lifetime calcium nutriture, particularly during the years of bone mineralization.[62]

Ninety-nine percent of the body's calcium is found in the skeleton. The remainder is in extracellular fluids, intracellular structures, and cell membranes. The body maintains calcium homeostasis in the extracellular fluids. If adequate calcium is not available from food, calcium is scavenged from the skeleton.

Low-calcium intake during adolescence is common and poses a particular problem in regard to achievement of genetically programmed peak bone mass. Poor calcium intake limits bone mineral accretion and thus leaves an individual with reduced skeletal reserve at menopause and when the involutional decline of old age begins.

Although many factors affect bone mass and strength (heredity, gonadal hormones, physical activity, other diseases, other life-style factors), investigations into maintenance of bone mineral mass have found that those individuals with higher lifetime calcium intake have greater bone mass as they age. The assumption has been made that those individuals who attain a higher peak bone mass can maintain a healthier level of bone density with age, even though bone loss still occurs.[62]

Unfortunately, calcium intake in women is less than optimal. According to the most recent U.S. Food Consumption Survey, the calcium intake of middle-aged and elderly women is about 75% of the RDA.[84] With the recognized decline in intestinal calcium absorption with age, this marginal calcium intake is of concern. Moreover, the 1989 RDA of 1200 mg/day of calcium for women 25 years and younger and 800 mg/day for those older than 25 years is less than the 1000 mg/day for premenopausal and estrogen-treated women and 1500 mg/day for postmenopausal women not being treated recommended by the NIH Consensus Development Conference on Osteoporosis[61] (see Chapter 22 for information on calcium toxicity).

Calcium is most bioavailable from foods, rather than supplements, and is found in significant amounts almost exclusively in milk and milk products. Calcium is not always available from plant sources (see Chapter 22). Daily consumption of low-fat or nonfat milk products is essential for the adequate consumption of calcium from foods (see Table 24-5; also see Chapter 25 for nondairy sources of calcium).

Table 24-5. Nutrient content of 1 cup servings of selected dairy products*

	Calories	Fat (g)	Cholesterol (mg)	Protein (g)	Calcium (mg)
Milk					
Lactaid	102	3.0	10	8.0	300
Whole 3.3%	150	8.2	33	8.0	291
Low-fat 2%	121	4.7	18	8.1	297
Low-fat 1%	102	2.6	10	8.0	300
Skim	86	0.4	4	8.4	302
Yogurt					
Nonfat plain	127	0.4	4	13.0	452
Low-fat plain	144	3.5	14	11.9	415
Low-fat coffee/ vanilla	194	2.8	11	11.2	389
Low-fat with fruit	225	2.6	10	9.0	314
Cottage cheese					
Creamed	217	9.5	31	26.2	126
Dry curd	123	0.6	10	25.0	46
Low-fat 2%	203	4.4	19	31.1	155

*Nutrient values from Pennington JAT: *Food values of portions commonly used,* ed 15, New York, 1989, Harper & Row.

If sufficient calcium is not consumed in the diet, supplementation to reach the recommended intake should be considered. Calcium carbonate is the most widely used calcium supplement and has the highest calcium content (40%) compared to other salts.

The solubility of calcium supplements is an important consideration when recommending supplementation. Many calcium supplements do not meet the United States Pharmacopeia (USP) standards for quality because the tablets are not formulated in a way that enhances their solubility. Insoluble calcium tablets may pass through the gastrointestinal (GI) tract intact with little if any calcium being absorbed. Patients should be advised to purchase calcium supplements that meet USP standards.[81]

Supplements should be taken with meals to increase absorption. The solubility of calcium carbonate and tribasic calcium phosphate is pH-dependent, being enhanced by normal gastric acidity. Calcium carbonate can cause gas or GI upset, but the symptoms can be alleviated by changing to another form, such as calcium citrate. On rare occasions, excessive calcium intake in conjunction with use of antacids has been reported to cause the milk-alkali syndrome.[81]

REFERENCES

1. Anderson JW, Chen W-JL, Sieling B: Hypolipidemic effects of high-carbohydrate, high-fiber diets, *Metabolism* 29:551-558, 1980.
2. Anderson JW et al: Hypocholesterolemic effects of oat-bran or bean intake for hypercholesterolemic men, *Am J Clin Nutr* 40:1146-1155, 1984.
3. Anderson JW et al: Lipid responses of hypercholesterolemic men to oat-bran and wheat-bran intake, *Am J Clin Nutr* 54:678-683, 1991.
4. Aravanis C et al: The Greek islands of Crete and Corfu, *Circulation* 42(suppl I):1-88, 1970.
5. Bendich A: Antioxidant vitamins and their role in immune response. In Antioxidant nutrients and immune function, *Adv Exp Med Biol* 262:39-55, 1990.
6. Bouchard C et al: The response to long-term overfeeding in identical twins, *N Engl J Med* 322:1477-1482, 1990.
7. Bowman WC, Rand MJ: *Textbook of pharmacology,* ed 2, Oxford, 1980, Blackwell Scientific.
8. Bray GA: Overweight is risking fate: definition, classification, prevalence, and risks. In Wurtman RJ, Wurtman JJ, editors: Human obesity, *Ann NY Acad Sci* 499:14-28, 1987.
9. Cambien F, Ducimetiere P, Richard J: Total serum cholesterol and cancer mortality in a middle age population, *Am J Epidemiology* 112:388-394, 1980.
10. Chandra RK: 1990 McCollum Award Lecture. Nutrition and immunity: lessons from the past and new insights into the future, *Am J Clin Nutr* 53:1087-1101, 1991.
11. Clark N: Eating right with type II diabetes, *Physician Sports Med* 20(9):17-18, 1992.
12. Colvin RM, Olson SB: Winners revisited: an 18-month follow-up of our successful weight losers. *Addict Behav* 9:305-306, 1984.
13. Committee on Diet Nutrition and Cancer. Assembly of Life Sciences. National Research Council: *Diet, nutrition, and cancer,* Washington DC, 1982, National Academy Press.
14. Correa P et al: A model for gastric cancer epidemiology, *Lancet* 2:58-60, 1975.
15. Dalton S: Eating management: a tool for the practitioner: yo-yo syndrome. In Frankle RT, Yang M-U, editors: *Obesity and weight control: the health professional's guide to understanding and treatment,* Rockville, Md, 1988, Aspen Publishers.
16. Dattilo AM: Dietary fat and its relationship to body weight, *Nutrition Today* 27:13-19, 1992.
17. *Diabetes mellitus,* ed 7, Indianapolis, 1973, Lilly Research Laboratories.
18. *Diet and health: 1989 implications for reducing chronic disease risk,* Washington DC, 1989, National Research Council, National Academy Press.
19. Dishman RK, editor: Exercise adherence: its impact on public health, Champaign, Ill, 1988, Human Kinetics Press.
20. Domel SB et al: Weight control for black women, *J Am Diet Assoc* 92:346-348, 1992.
21. Dwyer J et al: Unproven nutrition therapies for AIDS: what is the evidence? *Nutr Today* 23(2):25-33, 1988.
22. Foreyt JP: Predictors of Success and failure for long-term weight maintenance. In Issues in weight control, *J Am Diet Assoc* 92(1):17-22.
23. Forster JL et al: Preventing weight gain in adults: a pound of prevention, *Health Psychol* 7:515-525, 1988.
24. Fox SA: *Human physiology,* ed 2, Dubuque, Iowa, 1987, William C. Brown.
25. Gelb A, Miller S: AIDS and gastroenterology, *Am J Gastroenterol* 81:619-621, 1986.
26. Geppert J, Splett PL: Summary document of nutrition intervention in obesity, *J Am Diet Assoc* Suppl:S-31-S35, 1991.
27. Goldman L, Cook EF: The decline in ischemic heart disease mortality rates: an analysis of the comparative effects of medical interventions and changes in lifestyle, *Ann Intern Med* 101:825-836, 1984.
28. Gortmaker SL et al: Increasing pediatric obesity in the United States, *Am J Public Health* 141:535-540, 1987.
29. Graham S et al: Dietary factors in the epidemiology of cancer of the larynx, *Am J Epidemiol* 113:675-680, 1981.
30. Greenwood MRC, Pittman-Waller VA: Weight control: a complex, various, and controversial problem. In Frankle RT, Yang M-U, editors: *Obesity and weight control: the health professionals guide to understanding and treatment,* Rockville, Md, 1988, Aspen Publishers.
31. Grover SA et al: The benefits of treating hyperlipidemia to prevent coronary heart disease: estimating changes in life expectancy and morbidity, *JAMA* 267:816-822, 1992.
32. Guyton AC: *Textbook of medical physiology,* ed 5, Philadelphia, 1976, WB Saunders.
33. Harris WS: Fish oils and plasma lipid and lipoprotein metabolism in humans: a critical review, *J Lipid Res* 30:785, 1989.
34. Helmrich SP et al: Physical activity and reduced occurrence of non-insulin dependent diabetes mellitus, *N Engl J Med* 325(3):147-152, 1991.
35. Henry HJ et al: Increasing calcium intake lowers blood pressure: the literature reviewed, *J Am Diet Assoc* 85:182-185, 1985.
36. *HIV Nutrition Guidelines Committee,* Cleveland, Ohio, 1992, Health Action Task Force.
37. Hoeg J, Gregg RE, Brewer HB Jr: Special communication: an approach to the management of hyperlipoproteinemia, *JAMA* 225:512, 1986.
38. Jain M et al: A case control study of diet and colo-rectal cancer, *Int J Cancer* 26:757-768, 1980.
39. Karanja N, McCarron DA: Calcium and hypertension, *Annu Rev Nutr* 6:475-495, 1986.
40. Kark JD, Smith AH, Hames CG: The relationship of serum cholesterol to the incidence of cancer in Evans County, Georgia, *J Chronic Dis* 33:311-322, 1980.
41. Keys A et al: The diet and 15-year death rate in the Seven Countries Study, *Am J Epidemiol* 124:903, 1986.
42. Koda-Kimble MA, Rottblatt MD: *Diabetes mellitus.* In Young LY, Koda-Kimble MA, editors: Applied therapeutics: the clinical use of

drugs, ed 4, Vancouver, Wash, 1988, Applied Therapeutics.

43. Kolonol LN et al: Nutrient intake in relationship to cancer incidence in Hawaii, *Br J Cancer* 44:332-339, 1981.

44. Kris-Etherton PM, editor: *Cardiovascular disease: nutrition for prevention and treatment,* Chicago, Ill, 1990, Sports and Cardiovascular Nutritionists, The American Dietetic Association.

45. Kritchevsky D: Antioxidant vitamins in the prevention of cardiovascular disease, *Nutr Today* 27:30-33, 1992.

46. Levine AS et al: Effect of breakfast cereals on short-term food intake, *Am J Clin Nutr* 50:1303-1307, 1989.

47. Lipid Research Clinics Program: The Lipid Research Clinics Coronary Primary Prevention Trial Results. I. Reduction in incidence of coronary heart disease, *JAMA* 251:351-364, 1984.

48. Lipkin M, Newmark H: Effect of added calcium on colonic epithelial proliferation in subjects at high risk for familial colonic cancer, *N Engl J Med* 313(22):1381-1384, 1985.

49. Lubin JH et al: Dietary factors and breast cancer risk, *Int J Cancer* 28:685-689, 1981.

50. MacLennon R et al: Diet, transit time, stool weight, and colon cancer in two scandinavian populations, *Am J Clin Nutr* 31:S239-S242, 1978.

51. Malhotra SL: Dietary factors in a study of cancer colon from cancer registry with special reference to the role of saliva, milk and fermented milk products and vegetable fibre, *Med Hypotheses* 3:122-126, 1977.

52. Malone W: Studies evaluating antioxidants and B carotenes as chemopreventatives, *Am J Clin Nutr* 53:S305-S313, 1991.

53. McCarron DA: The calcium deficiency hypothesis of hypertension, *Ann Intern Med* 107:919-922, 1987.

54. Mettlin C, Graham S, Swanson M: Vitamin A and lung cancer, *J Natl Cancer Inst* 62:1435-1438, 1979.

55. Mettlin C et al: Diet and cancer of the esophagus, *Nutr Cancer* 2:143-147, 1981.

56. Mirvish SS: Inhibition of the formation of carcinogenic N-nitroso compounds by ascorbic acid and other compounds. In Burchenal JH, Oettgen HF, editors: *Cancer: achievements, challenges and prospects for the 1980s,* vol 1, New York, 1981, Grune and Stratton.

57. National Cholesterol Education Program: *Report of the expert panel on detection, evaluation and treatment of high blood cholesterol in adults,* Bethesda, Md, 1988, NIH publication no 88-2925, National Institutes of Health.

58. National Cholesterol Education Program: *Report of the expert panel on population strategies for blood cholesterol reduction.* Bethesda, Md, 1990, NIH publication no 90-3046, National Institutes of Health.

59. National Cholesterol Education Program Expert Panel: Report on detection, evaluation and treatment of high blood cholesterol in adults, *Arch Intern Med* 148:36, 1988.

60. NCI (National Cancer Institute): Diet, nutrition, and cancer prevention: a guide to food choices, Washington DC, 1987, NIH Publ No 87-2878. National Institutes of Health, Public Health Service, US Department of Health and Human Services. US Government Printing Office.

61. NIH (National Institutes of Health): Osteoporosis. Consensus Development Statement, 5 (3), 1984.

62. National Research Council: Recommended dietary allowances, ed 10, National Academy Press. Washington, DC, 1989.

63. Nutrition and HIV infection, *Nutrition in Clinical Practice,* 6:1-94, 1991.

64. Phillips RL: Role of lifestyle and dietary habits in risk of cancer among Seventh Day Adventists, *Cancer Res* 35:3513-3522, 1975.

65. Piquet J, Tison: Alcool et cancer de l'oesophage, *Bull Acad Med (Paris)* 117:236-239, 1937.

66. Prochaska HJ, Santamaria AB, Talay P: Rapid detection of inducers of enzymes that protect against carcinogens, *Proc Natl Acad Sci* 89:2394-2398, 1992.

67. Ravussin E et al: Reduced energy expenditure as a risk factor for body-weight gain, *N Engl J Med* 318:467-472, 1988.

68. Redard CL, Davis PA, Schneeman BO: Dietary fiber and gender: effect on postprandial lipemia, *Am J Clin Nutr* 52:837-845, 1990.

69. Resnick LM: Dietary calcium and hypertension, *J Nutr* 117:1806-1808, 1987.

70. Rivers JM, Collins KK: *Planning meals that lower cancer risk: a reference guide,* Washington, DC, 1984, American Institute for Cancer Research.

71. Schramm MM et al: Lack of an association between calcium intake and blood pressure in postmenapausal woman, *Am J Clin Nutr* 44:505-511, 1986.

72. Sharlin J et al: Nutrition and behavioral characteristics and determinants of plasma cholesterol levels in men and women, *J Am Diet Assoc* 92:434-440, 1992.

73. Shekelle RB et al: Dietary vitamin A and risk of cancer in the western electric study. *Lancet* 2:1185-1189, 1981.

74. Sherman C et al: *Quality food and nutrition services for AIDS patients,* Rockville, Md, 1990, Aspen Publications.

75. Sjoberg L, Persson L: A study of attempts by obese persons to regulate eating, *Addict Behav* 4:349-359, 1979.

76. Sorenson AW, Slatterly ML, Ford MH: Calcium and colon cancer: a review, *Nutr Cancer* 11:135-145, 1988.

77. Stunkard AJ et al: The body-mass index of twins who have been reared apart, *N Engl J Med* 322;1483-1487, 1990.

78. Surgeon General's Report on Nutrition and Health. 1988. US Department of Health and Human Services, Public Health Service, DHHS Publication No 88-50210, Washington, DC, 1988, US Government Printing Office.

79. Taylor WC et al: Cholesterol reduction and life expectancy: a model incorporating multiple risk factors, *Ann Intern Med* 105:605-614, 1987.

80. The Multiple Risk Factor Intervention Trial Research Group: Multiple risk factor intervention trial: risk factor changes and mortality results, *JAMA* 248:1465-1477, 1982.

81. Tolstoi LG, Levin RM: Osteoporosis-the treatment controversy. *Nutr Today* 27:6-12, 1992.

82. Tubiana, M: Human carcinogenisis- introductory remarks, *Am J Clin Nutr* 53:S223-S225, 1991.

83. Weisberger JH: Nutritional approach to cancer prevention with emphasis on vitamins, antioxidants and caratonoids, *Am J Clin Nutr* 53:S226-S237, 1991.

84. Wright HS et al: The 1987-88 nationwide food consumption survey: an update on the nutrient intake of respondents, *Nutr Today* 26:21, 1991.

85. Wylie-Rosett J: Evaluation of protein in dietary management of diabetes mellitus, *Diabetes Care* 11:143-148, 1988.

86. Wynder EL, Bross IJ: A study of etiological factors in cancer of the esophagus, *Cancer* 14:389-413, 1961.

87. Yang Mei-Uih: Body composition and resting metabolic rate in obesity. In Frankle RT, Yang M-U, editors: *Obesity and weight control: the health professionals guide to understanding and treatment,* Rockville, Md, 1988, Aspen Publishers.

88. Zeigler R: Vegetables, fruits and caratenoids and the risk of cancer, *Am J Clin Nutr* 53:S251-S259, 1991.

89. Zhang Y et al: A major inducer of anticarcinogenic protective enzymes from broccoli: isolation and elucidation of structure, *Proc Natl Acad Sci* 89:2399-2403, 1992.

■ RESOURCES ■

American Heart Association, National Center, 7320 Greenville Avenue, Dallas, TX 75231. Local chapters are the best resources. Provides patient, nurse, and physician education materials and programs. An excellent source for diet plans, guidelines, and food information, important for dietary counseling.

National Cholesterol Education Project, Department of Health and Human Services, Public Health Service, National Institutes of Health, National Heart, Lung, and Blood Institute, Bethesda, MD 20892. Provides research data and information; patient and practitioner education materials and programs.

National Cancer Institute. Provides consumer cancer prevention and treatment information.

Consumer Information Center, Pueblo, CO 81009.

Many USDA publications on diet and health.

National Center for Nutrition and Dietetics, Toll-free consumer hotline, 1-800-366-1655.

Pennington JAT: *Food values of portions commonly used,* ed 15, New York, 1989, Harper & Row. Provides complete nutrient content of foods, including many prepared and fast foods.

American Cancer Association, 1-800-562-2623.

American Diabetes Association, 1-800-232-3472.

National Kidney Foundation, 1-800-542-4001.

USDA Meat and Poultry Hotline; 1-800-535-4555; Information on food safety.

Centers for Disease Control AIDS Hotline, Atlanta, GA, 30301; 1-800-447-AIDS. In Atlanta 329-1295.

National Association of People with AIDS; (202) 483-7979.

Chapter 25

NUTRITION SCREENING AND ASSESSMENT

Susan M. Kleiner

According to Michener, "As the incidence of previously common debilitating diseases has declined, the benefits of incorporating preventive services into medical practice have become increasingly apparent."[21] The cholesterol screening and education initiatives have contributed to the decreasing incidence of heart disease. Prenatal screenings and assessments clearly affect pregnancy outcome.

In 1972, the Ten-State Nutrition Survey and the Health and Nutrition Examination Survey (HANES-Phase I) conducted by the National Center for Health Statistics reported the detection of groups and individuals in different parts of the country who were vulnerable to hunger and clinical and subclinical malnutrition.[11] Population groups that are deprived socially, economically, educationally, or medically were found to be at nutritional risk. Undernutrition was associated with growth cessation and developmental handicaps, poor outcomes of pregnancy, susceptibility to infectious diseases, delayed recovery from illness, and shortened life expectancy.[17]

After this recognition of the prevalence of malnutrition among Americans, Bistrian et al. documented the prevalence of malnutrition among hospitalized surgical and medical patients.[6,7] Today, even with nutrition intervention techniques available for those at risk of protein-malnutrition caused by primary illness,[32] the failure to identify and treat malnourished patients in hospitals continues.[16] For these reasons, groups targeted for nutritional surveillance and screening often include pregnant females, infants and children, hospitalized patients, and the elderly.

The publication of the *Surgeon General's Report on Nutrition and Health* in 1988 adjusted the focus of the nation's primary health care providers from disease treatment to disease prevention and treatment.[33] The recognition that diet plays a prominent role in five of the top 10 causes of death has shown that any American may fall into one or more high-risk groups for some type of malnutrition: that associated with underconsumption and conventional issues previously mentioned, and/or that associated with overconsumption and the relationship to several chronic diseases.

These risks are solid support for the nutritional assessment of patients by primary care physicians. The publication of the *Dietary Guidelines for Americans* (see the box on p. 442) has given primary care physicians a dietary model to follow while counseling patients.[26]

These dietary guidelines emphasize the positive, rather than negative, aspects of eating behavior. Instead of stating "avoid" or "do not eat" certain foods, the guidelines suggest that all foods can be eaten, but in moderation. This positive approach is more successful in promoting behavior change.

The dietary guidelines have been developed for educational use with healthy adult Americans. They may not be appropriate for patients with a diagnosed disease. For example, guideline 4, which advocates use of sugar in moderation, would be inappropriate for an insulin-dependent diabetic. Guideline 5, recommending salt and sodium only in moderation, would be inappropriate for a patient taking antihypertensive medication.

These guidelines should be used as a starting point for patient education. Patients with little nutrition knowledge will need more specific dietary advice to modify their diets and food behaviors.

BASIC PRINCIPLES OF NUTRITION ASSESSMENT AND SCREENING

The first nutrition assessment procedures were surveys used to describe the nutritional status of national populations. Classical nutrition assessment is defined as[16]:

The interpretation of information obtained from dietary, biochemical, anthropometric and clinical studies.

U.S. dietary guidelines (revised 1990)

Eat a variety of foods.

3-5 Servings vegetables (especially dark green and yellow)
2-4 Servings fruits (especially citrus)
6-11 Servings breads, cereals, rice, pasta
2-3 Servings milk, yogurt, cheese
2-3 Servings meats, poultry, fish, dry beans and peas, eggs, nuts

Maintain healthy weight.

Choose a diet low in fat, saturated fat, and cholesterol.
<30% of daily calories from fat
<10% of daily calories from saturated fat
<300 mg cholesterol per day

Choose a diet with plenty of vegetables, fruits, and grain products.

1 serving vegetable/fruit = 1 c raw, ½ c cooked, 1 medium piece
1 serving grain = 1 slice bread, ½ bun, bagel, English muffin, 1 oz cold cereal, ½ c cooked cereal, rice, pasta, grains

Use sugars in moderation only.

Examples of sugars include table sugar, brown sugar, raw sugar, glucose, fructose, maltose, lactose, honey, syrup, corn sweetener, high-fructose corn syrup, molasses, fruit juice concentrate

Use salt and sodium in moderation only.

1100-3300 mg sodium daily

If you drink alcoholic beverages, do so in moderation.

<1 drink/day for women, <2 drinks/day for men
1 drink = 12 oz beer, 5 oz wine, 1.5 oz liquor (80 proof)

From US Department of Agriculture, U.S. Department of Health and Human Services: *Nutrition and your health: dietary guidelines for Americans,* ed 3, Home and Garden Bulletin No. 232. Washington, DC: 1990, U.S. Government Printing Office.

Today we are interested in the nutritional assessment of populations and individuals, and different types of data-collection techniques are used, depending on the subject of investigation.

In the primary care setting, we need practical and reliable methods to quickly assess a patient's nutritional status and to solve common problems. The primary care practitioner should address common nutritional problems so that patients understand the importance of the diagnosis and recommended intervention. Preventive nutrition assessment and counseling should also be part of the physician's daily practice.

When uncommon or more complicated disease-oriented situations are detected (such as diabetes or heart disease), the busy primary physician may need to utilize the team approach for comprehensive health care. Referrals to specialists such as registered dietitians and nurse educators, who have the specialized training and time to devote to the patient's specific needs, can complement the care of the primary physician, resulting in improved patient compliance and case outcome.

Nutrition screening tools are useful for the rapid detection of glaring problems in an individual's diet. Several screening tools have been developed based on population studies, and they are generally focused toward specific population groups based on such factors as age, socioeconomic status, and race. A primary care physician could use these tools as a quick screen for patients, but they do not qualify as a method of nutrition assessment. Some of the nutrition screening tools available are included in this chapter.

Nutrition assessment tools

There are four parts to a complete nutritional assessment:

1. Dietary
2. Biochemical
3. Anthropometric
4. Clinical

All dietary assessment tools have strengths and weaknesses, yet the collection of food intake data is critical to the complete nutritional assessment of patients. The collection of dietary data is also important for the development of an intervention strategy and follow-up evaluation.

The following dietary assessment tools can be universally applied and can be adapted for each specific age group.[17] Examples of each tool follow. Two or more tools may be utilized to provide additional information about the dietary intake of a patient.

Generic nutrition questionnaire. The generic nutrition questionnaire (Table 25-1) is a universal questionnaire. Practitioners can select those questions that are appropriate for each situation then add others to elicit specific information required in their particular health care setting. If necessary, the questions can be phrased for the caregiver to answer; otherwise, questions can be answered by the patient.

24-Hour recall. The 24-hour recall (Table 25-2) is a dietary assessment tool that provides a historical window on food intake during a specific time. It can be used for any age group. The recall is based on the premise that information about foods and beverages that were consumed during the previous 24-hour period represents a broad picture of the client's food intake and habits. This assumption is flawed if the previous 24-hour period was not a typical day for the patient. It is therefore extremely important to determine whether the previous day's food intake was typical of the patient's diet. The 24-hour recall is best used with a second dietary assessment tool. It can also be useful

Text continued on p. 450.

Table 25-1. Generic nutrition questionnaire

Instructions for Practitioner:
  The generic nutrition questionnaire has been designed so that a nutrition questionnaire can be developed for any age or category. Questions have been listed under "generic" as well as under specific groupings. To develop a nutrition questionnaire for use with your clients, select those questions from the "generic" list and the specific lists (pregnancy, infancy, young child, and elderly) that are most appropriate to your group. Other questions can be added to make each questionnaire individualized to the needs of each setting.

Name: _____ Date: _____

This information will help us to give you more complete health care. It will be kept as a confidential part of your medical record.
  Please check answers to the following questions.

Data	Follow-up Required

I. Appetite
  a. How would you describe your appetite?
    ( ) Hearty   ( ) Moderate   ( ) Poor
  b. Do you enjoy eating?
    ( ) Yes   ( ) No   ( ) Sometimes
II. Eating pattern and attitudes about food
  a. Do you eat at approximately the same time every day?
    ( ) Yes   ( ) No   ( ) Sometimes
    If yes or sometimes, which meals, and how frequently?
  b. Do you skip meals?
    ( ) Yes   ( ) No
  If yes, at what times? _____
 	
  c. Are there any foods that you do not eat because you don't think they are good for you?
    ( ) Yes   ( ) No
  If yes, what? _____
 	
  d. Do you usually eat anything between meals?
    ( ) Yes   ( ) No
  If yes, name the two or three snacks (including bedtime snacks) that you have most often.
_____
 	
  e. During one week, where do you eat most of your food?
    Home _____   School _____
    Work _____   Restaurant _____
    Other _____ (identify)
  f. Are there any foods that you regularly eat because you think that they are good for you?
    ( ) Yes   ( ) No
  If yes, what? _____
 	
III. Food choices
  a. Is there any food you can't eat?
    ( ) Yes   ( ) No
  If yes, what food(s)?
  What happens when you eat this food?
_____
 	
  b. Are you allergic to any foods?	

Continued.

Table 25-1. Generic nutrition questionnaire—cont'd

Data

( ) Yes ( ) No

If yes, what food(s)? _____

What happens when you eat this food?

_____

_____

  c. Are there certain foods that you do not eat because you don't like them?

    ( ) Yes ( ) No

    If yes, what food(s)?

  d. Are there certain foods that you avoid eating because of your religious beliefs?

    ( ) Yes ( ) No

    If yes, what food(s)? _____

  e. Are there certain foods that you eat regularly because of your ethnic/cultural background?

    ( ) Yes ( ) No

    If yes, what food(s)? _____

  f. Are you on a special diet?

    ( ) Yes ( ) No

    Specify type of diet _____

    Who recommended the diet? _____

    If you have been on a special diet in the past, indicate what kind and how long _____

  g. How is your food usually prepared?

    ( ) Baked   ( ) Broiled   ( ) Fried

    Other _____

  h. Do you drink milk?

    ( ) Yes ( ) No

    If yes:

    ( ) Whole milk   ( ) Skim milk

    ( ) Other; specify _____

  i. List five of your favorite foods:

    _____

  j. List five of your least favorite foods:

    _____

IV. Weight history

  a. Have you ever had any problems with weight?

    ( ) Yes ( ) No

  b. If yes, what?

    ( ) Underweight   ( ) Overweight

    ( ) Other _____

  c. Are you now on a diet to lose weight?

    ( ) Yes ( ) No

    If yes, what kind? _____

    _____

    How long? _____

    Who recommended it? _____

  d. How do you feel about your weight?

    ( ) Too heavy   ( ) Too thin   ( ) Okay

  e. Do you ever vomit to keep your weight down?

( ) Every day   ( ) 3-4 Times/week

( ) Every week   ( ) Sometimes   ( ) Never

V. Supplements and medications

  a. Are you now taking any vitamin or mineral supplements:

    ( ) Yes   ( ) No

    If yes, what, how often, and what brand?

    _____

  b. Do you regularly take any medications prescribed by your doctor?

    ( ) Yes   ( ) No

    If yes, what? _____

  c. Do you regularly take any "over-the-counter" medications?

    ( ) Yes   ( ) No

    If yes, what? _____

VI. Smoking, alcohol, and substance use

  a. Do you smoke?

    ( ) Yes   ( ) No

    If yes, how many cigarettes per day?

    _____

  b. Do you drink any alcoholic beverages (liquor, wine, wine coolers, beer)?

    ( ) Yes   ( ) No

    If yes, what do you drink and how often?

    _____

    _____

  c. Do you smoke marijuana?

    ( ) Yes   ( ) No

    If yes, how often? _____

  d. How often do you use crack, cocaine, speed, or other street drugs?

    ( ) Every day   ( ) 3-6 times/week

    ( ) Every week   ( ) Sometimes   ( ) Never

VII. Exercise

  a. How often do you exercise?

    ( ) Every day   ( ) 3-6 times/week

    ( ) Once/week   ( ) Sometimes   ( ) Never

  b. List kinds of exercise you do most often _____

  c. How often do you get out of breath when you exercise?

    ( ) Often   ( ) Sometimes   ( ) Never

VIII. Household information

  a. Indicate the person who does the following in your household:

    Plans the meals _____

    Buys the food _____

    Prepares the food _____

  b. How much is spent on food each week for your household?

    $ _____   ( ) Don't know

    For how many people? _____

  c. Are there periods in the month when there isn't enough money for food or you run out of food?

    ( ) Yes   ( ) No

    If yes, when and how long are these periods? _____

    _____

Continued.

Table 25-1. Generic nutrition questionnaire—cont'd

Data	Follow-up Required
d. Indicate the types of kitchen equipment you have in your home. 　( ) Refrigerator　　　　( ) Working stove 　( ) Hot plate　　　　　( ) Piped water 　　　　　　　　　　　　( ) Sink IX. Food programs 　a. Are you receiving any of the following: 　　( ) Food stamps 　　( ) WIC vouchers 　　( ) Commodity foods 　b. Does your family use: 　　( ) Food co-ops　　　　( ) Food shelves 　　( ) Food pantries　　　 ( ) Soup kitchens 　　( ) Free or reduced-price school lunch and/or breakfast 　　( ) Summer feeding program 　c. How many hot meals do you have each week? 　　>7　　7　　6　　<6	

Pregnancy nutrition questionnaire

Select appropriate questions from the Generic Nutrition Questionnaire and then consider inclusion of the following questions:

Data	Follow-up Required
a. What was your weight before you became pregnant? 　_____ lb　　　　　　( ) Don't know b. During your last pregnancy, how much weight did you gain? 　_____lb　　　　　　 ( ) Don't know 　If known, in how many months? 　_____ c. How much weight do you expect to gain during this pregnancy? 　_____ lb　　　　　　( ) Don't know d. Has your weight changed by more than 10 lb within the past year before this pregnancy? 　( ) Yes　　　( ) No　　　　　　　　　　( ) Don't Know 　If yes, how much? _____ 　If yes, why? 　( ) Dieted　　　　　　( ) Began eating more 　( ) Illness. If so, what illness? _____ 　( ) Was pregnant or lactating 　( ) Change in lifestyle (for example, stress, increased exercise, or work) 　( ) Don't know　　　　( ) Other e. Has your eating pattern changed since you became pregnant? 　( ) Yes　　　( ) No 　If yes, how? _____ 　_____ f. Do you think that what you eat affects your health or the health of the baby? 　( ) Yes　　　( ) No	

Data	Follow-up Required
g. With this pregnancy, have you experienced either of the following? ( ) Nausea ( ) Vomiting If yes, when and how frequently? _____ h. Do you have any cravings for or eat such things as: ( ) Plaster ( ) Laundry starch ( ) Dirt or clay ( ) Other nonfood items i. How do you want to feed your baby? ( ) Breastfeed ( ) Formula ( ) Undecided	

Infant nutrition questionnaire

Select appropriate questions from the Generic Nutrition Questionnaire and then consider inclusion of the following questions:

Questions to be answered by parent or caregiver.

Data	Follow-up Required
a. Is the baby breastfed? ( ) Yes ( ) No If yes, does the baby also receive formula? ( ) Yes ( ) No If yes, what brand and kind? _____ b. Does the baby receive formula? ( ) Yes ( ) No If yes: ( ) Ready-to feed ( ) Concentrated liquid ( ) Other How is the formula prepared (especially dilution)? _____ Is the formula iron-fortified? ( ) Yes ( ) No c. Does the baby drink milk? ( ) Yes ( ) No If yes: ( ) Whole milk ( ) 2% milk ( ) Skim milk ( ) Other _____ Specify _____ d. How many times does the baby eat each day, including milk or formula?_____ e. If the baby drinks formula or milk, what is the usual amount in a day? ( ) Less than 16 oz ( ) 16 to 32 oz ( ) More than 32 oz	

Continued.

Table 25-1. Generic nutrition questionnaire—cont'd

Data	Follow-up Required
f. Does the baby usually take a bottle to bed? （　）Yes　　　　　（　）No If yes, what is usually in the bottle? _____ g. What was the infant's birthweight? _____ h. Was the infant premature? （　）Yes　　　　　（　）No i. Do you give your infant extra fluids? （　）Yes　　　　　（　）No If so, what and how much? _____ _____ j. At what age did you start cereal? _____ Is it iron-fortified? （　）Yes　　　　　（　）No Vegetables? _____ Fruit/juice? _____　　　　Egg yolk? _____ Meat and other protein? _____ Table food? _____　　　　Finger foods? _____ k. Do you make your own baby food? （　）Yes　　　　　（　）No Or do you use commercial foods? （　）Yes　　　　　（　）No l. Does your infant spit up often or have loose or hard stools? _____ m. Do you think the child has a feeding problem? （　）Yes　　　　　（　）No If yes, describe _____ _____	

The young child nutrition questionnaire

Select appropriate questions from the Generic Nutrition Questionnaire and then consider inclusion of the following questions:

Questions to be answered by parent or caregiver

Data	Follow-up Required
(For children more than 1 year of age but less than 4 years of age) a. Does the child drink anything from a bottle? （　）Yes　　　　　（　）No If yes: （　）Milk　　　　　（　）Other Specify _____ _____ b. Does the child take a bottle to bed? （　）Yes　　　　　（　）No If yes, what is usually in the bottle? _____	

Data

c. How would you describe the child's appetite?

( ) Good   ( ) Fair   ( ) Poor

Other (specify) _____

_____

d. Does the child eat clay, paint chips, or anything else not usually considered food?

( ) Yes   ( ) No

If yes: What? _____

How often? _____

The elderly nutrition questionnaire

Select appropriate questions from the Generic Nutrition Questionnaire and then consider inclusion of the following questions:

For questions with numbered answers, circle the number beside the answer given by the respondent.

Data   **Follow-up Required**

a. How do you buy your food?

1. Buy it myself.
2. Go food shopping with a relative or friend.
3. Have the food bought for me.
4. Don't need to buy food at a store because I eat in a restaurant.
5. Don't need to go food shopping because I eat with my family.

b. If you buy food at a store, which of the following foods do you buy every week?

1. Milk
2. Eggs
3. Cheese
4. Meat
5. Fruit juice
6. Fresh fruit
7. Cereal

8. Canned or frozen fruit
9. Fresh vegetables
10. Canned or frozen vegetables
11. Bread
12. Crackers
13. Canned soup
14. Canned fish

c. Do you need assistance with food shopping?

( ) Yes   ( ) No

If yes, do you get the assistance you need?

( ) Yes   ( ) No

d. Are there days in the week when you don't eat?

( ) Yes   ( ) No

If yes, which of the following reasons best describes your reason for not eating?

1. I don't have any food in the house.
2. I feel too sick to eat.
3. I feel too depressed to eat.
4. Other (give reason) _____

e. How many hot meals do you usually have each day?

More than 3   3   2   1   Less than 1

f. how many times in a day do you usually eat?

More than 3   3   2   1   Less than 1

Continued.

Table 25-1. Generic nutrition questionnaire—cont'd

Data	Follow-up Required
g. Do you eat meals at a congregate feeding site? ( ) Yes ( ) No If yes, how many meals do you get there per week? 7 6 5 4 3 2 1 h. Do you get home-delivered meals? ( ) Yes ( ) No More than 7 7 6 5 4 3 2 1 i. If you are not getting home-delivered meals, are you on a waiting list? ( ) Yes ( ) No If yes, how long have you been on the waiting list? 1. Less than a month 2. 1-3 months 3. More than 3 months	

Modified from: nutrition questionnaire in *Nutrition during pregnancy and lactation* (California Department of Health, 1975); Fomon SJ: *Nutritional disorders of children: prevention, screening and follow-up,* DHEW Publication No. (HSA) 77-5104 (US Department of Health, Education, and Welfare, Public Health Services Administration, reprinted 1977); Wong D, Whaley, LF: *Clinical handbook of pediatric nursing,* ed 2, St Louis, 1986, Mosby; and questionnaires contributed by Irene Alton, Janet King, and Daphne Roe. From Simko MD, Cowell C, and Hreha MS, editors: *Practical nutrition,* Rockville, MD, 1989, Aspen Publishers.

during follow-up visits to determine whether the patient is adapting to dietary recommendations.

Food frequency form. The food frequency form (Table 25-3) is a checklist that elicits data regarding the kinds of food eaten and the frequency of intake over a period of time. It can help to confirm the adequacy or deficiency of a patient's diet and is best used with a second dietary assessment tool.

Food diary. The food diary (Table 25-4) is a patient-recorded description of intake over a period of days (usually 3 to 7). Different from a recall, which is a historical record based on the patient's memory of the past 24 hours, the food diary is recorded by the patient or caregiver immediately after the patient eats. The patient or caregiver is given instructions on how to complete the diary at the first visit and returns the diary at the follow-up visit. The food and activity record (Table 25-5) describes food intake, activity, and mood. Each of these tools may be used as it appears or each may be adapted to specific situations.

The biochemical assessment of a patient through laboratory methods is an essential component to a complete nutrition assessment. Laboratory measures can identify the state or stage of a nutritional deficiency or degree of diet-related disease risk. Tissue stores, nutrient metabolites, and/or the activity of nutrient-dependent enzymes can be measured as part of the biochemical assessment. Tests that measure physiological or behavioral functions dependent on specific nutrients are described as functional, rather than biochemical, indices of nutritional status.[16] Examples of such functions include dark adaptation (vitamin A), taste acuity (zinc), capillary fragility (vitamin C), and cognitive function (iron).

According to Pi-Sunyer and Woo, the tests for different nutrients are not equally valuable, and therefore diagnostic weight cannot be placed equally.[27] For example, direct tests of water-soluble vitamins in the blood are more sensitive than indirect tests of the excretion of a metabolite in the urine. Precision and accuracy of tests must also be considered.

We are still discovering how certain nutrients travel between tissues and how they are utilized during activity. For instance, there is no single reliable biochemical index of zinc status in humans. Serum and plasma zinc levels have been used to assess status. Although circulating zinc may in some instances reflect the body's zinc status, it also may reflect zinc from a body storage pool that is available as necessary for metabolically active tissues. Zinc is mobilized under stress conditions of exercise, infection, or inflammation. Functional tests, including neuropsychological function, immune response, reproductive competence, and work capacity, might be more accurate for the assessment of zinc status.[4]

This is a particularly good demonstration of the importance of conducting a complete nutritional assessment, examining all four phases of the assessment strategy. Under these circumstances it would be appropriate to check circulating zinc, but no definitive diagnosis should be made based on this test alone.

Table 25-2. 24-hour recall

Name _____   Date of Birth _____ $\frac{\quad\quad}{\text{month}}$ / $\frac{\quad\quad}{\text{date}}$ / $\frac{\quad\quad}{\text{year}}$

ID# _____   Sex _____

| Time | Place | Food | Amount | For Practitioner Use | |
				Code Food Group	Summary

a. This is a typical day. Yes _____ No _____
b. I take a vitamin/mineral supplement. Yes _____ No _____
    If yes, name the brand _____
c. I have been on a special diet during the past 3 months. Yes _____ No _____
    If yes, the kind of special diet _____

Instructions:

1. Record time of day or night when you ate food or drank beverages (8 AM, 9 PM, etc.).
2. Indicate the place where you ate (home-kitchen, home-living room, restaurant, etc.).
3. Describe the specific food eaten or drunk during a 24-hour period, beginning with the first meal or snack (e.g., fried chicken, plain yogurt); use brand names.
4. Indicate the amount of food or beverage (e.g., ½ cup, 1 slice, 1 chicken leg, etc.).

Modified from Simko MD, Cowell C, and Gilbride JA: *Nutrition assessment: a comprehensive guide for planning intervention*, Rockville, Md, 1984, Aspen Publishers.

Table 25-3. Food frequency form

Client's Name: _____ Date: _____

Interviewer: _____

Food	Don't Eat	Do Eat	Serving Size	Number of Servings Per Week
I. Animal and vegetable protein foods Chicken				
Beef, hamburger, veal				
Liver, kidney, tongue, etc.				
Lamb, goat				
Cold cuts, hot dogs				
Pork, ham, sausage				
Bacon				
Fish				
Kidney beans, pinto beans, lentils				
Soybeans				
Tofu				
Eggs				
Nuts or seeds				
Peanut butter				
II. Milk and milk products Milk, fluid: Type: _____				
Milk, dry				
Milk, evaporated				
Condensed milk				
Cottage cheese				
Cheese (all kinds except cottage)				
Yogurt				
Pudding and custard flan				
Milkshake				
Sherbert				
Ice cream				
Ice milk				

Food	Don't Eat	Do Eat	Serving Size	Number of Servings Per Week
III. Grain products				
Whole grain bread				
White bread				
Rolls, biscuits, muffins				
Crackers, pretzels				
Pancakes, waffles				
Cereals: Brand: _____				
White rice				
Brown rice				
Noodles, macaroni, grits, hominy				
Tortillas (flour)				
Tortillas (corn)				
Bulgar				
Popcorn				
Wheat germ				
IV. Vitamin-C-rich fruits and vegetables				
Tomato, tomato sauce, or tomato juice				
Orange or orange juice				
Tangerine				
Grapefruit or grapefruit juice				
Papaya, mango				
Strawberries, cantaloupe				
White potato, yautia, yams, plantain, yucca				
Turnip				
Peppers (green, red, chili)				

Continued.

Table 25-3. Food frequency form—cont'd

Food	Don't Eat	Do Eat	Serving Size	Number of Servings Per Week
V. Leafy green vegetables				
Dark green or red lettuce				
Asparagus				
Swiss chard				
Bok choy				
Cabbage				
Broccoli				
Brussel sprouts				
Scallions				
Spinach				
Greens (beet, collard, kale, turnip, mustard)				
VI. Other fruits and vegetables				
Carrots				
Artichoke				
Corn				
Sweet potato or yam				
Zucchini				
Summer squash				
Winter squash				
Green peas				
Green and yellow beans				
Beets				
Cucumbers or celery				
Peach				
Apricot				
Apple				
Banana				
Pineapple				
Cherries				
VII. Snacks, sweets, and beverages				
Potato chips				
French fries				
Cakes, pies, cookies				
Sweet rolls, doughnuts				

Food	Don't Eat	Do Eat	Serving Size	Number of Servings Per Week
Candy				
Sugar or honey				
Carbonated beverages (sodas)				
Coffee: Type: _____				
Tea: Type: _____				
Cocoa				
Wine, beer, cocktails				
Fruit drink				
VIII. Other foods not listed that you regularly eat				

From Simko MD, Cowell C, and Hreha MS, editors: *Practical nutrition,* Rockville, Md, 1989, Aspen Publishers.

Table 25-4. Food diary

Name: _____ Date: _____

Please write down everything you eat for 3 days before your next appointment.

To do this:

1. Write down everything you eat or drink in the order in which it was eaten.
2. Include meals and snacks as well as gum and candy.
3. Write down the amount you eat. Use standard measuring cups and spoons. Record meat portions as ounces.
4. Write down items added to food (sugar on cereal, butter on bread, salad dressing to salad, etc.)
5. Write down the time you eat.
6. Write down how you prepared it (baked, fried, broiled, etc.).
7. Include a list of any vitamin and/or mineral supplements you take. Write down the name of the supplement, the amount of vitamins or minerals it contains, and the amount taken.

Examples:

Day 1: Time	Food and Preparation	Amount
12:30 PM	Peanut butter sandwich	1 tablespoon peanut butter 2 slices bread, whole wheat
	Milk, 2%	6 ounces

Make a separate sheet for each day.

From Simko MD, Cowell C, and Hreha MS, editors: *Practical nutrition,* Rockville, Md, 1989, Aspen Publishers.

Table 25-5. Food and activity record

Date _____   Name _____

Time	Food (quantity-type)	Activity and Length of Time	Where/with whom	Mood*	How hungry
Examples					
9:00 AM	Candy bar (1 large)	15 Min. in hall	School friend	Tired	Very
3:00 PM	Potato chips ½ medium bag	30 Min. watching TV	Home, alone	Bored	A little
5:30 PM	Cola (regular) 1 can	Thirsty	Work, another store clerk	"Down"	Thirsty
7:00 PM	Cookies (3 chocolate chip)	Late for dinner	Work, alone	Upset	Very

*Anxious, bored, content, depressed, "down," angry, tired, happy, relaxed, "up," celebrating, other.
From Simko MD, Cowell C, Hreha MS, editors: *Practical nutrition,* Rockville, Md, 1989, Aspen Publishiers.

To create efficient strategies for the assessment of biochemical/functional nutritional status of patients, population studies have identified specific nutrients considered to be the "high-risk nutrients" associated with certain population groups, based on life-cycle stage, as well as other population indices. In this chapter, recommendations for biochemical/functional assessments will be based on life-cycle stage.

The anthropometric assessment measures the physical dimensions and gross composition of the body.[16] It provides information about the nutritional history of the patient and can indicate undernutrition or overnutrition.

There are many methods of anthropometric measurement. Many are technical, technique-sensitive, and time-consuming, making them inappropriate tools for use in the busy practice of a primary care physician. After consulting with physicians, Simko, Hreha, and Cowell recommend the use of height and weight measurements and midarm circumference measurements to obtain anthropometric assessment data in a clinical office setting.[31]

Height and weight measures are indicators of growth. In infants, children, and adolescents, this is an extremely important indicator of health. Any significant departure from a child's own rate of growth should be investigated. In adults, weight-for-height measures may be predictors of disease. Significant increases or decreases in weight should be investigated.

Arm circumference measures are indicators of body fatness. This is an especially important tool for individuals whose height or weight measure is not valid (e.g., elderly who have lost height, amputees, individuals unable to stand, edematous patients) or does not conform to the height-weight standards (e.g., the muscular individual who may be overweight but not overfat).

To obtain the arm circumference, a nonstretchable cloth, flexible steel, or plastic measuring tape should be used. Insertion tapes (available from Ross Laboratories, Columbus, Ohio) are preferred because they have a "window" for taking readings. A more flexible tape may be preferable for use with infants, because their soft arm fat is easily indented by a stiff tape, resulting in measurement errors. The tape is applied lightly to the skin surface so that the tape is taut but not tight. This procedure avoids skin compression, which produces inaccurately low scores. Duplicate measures should be taken and the average used as the circumference score. The process for measuring upper arm circumference for young and older men and women is: arm straight; palm up, extended in front of the body, at a 90-degree angle; measure at the midpoint between the top of the acromion process of the scapula (shoulder) and the olecranon process of the ulna (elbow)[19,28] (Figs. 25-1 and 25-2).

Indices constructed from raw height and weight data, such as simple numerical ratios (weight/[height]^2) or weight or height to age, can add helpful information to the assessment process. Depending on the patient and clinical question, other measures of body circumference can be useful. More specific recommendations based on life-cycle stage will be included later in this chapter.

The medical history and clinical examination make up the clinical portion of a complete nutrition assessment. These methods are used to detect physical signs and symptoms of malnutrition. Because initial clinical signs and symptoms associated with malnutrition may be vague and

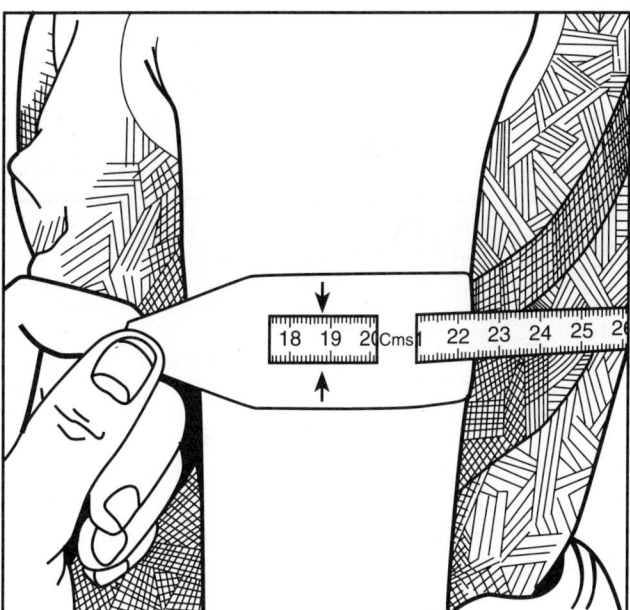

Fig. 25-2. Insertion tape. (From Robbins GE, Trowbridge FL: Anthropometric techniques and their application. In Simko MD, Cowell C, and Gilbride JA: *Nutrition assessment*, Rockville, Md, 1984, Aspen Publishers.)

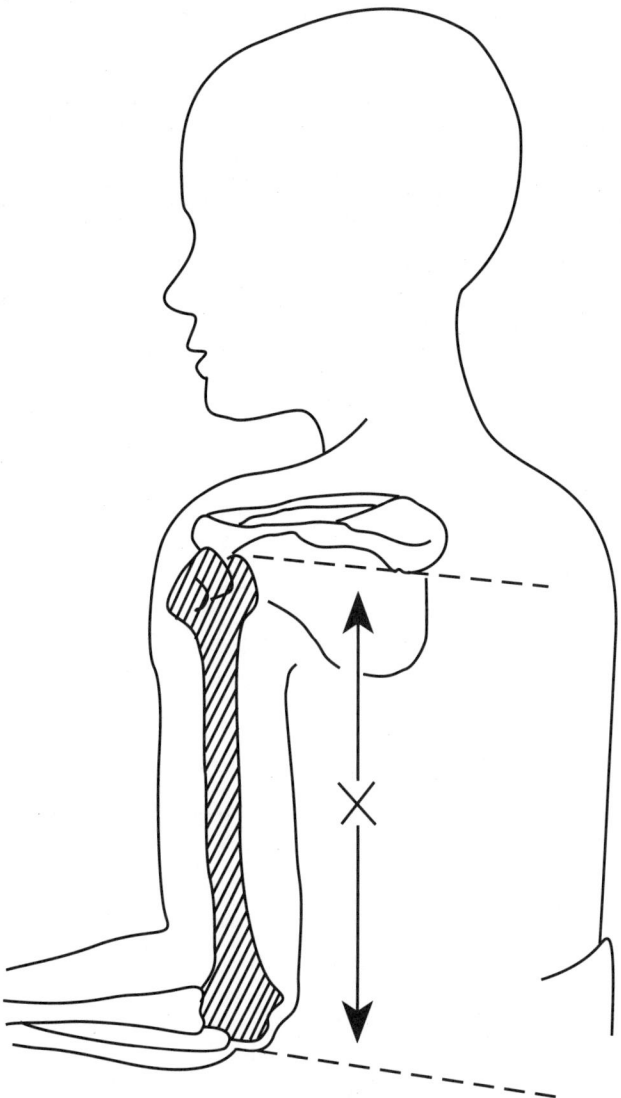

Fig. 25-1. Measuring mid-upper arm circumference. (From Simko MD, Cowell C, Gilbride JA: *Nutrition assessment, a comprehensive guide on planning intervention*, Rockville, Md, 1984, Aspen Publishers.)

do not usually occur specifically until the patient is in a frank state of nutrient depletion or overconsumption, the nutritional assessment should never rely exclusively on the results of a clinical assessment. It is desirable to detect marginal nutritional problems before clinical syndromes develop, and as a result, laboratory, dietary, and anthropometric methods should be included as an adjunct to clinical assessment.[16]

NUTRITION ASSESSMENT OF PREGNANT WOMEN

The nutritional assessment of a pregnant woman not only must consider her present nutritional status, but her lifetime nutritional status as well. The preconceptual period may be the most opportune time to concentrate on nu-

trition intervention, because the hope-to-be mother may be unusually receptive to dietary guidance.[3] Underweight women, women using oral contraceptives, and women with a history of prior poor outcomes of pregnancy should be targeted for such early assessment and intervention. Estrogen-containing oral contraceptives have been implicated in decreasing the level of serum folate and increasing the excretion of tryptophan metabolites associated with vitamin B_6 deficiency.[22]

Clinical assessment

The preconception history should include present height-weight status; weight-control activities and physical fitness programs currently and previously used; use of dietary supplements; alternative or unusual dietary practices (e.g., vegetarianism); medical risk factors that might affect nutritional status, especially diabetes, anemia, colitis, and any surgery on the GI tract, such as gastroplasty or intestinal bypass.[2]

A complete health and family history should also be collected as part of the nutritional data base established for each woman during the initial evaluation. This should include[3]:

- Pregravid weight
- Medical risk factors, including diabetes, anemia, hypertension, and cardiac, pulmonary, kidney, and thyroid disease
- Allergies
- Gallstones
- Pancreatitis

Table 25-6. Significant findings reflecting nutrient deficits during pregnancy

Nutrient deficit	Maternal	Fetal
Protein	Edema	Prematurity
	Hair loss	
	Change in hair color or texture	
Iron	Pallor	Low birthweight
B_{12}	Glossitis, pallor	
Folic acid	Glossitis	Neural tube defects
Calcium	Acceleration of osteoporosis	Decreased bone density
Zinc	Seborrheic dermatitis	Fetal malformation
	Alopecia	Neural tube defects
	Diarrhea	

Adapted from Moore MC: *Pocket guide to nutrition and diet therapy*, St. Louis, 1988, CV Mosby.

- Colitis
- Any previous GI surgery
- Methods of family planning, because oral contraceptives can decrease the levels of various nutrients in the blood.

Once pregnancy has been established, the health history should include assessment of the following:

- Medical risks affecting nutritional status, such as year from menarche if adolescent
- Percentage of ideal body weight for gestational age
- Infections
- Gestational diabetes
- Elevated blood pressure
- Generalized edema
- Hyperemesis
- Ptyalism (excessive saliva secretion)
- Severe heartburn
- Active gallstone
- Chronic diarrhea
- Inability to consume an adequate diet because of previous GI surgery

The physical examination of the pregnant woman includes an assessment of the health and well-being of the growing fetus as well as the mother. For specific physical manifestations associated with nutrient deficits, see Table 25-6.

Anthropometric assessment

The quantity and rate of maternal weight gain is the best anthropometric indicator of fetal growth and development. Different rates and amounts of weight gain are recommended during pregnancy for average, overweight, and underweight women, as well as for adolescent and multiple fetus pregnancies (Table 25-7). Prenatal weight should

Table 25-7. Estimating pregnancy weight status

Height (without shoes)		Weight* (without clothes)			
Feet	Inches	Underweight	Normal Weight	Overweight	Obese
4	8	< 89	89-109	110-129	>129
4	9	< 91	91-111	112-131	>131
4	10	< 94	94-114	115-135	>135
4	11	< 96	96-117	118-139	>139
5		< 99	99-121	122-143	>143
5	1	<102	102-124	125-147	>147
5	2	<105	105-128	129-152	>152
5	3	<109	109-133	134-157	>157
5	4	<112	112-137	138-162	>162
5	5	<116	116-142	143-167	>167
5	6	<120	120-146	147-173	>173
5	7	<123	123-151	152-176	>178
5	8	<127	127-155	156-183	>183
5	9	<130	130-159	160-188	>188
5	10	<134	134-163	164-193	>193
5	11	<137	137-167	168-197	>197
6		<140	140-171	172-202	>202
6	1	<143	143-175	176-207	>207

*Calculations of relative weight are based on the midpoint values by height for women with a "medium" frame at age 25, as given in the 1959 Metropolitan Life Insurance Table. Underweight is defined as a weight-for-height of <90% of the midpoint, normal weight as 90%-110%, overweight as 110%-130%, and obese as >130% of standard weight.
Adapted from Metropolitan Life Insurance Company, Statistical Bulletin No. 40, 1949, by J.E. Brown, University of Minnesota, October 1987. From Simko MD, Cowell C, Hreha MS, editors: *Practical nutrition,* Rockville, Md, 1989, Aspen Publishers.

be charted at the initial visit and all subsequent visits (Fig. 25-3).

Biochemical assessment

There are well-established guidelines for laboratory assessment of pregnant women (see Chapter 30). There are no specific nutrient-associated tests that should be routinely performed, aside from those to be mentioned here. Laboratory tests should be compared with standard values of pregnant, rather than nonpregnant, women, as pregnancy affects the laboratory standards of most of the biochemical indices.

At the initial visit, and then at each trimester, hemoglobin or hematocrit should be measured. Blood glucose determinations should be conducted at the initial visit for women at risk for diabetes, and at 24 to 28 weeks for all women. A urinalysis for protein and glucose should be conducted at every prenatal visit.[3]

Dietary assessment

It is common for physicians to inquire as to the quality of a pregnant woman's diet; however, unless diet seems to be an apparent risk, it is less common for a physician to collect true food intake data. It is assumed that patients eat well, but this is clearly not supported by national dietary surveys, and pregnant women are among the groups identified to be at nutritional risk.[11] A nutrition questionnaire should be administered at the initial visit to collect broad baseline data and evaluate the general nutrition practices of the patient. A 24-hour recall should be conducted at the initial visit and whenever indicated afterward, such as for follow-up evaluation or whenever a risk is identified.[3] If more complex dietary assessment, intervention, and education are necessary, referral to a registered dietitian specializing in obstetrics may be indicated.

NUTRITION ASSESSMENT OF INFANTS: BIRTH TO 2 YEARS

National nutrition surveys have identified infants as a group at particular risk of nutritional deficiency.[11] Therefore, health care practitioners cannot be satisfied with detection of nutritional disorders in infant patients. They must pursue the identification of individuals who are at increased risk of nutritional deficiencies or excesses.[14]

Clinical assessment

The health history includes information about the family and the infant's environment, the period of intrauterine development, and the events surrounding birth. Details of illnesses and abnormalities should be recorded.[14]

The physical examination should target clinical signs of specific nutritional deficiencies, although physical findings suggesting nutritional abnormality should be considered as only one part of the complete nutritional assessment. Biochemical, dietary, and anthropometric indices should be considered before establishing an exact diagnosis.

The hair, eyes, tongue, skin, neck, and skeleton are the most relevant sites for detecting the presence of nutritional abnormalities. Special attention should be paid to such general features as pallor, apathy, irritability, and the presence of petechiae, ecchymosis, dermatitis, or edema. The condition of the gums and teeth should be recorded. The possibility of cardiovascular, pulmonary, hepatic, or renal disease should be considered.[14]

Anthropometric assessment

Changes in length and weight are sensitive indicators of growth over time, and length and weight data with precise dates should be recorded diligently. However, the assessment of nutritional status using the growth charts published by the National Center for Health Statistics is somewhat misleading, as the individual's size at a specified age is compared with that of peers, rather than with the infant's own rate of growth. Growth rate, or changes in weight and length per unit of time, is more useful for the clinical nutrition assessment.

Only gross deviations from normal are usually detected solely by using these growth charts. Obesity, or excessive weight for height, is more readily detectable on the growth

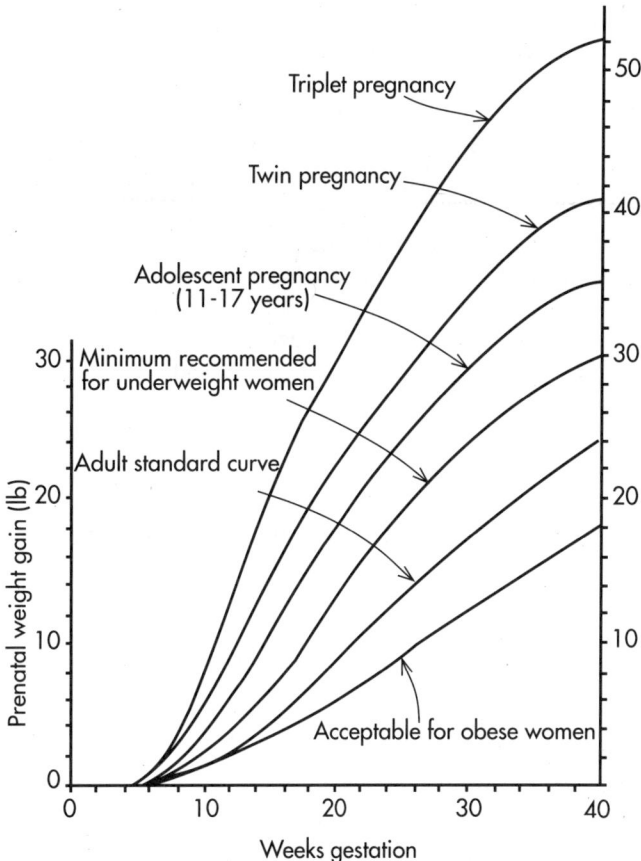

Fig. 25-3. Weight gain during pregnancy for selected subgroups of women. (From Williams SR, Worthington-Roberts B, editors: Nutrition through life cycle, St Louis, 1988, Mosby. In Simko MD et al: *Practical nutrition,* Rockville, Md, 1989, Aspen Publishers.)

chart than decreased rate of growth and potential nutritional deficiency.[14]

Clues to the identification of infants at nutritional risk are length for age below the 10th percentile and weight for length above the 90th or below the 10th percentile. Accuracy of measurement is essential, because measurement errors of 1 cm would place substantial numbers of patients with lengths between the 10th and 25th percentiles into a group meriting special attention. Conversely, infants with lengths less than the 10th percentile will be mistakenly thought to require no special attention.[14]

The measurement of head circumference is traditional in the anthropometric assessment of infants and is essential to the documentation of the presence of nonnutritional microcephaly and macrocephaly. However, in normal and malnourished infants, gain in head circumference closely parallels growth in length and adds little to assessment of nutrition status.[14]

Biochemical assessment

Suspicion of nutritional deficiency from the clinical assessment should be confirmed by laboratory tests. Tests are available for detecting nutritional abnormalities of protein, essential fatty acids, vitamins, and many minerals. Unless suspicion of dietary deficiency arises because of results of anthropometric, clinical, and dietary assessments, these laboratory tests need not be performed routinely.

The most prevalent nutritional deficiency among infants is iron deficiency.[14] Hemoglobin concentration and hematocrit should be routinely determined between 9 and 12 months of age in term infants and between 6 and 9 months of age in preterm infants. These lab values offer information relative to recent iron intake, but do not necessarily reflect iron storage. Between 9 months and 3 years of age, most anemia is the result of iron deficiency.[14]

If anemia is present, then iron stores have already been depleted. Laboratory tests useful in documenting the presence of iron deficiency are listed in Table 25-8. At least two or three of these tests should be conducted, because a normal value may be obtained in the presence of iron deficiency for any one of the tests, and abnormal values may be obtained in patients with good iron status.[14]

Dietary assessment

Obtaining the dietary history of infants is often easier than at any other age, because the caretaker is usually well informed regarding the child's usual intake and the variety of foods consumed is limited. In early infancy, the patient is breast- or formula-fed, and the only relevant information is quantity and quality of the liquid feedings. However, even at very early stages, some caretakers choose to give infants foods or liquids that are not normally recommended, and documentation of these practices is critical to the complete nutritional assessment of the infant.

Food intake information can be collected by a 24-hour recall method if daily intakes are consistent and regular. A 3-day to 7-day food diary can also be used to collect more complex dietary data. According to Austin, caretakers of underweight infants generally overestimate, and caretakers of overweight infants underestimate the amounts of food consumed.[5]

Common nutritional problems in infancy include feeding difficulties, overweight/obesity, nursing bottle caries, refusal to eat, and failure to gain weight.[5] If any of these problems requires more intervention than a busy primary

care physician can devote, a referral to a registered dietitian specializing in infant care should be considered.

NUTRITION ASSESSMENT OF CHILDREN

A thorough nutrition assessment of children at the time of routine health exams is important to identify the child that is at risk of either undernutrition or overnutrition. Undernutrition is the primary cause of growth retardation in children.[18] Obesity is the most common nutritional disorder of children in America.[12]

Clinical assessment

The pediatric health history should focus on present or current health concerns, as well as the child's past illnesses and family medical history. Acute or chronic diarrhea, infections, or other GI abnormalities, as well as the use of many medications, may be closely linked with symptoms of malnutrition. A history of weight gains and losses should be collected.

Frank protein-calorie malnutrition, or vitamin deficiency secondary to inadequate intake, is uncommon in the United States. However, children on restricted diets, such as strict vegetarian diets, have developed rickets, vitamin B_{12} deficiency, and riboflavin deficiency. Poor performance in school, lethargy, anorexia, and irritability may be symptoms of iron deficiency.[30]

Symptoms of food allergies may be manifested as GI disturbances, eczema, atopic dermatitis, bronchospasm, or failure to gain weight. A family history, combined with a physical examination for systemic symptoms of an IgE-mediated response, such as eye, skin, or lung manifestations after ingestion of specific foods, is helpful in making the diagnosis of food allergy vs food intolerance or food sensitivity. Virtually only a food allergy will exhibit such immune-system–associated responses. Food sensitivities and intolerances generally exhibit symptoms localized to the GI tract. If other symptoms arise, they are commonly secondary to the GI effects.

In young children, the physical assessment should focus on a few particular areas. Chronic diarrhea, when accompanied by poor weight gain, is an important indicator of

Table 25-8. Laboratory tests for the determination of iron status

Lab test	Iron deficiency state
Serum ferritin	<10 ng/ml
Transferrin saturation	<12%
Erythrocyte protoporphyrin	>70 μg/dl of packed erythrocytes
Mean corpuscular volume	<74 fl

Table 25-9. Drug-nutrient interactions of concern with young children

Drug type	Nutrient interaction
Anticonvulsants	Decrease absorption of vitamin D, folic acid, riboflavin
Antimicrobials	Decrease vitamin K synthesis; reduce level of intestinal lactose, folate, and vitamin B_{12}
Mineral oil laxatives	Interfere with absorption of vitamins A, D, E, and K

Table 25-10. Clinical signs associated with nutritional deficiencies

Body Area	Normal Appearance	Clinical Sign(s)	Nutritional Deficiency Indicated
Hair	Shiny, firm, not easily plucked	Hair dull and dry, lack of shine, thinness and sparseness, depigmentation (flag sign), straightness of previously curly hair, easy pluckability	Kwashirokor; less commonly, marasmus, protein-calorie
Face	Uniform skin color, smooth, healthy appearance, not swollen	Depigmentation: skin dark over cheeks and eyes, moon face	Protein-calorie, protein
		Scaling of skin around nostrils, nasolabial seborrhea	Riboflavin or niacin, pyridoxine
Eyes	Bright, clear, shiny, healthy, pink, moist membranes, no prominent blood vessels	Pale conjunctiva	Anemia: iron, folate, or B_{12}
		Bitot's spots, night blindness, conjunctiva and corneal xeroxis (drying), keratomalacia	Vitamin A
		Redness and fissuring of eyelid corners (angular palpebritis)	Ribaflavin, pyridoxine, niacin
Lips	Smooth, not chapped	Redness and swelling of mouth or lips, especially at corners of mouth (cheilosis) and angular stomatitis, angular scars	Riboflavin, niacin, iron, pyridoxine
Mouth		Ageusia, dysgeusia	Zinc
Tongue	Deep red in appearance, not smooth or swollen	Glossitis	Niacin, folate, riboflavin, iron, vitamin B_{12}
		Scarlet and raw	Nicotinic acid
		Magenta tongue	Riboflavin
Teeth	Bright, no cavities, no pain	Pitted, grooved teeth	Vitamin D
		Missing or erupting abnormally, gray or black spots (fluorosis) mottled	Fluoride
		Cavities	Poor hygiene and fluoride
		Mottled enamel	Excess fluoride
Gums	Healthy red, do not bleed, not swollen	Spongy, bleeding gums, swollen	Ascorbic acid (vitamin C)
Glands	Face not swollen	Thyroid enlargement	Iodine
		Parotid enlargement	Starvation (protein-calorie)
Skin	No signs of rashes, swelling, dark or light spots	Dryness of the skin (xerosis), sandpaper feel of skin (follicular hyperkeratosis)	Vitamin A or essential fatty acid
		Petechiae ecchymoses	Ascorbic acid and vitamin D
		Red, swollen pigmentation of exposed areas (pellagrous dermatosis)	Nicotinic acid and tryptophan
		Flakiness of the skin, lack of fat under skin	Kwashiorkor, essential fatty acid
		Increased fat	Obesity
		Scrotal and vulvar dermatosis	Riboflavin
Nails	Firm, pink	Nails spoon shaped (koilonychia)	Iron
Muscles and skeletal system	Good muscle tone, some fat under skin, can walk or run without pain	Muscle wasting	Starvation, Kwashiorkor marasmus
		Knock knees or bow legs	Vitamin D
		Thoracic rosary	Vitamin D, ascorbic acid
		Musculoskeletal hemorrhage	Ascorbic acid
Organ Systems			
Gastrointestinal	No palpable organs or masses	Hepatomegaly (fatty infiltration)	Protein
Cardiovascular	Normal heart rhythm, no murmur, normal blood pressure for age	Cardiac enlargement, tachycardia	Thiamine
Nervous system	Psychological stability, normal reflexes	Psychomotor changes, mental confusion	Kwashiorkor protein, thiamine, nicotinic acid
		Sensory loss, motor weakness, loss of vibration, loss of ankle movement, knee jerks, calf tenderness	Thiamine, vitamin B_{12} deficiency

nutrient malabsorption. A history of the illness episodes, including description of abdominal pain and flatus, and stool type and odors, will help distinguish the presence of carbohydrate or fat malabsorption. If episodes of diarrhea are persistent, conditions that need to be excluded are cystic fibrosis, celiac disease, postenteritis syndrome, milk protein intolerance, and giardiasis.[30]

Certain medications given to young children cause drug-nutrient interactions (Table 25-9).

In both young and school-aged children, fat distribution relative to obesity, or the presence of diminished subcutaneous fat and muscle-wasting indicative of undernutrition, should be inspected. Hydration status and condition of the skin, hair, head, eyes, ears, nose, and throat should be checked thoroughly for indications of malnutrition. A careful examination of the mouth and teeth is essential, as nutrition plays a prominent role in the development and acquisition of newly erupting teeth. The chest, abdomen, genitals, and cardiovascular, musculoskeletal, and neurologic systems should be examined and should conform to normal developmental standards. See Table 25-10 for a list of signs and symptoms associated with nutritional deficiencies.[18]

Anthropometric assessment

Height and weight should be assessed at all office visits, whether well-child or illness-related visits. A child's body size and rate of growth should be compared with reference standards; however, consistency in the child's own growth pattern is what is most important. Any loss of weight in a young child may be significant and may indicate malabsorption, anorexia secondary to chronic disease, or behavioral disturbances.

Height is the best indicator of long-term nutritional status. Regular linear growth is an important sign that a child's diet is adequate. However, if a child's height for age falls below the 5th percentile, it may indicate poor nutritional status. Of course, this could also be an inherent genetic trait. Any height-for-age measure between the 5th and 10th percentiles deserves further evaluation.[30]

Measurement of the weight index gives a quick but inexact indication of a child's relative leanness or fatness. It is the ratio of the actual weight to the ideal weight for age. A weight index of 0.9 to 1.1 is normal, less than 0.9 reflects leanness, greater than 1.1 indicates overweight, and greater than 1.2 indicates obesity. According to this index, muscular children will be classified as overweight, but a simple visual assessment of the child can rule out such a misclassification. If a more sophisticated method is necessary, a triceps skinfold measure can be taken.

Biochemical assessment

Because physical signs and symptoms of nutritional deficiency may not appear until a child is in a frank state of nutrient deficiency, laboratory analyses are essential at the earliest indication (from clinical history, dietary, and/or anthropometric assessment) of nutritional deficit. Nutrient levels and functional changes may be evaluated by examination of tissue, blood, and urine, and may occur while a patient is in marginal nutritional status (Table 25-11).

Hemoglobin or hematocrit should be used to screen for anemia. Because these tests are not indicative of iron stores, one should evaluate serum ferritin, transferrin, and total iron binding capacity (TIBC) to determine the cause of abnormal values. Common nutritional causes of anemia in children include iron deficiency, folate or vitamin B_{12} deficiency, and lead intoxication.

Atherosclerosis may begin during childhood and progress through young adulthood, although clinical manifestations usually do not appear until middle age or later. Cholesterol levels should be measured in obese patients, and in patients with a family history of heart disease, hypertension, diabetes mellitus, or gout.[18] According to epidemiological studies, in populations where the incidence of heart disease is low, mean levels of plasma cholesterol in children range from 100 to 150 mg/dl. Where there is a high incidence of adult coronary heart disease, cholesterol levels in children range from 150 to 200 mg/dl (see tables 25-12 and 25-13).

Dietary assessment

In young children (2 to 6 years) the nutrition history questionnaire and the 24-hour recall should be used to collect dietary intake data from the caregiver. In older children, both forms should be used, but data should be collected from the child and caregiver separately. This style of collection may yield different results and give the practitioner additional insight into the true diet of the child. Questions regarding the use of dietary supplements should be emphasized. The current diet of the child should be compared with the current height and weight status.

If anemia is present, the practitioner should ask specific questions about the type, amount, and frequency of meat consumption, and whether iron-fortified cereal is eaten daily. Children who are total vegans (eliminate all animal foods, including dairy and eggs), may be at risk of vitamin B_{12} deficiency. A dietary folate deficiency is associated with a vegetable-poor diet, especially when green leafy vegetables are lacking. Lead toxicity is most often associated with consumption of lead-contaminated water, paint chips, and severe air pollution.

Diet information should be evaluated in terms of the nutritional needs of each child. Food intake can quickly be compared with suggested foods and amounts listed in food group guides (see Chapter 22). Calorically excessive or deficient intakes, eating of bizarre or manufactured foods (such as so-called fruit leather or fruit roll-ups in place of fruit), or the omission of food groups should be identified

Table 25-11. Selected laboratory assessment and diagnostic implications

Laboratory test	Diagnostic implication	Comment
Hemoglobin and hematocrit	Used to screen for anemia; if present, further evaluation done to determine cause	Common nutritional anemias include iron, folate, or vitamin B_{12} deficiency Because of the increase in blood volume, iron requirements go up in growth; pubescence is a common time for anemia to be present
Lead	Measured in the serum; if present, further evaluation done to determine source Need careful investigation for practice of pica	Can occur in children from eating lead-based paint chips or unglazed pottery or from cigarette butts, batteries in mouth, inhaling gasoline fumes, or drinking water containing lead Found in old houses in paint
Total lymphocyte count	Used to screen for immune dysfunction Can occur secondary to severe malnutrition	Diminished cell-mediated immunity and diminished complement protein and hemolytic complement may indicate risk for recurrent and/or significant infection
Glucose	Measured in urine and blood; urine glucose will be positive only if the plasma glucose is markedly abnormal	Elevated in shock, burns, dehydration, and acidosis
Vitamins and minerals	Levels measured directly or by enzyme assay Important for normal cellular composition and function	Laboratory assessment suggested if clinical signs are demonstrated Water-soluble vitamins can be measured in the urine
Cholesterol	Elevated serum cholesterol in adults is a major risk factor for coronary heart disease; the incidence of coronary heart disease in adult populations correlates with the cholesterol levels of children in these populations; lower dietary cholesterol and saturated fat in populations correlates with lower plasma cholesterol levels and less coronary heart disease	200 mg/dl desirable blood cholesterol 200-239 mg/dl borderline high blood cholesterol 240 mg/dl high blood cholesterol
Lipoproteins	Low-density lipoprotein (LDL) and very low-density lipoproteins (VLDL) are highly correlated with total cholesterol and, like total cholesterol, are atherogenic High-density lipoproteins (HDL) are inversely correlated to total cholesterol and to the occurrence of arteriosclerotic vascular lesions	<130 mg/dl desirable LDL-cholesterol 130-159 mg/dl borderline high risk LDL-cholesterol >160 mg/dl high risk LDL cholesterol
24-hour urine creatinine excretion	Proportionally reflects amount of muscle mass Creatinine-height index calculated from mg creatinine/24 hour ÷ normal mg creatinine/24 hour × 100 = percentile	Careful collection of specimen is essential Elevation may reflect high-protein diet or exercise Creatinine-height index of less than 90% reflects muscle protein store depletion
Urinary urea nitrogen	Will drop with a deficiency of protein intake	Nitrogenous constituent of urine; mean daily excretion of 7-18 g
Delayed hypersensitivity skin antigen testing	Delayed response in malnourished patients	A risk factor for infection, sepsis, and mortality in debilitated patients
Plasma proteins Albumin	Low plasma levels reflect malnutrition, liver disease, kidney disease, or inflammation of the gut	Due to endogenous albumin synthesis, serum level stays up until very late in protein malnutrition
Transferrin	Decreased levels occur in protein-losing enteropathies, liver disease, and chronic infection; increased levels indicate severe iron deficiency	Transports circulating iron; measurement of transferrin alone is not a reliable index to assess protein nutrition
Thyroxine-binding prealbumin (PA) Retinol-binding protein (RBP)	PA-RBP complex is the most sensitive predictor to assess dietary protein deprivation	The serum levels of PA and RBP in children are approximately half those of adults

From Mammel KA: Nutrition assessment of the school age child. In Simko MD, Cowell C, Hreha MS, editors: *Practical nutrition,* Rockville, Md, 1989, Aspen Publishers.

Table 25-12. Plasma lipid concentrations in the first 2 decades of life (mg/dL)*

Age, years	No.	Serum total cholesterol (percentile)			Serum triglyceride (percentile)		
		5th	50th	95th	5th	50th	95th
White males							
0-4	238	117	156	209	30	53	102
5-9	1253	125	164	209	31	53	104
10-14	2278	123	160	208	33	61	129
15-19	1980	116	150	203	38	71	152
White females							
0-4	186	115	161	206	35	62	115
5-9	1118	130	168	211	33	57	108
10-14	2087	128	163	207	38	72	135
15-19	2079	124	160	209	40	70	136

Modified from *Pediatrics,* vol. 89, no. 3, part 2 (suppl), 1992. National Cholesterol Education Program: Report of the Expert Panel on blood cholesterol levels in children and adolescents.*All values have been converted from plasma to serum plasma value × 1.03 = serum value.

Table 25-13. Normal plasma lipoprotein concentrations in the first 2 decades of life (mg/dL)*

Age, years	LDL cholesterol				HDL Cholesterol			
	No.	Percentiles			No.	Percentiles		
		5th	50th	95th		5th	50th	95th
White males								
5-9	231	65	93	133	142	39	56	76
10-14	284	66	97	136	290	38	57	76
15-19	298	64	96	134	299	31	47	65
White females								
5-9	114	70	101	144	124	37	54	75
10-14	244	70	97	140	247	38	54	72
15-19	294	61	96	141	295	36	53	76

Modified from *Pediatrics,* vol. 89, no. 3, part 2 (suppl), 1992. National Cholesterol Education Program: Report of the Expert Panel on blood cholesterol levels in children and adolescents.*All values have been converted from plasma to serum plasma value × 1.03 = serum value. Note: The number of children age 0 to 4 years who had LDL and HDL cholesterol measured was too small to allow calculation of percentiles in this age-group. However, note that the percentiles for total cholesterol (Table 25-12) for ages 0-4 years and 5-9 years are similar.

through these methods. If a more detailed and time-consuming nutrient analysis is necessary, referral to a registered dietitian may be indicated.

Because obesity is a primary concern in children, a food and activity record may be useful in determining caloric expenditure, as well as when, where, and how a child eats.

Common nutritional problems in the young child include obesity/overweight, lactose intolerance, anemia, poorly balanced vegetarian diets, dietary intervention to control for heart disease, and refusal to eat.[13]

In the diets of school-age children, vitamins A, C, and B_6, minerals, calcium, and iron are most often at less than optimal intakes. Other common nutritional problems include[34]:

- Obesity/overweight
- Poorly balanced intake from vegetarian diets
- Eating disorders
- Inappropriate diets for athletic regimens
- Allergy
- Poor dental health and tooth decay
- Dietary intervention to control for heart disease

NUTRITION ASSESSMENT OF ADOLESCENTS

Contrary to the well-baby and well-child visits of younger patients, the usual office visits from adolescents are based on a physical complaint or other specific reason. Because eating habits of adolescents may range from healthy to very unhealthy, the physician should perform a nutritional assessment during these irregular visits. Such data may provide insight into the adolescent's general health behaviors, psychological health, and possibly the presenting symptoms leading to the office visit.

Clinical assessment

A written questionnaire may be used for the basis of the adolescent health history, but it should be followed by an oral history. Sometimes adolescents do not completely understand the relevance or importance of questions regarding their health history or family health history. They also may consider some of their own abnormal physical ailments as normal, because they have never experienced anything else.

Information on medications, both prescribed and over-the-counter, should be clearly solicited. Many people do not consider over-the-counter remedies as medications. Weight-loss, vitamin, and other dietary supplements, as well as laxatives and diuretics (or diet pills), should be included in this list of questions.

Allergy symptoms in relation to environmental or food stimuli should be queried. Wake-sleep patterns and activity patterns should be documented. A menstrual history should be completed on all girls.[20]

A physical exam is essential to the complete nutritional assessment of an adolescent, although physical findings are usually related to nonnutritional problems. Occasionally, nutrition-related symptoms do occur, and a careful differential diagnosis is necessary.

Anthropometric assessment

Regular height and weight measures are simple procedures to document growth patterns and identify possible nutritional problems. Serial measurements to follow rate of growth, rather than taking individual measurements for comparison with a reference standard, are more helpful in determining normalcy of growth.

Healthy weight and growth parameters, as well as body image concerns, should be discussed. Because the onset of puberty and development of secondary sex characteristics are closely linked with nutritional health, they should be sequenced using a sexual maturity rating, such as the Tanner scale. These life stages should be clearly explained to the adolescent patient, and the patient's feelings about his or her own sexual development and appearance should be discussed.[20]

Biochemical assessment

Routine hemoglobin and hematocrit measures are usually indicated for adolescents, because this life stage is associated with somewhat poor iron intake, rapid growth, and recurrent blood loss in girls. If these parameters are abnormal, serum ferritin, transferrin, or total iron binding capacity should be measured for adequacy of iron stores.

If the patient complains of fatigue or malaise, measures for anemia, white blood cell count, and differential, and the erythrocyte sedimentation rate may be useful.[20] If indicated by the family history or an anthropometric assessment of overweight or obesity, a cholesterol screening should be performed.[36]

Physical signs of malnutrition will lead the laboratory investigation. Hemoglobin/hematocrit, ferritin, and urinalysis are the most common laboratory tests. Other test results that may be helpful include those for TSH, T4, pregnancy, liver function, BUN, creatinine, carotene, folate, serum protein, and immunoglobulins.[20]

Dietary assessment

A nutrition history questionnaire combined with a food and activity record is the best method of collecting complete dietary information from an adolescent. Unfortunately, however, eliciting a complete and accurate recall and record of food intake is often difficult because the eating patterns of adolescents commonly have little routine. Many adolescents eat irregularly at different places and snack often, making accurate food recall and record-keeping difficult. Therefore one must assess the patient's ability and willingness to cooperate before evaluating the diagnostic strength of the dietary data.[1]

The interviewer may benefit by questioning the patient about the diet by using probing, but not leading, questions to jog the memory. A food frequency questionnaire may help validate the reliability of other dietary information.

The dietary intake data can be compared with the recommended intakes from the Daily Food Guide (see Chapter 22) and the Dietary Guidelines for Americans[26] to determine a gross estimate of nutritional quality. Caloric adequacy can be measured against the adolescent's activity and growth and weight patterns.

Nutrients of particular concern, such as minerals associated with musculoskeletal development and incremental increases in blood volume, should be considered in relation to the recommended dietary allowances according to age and sex.[23]

Adolescents commonly consume empty-calorie foods, such as carbonated beverages, and high-fat snack foods in place of a balanced diet. Encouraging an intake of calcium-rich and iron-rich foods, along with sufficient protein and vitamin C, should help significantly in creating a relatively well-balanced diet in an adolescent. More lean meats and citrus juices and fruits should be suggested.

Common nutritional concerns of the adolescent include overweight/obesity, underweight, eating disorders, pregnancy, substance abuse, prevention of cardiac disease, poorly designed vegetarian diets, and high physical activity from sports participation.[1] Any of these problems may

Table 25-14. Nutritional risk factors of chronic disease to be evaluated in the nutrition assessment of the adult

Disease	Dietary and health history	Clinical examination	Laboratory determination
Cardiovascular disease			
Coronary heart disease (CHD)	Family history of: Myocardial infarction Angina Elevated serum cholesterol Elevated triglyceride levels Diabetes mellitus Personal practices of: Smoking Excessive saturated fat and dietary cholesterol intake Inadequate polyunsaturated fat intake Inadequate dietary fiber intake	Obesity Xanthomas Electrocardiographic evidence of CHD Positive stress test Type A behavioral pattern	Elevated serum cholesterol, LDL cholesterol, triglycerides, uric acid Low HDL cholesterol Positive glucose tolerance test
Hypertension	Family history of: Hypertension Personal practices of: Excessive salt intake in salt-sensitive persons Inadequate calcium intake Inadequate potassium and magnesium intake	Obesity Elevated blood pressure	Protein urea Elevated blood urea nitrogen (BUN)
Diabetes	Family history	Obesity	Elevated fasting or postprandial blood sugar Glycosuria
Cancer (colon, breast, prostate)	Family history of cancer Personal Practices of: Smoking Inadequate unsaturated fat Excessive nitrosamine intake Inadequate dietary fiber Excessive caloric intake in women (uterine cancer) Excessive smoked foods Excessive alcohol	Obesity	

From Christakis G: Nutrition assessment of the adult. In Simko MD, Cowell C, Hreha MS, editors: *Practical nutrition,* Rockville, Md, 1989, Aspen Publishers. Copyright 1960, American Medical Association.

require more sophisticated time and counseling intervention than a busy primary care physician can devote. Referral to a registered dietitian specializing in the particular area of concern may be indicated.

NUTRITION ASSESSMENT OF ADULTS

Although certain adult subgroups in the United States clearly are still at risk for inadequate intakes of vitamin C, iron, folic acid, and calcium,[24] the major targets for nutritional assessment of adults in primary care are the dietary factors that influence chronic diseases, such as total calories, total fat, saturated fat and cholesterol, sodium, and fiber (Table 25-14).

Clinical assessment

The health history is a valuable portion of the complete nutrition assessment, not only for evaluating the nutritional status of the patient, but also for establishing a baseline of lifestyle and family history information that will be useful for later intervention and counseling. Lifestyle has a tremendous effect on food consumption, food behaviors, and subsequent health status. Also, the evaluation of the individual's history of disease has important implications in the analysis of the adult's nutritional status.

A complete physical examination is an important technique for assessing adult nutritional status. One should inspect the entire body, beginning with the head, hair, and face, including the eyes, ears, nose, lips, and oral cavity. A thorough inspection of the eyes, eyebrows, and eyelids for clinical signs of vitamin A deficiency is essential, especially in lower income subgroups. Clinical signs of hypertension, such as excessive straightening of the arteries, retinal hemorrhages, and exudates, or signs of diabetes, such as lesions of microaneurysms, are detectable upon physical

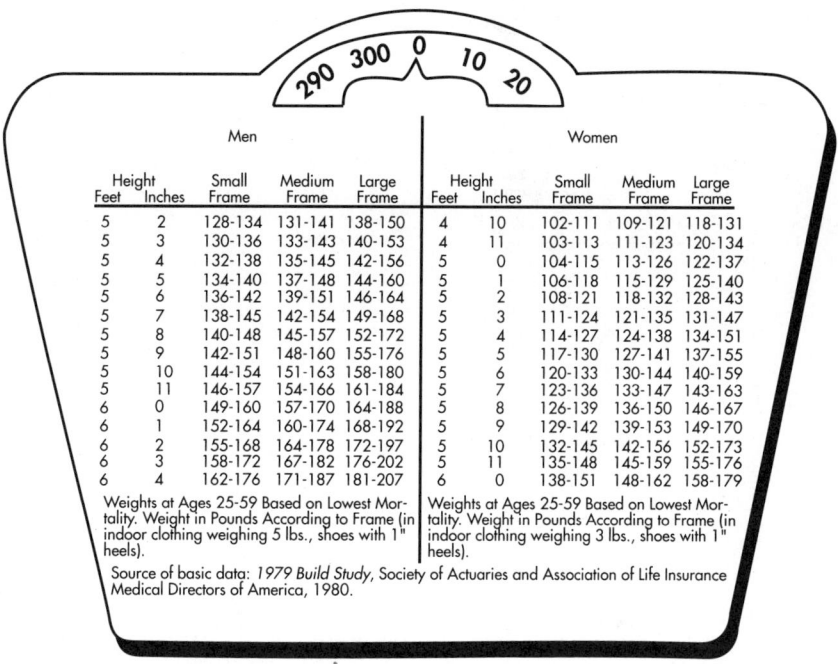

Men				Women			
Height		Small Frame	Medium Frame	Large Frame	Height		Small Frame	Medium Frame	Large Frame

Feet	Inches	Small Frame	Medium Frame	Large Frame	Feet	Inches	Small Frame	Medium Frame	Large Frame
5	2	128-134	131-141	138-150	4	10	102-111	109-121	118-131
5	3	130-136	133-143	140-153	4	11	103-113	111-123	120-134
5	4	132-138	135-145	142-156	5	0	104-115	113-126	122-137
5	5	134-140	137-148	144-160	5	1	106-118	115-129	125-140
5	6	136-142	139-151	146-164	5	2	108-121	118-132	128-143
5	7	138-145	142-154	149-168	5	3	111-124	121-135	131-147
5	8	140-148	145-157	152-172	5	4	114-127	124-138	134-151
5	9	142-151	148-160	155-176	5	5	117-130	127-141	137-155
5	10	144-154	151-163	158-180	5	6	120-133	130-144	140-159
5	11	146-157	154-166	161-184	5	7	123-136	133-147	143-163
6	0	149-160	157-170	164-188	5	8	126-139	136-150	146-167
6	1	152-164	160-174	168-192	5	9	129-142	139-153	149-170
6	2	155-168	164-178	172-197	5	10	132-145	142-156	152-173
6	3	158-172	167-182	176-202	5	11	135-148	145-159	155-176
6	4	162-176	171-187	181-207	6	0	138-151	148-162	158-179

Weights at Ages 25-59 Based on Lowest Mortality. Weight in Pounds According to Frame (in indoor clothing weighing 5 lbs., shoes with 1" heels).

Weights at Ages 25-59 Based on Lowest Mortality. Weight in Pounds According to Frame (in indoor clothing weighing 3 lbs., shoes with 1" heels).

Source of basic data: *1979 Build Study*, Society of Actuaries and Association of Life Insurance Medical Directors of America, 1980.

Fig. 25-4. Metropolitan height and weight tables, 1983. (Metropolitan Life Insurance Company, New York, 1983.)

exam. Skin around eyes should be examined for xanthelasma, or raised yellow or white lesions that contain cholesterol deposits identified as type II familial hyperlipoproteinemia.[9]

The exam should continue down the neck and thyroid gland, followed by the lungs, heart, abdomen, body skin, and nails. A brief neurological exam should also be included.

Anthropometric assessment

The standard adult anthropometric assessment is a measure of height and weight. These data, when compared with tables of height and weight (Fig. 25-4) or transformed into other indices that relate height and weight status, can be very useful in detecting undernutrition before signs of visible variations appear. More commonly in the United States, obesity can be detected, and an intervention program can be developed to help lower the risks of developing coronary artery disease, diabetes, and hypertension.

Weight/height ratios that are corrected for height are assumed to be better indices for the detection of obesity, compared with standard weight-for-height tables. These indices are called body mass indices, but they cannot differentiate overweight from overfat. A muscular individual would need to be assessed by either visual evaluation or skinfold measures.

Quetelet's Index, or the index most recently called the body mass index (BMI) is the ratio of weight in kilograms to height in centimeters squared (Fig. 25-5 and Table 25-

Table 25-15. Body mass index

Body mass index	Evaluation
Under 20	May be associated with health problems for some individuals
20-25	"Ideal" index range associated with the lowest risk of illness for most people
25-27	May be associated with health problems for some people
Over 27	Associated with increased risk of health problems such as heart disease, high blood pressure, and diabetes

From Classifications used for the Body Mass Index by Health and Welfare Canada (1988a).

15). Many investigators consider the BMI to be the best index for adult populations, as it is the least biased by height and is easily calculated. The BMI also correlates with many health-related indices such as mortality risk. Factors such as diet, smoking, and levels of physical activity confound this latter relationship, so that the range of acceptable values for the BMI varies among communities.[16]

Some investigators recommend measuring the waist:hip ratio, defined as the circumference of the waist divided by the circumference of the hips. This index measures fat distribution, is easier to determine and more precise than skinfold measures, and may be most helpful when com-

Nomogram for Body Mass Index

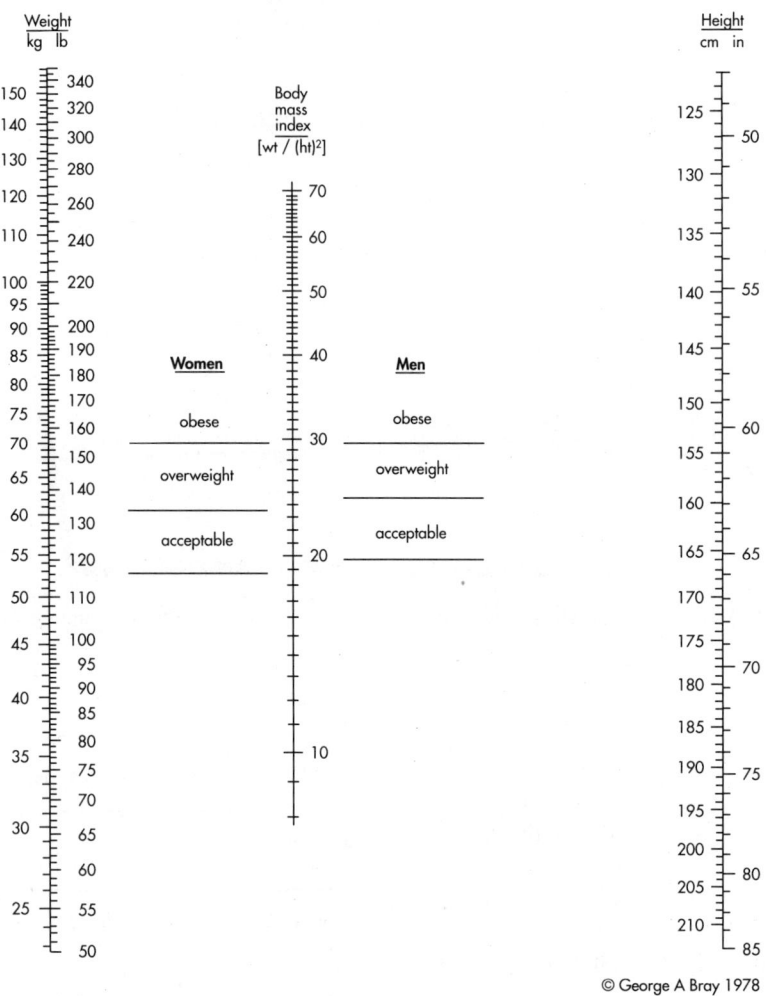

© George A Bray 1978

Fig. 25-5. Level one screen nomogram for body mass index. (From *Nutrition screening manual for professionals caring for older Americans,* Nutrition Screening Initiative, Washington, DC, American Academy of Family Physicians, American Dietetic Association, National Council on the Aging, 1991.)

bined with the BMI measure for assessing both subcutaneous and intraabdominal adipose tissue. Recent research suggests that waist:hip ratios greater than 1.0 for men and 0.8 for women indicate increased risk of cardiovascular complications and related deaths. However, more research is needed before specific waist:hip ratio standards can be recommended.[16]

Biochemical assessment

Serum cholesterol and iron status should be screened routinely. The physical, anthropometric, and dietary assessments will provide a basis for the rest of the biochem-

ical assessment. If protein/calorie nutrition needs to be evaluated, the following laboratory values are used: creatinine-height index, serum albumin, prealbumin or retinal binding protein, serum transferrin, total lymphocyte count, delayed skin hypersensitivity, and urinary urea nitrogen.[9]

Dietary assessment

As a matter of course, most physicians question patients about their smoking and drinking habits.[21] Eating habits sometimes are questioned, but rarely in any depth. Evaluating eating habits is an important key to determining the health of patients, because of the leading causes of death in the United States—heart disease, cancer, cerebrovascular disease, diabetes, and atherosclerosis—70% of the incidence has been associated with diet.[33]

Eating habits in the United States have changed significantly during the last 25 years. We eat fewer meals at home and rely more on restaurant meals, take-out foods, microwave meals, vending machine snacks, and many other prepared convenience foods. We eat fewer regular meals and more snacks.[35]

All of these changes require that the dietary assessment reflect the usual intake of all foods and beverages throughout the day, rather than targeting meals. Specific questions regarding vitamin-mineral supplementation and use of diet products should be included.

Age, socioeconomic status, ethnic group, and regional differences influence dietary consumption patterns. Nutrition screening and evaluation tools targeted toward specific subgroups may be helpful in evaluating the diets of these individuals.[2]

The nutrition history questionnaire in combination with a diet diary will give the most complete information about a patient's dietary regime. Patients must be instructed to complete the diary accurately. If a 24-hour recall is used, the previous 24 hours should clearly represent a usual day for the patient. It is best to use a 24-hour recall as a screening tool or for follow-up assessments. The food frequency form can give the physician an overall picture of the general food intake of the patient by food category. The history forms may be completed by patients before their office visit or while in the waiting room, but the physician should review the completed forms with the patient for accuracy and understanding.

Collection of dietary information is sometimes more complete when done by interview, because the interviewer can probe the patient's memory. The interviewer must use a matter-of-fact, nonjudgmental tone when asking questions, to create a noncritical atmosphere that promotes honest testimony by patients. Commentary or counseling regarding the dietary information must be saved until the initial diet interview is complete.[35]

The dietary data should be evaluated in terms of the patient's individual needs. Food intake can be compared with food group guides and dietary guidelines (see Chapter 22). These recommendations are for healthy adults and are designed to support general nutritional health and the prevention of disease. If patients are having difficulty complying with recommendations or are already ill with one or more diseases, a more sophisticated dietary assessment and treatment plan may be indicated. In this case, the physician should refer the patient to a specialized registered dietitian.

The common nutritional problems encountered during adulthood include overweight/obesity, high fat and cholesterol consumption, hypertension, low calcium intake and osteoporosis, abnormal dietary patterns associated with premenstrual syndrome, type II diabetes mellitus, and fad diets for weight loss.[35]

NUTRITION ASSESSMENT OF THE ELDERLY

The elderly population is actually subdivided into two groups: the healthy elderly and the frail elderly (or those who have health problems). The nutritional needs of the healthy elderly are the same as for any other healthy subgroup: health maintenance, optimal performance in cognitive and physical activities, and extended longevity. The nutritional needs of the elderly with health problems include therapy for disease management, prevention or cure of nutrient deficiencies, and avoidance of drug-nutrient interactions.[29]

The nutrition screening initiative

The nutrition screening initiative is a 5-year, multifaceted effort promoting routine nutrition screening and better nutrition care for older Americans. It is a joint effort of the American Academy of Family Physicians, The American Dietetic Association, the National Council on the Aging, and 33 other key health, aging, and medical organizations and professional associations. In 1991, a Consensus Conference of the Nutrition Screening Initiative (NSI), Nutrition Screening I: Toward a Common View, led to increased professional awareness of poor nutritional status and better definitions and standards for identification of risk factors and indicators of poor nutritional status in older Americans (Table 25-16).[37]

Out of this conference, *The Nutrition Screening Manual for Professionals Caring for Older Americans* was developed. The manual contains screens for both clinical-based and community-based professionals, including a self-administered nutritional health checklist and public awareness tool that describes the warning signs of poor nutritional status, similar to the warning signs used to assist in the early detection of cancer (Table 25-17).

The manual also contains two levels of nutrition screens to be administered by a professional. The level I screen can be administered by a health or social services professional and offers a simple method for separating those individuals who should be referred for evaluation and possible intervention from those who would benefit from other medical or community services. This screen includes questions regarding height, weight, eating habits, and lifestyle, and an assessment of socioeconomic and functional status.[25]

The level II screen is for those individuals whose checklist or level I screen indicated a potentially serious nutrition or medical problem. It provides more sensitive measures that can be taken by a health professional alone or as part of a complete physical exam. The level II screen includes a detailed history of weight change and laboratory and clinical indicators of protein-calorie malnutrition, obesity, and other nutrition-related disorders.[25]

Table 25-16. Risk factors and major and minor indicators of poor nutritional status in older Americans[31]

Risk factors	Major indicators	Minor indicators
Inappropriate food intake	Weight loss	Alcoholism
Poverty	Underweight/overweight	Cognitive impairment
Social isolation	Low serum albumin	Chronic renal insufficiency
Dependency/disability	Change in functional status	Multiple concurrent medications
Acute/chronic diseases or conditions	Inappropriate food intake	Malabsorption syndromes
Chronic medication use	Midarm muscle circumference	Anorexia, nausea, dysphagia
	<10th percentile	
Advanced age (80+)	Triceps skinfold	Fatigue, apathy, memory loss
	<10th percentile or >95th percentile	Poor oral/dental status, dehydration
	Obesity	Poorly healing wounds
	Nutrition-related disorders	Loss of subcutaneous fat and/or muscle
	Osteoporosis	Fluid retention
	Osteomalacia	Reduced iron, ascorbic acid, zinc
	Folate deficiency	
	B_{12} deficiency	

From *Nutrition screening manual for professionals caring for older Americans,* The Nutrition Screening Initiative, Washington, DC, 1991, American Academy of Family Physicians, American Dietetic Association, National Council on the Aging.

The manual also provides helpful tools for use in nutrition assessment, such as nomograms, U.S. dietary guidelines, activities of daily living guide, guides for anthropometric measures and calculations, and psychological tests and scales.

Clinical assessment

Depending on the health status of the individual, a caregiver, relative, or friend may need to be present to assist with the collection of a health history. A general medical history should include weight and appetite changes, gastrointestinal disturbances, newly acquired food intolerances, sensory abilities that may affect interest in food and eating patterns, and dental problems that may lead to eating difficulties or restricted choices.[29]

Determination of the patient's mental status is essential to the evaluation of the individual's ability to care for himself or herself independently. If unexplained mental deficits are noted, an investigation into alcohol abuse, anemia, vitamin B deficiency, polypharmacy, or dehydration may be warranted.

A physical examination of an elderly patient should include evaluation of skin and nails for elasticity, healing, ecchymoses or petechiae, and dermatitis. The lips and oral cavity should be completely examined for malocclusion, infection, membrane integrity, ability to chew and swallow, and adequate saliva production.[29] The classical signs of nutritional deficiency may not be as apparent and may be more nonspecific in the elderly than in younger populations (Table 25-18).

An assessment of ambulation and the activities of daily living is integral to the evaluation of the individual's ability to carry out food-related tasks. Visual and cognitive abilities must also be assessed relative to the use of cooking utensils and a stove or oven.

Formula for calculating stature from knee height[10]

Men: 64.19 (0.04 × age) + (2.02 × knee height)
Women: 84.88 − (0.24 × age) + (1.83 × knee height)

From Chumlea WC: *Nutritional assessment of the elderly through anthropometry,* Columbus, Ohio, 1984, Ross Laboratories.

Anthropometric assessment

Obtaining a standard height and weight measure is often not as easy in the elderly as with younger individuals. Loss of height and inability of the frail elderly to stand on a scale make even the most simple of measures difficult. If height and weight can be measured using standard techniques, the reference standards listed in Tables 25-19 and 25-20 should be used.

Estimated stature can be calculated from the measurement of knee height (see the box above) or directly from the measurement of armspan. For the frail elderly who cannot completely stretch out their arms, knee height is the preferable measurement. Measure knee height in inches from the bottom of the foot to the anterior of the knee with the ankle and knee at 90 degrees (Fig. 25-6). Unfortunately, these standards probably do not apply to nonwhites.[25]

For more complete anthropometric data, one can assess body fatness and lean body mass using the BMI, midarm circumference, and triceps skinfolds (Table 25-21).

Biochemical assessment

The laboratory assessment of the healthy elderly will focus on routine iron status and cholesterol screenings. In

Table 25-17. Determine your nutritional health

The warning signs of poor nutritional health are often overlooked. Use this checklist to find out if you or someone you know is at nutritional risk.

Read the statements below. Circle the number in the yes column for those that apply to you or someone you know. For each yes answer, score the number in the box. Total your nutritional score.

	Yes
I have an illness or condition that made me change the kind and/or amount of food I eat.	2
I eat fewer than two meals per day.	3
I eat few fruits, vegetables, or milk products.	2
I have three or more drinks of beer, liquor, or wine almost every day.	2
I have tooth or mouth problems that make it hard for me to eat.	2
I don't always have enough money to buy the food I need.	4
I eat alone most of the time.	1
I take three or more different prescribed or over-the-counter drugs a day.	1
Without wanting to, I have lost or gained 10 pounds in the last 6 months.	2
I am not always physically able to shop, cook and/or feed myself.	2
TOTAL	

Total your nutritional score. If it's—

0-2   **Good!** Recheck your nutritional score in 6 months.

3-5   **You are at moderate nutritional risk.** See what can be done to improve your eating habits and lifestyle. Your office on aging, senior nutrition program, senior citizens center or health department can help. Recheck your nutritional score in 3 months.

6 or more   **You are at high nutritional risk.** Bring this checklist the next time you see your doctor, dietitian, or other qualified health or social service professional. Talk with them about any problems you may have. Ask for help to improve your nutritional health. **Remember that warning signs suggest risk but do not represent diagnosis of any condition. See the next page to learn more about the warning signs of poor nutritional health.**

From *Nutrition screening manual for professionals caring for older Americans,* The Nutrition Screening Initiative, Washington, DC, 1991, American Academy of Family Physicians, American Dietetic Association, National Council on the Aging.

Disease

Any disease, illness, or chronic condition that causes you to change the way you eat or makes it hard for you to eat puts your nutritional health at risk. Four out of five adults have chronic diseases that are affected by diet. Confusion or memory loss that keeps getting worse is estimated to affect one out of five or more of older adults. This can make it hard to remember what, when, or if you've eaten. Feeling sad or depressed, which happens to about one in eight older adults, can cause big changes in appetite, digestion, energy level, weight, and well-being.

Eating poorly

Eating too little and eating too much both lead to poor health. Eating the same foods day after day or not eating fruit, vegetables, and milk products daily will also cause poor nutritional health. One in five adults skips meals daily. Only 13% of adults eat the minimum amount of fruit and vegetables needed. One in four older adults drinks too much alcohol. Many health problems become worse if you drink more than one or two alcoholic beverages per day.

Tooth loss/mouth pain

A healthy mouth, teeth, and gums are needed to eat. Missing, loose, or rotten teeth or dentures that don't fit well or cause mouth sores make it hard to eat.

Economic hardship

As many as 40% of older Americans have incomes of less than $6000 per year. Having less—or choosing to spend less—than $25 to $30 per week for food makes it very hard to get the foods you need to stay healthy.

Reduced social contact

One third of all older people live alone. Being with people daily has a positive effect on morale, well-being, and eating.

Multiple medicines

Many older Americans must take medicines for health problems. Almost half of older Americans take multiple medicines daily. Growing old may change the way we respond to drugs. The more medicines you take, the greater the chance for side effects such as increased or decreased appetite, change in taste, constipation, weakness, drowsiness, diarrhea, nausea, and others. Vitamins or minerals when taken in large doses act like drugs and can cause harm. Alert your doctor to everything you take.

Involuntary weight loss/gain

Losing or gaining a lot of weight when you are not trying to do so is an important warning sign that must not be ignored. Being overweight or underweight also increases your chance of poor health.

Needs assistance in self-care

Although most older people are able to eat, one of every five has trouble walking, shopping, and buying and cooking food, especially as they get older.

Elder years above age 80

Most older people lead full and productive lives. But as age increases, risk of frailty and health problems increase. Checking your nutritional health regularly makes good sense.

Continued.

Table 25-17—cont'd. Overview

We all recognize that many older Americans are at high risk of nutritional deficits, excesses, and imbalances that may negatively affect their health and well-being. The goal of the Nutrition Screening Initiative is to identify persons who are at risk before their health has deteriorated to the point that they must be medicated, institutionalized, or hospitalized. This level I screen has been designed to single out those older adults who need medical or nutritional attention and, just as important, to help health and social service workers determine what preventive action can be taken to ensure that the majority of older Americans do not become malnourished (Fig 25-5). Early identification of problems and appropriate intervention increase the likelihood that older people will live longer, more fulfilling, and more productive lives.

Carefully selected screening questions have been divided among four sections that correspond to the four most common types of action to be taken in assisting older adults to eat a healthy diet. The first section on body weight and change in weight is perhaps the most important because it will alert you as to whether the individual being screened should see a physician immediately. The next area screened examines the person's actual eating habits. Positive responses to these statements should flag the need to see a dentist, dietitian, or alcohol abuse counselor. The focus then shifts to problems in socioeconomic and functional status that would best be solved by a case manager, home health care service, social worker, or financial assistance. You might want to jot down names and telephone numbers of physicians (particularly those specializing in geriatric medicine), clinics, dietitians, dentists, psychologists, services, and agencies to have on hand when screening older adults.

Many of the questions on this screen are similar to those asked by home health care agencies and state-run community care programs. If you are familiar with this type of assessment, please rely on your prior training and experience when interpreting the responses that you receive from older adults. If you are a newcomer to this type of screening, take a conservative approach: If an individual gives you an ambiguous or vacillating response, assume he or she is at risk for that particular factor and place a check by the statement on the screen. Even if no serious problem currently exists, you will probably prevent the development of future problems, and a health care or social service professional will be able to determine what level of assistance is required to maintain or restore nutritional health.

If when you complete the level I screen it is apparent that the individual requires medical attention, you must determine whether the individual is able or willing to contact his or her own physician or whether an appointment should be made. If the individual indicates that he or she is willing to make an appointment, stress the importance of doing so soon. If the individual cannot or does not want to be responsible for scheduling a doctor's visit, then you or the person's case worker might want to assist the patient by scheduling an appointment.

A physician should be contacted if the individual has gained or lost 10 pounds unexpectedly or without intending to during the past 6 months. A physician should also be notified if the individual's body mass index is above 27 or below 24.

Living environment

☐ Lives on an income of less than $6000 per year (per individual in the household)

☐ Lives alone

☐ Is housebound

☐ Is concerned about home security

☐ Lives in a home with inadequate heating or cooling

☐ Does not have a stove and/or refrigerator

☐ Is unable or prefers not to spend money on food (<$25 to $30 per person spent on food each week)

Functional status

Usually or always needs assistance with (check each that applies):

☐ Bathing

☐ Dressing

☐ Grooming

☐ Toileting

☐ Eating

☐ Walking or moving about

☐ Traveling (outside the home)

☐ Preparing food

☐ Shopping for food or other necessities

If you have checked one or more statements on this screen, the individual you have interviewed may be at risk for poor nutritional status. Please refer this individual to the appropriate health care or social service professional in your area. For example, a dietitian should be contacted for problems with selecting, preparing, or eating a healthy diet, or a dentist if the individual experiences pain or difficulty when chewing or swallowing. Those individuals whose income, lifestyle, or functional status may endanger their nutritional and overall health should be referred to available community services: home-delivered meals, congregate meal programs, transportation services, counseling services (alcohol abuse, depression, bereavement, etc.), home health care agencies, day care programs, etc.

Please repeat this screen at least once each year—sooner if the individual has a major change in his or her health, income, immediate family (e.g. spouse dies), or functional status.

Table 25-17—cont'd. Activities of daily living (ADLs)

Bathing. Independent: assistance only in bathing a single part (back or disabled extremity) or bathes self completely. Dependent: assistance in bathing more than one part of body; assistance getting in or out of tub; does not bathe self

Dressing. Independent: gets clothes from closets and drawers; puts on clothes, outer garments, braces; manages fasteners (act of tying shoes is excluded). Dependent: does not dress self or remains partly undressed

Toileting. Independant: gets to toilet; gets on and off toilet; arranges clothes; cleans organs of excretion; may manage own bedpan used at night only; may or may not use mechanical supports. Dependent: used bedpan or commode or receives assistance getting to and using toilet

Transferring. Independent: moves in and out of bed independently; moves in and out of chair independently; may or may not use mechanical support. Dependent: assistance in moving in or out of bed and/or chair; does not perform one or more transfers

Continence. Independent: urination and defecation entirely self-controlled. Dependent: partial or total incontinence in urination or defecation; partial or total control by enemas, catheters, or regulated use of urinals and/or bedpans

Feeding. Independent: gets food from plate or its equivalent into mouth (precutting of meat and preparation of food, such as buttering bread, are excluded). Dependent: assistance in act of feeding; does not eat at all or parenteral feeding

Instrumental activities of daily living (IADLs)

Ability to Use Telephone

Shopping. Independent: takes care of all shopping needs; shops independently for small purchases. Dependent: must be accompanied on any shopping trip; completely unable to shop

Food Preparation. Independent: plans, prepares and serves adequate meals independently; prepares adequate meals if supplied with ingredients. Dependent: heats and serves prepared meals; prepares meals but does not maintain adequate diet; must have meals prepared and served

Housekeeping

Laundry

Mode of Transportation. Independent: travels independently on public transportation or drives own car; arranges own travel via taxi but does not otherwise use public transportation. Dependent: travels on public transportation when assisted or accompanied by another; travel limited to taxi or automobile with assistance; does not travel at all

Responsibility for Own Medication

Ability to Handle Finances

Summary

Most older adults with whom you interact will have a few existing or potential risk factors for poor nutritional status, but they will also probably be able to address these issues themselves with minimal (but appropriate) assistance. Many would benefit from an appointment with a registered dietitian, which may be a new concept to them. Others may need to see health care and social service professionals with whom they are accustomed to visiting, such as their dentist, their case worker, or a counseling service. Finally, some will need to see a physician for a complete examination. Many people don't think of poor diet or changes in body weight as a sufficient cause for seeking medical attention, but we hope to alert all Americans, particularly those who are older, to the critical role played by nutrition in maintaining good health and in preventing disease.

Table 25-18. Symptoms and signs with nutritional and nonnutritional etiologies in the elderly

Signs and symptoms	Nutritional etiology	Nonnutritional etiology
Night blindness	Vitamin A deficiency	Cataract
Congestive heart failure	Beriberi	Late effect of rheumatic, coronary, or alcoholic heart disease
Angular stomatitis	Ariboflavinosis	Oral candidiasis, drooling
"Phototoxic" dermatitis	Pellagra	Actinic reticuloid, thiazide photosensitivity
Peripheral neuropathy	Vitamin B_6 deficiencies (drug-induced)	Diabetic neuropathy
Purpura	Scurvy, vitamin K deficiency	Purpura, vasculitis, senile skin changes

From Roe DA: Nutrition assessment of elderly. In Simko MD, Cowell C, Hreha MS, editors: *Practical nutrition*, Rockville, Md, 1989, Aspen Publishers.

Table 25-19. Average height-weight table for men 65 years of age and over

Height in inches	Ages 65-69	Ages 70-74	Ages 75-79	Ages 80-84	Ages 85-89	Ages 90-94
61	128-156	125-153	123-151			
62	130-158	127-155	125-153	122-148		
63	131-161	129-157	127-155	122-150	120-146	
64	134-164	131-161	129-157	124-152	122-148	
65	136-166	134-164	130-160	127-155	125-153	117-143
66	139-169	137-167	133-163	130-158	128-156	120-146
67	140-172	140-170	136-166	132-162	130-160	122-150
68	143-175	142-174	139-169	135-165	133-163	126-154
69	147-179	146-178	142-174	139-169	137-167	130-158
70	150-184	148-182	146-178	143-175	140-172	134-164
71	155-189	152-186	149-183	148-180	144-176	139-169
72	159-195	156-190	154-188	153-187	148-182	
73	164-200	160-196	158-192			

Modified from *JAMA* 177:658, 1960.

Table 25-20. Average height-weight table for women 65 years of age and over

Height in inches	Ages 65-69	Ages 70-74	Ages 75-79	Ages 80-84	Ages 85-89	Ages 90-94
58	120-146	112-138	111-135			
59	121-147	114-140	112-136	100-122	99-121	
60	122-148	116-142	113-139	106-130	102-124	
61	123-151	118-144	115-141	109-133	104-128	
62	125-153	121-147	118-144	112-136	108-132	107-131
63	127-155	123-151	121-147	115-141	112-136	107-131
64	130-158	126-154	123-151	119-145	115-141	108-132
65	132-162	130-158	126-154	122-150	120-146	112-136
66	136-166	132-162	128-157	126-154	124-152	116-142
67	140-170	136-166	131-161	130-158	128-156	
68	143-175	140-170				
69	148-180	144-176				

Modified from *JAMA* 177:658, 1960.

the frail elderly, tests for malnutrition and dehydration are important. If indicated, bone scans for measurement of bone density may be performed.

Decreased serum albumin, serum transferrin, and lymphocyte count and a nonreactive skin may indicate protein-calorie malnutrition. Elevated hemoglobin, hematocrit, and BUN levels may indicate hypohydration.[29] Results from the clinical, anthropometric, and dietary assessments should lead the rest of the biochemical assessment.

Dietary assessment

An essential part of the dietary assessment of the elderly is the collection of data relative to the individual's ability to get food. Once this has been established, one can interview the patient regarding his or her diet. Questions relative to access to transportation and the following other areas are all integral to the patient's ability to eat:

- Do you drive?
- Do you have a car?
- Is someone available to drive you to the store when needed?
- Do you take public transportation?
- Are you able to open food packaging?
- Are you able to use the refrigerator?
- Are you able to reach into cupboards?
- Are you able to heat foods?
- What is your monthly financial situation?

A nutrition history questionnaire, a 24-hour recall, and a food frequency questionnaire will give the physician the

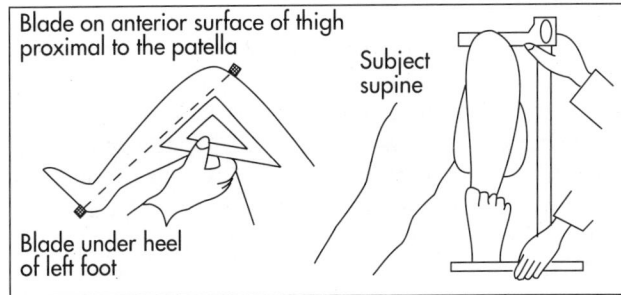

Fig. 25-6. Measurement of knee height. (From Chumlea WC, Roch AF, Mukherjee D: *Nutritional assessment of elderly through anthropometry,* Columbus, Ohio, 1984, Ross Lab.)

Table 25-21. Assessment of body composition in the elderly[15]

	Men		Women	
Percentile	Ages 55-65	Ages 65-75	Ages 55-65	Ages 65-75
Arm circumference (cm)				
10TH	27.3	26.3	25.7	25.2
50TH	31.7	30.7	30.3	29.9
95TH	36.9	35.5	38.5	37.3
Arm muscle circumference (cm)*				
10TH	24.5	23.5	19.6	19.5
50TH	27.8	26.8	22.5	22.5
95TH	32.0	30.6	28.0	27.9
Triceps skinfold (mm)				
10TH	6	6	16	14
50TH	11	11	25	24
95TH	22	22	38	36

*Arm muscle circumference = arm circumference in cm − 0.314 × triceps skinfold in mm.
From Frisancho AR: New norms of upper limb fat and muscle areas for assessment of nutritional status, *Am J Clin Nutr,* 34:2540-2545, 1981.

most practical and complete information generally available. Although the healthy elderly can usually maintain a diet diary, it is often too difficult to obtain a diary from someone who is not well.

It is best to use an interview style, rather than a self-administered style, of data collection to probe the client's memory. The interviewer must have patience in eliciting the needed information, because older individuals may take longer to remember the information required. Asking open-ended questions may jog the individual's short-term memory but will avoid suggesting an answer to the question.

Dietary data should be analyzed relative to the food group guides, dietary guidelines, and individual needs of the patient. This is a quick way to assess omissions of certain categories of foods, exceedingly high- or low-nutrient foods, and unusual diets.[8]

The recommended dietary allowances (RDAs)[23] separate the age categories through 50 years of age. All healthy people above 50 years are put into the same category, although a healthy 75-year-old may have different nutritional needs from his or her younger counterpart. The RDA may be an inappropriate standard for assessing the nutrient intakes of healthy Americans of advanced age. Clearly, the RDA is not recommended as a standard for use with the frail elderly.

Some common nutritional problems of the elderly are[8]:

- Obesity/overweight/fluid imbalance
- Osteoporosis
- Hypertension
- Oral problems
- Sensory changes that affect nutritional status
- Inadequate nutrient intake
- GI changes that affect nutritional status
- Polypharmacy
- Abuse of nutrient supplements

A physician may want to maintain a list of suggestions for some of these common problems. For instance, weight gain is a common problem with aging. Maintaining an ac-

tive lifestyle with regular exercise is important in slowing the decline in the metabolic rate. Otherwise, the rapid decline in metabolism with increasing age and loss of lean tissue leads to a smaller energy requirement, making it difficult to consume enough nutrients with the restrictive caloric intake.

Poor dentition is another common source of poor nutrient intake. Lack of dentition, inflammation, or poorly fitting prostheses will cause a patient to avoid many important foods, particularly meat, fruits, and vegetables. If the dental problems cannot be resolved, whole foods should be cooked until soft or mashed, so that all nutrients, including fiber, are available in the diet. If foods are not chewed well and are swallowed whole, nutrient absorption will not be optimal (see Chapter 23 for more discussion).

THE PRIMARY CARE PHYSICIAN AND COUNSELING

Effective counseling is a key to successful dietary change. Physicians must see themselves as expert consultants for patients who control their own health choices and develop a therapeutic alliance with patients to promote behavior changes toward healthful eating habits. All patients should receive the benefit of dietary counseling (see box).[21]

Eating behaviors are determined by biological, psychological, and sociocultural factors. Gut hormones, thermostatic mechanisms, and blood glucose levels are biological factors that influence eating behaviors and are the most familiar to physicians.[21]

Guidelines for nutrition counseling

- Develop a patient-physician partnership
- Counsel all patients
- Explain the relationship between behaviors and health
- Assess barriers to behavior change
- Obtain patient commitment
- Encourage patient participation
- Use a combination of strategies
- Design a behavior modification plan
- Monitor progress
- Involve other health professionals

From Michener JL: Nutrition counseling. Translating research into practice. Presented at the Opinion Leaders' Symposium for "Rx Nutrition: Good Health in Practice," Sponsored by University of Washington School of Medicine, Little Falls, New Jersey, 1989, Health Learning Systems.

Psychological factors are often more powerful in influencing eating behaviors than biological factors. These are many and varied, and include emotional conflict, self-image, and attitudes toward nutrition.[21]

Sociocultural factors also play a strong role in determining eating patterns and behaviors. Peer influence, time constraints, and lack of information, among many other factors, play a significant part in forming the eating behaviors of individuals.[21]

It is crucial for the physician-counselor to recognize that food is more than just a mode of transportation for nutrients into the body. Food is a very intimate and emotional component of our lives. It is at the center of many religious and cultural celebrations and is often linked to significant family memories, both good and bad. Food has been used for reward and punishment, and may represent a powerful emotional concept to some individuals.

The physician-counselor must recognize that although a patient may cognitively understand the benefits of changing his or her eating behaviors, the patient cannot do so until he or she overcomes the emotional barriers to that change. Instead of the physician designing a strategy for diet and behavior change, the patient must be involved in the process to set his or her own small goals for gradual change. This will help to secure the patient's commitment and ensure effective and permanent change.

Regular follow-up is essential to successful behavior change. If, by monitoring patient progress, the patient appears to be having difficulty in adhering to the jointly established plan for change, the physician should consider involving other health professionals, such as social and psychological counselors, registered dietitians, and nurse educators.[21]

SUMMARY

The publication of the *Surgeon General's Report on Nutrition and Health* in 1988 adjusted the focus of the nation's primary health care providers from disease treatment to disease prevention and treatment.[33] The recognition that diet plays a prominent role in five of the top 10 causes of death has led us to the realization that all Americans may fall into one or more high-risk groups for some type of malnutrition: that associated with underconsumption and/or that associated with overconsumption and its relationship to several chronic diseases. These issues have established solid evidence for the nutritional assessment and counseling of patients by primary care physicians.

A complete nutrition assessment is a four-part evaluation: clinical, anthropometric, biochemical, and dietary. Within these categories there are several different valid and reliable methods of collecting data. The appropriateness of the data collection method depends on the patient subgroup under examination.

Once the nutrition assessment is collected and analyzed, the physician should be intimately involved in the lifestyle modification counseling process. Regular follow-up for patient monitoring and support is necessary for the promotion of successful behavior change.

REFERENCES

1. Alton IR: Dietary assessment and management of the adolescent. In Simko MD, Cowell C, Hreha MS, editors: *Practical nutrition. A quick reference for the health care practitioner,* Rockville, Md, 1989, Aspen Publishers.
2. Ammerman AS et al: A brief dietary assessment to guide cholesterol reduction in low-income individuals: design and validation, *J Am Dietet Assoc* 91:1385-1390, 1991.
3. Anderson GD, Jacobson HN: Nutrition assessment of pregnant and lactating women. In Simko MD, Cowell C, Hreha MS, editors: *Practical nutrition. A quick reference for the health care practitioner,* Rockville, Md, 1989, Aspen Publishers.
4. Anderson RA, Guttman HN: Trace minerals and exercise. In Horton ES, Terjung RL, editors: *Exercise, nutrition, and energy metabolism,* New York, 1988, Macmillan Publishing.
5. Austin C: Dietary assessment of management of the infant. (Birth through two years.) In Simko MD, Cowell C, and Hreha MS, editors: *Practical nutrition. A quick reference for the health care practitioner,* Rockville, Md, 1989, Aspen Publishers.
6. Bistrian BR et al: Protein status of general surgical patients, *JAMA* 230:858-860,1974.
7. Bistrian BR et al: Prevalence of malnutrition in general medical patients, *JAMA* 235:1567-1570, 1976.
8. Chernoff R: Dietary assessment and management of the elderly. In Simko MD, Cowell C, Hreha MS, editors: *Practical nutrition. A quick reference for the health care practitioner,* Rockville, Md, 1989, Aspen Publishers.
9. Christakis G: Nutrition assessment of the adult. In Simko MD, Cowell C, Hreha MS, editors: *Practical nutrition. A quick reference for the health care practitioner,* Rockville, Md, 1989, Aspen Publishers.
10. Chumlea WC, Roch AF, Mukherjee D: *Nutritional assessment of the elderly through anthropometry,* Columbus, Ohio, 1984, Ross Laboratories.

11. Department of Health, Education and Welfare: *Ten-state nutrition survey in the United States, 1968-1970*, Atlanta, 1972, Centers for Disease Control.

12. Dietz WH: Childhood obesity: susceptibility, cause, and management, *J Pediatr* 103:676-686, 1983.

13. Endres JB: Dietary assessment and management of the young child. (Two through six years). In Simko MD, Cowell C, and Hreha MS, editors: *Practical nutrition. A quick reference for the health care practitioner*. Rockville, Md, 1989, Aspen Publishers.

14. Fomon SJ: Nutrition assessment of the infant. (Birth through two years). In Simko MD, Cowell C, and Hreha MS, editors: *Practical nutrition. A quick reference for the health care practitioner*, Rockville, Md, 1989, Aspen Publishers.

15. Frisancho AR: New norms of upper limb fat and muscle areas for assessment of nutritional status, *Am J Clin Nutr* 34:2540-2545, 1981.

16. Gibson RS: *Principles of nutrition assessment*, New York, 1990, Oxford University Press.

17. Gilbride JA, Cowell C, Simko MD: *The process of nutrition assessment*. In Simko MD, Cowell C, Gilbride JA, editors: *Nutrition assessment, a comprehensive guide for planning intervention*, Rockville, Md, 1984, Aspen Publishers.

18. Mammel KA: Nutrition assessment of the school age child. In Simko MD, Cowell C, Hreha MS, editors: *Practical nutrition. A quick reference for the health care practitioner*, Rockville, Md, 1989, Aspen Publishers.

19. McArdle WD, Katch FI, Katch VL: *Exercise physiology*, ed 2, Philadelphia, 1986, Lea & Febiger.

20. McKay C: Nutrition assessment of the adolescent. In Simko MD, Cowell C, and Hreha MS, editors: *Practical nutrition. A quick reference for the health care practitioner*, Rockville, Md, 1989, Aspen Publishers.

21. Michener JL: Nutrition counseling. Translating research into practice. Presented at the Opinion Leaders' Symposium for "Rx Nutrition: Good Health in Practice," Sponsored by University of Washington School of Medicine. Little Falls, New Jersey, 1989, Health Learning Systems.

22. Mycek MJ: Interaction of drugs with foods and nutrients. In Simko MD, Cowell C, and Gilbride JA, editors: *Nutrition assessment. A comprehensive guide for planning intervention*, Rockville, Md, 1984, Aspen Publishers.

23. National Research Council: Recommended dietary allowances, ed 10, Washington, DC, 1989, Subcommittee on the 10th Edition of the RDAs, Food and Nutrition Board, Commission on Life Sciences, National Academy Press.

24. Nutrition monitoring in the United States—a report from the Joint Nutrition Monitoring Evaluation Committee, Washington, DC, 1986, US Department of Health and Human Services and US Department of Agriculture.

25. *Nutrition screening manual for professionals caring for older Americans*, Nutrition Screening Initiative, Washington, DC, 1991, American Academy of Family Physicians, American Dietetic Association, National Council on the Aging.

26. *Nutrition and your health: dietary guidelines for Americans*, ed 3, Washington, DC, 1990, US Department of Agriculture, US Department of Health and Human Services.

27. Pi-Sunyer FX, Woo R: Laboratory assessment of nutrition status. In Simko MD, Cowell C, and Gilbride JA, editors: *Nutrition Assessment, a comprehensive guide for planning interventions*, Rockville, Md, 1984, Aspen Publishers.

28. Robbins GE, Trowbridge FL: Anthropometric techniques and their application. In Simko MD, Cowell C, and Gilbride JA, editors: *Nutrition assessment. A comprehensive guide for planning intervention*, Rockville, Md, 1984, Aspen Publishers.

29. Roe DA: Nutrition assessment of the elderly. In Simko MD, Cowell

30. Rosenthal SR, Padron CZ: Nutrition assessment of the young child. (Two through six years). In Simko MD, Cowell C, and Hreha MS, editors: *Practical nutrition. A quick reference for the health care practitioner*, Rockville, Md, 1989, Aspen Publishers.

31. Simko MD, Hreha MS, and Cowell C: How to use this reference. In Simko MD, Cowell C, and Hreha MS, editors: *Practical nutrition. A quick reference for the health care practitioner*. Rockville, Md, 1989, Aspen Publishers.

32. Steffee WP: Malnutrition in hospitalized patients, *JAMA* 244:2630-2635, 1980.

33. *The Surgeon General's report on nutrition and health*, Washington, DC, 1988, US Department of Health and Human Services, Public Health Service.

34. Thomas-Dobersen D: Dietary assessment and management of the school age child. In Simko MD, Cowell C, and Hreha MS, editors: *Practical nutrition. A quick reference for the health care practitioner*, Rockville, Md, 1989, Aspen Publishers.

35. Walsh JH: Dietary assessment and management of the adult. In Simko MD, Cowell C, and Hreha MS, editors: *Practical nutrition. A quick reference for the health care practitioner*, Rockville, Md, 1989, Aspen Publishers.

36. Weidman W et al: *Diet in a healthy child*. monograph, Dallas, Tex, 1983, The American Heart Association.

37. White JV et al: Nutrition Screening Initiative: Development and implementation of the public awareness checklist and screening tools, *J Am Dietet Assoc* 92:163-167, 1992.

━━━━━━━━━━ **RESOURCES** ━━━━━━━━━━

The Nutrition Screening Initiative, 2626 Pennsylvania Ave., NW, Suite 301, Washington, DC 20037.

Ross Laboratories, 625 Cleveland Ave, Columbus, OH 43215; for copies of growth charts and anthropometric standards for infants, children, adults, and the elderly.

Government resources

Health Information Center, Department of Health and Human Services, (800) 336-4797.

Health Resources and Services Administration, Department of Health and Human Services, Room 1445, 5600 Fisher's Lane, Rockville, MD 20857.

National Center for Education and Maternal Child Health, Department of Health and Human Services. 18-05 Parklawn Bldg., 5600 Fisher's Lane, Rockville, MD 20857.

National Institutes on Aging, Department of Health and Human Services, (800) 222-2225.

Select Committee on Aging, Subcommittee on Health and Long-Term Care, U.S. Congress. 377 Ford House Office Bldg., Washington, DC 20515.

Tufts/USDA Nutrition Center on Aging, Tufts University, 711 Washington St. Boston, MA 02111.

Chapter 26

PRACTICAL ISSUES
IN PATIENT CARE

Susan M. Kleiner

Permanent alteration of dietary habits is a matter of life-style change. Food plays a substantial and intimate role in our day-to-day activities and celebrations. To successfully change the way we eat, we must learn how to adapt our eating styles to new situations.

Many guides, guidelines, and recommendations offer nutrient standards to plan a healthy diet, but people shop for, choose, and eat food, not nutrients. Thus it is essential to offer patients practical food information so they can successfully adapt their food choices to dietary guidelines.

As nutrition becomes a major watchword of health promotion and disease prevention, patients and consumers need help and advice in deciphering the information deluge brought on by the media, medicine, and Madison Avenue. This chapter discusses the changing nutrition scene in the United States, including practical guidelines and suggestions to help patients move toward a healthier lifestyle.

NUTRITION, FADDISM, AND QUACKERY*

Nutrition and health fraud is commonplace, in no small part because of Madison Avenue advertising success. The Food and Drug Administration (FDA) conducted a study[12] to estimate the prevalence of advertising for possibly fraudulent health items during 1 month. A total of 435 questionable ads were identified in publications ranging from the smallest weekly newspapers to multimillion-circulation magazines. Not all of the nation's 10,000 daily and weekly newspapers and general-circulation magazines

were reviewed; 435 represents only a fraction of the number of questionable nutrition and health-care products and programs being peddled to the public each month.

It is only partially true that false advertising is unlawful and that nutrition and health claims are regulated by the government. The FDA does not have the money or staff to pursue the many claims that are made. Generally, only the most outrageous or life-threatening claims draw action. If a disclaimer accompanies a product or publication, a company or author generally cannot be held responsible even in cases that result in harm.

The FDA considers nutrition supplements as foods, not drugs. Therefore health claims made by the manufacturers of such items need not be proved before marketing, as is necessary for claims regarding drugs. Because the U.S. Postal Service requires truth in mail-order advertising, that agency is the primary avenue for regulation and control of mail-order health claims and nutrition supplements.

Nutrition quacks appeal to emotions, not logic. They want patients to believe in their "cures," and they rely on the emotional testimonials of their "cured" clients. They use sensational tabloids and other media to convey their messages. Nutrition and medicine are not religions; they are sciences, and the efficacy of treatments should be supported by scientific evidence, not by emotional testimony.

When qualified health professionals cannot offer a cure, purveyors of questionable therapies step in confidently. They usually are not certified or monitored by any regulatory agency or licensing board, so dissatisfied clients have little recourse.

A common strategy used by unqualified practitioners is to present a chronic disease as an external symptom of an internal or underlying dysfunction, disorder, or toxicity.

*Excerpted with permission from Kleiner SM: Beware of nutrition quackery, *The Physician and Sports Medicine* 18:46, 1990.

Cancer may be presented as a symptom, not the problem. "The problem is your immune system," states the practitioner. "Your body needs detoxification and these individually formulated vitamins."

Often a tremendous responsibility for the cure is placed on the patients. When a therapy doesn't work, the cure-seekers feel that they, and not the treatment, have failed. This protects unqualified therapists from their unhappy clients.

Weight-loss products are by far the most popular items promoted by fraud artists. Patients wish for a secret that will enable dieters to lose weight and keep it off. Promoters of diet books and products appear to some people to have found the secret. In addition to buying these magic foods and fad diets, people are lured by pills, potions, treatments, and devices that purportedly cause weight loss.

The bottom line on weight loss is basically the same: If calories consumed are less than calories expended, we lose weight, regardless of the creative way an author may tell the story. Equally important as losing weight is keeping it off. Without sound nutrition education and behavior modification, most attempts to maintain weight loss will fail.

Another form of fraud or quackery is the promotion of vitamin supplements and megadosing as the panacea for all ills. There are no data to support general megadosing of vitamins. Unless a person is vitamin deficient or has a recognized disorder in which pharmacologic doses of vitamin analogs are prescribed, megadosing will not be a benefit and will not make someone "super-well."

Complications caused by vitamin megadosing are an additional concern. Vitamin B_6 acts as an antagonist to L-dopa. Large vitamin C intakes may interfere with the results of clinical laboratory tests used to detect the presence of fecal and urinary occult blood.[3]

Nutrients interact in the body, so that larger intakes of one nutrient may negatively affect the absorption, metabolism, or excretion of others. For example, large doses of vitamin C will increase nonheme iron absorption from food, thereby decreasing intestinal absorption of copper. High intakes of zinc will also inhibit copper bioavailability. High-protein diets may increase calcium excretion.[3]

Dietary supplements are considered foods and not drugs and are therefore exempt from United States Pharmacopoeia standards. There is little quality control enforced on supplement manufacturers, and product contamination does occur. In 1982, the FDA warned physicians that certain bone meal and dolomite supplements, popular for their calcium content, were found to contain substantial amounts of lead. Commercial dietary algae supplements of spirulina were found to contain unhealthy amounts of mercury. Four major brands of fish oil capsules contained trace amounts of DDT metabolites and PCBs. Supplement dosages have been found to exceed the labeled dose amount, sometimes manifold, causing toxic reactions.[3]

To guard against health fraud and nutrition quackery,

Quackery criteria: Indications of nutrition fraud

- Treatment based on an unproved theory that usually calls for painless, nontoxic therapy.
- Credentials of author/purveyor aren't recognized in the scientific community.
- No reports published in scientific, peer-reviewed journals, but mass media is used for marketing.
- Purveyors claim the medical establishment is against them; they play on the public's paranoia about the phantom greed of the medical establishment.
- Treatment known only to author/purveyor; drugs and preparations manufactured according to a secret formula.
- Excessive claims that promise a dramatic, miraculous cure, including prolonging life or preventing disease.
- Emotional images rather than facts are used to support claims.
- Treatment calls for special nutritional support, such as vitamins, minerals, or health food products.
- Purveyors caution clients or readers against discussing the programs so that they don't get discouraged by those who are negative.
- Programs are based on drugs, treatments, or tests that have not been labeled for such uses.

Modified from Monaco GP: Primary care physician, *Med Times* 114(5):43-48, 1986.

---

one should measure purported treatments and cures against the "quackery criteria"—the hallmarks of unproved or worthless treatments (see box above).[13] The physician should suggest to patients that they seek advice from qualified and credentialed health-care professionals, and always get a second opinion.

When searching for nutrition information, the patient should go to a licensed or registered dietitian. Many, but not all, states have some sort of licensing standard for nutrition practitioners. If a state does not have such licensing, the physician should refer the patient to a registered dietitian. To find a registered dietitian, the patient can call a local hospital, a state or local dietetic association, or the American Dietetic Association.

In addition, consumer groups and government agencies help combat health fraud. For example, the American Council on Science and Health is a consumer education organization concerned with issues related to food, nutrition, chemicals, pharmaceuticals, lifestyle, environment, and health. The National Council Against Health Fraud investigates health claims, educates the public about untruths and deceptions, acts as a clearinghouse for individuals and organizations concerned with health misinformation, and supports legislation and legal action against health fraud. The FDA, listed in the telephone directory under U.S. Health and Human Services, can be contacted directly. In addition, each state has an attorney general and a consumer protection office that can be of service.

HEALTHFUL TRAVEL TIPS*

Many habits and familiar conditions are disrupted during travel, especially during a cross-country or overseas trip. Diet, exercise, clothing, sleep patterns, exposure to light and dark, noise, ambient temperature, and humidity all influence internal physiology and thus the way people feel and behave.

On a long trip going east or west across time zones, circadian rhythms are disrupted. This seems more apparent when going east, when we "lose time," than west, when we "gain time." North-south travel does not cause this problem. The following nutrition guidelines are intended to help make traveling a more comfortable, healthful experience.

Recommendations for the traveler

- Begin a light diet 12 hours before departure and maintain that style of eating throughout most of the trip. The patient will feel more comfortable initially, and if this strategy is followed throughout the trip, some dietary hazards may be avoided, especially hazards of overseas travel. Fancy diet planning is not necessary.
- A light diet emphasizes breads, cereals, vegetables, fruit, and low-fat dairy products. Fish, poultry, legumes, grains, and small amounts of eggs and cheese are good primary protein sources. Eat only small portions of beef and fat-laden foods, such as sauces and creams, fried foods, and rich desserts.
- Never travel hungry; it puts a person at the mercy of the fast-food snack vendors and the often poorly planned airplane meals. Light, healthful snack foods now can be purchased in many airports. Look for fresh or dried fruits, nuts, popcorn, low-fat fresh or frozen yogurt, or cheese and crackers. If planning ahead, bring such snacks from home including even homemade or deli sandwiches.
- Consider requesting special meals available on most airlines (such as seafood, fruit platters, low-fat/low-cholesterol and vegetarian meals); they are lower in fat and cholesterol than the regular fare. These meals must be requested through the ticket agent at least 24 hours before departure.
- Drink plenty of liquids. The controlled environment of the airplane cabin is very dry, and dehydration is the cause of many complaints, including headaches and mild constipation. Ask for the whole can of juice, seltzer, or soda that is offered instead of just a glassful. Water is always available. The extra fluid may necessitate more frequent voiding, but this also allows for ambulation and stretching during the flight.

- Caffeine and alcohol are both diuretics, and they will also disrupt the sleep-wake cycle. Avoid caffeine until the end of the flight. If alcohol is to be consumed, this should be limited to one drink, and optimally a light one such as a wine spritzer.
- Once at the destination, one should continue to eat as close to a normal diet as possible. To avoid problems with constipation, one should drink plenty of fluids and eat high-fiber foods like whole grains, fruits, and vegetables.
- When traveling to another country, one should beware of the water and food contamination problems. Always use bottled water, even for brushing teeth. Make sure that the bottle is well-sealed before drinking the water. In some parts of the world, empty bottles are refilled with tap water and sold at a lower price on street corners. Eat only cooked foods or peeled fruits and vegetables, because even though foods may have been washed, they were probably washed in local water.

DINING OUT SUCCESSFULLY

Dining out does not necessarily mean diet disaster. When going to a restaurant, the patient should be instructed to take control of the menu and meal. The patient should have a game plan before going to the restaurant (Table 26-1).

Recommendations for the patient eating out

- Choose a restaurant that offers nutritious choices. Avoid all-you-can-eat buffets and restaurants that offer only high-calorie, high-fat fare.
- Plan ahead. If dining out one evening, eat lighter during the day to allow some leeway with the evening meal.
- Before arriving at the restaurant, decide what type of food to order—chicken, fish, lean red meat, or a vegetarian entree.
- Watch for the hidden fat in restaurant cooking—sauces, condiments, butter, oil, mayonnaise, creams, and rich cheeses add a lot of fat to appetizers, entrees, and side dishes. The menu dictionary in the box on p. 481 is a helpful guide to hidden fats.
- Ask the server to leave out high-fat ingredients. Ask that sauces, salad dressings, and sour cream be served on the side so that the amount to be used can be controlled.
- Don't hesitate to make a substitution, such as a baked potato for French fries.
- Ask questions about foods on the menu. That's why the server is there. Be specific! How is the food prepared? What are the ingredients?

FAST FOODS

Eating at fast-food establishments is no longer a nightmare for those seeking healthy food choices. Whether one

*Excerpted with permission from Kleiner SM: Can't stomach long trips? Try these healthful tips, *The Physician and Sports Medicine* 18:41, 1990.

Table 26-1. Guide to healthy menu choices

Choose	Avoid
Appetizers	
Raw or steamed seafood: mussels, crabs, lobsters, shrimp; Raw or steamed vegetables, vegetable antipasto	Foods swimming in butter, clams, cheese
Soups	
Gazpacho, consommé, broth-type soups	Creamed soups
Entrees	
Broiled, poached, or grilled fish and shellfish; roasted, broiled, or grilled chicken (no skin); roasted turkey, pasta (with tomato sauce), stir-fry dishes, lean meats (round, sirloin, tenderloin, flank steak, filet mignon)	Fatty meat, fried and deep-fried foods, foods with cream sauces, gravies, or cheese
Vegetables	
Fresh vegetables, raw or steamed, baked potato	Fried vegetables, heavily buttered, creamed, or in cheese sauce
Breads	
Plain bread and breadsticks, hard rolls, bagels, English muffins	Baked with butter, shortening, or cheese; sweet rolls
Salads	
Oil and vinegar dressing, or a clear dressing; diet dressings without oil are excellent; use sparingly	Creamy dressings, meats, bacon, cheese, croutons
Sandwiches	
Tuna, chicken, turkey, seafood, lean cooked beef	Processed lunch meats, hard cheese, fried foods, sauces, gravies, mayonnaise, bacon
Desserts	
Fruit, sorbet, sherbet, frozen angel food cake, other pastries, specially made low-fat items	Commercial pies, cakes, yogurt, ice cream, candies

is on the road, in a hurry, or looking for a bargain, lower fat, healthier alternatives now are available at many fast-food restaurants (Table 26-2). However, consumers must beware of the pitfalls placed within their path.

Salad bars and salad plates are available at many establishments. However, people should be careful not to turn their low-fat salad into a replica of a high-fat cheeseburger by heaping it full of processed cheese, fried noodles, croutons, bacon bits, and creamy dressings. Instruct patients to use small servings of egg, turkey, cheese, and beans as protein sources. They should select the light, low-fat dressings, or use regular dressings sparingly.

Many fast-food restaurants have added chicken sandwiches to their menus. These are often the lowest fat sandwich selection. The chicken should be broiled or grilled, not fried, because any fried foods are high in fat.

Fish sandwiches are deceptively high in fat, because they are all fried. If searching for a low-fat alternative, one should avoid the fish sandwiches. Often, the small, regular burgers and cheeseburgers are much lower in fat than the fish or the double and triple burgers piled high with bacon and cheese.

Ethnic selections, such as chili, burritos, tacos, and

Menu dictionary

Some of the words commonly used on menus describe how high in fat the food will be.

Choose	*Avoid*
Steamed	Fried
In it's own juice	Sautéed
Boiled	Au gratin
Broiled	Buttery, buttered
Grilled	Creamed, cream sauce
Baked	Hollandaise
Roasted	Alfredo
Poached	Parmesan
Garden fresh	Marinated (in oil)
Tomato juice	Casserole
	Gravy
	Hash
	Potpie
	Crispy

Table 26-2. Fast food comparisons

	Calories	Fat grams
McDonald's		
Hotcakes with butter and syrup	410	9.2
English Muffin with butter	170	4.6
McLean Deluxe Sandwich	320	10.0
Hamburger	260	9.5
Cheeseburger	310	13.8
Quarter Pounder	410	20.7
Chef Salad	230	13.3
Burger King		
BK Broiler Chicken Sandwich	379	18.0
Wendy's		
Grilled Chicken Sandwich	340	13.0
Chili (regular serving)	240	8.0
Chili (large serving)	360	12.0
Plain baked potato	250	2.0
Salad bar (select low-fat items)		
Generic		
Burrito	392	13.6
Pizza with cheese, one slice	290	8.6
Pizza with pepperoni, one slice	306	11.5
Roast beef sandwich	347	13.4
Taco	187	10.4

Table 26-3. USDA food guide

Food group	Suggested servings
Vegetables	3-5 Servings
Fruits	2-4 Servings
Breads, cereals, rice, pasta	6-11 Servings
Milk, yogurt, cheese	2-3 Servings
Meats, poultry, fish, dry beans and peas, eggs, nuts	2-3 Servings

- One serving of vegetables is 1 cup of raw leafy greens or ½ cup of other vegetables. A ½ cup of cooked dry beans or peas may be counted as either one vegetable or serving or 1 oz of the meat group. Eat dark green leafy and deep yellow vegetables often.
- One serving of fruit is one medium piece of fresh fruit, ½ cup of small or diced fruit, or ¾ cup of juice. Have citrus fruits or juices, melons, or berries regularly.
- One serving of grain products is equal to one slice of bread; one half bun, bagel, or English muffin; 1 ounce of dry ready-to-eat cereal; ½ cup cooked cereal, rice, or pasta. Emphasize whole grain products daily.
- One serving of milk products is equal to 1 cup of milk or yogurt or 1½ oz of cheese. Choose skim or low-fat milk and fat-free or low-fat yogurt and cheese.
- One serving of meat and other protein products is equivalent to 2 to 3 oz of cooked lean beef, chicken without skin, or fish; or two medium eggs; or 1 cup of cooked dry beans or peas. Trim fat from meat and moderate the use of egg yolks and organ meats.

Modified from U.S. Department of Agriculture, U.S. Department of Health and Human Services: Preparing foods and planning menus using the dietary guidelines

pizza, are often nutritionally dense and lower in fat. Baked potatoes are always a low-fat selection, but high-fat cheese sauces and sour creams should be avoided.

Some restaurants now carry low-fat breakfast items, including cereal and low-fat milk, low-fat muffins, and more. English muffins and hotcakes are also good selections, as long as they are not drenched with butter. These items are better choices than the egg, cheese, and bacon sandwiches.

Many restaurants have nutrition information about their foods available at the counter. This information should be requested to help choose a meal.

If one cannot resist making a meal of high-fat foods, such as fries, shakes, and burgers with bacon and cheese, one should choose small portions rather than large or jumbo sizes. This will satisfy cravings and limit fat and calorie consumption.

One fast-food meal like this may contain nearly all the fat needed in a whole day. Light meals should be planned for the rest of the day to balance fat and calorie intake. These types of meals should not be eaten daily. Planning for and enjoying favorite high-fat foods once in a while helps one maintain an all-around healthy diet without feeling guilty or deprived.

HEALTHY DIET AND HEALTHY WEIGHT

The major nutritional problem facing most Americans is overconsumption of fat and calories. This has led to a na-

tional epidemic of obesity. If fat intake could be modified, however, weight control would be a far more manageable issue.

The first approach to practical weight loss and management is to educate patients about the components of a healthy diet. The *Dietary Guidelines for Americans*[4] are an excellent initial outline to follow and use as an educational tool. These guidelines emphasize moderation and avoidance of extremes in the diet:

Guideline 1: Eat a variety of foods

No single food provides all of the nutrients in the amounts needed every day. It is important to select foods from all food groups daily. Each food group contains foods high in specific categories of essential nutrients. But even within food groups, one must choose a variety of representative foods to ensure a nutritious and balanced diet.

The dietary guidelines group foods into five major categories. The USDA's Food Guide (Table 26-3) lists suggested serving numbers. Most people should have at least the lower number of servings suggested from each food every day. Those individuals with higher energy requirements based on body size and physical activity may need more than the suggested servings each day.

Guideline 2: Maintain healthy weight

Determining a healthy individual weight for a patient depends on how much body weight is fat, where the body fat is located, and whether a patient has weight-related medical problems, such as hypertension.

To achieve and maintain a healthy weight status, a healthy diet must be combined with a regular program of physical activity (see Chapters 18 and 19).

Guideline 3: Choose a diet low in fat, saturated fat, and cholesterol

Diets high in fat, saturated fat, and cholesterol clearly are linked with risk factors associated with the development of several chronic diseases. This style of diet is generally high in calories, leading to obesity, a separate risk factor for chronic disease.

To decrease the total fat, saturated fat, and cholesterol in a diet, suggest these tips:

- Use fats and oils sparingly in cooking.
- Use small amounts of salad dressings and spreads, such as butter, margarine, and mayonnaise. Try the new low-fat and fat-free products that replace many of these old high-fat favorites.
- Choose *liquid* vegetable oils most often, because they are lower in saturated fat.
- Check labels on foods to see how much fat and saturated fat are in a serving.

Guideline 4: Choose a diet with plenty of vegetables, fruits, and grain products

These foods are generally high in vitamins, minerals, complex carbohydrates, and fiber, and low in fat and calories. As emphasized in the first guideline, they should provide the majority of food servings every day.

People who follow diets high in vegetables, fruits, and grain products generally are healthier and have fewer problems with weight control.

Guideline 5: Use sugars only in moderation

There are two major problems with high sugar consumption.

1. Weight control. Individuals who consume large amounts of sugary foods yet maintain a healthy weight generally are replacing foods that offer high nutrient density with "empty-calorie" foods, thus maintaining caloric balance, but eliminating nutritionally essential foods in their diets. More commonly, individuals who consume large amounts of sweets are overweight.
2. Sugars can contribute to tooth decay, a major public health concern.

Therefore the advice from the USDA states that sugars should be used in moderation. If calorie needs are low, sugar should be used sparingly so as not to replace essential foods in the diet. Counsel patients to avoid excessive

---

Sugar terms	
Read food labels carefully. The presence of any of these ingredients means that there is sugar in the product.	
Table sugar (sucrose)	Honey
Brown sugar	Syrup
Raw sugar	Corn sweetener
Glucose (dextrose)	High-fructose corn syrup
Fructose	Molasses
Maltose	Fruit juice concentrate*
Lactose	

*This is generally a highly purified product that has little to no other nutritional value other than concentrated fruit sugar.

snacking and to brush and floss teeth regularly (see the box above).

Guideline 6: Use salt and sodium only in moderation

This guideline is included because of the association between high sodium intake and hypertension. When adults with hypertension restrict their sodium intake, their blood pressure usually decreases.

Although it is still not clear whether increased consumption of salt and sodium can lead to the development of hypertension universally, there may be some predisposed individuals in whom high sodium intakes may increase the risks of developing the disease.

Most Americans eat far more salt and sodium than necessary. The major source of sodium in our diets is processed foods, ready-to-eat foods, pickled foods, condiments, and salted snack foods. It is important to read food labels carefully. Choose those lower in sodium most of the time.

Guideline 7: If drinking alcoholic beverages, do so in moderation

Moderate drinking means:

Women: no more than one drink a day
Men: no more than two drinks a day
One drink equals:
- 12 oz of regular beer
- 5 oz of wine
- 1½ oz of distilled spirits (80 proof)

ESTIMATING FAT CONSUMPTION*

Controlling fat in the diet is clearly one of the major keys to weight management and disease prevention. The *Dietary Guidelines* recommend that we limit the total fat in our diets to 30% or less, the saturated fat to 10% or less, and cholesterol to 300 mg or less.

Some patients will thrive on a rigid plan that gives them

---

*Excerpted with permission from Kleiner SM: Have your cake—and enjoy it too, *The Physician and Sports Medicine* 19(5):15, 1991.

Table 26-4. Daily target fat rate formula

Total fat (TF)

Total daily calories × 30% = Daily calories from fat

$$\frac{\text{Daily calories from fat}}{9} = \text{Grams total fat}$$

(Example: 2000 calories × 30% = 600 600 ÷ 9 = 67 g TF)

Saturated fatty acids (SFA)

Total daily calories × 10% = Daily calories from SFA

$$\frac{\text{Daily calories from SFA}}{9} = \text{Grams SFA}$$

(Example: 2000 calories × 10% = 200 200 ÷ 9 = 22g SFA)

Daily target fat rate chart

Daily calorie level	Total (max g)	Saturated fatty acids (max g)
1200	40	13
1800	60	20
2400	80	27
3000	100	33

little leeway for choosing their own foods. Most patients, however, will not succeed on a dietary plan that does not allow occasional indulgence.

One way to include favorite treats in a healthy diet is to know the patient's estimated daily target fat rate. Then, recommend that the patient read labels and tally fat intake for the day until the target is reached. To calculate the daily target fat rate, a standard formula or chart can be used (Table 26-4).

Once daily target fat rate is calculated, food labels should be checked for the fat content per serving. The grams of total fat are listed on any food package that provides a nutrition label. Remind the patient that when tallying the grams of fat from one serving, only one serving of the food should be eaten.

The major sources of fat should be foods that are also dense in the nutrients needed daily for good health. Breads and cereals, low-fat dairy products, lean meats, poultry, fish, eggs, and vegetables are all sources of fat, yet they are packed full of other essential nutrients needed each day. Liquid vegetable oils and tub margarines contain unsaturated fats, are healthier than saturated fats, and, along with adding flavor and variety to food, can be part of a heart-healthy diet.

When a patient meets nutrient requirements for the day by following the serving numbers from the food guide, with extra calories and fat to spare, the patient can have a favorite snack or dessert. The patient should tally it against his or her target fat rate and consider it part of a healthy diet.

Other tempting options are some of the latest offerings from the food industry: new and lighter renditions of the original high-fat fare. Some foods have had some of the

fat and sugar removed; others offer artificial sweeteners, fat replacements, and fat substitutes, which may promise less fat and/or fewer calories. Also gaining in popularity are no-fat, no-cholesterol frozen desserts and baked goods.

People should not depend on the advertising hype on the front of the food label. To compare products, one must read the nutrition and ingredient labels of each product and compare the types and amounts of fat per serving.

By using the fat information on a nutrition label, one can also determine the percentage of calories from fat in the food. By limiting the majority of foods in the diet to those that have only 30% or less of their calories in fat, one can easily stay within the dietary guidelines. Fat is listed in grams (28 g = 1 oz) on the label, and 1 g of fat contains 9 calories. The following standard formula is used to calculate the percentage of calories from fat in food: Multiply the number of grams of fat per serving by 9, and divide that product by the total number of calories per serving:

$$\frac{\text{Grams of fat per serving} \times 9}{\text{Total calories per serving}} = \text{Percentage of calories from fat}$$

For example, if something has 6 g of fat per serving (per the nutrition label), multiply 6 by 9, which equals 54 fat calories. Divide the 54 fat calories by the 220 calories per serving (per the label), to determine that 24% of the calories for that food come from fat:

$$\frac{6 \text{ g Fat/serving} \times 9}{220 \text{ Calories/serving}} = \frac{54 \text{ fat calories}}{220 \text{ calories/serving}}$$
$$= 24\% \text{ of calories from fat}$$

Certainly some foods are more nutritious than others, but barring allergies or other medical conditions, no foods are forbidden. With planning, patients can include nearly any food in a healthy diet without feeling denied.

ARTIFICIAL SWEETS AND FATS

Artificial or synthetic sweeteners have been surrounded by controversy. Originally created to aid diabetics and to enhance the quality of other medically supervised diets, sweeteners such as the popular saccharin have found a much broader market with weight-conscious consumers. However, there is no evidence that the national increase in use of artificial sweeteners has spurred any permanent weight loss.

To meet the demand for variety, applicability, and better taste, many new artificial sweeteners have been created in the laboratory and introduced over the past few years. They include cyclamate, acesulfame-K, and by far the most popular, aspartame. All have passed the scrutinizing eye of the U.S. Food and Drug Administration (FDA), but again, not without their share of problems (Table 26-5).

Artificial fats constitute the latest "light" market entry, responding to research that indicates a positive correlation between fat in the diet and some types of cancer and heart

Table 26-5. Guide to fake fats and artificial sugars

Brand name	Calories/serving	Disadvantages
Artificial sweetener		
Sweet 'N Low Sugar Twin (Saccharin)	4	Bitter aftertaste; has been found to cause cancer in lab rats[8]
Equal Nutrasweet (Aspartame)	4	Destroyed during cooking; must be avoided by phenylketonurics; may cause reactions in people with hypersensitivity[8]
Sunette Sweet One Swiss Sweet (Acesulfame-K)	0	Least similar taste to sugar; has been found to cause cancer in lab rats; claims of inadequate testing for FDA approval[8]
Cyclamate	0	Lacks FDA approval; has been linked to cancer in lab rats[8]
Artificial fats		
Simplesse (microparticulated milk and egg protein)	1-2/g	Cannot be used for cooking
Olestra (sucrose polyester)	0	Lacks FDA approval, still in development because of safety questions

disease. One false fat product, Simplesse, is available as an ingredient in several foods, giving these foods the qualities that fats would otherwise provide (Table 26-5).

New food items that combine these artificial sweets and fat for the ultimate in low-calorie consumption are also being produced. What consumers do not know is that many of the FDA safety approvals are based on the assumption that no one will consume more than the recommended amount. These safety limits are extraordinarily high, and the average person is extremely unlikely to exceed them. However, an extremely calorie-conscious person, who may consume multiple servings of many different artificially sweetened products every day, could exceed these amounts. Additionally, children may be the most prone to overconsumption of artificially sweetened foods and beverages, particularly during the summer when higher volumes of liquid and frozen products are consumed.

The current FDA maximum safe amount of aspartame is 50 mg per kg of body weight per day. For a 132-pound person, this amounts to 80 packets of Equal or 15 soft drinks sweetened with Nutrasweet. Exceeding this amount might be possible when puddings, yogurts, frozen desserts, chewing gum, cereals, and gelatins are consumed, along with beverages.

The FDA's recommended maximum of 50 mg per kg body weight is high when compared with other world health recommendations. The World Health Organization sets its limit at 40 mg per kg of body weight in adults, and the Canadian Diabetes Association sets its more conservative limit at three to four packets of Equal or its equivalent in food per day.

Potential problems in setting safety limits may be compounded by the combination of artificial fats and sweeten-ers as ingredients in one food product. Because of their recent introduction and consequent lack of data on actual reactions, it is very hard to predict the effect different amounts or combinations may have on the human body.

Therefore the prudent recommendation for patients is that children and pregnant and lactating women should avoid the use of products containing artificial sweeteners and fats. All other individuals should be educated regarding the risks and benefits of the products, so that they may make their choices wisely (see Table 26-5).

FIBER*

One of the hottest topics in the area of diet and disease is fiber. Research has associated the amount of fiber in the diet with the development of dozens of medical conditions.[6] Many of these conditions are most prevalent in Western societies, where fiber consumption is significantly lower than in developing nations. The therapeutic and protective effects of fiber are strongest in reducing the risk of hyperlipidemia and coronary heart disease, cancer (especially colorectal cancer), diabetes, diverticulosis, and gallstones.[3]

The fiber story is complex. There are two types of fiber, and their functions and influence on risk factors for disease vary.

Water-soluble fibers

Fiber is an indigestible fraction of food and is classified by its ability to dissolve in water. The water-soluble fi-

---

*Exerpted with permission from Kleiner SM: Fiber facts. How to fight disease with a high-fiber diet, *The Physician and Sports Medicine* 18(10):19, 1991.

bers—gums, pectins, mucilages, and some hemicelluloses—are recognized for their ability to lower cholesterol levels and improve glucose tolerance. These fibers generally bind bile acids in the intestines and inhibit the recycling of cholesterol, thus reducing the body's total cholesterol pool. Water-soluble fibers are also effective in reducing the rise in serum glucose after meals and reducing the serum insulin response in diabetics. Good food sources of water-soluble fibers include barley, rice, corn, oats, legumes, apples and pears (the fleshy portions), citrus fruits, bananas, carrots, prunes, cranberries, seeds, and seaweed.

Water-insoluble fibers

Lignins, cellulose, and some hemicelluloses are water-insoluble fibers. These fibers are associated with improved gastrointestinal regularity and prevention of colon cancer. As bulk formers, they increase stool volume and weight, thereby decreasing transit time through the intestines. By decreasing the time that food remains in the intestines, the body's exposure to carcinogens in food products or as byproducts of digestion is markedly reduced.

Good food sources of water-insoluble fibers include root and leafy vegetables, whole grains (such as wheat, barley, rice, corn, and oats), legumes, unpeeled apples and pears, and strawberries.

The Expert Panel on Dietary Fiber of the Federation of American Societies for Experimental Biology recommends 20 to 35 g of fiber per day from water-soluble and water-insoluble fibers.[14] Most Americans consume only about 11 g per day. One benefit of eating high-fiber foods is that they are generally also low in fat, high in carbohydrate, and high in many vitamins and minerals, factors that are believed to protect against many chronic diseases.

Eating foods high in fiber is preferable to using dietary supplements. One should increase fiber intake gradually, to help prevent symptoms such as cramping, distension, and flatulence.

There are indications that diets too high in fiber may have adverse effects. Some studies[6,3] suggest that a diet supplemented with fiber to increase fiber intake may decrease absorption of calcium, iron, zinc, and other minerals. Obtaining fiber from food, rather than supplements, makes it difficult to consume fiber in amounts that could be nutritionally detrimental.

Consumers must beware of "high-fiber" nutrition claims on foods. One should read the nutrition label. A food should contain at least 2.5 to 3.0 g of dietary fiber per serving to be considered a good source of fiber (Table 26-6).

CAFFEINE

Coffee and tea account for approximately 20% of the daily caffeine consumed by adults in the U.S. Other important sources are soft drinks (5% of total adult caffeine intake) and chocolate (1.5% of total adult caffeine intake).

Table 26-6. Common fiber-containing foods

Food	Portion	Dietary fiber content (g)
Kidney beans, cooked	¾ cup	9.3
Cereal, all bran	⅓ cup	8.5
Fig, dried	3 medium	7.2
Prunes, dried	3 medium	4.7
Pear	1 medium	4.1
Apple	1 large	4.0
Potato, baked w/skin	1 medium	4.0
Banana	1 medium	3.8
Blackberries	½ cup	3.3
Carrots, cooked	½ cup	3.2
Barley, cooked	½ cup	3.0
Apple	1 small	2.8
Broccoli, cooked	½ cup	2.8
Strawberries	1 cup	2.8
Bread, whole wheat	1 slice	2.4
Cereal, wheat flaked	¾ cup	1.8
Oatmeal, cooked	¾ cup	1.6
Apricot	3 medium	1.4
Peach	1 medium	1.3
Bread, white	1 slice	0.6

Adapted from manufacturer's data; from Anderson JW, Bridges SR: Dietary fiber content of selected foods, *Am J Clin Nutr* 47:440, 1988; and from Pennington J, Church H: *Bowes and Church's food values of portions commonly used*, ed 14, Philadelphia, 1985, JB Lippincott.

Among teenagers, children, and infants, tea and soft drinks provide the greatest sources of caffeine[3] (Table 26-7).

The caffeine in coffee is not the only questionable substance. Coffee also contains mutagens, carcinogens, and toxic substances, including methylglyoxal, chlorogenic acid, atractylosides, kahweal palmitate, and cafestol palmitate.

Relationship to cancer

Much of the research regarding associations between cancer and caffeine have focused on coffee and tea consumption, as well as caffeine alone. In an exhaustive review of the epidemiologic and animal literature, the National Research Council concluded that, in general, there is extremely inconsistent data relating the incidence of coffee consumption to various types of cancers. Many confounding factors, such as diet, smoking, types of control subjects, and selection factors, further complicate the data. In general, the NRC committee concluded that there is no convincing evidence of an association between tea consumption and any type of cancer, and that there is very inconsistent data relating coffee consumption to bladder, colon, pancreatic, and ovarian cancers.[3]

Relationship to coronary heart disease

A positive relationship between coffee intake and elevated plasma total cholesterol was first identified by the

Table 26-7. Caffeine content of beverages, foods, and OTC drugs (mg)

Beverages

Carbonated beverages*

cherry coke, Coca-Cola—*12 fl oz (370 g)*	46
cherry cola, Slice—*12 fl oz (360 g)*	48
cherry RC—*12 fl oz (360 g)*	36
Coca-Cola—*12 fl oz (370 g)*	46
Coca-Cola Classic—*12 fl oz (369 g)*	46
cola—*12 fl oz (370 g)*	37
cola, RC—*12 fl oz (360 g)*	36
Mello Yello—*12 fl oz (372 g)*	52
Mr. Pibb—*12 fl oz (369 g)*	40
Mountain Dew—*12 fl oz (360 g)*	54
pepper type soda—*12 fl oz (368 g)*	37
Pepsi Cola—*12 fl oz (360 g)*	38

Carbonated beverages, low calorie*

diet cherry coke, Coca-Cola—*12 fl oz (354 g)*	46
diet cherry cola Slice—*12 fl oz (360 g)*	48
diet coke, Coca-Cola—*12 fl oz (354 g)*	46
diet cola, aspartame sweetened—*12 fl oz (355 g)*	50
diet Pepsi—*12 fl oz (360 g)*	36
diet RC—*12 fl oz (360 g)*	48
Pepsi Light—*12 fl oz (360 g)*	36
Tab—*12 fl oz (354 g)*	46

Coffee

brewed—*5 oz*	
Drip method	110-150
Percolator	64-124
instant	40-108
decaffeinated, brewed or instant	1-5
prep from inst powder—*6 fl oz water and 1 rd t powder*	
amaretto, General Foods—*6 fl oz water and 11.5 g powder (189 g)*	60
amaretto, sugar-free, General Foods—*6 fl oz water and 7.7 g powder (185 g)*	60
decaffeinated—*6 fl oz water and 1 rd t powder (179 g)*	2
francais, General Foods—*6 fl oz water and 11.5 g powder (189 g)*	53
francais, sugar-free, General Foods—*6 fl oz water and 7.7 g powder (185 g)*	59
irish creme, General Foods—*6 fl oz water and 12.8 g powder (190 g)*	53
irish creme, sugar-free, General Foods—*6 fl oz water and 7.1 g powder (185 g)*	48
irish mocha mint, General Foods—*6 fl oz water and 11.5 g powder (189 g)*	27
irish mocha mint, sugar-free, General Foods—*6 fl oz water and 6.4 g powder (184 g)*	25
orange cappuccino, General Foods—*6 fl oz water and 14 g powder (191 g)*	73
orange cappuccino, sugar-free, General Foods—*6 fl oz water and 6.7 g powder (184 g)*	71

Coffee—con't

suisse mocha, General Foods—*6 fl oz water and 11.5 g powder (189 g)*	41
suisse mocha, sugar-free, General Foods—*6 fl oz water and 6.4 g powder (184 g)*	40
vienna, General Foods—*6 fl oz water and 14 g powder (191 g)*	56
vienna, sugar-free, General Foods—*6 fl oz water and 6.7 g powder (184 g)*	55
w/chicory—*6 fl oz water and 1 rd t powder (179 g)*	38

Tea, hot/iced

brewed	
5 oz cup, major U.S. brands	20-90
5 oz cup, imported brands	25-110
instant powder—*1 t (0.7 g)*	31
with lemon flavor—*1 rd t (1.4 g)*	25
with sugar and lemon flavor—*3 rd t (23 g)*	29
with sodium saccharin and lemon flavor—*2 t (1.6 g)*	36
prep from inst powder	
1 t powder in 8 fl oz water (237 g)	31
Crystal Light—*8 fl oz (238 g)*	11
with lemon flavor—*1 rd t powder in 8 fl oz water (238 g)*	26
with sugar and lemon flavor—*3 rd t powder in 8 fl oz water (259 g)*	29
with sodium saccharin and lemon flavor—*2 t powder in 8 fl oz water (238 g)*	36

Candy and chocolate

baking choc, unsweetened, Bakers—*1 oz (28 g)*	25
chocolate	
german sweet, Bakers—*1 oz square (28 g)*	8
semi-sweet, Bakers—*1 oz square (28 g)*	13
choc chips	
Bakers—*¼ cup (43 g)*	12
german sweet, Bakers—*¼ cup (43 g)*	15
semi-sweet, Bakers—*¼ cup (43 g)*	14
milk choc, Cadbury—*1 oz (28 g)*	15

Frozen desserts

pudding pops, Jell-O	
choc—*1 pop (47 g)*	2
choc caramel swirl—*1 pop (47 g)*	1
choc fudge—*1 pop (47 g)*	3
choc van swirl—*1 pop (47 g)*	1
choc with choc chips—*1 pop (48 g)*	3
choc with choc coating—*1 pop (49 g)*	3
double choc swirl—*1 pop (47 g)*	2
milk choc—*1 pop (47 g)*	2
van with choc chips—*1 pop (48 g)*	1
van with choc coating—*1 pop (49 g)*	1

Data from: Whitney EN, Hamilton EMN, Rolfes SR: *Understanding nutrition,* ed 5, St Paul, Minn, 1990, West Publishing. and from Pennington JA: *Bowes and Church's food values of portions commonly used,* ed 15, Philadelphia, 1989, JB Lippincott.

*Caffeine-free carbonated beverages and most non-cola carbonated beverages contain no caffeine.

†Because products change, contact the manufacturer for updates.

Continued.

Table 26-7. Caffeine content of beverages, foods, and OTC drugs (mg)—cont'd

Pies		**Special dietary formulas, commercial and hospital**	
choc mousse, from mix, Jell-O—1/6 pie (95 g)	6	Ensure, choc, Ross Labs—8 fl oz (253 g)	8
Puddings, from instant mix		Ensure, coffee, Ross Labs—8 fl oz (253 g)	8
choc		Ensure HN, choc, Ross Labs—8 fl oz (253 g)	8
Jell-O—1/2 cup (150 g)	5	Ensure plus, choc, Ross Labs—8 fl oz (259 g)	10
sugar-free, D-Zerta—1/2 cup (130 g)	4	Ensure, plus, coffee, Ross Labs—8 fl oz (259 g)	12
sugar-free, Jell-O—1/2 cup (133 g)	4		
choc fudge		**Drugs†**	
Jell-O—1/2 cup (150 g)	8	cold remedies (standard dose)	
sugar-free, Jell-O—1/2 cup (135 g)	9	Dristan	0
choc fudge mousse, Jell-O—1/2 cup (86 g)	12	Coryban-D, Triaminicin	30
choc mousse, Jell-O—1/2 cup (86 g)	9	diuretics (standard dose)	
choc tapioca, Jell-O—1/2 cup (147 g)	8	Aqua-ban, Permathene H2Off	200
milk choc, Jell-O—1/2 cup (150 g)	5	Pre-Mens Forte	100
		pain relievers (standard dose)	
Milk beverages		Excedrin	130
choc flavor mix in whole milk—2-3 hp t powder in 8 fl oz milk (266 g)	8	Midol, Anacin	65
		Aspirin, plain (any brand)	0
choc malted milk flavor powder		stimulants	
in whole milk—3 hp t powder in 8 fl oz milk (265 g)	8	Caffedrin, NoDoz, Vivarin	200
with added nutrients in whole milk—4-5 hp t powder in 8 fl oz milk (265 g)	5	weight-control aids (daily dose)	
		Prolamine	280
choc syrup in whole milk—2 T syrup in 8 fl oz milk (282 g)	6	Dexatrim, Dietac	200
cocoa/hot chocolate, prep with water from mix—3/4 hp t powder in 6 fl oz water (206 g)	4		
Milk beverage mixes			
choc flavor mix, powder—2-3 hp t (22 g)	8		
choc malted milk flavor mix, powder—3/4 oz (3 hp t) (21 g)	8		
choc malted milk flavor mix with added nutrients, powder—3/4 oz (4-5 hp t) (21 g)	6		
choc syrup—2 T (1 fl oz) (38 g)	5		
cocoa mix powder—1 oz pkt (3-4 hp t) (28 g)	5		

Tromso Heart Study in 1983.[17] Since then, numerous epidemiologic studies have produced equivocal results.

As with the cancer research, confounding factors make comparing these studies very difficult. The well-known factors that might influence the incidence of coronary heart disease are:

- Diet
- Age
- Sex
- Body mass index
- Exercise
- Cigarette smoking
- Alcohol consumption
- Estrogen use
- Ethnicity
- Occupation
- Stress
- Drugs
- Baseline plasma total cholesterol level

In addition, the coffee-cholesterol relationship has been further confounded by the type of coffee used (origin of coffee beans), the method of preparation (instant, filtered, boiled, percolated), and the water. Research results have indicated that decaffeinated coffee may also be associated with a cholesterol-raising effect,[16] although dietary inconsistencies may account for this result.

In a 1990 review of the literature, Kris-Etherton reported that although a consensus appears to be emerging that coffee consumption can elevate plasma lipids, the evidence has so many inconsistencies that it would be premature to implicate coffee consumption as a coronary risk factor. "Practitioners are advised to assess the coffee consumption of their patients and to intervene when indicated. Coffee consumption may be of clinical importance for hypercholesterolemic patients."[9]

Even though the studies have had limitations, most cross-sectional studies have found a positive association between filtered and boiled coffee consumption and serum total cholesterol and low-density lipoprotein cholesterol (LDL-C) levels. Boiled coffee has consistently increased serum total cholesterol and LDL-C levels, but filtered coffee has not.[5]

A randomized controlled trial with an 8-week washout period followed by an 8-week intervention period was conducted on 100 healthy male volunteers. Subjects were assigned to one of four groups: 720 ml/day (3 cups) of caffeinated coffee, 360 ml/day (1.5 cups) of caffeinated coffee, 720 ml/day of decaffeinated coffee, or no coffee. Diet and activity were monitored and controlled statistically, and compliance was checked by urinary caffeine metabolites. Changes in plasma lipoprotein cholesterol concentrations were measured before and after washout and intervention.[5]

After the intervention period, men who consumed 720 ml of caffeinated coffee daily had mean increases in plasma levels of total cholesterol (0.25 mmol/L, p = .02), LDL-C (0.15 mmol/L, p = .17), and HDL-C (0.09 mmol/L, p = .12), after controlling for dietary changes, compared with the group that did not drink coffee.

This was a very well-designed study that demonstrated for the first time the effect of filtered, caffeinated coffee consumption on plasma total and LDL-C levels. The authors comment that the mechanism underlying the relationship between coffee drinking and plasma cholesterol levels is unknown. They speculate that the active substance is not caffeine, but some other substance that is removed partially by filter paper during the drip brewing process, or wholly by the decaffeinating process.

The amounts of coffee consumed by the subjects in this study are common to the diets of Americans. The authors concluded that the small changes in LDL-C and HDL-C observed in this study should not affect coronary heart disease risk.

Reproductive effects

Caffeine, given at high doses, clearly causes reproductive defects in rodents.[3] However, the evidence in humans is contradictory and inconclusive.

Several studies, after controlling for confounding factors such as maternal age, parity, father's occupation, maternal weight, and smoking, have related high coffee consumption with increased risks of low birth-weight infants.[7,11] Other studies have reported no such association.[2,10]

Because of the clear results of the animal data, and the slight, although equivocal human data, the prudent recommendation for patients who are planning for pregnancy or are pregnant is to limit caffeine and coffee consumption to a minimum, and avoid it if possible.

Caffeine as a drug

Caffeine, a stimulant, is one of the only drugs added to foods. The effects of caffeine differ for each individual depending on the amount of caffeine consumed, the length of

time for consumption, and the level of tolerance developed by the individual. A tolerance to caffeine is developed quickly.

Moderate consumption of caffeine (the equivalent of two cups of coffee per day) by healthy, nonpregnant adults appears to be relatively harmless. In larger amounts, caffeine can cause symptoms similar to anxiety. Complaints of dizziness, agitation, restlessness, recurring headaches, intestinal discomfort, and sleep difficulties have been reported by consumers of 8 to 15 cups of coffee per day.

Caffeine is addictive, and sudden abstinence causes a characteristic withdrawal headache. A common example of this is the office worker who consumes caffeinated coffee on the job but on the weekend and at home drinks little or no coffee. Headache and irritability may occur at midday on Saturday from lack of caffeine. In this situation or others where caffeine has been consumed long-term, even if use has been moderate, one should slowly cut back on consumption until intake is eliminated or significantly reduced to avoid the discomfort of withdrawal.

REFERENCES

1. Anderson JW, Bridges SR: Dietary fiber content of selected foods, *Am J Clin Nutr* 47:440, 1988; and Pennington J, Church H: *Bowes and Church's food values of portions commonly used*, ed 14, Philadelphia, 1985, JB Lippincott.
2. Berkowitz GS, Holford TR, and Berkowitz RL: Effects of cigarette smoking, alcohol, coffee, and tea consumption on preterm delivery, *Early Hum Dev* 7:239-250, 1982.
3. Committee on Diet and Health, Food and Nutrition Board, Commission on Life Sciences, National Research Council: *Diet and health: implications for reducing chronic disease risk*, Washington, DC, 1989, National Academy Press.
4. *Dietary Guidelines for Americans*, ed 3, Washington, DC, 1990, US Department of Agriculture, U.S. Department of Health and Human Services.
5. Fried RE et al: The effect of filtered-coffee consumption on plasma lipid levels, *JAMA* 267:811-815, 1992.
6. Gorman MA, Bowman C: Position of the American Dietetic Association: health implications of dietary fiber, *J Am Dietet Assoc* 88:216-221, 1988.
7. Hogue CJ: Coffee in pregnancy, *Lancet* 1:554, 1981.
8. Jacobson MF, Lefferts LY, and Garland AW: *Safe food: eating wisely in a risky world*, Venice, Calif, 1991, Living Planet Press.
9. Kris-Etherton PM, editor: *Cardiovascular disease: nutrition for prevention and treatment*, Chicago, 1990, American Dietetic Association.
10. Linn S et al: No association between coffee consumption and adverse outcomes of pregnancy, *N Engl J Med* 306:141-145, 1982.
11. Mau G, Netter P: Are coffee and alcohol consumption risk factors in pregnancy? *Geburtshilfe Frauenheilkd* 34:1018-1022, 1974.
12. Miller RW: *Critiquing quack ads*, Washington, DC, 1985, Federal Drug Administration, US Department of Health and Human Services No (FDA) 8885-4196, Government Printing Office.
13. Monaco GP: The primary care physician: the first line of defense in the battle against health fraud, *Med Times* 114(5):43-48, 1986.
14. Pilch SM, editor: *Physiological effects and health consequences of dietary fiber*, Bethesda, Md, 1987, Federation of American Societies for Experimental Biology.
15. U.S. Department of Agriculture, U.S. Department of Health and Human Services: Preparing foods and planning menus using the dietary guidelines, HG-232-8, 1989.

16. Superko HR et al: Lipoprotein and apolipoprotein changes during a controlled trial of caffeinated and decaffeinated coffee drinking in men, (abstract) *Circulation* 80:II-86, 1989.

17. Thelle DS, Arnesen E, and Forde OH: The Tromso heart study: does coffee raise serum cholesterol? *N Engl J Med* 308:1454, 1983.

18. Whitney EN, Hamilton EMN, Rolfes SR: *Understanding nutrition*, ed 5, St. Paul, Minn, 1990, West Publishing.

━━━━━━━━━━━━━━━━ **RESOURCES** ━━━━━━━━━━━━━━━━

Hotlines

American Institute for Cancer Research, Nutrition Hotline, (800) 843-8114.

National Cancer Institute, Cancer Information Service Hotline, (800) 4-CANCER.

National Center for Nutrition and Dietetics, toll-free consumer nutrition hotline, (800) 366-1655.

Government agencies

Environmental Protection Agency, 401 M St., SW, Washington, DC 20460.

Federal Trade Commission, Pennsylvania Ave. and 6th St., NW, Washington, DC 20580.

Food and Drug Administration, Department of Health and Human Services, 5600 Fishers Lane, Rockville, MD 20857.

U.S. Department of Agriculture, Fourth St. and Independence Ave., SW, Washington, DC 20250.

Other organizations

American Council on Science and Health, 1995 Broadway, 18th floor, New York, NY 10023.

American Dietetic Association, 216 W. Jackson Blvd., Chicago, IL 60606.

National Council Against Health Fraud, P.O. Box 1276, Loma Linda, CA 92354 (this organization has many local chapters).

Part VI

SPECIFIC APPROACHES TO DIFFERENT PATIENT GROUPS

Chapter 27

THE CHILD

Ruth Imrie
Richard Garcia
Douglas Moodie

The child is father of the man in his disease history as well as in other important respects. . . . Prevention in the eyes of the true physician is daily occupying a more and more important field, and surely in no sphere can more important results be obtained, than in checking the developing tendencies of child life (Black-lader, 1893).[13]

We can no longer divide life into segments such as fetal, neonatal, childhood, adolescence, adulthood and senescence. Rather, life is a dynamic continuum with the status at any one point in time being influenced by all that went before, and in turn, having an effect upon all that follows (Robbins, 1962).[55]

Prevention is the essence of the practice of those who provide health care for children. Members of the health care team, especially geneticists and obstetricians, have an opportunity to influence the well-being of the child even before the child exists. Preconceptional counseling allows health care choices to be made when the "influences that went before" are as unencumbered as they ever will be. The concern is to promote all aspects of the health of fetus, child, and adolescent in the most meaningful way as each new milestone of development is approached and attained. The hope is that each child will have the opportunity to develop to his or her full potential.

Great advances in the prevention of childhood diseases have been made since the turn of the century.[24] The infant mortality rate has dropped from 162/1000 to 9.1/1000 live births.[68] Fewer than 1 in 500 children die during childhood. In bygone years (and in some underdeveloped parts of the world at the present time) as many as half of all live born children died before the age of 5 years.[30] Infectious diseases, which used to be the leading cause of death, have been combated by a variety of measures including immunization programs. Now the leading cause of death in childhood is injuries; motor vehicle crashes account for the major proportion of mortality and morbidity. The last decade has seen a reduction in this area, and it is hoped that ongoing strategies will continue this encouraging trend (see Chapter 64).

The accompanying figures show the leading causes of death from infancy to adulthood (see Figs. 27-1 through 27-4).[69]

Since infectious diseases and other serious illnesses are less threatening to the health of children than in the past, attention can be focused on a newly emphasized group of childhood difficulties. R. J. Haggerty has identified behavioral, educational, and family-social problems as the "new morbidity" (1975).[33] Associated with the "new morbidity" are problems arising from changing patterns of life in this era, such as social and geographic mobility, divorce, overcrowding, and issues of employment, including an increasing number of mothers who work outside the home. The "new morbidity" has forced caregivers to respond by seeking "new prevention." In recent years the AAP manual *Guidelines for Health Supervision* has focused increasingly on areas of the well-child visit relating to the psychosocial status of the child, family, and environment and on developmental/behavioral assessment.[31] More time at each health supervision visit needs to be allotted for developmentally oriented anticipatory guidance, parent education, and counseling, so that issues related to both the "old" and the "new" morbidity can be addressed.

The vulnerable young child must rely on adults for nurturing and protection. Parents and health care providers need to collaborate as a team for the benefit of the child. As time passes, the child can be given the opportunity to be involved in his own health care decisions, often from the age of 4 or 5 years. In adolescence the young person will make his or her own decisions whether parents agree

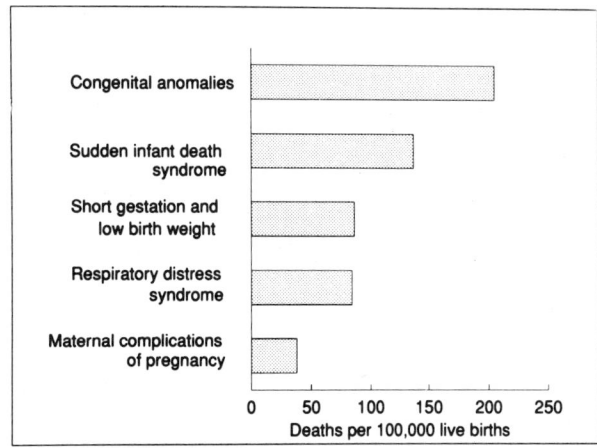

Fig. 27-1. Leading causes of infant mortality (1987). (From National Center for Health Statistics [CDC]: Health, U.S., 1989, and prevention profile. *Healthy people 2000*, DHHS Pub No [PHS] 50212, Dept of Health and Human Services.)

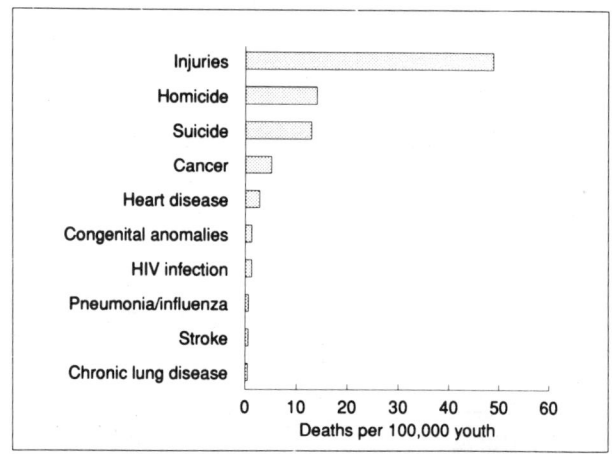

Fig. 27-3. Leading causes of death for youth age 15 through 24 (1987). (From *Monthly vital statistics report*, Supplement, Sept. 26, 1989. In *Healthy people 2000*, DHHS Pub No [PHS] 50212, Dept of Health and Human Services.)

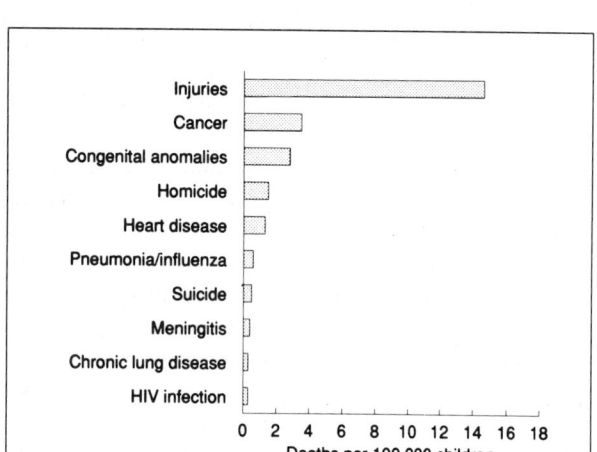
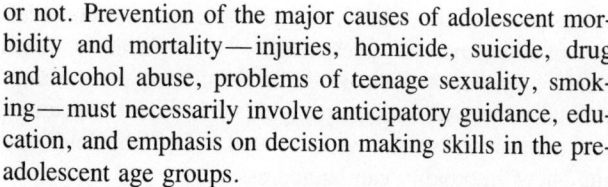

Fig. 27-2. Leading causes of death for children age 1 through 14. (From National center for health statistics [CDC]: *Healthy people 2000*, DHHS Pub No [PHS] 50212, Dept of Health and Human Services.)

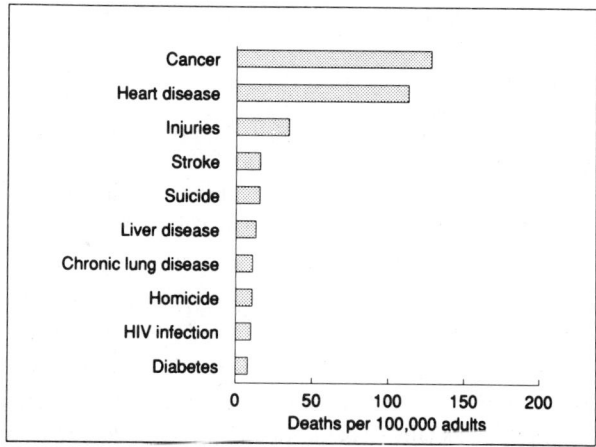

Fig. 27-4. Leading causes of death of adults age 25 through 64 (1987). (From National Center for Health statistics [CDC]: *Healthy people 2000*, DHHS Pub No [PHS] 50212, Dept of Health and Human Services.)

or not. Prevention of the major causes of adolescent morbidity and mortality—injuries, homicide, suicide, drug and alcohol abuse, problems of teenage sexuality, smoking—must necessarily involve anticipatory guidance, education, and emphasis on decision making skills in the preadolescent age groups.

Many adult conditions have their origins in childhood. Heart disease, cancer, stroke, and accidents cause 70% of deaths in American adults. Conditions with high morbidity include heart disease, obesity, hypertension, sexually transmitted diseases, mental and nervous disorders, and the results of violence. "Prospective" pediatrics (pediatric care that looks to the future) encourages the adoption of

healthy life-styles in preparation for adult life. "The goal of pediatrics is to keep an individual healthy during his adult life as well as during childhood."[30]

PREVENTIVE MEDICINE BEFORE BIRTH
Preconceptional counseling

In a society like that of the United States opportunities for preventive medicine exist even before conception.[26] Preconceptional counseling includes the following:

- Genetic counseling given after review of a careful family history of both prospective parents and any already existing children with special emphasis on genetically inherited diseases

- Testing for a disease carrier state or other risk factors, for example, Tay-Sachs disease and hemoglobinopathy screening, blood and Rh type determinations, serologic testing, rubella antibody titer determination, and testing for human immunodeficiency virus (HIV) infection if indicated
- Problems that can and should be resolved before pregnancy, for example, anemia or obesity
- Problems that are ongoing but may require extra care before or during pregnancy, for example, hypertension and diabetes
- A review of any complications that occurred in previous pregnancies, including congenital anomalies
- Anticipatory guidance about the possible effects of smoking, drugs, and alcohol on a developing fetus
- Emphasis on obtaining good early prenatal care once pregnancy has occurred

Prenatal and perinatal care

The value of good prenatal care in reducing the rates of infant death and low birth weight and their associated morbidity cannot be overemphasized. Maternal health and fetal growth are monitored at serial visits to the obstetrician and ongoing counseling and patient education offered. Maternal smoking, heavy alcohol consumption, drug use, and poor nutrition are all known to be associated with adverse effects on the fetus. Mothers less than 17 years are at particular risk of having low birth weight babies; mothers older than 35 years have an increased birth rate of babies with chromosomal abnormalities such as Down syndrome. Babies born to mothers of lower socioeconomic status are more likely to have higher mortality and morbidity rates.

Prenatal cytogenetic studies to detect genetic disorders, using techniques such as amniocentesis (at the sixteenth week of gestation) and chorionic villus sampling (at 9 to 12 weeks' gestation), may be offered in selected situations (see Chapter 38 on Genetics). Maternal serum α-fetoprotein (AFP) levels can be tested at 16 to 18 weeks' gestation to help identify open neural tube defects in the fetus. These anomalies are associated with high AFP levels. Low maternal serum AFP levels may be associated with fetal chromosomal abnormalities, particularly Down syndrome. When the serum AFP level is found to be abnormal, ultrasonography and amniocentesis (for amniotic AFP or cytogenetic abnormality) are performed.[26]

Ultrasonography can be used prenatally to diagnose hydrocephalus, neural tube defects, and renal, skeletal, and cardiac abnormalities. Pediatric subspecialists can be alerted so that appropriate interventions can be instituted in a timely fashion after the baby is born, perhaps preventing further complications of the condition. Alternatively, the ultrasound findings may furnish additional information required to make a decision regarding induced termination of pregnancy.

Skilled care during labor, delivery, and the postpartum period, best provided in the hospital setting, is vital to the reduction of perinatal and maternal morbidity and mortality. In recent years the infant mortality rate has declined from 29.2/1000 live births in 1950 to 9.1/1000 in 1990—a record low.[71] However, this is still higher than in many other developed countries and the mortality for black infants remains much higher than for whites.

As can be seen from Figure 27-1, four causes account for more than one half of all infant deaths: congenital anomalies, sudden infant death syndrome (SIDS), prematurity and low birth weight, and respiratory distress syndrome.[69] Infants who survive these conditions have an increased risk of permanent disabilities. Seventy-five percent of deaths in the first month and 60% of all infant deaths occur among low birth weight (less than 2500 g) infants. These infants, especially the very low birth weight infants (less than 1500 g), are also at risk for permanent developmental disabilities such as cerebral palsy and mental retardation. The incidence of prematurity and low birth weight is associated with poor prenatal care; maternal smoking, alcohol and drug use; and pregnancy before 18 years of age, all of which are preventable. Respiratory distress syndrome is usually a complication of prematurity.

Genetic factors cause about 25% of congenital anomalies. Therefore increased focus on genetic counseling, especially before conception, is an important preventive measure. Preconceptional counseling and AFP testing can be offered to families with a history of neural tube defects. Heavy maternal alcohol use may lead to the fetal alcohol syndrome (FAS), in which the infant shows typical features and long-term behavioral effects.

The causes of SIDS are unknown. The incidence is higher in males, premature babies, nonwhites, individuals in lower socioeconomic classes, and siblings of SIDS victims and in the winter season.

At the present an increasing number of babies are being affected by two other preventable diseases—HIV infection and cocaine addiction—with distressing implications for the future.

NEONATAL SCREENING

Early detection of inborn errors of metabolism such as phenylketonuria (PKU), galactosemia, and homocystinuria can be accomplished by neonatal screening so that treatment, dietary in type, can be instituted quickly, thus preventing mental retardation and other serious complications. Likewise neonatal screening for congenital hypothyroidism allows rapid initiation of therapy with L-thyroxine when indicated, preventing the onset of serious developmental and growth delays. Screening for a variety of hemoglobinopathies can also be a part of a newborn screen allowing for early planning for appropriate treatment strategies as needed.

The incidence of congenital hypothyroidism is 1 in 4000, PKU 1 in 15,000, galactosemia 1 in 50,000 and ho-

RECOMMENDATIONS FOR PREVENTIVE PEDIATRIC HEALTH CARE
Committee on Practice and Ambulatory Medicine

Each child and family is unique; therefore, these **Recommendations for Preventive Pediatric Health Care** are designed for the care of children who are receiving competent parenting, have no manifestations of any important health problems, and are growing and developing in satisfactory fashion. **Additional visits may become necessary** if circumstances suggest variations from normal. These guidelines represent a consensus by the Committtee on Practice and Ambulatory Medicine in consultation with the membership of the American Academy of Pediatrics through the Chapter Presidents. The Committee emphasizes the great importance of **continuity of care** in comprehensive health supervision and the need to avoid **fragmentation of care.**

A **prenatal visit** by first-time parents and/or those who are at high risk is recommended and should include anticipatory guidance and pertinent medical history.

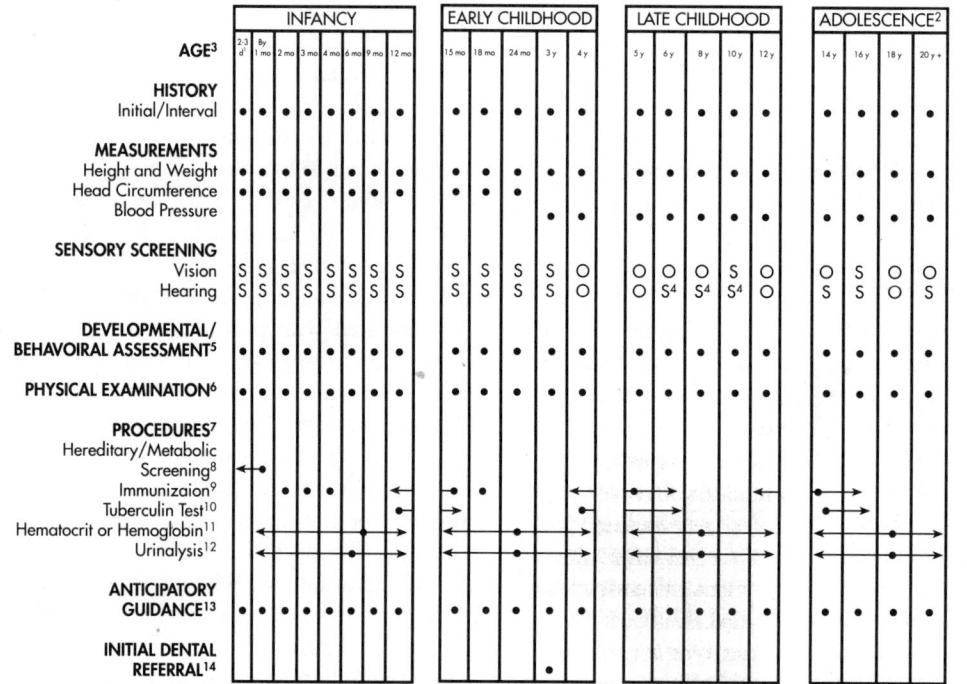

1. For newborns discharged in 24 hours or less after delivery.
2. Adolescent-related issues (eg, psychosocial, emotional, substance usage, and reproductive health) may necessitate more frequent health supervision.
3. If a child comes under care for the first time at any point on the schedule, or if any items are not accomplished at the suggested age, the schedule should be brought up to date at the earliest possible time.
4. At these points, history may suffice: if problem suggested, a standard testing method should be employed.
5. By history and appropriate physical examination: if suspicious, by specific objective developmental testing.
6. At each visit, a complete physical examination is essential, with infant totally unclothed, older child undressed and suitably draped.
7. These may be modified, depending upon entry point into schedule and individual need.
8. Metabolic screening (eg, thyroid, PKU, galactosemia) should be done according to state law.
9. Schedule(s) per *Report of the Committee on Infectious Diseases,* 1991 Red Book, and current AAP Committee statements.

10. For high-risk groups, the Committee on Infectious Diseases recommends annual TB skin testing.
11. Present medical evidence suggests the need for reevaluation of the frequency and timing of hemoglobin or hematocrit tests. One determination is therefore suggested during each time period. Performance of additional tests is left to the individual practice experience.
12. Present medical evidence suggests the need for reevaluation of the frequency and timing of urinalyses. One determination is therefore suggested during each time period. Performance of additional tests is left to the individual practice experience.
13. Appropriate discussion and counseling should be an integral part of each visist for care.
14. Subsequent examinations as prescribed by dentist.

NB: **Special chemical, immunologic, and endocrine testing** is usually carried out upon specific indications. Testing other than newborn (eg, inborn errors of metabolism, sickle disease, lead) is discretionary with the physician.

Key: ● = to be performed   S = subjective, by history   O = objective, by a standard testing method

The recommendations in this publication do not indicate an exclusive course of treatment or serve as a standard of medical care. Variations, taking into account individual circumstances, may be appropriate.

American Academy
of Pediatrics

Fig. 27-5. Recommendations for preventive pediatric health care. (From Committee on Practice and Ambulatory Medicine; *Recommenaations for preventive pediatric health care* July 1991, RE 9224, American Academy of Pediatrics.)

mocystinuria 1 in 200,000. Screening for PKU and congenital hypothyroidism is mandatory in all states.[25] Screening is performed by testing heel-prick blood specimens before the infant is discharged from the nursery and as close as possible to the time of discharge. If PKU testing is done within the first 24 hours of life, the test may yield an inaccurate result and should be repeated later, but before the third week of life. If an infant is sick or premature a blood specimen should be obtained at about 7 days of age.[26]

OFFICE VISITS FOR PREVENTIVE PEDIATRIC HEALTH CARE—CHILD-HEALTH SUPERVISION

It is estimated that pediatricians spend about 40% of their office time on child-health supervision—"well-child care."[20] Since 1967 the Academy of Pediatrics has published standards for periodic health supervision visits. These have been revised frequently. The most recent guidelines are reproduced in Figure 27-5. Twenty-two visits are suggested, beginning prenatally and extending through adolescence.

The chief objectives of these well-child visits are the following:

- To provide the opportunity for a relationship to form between the physician and/or nurse with the child and family so that care may be optimized
- To detect asymptomatic disease by examining the child and by performing screening tests such as those of vision, hearing, lead level, tuberculin, and phenylketonuria (PKU)
- To provide specific preventive measures such as immunizations and developmentally oriented anticipatory guidance[30]

Height and weight (and head circumference up to 2 years) of the child are measured at each visit and plotted on a growth chart (see Figs. 27-6 and 27-7). Isolated measurements are less helpful than repeated ones, which allow the pattern of the child's growth to be monitored. Several studies have shown that repeated frequent physical examinations are unlikely to reveal unexpected findings once an initial complete evaluation has been made.[27] Recommendations regarding physical examination at each visit may change in the future in order to allow more time for education.[20]

Blood pressure is measured at each visit from the age of 3 years. Blood pressure tables in Tables 27-1 and 27-2 and Figure 27-8 show the range of normal blood pressures at different ages for each gender. Information on the definition of hypertension is also included.[14]

Vision and hearing are assessed at each visit and formally tested at any age if an abnormality is suspected. Vision and hearing screening tests are performed in the office at 4 and 5 years and periodically thereafter. The AAP School Health Committee recommends that vision be

Table 27-1. Definition of hypertension in children

Normal blood pressure	Systolic and diastolic blood pressure <90th percentile for age and sex.
High normal blood pressure	Average systolic or average diastolic blood pressure between 90th and 95th percentiles for age and sex.
Hypertension	Average systolic or average diastolic blood pressure ≥95th percentile for age and sex with measurement on at least three occasions.

Table 27-2. Criteria for classification of hypertension by age group

Age	Hypertension
1-7 days	Systolic ≥ 96
8-30 days	Systolic ≥ 104
<2 years	Systolic ≥ 112
	Diastolic ≥ 74
3-5 years	Systolic ≥ 116
	Diastolic ≥ 76
6-9 years	Systolic ≥ 122
	Diastolic ≥ 78
10-12 years	Systolic ≥ 126
	Diastolic ≥ 82
13-15 years	Systolic ≥ 136
	Diastolic ≥ 86
16-18 years	Systolic ≥ 142
	Diastolic ≥ 92

screened annually, and hearing screening be performed in kindergarten and grades 1, 3, 6, 9, and 12 by school personnel.[47] Hearing and visual problems and asthma are the only physical conditions present in more than 1 in every 100 children.[30]

Tuberculin testing is routinely performed for low-risk populations in infancy, at school entry, and in adolescence.[50] Annual skin testing is recommended for high-risk groups (see the section, Tuberculosis Screening).

Immunizations are an important preventive feature of health supervision visits and are given according to the schedule in the section, Immunization.

Developmental and behavioral problems (the "new morbidity") are present in as many as one in five children.[30] Such problems may be diagnosed by parental interview and/or observation of the child during the health supervision visit.

Anticipatory guidance is given to encourage health promotion and disease prevention.[52] Imminent developmental milestones are discussed with emphasis on accompanying changes in behavior, parenting skills, and safety promo-

Text continued on p. 505.

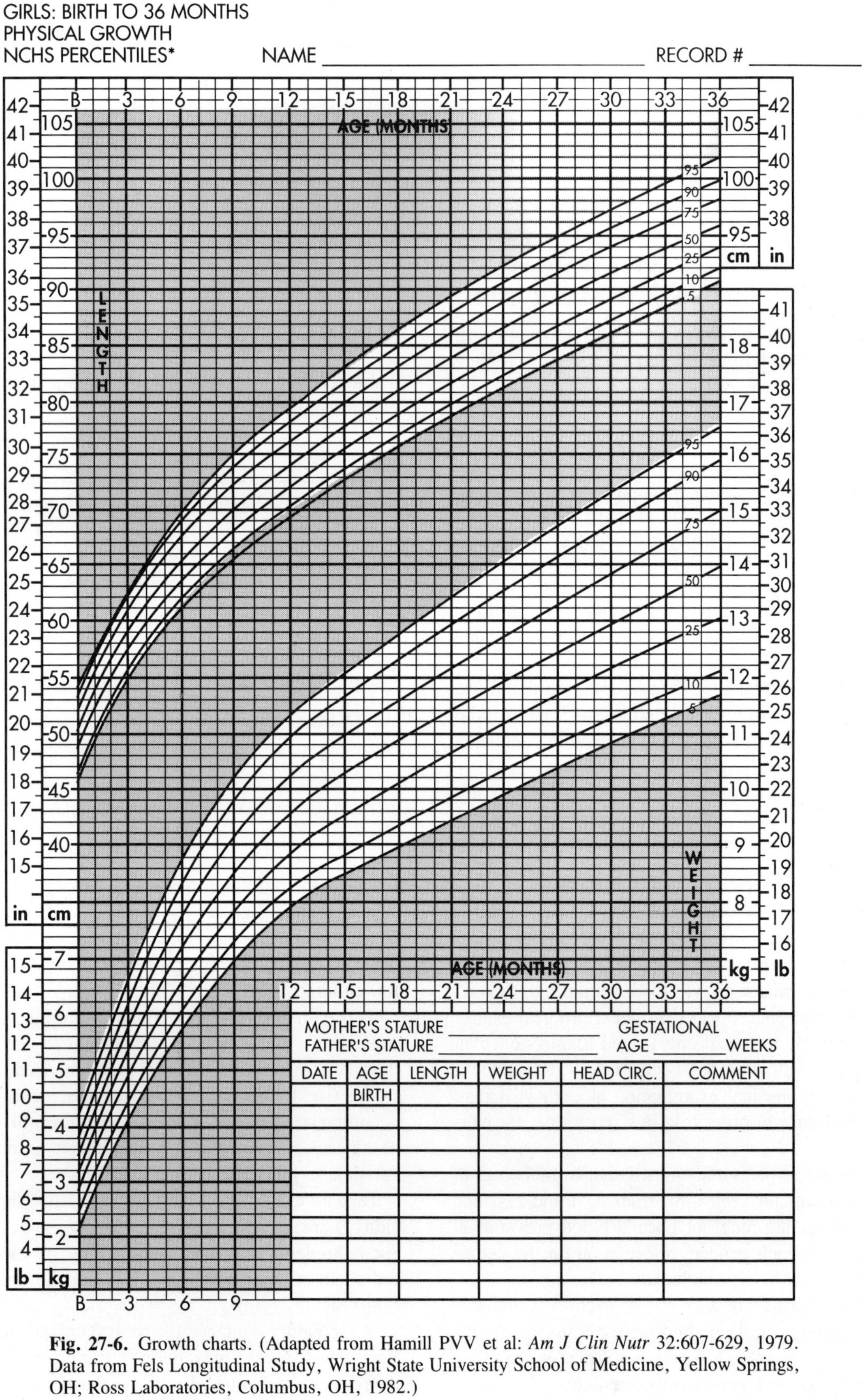

Fig. 27-6. Growth charts. (Adapted from Hamill PVV et al: *Am J Clin Nutr* 32:607-629, 1979. Data from Fels Longitudinal Study, Wright State University School of Medicine, Yellow Springs, OH; Ross Laboratories, Columbus, OH, 1982.)

GIRLS: BIRTH TO 36 MONTHS
PHYSICAL GROWTH
NCHS PERCENTILES*   NAME _____   RECORD # _____

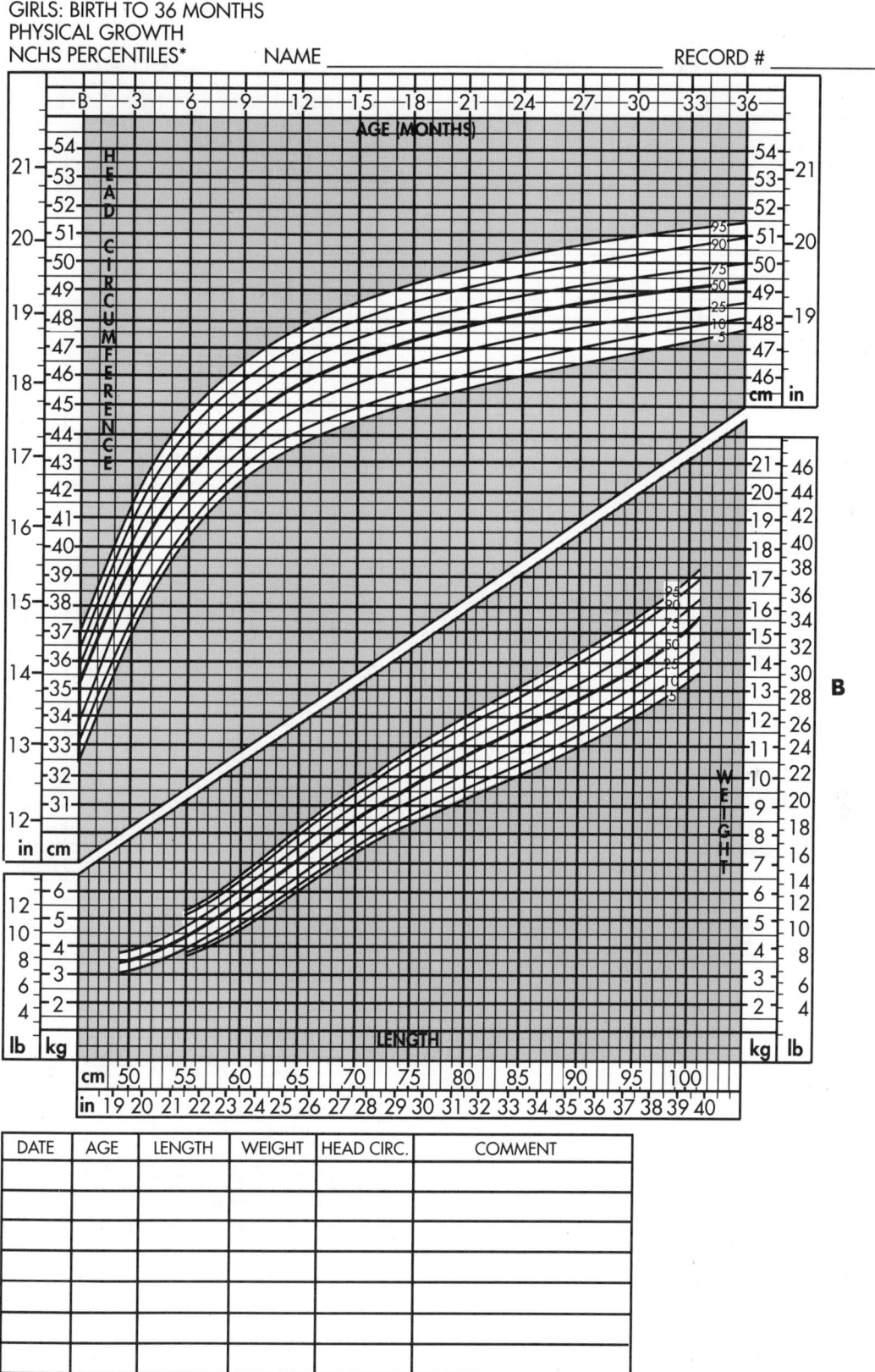

Fig. 27-6—cont'd. Growth charts.
Continued.

DATE	AGE	LENGTH	WEIGHT	HEAD CIRC.	COMMENT

GIRLS: 2 TO 18 YEARS
PHYSICAL GROWTH
NCHS PERCENTILES*   NAME _____   RECORD # _____

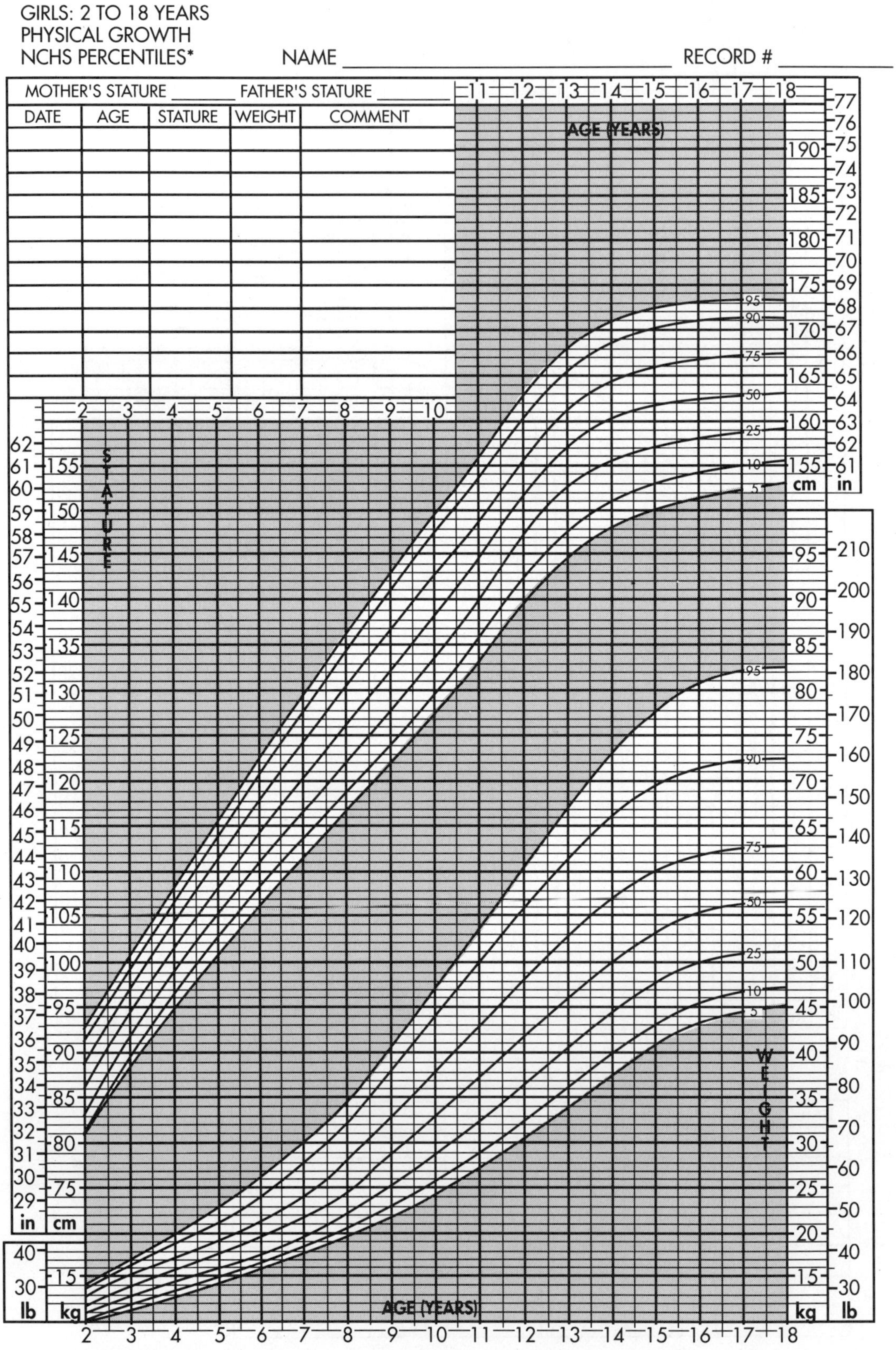

Fig. 27-6—cont'd. Growth charts.

BOYS: BIRTH TO 36 MONTHS
PHYSICAL GROWTH
NCHS PERCENTILES*   NAME _____ RECORD # _____

Fig. 27-7. Growth charts. (Adapted from Hamill PVV et al: *Am J Clin Nutr* 32:607-629, 1979. Data from Fels Longitudinal Study, Wright State University School of Medicine, Yellow Springs, OH; Ross Laboratories, Columbus, OH, 1982.)

Continued.

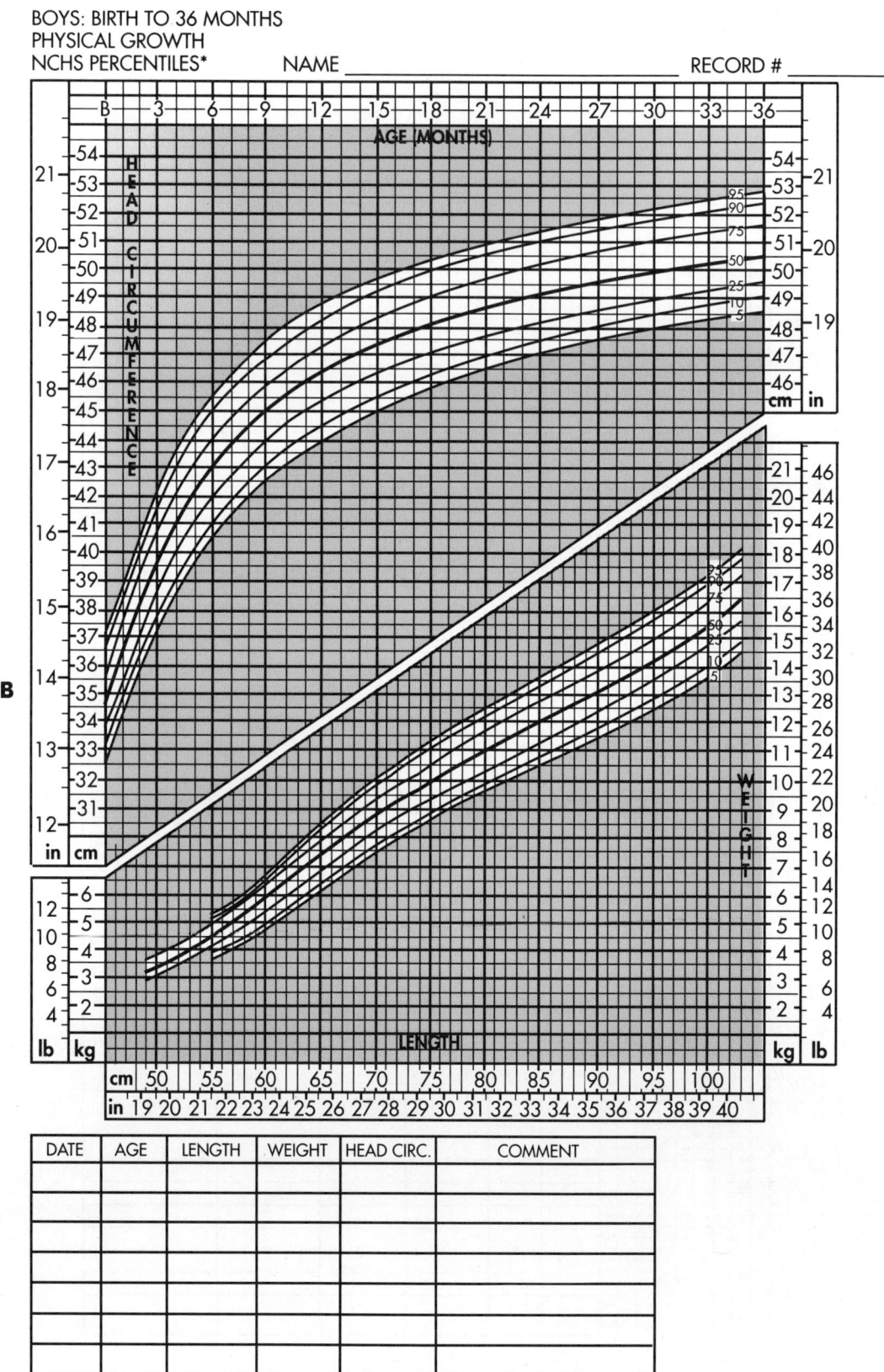

Fig. 27-7—cont'd. Growth charts.

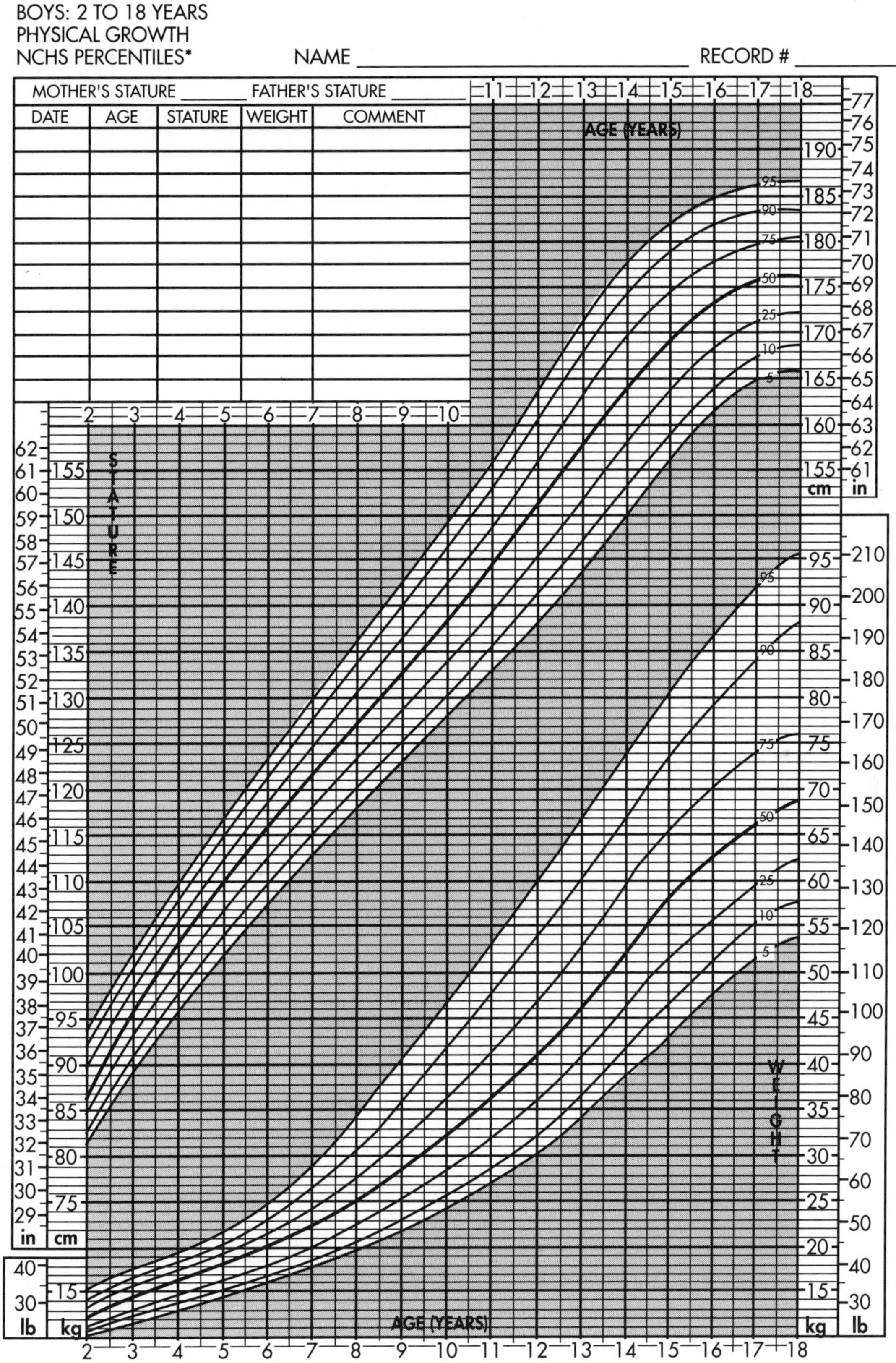

BOYS: 2 TO 18 YEARS
PHYSICAL GROWTH
NCHS PERCENTILES*   NAME _____   RECORD # _____

Fig. 27-7—cont'd. Growth charts.

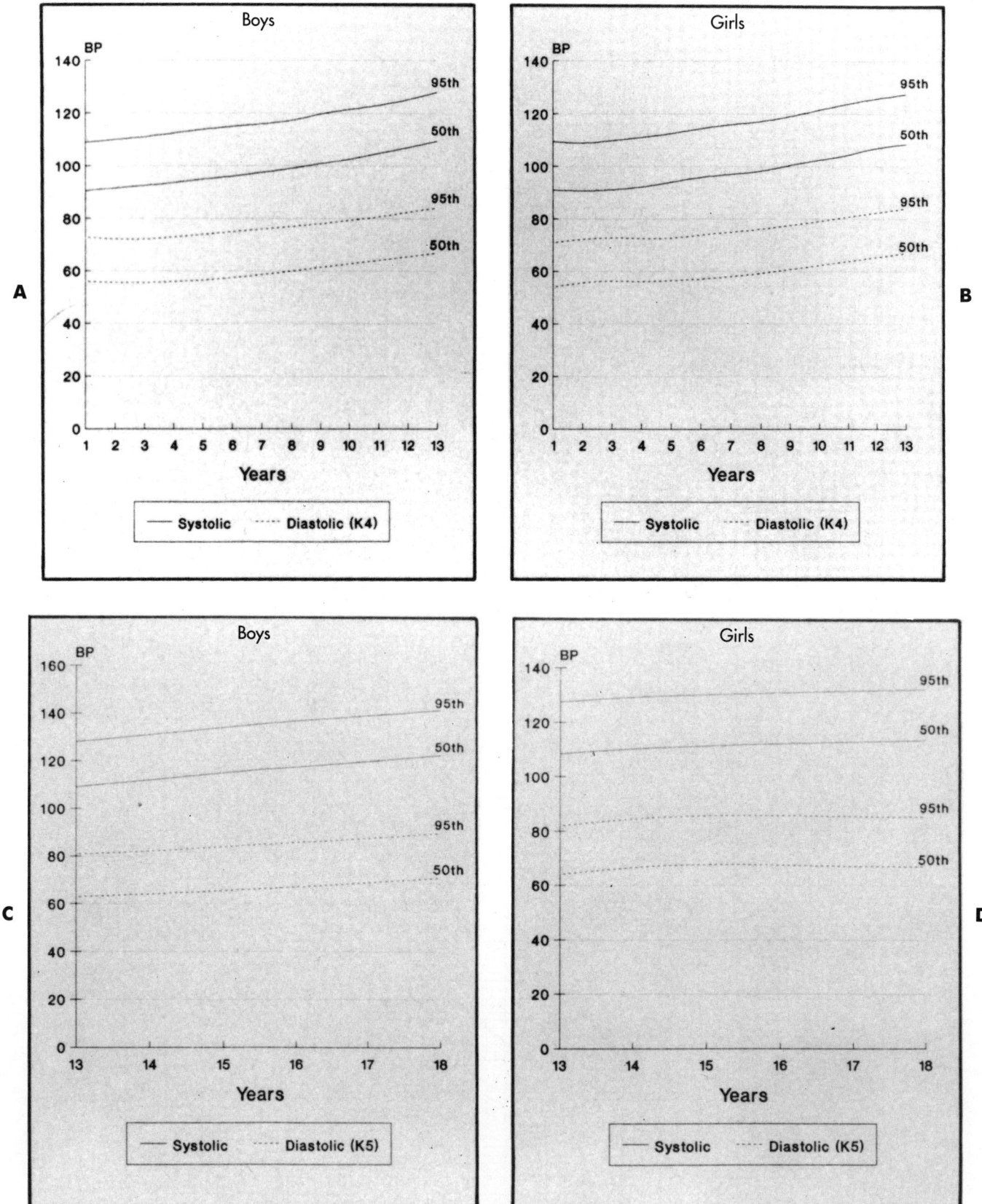

Fig. 27-8. Range of normal blood pressure by age and gender and definition of hypertension in children. **A,** Mean and 95th percentile values of systolic and diastolic blood pressure for boys 1 to 13 years of age. **B,** Mean and 95th percentile values of systolic and diastolic blood pressures for girls 1 to 13 years of age. **C,** Mean and 95th percentile values of systolic and diastolic blood pressure for boys 13 to 18 years of age. **D,** Mean and 95th percentile values of systolic and diastolic blood pressure for girls 13 to 18 years of age.

tion. Developmentally appropriate information regarding healthy life-styles is discussed.[31] Counseling related to family changes such as divorce or to problems such as learning difficulties may be offered.

The book *Guidelines for Health Supervision*, first published in 1985 by the AAP Committee on Psychosocial Aspects of Child and Family Health, is "a state-of-the-art manual intended to integrate the biomedical, psychosocial, and developmental aspects of preventive and health promoting care" for the recommended health supervision visits.[20] This handbook is invaluable for those involved in the ongoing care of children.[31]

Children with special needs, such as those with genetic disorders, congenital anomalies, very low birth weight, chronic medical conditions, "impaired" parents, or impoverished backgrounds, require more frequent visits for health supervision.[20]

"Group well-child visits" permit more time for anticipatory guidance and patient counseling than do individual visits.[20] A small group of parents and children can meet with a health care provider to discuss common developmental and behavioral concerns, health promotion, and disease prevention. The physical examination is performed but downplayed in importance.[48]

Many of the components of well-child visits are difficult to evaluate scientifically for their effectiveness. Success in health promotion seems to be a more likely outcome when there is a strong "therapeutic alliance" between the health care provider and the parents and child, and when the health care provider is person oriented as well as problem oriented. Continuity of care is vital so that different needs in health promotion may be addressed as the child continues to grow and develop.[31]

PRIMARY PREVENTION OF ATHEROSCLEROTIC CARDIOVASCULAR DISEASE

Those who provide health care for children can attend to issues that will increase the likelihood of full life expectancy and good quality of life during adulthood. The leading cause of death in the United States is cardiovascular disease resulting from atherosclerosis and hypertension.[7] There are 1.25 million myocardial infarctions each year in the United States. Approximately 20% occur in persons less than 55 years of age. Five hundred thousand deaths each year are attributable to coronary heart disease.[65] Atherosclerosis is a silent, progressive, lifelong process, which begins in early life. Pediatricians and other child health care deliverers are in a unique position to delay significantly and in many instances actually prevent the disease.

It is important to be aware of the truly multifactorial nature of atherosclerosis (see Fig. 27-9). Many risk factors interact to determine the incidence and progression of atherosclerosis. Major risk factors for coronary heart disease

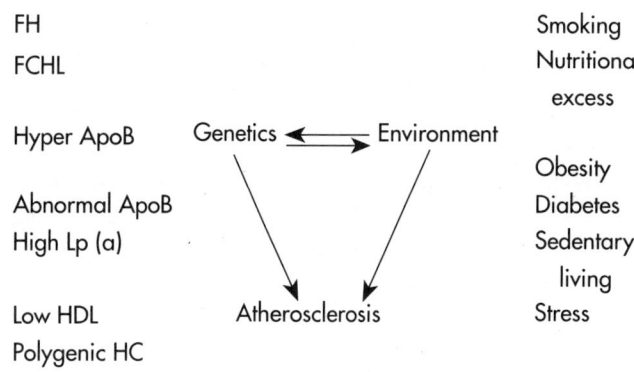

Key: FH = familial hypercholesterolemia; FCHL = familial combined hyperlipidemia; ApoB = apoprotein B100; Lp (a) = lipoprotein little a; HDL = high density lipoprotein; HC = hypercholesterolemia

Fig. 27-9. Multifactorial nature of atherosclerosis.

Risk factors for coronary heart disease*

Hypercholesterolemia
Hypertension
Cigarette smoking
Family history of premature CHD
Low levels of HDL cholesterol
High lipoprotein (a) levels
Obesity
Diabetes mellitus
Physical inactivity

---

*CHD, coronary heart disease; *HDL*, high-density lipoprotein.

include hypercholesterolemia, hypertension, and cigarette smoking. Other recognized factors include a positive family history for hypercholesterolemia or premature coronary heart disease, sedentary life-style, obesity, diabetes mellitus, low high-density lipoprotein (HDL) cholesterol level, and upper quartile lipoprotein(a) concentration (see box). Data from the Framingham Heart Study clearly demonstrate the importance of these risk factors and their additive character when several are present in individuals with respect to developing coronary heart disease.[16]

An individual's tastes, behavior, life-style choices, and approaches to management of life stresses are shaped in childhood. There is firm evidence that most recognized risk factors, if present in childhood, tend to persist into adult life. Several risk factors for future cardiovascular disease are present in American youth: Children in the United States consume too much salt.[53] Twenty percent of children are obese (5% are superobese).[28] Fifteen percent to 30% of adolescents are regular smokers.[58] Only 58% of American youth attain a level of physical activity that provides cardiovascular benefit regularly.[29] Children consume too much saturated fat and cholesterol habitually. Approximately 5% of children have a familial (genetic) dyslipidemia that may not be evident in primary relatives.

Environmental risk factors for coronary heart disease

Hypertension. Tracking studies show that adolescents who have persistently elevated blood pressure are far more likely to have hypertension as adults (see Tables 27-1 and 27-2 and Fig. 27-8).[12] It is estimated that 10% to 20% of U.S. society is salt sensitive and destined to become hypertensive if excessive salt is consumed.[53] Blood pressure increases with age in societies that have high salt intakes, and the converse is also true. The relative risk of hypertension increases fivefold if an individual is obese. The control of obesity, it is estimated, could prevent 50% of high blood pressure in whites and 30% in blacks.[12] The first steps in decreasing the incidence of hypertension are dietary modification, weight control, and establishment of regular patterns of exercise. Strong evidence indicates that hypertension persists into adulthood if it occurs after 10 years of age. Cardiovascular health education for families and schools is imperative for prevention of early onset coronary heart disease caused by hypertension.

Smoking. The risk of starting to smoke cigarettes increases between 6 and 12 years of age and is rare after age 20 years.[58] Cigarette smoking has been identified by the United States Surgeon General as the leading public health problem, the single most preventable cause of death, and the most important modifiable coronary risk factor.[70] If all smoking ceased, 25% fewer low birth weight babies, 33% less coronary heart disease, 85% less chronic obstructive lung disease, and 90% less lung cancer would result.[58] Cigarette smoking is responsible for 350,000 premature deaths in the United States each year.[66] Child health care providers should urge parents not to smoke since they are second only to peers in inducing adolescents to begin smoking.

Obesity. The prevalence of childhood obesity ranges from 10% to 30%.[56] Children of obese parents are at greatest risk as they are twice as likely to become obese adults. There are strong environmental and genetic influences on the incidence of obesity. The longer a child is obese, the greater the likelihood of his or her becoming an obese adult. An obese infant has double the risk of being an obese adult; an obese adolescent, six times the risk. The leading cause of hypertension in children is obesity. The obese individual is likely to have elevated blood cholesterol level, low HDL cholesterol level, a sedentary lifestyle, hypertension, and hyperinsulinism. Treatment and prevention of obesity involve increasing caloric expenditure through exercise, decreasing caloric intake through dietary change, and gaining psychological support through group effort and total family involvement.

Physical inactivity. The United States Surgeon General declared in 1980, "The fitness of our youth is a na-

---

Summary of American Heart Association Step One Diet

1. Nutritional adequacy should be achieved by eating a wide variety of foods.
2. Energy (calories) should be adequate to support growth and development and to reach or maintain desirable body weight.
3. The following pattern of nutrient intake is recommended:

   Saturated fats—less than 10% of total calories

   Total fat—an average of no more than 30% of total calories

   Dietary cholesterol—less than 300 mg/day

   Carbohydrates—about 55% of total calories

   Protein—about 15% to 20% of total calories

Modified from American Heart Association: *Dietary treatment of hypercholesterolemia: handbook for counselors.*

---

tional tragedy." Body fatness has gradually increased over the last two decades in the United States.[28] The likelihood of children's developing a healthy and lasting interest in regular physical exercise depends largely on parental example. It was estimated in the mid-1970s that nearly half of adult Americans did not engage in any form of exercise.

Physical inactivity is three to five times more prevalent in the United States than the other recognized coronary risk factors.[36] Fewer than half of U.S. children passed the fitness test of the President's Council on Physical Fitness and Sports in 1984.

Children should play when they go home from school, not snack, watch television, or do homework. Schools should be required to provide daily controlled and supervised physical education programs for their students.[38] Regular exercise results in less cardiovascular disease, high blood pressure, stress, obesity, and higher-HDL cholesterol levels.[54]

Lipid disorders in childhood. Lipid levels at birth are similar in all populations and the gene pool has not changed significantly. The observed incidence of coronary heart disease is largely due, therefore, to environmental influences. The incidence is highest in industrialized societies that have become largely sedentary; that consume diets too high in cholesterol, fat, and salt; and that have a high incidence of obesity and cigarette smoking.[39] American children currently receive 36% of total calories from fat, including approximately 14% from saturated fat. The National Cholesterol Education Program expert panel recommends the American Heart Association Step One Diet after 2 years of age for the entire population (see box).[44]

Diet is the most important variable affecting blood lipid levels within populations. Genetic influence determines the relative importance of recognized environmental factors. A significant number of inherited dyslipidemias are now rec-

Table 27-3. Serum lipid levels—children 3 to 19 years of age*

Lipid	5th percentile	Mean	95th percentile
TC	110 (3.1)	160 (4.1)	200 (5.2)
LDL-C	60 (1.7)	100 (2.6)	130 (3.4)
HDL-C	35 (0.9)	55 (1.4)	70 (1.8)
TG	30 (0.4)	60 (0.9)	110 (1.3)

*Values are milligrams/deciliter (mg/dl), those in parentheses millimoles per liter (mM/l). *TC,* total cholesterol; *LDL-C,* low-density lipoprotein cholesterol; *HDL-C,* high-density lipoprotein cholesterol; *TG,* triglycerides. (Modified from Lipid research clinics. Population studies data book. I. The Prevalence Study. Department of Health and Human Services 80:1527, 1980.

ognized and understood. Persons who consume a high-fat, high-cholesterol diet will have a markedly increased risk of coronary heart disease if a genetic lipid disorder is also present. The expected distribution of lipid levels in childhood and adolescence is seen in Table 27-3.

Genetic lipid disorders

Polygenic hypercholesterolemia. Polygenic hypercholesterolemia is a disorder thought due to a genetically determined sensitivity to dietary saturated fat that results in down regulation of low-density lipoprotein cholesterol (LDL) receptor site synthesis by the liver. The disease is estimated to affect 3% to 5% of the population and is manifested in childhood. LDL receptor synthesis is regulated by an LDL receptor gene. The incidence of hypercholesterolemia in relatives of an index individual is approximately half that which would be expected if inheritance were purely genetic in nature. The implication is that several genes interact with one another and the environment to produce disease.[44]

Familial combined hyperlipidemia. Familial combined hyperlipidemia is characterized by an overproduction of apolipoprotein B (ApoB) very low density lipoprotein (VLDL) particles by the liver. Of the population 1% to 2% is estimated to have the disorder. Simultaneous inheritance of several primary defects of lipoprotein metabolism may also play a role. Inheritance is often autosomal dominant and expression in childhood is not rare. More classically, however, the disease is not manifested until the second or third decade of life. In families with the disorder individuals may variably have hypercholesterolemia, hypertriglyceridemia, or both. Familial combined hyperlipidemia is responsible for approximately 10% of cases of premature coronary artery disease.[22,40] Occasionally individuals have abnormally high Apo protein B levels and relatively normal lipoprotein profiles otherwise. They are at increased risk for coronary heart disease. The disorder may be a variant of familial combined hyperlipidemia.

Familial hypercholesterolemia. Individuals with familial hypercholesterolemia (FH) have only half the normal number of LDL receptors; as a result LDL cholesterol is poorly cleared from the blood.[15] Tendon xanthomas, corneal arcus, or xanthelasmas found in primary or secondary relatives of a proband usually confirm the diagnosis. The incidence of FH is estimated to be 1 in 500 and it is responsible for 3% to 6% of premature myocardial infarctions.[40] Men with FH have a 50% likelihood of myocardial infarction by age 50 years and women by age 60 years. Individuals homozygous for the FH gene have essentially no LDL receptors. Their cholesterol levels are three to four times normal and survival beyond age 30 years is unlikely. Liver transplantation, plasmaphoresis, portocaval shunting, and hyperalimentation are treatment options for such individuals.

Familial defective ApoB100. A genetic defect in ApoB100 causing it not to be recognized by the LDL receptor affects 0.2% of the population.[40] The disorder is responsible for approximately one third of modest hypercholesterolemias. Techniques of molecular biology are necessary to make the diagnosis. The VLDL remnant is cleared well from blood because ApoE is normal.

When a child has a positive family history for premature coronary heart disease but no specific genotypic diagnosis, ApoB100, apolipoprotein A (ApoA), HDL subfractions, and lipoprotein(a) should be measured. Some families have an autosomal dominant inheritance of low HDL cholesterol concentration resulting in very increased risk of premature coronary artery disease. Persons who have lipoprotein(a) levels in the top quartile (greater than 30 mg/dl) have as much as a fivefold increased risk for coronary artery disease.[41] Elevated lipoprotein(a) level may well be the most prevalent inherited risk for atherosclerosis. Inheritance is autosomal dominant and appears to express itself in childhood. Lipoprotein(a) is a genetic variant of LDL and may act as a procoagulant.

Controversy surrounds routine versus selective screening of children for hypercholesterolemia. This author has a bias that universal screening of all children after 2 to 3 years of age for total cholesterol level is appropriate and productive. Children found to have a total cholesterol level above 200 mg/dl should then have a fasting lipoprotein profile made to define their lipid abnormality. The American Academy of Pediatrics Committee on Nutrition[1] and the expert panel of the National Cholesterol Education Program[44] recommend selective screening of children from families known to have a primary relative with hypercholesterolemia (>240 mg/dl) or premature coronary heart disease (<55 years of age). When there is a family history of hypercholesterolemia or premature coronary heart disease it is appropriate to consider a lipoprotein profile as the first screening test. Pharmacotherapy for children, except under unusual circumstances, is probably inappropriate before 10 to 12 years of age. The American Heart Association Step One diet is indicated and safe for all of the population above 2 years of age. The risk of coronary heart disease caused by hypercholesterolemia can be minimized by good general health habits. Greater emphasis by health care providers needs to be placed on avoidance of other coronary risk factors such as smoking, obesity, hypertension, and sedentary living. When there is a strong family history of premature coronary heart disease, referral to a pediatric preventive cardiology clinic or pediatric lipidologist may be considered for diagnosis and counseling.

Intensive dietary and often drug therapy of hypercholesterolemia in childhood is considered when the LDL cholesterol exceeds 190 mg/dl, or 160 mg/dl when there is a family history of premature coronary heart disease.[44] Careful, nutritionist supervised Step One and then Step Two American Heart Association (AHA) diets are first tried. If satisfactory reduction in LDL cholesterol level is not achieved, bile acid binding resins (cholestyramine or colestipol) and occasionally niacin are used. More severe and complex lipid disorders in childhood are best managed by the lipidologist.

Summary

Industrialized societies have an increased risk for atherosclerosis largely because of nutritional excess and unhealthy life-style choices such as smoking, sedentary living, and obesity. A population strategy directed by the National Cholesterol Education Program aims to lower total saturated fat and cholesterol intake for the entire country.[65] Physician involvement and direction involving prudent life-style choices such as regular aerobic exercise, nonsmoking, and diminution in salt intake are crucial. Hypertension surveillance and control along with direction regarding appropriate stress management can significantly reduce the likelihood of atherosclerotic cardiovascular disease. Early diagnosis of genetic dyslipidemias and their treatment can potentially eradicate premature coronary heart disease as long as such patients also make healthy life-style choices. Strategies suggested by the National Cholesterol Education Program Panel on Children and Adolescents[44] include the following:

- Be involved with school food service programs to encourage reduction of saturated fat and salt in school lunches.
- Be actively involved with school administration and parent/teacher programs to provide nutrition education at all grade levels.
- Encourage school athletic programs for all students on a regular basis.
- Provide aggressive nonsmoking messages. Take advantage of health maintenance visits to discuss risk factors for atherosclerosis.

- Encourage appropriate labeling for foods and provision of more low-fat foods and snacks for purchase.
- Be involved with mass media to provide public programming information regarding prudent nutrition, physical exercise, and nonsmoking.

IMMUNIZATIONS
Immunizations for healthy children

At the beginning of this century infectious diseases were the leading cause of death. Improvements in living conditions, for example, less crowding, safer food handling and water supplies, and development of antimicrobials and vaccines, have resulted in a marked reduction in the incidence and severity of infectious diseases.[24] Vaccines first became widely available in the United States in the 1940s and have steadily increased in number since then.

Figures show that at the present time, compared with the prevaccination era, there has been a greater than 90% reduction in the vaccine-preventable diseases—whooping cough, diphtheria, tetanus, poliomyelitis, measles, mumps, rubella, and congenital rubella syndrome. There is a 95% immunization rate for children entering school, largely because of state immunization requirements for school attendance.

Since 1985 vaccines have been developed to prevent invasive disease caused by *Haemophilus influenzae* type B (Hib). These diseases include meningitis, septic arthritis, osteomyelitis, epiglottitis, bacteremia, and cellulitis. About 75% of all serious infections with Hib occur in children less than 18 months of age. The first (polysaccharide) vaccine developed was recommended for administration to children 24 months or older. Subsequently newer conjugated vaccines have been developed, allowing effective administration at earlier ages. Since October 1990 immunization against this organism is commenced at 2 months of age.[51]

Measles vaccine became available in 1963. By 1983 the number of reported measles cases in the United States had fallen to an all time low of fewer than 1500. It was estimated that 52 million cases of measles had been prevented during this time and major complications of encephalitis and death had declined more than 99%.[73] Epidemics of measles became a problem again in late 1988 to 1990 though on a much smaller scale than in the prevaccination era.

The highest incidence of measles in 1989 was in the 15- to 19-year age group (high school and college students). Most of these young people had been vaccinated previously. Measles in this population represents, most commonly, primary failure to respond to the vaccine (prevalence estimated at 2% to 10%) or less commonly, secondary vaccine failure with waning immunity.[73] Children aged 0 to 4 years had the highest incidence rate of measles during 1990. Most of these children had never been immu-

Table 27-4. Recommended schedule for immunization of healthy infants and children (AAP October 1990*†)

Recommended age	Immunization
2 mo	DTP, TOPV, HbOC† or PRP-OMP‡
4 mo	DTP, TOPV, HbOC‡ or PRP-OMP‡
6 mo	DTP, HbOC‡
12 mo	PRP-OMP‡
15 mo	MMR, HbCV‡
15-18 mo	DTP, TOPV
4-6 yr	DTP, TOPV
11-12 yr	MMR§
14-16 yr (repeat q 10 yr)	Td

Modified from Peter G, editor: *Report of the Committee on Infectious Diseases,* ed 22, 1991, Elk Grove Village, Ill, American Academy of Pediatrics.
*For all products used consult manufacturer's package insert for complete details. *DTP,* diphtheria-tetanus-pertussis; *TOPV,* trivalent oral polio vaccine; *MMR,* measles-mumps-rubella; *Td,* adult tetanus and diphtheria toxoid.
†See the section Hepatitis B for AAP April 1992 recommendation regarding routine hepatitis B immunization schedules.
‡*H. influenzae* type B conjugate vaccines: HbOC, Hib titer, given at 2, 4, 6, and 15 months (total 4 doses); PRP-OMP, Pedvax HIB, given at 2, 4, and 12 months (total 3 doses); HbCV, any Hib conjugate vaccine (Hib titer, Pedvax HIB, or ProHIBit). For children less than 15 months the course of Hib immunization must be given with the same vaccine product. If Hib immunization is due at (or beyond) 15 months, any licensed conjugate vaccine may be given.
§ACIP recommends giving MMR reimmunization at 4-6 years.

nized. Measles vaccine, usually in combination with mumps and rubella vaccines, is recommended at 15 months. In view of the recent outbreaks high priority must be given to providing this first dose to as many children as possible. In addition since 1989 reimmunization is now recommended at 11 or 12 years (AAP) or at school entry (Advisory Committee on Immunization Practices [ACIP]).[17] Many colleges now require before enrollment that the student show proof of having received two measles containing vaccines after the age of 1 year. MMR is usually given for reimmunization to provide additional protection against mumps and rubella.[50] The primary vaccine failure rate for mumps and rubella is about 2% to 5%. Outbreaks of mumps have been reported in previously vaccinated young adults but this is not the case for rubella.

The following table (Table 27-4) outlines current recommendations for immunization of healthy children. The AAP *Red Book,* the report of the Committee on Infectious Diseases, gives extensive information on immunization practices and vaccines and should be read by health care providers responsible for the administration of immunizations.[50]

Since parents do not always present their children for immunization at the recommended times, it is helpful to refer to a schedule for children who have not been immunized in the first year of life. This is shown in Table 27-5.

Health care workers aim to provide comprehensive im-

Table 27-5. Recommended immunization schedules for children not immunized in first year of life

	Younger than 7 years but older than 15 months
First visit	DTP, TOPV, MMR
	HbCV—for children aged 15-59 mo
Interval after first visit	
2 mo	DTP, TOPV
4 mo	DTP
10-16 mo	DTP, TOPV
4-6 yr	DTP—not necessary if fourth dose was given after fourth birthday
(At or before school entry)	
	TOPV Not necessary if third dose was given after fourth birthday
11-12 yr	MMR At entry to middle school or junior high
10 yr after last tetanus immunization	Td Repeat q 10 yr

	7 years and older
First visit	Td, TOPV, MMR
Interval after first visit	
2 mo	Td, TOPV
8-14 mo	Td, TOPV
11-12 yr	MMR At entry to middle school or junior high
10 yr after last tetanus immunization	Td

Modified from Peter G, editor: *Report of the Committee on Infectious Diseases,* ed 22, 1991, Elk Grove, Ill, American Academy of Pediatrics.
*For all products used, consult manufacturer's package insert for complete details. *DTP,* diphtheria-tetanus-pertussis; *TOPV,* trivalent oral polio vaccine; *MMR,* measles-mumps-rubella; *Td,* adult tetanus and diphtheria toxoid.

munizations to all children. There are a variety of reasons why this does not occur. Low-income inner city children are less likely than others to receive immunizations in the recommended fashion. The Immunization Practices Advisory Committee (ACIP) investigated key barriers to immunizations. Many public programs are organized in such a way that it is difficult for families to obtain immunization for their children; inconvenient clinic hours, insufficient clinic staffing, or complicated appointment systems may be obstacles to the provision of good care.

Immunizations should not be deferred for unnecessary reasons such as minor afebrile upper respiratory infections. Instead of making several clinic visits, the child can receive many different vaccines simultaneously at different sites. For example, at 15 months a child may receive DTP, TOPV, MMR, and conjugate Hib vaccine at one visit. Many poor minority children do not receive ongoing care at one medical center but instead may use acute care clinics and emergency rooms, where immunizations are not offered. Occasionally immunizations are not given, or more seriously, a whole series is canceled, because the health care provider has misconceptions about vaccine contraindications.[50]

It is very important that parents and/or patients be informed about the benefits and risks of immunizations. The health care provider must also be familiar with common side effects of the various vaccines and of the selected adverse events that occur after immunization that are reportable. These are outlined in the National Childhood Vaccine Injury Act.[50]

Immunizations for premature infants

In clinical practice the question of when premature infants should start their series of immunizations often arises. The answer is that premature infants should be immunized at the usual chronological age and with the usual doses. The use of reduced volume, or divided doses of reduced volume, for DTP or other vaccine is not recommended for any child. No benefits have been shown in terms of reducing the frequency of associated adverse effects with DTP, and a diminished antibody response to reduced dosages of DTP in both term and premature infants has been reported.[50]

Immunization and pregnancy

Generally speaking immunization is avoided in pregnant women. Some, such as vaccines for tetanus, diphtheria, influenza, and hepatitis B, can be administered under special circumstances. All live virus vaccines should be avoided in pregnancy, however. There is theoretical risk but no definite evidence for injury to the fetus by a live virus vaccine. This is true even for congenital rubella syndrome after administration of rubella vaccine to women in the first trimester of pregnancy.[19] However, since there is a background rate of congenital anomalies in uncomplicated pregnancies, a defect might be attributed to a vaccine incorrectly. This is of practical importance when immunization using MMR is contemplated in adolescent females who may already be pregnant or sexually active; therefore, the theoretical risks of live vaccines in pregnancy should be pointed out to these young people. Preimmunization pregnancy testing is *not* felt to be necessary.[51] No fetal risk is posed by the administration of MMR to a child whose mother is pregnant.

Influenza vaccine

Influenza immunization should be offered yearly to children 6 months or older who have chronic pulmonary disease such as asthma, bronchopulmonary dysplasia, and cystic fibrosis; cardiac disease; sickle cell disease and other hemoglobinopathies; diabetes; chronic renal and metabolic diseases; immunosuppression; and long-term aspirin therapy (who may be at an increased risk of developing Reye syndrome as a complication of influenza).[50]

Close contacts of high-risk patients should also receive influenza immunization. These include families of high-risk children, adult hospital personnel in contact with pediatric patients, and children in households of high-risk adults.

A contraindication to the administration of the influenza vaccine is severe anaphylaxis to chicken or eggs (influenza vaccines are produced in eggs). If a high-risk child aged more than 1 year cannot receive the influenza vaccine for this reason, prophylactic amantadine (effective against influenza A infection only) may be offered.

Fever and/or local reactions may occur as side effects of the immunization but are not common.

The former concern about occurrence of Guillain-Barré syndrome after influenza immunization has disappeared. Ongoing studies have shown no increased risk of occurrence of this disease as an adverse effect.

Table 27-6 shows the recommended schedule for influenza immunization.

The antigenic characteristics of influenza viruses vary from year to year. New vaccines are prepared annually in anticipation of the strains that are expected to be prevalent, and only current vaccines can be used.

Children 8 years and younger receiving an influenza vaccine for the first time should be given two doses 4 or more weeks apart. Adults and children 9 years and older require only one dose. November is considered the optimal time for influenza immunization programs to be carried out.

Pneumococcal vaccine

The 23-valent pneumococcal vaccine should be given to certain children aged 2 years and older who fall into high-risk categories. These are children who have sickle cell disease, functional or anatomic asplenia, nephrotic syndrome or chronic renal failure, conditions associated with immunosuppression such as organ transplantation or cytoreduction therapy, cerebrospinal fluid (CSF) leaks, and HIV infection.[50]

Table 27-6. Schedule for influenza immunization

Age	Recommended vaccine	Dose	Number of doses
6-35 mo	Split virus only	0.25 ml	1-2
3-8 yr	Split virus only	0.5 ml	1-2
9-12 yr	Split virus only	0.5 ml	1
≥12 yr	Whole or split virus	0.5 ml	1

From Peter G, editor: *Report of the Committee on Infectious Diseases,* ed 22, 1991, Elk Grove Village, Ill, American Academy of Pediatrics.

Meningococcal vaccine

The quadrivalent meningococcal vaccine is used only in special circumstances: such as for children 2 years and older with functional or anatomic asplenia and certain immunosuppressed children, for control of outbreaks of meningococcal disease, for travelers to countries where meningococcal disease is prevalent, and for all American military recruits.[50]

Prevention of hepatitis B

Hepatitis B vaccine has been available since 1982. The vaccine is safe and 90% to 95% effective, yet the reported number of cases of the disease in the United States has increased. A general lack of awareness of the risks of the disease and the present cost of the vaccine are among the factors leading to inadequate vaccine use.[51]

The spectrum of disease caused by the hepatitis B virus (HBV) ranges from asymptomatic infection to acute fulminant fatal hepatitis. The risk of becoming a chronic carrier of hepatitis B surface antigen (HBsAg) is greater for individuals who become infected at an early age, so that infants in the perinatal period and the early months and years of life are particularly vulnerable. Any chronic carrier is at risk for developing cirrhosis or hepatocellular carcinoma many years later.

In the United States today infection in children and young people is most common in those from areas of high-risk HBV endemicity such as Alaska and Hawaii and immigrants from Southeast Asia and Africa. Children in institutions for the developmentally disabled; hemophilia patients and others receiving blood products; hemodialysis patients; and household contacts of HBV carriers are also at risk. Adopted children and immigrants from high-risk areas should be screened for HBsAg. Perinatal transmission to neonates may occur when mothers are HBsAg-positive. Routine screening is recommended for all pregnant women. Adolescents who are using illicit intravenous drugs, who are involved in heterosexual activity with several partners, or who are engaging in male homosexual activity are at high risk for acquiring HBV infection.[51]

Only selective immunization for high-risk individuals, as listed in the box, was formerly recommended.[50] This policy of selective immunization was difficult to implement from a practical point of view and in April 1992 routine universal immunization of infants became the recommended policy.[4] This immunization schedule is shown in Table 27-7.

Universal, rather than selective, immunization provides much better protection against hepatitis B in young children. In the future adolescents and young adults, if immunized as infants, will already be protected should they choose to become involved in high-risk behavior. However, the immunization of all high-risk groups needs to be encouraged as before, and as soon as it is feasible, routine immunization of all current adolescents should be implemented.[4]

As mentioned, routine screening of all pregnant women for hepatitis B continues to be standard policy.[50] Recommendations for the *postexposure* situation of the infant whose mother is HBsAg-positive are as follows:

- The infant should be bathed carefully by a gloved attendant as soon as possible after birth to remove maternal blood and secretions; the remainder of the in-

Table 27-7. Recommended routine hepatitis B immunization schedules

Maternal hepatitis B surface antigen status	Dose	Age
Negative*	1	0-2 days
	2	1-2 mo
	3	6-18 mo
Positive	1†	0 days
	2	1 mo
	3	6 mo

From Committee on Infectious Diseases: *Pediatrics* 89:4, 1992.
*Alternative schedule: Dose one at 1 to 2 months of age, dose two at 4 months, and dose three at 6 to 18 months.
†Hepatitis B immune globulin should also be administered.

High-risk groups who should receive hepatitis B immunization regardless of age

Hemophiliac patients and other recipients of certain blood products
Intravenous drug abusers
Heterosexual persons who have had several sex partners in the previous 6 months and those who have recently contracted sexually transmitted disease
Sexually active homosexual and bisexual males
Household and sexual contacts of HBV chronic carriers
Household members of adoptees from HBV-endemic high-risk countries who are HBsAg-positive
Specified infants, children, and other household contacts in populations of high HBV endemicity
Staff and residents of institutions for the developmentally disabled
Staff of nonresidential day care and school programs for developmentally disabled if attended by known HBV carrier; other attendees in certain circumstances
Hemodialysis patients
Health care workers and others at occupational risk
International travelers who will live for more than 6 months in area of high HBV endemicity and who otherwise will be at risk
Inmates of long-term correctional facilities

From Peter G, editor: Report of the Committee on Infectious Diseases, ed 22, 1991, Elk Grove Village, Ill, American Academy of Pediatrics.

fant's stay in the nursery requires no special precautions.

- Hepatitis B immune globulin (HBIG) should be given as soon as possible after birth, preferably within 12 hours.
- Hepatitis B vaccination should be initiated within 7 days of birth, preferably within 12 hours; second and third doses are given 1 and 6 months after the first (see Table 27-7). The later doses can be given concurrently with DTP but at a separate site and with a different syringe.
- Infants should be tested at 9 months of age or later for HBsAg and anti-HbsAg to determine whether immunity has been induced.
- Breast-feeding adds no risk for these infants who have started immunoprophylaxis.

Varicella (chickenpox)

For the great majority of children varicella is more a nuisance than a dangerous disease. However some children are at particular risk of developing severe and even life-threatening complications. Such children include those who are immunocompromised, premature infants less than 28 weeks' gestation or less than 1000 g in weight, and neonates whose mothers have had varicella less than 5 days before or 2 days after birth. A pregnant woman in whom varicella develops during the first trimester of pregnancy has a 2% to 3% risk of defects being produced in her fetus. When varicella occurs in adults it often takes a more severe form. Even in a healthy child the uncomplicated disease can cause much disruption in the lives of working parents.[43]

A live attenuated varicella vaccine was developed in Japan in 1974 and since then has been tested extensively in immunocompromised and healthy children in Japan, Europe, and the United States. The vaccine is awaiting licensing and is likely to be included in the routine immunization schedule in the near future, probably in combination with MMR.

Passive immunization using varicella-zoster immunoglobulin (VZIG) has been possible since the early 1970s. It can be used after significant exposure to an active case of chickenpox for the high-risk children mentioned. It may also be offered to susceptible adults, particularly pregnant women. It must be given to these high-risk, susceptible individuals as soon as possible and certainly no later than 96 hours after exposure. Complete details on the use of VZIG can be found in the *Red Book*.[50]

Immunodeficient and immunosuppressed children

Immunocompromised persons may receive inactivated vaccines, but protection from the vaccine may be reduced.

Live bacterial and viral vaccines (BCG, measles, mumps, rubella, and the oral polio vaccines; also typhoid and yellow fever vaccines) are totally contraindicated in patients with congenital disorders of immune function and are generally contraindicated in immunosuppressed chil-

dren. The live varicella vaccine, not yet generally available, may be used for susceptible children with cancer, since for these children the risk of the actual disease outweighs the risk of the attenuated vaccine virus.

Children infected with HIV may be given an almost routine immunization schedule. Inactivated polio virus (IPV) must be substituted for the live oral polio vaccine. Since measles in these children may be extremely severe, live attenuated measles vaccine can be used, because the benefits of immunization seem to outweigh the risks. These children should receive pneumococcal vaccine and influenza immunization should be considered. The administered vaccines may have reduced efficacy, however.

Oral polio vaccine should not be given to normal siblings and other household contacts of immunocompromised patients, since the vaccine virus is transmissible and may cause disease in the patients. The killed vaccine, inactivated polio virus, may be given safely. Measles, mumps, and rubella vaccine can be given to normal siblings and household contacts because transmission of these vaccine viruses does not occur.[50]

Vaccines of the future

New vaccines are already being developed to protect children against the diseases caused by rotavirus and respiratory syncytial virus. Vaccine manufacturers are attempting to combine vaccines so that fewer injections and perhaps fewer office or clinic visits will be necessary. This should result in more complete as well as less painful immunizations and would represent yet another improvement in pediatric preventive care.

INJURY PREVENTION AND SAFETY PROMOTION

Observers of the national medical scene have noted that the next great increase in life expectancy will result not from major medical breakthroughs but rather from changes in life style. Because preventable injuries are the major factor in number of productive years and lives lost, it is appropriate that pediatricians focus their attention on instituting these changes in life style at a critical time of life when life style is being molded.[27]

Injuries to children are a major concern since nearly half of all deaths in young people below the age of 24 years are caused by unintentional injury. Before the age of 14 years about half of the unintentional injuries are due to motor vehicle crashes, whereas in the age group 15 to 24 years three quarters of the deaths involve motor vehicles. The morbidity from injuries is also great: for every death there are about 100 injuries, some of which are disabling or disfiguring.[69]

Infections, which used to be the leading cause of death in children, have been greatly reduced by the success of immunization programs. In recent years advances have been made by the introduction and implementation of programs aimed at reducing injuries, which are a major threat to young people's health and happiness.

Curiosity and the urge to explore are characteristics of children that are regarded as signs of good health and development. Increasing independence is sought by the child; some risk taking must accompany this. Learning to make decisions is also a feature of growing up. Thus it is the inherent nature of the developing child to be vulnerable to injury.

While the child is young adult caregivers can provide protection from environmental dangers. Physicians, as part of the anticipatory guidance segment of the well-child visit, can emphasize the main hazards at different developmental stages, suggest preventive strategies, and hope for good compliance. As the child becomes older and begins to make independent decisions, safety promotion can be encouraged with the child directly. This anticipatory guidance is of utmost importance to young people, both before and during adolescence. Adolescents are at great risk from fatal and nonfatal injuries, both unintentional and intentional.

Figure 27-10 illustrates the model of interactive forces of injury causation and prevention strategies.[32]

Accidents are caused by injurious agents and interventions can be planned, just as with disease. This is contrary to the notion that accidents always happen by chance and are beyond control. The diagram depicts three main preventive strategies:

1. Education/persuasion: to modify behavior by making people aware of hazards and of ways to avoid or eliminate them
2. Legislation/enforcement: to acquire by law behavior or conditions that help ensure safety or at least do not endanger
3. Passive/automatic: to provide protection through product or environmental design

Studies show that passive/automatic safeguards offer the best injury prevention and that individuals are more compliant in injury prevention where a law is in effect. Education/persuasion is least successful.

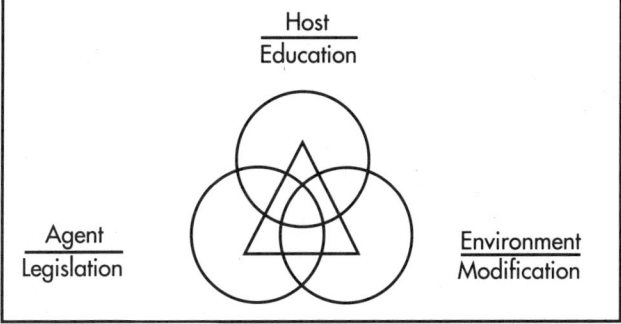

Fig. 27-10. Interactive forces of injury causation and prevention strategies. (From Interactive forces of injury causation and prevention strategies, *Pediatr Rev* 10:6, 1988.)

Motor vehicle accidents

As mentioned, motor vehicle accidents are the leading cause of death in the below 25-year-old age group and the major cause of disability.[69] Infants less than 6 months of age are especially vulnerable as passengers; the death rate is 9.1 per 100,000 compared to 4.8 per 100,000 for children older than 6 months.

The use of lap belts and shoulder harnesses by adults results in a 75% reduction in mortality.[42] Twenty-five states and the District of Columbia have state laws enforcing their use. However these restraint systems are ill suited to small children, and therefore child car seats were developed. The 1981 federal standards regulating child safety restraints were very specific in their requirements for design, installation, and use.

Different kinds of car seats are used at different ages:

- Infant safety seats for infants weighing less than 9 kg (20 lb) that face the rear of the car
- Convertible safety seats for infants and toddlers weighing 18 kg (40 lb) or less that face the rear for infants and the front for toddlers
- Booster seats for children weighing 13.5 to 27 kg (30 to 60 lb) that face forward

It is extremely important that the weight-appropriate car seat be used and correctly secured. Information on the different types of car seats and their purchase is included in the Resources section.

Children weighing more than 18 kg (40 lb) can use lap belts if they sit on a cushion, and when taller than 137.5 cm (55 inches) can safely use the three-point lap-shoulder restraints. Children are more likely to use seat belts themselves as they grow older if their adult role models regularly do so.

Children are safest when they are riding restrained in the back seat. An added advantage of safety restraints is that they prohibit movement around the car by the child, which in itself could prove distracting and dangerous to the driver.

For children below the age of 5 years the proper use of restraints can decrease deaths by 90% and injuries by 80%.[63] Such use has helped to reduce childhood mortality from motor vehicle crashes since 1970; continuing effort is required. Child passenger protection laws are in effect in all 50 states and the District of Columbia.

Cooperation by occupants of the car is obviously required in order for safety restraints to be effective. Since such cooperation is not always present, researchers and consumer advocates have pushed for passive restraint systems—automatic seat belts that wrap around the occupant when the door is closed and airbags that inflate automatically when a front end collision occurs. It is estimated that passive restraints will reduce injuries by more than 35% and save 10,000 lives annually. Currently passive restraints are being phased in as standard equipment by car manufacturers. The airbag is designed mainly for the driver, but some cars have two airbags, providing protection for the driver and front seat passenger. Lap belts should be used in addition.[32]

Controversy continues around the subject of seat belts for children in school buses. At present this is not required.

Alcohol abuse and driving

Blood alcohol concentrations of 0.10% or higher are found in drivers involved in more than half of all fatal motor vehicle crashes and in one third of serious injuries.[42] Other drugs may also be involved. This is especially true for adolescents. Current legislation and most substance abuse programs have not been very effective in counteracting this problem. Students Against Drunk Driving (SADD), however, shows encouraging results, and organizations like Mothers Against Drunk Driving (MADD) continue to lobby for more effective legislation.

Providers of health care to young people must continue to emphasize the risks of alcohol to driver and passenger alike, as part of driving safety counseling included in anticipatory guidance.[31]

Pedestrian injuries

Half of all children who die of motor vehicle injuries are pedestrians, not passengers.[63] For 5- to 9-year-old children pedestrian injuries are the most common cause of injury-related deaths. Nonfatal injuries are common. Most injuries occur when children are crossing streets. A variety of strategies are needed, including teaching of pedestrian safety at home and in school, supervised road crossing when possible, and use of light colored clothing with retroreflective panels for pedestrians at night.[32]

Bicycle injuries

Bicycle injuries are a more common cause of death in children than accidental poisonings, suffocation, firearm injuries, or falls. More than 500 bicycle related deaths occur each year, primarily in the 5- to 14-year age group. Adolescent deaths from bicycle injuries are on the increase. More than 300,000 children are treated for bicycle related injuries in emergency rooms each year. The majority of severe and fatal bicycle injuries involve head trauma. Most bicycle injuries do not involve collision with a car but occur because of the rider's loss of control, for example, skidding or hitting a bump.[37]

Preventive strategies include general measures such as buying a bicycle that is the correct size and knowing road safety rules. More specifically, since head trauma is important in bicycle injuries, care providers need to make parents aware of the importance of helmets, which may produce a 70% to 90% reduction in fatal head injuries.

The AAP includes bicycle safety in its TIPP program and the National Safety Council has published useful materials (see Resources).

All-terrain vehicles

The use of three- and four-wheeled motorized recreational vehicles by children has been associated with serious injuries, especially to the brain.[32] In 1988 the sale of three-wheeled models was banned and the sale of four-wheeled vehicles, which are considered less dangerous, restricted to riders 16 years and older. The AAP views these vehicles as major hazards to the safety of children.[42]

Fire, burns, and scalds

Burns and scalds are an important and common cause of death and nonfatal injury.[42] Children who survive injuries may face long hospitalizations, several surgical procedures, and disfigurement. The following are examples of important preventive measures:

- Smoke detectors in the home, ideally on each floor
- Flame-retardant children's sleepwear and clothing (Federal Flammable Fabrics Act, 1967)
- Counseling on keeping matches and lighters in an inaccessible place or ensuring their safe use
- Counseling of adults and teens who smoke not to smoke cigarettes in bed
- Teaching children what to do if a fire breaks out at home
- Reduction of water heater thermostat settings to 120° F to prevent tap water scalds (hot tap water at 150° F can cause a full-thickness burn in 2 seconds)
- Prevention of kitchen scalds by keeping children away from the stove and turning pot handles toward the back of the stove

Drowning

Drowning is a common cause of death in children, and in some areas of the United States, including the South, Southwest, and California, is the number one cause of death in children aged less than 5 years.[42] Drownings can occur in any body of water including a bathtub or pail. Alcohol and drug use have been found to be involved in nearly one half of all drowning deaths of adolescents and young adults.

Preventive strategies include the following:

- Never leave young children unattended in the bathtub.
- Pools should be fenced in on all four sides.
- Provide swimming instruction for children aged more than 4 or 5 years (this is not recommended for younger children).
- Make rules for swimming safety, including adult supervision and never swimming alone.
- Enclose bodies of water in the community such as water-filled quarries, which are dangerous to children.
- Counsel older children about the role of alcohol in drownings.

Falls

Falls are very common and more often result in nonfatal injuries than fatal ones. Anticipatory guidance might include some of the following points:

- Infants start rolling at about 4 months and therefore can fall off changing tables or beds.
- Safety gates should be installed at the top and bottom of stairwells in a home where there are infants and toddlers.
- Window guards help prevent window falls.

Baby walker injuries

Approximately 1 million baby walkers are sold yearly and are used by infants aged 5 to 15 months.[32] Unfortunately injuries associated with their use are common. The most severe are caused by tipping over and falling down stairs. Information about the dangers of walker use should be part of anticipatory guidance for young parents.[31]

Firearm injuries

Morbidity and mortality associated with firearms are increasingly distressing problems. In 1989 among young people aged 1 to 19 years 4000 firearm deaths occurred, including unintentional injuries, homicides, and suicides. Nonfatal injuries occur approximately five times more commonly than fatal injuries; about one quarter of these result in permanent, primarily neurologic, damage.[2,5]

Firearms are the fifth ranking cause of death resulting from unintentional trauma in the United States for children less than 18 years.[32] They account for about 500 deaths per year and about 8000 nonfatal injuries. Most of these injuries occur in the home. Guns kept in the home for "protection" appear to be much more likely to kill a member of the family than an intruder. Firearms are a major hazard and should be removed from the home environment. If this is impossible, they should be unloaded and locked up in a safe location.[2,5]

There is an escalation of violent and aggressive behavior in our society. One contributing factor may be that violent and aggressive behavior, including shooting, is commonplace on television programs. Children and young people may use an available firearm to try to settle an argument. Most homicides caused by firearms are the result of acts of rage involving relatives or acquaintances.[63] Seventy percent of teen homicides involve firearms, mostly handguns. Firearm homicides are the leading cause of death for urban black adolescents and young adults.

Firearms account for the majority of teen suicides in the United States.[2] Recently the most rapid increase in the suicide rate involving firearms has been among 15- to 24-year-old males.

Gun control is the subject of much debate at the present time.[2,5,21] Handguns pose the most risk to the health of children and adolescents. They account for approximately 20% of the firearms in use today yet are involved in 90% of criminal and nonintentional firearm misuse.[63]

Nonpowder firearms (air guns) such as BB and pellet guns cause few deaths but many injuries, especially to the eye, face, head, and neck. Health care providers should call for stricter regulation of these nonpowder weapons by the government.[2,32]

Poisonings

In children less than 5 years of age morbidity from poisoning is high, but fortunately mortality is low. Annually approximately 850,000 incidents of poison exposure are reported to poison centers. The mortality of approximately 400 in the 1960s fell to 55 in 1983.[63] The most significant factor leading to this decline in mortality was the Poison Prevention Packaging Act of 1970, which required that certain specified hazardous substances have child resistant packaging.

Poisonings in children less than 5 years almost always are acute accidental episodes that occur when an exploring child discovers a potentially toxic substance that he or she can ingest. In adolescents poisonings are most likely to result from suicide attempts. In 6- to 12-year-olds, who less commonly ingest poisons accidentally, the possibility of a purposeful overdose by the child should be considered. The most commonly ingested agents are medications (40%), plants, cosmetics, and cleaning substances. Fatal poisonings are caused by carbon monoxide inhalation (35%), medications (35%), pesticides (7%), and volatile petroleum distillates (7%). Salicylates and other analgesics, tricyclic antidepressants, and ferrous sulphate account for 75% of fatal accidental drug ingestions in children.

Important points about poison prevention include the following[27]:

- Encourage the purchase of products in child-resistant containers.
- Remind parents regularly about appropriate storage (out of sight, out of reach, childproof locks) and handling (proper use, continual observation while in use) of potentially harmful substances.
- Recommend the storage in every home where a young child lives or visits of a 30 ml (1 oz) bottle of ipecac syrup.
- Ensure that each family prominently displays the phone number of their local poison control center (or emergency room or doctor's office) to call in case of poisoning exposure.

Should a poisoning occur, in order to decrease morbidity and prevent mortality, caregivers should initiate immediate first aid steps:

1. Life support measures (cardiopulmonary resuscitation if needed)
2. Dilution and irrigation of toxins (see box) [63]

First aid for poison exposures

Inhaled poison

Immediately get the person to fresh air. Avoid breathing fumes. Open doors and windows wide.

Poison on the skin

Remove contaminated clothing and flood skin with water for at least 10 minutes.

Poison in the eye

Flood the open eye with lukewarm water for 15 minutes. Pour it from a large glass held 2 to 3 inches from the eye. Do not force the eyelid open. Remove contact lenses after immediate irrigation.

Swallowed poison

Unless the victim is unconscious, is having convulsions, or cannot swallow, give a small glass (2 to 4 ounces) of water, then determine whether the patient should vomit.

From Summitt RL, editor: *Comprehensive pediatrics,* St. Louis, 1990, Mosby–Year Book.

Ipecac syrup doseage

- 10 ml for a child 6-12 months followed by 120 to 180 ml clear fluid
- 15 ml for a child older than 1 year followed by 180 to 240 ml clear fluid
- 30 ml for child older than 12 years followed by 240 ml clear fluid or more

---

Emergency consultation should then be sought by calling a local poison control center or other source of medical help. Gastric evacuation at home using syrup of ipecac to induce emesis will be advised unless contraindications exist (see box).[10] Emesis should *not* be induced if:

- Patient is unconscious, is stuporous, exhibits seizure activity, has no gag reflex.
- Patient is less than 6 months.
- Patient ingested acid or alkali corrosive substances (such as drain cleaner, oven cleaner, toilet bowl cleaner).
- Patient ingested hydrocarbons (such as furniture polish, kerosene, gasoline, other petroleum products).
- Patient ingested rapid-acting central nervous system (CNS) depressant (such as tricyclic antidepressant, strychnine).

Emesis is usually induced within 15 to 30 minutes. For children older than 1 year these doses can be repeated once if no emesis occurs within this time.

After first aid measures the child should be transported to the emergency room if this is recommended. Gastric lavage is performed in selected cases. Activated charcoal may be given to retard toxin absorption further; to increase the rate of excretion, cathartics may be administered.

Other forms of treatment are given as indicated.

The following box lists substances of low toxicity if ingested.[10] Only mild gastrointestinal distress may be produced.

Nevertheless the ingestion of even a low-toxicity substance may indicate that the child is at risk for more serious problems and the incident provides an opportunity for further anticipatory guidance with the family.

Anticipatory guidance and injury prevention

Anticipatory guidance about the prevention of injuries is a very important component of each health promotion (well-child) visit. Since the type of injury to which children are susceptible varies according to developmental stage, Table 27-8, which classifies injuries by age, is helpful. It is included in the AAP TIPP program (see Resources).[42]

To highlight the importance of anticipatory guidance in injury prevention the Executive Board of the AAP issued the statement shown in the box on p. 518.

These five recommendations are related to major causes of childhood mortality and morbidity and are quite simple to implement.[42]

CHILD ABUSE, INCLUDING CHILD HOMICIDE: INTENTIONAL INJURIES

Although the rate of unintentional childhood injuries has been decreasing over recent years, this is not true of child homicide. Children may be killed, most often by a parent, as the result of a single act or repeated acts of physical abuse.[25] Annually 5000 deaths are attributed to child abuse. Another scenario is that of the murder/suicide situation in which an adult shoots family members and then commits suicide. Similarly a crazed individual may open fire on a group of unsuspecting and unknown victims and kill randomly, finally killing himself or herself. Newspaper reports of homicide that occurred after a child was abducted are sadly all too frequent and underscore the need for ongoing education about "stranger safety."[31]

Approximately 2 million cases of child abuse are reported annually; for every reported case many others escape detection. Child abuse includes physical abuse (75% of all cases), emotional abuse, sexual abuse (most frequently incest), and neglect. Any given child may suffer from a variety of these types of abuse. Prevention of child abuse may be possible when a health care provider can recognize an "at risk" situation. Parents of any socioeconomic background may have low frustration thresholds or personality disorders, may be living in particularly stress-

---

Low toxicity ingestions*

Abrasives	Hand lotions and creams
Adhesives	Ink (black, blue, indelible, felt-tip markers)
Antacids	Kaolin
Antibiotics	Lanolin
Baby product cosmetics	Linoleic acid
Ballpoint pen inks	Linseed oil
Bathtub floating toys	Lubricants and lubricating oils
Birth control pills	Newspapers
Calamine lotion	Paint (indoor and latex)
Candles (beeswax or paraffin)	Pencil (graphite)
Chalk (calcium carbonate)	Petroleum jelly (Vaseline)
Clay (modeling or Play Doh)	Polaroid picture coating fluid
Corticosteroids	Putty (less than 2 oz)
Cosmetics (most, except perfumes)	Sachets (essential oils, powder)
Crayons marked AP or CP	Shampoos and soap
Dehumidifying packets (silica)	Shoe polish (not containing aniline dyes)
Deodorants and deodorizers	Spackle
Etch-A-Sketch	Suntan preparations
Fabric softener	Sweetening agents (saccharin, cyclamate)
Fish bowl additives	Teething rings
Glues and pastes	Thermometers (mercury)
Greases	Tooth paste (without fluoride)
Gums	Vitamins without iron
Hair products (dyes, sprays, tonics)	Zinc oxide

From Barkin RM, editor: *Emergency pediatrics,* St. Louis, 1990, Mosby–Year Book.
*These materials generally do not produce significant toxicity except in large doses. Toxicity is altered if the patient is pregnant or has an underlying disease.

---

ful situations, or may be abusing alcohol or drugs. Children who are premature or handicapped are known to be at special risk for abuse; other children, for example, those who cry a great deal or who seem to be excessively active, may become abuse victims. Gentle, understanding inquiry about the possibility of these at risk situations during well-child visits may lead to the initiation of appropriate preventive interventions.

At other times prevention of further abuse must be addressed. In other words abuse has already occurred and recognition of the intentional injury is the issue.[30] If the history given for a particular injury seems implausible, given the type of injury and the developmental age of the child, then intentional (nonaccidental) injury must be suspected. An older child may have a history of new onset of difficulty sleeping, vague headaches, abdominal pains, anxious behavior, enuresis or encopresis as a result of abuse (especially sexual, where there is frequently no visible evidence of abuse).

Examination of an injured child may give rise to suspicion of abuse if there are bruises of unusual configuration, for example, that outline a belt strap or whip.[72] Cigarette burns to the skin or deliberate immersion scalds have a distinctive pattern. Findings on the skin of an abused child give the best clues leading to an accurate diagnosis. Fractures may occur; any fracture in a child less than 2 years old should arouse suspicion. If several fractures at different stages of healing are found, the child should be presumed to be a victim of abuse. Intracranial injuries may occur (especially in the "shaken child syndrome"); together with intraabdominal injuries they are the most frequent cause of fatal child abuse.

All states require that health professionals report suspected child abuse to the local Child Protective Service. Failure to do so is prosecutable in 37 states. Health care professionals are legally protected from liability if their suspicions turn out to be unfounded. Each abuse situation is investigated and strategies planned to ensure the ongoing safety of the child (and any siblings), either within the family's home or elsewhere, a foster home, for example. The child may need to be hospitalized briefly to provide a safe environment while the diagnosis of abuse is being investigated.

If a health care provider suspects child abuse, it is vital to remember that the factors leading to the abuse and the identity of the perpetrator should not be the concern of that provider. The only immediate concerns should be the well-being and safety of the child.

Policy statement on injury prevention approved by Executive Board of AAP

All children should grow up in a safe environment.

Anticipatory guidance for injury prevention should be an integral part of the medical care provided for all infants and children.

All physicians caring for children should advise parents to provide the following for their children's safety:

1. Currently approved child car restraints.
2. Smoke detectors in the home that would protect the child's sleeping area.
3. Safe hot-water temperatures at the tap.
4. Window and stairway guards/gates to prevent falls.
5. A 30 ml (1 oz) bottle of syrup of ipecac.

In addition, all physicians caring for children should counsel parents in age-appropriate, season-appropriate, and locality-appropriate prevention strategies that reduce common serious injuries. Medical records should reflect this counsel.

From McIntire M, editor: *Injury control for children and youth,* 1987, Elk Grove Village, Ill, American Academy of Pediatrics.

THE SCHOOL AS A PARTNER IN HEALTH PROMOTION

Since about one quarter of a child's time is spent in school, the school environment, both in and out of the classroom, can offer health promotion and disease prevention opportunities. Young people may start to use tobacco, alcohol, and marijuana by the time they are in grades six through eight; therefore education about the risks involved should begin in the elementary school.[69] Age-appropriate information about sexuality and sexually transmitted diseases, including acquired immunodeficiency syndrome (AIDS), should be made available in the preteen years. Likewise since violence is a part of life today, programs on conflict resolution and firearm risks are important for the same age group. The benefits of good nutrition and exercise habits can usefully be included in the health education curriculum and demonstrated in the school cafeteria, playground, gymnasium, and playing field.[20] The importance of motor vehicle, bicycle, and road safety can be stressed as part of the daily routine of traveling to and from school activities.

Early identification of learning, emotional, and behavioral problems may be prompted by the concerns of school personnel, thus helping to reduce or prevent long-term difficulties and secondary complications.

In some areas of the United States school-based health clinics provide preventive health education, counseling, and routine medical care to disadvantaged adolescents.[57]

School nurses, school physicians, and social workers play important roles on the team of health professionals working together to promote the well-being of children, both now and in the future.[47]

CHILDREN AND TELEVISION

The media could function as a powerful force for positive health habits and attitudes in America. Unfortunately, at the present time, they are mostly part of the problem and only rarely are they part of the solution.[60]

No one would argue in this day and age whether television plays a major role in family life. Children are often placed in front of a television set from infancy and become interested in following programs from the age of 2 years or so. We know that from then on most children spend 3 to 5 hours daily on television viewing.[59] The United States is the only Western nation that does not produce at least 1 hour per day of educational programming on its national networks. Rather our children are growing up with a daily opportunity to watch violent, aggressive behavior in the form of murders, rapes, armed robberies, assaults, and shootings; sexual behavior, obvious and inferred, apparently bereft of any harmful consequences; use of alcohol emphasized in "successful" socializing and as a part of stress reduction; and commercials between programs that encourage the purchase of beer and wine and use sexual overtones to promote the sale of all kinds of products. Music videos on MTV are often sexually suggestive and may be violent in addition. Overall people's problems on television programs seem to be resolved with "a quick fix"; instant gratification is the message.

It has been shown that growing up with these influences can lead to an effortless, passive absorption and acceptance by children of the behavior modeled on television.[49] A subtle shaping of attitudes and beliefs can occur as the child develops. Whereas most adults recognize that life in television programs is not "real," this may not be true for children, so that the effects of television on them may be more powerful.

What is learned in childhood may be played out in adolescence. The leading causes of death in adolescence are automobile accidents, homicides, and suicides. Many such deaths are alcohol related. Deaths from gunshot injuries are common. Associated morbidities are also high. The U.S. teen pregnancy rate is over 1 million/year and sexually transmitted diseases are common.

There is also a displacement effect, unhealthy in itself, brought about by television.[60] The hours spent watching television make less time available for worthwhile activities such as reading and other hobbies, playing with friends, or becoming involved in sports. In addition the lack of physical activity associated with watching television may lead to obesity. Paradoxically the tendency of television programs to overemphasize thinness may sway some teens toward the eating disorder of anorexia nervosa.

What can be done to help prevent the harmful effects of television viewing? How can television be used to transmit positive messages?

The AAP Committee on Communications issued the policy statement *"Children, adolescents and television"* in

Table 27-8. Childhood injuries and prevention methods, by age

Typical injuries	Normal behavioral characteristics	Parental precautions
First year Car crashes Falls Choking Fires Burns Drowning	At 3 months can wiggle, roll and reach, followed by creeping and standing. Puts any and everything in mouth. Helpless in water.	Use a safe car seat. Never leave infants alone on tables, beds, etc. Use safe cribs and gates. Keep small objects, hard foods, and harmful substances out of reach. Never leave alone in or near water, hot liquids, or any heat source. Install a smoke detector. Have syrup of ipecac in home. Know how to save a choking child.
Second year Poisoning Falls Burns Drowning Car crashes	Can walk, run, climb, jump, and explore. Likes "cooking" and other imitative behavior. Cannot swim but can learn "water confidence."	Use safety caps. Store all household products and medicines out of reach. Use window screens and gates. Keep toddlers in enclosed space when outdoors and not closely supervised. Install safety covers on electric outlets; keep electric cords, handles of pots and pans on stove out of reach, and hot foods away from edge of table. Never leave child in tub or pool. Lower hot water heater to 120°-130° F. Use toddler car seat.
2-4 years Falls Burns Poisoning Drowning Car crashes	Can open doors and drawers. Runs, climbs and rides a tricycle. Uses tools, plays with mechanical gadgets. Can throw ball and other objects. Interested in fire.	Keep doors locked in dangerous areas. Use screens, guards and gates. Teach about watching for autos in driveways and streets, and danger of following ball into street. Keep firearms locked up. Keep medicines, knives, electrical equipment and matches out of reach. Group swimming lessons after 3 years.
5-9 years Car crashes Bicycle accidents Drowning Firearms Burns	Daring and adventurous. Better control over large than small muscles. Loyal to group, willing to follow suggestions of leaders, takes dares.	Teach pedestrian, motor vehicle, and bicycle safety. No highway bicycling under age 10. Use seat belts. Continue swimming classes. Keep firearms locked up except when adults can supervise. Age 6 is the youngest for unsupervised play with dogs.
10-14 years Car crashes Bicycle accidents Firearms Drowning Burns Falls	Seeks strenuous physical activity, likes novel sites and plays in hazardous places. Need for approval and self-assertion leads to daring and hazardous feats.	Continue rules of bicycle, boat, and motor vehicle safety with good examples set by adults. Instruct in safe use of firearms and fireworks. Provide safe facilities for recreation and social activities. Stress the buddy system in all sports.

Modified from Shaffer TF: Accident prevention, *Pediatr Clin North Am* 1:426, 1954 and TIPP, American Academy of Pediatrics.

1990.[3] It recommends that parents monitor programs that their children watch, selecting those that carry more positive messages. Viewing television together as a family allows discussion and sharing of values. Limiting television watching to 1 hour daily modifies harmful effects and leaves time for other enjoyable healthy activities.

Television consumers in general and providers of care to children in particular can lobby for increased overall regulation of television by the Federal Communications Commission (FCC) and for increased educational programming. Cigarette companies voluntarily withdrew their advertisements from television when counteradvertising was threatened; children's caregivers can push for the disappearance of beer and wine commercials.[60] On the other hand a protest in favor of advertisements for birth control needs to be waged. Further ongoing research on the effects of television on children is needed.

LEAD SCREENING

The U.S. Public Health Service estimates that more than 3 million children below age 7 have elevated lead levels in their blood—one child in every six (17%).[25] No economic or social subgroup of children is safe from the risk of having blood lead levels high enough to cause adverse health effects. The risks are greatest, however, for poor inner city children living in older housing that contains leaded paint. One of 10 such children aged 6 months to 5 years has a level above 25 µg/dl and 2 of 3 have levels above 15 µg/dl.[67]

Children, especially those less than 6 years, are more sensitive to the toxic effects of lead than are adults, and since lead crosses the placenta, the fetus is at particular risk. Lead primarily affects the peripheral and central nervous systems, resulting in problems ranging from the now exceedingly rare acute lead encephalopathy (usually associated with levels above 80 µg/dl) to much more subtle effects. In the last decade researchers such as Needleman have shown that blood lead levels as low as 10 to 25 µg/dl can have deleterious effects on behavior, learning, and development ("subclinical poisoning").[46] This is depicted in Figure 27-11.[67]

In 1970 the CDC defined lead poisoning as a blood lead level of 30 µg/dl or more; in 1985 as a result of later studies the toxic level was lowered to 25 µg/dl. New guidelines from the CDC in 1991 specify 10 µg/dl as the level above which action should be taken.[18,45]

The major source of lead is lead based paint. Recently it has been recognized that a child need not eat paint chips to cause an elevated lead level; ingestion of lead dust generated by everyday wear and tear on lead painted surfaces is a greater threat. Removing lead based paint by scraping or sanding creates high concentrations of lead dust that can be dangerous.[68] Lead dust settles on household objects and surfaces or in soil and is ingested by children's mouthing of contaminated items or by hand-to-mouth transfer. Other sources of lead include lead related industries, water from leaded pipes or pipes with lead solder, and automobile emissions. Lead from auto exhausts may be inhaled or deposited in soil. Less common sources are certain imported ceramic dishes, various folk remedies, and unusual ethnic cosmetics.

The amount of lead permitted in gasoline was reduced in 1987. Paint manufacturers removed much of the lead from paint in the 1950s, and the lead content of paint was regulated in 1977. However 74% of all private housing built before 1980 contains some lead paint and 3 million tons of old lead line the walls and fixtures of 57 million American homes (U.S. Department of Housing and Urban Development 1990). This is why the lead problem persists.

In an effort to prevent lead poisoning the new CDC recommendations include universal screening of all children less than 6 years, rather than the more selective testing previously suggested (CDC 1985; AAP 1987). Free erythrocyte protoporphyrin (FEP), commonly assayed as zinc protoporphyrin (ZPP), until now the test of choice for lead screening, is not sensitive at the lower levels of lead poi-

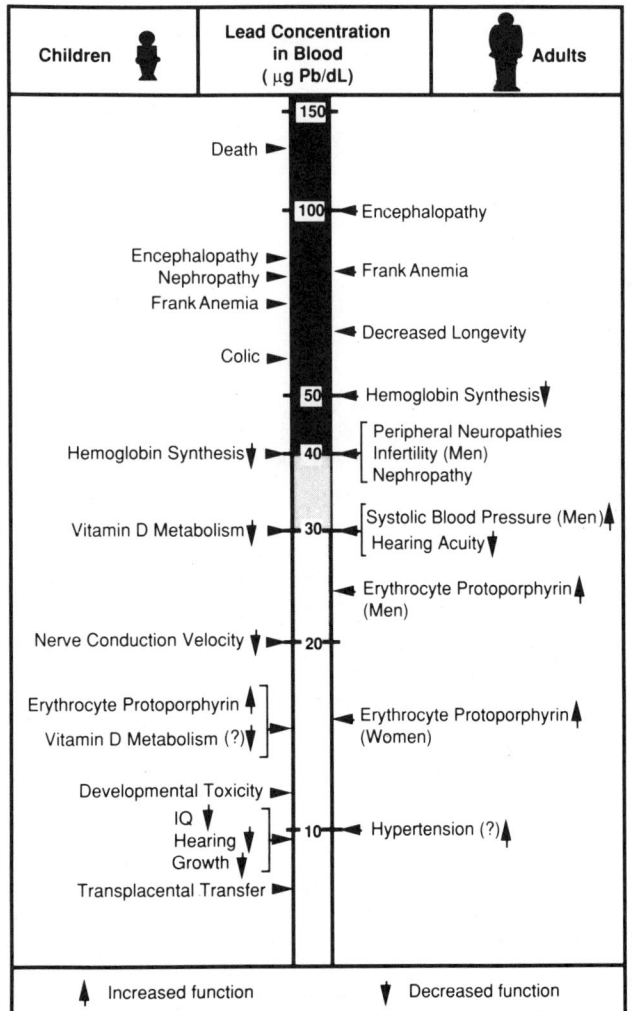

Fig. 27-11. Effects of inorganic lead on children and adults—lowest observable adverse effect levels. (Adapted from AISDR: *Case studies in environmental medicine, lead toxicity,* U.S. Dept. of Health and Human Services, Public Health Service, June 1990.)

soning; blood lead level should be determined instead.[67] Local health departments can identify sources of lead in or around the home and can provide families with information on how to remove or cover up lead based paint safely.[68] Suburban owners of older homes need to be aware of lead poisoning dangers before renovations are carried out, since they may not realize that problems with lead can be associated with dwellings other than inner city dilapidated housing. Iron and calcium deficiencies should be prevented because the quantity of lead absorbed increases significantly in these conditions.

Neurologic consequences of chronic exposure to lead are irreversible. The aim of society must be to remove lead from the environment and thus eliminate one of the most common environmental hazards to U.S. children.[45] In practice this is a difficult and expensive task.[9]

SCREENING FOR TUBERCULOSIS

The incidence of tuberculosis (TB) has recently increased after showing a decline from 1963 to 1985.[25,35] The disease is particularly common in the aged, the homeless, minority groups, those living in poverty, and individuals infected with HIV. Children of all ages, especially infants and adolescents, are susceptible.

Screening is performed by the Mantoux test or multiple puncture tests (tine, Heaf, Mono-Vacc).[50] The Mantoux test, in which 5 units (5 TU) of tuberculin purified protein derivative (PPD) is injected intradermally, is the most accurate tuberculin skin test. A positive test result, read at 48 to 72 hours, consists of induration (not erythema alone) of more than 10 to 15 mm diameter. For children at high risk induration of 5 to 9 mm diameter should be considered positive. Multiple puncture tests are less accurate, though easier to administer. Positive reactions to a multiple puncture test should be confirmed by a Mantoux test.

Annual tuberculin testing of high-risk children is recommended. High-risk groups include poor and minority children, those who live with a tuberculous adult, and those who have a cellular immune deficiency such as HIV infection.[35] For low-risk groups testing is recommended at 12 to 15 months, before school entry, and in adolescence.

Children who have a positive Mantoux test result should have a chest roentgenogram and clinical evaluation for TB. If active disease is present, treatment guidelines should be followed. If no evidence of active disease is found, a course of isoniazid (INH) should be given to protect against its development. The recommended dose of INH is 10 mg/kg (maximum 300 mg) once daily in a single dose. This should be continued for 9 months in infants and children. Children with HIV infection should have preventive therapy for at least 12 months. The incidence of INH-induced hepatitis in otherwise healthy infants and children is extremely low.

BCG vaccination

Bacille Calmette-Guerin (BCG) vaccine is a live vaccine derived from attenuated strains of *Mycobacterium bovis*. BCG vaccination is rarely required in the United States, where the risk of acquiring tuberculosis is relatively low.[50] However BCG vaccination should be considered for the following groups of tuberculin-negative children when compliance or success with INH prophylaxis is unlikely: Children who live in households where they have repeated exposure to untreated or ineffectively treated patients with active disease; children continuously exposed to patients with TB resistant to INH or rifampin; children living in communities where the rate of new infections is greater than 1% per year and where usual screening and treatment programs are not feasible; children with asymptomatic HIV infection who are at high risk of exposure to active TB.

Prior BCG vaccination usually induces a positive tuber-culin skin test result. As time goes by, skin test reactivity diminishes. Most children show less than 10 mm of induration if skin testing is carried out more than 10 years after BCG vaccination. BCG is unlikely to produce more than 15 mm of induration at any time. Since there is no method of distinguishing a positive skin test result caused by BCG from that caused by *M. tuberculosis,* a positive result in a BCG recipient may indicate the need for preventive chemotherapy with INH.

PREVENTION OF DENTAL DISEASE

The 20 deciduous teeth normally erupt between the age of about 6 months to 2 years and the permanent teeth (32 in number, including the "wisdom teeth," the third molars) normally erupt between 6 and 22 years of age. When sugar is eaten the bacteria in plaque produce acids that attack tooth enamel. Eventually the enamel may break down and a cavity may form. Recent studies show that 58% of children aged 6 to 8 and 78% of 15-year-olds have caries.[69] The average adult in the United States has 10 to 17 decayed, missing, or filled permanent teeth. Periodontal diseases are also common in adults.

The following points are important in the prevention of dental caries and periodontal disease[23]:

- Fluoridate community water supplies.
- Give fluoride supplements for infants and children where water fluoridation is not available. This is given from birth to 13 years of age. The dosage of fluoride supplements is shown in Table 27-9.
- Prevention of nursing bottle tooth decay by discouraging the practice of putting a baby to bed with a bottle containing fruit juice, milk, or formula.
- At age 1½ to 2 years the child mimics adult behavior by brushing his or her own teeth.[31]
- At this age encourage the child to brush his or her teeth daily; add flossing when feasible.
- Use of fluoride-containing toothpaste.
- Avoid an excess of sugary foods.
- Arrange the first dental visit at age 3 years.
- Encourage the school-aged child to brush his or her teeth at least once daily; add flossing when feasible.
- Arrange dental check-ups at least once every year for school-aged children.

Table 27-9. Dosage of fluoride supplements

Age	Water fluoride <0.3 ppm*	Water fluoride 0.3-0.7 ppm	Water fluoride >0.7 ppm
2 wk-2 yr	0.25 mg/day	—	—
2-3 yr	0.5 mg/day	0.25 mg/day	—
>3 yr	1 mg/day	0.5 mg/day	—

From Crawl JJ: *Pediatr Clin North Am* 33:4, 1986.
ppm, parts per million.

Table 27-10. Prophylactic regimens for neonatal gonococcal ophthalmia, recurrent otitis media, recurrent urinary tract infections

Infection	Prevention	Length of treatment
Neonatal gonococcal ophthalmia	1% silver nitrate drops or 0.5% erythromycin ointment or 1% tetracycline drops or ointment	Topically into each eye, one time
Recurrent otitis media	Amoxicillin 20 mg/kg up to 250 mg or Sulfisoxazole 50-75 mg/kg/day in 2 divided doses up to max of 3 g/day 50-75 mg/kg/bid up to maximum of 3 g/day	Once daily for weeks/months po Two doses daily for weeks/months po
Recurrent urinary tract infections	Trimethoprim-Sulfa (TMP) 2 mg/kg/24 hr or Nitrofurantoin 1-2 mg/kg up to 100 mg	Once daily at night for weeks/months po Once daily at night for weeks/months po

Modified from Peter G, editor: *Report of the committee on infectious diseases,* 1991, Elk Grove Village, Ill, American Academy of Pediatrics.

- Apply topical fluoride in the form of mouth rinses, solutions, or gels that act at the surface of the teeth to help prevent decay; many schools offer weekly fluoride mouth rinse ("swish") programs.
- Apply topical plastic sealants to the chewing surfaces of premolars and molars to provide the teeth a barrier to plaque and acid.
- Avoid smoking and alcohol use, which jeopardize oral health.

The incidence of dental caries among children has declined in recent years, yet many, especially individuals in lower socioeconomic groups, still obtain no regular dental care.

CHEMOPROPHYLAXIS

Chemoprophylaxis in children is used to prevent neonatal gonococcal ophthalmia, bacterial endocarditis, recurrent otitis media, recurrent urinary tract infection, recurrent rheumatic fever, and, in asplenic children, fulminant bacteremia.[50]

Table 27-10 outlines prophylactic regimens for neonatal gonococcal ophthalmia, recurrent otitis media, and recurrent urinary tract infections.

Prevention of bacterial endocarditis

Prophylaxis is recommended for the following cardiac conditions: (1) most congenital cardiac malformations, (2) previous history of bacterial endocarditis, (3) rheumatic and other acquired valvular dysfunction, (4) hypertrophic cardiomyopathy, (5) mitral valve prolapse with insufficiency, (6) prosthetic cardiac valves.

Prophylaxis should be given to such patients undergoing the following procedures: (1) all dental procedures likely to induce gingival bleeding, (2) tonsillectomy and/or adenoidectomy, (3) surgical procedures or biopsy involving respiratory mucosa, (4) bronchoscopy, (5) incision and

Table 27-11. Prevention of recurrences of rheumatic fever

Drug	Patient weight >60 lb (27.3 kg)	Patient weight <60 lbs
Benzathine penicillin G or	1,200,000 U IM once every 3-4 weeks	
Penicillin V or	250 mg (400,000 U) twice a day po	125 mg (200,000 U) twice a day po
Sulfadiazine	1 g once a day po	0.5 g once a day po

Modified from Peter G, editor: *Report of the Committee on Infectious Diseases,* 1991, Elk Grove Village, Ill, American Academy of Pediatrics.

drainage of infected tissue, (6) a variety of genitourinary and gastrointestinal procedures.

Figure 27-12 represents a patient information card printed by the American Heart Association, outlining prophylaxis for dental/oral/upper respiratory tract and genitourinary/gastrointestinal procedures. Pediatric dosages are described.[8]

Prevention of recurrences of rheumatic fever

Antibiotics are given long-term, perhaps for life, to prevent group A streptococcal infections, which could lead to a recurrence of rheumatic fever (secondary prophylaxis).[50]

Table 27-11 shows antibiotic dosages for the prevention of recurrences of rheumatic fever.

Prophylaxis of fulminant bacteremia in asplenic children

Asplenic individuals, regardless of age, have an increased risk of fulminant bacteremia.[50] Organisms responsible for such bacteremia are *Streptococcus pneumoniae*

Name: _____

needs protection from
BACTERIAL ENDOCARDITIS
because of an existing
HEART CONDITION

Diagnosis: _____

Prescribed by: _____

Date: _____

For Dental/Oral/Upper Respiratory Tract Procedures

I. Standard Regimen In Patients At Risk (includes those with prosthetic heart valves and other high risk patients):

Amoxicillin 3.0 g orally one hour before procedure, then 1.5 g six hours after initial dose.*

For amoxicillin/penicillin-allergic patients:

Erythromycin ethylsuccinate 800 mg or erythromycin stearate 1.0 g orally 2 hours before a procedure, then one-half the dose 6 hours after the initial administration.*

—OR—

Clindamycin 300 mg orally 1 hour before a procedure and 150 mg 6 hours after initial dose.*

II. Alternate Prophylactic Regimens For Dental/Oral/Upper Respiratory Tract Procedures In Patients At Risk:

A. For patients unable to take oral medications:

Ampicillin 2.0 g IV (or IM) 30 minutes before procedure, then ampicillin 1.0 g IV (or IM) OR amoxicillin 1.5 g orally 6 hours after initial dose.*

—OR—

For ampicillin/amoxicillin/penicillin-allergic patients unable to take oral medications:

Clindamycin 300 mg IV 30 minutes before a procedure and 150 mg IV (or orally) 6 hours after initial dose.*

B. For patients considered to be at high risk who are not candidates for the standard regimen:

Ampicillin 2.0 g IV (or IM) plus gentamicin 1.5 mg/kg IV (or IM) (not to exceed 80 mg) 30 minutes before procedure, followed by amoxicillin 1.5 g orally 6 hours after the initial dose. Alternatively, the parenteral regimen may be repeated 8 hours after the initial dose.*

For amoxicillin/ampicillin/penicillin-allergic patients considered to be at high risk:

Vancomycin 1.0 g IV administered over one hour, starting one hour before the procedure. No repeat dose is necessary.*

*Note: Initial pediatric dosages are listed below. Follow-up oral dose should be one-half the inital dose. Total pediatric dose should not exceed total adult dose.

Amoxicillin:†	50 mg/kg	Vancomycin:	20 mg/kg
Clindamycin:	10 mg/kg	Ampicillin:	50 mg/kg
Erythromycin ethylsuccinate		Gentamicin:	2.0 mg/kg
or stearate:	20 mg/kg		

† The following weight ranges may also be used for the initial pediatric dose of amoxicillin:
<15 kg (33 lbs), 750 mg
15–30 kg (33–66 lbs), 1500 mg
>30 kg (66 lbs), 3000 mg (full adult dose)

Kilogram to pound conversion chart: (1 kg = 2.2 lb)

Kg	Lb
5	11.0
10	22.0
20	44.0
30	66.0
40	88.0
50	110.0

For Genitourinary/Gastrointestinal Procedures

I. Standard regimen:

Ampicillin 2.0 g IV (or IM) plus gentamicin 1.5 mg/kg IV (or IM) (not to exceed 80 mg) 30 minutes before procedure, followed by amoxicillin 1.5 g orally 6 hours after the initial dose. Alternatively, the parenteral regimen may be repeated once 8 hours after the initial dose.*

For amoxicillin/ampicillin/penicillin-allergic patients:

Vancomycin 1.0 g IV administered over 1 hour plus gentamicin 1.5 mg/kg IV (or IM) (not to exceed 80 mg) one hour before the procedure. May be repeated once 8 hours after initial dose.**

II. Alternate oral regimen for low-risk patients:

Amoxicillin 3.0 g orally one hour before the procedure, then 1.5 g 6 hours after the initial dose.**

**Note: Initial pediatric dosages are listed below. Follow-up oral dose should be one-half the initial dose. Total pediatric dose should not exceed total adult dose.

Ampicillin:	50 mg/kg	Gentamicin:	2.0 mg/kg
Amoxicillin:	50 mg/kg	Vancomycin:	20 mg/kg

Note: Antibiotic regimens used to prevent recurrences of acute rheumatic fever are inadequate for the prevention of bacterial endocarditis. In patients with markedly compromised renal function, it may be necessary to modify or omit the second dose of gentamicin or vancomycin. Intramuscular injections may be contraindicated in patients receiving anticoagulants.

Adapted from *Prevention of Bacterial Endocarditis: Recommendations by the American Heart Association* by the Committee on Rheumatic Fever, Endocarditis, and Kawasaki Disease. *JAMA* 1990;264:2919–2922, © 1990 American Medical Association (also excerpted in *J Am Dent Assoc* 1991;122:87–92).

Please refer to these joint American Heart Association–American Dental Association recommendations for more complete information as to which patients and which procedures require prophylaxis.

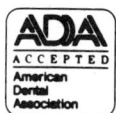 **American Heart Association**

National Center
7320 Greenville Avenue
Dallas, Texas 75231

78-1003 (CP)
90-100M
4-91-511.2M
90 06 19 B

The Council on Dental Therapeutics of the American Dental Association has approved this statement as it relates to dentistry.

Fig. 27-12. Patient information care, bacterial endocarditis handout (From Committee on Rheumatic fever, Endocarditis, and Kawasaki Disease; Prevention of bacterial endocarditis: recommendations by the American Heart Association, *JAMA* 264:2919-2922, 1990.)

Table 27-12. Prophylactic regimen for asplenic children

Drug	Child >5 years of age	Child <5 years of age
Penicillin V or	250 mg bid po	125 mg bid po
Amoxicillin or		20 mg/kg/day po
Trimethoprim-sulfamethoxazole (TMP)		TMP 4 mg/kg/day

Adapted from Peter G, editor: Report of the Committee on Infectious Diseases, 1991, Elk Grove Village, Ill, American Academy of Pediatrics.

(most common), *Neisseria meningitides, Haemophilus influenzae* type B, and *Escherichia coli.* The risk of dying of such sepsis depends on the cause of asplenia. The mortality rate is much higher in thalassemia than in sickle cell disease, which in turn carries a much greater risk than splenectomy after trauma.

Daily prophylaxis given to children with sickle cell disease has been shown to be effective in reducing the incidence of severe bacterial infection by 84% in comparison to that in placebo treated children. Authorities feel that prophylaxis should be strongly considered for all asplenic children less than 5 years of age and considered for older children (Table 27-12). It is not clear at what age prophylaxis should be discontinued.

In addition pneumococcal vaccine and meningococcal vaccine should be administered to asplenic children 2 years and older. Routine immunization against *Haemophilus influenzae* type B should be given from 2 months of age.

SUMMARY

The responsibility of promoting health and preventing disease in children is a shared one. Persons in many different disciplines—teachers and other school personnel, nurses, social workers, physicians, dentists, allied health workers, church officials, community leaders, politicians, law enforcement officers, and housing officials, as well as parents—all play a role. Despite the successes of health promotion during this century, problems remain.

The number of children and young adults infected with HIV continues to increase. Especially rapid increases are occurring in babies born to women in high-risk groups.[50] Long-term implications of these trends are alarming, in terms of both human suffering and treatment costs.[69] Intense research with the hope of development of a vaccine continues. Prevention is crucial and public education regarding high-risk behavior is mandatory.

Nearly 25% of children less than 6 years of age are members of families whose income is below the federal poverty level. Low socioeconomic status is a major risk factor for poor health in all age groups.[30] Children in poor families are more likely to suffer frequent illness and more resulting disability and complications than other children. The death rate of poor children is higher in all age groups.[69] They are more likely to live in unsafe, overcrowded conditions and to be exposed to environmental hazards such as lead poisoning. Such children are less likely to have positive educational experiences and their families frequently lack social support. If and when health care providers have contact with these children, an awareness of their problems should intensify efforts to provide needed health care.

More than 30 million Americans have no form of health insurance.[1] This figure includes one of every six children and one of every four pregnant women. Even when families carry insurance, preventive care is often not covered. Lack of health insurance, total or relative, is the most significant barrier to health care access in the United States. Currently the AAP is campaigning for a national health plan so that all children less than 21 years and all pregnant women can receive necessary care.[34] Legislative action is actively being sought.

The challenge of meeting the health care needs of young people continues. When interacting with children and their families we must all take full advantage of the opportunity to discuss prudent life-style choices, effective coping skills, and preventable types of morbidity and mortality. Whenever possible genetic predisposition to certain diseases must be diagnosed early and appropriate interventions provided.

The aim of pediatrics is to assist each boy and girl to reach maturity equipped physically, mentally, and socially to function as responsible members of society within the limits approaching his/her own potential, and to have the opportunity of thoroughly enjoying the years of getting there. (Dr. Waldo Nelson 1972)

REFERENCES

1. American Academy of Pediatrics: *Children first . . . access to health care, a legislative proposal,* Washington DC, 1990, Department of Government Liaison.
2. American Academy of Pediatrics: Committee on Adolescence: Firearms and adolescents, *Pediatrics* 89(4):784-787, 1992.
3. American Academy of Pediatrics: Committee on Communications: *Policy statement: update: children, adolescents and television,* Elk Grove Village, IL, 1990, American Academy of Pediatrics.
4. American Academy of Pediatrics: Committee on Infectious Diseases: Universal hepatitis B Immunization, *Pediatrics* 89(4):795-799, 1992.
5. American Academy of Pediatrics: Committee on Injury and Poison Prevention: Firearm injuries affecting the pediatric population, *Pediatrics* 89(4):788-789, 1992.
6. American Academy of Pediatrics, Committee on Nutrition: Indications for cholesterol testing in children, *Pediatrics* 83:141-142, 1988.
7. American Heart Association: 1987 *heart facts,* Dallas, TX, 1987, American Heart Association.
8. American Heart Association: Prevention of bacterial endocarditis: recommendation, Committee on rheumatic fever, endocarditis, and Kawasaki disease, *JAMA* 264:2929-2922, 1990.

9. Amitai Y et al: Residential deleading: effects on the blood lead levels of lead-poisoned children, *Pediatrics* 88:893, 1991.

10. Barkin RM, editor: *Emergency pediatrics,* ed 3, St. Louis, 1990, Mosby-Year Book.

11. Berenson GS et al: Review: atherosclerosis and its evolution in childhood, *Am J Med Sci* 294:429-440, 1987.

12. Berenson GS et al.: Risk factors in early life as predictors of adult heart disease: the Bogalusa Heart Study, *Am J Med Sci* 298:141-151, 1989.

13. Blacklader AD: The president's annual address, *Trans Am Pediatr Soc,* 5:8-16, 1893.

14. Bock GH, editor: Hypertension in infancy and childhood, *Pediatr Ann* 18:529, 1989.

15. Brown MS, Goldstein JL: A receptor-mediated pathway for cholesterol homeostasis, *Science* 232:34-47, 1986.

16. Castelli WP: Epidemiology of coronary heart disease: the Framingham study, *Am J Med* 76(2A):4-12, 1984.

17. Centers for Disease Control: Measles prevention: recommendations of the Immunization Practices Advisory Committee (ACIP), *MMWR* 38:1, 1989.

18. Centers for Disease Control: Preventing lead poisoning in young children: a statement by the Centers for Disease Control, Atlanta, CA, 1991, US Dept of Health and Human Services.

19. Centers for Disease Control: Rubella vaccination during pregnancy—United States—1971-1988, *MMWR* 38:289, 1989.

20. Charney E, editor: *Well-child care, report of the Seventeenth Ross Roundtable on critical approaches to common pediatric problems,* Columbus, OH, 1986, Ross Laboratories.

21. Christoffel KK: Toward reducing pediatric injuries from firearms: charting a legislative and regulatory course, *Pediatrics* 88:294, 1991.

22. Cortner JA, Coates PM, Gallagher PR: Prevalence and expression of familial combined hyperlipidemia in childhood, *J Pediatr* 116:514-519, 1990.

23. Crall JJ: Promotion of oral health and prevention of common pediatric dental problems, *Pediatr Clin North Am* 33:4, 1986

24. Eisenberg L: Preventive pediatrics: the promise and the peril, *Pediatrics* 80:415, 1987.

25. Fisher M, editor: *Guide to clinical preventive services, report of U.S. Preventive Service Task Force,* Baltimore, 1989, William and Wilkins.

26. Frigoletto FD, Little GA, editors: *Guidelines for perinatal care,* ed 2, Elk Grove Village, IL, 1988, American Academy of Pediatrics.

27. Fulginiti VA: Pediatric patient education: challenge for the '80s, *Pediatrics* Suppl 74:913, 1984.

28. Gertmaker SL, Dietz WH: Increasing pediatric obesity in the United States, *Am J Dis Child* 141:535-559, 1987.

29. Gilbert GG, Montes JH, Ross JG: *Summary of findings from the National Children and Youth Fitness Study,* Washington DC, 1984, Office of Disease Prevention and Health Promotion. Public Health Service, U.S. Department of Health and Human Services. Government Printing Office.

30. Green M, Haggerty RJ: *Ambulatory pediatrics III,* Philadelphia, 1984, WB Saunders.

31. Green M, editor: *Guidelines for health supervision II,* Elk Grove Village, IL, 1988, American Academy of Pediatrics.

32. Greensher J: Recent advances in injury prevention, *Pediatr Rev* 10:171, 1988.

33. Haggerty RJ, Roghmann KJ, Pless IB: *Child health and the community,* New York, 1975, Wiley.

34. Harvey B: Special report: a proposal to provide health insurance to all children and all pregnant women, *N Engl J Med* 323:1216, 1990.

35. Inselman LS: Tuberculosis in children: an unsettling forecast, *Contemp Pediatr* 7:10, 111-130, 1990.

36. Jopling RJ: Health related fitness as preventive medicine, *Pediatr Rev* 10(5):141-148, 1988.

37. Karp S: A 10-point program for bicycle safety, *Contemp Pediatr* 4:16, 1987.

38. Kraus: Unfit kids, *Contemp Pediatr* 5:18-47, April 1988.

39. Kwiterovich PO Jr: Biochemical, clinical, epidemiological, genetic and pathologic data in the pediatric age group relevant to the cholesterol hypothesis, *Pediatrics* 78:349-362, 1986.

40. Kwiterovich PO Jr: Diagnosis and management of familial dyslipoproteinemia in children and adolescents. *Pediatr Clin North Am* 37(6):1489-1523, 1990.

41. Lawn RM, Berg K: Lipoprotein(a) and atherosclerosis - Davis Conference. Angelo N. Scaner: Moderator. *Ann Intern Med* 115:209-218, 1991.

42. McIntire M, editor: *Injury control for children and youth,* Elk Grove Village, IL, 1987, American Academy of Pediatrics.

43. Moffitt JE, Feldman S: Chickenpox: new dangers, new therapies, *Contemp Pediatr* 8:13, 1991.

44. National Cholesterol Education Program: Report of the Expert Panel on Blood Cholesterol Levels in Children and Adolescents, NHLBI Information Center, Draft Report 4/17/91.

45. Needleman HL, Jackson RJ: Lead toxicity in the 21st century: will we still be treating it? *Pediatrics* 89(4):678-680, 1992 (commentary).

46. Needleman et al: The long-term effects of exposure to lead in childhood: an 11-year follow-up report, *N Engl J Med* 322:83, 1990.

47. Newton J, editor: *School health: a guide for health professionals,* Elk Grove Village, IL, 1987, American Academy of Pediatrics.

48. Osborn LM, Woolley FR: The use of groups in well-child care, *Pediatrics* 67:701, 1981.

49. Pearl D, Bouthilet L, Lazar J, editors: Television and behavior: ten years of scientific progress and implications for the eighties. DHHS Publication ADM 82-1195, 1 and ADM 82-1196, 2. Washington DC US Government Printing Office, 1982.

50. Peter G, editor: *Report of the committee on infectious diseases,* ed 22, Elk Grove Village, IL, 1991, American Academy of Pediatrics.

51. Phillips CF: Keeping up with the changing immunization schedule, *Contemp Pediatr* 8:20, 1991.

52. Reisinger K, Bires J: Anticipatory guidance in pediatric practice, *Pediatrics* 66:889, 1980.

53. Ringel RE: Essential hypertension and the role of dietary salt. American Academy of Pediatrics National Meeting, Chicago, October 24, 1989.

54. Riopel DA et al: Coronary risk factor modification in children: exercise. *Circulation* 74(5):1189A-1192A, 1986.

55. Robbins FC: The long view, *Am J Dis Child* 104:99, 1962.

56. Rosenbaum M, Leibel RL: Obesity in childhood, *Pediatr Rev* 11(2):43-55, 1989.

57. School-Based Clinics: *A guide for advocates,* Houston, 1988, Support Center for School-Based Clinics.

58. Silvis GL, Perry CL: Understanding and deterring tobacco use among adolescents, *Pediatr Clin North Am* 34(2):363-376, 1987.

59. Singer DG, Benton W: Caution: television may be hazardous to a child's mental health, *J Dev Behav Pediatr* 10:259, 1989.

60. Strasberger VC: Television and adolescents: sex, drugs, rock'n'roll. In *Adolescent medicine: state of the art reviews,* Philadelphia, 1990, Hanley and Belkus, Inc.

61. Strong WB, Dennison BA: Pediatric preventive cardiology: atherosclerosis and coronary heart disease, *Pediatr Rev* 9:303-314, 1988.

62. Strong WB: The Child: when to begin preventive cardiology, *Curr Probl Pediatr* 14(6): 1984.

63. Summitt RL, editor: *Comprehensive pediatrics,* St. Louis, 1990, Mosby–Year Book.

64. Task force for blood pressure control in children, *Pediatrics* 79(1):1-25, 1978.

65. The Expert Panel: Report of the National Cholesterol Education Program: expert panel of detection, evaluation and treatment of high blood cholesterol in adults, *Arch Intern Med* 148:36-61, 1988.

66. The health benefits of smoking cessation: a report of the Surgeon General, Centers for Disease Control, U.S. Department of Health and Human Services Publication, 90-8416, 1990.

67. U.S. Department of Health and Human Services: *Case studies in environmental medicine—lead toxicity,* 1990.

68. U.S. Consumer Product Safety Commission Safety Alert: *What you should know about lead-based paint in your home,* 1990.

69. U.S. Department of Health and Human Services: Healthy people 2000, Washington DC, 1990.

70. U.S. Public Health Service: *Teenage smoking: national patterns of cigarette smoking, ages 12 through 18, in 1972 and 1974,* U.S. Department of Health, Education and Welfare No (NIH) 76-931, 1976.

71. Wegman ME: Annual summary of vital statistics, *Pediatrics* 88:1081, 1991.

72. Wissow LS: Child advocacy for the clinician, an approach to child abuse and neglect, Baltimore, 1990, Williams and Wilkins.

73. Wittler RR et al: Measles revaccination response in a school-age population, *Pediatrics* 88:1024, 1991.

74. Wynder EL: Cholesterol: a pediatric perspective, American Health Foundation Monograph, Coronary Artery Disease Prevention. *Prev Med* 18:323-409, 1989.

RESOURCES

Prenatal care

American College of Obstetricians and Gynecologists (ACOG), 409 12th Street SW, Washington DC 20024-2188.

Healthy Mothers, Healthy Babies Coalition, 409 12th Street SW, Washington DC 200024-2188.

National Pregnancy Hotline, 1-800-852-5683; 1-800-831-5081 (California). Provides counseling and referral to pregnant women.

National Down Syndrome Society, 1-800-221-4602.

Spina Bifida Hotline, 1-800-3141.

March of Dimes Birth Defects Foundation, 1275 Mamaroneck Ave, White Plains, NY 10605.

Child-health supervision—well-child care

Caring for your baby and young child—birth to age 5. A parenting guide. Published by American Academy of Pediatrics.*

Caring for your adolescent ages 12-21. Published by American Academy of Pediatrics.*

Healthy kids (birth-3 years) and *Healthy kids (4-10 years).* Magazines for parent education available by order from American Academy of Pediatrics.*

Primary prevention of atherosclerotic cardiovascular disease
Life-style management

American Alliance of Health, Physical Education, Recreation and Dance (AAHPERD), Health-Related Physical Fitness Test Manual, 1900 Association Drive, Reston VA 22091.

Manuals to assist physicians in specific assessment of youth health and fitness.

Governors Council of Health and Physical Fitness Family FUN Award, c/o Primary Children's Center, 320 12th Ave., Salt Lake City, UT 84103. *Fitness Unity* (stress management) *Nutrition.* Resource for families to enjoy healthful life style management.

Hall D, Gabble JE, Hawley D: *A resource for wellness planning: lifeguide,* Clackamus, OR, 1988, Wellsource. Excellent and complete resource for life-style management. "Wellness profile."

Jopling RT: Health related fitness as preventive medicine, *Pediatr Rev* 10(5):141-148, 1988. A thoughtful summary of the importance of family fitness written for the practicing physician.

Kuntzleman CT: *The well family book.* Contact Fitness Finders, 133 Taft Road, Spring Arbor, MI, 49283-057. Specifics of family fitness, nutrition, and management of stress.

Kwiterovich PO: *Beyond cholesterol,* Baltimore and London, 1989, Johns Hopkins University Press. Excellent resource to help lay public understand cholesterol, fat, and atherosclerosis.

Lorin MI: *The parents' book of physical fitness for children,* New York, 1978, Atheneum.

Better health through fitness. Guidelines for teens on physical fitness—educational leaflets. Available by order from American Academy of Pediatrics.*

Smoking programs

Glynn TJ: *School programs to prevent smoking: the National Cancer Institute guide to strategies that succeed,* Washington, DC, US Dept Health and Human Services, PHS, NIH, DHHS Public No (NIH) 1990.

Smoking and heart disease—educational leaflets. Available by order from American Heart Association National Center. 7320 Greenville Avenue, Dallas TX 75231.

Dietary management

American Heart Association diet: an eating plan for healthy Americans. American Heart Association National Center, 7320 Greenville Ave, Dallas TX 75231.

Dietary treatment of hypercholesterolemia: a manual for patients. AHA, National Heart Lung and Blood Institute, 1988.

Healthy start—food to grow on. Information and education leaflets that promote healthful eating habits for children 2 years and older. Available by order from American Academy of Pediatrics.*

Children and television

Television and the family. Educational leaflet for parents available from American Academy of Pediatrics.*

Lead screening

What you should know about lead-based paint in your home. Practical information from U.S. Consumer Product Safety Commission, Washington DC, 20207.

Prevention of dental disease

Tooth decay.

Educational leaflet available by order from National Institute of Dental Research, Public Inquiries and Reports Section, National Institute of Dental Research, Bethesda, MD 20892.

Fluoride helps prevent tooth decay and *Seal out decay.*

Educational leaflets available by order from American Dental Association, Bureau of Health Education and Audiovisual Services, 211 East Chicago Ave, Chicago IL 60611.

Chemoprophylaxis—sickle cell disease

National Association for Sickle Cell Disease 1-800-421-8453. Offers genetic counseling and an information packet.

Immunizations

Protecting your child against diphtheria, tetanus and pertussis. Educational leaflet about immunizations with new revised schedule. Available by order from American Academy of Pediatrics.*

Injury prevention and safety promotion

TIPP—the injury prevention program. Age-related safety educational materials available by order from the American Academy of Pediatrics.*

Shopping guide for car seats. Annually updated guide on the different types of car seats and how to use them. Available by order from American Academy of Pediatrics.*

National Highway Traffic Safety Administration Auto Safety Hotline 1-800-424-9393. Information on use of safety belts, child safety seats, and so on.

National Safety Council 444 N. Michigan Ave., Chicago IL 60611. Provides educational materials, including videos, on safety and accident prevention. *The bike book* is one example.

Burn prevention tips. Booklet available by order from Shriner's Burns Institutes, Public Relations Department, Shrine International Headquarters, P.O. Box 31356, Tampa, FL 33631-3356.

What about plants? Educational leaflet about poisonous plants. Available by order from American Association of Poison Control Centers (AAPCC), 3800 Reservoir Road NW, Washington DC 20007.

Mothers Against Drunk Driving (MADD) P.O. Box 541688 Dallas, TX 75354-1688.

Students Against Drunk Driving (SADD) P.O. Box 800, Marlboro, MA 01752.

Child abuse

National Child Abuse Hotline 1-800-422-4453. Information and professional counseling on child abuse. Referrals to local social service groups offering counseling on child abuse.

Parents Anonymous Hotline 1-800-421-0353 (1-800-352-0306 California). Information on self-help groups for parents involved in child abuse.

Clearinghouse on Child Abuse and Neglect Information. P.O. Box 1182, Washington DC 20013.

Child sexual abuse. What It Is and How to Prevent It. Educational leaflet available by order from American Academy of Pediatrics.*

AIDS

National AIDS Hotline 1-800-342-AIDS. Information on the prevention and spread of AIDS.

Drug and alcohol information and counseling

National Cocaine Hotline 1-800-COCAINE.

National Institute on Drug Abuse 1-800-662-HELP.

National Council on Alcoholism 1-800-NCA-CALL. Referrals to local affiliates; provides written information on alcoholism.

---

*American Academy of Pediatrics, P.O. Box 927, Elk Grove Village, IL 60009-0927, 1-800-433-9016, Fax: 708-228-1281.

Chapter 28

THE ADOLESCENT

Kurt W. Jensen
Vanessa K. Jensen

SOCIOBEHAVIORAL MORBIDITIES AND MORTALITIES OF ADOLESCENCE

The adolescent stage of development has been described as both the best and the worst of times.[95] Major morbidities and mortalities for the teen years reflect this paradox, with new-found freedoms and privileges providing the gateway to participation in high-risk, potentially life-threatening behaviors. Accidents (primarily automobile), homicide, and suicide account for more than 80% of adolescent mortality.[131] All stem at least in part from volitional behaviors and are arguably the three most preventable health hazards facing youth today. Major morbidities of adolescence include the consequences of adolescent sexual behavior (e.g., sexually transmitted diseases and teen pregnancy) and the effects of adolescent mental illness. Because adolescent morbidities have a high co-variance, each risk behavior must be considered both individually and in the context of other risk behaviors.[77]

In the teenage years sexual activity, alcohol/drug use, and motor/recreational vehicle use often increase; each potentially high-risk behavior significantly impacts mortality rates[77,100] (Fig. 28-1). Three quarters of those killed between the ages of 15 and 24 die in motor vehicle accidents.[153] Homicide is the second leading cause of death for this age group; 1988 figures show 14.2 deaths per 100,000.[144] Suicide is the third leading cause; in the last four decades suicide rates have increased substantially to a rate of 12.8 per 100,000 youths in 1988.[105] Comparison of two age groups, 10 to 14 versus 15 to 19, shows that the latter will experience a *400%* increase in the number of homicides and motor vehicle accidents and a *600%* increase in suicide rates.[77] Alcohol or drug use will be a factor in at least 50% of these disasters.

Data regarding behavioral excesses among teenagers (e.g., sexual activity and use of tobacco, alcohol, and illicit drugs) forebode an onslaught of later afflictions ranging from acquired immunodeficiency syndrome (AIDS) to lung cancer. A recent report on alcohol use among teens and young adults showed that 90% of high school seniors had tried alcohol, and 32% reported heavy use (five or more consecutive drinks) within the past 2 weeks.[82] Although in recent years the use of illicit drugs has gradually but steadily declined, figures for 1990 indicate that 33% of high school seniors and college students reported using an illicit substance within the past year.[82] In a 1990 survey of students in grades 9 through 12, 36% reported tobacco use within the past 30 days.[82] Adverse developmental consequences may accompany adolescent sexual behavior; recent data show a pregnancy rate of 92.9/1000 for white teens and 185.8/1000 for black teens.[70] Each year one in five sexually active 15- to 19-year-olds becomes pregnant.[108] The risk of sexually transmitted diseases puts teens further at risk.[26]

Negative media stereotypes portraying teens as narcissistic, moody, and rebellious[137] may lead many to feel justified in "blaming the victim" for the consequences of their behavior. But teen participation in high-risk behaviors is rarely, if ever, the sole result of willful, predetermined actions. Instead diverse cognitive, environmental, and biologic elements are likely to influence teen behavior. Primary adolescent developmental goals include emancipation and autonomy, and realization of these objectives requires experimentation and exploration.[74] Developing teens may find that Western culture's long-standing reinforcement of independence, self-indulgence, and "radical" behaviors has left only the most extreme (and often dangerous) mores to challenge.

Although the majority of adolescents will emerge from

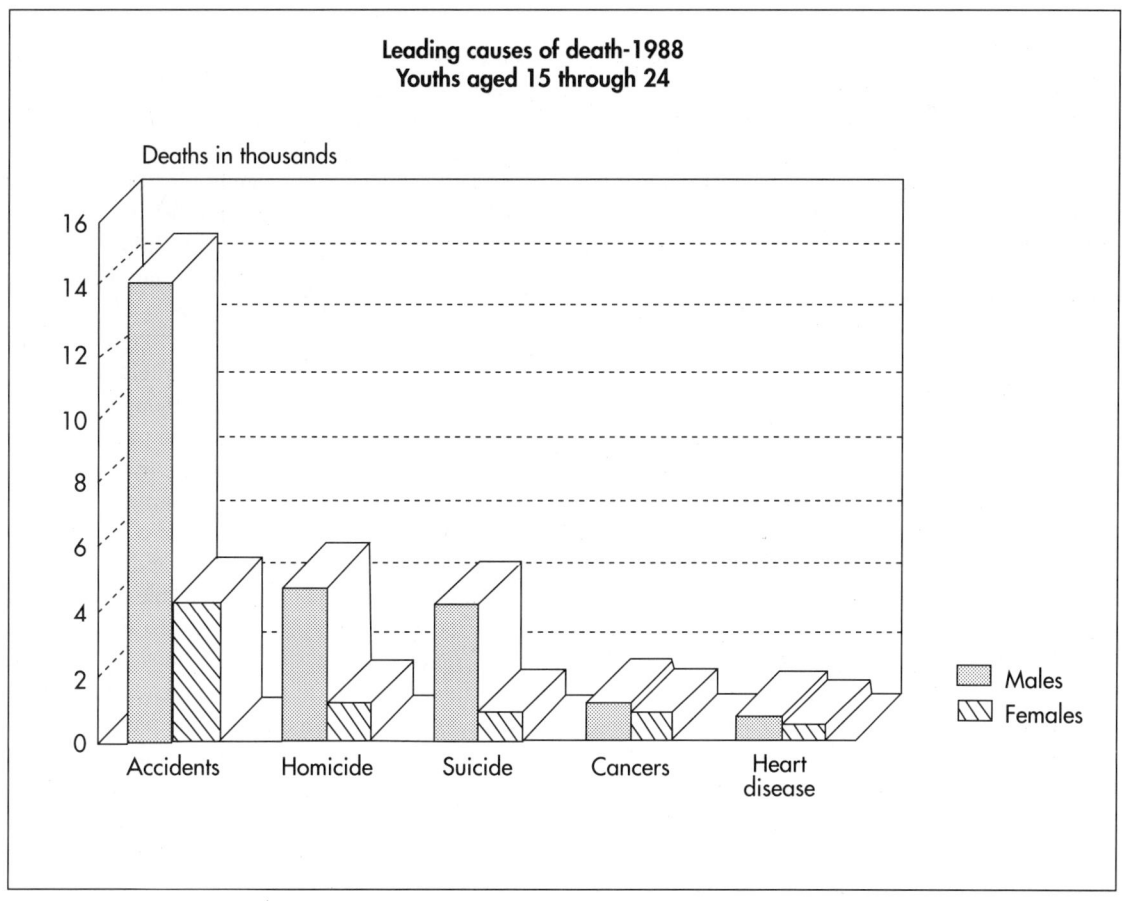

Fig. 28-1. Leading causes of death among 15- to 24-year-olds, 1988. (From US Bureau of Census: *Statistical abstract of the United States 1991*, ed 111, Washington DC, 1991, US Department of Commerce.)

this developmental period intact,[116] many are clearly "at risk." Patients engaging in high-risk behaviors may come to physicians' attention when seeking treatment for associated physical trauma and/or disease (e.g., sexually transmitted diseases, gunshot wounds, chemical addictions). Others experiencing less overt symptoms may fail to receive treatment from health care professionals for a variety of reasons. A third group, those not yet engaging in high-risk health behaviors, may go unnoticed and unattended. Despite variability in presentation all three groups are at some degree of risk and would likely benefit from preventive health care efforts.

As the primary health care providers for adolescents physicians can have considerable impact on the health-related behaviors of this population.[104,143] This chapter will review the physician's role in preventive health care for the adolescent patient and will discuss general issues related to the prevention of high-incidence mortalities and morbidities for adolescents. Primary areas of risk will be reviewed, examining problem scope, risk factors, assessment issues, and preventive interventions for each.

ISSUES IN PREVENTION

Research examining the efficacy of prevention programs with adolescents shows that only the most time- and labor-intensive interventions have been successful, and positive effects generally have been limited to short-term behavioral changes.[118] Effective prevention programs are typically multifactorial, involving strategies such as parent/family participation, social-skills training, and education. When compared to such programs, the preventive efforts of the practicing physician are likely to be far less comprehensive and may have less measurable impact on adolescent patients' behaviors. However to the degree that the physician's interventions complement and corroborate other preventive and/or educational efforts they may further reduce the morbidity and mortality stemming from adolescent involvement in high-risk behaviors.

Physician use of prevention strategies involves four steps: (1) identification of risk factors and high-risk behaviors for the adolescent population; (2) assessment of the beliefs, knowledge, and behaviors of the patient and family related to these factors; (3) implementation of prevention activities including education of patients and families regarding high-risk behaviors; and (4) intervention as necessary for those engaging in (or suffering the consequences of) high-risk behaviors. Before implementing these steps the physician should establish a trusting relationship with the patient and his or her family, thereby increasing the likelihood of a positive response to prevention and anticipatory guidance efforts.

Setting the stage: the physician-patient relationship

The routine health care visit for the adolescent patient provides an excellent opportunity for the primary care physician to assess more than the absence or presence of disease, focusing as well on patient attitudes, beliefs, and behaviors that may significantly influence medical status.[99,100,131] Consideration of social, psychological, nutritional, and sexual issues and concerns can considerably expand the physician's understanding of the teenage patient's health status, at the same time highlighting potential problem areas.

Consideration of the teenage patient's cognitive limitations and "worldview" can assist in the planning and execution of prevention strategies. Though adolescents are not as unruly or temperamental as is often assumed,[116] they are likely to appear more immature, impulsive, and egocentric than adult patients.[74] Teen patients' cognitive abilities are limited by the extent of their neurologic development and depth of life experience. Thus one can rightfully expect early and middle adolescents to act in a more naive, irresponsible manner than older teens, though neither group is likely to display "mature" attitudes or behaviors. Because of these developmental realities prevention efforts that emphasize the long-term consequences of behavior and fail to address teens' here-and-now focus are likely to prove inadequate.

The success of prevention efforts also depends on the physician's comfort level in dealing with a variety of potentially sensitive subjects.[137] Morals, values, and social expectations become fundamental issues, and the physician may find that "being heard" depends more on process than content. The patient's ability to "open up" and effectively explore health-related issues will be influenced by the physician's style of communication and ability to gain the teenager's trust and confidence. Establishing an effective working relationship with the adolescent patient is by no means an easy task and requires a different demeanor and set of skills than are required with other age groups.

A study examining adolescent beliefs about the doctor-patient relationship and privileged information indicated that a majority of teens presumed that physicians would breach confidentiality[30]; most could recall at least one experience in which a physician had shared information with parents without patient permission. Concerns about confidentiality may diminish the patient's willingness to share pertinent information with the physician. Failure to ad-

dress adolescent skepticism regarding privileged communication may severely limit the efficacy of any preventive intervention.

Conversely, parents may be hesitant to have the physician forge a confidential relationship with their child. They may have strong feelings and beliefs regarding "appropriate" teenage behavior and may be concerned about how the physician will influence their child. To avoid conflict around this issue it is helpful to start by meeting jointly with the adolescent patient and his or her family to discuss the importance of confidentiality.[137] "Ground rules" can be outlined, informing all participants that doctor-patient dialogue is generally confidential, though confidentiality is not an absolute right for the teenage patient. Limits of confidentiality should be discussed openly, informing both patient and parents that privileged communication will not be shared except when legal or ethical codes mandate disclosure.[96,131] Patients and parents should also be informed of policies regarding who is responsible for payment of fees when the adolescent patient requests an appointment without parental consent, a situation most likely to arise when the patient is trying to prevent parental involvement.

In anticipation of the adolescent patient's needs and circumstances it behooves the physician to spend some "one-to-one" time during routine visits with younger patients.[30] This helps to normalize time spent alone with the physician and can circumvent parent or patient anxiety when teenage issues and concerns later necessitate "private" discussions. As early as age 5 children can respond to questions about school, peer relationships, and leisure activities with minimal parental assistance. Children should be included in the process of diagnosis, treatment, and prevention as early as possible,[30] using dialogue to highlight patients' capacity to make healthy choices in everyday living. This approach can begin to communicate the "metamessage" that individual patients' beliefs, attitudes, and behaviors are critical components to ongoing health. Children familiar with this style of interaction may be more likely later to share personal information regarding potentially sensitive issues such as sexuality and alcohol use.[30] Physicians' attempts to empower patients in this manner may be the most effective prevention strategy employed.

How the physician presents prevention-related materials will significantly influence teens' ability and willingness to accept and use information. For example prevention programs addressing adolescent substance abuse have found that straightforward educational strategies are most often ineffective, whereas those designed to improve adolescent social skills and self-esteem have met with greater success.[15] Though adolescents identify physicians as their "preferred and most used source of health information,"[125] they may disregard communications rendered in the customary "doctor-to-patient" fashion. Information provided should be delivered in a succinct, nonjudgmental man-

Table 28-1. Recommended screening and examination for adolescents ages 13-18 schedule

Screening	Counseling	Immunizations & chemoprophylaxis
History Dietary intake Physical activity Tobacco/alcohol/drug use Sexual practices	**Diet and exercise** Fat (especially saturated fat), cholesterol, sodium, iron,[‡] calcium[‡] Caloric balance Selection of exercise program	Tetanus-diphtheria (Td) booster[**] ***High-risk groups*** Fluoride supplements (HR15)

Physical exam
Height and weight
Blood pressure
High-risk groups
Complete skin exam (HR1)
Clinical testicular exam (HR2)
	Substance use
	Tobacco: cessation/primary prevention
	Alcohol and other drugs: cessation/primary prevention
	  Driving/other dangerous activities while under the influence
	  Treatment for abuse
	High-risk groups
	Sharing/using unsterilized needles and syringes (HR12)
		This list of preventive services is not exhaustive. It reflects only those topics reviewed by the U.S. Preventive Services Task Force. Clinicians may wish to add other preventive services on a routine basis, and after considering the patient's medical history and other individual circumstances. Examples of target conditions not specifically examined by the Task Force include developmental disorders, scoliosis, behavioral and learning disorders, and parent/family dysfunction

Laboratory/diagnostic procedures ***High-risk groups*** Rubella antibodies (HR3) VDRL/RPR (HR4) Chlamydial testing (HR5) Gonorrhea culture (HR6) Counseling and testing for HIV (HR7) Tuberculin skin test (PPD) (HR8) Hearing (HR9) Papanicolaou smear (HR10)[1]	**Sexual practices** Sexual development and behavior[§] Sexually transmitted diseases: partner selection, condoms Unintended pregnancy and contraceptive options	**Remain alert for:** Depressive symptoms Suicide risk factors (HR11) Abnormal bereavement Tooth decay, malalignment, gingivitis Signs of child abuse and neglect.
	Injury prevention Safety belts Safety helmets Violent behavior[‖] Firearms Smoke detector	
	Dental health Regular tooth brushing, flossing, dental visits	
	Other primary preventive measures ***High-risk groups*** Discussion of hemoglobin testing (HR13) Skin protection from ultraviolet light (HR14)	

*One visit is required for immunizations. Because of lack of data and differing patient risk profiles, the scheduling of additional visits and the frequency of the individual preventive services listed in this table are left to clinical discretion (except as indicated in other footnotes).

†Every 1-3 years.

‡For females.

§Often best performed early in adolescence and with the involvement of parents.

‖Especially for males.

**Once between ages 14 and 16.

From U.S. Preventive Services Task Force: *Guide to clinical preventive services: an assessment of the effectiveness of 169 interventions*, Baltimore, Williams & Wilkins, 1989.

HR1, Persons with increased recreational or occupational exposure to sunlight, a family or personal history of skin cancer, or clinical evidence of precursor lesions (e.g., dysplastic nevi, certain congenital nevi). *HR2*, Males with a history of cryptorchidism, orchiopexy, or testicular atrophy. *HR3*, Females of childbearing age lacking evidence of immunity. *HR4*, Persons who engage in sex with multiple partners in areas in which syphilis is prevalent, prostitutes, or contacts of persons with active syphilis. *HR5*, Persons who attend clinics for sexually transmitted diseases; attend other high-risk health care facilities (e.g., adolescent and family planning clinics); or have other risk factors for chlamydial infection (e.g., multiple sexual partners or a sexual partner with multiple sexual contacts). *HR6*, Persons with multiple sexual partners or a sexual partner with multiple contacts, sexual contacts of persons with culture- proven gonorrhea, or persons with a history of repeated episodes of gonorrhea. *HR7*, Persons seeking treatment for sexually transmitted diseases; homosexual and bisexual men; past or present intravenous (IV) drug users; persons with a history of prostitution or multiple sexual partners; women whose past or present sexual partners were HIV-infected, bisexual, or IV drug users; persons with long-term residence or birth in an area with high prevalence of HIV infection; or persons with a history of transfusion between 1978 and 1985. *HR8*, Household members of persons with tuberculosis or others at risk for close contact with the disease; recent immigrants or refugees from countries in which tuberculosis is common (e.g., Asia, Africa, Central and South America, Pacific Islands); migrant workers; residents of correctional institutions or homeless shelters; or persons with certain underlying medical disorders. *HR9*, Persons exposed regularly to excessive noise in recreational or other settings. *HR10*, Females who are sexually active or (if the sexual history is thought to be unreliable) aged 18 or older. *HR11, Recent divorce, separation, unemployment, depression, alcohol or other drug abuse, serious medical illnesses, living alone, or recent bereavement. HR12*, Intravenous drug users. *HR13*, Persons of Caribbean, Latin American, Asian, Mediterranean, or African descent. *HR14*, Persons with increased exposure to sunlight. *HR15*, Persons living in areas with inadequate water fluoridation (less than 0.7 parts per million).

ner,[99] and the adolescent patient should be invited to discuss and question data presented. The physician should try to use the patient's language and terminology wherever possible, remembering that excessive efforts to do so may be viewed as insincere. The physician should attempt to validate the adolescent's concerns and beliefs, even when physician recommendations run counter to the patient's attitude and behavior.

In routine adolescent health care visits physicians spend an average of 11.6 minutes in face-to-face contact with each patient.[76] Although this may allow adequate time to address patients' medical problems and complaints, it leaves little opportunity for a comprehensive evaluation of health risks or a discussion of prevention-related issues.[131] The physician planning to provide these services may need to alter office protocols significantly, allowing more time per visit, encouraging parental involvement, and gradually reshaping patient expectations. The increased time spent on each case may also necessitate adjustments in fee structure,[100] with higher fees passed along to third-party payers and/or the families receiving care.

Assessment issues

Before designing prevention strategies for a particular adolescent patient the physician should attempt to assess areas of risk. Complete medical, family, and social histories can provide considerable insight into potential problem areas for the teenage patient. Background questionnaires, screening devices, and family interviews allow the physician to gather more than the limited information generally procured during the patient interview.[100] For example concise screening devices used to assess depression/suicidality and parent-adolescent conflict have proved useful in adolescent medicine.[132] Computer-assisted screenings have also been well accepted and effective in identifying adolescent problem areas and may be the next major tool used to evaluate teens.[111]

Segments of the physical examination can be used to initiate conversation about related high-risk behaviors. For example, while assessing lung strength and condition the physician might inquire about cigarette or tobacco use. Discussing components of the physical exam and the rationale for each step may ease patient anxiety and help educate the adolescent regarding typical medical evaluation procedures. The physician may use this time to address patient questions and to encourage the teenager to become a more critical and informed health care consumer. However when major concerns arise, it may be appropriate to complete the examination and allow the adolescent to dress before engaging in in-depth dialogue. A thorough prevention examination for the adolescent patient is outlined in Table 28-1, following guidelines from the U.S. Preventive Services Task Force.[156]

In evaluating adolescent patients' psychosocial functioning the physician should consider progress made toward three key maturational objectives: (1) emotional independence, particularly from family; (2) comfort with gender identity and sexuality; and (3) recognition and acceptance of one's role as an adult member of society.[99] Inquiry regarding adolescents' peer relationships and social life may help to illustrate their success or failure along these dimensions and serve as an entry point to discussion of more sensitive issues.

GENERAL HEALTH/LIFE-STYLE

General physical health issues should be fully addressed during the adolescent patient's visit, keeping in mind that the majority of teenage morbidity stems from preventable biobehavioral factors. Relevant topics may include immunizations, nutrition, weight status, exercise and fitness, and effects of television viewing.

Immunizations

As with younger children, up-to-date immunizations will be part of the treatment regimen during routine adolescent medical visits.[100] For new patients copies of immunization records should be obtained whenever possible. The immunization schedule outlined in Chapter 27 may be appropriate for the majority of teen patients. In addition, the physician should discuss the need for later immunizations with adolescents approaching adulthood.

Nutrition and weight

Many "life-style" habits and behaviors have been shown to have significant influence on both physical and mental health: diet and exercise are two of the most important. These habits often begin in childhood[35] and may be firmly entrenched by the teenage years.

It is estimated that between 15% and 30% of all adolescents are obese,[51] generally defined as greater than 120% of ideal body weight for sex and height or triceps skinfold measures greater than 85th percentile.[33] The prevalence of obesity among adolescents increased dramatically between the mid-1960s and 1980: The incidence of teenage obesity increased from 15% to 18% among males and from 16% to 25% among females.[43] The prevalence of "superobesity" (above the 95th percentile triceps skinfold) increased substantially during the same period.[43] The number of children and teenagers becoming obese is rising, as is the percentage of excess weight carried by each individual child.[41]

The cause of obesity is multifactorial, involving genetic, nutritional, psychologic, social, and cultural factors.[41,112] Most experts agree that heredity plays a key role by predisposing children to gain or maintain a certain weight range.[20,47] However for many children the home environment is likely to be the primary causal factor.[41] Parental obesity, family size, socioeconomic status, and parental education have all been found to correlate with childhood obesity. Adolescent television viewing is another strong influence: increased viewing time coincides with greater weight gain[42] and greater caloric intake.[146]

The longer a child remains obese, the less likely he or she is to eventually attain and maintain appropriate weight status as an adult.[20] The odds of an obese adolescent's becoming an average weight adult have been estimated at 28:1.[32] Hence efforts to prevent obesity throughout the life span rely substantially on child/adolescent prevention efforts. Early intervention is particularly critical for adolescent patients with a strong family history of weight-related health problems. Children and adolescents who engage in behaviors that facilitate weight maintenance efforts may be less likely to become obese in adulthood.

Success rates for long-term weight reduction are low,[41] particularly for the morbidly obese. Effective weight reduction and weight management programs for adolescents generally involve a combination of interventions, including nutrition education, behavior modification, and exercise.[33] Self-esteem and psychosocial issues should also be addressed as cognitive and/or emotional factors may contribute to the "cycle" of overeating.

The benefits of and mechanisms for appropriate weight maintenance should be reviewed with all adolescents. Teens should be warned about the potential dangers of "fad" diets. Patients following such diets without supervision may experience a number of mental and physical consequences, including headaches, dizziness, fatigue, poor concentration, and/or menstrual difficulties.[98]

Exercise and physical activity

The rising rate of obesity for American teens appears to result in part from their decreased participation in exercise and physical activity.[155] Despite the physical fitness craze of the 1980s a high percentage of children and adolescents are not involved in regular physical activity and continue to be overweight.[127] As early as for students in fourth grade, schools begin to limit children's physical education to participation in competitive sports, the very activities that overweight and out-of-shape children are least likely to engage in.[127] Physical education classes may not provide the intensity of activity necessary for good health; the 1990 Youth Risk Behavior Survey found that although approximately half of all high school students were involved in physical education classes, fewer than one fourth attended such classes daily.[27] In addition nearly one fourth of the adolescents enrolled in these classes engaged in fewer than 20 minutes of physical activity per class.

Children and adolescents should be encouraged to engage in regular physical activity to help maintain ideal body weight and increase cardiovascular fitness.[44] Early development of healthy exercise habits may foster long-term commitment to regular physical activity. Consistent participation in moderate levels of exercise may improve patient affect, mood, and self-esteem. Involvement in competitive sports may enhance adolescents' social skills[45]; however, parents should closely monitor these programs as pressure to perform and use of harsh consequences may have negative physical and psychologic repercussions.[45] Parents and patients should be encouraged to weigh the costs and benefits of participation before enrolling in competitive athletics. The physical risks associated with any given sport should be reviewed a priori; physicians can provide information on accident prevention to those electing to participate.

Although competitive sports may play an important role in some adolescents' development, children at risk for obesity are more likely to benefit from "life-style" exercise or activity.[48] Life-style exercises include any physical activity that occurs as part of normal, daily routine; common examples are walking, playing with pets, or doing chores. These are generally low-cost activities, requiring little in the way of supplies or equipment. Because patients typically find these exercises enjoyable and easy to work into a daily schedule, they may be well suited for obese or at-risk adolescent patients who might otherwise avoid exercise altogether. Adolescent participation may be further enlisted by highlighting the immediate benefits associated with exercise (e.g., improved appearance and mood). In addition acknowledgment of the obstacles to engaging in exercise (e.g., it sometimes feels like work) may help the patient to overcome these impediments.

Television

Television and the media in general have been described as "the most important and unrecognized influence on adolescent behavior in American society today."[142] For many adolescents television and video games become the primary source of entertainment and interfere with peer-group involvement and related social-skill development. Indiscriminate and/or extensive television viewing by children has been shown to contribute to increased aggression[28,94,142] and decreased creativity.[94] Television's inaccurate and unrealistic portrayal of life may at times significantly influence the behaviors of an impressionable adolescent audience. Increased teenage sexuality,[142] suicide,[63,64] and obesity[42] are morbidities and mortalities reflecting these dynamics.

The American Academy of Pediatrics recommends that television viewing be limited to 1 to 2 hours per day and that parents closely monitor program selection for children and adolescents.[3] Although parents may exercise less control over children as they enter the teenage years, limitations on the duration and type of shows watched should be strongly encouraged. Parents should be especially urged to prohibit the viewing of excessively violent or graphic shows, the shows that teens may be most adamant about seeing. Adolescents and parents may initially see these limitations as severe or overly strict. However parents provided with information about the risks of excessive televi-

---

Television guidelines for parents

Adolescent viewing

- Limit television to 1-2 hours per day, especially during the school week
- Monitor all television/movies; restrict shows with excessive violence or sexual behavior
- Use "co-viewing" as an opportunity to teach teens about critical television viewing
- Talk with teens about questionable shows or shows that endorse values far different than the values of the family or community
- Be firm, even if it requires removing television from the teen's bedroom; limit the amount of "family time" spent watching television

---

Substance abuse in adolescence

Risk factors

ADOLESCENT FACTORS	FAMILY FACTORS
School failure	Family history of drug or alcohol problems
Tobacco use	
Association with peers who use alcohol/drugs	Family history of criminal or antisocial problems
	Parental permissiveness about chemical use
	Family dysfunction
	Discipline problems in the home

---

sion viewing are more likely to agree with and follow recommended guidelines (see box).

SUBSTANCE USE AND ABUSE
Background information and risk factors

Alcohol and/or drug use is a contributing factor in more than half of all adolescent auto accidents, suicides, and homicides, the three leading mortalities for this age group.[153] Despite the recent proliferation of educational and prevention programs dealing with this issue alcohol and drug abuse continues to be the major health care problem for adolescents. Although statistics reported by the National Institute on Drug Abuse [82] indicate that the use of alcohol and illicit drugs by teens is slowly declining, the number using remains alarmingly high. For example, a recent survey of high school seniors showed that 90% had tried alcohol, 57% had used it within the past month, and almost 4% were drinking daily[82] (Fig. 28-2). In addition 19% of high school seniors reported daily cigarette smoking,[82] the single most preventable cause of death.[115]

"Adolescent patterns of alcohol and drug use vary considerably, though the first episode often occurs during late elementary or early high school years."[1] For the adolescent population as a whole increasing age is accompanied by greater numbers using, increased frequency of use, and a wider range of drug choice.[2] Although some teens will discontinue drug use after a brief period of experimentation, the majority will continue to use with varying frequency and intensity.[96]

In identifying adolescents at risk for alcohol or drug-related problems the physician must distinguish between age-appropriate experimentation and the abuse of drugs. Recognizing the difference between use and abuse may be critical to working with the adolescent just beginning to experiment with alcohol or drugs. The vast majority of teens have tried drugs at one time or another, and most will never experience significant use-related problems.[2] Progression from "licit" to illicit drugs is not imminent, as

the vast majority of teens stop use long before they approach dependence.[84] Teenage alcohol use might be better be viewed as a "rite of passage" than a pathologic indicator.

Identifying all youth who drink or use drugs as "chemically dependent" may serve only to alienate the adolescent patient and sabotage any preventive measures. At the same time the physician who ignores or overlooks adolescent drug abuse may unknowingly provide what is taken as tacit approval. The American Academy of Pediatrics cautions against either position:

Alcohol consumption, by virtue of its longstanding social acceptance, is considered to be drug abuse only when carried to an extreme form. Usage of other drugs, cannabis and its derivatives, for example, is considered by most societies to be so dangerous that any usage, however innocent, is drug abuse. Both attitudes are faulty, and potentially dangerous.[4]

Appropriate assessment, prevention, and treatment of drug abuse are contingent on the physician's knowledge and awareness of the dynamics associated with chemical abuse.[2] Children suffering from poverty, oppression, or abuse are perhaps the most likely to use drugs as a means of coping or escape.[2] However, children and adolescents experiencing any form of deprivation—be it inadequate supervision, disrupted family structure, or other difficulties—may turn to substance use or abuse to help them cope with less than ideal circumstances. Research has shown that teens of every socioeconomic and cultural background are at risk to develop substance abuse problems,[133] though several factors have demonstrated predictive value in identifying high-risk adolescents.

A variety of indices related to family history and behavior are associated with adolescent smoking and substance abuse, including (1) presence of an alcoholic or chemically dependent parent, (2) family history of criminal or antisocial behavior, (3) parental problems with disciplining or controlling children, and (4) parental use or permissive at-

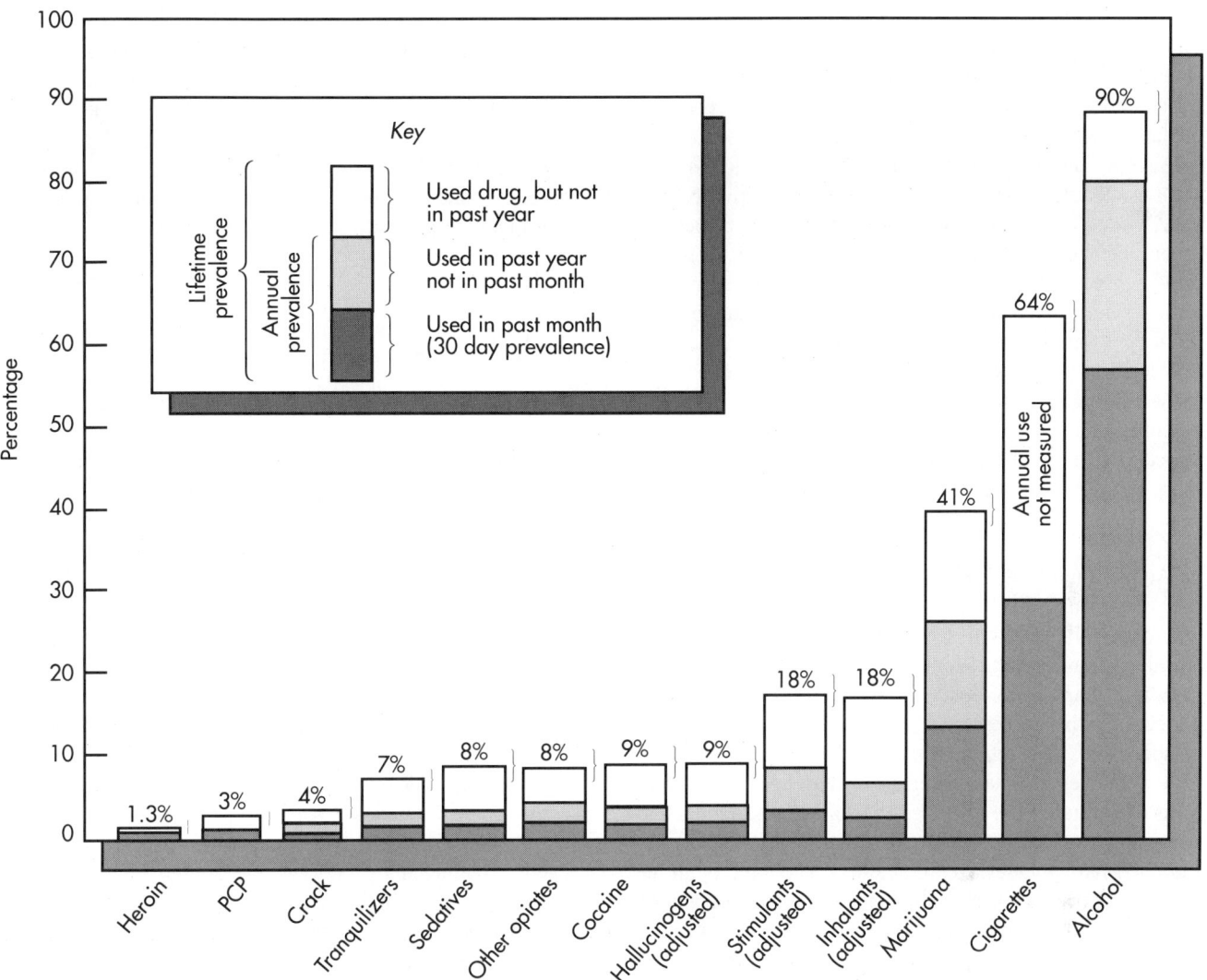

Fig. 28-2. Prevalence and recency of drug use, class of 1990. (From Johnston LD, O'Malley PM, Bachman JG: *Drug use among American high school seniors, college students and young adults, 1975-1990,* vol 1, Rockville, MD, 1991, National Institute on Drug Abuse, U.S. Department of Health and Human Services.)

titudes about alcohol and/or other controlled substances.[67] Primary factors associated with adolescent hard liquor and illicit drug use include parental drug use[161] and quality of parent-child relationships.[59] Children of alcoholics are more likely to exhibit hyperactivity, delinquent behavior, psychosomatic complaints, and a variety of school-related problems.[128] They are four times more likely to become alcoholic than children with nonalcoholic parents (see box).[61,62]

Peer group behavior and attitudes regarding substance abuse may at times be the most critical factor affecting adolescent drug use. Drug-using friends are the most powerful model and are most likely to serve as the initial contact with or provider of illicit chemicals.[133] Adolescents are more likely to be alcohol and/or drug abusers if they place high value on independence and autonomy, have low ex-

pectations regarding achievement, and demonstrate a greater proneness to engage in delinquent behaviors.[50]

Academic performance is generally inversely correlated with chemical abuse: Failure in school, regardless of cause, is associated with earlier onset of drug use and continued use thereafter.[15] Failure in elementary and junior high schools is often a precursor to problems with substance abuse.[133] Adolescents expressing a lack of interest in academics are much more likely to be users,[50] though at present college students consume more alcohol than their noncollege counterparts.[82]

When drug use goes beyond experimentation, the adolescent may telegraph this progression through behavioral cues, including: (1) a sudden and significant reduction in family interactions, (2) "undesirable" behaviors such as lying and excessive expression of anger, (3) affective distress such as depression or irritability, (4) delinquent behaviors such as stealing and truancy, and (5) academic problems.[50] Earlier onset of drug use[15,67] and use of tobacco and hard liquor in combination[84] have also been associated with progression to illicit drug use.

Several authors have identified stages of alcohol and drug use that teenagers may experience in a stepwise fashion.[84,96,133] Teens generally follow a four-step progression when intensified use is observed: (1) nonuse, (2) beer and/or wine, (3) marijuana, and (4) other illicit drugs.[84] Other stage conceptualizations vary somewhat, but all identify a variety of behavioral, academic, psychosocial, and legal consequences associated with adolescents' progressive drug use. In recent years the ready availability of cocaine, crack, and similarly acting psychoactive drugs appears to have altered this pattern for many teens, as these drugs provide the entry point to substance abuse.

Assessment

As the routine adolescent medical visit is multipurpose, general discussion about the patient's physical, mental, and behavioral status is likely the best first step in performing an assessment, followed by a review of any outstanding symptoms or concerns. Relaxed, informal inquiry concerning the adolescent's academic performance, peer relationships, leisuretime activities, and family can provide valuable information regarding the signs and symptoms of substance use.[2,96,133] The adolescent's alcohol and drug use/abuse may be assessed while questioning the patient and family about overall health.[96] The topic might be introduced by asking about alcohol and drug use among the patient's peers, family members, and so on.[2] A calm, nonjudgmental, and supportive style of interaction may enhance the adolescent's capacity to self-disclose,[2,96,128] as will the physician's depiction of drug abuse as a health problem rather than a weakness or moral failing.[96]

When adolescents do not volunteer information about their drug use in the course of general inquiry or discussion, questions about tobacco use can serve as a "gateway" topic. Information regarding tobacco use can be important for three reasons: (1) more than 90% of alcohol addicts and abusers smoke heavily,[106] (2) use of tobacco and hard liquor is often a precursor to use of illicit drugs other than marijuana,[84] and (3) tobacco use is the largest contributor to premature death in this country, with three quarters of adolescent users continuing into adulthood.[156] Although in-depth discussion of tobacco use and related prevention strategies is beyond the scope of this section, relevant assessment and education should be performed with every adolescent patient.

Direct questions regarding alcohol and drug use may only lead to denial, particularly if the examiner is not perceived as having the teen's best interests in mind. The majority of adolescents using drugs do not view it as a problem behavior.[150] Even patients experiencing significant hardships caused by chemical use may be unwilling or unable to recognize or admit that drug use is a problem.[133,150] Denial is generally recognized as the most predominant defense mechanism used by alcohol and chemically dependent patients,[96,133] as well as family members.[133]

By first normalizing adolescent substance use, the following example demonstrates a style of questioning that may facilitate patients' self-disclosure:

Mary, most people have at least experimented with alcohol by the time they're your age. They've usually tried beer or wine, and many have been drunk a time or two. I'm wondering, when's the last time you had something to drink?

In identifying patients with drinking problems, direct questions such as "How much and how often do you drink?" have been found significantly less sensitive than screening devices such as the Michigan Alcoholism Screening Test.[36] As the effectiveness of any preventive strategy in part depends on accurate assessment, this shortcoming may significantly impede prevention efforts.

To enhance assessment accuracy the physician should attempt to perform a multimodal evaluation, using interviews of both patient and family, as well as results from one or more screening devices.[156] At the same time the physician should keep in mind that the accuracy of the adolescent patient's self-report may be jeopardized by fears that sensitive, personal, and perhaps self-incriminating information will be shared with parents, school officials, or legal authorities.[30,160] Clarification regarding the privileged communication between the adolescent and physician may help to minimize these concerns.[2,96,156]

A family interview should be part of the assessment process whenever possible. Although family members, particularly parents, rarely have direct knowledge of the extent of drug use, the information they provide about associated factors (e.g., academic performance and leisure activities) may be helpful. The family interview gives the physician an opportunity to examine parental attitudes and behaviors with regard to drug use and provides a chance to educate parents regarding their role as models.[1,160] Patient prognosis is significantly improved when families are involved in the assessment process and when the family or patient (rather than the physician) is the first to acknowledge that drug use is a problem.[96,156]

Screening devices can be used to verify or augment the assessment process. Though questionnaires such as the Michigan Alcoholism Screening Test (MAST),[134] the CAGE questionnaire,[49] and the Addiction Severity Index[102] are designed for adult populations, these and other research-validated instruments can be used to supplement information provided by the patient and family.

Prevention strategies

One comprehensive study examining adolescent alcohol abuse found that excessive drinking is only one of many problem behaviors that are consistently observed in delinquent or oppositional youth.[50] A number of environmental, personality, and behavioral factors appear to contribute to alcohol and drug abuse, and simplistic unidimensional prevention efforts are unlikely to deter problem development. To date even the most comprehensive, intensive prevention programs addressing adolescent chemical dependency have been only partially successful.[15] Efficacy has depended in part on the preventive strategies employed as well as program duration and intensity. For example studies employing psychosocial skills training to reduce tobacco use among adolescents have shown short-term success; however the interventions used in these programs were generally labor- and time-intensive, and long-term success (i.e., beyond 1 year) is believed to be low.[15]

Though a necessary prerequisite, knowledge alone is not sufficient to change adolescent attitudes or behavior regarding alcohol/drug use.[156] Prevention programs using educational strategies alone have proved insufficient: "Although programs utilizing information dissemination/fear-arousal approaches as well as those emphasizing affective education have proliferated for at least a decade and a half, the available evidence suggests that neither approach is effective."[15] Programs have been able to increase subjects' knowledge of the negative effects of drug use and have influenced students' attitudes, but behavioral changes have been minimal at best.[15,60]

To the degree that the individual physician's prevention strategies are comprehensive in scope, are time-intensive, and are consistent with other prevention efforts, they can at least partially overcome the limitations of previously described prevention programs. To meet these criteria the strategies used must be well organized and planned. Exclusive reliance on educational interventions will probably have little effect on adolescent behaviors, even when patients appear receptive and eager for information. However when significant others (e.g., parents and teachers) work in concert with the physician and adolescent patient to plan and implement ongoing prevention activities, the potential impact is significantly greater.[156]

After determining the degree to which an adolescent is using or abusing chemicals appropriate prevention strategies can be executed. For teens just beginning to experiment with drugs, the physician should attempt to educate both patient and family concerning the range of potential problems they might incur.[1] Although patients in this category are rarely concerned about the potential problems associated with drug use, their families may be apprehensive and interested in learning more. Preventive efforts should focus in part on teaching parents about the risks associated with tobacco, alcohol, and drug use and alerting them to the signs and symptoms of abuse or addiction.[156,160] The physician should emphasize to parents the importance of appropriate modeling, urging them to use only moderate amounts of alcohol in a safe, controlled manner.[1]

The physician can empower parents by supporting their attempts to enforce appropriate rules and regulations. Parents may need counsel and reassurance in outlining appropriate behavioral guidelines and disciplinary strategies.[160] The physician might recommend that parents organize "family meetings" during periods when the adolescent is at particularly high risk to begin using chemicals (e.g., new school, family changes, moves).[2,96] Parents should be encouraged to routinely discuss behavioral alternatives to driving while intoxicated or traveling with intoxicated peers.[2] They should be reminded that they ultimately have the right and responsibility to decide what is best for their children but should be warned of the limitations of advice giving to adolescents.[160]

When appropriate, adolescents should be encouraged to discuss alcohol- and drug-related issues with their parents. When high-risk signs and symptoms (e.g., family history of alcohol problems, drug-abusing friends) are evident, both patient and family should be alerted to these unfavorable conditions and the dangers associated with continued chemical use.[156]

Another effective preventive strategy involves encouraging teens to increase their involvement in peer activities. Adolescents identify "boredom" as one of the major reasons why they turn to alcohol and drugs.[160] In addition teens may initially use chemicals to reduce the psychological pain ensuing from poor peer relations and the low self-esteem that often follows.[134] Continued efforts to establish positive peer relationships and age-appropriate social activities are key to a favorable outcome for this developmental predicament. To aid in these efforts the physician can assist parents in structuring the home environment so that privileges are contingent on appropriate use of leisure time (for example, making use of the car on weekends contingent on participation in at least one organized after-school activity each quarter). This strategy is consistent with research showing that social pressure can significantly reduce alcohol/drug use.[107]

Adolescent patients' perceptions of the prevalence of drug use by both peers and adults can have a major influence on their own use.[135] In prevention programs two major factors leading to decreased drug use have been (1) adolescents' beliefs regarding the prevalence of drug use by peers and (2) their expectation that friends would react negatively if they were to use drugs.[80] The physician may shift patient perceptions by "mentioning" that almost half of all adolescents do not routinely drink or use drugs, and that these behaviors are becoming less and less popular among this age group. Discussion of the media's attempts to profit at teenagers' expense by glorifying chemical use may further alter patient beliefs and help curb susceptibility to these messages.

Parents who suspect drug abuse may ask physicians for suggestions about what they should do. The physician can advise parents to discuss their concerns with the teenager and to use "search and seizure" procedures if they have strong suspicions and evidence of drug use.[133] When the patient denies use and verification proves difficult, parents should be advised to set appropriate limits and continue to watch for signs and symptoms of drug use/abuse. Written contracts that clearly communicate parental expectations regarding drug use and specifically outline the consequences for violation can be drafted. A variety of disciplinary measures can be used to reduce drug use and related activities[133]; for example, driving privileges might be contingent on alcohol-free driving and compliance with certain household rules. At the same time the physician should warn parents that overreliance on disciplinary tactics may exacerbate parent-child conflict and have little effect on adolescent drug use.

Parents should be cautioned concerning the emotional trauma they may experience on discovering that their child is using illegal drugs. Anger, guilt, fear, and frustration (often paradoxically accompanied by denial) are common reactions to this realization.[2,96,133] Despite their affective distress parents should be encouraged to emulate the physician's demeanor in confronting the adolescent, using a calm, nonjudgmental approach that underscores the teenager's responsibility for his or her own behavior.

Given the constellation of symptoms typically accompanying chemical abuse (e.g., family discord, poor academic performance), referral for psychologic services may be appropriate.[1,156] Research supports the efficacy of counseling when problem drinking is a part of the presenting problem[29,93]; additional psychiatric problems (e.g., dual diagnosis) may necessitate referral for more in-depth treatment.

Finally the physician who works with adolescent patients needs to consider the degree to which he or she serves as an appropriate role model.[156] The malleable teenager is much more likely to emulate the behaviors of adults than to heed their advice, and the physician's status as a health care expert may amplify his or her potential impact. Physicians' efforts to assist in the development and promotion of prevention programs in schools, churches, and community agencies can further expand their scope of influence with both individual patients and the community.[1]

ADOLESCENT SEXUALITY

The primary goals of preventive adolescent health care related to sexuality should be to assist the teenage patient (1) to develop a healthy sexual identity and responsible sexual behavior, (2) to prevent sexually transmitted diseases (STD), and (3) to prevent premature pregnancy.

Background information and risk factors

Despite parental worries, warnings, and wishes to the contrary, adolescents are prone to engage in sexual behaviors. National studies show that 60% of white males and females engaged in sexual intercourse by age 18 and 19, respectively.[23] For black adolescents sexual activity begins earlier: 60% of black males experience sexual intercourse by age 16 and 60% of black females by age 18.[23] Approximately 7% of all females aged 15 to 19 become pregnant and 18% of all sexually active teenage females conceive each year.[97] Although the age of first sexual activity appears to be leveling off, the percentage of adolescent girls engaging in intercourse is increasing[153] (Fig. 28-3).

Parents, schools, and community organizations have tried for decades to thwart adolescent sexual activity, though efforts to date appear to have had minimal impact. For example increased publicity regarding human immunodeficiency virus (HIV) infection has not significantly altered adolescent sexual behavior.[114,145] In fact at present the AIDS virus may be spreading among segments of the teen population faster than any other age group[120]; in addition adolescents continue to experience significant rates of STD[26] and unplanned pregnancies.[97]

As noted previously, teenagers often have difficulty recognizing their own shortcomings or assessing the long-range impact of their behaviors. These developmental limitations may restrict the adolescent patient's ability to make healthy choices regarding sexual behavior.[74] In making decisions about sex the adolescent patient's options and outcome will in part be determined by a convergence of sociodemographic, biologic, environmental, psychosocial, and behavioral variables.

Sexually transmitted diseases. The incidence of STDs is high among adolescents: teen rates are second only to those in the 20- to 25-year age group.[21] The most common STDs are likely to be chlamydia and human papilloma virus (HPV),[120] though adolescents are also at risk for gonorrhea, syphilis, and genital herpes.[26] Exact numbers are difficult to determine as some infections, including HPV and chlamydia, are not reportable diseases.[125]

It is estimated that one in six Americans is infected with genital herpes simplex virus.[25] Data on gonorrhea show that although the number of cases of gonorrhea among all age groups declined between 1975 and 1989,[122] the incidence of gonorrhea increased during the 1980s for all males and for black females aged 15 through 19.[26] Although infrequent, syphilis is also on the rise in some parts of the United States, and overall rates were higher in 1989 than at any point since World War II.[26] Congenital syphilis is widespread among black heterosexuals and minority teenage females, and rates are currently on the rise.[25]

To date the incidence of HIV in adolescents is comparatively low. As of 1989 fewer than 1% of all reported cases of acquired immunodeficiency syndrome (AIDS) were among 15- to 19-year-old patients.[37] However these statistics may be misleading for two reasons: (1) the number of infected adolescents is often underestimated, as data for this age group are not always included in either pediatric or adult statistical analyses,[147] and (2) these rates of infection only reflect patients diagnosed during the teenage years; HIV may remain nonsymptomatic for 5 to 10 years

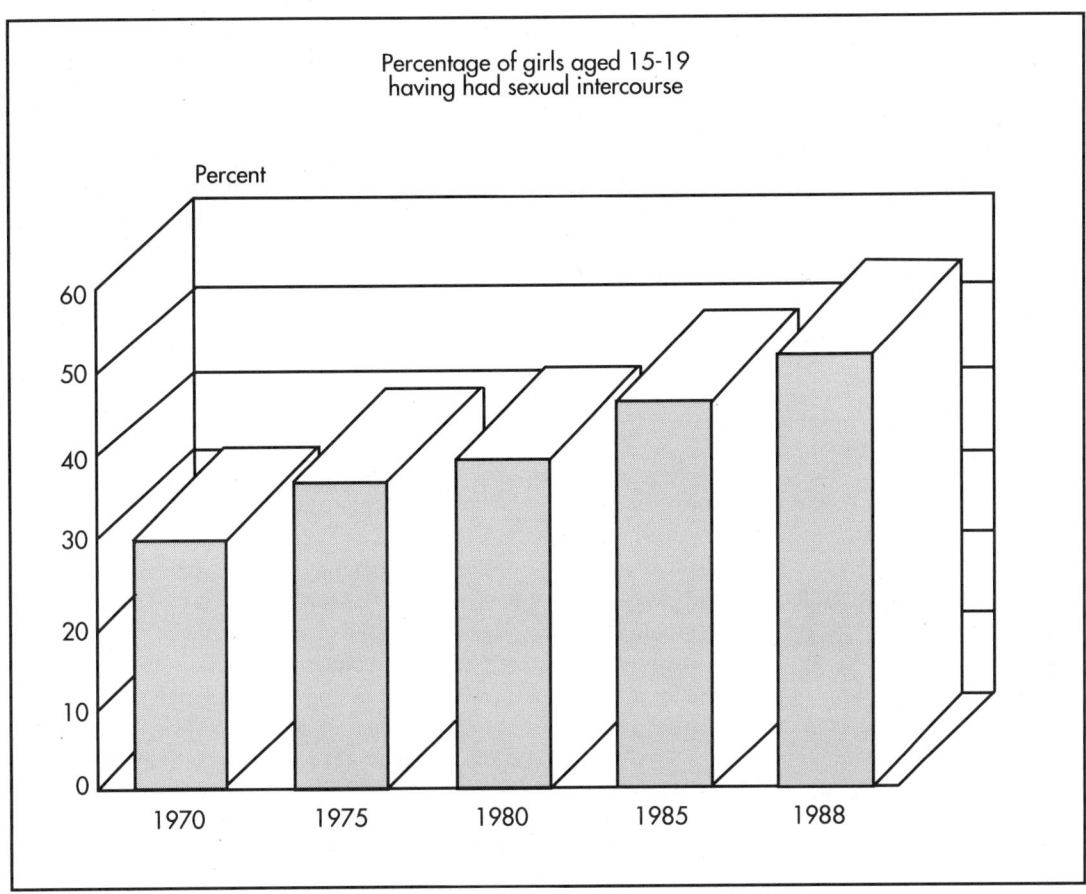

Percentage of girls aged 15-19
having had sexual intercourse

Fig. 28-3. Percentage of 15- to 19-year-old females having had sexual intercourse 1970-1988. (From U.S. Department of Health and Human Services, Public Health Service: *Healthy people 2000, national health promotion and disease prevention objectives,* Washington DC, 1991, Department of Health and Human Services.)

after exposure and many persons identified as seropositive in early adulthood are likely to have acquired the virus during adolescence.[90,154] Despite the relatively low rates of HIV infection among adolescents AIDS was the sixth leading cause of death for persons in the 15- to 24-year age group in 1988.[108]

Widespread screening of teenagers for HIV has not been encouraged; instead most recommendations have suggested that high-risk adolescents be identified and tested, using concomitant pretest and posttest counseling.[90] Accurately distinguishing those at risk for acquiring HIV, however, has proved difficult. Teens identified as at high risk may include: (1) males with a history of same-gender sexual activity; (2) teens with a history of parenteral drug use; (3) partners of persons in these two groups; (4) teens who have a history of syphilis or two or more other STDs; (5) females with pelvic inflammatory disease (PID); and (6) teens with history of transfusion or receipt of blood products.[37] A recent study found that the rate of HIV infection among patients meeting one or more of these criteria was 41/1000, whereas the rate for adolescent controls was 3.7/

1000.[37] The same study found that screening only "high-risk" teens (as previously defined) identified only 38% of patients infected with HIV in this population. Hence limited testing may miss a large percentage of HIV infected adolescents. Nevertheless mandatory screening without proper preparation and follow-up services is not recommended[68] because of the potential psychologic and social consequences.

The majority of adolescents infected with HIV acquire the virus through sexual activity; highest rates of infection are among minority group members and males.[90] Gay males may be at particular risk for HIV because of its high prevalence among homosexual men.[90,120] High-risk behaviors associated with HIV (and other STD) infection include unprotected intercourse (particularly anal intercourse), intercourse with multiple partners, intravenous drug use, and sexual activity with a high-risk person.[90] Drug or alcohol use increases the risk of STD infection because users often experience diminished impulse control and are less likely to adhere to safe-sex practices (see box on p. 540).[71]

STDs in adolescence

Risk factors

BEHAVIORAL/ PSYCHOLOGICAL	SOCIODEMOGRAPHIC
Early onset of sexual activity	Member of a minority group (particularly for males)
Multiple partners	
Exposure to high-risk sex practices (e.g., anal sex)	Inner city residence
Same-sex sexual activity (particularly for males)	
Low self-esteem	

Teen pregnancy. Despite a recent downward trend in teen pregnancy[97] the United States continues to have one of the highest rates in the developed world.[83] Estimates are that 40% of white females and more than 60% of black females will become pregnant by age 20.[153] Nearly one half of all adolescent females aged 15 to 19 have engaged in sexual intercourse; nearly one third of the sexually active females in this group have one or more premarital pregnancies.[39]

Adolescent mothers are likely to experience significant hardships: Even when compared to females with similar socioeconomic backgrounds, teenagers who become mothers are likely to have less education, lower job status, and less satisfactory marital relationships.[54,55,163] Though ongoing financial status is marked by significant variability,[55] the pregnant teen and her child are at greater risk for long-term poverty.[149] Children born to teen mothers are at increased risk for a variety of developmental and environmental difficulties.[97,163]

The causative factors contributing to unplanned teen pregnancies are likely to include a medley of sociocultural, family, and individual components.[153] High pregnancy rates in some schools or communities may lead some adolescents to view pregnancy as "normal" or expected behavior. For adolescents living in impoverished or undesirable environments pregnancy and childbirth may be viewed as "a way out." Adolescent girls with a history of school failure are at high risk for teen pregnancy.[54] As noted previously, alcohol and drug use may lead to decreased use of contraception, thus increasing risk of pregnancy.[71]

Assessment issues

Sexuality should be addressed as part of the routine medical visit, before the onset of puberty whenever possible.[65] Unless otherwise requested, discussion of related issues should be conducted privately with the adolescent, providing reassurance that information discussed is confidential and will not be shared with parents. As in other areas assessment can begin by reviewing the adolescent's social activities and peer relationships, gradually progressing

to issues of dating and sexual behavior. As the patient becomes more comfortable discussing sex-related issues with the physician, concerns may be raised about feelings, thoughts, and behaviors related to this topic.[22] Most adolescent concerns are likely to be relatively "normal," and reassurance about age-appropriate apprehensions may prove adequate intervention. For sexual problems or concerns beyond the physician's expertise referral to a health specialist with relevant training may be necessary.

In assessing patient sexual behavior the physician should ask about types of sexual activity engaged in, number of partners, and involvement in high-risk sex practices (e.g., anal intercourse, prostitution, group sex).[90] Adolescents should be specifically asked about type and frequency of contraceptive use, and a complete history of STDs and pregnancies should be obtained.[22]

The topic of alcohol/drug use should be addressed when discussing sexual activity as these behaviors often are associated.[135] Teens who use drugs are more likely to engage in intercourse at an early age[152] and are less likely to use adequate contraception.[71]

When discussing sexual activity the physician should not assume that all activity involves a partner of the opposite sex. Same-gender sexual activity is relatively common in early adolescence, particularly for males: estimates suggest that as many as 10% of males and 5% of females are homosexual.[138] The process of realizing and accepting that one is homosexual (or bisexual) takes place gradually over time,[40,100,121] and adolescent patients may vary considerably in their awareness of and comfort with this issue.

For gay males or males engaging in same-gender sexual activity, open discussion of these behaviors and associated risks is essential to optimal health maintenance. Adolescents involved in homosexual behavior may be at greater risk for physical afflictions such as STDs, enteric diseases, and sexual-activity-related trauma.[100,109] They may also be more susceptible to a variety of psychosocial problems such as disrupted family relations, substance abuse, and academic difficulties.[120] Psychologic intervention may help the patient and/or family to understand and accept the adolescent's evolving sexual identity.[40,121] Psychotherapeutic treatment, however, should not be identified as a way to alter the patient's sexual orientation.[40]

Given the high incidence of sexual abuse and its potential impact on sexual identity and overall mental health, every adolescent patient should be considered at risk and screened accordingly.[40] In one study 6.7% of white females and 8.8% of black females reported having sexual intercourse by age 14[152]; however only 2.3% percent of white and 5.7% of black females identified this experience as consensual. Sexual abuse in the home can continue through adolescence, and health care professionals should be alert to the possibility of incest or abuse.[6,40] Females in particular should be assessed for sexual coercion and/or date rape and ongoing risk should be discussed. The physician should encourage female patients to report any instances of forced sexual activity.

In assessing the adolescent's general sexual functioning the physician should focus in part on overall self-esteem and self-concept. Low self-esteem has been identified as one possible risk factor in the development of STDs among teens.[16] Positive self-esteem and beliefs about competence may enhance the teenager's ability to fend off unwanted sexual advances or insist on the use of appropriate contraception. Questions used to evaluate teenagers' self-confidence as it relates to sexual behavior might include "If your partner wanted to make love and you did not have a condom available, what would you do?;" or "If you and your new girlfriend wanted to have sex but she had recently broken up with a guy she thought had some kind of sexually transmitted disease, what would you do?"

STD screening should be used to assess high-risk adolescents[156] (Table 28-1) but should be viewed as only a part of the overall prevention effort. Screening can allow early identification of STDs but may provide adolescent patients with a false sense of security when test results are negative. In the case of negative screenings adolescent patients should be explicitly cautioned about the time-limited utility of these results and should be encouraged to abstain from intercourse or restrict sexual activity to "safe sex" practices.

Prevention strategies

Efforts to prevent sexually related morbidity (primarily STDs and teen pregnancy) can begin when reviewing developmental issues and concerns with parents of preadolescent children. Parents should be reminded that sexuality is a normal part of adolescence, highlighting the important role that parental guidance and support play in helping children to understand their sexual development and adopt healthy behavioral standards. Parents should be encouraged to maintain open lines of communication with their adolescent children. Teens are more likely to delay onset of sexual intercourse when they are more socially connected with or receive greater supervision from a parent.[23,75,79]

Counseling adolescents on appropriate contraceptive use can be an uncomfortable procedure for physicians and parents alike. Nevertheless the sexually active adolescent needs confidential access to contraception.[110,139] If the physician is uneasy about or unwilling to provide these services, the patient should be referred to another professional or organization for follow-up. "Dual methods" of contraception, including the use of oral contraceptives along with a barrier method (i.e., latex condoms and spermicides containing nonoxynol 9), are recommended to assist in the prevention of pregnancy and STD infection.[153,156]

Though rarely the favored choice among adolescent patients, abstinence from sexual intercourse is the most ef-

fective method of preventing STD and pregnancy.[156] Unfortunately the use of scare tactics, threats, and "plea bargains" by adult caregivers and professionals may undercut the credibility of this position. Physicians can avoid this faux pas by candidly discussing both the risks and the rewards associated with teen participation in sexual intercourse. Adolescents should be urged to consider abstinence as the most effective means of preventing STD and pregnancy[156]; candid discussion of contraceptive use should always follow, even when teens deny participation or interest in sexual activity. The use of "outercourse" (e.g., masturbation, sexual touching, massage) can be reviewed as a healthy (and much safer) alternative to intercourse.[68]

The degree to which overall mental health and self-esteem influence adolescent sexual behavior has received little attention in the literature but should not be underestimated. The more a teenager participates in healthy, age-appropriate activities, the less likely he or she may be to engage in high-risk or irresponsible sexual practices. The more positive the relationships between the teenager and the family and community, the less likely that sexual activity will serve as compensation for lack of affection, attention, or pleasure, real or imagined.

Sexually transmitted diseases. To date STD prevention programs have been based largely on the assumption that increased knowledge would lead to behavior change. Preventive strategies have encouraged teens to abstain from sex, limit sex partners, "know" their partners, or be monogamous.[68] For the adolescent patient however these are not "useful" concepts. The adolescent's egocentric thought processes and sense of invulnerability may dilute the impact of any incoming message inconsistent with current cognitive schema. Defiant, oppositional teens are the most likely group to engage in high-risk behaviors but the least likely group to assimilate cautionary messages.

As with other preventive efforts the physician should attempt to communicate in an empathic, caring manner. Prevention strategies should be "in sync" with the teenager's developmental level and should attempt to solicit maximum patient participation. Adolescents must understand that all sexually active persons are at risk for STDs[26]; the myth that only prostitutes and drug abusers have STD must be discussed as part of an overall prevention effort.

Boyer outlines a comprehensive approach to STD prevention for adolescents, incorporating both skill development and educational strategies[16] (Fig. 28-4). Boyer's recommendations include strategies for implementation at the family, physician, school, and community levels.[16] Methods of prevention should take into account the social and cultural environment in which adolescents live; programs should be sensitive to prevailing cultural norms and values. Prevention program efficacy may be further enhanced when services are conveniently located and easily accessible to adolescent patients.[16]

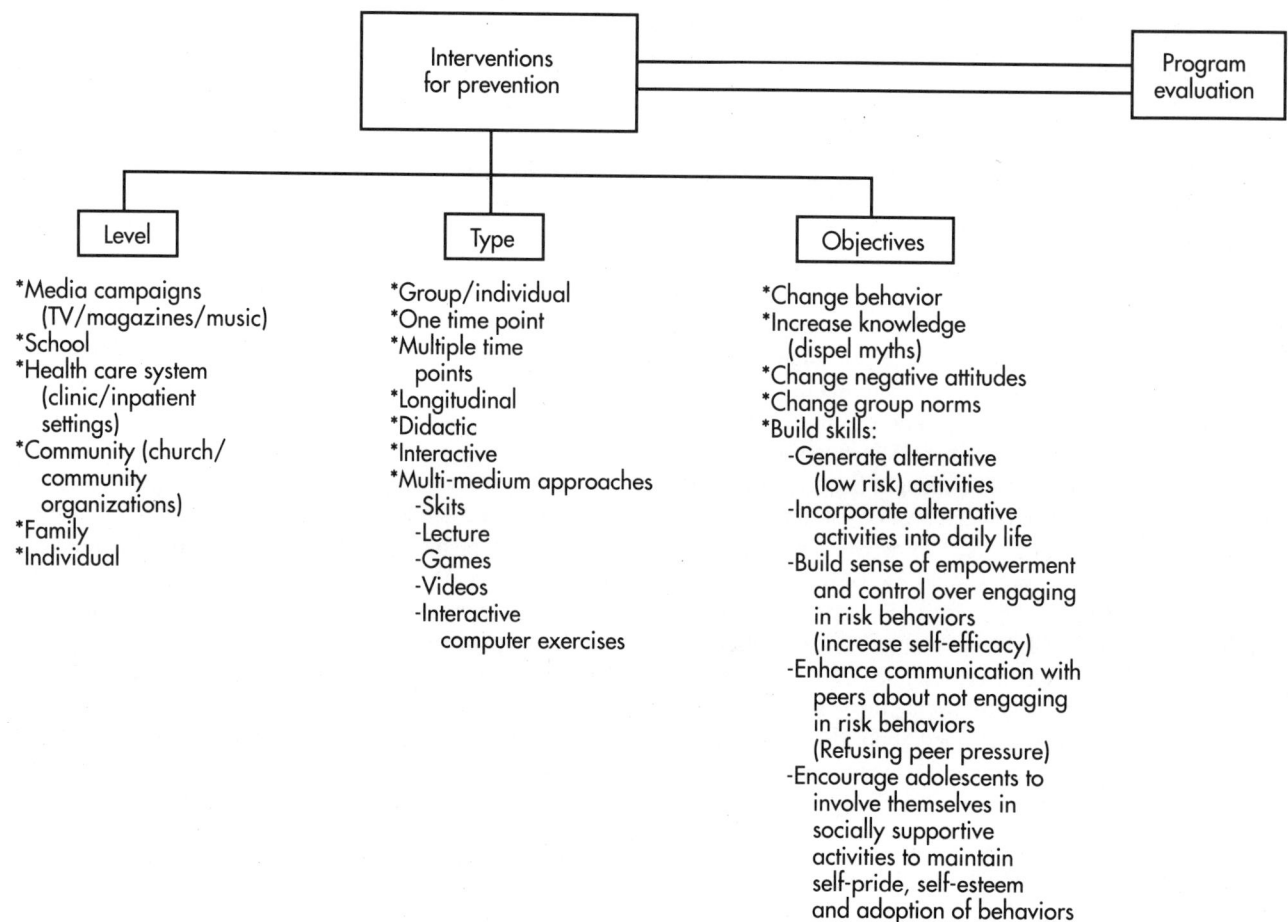

Fig. 28-4. Strategies for education and prevention of STDs in adolescents. (From Boyer CB: *Adolesc Med State of the Art Reviews* 1(3):597-614, 1990.)

Because of the limited duration and scope of sex education classes offered in high school they are unlikely to prove adequate in preventing STDs. In light of this deficit physicians should be prepared to discuss alternatives to sexual intercourse with adolescent patients, recognizing that sexual behavior during adolescence is by no means atypical. Safe sex practices and the risks associated with specific sexual behaviors should be discussed with all sexually active teens. Regardless of individual physicians' beliefs regarding adolescent sexual activity, teens need adequate information and access to services along with home, school, and community support.[139]

Teen pregnancy and contraception. The majority of children in the United States receive some type of formal sex education, generally covering issues of reproduction and contraception.[39,162] However the quality of this information varies considerably, and it is usually not presented until junior high or high school.[39] Few children receive comprehensive education regarding the use of contraceptives before high school,[129] though, contrary to myth, re-

search has shown that education does not lead to increased sexual activity.[39,162]

The provision of comprehensive sex education programs and contraceptive/family planning services can help to significantly reduce teen pregnancy.[54,130,157] Cognitive-behavioral programs designed to teach problem-solving/decision-making skills and increase knowledge regarding sex and contraception have demonstrated positive effects.[130]

School-based clinics designed to provide sex education and access to contraceptives have been successful in decreasing teen pregnancy rates.[38] However, traditional school-based sex education programs may have little effect on teens' sexual behavior, incidence of STD, or pregnancy rates.[141] The problem may be one of too little, too late: For example before age 14 less than 10% of children enrolled in U.S. urban schools participate in comprehensive sex education programs with at least 1 hour of discussion regarding contraception.[129] Effective prevention may depend on early provision of age-appropriate sex educa-

---

Adolescent depression and family conflict

Screening questions

- Have you seriously considered killing yourself recently?
- Do you feel tired much of the time?
- Do you feel sad, down, or depressed much of the time?
- Are you able to talk to your family easily?
- Are you currently having conflicts with your family?
- Do you and your family generally solve problems without a hassle?
- Do you often feel hatred for your family?

From Schubiner H, Robin A: *Pediatrics* 85:813-818, 1990.

Behavioral/emotional disorders

Risk factors

ADOLESCENT FACTORS	FAMILY FACTORS
Lower cognitive/academic ability	Lower socioeconomic status
Lower self-esteem	Single- parent home
History of abuse/neglect	Family dysfunction
Physical illness	Family history of mental illness
Poor peer socialization	Family history of substance abuse
	Poor parental supervision

---

tion[110] and timely access to appropriate contraceptive services for sexually active teens.[110,139]

ADOLESCENT MENTAL HEALTH

Although entry into adulthood may be mitigated by continued support from parents and family, increased responsibilities and obligations may try adolescent coping skills and adversely affect overall mental health. Individual, interpersonal, and environmental factors simultaneously contribute to the adolescent's level of stress and emotional/behavioral adjustment. Biologic and genetic factors may predispose the adolescent to react to stressors in nonadaptive ways. Nevertheless despite the multitude of physiologic, psychologic, and environmental changes faced by adolescents the vast majority of teenagers do not develop significant mental illness or behavioral disturbances.[116] Rates of mental health disorders in adolescents parallel rates in the adult population of approximately 10% to 20%[116]; the incidence of more severe conditions is somewhat lower.[8]

The range of factors contributing to or predisposing an adolescent to mental health disorders is broad and complex. For example the incidence of behavioral/emotional disorders is higher for children and adolescents with communication disorders,[119] for late-maturing males and early-maturing females,[77] for children of alcoholics,[10,81] and for those living in poverty.[6]

Additional factors that place a child at greater risk for behavioral or emotional disorders include low cognitive abilities, poor physical health, socialization deficits, low self-esteem, and school failure.[34] Family factors may play a key role in the development of psychiatric disturbances. Children of dysfunctional families are generally at greater risk; for example when a parent is mentally ill or has an arrest record the children are more likely to suffer from a psychiatric disorder.[34] In general primary risk factors for psychiatric/emotional disorders encompass biologic/genetic, environmental, and social domains (see box).

The prevention of adolescent mental health problems (or, phrased more positively, the promotion of good mental health) has received relatively little attention in the literature to date. Few programs addressing the stressors and psychiatric problems experienced by this population have been implemented, and fewer still have reported outcome data. The physician's prevention efforts should generally follow the model of prevention described above, with identification and assessment of risk factors leading to design and implementation of appropriate prevention strategies.

General assessment

Data used to assess the adolescent patient's mental health are generally limited to the physician's observations during patient and family interviews. Psychologic tests and questionnaires can be used to supplement this information. Screening measures for school-age populations (e.g., the Pediatric Symptoms Checklist[78]) have shown some utility in identifying children at risk for psychosocial difficulties; however, assessment tools specific to the adolescent population have received less attention in the literature and may be underused.

Schubiner and Robin describe a brief seven-item questionnaire that can be used to screen for patient depression and parent-adolescent conflict (see box).[132] Outcome data suggest that this questionnaire has a "hit rate" better than that obtained through physician observation/interview alone. Computerized screening instruments have also been used to obtain supplemental information from adolescent patients.[111]

Because it is a multidimensional attribute, adolescent mental health should be evaluated in terms of cognitive, affective, and behavioral manifestations. Psychologic distress may be evidenced by physical complaints, behavioral changes, and/or significant changes in affect.[6] The full range of behavioral and learning disturbances should be assessed as part of the adolescent patient's interview, ruling out primary problem areas such as oppositional behaviors, attentional problems, and developmental delays.

A history of physical and/or sexual abuse should always be considered when assessing possible emotional or behavioral difficulties. Adolescents are as likely or more likely to be the victims or perpetrators of violence at home than younger children.[57] Particularly when teenagers display oppositional behaviors, parents may resort to physical means of discipline. The guidelines used in reporting child abuse also apply to adolescents; physical indicators (e.g., unexplained bruises, welts, or scars) and/or direct report of the use of excessive force require follow-up with child protective services.[57]

Though far beyond the scope of this chapter, there is a clear overlap between the physiologic and psychologic components of many mental health disorders.[56] Approximately 25% to 35% of adolescent patients' initial complaints to their physicians (excluding acne) are related to functional problems.[6] The physician must always be aware of the extensive interplay of the biologic, psychologic, social, and cultural aspects of adolescent development as they relate to mental health and illness.[116]

In talking with the adolescent patient about emotional distress and mental health the physician should attempt to follow the "style" and "content" recommendations described previously. Confidentiality should be reviewed beforehand and a caring, concerned (versus authoritarian) demeanor should be employed. In cases in which an ongoing positive relationship with a patient has been established the physician may find that direct questions yield accurate information about the adolescent's emotional functioning. When the patient-physician relationship is less "reliable," indirect lines of questioning such as those used to assess chemical use/abuse may prove more effective. For example, questions regarding the physical symptoms associated with depression and anxiety are likely to meet with less resistance than purely "psychologic" or "feelings-based" questions.

Adolescent stress and the family

Normal adolescent efforts to achieve separation/individuation typically accelerate for a 6 to 12 month period between the ages of 13 and 17.[56] The degree of trauma that results from this process varies considerably, as biologic, psychologic, social, and cultural factors play key roles in the outcome.[116] Problematic parent-adolescent relations may become more salient during any of a number of developmental or family changes including divorce, birth of a new child, physical or emotional illness in a parent, or parental job changes. Adolescent strivings for independence and autonomy may trigger family conflict.[53] Academic problems, alcohol/drug abuse, depressed or angry affect, and illegal activities can all reflect problems in family relations or difficulties in management of family stressors.[56]

The adolescent patient witnessing parental divorce may display both behavioral and emotional sequelae. Despite a recent leveling off of the divorce rate in the United States, nearly one half of all children born since the 1970s have or will have divorced parents.[58] Most divorced adults eventually remarry and children may be exposed to a series of parental configurations throughout childhood.[69] Adolescent children may initially react to family division with anger and depression and may side with one parent over the other.[89] Some teens experience long-term consequences, including problems with commitment and an ongoing fear of relationship failure.[56] Others emerge from the divorce relatively unscathed, perhaps more mature and independent for having lived through it.[56,69]

The physician's efforts to prevent family disruption can begin a priori, educating parents about the changes they can expect in their prepubescent child and offering suggestions for age-appropriate parenting techniques. Physicians can support parents' attempts to establish realistic rules and guidelines for their adolescent to follow, at the same time advocating adolescent participation in this process.[56] The physician can encourage parents to respect the child's increasing need for privacy and suggest ways to avert hostile interactions with the adolescent. Recommended readings can be made available in the office or a reading list can be offered to parents interested in learning more about these issues.

When sibling rivalry is a source of family distress, the physician's attempts to normalize sibling conflict may significantly reduce parental anxiety.[56] Parents should be given guidelines to assist them in managing disagreements, encouraging them to use fair, consistent, and firm disciplinary measures when adult intervention becomes necessary. Physical assault or sexual acting out requires more directive action, and families should be referred to appropriate professional resources as needed. Although the physician may accurately identify factors contributing to family unrest (e.g. parental alcoholism, marital discord), significant problems may warrant referral to a mental health professional or agency with expertise in dealing with specific problems.

School performance in the adolescent

Children with a history of attentional, learning, or behavioral problems are clearly at risk for academic shortcomings. Children and adolescents who have a family history of such problems or have medical or psychological problems may also be at increased risk for difficulties in school.[56] Statistics show that 5% to 15% of all school age children have learning disabilities,[148] 1% to 3% are mentally retarded,[124] and approximately 3% have attention-deficit hyperactivity disorder,[7] all of which increase the risk of academic difficulties.

At-risk adolescents may benefit from early intervention; the school, the community, and/or private resources can provide assessment, counseling, and prevention services. If unrecognized, attention and learning problems may escalate and place an adolescent at even greater risk for later school failure and/or conduct problems.[12]

In assessing school-related problems and recommending interventions the physician can enhance his or her role as facilitator by enlisting the expertise of parents and school officials. The physician should begin by pooling all available resources, including school evaluations, academic records, and interviews with parents, teachers, and adolescent patients. When long-standing academic problems are noted or a learning disability is suspected, a psychoeducational evaluation should be obtained.[56] Although many children's learning and attention problems are identified during or before elementary school, many problems (e.g., specific learning disabilities or attention deficit disorder without hyperactivity) may remain undetected until middle or high school.[56]

If significant emotional disorders or conduct problems are noted, referral for psychologic and/or psychiatric assessment and treatment is warranted. Referral for neurologic consultation is unlikely to provide useful information regarding behavioral disorders unless a tic disorder, seizure disorder, or other underlying neurologic syndrome is suspected.[56]

Oppositional and delinquent behavior

Parental concerns about adolescent acting-out behaviors may be brought to the physician's attention during routine medical visits. Empathizing with parental frustration and anger may be the best start in addressing complaints about a teen's problem behaviors. Reminding parents that adolescent "rebellion" and nonconformity are in part developmental milestones can significantly reduce parental distress. When adolescent behavioral problems are subclinical (i.e., do not substantiate a psychiatric diagnosis), suggestions regarding effective, age-appropriate disciplinary measures may prove helpful.[56]

The prevalence of conduct disorders among adolescents has been estimated at between 1.5% and 5.4%.[34] Primary risk factors for conduct disorders include male gender, age, poverty,[34] low academic performance, association with "acting-out" youth,[113] and parental history of arrest.[56] Parental inconsistency, disciplinary problems in the home, and poor parental supervision have been associated with early antisocial behavior and delinquency.[7,113] Criteria for diagnosis and treatment of conduct disorder include aggressive/assaultive behavior toward persons or animals, stealing, repetitive lying, fire setting, running away, involvement in illegal activities, and destruction of property.[7] In looking at prognosis and course, antisocial behavior in childhood frequently appears to continue into adolescence and adulthood.[113]

Less extreme forms of oppositional behavior are common among adolescents. However parents may react strongly to a number of teen indiscretions, including frequent lying, defiance toward parents and other figures in authority, poor academic performance with a history of previously good school work, excessive swearing, and refusal to do routine tasks. Although distressing to parents these behaviors may be "normal" reactions to stress or simply age-appropriate limit testing.[56] Parental efforts to control adolescent behavior via random or inconsistent means may further increase parent-child conflict.[117] Talking with parents about the high incidence of these behaviors and asking them to recall some of their own misbehaviors may help to ease family tensions.

In many families parents have come to rely exclusively on lectures and punishments (e.g., "grounding") in their attempts to control adolescent misbehavior. At times these "solutions" may become part of the problem,[158] as continued punishment exacerbates the parent-child conflict. Exploring alternative disciplinary tactics may help to break the cycle that has developed; for example parents could be encouraged to emphasize "rewards" rather than "punishments," making privileges (watching television, using the car, going out with friends) contingent on task performance (completing homework assignments, finishing chores). Parents may need reassurance that such reinforcement paradigms are appropriate and may benefit from suggestions on how to discipline with minimal anger and/or lecturing. The physician can help parents to design and implement "contracts" that clearly articulate behavioral expectations and often improve adolescent compliance.

Although conduct disorders almost invariably require professional and/or legal intervention, milder oppositional behaviors may be remedied by firm limit setting, increased communication between parent and adolescent, and the adolescent's continued maturation.[56] Early recognition of oppositional behaviors and appropriate use of "low-level" interventions (e.g., behavioral contracting, privilege restriction) should prove adequate in dealing with the majority of adolescent infractions. Prevention strategies may include the recommendation of parenting books or provision of handouts that summarize effective disciplinary strategies.

To maximize efficacy, efforts to prevent oppositional behavior should begin long before the adolescent reaches puberty. Parent training has proved effective when used with preadolescent antisocial youth.[113] Parents well versed in the use of behavioral parenting techniques are likely to fare better when adolescent limit testing occurs. Physicians should target families with inconsistent rule enforcement or chaotic home environments for early preventive efforts, providing guidance during or before preadolescence whenever possible. Prevention programs that target high-risk youth may be the most cost-effective method of deterring adolescent behavior problems.[17]

Eating disorders

Eating disorders, including anorexia nervosa, bulimia nervosa, and atypical eating disorders, are increasingly common among adolescents and young adults, particularly females.[6,52] *Anorexia* is generally defined as (1) an intense drive for thinness with a refusal to maintain appropriate body weight; (2) an intense fear of gaining weight, (3) a disturbance in body perception, and (4) for females, a cessation of normal menses.[7] *Bulimia* is characterized by (1) recurrent binges of eating, (2) feelings of lack of control over eating, (3) the use of purging methods, and (4) a persistent concern over body shape and weight.[7] Eating disorders affect an estimated 5% to 15% of adolescent girls and young women, with mortality rates as high as 9%.[6,11]

A number of personality, family, and environmental factors have been associated with eating disorders. The disorders are more common in females of middle- and upper-middle-class background, leading some to hypothesize that a family/societal influence is involved.[11] Women who have eating disorders have been anecdotally described as perfectionistic, rigid-thinking, and hard-driving; symptoms related to food restriction have been labeled as control issues for many patients.[11] In addition some speculate that Western society's emphasis on body image and thinness, particularly for females, may have a significant impact on the rates of eating disorders in this culture.[11,31,52]

Effective prevention of eating disorders requires early identification of patients with inappropriate expectations for body weight and/or excessive concerns about thinness.[5] Although only a small percentage of females with such concerns may become anorexic, prevention efforts may be justified by this disorder's high mortality and morbidity rates, as well as its resistance to treatment.[11,52] As with other areas of health risk early recognition and prevention tactics may significantly improve patient outcome.[33] Hence physicians should ask every female patient how she feels about her overall physical appearance, at the same time recognizing that the majority of females will express at least minimal concern about body image. If discontent appears greater than expected (given patient's age, developmental level, and so forth), referral for further psychologic/psychiatric evaluation and treatment should be considered. The physician should remain sensitive to potential medical complications and remain an active part of the ongoing treatment regimen.[5,11]

In working with preadolescent female patients the physician should discuss upcoming physical changes and outline the expected range of growth and development.[137] The importance of a balanced diet and moderate exercise regimen should be highlighted.[153] In discussing these issues, early signs of food obsessions or overly rigid meal planning should be noted and addressed. Patient worries and concerns about food and/or weight should be reviewed and follow-up treatment or referral provided as needed. Parents should be counseled regarding typical adolescent changes in eating habits and informed of any potential problems. However, as parental criticism and overinvolvement may exacerbate adolescent limit testing, parents should be encouraged to provide nurturance and guidance while respecting the teen's need for some self-direction in diet/activity planning.

Depression/affective disorders

In the past decade adolescent affective disorders have received increasing attention in the literature.[91] Adolescent manifestations of emotional distress were previously viewed as a developmental milestones,[116] experiences that teens would "outgrow." However recent studies have shown that childhood and adolescent depression can have a significant and ongoing impact on an individual's social skills, academic performance, and overall development.[91] Although adolescent mania and bipolar disorders are less prevalent and less extensively studied, patients experiencing related disorders are at risk for suicidal ideation and a host of other psychosocial problems.[92,159]

The prevalence of major depression and dysthymia within the general adolescent population has been reported as somewhere between 2% and 6%.[8,34,86] Adolescents experiencing major depression are at risk for other emotional disorders as well, particularly anxiety disorders.[86,92] A somewhat larger number of adolescents (between 10% and 20%) report symptoms of depression or depressed mood.[72,85] Thus although the number of teens meeting diagnostic criteria for an affective disorder is small, the larger number experiencing related symptoms may also need assistance.

Teen depression may be evidenced by somatization (e.g., headaches, stomachaches, unexplained aches and pains), delinquency (e.g., drug abuse, acting out behavior), or other behavioral/emotional manifestations.[10] Teens with a family history of affective disorder are at greater risk for depression,[7,10] as are those with a family history of substance abuse.[81] Children and adolescents living in stressful environments,[10] those of lower socioeconomic status,[85] and those experiencing chronic physical illness[7] may also be at increased risk for depression.

Determining the character and intensity of an adolescent patient's depression may prove difficult. Like their adult counterparts, depressed teens may employ defense mechanisms (i.e., denial, displacement, and repression) that restrict the utility of straightforward diagnostic procedures such as direct questioning. For this reason multiple assessment tools should be used to evaluate a patient for depression, including interviews with the patient and family members, screening questionnaires, school reports, and psychologic test data.[10] Depressed adolescents may display a variety of symptoms, including dysphoric mood, changes in appetite and sleep patterns, anhedonia, psychomotor retardation, agitation, or concentration problems.[6,7,10] As depressive symptoms may also indicate the presence of suicidal ideation, the physician should be prepared to assess and refer as needed (see box).

Quantitative measures of affective distress can provide further data regarding the presence or absence of a psychi-

<table>
</table>

Symptoms of depression in adolescents	
Behavioral/psychological	*Physical*
Helplessness/hopelessness	Change in appetite
Loss of interest in usual activities	Weight loss or gain
Decreased concentration	Loss of energy or hyperactivity/agitation
Poor academic performance	Change in sleep patterns
Change in mood/sadness	Physical complaints without medical cause
Tearfulness	Headaches/abdominal pain
Change in socialization	
Drug/alcohol use or abuse	
Increased risk-taking behavior	
Suicidal thoughts/behaviors	

Adolescent suicide

Risk factors

ADOLESCENT FACTORS	FAMILY FACTORS
White male	Poor family support
Alcohol or drug use/abuse	Family history of psychiatric illness
Depression/affective disorder	Availability of firearms in the home
Previous suicide attempt	
Recent exposure to suicide	
Recent personal crisis	
History of physical/sexual abuse	

atric disorder. Screening questionnaires such as the Beck Depression Inventory or the Children's Depression Inventory can be used to screen adolescent patients for depression.[101] The screening questionnaire outlined by Schubiner and Robin (see box above) can be used to highlight psychosocial problems that may contribute to emotional distress.[132] Structured interviews may be used to obtain information regarding the degree and kind of depression a patient may be experiencing, though time and labor demands may limit their use to patients identified as high-risk.

Academic records and school-related data can further help the physician in assessing affective disorders. Declining grades, social withdrawal, and other factors associated with the school milieu are critical cues to adolescents' emotional disposition. Input from teachers, counselors, and related personnel can highlight the patient's behavior during a significant portion of his or her daily schedule.[87]

Adolescents who have vague complaints, a high-risk profile, or an ambiguous clinical picture might be referred to a mental health specialist (e.g., child/family psychologist or psychiatrist) for follow-up evaluation and/or treatment. Contributing factors that are amenable to treatment (e.g., family conflict) can be further addressed in this setting. Left unattended an otherwise treatable disorder can have long-lasting impact on the adolescent's cognitive and behavioral functioning.[73]

Little research has been published regarding the prevention of depression and other affective disorders in children and adolescents. Routine screening for depression in adults has not been shown to improve the rate of identification.[24,156] Comparisons of early intervention versus later treatment of depression have shown little difference in long-term outcome.[24,156] Thus routine screening for depression in asymptomatic adults is likely to be of limited benefit. However for adolescent patients early identification and treatment are warranted because of the significant consequences (e.g., suicide) that may accompany affective disorders.[156]

ADOLESCENT SUICIDE
Background information and risk factors

Suicide is currently the third leading cause of death among adolescents and young adults in the United States, at a yearly rate of 11.3/100,000 for 15- to 19-year-olds and 15.0/100,000 for 20- to 24-year-olds.[151] Suicide is the second leading cause of death for white males aged 15 to 24 (23/100,000)[153]; the suicide rate for black males in this age group is significantly lower, at about 15/100,000.[151] Adolescent females, both black and white, *attempt* suicide much more frequently than adolescent males (2:1 vs 3:1)[46]; they generally use less lethal methods and are less often "successful."[46,100,153] Idiosyncratic variables influence each individual's susceptibility, and every adolescent patient should be considered at risk and screened for suicidal ideation.

For adults the diagnosis of affective disorder, depressed, is considered a major precursor to suicidal ideation or behavior.[13] Kovacs reports that by adolescence the relationship between significant affective disturbance and suicidal behavior begins to emerge.[91] One comparison of adolescents who committed suicide with adolescents hospitalized for treatment of suicidal ideation showed that "successful suicides" experienced a significantly higher rate of bipolar disorder.[19] Adolescents diagnosed and treated for depression are at high risk for later episodes of depression[92]; these patients should be regarded as at risk for suicide during and after treatment, and parents should be informed accordingly.[9,91]

Other risk factors for suicidal ideation and behavior include (1) drug/alcohol use or abuse,[9,136] (2) history of previous suicide attempt,[9,136] (3) family history of suicide attempt,[136] (4) recent crisis or stressor,[9] (5) poor family support,[9] (6) recent suicides described in the media,[63,64] (7) availability of firearms in the home,[18,19] and (8) history of impulsive behavior.[9] Adolescents with low self-esteem, rigid thinking, somatization disorders, conduct disorders, or a history of reckless or delinquent behaviors are also at higher than average risk for suicide.[9] In addition adolescents with a history of physical or sexual abuse are more likely to act on suicidal ideation[123,136]; such abuse also increases the likelihood that teens will engage in other health-risk behaviors such as alcohol/drug use, use of tobacco, and self-induced vomiting[123] (see box).

Assessment issues

Adolescents should be screened for depression and suicidal ideation during each medical visit.[73] This will in part involve direct questioning of the patient, as in the following example:

Cathy, you tell me that you've been experiencing some down periods lately, and often when people feel this way they think about hurting themselves in some way. I'm wondering, *when was the last time* you thought about or felt like hurting yourself in some way?

Physicians may not routinely inquire as to a family's history of mental illness and/or suicidal behavior. However, the health risks associated with these disorders may be as great as or greater than those of other diseases with a strong hereditary component that are routinely included in medical screenings (e.g., heart disease, diabetes). Questions about family relations and recent personal and family stressors should be asked to highlight additional factors associated with teen depression and suicide.[9]

Acute factors potentially fostering suicidal ideation include breakup with a significant other,[9] drug intoxication,[9,73] and feelings of hopelessness.[72] Both physician and family should be alert to warning signs including the communication of suicidal intent and the giving away of personal items.[72] Although the adolescent patient may show no interest or commitment, referral to appropriate mental health professionals should be pursued when significant signs of depression and/or suicidal ideation appear evident.

Prevention strategies

Early detection and intervention with depressed and/or suicidal adolescents is clearly the most effective method of preventing self-injurious behavior.[153] As with mental illness, suicidal behavior results in part from patients' affective distress, negative environmental circumstances, and inadequate coping skills. Hence prevention of suicide may best be viewed as part of an overall effort to prevent severe emotional distress and psychiatric illness.

Adolescents should be directly questioned about self-destructive thinking,[72] and both patient and family should be informed when significant risk factors are observed, particularly when a history of affective disorder or suicidal behavior is present. Broad-based media efforts to educate adolescents about suicide have not proved useful and may paradoxically increase teen suicidal behaviors.[64] The physician should ask about the presence of firearms in the

---

Adolescent violence/homicide

Risk factors

ADOLESCENT FACTORS	FAMILY FACTORS
Black male	Low socioeconomic status
Age 15 to 24	Family history of violence/abuse
History of abuse	
Association with violent peers	

---

home, as the presence of such weapons significantly increases the risk of teen suicide, regardless of how the weapons or ammunition are stored.[18]

ADOLESCENT HOMICIDE AND VIOLENCE
Background information and risk factors

Homicide is the second leading cause of death for those age 15 to 24, and the leading cause of death for blacks in this age range.[151,153,156] Most of these murders are forms of "expressive violence," acts of anger and emotion directed against friends, relatives, or acquaintances.[153] In 1980 homicides and assaults accounted for 23,970 deaths, 350,000 hospitalizations, 1.5 million hospital days, and at least $638 million in health care expenditures[126]; child/adolescent homicide alone costs an estimated 93,000 years of potential life.[6] Fueled in part by socioeconomic factors U.S. rates of adolescent homicide and assault are currently on the rise.[153]

Several factors correlate highly with increased violence among youth. Poverty is a primary factor, as homicides occur more often in densely populated, lower socioeconomic status (SES) urban areas.[153] Although the risk of death by homicide is significantly greater for blacks, much of this difference disappears when SES is accounted for.[153] Consistent with general cultural norms regarding physical aggression and gender, males are much more likely than females to be the victims of homicide or other assault.[66] However continued gender role diffusion[140] and female adolescents' increased involvement in the illegal drug trade may narrow this difference significantly.

Adolescents' participation in and exposure to violence are also influenced by cultural and familial norms regarding violent behavior. A history of abuse in childhood is found more frequently than would be expected among both victims and assailants of homicide.[88] When adolescents are reared in family and sociocultural environments where violence is endorsed as an effective problem-solving strategy, complicity is hardly surprising[103] (see box).

Adolescents' participation in gangs appears to increase both teen violence and the public's awareness of these acts. Although urban gangs have been a concern for generations, the illegal drug trade and the growing availability of firearms amplify the potential menace posed by these groups.[66] Youth gangs are common: It has been estimated that one in five adolescent males in U.S. communities of 10,000 or more has joined an organized group involved in substance use and/or delinquent activity.[14] Such gangs are likely to exist in cities with a large minority population where members are not integrated into the predominant culture.[66]

Assessment issues

Health care personnel should question teens about exposure to and participation in violent acts as part of routine history taking.[144] Inquiry should explore potential areas of conflict within the teen's environment, including physical aggression among family members, neighborhood violence, and fighting at school. The patient and family should be asked about the presence of firearms in the home, the storage of weapons and ammunition, and teens' accessibility to these items. Teens should also be questioned about the relationship between violence/aggression and sexual behavior. Both males and females should be asked about times when they were coerced or forced into a sexual relationship, with or without violence.

Youth involvement in gangs should be routinely assessed, especially when changes in social behavior have been observed or reported. Gang membership may be conveyed through style of dress and language,[66] with paraphernalia and markings varying by locale. Many youth gangs use the trappings of professional sports teams and brand-name sportswear to convey their alliance. Parents should be asked about signs of gang involvement; common indicators include (1) an alteration in clothing preference, (2) a sudden change in friends and activities, (3) unexplained bruises, (4) tattoos or other body markings, (5) availability of money without explanation, (6) new nicknames, (7) interest in weapons, and (8) unfamiliar graffiti or "doodling."

Prevention strategies. Large-scale prevention programs targeting violence among adolescents are under way in many cities throughout the United States; Boston's Violence Prevention Project of the Health Promotion Program for Urban Youth is one example.[140] Programs typically use a variety of culturally sensitive and age-appropriate materials to help teens explore alternatives to violent behavior. The underlying assumption is that if teens learn other methods of problem solving and conflict resolution, the overall rate of violent behavior will decrease.[153] As with other prevention efforts, programs addressing teen violence target high-risk youth and attempt to intervene early.[66] They employ a variety of cognitive, behavioral, and social learning strategies intended to "inoculate" youth against participation in violent behaviors. As these efforts are a fairly recent development, outcome studies are not yet available as to program efficacy.[66]

The physician working with individual adolescent patients may find little research to draw from in developing violence-prevention strategies. Stringham and Weitzman have outlined tactics that primary care physicians may employ in assessing and counseling at-risk youth.[144] They recommend that all children and adolescents be questioned regarding violence at home and school, and anticipatory guidance offered to patients and parents in need.

Physicians should be familiar with the "colors" of youth gangs in their area and should consult local resource centers or police organizations to identify characteristic problem behaviors. Local universities and health care organizations may be implementing programs to address youth violence and may provide further assistance. Parents should be provided with relevant information, alerting them to possible signs of participation in these groups.

As is true of many sociocultural problems, knowledge is a necessary but not sufficient component to the prevention of teen violence. The most promising strategies for idiopathic prevention are likely to involve the training of preadolescents in nonviolent problem solving, conflict resolution, and stress management skills. However the efficacy of broader-based prevention programs will no doubt depend on their capacity to address larger social issues such as poverty, social inequity, and racism.[66] Adolescents' involvement in youth gangs can only be prevented by addressing the underlying needs that lead to gang affiliation: desire for "status, a place of acceptance, and a sense of self-worth."[66]

Physicians can perhaps best help individual families by alerting parents to the risk factors associated with adolescent violence. Parents should be made aware of the early signs of gang involvement, drug use, and criminal activity. Families in high-risk neighborhoods should be encouraged to use community and school resources designed to mitigate teen violence. Parents should be reminded that the best defense is a good offense, as a supportive, structured, and caring home environment may be the most compelling preventive measure available.

SUMMARY

Historically a segment of the teenage population has always engaged in rebellious, defiant behaviors. The adolescent stage of development is often accompanied by participation in high-risk behaviors such as alcohol/drug use, gang involvement, and sexual activity. Although the majority of teens emerge from this developmental period relatively intact, a substantial minority suffer physical and/or psychologic consequences of their actions. Participation in high-risk behaviors has become increasingly life-threatening, though the three leading causes of adolescent death (injuries/accidents, homicide, and suicide)[153,156] are perhaps the most preventable.

The arguments in favor of prevention are clear, and savings in dollars, lives, and human suffering are substantial. Although prevention programs may require considerable financial investment, the cost of ignoring these problems may be far greater. For example Strasburger estimates that the cost of providing family planning services to sexually active girls would be less than 3% of the cost a community would bear if such services were withheld.[143] Over time the financial burden of *not* providing preventive health care services is staggering, and "hidden costs" (e.g., welfare payments to pregnant teens, foster care for infants born with HIV) are often formidable. When the potential lives and productivity lost are taken into account, the argument for prevention becomes even more convincing.

Successful prevention programs have several features in common: They target a specific problem area, attempt to promote long-term changes in behavior, focus on skill development, and emphasize the importance of building on social networks.[118] During a standard office visit the brief duration of patient contact and limited resources available generally restrict the individual practitioner's ability to fulfill these criteria. However to the degree that the physician's work is consistent with these guidelines and supports the objectives of related prevention efforts, decreased adolescent morbidity and mortality should result. The clinician's potential impact may be further broadened by participation in prevention programs at local, state, and federal levels.

REFERENCES

1. American Academy of Pediatrics, Committee on Adolescence: Alcohol use and abuse: a pediatric concern, *Pediatrics* 79:450-453, 1987.
2. American Academy of Pediatrics, Committee on Adolescence: The role of the pediatrician in substance abuse counseling, *Pediatrics* 72:251-252, 1983.
3. American Academy of Pediatrics, Committee on Communications: Children, adolescents and television, *Pediatrics* 85:1119-1120, 1990.
4. American Academy of Pediatrics, Committee on Youth and Committee on Adolescent Medicine, Canadian Paediatric Society: Alcohol consumption: an adolescent problem, *Pediatrics* 55:557-559, 1975.
5. American College of Physicians, Health and Public Policy Committee: Eating disorders: anorexia nervosa and bulimia, *Ann Intern Med* 105:790-794, 1986.
6. American Medical Association: *White paper on adolescent health*, Washington DC, 1987, American Medical Association.
7. American Psychiatric Association: *Diagnostic and statistical manual of mental disorders*, ed 3, Washington DC, 1987, American Psychiatric Association.
8. Anderson JC et al: DSM-III disorders in preadolescent children: prevalence in a large sample from the general population, *Arch Gen Psychol* 44:69-76, 1987.
9. Atala KD, Baxter RF: Suicidal adolescents: how to help them before it's too late, *Postgrad Med* 86(5):223-230, 1989.
10. Aylward GP: Understanding and treatment of childhood depression, *J Pediatr* 107:1-9, 1985.
11. Balaa MA, Drossman DA: Anorexia nervosa and bulimia: the eating disorders, *Dis Mon* 31(6):1-52, 1985.
12. Barkley RA: *Attention-deficit hyperactivity disorder*. In Mash EJ, Barkley RA, editors: *Treatment of childhood disorders*, New York, 1989, The Guilford Press.
13. Bennets M: *Depression*. In Matzen R, Lang R, editors: *Clinical preventive medicine*, St. Louis, 1992, Mosby–Year Book.
14. Berland DI, Homlish JS, Blotcky MJ: Adolescent gangs in the hospital, *Bull Menninger Clin* 53:31-43, 1989.
15. Botvin GJ: Drug abuse research: second triennial report to Congress, Washington DC, 1987, National Institute on Drug Abuse, U.S. Department of Health and Human Services.
16. Boyer CB: Psychosocial, behavioral, and educational factors in preventing sexually transmitted diseases, *Adol Med State of the Art Reviews*1(3):597-614, 1990.
17. Boyle MH, Offord DR: Primary prevention of conduct disorder: issues and prospects, *J Am Acad Child Adolesc Psychiatry* 29:227-233, 1990.
18. Brent DA et al: The presence and accessibility of firearms in the homes of adolescent suicides, *JAMA* 266:2989-2995, 1991.
19. Brent DA et al: Risk factors for adolescent suicide: a comparison of adolescent suicide victims with suicidal inpatients, *Arch Gen Psychiatry* 45:581-588, 1988.
20. Brone RJ, Fisher CB: Determinants of adolescent obesity: a comparison with anorexia nervosa, *Adolescence* 23(89):155-168, 1988.
21. Brookman RR: *Infections of the male and female reproductive tracts*. In Hofman AD, Greydanus DE, editors: *Adolescent medicine*, Norwalk, CT, 1989, Appleton & Lange.
22. Brookman RR: *Reproductive health assessment of the adolescent*. In Hofman AD, Greydanus DE, editors: *Adolescent medicine*, Norwalk, CT, 1989, Appleton & Lange.
23. Brooks-Gunn J, Furstenberg FF, Jr: Adolescent sexual behavior, *Am Psychol* 44:249-257, 1989.
24. Canadian Task Force on the Periodic Health Examination: Periodic health examination, 1990 update: 2. Early detection of depression and prevention of suicide, *Can Med Assoc J* 142:1233-1238, 1990.
25. Cates W Jr, Hinman AR: Sexually transmitted diseases in the 1990s, *N Engl J Med* 325:1368-1369, 1991.
26. Cates W Jr: The epidemiology and control of sexually transmitted diseases in adolescents, *Adolesc Med State of the Art Reviews* 1(3):409-428, 1990.
27. CDC: Participation of high school students in school physical education—United States, 1990, *MMWR* 40(35): 607,613-615, 1991.
28. Centerwall BS: Exposure to television as a risk factor for violence, *Am J Epidemiol* 129:643-652, 1989.
29. Chick J, Lloyd G, Crombie E: Counselling problem drinkers in medical wards: a controlled study, *Br Med J* 290:965-967, 1985.
30. Cogswell BE: Cultivating the trust of adolescent patients, *Fam Med* 27:254-258, 1985.
31. Collins ME: Education for healthy body weight: helping adolescents balance the cultural pressure for thinness, *J School Health* 58:227-231, 1988.
32. Comerci GD, Kilbourne KA, Harrison GG: *Adolescent nutrition*. In Hofman AD, Greydanus DE, editors: *Adolescent medicine*, Norwalk, CT, 1989, Appleton & Lange.
33. Comerci GD, Kilbourne KA, Harrison GG: *Eating disorders: obesity, anorexia nervosa, and bulimia*. In Hofman AD, Greydanus DE, editors: *Adolescent medicine*, Norwalk, CT, 1989, Appleton & Lange.
34. Costello EJ: Developments in child psychiatric epidemiology, *J Am Acad Child Adolesc Psychiatry* 28:836-841, 1989.
35. Cresanta JL et al: Prevention of atherosclerosis in childhood, *Pediatr Clin North Am* 33(4):835-858, 1986.
36. Cyr MG, Wartman SA: The effectiveness of routine screening questions in the detection of alcoholism, *JAMA* 259:51-54, 1988.
37. D'Angelo LJ et al: Human immunodeficiency virus infection in urban adolescents: can we predict who is at risk? *Pediatrics* 88:982-986, 1991.
38. Davis SM: Preventing adolescent pregnancy, *Adolesc Med State of the Art Reviews* 1(1):113-126, 1990.

39. Dawson DA: The effects of sex education on adolescent behavior, *Fam Plann Perspect* 18(4):162-170, 1986.

40. Deisher RW, Remafedi G: *Adolescent sexuality.* In Hofman AD, Greydanus DE, editors: *Adolescent medicine,* Norwalk, CT, 1989, Appleton & Lange.

41. Dietz WH: Prevention of childhood obesity, *Pediatr Clin North Am* 33(4):823-834, 1986.

42. Dietz WH Jr, Gortmaker SL: Do we fatten our children at the television set? Obesity and television viewing in children and adolescents, *Pediatrics* 75:807, 1985.

43. Dietz WH et al: Trends in the prevalence of childhood and adolescent obesity in the United States, *Pediatr Res* 19:198A, 1985.

44. Dwyer J: Promoting good nutrition for today and the year 2000, *Pediatr Clin North Am* 33(4):799-822, 1986.

45. Dyment PG: *The adolescent athlete.* In Hofman AD, Greydanus DE, editors: *Adolescent medicine,* Norwalk, CT, 1989, Appleton & Lange.

46. Eisenberg L: The epidemiology of suicide in adolescents, *Pediatr Ann* 13(1):47-54, 1984.

47. Epstein LH, Cluss PA: Behavioral genetics of childhood obesity, *Behav Ther* 17:324-334, 1986.

48. Epstein LH et al: A comparison of lifestyle exercise, aerobic exercise, and calisthenics on weight loss in obese children, *Behav Ther* 16:345-356, 1985.

49. Ewing JA: Detecting alcoholism: the CAGE questionnaire, *JAMA* 252:1905-1907, 1984.

50. Filstead WJ, Mayer JE: *Adolescence and alcohol: an overview and introduction.* In Filstead WJ, Mayer JE, editors: *Adolescence and alcohol,* Cambridge MA, 1980, Ballinger.

51. Foreyt JP, Cousins JH: *Obesity.* In Mash EJ, Barkley RA, editors: *Treatment of childhood disorders,* New York, 1989, The Guilford Press.

52. Foreyt JP, McGavin JK: *Anorexia nervosa and bulimia nervosa.* In Mash EJ, Barkley RA editors: *Treatment of childhood disorders,* New York, 1989, The Guilford Press.

53. Foster SL, Robin AL: *Parent-adolescent conflict.* In Mash EJ, Barkley RA, editors: *Treatment of childhood disorders,* New York, 1989, The Guilford Press.

54. Furstenberg FF Jr, Brooks-Gunn J, Chase-Lansdale L: Teenaged pregnancy and childbearing, *Am Psychol* 44(2):313-320, 1989.

55. Furstenberg FF Jr, Brooks-Gunn J, Morgan SP: Adolescent mothers and their children in later life, *Fam Plann Perspect* 19(4):142-151, 1987.

56. Gabriel HP, Hofman AD: *Behavioral problems.* In Hofman AD, Greydanus DE, editors: *Adolescent medicine,* Norwalk, CT, 1989, Appleton & Lange.

57. Gelles RJ: Family violence and adolescents, *Adolesc Med State of the Art Reviews* 1(1):45-54, 1990.

58. Glick PC, Lin S: Recent changes in divorce and remarriage, *J Marriage Fam Ther* 48:737-747, 1986.

59. Glynn TJ: From family to peer: a review of transitions of influence among drug-using youth, *J Youth Adolesc* 10:363-383, 1981.

60. Goodstadt MS, Sheppard MA: Three approaches to alcohol education, *J Stud Alcohol* 44:362-380, 1983.

61. Goodwin DW et al: Alcohol problems in adoptees raised apart from alcoholic biological parents, *Arch Gen Psychiatry,* 28:238-243, 1973.

62. Goodwin DW et al: Drinking problems in adopted and nonadopted sons of alcoholics, *Arch Gen Psychiatry* 31:164-169, 1974.

63. Gould MS, Davidson L: Suicide contagion among adolescents, *Adv Adolesc Mental Health* 3:29-59, 1988.

64. Gould MS, Shaffer D: The impact of suicide in television movies: evidence of imitation, *N Engl J Med* 315:690-694, 1986.

65. Grant LM, Demetriou E: Adolescent sexuality, *Pediatr Clin North Am* 55:1271-1289, 1988.

66. Greydanus DE et al: The gang phenomenon and the American teenager, *Adolesc Med State of the Art Reviews* 1(1):55-70, 1990.

67. Hawkins JD, Lishner DM, Catalano RF Jr: *Childhood predictors and prevention of adolescent substance abuse.* In Jones CL, Battjes RJ, editors: *Etiology of drug abuse: Implications for prevention,* Washington, DC, 1985, National Institutes of Drug Abuse, U.S. Department of Health and Human Services.

68. Hein K: Risky business: adolescents and human immunodeficiency virus, *Pediatrics* 88:1052-1054, 1991.

69. Hetherington EM, Hagan MS, Anderson ER: Marital transitions: a child's perspective, *Am Psychol* 44:303-312, 1989.

70. Henshaw SK, Van Vort J: Teenage abortion, birth and pregnancy statistics: an update, *Fam Plann Perspect* 21:85-88, 1989.

71. Hingson RW et al: Beliefs about AIDS, use of alcohol and drugs, and unprotected sex among Massachusetts adolescents, *Am J Public Health* 80(3):295-299, 1990.

72. Hodgman CH: *Depression, suicide, out-of-control reactions, and psychoses.* In Hofman AD, Greydanus DE, editors: *Adolescent medicine,* Norwalk, CT, 1989, Appleton & Lange.

73. Hodgman CH: Adolescent depression and suicide, *Adolesc Med State of the Art Reviews* 1(1):81-96, 1990.

74. Hofman AE: Clinical assessment and management of health risk behaviors in adolescents, *Adolesc Med State of the Art Reviews* 1(1):33-44, 1990.

75. Inazu JK, Fox GL: Maternal influence on the sexual behavior of teen-age daughters, *J Fam Issues* 1:81-102, 1980.

76. Irwin CE Jr: Why adolescent medicine? *J Adolesc Health Care* 7:2S-12S, 1986.

77. Irwin CE Jr: The theoretical concept of at-risk adolescents, *Adolesc Med State of the Art Reviews* 1(1):1-14, 1990.

78. Jellinek MS et al: Pediatric symptom checklist: screening school-age children for psychosocial dysfunction, *J Pediatr* 112(2):201-209, 1988.

79. Jessor SL, Jessor R: Transition from virginity to nonvirginity among youth: a social-psychological study over time, *Dev Psychol* 11:473-484, 1975.

80. Johnson CA et al: Relative effectiveness of comprehensive community programming for drug abuse prevention with high-risk and low-risk adolescents, *J Clin Consult Psychol* 58:447-456, 1990.

81. Johnson JL, Boney TY, Brown BS: Evidence of depressive symptoms in children of substance abusers, *Int J Addict* 25:465-479, 1990-1991.

82. Johnston LD, O'Malley PM, Bachman JG: *Drug use among American high school seniors, college students and young adults, 1975-1990,* vol 1, Rockville MD, 1991, National Institute on Drug Abuse, U.S. Department of Health and Human Services.

83. Jones EF et al: Unintended pregnancy, contraceptive practice and family planning services in developed countries, *Fam Plann Perspect* 20(2):53-67, 1988.

84. Kandel D, Faust R: Sequence and stages in patterns of adolescent drug use, *Arch Gen Psychiatry* 32:923-932, 1975.

85. Kaplan SL, Hong GK, Weinhold C: Epidemiology of depressive symptomatology in adolescents, *J Am Acad Child Psychiatry* 23:91-98, 1984.

86. Kashani JH et al: Depression, depressive symptoms, and depressed mood among a community sample of adolescents, *Am J Psychiatry* 144:931-934, 1987.

87. Kazdin A: *Childhood depression.* In Mash EJ, Barkley RA, editors: *Treatment of childhood disorders,* New York, 1989, The Guilford Press.

88. Kazdin AE: Treatment of anti-social behaviors in children: Current status and future directions, *Psychol Bull* 102:187-203, 1987.

89. Keshet JK, Mirkin MP: *Troubled adolescents in divorced and remarried families.* In Mirkin MP, Koman SL, editors: *Handbook of adolescents and family therapy,* New York, 1985, Gandner Press.

90. Kipke MD, Hein K: Acquired Immunodeficiency Syndrome (AIDS) in adolescents, *Adolesc Med State of the Art Reviews* 1(3):429-450, 1990.

91. Kovacs M: Affective disorders in children and adolescents, *Am*

Psychol 44(2):209-215, 1989.

92. Kovacs M, Gatsonis C: *Stability and change in childhood- onset depressive disorders: longitudinal course as a diagnostic validator,* In LN Robins, JE Barrett, editors: *The validity of psychiatric diagnosis,* New York, 1989, Raven Press.

93. Kristenson H: Methods of intervention to modify drinking patterns in heavy drinkers, *Rec Dev Alcohol* 5:403-423, 1987.

94. Liebert RM, Sprafkin J: The early window—effects of television on children and youth, ed 3, New York, 1990, Pergamon Press.

95. Leiman AH, Strasburger VC: Counseling parents of adolescents, *Pediatr* 76(4):664-667, 1985.

96. Macdonald DI: *Substance abuse, Pediatr Rev* 10(3):89- 95, 1988.

97. Maciak BJ et al: Pregnancy and birth rates among sexually experienced US teenagers—1974, 1980, and 1983, *JAMA* 258(15):2069-2071, 1987.

98. Mallick HJ: Health hazards of obesity and weight control in children: a review of the literature, *Am J Public Health* 73:78-87, 1983.

99. Marks A: Aspects of biosocial screening and health maintenance in adolescents, *Pediatr Clin North Am* 27:153-161, 1980.

100. Marks A, Fisher M: Health assessment and screening during adolescence, *Pediatrics* 80(1):135-158, 1987.

101. Matsen JL: *Treating depression in children and adolescents,* New York, 1989, Pergamon Press.

102. McLellan AT et al: An improved diagnostic evaluation instrument for substance abuse patients: The Addiction Severity Index, *J Nerv Ment Dis* 168:26-33, 1980.

103. Resilience can be fostered through interventions, *Ment Health Weekly* 1(15):1-3, 1991.

104. Millstein SG et al: Health-risk behaviors and health concerns among young adolescents, *Pediatrics* 3:422-428, 1992.

105. Monthly vital statistics report 37(13), Hyatsville, MD, 1989, National Center for Health Statistics.

106. NCADD fact sheet: alcoholism and alcohol-related problems, New York, 1990, National Council on Alcoholism and Drug Dependence.

107. Nordstrom G, Berglund M: Successful adjustment in alcoholism: relationships between causes of improvment, personality, and social factors, *J Nerv Mental Dis* 174:664-668, 1986.

108. Novello O: *Report of the secretary's work group on pediatric AIDS infection and diseases,* Washington DC, 1988, Department of Health and Human Services.

109. Owen WF Jr: Medical problems of the homosexual adolescent, *J Adolesc Health Care* 6:278-285, 1985.

110. Panel on Adolescent Pregnancy and Childbearing, Committee on Child Development Research and Public Policy: *Risking the future, Adolescent sexuality, pregnancy, and childbearing,* vol 1, Washington DC, 1987, National Academy Press.

111. Paperny DM et al: Computer-assisted detection and intervention in adolescent high-risk health behaviors, *J Pediatr* 116:456-462, 1990.

112. Parry-Jones WLL: *Obesity in children and adolescents.* In Burrows SGD, Beumont PJV, Casper RC, editors: *Handbook of eating disorders,* pt 2, *Obesity,* Amsterdam, 1988, Elsevier Science Publishers.

113. Patterson GR, DeBarsyshe BD, Ramsey E: A developmental perspective on antisocial behavior, *Am Psychol* 44:329-335, 1989.

114. Petosa R, Wessinger J: The AIDS education needs of adolescents: a theory-based approach, *AIDS Educ Prev* 2:127-136, 1990.

115. Pollin W: Drug abuse, USA: How serious? How soluble? *Issues Sci Technol* Winter, 20-27, 1987.

116. Powers SI, Hauser ST, Kilner LA: Adolescent mental health, *Am Psychol* 44:200-208, 1989.

117. Preto NG, Travis N: *The adolescent phase of the family life cycle.* In Mirkin MP, Koman SL, editors: *Handbook of adolescents and family therapy,* New York, 1985, Gandner Press.

118. Price RH et al: The search for effective prevention programs: What we learned along the way, *Am J Orthopsychiatr* 59(1):49-57, 1989.

119. Prizant BM et al: Communication disorders and emotional/behavioral disorders in children and adolescents, *J Speech Hear Dis* 55:179-192, 1990.

120. Remafedi G: Sexually transmitted diseases in homosexual youth, *Adolesc Med State of the Art Reviews* 1(3):565-581, 1990.

121. Remafedi G, Blum R: Working with gay and lesbian adolescents, *Pediatr Ann* 15:773-785, 1986.

122. Rice RJ et al: Gororrhea in the United States 1975-1984: is the giant only sleeping? *Sex Transm Dis* 14:83-87, 1987.

123. Riggs S, Alario AJ, McHorney C: Health risk behaviors and attempted suicide in adolescents who report prior maltreatment, *J Pediatr* 116(5):815-821, 1990.

124. Robinson NM, Robinson HB: *The mentally retarded child,* ed 2, New York, 1976, McGraw Hill.

125. Rosen DS, Xiangdong M, Blum RW: Adolescent health: Current trends and critical issues, *Adolesc Med State of the Art Reviews* 1(1):15-32, 1990.

126. Rosenberg ML et al: *Violence, homicide, assault, and suicide.* In RW Amler, HB Dull, editors: *Closing the gap: the burden of unnecessary illness,* New York, 1987, Oxford University.

127. Ross JG, Pate RR: A summary of findings: The national children and youth fitness study II, *J Phys Educ Recreation Dance* 58:51-56, 1987.

128. Russel M, Henderson C, Blume B: *Children of alcoholics: a review of the literature,* New York, 1985, Children of Alcoholics Foundation.

129. Scales P: The changing context of sexuality education: paradigms and challenges for alternative futures, *J Fam Relations* 34:265-274, 1986.

130. Schinke SP, Blythe BJ, Gilchrist LD: Cognitive-behavioral prevention of adolescent pregnancy, *J Counsel Psychol* 28:451-454, 1981.

131. Schubiner HH: Preventive health screening in adolescent patients, *Primary Care* 16(1):211-230, 1989.

132. Schubiner H, Robin A: Screening adolescents for depression and parent-teenager conflict in an ambulatory medical setting: a preliminary investigation, *Pediatrics* 85:813-818, 1990.

133. Schwartz RH, Cohen PR, Bair GO: Identifying and coping with a drug-using adolescent: some guidelines for pediatricians and parents, *Pediatr Rev* 7(5):133-139, 1985.

134. Selzer ML: The Michigan Alcoholism Screening Test: The quest for a new diagnostic instrument, *Am J Psychiatr* 127:1653- 1658, 1971.

135. Shafer M, Boyer CB: Psychosocial and behavioral factors associated with risk of sexually transmitted diseases, including human immunodeficiency virus infection, among urban high school students, *J Pediatr* 119:826-833, 1991.

136. Shafii M et al: Psychological autopsy of completed suicide in children and adolescents, *Am J Psychiatry* 142:1061- 1064, 1985.

137. Silber TJ: Approaching the adolescent patient: pitfalls and solutions, *J Adolesc Health Care* 7:31S-40S, 1986.

138. Sladkin KR: Counseling the sexually active teenager: reflections from pediatric practice, *Pediatrics* 76(4):681-684, 1985.

139. Society for Adolescent Medicine: Positions papers on reproductive health care for adolescents, *J Adolesc Health Care* 4:208-210, 1983.

140. Spivak H, Hausman AJ, Prothrow-Stith D: Practitioners' forum: public health and the primary prevention of adolescent violence—the violence prevention project, *Violence Victims* 4(3):203-212, 1989.

141. Stout JW, Rivara FP: Schools and sex education: does it work? *Pediatrics* 83:375, 1989.

142. Strasburger VC: Television and adolescents: sex, drugs, rock'n'roll, *Adolesc Med State of the Art Reviews* 1(1):161-194, 1990.

143. Strasburger VC: Sex, drugs, rock'n'roll: are solutions possible? A Commentary, *Pediatrics* 76(4):704-712, 1985.
144. Stringham P, Weitzman M: Violence counseling in the routine health care of adolescents, *J Adolesc Health Care* 9:389-393, 1988.
145. Strunin L, Hingson R: Acquired immunodeficiency syndrome and adolescents: knowledge, beliefs, attitudes, and behaviors, *Pediatrics* 79:825-828, 1987.
146. Taras HL et al: Television's influence on children's diet and physical activity, *J Dev Behav Pediatr* 10:176-180, 1989.
147. Task Force on Pediatric AIDS, American Psychological Association: Pediatric AIDS and human immunodeficiency virus infection: psychological issues, *Am Psychol* 44(2):258-264, 1989.
148. Taylor HG: *Learning disabilities*. In Mash EJ, Barkley RA, editors: *Treatment of childhood disorders*, New York, 1989, The Guilford Press.
149. Testa M, Wulczyn F: *The state of the child, vol 1, Children's Policy Research Project*, 1980, University of Chicago.
150. Turanski JJ: Reaching and treating youth with alcohol related problems: a comprehensive approach, *Alcohol Health Res World* 7(4):3-9, 1983.
151. US Bureau of the Census: *Statistical abstract of the United States 1991*, ed 111, Washington DC, 1991, US Department of Commerce.
152. US Department of Health and Human Services, Public Health Service: Center for population research, 1990 progress report, Bethesda MD, 1990, National Institutes of Health.
153. US Department of Health and Human Services, Public Health Service: *Healthy people 2000: national health promotion and disease prevention objectives*, Washington DC, 1990, Department of Health and Human Services.
154. US Department of Health and Human Services, Public Health Service: *Health United States 1988*, Hyattsville, MD, 1989, Department of Health and Human Services.
155. US Department of Health and Human Services: *Summary of findings from National Children and Youth Fitness Survey*, Washington DC, 1985, Office of Disease Prevention and Health Promotion.
156. US Preventive Services Task Force: *Guide to clinical preventive services: an assessment of the effectiveness of 169 interventions*, Baltimore, 1989, Williams & Wilkins.
157. Vincent ML, Clearie AF, Schluchter MD: Reducing adolescent pregnancy through school and community-based education, *JAMA* 257(24):3382-3386, 1987.
158. Watzlawick P, Weakland JH, Fisch R: *Change: principles of problem formation and problem resolution*, New York, 1974, WW Norton.
159. Weller RA et al: Mania in prepubertal children: has it been underdiagnosed? *J Affective Disorders* 11:151-154, 1986.
160. Wodarski JS: Adolescent substance abuse: practice implications, *Adolescence* 25:667-688, 1990.
161. Wodarski JS, Hoffman SD: Alcohol education for adolescents, *Soc Work Educ* 6(2):69-92, 1984.
162. Zelnik M, Kim YJ: Sex education and its association with teenage sexual activity, pregnancy and contraceptive use, *Fam Plann Perspect* 14(3):117-126, 1982.
163. Zuckerman BS et al: Adolescent pregnancy: biobehavioral determinants of outcome, *J Pediatr* 105(6):857-863, 1984.

RESOURCES

Adolescent Sexuality (including Contraception, STDs, and AIDS)

American Social Health Association, (Information on STDs), (800) 982-5883.

Federation of Parents and Friends of Lesbians and Gays, PO Box 20308, Denver, CO 80220.

National Abortion Federation Hotline, (800) 772-9100.

National AIDS Hotline, Centers for Disease Control, Atlanta GA 30333, (800) 342-AIDS.

National AIDS Hotline for Teens, (800) 234-TEEN.

National Gay and Lesbian Task Force, 1517 U Street NW, Washington, DC 20009.

Planned Parenthood National Headquarters, 810 Seventh Ave, New York, NY 10019.

How to talk to your children about sexuality, Planned Parenthood Federation of America, Inc. New York: Doubleday, 1986.

Parent's guide to teenage sexuality, New York, Henry Holt & Co, 1989.

Gale J: *A young man's guide to sex*, Los Angeles, 1988, The Body Press.

Fiedler J, Fiedler H: *Be smart about sex: facts for young people*, Hillside NJ, 1990, Enslow Publishers.

Voss J, Gale J: *A young woman's guide to sex*, Los Angeles, 1986, The Body Press.

Hopper CE, Allen WA: *Sex education for the physically handicapped youth*, Springfield, IL, 1980, Charles C Thomas Publishers.

Raising adolescents/parenting

Step Family Foundation, 333 West End Ave, New York, NY 10023.

ToughLove, PO Box 1069, Doylestown, PA 18901.

Winn M: *The plug-in drug*, New York, 1985, Viking Penguin.

Steinberg L: *You and your adolescent: a parent's guide for ages 19-20*, New York, 1990, Harper & Row.

Rosemond J: *John Rosemond's six point plan for raising happy healthy children*, Kansas City, 1989, Andrews & McMeel.

Canter L: *Homework without tears*, New York, 1987, Harper and Row.

Canter L, Canter M: *Assertive discipline*, New York, 1988, Harper and Row.

Alcohol and drug use in adolescence

Al-Anon Family Group Headquarters, 1372 Broadway, New York, NY 10018.

Alcoholics Anonymous World Services, PO Box 459, Grand Central Station, New York, NY 10163.

National Clearinghouse for Alcohol and Drug Information (NCADI), PO Box 2345, Rockville MD 20852.

Hodgson HW: *A parent's survival guide: how to cope when your kid is using drugs,* San Francisco, 1986, Harper & Row.

Mental health

American Psychological Association, 750 First St. NE, Washington, DC 20002-4242.

American Society for Adolescent Psychiatry, 5530 Wisconsin Ave NW Suite 1149, Washington, DC 20815.

American Anorexia/Bulimia Association, Inc., 133 Cedar Lane, Teaneck, NJ 07666.

Association for Children and Adults with Learning Disabilities, 4156 Library Road, Pittsburgh, PA 15234.

National Committee on Youth Suicide Prevention, 825 Washington St, Norwood MA 02062.

National Association of Anorexia Nervosa and Associated Disorders, Box 7, Highland Park, IL 60035.

National Alliance for the Mentally Ill, 11323 West Eighteenth Ave, Lakewood CO 80215.

National Anorexia Aid Society, 5796 Karl Road, Columbus, OH 43229.

National Consortium for Child Mental Health Services, 3615 Wisconsin Ave NW, Washington, DC 20016.

National Runaway Switchboard and Suicide Hotline, 3080 North Lincoln Ave, Chicago, IL 60657, (800) 621-4000.

Runaway Hotline, (800) 231-6946.

Harris SO, Reynolds EN: *When growing up hurts too much: a parent's guide to knowing how to choose a therapist with your teenager,* New York, 1990, Lexington Books.

Adolescent/child advocacy

Children's Defense Fund, 1520 New Hampshire Ave NW, Washington, DC 20036.

National Black Leadership Council, 250 West Fifty-fourth St Suite 800, New York NY 10019.

Chapter 29

CAREER DEVELOPMENT

Barbara Gould Pelowski
Kathleen FitzSimons

RATIONALE

Sigmund Freud suggested that maturity is the capacity to love and to work 60 years before Gail Sheehy published *Passages* (1976)[18] describing the developmental crises of adulthood. During more than a half century, interest in adult development emerged as an area of intense popularity as writers and social scientists published such titles as, *The Seasons of a Man's Life* (Levinson, 1978),[13] "Woman's Place in Man's Life Cycle" (Gilligan, 1979),[6] and *Work and Love: The Crucial Balance* (Rohrlich, 1980).[17]

During the 1980s the increase in publications dealing with adult development continued at an even greater rate. In fact, more than one half of the literature reviewed in preparation for this chapter was published in the past 10 years. Included in the writing related to adult development are several ideas that reinforce why the subject of career development is a relevant topic in a book about preventive medicine.

The impact of stress on health

The first notion is that any change, positive or negative, including a change related to career, contributes to stress that affects health.[11] As Holmes and Rahe developed their theory of the relationship of stress to illness, they created The Social Readjustment Rating Scale in which the effects of specific changes common in adults' lives were measured and quantified. Results of their research indicate that the magnitude of life change, including career change, is significantly related to time of disease onset and seriousness of the illness. A major change in employment, including a promotion or loss of employment or other career transition, is perceived as a stressor of relatively high magnitude.

Career satisfaction and health

The second idea relating career development and health is that the more satisfied people feel about their lives, their main roles, or their careers, the better is their health.[22] In a 1978 study assessing role responsibilities, role burdens, and physical health, Verbrugge determined that the more roles men and women occupy, the better their health. Identifying worker, spouse, and parent as the three major roles of adults, Verbrugge concluded that the link between high role involvement and good health comes from having the opportunity to express diverse skills and to access social supports, resources, and social stimulation. These in turn can serve to maintain physical and mental health.[22] Conversely, as general contentment with life and career declines, health drops sharply.

Physicians as resources

A third consideration is the fact that adults in life transition consult physicians as resources in the process of making decisions about next steps in their lives. In a study published by Pelowski (1981) regarding the decision-making processes of 200 mid-life adults, physicians and other professional resource people are cited by 12% of the men and 25% of the women as helpful in the process of making a change in their lives.[16] In a study published by the College Board (1980), indications were that 36% of the population in the United States between the ages of 16 and 65 were in career transition.[20] Two thirds of the adults studied said they were experiencing or anticipating problems in the process of change. Considering the above three ideas, it becomes clear why practitioners of preventive medicine need to concern themselves with issues related to career development.

CAREER DEVELOPMENT: A HISTORICAL PERSPECTIVE
Early contributions

Career development, as the theory and practice of occupational choice and change is currently known, evolved during a century of study concerning individual differences. As early as 1909 with the publication of Frank Parsons' major work, *Choosing a Vocation,* scientists of human behavior were influenced by the concept that an individual chooses a career based upon a three-part framework[12]:

"First, a clear understanding of yourself, aptitudes, abilities, interests, resources, limitations, and other qualities. Second, a knowledge of the requirements and conditions of success, advantages and disadvantages, compensations, opportunities, and prospects in different lines of work. Third, true reasoning on the relations of these two groups of facts."

From the contributions of Parsons and others, a national career guidance movement began. The first National Conference on Vocational Guidance was held in 1910, followed 3 years later by the founding of an organization now known as the National Career Development Association.

Development in testing

At the same time that the guidance movement was earning national recognition, an interest in measuring individual differences emerged. Standardized tests were developed as a means of identifying what is representative of a population. Through experimentation and analysis, norms were established to describe "normal" ranges of measurement. One such test was the Stanford-Binet measurement of IQ that was first used in the assessment of armed service personnel in World War I. As an assessment device, the Stanford-Binet could "discriminate among the aptitudes of (military personnel) capable of implementing the increasingly bureaucratic organization and technological weapons systems of the armed forces of the day."[12]

Later, aptitude tests and interest inventories were developed to aid in the prediction of job satisfaction and success. Achievement testing in public schools also became popular, supported by federal legislation that provided for a national vocational education program and the initiation of graduate programs in counselor education at land-grant universities.

Development of counseling theory

As various kinds of assessment instruments developed and more people educated themselves as counselors, different counseling methods evolved. In the 1940s two distinct approaches to individual counseling were identified. Both *directive* and *nondirective* counseling approaches had an impact on the career guidance movement. *Directive counseling* assumes that career choice is a cognitive process that involves matching personality with job requirements. It seeks to maximize the use of valid tests and appropriate information without emphasis on the decision-making process. *Nondirective counseling* suggests that an individual's self-concept and affective and motivational behavior must also be considered in determining appropriate career choice. Nondirective counselors emphasize the client and the counseling process with less attention given to tests and records. Eventually these two perspectives blended, resulting in much of the current career counseling focus on human development and life experience.

With the influx of World War II veterans to American colleges and universities, more guidance services were needed. Training programs in industrial psychology, educational psychology, counseling psychology, and school psychology incorporated courses in tests and measurements. Organizations such as the College Entrance Examination Board (CEEB) and the American College Testing Program (ACT) expanded their test usage to predict success at the college level.

In the 1950s several theorists emerged who contributed to career education by providing insights into developmental stages and tasks associated with life transitions, as well as the more commonly understood issues of personality and work environment factors, and decision-making processes. The 1960s, with its focus on the status of women and minorities, challenged the counseling profession to reexamine the role and meaning of work. Black Americans found support for vocational growth in such federal programs as the Job Corps. Women discovered opportunities for career development in expanded career education programs that emphasized career awareness, career exploration, value clarification, and decision-making skills. An aging population found increased federal support for geriatric services, including retirement planning and leisure time programming.

Since the late 1970s, career guidance programs have placed greater emphasis on a humanistic approach designed to increase a person's self-awareness of possibilities, both in oneself and in the changing work world. Within this historical framework several theories of career counseling were developed.

Summary of theories

According to Zuncker (1990), theories of career development are conceptual systems designed to delineate relationships between a sequence of events that lead to causes and effects. They represent attempts to understand vocational behavior, as well as the priorities in career counseling today. A brief overview of the theories provides a context within which career issues and concerns may be further discussed. A more complete explanation of each theory is found in Zuncker.[24]

- *Trait and factor theory,* as postulated by Parsons in 1909, assumes that individuals have unique patterns of ability or traits that can be measured and subsequently matched to the needs of the workplace.

- *Developmental approaches,* defined by Ginzberg in 1972 and more recently in 1984, by Super in 1972; by Tiedeman and O'Hara in 1963; by Gottfredson in 1981; and by Knefelkemp and Slepitza in 1976, vary in focus but essentially emphasize the stages and/or tasks of human development over the life span.
- The *needs approach,* presented by Roe in 1956, underscores the importance of early childhood experiences in generating the needs, interests, and attitudes that are later reflected in the choice of a career.
- The *typological approach,* formulated by Holland in 1973, suggests that career choice is an expression or extension of personality types that fit with specific occupational profiles. Congruence between personal orientation and occupational environment is key to career satisfaction.
- *Decision theory,* as exemplified by Gelatt in 1962, is used to explain the process of career planning as a series of decisions or choices and provides a framework for a counseling program.
- *Social-learning theory,* as defined by Krumboltz, Mitchell, and Gelatt in 1975, postulates that career development involves four factors: (1) inherited abilities, (2) environmental circumstances, (3) learning/educational experiences, and (4) task-approach skills such as problem-solving, decision-making, work habits, and the like.
- *Psychoanalytic approaches,* such as that postulated by Osipow in 1983, focus (inward) on a framework in which work is perceived as a method of satisfying impulses and providing an outlet for sublimated wishes.
- *Sociological or situational theory,* as presented by Blau-Gustad-Jessor-Parnes and Wilcox in 1956, focuses on the interrelationship among biologic, psychologic, economic, and sociologic factors that determine occupational choice and development. Such a perspective is useful in clarifying situational elements in the career development process.
- *Learning theory,* as described by O'Hara in 1968 and by Miller in the same year, stresses learning principles, including behaviors involved in decision-making, as the basis for effective career decisions.

Implications

Although the aforementioned theories have a variety of labels, they are all in some way concerned with the relationship between individuals and their unique characteristics or pattern of development, and the society in which they develop. The major difference, according to Zuncker (1990), is the nature of the factors that influence the career decision-making process.[24] Although most of the research regarding career development is based on white male samples, there are, nonetheless, common implications that are useful to the physician or other professional consulting on career issues. Zuncker's thinking is summarized at right.[24]

CURRENT PERSPECTIVES ON CAREER PLANNING: AN OVERVIEW
Significant trends and influences

During the past few years, increasing numbers of people within our society have indicated a need for career life planning opportunities and programs. The factors precipitating this interest are indeed complex. Some would say it has to do with job-related stress, whereas others emphasize dissatisfaction with the work itself and organizational life as it exists today. In addition, more and more workers are finding themselves out of sync with job requirements as they fail to continue their self-development at a rate consistent with technologic changes in the workplace. Economic issues also continue to force layoffs of experienced personnel, both from blue collar manufacturing and white collar middle management jobs. Many of these workers find it nearly impossible to reenter the ranks of the "gainfully employed" even though they have years of professional, technical, or managerial qualifications and experience. The psychologic ramifications of these workforce changes are not to be minimized.

Dramatic demographic shifts have resulted in a diverse, multicultural, older, and more female workforce in which

---

Summary of theories of career development

- Career development is a lifelong process that takes place in stages.
- Individuals may be helped to cope with the transitions that occur at various stages.
- Career maturity is acquired through successfully accomplishing developmental tasks within each life stage.
- From each individual's uniqueness come certain values, interests, abilities, and behavioral tendencies that shape career development.
- Self-concept as an ongoing process affects career decisions.
- A match between an individual's personality and the work environment is key to job satisfaction.
- Individual characteristics and traits can be measured through standardized instruments and may be used to predict future adjustment.
- Identifying what an individual believes on the basis of his observations and experience is important in shaping counseling strategies.
- Occupational information resources must be introduced over the life span.
- Career choice involves learning effective decision-making and problem-solving skills.
- Career choice is affected by both internal and external limits such as fear and lack of confidence or economic constraints and discrimination.
- Career development must be viewed in relation to such cognitive factors as gender and occupational roles.

culture, race, gender, and lifespan development issues take on new meaning. Growing numbers of minorities and women are competing for jobs within a shifting, uncertain economy where many levels of jobs are being eliminated. Although more people have moved into middle-income levels, the number of disenfranchised and disadvantaged has increased as well. The escalation of costs related to standard of living has more than doubled, thereby widening the gap between the "haves" and the "have nots." Issues pertaining to "dual career couples" have emerged, as both partners choose, or feel compelled to choose, jobs outside the home. Because many businesses are contracting rather than expanding, some people must accept jobs at much lower levels than they might have expected years ago. The global economy brings with it a rich diversity that has precipitated concerns around equal opportunity and affirmative action. Reassessment and redirection of career and life goals has become common among individuals in midlife who are questioning their commitment to organizations, while organizations are reassessing and realigning their goals to stay competitive.

Simultaneously, high school and college age youths, as well as young adults who are out of school and preparing to enter the workforce, are experiencing difficulties in securing their niche in the workforce, either because they are competing for the same jobs as the older, more experienced worker or, because of high expectations, they are unwilling or ill-prepared to accept available jobs. In either case, there are potentially valuable people of all ages "floundering for lack of sound advice on choosing the right career in the first place and, later adapting when necessary to changing circumstances. . . ."[15] Clearly a need exists for effective career planning over the whole life span. Although a number of programs and services have, in fact, been launched over the years, many fall short of meeting the needs and expectations of individuals, young and old.

Among the responsibilities of physicians as counseling professionals is the need to be cognizant of the job market changes that affect career choice and development. Understanding the context in which a person may be making a career decision and being sensitive to accompanying emotional and physiologic stress is key to helping the individual maintain good health. Conversely, good health is critical to an individual's career development.

Hall[8] further summarizes the trends that take into account technologic, organizational, and individual/societal changes that employees will face in the 1990s. These trends are listed in the following:

- More and different kinds of specialists with different values, career insights, and technical languages
- More people working away from the traditional office setting
- More flexible approaches to work (such as flexible hours, job sharing, and part-time employment)

- Decreased loyalty to companies (people will change jobs and careers more often)
- Formal organizational structure giving way to project teams, task forces, matrix structures, and interdependent units
- An increasing need to train and retrain people at different career stages to maintain job security
- Changes in how people relate to each other (e.g., communication via computer) lack nonverbal cues and display no emotion
- More collaborative and cooperative work, including involvement in decision making
- Pressure to increase job satisfaction by changing job content

Impact of societal changes

In addition to changes anticipated in the work force, physicians dealing with career issues must be aware of changes in the perceptions of adults toward their lives in general. In recent years, many Americans have begun to see their social environment, work world, and themselves in a new light. As a result of numerous socioeconomic changes, many beliefs and values have altered—some dramatically and others less so. Nonetheless, many of the traditional paradigms, particularly with regard to work, are being reevaluated.

Montana and Higginson suggest that our cultural understanding of the organization of work is undergoing change.[15] Although occupational achievement is still considered important, work is no longer considered virtuous in the moral sense that it once was. It has become, for many, a means to personal satisfaction through the direct acquisition of material goods. Although most Americans still aspire to the prestige that high income and high status signify, an increasing number of people are questioning the validity of such goals. Many are entering the workforce with different expectations, which is precipitating a reexamination of the concepts of motivation and success. There is a growing awareness that, in many ways, America's material progress has had harmful effects on its human and natural resources. With so many technologic, social, and economic changes occurring so rapidly, many people are becoming acutely conscious of the need for meaning and security in their lives. This does not mean that meaningful work is an anomaly; it simply means that the emphasis in the career planning process needs to be on work within the full context of our lives. Perhaps the most important reason for the significance of career is that it represents a person's entire life in the work setting ". . . . and work, for most people, is a primary factor in determining the overall quality of life."[8] Conceivably it could be said, therefore, that planning for a career is actually planning for life; hence, the references to career life planning.

Significant changes and new attitudes have developed in

the educational domain as well. As more people have the opportunity to become better educated, traditional beliefs of parents and of preceding generations about work are being questioned. All agree that more education means more options, and yet there appears to be a growing mismatch between individual and organizational needs and expectations. In addition, there is a growing concern as to whether the type of learning being offered through public education is, indeed, relevant in preparing people for productive lives. The call for school reform is ongoing while the debate over the purpose of schooling and who and what is responsible for the breakdown of public school systems continues. Nonetheless, the changes have led to education being viewed as a lifelong process.

"At a time when so many old rules no longer apply, when established structures have a diminished importance in the world at large, when opportunities for growth and life enhancement abound, the need for new and resilient guidelines at the personal level is more urgent than ever." [15] Being resilient and adaptable, managing uncertainty and ambiguity, and being innovative in career and family management are going to be the foundation for a meaningful career.

Finally, Feldman[5] summarizes some of the substantial ways that career perspectives have changed over the last few years:

- The term career no longer pertains only to individuals in high-status or rapid advancement occupations.
- The term career no longer refers only to vertical job changes.
- The term career is no longer synonymous with employment in one occupation or in one organization.
- No longer is it assumed that the organization has unilateral control over the individual.
- No longer is it assumed that the organization will take care of its employees in a paternalistic manner.
- No longer is it assumed that careers in management are the province of (white) men alone.
- No longer is it assumed that career success should be measured by high salary and high occupational status alone. Today career success is personally defined.
- No longer do we assume an individual's career aspirations will remain stable over a many year period.

Prevailing myths

In addition to new perspectives on careers, career life planning must be concerned with beliefs and misconceptions that influence our thinking and get in the way of our making informed decisions around work. Montana and Higginson point out the irony of how we live in a nation that offers access to vast amounts of information and knowledge and yet many of us lack the facts we need to understand ourselves and others and to cope successfully with the changes around us.[15] They note that the reason for this is twofold. On one hand we don't seek out information pertinent to our well-being; on the other hand, we often resist accepting facts and ideas that may be counter to our own because it may be upsetting or simply inconvenient to do so. We are seldom conscious of this resistance and the flaws in our reasoning that influence our perceptions.[15]

The following myths represent nine of the more commonly held misconceptions that strongly influence our attitudes about other people as well as ourselves:

1. All individuals go through a lockstep sequence of education/work/retirement during the three stages of life.
2. People with initiative and ingenuity have unlimited opportunities and can do anything they set out to do.
3. If individuals work hard, they will gain recognition, receive increased compensation, and will be promoted.
4. The more schooling individuals obtain, the more capable they are.
5. Childhood is the developmental stage of life; adulthood is the time when individuals peak and plateau; and old age is a period of decline.
6. People who make the correct choices when they are young adults will be happy and fulfilled the rest of their lives.
7. It is a sign of instability when an individual wants to change career direction during midlife.
8. Individuals are as old physiologically and psychologically as they are chronologically.
9. There is "one best career" that is most suitable for each individual.

The most damaging aspect of myths is that they do, in fact, become self-fulfilling. People believe they are facts and behave accordingly. For example, an older person may engage in behavior that benefits the stereotype about being forgetful, senile, or inactive. It behooves each person to reflect on his or her belief systems and be aware of the influence each has in projecting them onto self and others.

Key issues

In addition to the influence of prevailing myths, key issues in career life planning need to be considered and understood for their impact on the process. Montana and Higginson offer profound insight on the following six major issues.[15]

Need for information. The need for appropriate, accurate, and updated information about virtually everything that affects our choices is key. And in this day of complex technologic developments and sophisticated communication systems, the challenge of obtaining such information can be quite intimidating. Although seeking professional consultation is appropriate, *there is often a tendency to rely on the advice or insight of an external authority fig-*

ure, which may or may not be accurate.[15] The task of professionals is to acknowledge the limitations of their knowledge base and to support and empower individuals to assume ownership for the choices they make. It is imperative that individuals develop their own critical thinking as they become their own "experts" in the career decision-making process.

Concept of lifelong learning. The emphasis on education and lifelong learning is also related to the nature and pace of changes taking place in our society. No one can or should expect to get by without acquiring new skills and knowledge. And yet, *too few adults are committed to lifelong education and strongly resist the idea of returning to formal schooling.*[15] This idea contradicts the traditional concept in which it was expected that all of the education needed for life would be acquired in the early years. This is not so anymore. As a result, many older adults feel deceived, angry, (and even embarrassed) when it is suggested that, despite their many years of experience, they may need to return to school. Indeed, for many occupations, a bachelor's degree is now the minimum level of required education (Fig. 29-1). For young adults this attitude toward education plays itself out in a different yet equally limiting way. They often naively expect that their vocational training or college education entitles them to the job of their choice, even if they have had virtually no related experience. To complicate matters even more, the type of relevant education and training that people may need may

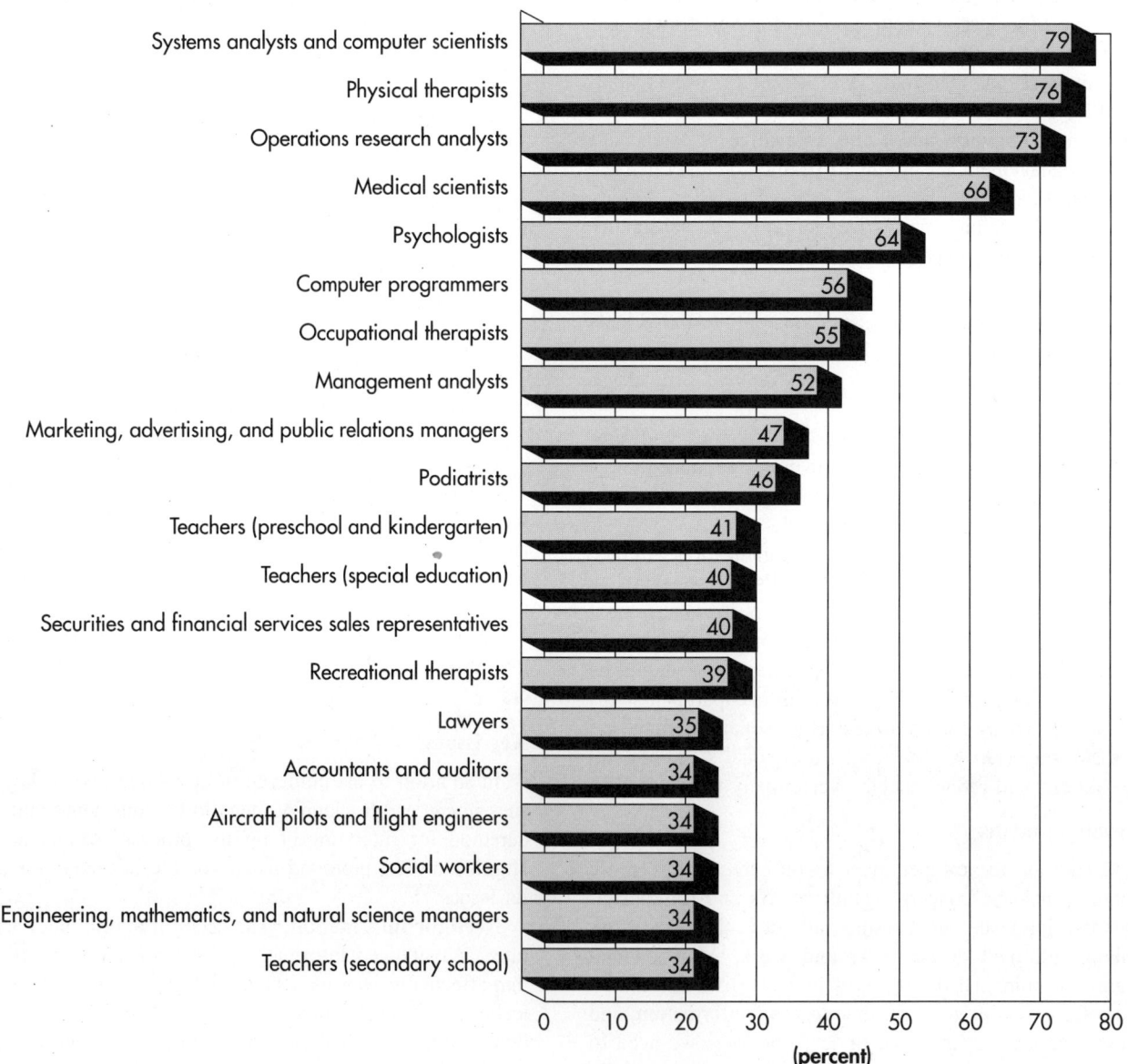

Fig. 29-1. Fastest growing occupations requiring a college degree or more education (projected 1990-2005) in percent. (From *Occupational Outlook Quarterly*, Fall 1991.)

not be available or easily accessible. How unfortunate when such shortsightedness and limited vision get in the way of adult development. The task of professionals serving in the role of advocate, guide, or counselor is to encourage a broader outlook toward education and to support a quest for new knowledge (Fig. 29-2).

Opportunities and options. The number of work opportunities available to individuals is often a matter of researching the kinds of options that are available while being realistic and recognizing the barriers and constraints that exist. On the one hand, it is naive to assume that there are unlimited opportunities to which people are entitled; on the other hand, an increasing number of new careers and work options are evolving with ongoing advances in technology. Access to opportunities requires more than persistence, eagerness, and tenacity; factors such as age, sex, family background, education, appearance, personality, intelligence, ability, and experience do, in fact, come into play. Montana and Higginson point out one of the lessons learned in the past few years is that *no one is immune from unemployment.*[15] People at all levels of organizations have been laid off, fired, or encouraged to retire early. People should learn as much as they can about the range of opportunities in the job market, to become expert, so to speak, about their areas of interest, so that we can prepare and

position themselves to take advantage of them. The task of guiding professionals is to encourage such a realistic approach.

Change and uncertainty. Although resistance to change is a common reaction among most people, scientific, technologic, social, global, and economic changes are here to stay. The barrage of new ideas and images has made us acutely aware of the impermanence of knowledge and uncertainty of life. Most of us experience some degree of anxiety in response to perceived or expected changes, particularly when they are threatening to our life or our security (i.e., jobs). *Nonetheless, flexibility and adaptation to change may be one of the most important strengths an individual can bring to the job market.*[15] The aim in career planning is to encourage individuals to understand and come to terms with the uncertainty in their personal and work lives and to actually embrace change, thereby reducing anxiety and stress.

Personal problems. Although lack of information or knowledge about job prospects, occupational options, and the general state of the economy can seriously impede an individual's progress in career/life planning, lack of awareness about oneself and insight into one's personal strengths and weaknesses can be just as serious. Personal problems can seriously handicap an individual's effectiveness in making appropriate career choices. At the heart of this issue is self-esteem and the ability to control emotions, desires, and inner conflicts without repressing them. Montana and Higginson[15] cite Parker's list of factors that cause some of the most common stressful circumstances of daily living:

1. Separation from a loved one (through death or divorce)
2. Economic difficulties caused by inflation and high standards
3. Fatigue caused by excessive employment or household demands
4. Loss of self-esteem caused by work- or role-related issues
5. Illness that is neglected or handled inappropriately
6. Lifestyle inconsistent with temperament
7. Traumatic past or present experiences
8. Continued interpersonal or work-related conflicts

Many of these stressors are related to goals, values, boundaries, and sense of self. According to Rohrlich (1980), work is the most visibly structured and bounded area of our lives.[17] It not only offers a sense of purpose and direction, but it meets our need for order and self-definition. When people are defined by roles, titles, earning levels, and/or technical skills, it is because these factors are precise and unambiguous. Of course, when carried to the extreme it may be limiting to define oneself by a job title; but on the other hand, *the more precisely defined the categories we feel we belong in, the greater is our sense of*

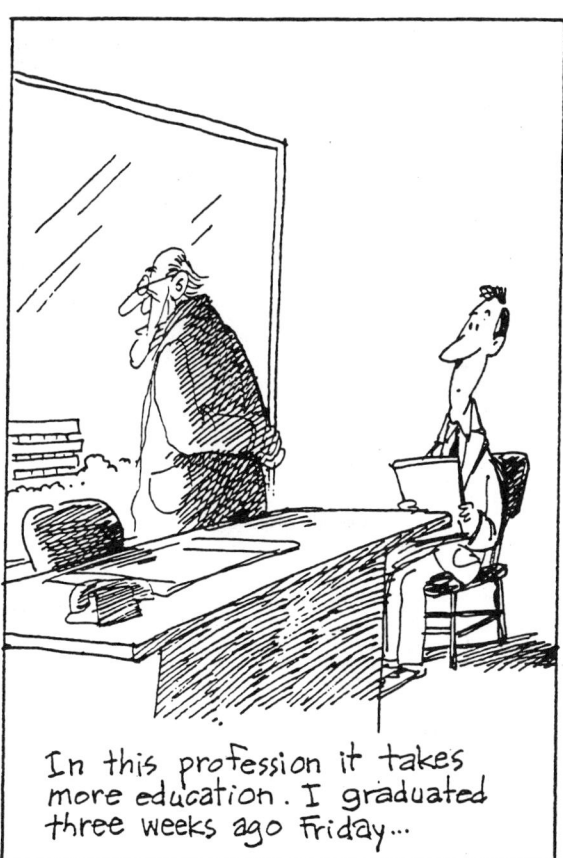

In this profession it takes more education. I graduated three weeks ago Friday...

Fig. 29-2. (From Shingleton J: *Which niche?*)

self-definition.[15] Our values help us determine our aspirations, as well as the scope of our commitment to, and what we want from, work. The aim is to set goals accordingly.

Need for planning. Just as organizations have recognized the critical need for strategic planning and sound managerial practices in these uncertain times, individuals also need to develop a career plan with short-term and long-term goals that serve as a framework within which informed decisions can be made and problems solved. "Career planning is a deliberate process of (1) becoming aware of self (strengths and weaknesses), opportunities, constraints, choices, and consequences, (2) identifying career-related goals, and (3) programming work, education, and related developmental experiences to provide the direction, timing, and sequence of steps to attain a specific career goal."[8] Unfortunately, more often than not, individuals abdicate responsibility for managing their lives and their careers. They need to be encouraged to take on the task.

THE CAREER LIFE PLANNING PROCESS
A three-step framework

As indicated above, career life planning is the process of defining career goals, based on a thorough assessment of values, interests, skills and experience, researching related work options, and developing an action plan—an explicit, point-by-point framework and timetable for putting a decision into action. Career life planning today continues to be essentially a three-step process: (1) self assessment; (2) research/assessment of occupation, careers, and job options; and (3) goal-setting within the context of a life plan.

Self-assessment. The basic self-assessment process begins with responses to such questions as "who am I?" "what do I want?" "where do I go from here?" "what are

my strengths and weaknesses?" "what am I interested in doing?" "what is important in my life; i.e., what do I value?" "what are my short- and long-term goals?" Regardless of age or stage in life, these are the core questions that must be addressed. As noted earlier, it is ironic that with all the information that is available to us on just about any subject in the world, we typically have very little information or insight about ourselves. From early in life people are programmed to look outside themselves for answers to life's questions (i.e., teachers, parents, physicians, counselors, government officials, bosses, and coaches become the authority figures that provide answers). Thus it is not surprising that they become the sources for self knowledge as well. In this regard, there are numerous resources available, including a wide range of inventories on interests, values, skill/abilities, aptitude, and personality traits, as well as books, services, professionals, and programs to help put together a personal profile. (Please refer to Resources at the end of this chapter.) The goal, however, is for individuals to become grounded and secure in their own abilities to make informed and appropriate decisions (Fig. 29-3).

Assessment of job market. Being well informed about occupational options is equally essential to the process of career life planning. In fact, lack of awareness of the available options is probably more limiting than lack of skills or jobs. This information may be obtained through a variety of means, including books, computerized programs, informational interviews, volunteer work, internships, temporary projects, workshops, and coursework. It is not unlike an independent research project in which all past and current references are explored. The goal of researching careers is to expand the notion and broaden a

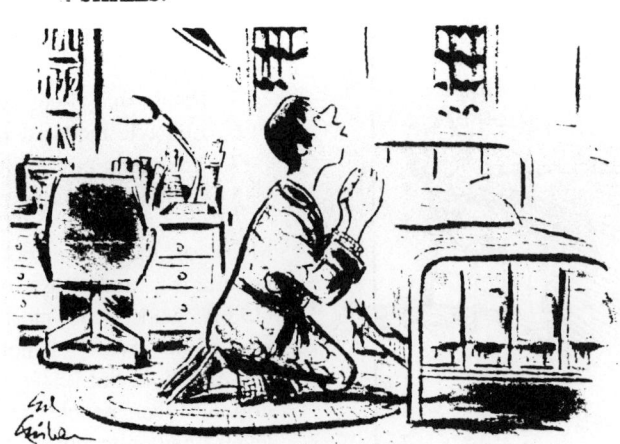

"... and give me good abstract-reasoning ability,
interpersonal skills, cultural perspective, linguistic comprehension,
and a high sociodynamic potential."

Fig. 29-3. (From *The New Yorker*, 1981. Drawing by Ed Fisher.)

perspective on what's possible in terms of work and to identify options that fit in terms of values, interests, and skills (Fig. 29-4). This means getting to know the core characteristics of the fields being considered, including the following:

- The nature of the work
- Working conditions
- Required training, education, or other qualifications
- Job outlook
- Pay range
- Related occupations

In many respects, this information-gathering step is the most challenging because there are no short-cuts or parameters, except those imposed by the individual whose task is to analyze and prioritize the data. It is tedious, time-consuming, and oftentimes discouraging. It is also rewarding, revealing, and well worth the effort. See Figs. 29-5 and 29-6 for the fastest-growing occupations and for occupations with the largest job growth.

The informational interview deserves added attention. It is often the best source of career/job information. Asking people directly about an occupation provides first-hand information that is current and personal. It affords an individual the opportunity to express issues and concerns that are personally important. One of the indirect benefits of informational interviews is the network of contacts it produces. It is clearly a critical strategy in career planning.

Development of a plan. Integrating personal information with career information is the next step in the process; that is, putting together the information that has been gleaned and making sense out of it in the form of a plan. The facts must be weighed against the factors that are personally important to the individual. They serve as a kind of framework for putting a plan into place, with short- and long-term goals, a timeline, and expected outcomes. The key to developing a framework on careers is not found in the individual, the organization, or the work itself, but rather "in the ways in which cultural, organizational, occu-

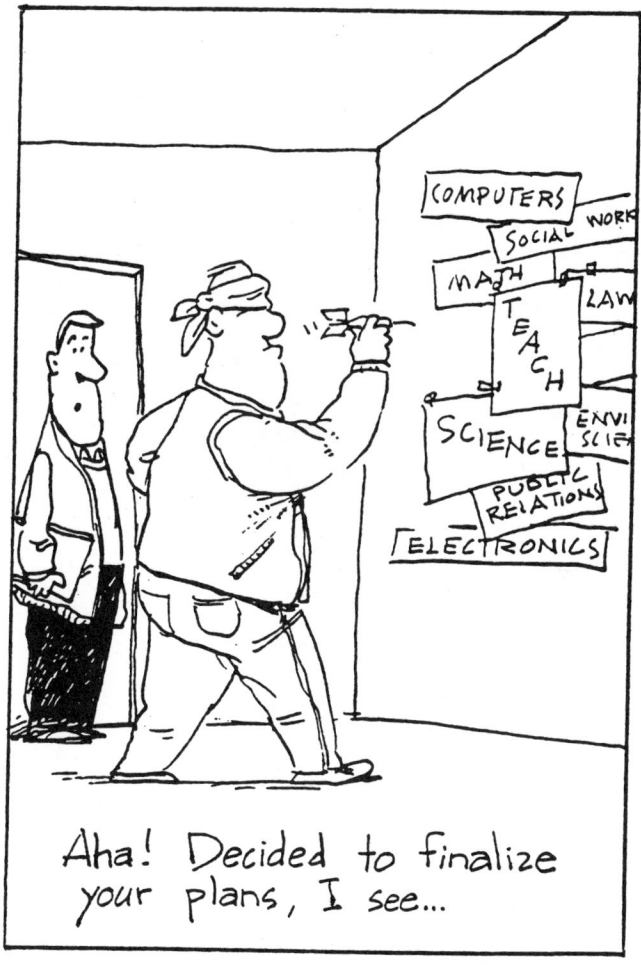

Fig. 29-4. (From Shingleton J: Which niche?, illustrated by Phil Frank, 1989, Bob Adams.)

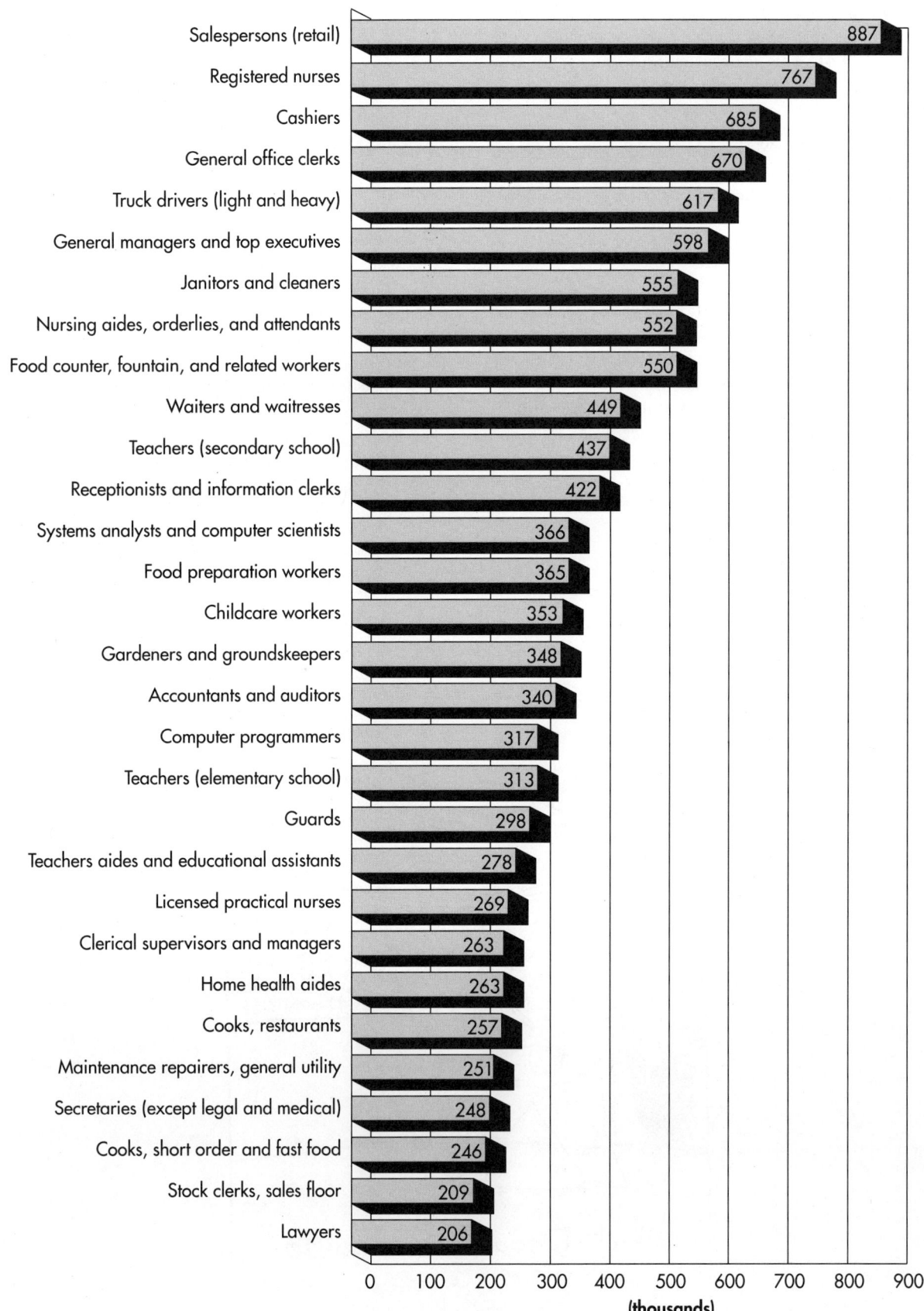

Fig. 29-5. Occupations with the largest numerical increases (projected 1990-2005) in thousands. (From *Occupational Outlook Quarterly*, Fall 1991.)

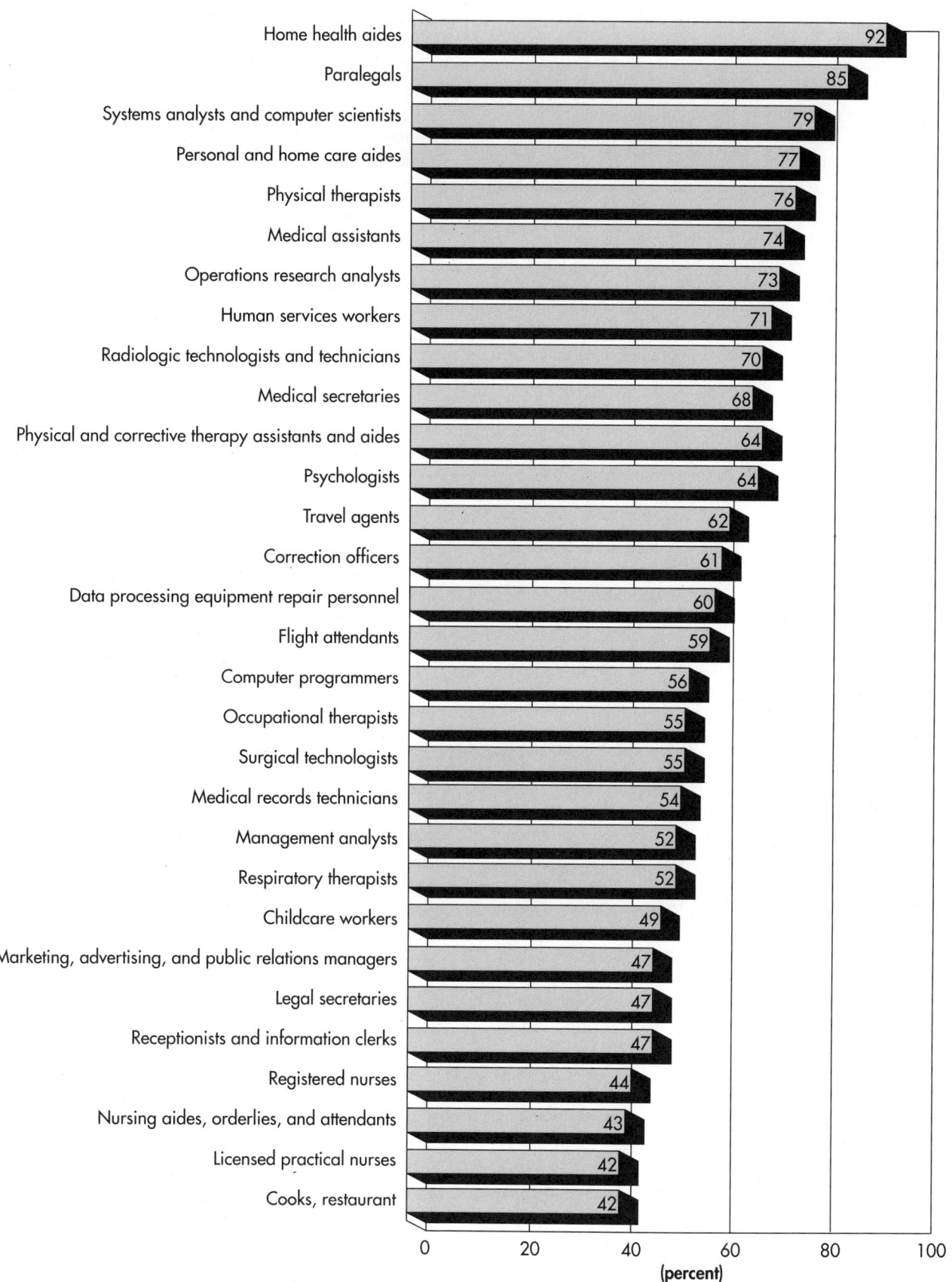

Fig. 29-6. Fastest growing occupations (projected 1990-2005) in percent. (From *Occupational Outlook Quarterly*, Fall 1991.)

pational demands interact with individual aspirations, family concerns, and work demands across time."[21]

Look at the future

One last note of caution: the traditional approach to career planning has not been unlike the traditional approaches to planning in organizations. A career was initially conceptualized as an individual phenomenon; the planning for which was a rational, patterned process that eventually led to the achievement of stated goals and objectives. Today the actual planning process must factor in the nonrational and allow for a great deal of uncertainty, ambiguity, and change. Planning for future change continues to be essential to goal achievement, but intuition, flexibility, innovation, and communion are concepts that need to be fully integrated into the process.

ASSESSMENT
Expectations

Early and continuous career planning increases the likelihood that an individual's values, interests, skills, and goals will be meshed with appropriate career choices. Because the average adult spends more than 2000 hours per year at work,[4] finding an enjoyable and satisfying career is paramount to a sense of self-worth and fulfillment. Career exploration ideally begins in high school with thoughtful course selection, some work experience, and career research, part of which is self- assessment. However, many schools have limited resources and/or place a low priority on career guidance. Consequently, many high school students graduate with only a superficial awareness of what their goals and interests are or how these would mesh with a career. Without that self-knowledge, an individual is likely to seek education, training, or employment that meets immediate needs but does not lead toward lifelong career development. Even when career guidance is available in the high school setting, services are often limited to large group administration of standardized tests or the unguided use of computerized information systems. Furthermore, tests assessing individual values, interests, and abilities are often interpreted in such general terms in a group setting that the potential usefulness is lost. Computer programs offered as an isolated source of information can be very misleading.

Fortunately, adolescents who go on to college or training programs usually will find a career development program available to help direct their curricular and career choices. Assessment is often a central methodological tool in such a service. Nevertheless, it is important to note that there is no one "best" assessment instrument for everyone. Whether the need is to predict success in a particular career, to determine how compatible a person would be in a certain work culture, to monitor individual readiness to choose a career, or to evaluate how well the goals of career guidance have been achieved, there are numerous in-

struments from which to choose. The goal in identifying an appropriate career assessment instrument should be to find a usable test that by reputation seems to measure what the individual wants to know. Additional considerations in the choice of a test are the age and reading level of the individual, the length of time needed to administer the instrument, equipment needed, cost, ease of scoring, types of scores available and the competencies of the interpreter.

Types of assessment instruments

Formal assessment can, and often does, include measures of interests, ability, achievement, aptitude, personality, and career maturity.

- **Interest assessment** is used to identify an individual's areas of inclination or preference.
- **Aptitude assessment** is used to predict success in a job role or in an educational program.
- **Personality assessment** measures individual characteristics that affect work behaviors, perceptions, and attitudes.
- **Achievement assessment** is used to determine whether a person has the basic academic skills necessary to enter a specific educational program or to measure the level of accomplishment in a prior or current occupation.
- **Career maturity assessment** determines an individual's readiness to make a career decision.
- **Computer-assisted assessment** includes both information retrieval systems and career decision-making programs.

Interest assessment. Assessment of career interests is an integral part of the overall assessment of an individual's career needs. Levinson and Folino note that "interests have been found to be a major determinant of college major and occupational choice, and to exert a greater influence on occupational choice than do aptitudes."[14] Traditional measures of interests used to predict vocational behaviors, focus on how well an individual may be expected to achieve occupationally, and how long and how well-satisfied the person will be in different careers. Some commonly used tests of this nature are the Kuder Occupational Interest Survey, the Strong-Campbell Interest Inventory, and Holland's Self-Directed Search.

Kuder Occupational Interest Survey form DD, revised (designed by Kuder and Diamond, 1985). Used with adolescents and adults, grades 11 and above, the Kuder Occupational Interest Survey evaluates occupational and college major interests. The 100-item paper-pencil test measures interests in 10 occupational areas: outdoor, mechanical, scientific, computational, persuasive, artistic, literary, musical, social science, and clerical. It is self-administered in approximately 30-40 minutes and is computer scored. Costs include: Materials and scoring for 20 persons $70; audiocassette "Expanding Your Future" (a guide to help individuals interpret and use their scores) $11.50; "Counseling with KOIS" (a handbook for counselors) $5; no charge for general manual if requested when ordering. Order from Science Research Associates, Inc.

Strong-Campbell Interest Inventory (designed by Campbell and Hansen, 1985). Used with adolescents and adults, grades 8 and above, this test measures occupational interests in a wide range of career areas. A 325-item paper-pencil multiple-choice test, it requires the individual to respond either "like," "indifferent," or "dislike" to items covering a broad range of familiar occupational tasks and day-to-day activities. Responses are analyzed by computer to yield a profile that presents scores on 23 basic interest scales and 207 occupational scales reflecting degree of similarity between respondent and people employed in particular occupations. Occupations are divided into six primary interest areas: realistic, investigative, artistic, social, enterprising, and conventional (based on John Holland's research). The Strong-Campbell is self-administered, takes approximately 25-30 minutes, and is computer-scored. The Strong-Campbell is available in French, Spanish, Hebrew, German, and Slovak, in addition to English. Costs include: Profile only, $2.15-$3.35, depending upon quantity; profile and interpretation, $3.60-$5.60, depending upon quantity; or scoring via microcomputer: profile only, $1.55-$2.00; profile and narrative, $3.10-$4.00. Order from: Stanford University Press; distributed by Consulting Psychologists Press, Inc.

The Self-Directed Search (designed by Holland, 1985). Used with adolescents and adults, ages 15-70, the SDS assesses interests, occupational preferences, competencies and self concepts. It is available in both paper-pencil and computerized forms and yields six interest scores (realistic, investigative, artistic, social, enterprising, and conventional) as well as a three-letter occupational code used for exploring occupational possibilities. Form E ("easy") is available for people at a fourth-grade reading level or for reading deficient high school students. The SDS is also available in French, Dutch, Chinese, Vietnamese, Japanese, Arabic, Afrikaans, and Danish, in addition to English. According to Martin Jaffe, Director of InfoPLACE, Cuyahoga County Regional Public Library, the Self-Directed Search is often the assessment of choice because it is self-administered in only 30-45 minutes, is self-scored, self-interpreted, and inexpensive. Costs include: Professional kit (manual, 25 booklets, and Occupational Finders), and 10 "You and Your Career" booklets $44; or 50 uses of the computer version $150. Order from: Psychological Assessment Resources, Inc.

Aptitude assessment. Assessment of aptitude is the oldest form of individual assessment. Popular as an investigative tool in early adolescence, instruments such as the Differential Aptitude Test (DAT) are used to help students plan their secondary school program. Other aptitude tests such as the General Aptitude Test Battery (GATB) and the Wechsler Adult Intelligence Scale—Revised (WAIS-R) are used to help adults predict future job performance. Nevertheless, it should be noted that correlations between aptitude tests and occupational performance have not been particularly high.[3]

Differential Aptitude Test (designed by Bennett, 1982). Used with junior and senior high school students, the DAT is a multiple-item paper-pencil test of eight abilities: verbal reasoning, numerical ability, abstract reasoning, clerical speed and accuracy, mechanical reasoning, space relations, spelling, and language usage. A ninth score, an index of scholastic ability, is obtained by adding the verbal reasoning and numerical ability scores. Poor readers and students with various disabilities will find the DAT a poor predictor. The DAT is completed in three hours or longer and is hand, machine, or computer scored. Costs include: Specimen set (test, directions, administrator's handbook, answer documents, list of correct answers, order for scoring service, sample profile forms) $11.00; Career Planning Service Information Packet (counselor's manual, directions, glossary, sample career planning report, explanation of school summary report, answer document, orientation booklet) $8.00. Order from The Psychological Corporation.

General Aptitude Test Battery (designed by the United States Employment Service). The GATB is "the most widely used test of multiple aptitudes with over 500 studies documenting the extent to which it predicts future job performance."[3] Use must be authorized by State Employment Service Agencies. The GATB is a 434-item paper-pencil test consisting of 284 multiple-choice questions, 150 dichotomous choice questions, and two dexterity form boards. Twelve subtests measure nine vocational aptitudes: general learning ability, verbal, numerical, spatial, form perception, clerical perception, motor coordination, finger dexterity, and manual dexterity. Results indicate the individual's likelihood of success in various occupations. Used for older adolescents and adults, the GATB takes approximately two-and-a-half hours to administer, and is hand or computer scored. Costs are available from State Employment Service Agencies only. Order from the U.S. Department of Labor.

Wechsler Adult Intelligence Scale, revised (designed by Wechsler). The WAIS-R is used with adolescents and adults, ages 16 and older, as a measure of intellectual ability. It is widely used in counseling as a valid measure of vocational aptitude. The WAIS-R contains both a verbal and a performance section, the scores from which yield a measure of IQ. It is available in Spanish. The WAIS-R is completed in approximately 75 minutes and must be evaluated by a trained examiner. Costs include: complete set (all necessary equipment, manual, 25 record forms with attache case) $175.00; complete without attache case $155.00. Order from The Psychological Corporation.

Personality assessment. Personality assessment in career counseling is helpful in providing self-knowledge relevant to career choice and to career adjustment. Personality factors not only influence the work environment an individual finds satisfactory, but personal characteristics affect an individual's interaction with others. " . . . *There is clear evidence that more people lose their jobs because of an inability to get along with other colleagues than for any other reason.*"[2] However, personality assessment has its limitations in career counseling because there are no inventories of work personality, *per se,* and personality instruments developed for other purposes are indirect applications.[2]

From the hundreds of personality instruments available, two of the most commonly used in career counseling are The Myers-Briggs Type Indicator and The Sixteen Personality Factor Questionnaire.

Myers-Briggs Type Indicator (Myers and Briggs, 1975). The MBTI is based on the theory of psychologic types created by Carl Jung in which an individual shows a disposition toward four bipolar aspects of personality: extroversion-introversion; sensing-intuition; thinking-feeling; and judging-perceptive. The instrument is a 166- to 126-item paper-pencil or computer-administered test that yields a profile with an interpretation of scores and a chart explanation of each of the 16 MBTI types. These types, in turn, can be matched with career requirements. The MBTI, appropriate for sixth graders through adults, is self-administered in 20-30 minutes and may be hand or computer scored and interpreted. Costs include: Counselor's kit (specify Form F, 166 items or Form G, 126 items: manual, key, "Introduction to Type," 5 tests, 25 answer sheets) $27.50. Order from Consulting Psychologists Press, Inc.

Sixteen Personality Factor Questionnaire (Cattell, 1969). Appropriate for adults and older adolescents, the SPFQ uses factor analysis to measure 16 primary personality traits, including levels of assertiveness, shrewdness, self-sufficiency, tension, anxiety, neuroticism, and rigidity. The SPFQ predicts job-related criteria, such as length of time an individual is likely to remain with a company, sales effectiveness, work efficiency, and tolerance for routine, or may be used to provide information about individual strengths, behavioral attitudes, and gratifications. There are five equivalent forms with 105 to 187 items each, including forms created for individuals with a below sixth-grade reading level. Testing time is 30-60 minutes, and the SPFQ can be hand or computer scored. Interpretation can be presented in a profile analysis or through more complex statistical methods. Costs include: 25 reusable test booklets $16.50; 25 machine-scorable answer sheets $5.50; 50 hand-scorable answer sheets $6.50; 50 profile sheets $6.50; 50 hand-scorable answer-profile sheets $7.50. Order from the Institute for Personality and Ability Testing, Inc.

Achievement assessment. "Achievement assessment is probably the least commonly used type of formal assessment measure in the career assessment process."[10] It is apt to be specifically related to a particular field of interest to measure whether an individual has the skills and education to succeed in that career. For example, The Ohio Vocational Achievement Test Program assesses high school students in eleven vocational areas. The complete battery reveals the correlation of student academic aptitude and vocational achievement. Thirty-nine individual tests are available to evaluate and diagnose achievement for instructional improvement in specific vocational areas, such as farm management, clerk-stenographer, construction electricity, and food service personnel. More information is available from the Instructional Materials Laboratory, Ohio State University.

Career maturity assessment. Crites points out that traditional measures of aptitude, interests, personality, and achievement are mediocre predictors of success in specific careers.[7] Rather than trying to use such tests alone, Crites argues that there is greater value in career maturity assessment, or the measure of an individual's readiness to make a career decision. He sees the career choice process as being more important than the content. According to this perspective, descriptive data are more important than predictive information; how individuals make choices is more important than what choices are made. Two measures of career maturity which can be administered either individually or in groups are The Career Maturity Inventory (CMI) and The Career Development Inventory (CDI).

Career Maturity Inventory (Crites, 1973). Used with adolescents, grades 6-12, the CMI consists of two paper-pencil inventories that measure a student's maturity regarding attitudes and competencies toward career decisions. The Attitude Scale specifically measures the student's maturity with respect to decisiveness, involvement, independence, orientation, and compromise when it comes to making a career choice. The Competency Test contains five subtests measuring self-appraisal, occupational information, goal selection, planning, and problem solving. The value of the CMI is that the results may be used to identify the two principal problems individuals encounter in career decision-making: indecision and unrealism.[7] According to Crites, the CMI can be used not only for diagnosis of these two general decisional problems but also for finer pinpointing of the factors producing the problems. Although the CMI is untimed, administrators allow 25 minutes for the screening form and 35 minutes for the counseling form. It is hand-keyed but may be computer scored. Thirty-five test books, a manual, and a key may be ordered for $26.25 from CTB/McGraw-Hill.

Career Development Inventory (Super, Thompson, Lindeman, Jordaan, & Myers, 1960 and 1982). Used with adolescents, grades 10-12 (school form) or college students (college and university form), the CDI is a multiple-item paper-pencil inventory that assesses knowledge and attitudes about career choices. The value of the CDI is that the results may be used to select a counseling strategy through problem diagnosis, to determine the individual's readiness for choice making, and to focus on the attitudes, behaviors, and knowledge needed to make good choices. Although the CDI is untimed, administrators allow 55 to 65 minutes. It is computer scored.

The school form, including a specimen set (test booklet, answer sheet, and manual) may be ordered for $12.50; computer scoring is $2.00 each. For the college and university form, 25 test booklets cost $17.00; the user's manual $11.00; the technical manual $13.50; and 10 answer sheets $24.00. Both may be ordered from Consulting Psychologists Press, Inc.

Computer-assisted assessment. Computer-assisted career guidance (CACG) has gained considerable acceptance as public secondary schools, colleges and universities, library systems, and other organizations acquire CACG systems, and as computers in general become common in homes and work places. Because the systems are interesting, enjoyable, and valuable, *students who have access to computer-assisted programs prefer them over other career information resources.*[9]

There are two types of computer-assisted systems: (1) information systems and (2) complete career guidance systems. Some provide straightforward information on occupations and education, e.g., the Guidance Information System (GIS). Others are closer to interactive career counseling; e.g., DISCOVER and the System of Interactive Guidance and Information (SIGI). Both types of systems serve the purpose of providing vast amounts of occupational information to an individual while at the same time providing a resource that is attentive to individual differences, as well as responsive to distinctive needs and content without biases or prejudice. Using computer programs for the purpose of information gathering, a task that is routine and repetitive for most counselors, provides more time for interaction between individuals seeking career assistance and a helping professional. Other advantages of computer-assisted guidance systems are the cost-effectiveness and sophistication of available programs. Reliability and validity are still in question.

DISCOVER (American College Testing Corporation). DISCOVER combines career guidance and search strategies to provide the user with self-knowledge and to link that knowledge with occupational and educational information. There are three versions of DISCOVER:

1. For post-secondary students and adults in career transition
2. For secondary school students
3. For junior high and middle school students (grades 6-9)

Post-secondary students and adults. The adult system of DISCOVER allows the individual to use either the "Information Only" approach to retrieve data from various files or the "Guidance" approach to work through the nine modules of the program. The latter introduces the user to the ACT world of work design as it relates to the individual's interests, abilities, experience, and values. Then specific careers are displayed in order of the number of matches found between the user's characteristics and those of the occupation. Information about selected occupations appears, after which the user narrows the list of careers to ten or fewer. Finally, training paths are identified and next steps are outlined, such as listings of specific schools or institutions offering training, information concerning job hunting skills, financial aid recommendations, and information about nontraditional methods of acquiring credit. The cost for leasing DISCOVER is $1750.00/year, first copy; cost decreases with additional copies. Order from the American College Testing Program.

Secondary school student. The high school version of DISCOVER is similar to the adult version, but it also includes identification of fields of study that may lead to employment in desired areas. Students may also use results of interest inventories such as the Self-Directed Search, and/or aptitude tests such as the Differential Aptitude Test. The occupational files in DISCOVER include information on 2921 vocational/technical schools, 1458 two-year colleges, 1731 four-year colleges, 1241 graduate schools, 144 external degree programs and 212 military programs. Data files are updated yearly to provide current information. DISCOVER may be used in 2 to 4 hours, although work sessions can easily be broken up into 30 to 45 minute segments. The cost for leasing DISCOVER for high schools is $1750.00 for the first copy.

Junior high and middle school students. DISCOVER for junior high and middle school students has only three parts: (1) You and the World of Work, (2) Exploring Options, and (3) Planning for High School. As students explore their interests and learn more about work choices, one option is to run parts 1 and 2 in seventh grade, saving part 3 for eighth grade. Unlike the high school or adult versions, the middle school program uses "Moxey the Mouse" in a maze, presenting the program as a game in which the student tries to help Moxey reach the goal of a piece of cheese by answering questions about worker tasks. In the third component, "Planning for High School," DISCOVER takes students from the concept of work on to self assessment and into the planning stage, including consideration of graduation requirements and courses that may meet those needs. Bronk, in his review of the middle school DISCOVER program, observes that it is "the relationship of careers to the individual school program that makes DISCOVER a real success."

SIGI-Plus (Educational Testing Service). This system is another comprehensive career planning program that is divided into nine separate but interrelated sections, each of which relates to a stage of the career decision making process. Unlike DISCOVER, this program allows the user to choose desirable and undesirable work characteristics and provides specific occupational information, such as skills required, possibilities for advancement, and potential income. When presenting occupational skills, the SIGI-Plus program allows the user to rate himself on these skills. Other areas covered are: career preparation (including finding time and money and arranging care for others), and what steps to take next. Data is updated annually and can be adapted to include local employment conditions. SIGI-Plus may be completed in approximately three hours, although the user may stop at any time and continue later. Included in the annual license fee of $1,075 - $1,375 is a Guide to Further Resources. Order from: Educational Testing Service.

The Guidance Information System (GIS) (Houghton Mifflin Company). GIS is another computer-assisted guidance program, often used by career guidance centers in schools and colleges. GIS consists of six major filing systems: (1) Occupational Information, (2) Armed Services Occupational Information, (3) Two-Year College Information, (4) Four-Year College Information, (5) Graduate and Professional School Information, and (6) Financial Aid Information. These files are updated semi-annually by the publisher. An individual may use SIGI-Plus to look up information about known or previously chosen career areas, schools, or financial aid programs, or may develop an index in any of the files based on the user's personal preferences and choices. The program and its support guides cross-reference selections to other commonly used encyclopedia resources. It does not provide options for self-exploration other than through choices based on job characteristics. SIGI-Plus is available to universities and schools for an annual license fee of $1,950; the Career Decision Making System (on-line interest inventory) is available for an additional $399.

Issues regarding assessment. One of the criticisms of the use of assessment instruments in career counseling is that too much validity may be placed on the "objective" instrument. The fear is that by the content included or excluded in a test or a computer program, goals may be defined and decisions made that may not be appropriate for the individual using the instrument. With most people looking for a cut-and-dried solution to their career needs, assessment provides a simple and direct means of gathering information that is bound to be insufficient by itself. It is particularly tempting for counselors with limited time to offer computer-assisted assessments such as "Discover" and "SIGI-Plus" without accompanying guidance.

Another concern is that because most assessment tools have been developed by and validated on predominantly white middle class male populations whose cultural, edu-cational, and economic backgrounds are different from Black, female, or other groups, that the test norms may not be valid for everyone.

A third concern is that assessment instruments might not be used by properly trained personnel. Less skilled counselors, or those with insufficient time, may be tempted to use assessment as the major technique of advisement when it should be only a part of the career development process. Assessment instruments are most effectively used in career counseling when combined with other methods. Discussion with a knowledgeable adult, both individually and in groups, as well as reading and research, contribute to an effective career exploration process. Resource people may include parents, teachers, school guidance counselors, counseling psychologists, library specialists, vocational counselors, and medical and rehabilitation personnel.

With the growing number of assessment tools, particularly computerized career assessments, professional organizations are educating their members regarding the competencies needed to use computer-based systems for career information and exploration. There also is increased attention to promoting an awareness of ethical codes and practices.

SUMMARY

Career development is a lifelong process of self-assessment meshed with occupational awareness. No matter what theoretical perspective is considered, the goal is to achieve satisfaction in one's work. Because research indicates that satisfaction with career role significantly influences health; that change in career is a major source of stress; that stress adversely affects health; and that in times of change and stress physicians are likely to be consulted by adults, it is essential that career development be understood by physicians dealing with preventive medicine.

Knowledge of current perspectives and key issues affecting career life planning will be helpful in understanding the social, economic, and emotional factors affecting an individual in career transition. Knowledge of assessment instruments available to measure interests, aptitude, personality, achievement, and career maturity will help the physician suggest appropriate tests. Awareness of additional resources, including computer software, publications, and national and community organizations, adds to the physician's competency in being able to guide an individual through a career planning process or refer to an appropriate professional.

Given the limitations of time and space, this chapter does not deal with such specific career related issues as "burn out" or mid-life career change. The authors wish to acknowledge the importance of these and other issues by including several references for the physician's further study.

REFERENCES

1. Brown D, Brooks L et al: *Career choice and development: applying contemporary theories to practice* (2nd edition), San Francisco, Oxford, 1990, Jossey-Bass.
2. Brown MB: Personality assessment in career counseling, *Career Planning and Adult Development Journal* 6(4):22-26, 1990-91.
3. Capps FC, Heinlein WE, Sautler SW: Aptitude testing in career assessment, *Career Planning and Adult Development Journal* 6(4), 1990-91.
4. Careers Sourcebook: *An information guide for career planning*, ed 2, Detroit, NY, Ft. Lauderdale, London, 1992, Gale Research.
5. Feldman DC: *Managing careers in organizations*, Glenview, Ill., 1988, Scott Foresman and Co.
6. Gilligan C: Woman's place in man's life cycle, *Harvard Educational Review* 49(4): 431-446, 1979.
7. Gysbers NC et al: *Designing careers*, San Francisco, Washington, London, 1984, Jossey-Bass.
8. Hall DT, et al: *Career development and organizations*, San Francisco, 1986, Jossey-Bass.
9. Haring-Hidore M: In pursuit of students who do not use computers for career guidance, *Journal of Counseling and Development* 63(3):139-140, Nov. 1984.
10. Hohenshil TH, Solly DC: An overview of career assessment methods and models, *Career Planning and Adult Development Journal* 6(4), 1990-91.
11. Holmes TH, Rahe RH: The social readjustment rating scale, *Psychosom Res* 11:213-218, 1967.
12. Kapes JT, Moran Mastic M: *A counselor's guide to career assessment instruments*, Alexandria, Va, 1988, The National Career Development Association (Division of the American Association for Counseling and Development).
13. Levinson DJ: *The seasons of a man's life*, New York, 1978, Ballantine Books.
14. Levinson EM, Folino L: Career interest assessment techniques, *Career Planning and Adult Development Journal* 6(4), 1991.
15. *Planning for Americans*, New York, 1978, National Center for Career Life Planning (Division of American Management Association).
16. Pelowski BG: *Decision-making at mid-life: graduate school as an alternative for effecting change in the lives of men and women, ages 35 and older*, East Lansing, 1981, Michigan State University.
17. Rohrlich JB: *Work and love: the crucial balance*, New York, 1980, Summit Books.
18. Sheehy G: *Passages: predictable crises of adult life*, New York, 1976, E.P. Dutton and Company.
19. Sweetland RC, Keyser DJ, editors: *Tests: a comprehensive reference for assessments in psychology, education, and business*, Kansas City, Kan., 1986, Test Corporation of America.
20. Aslanian CB, Brickell HM: *Transition: life changes as reasons for adult learning*, New York, 1980, College Entrance Examination Board.
21. Van Maanen JV, Schein EH, Bailyn L: *The shape of things to come: a new look at organizational careers*. In Hackman JR, Lawler EE, Porter LW, editors: *Perspectives on behavior in organizations*, New York, 1977, McGraw Hill.
22. Verbrugge LG: *Role responsibilities, role burdens, and physical health*. In Crosby FJ, editor, *Spouse, parent, worker*, New Haven and London, 1976, Yale University Press.
23. Walz GR, Blever JC, Maze M: *Counseling software guide: a resource for the guidance and human development professions*, Alexandria, Va., 1989, American Association for Counseling and Development.
24. Zuncker VG: *Career counseling: applied concepts of life planning*, ed 3, Pacific Grove, Calif., 1990, Brooks/Cole.

SUGGESTED READINGS

Arthur MB, Hall DT, Lawrence BS: *Handbook of career theory*, New York, 1989, Cambridge University Press.
Bolles RN: *The three boxes of life*, Berkeley, Calif., 1978, Ten Speed Press.
Bolles RN: *What color is your parachute?*, Berkeley, Calif., 1990, Ten Speed Press.
Campbell D: *If you don't know where you're going, you'll probably end up somewhere else*, Niles, Ill., 1974, Argus Communications.
Gould RL: *Transformations: growth and change in adult life*, New York, 1978, Simon and Schuster.
Hall DT: *Careers in organizations*, Pacific Palisades, Calif., 1976, Goodyear.
Hecklinger FJ, Curtin BM: *Training for life: a practical guide to career and life planning*, ed 3, Dubuque, Iowa, 1987, Kendall/Hunt.
Hirsh SK, Kummerow J: *Life types*, New York, 1989, Warner Books.
Kanter RM: *Work and family in the United States*, New York, 1977, Russell Sage Foundation.
Krannich RL: *Careering and re-careering for the 1990's: the complete guide to planning your future*, Woodbridge, Va, 1989, Impact Publications.
Maccoby M: *Career and self-fulfillment: are they compatible?*, Lifelong Learning Conference, Akron, Ohio, 1980, University of Akron.
McCoy VR: *Adult career development and the importance of the dream*, Presented at Kansas City Community College, Kansas City, Kan., 1979.
McDaniels C: *The changing workplace: career counseling strategies for the 1990's and beyond*, San Francisco, London, 1989, Jossey-Bass.
Neugarten BL: *Time, age, and the life cycle*. In McCoy VR, Ryan C, Sutton R, Winn N, editors: *A life transitions reader*, Lawrence, Kan., 1980, University of Kansas.
Pearlin LI: *Life strains and psychological distress among adults*. In Smelser NJ, Erikson EH, editors: *Themes of work and love in adulthood*, Cambridge, Mass., 1980, Harvard University Press.
Savage KM: *The sourcebook*, Cleveland, Ohio, 1991, Cuyahoga County Public Library.
Seltz NC, Collier HV, editors: *Meeting the educational and occupational planning needs of adults*, Bloomington, Ind., 1977, Indiana University.
Stoodley M: *Information interviewing: what it is and how to use it in your career*, 1990, Garrett Park Press.
Terkel S: *American dreams: lost and found*, New York, 1980, Pantheon Books.

═══ RESOURCES ═══

Organizations and their publications

American Association for Counseling and Development (AACD) 5999 Stevenson Ave., Alexandria, VA 22304. For counseling and human development professionals. Maintains special library of 5,000 books and pamphlets. Among publications: *Journal of Counseling and Development,* bimonthly; *Journal of Employment Counseling,* quarterly; *Vocational Guidance Quarterly.*

National Career Development Association. A division of AACD. Publishes *Career Development Quarterly.*

Career Planning and Adult Development Network, 4965 Sierra Road, San Jose, CA 95132. For human resource professionals, career counselors, educators, and researchers. Publishes *Career Planning and Adult Development Journal,* quarterly.

College Scholarship Service, C.N. 6335, Princeton, NJ 08541. Publishes the Financial Aid Form (FAF) for use in applying for financial aid to U.S. colleges and universities.

InfoPLACE services, Cuyahoga County Public Library, 5225 Library Lane, Maple Heights, OH 44133-1291. Professional career guidance, job search assistance, and educational information and referrals.

National Learning Corporation, 212 Michael Drive, Syosset, NY 11791. Publishes a series of study guides with multiple-choice examination questions and solutions for various careers.

Other resources

Dictionary of Occupational Titles, ed 4, 1977. U.S. Government Printing Office, Washington, DC 20402. Fourth Edition Supplement, 1986. Defines 20,000 job titles. Includes an industry-occupation cross index. Each description lists job duties, indicates the industry where the job is done, and what equipment or tools are used. The description is useful as a skill checklist in resume writing.

Occupational Outlook Handbook, biennial. Superintendent of Documents. U.S. Government Printing Office, Washington, D.C. Lists occupations and comprises about 86% of all jobs in the economy. Includes information regarding what the worker does, working conditions, education and training required, advancement, job outlook, earnings, and sources of additional information.

The Encyclopedia of Careers and Vocational Guidance, 1990. William E. Hopke, editor-in-chief. J.G. Ferguson Publishing Co., 200 W. Monroe, Suite 250, Chicago, IL 60601. Four volume set that provides 900 occupations and describes job trends in 71 industries.

Jobs Rated Almanac: Ranks the Best and Worst Jobs by More than a Dozen Criteria, 1988. Les Krantz, editor. World Almanac, 200 Park Ave., New York, NY 10166. Ranks 250 jobs by environment, salary, outlook, physical demands, stress, security, travel opportunities, and geographic location. Includes jobs the editor feels are the most common, most interesting, and the most rapidly growing.

Kennedy's Career Strategist: a monthly guide to career planning success and job satisfaction. Marilyn Moats Kennedy. 1153 Wilmette Ave., Wilmette, IL 60091.

National Business Employment Weekly. Tony Lee, editor, Dow Jones Company, Inc., 420 Lexington Ave., New York, NY 10170. Weekly newspaper with articles related to employment activities and advertisements of jobs available. A "Calendar of Events" lists job clubs, seminars, and workshops offered nationwide.

Mature/Older Job Seeker's Guide, Brenda Crawley, National Council on Aging, Inc., 600 Maryland Avenue, SW, West Wing 100, Washington, DC 20024. Information and exercises geared to the realities of the mature/older person's job search needs.

Community organizations

Many organizations common to communities throughout the United States are likely resources for information regarding jobs and careers, education, and counseling. Such community resources include:

The Forty Plus Club of New York, 15 Park Row, New York, NY, 10038. A national organization that helps unemployed executives over 40-years-old to organize their job searches. Has clubs in seventeen U.S. cities.

United Way Services for "info lines."

Public libraries for reference materials and educational programs, and sometimes career counselors.

Local college and university career centers for counselors and information about educational opportunities.

Churches for counselors and support groups.

YMCA's for educational programs.

Hospitals and clinics for health evaluations.

County cooperative extension services for information about the community.

Chamber of Commerce for information about community resources.

Local newspapers for information about current educational programs and available jobs.

Local telephone books for listings of community organizations.

Federal Job Opportunity listing.

Testing resources

American College Testing Program, 230 Schilling Circle, Schilling Plaza South, Hunt Valley, MD 21031. To order the DISCOVER computer system.

Consulting Psychologists Press, Inc., 577 College Avenue, P.O. Box 60070, Palo Alto, CA 94306. To order the Strong-Campbell Interest Inventory, the Myers-Briggs Type Indicator, the Career Development Inventory.

CTB/McGraw-Hill, Publishers Test Service, Del Monte Research Park, 2500 Garden Road, Monterey, CA 93940. To order the Career Maturity Inventory.

Educational Testing Service, Rosedale Road, Princeton, NJ 08541, To order the SIGI-Plus computer system.

Houghton Mifflin Co., Educational Software Division, 1 Beacon Street, Boston, MA 02108. To order the GIS computer system.

Institute for Personality and Ability Testing, Inc., P.O. Box 188, 1602 Coronado Drive, Champaign, IL 61820. To order the Sixteen Personality Factor Questionnaire.

Instructional Materials Laboratory, The Ohio State University, 1885 Neil Avenue, Columbus, OH 43210. The Ohio Vocational Achievement Test Program.

The Psychological Corporation, A Subsidiary of Harcourt Brace Jovanich, Inc., 555 Academic Court, San Antonio, TX 78204. To order the DAT and the WAIS-R.

Psychological Assessment Resources, Inc., P.O. Box 98, Odessa, FL 33556. To order the Self-Directed Search.

Science Research Associates, Inc., 155 North Wacker Drive, Chicago, IL 60606. To order the Kuder Occupational Interest Survey.

U.S. Department of Labor, Division of Testing, Employment and Training Administration, Washington, DC 20213. To order the GATB.

Chapter 30

THE ADULT FEMALE

Contraception and preventive services in pregnancy

Linda Bradley

PRECONCEPTUAL CARE

Pregnancy is just one part of a woman's long reproductive life cycle. It should be considered to last 12 months rather than the traditional 9 months. As women and couples "plan" to have babies, they will seek advice and care from family physicians and obstetrician/gynecologists before becoming pregnant.

Patients at this time are concerned with high expectations for a "perfect baby." Less than 50 to 75 years ago, a woman's greatest concern was her ability to be alive after the birth of her child. In fact, today in some parts of the world, such as Africa, one out of 150 women die in childbirth, compared with the United States, where less than one out of 10,000 women will die as a result of delivery. In essence, over the past 50 years, the maternal mortality has decreased 50-fold, and perinatal mortality has decreased threefold.[138,229]

Epidemiology and risk factors

As women have come to expect a safe and pain-free delivery experience, they have shifted their attention from the actual birthing process to concerns about the possible benefits of preconceptual care. The basic tenets of preconceptual care involve: assessing risk factors before pregnancy, establishing and maintaining a healthy lifestyle, and when necessary making adjustments in the medical psychosocial mileu.[10]

Many patients do not seek prenatal care until the seventh to twelfth week of gestation, by which time organogenesis has occurred. Many lifestyle habits could be modified before conception, such as smoking, alcohol intake, drug use, over-the-counter drug use, and nutrition. Patients with chronic illnesses, such as hypertension, diabe-

tes, or obesity, should attempt to have their illness under the best possible control before an anticipated pregnancy.[10]

Although many women have consciously elected to pursue their education, career goals, and economic independence, many have not chosen reliable means of contraception. Many women think that "if it happens, it will just happen," regarding their ability to have a child. In fact, statistics from 1982 revealed that 54% of pregnancies are unintended.[211] Of the 6.1 million women who became pregnant, 1.3 million had births that were unintended, 0.4 million had a spontaneous miscarriage, and 1.6 million abortions were performed.[211] Women between the ages of 15 and 44 experienced a 29.1% incidence of "mistimed" pregnancies, and 10.5% of these pregnancies were unwanted. Higher rates of unintended pregnancy are seen in unmarried women, minorities, and teenagers.[211]

Therapeutic interventions

How can health care providers provide preconceptual counseling when so many pregnancies are unintended or unplanned? Patients may be educated about the importance of preconceptual care at premarital exams (which are required by some states), women's shelters, and when patients present for a pregnancy test and the results are negative. In addition, health classes during high school and science courses in college should emphasize the need for preconceptual care.

Screening

In 1989, the Federal Expert Panel on the Content of Prenatal Care recommended that preconceptual care be considered an integral part of prenatal care for all women.

This task force recommended that all women be comprehensively assessed for risk factors related to poor outcome and that these risk factors be identified preconceptually, when modifications and lifestyle changes could be made.[51,214] Tests to be conducted during preconceptual care should demonstrate efficacy and effectiveness in identifying conditions before they might otherwise be recognized. Also, tests should be performed economically, cause minimal discomfort, and have few side effects. In addition, modification of treatment plans and intervention should be available if a condition is identified.[51]

The American College of Obstetricians and Gynecologists guidelines recommend that the following risk factors be identified during a preconceptual care visit.[10]

- Medical history (including a narrative description of the patient's sociodemographic information, menstrual history, obstetrical history, contraceptive history, sexual history, infectious disease history, and family and genetic history)
- Psychological history (including information regarding social supports, stress levels, physical abuse, sexual abuse, mental status, pregnancy readiness)
- Nutrition
- Substance abuse

Some institutions employ risk-modification checklists in their prenatal clinic. Common forms include those developed by Hobel, Sokal, and Morrison.[123,181,242]

Antepartum surveillance. Antepartum care begins with the first prenatal visit and continues until the patient enters labor. Patients should be strongly urged to present for antepartum care as soon as their pregnancy is established. This enables the physician to identify risk factors for the pregnancy that may need to be modified to improve pregnancy outcome. At the first physical examination, risk factors, as mentioned previously, must be identified. These factors can be tabulated on any of the currently available risk-factor score sheets, including those by Hobel, Sokal, or Hollister[123,242] (see the box above).

Follow-up visits will depend on the patient's identified risk factors. For the low-risk patient, ideally visits are every 4 weeks during the first 28 weeks of the pregnancy, followed by every 2 weeks until the thirty-sixth week, and weekly thereafter. Once a patient is postdates, visits may be scheduled more often for biophysical profile studies until labor commences or is induced.[10] Patients with high-risk factors, such as diabetes, hypertension, or multiple gestation, may require surveillance more frequently.[10]

Each antepartum visit should be educational for both the patient and physician. The patient needs to inform the physician of any new risk factors or problems that she has encountered. Likewise, the physician should provide positive feedback when possible, update the patient regarding dietary guidelines, weight gain, and blood pressure, determine whether the patient has any questions, and deliver re-

---

Preconception risk modification check list

1. Discontinue alcohol.
2. Discontinue recreational drugs.
3. Discontinue smoking.
4. Use effective contraception until pregnancy is desired.
5. Before pregnancy, patient should know Rubella status; if nonimmune, patient should be vaccinated before pregnancy and advised not to become pregnant for two menstrual cycles after vaccination.
6. Patients with longstanding medical problems, such as hypertension, diabetes, collagen vascular disease, should have the best possible control of their illness before planning pregnancy and should consider:

    Is this the best time for the patient to be pregnant?
    Are the medical risks, mortality, and morbidity acceptable to the patient and family?

    Patients with significant medical problems should be offered preconceptual counseling with a knowledgeable obstetrician or perinatologist. This consultation will help determine whether therapeutic interventions are worthwhile.
7. Genetic counseling should be offered to all patients with prior affected pregnancies, including sickle cell disease, Tay-Sachs disease, and cystic fibrosis.

---

sults of any tests that have been performed. At each visit, blood pressure, weight, fundal height, urinalysis, and fetal heart rate should be recorded. Once quickening occurs (after the twentieth week of pregnancy), the physician should ask about fetal movement. A fetal movement kick-count often is recommended as a measure of fetal well-being after the thirty-sixth week of pregnancy.[10] Fetal position is also noted on each visit; however, if the fetus is noted to be in the breech position after the thirty-sixth week, the obstetrical team may consider external cephalic version.[10]

Antepartum Screening Tests. The American College of Obstetrician and Gynecologists has mandated that certain tests be automatically performed on all patients presenting for prenatal care. Additional tests may be necessary, depending on the history and physical examination of the patient.

Currently, the following tests are recommended to be performed at the first prenatal examination: hemoglobin, hematocrit, and urinalysis (including the microscopic examination and culture). Additionally, blood group and Rh typing, antibody screen, Rubella antibody titer measurement, syphillis screening, Pap smear, and hepatitis B virus screen should be performed on all patients.[10]

The estimated date of delivery (estimated date of confinement; EDC) is of paramount importance in managing a pregnancy. Complications related to pregnancy, such as intrauterine growth retardation, postdates, prematurity, and evaluation of abnormal bleeding during pregnancy can best be managed by knowing the EDC.[10] If a patient begins her pregnancy and does not know the date of her last menstrual period, it would be important to perform an ultrasound early in the first trimester. A first-trimester ultrasound is the most accurate method of determining the EDC. In addition, estimating an appropriate EDC is important for patients who will undergo an elective cesarean section to prevent iatrogenic prematurity.[10]

Additional prenatal screening tests that may be offered to a patient, depending on her medical risk factors, are ultrasound, amniocentesis, or chorionic villus sampling.[10]

All women should be offered a screening test for maternal serum alpha-fetoprotein (MSAFP) between the sixteenth and eighteenth weeks of pregnancy.[10]

Between the twenty-sixth and twenty-eighth weeks of pregnancy, patients should be screened for diabetes, and a repeat hemoglobin and hematocrit should be performed.

Prevention of hemolytic disease and isoimmunization in the newborn represents a triumph for modern obstetrics. Patients who are Rh negative and Du negative should receive RhoGAM to prevent sensitization in the fetus. Gorman et al,[103] proved that passive immunization could prevent hemolytic disease in the newborn. Candidates for RhoGAM are any pregnant patient who is Rh negative and Du negative and who is not already isoimmunized. Factors that increase the risk of a maternal fetal bleed warrant RhoGAM administration. In general, RhoGAM should be

administered within 72 hours of a maternal-fetal blood exchange.

Usually, 300 mcg of RhoGAM is administered after the first trimester. This amount will neutralize 15 mg of packed cells or 30 ml of whole blood. Fetal bleeding exceeding this amount is rare.[51] Additionally, patients who have a first-trimester miscarriage or abortion should receive 50 mcg of RhoGAM.

Patients who have second- or third-trimester bleeding, amniocentesis, external cephalic version, or antepartum fetal demise routinely should receive 300 mcg of RhoGAM intramuscularly. Several authors have confirmed that patients who received immunoprophylaxis had a sensitization rate of 0.18%, compared with untreated patients whose risk was 6.9%.[31] Therefore, RhoGAM prophylaxis should be offered to all patients who meet the criteria for treatment (see the box below).

At the twenty-eighth week, a repeat antibody test for Rh-negative unsensitized patients should be performed. These patients should receive prophylactic administration of RhoGAM if this test is negative. RhoGAM should be given to any Rh-negative unsensitized patient after an amniocentesis, chorionic villous sampling (CVS) or episodes of placental bleeding.

Between the thirty-second and thirty-sixth weeks of pregnancy, an ultrasound may be warranted if there is evidence of growth discrepancy or poor maternal weight gain. Patients should be retested for sexually transmitted diseases, and hemoglobin or hematocrit tests should be repeated.[10]

Additionally, the expert panel on the content of prenatal care notes that HIV testing should be considered in patients with high-risk factors or behaviors that increase the risk for acquiring HIV.[46,214] In 1986, one out of five patients presenting for maternity care at a local New York Hospital was infected with the HIV virus.[148] Risk factors such as prostitution, multiple sex partners, blood transfusions (received between 1978 and 1986), and sex partners who are drug users are indications for periodic HIV testing during pregnancy.[46,148] It is well known that infants acquire HIV transplacentally and ultimately have prolonged morbidity and risk of death if HIV is contracted. All HIV-positive patients are advised not to become pregnant. HIV-infected women should not breastfeed.

Routine testing for toxoplasmosis, varicella, herpes simplex, and cytomegalovirus currently is not performed unless the clinical history or physical exam warrants it.[266]

Screening tests for genetic birth defects. All patients who will be 35 or older at the time of the birth of their child should be offered chromosomal analysis to detect congenital birth defects.[99]

As women age, infertility, miscarriage, and congenital malformation risk also increase. Definite biochemical, environmental, or aging factors may affect the quality of the ovum. The estimated rate of significant cytogenetic abnormalities increases with age, such that approximately one

---

Candidates for RhoGAM

Any Rh-negative, Du-negative patient who is pregnant and potentially has suffered a maternal fetal bleed. This includes

1. In the first trimester of pregnancy, women with:
   a. Elective abortion
   b. Missed abortion
   c. Spontaneous abortion
   d. Ectopic pregnancy
   e. Preceeding chorionic villus sampling
   Rx: Minidose RhoGAM, 50 mcg IM administered within 72 hours of the event/bleed.
2. In the second trimester of pregnancy, women with:
   a. Spontaneous abortion
   b. Induced abortion
   c. Preterm delivery
   d. Amniocentesis
   e. Second-trimester bleeding
   Rx: RhoGAM, 300 mcg IM.
3. In the third trimester of pregnancy, women with:
   a. Third-trimester bleeding
   b. Delivery
   c. External version
   d. Antepartum fetal demise
   Rx: RhoGAM, 300 mcg IM after delivery, procedure, or demise.

out of 2000 births at the age of 20 are affected, one out of 300 births at age 35 are affected, one out of 100 births at age 40, one out of 40 at age 45, and one out of 10 at age 49 are affected by a cytogenetic abnormality.[125]

Women over the age of 35 have an increased risk of spontaneous abortion, more aneuploid conceptions, and increased rate of miscarriage of euploid conceptions than do younger women.[77] In addition, the incidence of congenital malformations increases with maternal age independent of birth order. Congenital malformations represent the sum of nonlethal chromosomal abnormalities, plus teratogenic influences from the environment, plus developmental problems from the intrauterine environment.[77] Because of these increased risks, women who will be 35 years of age or older at the birth of their child should be offered chromosomal analysis in the form of chorionic villus sampling or genetic amniocentesis.

Patients with a prior chromosomally affected child or habitual abortions should be offered genetic testing. In addition, all patients between their sixteenth and eighteenth weeks of pregnancy should be offered maternal serum alpha fetoprotein determination if reliable laboratories and counseling are available to the patient. One should document that the test was offered and accepted or declined.

Routine ultrasound currently is not recommended for all patients to detect congenital birth defects.[10] However, in patients with many risk factors, which may complicate a pregnancy, routine use of ultrasound is highly recommended. These factors can include maternal conditions such as diabetes, obesity, or hypertension; renal, cardiac, or severe gastrointestinal disease; collagen vascular disease, and prior complications of pregnancy. Other factors, including lifestyle conditions such as smoking, drug use, alcohol ingestion, and poor nutrition, may also increase a woman's need for early ultrasound screening. In addition, patients who present with an uncertain last menstrual period should routinely be offered an obstetrical ultrasound to determine the estimated date of confinement and thereby help to prevent the tragedies of postdatism, which include stillbirth, macrosomia, oligohydramnios, and intrauterine growth retardation.

Patients presenting in the first trimester with irregular bleeding or uncertain last menstrual period should be offered a level-one ultrasound examination. This exam includes measurements of the biparietal diameter (BPD) and femur length. In addition, the placenta can be localized and the number of fetuses can be determined. In the event that the level-one ultrasound is abnormal, a level-two ultrasound is recommended. This allows for a higher resolution scan of fetal small parts and a more detailed analysis of the hands, bladder, cerebral hemispheres, facial contours, and spine. In addition, patients with multiple pregnancies are offered a level-two scan. Many studies have shown that approximately 10% to 60% of pregnancies can be labeled high risk, thereby necessitating an obstetrical

ultrasound. Obstetrical ultrasounds are also used before amniocentesis and choronic villus sampling to decrease complication rates.[136]

First-trimester ultrasound is most accurate for dating a pregnancy.[126] First-trimester ultrasound includes measurement of the crown-rump length (CRL). With growth of the fetus, structural details are better appreciated during the second and third trimester. A second- or third-trimester ultrasound will include measurements of fetal length, abdominal circumference, biparietal diameter, and head circumference. It is possible by extrapolation of this data to calculate fetal weight and age.[126] Current cost for obstetrical ultrasounds range from $150 to $190 per scan.

Expected outcome of screening. Approximately 3% of all newborns in this country have a birth defect.[184] Some of these are minor defects, and others are major defects that are incompatible with life. In 1985, 6300 infants died as a result of congenital anomalies.[184] Birth defects are the leading cause of infant mortality and result in more than three fourths of all physical handicaps suffered by children.[99] Many birth defects, such as neural tube defects and chromosomal aneuploidy (e.g., Down's syndrome), can be detected prenatally.[76]

Women over the age of 35 have a higher incidence of delivering an anomalous child with Down's syndrome. Most studies show that the risk of Down's syndrome is 1 in 2000 at the age of 20, 1 in 375 at age 35, 1 in 100 at age 40, 1 in 30 at age 45, and 1 in 9 at age 49.[66]

Effectiveness of early detection

Screening tests for Down's syndrome include chorionic villus sampling, amniocentesis, measurement of maternal serum alpha fetoprotein (MSAFP), and ultrasound imaging.[7]

Assuming that all women over the age of 35 underwent amniocentesis, extrapolating the available data would predict that 200 to 300 normal fetuses would be exposed to an amniocentesis for every one case of Down's syndrome that would be detected.

Other tests that have been used, but that are not routine screening tests for Down's syndrome, include ultrasonography determination of skin folds and femur length, serum estriol, and quantitative measurements of serum HCG values.

Some researchers have found ultrasonographic changes including a thickened nuchal fold and short femur present in some pregnancies affected with trisomy 21.[29] Benacerraf found that if these two findings were present, a sensitivity of 75% and a specificity of 98% were noted.[29] Other researchers have failed to duplicate these studies to date.

Chorionic villus sampling (CVS) is one of the newer diagnostic methods used to detect genetic chromosomal abnormalities. Benefits include rapid results, which are obtainable within 72 to 96 hours. A small amount of fetal tissue (5 to 40 mg) or chorionic villi can be obtained transcervically or transabdominally.[35] Patients with a severely displaced uterus (retroverted or anteflexed), uterine myomas, cervicitis, or multiple pregnancies may have more difficulty in undergoing this test. Determining the chromosomal, enzymatic, and DNA status of the fetus is possible with this test.[9] The same indications for genetic amniocentesis also apply to the CVS test. The procedure-related risks of this test are slightly higher than those of the amniocentesis.[9] Operator experience and special laboratory facilities are necessary to adequately perform this test.[35] Patients who have a normal CVS but an elevated MSAFP test during the middle trimester may still need an amniocentesis to determine amniotic fluid alpha fetoprotein levels and acetylcholinesterase values.[9]

Amniocentesis

Genetic amniocentesis has been the gold standard for detecting genetic chromosomal abnormalities in the fetus. This test can be performed as early as the twelfth week of pregnancy; however, it is usually performed between weeks 15 and 17. The procedure is performed through ultrasound-guided, transabdominal insertion of a needle into the amniotic fluid. Continuous ultrasound guidance decreases the risk of fetal injury, placental injury, and complications. Many genetic and biochemical analyses can be performed on the amniotic fluid and are accurate 99% of the time.[9] Complications occur in 0.5% of pregnancies tested.[9]

These complications include bacterial infection and fetal injury. With continuous ultrasound guidance, complication rates are minimal. Most collaborative studies in the United States revealed that the rate of fetal loss after an amniocentesis was 3.5%. Patients without the procedure have a pregnancy loss of 3.2%. Approximately 1 ml of amniotic fluid is removed for each week of gestation. Thus an early amniocentesis performed at 9 to 10 weeks' gestation would require 9 to 10 ml of amniotic fluid; at 15 weeks' gestation approximately 15 ml is withdrawn. Viable cells require approximately 2 to 2½ weeks to grow and to be analyzed chromosomally.

Chorionic villus sampling

Chorionic villus sampling offers earlier genetic testing for patients who are at risk for congenital anomalies. Chorionic villus sampling can be performed transcervically or transabdominally under ultrasound guidance between the ninth and twelfth weeks of pregnancy. Approximately 10 to 25 mg of chorionic villi are extracted. Because the sampled cells are derived from the fetus, this procedure is similar to taking a cell sample from the fetus. Within 2 to 4 days of obtaining the sample, the tissue actively grows and can be analyzed for cytogenetic, enzymatic, and DNA restriction enzyme assays.[36]

Candidates for chorionic villus sampling. Any patient who is at increased risk of having a child with con-

genital birth defects based on the maternal age or past obstetric indicators would be a candidate for chorionic villus sampling. Patients who want a first-trimester diagnosis of chromosomal aberrations are candidates. Common indicators include the following:

- Maternal age over 35
- Previous child with trisomy
- Mother who is a carrier of an X-linked gene (e.g., Duchenne muscular dystrophy)
- Parents who are carriers of a recessive gene (e.g., Tay-Sachs, sickle cell anemia, cystic fibrosis)
- Parents who are carriers of a chromosome rearrangement[36]

Risks associated with chorionic villus sampling. Chorionic villus sampling was first performed in 1968 by the transcervical route. An International Registry confirms that chorionic villus sampling rates have increased in the past 5 to 10 years. Approximately 80,000 procedures have been performed worldwide. A trained maternal-fetal physician-specialist usually performs the procedure under ultrasound guidance. Reported complication rates include cramping, 10.6%; maternal bleeding, 9.8%; infection, 0.50%; and spontaneous miscarriage, 2.6%. Remote potential risks include risk to the fetus, such as injury leading to malformations or limb deformities, Rh sensitization, puncture of the uterus, and septic shock.

Spontaneous miscarriage is greater during the first trimester (when the CVS is performed). Thus the miscarriage rate appears to be slightly higher than that associated with amniocentesis. Published reports reveal that the risk for fetal loss after chorionic villus sampling is approximately 2% to 4%. Clearly, patients with acute cervicitis, pelvic inflammatory disease, or large lower-uterine-segment fibroids should not undergo the transcervical approach. The transabdominal route may be offered to these patients.

Chorionic villus sampling has the advantage of diagnosing a congenital birth defect earlier, enabling the physician and patient to decide whether termination of pregnancy is desired. First-trimester terminations are safer, technically easier to perform, and less costly.

Conventional amniocentesis, which is performed between the fifteenth and sixteenth weeks of pregnancy and requires approximately 2½ to 3 weeks before results are available, allows enough time to elapse for the patient to notice fetal movement and activity. If the results are abnormal, many women find it difficult to terminate a pregnancy after they note fetal activity and bond with the fetus.

Patients who undergo chorionic villus sampling require a follow-up ultrasound at approximately 16 to 18 weeks' gestation. This ultrasound will determine the presence of central nervous system abnormalities such as spina bifida or other neural tube defects. A patient needs to understand that if her maternal serum alpha fetoprotein level is elevated, amniocentesis may be needed so that the amniotic fluid alpha fetoprotein and acetylcholinesterase levels can be tested.

The approximate cost of chorionic villus sampling in 1992 is $1500 to $1700. This includes the physician cost, processing charges, room charges, and genetic studies.

Screening for neural tube defects

The American College of Obstetrics and Gynecology strongly recommends that all pregnant women be offered a screening test for neural tube defects known as the maternal serum alpha fetoprotein assay (MSAFP).

The MSAFP test is a serum assay performed between the fifteenth and eighteenth weeks of pregnancy. When the level is "elevated" (usually 2.5 times the median value), 56% to 90% of affected fetuses can be detected when this modality is combined with ultrasound and measurement of amniotic AFP levels.[218]

Elevated levels have been associated with increased risk of neural tube defects but also have been noted in patients with multiple gestations and congenital anomalies such as omphalocele, congenital nephrosis, Turner's syndrome, fetal bowel obstruction, and teratomas. In addition, higher levels have been seen in pregnancies that later were associated with preterm labor, intrauterine growth retardation, fetal demise, and preeclampsia.[218] This caveat is important, because modifications in obstetrical management may occur in the event of an abnormal assay. This may include more frequent antepartum visits and use of intrapartum fetal monitoring during labor.

Because elevated maternal serum alpha fetoprotein levels can be associated with neural tube defects as well as other abnormalities such as fetal demise, preeclampsia, and intrauterine growth retardation, additional studies have been sought to confirm the etiology of abnormal levels. A second test, of acetylcholinesterase (AChE), was devised for this purpose.

Acetylcholinesterase is present in neural tissue. In patients with neural tube defects, this enzyme leaks from the affected tissue, and its concentration increases within the amniotic fluid. This test is performed only when the maternal serum alpha fetoprotein is elevated. In addition to being increased in neural tube defects, AChE levels are elevated in approximately 67% of fetuses with an omphalocele or gastroschisis, and 57% of fetuses with cystic hygroma. Therefore, in the event of an elevated maternal serum alpha fetoprotein level, a high-resolution ultrasound be performed of the spinal column and ventral abdominal wall is recommended to detect fetal abnormalities.[240]

Although not all open neural tube defects are associated with elevated serum AFP levels, the amniotic fluid AFP and acetylcholinesterase always will be elevated.[218] In addition, closed neural tube defects may not be associated with elevated AFP findings. Low levels of maternal serum AFP have been associated with an increased risk of Down's syndrome.[66]

Counseling and compliance. Patients who are currently pregnant but have had a previously affected child or first-degree relative, or are using valproic acid, should be advised to have a MSAFP.

The laboratory services provided to the physician play an important role in the interpretation of abnormal MSAFP values. Each lab should provide results, including a range of normal values for the patient's population, and also provide consultative services to the physician. Calculation of MSAFP must consider the maternal age, weight, number of fetuses, race, and presence of insulin-dependent diabetes mellitus. For instance, black patients generally have a higher level of serum AFP than the white population.[10]

Other patients who would benefit from genetic screening include Eastern European Jews, who should be screened for Tay-Sachs disease; blacks, for sickle cell anemia; Phillipinos and Southeast Asians, for alpha thalassemia; and Greeks and Italians, for beta thalassemia.[9]

In addition, patients who have an affected relative with Huntington's disease, hemophilia, or sickle cell disease also should consider genetic testing. The DNA sequence of the cystic fibrosis gene is known, but general population screening for cystic fibrosis currently is not recommended.[267]

Therapeutic interventions. Therapeutic interventions are highly probable in the case of patients who have had a history of a child with a neural tube defect. Since the end of World War II many scientists have linked folic acid deficiency with the later development of neural tube defects such as spina bifida, anencephaly, and encephalocele. Most recently the British Medical Research council (MRC) vitamin study reported the results of a prospective randomized trial of patients who were planning a pregnancy and who had had an infant or fetus with a neural tube defect. The study began in July, 1983 and was halted in 1991 when preliminary results showed a significant reduction in the incidence of neural tube defect in patients who used 4 mg per day of a folic acid supplement.[183] At this time, the Centers for Disease Control has issued an "interim" recommendation for folic acid supplementation during pregnancy, pending further research.[183] Because multivitamins and over-the-counter prescriptions contain folic acid but also contain vitamins A and D, it is recommended that the 4 mg of folic acid be obtained only under a physician's guidance and prescription. The folic acid should be supplied as a 4 mg supplement. A patient attempting to achieve the total 4 mg dose by ingesting multiple doses of a multivitamin complex may overingest other vitamins, particularly vitamins A and D, which can lead to harmful complications.[48,183]

At this time, the only patients who are advised to use 4 mg of folic acid daily are those who have had a prior pregnancy with a child with a neural tube defect. These recommendations currently are not intended for women who have never given birth to an anomalous child, who have relatives who have had an affected infant, who themselves have had spina bifida, or who take the anticonvulsant valproic acid—a known cause of spina bifida.[48,183]

Screening recommendations for chronic medical illnesses

As obstetric outcomes have been improved, many women with chronic medical conditions have elected to become pregnant. A recent study by Lehmann noted that 27.2% of women over the age of 40 attempting pregnancy had medical conditions that predated the pregnancy.[51,152]

Patients presenting with medical problems before pregnancy should receive preconceptual care to optimize pregnancy outcome. Some medical problems that may predate pregnancy include cardiovascular disease with chronic hypertension, diabetes mellitus, a history of phenyketonuria (PKU), a history of Graves' disease, immune thrombocytopenia, or lupus erythematosus.[115]

Therapeutic interventions for high-risk pregnancy behaviors

Smoking. The proportion of women who smoke has increased from 1940 until the present. Lung cancer currently has replaced breast cancer as the number one cause of cancer death in women.[92] Smoking is seen more frequently among blacks and persons of low socioeconomic status. Although pregnancy often presents the first opportunity for patients to go "cold turkey" and stop smoking, reports reveal that 25% to 40% of female smokers do not quit smoking during pregnancy.[269]

Approximately 5% of perinatal deaths and 14% of all preterm deliveries in the United States have been attributable to maternal smoking. In addition, approximately 12% to 15% of children experiencing sudden infant death are born to mothers who smoke.[269]

Associated risk factors attributable to smoking include increased incidence of fetal loss, intrauterine growth retardation, congenital anomalies, abruptio placenta and placenta previa, and preeclampsia.

Additional postnatal complications include increased problems with respiratory distress syndrome, sudden infant death, low birth weight, and stillbirth.[96]

Cigarettes are known to contain many hazardous components. In patients who are preparing for pregnancy, it is maintaining a healthy lifestyle is advisable. This includes decreasing the consumption of cigarettes. Currently, no guidelines are available to suggest how soon a person should stop smoking before conception. In animal models, nicotine has been shown to produce a decrease in uterine blood flow, an increase in uterine vascular resistance, and an increase in levels of placental epinephrine and norepinephrine. In addition, several components of cigarette smoke have been associated in the animal model with depleting or destroying the oocyte.[156] Additionally, patients who smoke will enter menopause an average of 1.8 years sooner than their nonsmoking counterparts.

The physician should provide prudent information to assist the patient to stop smoking. She should be counseled that smoking cessation will help reduce the problems and complications listed above (see Chapter 16).

Without discovery, there is no recovery. If the patient discovers in advance, or is educated in advance, about the sequelae of continued smoking during pregnancy, she may have additional motivation to stop this unsafe practice.

Effective early screening would be helpful in modifying behavior patterns of patients who smoke. Many women begin smoking in the adolescent period, when a risk-reduction and education program may have marked success. In a recent study, 34% of women who smoked were unaware that smoking increased the risk of miscarriage, stillbirth, premature birth, or low birth weight.[96]

The effectiveness of an intervention program depends on frequency of contact with the patient, the number of months of intervention, the use of face-to-face counseling, and the personality of the counselor. The doctor-patient relationship of a pregnancy presents an optimal opportunity for intervention. The patient must also be willing and motivated to change her personal habits.[67]

Screening for alcohol abuse during pregnancy

Approximately 50% of all American adults consume alcohol. Most studies indicate that 11% of Americans drink alcohol daily, 10% have a dependence on alcohol, and 8% have reported a recent drinking binge.[30] In addition to such alcohol-related complications as excess death from motor vehicle accidents and cirrhosis, pregnancy-related complications have also been noted.[30] Approximately 1 out of 750 newborns is affected by the fetal alcohol syndrome.[114] This syndrome is associated with intrauterine growth retardation, organ anomalies, mental retardation, and neural sensory problems.[114] The fetal alcohol syndrome is the leading cause of mental retardation in the United States today.[114]

About 3% of women in United States drink three or more glasses of alcohol per day. These women are less likely than others to decrease their alcohol consumption once they become pregnant.[51] Only one third of patients who consumed more than three drinks per day reduced their consumption, and only 17% stopped drinking entirely during their pregnancy.[210] No safe level of alcohol consumption currently is known for pregnant women.[10] Most studies suggest that women who have two to four drinks per week in the first trimester are at increased risk of spontaneous abortion. At three or more drinks per week, an infant's IQ may be expected to decrease by five points and the incidence of an IQ less than 85 is tripled.[51,247]

The responses to direct questioning regarding alcohol ingestion are notoriously inaccurate. The CAGE questionnaire represents a good means of detecting alcohol abuse. These questions are easily adaptable in the primary care setting and have excellent sensitivity and specificity.[86]

A preconceptual early-detection program, identifying

Fetal complications of drug use in pregnancy

Cocaine

Spontaneous abortion
Abruptio placenta
Preterm birth
Intrauterine growth retardation (IUGR)
Acute hypertensive disorders of pregnancy
Congenital defects
Maternal respiratory or cardiovascular arrest
Generalized seizures
Cardiac dysrhythmias
Rupture of descending aorta
Postnatal neurodevelopmental aberrations
Skeletal defects
Ocular malformations
Urologic malformations:
  Hypospadias
  Hydroureter
  Hernias
Maternal risks:
  Increased risk for polydrug abuse
  HIV
  Violence/abuse
  Hepatitis
  Poor prenatal care
  Sexually transmitted diseases

Marijuana

Often associated with other illicit drug use
Inadequate weight gain
Hyperemesis
Low birth weight
Increased meconium aspiration

Smoking[122]

Preterm birth
Low birth weight
Early fetal loss
Preeclampsia
Abruptio placenta
Placenta previa
Increased incidence of acute respiratory infections postnatally
Sudden infant death
Increased cancer risk in mother (lung) and increased risk of cardiovascular disease
Unknown long-term effects of passive smoking

Heroin

Spontaneous abortion
Abruptio placenta
Intrauterine growth retardation
Congenital defects

Alcohol[1]

Fetal alcohol syndrome
Mental retardation
Facial dysmorphology
Septal heart defects
Hip dislocations
Hernias
Hemangiomas
Abnormal oral cavities
Low birth weight
Preterm birth
Maternal risk:
  Liver disease
  Suicide
  Affective disorders
  Sleep disorders
  Poor parenting/coping skills

Himmelberger D, 1978[122]
Abel EL, 1986[1]

women drinkers, can lead to lower alcohol consumption and subsequently fewer neonatal complications. This intervention also allows for alliance with Alcoholics Anonymous centers and enlistment of family support for treating this problem. Although some patients must reach "rock bottom" before terminating their drinking habits, social pressures are the principal stimulus to changing drinking behavior in the majority of patients.[30]

Pregnant women who drink are also at risk for illicit use of other drugs such as cocaine, marijuana, and heroin. The use of these agents has been associated with increased risk of spontaneous abortion, intrauterine growth retardation, mental retardation, placental abruption, congenital birth defects, and low birth weight (see box above).

In addition, women in labor who are cocaine users are at increased risk for intrapartum fetal distress, meconium aspiration, and other neonatal complications.[50] The same guidelines for early detection and screening mentioned previously are recommended for patients who are abusing illicit drugs (see box above).

Nutrition (See also Chapters 22-26)

Nutritional needs and requirements are modified during pregnancy because of the physical changes occurring

within the growing fetus. The growing fetus develops gradually over a period of 280 days while in utero. The most rapid growth occurs during the second and third trimesters. Fetal weight approximates 500 g at week 20 and is 1500 g by the thirtieth week.

The nutritional status of the patient is important during pregnancy and may modify the outcome of the fetus.[273] Natural experiments in Russia in 1942 during the war and findings noted from women pregnant in the winters of 1944 and 1945 in Holland showed an increased risk of perinatal mortality and morbidity in women who experienced mild episodes of starvation.[273] Studies of these incidents revealed that "poor nutrition in the latter part of pregnancy affects fetal growth, whereas poor nutrition in the early months affects development of the embryo and its capacity to survive.[273]

In general, scientific studies have confirmed what the average patient tends to know regarding nutrition and pregnancy. That is, infants born to mothers who are overweight are larger than infants born to smaller mothers. In addition, the fetal outcome is poorer if a women enters pregnancy at 10% or more below her ideal weight.[273] Underweight women have more low-birth-weight babies, a higher incidence of prematurity, and infants with a low

---

Dietary guidelines in pregnancy

1. Pregnancy requires an additional 300 calories.
2. Protein requirements are 60 to 75 g: four servings daily.
3. Green leafy and yellow vegetables: three servings daily.
4. Fluids: 8 oz daily.
5. Calcium foods: four servings daily.
6. Vitamin C: two servings daily.
7. Whole grain and legumes: five servings daily.

Prenatal multivitamin mineral supplementation

Iron, 30 mg	Vitamin B$_6$, 2 mg
Zinc, 15 mg	Folic acid, 300 mcg
Copper, 2 mg	Vitamin C, 50 mg
Calcium, 250 mg	Vitamin D, 5 mg

Apgar score at birth. In addition, women who are underweight have a higher incidence of anemia.[273]

Entering her pregnancy at the ideal weight (for height and age), a patient should gain approximately 26 to 35 lb. A patient with twins should expect to gain 35 to 45 lb.[10]

Therapeutic interventions. Patients need an additional 300 Kcal per day and a total of 60 g of protein per day while pregnant.[10] If a patient's diet is adequate in the fat-soluble and water-soluble vitamins, supplementation is not necessary. If there is a doubt about a patient's diet, the patient can be safely advised to purchase a vitamin and mineral supplement that provides the RDA requirements for pregnancy[10] (see box above). Patients who are heavy smokers, alcoholics, drug abusers, or carrying more than one fetus, or who have a poor diet may benefit from a nutritional supplement. This supplement should be taken between meals or at bedtime to promote absorption of the nutrients.[10,273]

Folic acid. Folic acid requirements increase in pregnancy. In a nonpregnant state, women require 50 to 100 mcg of folic acid daily. The demands of pregnancy require a minimum of 100 to 400 mcg per day. Without folic acid supplementation, the body's store will become deficient or depleted within approximately 6 weeks. Resultant megaloblastic anemia occurs in 1% to 4% of pregnancies. Some studies have suggested that severe folic acid deficiency may cause complications in the third trimester, such as abruptio placenta and bleeding; however, other studies do not confirm these complications.

For these reasons, women generally receive folic acid supplementation during pregnancy,[121] provided by a multivitamin containing 300 mcg of folic acid per day.

Iron. In preparation for blood loss that occurs at delivery (approximately 300 to 500 ml with vaginal birth and 1000 ml at cesarean section), and because of the increased red blood cell volume of pregnancy, additional daily iron is needed. Red cell volume increases approximately 26% or 345 ml over the nonpregnant state. Iron-deficiency anemia is the most common anemia of pregnancy occurring in 15% to 50% of pregnancies in the United States. The pregnant state requires 700 to 1150 mg of iron throughout gestation. Iron requirements are the greatest during the second trimester. To prevent iron-deficiency anemia, pregnant women are currently advised to ingest 300 mg of ferrous sulfate daily, which contains 60 mg elemental iron. In addition, women are encouraged to ingest foods with high iron content, such as legumes, collards, turnip greens, beef, spinach, and dried fruits (see also Chapters 22-26).

Complications of pregnancy or increased incidence of perinatal mortality are very rare in iron-deficient pregnancies. Isolated case reports have documented complications only with severe anemia in which hemoglobin levels are below 6 g.[26]

Vitamin D. The recommended dietary allowance of vitamin D is 10 mcg per day. Excessive amounts have been associated with infantile hypercalcemia. Conversely, patients have also been known to have complications from inadequate levels of vitamin D. Specifically, in climates where sunlight is minimal, some babies have been noted to have enamel hypoplasia and neonatal hypocalcemia.[272]

Vitamin A. The recommended dietary allowance of vitamin A for pregnant women is 800 IU per day. Women who have used excessive amounts of vitamin A (greater than 25,000 IU per day) and women who have used an analog of vitamin A known as isotretinoin in the treatment for cystic acne have been reported to have increased risk of congenital malformations in the fetus.

Although the number of case studies is small, reported abnormalities have included malformations of the nervous system, cranium, face, thymus, and heart.[225]

Special situations. Patients who are complete vegetarians should have the following daily supplements: vitamin D, 400 IU; calcium, 600 mg; and vitamin B$_{12}$, 20 mcg. Severely anemic patients receiving supplemental iron should also take 15 mg of zinc and 2 mg of copper because the iron may interfere with the aborption and utilization of these elements.[10,273]

Summary. If a multivitamin and mineral supplement is recommended to a patient, the American College of Obstetrics and Gynecology suggests components for the supplement to be as listed in the box above.[10]

Preconceptual counseling should encourage patients to maintain their ideal body weight for age and height. Once the patient has become pregnant, diet modifications and supplemental minerals and vitamins should be ordered as necessary. Patients should be encouraged to discuss nutritional concerns with a physician or a nutritionist. Ideal

Teratatogens: drugs to avoid in pregnancy[9,141]

Gold	Diazepam
Lithium	Disulfiram
Isotretinoin	Etretinate
Folate antagonists	Methimazole
Valproic acid	Streptomycin
Warfarin	Sodium Iodide-131
Phenytoin	Cocaine
Trimethadione	Phencyclidine
Tetracycline	
Thalidomide	
DES (diethylstilbestrol)	
Chloramphenicol	

Guidelines for use of over-the-counter drugs

Over-the-counter drugs to avoid:

Cigarettes
Alcohol

Guidelines:

Although potential teratogenic effects of over-the-counter drugs have been described, very few have been shown to have actual adverse outcomes. Nonetheless, over-the-counter medications should be minimized, and alternative treatments should be used, such as physical therapy and exercise.

weight gain during pregnancy should be encouraged.[10] Pregnancy is not the time for "dieting," joining Weight Watchers, or, conversely, "eating for two." Ideal weight gain is 35 pounds in an average pregnancy.

Medications in pregnancy

Epidemiology and risk factors. Each year approximately 6000 children (3% of births) will be afflicted with a serious birth defect. Drugs are thought to account for 4% to 5% of malformations. Most birth defects cannot be traced to a single etiology. The average patient ingests 4 to 11 drugs during pregnancy (see box above). Approximately 40% of these are taken during the first trimester.[9]

Patient education is important. Many physiologic changes in pregnancy are normal and should be anticipated. Drugs will not cure these adaptive changes of pregnancy. Labor and delivery will! Reassurance is usually all that is necessary.

Therapeutic interventions. Patients should be advised to discuss routine use of over-the-counter medications with their physicians (see box above, right). Risks and benefits of drug use should be discussed. Nonpharmacologic treatments are possible for many minor discomforts. In addition, physicians should not prescribe known teratogenic drugs.

Physicians prescribing drugs during pregnancy should adhere to the FDA's drug package insert, as well as rely on textbooks, references, regional teratogen registries, and data supplied by drug manufacturers about the teratogenic possibilities of exposure to drugs during pregnancy.[228] Consultative services with a perinatologist should be sought when in doubt.

Exercise during pregnancy

Epidemiology and risk factors. Tremendous physiologic changes occur in the human female during pregnancy. These changes occur in the cardiovascular, respiratory, and musculoskeletal systems.

Although exercise counseling of women in a nonpreg-

General guidelines for exercise in pregnancy

1. Review exercise regimen with physician before embarking on exercise program.
2. Limit strenuous exercise, in which the heart rate increases to 140, to no longer than 15 minutes.
3. Include warm-up and cool-down periods.
4. Drink one glass of water for every 30 minutes of exercise.
5. Wear loose-fitting, nonconstrictive clothes.
6. Never use hot tubs, saunas, or steam rooms.
7. Good exercises for the novice to consider are walking, stationary bike riding, swimming, Kegel's exercises, and aerobic programs designed for pregnancy.
8. Exercises to avoid during pregnancy are ice skating, diving into swimming pools, scuba diving, contact sports, jogging more than 2 miles per day, downhill skiing, high-altitude (10,000 feet) climbing, cross-country skiing, or horseback riding.
9. The standard rule for highly athletic women who desire to continue their exercise regimen during pregnancy is to contact their personal physician for guidelines, management, and recommendations.

nant state encourages a program of vigorous cardiovascular activity, less objective information is available for physicians treating the pregnant patient who wants to exercise. How much exercise is safe, required, or necessary is only partially known. The American College of Obstetricians and Gynecologists has succinctly outlined in its recent *Guidelines for Prenatal Care* recommendations for patients who desire to exercise during pregnancy.[10] Pregnancy is not a time for patients who lead otherwise sedentary lives to become marathon joggers in the hope of improving pregnancy or shortening labor. In general, exercise programs should be tailored to the patient[10] (see box above).

Higher levels of elastin and progesterone result in increasing laxity of the musculoskeletal system. Increased lordosis, accumulation of fluid in the lower extremities, and decreased joint stability all may be seen during pregnancy.[15] These musculoskeletal changes theoretically may place the patient at increased risk of injury.

Major cardiovascular adaptations are seen, including a 40% increase in cardiac output and a heart rate increased by 16 beats per minute by midpregnancy. Because of the enlarging uterus, which includes the weight of the fetus, amniotic fluid, and placental structures, hypotension is seen more frequently after pregnant women undergo prolonged standing or recumbency in the supine position.[205] These cardiac manifestations have important implications for exercise in pregnancy.

The respiratory system also undergoes several adaptive changes during pregnancy, including an increased inspiratory capacity, reduced functional residual capacity, and increased oxygen consumption, minute ventilation, and tidal volume. Notably, the pco_2 is reduced, but the arterial Ph is maintained at 7.44. Thus maternal alkalosis occurs during pregnancy, which facilitates placental gas exchange.[15]

There is limited human data on the effects of exercise on blood flow to visceral organs and the uterus. Some studies show that the exercising female can expect to redistribute blood supply to the exercised muscle, with a decreased perfusion to the placenta. Each minute 500 to 600 ml is delivered to the uterus. Of this blood flow, 90% will go to the placenta and 10% to the myometrium.[15] Blood flow through the placenta is estimated to decrease by 25% during exercise.[180] Although additional studies are not currently available, patients whose pregnancies are compromised by intrauterine growth retardation should be advised to limit their participation in vigorous athletic programs.[10]

Fetal response to exercise is difficult to study and measure objectively in the human model. Most studies have attempted to measure the fetal heart rate patterns, breathing responses, and Doppler flow of blood through the umbilical cord. These parameters are technically difficult to measure in the exercising patient, so most observations are limited to the immediate preexercise and postexercise periods, when fetal homostasis may have occurred.[16] If we extrapolate the events that are commonly seen during active labor, certain patterns are noted. Fetal tachycardia and an increase in fetal blood pressure is noted during episodes of transient hypoxemia. This is an adaptive mechanism whereby the fetus can facilitate the transfer of oxygen and decrease the CO_2 tension across the placenta.[16]

There has been a paucity of well-controlled studies of intensely athletic women who exercise throughout pregnancy.[15] Over the years, many have feared that strenuous exercise is related to the potential development of intrauterine growth retardation caused by the decrease in placental blood flow that occurs during exercise. Most studies on athletic women have focused on an elite population. These pregnancies in general have been associated with minimal complications. In one uncontrolled study, very athletic women delivered babies weighing 2600 to 3000 g, with few babies weighing over 3500 g.[15] Animal studies have clearly shown that animals subjected to strenuous activities will have smaller babies than their sedentary counterparts.[15]

During pregnancy, the basal body temperature increases by 0.5° C until the second trimester. Patients should be advised not to become hyperthermic during exercise. The fetus has minimal ability to dissipate heat. Hyperthermia can be a teratogen.[10]

Guidelines for exercise in pregnancy: therapeutic interventions. Exercise during pregnancy offers many of the same benefits as in the nonpregnant state. These include improved mental health, improved quality of sleep, decreased stress, and improved muscular tone. However, because of the many physiologic and adaptive changes during pregnancy, modifications in the exercise program have been recommended by the American College of Obstetrics and Gynecology (ACOG).[10] Ideally, healthy patients should continue to exercise moderately. Activities such as swimming, stationary bike riding, dancing (low-impact aerobic), or walking are recommended.

An exercise program can be considered in pregnant patients who do not have the following contraindications: active myocardial disease, congestive heart failure, rheumatic heart disease (class II and above), risk factors for premature labor, incompetent cervix, multiple pregnancies, ruptured membranes, vaginal bleeding of unknown origin, history of fetal distress, hypertension, or IUGR.[10]

Counseling. The essentials of exercise during pregnancy for patients without risk factors is summarized as follows[10]:

1. Patients engaging in exercise should include brief warm-up and cool-down periods to prevent musculoskeletal strains during exercise.
2. Increased fluid and caloric intake during exercise is recommended to prevent dehydration and hypoglycemia. Patients should wear loose-fitting clothing to decrease their risk for hyperthermia.
3. Patients should minimize the amount of jerky movements, exercises in the supine position, and exercises that require a Valsalva maneuver.
4. The most strenuous part of the exercise activity should not last more than 15 minutes. After a brief cool-down period, resumption of the exercise may be considered.
5. The patient's heart rate should not exceed 140 beats per minute.
6. Patients who have been sedentary for most of their lives can participate in exercise but should proceed at their own pace.
7. Benefits from exercise can be seen in improved muscle tone and decreased backache and strain.
8. When in doubt, the patient should always err on the

side of conservatism. The motto "no pain—no gain" should not be incorporated into the exercise regimen during pregnancy. If the patient becomes uncomfortable or experiences increased uterine contractions or pain, the activities should stop. The patient then should increase fluid intake and rest.

Aquatic exercise programs may produce additional benefits, including a decreased incidence of joint stress, decreased muscle aches, and decreased risk of hyperthermia.

Summary. The medical literature currently does not prove that labor is shorter or quicker in women who exercise during pregnancy. However, other health benefits, such as improved muscle tone, increased sense of well-being, and increased endurance, may be seen in women who exercise during pregnancy. These patients may also be more motivated to continue an exercise program postpartum. Notable trends among women who exercise include decreased maternal weight gain, smaller babies, and low incidence of fetal injury.

CONTRACEPTION
Epidemiology and risk factors

Data recently released from the Allen Guttmacher Institute reported that 47% of all pregnancies in the United States were unintended in 1987.[182] The social, economic, and personal cost of these unintended pregnancies is staggering. Unintended pregnancy and lack of adequate contraceptive practices cross all social, economic, and racial lines. As health care providers, we have daily contact with a huge patient population at risk for unintended pregnancy. Our ability to inspire, counsel, and educate patients about effective contraceptive practices could have a significant public health effect if fulfilled. Mosher has estimated that as many as one third of all unintended pregnancies and 500,000 abortions could be prevented if the proportion of women not using contraception were reduced by half.[182]

In a recent editorial, Barber said there is an "urgency to devise more and better contraceptive options. The world population is now topping 5 billion and if this growth rate continues, the total will be 10 billion by the year 2030. There are 600,000,000 women of reproductive age in the world today and three trillion acts of intercourse annually, 12,000 ejaculations per second and 60,000,000 sperm released per ejaculation—equaling seven hundred and twenty trillion sperm released worldwide!"[21]

Teenage pregnancies have reached epidemic proportions. In fact the United States has one of the highest teenage pregnancy rates of any industrialized nation. Each year in the United States, one million adolescent females age 15 to 19 (about 8% to 10% of this age group) and nearly 30,000 girls under age 15 become pregnant.[164,255] Of this group, approximately 40% of pregnant females age 15 to 19 will electively undergo an induced abortion.[164,255]

Teenagers account for 27% of all induced abortions in the United States; the abortion rate in women age 18 and 19 is higher than in any other age group.[255] Nearly 490,000 females age 15 through 19 give birth each year, and a third of these mothers are 17 or younger.[255] Each year 10,000 women under the age of 15 give birth.[255]

The rates of sexual activity continue to increase in American teens. More than 50% of unmarried U.S. adolescents report having had sexual activity by age 18. As teens mature, the percentage of sexual activity per age group also increases. The data from the Allen Guttmacher Institute has noted that 18% of women at age 15 have been sexually active, 29% at age 16, 40% at age 17, 54% at age 18, and 66% by age 19 have been sexually active.[213] Our national health objectives call for reducing the proportion of teens that are sexually active by the year 2000. The aim is to decrease intercourse rates to less than 15% by age 15 and less than 40% by age 17. Another goal is to persuade 90% of adolescents under age 19 to use contraception.[47]

The need for effective and reliable contraception among teens and adults is apparent when one realizes that without contraception, 89% of heterosexual couples who engage in regular sexual activity will conceive within 1 year.[252]

Without effective contraception, there will be one million teenage pregnancies per year in the United States, and 75% of these pregnancies will have been "mistakes." The numbers are staggering. However, data reveal that 20% of pregnancies will occur within the first month of coitus and 50% will occur within the first 6 months of intercourse.[135] With regard to teen pregnancy, more than half of these pregnancies are carried to term, and approximately 45% end in abortion, the highest rate in the industrialized world.

Not only are teenage women having unintended pregnancies, but 18% of births to women age 35 to 44 are thought to be unwanted also.[135] It is not unusual for practitioners to discover that a perimenopausal patient is pregnant. Pregnancy is possible for a year after the last menses.

Many contraceptive options are available today. At no time in history have women had as many safe, effective, economical, and reliable choices for contraception. Some of these choices include the Norplant implant, oral contraceptive pills, diaphragm, vaginal sponge, IUD, tubal ligation, and spermicides (see Table 30-1).

Norplant

More than 30 years have passed since the American public has been offered a new, reversible, safe, and effective means of contraception. After worldwide tests in more than 20 countries and in clinical trials involving more than 300,000 women, the FDA approved the use of the Norplant device in January 1991. Research has confirmed the effectiveness, ease, and safety of this device.[274]

Description. Currently, more than 100,000 U.S. women have opted to have the match-stick size device inserted into their upper arm. The Norplant system, devel-

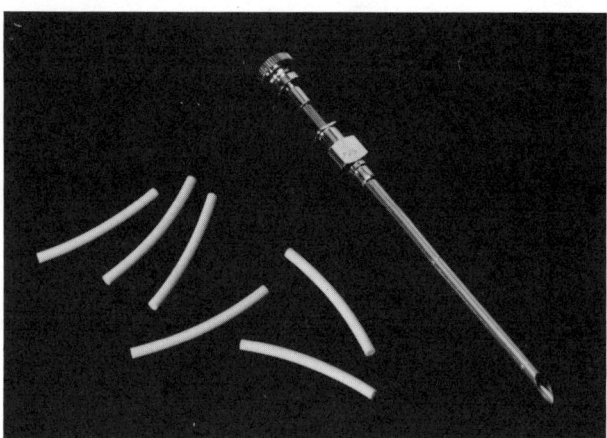

Fig. 30-1. Norplant device (six silastic capsules) and inserting trocar.

oped by Wyeth-Ayrest Company, provides daily and continuous delivery of levonorgesterel, a synthetic progesterone, for 5 years[155] (Fig. 30-1).

This device is easily inserted in the outpatient setting. Six nonreactive silastic capsules are placed subdermally on the inside of the upper arm through a 2 mm incision. Each capsule is made of a copolymer of dimethylsiloxane and methylvinylsiloxane. This copolymer has been used in many other medical devices, including ventricular peritoneal shunts and heart valves. Scientific studies reveal that the capsules are permeable, allowing the levonorgesterel to freely diffuse through tissue. Furthermore the capsules are nontoxic, noncarcinogenic, and nonbiodegradable.[274]

Ideally, the Norplant device should be inserted during the menstrual cycle and no later than day 7 of the menses. It can be inserted immediately after abortion, miscarriage, or pregnancy, or at the 6-week postpartum visit after delivery. Each capsule contains 36 mg of crystalline levonorgesterel. Contraception effectiveness begins immediately. On the first day of insertion, 80 to 85 mcg of levonorgesterel is released, and 30 to 50 mcg is released each day over the next 5 years.[155,236]

Levonorgesterel is the progesterone component found in many oral contraceptives pills used today. The amount of medication secreted daily in the Norplant equals one-half to one-quarter of the progesterone dose used in combined oral contraceptives. Levonorgesterel is highly progestational and is not converted to estrogen. Because of the lipophilic attraction of levonorgesterel to fat content, steady-state levels in the blood can be achieved. It is 100% bioavailable in the body, with no first-pass effect on the liver.[274] The current cost, including the device, office fees, insertion fees, and removal, averages $500 to $700. This device can remain in place for 5 years.

Mechanism of action. As a hormone, progesterone alone does not inhibit ovulation. More recent data reveal

that ovulation can be expected to occur in 50% to 60% of menstrual cycles in which Norplant is used. The dominant mechanism of action appears to be related to the thick, tenacious cervical mucus that is produced continuously. This creates a hostile environment and an impermeable barrier to sperm. In addition, endometrial atrophy is noted. A less-hospitable intrauterine environment is created, preventing implantation of the fertilized egg. Therefore contraceptive efficacy is mainly provided by the thickened mucus, which prevents sperm migration and suppresses tissue and growth within the endometrial cavity.[236]

Efficacy. Most studies have shown that, once the Norplant device is removed, 50% of those patients desiring pregnancy conceive within 3 months and 86% within 1 year.[236]

Considering all current reversible means of contraception, the Norplant implant has the lowest pregnancy rate. Its pregnancy-preventing effectiveness is better than that of the IUD, diaphragm, spermicides, and oral contraceptive pill. It is better than the oral contraceptive pill because patient motivation or compliance is not a factor in its effectiveness. Many pregnancies occur with oral contraceptives because of patient noncompliance (forgetting to take the pill). The failure rate for Norplant in about 1000 users was four or five per thousand users a year; for oral contraceptives the rate is 20 to 50 per thousand per year.[23]

Combining worldwide studies in which compounded data included body size and divergent patient populations, the pregnancy rates for Norplant have been impressive. For the first 3 years, the rates were 0.2 to 0.5 per 100 women years, and 1 to 2 per 100 women years during the fourth and fifth years of use. In one study, the 5-year pregnancy rate for women weighing less than 110 lb (50 kg) was .2 per 100 women years. For women weighing more than 154 lb (70 kg) the pregnancy rate was 1 per 100 women in the second year, 4 per 100 women in the third year, and about 7 per 100 women in the fifth year.[71]

Effectiveness is lower in patients who may be on other medications. Specifically, patients using rifampin, carbamazepine, isoniazid, barbiturates, or phenytoin may have decreased effectiveness.[239] This same trend is also seen in oral contraceptive users.

Metabolic effects. The amount of levonorgesterel released approximates 30 mcg per day over a period of 5 years. This amount of levonorgesterel is less than the amount the patient would receive by using a 50 mcg oral contraceptive pill daily, such as Levlen. Consequently, no adverse effects on lipoproteins, glucose tolerance, or blood pressure have been noted.[71] In addition, no adverse coagulopathies or fibrinolytic changes have been noted with Norplant. This makes Norplant ideal for patients who may not be candidates for the oral contraceptive pill because of medical history of coagulopathy.

Adverse reactions to the Norplant device can be divided into those related to the technical aspects of insertion and removal of the device, and those related to menstrual irregularities or changes in the quantity and quality of menstrual flow. Because Norplant is surgically inserted, it is not unusual that complications from insertion and removal have been reported. Insertion takes place in the office. Most physicians can insert it within 10 to 20 minutes. Pain, itching, and local infection have been noted. If questioned after placement, patients describe a "soreness" related to the insertion of the device that may last for 1 to 2 days. Approximately 3.7% of users complained of pain and itching.[236] Most patients state that they suffered less pain and discomfort than they had anticipated. The infection rate is approximately .7%, and infection has occurred when unsanitary means of insertion or poor surgical technique have been used. About 6.2% of physicians have noted difficulty in removal of the Norplant device. This may result because the silastic capsule develops a fibrinous sheath within 1 to 3 months of insertion. This may make removal more difficult.[71]

Adverse reactions. The biggest complaint from patients using Norplant has been menstrual irregularity. Most surveys have revealed a 60% to 70% incidence of changes in the menstrual cycle. Patients will note longer periods and longer intervals between periods. The total number of days of menstruation usually increases, but the amount of bleeding decreases over time.[4]

The good news is that most bleeding abnormalities improve within 8 to 12 months of Norplant use. Because progesterone is the only hormonal component of the Norplant, the lack of estrogen causes fragility of the endometrial tissue. Thus menstrual irregularity is common. Bleeding irregularities have been categorized in the following way: 27.6% of patients complain of prolonged bleeding, 17.1% of spotting, 9.4% of amenorrhea, 7.6% of irregular onset of bleeding, 7% of frequent onset of bleeding, and 5.2% of scanty bleeding. To describe the irregularities another way, about 44% of the patients will experience at least one episode of bleeding lasting 8 or more days, and 15% will report at least one episode of bleeding lasting 15 or more days. After 3 years of use, these percentages fall to 24% and 7% respectively.[4]

Other rare side effects may be related to formation of ovarian cysts. As mentioned earlier, 50% to 60% of patients will ovulate while using Norplant. Most of these cysts are follicular cysts and have been noted to resolve spontaneously.[4]

Other adverse reactions reported include breast discharge, cervicitis, increased vaginal secretions, vaginitis, musculoskeletal pain, weight gain, nausea, and dizziness. Of patients who ask that the device be removed (who do not want a pregnancy), 90% do so because of aberrations in the menstrual cycle. The attrition rate has been calculated to be approximately 20 per 100 years per year. This is comparable to or less that seen with patients using oral contraceptives.[274]

Contraindications. There are five absolute contraindications to Norplant use. These are undiagnosed genital bleeding, pregnancy, active thrombophlebitis or thromboembolic disorders, acute liver disease or liver tumors, and known or suspected breast carcinoma. Unlike oral contraceptives, Norplant is not contraindicated with known or suspected estrogen-dependent neoplasia, cerebrovascular disease, or coronary artery disease. In addition, women over the age of 35 can use Norplant effectively.[71,236]

Summary. Norplant offers a new means of reversible contraception for women throughout the world. This new device produces low pregnancy rates through constant production of levonorgesterel. Patient compliance is not a factor in the efficacy. In addition, minimal metabolic effects have been seen. This device is not for all patients. A well-informed patient who has been educated about the side effects of this device (bleeding abnormalities) will best appreciate, tolerate, and continue to use the device. Quick return of fertility has been documented, and patient acceptance of this new device is increasing.

Diaphragm

Historical perspectives. The use of diaphragms has waxed and waned over the years. When there was heightened concern about the safety of IUDs and oral contraceptives, many women elected to use this reversible means of contraception. Currently, 6% to 8% of U.S. women use the diaphragm as a contraceptive.

The current diaphragm is made of latex rubber and covers the opening to the cervix. One can find many similar devices used in history to occlude or block the cervical os. Egyptian drawings dating to 1850 BC reveal pictures of women placing crocodile excrement and honey in the vagina to decrease sperm penetration.[231] The Europeans used linen cloths and wafers of molded wax placed inside the vagina to decrease the risk of unplanned pregnancy in the same way. Other studies have shown that women used other objects, such as half of a lemon rind, and inserted this into the vagina, effectively covering the cervical os.[231] These women did not realize that they were perhaps changing the pH of the vagina and creating an environment more hostile to sperm. For centuries, other mechanical barriers have been used, such as leaves, sea sponges, pieces of wool soaked in oil, and fig pulp, to block the millions of sperm released with each act of coitus.[90]

In the early 1900s providing contraceptive services to women was illegal in this country. Margaret Sanger, an ardent feminist, had established her Brooklyn Birth Control Clinic. She was imprisoned for 30 days in 1916 for selling diaphragms. Her sister followed in her footsteps. She also was incarcerated in 1916 for selling diaphragms, which had been illegally imported from Germany.[57]

Description. The diaphragm is a latex rubber device made in the shape of a shallow dome. There are 11 sizes, ranging from 65 mm to 105 mm (3 to 5 inches). Three dif-

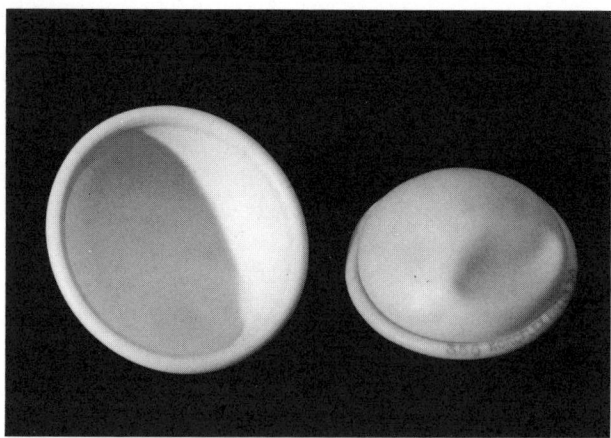

Fig. 30-2. The modern diaphragm.

ferent rim styles are produced. To obtain the correct size, the patient must be fitted individually. A physician, midwife, or physician's assistant can be taught to fit the device. When the diaphragm is properly fitted, it will completely encircle the cervical os, adhere to the lateral vaginal sidewalls, be tucked behind the symphis pubis, and be unnoticeable to the patient and her partner. The patient should be fitted with the largest diaphragm that is comfortable, to ensure that the diaphragm does not become dislodged[57] (Fig. 30-2).

Modern diaphragms are available in three types, the coil spring, flat spring, and arcing spring types. In the U.S., the coil spring has been most popular. The rim is made of a cadmium-plated coil shaped like a spring and encased in latex. This material is compressible and flexible when squeezed. The Ortho diaphragm and the Koromex coil spring are two examples of the coil-spring-type diaphragm. Candidates for the coil spring diaphragm include the average woman with strong vaginal muscles, a high arch behind the symphysis pubis, a normally positioned uterus, and a normal size and contour of the vagina. This is probably the ideal diaphragm for the nulliparous patient.[57,231]

The flat spring also is covered by latex, and its design allows it to be compressed in only one plane. Some patients prefer this characteristic because the device tends to be less slippery and therefore less likely to have a "frisbee" type of effect. The Ortho (coil spring) diaphragm is an example of this type. This diaphragm is also suitable for nulliparous patients and may be advisable in a woman with a shallow pubic arch, strong vaginal muscles, and normal vaginal length.[57,231]

The arcing spring diaphragm has a double spring in the rim and exerts more pressure against the vaginal walls. This device works better in women who have lost vaginal tone as a result of childbirth and have a mild-degree cystocele, rectocele, or uterine prolapse. Other women benefit-

ting from this type of device are those who have marked degrees of uterine displacement, including those with retroverted or severely antiverted uterus. Physicians who have a patient with these problems may find an Ortho All Flex or coil flex arcing diaphragm to be a better choice.[57,231]

Effectiveness. The diaphragm is extremely effective in women who are motivated and mature, and who have been properly fitted. The effectiveness of three types of diaphragms currently on the market (arcing, coiled, and flat) have never been compared in a study. However, most medical studies quote pregnancy rates between 13 and 20 per 100 women years. In well-motivated women, this may improve to 2.4 per 100 women years. Most studies show that older women, longer users of diaphragms, and women who have had as many children as they wanted have a lower pregnancy rate associated with diaphragm use.[74,233,249]

For the diaphragm to prevent pregnancy, patients must also use a spermicide. A spermicidal agent containing nonoxynol-9 must be placed around the rim and covering the inner dome and outer aspect of the diaphragm. Approximately 1 to 2 tablespoons of contraceptive cream or jelly should be used as directed. The diaphragm coated with the spermicide should be placed into the vagina no more than 6 hours before having intercourse.[249] After coitus, the diaphragm should be left in place for a minimum of 6 hours. Each act of intercourse should be preceded by application of contraceptive cream or jelly into the vagina via an applicator. If the diaphragm is correctly fitted into the vagina, the patient and her partner should not be able to feel the diaphragm.[57] The patient should be instructed to bring the edge of the rim together and insert the diaphragm upward and backward into the vagina as far as her fingers can place it. The fingers should be removed, and at that point, the diaphragm opens spontaneously. The patient should then be instructed to feel the rim or edge of the diaphragm and tuck it securely behind the symphysis pubis. She should also ensure that the cervix (which "feels like the tip of your nose") is covered by the latex.

Once the last act of coitus has occurred, the diaphragm should be left in place for a minimum of 6 hours and not longer than 24 hours. All patients should be informed that the diaphragm should never be left in the vagina for more than 24 hours continuously, to decrease the risk of toxic shock syndrome (TSS).[57] It should then be removed, washed, and placed in a dry container near her bed. The patient should always be instructed to hold the diaphragm up to light and carefully check for holes or tears within it. The diaphragm should be replaced every 2 years because the latex may begin to pucker or tear. In addition, the diaphragm should be refitted after a vaginal delivery, change in weight of more than 20 pounds, or a second-trimester abortion.[57]

An additional advantage of the diaphragm is the decreased incidence of sexually transmitted diseases in women using this method. One mechanism of action is that the diaphragm acts as a physical barrier, preventing the ascent of abnormal pathogens into the cervix. In addition, the spermicide nonoxynol-9 has been shown to be helpful in killing or inactivating organisms, such as those involved in gonorrhea, syphilis, chlamydia, genital herpes, trichomoniasis, and genital warts. Some studies reveal that hepatitis B and the AIDS virus may also be inactivated by nonoxynol-9.[249]

Many researchers believe that cancer of the cervix or its precursors may be linked by a sexually transmitted virus known as human papilloma virus (HPV). In this vein, we can find a decreased incidence of abnormalities in the Pap test in women using the diaphragm. The diaphragm offers mechanical barrier against the acquisition of HPV, which may explain the decreased incidence of abnormal Pap tests in women who use the diaphragm.

Advantages of the diaphragm. The diaphragm for most women provides a safe, reversible, and economic means to prevent pregnancy. Most diaphragms cost $15 to $20 in 1992. The contraceptive cream or gel costs approximately $8 to $10 per tube at retail drug stores. Each spermicidal tube contains enough spermicide for 10 acts of intercourse. Women who do not like the idea of having "hormones" in their body may find this device particularly appealing. In addition, women desiring pregnancy can conceive immediately after discontinuing the diaphragm. No waiting period is needed, unlike the birth control pill. The patient's partner can provide additional motivation as well as assist with placement of the device. In addition, women over the age of 40 who do want to continue using oral contraceptives and women in the perimenopausal period may prefer this method. Some couples report that foreplay can include inserting the diaphragm, thereby making sexual activity more spontaneous. Women with complaints of decreased lubrication notice an advantage because the spermicide also functions as a lubricant.[249]

Disadvantages. Women who are reluctant to touch their genital area or feel embarrassed with a health care provider performing frequent pelvic examinations to achieve a proper fit may not like the diaphragm. In addition, patients who are virginal may find the first fitting with placement and retrieval slightly uncomfortable. Often these patients can be encouraged to use a condom or spermicidal cream until penetration has been achieved and then return to the office for a fitting. Other women who may not successfully use a diaphragm include those with severe genital prolapse, such as a rectocele or cystocele. Patients with significant pelvic relaxation may be unable to achieve a proper and snug fit. Some patients and their partners find the vaginal cream or contraceptive gel messy and repulsive. For patients who engage in oral-genital contact, the presence of the spermicide may be asthetically unpleasing. In addition, some patients complain that spontaneity of in-

tercourse is decreased because of the need to place the diaphragm before intercourse. This group of patients could be counseled to wear the diaphragm every night so that intercourse can be more spontaneous.

In addition, some women report more frequent urinary tract infections because of diaphragm use. Several studies have reviewed the incidence of urinary tract infections (UTIs) in women using diaphragms compared with rates among those who were using oral contraceptives or other means of contraception. Bladder infections occur twice as often in diaphragm users compared with patients using oral contraceptive pills. The incidence of primary and secondary UTIs is greater for women using diaphragms.[90] One may note that the urethra is compressed and may become partially obstructed when the diaphragm is in place. Some patients are unable to completely empty the bladder and stagnant urine accumulates, leading to an excellent culture medium and higher chance of urinary tract infection. Additional studies have shown if a smaller diaphragm is placed, the incidence of urinary tract infection may decrease significantly.

From 2% to 4% of patients may experience an allergic reaction to the rubber latex found in the diaphragm. Symptoms include itching, burning, or rash. When this occurs, the device should be discontinued.

Summary. The diaphragm is an extremely important and effective barrier contraceptive method. When it is fitted correctly in a highly motivated patient with concurrent use of a spermicidal cream or jelly and a condom, pregnancy rates can be extremely low. Additional benefits include a decreased incidence of sexually transmitted diseases and abnormal Pap tests.

Condoms

Historical perspectives. The condom was invented about 400 years ago, and it remains the only reversible form of male contraception available. The first male contraceptive was developed by Gabriele Fallopius. Although this first device was developed primarily for the prevention of transmission of sexual diseases, the contraceptive benefits were later noted. In his early writing, Fallopius states[39]:

"As often as man has intercourse, he should (if possible) wash the genitals, or wipe them with a cloth; afterwards he should use a small linen cloth made to the glans and draw forward the prepuce over the glans; if he can do so. It is well to moisten it with saliva or with a lotion; however: it does not matter; if you fear lest syphilis be produced in the canal, take the sheath of this linen cloth and place it in the canal; I tried the experiment on 1100 men, and I call immortal God to witness that not one of them was infected."[39]

During the eighteenth century, men became more creative in their attempts to develop the perfect condom. Many materials were used, including the intestine of lambs, sheep, and goats, and fish bladders. Until the nineteenth century, when latex rubber condoms were mass produced, condoms were fairly expensive. In many instances, only the very wealthy and noble could afford to use them. Although designed to decrease the risk of sexually transmitted diseases, men in the early eighteenth century reused condoms many times during sex with spouses or prostitutes. As reproductive biology advanced, the contraceptive benefits attributable to the use of condoms became apparent.[39]

Description. Mass marketing, consumer demand, and the increased incidence of sexually transmitted diseases have made condom sales increase dramatically. In the 1970s, approximately 30 million condoms were sold; today sales of 45 to 50 million have been recorded. Condoms are the most preferred means of reversible contraception in Japan, China, and Scandinavia.[233] It is the third most popular means of contraception in the United States.[233]

No longer relegated "behind the counter," the condom can be found brightly packaged and located in the aisles and shelves of most drug stores. Exotic names have been given to condoms, such as the Hugger, Excita, Rough Rider, and Tahiti. Condoms are sold individually and in packages of three or 12. They can be found in men's and women's locker rooms, high school bathrooms, and truck stops. Various shapes, textures, and colors of condoms are available. In addition, patients also have the choice of lubricated or nonlubricated condoms. In a special edition, the 1989 *Consumer Reports* magazine found that the preference in condoms was higher for lubricated condoms with a reservoir tip, although some persons liked extra-thin, extra-strong, or lubricated spermicidal condoms.[231]

In the mid-1800s condoms were made of latex rubber with a seam from the tip to the ring. The modern condom is made of latex rubber that is stretchable and seamless. At the tip of the condom is a reservoir or a plain end.

The quality control and production of condoms have improved tremendously. It is rare for a condom produced in the United States to break or tear. Less than one in 300 condoms will rupture at the time of use. However, the latex can deteriorate if left in warm places (e.g., glove compartment or back pocket), and the condom should not be used with lubricants such as baby oil, vaseline, or mineral oil. When these products were added to the condom and the condom was scientifically tested, damage was noted, and HIV virus readily leaked from the condom.[57]

Advantages. Condoms have many advantages. These include excellent contraceptive effectiveness when used correctly, easy availability, low cost, nonprescription use, and decreased risk of transmission of sexually transmitted diseases in users. One dozen condoms cost approximately $7 to $9. If used correctly, condoms are theoretically effective in preventing pregnancy 97% to 98% of the time; actual effectiveness is 80% to 85%.[57] In addition, the acceptance rate has grown recently because of the concern about sexually transmitted diseases, especially AIDS;

more men and women are motivated to use them. Many couples are using a "back-up" method, using condoms with another contraceptive modality (e.g., IUD, pill, Norplant). This strategy is used to decrease the risk of STDs. Condoms have a decreased incidence of discontinuance compared with other methods, such as the IUD or oral contraceptives.

Since 1981 and the discovery of AIDS, many studies have demonstrated that the HIV virus is less likely to penetrate a latex condom than condoms made of other materials. Some studies have suggested that animal-membrane condoms do not protect against HIV or hepatitis. In addition, other benefits have been seen in partners of patients who use condoms. Specifically, there is a decreased incidence of pelvic inflammatory disease, cervical carcinoma, human papilloma virus transmission, hepatitis B, and genital herpes.[57]

Condoms do not require a visit to a health care provider. They are readily accessible and available without a doctor's prescription. Both men and women can feel free to purchase condoms and keep them safely stored until needed. To achieve maximum effectiveness, Elizabeth Connell advocates the following[57]:

- Use a new condom every time you have sexual intercourse or other acts between partners that involve contact with the penis.
- Put a condom on after the penis is erect and before intermittent contact because lesions, preejaculate secretions, semen, vaginal secretions, saliva, urine, and feces can contain certain STD organisms.
- Place condom on the head of the penis and unroll or put it all the way to the base.
- Leave an empty space at the end of the condom to collect semen. Remove any air remaining in the tip of the condom by gently pressing air out toward the base of the penis.
- If a lubricant is desired, use water-based lubricants such as KY jelly. Do not use oil-based lubricants, such as those made with petroleum jelly, mineral oil, vegetable oil, or cold cream because these may damage the condom.
- After ejaculation, carefully withdraw the penis while it is still erect. Hold on to the rim of the condom as you withdraw so that the condom does not slip off.
- Store condoms in a cool, dry place.
- If the rubber material is sticky, brittle, or obviously damaged, do not use.
- Do not reuse condoms.[57]

Disadvantages. The majority of complaints from patients using the condom arise from the lack of spontaneity or the need to interrupt sexual activity to put the condom on. For the condom to be effective, it must be used with every act of intercourse. This requires a highly motivated couple. For patients complaining of this interruption problem, one may suggest that the couple include placement of the condom on the penis in foreplay. In addition, some patients complain of the condom slipping off before completion of coitus. To decrease this risk, the patient should be counseled to withdraw the penis while still erect and dispose of the condom. In addition, some men complain of decreased tactile sensitivity. Latex condoms may impede the transmission of heat from the vaginal mucosa to the penis. Men complaining of this problem may find that purchasing the thinner condoms may be beneficial. In addition, condoms made from the skin or intestine of lambs are ultrathin, and men complaining of decreased sensation may find these helpful. However, this type of contraception does not decrease the transmission of sexually transmitted diseases.

A few patients or partners may have a true latex allergy manifested by a rash on the scrotum, vulva, or thigh. Patients experiencing these problems may benefit from a condom made of natural lamb. In addition, the spermicidal gel, nonoxynol-9, may cause a chemical vulvitis, vaginitis, or penile inflammation.

Summary. Although the condom was introduced to the world 400 years ago, many subtle changes have been made in its appearance. Much has been learned about its effectiveness in preventing pregnancy and transmission of sexually transmitted diseases. The simultaneous use of the condom and other contraceptive methods will continue to be strongly advocated so the disease-preventing potential of the condom can be achieved. Condoms are affordable and effective when used by a well-motivated couple.

Contraceptive sponges

Since the days of antiquity, women have sought creative ways to prevent pregnancy. Sea sponges, fruit, lemon rinds, and other objects have been inserted into the vagina to prevent pregnancy.[90] In 1983, the Today contraceptive vaginal sponge was introduced by Whitehall Laboratories, New York. The modern device is made of a disposable polyurethane component. The device is small, produced in one size of approximately 2 inches in diameter and 1.2 inches thick.[57] It has a "dimple" or concave side, which is applied to the cervix. The outer covering contains a woven polyester strap to facilitate removal of the device. Each sponge is disposable and contains 1 g of nonoxynol-9. Within 24 hours, 125 to 150 mg of nonoxynol-9 is released. Three contraceptive modes of action have been described. It functions as a physical barrier, blocking the cervical os, it constantly releases nonoxynol-9, and it absorbs semen.[173]

Advantages. Distinct advantages of the Today Contraceptive Sponge are that it can be purchased over the counter and does not require fitting. Unlike the diaphragm, which must be fitted by a health care provider, an individual can purchase at a drug store a box of three, six, or 12 sponges. In addition, the sponge can be left in place up to 24 hours and does not require the addition of more contraceptive cream or gel for multiple acts of intercourse. As previously mentioned, patients using the diaphragm must add contraceptive cream or gel for each act of intercourse. Many patients enjoy the spontaneity of intercourse when using the Today Sponge. In addition, nonoxynol-9 has been shown to have bactericidal and virucidal activity against gonorrhea, trichomonas, staphylococcus aureus, herpes, syphilis, and chlamydia.[57]

Patients also state that the contraceptive sponge is not as messy as the diaphragm. To activate the nonoxynol-9–impregnated device, patients must apply approximately 2 tablespoons of water to the sponge and insert the sponge into the vagina so that it covers the cervical os. Once intercourse has been completed, the sponge should be left in place for 6 to 8 hours to effectively immobilize and inhibit sperm activity. After that, the contraceptive sponge should be removed and discarded.

Disadvantages. Very few serious side effects have been reported with the Today Sponge. However, some patients have had allergic reactions to the nonoxynol-9. A minority of patients develop vulvar irritation, vaginitis, or a rash. Some patients have stated that sexual intercourse is more uncomfortable because vaginal secretions are minimal and less lubrication is felt. The sponge may absorb some vaginal secretions. Some multiparous patients may complain that the sponge dislodges during intercourse. For these patients with lax vaginal tone from childbirth, a larger size is currently not available; the Today Sponge is manufactured in one size only. The cost of the Today Sponge may be prohibitive if patients have frequent coitus. Each Today Sponge costs approximately $1.25 to $1.75. They may be sold individually, or in cases of three, six, or 12. Some patients have also had difficulty removing or retrieving the sponge. In one study, about 6% of patients discontinued use of Today Sponge because of difficulty retrieving or removing it. Some patients have had the embarrassment of seeking medical attention to have it removed.

Effectiveness. Most studies have shown that the Today Sponge is not as effective in preventing pregnancy as the diaphragm or other methods. In general, most pregnancy rates after 12 months of use vary from 20% to 27%.[173]

Summary. The contraceptive Today Sponge offers an alternative barrier method for women wishing to prevent pregnancy. A well-motivated patient who is comfortable inserting the Today Sponge may find that this method is less messy, allows for more spontaneous intercourse, and is reversible. In adolescents, this method allows for more privacy and is certainly better than not using any method at all. In addition, this method produces a decreased incidence of sexually transmitted disease. When combined with the condom, lower pregnancy rates can be achieved.

Spermicides

Today, three types of contraceptive spermicides are available. All of them can be purchased without a prescription. All of these spermicides contain nonoxynol-9, which effectively acts as a surfactant, attacking the membrane covering the head of the sperm, immobilizing and destroying the sperm. The three types of spermicides are vaginal suppositories or vaginal inserts, creams or jellies, and foamy aerosols. All three types of spermicides use the same mechanism of immobilizing and destroying the sperm.

Description

Vaginal suppositories. Vaginal suppositories are made in the shape of a small bullet and must be inserted into the vagina at least 10 to 20 minutes before intercourse. This is necessary so that the insert can dissolve, allowing the spermicide to coat the upper vagina and cervical os. Some vaginal suppositories contain a foaming agent that releases carbon dioxide, producing small bubbles that disperse in the vagina, which allows the medication to mix in the upper vaginal walls.[231] After each act of intercourse, an additional suppository must be inserted. Patients are advised not to douche or shower for at least 6 hours after the last act of intercourse.[57]

Contraceptive foams. Contraceptive foams are available in a small aerosol can. Most directions call for the patient to shake the can approximately 20 times before inserting the foam into an applicator. Using the applicator, the patient should put the foam into the vagina no more than 1 to 2 hours before intercourse. More foam must be inserted before additional acts of intercourse.[57]

Contraceptive creams. Contraceptive creams or jellies are inserted with an applicator and placed high into the vagina. This medication melts rapidly because of the high body temperature. After each act of intercourse, additional spermicidal jelly or cream must be applied.

Disadvantages. Disadvantages of the spermicides include the need to plan for intercourse and to have the medication readily available. In addition, patients engaging in oral-genital contact may find this method unpleasant. Some patients complain of a heavier vaginal discharge or increased messiness with these products. These medications do not require a prescription and are relatively inexpensive. Currently, patients may expect to pay about 50 cents for each act of intercourse if a spermicide is used. This method used alone is not particularly effective. Most studies quote the effectiveness at 80% to 95%; however, this can be improved if a condom is used concomitantly.

IUDs

Arab camel drivers reportedly were the first individuals to have used IUDs. The IUDs were made of stone or rocks and were placed into the endometrial cavity of camels. Thus camels could not become pregnant during their long trip across the desert.[90] These camel drivers were the first to note that insertion of a foreign device would prevent pregnancy. Since 1920, we have seen many devices inserted within the uterine cavity of women throughout the world to prevent pregnancy. More than 40 types of devices have been invented.

In the early twentieth century, German physicians creatively made silk worm gut into the shape of a ring and inserted it in the uterine cavity. The Japanese, Chinese, and Germans in the 1920s and 1930s used devices made of silk worm gut, gold, and silver. Because of high infection rates, these devices were later removed.[39,109]

The 1960s and 1970s brought a renewed interest in the IUD. Many different IUDs were invented during this era. Frequently the device was named after the gynecologist inventing it, such as the Grafenberg Ring, Lippes Loop, Birnberg Bow, and Tatum IUD. The name *Dalkon Shield* was derived from parts of the surnames of its discovers.[213] During the last 30 years more than 27 different devices have been used worldwide.

Currently only two IUDs are approved by the FDA for use in this country. These are the Paragard device and Progestasert IUD. Because of the malpractice lawsuits brought against several companies, earlier IUDs have been withdrawn from the market. Many well-tested and well-accepted devices, such as Copper 7, were removed from the marketplace because of a company's inability to obtain liability insurance.[95]

Description. Women in this country have two choices in IUDs. These are the Copper T 380 A (Paragard IUD) and Progestasert IUD. Many other types are available in the worldwide IUD market, but these are not available in the United States. Women seeking other alternatives have traveled to Canada for additional choices. Worldwide, more than 60 million women are reportedly using the IUD.[251]

The copper T 380 (Paragard-Gyno Pharmaceutical) was introduced in the United States in 1988. This device is made in the shape of a T and is encased in copper. The device contains 380 mm^2 of exposed copper and polyethlyene. Barium has been added within the device to increase its radiopacity. The tail is made of two monofilament strings that are extruded through the cervix. The device is easily inserted within the uterus by using a plunger tube, after securing the arms of the T into the plunger.[251] It has been used in other countries since 1982. The device is marketed in this country to be used for 8 years (Fig. 30-3).

The Progestasert (Alza Corporation, Palo Alto, California) was approved by the FDA as a contraceptive in 1976. It is a small device measuring 36 mm in length. It is T-shaped, and the device is made of ethylenevinyl acetate copolymer. The device has 38 mg of progesterone in silicon oil, and it is encased in barium sulfate to increase its radiopacity. Each day 65 mg of progesterone is released. The device must be removed after 1 year. Efficacy declines thereafter. In France, the device is approved for placement for 18 months.[251] Patients using the Progestasert have noticed a decreased incidence in primary dysmenorrhea and menstrual blood loss because of the presence of progesterone.

Mechanism of action. There have been many theories

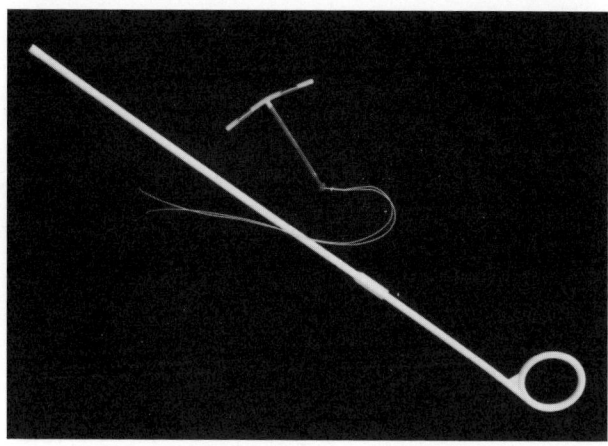

Fig. 30-3. Paragard IUD device and inserter.

about the mechanism of action of the IUD. Scientists thought incorrectly for many years that the IUD prevented the embryo from implanting. Newer studies indicate that the IUD works by stimulating a mild inflammatory reaction within the uterus, causing an increased circulation of prostaglandins, chemotactic enzymes, polymorphonuclear leukocytes, plasma cells, and macrophages, and increased foreign giant cell reactions. These foreign giant cell reactions are probably toxic to sperm. In addition, we know that fluid from the uterine cavity can reflux into the tubes, thereby carrying this spermicidal and contraceptive activity into the tubal ostia. This environment is hostile to sperm activity. Whatever the mechanism of action, the pregnancy rates with the IUD are extremely low.[271]

Advantages. The main advantages of the IUD are its reliability and convenience. Lack of patient compliance does not compromise the effectiveness of the IUD. In addition, women who desire spontaneity with intercourse and who wish to avoid hormones in their body will find the IUD acceptable. There are minimal changes in the menstrual cycle in women using the IUD. There is no effect on ovulation, and the IUD is reversible. Approximately 50% to 85% of patients who have an IUD inserted elect to continue using it after 1 year. Patients with strong risk factors prohibiting the use of oral contraceptives will find excellent contraception with the IUD. Grimes noted that in 1982, among IUD users, 83% had previously used oral contraceptives, and of these 36% had been advised by a physician to stop taking the pill. About 60% of IUD users in the United States are not candidates for oral contraception because of smoking or other risk factors.[109]

In most clinical contraceptive trials, the pregnancy rate in IUD users appears to be 1 to 3 pregnancies per 100 women per year.

Disadvantages. The main disadvantages with IUD use are the high initial cost and subjective symptoms of pain and bleeding at the time of insertion. Most private insur-

ance companies do not cover the cost of an IUD. These costs may range from $150 to $290 for insertion, removal, and office visits. Amortized over 8 years, however, the Paragard IUD is less expensive than the oral contraceptive pill, which costs approximately $20 per month. The high initial cost of the Paragard IUD, however, may be prohibitive for some patients. The Progestasert IUD also is expensive because it must be inserted and removed each year, with average fees ranging from $120 to $175 for reinsertion of this device.

Approximately 5% to 15% of patients will ask to have their IUD removed because of pain and bleeding. If a patient complains of menorrhagia or dysmenorrhea, a prostaglandin synthetase inhibitor (such as ibuprofen, meclofenamate, or naproxen) may relieve menstrual cramps and decrease bleeding. If these fail to control the patient's bleeding, the IUD may need to be removed. Some patients also note slightly heavier menstrual cycles, especially patients using the Paragard IUD; however, this bleeding may also be improved with prostaglandin synthetase inhibitor. Iron supplementation should be recommended in patients with very heavy menstrual periods.

Patients should have the IUD inserted while on their menstrual cycle because this ensures that the patient is not pregnant and facilitates insertion as the cervical os is dilated during menses. The newer IUD devices have a simplified means of insertion. The uterus is sounded, and the appropriate depth of the uterine cavity is noted. The plunger, which holds the IUD, gently releases the IUD into the uterine cavity. The risk for uterine perforation is minimal. The complication rate is 1 to 3 per 1000 insertions and tends to decrease as the operator gains experience.[271] If complications occur, a surgical procedure may be required to remove the device. If the IUD is lost, the uterine cavity should be sounded or hysteroscoped gently to determine if the IUD is present within the uterine cavity. If this cannot be ascertained, the patient should be sent for an ultrasound or anteroposterior and lateral x-rays of the pelvis. The barium-sulfate–impregnated IUD can be located on x-ray.[109]

Patients using the IUD can expect a pregnancy rate of 1 to 3 pregnancies per 100 women per year. Women becoming pregnant with the IUD are at risk for septic abortion and ectopic pregnancy.[81] All patients should be told before the insertion of the IUD that, if there is an episode of amenorrhea, an early pregnancy test is warranted. If a patient becomes pregnant, the IUD should be removed immediately to decrease the risk of septic or spontaneous abortion. Many studies have shown that the high rate of spontaneous abortion can be reduced if the device is removed promptly. The risk of prematurity, premature rupture of the membranes, and premature labor can be reduced safely if the IUD is removed before the second trimester. Women using the Progestasert IUD have a slightly higher risk of ectopic pregnancy if a failure occurs.

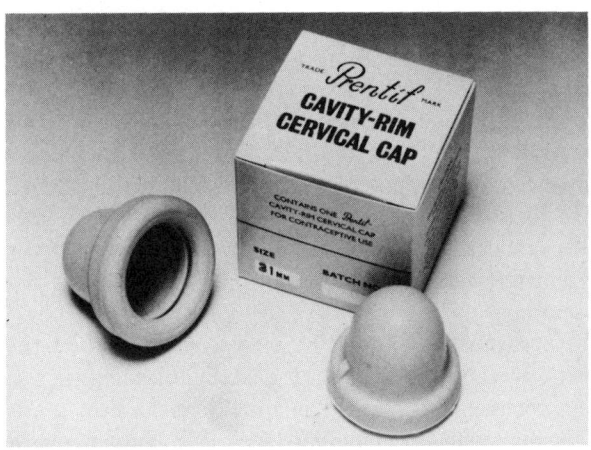

Fig. 30-4. The Prentif cervical cap.

Summary. Most epidemiologic data support the safety and effectiveness of the IUD. Patients who are in a monogamous relationship and carefully selected, counseled, and fitted will find years of excellent contraception.

Cervical cap

In 1988 the Food and Drug Administration approved the use of the cervical cap. The cervical cap is made of natural rubber and is held in place by a suction-like seal that covers the cervix. Currently, there are three cervical caps available worldwide, the Dumas, Vimul, and Prentif caps. The only cervical cap approved in the United States is the Prentif cervical cap[174] (Fig. 30-4).

Mechanism of Action. The Prentif cervical cap acts as a barrier to sperm by covering the cervical os. The cap must be fitted by a health care professional. The cervical cap is currently available in four sizes: 22, 25, 28, and 31 mm diameters, and is approximately 1¼ to 1½ inches long.[57] The cervical cap, when fitted correctly, creates a suction seal. It covers only the cervix and reaches up close to the vaginal fornix. A spermicidal agent also must be used to prevent pregnancy. The cervical cap should be filled one half to one third full with a spermicidal cream or jelly.[174]

Effectiveness. The cervical cap appears to be as effective as the diaphragm in preventing pregnancy. Currently, there have been few randomized multicenter trials comparing the effectiveness of the cap and the diaphragm. However, in several unpublished studies, the effectiveness was approximately 83% to 93%.[57] Patients who are well motivated, are comfortable with touching their genitals, and have not had cervical trauma or obstetrical lacerations to the cervix appear to fare well with the cervical cap. Patients who have a shortened cervix may find the Prentif cap less effective.

Advantages. Many patients prefer the cervical cap to the diaphragm. Patients often note that the cervical cap is less messy than the diaphragm, is more economical, and can be left in place for up to 48 hours. In addition, because the cervical cap fits only on the cervix, it is less likely to put pressure on the bladder (than the diaphragm) and therefore it carries less chance of urinary tract infections.[174] In addition, sexual activity can be more spontaneous because the cap can be inserted up to 6 hours before intercourse and left in place for 24 to 48 hours after intercourse before removal is necessary. If a couple has intercourse sessions less than 6 hours apart, additional spermicide is not necessary. The cap should be left in place for at least 8 hours after the last act of coitus and then removed.

Disadvantages. The cervical cap must be fitted by health professionals to ensure a proper fit. Currently, only four sizes are available, so some patients with unusual cervical shapes or history of cervical trauma may not find a cap that fits.[57] The average time to properly fit, educate, and practice placing the cervical cap is approximately 30 to 60 minutes. There is also the theoretical risk of toxic shock.[57] The cervical cap currently is not recommended for women on their menstrual cycle. Early multicenter trial studies suggest that patients who use the cervical cap were at slightly increased risk of having an abnormal Pap test. The FDA recommends that patients who have been fitted for a cervical cap return for a repeat Pap test 3 to 6 months after the original fitting. Patients who have had a history of an abnormal Pap test should not use a cervical cap because of this potential complication. In addition, some patients have complained of a malodorous, foul discharge when the cervical cap is left in place longer than 24 to 48 hours.

The Prentif cervical cap offers an alternative barrier method for women who are motivated, who are comfortable with their genital anatomy, and who desire a reversible means of contraception. To increase the effectiveness of the cervical cap, proper fitting is essential.

Postcoital contraception

Despite a patient's best attempts to prevent pregnancy, contraceptive failures do occur. A condom may slip off or tear, a patient may forget to place her contraceptive cream, or the cervical cap or diaphragm may be left in the dresser drawer. The patient may forget to take her oral contraceptives for more than 2 days, or the patient simply may forget to insert her reliable method of contraception because she was not planning to have intercourse. There are also those unfortunate patients who are raped and who seek medical care after this devastating event. Practitioners should be aware of effective postcoital, "morning after" contraception for patients fitting these profiles.

A patient's chance for pregnancy after an episode of unprotected intercourse will depend on the time of her menstrual cycle in which sexual intercourse occured. Jay Trussel estimates that if unprotected intercourse occurs 3 days before ovulation, the pregnancy rate is approximately 20% in that cycle; about 25% for intercourse 1 day before ovulation, and about 15% on the day of ovulation. Pregnancy is extremely rare if intercourse occurs more than 2 days after ovulation.[252]

Ovral, an oral contraceptive that contains .05 mg of ethinyl-estradiol and .5 mg of norgestrel, is often used as a postcoital means of contraception by physicians in the United States. A patient should take four Ovral tablets no later than 72 hours after unprotected intercourse. The patient is advised to take two Ovral tablets at one time and a repeat dose (additional two tablets) 12 hours later. The administering physician should prescribe additional tablets in case nausea or vomiting occur with this medication. Presumably, the oral contraceptive functions as an interceptor, by preventing implantation of the egg after fertilization has taken place. The endometrial lining becomes inhospitable to the fertilized egg because of the higher estrogen/progesterone mileu and decreases the likelihood of successful implantation. Patients using Ovral should also be cautioned that tubal pregnancy is possible, and these patients should be evaluated if pregnancy occurs.[87]

Patient education is very important when administering this medication. Repeated use of this means of pregnancy prevention should be discouraged. The patient should be made aware that this medication is being administered only because of the urgent nature of her situation. In addition, side effects from high doses of oral estrogen should be mentioned. Approximately 70% of users develop nausea, and approximately 19% develop vomiting. An antiemetic should therefore be prescribed with Ovral.[252] The patient should be advised to take an antiemetic approximately 1 hour before taking each Ovral tablet. The patient should also be told that if she vomits within 4 hours of taking Ovral, she should take additional Ovral tablets.

Other side effects include headaches, dizziness, menstrual irregularities, and breast tenderness. Approximately 20% of patients taking Ovral may experience change in their menstrual cycle. If this occurs, early pregnancy testing should be performed.[252]

Effectiveness. Studies evaluating patients who have used Ovral as a means of postcoital contraception revealed a pooled failure rate of 1.8%.[87]

Summary. In conclusion, a patient experiencing unprotected midcycle intercourse should consider using four tablets of Ovral as a means to prevent an unplanned pregnancy. The patient should be counseled regarding the effectiveness of this modality and the need for a very early but sensitive pregnancy test at the conclusion of her menstrual cycle to confirm that pregnancy has not occurred.

Tubal sterilization

Tubal ligation is emerging as one of the more popular means of permanent contraception for couples who do not want more children. It is estimated that by the year 2000 one out of four couples will use tubal sterilization as a permanent means of contraception.[207]

In 1987, female sterilization was practiced by 19.1% of couples who had completed their child bearing, and male sterilization accounted for 13.4% of total contraceptive practices in the United States. When one combines these numbers, at least 32.5% of couples use sterilization as a means of contraception, making this the number one contraceptive choice in the United States.[19]

In 1987, 640,000 women in the United States were sterilized. Most of the sterilizations occurred in the immediate postpartum period, and other patients had interval procedures. On the average, 1.15 million male and female sterilizations are performed annually in the United States.[19]

Efficacy and hazards. Despite our best intentions, no contraceptive practices currently available have a 0% risk of pregnancy except for hysterectomy. Patients who decide to undergo a tubal ligation should understand that the overall failure rate is approximately 1 in 250 to 300 patients.[252]

Tubal ligation is a very effective means of contraception and should be considered a permanent procedure. Many patients mistakenly believe that "the tubes can be untied." It is very important that patients be told that generally this method is permanent and nonreversible. Although reversal procedures are possible, only 30% to 70% of patients are candidates for the reversal procedure, and of these, 70% to 80% may successfully achieve an intrauterine pregnancy.[207] Although most commercial insurers will pay for tubal ligations, many will not pay for the "elective" reversal procedure.

Patients who have had a tubal ligation and who conceive after the procedure have a 15% to 20% chance of an ectopic pregnancy. Any patient experiencing signs or symptoms of pregnancy after a tubal ligation, such as episodes of amenorrhea or irregular bleeding, should be thoroughly evaluated to rule out tubal pregnancy. This is a very important medical caveat to tubal ligation.

Most tubal ligations in this country are performed in the postpartum period or as an interval procedure. When performed by a trained physician, the morbidity and mortality of the procedure are low. The fatality rate is approximately 3 to 4 per 100,000 cases. Causes of death often are related to hemorrhage, infection, or anesthetic complications.[202]

Methods of tubal ligation. There are three basic ways to occlude the fallopian tubes. These are electrocauterization; placement of silastic bands, rings, or clips on the tubes; and removal of a portion of the distal fallopian tube. In China, most patients are sterilized by the placement of caustic fluid hysteroscopically through the proximal or cornual portion of the fallopian tube. Postpartum sterilization is generally performed in the U.S. through a small, 2 to 4 cm subumbilical incision. With the rapid involution of the uterus immediately after delivery, the tubes are identified beneath the umbilicus, thereby making the postpartum sterilization procedure very easy. Most patients having the tubal ligation months after delivery will have it performed as a diagnostic laparoscopy, with occlusion of the fallopian tubes by silastic bands, and less commonly as a minilaparotomy, or vaginal tubal ligation.

When amortized, the cost of a tubal ligation is significantly less than other means of contraception. In this country, the average outpatient cost for this procedure, including surgical fees, operating time, and anesthesia, is approximately $2500 to $3500.

Importance of counseling before sterilization. Unfortunately, approximately 3% to 25% of sterilized women later regret their decision.[151] How can we as health care providers decrease the number of patients who later regret their decision to undergo permanent sterilization? Many common characteristics are seen in patients who later regret their decision to undergo permanent sterilization. They are under the age of 30 at the time of the procedure, have less than 12 years of formal education, are single, separated, divorced, or widowed at the time of their procedure; had a change in marital status after their sterilization, or are under severe social, financial, or emotional distress at the time of the sterilization. Approximately 3% to 25% of sterilized women will later regret their decision, and approximately 1% to 2% will actually have a reversal procedure.[151]

The leading reason for requesting a reversal procedure is the desire for children in women who later remarry or have a change in their marital status. Nine of 115 women who were questioned by Leader et al. requested reversal procedures because of remarriage.[151]

Patients who are covered by Medicaid must undergo extensive counseling, as well as sign a lengthy consent form before sterilization can be performed. Patients must be at least 21 years of age and must have signed a consent form at least 30 days before the procedure. The form is valid for 6 months. In the event of a preterm delivery, the consent form can be waived by signature given at least 72 hours before sterilization is performed. Physicians in private practice using commercial insurers do not have these cumbersome rules to follow.[57]

Patients should always be offered the option of a prescription for a reversible means of contraception. Also, the patient should be informed that her partner has the option of having a vasectomy. One must ensure that all patients realize that the procedure is essentially irreversible. The patient should also be told of other available long-term contraceptive methods, including the Paragard IUD (which is effective for 8 years) and the Norplant (which is effective for 5 years).

Summary. It is critical for physicians and health care providers to counsel patients regarding the permanence of sterilization, the technical aspects of the surgical procedure, and the alternative contraceptive modalities. Tubal ligation is an excellent choice for individuals who are certain that they do not want any more children. Women who have had a tubal ligation and present with symptoms of pregnancy, including episodes of amenorrhea, should be evaluated for pregnancy.

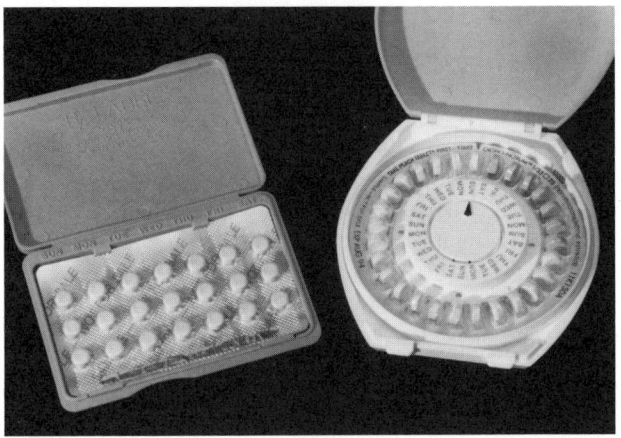

Fig. 30-5. Examples of oral contraceptive pills used today.

Oral contraceptives

Historical perspectives. It has been more than 30 years since the development of the oral contraceptive pill (Fig. 30-5). In 1960 the FDA formally approved the use of oral contraceptive pills. Since then, more than 100 million women have used the oral contraceptive pill. Currently, birth control pills rank as the number one method of reversible birth control among women aged 15 to 44. Today, 60 million women use birth control pills worldwide, with 11 million of these women in the United States. The development of the oral contraceptive pill was a monumental advance in scientific medicine.[207]

When Pincus and Rock introduced the birth control pill in the 1960s, very large amounts of estrogen and progesterone were used. In fact, one of the first pills was Enovid, which contained a combination of 10 mg of norethynodrel and 150 mg of mestranol. It later became obvious that the high doses of progesterone and estrogen were associated with side effects, including thromboembolic events, heart attacks, stroke, nausea, and vomiting, and were not well tolerated by patients. However, in the ensuing 30 years, major modifications in the birth control pill have been made. In addition, not only are the total dosages of estrogen and progesterone lower, but distinct benefits of the birth control pill have been recorded. Today, birth control pills contain no more than .03 to .05 mg estrogen, and most contain less than 1 mg progesterone. The safety, efficacy, and contractive benefits of the birth control pill now are established (Fig. 30-5).

Mechanism of action. Simply stated, oral contraceptives are synthetic hormones that act to replace and suppress hormones that are made by the ovary. Birth control pills function at the level of the hypothalamus, altering pituitary function and suppressing follicle stimulating hormone (FSH) and luteinizing hormone (LH) levels. Because the pills are administered daily, ovulation does not occur, tenacious cervical mucus is produced, and alteration in the tubal transport mechanism is noted, as well as alteration in the endometrial integrity, creating an environment more hostile to implantation. Compliance with the birth control pill schedule is necessary at all times but is more important during the first 14 days of the menstrual cycle to prevent the dominant follicle from developing, thereby preventing pregnancy.[208]

Health benefits from oral contraception. Oral contraception was developed to prevent pregnancy. However, over the ensuing 30 years, additional noncontraceptive benefits have been noted, including decreased incidence of dysmenorrhea, decreased blood loss during menses, lighter menstrual flow, decreased risk for endometriosis, decreased risk of ovarian and uterine cancer, increased bone mass, and the socioeconomic benefits that result from delayed childbearing and avoidance of unintended pregnancy.[191]

The news media have not enthusiastically spread the good news about birth control pills and these noncontraceptive benefits. In fact, the FDA took longer than 10 years to insert the noncontraceptive benefits into the oral contraceptive informational packet. Health care providers not only should counsel patients about the effectiveness of the pill in preventing pregnancy, but also about the non-contraceptive benefits.

Gynecologic benefits of the pill. Two gynecologic malignancies have been shown to be decreased in patients who ever used oral contraceptives. These are endometrial cancer and ovarian cancer. A large study by the Oxford Family Planning Association compared at least 13 case control studies and noted a 40% reduction in the risk of epithelial ovarian cancers in users of oral contraceptive pills versus nonusers.[257]

The Centers for Disease Control and the National Institute of Child Health and Human Development (CASH) study revealed the important factor that the gynecologic malignancy protective benefits of the pill lasted from 5 to 10 years after the last pill was taken. The mechanism of action is through suppression of the hypothalamic pituitary ovarian axis and decreased incidence of recurrent and incessant ovulation that has been associated as a risk factor for ovarian cancer. Perhaps the oral contraceptive pill replaces the "natural" patterns that have characterized human reproduction over time.[208] Centuries ago most women did not begin menstruation until age 18 or 20 and breastfed their children for several years; each birth led to long periods of anovulation, which is associated with decreased risk of ovarian cancer. Many of our ancestors may have had only 20 to 50 menstrual cycles in a lifetime (the remainder of the time they were pregnant or lactating). Today's woman may have 250 to 350 episodes of menstruation during her lifetime.[208] The pill may therefore help to restore the natural reproductive cycle, closer to that of our ancestors.

Endometrial cancer rates have also been shown to be decreased in two studies conducted by CASH and the World Health Organization collaborative study in 1988.[44,270] These studies show that there is a 50% lower chance of developing endometrial cancer among ever users than among never users. These benefits increase if a patient uses the pill longer than 1 year. There was no reduction in the incidence of uterine sarcoma or leiomyosarcoma in patients who have used birth control pills.[44]

Because birth control pills effectively suppress the hypothalamic-pituitary-ovarian axis, clinicians can also expect to find a decreased risk of functional cysts in users. In fact, "corpus luteum cysts decreased by 80% and follicular cysts are also decreased by 50%."[257] At least several thousand admissions and unnecessary surgeries are thought to have been avoided by use of the birth control pill. Clinically, ruptured follicular or hemorrhagic corpus luteum cysts may cause acute abdominal pain, necessitating further diagnostic testing such as ultrasound, hospitalization, and possible surgical procedures. Functional cysts are less frequent in patients using the birth control pill. The pill has not been shown to decrease the risk of benign dermoid cysts (teratomas) or cyst adenomas.[257]

An additional gynecologic benefit of oral contraceptives is the reduction of menstrual blood loss. The menstrual cycle in a woman using the birth control pill is often described as a lighter flow with associated fewer menstrual clots, as well as decreased incidence of dysmenorrhea. As a result, iron deficiency anemia is rarely seen in users. The treatment of menorrhagia may involve use of the oral contraceptive in such a way as to induce a "chemical dilation and curettage." Patients experiencing excessively heavy uterine bleeding (who are not pregnant) may benefit from a short course of an oral contraceptive containing .035 mg of estrogen, taken qid for 4 days. This will induce endometrial atrophy and result in hemostasis. In some patients, the birth control pill may also rapidly improve primary dysmenorrhea and occasionally improve premenstrual tension syndrome.[191]

Patients on the birth control pill have a decreased rate of pelvic inflammatory disease (PID). Birth control pills have also been shown to decrease the incidence of salpingitis by preventing the spread of pathologic bacteria into the endometrial cavity. The pill causes the cervical mucus to become tenacious, thereby, it is thought, impeding the spread of abnormal bacteria through the cervix. Each year, approximatley 1 million women in the U.S. experience acute salpingitis. The CDC indicates that women using the birth control pill for at least 1 year have a 50% lower chance of being hospitalized for an acute episode of pelvic inflammatory disease. This is a distinct gynecologic benefit in the younger population (ages 15 through 24), in which this disease is most likely to occur.[191]

Patients using the pill also have a decreased risk of ectopic pregnancy when compared with women choosing other methods of contraception. The mechanism of action of oral contraceptives is the inhibition of ovulation. Without ovulation, ectopic pregnancy is less possible; therefore the morbidity and mortality associated with this illness are also decreased.[191]

Metabolic benefits. Recent studies by Hannaford revealed that women using oral contraception have a decreased risk of rheumatoid arthritis. His study compared more than 20,000 patients using oral contraception with nonusers and noted a 20% lower chance of developing rheumatoid arthritis.[113] Patients who were approximately age 40 to 44 benefitted from the use.[113] In addition, patients from families with strong risk factors for rheumatoid arthritis seemed to benefit more. Oral contraceptive pill use appears to help prevent progression of rheumatoid arthritis and reduce the aggressiveness of the disease.

Women using oral contraception also have a relative increase in bone mass of 1% to 3% during the menstrual lifetime of the user. By extrapolating these data, we may find that this increased bone mass may be associated with decreased risk of osteoporosis in later life. The bone mass that is the most increased in concentration is the vertebral bone and not the peripheral bone.[154]

Cardiovascular benefits. During the past 35 years, clinicians have seen a decreased risk of cardiovascular-induced disease in women using oral contraception as the total estrogen dose has decreased.[64] The risk of myocardial infarction, hemorrhagic stroke, and venous thrombosis has markedly decreased. In fact, women who are nonsmokers and without hypertension or diabetes can be reasonably confident that they will not suffer a negative cardiovascular event because of the birth control pills. Women over the age of 35, without risk factors, and who are nonsmokers, can use the pill safely.[64]

Earlier cardiovascular complications related to the pill were thought to be the result of the high progesterone levels, causing a decrease in HDL, increase in LDL lipoproteins, and high estrogen levels. Prior studies revealed that the cardiovascular death rate was one in 10,000 women over the age of 35 who smoked and was less than one in 50,000 in women under the age of 35 who were nonsmokers. Cardiovascular morbidity was related to cigarette smoking itself as well as to hypertension and diabetes. Current FDA guidelines support the use of oral contraceptives in women over the age of 35 who are not hypertensive, diabetic, and smokers. Current low-dose (less than 50 mcg of estrogen) preparations essentially have a neutral or minimal effect on the coagulation system.[64]

A recent study by Adams compared the effect of atherosclerotic changes in the cardiovascular system in the macaque monkey. These monkeys were fed high-fat diets and were placed on a 50 mcg estrogen preparation. The control group was also fed a high-fat diet but was not placed on oral contraception. At autopsy, the monkeys who used oral contraception had a decreased risk of coronary artery disease despite their high-fat diet.[3] This has significant implications in the human model, if in the future we can discover that women using birth control pills

have a decreased risk of atherosclerosis and subsequent coronary artery disease.[3] More than 50% of the deaths in this country are associated with events related to atherogenic changes within the cardiovascular system. We currently cannot draw conclusions about the human model, but certainly this research model appears promising.

Socioeconomic benefits. Women using oral contraception have a much lower risk of an unintended pregnancy than a nonuser. This has special implications for women and couples desiring to "space" their pregnancies or coordinate them with career and education. The emotional and financial cost of an unintended pregnancy has dramatic implications for the adolescent, single, career, or married individual.[191]

We must not forget that childbirth can be hazardous to a woman's health. Especially in third-world countries, maternal mortality is staggering. For instance, in Africa one out 150 women who are pregnant will die from child birth, compared with 1 out of 10,000 women delivering in the developed countries. As Malcom Potts states, "One woman each minute dies somewhere in the third world from child birth or the consequences of abortion."[208] Birth control pill use in these countries can have a positive effect on the general health of users compared with nonusers.

Breast disease. The incidence of benign breast disease is decreased in women using birth control pills. This includes a decreased risk of fibroadenomas and chronic cystic disease. In addition, many women note fewer episodes of mastalgia when using birth control pills.[37]

After 1 to 2 years of oral contraceptive use, a decreased incidence of benign breast disease occurs. This effect is seen among women of all ages, and this protection is conferred for 1 year after discontinuing the use of birth control pills. The mechanism of action has been thought to be related to the manner in which progesterone decreases breast cell proliferation that is normally seen in the first half of the menstrual cycle.[37]

The incidence of breast cancer in U.S. women approximates one in nine. An excellent review by Richard Edgren in 1991 evaluated the effects of oral contraception on breast cancer.[82] He concluded that there appeared to be no significant increased risk for breast cancer in users. There is perhaps a small subgroup of women (very young women using birth control pills for extended periods of time before the birth of their first child) that may have increased risk of breast cancer; however, the data appear to be inconclusive. His general conclusion is that oral contraceptives do not induce or cause breast cancer.[82]

This question of whether oral contraceptive use causes breast cancer remains very emotional, personal, and charged. Certainly we know that oral contraceptive users are less likely to develop benign breast disease. They are also more likely to undergo periodic breast examinations and mammography. Thus with more physician contact, breast disease may be more likely to be detected. In fact, breast cancer in oral contraceptives users is usually detected earlier than in nonusers. Recent reports by the CDC[45] have analyzed oral contraceptive pills in subsequent development of breast cancer. No increased risk for breast cancer was found when the variables of first full-term pregnancy, use of oral contraceptive pills for 4 to 6 years, younger than 20, lack of family history, or prior risk of benign breast disease were considered. Additional studies are being conducted.[45]

Until further reports are published I feel very confident in prescribing oral contraceptive pills to my young patients who have a family history of breast cancer or who have not achieved their first full-term pregnancy.

Cervical cancer. Cervical cancer is more frequent in women who are sexually active than in virgins. There is also growing evidence that cervical cancer is a sexually transmitted disease, related to the human papilloma virus (HPV). Many epidemiologic studies have reported an increased risk of cervical cancer in women using the birth control pill.[256] However, many confounding variables, often known as the "sexuality index," have not been included in the methodology of these scientific studies. This index includes an estimation of the age of first intercourse, number of sexual partners, exposure to HPV, history of smoking, use of barrier methods, and economic status. There does appear to be a twofold to threefold increased risk of carcinoma-in-situ in women who are using oral contraceptives, however, in many of the scientific studies, the "sexuality index" has often not been studied significantly.[256] Patients who use oral contraception also have more office visits and more frequent Pap smears than nonusers. Women who are using barrier methods, such as diaphragms or condoms, are at decreased risk of acquiring sexually transmitted diseases, such as HPV, and subsequently have less risk factors for the development of cervical neoplasia.[256]

Other malignancies. When oral contraception was introduced in this country in the 1960s, there were concerns that its use was associated with increased risk of hepatic carcinoma and malignant melanoma. A recent review of the literature reveals that most of these reports were anecdotal and flawed in their design. In general, the risk of hepatic carcinoma or malignant melanoma is not increased in oral contraceptive users.[82]

Uterine fibroids. In 1986, the Oxford Family Planning Association noted a decreased risk of uterine fibroids of 30% in patients who had used oral contraceptives for at least 10 years.[227] Obese women in the study had less risk reduction than women with ideal body weight. Women who smoked also had an increased risk for uterine fibroids. The biological mechanism behind these effects may be related to the progestin-dominant effect of the birth control pills and the decreased risk of unopposed estrogen (which has been related to increased risk of fibroids).[227] Because pelvic fibroids are the most common pelvic tumor in women, the decreased risk of uterine fibroids in women using birth control pills may also be considered a major protective benefit of birth control pills. Uterine fibroids are often associated with heavier menstrual blood flow, pelvic pain, and need for surgical procedures. If this protective effect proves to be true, the quality of life for many women can thereby be improved.[227]

Toxic shock syndrome. In the early 1980s, a plethora of medical studies suggested an increased risk of toxic shock syndrome in menstruating women. Toxic shock syndrome was originally reported in women using superabsorbent tampons. More recent data by Gray suggest that an indirect benefit of oral contraceptives is decreased menstrual blood flow and decreased menstrual blood loss, thereby lowering the need for women to use superabsorbent tampons. If there is less blood loss, a slender or light tampon could be used, thereby indirectly decreasing the risk for toxic shock.[107]

Improving patient compliance. The birth control pill is an excellent means of contraception. However, most studies reveal that the discontinuation rate of the birth control pill in the first year may approximate 25% to 30%.[212] A study by Grady found that one third of married women between ages 15 and 44 discontinue birth control pills in 1 year. Many of these women who did discontinue the birth control pill failed to use any other effective means of contraception during that subsequent year.[105]

The most common reason women discontinue the birth control pill may be lack of education regarding frequent but often reversible and temporary side effects of the pills.[105] Some women become dissatisfied with the pill because of related physical problems or aberrations in the menstrual cycle that may occur initially. A survey by Pratt revealed that of the patients who quit the birth control pill, 98% do so because of perceived physical problems, including weight gain, nausea, headache, or menstrual abnormalities that are related to the use of the pill.[212] Less frequently, women discontinue the pill because they develop hypertension or heart disease while on the pill.[212] Adolescent patients more frequently discontinue the pill because of concerns about their future fertility, possible birth defects associated with the pill, risk of cancer, or the interaction with cigarettes.[84]

The modern oral contraceptive pill is generally safe and patients should be advised of this. The modern pill of the 1990s bears little resemblance to its early predecessor. However, the memories of the media, public, and patient take years to fade. Yes, the early pill had problems, but the new monophasic or triphasic preparations are safe for most patients.

Patients should be informed of the following:
- Hypertension rarely occurs in oral contraceptive users; less than 5% of patients develop this idiosyncratic phenomenon.
- Only cigarette smokers over the age of 35 using oral

contraceptives have an increased risk of dying from myocardial infarction and stroke. Women on oral contraceptives under the age of 35 do not share this increased risk if they are smokers.

- The risk of atherosclerosis appears to be lower in oral contraceptive pill users than in nonusers. Young women on oral contraceptives dying from myocardial infarction have less extensive atherosclerotic changes in their blood vessels when compared with nonusers.
- Pregnancy rates are .1 to 3% per year in highly motivated patients.
- Oral contraceptive pills cost approximately $15 to $22 per cycle.
- Fertility is not decreased in previous oral contraceptive users. There is a slight delay in achieving pregnancy in previous oral contraceptive users compared with non-users. This is due to the suppressive effects on the hypothalamic pituitary axis.

It is extremely important to counsel patients not only about the contraceptive benefits, but also about the noncontraceptive benefits that result from using birth control pills. All patients should be educated thoroughly at their first visit about usual nuisance side effects, such as irregular bleeding, breakthrough bleeding, mild weight gain, or nausea. These side effects should be discussed in relation to the overall benefits of the pill. In addition to verbal instruction, written material may be helpful to the patient to keep at home, including instructions on when to start the pill, what to do if she forgets to take the pill, and anticipated side effects. It is extremely helpful to show the patient the actual package of birth control pills she will be taking, explain the approximate cost of the pill, and give helpful hints on how to remember to take the pill. This can include suggesting that the patient take the pill at the same time each day, such as when she brushes her teeth or goes to bed.

If the patient experiences a side effect, she should be informed that more than 20 different brands of birth control pills are available. Usually making slight adjustments in the estrogen or progesterone component will identify a suitable alternative. The patient should always be informed that she should telephone you or your designated assistant before discontinuing the birth control pills. Especially in adolescent patients, a follow-up visit 6 weeks to 3 months later will aid in improving patient compliance, allay any fears regarding the use of the pill, and encourage continued use of the pill.

To minimize nuisance side effects, it is important to select the birth control pills containing a .030 to .035 mg estrogen preparation. The progestin dose of the birth control pill may need to be altered if nausea, breakthrough bleeding, or breast tenderness occur.

Summary. The formulation of the oral contraceptive pill have evolved greatly over time. Oral contraceptive pills reduce the incidence of many common and often disabling gynecologic conditions. It has been estimated that more than 50,000 hospitalizations are prevented by birth control pills each year.[191] Patients should be assured that not only do birth control pills provide excellent contraceptive benefits and the resulting peace of mind, but also at least nine noncontraceptive benefits are associated with birth control pill use. These include a decreased risk of an ectopic pregnancy, decreased risk of dysmenorrhea, less blood loss and subsequently less chance for developing anemia, decreased risk of pelvic inflammatory disease, decreased incidence of uterine and ovarian cancer, decreased risk of benign breast disease, and decreased risk of rheumatoid arthritis.[191] Additionally, we await further scientific study to determine whether uterine fibroids, toxic shock syndrome, and osteoporosis will also be reduced. Women should be reassured that by choosing the birth control pill, they have chosen a very effective and reversible means of contraception.

HOME PREGNANCY TESTING

The earliest means of pregnancy detection relied on the patient's subjective symptoms of pregnancy, missed menstrual periods, and physical examination confirming enlargement of the uterus. In the 1900s physicians relied solely on Hegar's sign—a differential softness between the uterus and cervix.[149] These variables may not be present until the third month of pregnancy. It is advantageous in certain medical conditions, such as hypertension, diabetes, or history of ectopic pregnancy, to know early if the patient is pregnant.

Tracing the historical development of pregnancy tests, one can see the evolution of improvements in methodology, less time needed to perform the test, improved accuracy of the test, animal-free testing, and development of a testing mechanism that could be performed by the patient.

The first bioassay was developed in 1928, the Ascheim-Zondek (A-Z) test.[98] This test took 96 hours to perform and required multiple injections of human chorionic gonadotropin (HCG) into a rat, which was later sacrificed. This test was sensitive after 1 to 2 weeks of a missed menstrual period, or 3 to 4 weeks after conception.[60] In 1931 the Friedman test was developed, followed by the "South African Frog" bioassay in 1942.[149] In 1960, in vivo bioassays were developed. This was a major advance because animals were no longer necessary. In the 1970s, home pregnancy tests became available.

A new concept in health care has emerged. Consumers increasingly demand that they be involved in decisions about their health and testing. Many self-diagnostic home tests are emerging, including home monitoring for blood pressure, evaluation of hematuria, glucose testing, hemoccult stool testing, pregnancy testing, ovulation prediction, strep throat testing, urinary tract infection tests, and visual acuity tests.[226]

The sales of home self-testing products have increased

Table 30-1. Comparison of various contraceptive methods[32,155,249]

Method	Pros	Cons	Cost

Oral contraceptives	Decreased incidence of dysmenorrhea
	Decreased menstrual blood loss
	Less risk of anemia
	Decreased risk of ovarian and endometrial cancer
	Decreased risk of functional ovarian cysts, endometriosis, fibroid uterus, and benign breast disease
	Increases bone density
	Decreased risk of pelvic inflammatory disease
	Improves acne
	Excellent contraceptive effectiveness
	Low failure rate of 0.1% to 3.0%/yr
	Less need for abortions
	Less need for sterilization
	Less risk for ectopic pregnancy
	Decreased risk of rheumatoid arthritis
	May be used in women over the age of 35 and extending to menopause in women without risk factors
		Requires compliant patient for method to be effective
		Must be used daily
		Menstrual irregularities possible (1%-5%):
		  Amenorrhea
		  Breakthrough bleeding
		Headaches, migraine, depression, decreased libido possible
		Drug interactions possible, with carbamazepine, primidone, phenytoin, phenobarbital, and rifampin; alternative contraception should be used in patients taking these drugs
		Should not be used in
		  Women >35 who smoke and/or with
		  Liver disease
		  Breast cancer
		  Prior history of thromboembolic events, MI, cerebrovascular accidents
			$18-$25 per month

Cervical cap	May remain in place 24-48 hours after intercourse Less spermicide needed than with diaphragm Less noticeable to partner Not a systemic form of contraception Less risk of bladder infections Does not affect menstrual blood flow	Patients with distorted cervix cannot be fitted More difficult to teach insertion techniques to patient Potentially may dislodge from cervix during coitus Possible vaginal discharge Requires Pap test after 3 months' use, then annually there after Patients with history of toxic shock syndrome should not use Requires fitting by health care worker or physician	$29-$35 for cap Additional costs for office visit and fitting charges

Norplant	Patient compliance not necessary to achieve effectiveness
	Long-term sustained effectiveness (5 years)
	Not associated with metabolic changes in carbohydrate, lipid, coagulation, liver, kidney, or immunoglobin levels
	Highly effective contraception (less than 0.2% pregnancy rate/yr)
		Requires office visit for insertion and removal
		Menstrual irregularities possible
		Implants may be visible in thin woman
		Women with darker complexions may notice increased pigmentation near the implants
		Not suitable for use in woman with:
		  Active thromboembolic disease
		  Undiagnosed genital bleeding
		  Acute liver disease
		  Liver tumors
		  Known or suspected breast cancer
		Does not protect against STDs
			$500-$700/5 years; includes office visit and removal

Continued.

Table 30-1. Comparison of various contraceptive methods[32,155,249] —cont'd

Method	Pros	Cons	Cost
Diaphragm	Decreased risk of STDs Provides increased lubrication during coitus Decreased risk of abnormal Pap smear	Failure rate < 18%-20% Vaginal irritation in 1% of patients Requires fitting by health care professional UTIs approximately twice as common as in oral contraceptive users Should not be prescribed in patients with history of toxic shock syndrome	$20/diaphragm Additional costs for office visit and fitting charges
Condoms	Decreased risk of transmission of STDs Can be purchased over the counter Are usable for 5 years if stored properly	Less effective if oil-based lubricants used Breakage of condoms 1-12 per 100 acts of vaginal intercourse Requires motivation and compliance by the patient and partner Higher breakage rate of condoms with anal intercourse	$8-$12/dozen
Contraceptive sponge	Can be purchased over the counter May be left in place for 24 hours after placement and does not have to be removed after each act of coitus during this time	Allergic reaction noted in 4% 8% of patients complain of decreased lubrication Patients with marked pelvic relaxation may find insertion and retention of the sponge difficult Only one size currently available Occasionally difficult to remove	Three for $5
Spermicides	Offers protection against STDs Inexpensive Easy to insert Does not require prescription	Failure rate 20%/yr Must be placed intravaginally 10-30 minutes before coitus Must be reapplied after each act of coitus 1%-5% develop an allergic reaction	$7-$10/tube
IUD	Paragard IUD (may remain in situ for 8 years) Pregnancy rate 0.5%-1%/yr Continuation rate is greater than other reversible methods Does not require patient motivation for success	Progestasert IUD must be removed yearly 5%-15% of IUDs removed within 1 year because of pain or bleeding May be associated with increased incidence of dysmenorrhea or menorrhagia Cannot be used in woman with prior history of endocarditis, rheumatic heart disease, or prosthetic heart valves IUDs must be inserted by health professional Not advised for patients with multiple sexual partners or uterine anomalies (bicornuate uterus, fibroids, or cervical stenosis) Immunocompromised patients should not use IUD	Paragard $200/8 years Progestasert: $175/yr Additional fees for insertion and removal
Sterilization	Safest of all contraceptive methods Low failure rate of 1-3 in 500 patients Should be considered a permanent procedure	Mortality 1.5/100,000 procedures Usually requires ambulatory hospital setting and anesthesia If pregnancy occurs 20% incidence of ectopic Approximately 2-5/1000 sterilized woman regret their decision	$500-$1000 plus additional costs of ambulatory facility and anesthesia

Table 30-2. Home pregnancy tests

Test kit	Concentration sensitivity HCG mIU/ml	Sensitivity %	Specificity %	Approximate cost
Accutest	400-800	51.7	88.9	$10
Advance	50-150	91.2	100	$11
Answer-2	200	100	93.5	$12
EPT-Plus	1000	94.6	100	$12
Fact	50-150	100	93.5	$13
First Response	50	92.9	100	$13
Predictor	600-900	100	76.7	$10

(Adapted from Latman N et al: Evaluation of home pregnancy test kits, *Biomed Instrument Tech* 23:144, 1989.)

from $515 million in 1986 to $1.4 billion in 1992, with an average growth rate of 18% per year projected over the next 5 years.[124]

Sales for home pregnancy testing grew to $72 million in 1987 from $35 million in 1984. It is estimated that one out of 10 pregnancy tests now is performed at home. The largest competitors in home pregnancy testing, Ortho Pharmaceutical and Warner-Lambert, spent $8 million on consumer advertising in 1986.[59]

Monoclonal antibody testing

Monoclonal antibody testing has replaced the earlier hemagglutination inhibition test. The monoclonal antibody test offers great sensitivity, which approaches that of the serum radioimmunoassay, and is as economical as the latex hemagglutination-inhibition slide test.[33] In his excellent review, Bluestein states that "monoclonal antibodies are produced by hybridomas. These cell culture lines are manufactured by fusion of B-lymphocytes and myeloma cells, uniting the specificity of the antibody production by B-lymphocytes with high production capacity of myeloma cells."[33] Because the antibody is specific and uniform for one part of the hormone, these antibodies will bind only to a single antigenic site on the HCG molecule.[33] This will prevent cross reactivity with antigens that are not related to HCG and will allow greater specificity and sensitivity of monoclonal antibody testing.[40]

Pregnancy test kits are based on the premise that HCG is secreted in the urine and can be detected by monoclonal antibody testing. HCG is detected approximately 8 days after fertilization or 1 to 2 days after implantation. Most home test kits require that at least 0.2 IU/ml HCG or greater be present for pregnancy to be detected. Generally, this corresponds to the quantity of HCG that is detected at the time of the first missed menstrual cycle, or 24 to 27 days following the end of the previous menstrual period.[18,89]

Most monoclonal antibody tests become positive when the HCG values are 20 to 50 mIU/ml. Urine is placed on a membrane with antialpha monoclonal antibodies; HCG and the urine bind to the membrane. A solution is then added that reacts with a beta subunit, creating an antibody-HCG antibody complex.[89]

Next, the second antibody attaches to the complex, which will form a blue dot created by an enzymatic reaction with alkaline phosphatase. A blue dot indicates a positive pregnancy test.[89] The reliability and accuracy of a home pregnancy test depend on the patient, her comfort in interpreting the instructions, and her care in following the instructions. Most studies have shown that patients with higher incomes, older patients, and those with more formal education have consistently more accurate results.[89]

The FDA requires that home pregnancy testing have a 95% or greater accuracy when performed correctly. Translated, this means that one must determine both the sensitivity and the specificity of the pregnancy test kit. The sensitivity of a pregnancy test is the percentage of pregnant women who obtain positive results (true positives); the specificity is the percentage of women who are not pregnant and obtain negative results (true negatives).[60]

The modern monoclonal antibody urine pregnancy tests are less prone to false-positive results. However, false positives have been reported in women with staphylococcal urinary tract infections, abortion, miscarriage, lung cancers (small cell), choriocarcinoma, and ovarian cancer[33]; and false-negative results have been seen if the urine or pregnancy test kit is chilled, if the test is done too early in the menstrual cycle, or if instructions are not followed sequentially.[33]

More than 10 products are marketed for home pregnancy testing. They differ in several qualities, including cost, ease of use, time required to perform the test, and how early the test can be performed after missing a menstrual cycle. For instance, the Q Test (Becton-Dickson) can be performed 1 day after a missed menstrual cycle and requires 5 to 15 minutes after the test is performed to produce results; the product Answer (Carter Products) cannot be performed until 3 days after a missed menstrual period, and it takes approximately 60 minutes to perform.[215]

Nine pregnancy test kits were evaluated for optimal accuracy, sensitivity, ease of operation, and definitude of results.[149] The optimal accuracies of nine pregnancy test kits range from 97.1% to 69.6%.[149] Certain individual brands of home pregnancy tests show tendencies toward false-positive results (these included Predictor and Daisy brands) or false-negative results (Accutest). The EPT plus, First Response, and Advance tests seem to yield very definitive results, with the most sensitive test being the revised First Response test.[149] Tests that use a change in the color to indicate a positive pregnancy test were preferred by 86.2% of patients vs. 12.3% for a precipitate response. The EPT test consistently detected at least 150 mIU/ml of HCG, and the revised First Response detected 112 mIU/ml in the urine 100% of the time.[149] A Latman and Bruot[224] study appears to show that the optimal accuracy, specificity, detection, sensitivity, and human factor variations were wide among the home pregnancy test kits that were evaluated.[149] Because the HCG values double every 48 hours in a normal pregnancy,[224] a test may be more accurate if the patient waits 2 to 4 days from her missed menses before performing the test. This may decrease the need for repeat testing that is often seen in patients performing the test too early.

Several enzymatic reactions are necessary to perform the monoclonal antibody urine testing. These enzymatic reactions are both time and temperature dependent. If the specimen or test solution is cold, the enzymatic reactions may be reduced, and this may lead to a false-negative reading.[18]

Who purchases home pregnancy tests

In the 1988 National Maternal Infant Health Survey, Jeng et al. studied 4700 women from varying sociodemographic backgrounds who used home pregnancy testing. They found that the most frequent users were white, married, over the age of 35, and highly educated, and had high family income.[134] She concluded that this patient population was more likely to use home pregnancy tests because of several factors. The current cost of the urine pregnancy home test kit ($12 to $17) may make this modality unaffordable to patients from lower socioeconomic classes. In addition, older women may have a higher frequency of use because of their increased risk of infertility and because older women may feel more comfortable performing the tests and interpreting the results.[134]

College students are also frequent users of home pregnancy tests. In 1987 Coons et al. studied college students entering a student health center and found that one of six females seeking pregnancy testing had used a pregnancy test kit before coming to the student health clinic for pregnancy testing. Approximately 64.3% of these had used this kit only once. They purchased the kit because they often thought that they might be pregnant. In 40% of the cases, the student had a cluster of pregnancy-related symptoms, (breast tenderness, nausea, vomiting); 67.2% of students had missed a period; and 25% had "intercourse and wor-

ried and wondered if they were pregnant and 19% had indicated that they had not used or misused birth control measures."[60] In addition, other primary reasons for using a home pregnancy test included the speed of obtaining results, confidentiality, convenience, and accuracy.[60] More than 90% of the students in this study felt that they had confidence in performing the test and were comfortable with the accuracy of the results they had obtained.

Most patients purchasing home pregnancy tests do so at a pharmacy or a drug store. Major factors influencing the selection of a specific brand of home pregnancy test are advertisements, price, and information on the package. Less than 3% of patients use the advice from their physician, and less than 6% rely on recommendations made by the pharmacist. Rarely do patients identify cost as a factor in selecting the test.[59]

Patients who benefit from home pregnancy testing

Patients can be notoriously inaccurate in their determination of their risk for pregnancy. Ramoska studied three historical variables that might be associated with pregnancy. He found that even if the last menstrual period was on time, the patient thought she was not pregnant, and the patient said there was "no chance" that she could be pregnant, there was still at least a 10% chance that she was pregnant.[216] Therefore home pregnancy testing can provide helpful early information to allow women to accurately know whether they are pregnant.

In addition, a patient at high risk for ectopic pregnancy, such as a patient who has had previous tubal surgery or a prior ectopic pregnancy, may be advised to have a very early pregnancy test when her menstrual period is more than 2 or 3 days late.[217] Urine monoclonal antibody testing can detect urinary HCGs when corresponding serum levels are between 20 and 50 mIU/ml, and the quantitative serum can detect HCG concentrations of less than 10 mIU/ml. Less than 3% of patients with ectopic pregnancies have serum HCG concentrations below 40 mIU/ml, and very few would be missed by a urine monoclonal test.[224] Ectopic pregnancies that produce HCG of less than 40 mIU/ml are not as likely to undergo rupture and are more likely to undergo spontaneous reabsorption of the pregnancy. These patients can be treated with serum quantitative HCG every 48 hours.[34]

Other patients likely to benefit from early pregnancy testing include women over the age of 35 and women who have a history of an abnormal fetus and who may be candidates for early chorionic villus sampling (CVS) for genetic studies. A patient with these characteristics who was able to confirm an early pregnancy should be seen within the first several weeks of her pregnancy so that the early CVS could be scheduled.[217]

In addition, patients with diabetes should have early pregnancy tests to optimally manage their glucose. Because pregnant diabetics are at increased risk of congenital abnormalities, tight glucose control is recommended pre-conceptually and in the early first trimester. In addition, patients with hypertension and uterine anomalies may benefit from early urine testing.[15] Infertility patients using Clomiphene to induce ovulation may experience late or scanty menstrual cycles. Before one adjusts the dose of Clomiphene, a patient with a slight irregularity of her menstrual cycle may benefit from home pregnancy testing, to ensure that the Clomiphene is not restarted when she is pregnant.[217]

In addition, some patients have episodes of oligoamenorrhea and are uncertain whether they are pregnant. A home pregnancy test may be helpful to patients who are more than 40 to 60 days late for their menstrual cycle and who have had unprotected intercourse. In addition, patients who are on oral contraceptive pills and who complain of a scanty menstrual cycle may consider taking a home pregnancy test. If a patient has missed more than two or three pills during the month, the patient has been on antibiotics, or patient compliance is a concern, a pregnancy test should be offered to ensure that pregnancy has not occurred[217] (see the box at right).

Basal body temperature

Another method of home pregnancy testing is measurement of basal body temperature (BBT). Some patients may be candidates for taking their basal body temperature.

Many years ago, before home pregnancy testing, patients and physicians alike relied on the basal body temperature chart to detect ovulation and possible pregnancy. Today, this is called the symptothermal method. This method requires a woman to take her temperature before arising from bed each morning. This is necessary because activity and movement will alter metabolism and temperature. Any thermometer will suffice, including a digital thermometer, rectal thermometer, or oral thermometer. The medical literature has widely shown that progesterone that is secreted after ovulation is thermogenic and thus causes a slight rise in temperature. In fact, before ovulation, basal body temperature is slightly lower than normal basal body temperature. Once ovulation has occurred, the basal body temperature increases by 0.4° to 0.8° F or 0.2° to 0.4° C until just days before menstruation. A basal body temperature consistently above 98.2° F for 7 to 10 days in a row can correlate with early pregnancy.[217] However, approximately 10% to 15% of patients who ovulate will not demonstrate a biphasic BBT. Many pregnant woman complain of feeling warm or hot all the time. This may be caused by the increased blood flow, supply, and volume that occur with pregnancy, or also by the slight increase in temperature caused by higher levels of progesterone.

Summary

Home diagnostic urine pregnancy tests will continue to be an important component of the expanding self-testing

---

> **Candidates for home pregnancy testing**
>
> Any patient without reliable contraception with a missed menses can be offered home pregnancy testing. Additional patient groups include:
> 1. Infertility patients
> 2. Patients who misuse/disuse of contraception
> 3. Missed menses in patient with history of ectopic pregnancy
> 4. Patients 35 years of age or older
> 5. Diabetic patients planning pregnancy
> 6. Patients using Clomiphene with scanty or irregular menses
> 7. Patients with oligoamenorrhea
> 8. Hypertensive patients
> 9. Women with uterine anomalies (biscornuate or septate uterus)
> 10. In women before elective radiography procedures

product market. Patients with risk factors for ectopic pregnancy, history of recurrent miscarriages, infertility problems, or misuse of contraception will be ideal candidates for home testing. Patient involvement, motivation, education, and formal training may influence test results. Prompt office follow-up is essential for patients who may have "at-risk pregnancies."

Osteoporosis and menopause

Holly L. Thacker

Menopause begins with the onset of the last menstrual period. A woman is born with a limited number of ovarian follicles available for ovulation. After approximately 400 ovulations, the reproductive capacity is exhausted and endogenous estrogen levels decline. The decline of ovarian function is gradual and begins around age 35. The average age range of menopause is 40 to 55, with the median approximately 51 years. Mature women are defined as women who are past the age of childbearing. Cigarette smokers undergo menopause a few years earlier than nonsmokers because of faster estrogen metabolism in the liver.

The average age of menopausal onset has not changed much in the last century; however, the average life span of a woman has lengthened. Therefore the amount of time a woman spends in an estrogen-deficient state is increasing, with certain physiologic and metabolic consequences. The climacterium is the period of prolonged estrogen deficiency.

The onset of the menopause is an excellent time to reassess a woman's overall health and need for health maintenance, including the need for estrogen-replacement therapy. Menopause can be medically viewed as an adult-onset primary hypogonadism, with five target areas primarily affected. These effects are skin and hair changes, genitourinary atrophy, neuroendocrine and vasomotor changes, skeletal bone loss, and most important, an increase in cardiovascular disease. These changes may affect women differently and occur over a variable time span. Constitutional factors, genetic predisposition, and the level of endogenous estrogen production from nonovarian sources play a role in this variability. Adrenal androstendione is converted peripherally into estrone in adipose tissue; therefore obese women tend to have higher estrogen levels and less problems with osteoporosis. However, obese women tend to have problems from this unopposed estrogen. Unopposed estrogen may lead to endometrial hyperplasia and an increased risk of endometrial cancer. Obesity, particularly android obesity, is associated with increased rates of hyperlipidemia, diabetes mellitus, cardiovascular disease, and some types of cancer.

SKIN AND HAIR CHANGES

The lack of ovarian follicle production of estrogen coupled with the continuous production of androgens from remaining ovarian stroma lead to some skin and hair changes in many postmenopausal women. These changes result from both the estrogen deficiency and the relative androgen excess. The estrogen deficiency skin changes include loss of elasticity and decreased collagen. Dryness of mucosal surfaces may occur. Relative androgen excess symptoms include minor facial hirsutism, deepening of the upper voice register, and an androgenic-pattern alopecia in women who are genetically predisposed to this pattern.

Women who undergo surgical menopause, that is, bilateral oophorectomy, tend to experience less androgen-excess skin and hair problems, as approximately half of all androgens are produced in the ovary. The remaining endogenous androgens in women are produced in the adrenal gland.

UROGENITAL CHANGES

Urogenital atrophy can be manifested by dyspareunia, blood-tinged vaginal discharge from atrophic vaginitis, irritable bladder with urinary frequency and urgency, and pruritis vulvae. Pelvic relaxation may also be accentuated. Urogenital atrophy can be treated with topical estrogen therapy or with systemic estrogen-replacement therapy. Topical estrogen is well absorbed from the thin, atrophic vaginal mucosa; however, once the integrity of the vaginal mucosa is improved, the systemic absorption diminishes, and therefore the systemic effects of estrogen replacement are not maintained. Lubrin and Replens are two nonhormonal, over-the-counter products that can provide vaginal lubrication.

Sexual function can be affected as a direct consequence of urogenital atrophy and resultant dyspareunia. Sexual function may be secondarily affected if a woman is having vasomotor symptoms and sleep disturbance. Women who undergo surgical menopause may, in addition, report decreased libido resulting from a decreased level of endogenous testosterone.[234] These women may be candidates for hormone replacement that includes small doses of testosterone as in Estratest and Estratest HS (half strength).

NEUROENDOCRINE CHANGES

Neuroendocrine changes include the well-known vasomotor symptoms that affect at least half of all menopausal women. The hot flash (sensation of warmth) and the hot flush (sensation of warmth coupled with the appearance of facial erythema) can range from a minor inconvenience in some women to a debilitating symptom in others. The sensation typically begins around the upper torso and neck and spreads to the face and head. It may be accompanied by diaphoresis. This phenomenon is more likely to occur at night, in warm environments, after ingesting warm beverages, or after alcohol or caffeine ingestion. If the hot flashes occur at night they can lead to a sleep disturbance, with consequent fatigue and depression. Psychiatric disease is not increased in menopausal women; however, women with a history of poor coping patterns and/or depression may have preexisting psychiatric disturbances exacerbated if they have hot flashes and an associated sleep disturbance.[264]

The physiology of the hot flash/flush is not clearly defined; however, it is thought to involve hypothalamic involvement with pulses of gonadotropin-releasing factors, which affect the autonomic nervous system and lead to vasomotor instability. Untreated hot flashes may last for 2 to 3 years; however, some women experience these uncomfortable sensations for decades. For some women, these symptoms can interfere with the quality of life.

ACCELERATION OF BONE LOSS

Estrogen deficiency affects the musculoskeletal system by accelerating bone loss over bone formation. Estrogen receptors are present in bone tissue. Type I osteoporosis, primarily trabecular bone loss, is accelerated in menopausal women. The spine is composed primarily of trabecular bone. The average woman reaches peak bone mass at around 30 to 35 years of age. Approximately 1% of bone is lost per year, with the percentage rising to as much as 4% to 5% per year in the face of estrogen deficiency for the 10 to 15 years after menopausal onset. Estrogen replacement retards this loss and stabilizes bone mass in the vast majority of women receiving estrogen. Both oral estrogens and transdermal estrogen are approved by the FDA for both the prevention and treatment of postmenopausal osteoporosis. The prior use of estrogen-replacement therapy in postmenopausal women has been shown to protect against fractures, including the potentially deadly hip fracture.[139]

Calcium alone will not prevent the accelerated loss of trabecular bone; however, calcium is needed as a substrate for estrogen's beneficial effect on bone. In addition, calcium supplementation alone may help prevent the type II senile osteoporosis of cortical bone. The hip is primarily composed of cortical bone.

A menopausal woman needs to understand that calcium and exercise, while important for a number of reasons, are not a substitute for estrogen replacement. Aging and estrogen deficiency are associated with a decrease in calcium absorption from the gut. Therefore, it is recommended that women over the age of 55 years ingest a total of 1500 mg of calcium a day and that women under the age of 55 years ingest 1200 mg of calcium per day in the absence of abnormal calcium metabolism; however, osteopenic women need estrogen replacement to protect against further bone loss.

RISK FACTORS FOR OSTEOPOROSIS

Risk factors for osteoporosis include: underweight for height; small bone structure; white (especially Northern European descent) or Asian; tobacco, alcohol, and caffeine excess; and a diet low in calcium (which is typical of the U.S. high-fat, high-protein, low-fiber diet). The medical conditions that predispose to osteoporosis include: primary hyperparathyroidism, endogenous hypercortisolism or exogenous glucocorticoid use, multiple myeloma, and hyperthyroidism. Even slight overreplacement of thyroid hormone has been shown to accelerate bone loss.[244] Many perimenopausal women are receiving thyroid hormone for primary hypothyroidism. These women may be clinically euthyroid; however, they may be biochemically slightly overreplaced, which is reflected in a suppressed supersensitive TSH (thyroid stimulating hormone) level.

It is not possible to clinically predict with accuracy which women will develop osteoporosis. Bone densitometry of the lumbosacral spine and hips helps determine which women are at increased risk for fractures based on a degree of osteopenia compared with age-matched controls. However, bone densitometry is expensive and provides information only about the current, not future, status of the bone.

Half of all white women have osteopenia by age 60 to 65. Hip fractures may be one end result of osteoporosis and are associated with a significant morbidity and mortality. Furthermore, hip fractures contribute significantly to health care expenditures. Both the individual and societal benefits of preventing or at least delaying the onset of osteoporotic medical complications are clear. Wrist fractures (particularly Colles' fracture) and thoracic spinal compression fractures causing the so-called "dowager's hump" are also well-recognized complications of osteoporosis that at the very least affect a woman's quality of life.

TREATMENT OF OSTEOPOROSIS

Once osteoporosis is established, it is very difficult to treat, and therefore supportive care with palliative measures is often required. The medical treatment goals are to prevent further bone loss and to lessen resultant pain that may result from spontaneous fractures. There are no known medical treatments that will completely restore both normal bone mass and architecture in trabecular and cortical bone. Because of the difficulties encountered in treating established osteoporosis, the patient and the clinician must give preventive measures utmost consideration.

Prevention of osteoporosis clearly is key, as treatment of osteoporosis is generally unsatisfactory. Fluoride can increase trabecular bone mass but has not decreased fracture incidence. Fluoride treatment is frequently fraught with side effects and is mentioned primarily as a historical footnote. Calcitonin can stabilize bone mass for about 2 years and has been noted to be analgesic for the bone pain in some patients. Calcitonin acts directly through receptors in osteoclasts to decrease osteoclastic activity. It is expensive and administered by subcutaneous injection. The salmon calcitonin can cause allergic reactions. Intranasal administration of calcitonin is available in Europe and, one hopes, will be available in the United States soon. Calcitonin's effects unfortunately may last for only approximately 2 years, and this is a limiting factor.

Didronel (etidronate), a bisphosphonate, has been shown to stabilize and actually improve trabecular bone mass in a 2-year study.[260] A decrease in vertebral spinal fractures was noted. This compound inhibits osteoclast-mediated bone resorption. This medicine is administered daily on an empty stomach for adequate absorption for 2 weeks out of every 3 months. Diarrhea and gastrointestinal upset may occur in some patients. Calcium supplementation is given during the Didronel-free periods. Didronel has been studied in postmenopausal osteoporosis for only a few years. The long-term effects and the continued benefit for bone are not known.

OSTEOPOROSIS PROPHYLAXIS FOR THE WOMAN WITH BREAST CANCER

For the woman with breast cancer, the issue of osteoporosis prophylaxis is challenging, as most clinicians consider a personal history of breast cancer an absolute contraindication for estrogen-replacement therapy. Tamoxifen is a nonsteroidal mixed estrogen agonist and antagonist. Tamoxifen has an antiestrogen effect on breast tissue and is used clinically to treat women with breast cancer.

Tamoxifen has agonist activity on trabecular bone and may preserve bone mass in women with breast cancer who are not thought to be candidates for estrogen replacement. A recent study demonstrated that postmenopausal women treated with tamoxifen had preservation of the bone density of the lumbar spine.[157] Whether the favorable effect on bone density is accompanied by a decrease in fracture risk is yet to be proven. Tamoxifen also exerts an agonist effect on the uterus. Therefore any postmenopausal bleeding in a woman on tamoxifen needs to be carefully evaluated.

Tamoxifen, which may protect bone, will not lessen vasomotor reactions. Therefore other agents used to treat hot flashes need to be considered in the woman who cannot or will not use estrogen replacement. Clonidine, a centrally acting alpha-2 agonist, will relieve vasomotor symptoms in some women and is available in a patch in three strengths. Naproxen, a nonsteroidal antiinflammatory medicine, has also been found to be helpful in reducing vasomotor symptoms. Bellergal, a combination medicine with the barbiturate phenobarbital, has also been used with some success; however, care needs to be exercised when using a potentially addictive drug.

Intermittent, cyclical Didronel therapy might also be considered for women with a history of breast cancer to preserve trabecular bone mass; however, further study is needed. Calcitonin, as described previously, is another agent to consider.

CARDIOVASCULAR SYSTEM CHANGES

Calculations have shown that a 50-year-old white woman is 10 times more likely to die from cardiovascular disease than from either hip fractures or breast cancer.[68] Deaths from premature cardiovascular disease are at least as likely for black women. Because cardiovascular disease is the number-one cause of death in mature women, strategies to reduce cardiovascular morbidity and mortality need to be addressed as vigorously in women as in men. However, in women, surgical menopause and premature menopause are significant risk factors for coronary artery disease, in addition to the traditional risk factors of tobacco use, diabetes mellitus, hyperlipidemia, family history, and advancing age. Even "natural" menopause may be a risk factor for coronary artery disease.[169]

Recent observational epidemiologic studies have strongly suggested that estrogen-replacement therapy in women reduces cardiovascular deaths significantly.[24,85] One study of more than 8800 postmenopausal women found that the death rate from all causes in women who had been on estrogen-replacement therapy for more than 15 years was reduced by 40%.[117] The Boston Nurses' Health Study found that the risk for heart disease was reduced by 70% in current users of estrogen-replacement therapy and that the risk was reduced by 50% for women who had ever received estrogen replacement therapy.[245] The marked reduction in cardiovascular mortality seen in women who have received estrogen-replacement therapy strongly suggests that the majority of mature women, particularly those with atherosclerotic heart disease or at risk for atherosclerotic heart disease, should be considered for estrogen replacement on this basis alone.

The cardioprotective effect of estrogen-replacement therapy is in part thought to be related to the effects on lipoprotein ratios. Oral conjugated estrogens decrease total cholesterol, decrease LDL-cholesterol, and increase HDL-cholesterol levels. Transdermal estradiol (Estraderm) decreases both total cholesterol and LDL-cholesterol and does not increase triglycerides (which may occur with oral estrogen in some predisposed women). Elevated triglyceride levels are usually inversely associated with HDL-cholesterol levels. The Lipid Research Clinic study demonstrated that a 1% reduction in total cholesterol leads to a 2% reduction in the risk of coronary disease. Analyses examining the complex association between estrogen use and cardiovascular mortality suggest that the cardioprotective effect of estrogen is mediated in significant part through the increase in HDL-cholesterol.[41]

Other investigators have suggested that the favorable lipid effects constitute only part of the cardiovascular benefit of estrogen replacement. Estradiol improves smooth muscle tone and has a direct beneficial effect on vessel wall physiology. Low doses of conjugated estrogen are not associated with the increases in the coagulation system that are seen with oral contraceptive doses of estrogen. Renin substrate is not increased in women who receive transdermal estradiol (which avoids enterohepatic metabolism).[52] Blood pressure is not adversely affected by estrogen replacement; rather, there is a small, statistically significant decrease in mean blood pressure for women on estrogen replacement therapy. A very small percentage of women may have an idiosyncratic reaction to oral estrogen with subsequent elevation of the blood pressure. However, these women can usually tolerate the estrogen patch, which avoids enterohepatic metabolism and thus has no effect on the renin-angiotensin system.

ESTROGEN REPLACEMENT AND THE BREAST

The effect of estrogen replacement on the breast is somewhat controversial. Estrogen is a trophic growth hormone and therefore may promote the growth of existing breast cancer. However, estrogen is not thought to be a carcinogen. A recent metaanalysis of the major breast cancer studies does not show any increased risk of breast cancer in ever users of estrogen vs. never users of estrogen replacement; however, this is a controversial area. The results of studies published before 1985 can be summarized as showing perhaps a small increase in breast cancer risk after many years of estrogen use, but even this conclusion has been debated.[128] The prospective Boston Nurses' Health Study notably concluded that many years of past estrogen use did not increase the risk of breast cancer, but that current use may modestly increase the risk for breast cancer.[54]

However, it appears that even if there is an increased risk for breast cancer associated with the use of estrogen replacement, the risk is small and is offset by the apparent cardioprotection afforded to most women. Unwarranted fear of breast cancer alone should not dissuade a woman from receiving estrogen replacement if she is otherwise a good candidate. However, women at high risk for breast cancer may be a different subgroup. Fibrocystic breasts are not a contraindication for estrogen replacement. However, women with dysplasia on breast biopsy are at increased risk for breast cancer, and one must exercise care when prescribing any hormone replacement. Women with a family history of a first-degree relative with premenopausal breast cancer are also at increased risk for breast cancer.

CONTRAINDICATIONS TO HORMONE REPLACEMENT

Absolute contraindications to estrogen replacement have included primarily estrogen-receptor-positive breast cancer. Recently, some physicians have suggested that this may be too dogmatic.[63] Some women with presumably cured breast cancer may be more likely to expire from heart disease and/or suffer the consequences of osteoporosis. Tamoxifen may be the answer to both bone protection and decreased cardiovascular risk in the woman with breast cancer; however, further study is needed. Because tamoxifen may cause stimulation and proliferation of the endometrium, any postmenopausal bleeding in a woman on tamoxifen needs to be evaluated.

Pregnancy is an obvious absolute contraindication to hormone replacement therapy. Occasionally, a perimenopausal woman with amenorrhea may be pregnant, and one should rule this out before starting hormone replacement therapy. Women who have practiced birth control should be advised to continue to do so for 1 year after the onset of menopause, as occasional ovulation can occur after the apparent cessation of natural menses.

Undiagnosed vaginal bleeding is another absolute contraindication to estrogen-replacement therapy. Postmenopausal bleeding must always be evaluated because 10% of women with bleeding will be diagnosed with abnormalities such as adenomatous hyperplasia or endometrial carcinoma. The remainder of women with postmenopausal bleeding will have a proliferative endometrium from lack of progesterone (caused by anovulation), endometrial polyps, cervical or vulvar lesions, or atrophic vaginitis. In the older woman, the vaginal bleeding often is due simply to thin, atrophic vaginitis with resultant tearing and bleeding of the friable vaginal mucosa.

An estrogen-dependent cancer, such as uterine cancer, is not a contraindication for estrogen-replacement therapy provided that the uterine cancer is considered cured either by surgical excision of a low-grade, early-stage cancer, or by lack of evidence of recurrence after 5 years from initial treatment. When progestins are prescribed to women with intact uteri, the increase in endometrial cancers associated with estrogen use alone can be prevented.[199] Ovarian cancers are generally not thought to be estrogen dependent and therefore do not constitute a contraindication to hormone replacement.

Uterine leiomyomata (fibroids) are not an absolute contraindication to estrogen replacement. Fibroids generally shrink in the menopause because of estrogen deficiency. The low doses of estrogen replacement used in the climacterium generally do not cause problems with uterine fibroid enlargement. Lymphangioleiomyomatosis and benign metastasizing leiomyoma are rare conditions that occur in women primarily of the childbearing years. Both of these conditions, which cause fibroid growth in the lung, appear to have hormonal dependence and may therefore be contraindications for estrogen-replacement therapy.

A remote history of deep venous thrombosis is not a contraindication to estrogen replacement therapy. Low doses of conjugated estrogens have not been found to significantly affect hepatic coagulation proteins. In addition, the Estraderm patch, which avoids enterohepatic metabolism altogether, has not been found to change baseline hepatic coagulation proteins at various doses. Therefore this may be an advantage for the woman with a history of prior thromboembolism. The patch may also be more advantageous to women prone to nausea with oral preparations and in smokers who have altered hepatic metabolism of estrogen.

Migraineurs may enjoy relief of their headaches at the onset of menopause. Conversely, they may have worsening of their headaches. Because migraine headaches are thought in part to be due to a hypersensitivity state, selecting an estrogen product that contains only a single substance, such as Estraderm patch (pure 17-B estradiol) or Ogen (estrone), rather than premarin, which is a combination of estrogens including equilenin, equilin, and estrone (obtained from purifying pregnant-horse urine), is thought to be clinically more helpful. To date, this has not been proven by a clinical study. Active liver disease and symptomatic cholelithiasis are relative contraindications to hormone replacement.

MEDICAL EVALUATION OF THE HEALTHY, MATURE WOMAN

The medical evaluation of the healthy mature woman begins with a focused history and physical. One should ask about symptoms of estrogen deficiency, including hot flashes, sleep disturbance, mood and memory changes, skin or hair changes, urinary urgency and frequency, exacerbation of stress urinary incontinence, dyspareunia, pruritis of the vulva, and sexual dysfunction. The medical and gynecologic history along with the drug, dietary, and exercise habits provides the initial basis for risk assessment of the mature woman.

The physical exam should include height, weight, blood pressure, attention to the skin, thyroid, and abdominal, rectal, and pelvic exam, including Papanicolau smears of the endocervix and ectocervix. Signs of pelvic relaxation, including cystocele and rectocele, should be noted. Breast exam with instruction in patient self-examination is important.

Laboratory tests should include a baseline cholesterol level. Follicle stimulating hormone (FSH) and estradiol levels are usually not needed to diagnose the menopausal state but can occasionally be helpful. An FSH greater than

Table 30-3. Approximate relative estrogen potency doses

Medication	Route	Dosage range				
Premarin (conjugated equine estrogens)	PO Vaginal	0.3 mg	0.625 mg* 2-4 g*	0.9 mg	1.25 mg	2.5 mg
Estratab (esterified estrogen)	PO	0.3 mg	0.625 mg*		1.25 mg	2.5 mg
Ogen (estrone)	PO Vaginal		0.625 mg* 2-4 g*		1.25 mg	2.5 mg
Estrace (micronized estradiol)	PO Vaginal		1.0 mg* 1-2 g*		2.0 mg	
Estraderm (17-B-estradiol)	Percutaneous		0.05 mg patch*		0.10 mg patch	

*Recommended minimum dose.

Table 30-4. Approximate relative progestin potency doses

Medication	Route	Dosage range		
Provera (medroxyprogesterone acetate)	PO	2.5 mg*	5.0 mg**	10 mg
Amen, Cycrin (medroxyprogesterone acetate)	PO			10 mg (scored)
Micronor or Nor Q.D. (norethindrone)	PO		0.35 mg**	0.35 mg BID
Norlutate (norethindrone acetate)	PO			One half of scored 5 mg tab = 2.5 mg, which is approximately equal to 15 mg of medroxyprogesterone acetate

*Recommended minimum daily dosage.
**Recommended minimal cyclic dosage.

40 IU/ml and an estradiol level less than 20 pg/ml confirms the primary gonadal failure state. A supersensitive thyroid stimulating hormone (TSH) level can be helpful in detecting possible overreplacement in women on thyroxine replacement who may be at increased risk for bone loss.

A screening mammogram should be obtained yearly in women over the age of 50 years. Bone densitometry with dual energy x-ray absorptiometry (DEXA) should generally be reserved for selected healthy, mature women, particularly those women in whom the results of bone densitometry would affect the decision to institute hormone-replacement therapy. Other health maintenance activities such as immunizations need to be addressed.

HORMONE-REPLACEMENT REGIMENS

The goal of estrogen replacement therapy is not to normalize the FSH value, but rather to use the minimum effective replacement dose to suppress vasomotor reactions, treat urogenital atrophy, prevent bone loss, and provide cardioprotection. This dose for postmenopausal women is generally equivalent to 0.625 mg of conjugated estrogens (Table 30-3). Younger women and women who have undergone surgical menopause may need at least twice this replacement dose to suppress vasomotor symptoms.

Ogen (estrone) is slightly weaker than Premarin by milligram, and therefore this agent may be helpful in the woman prone to breast tenderness. Conversely, breakthrough vasomotor symptoms may occur with Ogen in the woman with little endogenous estrogen production, and therefore 1.25 mg of estrone may be needed. The Estraderm 0.05 mg patch is equivalent to 0.625 mg of conjugated equine estrogens, and the 0.10 patch is equivalent to 1.25 mg of conjugated equine estrogens. The equivalent dose of Estrace (micronized estradiol) is 1 mg to 0.625 mg of conjugated equine estrogen. Estrace may increase sex-binding globulin the most and therefore be of benefit in the mature women with androgen-excess-related skin and hair complaints. Estratab (a combination of estradiol and estrone) is equivalent to Premarin by milligram.

For the woman with an intact uterus, either cycled or continuous progestin therapy is needed to prevent endometrial hyperplasia associated with continuous daily estrogen.

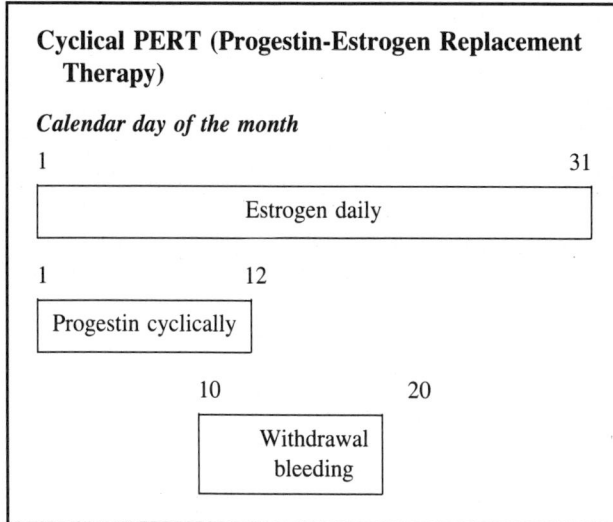

Cyclical PERT (Progestin-Estrogen Replacement Therapy)

Calendar day of the month

1   31

| Estrogen daily |

1   12

| Progestin cyclically |

        10   20

| Withdrawal bleeding |

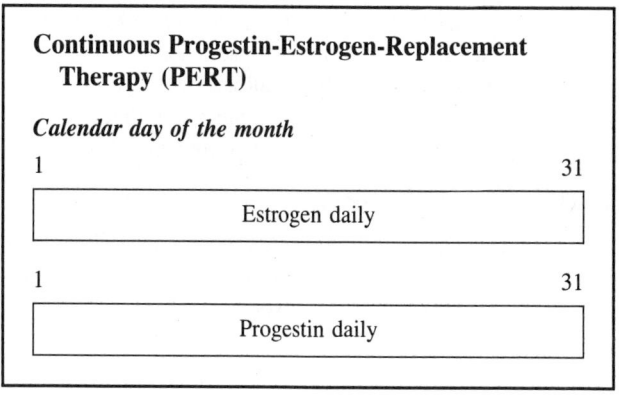

Continuous Progestin-Estrogen-Replacement Therapy (PERT)

Calendar day of the month

1   31

| Estrogen daily |

1   31

| Progestin daily |

Cyclic, progestin-opposed estrogen therapy actually appears to be associated with a lower risk for endometrial carcinoma compared with the postmenopausal woman who receives no hormone replacement.[199] The recommended regimen of hormone replacement includes the use of conjugated estrogens (0.625 mg) daily with the addition of medroxyprogesterone acetate (Provera 5 mg) for the first 12 days of the calender month (See Table 30-4 and the box above). There is no reason to cycle the estrogen replacement, because many women who stop the estrogen replacement for even a few days have resumption of estrogen deficiency symptoms such as hot flashes. Twice the amount of progestin is usually needed to cause maturation of the endometrium from a proliferative phase to a secretory phase in younger women and in heavier women. The latter tend to have higher endogenous levels of estrogens from peripheral aromatization of adrenal androgens.

On the cycled program of Provera for the first 12 calender days, absence of withdrawal bleeding is fine; however, mild uterine bleeding usually occurs midmonth. In the absence of cervical os stenosis/occlusion, absence of withdrawal bleeding simply indicates that there is no endometrial lining to be shed. Uterine bleeding that occurs before day 10 of the calender month needs to be investigated, as this is an indication that the endometrium may be abnormal.[195] There is no reason that cyclic uterine bleeding (on hormone replacement) should be any more confusing to the mature woman or her physician than the cyclic bleeding associated with the previous regular menstrual cycles in the premenopausal woman. In either case, it is the unexpected heavy flow with clots or the intermenstrual or postcoital spotting that needs to be evaluated.

Some women will object to the resumption of monthly uterine bleeding; however, it is generally a small inconvenience for benefits of relieving vasomotor symptoms, reversing urogenital atrophy, preventing the accelerated bone loss associated with estrogen deficiency, and dramatically reducing cardiovascular risk.

A continuous, combined program of daily estrogen and daily progestin can be offered to women who object to monthly menses (see the box above). Little has been published regarding the continuous combined PERT (progestin-estrogen-replacement therapy) regimen; however, the regimen has the advantage of inducing amenorrhea within 6 to 9 months. Progestins work by down regulating the estrogen receptors in the endometrium. The dose of progestin prescribed daily is generally half of the cycled dose, that is 2.5 mg of Provera daily. Using the 5 mg dose of Provera daily for the first few months, followed by the 2.5 mg dose, may induce anenorrhea sooner. Because this is not a cycled program, it is impossible to tell whether uterine bleeding that may occur in the first 9 months is normal or not. Therefore one of the disadvantages of this regimen is the need for outpatient endometrial biopsy at the onset of any uterine bleeding (which is likely to occur in the first few months of noncycled therapy). Furthermore, more research is needed on progestin's effects on lipoprotein metabolism and cardiovascular risk before this program can be recommended for widespread use. Progestins somewhat blunt the favorable lipid changes imparted by estrogen. This continuous combined regimen may become the regimen of choice in the future if cardiovascular benefit is equal compared with the cycled program.

Some women are intolerant of progestins because of premenstrual-like symptoms with mood changes and irritability. Sometimes these women respond to a change in the progestin. The lowest possible dose of progestin should be used to prevent adverse metabolic and psychologic effects. Women without a uterus do not need a progestin (unless they have a recent history of significant endometriosis). Current epidemiologic studies do not support the addition of progestins to estrogen for the purpose of bone or breast protection.[58] For the woman who cannot tolerate progestins and has an intact uterus/endometrium, estrogen-replacement therapy can be prescribed alone as long as both the patient and physician realize that this is a departure from standard practice, that the risk for endometrial cancer from unopposed estrogen-replacement therapy continues for many years after the treatment, and therefore that these women need to be carefully monitored with yearly endometrial biopsies. Cycling the estrogen alone does not protect the endometrium and is not recommended.

ENDOMETRIAL BIOPSY

Endometrial biopsy is indicated in women with a history of unopposed estrogen therapy (on at least a yearly basis). Endometrial biopsy is also indicated for any menopausal woman not on hormone replacement who has any postmenopausal bleeding more than 6 months after cessation of the natural menses. Biopsy is also indicated in women who are on hormone-replacement therapy and have bleeding that is off schedule. A normal bleeding pattern that occurs at the expected time, that is, after the tenth of the calender month, does not need to be investigated with endometrial biopsy. Contraindications to outpatient endometrial biopsy include pregnancy and cervical, uterine, or pelvic infections. Cervical os (internal os and/or external os) stenosis is a relative contraindication.

Most women, particularly parous women without cervical stenosis or atrophy, tolerate the outpatient, pipelle suction endometrial biopsy without much discomfort or need for analgesia. The 3.1 mm flexible, plastic pipelle or 3.0 mm Z-sampler catheter is inserted into the endometrial cavity under aseptic technique. The endometrial tissue is aspirated and curetted by the catheter alone. This mode of endometrial biopsy is simple to perform and represents an improvement over the Vabra technique in terms of patient acceptance and ease of performance (Fig. 30-6, *A-E*). Medical physicians managing menopausal women should become proficient with this outpatient technique.

Women should be referred to a gynecologist for a surgical dilation and curettage (D & C) if any abnormal endometrial tissue is detected by the endometrial sampling. Women who continue to have abnormal bleeding or in whom the pipelle biopsy is unsuccessful should also be referred to a gynecologist. However, the vast majority of mature women on hormone replacement can be successfully managed by the woman's principal medical physician.

SUMMARY

Overall, in the majority of mature women the benefits of estrogen replacement outweigh the risks. However, the majority of mature women presently do not receive hormone-replacement therapy. Unfortunately, the combination of myths and misunderstandings, the nuisance of withdrawal bleeding, and the fear of breast cancer prevents many mature women who are appropriate candidates from receiving estrogen-replacement therapy.

Other times, it is the physician who fails to consider and recommend estrogen-replacement therapy by mistakenly equating contraceptive doses of synthetic estrogens

and their associated cardiovascular/thrombotic effects with the estrogen doses used for hormone replacement. Because a woman was not a candidate for oral contraceptives because of the presence of smoking, hypertension, diabetes, or hyperlipidemia, it does not mean she is not a candidate for estrogen-replacement therapy. Actually, women with these cardiovascular risk factors are excellent candidates for estrogen replacement along with other appropriate medical measures to reduce cardiovascular risk.

Recommended health maintenance guidelines from the 1989 U.S. Preventive Services Task Force include the discussion of estrogen-replacement therapy for female patients who are at "high risk" for osteoporosis.[253] It can be difficult at best to determine an individual woman's risk for osteoporosis on clinical grounds alone, and bone densitometry is currently an expensive tool that many insurance carriers do not cover. By following these guidelines, some women who are not considered "high risk" for osteoporosis will not be counseled and may go on to develop osteoporosis or other complications of prolonged estrogen deficiency. Even with the important issue of osteoporosis prophylaxis aside, I believe that all mature women should be counseled on the benefits and risks of estrogen-replacement therapy, especially in light of the apparent significant cardioprotective advantages of estrogen, as well as the improved quality of life for those women who experience the symptoms of estrogen deficiency.

Urinary incontinence

Richard Troy

Simply stated, *urinary incontinence* is the involuntary loss of urine. Only when urine loss becomes severe or unmanageable does the patient seek medical care. For this reason, the true prevalence of urinary incontinence is unknown. It has been estimated that presently 10 million people suffer from urinary incontinence in the United States. The estimated cost of care for these patients is 10.3 billion dollars annually.[185a] Urinary incontinence affects all age groups but is more common in the elderly than young and more common in females than males. The prevalence of urinary incontinence in institutionalized patients is especially high.

Urinary incontinence threatens both the medical and mental health of the unfortunate patient. Involuntary urine loss may predispose a patient to urinary tract infections, pressure sores, and skin rashes. Urinary incontinence can have a devastating effect on the psychosocial well-being of patients, leading to isolation from their community, family and friends, caretakers, and even spouse. It is therefore necessary that urinary incontinence be recognized as a major source of morbidity that is potentially curable and preventable.

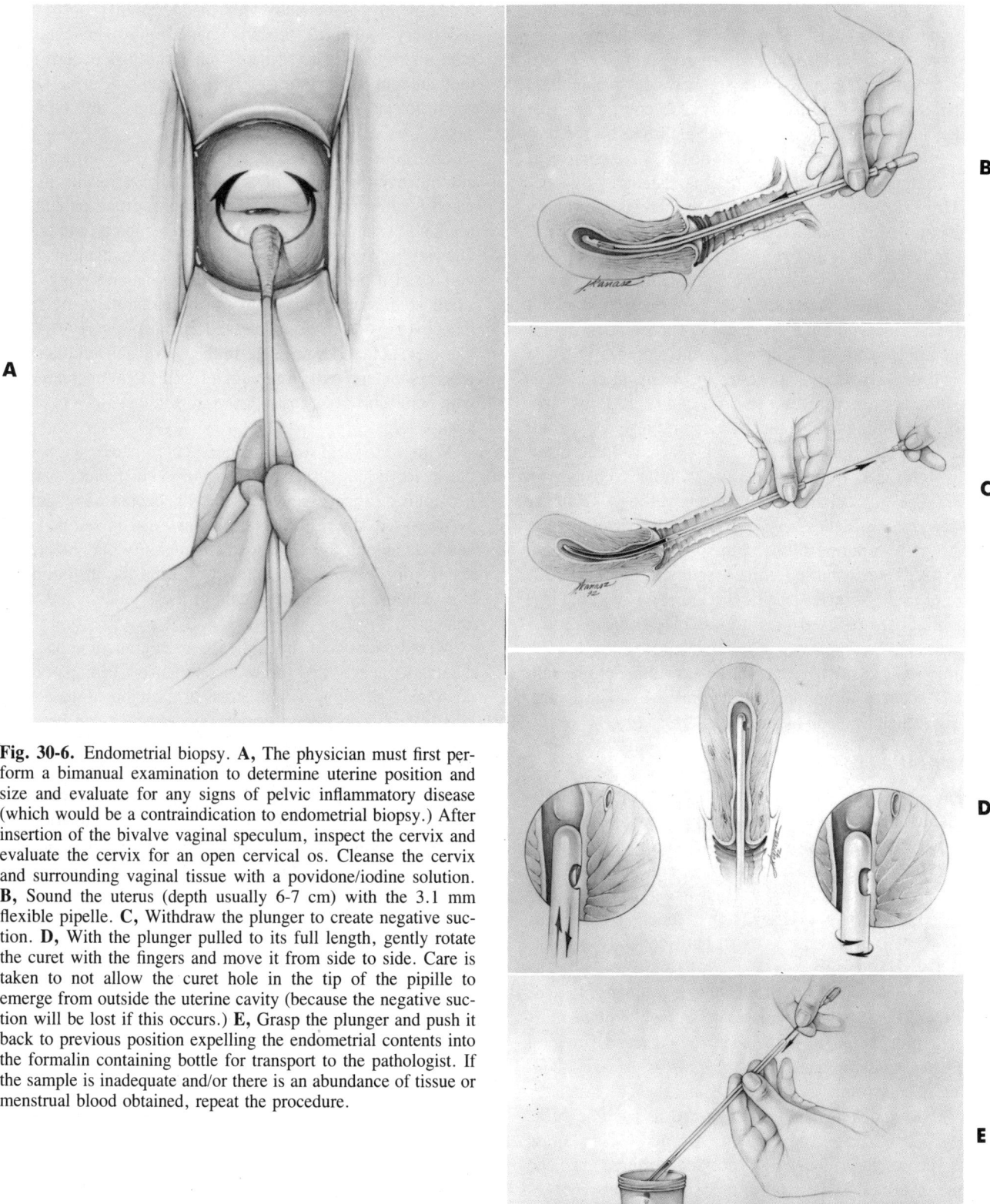

Fig. 30-6. Endometrial biopsy. **A,** The physician must first perform a bimanual examination to determine uterine position and size and evaluate for any signs of pelvic inflammatory disease (which would be a contraindication to endometrial biopsy.) After insertion of the bivalve vaginal speculum, inspect the cervix and evaluate the cervix for an open cervical os. Cleanse the cervix and surrounding vaginal tissue with a povidone/iodine solution. **B,** Sound the uterus (depth usually 6-7 cm) with the 3.1 mm flexible pipelle. **C,** Withdraw the plunger to create negative suction. **D,** With the plunger pulled to its full length, gently rotate the curet with the fingers and move it from side to side. Care is taken to not allow the curet hole in the tip of the pipille to emerge from outside the uterine cavity (because the negative suction will be lost if this occurs.) **E,** Grasp the plunger and push it back to previous position expelling the endometrial contents into the formalin containing bottle for transport to the pathologist. If the sample is inadequate and/or there is an abundance of tissue or menstrual blood obtained, repeat the procedure.

PATHOPHYSIOLOGY

Urinary incontinence is a symptom of lower urinary tract dysfunction; it is not a disease. The lower urinary tract consists of the bladder and urinary sphincter. Continence requires coordinated activity between a compliant bladder and a competent sphincter. The coordination of bladder and sphincter activity is accomplished by the nervous system. Maintenance of continence, i.e., control of reflex voiding, is a learned skill that is demanded by society. Urine loss may occur whenever there is a primary dysfunction of the bladder, sphincter, or nervous system. Frequently pathology in two or all three components of the continence mechanism will result in urine loss.

The two primary functions of the lower urinary tract are the storage and volitional evacuation of urine. Urinary incontinence is seen as a failure of urine storage.[23a] Urine loss will occur whenever pressure in the bladder exceeds the pressure exerted by the urinary sphincter. Low pressure bladder filling and storage occurs primarily as a result of the viscoelastic properties of the bladder wall that result in small changes in bladder pressure with large changes in volume (i.e. compliance).[185a] During filling, sphincter pressure rises as bladder capacity is near. The role of the nervous system during filling is to suppress reflex voiding and to facilitate increased urinary sphincter resistance. A failure of urine storage secondary to either a rise in bladder pressure above sphincter pressure (as may occur with decreased bladder compliance or uninhibited bladder contractions) or a fall in sphincter pressure below bladder pressure (as may occur with uninhibited urethral relaxation or urethral dysfunction) leads to urine loss.

CLASSIFICATION

Many different classification systems have been developed in an attempt to categorize urinary incontinence. Frequently these classification systems become cumbersome and clinically unuseful. The majority of adult patients with urinary incontinence can be grouped into four major subtypes: stress, urge, overflow, and functional incontinence.[185a] Mixed patterns do exist, but frequently one pattern will predominate.

Stress urinary incontinence is the involuntary loss of urine that occurs when increases in intraabdominal pressure are transmitted to the bladder and exceeds urethral closure pressure (sphincter pressure). Stress urinary incontinence occurs primarily in women and, when associated with pelvic floor relaxation, is described as genuine stress urinary incontinence. Incontinence occurs during stress maneuvers such as coughing, sneezing, lifting, etc. The volume of urine loss is small to moderate and postvoid residual is typically small.

Urge incontinence occurs when an uninhibited or involuntary bladder contraction is of sufficient magnitude to overcome urethral pressure. Urge incontinence occurs in both men and women. In women it may be an isolated finding or associated with pelvic floor relaxation. In men it is frequently associated with bladder outlet obstruction secondary to benign prostatic hypertrophy. Patients will note a strong urge to urinate with urine loss occurring as they attempt to get to a toilet. The volume of urine loss is small to moderate and postvoid residuals are typically small.

Overflow incontinence is the result of an acute or chronic overdistension of the bladder that results in elevated bladder pressures. In the chronic setting patients do not have an urge to urinate and are frequently completely unaware of the overdistended state of their bladders. The volume of urine loss is variable. Some patients report only small volume urine loss that can be precipitated by stress maneuvers (i.e. rises in intraabdominal pressure will further elevate bladder pressure in the overdistended bladder), whereas others will complain of near total incontinence with persistent urine loss. Postvoid residuals, as a rule, are always large.

With functional incontinence, coordinated activity of the lower urinary tract remains intact but factors such as immobility, inaccessible toilets, or decreased cognitive awareness result in urine loss. Functional incontinence is common among the elderly whose mobility may be significantly impaired, the chronically ill, and the institutionalized patient. Postvoid residuals in these patients are variable.

Mixed patterns of incontinence are not uncommon. Frequently urgency and urge incontinence accompany the complaints of females with stress urinary incontinence. As noted previously, stress urinary incontinence can be associated with overflow incontinence as in males with bladder outlet obstruction and urinary retention. It should be remembered that the marginally continent patient frequently has developed strategies to avoid settings and situations in which incontinence occur. Once removed from a familiar environment, urinary incontinence may result.

EVALUATION

The evaluation of the incontinent patient begins with a thorough history and physical examination. During history taking, it is important not only to focus on the patient's description of their incontinence but to obtain pertinent details from the patient's past medical and surgical histories. A complete list of medications, both prescribed and over-the-counter, should be obtained from all patients. The times at which medications are taken is to be noted. It is not uncommon to find that in patients with nocturnal frequency and incontinence that they are taking diuretics before going to bed. Information regarding the patient's current social and residential situation is also helpful in better appreciating complaints of urine loss. A review of symptoms should include information on new or residual neurologic defects and bowel function. In female patients, a gynecologic review of symptoms is essential, including par-

Table 30-5. Categorization of urinary incontinence

Type of incontinence	Setting	Urgency	Volume loss	Degree bladder empty	Corroborating information on physical exam
Stress	Stress maneuver	−	Small-moderate	Complete	Pelvic floor relaxation
Urge	Attempting to get to bathroom	+	Small-moderate	Complete	Normal exam
Overflow	Stress maneuvers/ persistent	−	Variable	Incomplete	Distended bladder
Functional	Variable	N/A	Moderate-large	Not aware	Altered mental status

ity, route of delivery, onset of menopause, and presence of vaginal irritation or infection.

With reference to the patient's specific complaints of urinary incontinence, the treating physician should ascertain the duration, frequency, and progressive nature of urine loss. The key to understanding symptoms of urine loss is to establish the setting in which urine loss occurs and whether a sense of urgency (the feeling of the need to urinate) occurs before urine loss. The volume of urine loss and the degree to which patients feel they empty their bladders with urination are two additional important pieces of information.

A physical examination should be performed in the incontinent patient, with special attention directed toward the neurologic, genitourinary, and rectal examination. A neurologic examination includes an assessment of the patient's mental status, motor strength, sensation, and deep tendon reflexes in the lower extremities. Genitourinary examination should include palpation of the abdomen to detect the presence of a distended bladder and an examination of the male and female external genitalia and perineum. During rectal examination, one should note the presence of anal fissures, excoriations, rectal tone and in males assessment of the size and consistency of the prostate gland. Once information from the history and physical has been obtained, it is frequently possible to group patients into one of the four main subtypes of incontinence (Table 30-5).

Those patients who cannot be accurately categorized or those who have failed empiric trials of therapy require further evaluation. A urinary pressure flow study with the use of fluoroscopy and video monitoring represents the state-of-the-art in the evaluation of the incontinent patient. The components of this study include a cystometrogram, electrophysiologic monitoring of sphincter activity, fluoroscopic imaging of the bladder recorded on a video monitor, urethral pressure profilometry, and uroflowmetry. Information that can be obtained with this study includes pressure within the bladder and urethra during filling and evacuation; electrical activity of the urinary sphincter during filling and evacuation; and visualization of the bladder outlet during filling and evacuation. The individual components of this elaborate study can be used separately to assess bladder filling or emptying, but in difficult diagnostic situations the most information can be obtained by careful monitoring through a complete filling and emptying cycle.

RISK FACTORS AND PRIMARY PREVENTION

For a successful preventive strategy to be implemented, two things must occur. First, health care professionals must realize that urinary incontinence is a significant source of morbidity and that many forms of urinary incontinence can be successfully treated and possibly prevented. Second, risk factors involved with urinary incontinence must be identified. At present, patient's age, gender, and parity have been established as risk factors for urinary incontinence. Other risk factors that have been suggested are those of menopause, chronic illness, and various medications.[185a] Once identified, efforts at prevention should be directed toward these high-risk groups. Preventive measures may take the form of life-style and environmental changes such as decreasing fluid intake when toilets are not available or in improving access to toilet facilities. Avoidance of medication, which may contribute to urinary incontinence and the prevention of urinary tract infections, are two additional measures that may reduce episodes of urine loss.

SECONDARY PREVENTION AND MANAGEMENT

All patients with urinary incontinence should be considered for evaluation and treatment. Although a cure is not always possible, the majority of patients will benefit from treatment, in so far as the frequency and volume of urine loss typically diminish. Even in those patients whose incontinence is not improved with therapeutic intervention, the heightened awareness of the patient and caretakers, both professional and nonprofessional, results in fewer complications related to urinary incontinence. The timely use of absorbent pads and diapers as part of a management program may eliminate many social constraints burdening the patient.

Multiple modalities have been developed for the treatment of urinary incontinence. In selected cases, a single modality may provide a cure, but the majority of times a combination of different modalities provides the best chance of effecting a positive result. Therapeutic strategies most commonly employed are behavioral techniques, pharmacologic intervention, and surgical intervention. The treatment of any patient must be individualized, taking into account the patient's perception of the problem, expectations of intervention, environment, and clinical status. Therapy should usually begin with the most noninvasive procedures and those associated with the fewest side effects and then progresses to more invasive treatment options as are necessary.

Behavioral techniques

Successful implementation of behavioral techniques for management of urinary incontinence requires a well-motivated patient without cognitive deficits. Bladder training (timed voiding), pelvic floor muscle exercises (Kegel exercises), and biofeedback are all forms of behavioral modification techniques designed to improve continence.

Bladder training, also known as timed voiding or toileting, heightens the patient's awareness of the need to void and aims to keep bladder volumes relatively small. Patients are instructed to void initially at 30 to 60-minute intervals whether or not they have the urge to urinate. If the urge to urinate arises before the scheduled void, the patients are instructed to attempt to suppress this urge. If they are unable to, the patients are permitted to void but still should adhere to the voiding schedule. Voiding intervals are gradually increased until the patient is voiding every 3 to 4 hours. Studies have indicated cure rates of 10% to 15% and improvement in the majority of patients with the use of bladder training.[86a]

Biofeedback is also designed to heighten the patient's awareness of the state of the bladder and urinary sphincter. With the use of monitoring equipment, the patient learns to relax the bladder and abdominal wall musculature and to contract the urinary sphincter and pelvic floor muscles during bladder filling. The patient receives cues from the monitoring equipment as to the effectiveness of the appropriate relaxation and contraction. The goal of therapy is to have the patient eventually use these maneuvers automatically without the aid of monitoring equipment, thus preventing incontinence. Studies indicate that approximately 25% of patients are cured and an additional 30% are improved when biofeedback is used in the treatment of stress and/or urge incontinence.

Pelvic floor muscle exercises are done to strengthen the voluntary muscles of the urinary sphincter, the periurethral muscles, and pelvic floor muscles. The heightened awareness of the muscles involved in the maintenance of continence is another benefit of these exercises. These exercises have been used in treatment of both stress and urge incontinence but are most effective in the treatment of mild forms of genuine stress urinary incontinence (Fig. 30-7).

Pharmacologic treatment

Medications used in the treatment of urinary incontinence are chosen because of the ability to decrease the frequency and strength of uninhibited contractions or increase resistence of the urinary sphincter. While this form of therapy is relatively "noninvasive," significant side effects can be encountered. The most bothersome side effects of those drugs meant to decrease uninhibited contractions are related to anticholinergic effects, such as dry mouth, dry eyes, blurred vision and constipation. Also, these medications may put the patient with poor detrusor contractility or significant bladder outlet obstruction (as may occur with benign prostatic hypertrophy) into urinary retention. Medications used to increase the resistance of the urinary sphincter are generally well tolerated but can be associated with significant side effects. Therefore these medications should be used cautiously.

Because acetylcholine is the final neurotransmitter of the parasympathetic nervous system, and because parasympathetic input is believed to play a major role in a voluntary bladder contraction, many anticholinergics have been used in an attempt to control uninhibited bladder contractions. As a class, these medications increase the volume to the first involuntary contraction, decrease the strength of the contraction, and increase total bladder capacity.[23a] They do not increase the time the patient has to void, and if an uninhibited contraction occurs, urgency and urge incontinence may persist. The goal of therapy is to decrease the frequency of these episodes. The most commonly used anticholinergic medication is propantheline 15-30 mg by mouth every 4 to 6 hours. Significant anticholinergic side effects, especially with the higher doses and more frequent administration schedules, tend to occur.

The second class of medications used to inhibit involuntary bladder contractions is the direct smooth muscle relaxants: oxybutynin (Ditropan), dicyclomine (Bentyl), and flavoxate hydrochloride (Urospas). Associated with their direct smooth muscle relaxant properties are mild to moderate anticholinergic effects, and in the cases of oxybutynin and flavoxate, a local anesthetic effect is also encountered. The effect of these medications on the bladder is similar to that of propantheline and side effects are primarily related again to their anticholinergic properties. These direct smooth muscle relaxants can be used in combinations with anticholinergic medication for an additive effect in the control of uninhibited contractions.

Medications intended to increase resistance of the urinary sphincter are primarily the alpha-agonists; ephedrine, pseudoephedrine, and phenylpropanolomine. Phenylpropanolomine has been the most commonly used medication because its peripheral action with alpha-receptors is similar to ephedrine and pseudoephedrine while centrally it causes less stimulation. These medications bind to smooth muscle

Managing incontinence

Pelvic floor muscle exercises
Special pelvic floor muscle exercises were developed by a doctor named Kegel (so they are sometimes called "Kegels"). They work in mild cases of stress incontinence because incontinence is often related to weak pelvic floor muscles. Since these inner muscles are under our voluntary control, we can exercise them to build up their strength and bulk, like a body builder builds up outer muscles.

Why do the exercises
The pelvic floor muscles act as a sling to keep the bladder and bladder neck lifted; they also form the external sphincter. Sometimes these muscles weaken, allowing pelvic organs to drop down. By doing specific exercises **over a period of time,** you can tighten up and strengthen the pelvic floor and sphincter muscles.

How to do them
1. Sit on the toilet and start to urinate. Try to stop the flow of urine midstream by **contracting** (tightening) your pelvic floor muscles. These are the same muscles used to stop a bowel movement.

2. Repeat several times, until you are sure of the action and sensation of consciously contracting these muscles. Do not tighten your abdominal, leg, or buttock muscles.

3. An alternate way to exercise the pelvic floor muscles is with a small vaginal weight, which you insert briefly in the vagina. Holding the weight in makes you contract the right muscles.

When to do them
For stress incontinence, repeat the exercise four times, holding each contraction for a count of four. Do this every hour, whether at your desk or watching TV. They must be performed daily for at least 2 to 3 months to be effective.

Day 1

3 months later

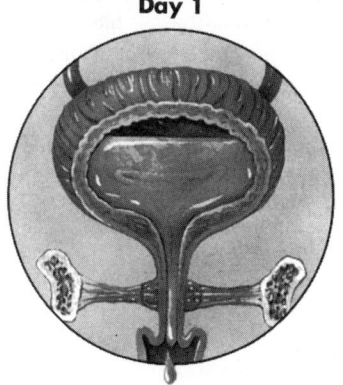 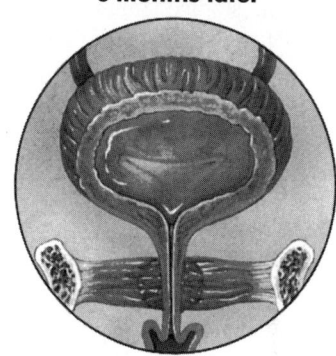

Before: Weak, thin pelvic floor muscles can't support bladder neck. Sphincter is weak and leakage occurs.

After: Stronger, thicker pelvic floor muscles restore sphincter strength. No more leakage.

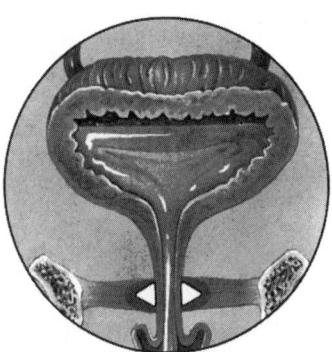 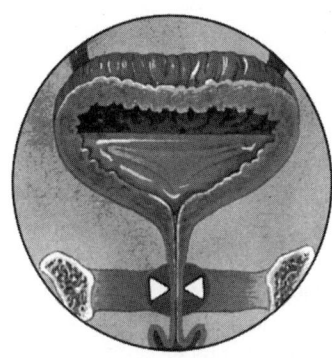

Practice pelvic floor muscle exercises while urinating. When you relax the muscles, they let urine out.

Tightening the pelvic floor muscles stop the flow midstream. Repeat the relaxation and contraction.

Bladder drill
For urge incontinence, the same exercise can be used to do a "bladder drill" that retrains your bladder. When the external sphincter contracts, it signals the bladder to relax, so the urge eventually subsides. Every time you feel urinary urgency, try to stop the feeling by contracting the pelvic floor muscles. Try to hold your urine a little longer each time, gradually increasing the time between urinating to 2, 3, or _____ hours. You should start to see improvement in 2 to 3 weeks.

Fig. 30-7. Pelvic floor muscle exercises for managing urinary incontinence. (From *Incontinence,* San Bruno, CA, 1987, Krames Communications.)

alpha-receptors at the bladder neck, which cause contraction of these muscle fibers and therefore increase outlet resistence. These medications have been used most successfully in women with mild to moderate stress urinary incontinence and with some benefit in males with postprostatectomy stress urinary incontinence. These medications need to be used with caution in those patients with a history of hypertension, cardiovascular disease, or hyperthyroidism.

The tricyclic antidepressant imipramine has been used to facilitate urine storage. Imipramine has a direct smooth muscle relaxant, local anesthetic, and mild anticholinergic effects on the bladder. Also, by inhibiting the reuptake of norepinephrine, urinary sphincter resistance increases. Potential side effects of this medication include postural hypotension, sedation, and the spectrum of anticholinergic effects noted earlier. The usual adult dosage is 25 mg 4 times daily, with dose reduction for both young and elderly patients.

Because urinary incontinence is common in postmenopausal female patients and atrophic vaginitis frequently accompanies urinary incontinence in these patients, replacement therapy with estrogen has been used. While estrogen replacement therapy has little objective effect on stress urinary incontinence, it can improve the urgency and at times the urge incontinence experienced by these women. The combination of estrogen therapy with an alpha-agonist may be most beneficial.

Surgical intervention

The role of surgery in the management of urinary incontinence has evolved during the past 50 years. Surgery may be considered when less invasive forms of therapy have failed. Surgery is indicated only after a complete urologic evaluation of the patient has been performed, including radiographic and urodynamic studies when indicated. A clear understanding of the pathophysiology of a patient's urinary loss and the selection of an appropriate operation are the keys to successful surgical correction of urinary incontinence. Surgery has been most successful in the treatment of genuine stress urinary incontinence, overflow incontinence secondary to prostatic enlargement and certain forms of urge incontinence.[251a]

Moderate to moderately severe stress urinary incontinence associated with pelvic floor relaxation (genuine stress urinary incontinence) can be surgically corrected by a number of transabdominal or transvaginal procedures. The goal of surgery is to relocate the bladder neck and proximal urethra to a relatively fixed intraabdominal location. Regardless of the type of surgical approach used, success rates in the range of 85% to 95% can be expected. Patients with severe stress urinary incontinence related to a damaged urethra and urinary sphincter, as may occur in women secondary to previous vaginal or urethral surgery, or in men after a transurethral or radical prostatectomy, require a more extensive operative procedure designed to compress the urethra and thereby increase urethral resistance. In women this may be achieved with a pubovaginal sling. In males the use of an artificial urinary sphincter achieves this goal. The success rates are not as great as those associated with surgical treatment of genuine stress incontinence.

In the past, patients with intractable uninhibited contractions of the bladder were frequently treated with urinary diversion in the form of an ileal conduit. While this eliminated the lower urinary tract as a cause of incontinence, the need to wear an external urinary collection device and then long-term detrimental effect on kidney function has limited its usefulness. At present the use of various intestinal segments to augment the bladder, thereby increasing capacity and decreasing pressure, is viewed as a more acceptable surgical alternative. The long-term effects of these procedures on the metabolic status and kidney function of the patient remain to be realized.

Cancers of the female genital tract

Jerome L. Belinson

The National Cancer Institute estimates that cervical, uterine, and ovarian carcinoma will account for 12% of the reported cancers in women in 1992.[7] The National Center for Health Statistics estimates the same three malignancies will account for 9% of the cancer deaths in women in 1992.[7] Detecting these malignancies when they are localized, rather than when they are demonstrating regional or distant spread, clearly translates into less morbidity and lower mortality. Our patients often find it difficult to understand how diseases so devastating can escape detection. In addition, the tests that are effective in diagnosing cancers are also so costly and so insensitive that, when applied to large segments of the population, drive up medical costs and result in unacceptable morbidity associated with the work-up of false-positive tests.

A distinction should be made between a screening test and a diagnostic test. A screening test is designed to classify an individual as likely or unlikely to have the disease in question. To be effective, a screening test should be easy to perform, acceptable to the patient, and inexpensive. The disease screened, on the other hand, should have a treatment that, if applied early, will improve outcome. In addition, the disease should have a preclinical phase, a high prevalence in the screened population, and a long enough duration to make the test cost effective. A diagnostic test, on the other hand, is applied to individuals who present with symptoms. Diagnostic tests should be highly specific with a high positive predictive value.[127]

CANCER OF THE ENDOMETRIUM

It is estimated in 1992 that 32,000 new cases of uterine cancer will be diagnosed, resulting in 5600 deaths in the United States.[7] The incidence of endometrial cancer was stable between 1940 and 1970 at approximately 70 cases per 100,000 women per year. Between 1970 and 1975, the incidence of endometrial carcinoma dramatically increased to 134 cases per 100,000 women per year. This increase primarily reflected the rise in postmenopausal estrogen replacement therapy. By 1978, likely secondary to recognition of the risk imparted by unopposed estrogen therapy, the rate of endometrial cancer in the 50-to-59-year-old age group had fallen back to 1970 levels. However, without explanation, the incidence in older women has continued to rise. The average age of diagnosis of endometrial cancer is 58 years, with less than 4% of cases occurring before the age of 40. White women in the United States are nearly twice as likely to develop endometrial carcinoma as black women.[259]

Risk factors

Obesity is an important constitutional risk factor for the development of endometrial carcinoma.[72,275] Women who are more than 50 pounds over ideal body weight appear to have a nine times greater risk of developing endometrial carcinoma. This is basically an effect of unopposed estrogen. In the postmenopausal woman, the primary circulating estrogen is estrone. Androstendione produced by the adrenal glands is peripherally aromatized in fatty tissue, resulting in estrone. Increased conversion as occurs in obesity increases the blood levels of estrone.[163] This, combined with the decrease in sex hormone binding globulin in obese individuals, results in elevated circulating estrogen levels.

The risk of developing endometrial carcinoma because of unopposed estrogen can also occur endogenously secondary to estrogen-producing neoplasms. These tumors, such as granulosa-theca tumors, are uncommon and are therefore not helpful in identifying high-risk patients. More frequently, the patient presents with abnormal uterine bleeding, which leads to a diagnosis of pelvic masses. Exogenous estrogens have now been quite clearly implicated as increasing the risk of uterine carcinoma.[165,170,231,241,276] It is interesting that women with no other constitutional risk factors appear to be at the highest risk because of estrogen replacement therapy.[72] The risk of developing endometrial carcinoma from unopposed estrogen therapy appears to increase with dose and duration of therapy, and decrease on stopping therapy over a period of several years. Women with Turner's syndrome who received DES for feminization,[69] as well as women taking a sequential oral contraceptive, also had an increased risk of endometrial carcinoma.[238] The particular oral contraceptive was unique in that the progesterone was extremely weak and the patients were essentially receiving unopposed estrogen. The drug is no longer sold.

Non–estrogen-producing ovarian tumors apparently may induce increased androgenic activity in the ovarian stroma by their presence. In addition, the ovarian stroma will occasionally become hyperactive in the absence of an associated tumor (stromal hyperplasia), also resulting in increased ovarian androgens. Both of these circumstances result in an increased "prehormone" that becomes peripherally converted (aromatized), resulting in elevated unopposed estrogens in the postmenopausal woman.[163]

Patients with polycystic ovarian disease have an increased risk of endometrial cancer. These patients account for a significant percentage of patients developing ovarian cancer under the age of 40.[72] In these women, anovulation results in unopposed estrogen stimulation of the endometrium. This effect may be accentuated by peripheral conversion of ovarian stromal androgens.

Diabetes is another constitutional risk factor for developing endometrial carcinoma. After controlling for age, weight, and socioeconomic status, the relative risk appears to be 2.8.[166,230]

Patients who have received radiation therapy to the pelvis are also at increased risk for developing endometrial cancers.[223] In former times, patients often received low doses of radiation to stop menstrual periods by inducing ovarian failure. This low dose of radiation has been associated with an increased risk of uterine sarcomas as well as more common types of endometrial cancers. Standard therapeutic doses of pelvic radiation therapy as delivered for carcinoma of the cervix also appear to be associated with an eight times relative risk of developing carcinoma of the endometrium. These cases are often advanced when diagnosed. The cervical stenosis resulting from the radiation therapy prevents the bleeding symptoms that often lead to the diagnosis while the tumor is still confined to the uterus. Nulliparity also appears to increase one's risk relative to multiparity, depending on the number of deliveries, from two to five times. This risk factor is quite complex to evaluate because it is influenced by the multiple causes of infertility, among them the variety of causes of anovulation. Finally, 50% of women with endometrial carcinoma have none of the known risk factors.[166,230]

Modification of risk factors

The most important risk factor is unopposed estrogen stimulation of the endometrium. The administration of a progestin (e.g., medroxyprogesterone acetate, 10 mg, 10 to 12 days each month) appears to eliminate the increased risk of estrogen administration or anovulation.[101,200] This medication is usually begun on day 16. Users of combination oral contraceptives also appear to have a lower risk of developing endometrial cancer. A 50% reduction in risk was greatest in nulliparous women. This protection seemed to last for many years upon stopping the oral contraceptives. The protective effect is eliminated by the use of unopposed menopausal estrogen replacement.[44,190,263]

Even in ovulating women or women on estrogen replacement as well as progestin therapy, the endometrium may demonstrate focal insensitivity to progesterone. As a result, an occasional patient may still develop an endometrial carcinoma.

Weight reduction with the consequential reduction in peripheral conversion of adrenal androgens will result in a decrease in the circulating levels of estrone and an increase in steroid-binding globulin. The presumption is that this will decrease the risk of endometrial hyperplasia and endometrial carcinoma.

Presenting symptoms

The most important presenting symptom of endometrial carcinoma is vaginal bleeding. Endometrial carcinomas present with abnormal uterine bleeding in 90% of cases. In addition to the high suspicion associated with postmenopausal bleeding (13% to 16% incidence of endometrial carcinoma), abnormal uterine bleeding in the premenopausal woman can likewise be secondary to an endometrial carcinoma or endometrial hyperplasia. This is especially true in anovulatory younger women or women in the perimenopausal years. The older the patient, the greater is the risk that her postmenopausal bleeding is secondary to an endometrial carcinoma. Hawwa et al. in 1970 reported that atrophic changes in the vagina were the most likely explanation for a single episode of postmenopausal bleeding. However, 7% of these patients had carcinoma. Hawwa's studies also suggested that increased volume of postmenopausal bleeding did not correlate with increased likelihood of malignancy.[49,116,193]

The endometrial hyperplasias are important. They may be the etiology of abnormal uterine bleeding. They may be the result of anovulation and associated with infertility. They may result from exogenous estrogens. They can be associated with estrogen-producing ovarian neoplasms. Most important, they may be precursors to endometrial carcinomas. The risk of endometrial hyperplasia progressing to endometrial carcinoma relates to the severity of the lesion, primarily indicated by the degree of cytologic atypia. Cystic hyperplasia has a low risk of malignant progression, and adenomatous hyperplasia has an increasing neoplastic potential based on the degree of cytologic atypia. The literature supports a 10% to 30% progression rate for these lesions. In general, atypical adenomatous hyperplasia is treated like a well-differentiated adenocarcinoma. In fact, in 12% to 15% of the hysterectomies on patients who have atypical adenomatis hyperplasia, a concomitant endometrial carcinoma is found.[146,178,265]

Some patients will present with a purulent vaginal discharge that may be slightly blood tinged. This may signal a hematometria secondary to an endometrial carcinoma in a patient with some cervical stenosis. Endometrial polyps are found in 7% to 23% of patients who present with postmenopausal bleeding. In up to 30% of cases of endometrial cancer, benign endometrial polyps also exist. Therefore finding a polyp in a postmenopausal woman should arouse the suspicion of a concomitant uterine malignancy or the potential development of such in the future.[14,203]

Screening recommendations

The American College of Obstetricians and Gynecologists suggests that total population screening for endometrial cancer and its precursors is neither cost effective nor warranted. The college suggests that high-risk patients may require endometrial sampling.[2] The American Cancer Society states that women should report postmenopausal bleeding. High-risk women should have an endometrial tissue sample at menopause.[6] The high-risk group mentioned by both the American College of Obstetricians and Gynecologists and the American Cancer Society recommendations should include the following categories:

- Women receiving postmenopausal estrogen therapy.
- Women with a history of endometrial hyperplasia.
- Women more than 50 pounds over ideal body weight.
- Premenopausal women with chronic anovulation and/or infertility.

Many devices are available for cytologic as well as histologic sampling of the endometrium. Many papers have carefully analyzed each of these techniques and compared them with each other. No technique is currently available that when applied to large populations of women adequately screens for endometrial cancer and the hyperplasias.[131,137,144,258]

Currently, this author prefers a suction histologic technique for obtaining an endometrial sample. The newest devices are simple, easy to use, and well accepted by the patients, and they reliably diagnose hyperplasias as well as cancers.[137]

To understand the rationale for the screening recommendations, one must consider a variety of factors. The Pap smear is positive in less than 50% of patients who have adenocarcinoma of the endometrium.[12,277] Ng demonstrated that the presence of normal endometrial cells after the twelfth day of the menstrual period or after the menopause suggests the presence of polyps, hyperplasia, or endometrial adenocarcinoma.[187] Obviously any patient who presents with symptoms needs a diagnostic test, not a screening procedure. However, the current suction curettage devices serve as an excellent initial step for both screening and diagnostic modes.[137] A formal fractional curettage is still considered the gold standard and is now generally accompanied by hysteroscopy. However, less than 3% of the time will an office suction endometrial biopsy miss the diagnosis of cancer.[110]

In reviewing the many devices designed for cytologic

and histologic sampling of the endometrium, most studies have arrived at similar conclusions. Whether one washes, brushes, scrapes, or aspirates to obtain a cytologic sample from the endometrium, it is generally extremely well tolerated. This is primarily because of the small size of the instruments. The cost is usually lower than for histologic techniques because the pathology charges are similar to the handling of Pap smears.

Cytologic screening, however, has its shortcomings. Although the reported accuracy of cytologic screening compared with dilation and curettage (D&C) ranges from 75 to 100% in diagnosing endometrial cancers, the studies range from 31% to 100% in diagnosing endometrial hyperplasias.[258] Additionally, the series that have the best results tend to be quite small. Perhaps more important is the difficulty in the interpretation of endometrial cytology. Cervical cytology has taken 5 decades to reach its current level, and still we find tremendous variation in laboratory expertise. Endometrial cytology is difficult, and because of the general lack of experience, laboratory variation can be extreme.[132,176]

Histologic sampling devices, on the other hand, perform extremely well compared with D & C in the diagnosis of adenocarcinomas and precursor lesions.[137,194,258] In addition, endometrial polyps are more likely detected. The fact that it is a histologic specimen tends to make the diagnostic interpretation more reproducible. The "pipelle," a modern version of the older suction curettage instruments, is easy to use and approaches the cytologic instruments in patient acceptance.[137] The cost is a problem, however, because the pathology department handles the specimen as a standard histology.

Several interesting problems have prevented the acceptance of endometrial screening within the medical community and by patients. First, endometrial cancer is a highly curable malignancy in the absence of screening.[27] Second, the most likely patients to be screened are those patients who are obese, with chronic anovulation, or on estrogen replacement therapy. These estrogen-related endometrial cancers, although similar in outcome when compared by stage and grade, as a group tend to be lower stage and lower grade at diagnosis. One therefore finds that patients who are the most curable are the ones screened.

Third, there is no doubt that the various cytologic methods or the office suction biopsy techniques could save millions of dollars in patient charges for hospital based D & C procedures. However, undoubtedly this would be negated by a rise in hysterectomies for "precancerous endometrial lesions." No matter how mild the hyperplasia may be, once a patient hears the term "precancerous" whether appropriately or inappropriately applied, the fear engendered usually leads rapidly to a hysterectomy with mutual agreement. Clearly the need for most of these hysterectomies, based on the true cancer risk, is highly questionable.

Fourth, with the age-specific incidence of endometrial cancer rising with increasing age, one discovers that the inability to perform an office endometrial sampling also increases with age. In Koss' study of 1280 asymptomatic women, 17% of women over 70 years of age could not be sampled.[144]

Whenever one is investigating abnormal uterine bleeding or a patient is being evaluated who has a known endometrial carcinoma or precursor lesion, a thorough pelvic examination is indicated. This should include visual inspection of the external genitalia, a speculum examination of the vagina, a careful bimanual and rectovaginal exam, and careful assessment of the inguinal nodes. An occasional patient will have a pelvic mass related to the endometrial cancer or precursor lesion. In addition, often in the obese patient, most of the information gained from a pelvic examination comes from careful palpation of the cul-de-sac on rectovaginal examination. Often, only on this portion of the examination does one delineate the size of the uterus, the presence of a pelvic mass, or the presence of cul-de-sac nodularity.

Short of sampling the endometrial cavity, the progesterone challenge test has been promoted as a preliminary screen.[102,112] The test involves administering to postmenopausal women with an intact uterus 13 days of 10 mg medroxyprogesterone acetate. If there is no withdrawal bleeding, the assumption is the absence of any proliferative activity within the endometrium and therefore low risk for carcinoma or precursor lesions. Withdrawal bleeding in the postmenopausal woman should be followed by proper endometrial sampling. The ultimate effect of this form of management on morbidity and mortality from endometrial carcinoma awaits further studies.

OVARIAN CANCER

Ovarian cancer accounts for 4% of cancers in women and will cause 5% of the deaths from cancer in women in 1992. The National Cancer Institute predicts 21,000 new cases will occur in 1992, with 13,000 deaths.[7] Since 1930, the age specific incidence apparently has been very slowly increasing. The explanation for this is unclear. Comparing the years 1979 to 1980 with the previous decade appears to show a decrease in overall death rate, primarily accountable to a 33% decrease in death rate in patients under the age of 50.[172]

The problem is quite clear. Ovarian cancer is a highly curable disease when diagnosed early and difficult to cure once it has spread beyond the ovary.[100] Unfortunately, in 80% of patients presenting with ovarian cancer, the cancer already has spread beyond the ovary. While working to develop new forms of therapy for advanced disease, we also need to strengthen our research efforts toward early diagnosis.[28,222]

Ovarian cancer is a heterogeneous group of cancers that occur in four major categories. First are the epithelial tumors, which include tumors that are predominantly glandular and resemble the müllerian-derived epithelium of the genital tract. The apparent invagination of the surface of the ovary, which embryologically resembles the surface of the entire peritoneal cavity, places totipotential mesothelial cells within the structure of the ovary. If the cells differentiate to resemble fallopian tube epithelium, serous tumors are formed. If they form endometrial epithelium, this leads to endometrioid tumors. If the cells differentiate toward the endocervix, mucinous tumors are the result.[118] This group also includes clear cell tumors, the Brenner tumor consisting of transitional type epithelium, and other mixed and undifferentiated types. The epithelial tumors are the category of ovarian tumors generally referred to when one speaks generically about ovarian cancer. They are the dominant tumor, accounting for 85% of all ovarian cancers, and are less frequent only in women under the age of 20, in whom germ cell tumors dominate.

The germ cell category includes such tumors as the dysgerminoma, the endodermal sinus tumor, embryonal carcinomas, and malignant teratomas. The third category is the sex cord stromal tumors. This category includes the granulosa-theca cell and the Sertoli-Leydig cell tumor. The tumors in this category have the ability to produce predominantly female or male hormones, or occasionally corticosteroids. The final category is the stromal tumors (nonfunctioning), which include tumors such as ovarian fibromas. Most discussions on ovarian cancer focus on the epithelial tumors.

Risk factors

A variety of risk factors have been identified for carcinoma of the ovary. They can be divided into four major categories: genetic, environmental, hormonal, and viral.

Genetic. Epithelial tumors of the ovary are more common in women over the age of 45 and in white women with Northern European ancestry.[237] Jewish women in particular appear to have an increased incidence of ovarian cancer.[108,262]

Several high-risk family syndromes have been identified. First, inherited site-specific epithelial ovarian cancer is known.[153,161] The familial ovarian cancer syndromes appear to occur at a younger age, by 10 to 15 years. The predominant histologic variety is a serous tumor, making up 98% of the cases, as opposed to under 70% outside of the familial syndrome.[159] The familial syndromes also seem to be more frequently higher grade and more frequently bilateral.

There appears to be also a familial breast-ovary syndrome.[161] It is possible that this may be the most important of the familial ovarian syndromes, with individuals showing both an increased occurrence of breast and ovarian cancers. Having two first-degree relatives with either the site-specific or breast ovary syndromes appears to increase the risk of developing ovarian cancer from baseline (1 out of 70 after age 40) to a 50% risk.

Cancer of the ovary is also a component of the cancer family syndrome, which includes primarily carcinomas of the colon, endometrium, breast, and ovary.[162] Turner's syndrome with XO/XY mosaicism is also associated with dysgerminomas and gonadoblastomas.[250] Peutz-Jeghers syndrome leads to a 14% risk of granulosa theca cell tumors as well as papillary adenocarcinomas.[160] Multiple nevoid basal cell carcinoma syndrome gives rise to ovarian fibromas.[160] Finally, the ovarian fibromata syndrome gives rise to ovarian fibromas.[78]

In the process of evaluating patients with a suspected pelvic mass, one must rely on well-documented pedigree findings, because physical stigmata associated with a particular syndrome (e.g., Peutz-Jeghers, Turner's) are generally not present. One should look for the cardinal features of hereditary cancer, which are early age of onset, multiple primary sites and vertical transmission following a mendelian inheritance pattern. Late onset in a family may be due to a chance occurrence or the phenomenon known as variable penetrance, which causes a variable age of onset. This is seen in essentially all autosomal dominant diseases. Variable penetrance makes the identification of high-risk individuals especially difficult in small families.[160] Less than 5% of women who develop ovarian cancers have a family history of the disease, adding to the difficulty.

Environmental. Ovarian cancer appears to be more common in the industrialized nations. The one prominent exception to this is Japan. However, Japanese women have an increased incidence of ovarian cancer on immigrating to the United States.[70]

The literature has been inconclusive on the risks of talc exposure. Asbestos contamination of talc has been suspected as the culprit.[62] A study from England suggested an excess risk among cosmetic workers.[186] All the talc discussions show that the peritoneal cavity of women is well recognized as distinctly different from men in its accessibility to environmental exposure.[83]

Radiation has been implicated as increasing the relative risk 1.6 times for developing ovarian cancer in women therapeutically irradiated for carcinoma of the cervix. As in most radiation-induced lesions, this appears to occur 20 years on average after therapy.[142]

Hormonal. Nulliparity, low parity, and infertility are risk factors for the development of ovarian carcinoma. A woman with no pregnancies versus a woman with multiple pregnancies has a three to five times increased relative risk of developing ovarian cancer. The issue appears to be infertility, and there is a recurring theme of uninterrupted gonadotropin stimulation of the ovaries in women who develop ovarian cancer. Women who have a late menopause and who experience more than 40 years of menses are likewise at increased risk.[68] Further support is given to this theory of "incessant ovulation" by the fact that oral contraceptives appear to reduce the risk of developing ovarian carcinoma. Their effect is proportional to the duration of use after a minimum of 3 months, and if used longer than 5 years the relative risk appears to be .4.[61,75] There is no evidence for exogenous estrogen therapy in the postmenopausal woman causing an excess of ovarian cancer at this time. Some investigators have noted that a slight increase of endometrioid carcinomas appears to occur in women on replacement estrogens. Overall, however, the number of ovarian cancer cases was not increased.[216]

Viral. Much discussion over the years has been devoted to an increased risk of ovarian cancer associated with rubella and subclinical mumps infections.[171] The issue becomes confusing because mumps oophoritis is so rarely clinical that the primary focus is on viral titers. Childhood mumps may, in fact, be ovarian protective. The complexities of epidemiologic investigations are demonstrated by this observation, which has been viewed by some as a surrogate measure of family size. Children growing up in large families were more likely to develop childhood mumps and grow up to have large families.[108]

Modification of risk factors

As mentioned previously, oral contraceptives do appear to affect the risk of developing ovarian carcinoma. How familial risk is modified by taking oral contraceptives is unknown. Avoidance of exposure to talc may have some significance. Many women tend to use talc quite heavily on their perineum, occasionally placing it on diaphragms and sanitary pads. This practice is probably reasonable to avoid until this issue is clarified. There is some controversial evidence that obesity may be a risk factor for the development of ovarian carcinoma.[192] At any rate, it is far more difficult to diagnose early ovarian cancer in an obese woman than in a thin woman. An accurate examination is frequently prevented in the obese patient.

Presenting symptoms

The fact that over 80% of patients with ovarian carcinoma are first diagnosed after the disease is spread beyond the ovary indicates that reliance on symptoms will never work for early diagnosis. The presenting symptoms of patients with ovarian cancer are unfortunately frequently the symptoms of a space-occupying mass or fluid, or the effects of catabolism. Such symptoms as abdominal discomfort, gastrointestinal bloating from a large mass or fluid, or some intestinal constriction by metastatic disease are frequent. Patients often experience urinary frequency and pelvic pressure, or backache from the direct pressure of a pelvic mass. Abnormal bleeding can occur related to a hormonally active tumor or excessive androgenic activity in the ovarian stroma surrounding the tumor. In addition, metastatic disease to the endometrium can also result in abnormal bleeding. Weight loss, unfortunately, is a presenting symptom in many patients and is generally indicative of advanced disease.

On examining patients, one must perform not only a careful examination of the supraclavicular nodes, chest, and abdomen, but also a thorough pelvic exam. As a component of that pelvic exam, a thorough rectovaginal exam is essential. Careful assessment of the cul-de-sac on rectovaginal examination is frequently the key to determining the presence or absence of a pelvic mass and possibly a pelvic malignancy. Occasionally, because of torsion or hemorrhage into a mass, a patient may develop acute symptoms of pain. One hopes that when these patients are taken to the operating room under emergency conditions, there is access to a pathology laboratory, so that an accurate intraoperative diagnosis can be made and the proper operation performed.

Screening recommendations

The silent occurrence of ovarian carcinoma and its resulting spread well before diagnosis in most cases frequently create an insurmountable condition for current therapy. Clearly, early diagnosis is a key to controlling this disease, and therefore the issue of population screening again surfaces. Unfortunately, a recognizable preinvasive stage has not been described, except Stenback's observation that ovarian cancer may arise from malignant transformation of benign ovarian tumors.[246]

Clearly the routine pelvic examination is unsatisfactory. Even the concept of the postmenopausal palpable ovary has added little to the overall management and outcome.[22] This concept states that a palpable ovary in a woman more than 3 years postmenopausal should be viewed as suggestive of carcinoma. This finding obviously varies greatly, depending on the patient and the examiner. In general, any defined ovarian enlargement in the premenarchal or postmenopausal woman requires investigation. During the reproductive years, functional cystic enlargements dominate, and reexamination after a menstrual cycle is warranted.

Currently, attempts at screening for ovarian cancer all lack the specificity (considering the prevalence of the disease) to have a positive predictive value that is acceptable. Because the finding of a positive test would ultimately result in laparoscopy or laparotomy, most physicians would be unwilling to accept a screening test with a positive predictive value of less than 10% to 20%. Screening currently is focused on the areas of serum markers and ultrasound.

Bast et al. reported on the most useful marker to date, the CA-125. A murine monoclonal antibody detects the tumor-associated antigen, CA-125, in 80% of nonmucinous epithelial ovarian cancers.[25] In a Swedish study, 1082 women over the age of 40 were screened for the CA-125, and 3.3% were greater than 35 units/ml and 1% greater than 65 units/ml. Of the 36 patients who had an initial elevation of greater than 35 units/ml, one patient showed a sustained doubling, and she had a stage 3 ovarian carcinoma. She was ultimately diagnosed 21 months after her first CA-125 and 15 months after the first doubling.[279] Obviously, this is an early application, and new markers or a combination of markers may ultimately be of adequate specificity.

Dembo et al. reported that another marker NB/70K was elevated in 50% of patients with mucinous ovarian carcinoma. The combination of this marker with CA-125 is complementary in monitoring patients; however, they currently have had no role in a screening mode.[73] A variety of other markers have been reported, none of which yet appears to approach the clinical usefulness of CA-125. Most recently, Cole reported that a portion of the beta subunit of human chorionic gonadotropin (HCG) with a molecular weight of 28% of beta HCG was detectable in the urine of patients with ovarian cancers. This marker appears more useful than CA-125 in detecting early disease, but further trials of single and combined assays are needed.[55]

There are a variety of protein markers that have no application in screening but are currently extremely useful when applied appropriately in the follow-up monitoring of a patient known to have specific ovarian tumors. Examples of these are the beta HCG (embryonal tumors, choriocarcinomas, teratomas), alpha-fetal protein (AFP) (endodermal sinus tumors), and carcinoembryonic antigen (CEA) (mucinous tumors).[143]

Campbell was one of the first to propose the use of a pelvic ultrasound to screen for ovarian carcinoma. He observed that 94% of all ovarian cancers have cystic spaces and nearly all epithelial tumors are partially cystic.[42] Finkler evaluated CA-125 and pelvic ultrasound as well as clinical examination in combination for ability to differentiate malignant from benign ovarian masses. When used by itself in premenopausal women, CA-125 had a positive predictive value of 36%; in postmenopausal women it had a 94% positive predictive value. When CA-125 was combined with a positive pelvic ultrasound, the results in postmenopausal women approached 100%. Finkler also demonstrated that in postmenopausal patients with a pelvic ultrasound not suggestive of cancer and a CA-125 less than 35 units/ml, the negative predictive value was 91%.[91]

A group at the University of Kentucky using vaginal ultrasound[120] and two British investigators using primarily abdominal ultrasound[104,133] have applied these techniques in a screening mode. The criteria and descriptive findings are as follows: The ovaries are sized by using one of several comparable formulas, such as the prolate ellipse formula (width of the ovary × height × thickness × .523 expressed in cubic centimeters).[188] Premenopausal ovaries are described as normal in size if they are less than or equal to 18 cc and morphologically uniformly hypoechogenetic with sharp borders or entirely cystic.[188] Postmenopausal ovaries are considered normal in size if they are less than or equal to 8 cc and uniformly hypoechogenetic with sharp borders.[104,133] Fleisher also described two additional morphologic categories: complex or purely solid.[93] The interobserver variation using transvaginal sonography

is very small, making the technique, in the opinion of Higgins, applicable to screening.[119] Higgins screened 506 asymptomatic women over the age of 40, and 2.4%, or 12 women, had abnormal scans. Of these, 10 agreed to surgery, and all 10 had tumors, one of which was a malignancy.[120] Their studies have expanded, and combining them with the European experience appears to show that about .1% of postmenopausal women on initial screen will have an ovarian cancer diagnosed. All of the primary ovarian lesions detected in asymptomatic women have been stage 1 tumors.

Clearly age is the most useful characteristic of a high-risk population.[133] For screening, postmenopausal status, a positive family history, and possibly longstanding infertility apparently should be the focus. The largest series to date of postmenopausal women was reported preliminarily, with incomplete 1-year follow-up on 20,000 postmenopausal women.[189] The study protocol uses CA-125 as the initial screen, with a follow-up in 1 year if it is less than 30 units/ml and an ultrasound if it is abnormal. Oram reports the following:

Test	Specificity
CA-125	98.3
Vaginal exam	97.7
Vaginal exam/ultrasound	99.4
CA-125/ultrasound	99.9
CA-125/vaginal exam ± ultrasound	100.0

Oram reports three false-negative cases. A stage III germ cell tumor with a CA-125 level of 10 units/ml was diagnosed 8 months after the initial screening. A stage III serous carcinoma, with CA-125 of 22 units/ml, was diagnosed 13 months after the initial screening. A stage III clear cell carcinoma, with CA-125 of 85 units/ml and who refused the ultrasound per protocol, was diagnosed 6 months after initial screening. There were 11 false positives out of 20,000 screened.[189] As stated earlier, an acceptable positive predictive value is arbitrary, depending on the diagnostic procedure that follows. In ovary, the diagnostic procedure required is an operation (i.e., laparoscopy or laparotomy). Therefore the positive predictive value must be high to reduce the number of negative operations as much as possible.

The Familial Ovarian Cancer Registry at the Cleveland Clinic Foundation was established to address this issue of screening and to help identify a high-risk group in which to focus screening efforts and investigations more effectively. As previously stated, this discussion has focused by necessity on the epithelial tumors of the ovary. However, functioning ovarian tumors, although uncommon, present dramatically in the premenarchal woman and often in the menstruating or postmenopausal woman with abnormal bleeding or defeminization. Finally, in terms of the frequency of malignant growths within the ovary, metastatic disease to the ovary is more common than all categories of primary ovarian cancers, with the exception of epithelial tumors. This occurs principally from the breast, colon, or uterine endometrium.

CERVICAL UTERINE CANCER

It is estimated that, in the United States, 13,500 women will develop invasive carcinoma of the uterine cervix in 1992. If one adds to this an estimated 50,000 new cases of carcinoma in situ of the cervix, the magnitude of this problem is evident. It is estimated that 4400 women will die from carcinoma of the uterine cervix in 1992. Data from 1988 demonstrated that only 50% of women diagnosed as having cervical cancer had localized disease.[7] For a tumor so readily diagnosed, this amplifies the need for proper surveillance. The world-wide incidence of cervical cancer is second to breast cancer, but it is the most common cancer in developing countries, where screening programs are poorly developed.[158,168]

Risk factors

Socioeconomic status is inversely related to the incidence of cervical carcinoma. This relationship does not account for the racial difference in the incidence of the disease.[168] The most compelling risk factors clearly make a convincing argument for carcinoma of the cervix being a sexually transmitted disease. Women who initiate coitus less than 1 year after menarche have a 26 times relative risk of developing cervix cancer. Initiation from 1 to 5 years after menarche carries a seven times relative risk. First intercourse at less than age 16 is associated with a 16 times relative risk. Having more than four sexual partners vs. one or zero has a 3.6 relative risk, and having more than one sexual partner before age 20 has a relative risk of 7. Women who have had genital warts vs. those who have never had genital warts have a 3.2 relative risk.[201] Women whose husbands have previously been married to a woman who developed a cervix cancer have an increased risk of developing cervix cancer themselves. If the husband had penile or prostatic cancer, their risk appears likewise increased.[106] A woman who may have had only one partner but whose husband has had multiple partners is likewise at increased risk.[201,278] Smoking more than five cigarettes per day (more than 20 years vs. less than 1 year) has a relative risk of four for the development of carcinoma of the cervix.[201]

The common etiologic thread of carcinoma of the cervix appears to be an infectious agent. Over the years, numerous theories have been proposed, with a strong effort to implicate the herpes virus.[254] The initial enthusiasm for the potential role of the herpes virus and other infectious agents such as trichomonas or chlamydia trachomatis appears to be misplaced, because these agents appear to be associated with the sexual activity of the high-risk population rather than causative.

Recently, beginning with the observation of Meisels, an enormous amount of convincing data has accumulated linking human papilloma virus with cervical carcinoma.[175] Shope in 1933 documented the ability of the papilloma virus to induce epithelial growths.[235] The papilloma virus primarily infects epithelial tissue. These are DNA viruses that are highly prevalent in mammalian species, and they produce a wide variety of papillary growths. Numerous strains of the human papilloma virus have been identified through DNA hybridization techniques. HPV-1 is associated with plantar warts, HPV-2 with cutaneous warts, and HPV-3, HPV-5, and HPV-EV with epidermodysplasia verruciformis. HPV-6, 11, 16, 18, 31, 33, and 35 currently appear to be identified most frequently associated with genital disease. HPV-6 and 11 are associated with condyloma accuminata, and HPV-16 and 18 most frequently with higher grades of dysplasia and invasive carcinoma. Reed demonstrated that HPV-6 and 11 were found in 33% of patients with mild dysplasia (cervical intraepithelial neoplasia; CIN I). Of CIN I lesions, 15% contained HPV-6 and 11; and of CIN III, 4.5%.[219] The presence of HPV-16 varies directly with the severity of CIN, ranging from 10% to 25% in CIN I lesions to 50% to 75% of CIN III lesions.[145]

Currently it is not clear whether all cervix cancer is HPV associated. More than 60 viral types have been identified, and possibly types yet to be identified will be responsible for those apparent nonviral-associated lesions observed today. Some tumors may contain copy numbers of a known HPV type too low to detect with current techniques. On the other hand, a variety of issues of viral latency, persistence, and reactivation must be addressed in the future, because some studies suggest 10% to 50% of apparently healthy women are infected with genital human papilloma viruses. The primary evidence that HPV is etiologically related to cervical cancer is summarized as follows.

- HPV infections induce cervical lesions that are histologically identical to CIN.
- Most invasive lesions contain HPV, and CIN lesions contain HPV, with their viral profile changing with increasing grade.
- Cell lines derived from cervical cancer contain integrated HPV DNA.
- HPV DNA appeared to be stable in fresh biopsy material and established transformed cell lines.*

There appears to be a high rate of spontaneous regression of HPV lesions because of the prevalence of infectious nonneoplastic lower-genital-tract HPV. This suggests that immunocompromise or cofactors are required for premalignant and malignant conversion.[111,177] Cytologists often describe koilocytosis on pap smear reports as the cytopathic change that is associated with the presence of the

*References 38, 65, 88, 94, 129, 140, 220.

human papilloma virus infection. As cells become more immature, as in higher grade dysplasias and carcinoma in situ, they are less likely to demonstrate this change. One of the current unresolved challenges is to identify those patients whose HPV infection is likely to progress as opposed to those that will spontaneously regress. We hope future studies will determine whether the ability to identify the viral type will enable one to select the appropriate subset of patients for therapy and the majority for observation. Apparently one can classify HPV types according to their malignant potential. HPV 6, 11, 42, 43, and 44 represent the low-risk viruses. Intermediate risk viruses include HPV 31, 33, 35, 45, 51, 52, and 56. HPV 16 and 18 are high-risk viruses. HPV 18 is of particular interest in that it is detected in very few cases of CIN but in 22% of invasive squamous cell cancers. HPV 18 has been suggested as the cause of rapidly progressive cervical carcinoma. Possibly the lesions pass through CIN so quickly that they are not detected.[147,268] HPV has also been described in up to 55% of cases of adenocarcinoma. Again, HPV 18 might be the far more prevalent type.[248]

In the short term, well-established techniques for the prevention of sexually transmitted diseases, such as the condom, may decrease the risk of papilloma virus infection. With early educational programs, a better understanding may result in improved control of sexually transmitted diseases.

Presenting symptoms

A combination of postmenopausal bleeding, irregular menses, and postcoital bleeding account for the presenting symptom in the majority of patients with cervical carcinoma. Approximately 9% of patients present with vaginal discharge, some 6% with pain, and 8% of patients are asymptomatic.[196] Problems of bleeding, pain, and discharge are more common with advanced disease, whereas the abnormal Pap smear at the time of routine examination is more common with early disease. Of particular interest is the patient who is asymptomatic and who on examination has a friable cervix that bleeds easily with the performance of a Pap smear. The Pap smear in these patients may show inflammation. Such a Pap smear report should warn the clinician to review his or her examination findings and be particularly careful not to misinterpret a result reflecting the inflammatory exudate on the surface of a tumor. In general, one should biopsy a cervix that looks abnormal rather than rely on the Pap smear alone.

Screening recommendations

Papanicolaou introduced the Pap smear as a screening test for cervical cancer 50 years ago. Well-organized screening programs have demonstrated that the incidence of invasive cancer and the site-specific mortality have benefitted from these programs. The British Columbia Cervical Cancer Screening Program demonstrated a 78% de-

crease in incidence and a 72% decrease in mortality since the program was initiated in 1955.[13] The Alameda County data from 1960 to 1974 demonstrated a 40% reduction in the incidence and mortality among white women in the country. The study also reported that 29% of women diagnosed as having invasive cervical cancer had a history of a recent negative cytology.[79] The Kentucky Screening Program reported by Christopherson noted more than a 50% decrease in the death rate from cervical cancer, comparing the years 1973-1977 with 1953-1957.[53]

These results from successful screening programs would seem to settle the issue of annual screening. However, in 1976, the Canadian Task Force (The Walton Report)[43] recommended that a woman should begin having Pap smears at the onset of sexual activity. They recommended that, after two negative Pap smears, Pap smears be done every 3 years, and high-risk women continue to have annual Pap smears. High risk was defined as early onset of sexual activity or multiple sexual partners. A number of papers followed the Walton Report, capped off by a recommendation by the American Cancer Society in 1980 endorsing screening every 3 years. This was strongly countered by the American College of Obstetricians and Gynecologists, holding to a position of annual screening, and the lines were therefore drawn for the continuing controversy.

The American Cancer Society and the American College of Obstetricians and Gynecologists, in an attempt to decrease some of the confusion about cervical cancer screening, issued joint guidelines in 1988.[8,11] Both suggested that screening should commence at the onset of sexual activity and should begin with three negative annual tests. After the initial three annual screens, screening should continue every 3 years. Both organizations recommend that screening should continue for the lifetime of the person. More frequent screening is recommended for high-risk individuals, defined as those with onset of sexual activity before age 18, DES exposure in utero, multiple partners (two or more), or partners with multiple other partners. If an individual is in a high-risk group, the decision about screening interval needs to be an informed decision involving the doctor and the patient.[11]

The current guidelines, especially from the American College of Obstetricians and Gynecologists' standpoint, represent a modification of the earlier stance adhering to annual screening. Beginning with the Walton Report and the more recent writings of David Eddy, the population-based screening programs clearly must be viewed differently from privately funded screening for individuals based on their needs and desires.[80]

Day, at the International Agency for Research on Cancer, analyzed data from several population-based screening programs in North America and Europe on the incidence of invasive cervical cancer related to screening frequency. The data reported assumed that screening began at age 35 and that each woman had had a previous negative Pap smear. The model looked at screening between the ages of 35 and 64 years.[130] The American Cancer Society developed a mathematical model to estimate the relative effectiveness of different screening frequencies. The mathematical predictions were within 1% of the empirical data from Day's analysis.[79] The greatest difference between the model and Day's data was that the model overestimated the benefits of annual examination compared with biannual or triannual exams.

Based on newer empirical data, especially in regard to the average duration of the preinvasive stage of cancers that progress rapidly and further analysis of the sources of the false-negative Pap test, the model was recalibrated to improve its accuracy. The revised model demonstrates that the cumulative rate of invasive cancers of the cervix will be reduced 91% with triannual screening. This would require 10 tests between the ages of 35 and 64 years. If one moved to annual screening, requiring a total of 30 tests during that same interval, the improvement in the reduction of cervical cancer would be less than 3%. This would result in more than four times the cost.[79] The effectiveness of screening at different frequencies is determined primarily by four parameters:

1. The proportion of cervical cancers having a long preinvasive stage
2. The duration of the preinvasive stage
3. The duration of preinvasive stage for cases that progress rapidly
4. The false-negative rate of the Pap smear.

A variety of studies have documented the false-negative rate ranging from 5% to more than 55%.[179] In general, the false-negative rate is lower for patients with invasive disease than with milder grades of CIN. Highly specialized labs clearly are the exception, and a false-negative rate of 20% to 30% for a single smear in routine practice is to be expected. The false-negative rate will depend on the ability of the individual taking the smear, the location and grade of the lesion, the accuracy of interpretation, and the age of the patient. It is important to know that the false-negative Pap was included in the mathematical model. However, when it comes to the individual patient and her individual risk factors, the screening interval may be appropriately different from population-based recommendations. Still, the most important step is to screen the unscreened. Women who have never had a Pap smear have a four times greater risk of cervical cancer compared with women from a screened population.[150]

Many of the cancer screening efforts have neglected the older population of women. Between 1974 and 1986, cervical cancer mortality declined only 17% among women aged 50 and older, compared with 43% for women under the age of 50. Women age 65 and older account for nearly half of the deaths from cervical cancer.[167] Most of this poor outcome is attributable to lack of screening; however, the difficulty in obtaining an accurate smear from some elderly patients, as well as the potential influence on progression rate from the altered immune status in the elderly, may also affect these data. There currently is no data looking specifically at the behavior of HPV in an elderly population.

There are a variety of other issues concerning Pap screening. As mentioned previously, some suggest that HPV 18 may be associated with a more rapidly developing variety of cervical cancer. If the character or rate of progression of CIN begins to change, screening frequencies will need to be reevaluated. Unless high-risk individuals can be shown to have a high risk of acquiring an HPV subtype that has a more rapid progression, simply being high risk does not necessarily mean the individual needs to be screened more frequently. The individual only needs to be screened. There is no evidence to promote frequent Pap smear screening for the detection of other malignancies by pap smear or by pelvic exams. Population-based data demonstrate no evidence to support this practice.[43] There is some concern that, whatever the final recommendation, the actual screening interval tends to be longer. Again, on a population-based program, this requires education rather than adjusting the entire program.

Women who have had a hysterectomy often ask whether they need continued Pap screening, especially if the ovaries have been removed at the time of the hysterectomy. The primary determinant of the need for continued screening is the individual woman's risk, based especially on the reason the hysterectomy was performed. If the hysterectomy was performed for preinvasive or invasive cervical cancer, follow-up screening is vitally important. A woman who has had negative smears her whole life and then has a hysterectomy for reasons unrelated to preinvasive or invasive cervical cancer likely will obtain minimal benefit from future screening.

It is also important to note that, regardless of the screening interval, when an abnormal result is obtained on a Pap smear, the results must be appropriately followed. On retrospective review, 15% of cervical cancers apparently reveal inappropriate follow-up of prior abnormal Pap smears.[168,179]

Over the past several years, the many discussions about screening interval primarily have focused on money. The screening process has minimal morbidity and is well accepted by patients. It is important that the individual patient understands that she can make a decision for herself with her physician to be screened at more frequent intervals based on her personal risk. In a private pay system, this would be especially true. However, as stated before, the most common reason women with cervical cancer escape detection is that they have never been screened. The majority of these cases occur in older women.[168] Screening the unscreened must be the priority because primary

Table 30-6. Summary

	Risk factors	Screening recommendations
Endometrial cancer	Obesity Unopposed estrogen (exogenous and endogenous) Diabetes Nulliparity Pelvic radiation	Not cost-effective Nor warranted

Ovarian cancer	Genetic
	  Northern European ancestry
	  Site-specific
	    Ovarian syndrome
	    Breast/ovarian syndrome
	    Lynch II syndrome
	Environmental
	  Industrialized nations
	  Talc?
	  Pelvic radiation
	Hormonal
	  Infertility
	Viral?
	  Rubella
	  Subclinical mumps (non-childhood)
		Women from high risk families should have:
		  vaginal ultrasounds, CA-125, and pelvic exams q 6
		  mos.

Cervical cancer	Coitus before age 18
	Multiple sexual partners (or a partner with multiple
	  contacts)
	Cigarette smoking
	DES exposure
		Annual Pap smear beginning with onset of sexual ac-
		  tivity
		If *low risk* then every 3 years after 3 negative annual
		  screens

Vulvo-vaginal	Same as cervical cancer	Specific screening not warranted

---

The Bethesda system
Atypical squamous cells
Squamous intraepithelial lesions (cellular changes consistent with HPV)
Low grade
HPV
Mild dysplasia/CIN 1
High grade
Moderate dysplasia/CIN 2
Severe dysplasia/CIN 3
Carcinoma in situ/CIN 3
Squamous cell carcinoma

prevention unfortunately is often most appreciated by those at low risk.

The Pap smear should be performed with good visualization of the cervix and before wiping any mucus from the cervix. The Pap smear should consist of an endocervical sample as well as an exocervical scrape. Both may be placed on the same slide, and they should be either placed in alcohol or sprayed with spray fixative within 10 to 15 seconds of placing them on the slide. In the postmenopausal woman, drying artifact will occur much more quickly than the younger woman at midcycle. An adequate endocervical sample is essential, and the current brush technique appears to satisfy issues of quality, as well as ease of performance and patient satisfaction.

In 1988 the Bethesda system for reporting cytologic diagnosis of squamous cell abnormalities of the cervix was published (see box at left). The attempt, as with previous classifications, is designed to simplify the reporting system as well as recognize current theories of pathogenesis.[185]

VULVAR AND VAGINAL MALIGNANCIES

Vulvar and vaginal cancers combined account for less than 5% of the malignant lesions of the female reproductive tract. The majority of cases are associated with many of the same risk factors as squamous carcinoma of the cervix, except the diseases tend to occur 16 to 20 years later.[204] Screening specifically for either vulvar or vaginal cancers is unjustified. However, two points concerning early diagnosis are vital.

Vulvar cancers usually present with vulvar itching or pain. Any time a woman has a pelvic exam, the examiner should carefully inspect the vulva. Unless the lesion is moist, a pap smear will likely not be accurate. A painful ulcer that resembles a herpetic lesion may be watched for a week to 10 days, but then biopsy is essential without improvement. All other ulcerative lesions, as well as white lesions and pigmented lesions, should be biopsied. The easiest way to biopsy the vulva is to use a small amount of local anesthesia and a 3 mm Keys dermal punch.

Carcinoma of the vagina most frequently occurs in the posterior wall, upper-third, and anterior wall, distal-third. As one removes the speculum from the vagina, the posterior blade, which would have covered the upper-third posterior wall lesion, is replaced by the cervix moving posteriorly. Therefore, unless one is careful, a small early vaginal lesion could be missed. Likewise, examiners frequently remove the speculum quickly as it reaches the outer third of the vagina and could easily fail to notice an anterior distal-third lesion. If any abnormalities are seen or palpated, they should be sampled with a Pap test and biopsied. For this, a standard cervical biopsy instrument is most appropriate. Most commonly, we are seeing multifocal, nonneoplastic papilloma virus lesions in the vagina with a somewhat lower incidence of accompanying vaginal dysplasia. These lesions, when viewed through the colposcope and biopsied, are generally treated by topical chemotherapy,[20] excision, or laser ablation[243] (Table 30-6).

REFERENCES
1. Abel EL, Sokol RJ: Fetal alcohol syndrome, *Lancet* 2(8517):1222-1223, 1986.
2. ACOG Committee opinion 68: Report of task force on routine cancer screening, 97, April, 1989.
3. Adams MR et al: Contraceptive steroids and coronary artery atherosclerosis in cynomolgus macaques, *Fertil Steril* 47:1010, 1987.
4. Affandi B et al: Five year experience with Norplant, *Contraception* 36:417-428, 1987.
5. American College of Obstetricians and Gynecologists: *Alpha-fetoprotein,* ACOG Technical Bulletin *154,* Washington, DC, 1991, The College.
6. American Cancer Society: ACS report of the cancer related health check-up, *CA* 30:194-240, 1980.
7. American Cancer Society: Cancer factors and figures, 92:425, 1992.
8. American Cancer Society: Statement by Dr. Harmon Eyre, National President, New York, 1988, the Society.
9. American College of Obstetricians and Gynecologists: *Antenatal diagnosis of genetic disorders,* ACOG Technical Bulletin *108,* Washington, DC, 1987, the College.
10. American College of Obstetricians and Gynecologists: *Guidelines for perinatal care,* ed 3, Washington, DC, 1992, the College.
11. American College of Obstetricians and Gynecologists: Statement of George Morley, M.D., president ACOG, Washington, DC, Jan 19, 1988, the College.
12. An-Foraker SH: Cytologic detection of adenocarcinomatous lesions by routine gynecologic sample, *Can J Med Tech* 38:84, 1976.
13. Anderson GH et al: Organisation and results of the cervical cytology screening programme in British Columbia, 1955-1985, *Br Med J* 296:975-978, 1988.
14. Armenia CS: Sequential relationship between endometrial polyps and carcinoma of the endometrium, *Obstet Gynecol* 30:524, 1967.
15. Artal R: Exercise in pregnancy. In Cherry S, Merkatz I, editors: *Complications of pregnancy: medical, surgical, gynecologic, psychosocial and perinatal,* ed 4, Baltimore, 1991, Williams and Wilkins.
16. Artal R et al: Fetal responses to maternal exercise. In Artal R,
Wisell RA, editors: *Exercise in pregnancy,* ed 2, Baltimore, 1990, Williams and Wilkins.
17. Artal R et al: Pulmonary responses to exercise in pregnancy, *Am J Obstet Gynecol* 154:378-383, 1986.
18. Asch RH et al: Performance and sensitivity of modern home pregnancy tests, *Int J Fertil* 33(3):154-161, 1988.
19. Attico NB: Contraception update, *IHS Primary Care Provider* 14:77-85, 1989.
20. Ballon STC, Roberts JA, and Logasse LD: Topical 5-Fluorouracil in the treatment of intraepithelial neoplasia of the vagina, *Obstet Gynecol* 54:163-166, 1979.
21. Barber H: New options for contraception, *The female patient,* vol 16, Belle Mead NJ, 1991, Core Publishing.
22. Barber HRK, Garber EA: The PMPO syndrome (post menopausal palpable ovary syndrome), *Obstet Gynecol* 38:921, 1971.
23. Barden CW: Contraceptive choices, *Int J Fertil* 34(suppl):88, 1989.
23a. Barrett D, Wein A: Voiding dysfunction: diagnosis, classification, and management. In Gillenwater J, et al (editors): *Adult and pediatric urology,* St. Louis, 1991, Mosby–Year Book.
24. Barrett-Connor E, Bush TL: Estrogen and coronary heart disease in women, *JAMA* 265:1861-1864, 1991.
25. Bast RC et al: A radioimmunoassay using a monoclonal antibody to monitor the course of epithelial ovarian cancer, *N Engl J Med* 309:883, 1983.
26. Beischer, NA: The effects of maternal anemia upon the fetus, *J Reprod Med* 6:262-265, 1971.
27. Belinson JL et al: Clinical stage I endometrial carcinoma: a management plan with long term follow-up (Submitted to Surgery, Gynecology and Obstetrics, 1991).
28. Belinson JL et al: Management of epithelial ovarian carcinoma using a platinum based regimen—a ten year experience, *Gynecol Oncol* 37:6673, 1990.
29. Benacerraf BR et al: Sonographic diagnosis of Down's syndrome in the second trimester, *Am J Obstet Gynecol* 153:49, 1985.
30. Berkelman RL et al: Patterns of alcohol consumption and alcohol related morbidity and mortality, *MMWR CDC Surveill Summ* 35:155-555, 1986.
31. Berkowitz RL: Intrauterine transfusion. Antepartum symposium on high-risk pregnancy, *Clin Perinatol* 7:2-9, 1980.
32. Berol V et al: Oral contraceptive use and malignancies of the genital tract, *Lancet* 11:1331-1334, 1988.
33. Bluestein D: Monoclonal antibody pregnancy tests, *Am Fam Phys* 38(1):197-204, 1988.
34. Bluestein D: Should I trust office pregnancy tests, *Postgrad Med* 87:(6):57-64, 1990.
35. Brambati B et al: Chorionic villus sampling: an analysis of the obstetric experience of 1000 cases, *Prenat Diagn* 7:157-169, 1987.
36. Brambati B, Lanzani A: Transabdominal and transcervical chorionic villus sampling; efficiency and risk evaluation of 2411 cases, *Am J Med Genet* 35:160-164, 1990.
37. Brinton LA et al: Risks factors for benign breast disease, *Am J Epidemiol* 113:203-214, 1981.
38. Buckley JD et al: Case control study of the husbands of women with dysplasia or carcinoma of the cervix uteri, *Lancet* 2:1010, 1981.
39. Bullough V: *Contraction: a guide to birth control methods.* Buffalo, NY, 1990, Prometheus Books.
40. Burdon RH et al: *Laboratory technique in biochemistry and molecular biology,* New York, 1987, Elsevier.
41. Bush TL et al: Cardiovascular mortality in noncontraceptive use of estrogen in women: results from the Lipid Research Clinics Program follow-up study, *Circulation* 75:1102-1109, 1987.
42. Campbell S et al: Real-time ultrasonography for determination of ovarian morphology and volume, *Lancet* 425:6, 1982.
43. Canadian Task Force, cervical cancer screening programs: Epidemiology and natural history of carcinoma of the cervix, *Can Med Assoc J* 114:1003-1033, 1976.

44. Cancer and Steroid Hormone Study of the Centers for Disease Control and the National Institute of Child Health and Human Development: Combination contraceptive use and the risk of endometrial cancer, *JAMA* 257:796-800, 1987.

45. Cancer and Steroid Hormone Study of the Centers for Disease Control and the National Institute of Child Health and Human Development: Oral contraceptive use and the risk of breast cancer, *N Engl J Med* 315:405, 1986.

46. Centers for Disease Control: Public health service guidelines for counseling and antibody testing to prevent HIV infection and AIDS, Public Health Sem *MMWR* 36:509-515, 1987.

47. Centers for Disease Control: Sexual behavior among high school students, *MMWR* 40:885-888, 1992.

48. Centers for Disease Control: Use of folic acid for prevention of spina bifida and other neural tube defects, 1983-1991, *MMWR* 40:513-516, 1991.

49. Chamlian DL, Taylor HB: Endometrial hyperplasia in young women, *Obstet Gynecol* 36:659, 1970.

50. Chasnoff IJ: Cocaine use in pregnancy: perinatal morbidity and mortality, *Neurotoxicol Teratol* 9:291-293, 1990.

51. Cherry S, Merkatz I, editors: *Complications of pregnancy: medical, surgical gynecology, psychosocial and perinatal,* ed 4, Baltimore, 1991, Williams & Wilkins.

52. Chetkowski RJ et al: Biologic effects of transdermal estradiol, *N Engl J Med* 314:1615-1620, 1986.

53. Christopherson WM: Cytologic detection in diagnosis of cancer. Its contributions and limitations, *Cancer* 51:1201, 1983.

54. Colditz GA et al: Prospective study of estrogen replacement therapy and risk of breast cancer in postmenopausal women, *JAMA* 264:2648-2653, 1990.

55. Cole LA, Nam JH: Urinary gonadotropin fragment (UGF) measurements in the diagnosis and management of ovarian cancer, *Yale J Biol Med* 62:367-378, 1989.

56. Collins WP: Early pregnancy tests, *Br J Obstet Gynecol* 97:204-207, 1990.

57. Connell E: Barrier contraceptives, *Clin Obstet Gynecol* 32:2, 1989.

58. Consensus Conference: Progestagen use in postmenopausal women, *Lancet* 2:1243-1244, 1988.

59. Coons S: A look at the purchase and use of home pregnancy-test kits, *Am Pharm* (4):46-48, 1989.

60. Coons SJ et al: The use of pregnancy test kits by college students, *J Am Coll Health* 38:171-175, 1990.

61. Cramer DW et al: Factors affecting the association of oral contraceptives and ovarian cancer, *N Engl J Med* 307:1047-1057, 1982.

62. Cramer DW et al: Ovarian cancer and talc: a case-control study, *Cancer* 50:372-376, 1982.

63. Creasman WT: Estrogen replacement therapy: is previously treated cancer a contraindication? *Obstet Gynecol* 77:308-312, 1991.

64. Croft P et al: Risk factors for acute myocardial infarction in women: evidence from the Royal College of General Practitioners' oral contraceptive study, *Br Med J* 298:165-168, 1989.

65. Crum CP et al: Human papilloma virus type 16 and early cervical neoplasia, *N Engl J Med* 310:880, 1984.

66. Cuckle HS et al: Estimating a woman's risk of having a pregnancy with Down's syndrome using her age and serum AFP level, *Br J Obstet Gynecol* 94:387, 1987.

67. Cummings KM: Factors influencing success in counseling patients to stop smoking, *Patient Educ Counsel* 8:189-200, 1986.

68. Cummings SR, Black DM, and Rubin SM: Lifetime risks of hip, Colles', or vertebral fracture and coronary heart disease among white postmenopausal women, *Arch Intern Med* 149:2445-2448, 1989.

69. Cutler BS et al: Endometrial carcinoma after stilbestrol therapy in gonadal dysgenesis, *N Engl J Med* 287:628, 1972.

70. Cutler SJ, Young JL, editors: Third national cancer survey: incidence data, *National Cancer Institute Monograph No 41,* DHEW publication (NIH) 75-787, Washington, DC, 1975, US Government Printing Office.

71. Darney P et al: Sustained-release contraceptives, *Curr Prob Obstet Gynecol Fert* 13(3):96-125, 1990.

72. Davies JL et al: A review of the risk factors for endometrial carcinoma, *Obstet Gynecol Surv* 36:107-116, 1981.

73. Dembo AJ, Cheng PL, and Urbach GI: Clinical correlations of ovarian cancer antigen MB/70K: a preliminary report, *Obstet Gynecol* 65:710, 1985.

74. Dent T, Brueschke E: Barrier contraceptives, *Female Patient* (6):57-62, 1981.

75. Dicker RC et al: Oral contraceptive use and the risk of ovarian cancer, *JAMA* 249:1596-1599, 1983.

76. Donnenfeld AE et al: Sonographic findings in fetuses with chromosome abnormalities, *Clin Obstet Gynecol* 31:80-96, 1988.

77. Dorfman S: Pregnancy for older parents. In Cherry S, Merkatz I, editors: *Complications of pregnancy: medical, surgical, gynecologic, psychosocial and perinatal,* Baltimore, 1991, Williams & Wilkins.

78. Dumont-Herskowitz RA, Safaii HS, and Senior B: Ovarian fibromata in four successive generations, *J Pediatr* 93:621, 1978.

79. Dunn JE, Schweitzer V: The relationship of cervical cytology to the incidence of invasive cervical cancer and mortality in Alameda County, California, 1960-1974, *Am J Obstet Gynecol* 139:868, 1981.

80. Eddy DM: Screening for cervical cancer, *Ann Intern Med* 113:214-226, 1990.

81. Edelman DA et al: The intrauterine device and ectopic pregnancy, *Contraception* 36:85, 1987.

82. Edgren RA: Oral contraceptives and cancer, *Int J Fertil* 36(suppl)(3):37-50, 1991.

83. Egli GE, Newton M: The transport of carbon particles in the human female reproductive tract, *Fertil Steril* 12:151, 1961.

84. Emans SJ: Adolescent compliance with the use of oral contraceptives, *JAMA* 257:3377, 1987.

85. Ettinger B: Hormone replacement in coronary artery disease, *Obstet Gynecol Clin North Am* 17:741-757, 1990.

86. Ewing JA et al: Detecting alcoholism: CAGE questionnaire, *JAMA* 252:1905-1907, 1984.

86a. Fantl JA et al: Efficacy of bladder training in older women with urinary incontinence, *JAMA* 265:5.

87. Fasoli M et al: Post coital contraception, *Contraception* 39:459, 1989.

88. Fenoglio CM, Ferenczy A: Etiologic factors in cervical neoplasia, *Semin Oncol* 9:349, 1982.

89. Fields S et al: Pregnancy testing—home and office, *West J Med* 154(3):327-328, 1991.

90. Finch BE: *Balls, feathers and caps. Contraception through the ages,* Springfield, Ill, 1964, Charles C. Thomas.

91. Finkler NJ et al: Comparison of serum CA-125, clinical impression and ultrasound in the preoperative evaluation of ovarian masses, *Obstet Gynecol* 72:659-664, 1988.

92. Fiore MC et al: Trends in cigarette smoking in the United States: the changing influence of gender and race, *JAMA* 261:49-55, 1986.

93. Fleisher AC et al: Differential diagnosis of pelvic masses by gray scale sonography, *Am J Roent* 131:469, 1978.

94. Foo YS, Reagan J, Richart RM: Definition of precursors of cervical cancer, *Gynecol Oncol* 12:220s, 1981.

95. Forrest JD: The end of IUD marketing in the United States: what does it mean for American women? *Fam Plann Perspect* 18:52, 1986.

96. Fox SH: Perceptions of risks of smoking and heavy drinking during pregnancy: 1985 NHIS findings, *Public Health Rep* 102:73-79, 1987.

97. Foxman B, Frerichs R: Epidemiology of urinary tract infection: I. Diaphragm use and sexual intercourse, *Am J Public Health* 75:1308, 1985.

98. Friedman MH, Lapham ME: A simple, rapid procedure for laboratory diagnosis of early pregnancies, *Am J Obstet Gynecol* 21:405, 1931.

99. Galjaard H: Early diagnosis and prevention of genetic disease. In Galjaard H, editor: *Aspects of human genetics,* Basel, Switzerland, 1984, Karger.

100. Gallion HH et al: Adjuvant oral alkylating chemotherapy in patients with stage I epithelial ovarian cancer, *Cancer* 63:1070-1073, 1989.

101. Gambrell RD: Prevention of endometrial cancer with progestogens, *Maturitas* 8:159-160, 1986.

102. Gambrell RD et al: Use of the progestogen challenge test to reduce the risk of endometrial cancer, *Obstet Gynecol* 55:732, 1980.

103. Gorman JC et al: Intramuscular injections of a new experimental gamma globulin preparation containing high levels of anti-Rh antibody as a means of preventing sensitization to Rh, *Proceedings of the Ninth Congress of the International Society of Hematology* 2:545-552, 1962.

104. Goswamy RK, Campbell S, and Whitehead MI: Screening for ovarian cancer, *Clin Obstet Gynecol* 10:621-643, 1983.

105. Grady WR et al: Contraceptive discontinuation among married women in the United States, *Studies Fam Plann* 19:227, 1988.

106. Graham S et al: Genital cancer in wives of penile cancer patients, *Cancer* 44:1870, 1989.

107. Gray RH: Toxic shock syndrome and oral contraception, *Am J Obstet Gynecol* 156:1038, 1987.

108. Green MH, Clark JW, and Blayney DW: The epidemiology of ovarian cancer, *Semin Oncol* 11:209-226, 1984.

109. Grimes D: "Whither the intrauterine device?" *Clin Obstet Gynecol* 32:6, 1989.

110. Grimes DA: Diagnostic dilation and curettage: a reappraisal, *Am J Obstet Gynecol* 142:1-6, 1982.

111. Halpert R et al: Human papilloma virus and lower genital neoplasia in renal transplant patients, *Obstet Gynecol* 68:251, 1986.

112. Hanna JH et al: Detection of postmenopausal women at risk for endometrial carcinoma by a progestogen challenge test, *Obstet Gynecol* 147:872, 1983.

113. Hannaford P: Oral contraceptives and rheumatoid arthritis: new data from the Royal College of General Practitioners' oral contraceptive study, *Ann Rheum Dis* 49(10):744-746, 1991.

114. Hanson JW: The effects of moderate alcohol consumption during pregnancy on fetal growth and morphogenesis, *J Pediatr* 92:457-460, 1978.

115. Harrison EA: Preconception and postconception care of women with medical illness. In Merakatz IR, editor: *New perspectives on prenatal care,* New York, 1990, Elsevier.

116. Hawwa ZM, Nahhas WA, and Copenhaver EH: Postmenopausal bleeding, *Lahey Clin Found Bull* 19:61, 1970.

117. Henderson BE, Paginini-Hill A, and Ross RK: Decreased mortality in users of estrogen replacement therapy, *Arch Intern Med* 151:75-78, 1991.

118. Hertig AT, Gore H: Ovarian cystomas of germinal epithelial origin–a histogenetic classification, *Rocky Mt Med J* 55:47-55, 1958.

119. Higgins RV et al: Intraobserver variation in ovarian measurements using transvaginal sonography, *Gynecol Oncol* 39:69-71, 1990.

120. Higgins RV et al: Transvaginal sonography as a screening method of ovarian cancer, *Gynecol Oncol* 34, 402, 1989.

121. Hill FG: Hematologic disorders, *Clin Obstet Gynecol* 9:75, 1982.

122. Himmelberger D et al: Cigarette smoking during pregnancy and the occurrence of spontaneous abortion and congenital abnormality, *Am J Epidemiol* 108:470, 1978.

123. Hobel CJ et al: Prenatal and intrapartum high-risk screening II. Risk factors reassessed, *Am J Obstet Gynecol* 135:1051, 1979.

124. Home test market expected to top $1 billion by 1992, *Drug Top* 131(18):58, 1987.

125. Hook EB: Rates of chromosome abnormalities at different maternal ages, *Obstet Gynecol* 58:282-283, 1981.

126. Horenstein J: Ultrasound assessment of fetal growth and fetal measurements, *Semin Perinatol* 12:23-30, 1988.

127. Hulka BS: Cancer screening: degrees of proof and practical application, *Cancer* 62:1776-1780, 1988.

128. Hulka BS: Hormone-replacement therapy and the risk of breast cancer. *CA* 40:289-296, 1990.

129. Hulka BS: Risk factors for cervical cancer, *J Chron Dis* 35:3, 1982.

130. IARC Working Group on Evaluation of Cervical Cancer Screening Programs (Day NE): Screening for squamous cervical cancer: duration of low risk after negative results of cervical cytology and its implication for screening policies, *Br Med J* 293:659-664, 1986.

131. Iversen OE, Segadal E: The value of endometrial cytology. A comparative study of the Gravlee Jet-Washer, Isaacs Cell Sampler and Endoscann versus curettage in 600 patients, *Obstet Gynecol Surv* 40:14-20, 1985.

132. Jaber R: Detection of and screening for endometrial cancer, *J Fam Pract* 26:1, 1988.

133. Jacobs I, Stabile I, and Bridges J: Multimodal approach to screening for ovarian cancer, *Lancet* I(8580):268-271, 1988.

134. Jeng L et al: How frequently are home pregnancy tests used? Results from the 1988 National Maternal and Infant Health Survey, *Birth* 18:1, 1991.

135. Jones EF et al: Unintended pregnancy, contraceptive practice and family planning services in developed countries, *Fam Plann Perspect* 20:53-67, 1988.

136. Kafe S: Topics in prenatal diagnosis. In Cherry S, Merkatz I, editors: *Complications of pregnancy: medical, surgical, gynecologic, psychosocial and perinatal,* Baltimore, 1991, Williams & Wilkins.

137. Kaunitz AM et al: Comparison of endometrial biopsy with the endometrial Pipelle and the Vabra aspirator, *J Reprod Med* 33:427-431, 1988.

138. Kaunitz MA et al: Causes of maternal mortality in the United States, *Obstet Gynecol* 65:605, 1985.

139. Kiel DP et al: Hip fracture and the use of estrogens in postmenopausal women, *N Engl J Med* 317:169, 1987.

140. Kessler II: Cervical cancer: social and sexual correlates. In Peto R, zurHausen H, editors: *Viral etiology of cancer,* New York, 1986, Cold Spring Harbor Laboratory.

141. Kleinberg F et al: Effect of drugs and chemicals on the fetus and newborn, *Mayo Clin Proc* 59:707, 1984.

142. Kleinerman RA et al: Second cancers following radiotherapy for cervical cancer, *J Natl Cancer Inst* 69:1027-1033, 1982.

143. Knapp RC, Bertowitz RS: *Gynecologic oncology* New York, 1986, Macmillan.

144. Koss LG et al: Screening of asymptomatic women for endometrial cancer, *CA* 31:300-317, 1981.

145. Koutsky LA, Galloway DA, and Holmes KK: Epidemiology of genital human papillomavirus infection, *Epidemio Rev* 10:122-163, 1988.

146. Kurman RJ, Kominski PF, and Norris HJ: The behavior of endometrial hyperplasia. A long term study of "untreated" hyperplasia in 170 patients, *Cancer* 56:403, 1985.

147. Kurman RJ et al: Analysis of individual human papilloma virus types in cervical neoplasia. A possible role for type 1 in rapid progression, *Am J Obstet Gynecol* 159:293, 1988.

148. Landsom S et al: Serosurvey of HIV infection in parturients, *JAMA* 258:2701-2703, 1987.

149. Latman N, Bruot B: Evaluation of home pregnancy test kits, *Biomed Instrument Tech* 23:144-149, 1989.

150. LaVecchia C, Francschi S, and DeCarli A: Pap smears and the risk of cervical neoplasia: quantitative estimates from a case controlled study, *Lancet* 2:779, 1984.

151. Leader A et al: A comparison of defineable traits in women requesting reversal of sterilization and women satisfied with sterilization, *Am J Obstet Gynecol* 145:198-202, 1983.

152. Lehmann DK: Pregnancy outcome in medically complicated and uncomplicated patients aged 40 years or older, *Am J Obstet Gynecol* 57:738-742, 1987.

153. Lewis ACW, Davison BCC: Familial ovarian cancer, *Lancet* 2:235-237, 1969.

154. Lindsay R et al: The effect of oral contraceptive use on vertebral bone mass in pre- and post-menopausal women, *Contraception* 34:333, 1986.

155. Liskin L et al: Hormonal contraception: new long-acting methods, *Popul Rep* 15:57, 1987.

156. Longo LD: The biologic effects of carbon monoxide on the pregnant woman, fetus, and newborn infant. *Am J Obstet Gynecol* 129:69, 1977.

157. Love RR et al: Effects of tamoxifen on bone mineral density in postmenopausal women with breast cancer, *N Engl J Med* 336:852-856, 1992.

158. Lunt R: Worldwide early detection of cervical cancer, *Obstet Gynecol* 63:708, 1984.

159. Lurain JR, Piver MS: Familial ovarian carcinoma, *Gynecol Oncol* 8:185, 1979.

160. Lynch HT et al: Surveillance and management of patients at high genetic risk for ovarian carcinoma, *Obstet Gynecol* 59:589-596, 1982.

161. Lynch HT et al: Familial association of breast/ovarian carcinoma, *Cancer* 41:1543-1549, 1978.

162. Lynch HT, Lynch PM: Tumor variation in the cancer family syndrome: ovarian cancer, *Am J Surg* 138:439, 1979.

163. MacDonald PC et al: Effect of obesity on the conversion of plasma androstenedione to estrone in postmenopausal women with and without endometrial cancer, *Am J Obstet Gynecol* 130:448-455, 1978.

164. Maciak BJ et al: Pregnancy and birth rates among sexually experienced U.S. teenagers—1974, 1980, 1983, *JAMA* 258:2069-2071, 1987.

165. Mack TM et al: Estrogens and endometrial cancer in a retirement community, *N Engl J Med* 294(23):1262-1267, 1976.

166. MacMahon B: Risk factors for endometrial cancer, *Gynecol Oncol* 2:122, 1974.

167. Mandelblatt J et al: Clinical implications of screening for cervical cancer under Medicare, *Am J Obstet Gynecol* 164:644-651, 1991.

168. Mandelblatt J: Cervical cancer screening primary care: issues and recommendations, *Prim Care* 16:133-155, 1989.

169. Matthews KA et al: Menopause and risk factors for coronary heart disease, *N Engl J Med* 321:641-646, 1989.

170. McDonald TW et al: Exogenous exposure to estrogen and endometrial carcinoma: case control and incidence study, *Am J Obstet Gynecol* 127:572-580, 1977.

171. McGowan L et al: The woman at risk for developing ovarian cancer, *Gynecol Oncol* 7:325, 1979.

172. McKay FW, Hanson MR, and Miller RW: *Cancer mortality in the United States: 1950-1977*, NCI Monograph 59, NIH Publication 82:2435, 1982.

173. A vaginal contraceptive sponge, *Med Lett Drugs Ther* 25(642):78-84, 1983.

174. Cervical cap, *Med Lett Drugs Ther* 30(776):93-94, 1988.

175. Meisels A, Fortin R, and Roy M: Condylomatous lesions of the cervix II. Cytologic colposcopic and histopathologic study, *Acta Cytol* 21:379-390, 1977.

176. Meisels A, Jolicoeur C: Criteria for the cytologic assessment of hyperplasias in endometrial samples obtained by the Endopap endometrial sampler, *Acta Cytol* 29:297, 1985.

177. Meisels A, Morin C: Human papilloma virus and cancer of the uterine cervix, *Gynecol Oncol* 12:111s, 1981.

178. Mencaglia L et al: Endometrial carcinoma and its precursors: early detection and treatment, *Int J Gynecol Obstet* 31:107-116, 1990.

179. Morell ND et al: False-negative cytology rates in patients in whom invasive surgical cancer subsequently developed, *Obstet Gynecol* 60:41-45, 1982.

180. Morris N et al: Effective uterine blood flow during exercise in normal and pre-eclampsia pregnancies, *Lancet* 2:481-484, 1956.

181. Morrison I et al: Perinatal mortality and antepartum risk scoring, *Obstet Gynecol* 53(3):362, 1979.

182. Mosher W: Fertility and family planning in the U.S.; insights from the National Survey of Family Growth, *Fam Plann Prospect* 20:207-217, 1988.

183. MRC Vitamin Study Research Group: Prevention of neural tube defects: results of the medical research council vitamin study, *Lancet* 338:131-137, 1991.

184. National Center for Health Statistics: *Vital statistics of the United States, 1985*, vol 2, part A, Washington, DC, publication no DHHS (PHS) 88-110.

185. National Cancer Institute Workshop: The 1988 Bethesda system for reporting cervical/vaginal cytological diagnoses, *JAMA* 262:931-934, 1989.

185a. National Institutes of Health Consensus Development Conference Statement, Urinary Incontinence, 7(5), 1988.

186. Newhouse ML: Cosmetic talc and ovarian cancer, *Lancet* 1:528, 1979.

187. Ng ABP et al: Significance of endometrial cells in the detection of endometrial carcinoma and its precursors, *Acta Cytol* 18:356, 1974.

188. Nicolini U, Ferrazzi E, and Bellotti M: The contribution of sonographic evaluation of ovarian size in patients with polycystic ovarian disease, *J Ultrasound Med* 4:347-351, 1985.

189. Oram DH, Jacobs IJ, and Brady JL: Early diagnosis of ovarian cancer, *Br J Hosp Med* 44:320-324, 1990.

190. Ory HW: Oral contraceptive use and the risk of endometrial cancer, *JAMA* 249:1600, 1983.

191. Ory HW: The non-contraceptive health benefits from oral contraceptive use, *Fam Plann Perspect* 12:182-184, 1982.

192. Ossler M: Obesity and cancer: a review of epidemiological studies on the relationship of obesity to cancer of the colon, rectum, prostate, breast, ovaries, and endometrium, *Dan Med Bull* 34:267-274, 1987.

193. Pacheco JC, Kempers RD: Etiology of postmenopausal bleeding, *Obstet Gynecol* 32:40, 1968.

194. Padawer MJ, Weir JH: Evaluation of a preevacuated endometrial suction apparatus in general obstetric-gynecologic practice, *NY State J Med* 76:885-888, 1976.

195. Padwick MI, Davies JP, and Whitehead MI: A simple method for determining the optimal dosage of progestin in postmenopausal women receiving estrogens, *N Engl J Med* 315:930-934, 1986.

196. Pardanani NS, Tischler LP, and Brown WH: Carcinoma of the cervix: evaluation of treatment in a community hospital, *NY State J Med* 75:1018, 1975.

197. Paul C et al: Oral contraceptives and risk of breast disease, *Int J Cancer* 46:366, 1990.

198. Percical-Smith R et al: Vaginal colonization of E. coli and its relation to contraceptive methods, *Contraception* 27-497, 1983.

199. Persson I et al: Risk of endometrial cancer after treatment with estrogens alone or in conjunction with progestagens: results of a prospective study, *Br Med J* 298:147-151, 1989.

200. Persson IR et al: The risk of endometrial neoplasia and treatment with estrogens and estrogen-progesterone combinations, *Acta Obstet Gynecol Scand* 65:211-217, 1986.

201. Peters RK et al: Risk factors for invasive cervical cancer among Latinos and non-Latinos in Los Angeles County, *J Natl Cancer Inst* 77(5):1063-1077, 1986.

202. Peterson H et al: Mortality risk associated with tubal sterilization the United States hospitals, *Am J Obstet Gynecol* 143:125, 1982.

203. Peterson WF, Novak ER: Endometrial polyps, *Obstet Gynecol* 8:40, 1956.

204. Pettersson, F, editor: Annual report on the results of treatment in gynecologic cancer, *Int J Gynaecol Obstet* (suppl) 36:1-313, 1991.

205. Pivarnik JM et al: Cardiac output responses of primigravid women during exercise determined by the Fick technique, *Obstet Gynecol* 75:954-959, 1990.

206. Pollack W et al: Rh immune suppression: past, present, and future.

In Frigoletto D Jr, Jewett J, Konugres A, editors: *Rh hemolytic disease,* Boston, 1982, GK Hall Publishers.

207. Potts M: Birth control methods in the United States, *Fam Plann Perspect* 20:388, 1988.

208. Potts M: The future of hormonal contraception, *Int J Fertil* (suppl) 3:57-63, 1991.

209. Potts M: World population problems: an overview, *Clin Obstet Gynecol* 32(2):329, 1989.

210. Prager K et al: Smoking and drinking behavior before and during pregnancy of married mothers of live-born infants and stillborn infants, *Public Health Rep* 99:117-127, 1984.

211. Pratt WF et al: Understanding U.S. fertility: findings from the National Survey of Family Growth Cycle III, *Popul Bull* 39:1-42, 1984.

212. Pratt WF, Bachrun CA: What do women use when they stop using the pill? *Fam Planning Perspect* 19:257, 1987.

213. Pratt WF et al: Understanding U.S. fertility: findings from the National Survey of Family Growth, Cycle III, *Popul Bull* 39:1-42, 1984.

214. Public Health Service Expert Panel on the Content of Prenatal Care: *Caring for our future: the content of prenatal care,* Washington, DC, 1989, Department of Health and Human Services.

215. Quattocchi E: Helping patients understand home testing devices, *Drug Topics* 132(9):65, 1988.

216. Ramoska E: Reliability of patient history in determining the possibility of pregnancy, *Ann Emerg Med* 18:48-50, 1989.

217. Rebar R: Practical applications of home diagnostic products: a symposium, *J Reprod Med* 32(9) (suppl):705-727, 1987.

218. Reed BD et al: Maternal serum alpha-fetoprotein screening, *J Fam Pract* 27:20-23, 1988.

219. Reed R et al: Sexually transmitted papilloma viral infections I. The anatomic distribution and pathologic grade of neoplastic lesions associated with different viral types, *Am J Obstet Gynecol* 156:212-222, 1987.

220. Reeves WC, Rawls WE, and Brinton LA: Epidemiology of genital papilloma virus and cervical cancer, *Rev Infect Dis* 11:426-439, 1989.

221. Rietmejer C et al: Condoms as physical and chemical barrier agents against HIV, *JAMA* 1851, 1988.

222. Richardson GS et al: Common epithelial cancer of the ovary, *N Engl J Med* 312:474, 1985.

223. Rodriguez J, Hart WR: Endometrial cancers occuring 10 or more years after pelvic radiation, *Int J Gynecol Pathol* 1:135, 1982.

224. Romero R et al: The value of serial human chorionic gonadotropin testing as a diagnostic tool in ectopic pregnancy, *Am J Obstet Gynecol* 155(2):392-394, 1986.

225. Rosa FW et al: Vitamin A, *Teratology* 33:355-364, 1986.

226. Rosendahl I: Self-care continues to fuel OTC drug market, *Drug Topics* 130:(9):60-63, 1986.

227. Ross RK et al: Risk factors for uterine fibroids: reduced risk associated with oral contraceptives, *Br Med J* 293:359, 1986.

228. Ruggiero RJ: Teratogenic drugs. In Parer J, editor: *Antepartum and intrapartum management,* Philadelphia, 1989, Lea and Febiger.

229. Sacks PS et al: Reproductive mortality in the U.S., *JAMA* 247:27-89, 1982.

230. Schwartz Z et al: A novel approach to the analysis of risk factors in endometrial carcinoma, *Gynecol Oncol* 21:228, 1985.

231. Shapiro H: *The new birth control book,* New York, 1988, Prentice Hall Press.

232. Shapiro S et al: Risk of localized and widespread endometrial cancer in relation to recent and discontinued use of conjugated estrogens, *N Engl J Med* 313:969-972, 1985.

233. Sherris JD: Update on condoms—products, protection, promotion, *Popul Rep* (H) 6:36, 1982.

234. Sherwin BB, Gelfand MM: The role of androgen in the maintenance of sexual function in oophorectomized women, *Psychosom Med* 49:397-409 1987.

235. Shope RE: Infectious papillomatosis of rabbits, *J Exp Med* 58:607-624, 1933.

236. Shoupe D, Mishell DR: Norplant: subdermal implant system for long term contraception, *Am J Obstet Gynecol* 160:1286-1292, 1989.

237. Silverberg E: *Statistical and epidemiological information on gynecological cancer,* New York, 1986, American Cancer Society.

238. Silverberg SG, Makowski EI: Endometrial carcinoma in young women taking oral contraceptives, *Obstet Gynecol* 46:503, 1975.

239. Sivin I: International experience with Norplant and Norplant-2 contraceptives, *Stud Fam Plann* 19:81-94, 1988.

240. Smith AD et al: Amniotic-fluid acetylcholinesterase as a possible diagnostic test for neural-tube defects in early pregnancy, *Lancet* 1:685-688, 1979.

241. Smith DC et al: Association of exogenous estrogen and endometrial carcinoma, *N Engl J Med* 293:1164, 1975.

242. Sokal R et al: Clinical application of high risk-scoring on an obstetrics service, *Am J Obstet Gynecol* 128(6):652, 1977.

243. Stafl A, Wilkinson E, and Mattingly RF: Laser treatment of cervical and vaginal neoplasia, *Am J Obstet Gynecol* 128:128-136, 1977.

244. Stall GM et al: Accelerated bone loss in hypothyroid patients overtreated with L-thyroxine, *Ann Intern Med* 113:265-269, 1990.

245. Stamfer MJ et al: A prospective study of postmenopausal estrogen therapy and coronary heart disease, *N Engl J Med* 313:1044-1049, 1985.

246. Stenback F: Benign, borderline and malignant serous c cystadenomas of the ovary, *Pathol Res Pract* 172:58-72, 1981.

247. Streissgut AP et al: IQ at age 4 in relation to maternal alcohol use and smoking during pregnancy, *Develop Psych* 25:3-11, 1989.

248. Tase T et al: Human papilloma virus types and localization in adenocarcinoma and adenosquamous carcinoma of the uterine cervix: a study by in situ DNA hybridization, *Cancer Res* 48:993-998, 1988.

249. Tatum HJ, Connell E: Barrier contraception: a comprehensive overview, *Fertil Steril* 36:1, 1981.

250. Teter J, Boczkowski K: Occurrence of tumors in dysgenetic gonads, *Cancer* 20:1301, 1967.

251. Treiman K, Liskin L: IUDs—a new look, *Popul Rep* (B) 5:1, 1988.

251a. Troy R, Siegel S: Surgical management of urinary incontinence. In Doughty D (editor): *Urinary and fecal incontinence,* St. Louis, 1991, Mosby–Year Book.

252. Trussell J, Kost K: Contraceptive failure in the United States: a critical review of the literature, *Stud Fam Plann* 18(5):237-283, 1987.

253. United States Preventive Services Task Force: *Guide to clinical preventive services. An assessment of the effectiveness of 169 interventions,* Baltimore, 1989, Williams & Wilkins.

254. Vass-Sorensen M et al: Prevalence of antibodies to herpes simplex virus and frequency of HLA antigens in patients with preinvasive and invasive cervical cancer, *Gynecol Oncol* 18:39, 1984.

255. Ventura SJ et al: Estimates of pregnancies and pregnancy rates for the United States, 1976-1985, *Am J Public Health* 78:507-511, 1988.

256. Vessey M, Grice D: Carcinoma of the cervix and oral contraceptives: epidemiological studies, *Biomed Pharacother* 43:157, 1989.

257. Vessey MP et al: Ovarian neoplasms, functional ovarian cysts, and oral contraceptives, *Br Med J* 294:1518-1520, 1987.

258. Vuopala S: Diagnostic accuracy and clinical applicability of cytological and histological methods for investigating endometrial carcinoma, *Acta Obstet Gynecol Scand* (suppl) 70:1-72, 1977.

259. Walker AM, Jick H: Declining rates of endometrial cancer, *Obstet Gynecol* 56:733-736, 1980.

260. Watts NB et al: Intermittent cyclical etidronate treatment of postmenopausal osteoporosis, *N Engl J Med* 323:73-79, 1990.

261. Weiss NS et al: Noncontraceptive estrogen use and the occurrence of ovarian cancer, *J Natl Cancer Inst* 68:95-98, 1982.

262. Weiss NS, Peterson AS: Racial variation in the incidence of ovarian cancer in the United States, *Am J Epidemiol* 107:91-95, 1978.

263. Weiss NS, Sayvetz TA: Incidence of endometrial cancer in relation to the use of oral contraceptives, *N Engl J Med* 302:551, 1980.

264. Weissman MM: The myth of involutional melancholia, *JAMA* 242:742-744, 1979.

265. Welch WR, Scully RE: Precancerous lesions of the endometrium, *Hum Pathol* 8:503, 1977.

266. Whitley RJ: Infectious disease in the prenatal period and recommendations for screening. In Merkatz IR, editor: *New perspectives on prenatal care*, New York, 1990, Elsevier.

267. Wilfond BS: The cystic fibrosis gene: medical and social implications for heterozygote detection, *JAMA* 263:2777-2783, 1990.

268. Willett GD et al: Correlation of histologic appearance of intraepithelial neoplasia of the cervix with human papilloma virus types. Emphasis on low grade lesions including so-called flat condyloma, *Int J Gynecol Pathol* 8:18, 1989.

269. Williamson DF et al: Comparing the prevalence of smoking in pregnant and nonpregnant women, 1985 to 1986, *JAMA* 261:70-74, 1989.

270. World Health Organization collaborative study of neoplasm and steroid contraceptives: Endometrial cancer and combined oral contraceptives, *Int J Epidemiol* 17:263-269, 1987.

271. World Health Organization: *Mechanism of action, safety and efficacy of intrauterine devices*, Technical report series 753, Geneva, 1987, World Health Organization.

272. Worthington-Roberts B: Nutritional deficiencies and excesses: impact on pregnancy, part 2, *J Perinatol* 5:12-21, 1985.

273. Worthington-Roberts B: Nutrition and pregnancy. In Cherry S, Merkatz I, editors: *Complications of pregnancy: medical, surgical, gynecologic, psychosocial and perinatal*, ed 4, Baltimore, 1991, Williams and Wilkins.

274. Woutersz T: The Norplant device, *Int J Fertil* 36(suppl)(3):51-56, 1991.

275. Wynder E, Escher G, and Mantle N: An epidemiologic investigation of cancer of the endometrium, *Cancer* 19:489-520, 1966.

276. Ziel HK, Finkle WD: Increased risk of endometrial carcinoma among users of conjugated estrogens, *N Engl J Med* 293:1167-1170, 1975.

277. Zucker PK, Kasdon EJ, and Feldstein ML: The validity of Pap smear parameters as predictors of endometrial pathology in menopausal women, *Cancer* 56:2256-2263, 1985.

278. Zunzunegui MV et al: Male influences on cervical cancer risk, *Am J Epidemiol* 123:302, 1986.

279. Zurawski VR et al: Prospective evaluation of serum CA 125 levels in a normal population, phase I: the specificities of single and serial determinations in testing for ovarian cancer, *Gynecol Oncol* 36:299-305, 1990.

RESOURCES

Reproductive organ cancers

American Cancer Society (ACS), (800) ACS-2345; Offers information about risk factors and early detection.

American College of Obstetricians and Gynecologists (ACOG), 409 12th St, SW, Washington, DC 20024-2188; educational pamphlets are available (for a fee) on subjects related to women's health.

National Cancer Institute (NCI)

Publications: Free; order by calling (800) 4-CANCER.

What You Need to Know About Cancer in the Uterus (NCI Pub. #91-1562)

What You Need to Know About Cancer of the Cervix (NCI Pub. #91-2047)

What You Need to Know About Cancer of the Cervix (NCI Pub. #91-2047)

What You Need to Know About Ovarian Cancer (NCI Pub. #91-1561)

Cancer Information Service (CIS):

CIS is a nationwide telephone service set up by NCI to respond to questions from cancer patients and their families, health professionals, and the public. CIS information specialists give callers information and publications free on all aspects of cancer and local cancer-related services. All calls are confidential. Spanish-speaking staff is also available. By dialing the CIS number, you will be connected to the CIS office serving your area.

PDQ (Physician Data Query):

PDQ is a computerized listing of up-to-date and accurate information for patients and health professionals on:

- The latest types of cancer treatments
- Organizations and doctors involved in caring for people with cancer

To access PDQ, doctors may use an office computer or the services of a medical library. Doctors and patients can retrieve information stored in PDQ and learn how to use the system by calling the CIS number, (800) 4-CANCER. To get information from PDQ, the caller needs to know the exact medical name and the stage of the cancer.

Menopause

Utian WH, Jacobowitz RS: *Managing your menopause*, New York, 1990, Prentice Hall.

Greenwood S: *Menopause, naturally: preparing for the second half of life*, San Francisco, 1989, Volcano Press.

Nachtigall L: *Estrogen: the facts can change your life*, Tucson, 1987, Body Press.

Brown Doress P, Laskin Siegel D: *Ourselves growing older: women aging with knowledge and power*, New York, 1987, Simon and Schuster.

The North American Menopause Society. Provides a complete list of recommended reading plus names of menopause specialists in the United States. Write: University Hospitals of Cleveland; Department of OB GYN, Box MC; 2074 Abington Rd; Cleveland, OH 44106.

Preconceptual care

Maternal and Child Health Center. Up-to-date information and guidelines for pregnancy and child-related issues.

Healthy Mother, Healthy Babies Coalition: *What's safe in pregnancy? How to prevent accidents*, 409 12th St. SW, Washington, DC.

National Council on Alcoholism. Pertinent, helpful information and materials on recognizing the alcoholic, and strategies in helping the addicted; 468 Park Ave South, New York, NY 10016.

National Library of Medicine. Over 300 health hotlines are listed. 8600 Rockville Pike, Bethesda, MD 20894; Attn: Health Hotlines.

Urinary incontinence

Agency for Health Care Policy and Research, *Urinary In-continence Patient Guide,* Publications Clearinghouse, P.O. Box 8547, Silver Spring, MD 20907.

Alliance for Aging Research, 2021 K Street, NW, Suite 305, Washington, D.C. 20006.

The Bladder Health Council, American Foundation for Urologic Disease, 1120 N. Charles Street, Baltimore, MD 21201.

HIP, Help for Incontinent People, P.O. Box 544, Union, SC 29379.

The National Institute on Aging Information Center, P.O. Box 8057, Gaithersburg, MD 20870-8057.

The Simon Foundation for Continence, P.O. Box 835, Wilmette, IL 60091.

Chapter 31

THE ADULT MALE

Benign Diseases of the Prostate

Todd Cohen
Steven Siegel

BENIGN PROSTATIC HYPERPLASIA

Benign prostatic hyperplasia (BPH) is a urologic disease that affects nearly all men. Although its presence has been known since the time of the ancient Egyptians, the cause of the disease still eludes doctors and researchers today. Several theories try to explain the development of prostatic enlargement with age, but all are still speculative. As the age of the general population steadily increases, the number of men who will suffer from the clinical manifestations of BPH will also increase. Unfortunately, no satisfactory preventive measures are currently available. Researchers are continually conducting studies seeking some answer that will retard or prevent the growth of the prostate, in order to reduce one of the most common diseases afflicting men today.

Anatomy

The prostate gland begins to develop at the end of the 11th week of fetal growth from the multiple endodermal buds arising from the urothelial epithelium above and below the mesonephric duct. These buds undergo multiple cycles of branching and eventually protrude into the surrounding mesenchyme of the urogenital sinus. This mesenchyme differentiates into the muscular stroma and connective tissue of the gland. By the fifth month, the gland is well developed and continues to grow throughout fetal life. The normal growth and development of the prostate depend on the presence of testosterone and its conversion to dihydrotestosterone.[36,91] Coffey[23] has described the presence of 5-α-reductase in the epithelium and stroma of the urogenital sinus, which catalyzes this conversion.

The prostate develops into a conical shaped gland that lies in the true pelvis behind the inferior border of the symphysis pubis. The base of the gland is that part that contacts the bladder neck, while the apex, inferior to the base, abuts the urogenital diaphragm. The prostate measures approximately 4 cm in transverse diameter at the base, measures 2 cm at the apex, and is between 3 and 4 cm in length.[36,86,129] The average weight of the normal gland is between 12 and 20 grams.[36,86]

Early investigators described the prostate gland as having a lobar configuration. They termed these the anterior, posterior, middle, right, and left lateral lobes. More recent studies of the architecture of the gland reveal a more complex design. McNeal[73] describes the presence of three major glandular regions of the prostate and an anterior region that is primarily fibromuscular (Fig. 31-1). In this schema, the prostatic urethra acts as an anatomic landmark. It is divided into proximal and distal sections midway through the gland where the verumontanum lies on the posterior wall.[73] At this point there is an acute angulation to the urethra of approximately 35 degrees anteriorly. McNeal has shown that the posterior portion of the urethra receives the ejaculatory ducts and the great majority of the prostatic ducts.[73] The glandular portions of the prostate are divided into the peripheral, central, transitional, and periurethral zones. The peripheral zone accounts for nearly three quarters of the glandular tissue. It lies in the posterior aspect of the prostate extending from the base to the apex and laterally to the neurovascular bundles on either side. This is the portion of the gland that is palpable on digital rectal examination. Nearly 70% of all prostatic cancers arise in this region.[116] The central zone comprises about 20% of the glandular tissue and is situated at the base of the gland posterior to the bladder neck and urethra. The ejaculatory ducts traverse this portion of the prostate. The transitional and periurethral zones comprise the remainder of the gland, and although these account for a minor amount of the normal prostatic tissue, benign adenomas arise exclusively from these two areas.[74] The transitional zone surrounds the proximal portion of the prostatic urethra from the bladder neck to an area just proximal to the verumontanum. The periurethral glands lie within the prostatic sphincter, accounting for minimal amounts of normal glandular tissue.[36,73,74,121]

Pathology

The tissue that develops into BPH derives from two specific zones. The transitional zone is the larger of the two; the periurethral areas constitute the remainder. All BPH nodules arise from these areas. The prostate is composed of several different tissue types, including glandular, stroma, and smooth muscle. Adenomatous growths can be composed of any of these alone but most commonly are found to contain a combination of all three elements. Franks[32] described the five most common structures:

1. Pure stromal
2. Fibromuscular
3. Muscular
4. Fibroadenoma
5. Fibromyoadenoma

Grossly these lesions appear to be well encapsulated; however, a true capsule is not present. As the adenoma grows, the surrounding normal tissue is compressed, giving the impression of a "pseudocapsule." The macroscopic and microscopic appearance of the adenoma varies, depending on composition. The more glandular nodules tend to be more yellow-white; an abundance of fibromuscular tissue promotes a gray hue.[25] The weight of the adenoma can vary from a few grams to several hundred.

When the glandular element is most abundant a proliferation of glands of various sizes is seen microscopically. These glands maintain the normal morphologic characteristics of prostatic glands in that they retain a dual cell layer, an inner columnar layer, and an outer cuboidal layer.[25,36] These hyperplastic glands usually have a more papillary configuration than the normal prostatic glands. Adenomas that arise in the transition zone tend to contain more glandular elements; fibromuscular predominance is more commonly seen in the periurethral regions.[74,103] Areas of squamous metaplasia and infarction are also commonly seen.

Epidemiology

The true incidence of benign prostatic hyperplasia is difficult to ascertain for the general population, because both the clinical and pathologic aspects of the disease

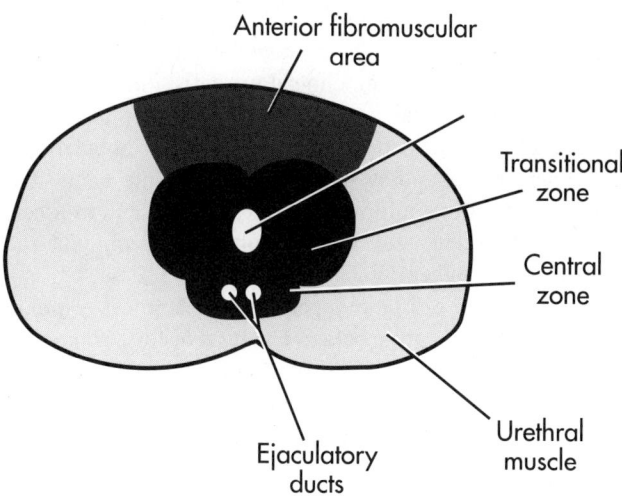

Fig. 31-1. Cross-section of the prostate gland.

merit consideration. Usually only those patients with clinical symptoms seek medical attention. Thus, those men who have morphologic evidence of BPH may never be seen. Autopsy studies have demonstrated men with markedly enlarged glands or large adenomas who had been free of bothersome symptoms.

Berry et al.[6] compiled the results of several autopsy studies to determine the presence of histologic BPH with advancing age. They found the average weight of a "normal" prostate to be 20 ± 6 g, regardless of age, when no evidence of BPH was present. They determined the prevalence of pathologic BPH in the age range of 31 through 40 to be only 8%. However, by the age of 51 to 60 years 50% of the male population showed evidence of BPH. The average weight of the diseased prostate was 33 ± 16 g, a significant increase from that of unaffected glands. Further statistical analysis of their data reveals that pathologic evidence of BPH likely begins before the age of 30. The adenoma then undergoes many phases of growth. Between the ages of 31 and 50 the prostate adenoma grows with a doubling time of approximately 4.5 years. During the second phase, the doubling time slows to about 10 years. In the final phase, the growth is substantially slower, with doubling occurring every 100 years. This and other studies determine the overall incidence of pathologic BPH to be in the range of 75% to 85% of all white and black males.[102]

Studies from the Baltimore Longitudinal Study of Aging (BLSA) have shown a correlation between the prevalence of clinical and pathologic BPH over time. Guess et al.[41] analyzed the data over a 30-year follow-up period on 1057 men and showed that the prevalence of clinically diagnosed BPH was within one standard error of the prevalence of pathologic BPH as determined in autopsy studies. These findings held true over each of five decade-long intervals. They concluded that "when averaged over a large population, the age-related factors responsible for triggering pathological BPH may be more closely related to those responsible for triggering clinical prostatism than the large amount of individual variation might lead one to expect. Whatever the explanation, it appears that, for populations, clinicians and pathologists are measuring the same disease".[41] From this information, one may be able to ascertain the prevalence of BPH simply by determining the prevalence of either clinical or pathologic disease.

Even though prostatic hyperplasia is the most common disease treated by urologists, the natural history or prognosis of clinical symptoms remains poorly understood. Urologists are still unable to determine who will eventually require treatment when patients have early complaints. Perhaps the best way to examine the progression of disease is to determine the probability that an individual will undergo definitive treatment. Lytton et al.[66] predicted the incidence rates of prostatectomy in various age groups in New Haven between 1953 and 1961. They assumed that symptomatic men would choose to have surgery locally. Using this information together with the population characteristics in New Haven and the number of prostatectomies performed, they found the probability of a 50-year-old man's undergoing prostatectomy in his lifetime to be 10%. One of the most significant findings of their study was that the incidence of prostatectomy increases with age, suggesting that clinical BPH also increases with age.

Birkhoff[7] using Lytton's assumptions and calculations, reevaluated the incidence of prostatectomies using new surgical rates from 1978 and found the probability of a 50-year-old's undergoing prostatectomy to be between 20% and 25%. The Normatice Aging Study of 2036 men confirmed this increased incidence rate, reporting a 29% chance of prostatectomy if a 40-year-old would live to the age of 80 years.[39]

Ball and associates[2] reviewed the outcome after a 5-year follow-up period for 107 men who initially had symptoms of prostatic obstruction. Only 10 patients eventually required surgery, 2 for acute urinary retention and 8 for severely worsening symptoms. The remaining 97 continued without treatment. Of the untreated patients, 50 experienced no changes in their symptoms, 31 improved, and only 16 worsened. Urodynamic studies performed at presentation and on follow-up evaluation showed no significant changes. None of the data at the initiation of the study were helpful in predicting who would eventually require treatment.[2] Birkhoff and associates, following patients prospectively, also showed that no objective or subjective parameters, including prostatic size, correlate with deterioration of symptoms or development of acute urinary retention.[8]

The finding that not all men who show pronounced histologic changes of BPH require treatment clearly suggests that factors other than prostatic bulk contribute to symptoms. Caine has proposed that factors leading to bladder

outlet obstruction have a static and a dynamic component.[14,15] The static component of obstruction is primarily a determinant of the size of the prostate; the dynamic component is a function of the tone of the prostatic smooth muscle.[14,15] Current treatment modalities are aimed at either or both of these components. Any factors that may affect either of these areas could conceivibly alter the clinical picture of BPH. For example, many common cold remedies have been implicated in worsening of obstructive symptoms. Several of these contain agents that enhance sympathetic tone, which in turn could lead to contraction of the prostatic smooth muscle. Inflammation, as occurs with prostatis, produces swelling of the gland and relative increase in prostatic size. Simple changes can dramatically alter the clinical course of BPH. Some of these are even implicated in the onset of acute urinary retention.

Acute retention is the inability to pass urine effectively by normal means and often occurs as a consequence of BPH. Ball's series described a less than 2% incidence (2/107) of retention in those who initially had obstructive symptoms.[2] However, most other reports find the occurrence more common.[7,39,66] Lytton reported that 10% to 15% of those men who underwent prostatectomy experienced retention.[66] Birkhoff's group related that 10 of 53 (19%) of their patients followed for clinical symptoms ultimately developed acute retention.[39] They noted that these patients were actually less symptomatic both subjectively and objectively before this presentation. It may be that some precipitating event causes acute retention to develop in men with "prostatism."

Spiro et al. studied the role of prostatic infarction tn causing acute retention.[115] They compared two groups of 100 men undergoing prostatectomy. The first group suffered from acute retention; the second had symptomatic BPH. Those with retention had an incidence of infarction of 85% compared to only 3% in the other group. It is possible that prostatic infarct affects the static component, dynamic component, or both. However, the actual mechanism leading to acute retention, even in the presence of infarction, remains unknown.

Risk factors

BPH does not occur in men castrated before the age of 40. The testes are believed necessary, at least, for the induction of BPH.[34,36,87] This is most likely a result of the hormones produced by the testes. Testicular androgens are responsible for normal prostatic growth but have not yet been determined to be the cause of BPH.

Other than the presence of testicular androgens, age is the only other uncontroversial risk factor for BPH.[3,6,29,36,39,102] BPH is rarely diagnosed before the age of 40; by age 80, the prevalence is approximately 75% to 85%.[39,87] As has been described, the risk of an individual's undergoing prostatectomy increases with increasing age,[7,66] as does the incidence of pathologic disease.[6] Several investigators believe that intraprostatic levels of the testosterone metabolite dihydrotesterone (DHT) increase with age, and DHT is thought to be responsible for the changes in incidence of BPH.[34,45,108,130] Siiteri and Wilson described DHT levels that were higher in BPH tissue than in normal tissue.[34,111] This was accepted and confirmed by several authors[34] until Walsh and associates contradicted this finding.[128] They determined that the low levels of DHT in normal glands of autopsy specimens could be secondary to degradation of DHT with cooling.[128] Bolton and his group performed studies on surgically resected prostates and showed only minor decreases in DHT levels with cooling.[10] Thus, as Geller[34] states, DHT levels are higher in BPH than in normal individuals but not as high as previously thought. Increased hormone levels still after a plausible explanation for higher incidences of BPH with age.

No studies have supplied conclusive evidence that race is a risk for development of BPH. Lytton[65] stated that early in this century investigators believed that BPH is rare among blacks, but subsequent studies actually found the incidence higher among this group than in whites. He concluded that in the United States, the incidence among blacks and whites is about equal and likely to be lower in African blacks.[65] Asians are known to have lower incidence rates than whites.[29,65] However, American (and Westernized) Asians have a much higher incidence than their Asian counterparts.[29,65] Whether this finding is due to environmental factors, diet, or other influences is still unknown. Lytton also noted the operative incidence among Jews to be about three times higher than among Catholics and Protestants, suggesting higher incidence rates.[66] Glynn et al. describe similar findings.[39]

Environmental pollution, water purification, and lifestyle are thought to be possible risks, but have not been definitively proved to be. Diet has been implicated, but again, no particular foods or beverages are known to alter prostatic growth. Other diseases are also associated with BPH, including diabetes, cirrhosis, and coronary artery disease. The incidence of each of these increases with age, and thereby age could be the sole explanation for this association.

Symptoms

The symptoms of BPH are usually divided into two groups. The *obstructive* symptoms are those caused by the physical narrowing of the prostatic urethra. These include weakened size and force of the stream, hesitancy, intermittency, postvoid dribbling, and straining. As bladder outlet obstruction increases, urethral resistance also increases. Greater pressures are needed to initiate a stream, often necessitating straining (Valsalva maneuver) to overcome the resistance; more time is required to generate these pressures resulting in hesitancy. Intermittency and dribbling occur when the bladder is unable to maintain the higher

pressures for long enough periods to complete voiding. *Irritative* symptoms occur secondary to bladder instability. As the bladder is unable to empty completely, frequency and nocturia result. Irritation of the bladder enhances the sense of urgency, and urge incontinence is a common sequela. Finally, if the detrusor decompensates further, overflow incontinence or acute retention may occur.

Other problems can accompany the presence of BPH. BPH is the most common cause of gross hematuria in men over the age of 60.[36] Initial or terminal bleeding is most common; however severe hemorrhages are also seen. Urinary tract infections may develop as a result of BPH, causing significant postvoid residuals and stasis of urine. When this urine is not evacuated, it becomes a good culture medium for bacteria. Later in the disease process, the degree of obstruction may worsen and the bladder can become chronically overdistended. Vesicoureteral reflux and/or upper tract obstruction with subsequent hydroureteronephrosis is a possible consequence.

Several seemingly benign actions and medications can actually lead to worsening of obstructive symptoms. The most common of these is the consumption of large amounts of fluids. When more fluids are consumed, more are excreted. This can result in increased frequency or other symptoms. To prevent this problem, fluid intake should be lessened at those times when frequent voids become more irritating (i.e., at or near bedtime or before traveling).

Diuretics increase urine by a variety of different mechanisms. Their use mimics the problems of increased fluid consumption as previously described. Patients on diuretics often report symptoms of BPH or worsening of their prior symptoms while taking diuretics. When evaluating a patient with voiding complaints this should always be remembered as discontinuation of the diuretic often alleviates these symptoms.

Common cold remedies such as pseudoephedrine and diphenhydramine can also exacerbate symptoms of BPH. These medications all exhibit some α-adreneric properties. The prostate contains variable amounts of smooth muscle that respond to α-adrenergic stimulation by increasing the tone of the gland (see the Treatment section). This increase in tone can physically worsen the obstruction. It is common to see men with BPH in the emergency room in complete retention after taking cold tablets. These over-the-counter medications should be avoided when possible by this population.

Screening and evaluation

Screening for benign prostatic hypertrophy is not generally indicated because the condition may be present and not cause symptoms or sequelae, whereas at other times it may be present and lead to problems. Indirectly, screening is done by performing digital rectal examination, traditionally performed as part of the general medical examination and also as a screening maneuver for colon and rectal cancer. Evaluation for and of benign prostate enlargement is indicated only when symptoms that suggest that this condition is present arise. Evaluation of benign prostate enlargement includes history, physical examination, and studies to determine the significance of the symptoms experienced.

A careful history is perhaps the most important aspect of the evaluation of BPH. Through it the physician may be able to ascertain the severity of the patient's symptoms and determine whether further evaluation or treatment is warranted. Each symptom should be addressed individually. If the patient is experiencing the symptom, the physician should assess the degree of the problem. This can be recorded as a severity score (i.e., on a 0 to 4 scale) or by descriptive terms in the physician record. In this way, the progression of symptoms can best be followed.

Physical examination of the patient to assess BPH includes more than simple palpation of the prostate gland. A proper abdominal examination is necessary to evaluate the presence of bladder distention, costovertebral angle tenderness, pain, presence of masses, or any other abnormalities that may accompany BPH or cause similar symptoms. The genitalia should be carefully inspected and palpated. Meatal strictures, penile defects, and urethral abnormalities that may help elucidate the patient's symptoms can often be identified. Finally a digital rectal examination should be performed. Care should be taken to note the size, texture, position, and tenderness of the gland.

Uroflow studies are often used as a screening procedure to determine the severity of outlet obstruction. It is believed that flow rates of 10 cm^3/sec or less are consistent with obstruction; those with rates above 15 cm^3/sec indicate the absence of obstruction. However, many patients with significant outlet obstruction generate bladder pressures that are able to overcome the outlet resistance and create flow rates above 15 cm^3/sec.[9,42] Hald reports on Gerstenberg's finding that patients with this situation are significantly younger than those patients with lower flow rates and prostatism.[42] He proposes that these patients will progress to the typical situation of low flow/high pressure.[42] Therefore, voiding flow rates should not be used as a solitary test to evaluate the degree of obstruction.

Pressure/flow studies monitor the detrussor pressure with respect to flow rates during voiding. These studies are more useful in that they provide information about the pressure that the bladder must generate to produce a particular flow. This will aid in differentiating between a weakened bladder and obstruction (i.e., a weak bladder may generate a low flow rate because of low pressure).

Renal function should be assessed by measurement of blood urea nitrogen (BUN) and creatinine levels. BPH alone can cause worsening of renal function reflected by elevation of BUN and creatinine levels. This finding in the absence of other causes of renal insufficiency should lead

the physician to evaluate the patient's upper urinary tracts for evidence of hydronephrosis.

The kidneys and ureters can be examined by a number of different studies. Intravenous urogram (IVU) provides information on the anatomy as well as the function of the kidneys. Hydroureteronephrosis can easily be detected by the IVU. Bilateral "hydro" is present if obstruction is present, whereas a unilateral process generally indicates a cause other than bladder outlet obstruction. When IVU is performed, a postvoid film is helpful to determine the degree of bladder emptying. Renal ultrasound may be substituted for IVU in cases where the use of intravenous contrast is contraindicated (i.e., elevated creatinine level). Ultrasound provides an excellent determination of the presence of hydronephrosis but does not provide functional information. A bladder ultrasound can evaluate the amount of residual urine after voiding.

Cystoscopy can be performed as a diagnostic procedure especially if the cause of the patient's symptoms remains equivocal. Visual inspection of the urethra may help confirm the diagnosis of BPH or may reveal other abnormality. Like the actual size of the prostate, the appearance of urethral obstruction does not correlate well with the severity or even presence of symptoms. Thus if BPH is suspected, and surgical treatment is planned, cystoscopy is generally performed at the time of treatment.

Prevention and treatment

Intervention for benign prostate enlargement is indicated only when symptoms are present. Primary prevention therefore is not employed. Secondary prevention depends on the degree of symptoms and results of the evaluation performed. Options for secondary prevention or treatment have greatly expanded in recent years and now include surgery, balloon dilation, microwave hyperthermia, ureteral stents, and medications.

Certain indications necessitate surgical intervention for BPH. These include the following:

1. Complete urinary retention
2. Severe gross hematuria
3. Hydronephrosis and concomitant azotemia

Less severe complications also indicate the need for treatment, but urgent intervention is usually not necessary. These include the following:

1. Severe obstructive or irritative symptoms that interfere with one's quality of life
2. Large residual volumes with or without recurrent infections
3. Presence of bladder calculi
4. Low flow rates with high detrussor pressure

Surgical prostatectomy, usually transurethral resection of the prostate (TURP), remains today the most common treatment for symptomatic BPH and is the *gold standard* by which all other treatment modalities are judged. Approximately 400,000 prostatectomies are performed each year in the U.S. for a variety of indications. The operative morbidity and mortality are generally reported to be 18% and less than 1%, respectively.[78] Although morbidity rates have remained relatively stable, mortality rates have decreased significantly, from 2.5% in the 1960s.[74] According to the cooperative study and other reports, the major risks contributing to perioperative mortality included age over 66 years, chronic renal insufficiency (preoperative creatinine level greater than 1.5 mg/dl), and glands of 60 g or greater.[78,81,91] These same parameters together with resection times of greater than 90 minutes, preoperative acute urinary retention, age over 80, and black race increase risk of morbidity.[78,81,91]

Common complications following TURP include failure to void, infections, and bleeding. The cooperative study found failure to void to occur most often (6.5%).[78] Some investigators find the incidence of genitourinary infection to be in the area of 20%;[21] however, this may be an overestimation. Operative morbidity is usually caused by excessive bleeding, perforation of the surgical capsule of the gland, and absorption of large quantities of irrigant. Nonhemolytic irrigation solutions, most commonly 1.5% glycine, are used during resections. Glycine has a lower osmolality than serum (approximately 200 mOsm/kg versus 280 to 300 mOsm/kg); absorption of large quantities of this fluid can result in dilutional hypernatremia.[77] Metabolites of glycine and glycine itself may also have direct neural toxicity.[100] The risk of this *TUR syndrome,* or dilutional hyponatremia, increases with increasing operative time and size of glands, where the absorptive surface is greater.

Sexual dysfunction and retrograde ejaculation are possible adverse consequences of TURP. Rates of post-TURP sexual dysfunction have been reported to be as high as 40%.[43,78] Hargreave and Stephenson[43] carefully evaluated over 250 men and found that of those patients who were potent before surgery only 4% became impotent and 3% became partially impotent. Retrograde ejaculation or decreases in preoperative ejaculates occur in about 75% of post-TURP patients.[48,92] The risk of incontinence after surgery is small yet is a definite consideration. Several authors report this risk to be on the order of 1%.[21,77,78,91] Bladder neck contractures and urethral strictures are two possible sequelae of TURP. Most reports describe a 2% to 4% incidence of these complications.[1,21,36,43,46,77-79,81,91]

The results of prostatectomy for benign disease demonstrate rates of improvement of symptoms to be in the range of 85% to 95%.[1,21,36,43,46,77-79,81,91,121] Subjective improvements tend to occur more frequently than do objective measures, which make follow-up urodynamic studies less necessary. Chilton et al. found that only 5.1% of their patients required reresection over a 5-year period.[21] Other studies report similar results.[46,78,79]

Open prostectomy is another manner in which the ade-

noma may be removed. This requires an open operation resulting in longer hospital stays and greater morbidity and mortality than TURP. It is especially useful in situations where the adenoma is so large that the time required for TURP would significantly enhance the risk of operative complications. The results of open prostatectomy with respect to subjective parameters are similar to those of TURP.[36,78,91]

Transurethral incision of the prostate (TUIP) is a surgical alternative to TURP. In this procedure grooves are cut into the prostate gland from the bladder neck to the verumontanum by an electric knife. No tissue is actually resected. Patients require anesthesia and are generally hospitalized for 2 to 3 days postoperatively. Patients best suited for this technique have smaller glands, in the range of 20 g, and have minimal median lobe enlargement.[46,79] Advantages include a short operative and anesthetic time, decreased blood loss and fluid absorption, and lower risk of postoperative complications of vesical neck contracture and retrograde ejaculation. The major disadvantage of TUIP is the lack of tissue obtained for analysis. A diagnosis of stage A adenocarcinoma of the prostate may be made in up to 10% of TURP specimens. Transurethral incision of the prostate is not well suited for larger glands, primarily because of technical difficulty,[91] but results in properly selected patients are equal to those of TURP.[22,74,92]

Balloon dilation is a nonsurgical technique that is performed transurethrally, usually with local anesthesia with intravenous sedation. Many centers however, use regional blockades or general anesthesia.[28,40,98] Placement of the balloon is accomplished under direct vision endoscopically, fluoroscopically, or through transrectal digital palpation. The exact mechanism by which dilation alleviates obstructive symptoms is unknown. Several proposals include simple compression of the adenoma, stretching of the elastic capsule, disruption of the capsule, and fracture of the anterior commissure.[28] To date, little information is available in the literature regarding long-term results in properly controlled clinical trials using this technique. Goldenberg and associates performed balloon dilation on 28 men with BPH and studied its efficacy over a 12-month period.[40] Initially between 25% and 30% of the patients showed improvement in both subjective and objective criteria (including peak flow rates). However, on review of these same patients, both subjective and objective improvements decreased to 7% and 6%, respectively. Results seen to date are generally temporary[28] and not as impressive as those of TURP and TUIP. However, the procedure's advantages include simplicity and safety, and decreased need for anaesthesia, along with limited postoperative hospitalization and cost.[28,40,97,98] Like that of TUIP, the major disadvantage is the possibility of missing an occult malignancy.[40,97] Relative contraindications include presence of a large median lobe, presence of chronic obstructive changes in the lower urinary tract such as a large residual volume or urinary retention, known prostate cancer, prostatis, and poorly compliant bladders.

A metallic coil, inserted endoscopically, has been used to stent or hold open the prostatic urethra in chronically ill patients who had previously managed with chronic indwelling Foley catheters. In a prospective study, Vincente et al.[126] were able to obtain normal voiding in a significant proportion of their patients with negligible postvoid residual volumes. This form of management is also being tried in conjunction with balloon dilation, during which a titanium mesh stent is positioned over the dilating balloon and left in place after the balloon is removed. These procedures offer an attractive alternative to the high-risk surgical patient because of the ability to regain normal voiding function and obviate the need for urethral catheter with associated risks of urinary tract infection. Potential disadvantages include infection and migration of the stent, and possible incontinence secondary to improper placement of the stent across the external sphincter.

Another treatment modality is transurethral microwave hyperthermia, which involves heating the prostate via several microwave antennae attached to a Foley catheter. The Foley catheter is positioned against the bladder neck so that the antennae are located in the prostatic urethra. These treatments are performed on an outpatient basis under local anesthesia.[103] Initial studies have shown subjective improvement in nocturia and force of the urinary stream. Adverse effects were temporary; they included bladder spasms, hematuria, dysuria, and urethral pain immediately after the treatments. Clinical trials are now being conducted in the United States and no long-term data have yet been reported.

Many studies have been done in recent years to determine the precise autonomic innervation of the prostate and bladder. Caine and others[14-16] have demonstrated that isolated human prostatic tissue contracts in the presence of norepinephrine. In further studies[16] they reported that this response was negated when the tissue was pretreated with phenoxybenzamine, a nonselective α-adrenergic antagonist. In contrast to this finding, the contractive response of the bladder to α-adrenergic stimulation was found to be 40-fold less than that of the prostate.[56] Using histochemical, immunofluorescent, and pharmacologic techniques, α_1-adrenergic receptors were found to be the predominant type in normal prostatic stroma and capsule as well as within prostatic adenomas.[15] Additionally, the density of these α_1-adrenergic receptors is high in the bladder neck and prostate as compared to the bladder body.[57] Thereby, selective blockage of the α_1 receptors should promote decreased prostatic smooth muscle tone without affecting bladder function, thus affecting the dynamic component of bladder outlet obstruction.

Initial clinical trials using α-adrenergic blockade were made by Caine and associates in 1976 using phenoxybenzamine.[17] They found that in five of eight men with urinary retention, voiding was restored. They also stated that treatment was effective for other symptoms of prostatism. In 1978, Caine and his group also reported results of a double-blind placebo study using phenoxybenzamine in men with BPH.[16] Peak urinary flow rates in their patients increased in the placebo group and the phenoxybenzamine group by 1.2 and 6.2 cm^3/sec, respectively. However, a significant proportion of these patients reported side effects including tiredness, dizziness, impaired ejaculation, nasal stuffiness and dryness, and difficulty with visual accommodation. Side effects, secondary to the nonselective blockade effect, along with potential concerns about gastrointestinal malignancies in laboratory animals associated with the use of this drug, have made its use unattractive.

Prazosin, a selective α_1, adrenergic antagonist, was introduced in 1977.[59] Several investigators have studied the efficacy of this drug for BPH.[15,56,57,59] These showed that prazosin treatment resulted in significant increases in maximum and average flow rates as well as reduction in residual volumes. Side effects compared to those in phenoxybenzamine were vastly decreased. Significant improvements in urinary flow rates have been documented with use of this agent.[56] More recent studies have focused attention on longer-acting agents such as terazosin. These medications have the advantage of once per day dosing. Clinical studies in normotensive males with symptomatic BPH have shown that peak and mean urinary flow rates significantly improved and subjective obstructive and irritative voiding symptom scores were substantially reduced in patients treated with prazosin.[58,59] No mean changes in blood pressure were demonstrated in this normotensive study population. Although management with α-adrenergic blocking agents does not prevent progression of BPH, it may be beneficial in providing relief of symptoms in those men who cannot or opt not to have surgery. The use of these agents is best confined to men without changes of urinary tract decompensation, such as significant postvoid residual, chronic urinary tract infection, or hydronephrosis. These drugs may also prevent or reverse episodes of acute urinary retention. Dosing of these agents is usually accomplished by a titration method. The patient is begun on an initial dose of 1 mg of prazosin once to twice per day. This dose can be increased up to 5 mg bid depending on symptomatic relief and onset of any adverse reactions such as hypotension, orthostasis, or lethargy.

Normal prostatic growth and development are dependent on androgens and most specifically dihydrotestosterone (DHT), a reduction product of prostatic testosterone by the enzyme 5-α-reductase. The size of the prostate decreases when the level of prostatic androgens falls below a critical level.[12,70,71] If a critical level of prostatic antigen is required to cause or maintain BPH, then androgen withdrawal should result in diminution of prostatic size and obstructive symptoms.

Development of a number of antiandrogenic agents for management of prostate cancer has prompted use of these agents for BPH. In a recent study, Bosch and associates evaluated 12 patients, 6 receiving the gonadotropin releasing hormone (GnRH) agonist buserelin and 6 receiving the androgen cyproterone acetate.[12] After 12 weeks of therapy, the average decrease in prostatic volume was 29% by ultrasound determination; however, the urodynamic changes were minimal and relief of clinical symptoms was not obtained. After discontinuation of the drugs, the prostates returned to pretreatment size within 6 to 36 weeks. Nearly all patients experienced impotence and hot flashes on these medications, but symptoms were largely reversed after discontinuation of the treatment. In another study, Peters and Walsh[96] examined the influence of nafarelin acetate (GnRH agonist) on prostatic weight, histologic characteristics, voiding symptoms, and flow rates. The prostate gland was observed to decrease by a mean volume of 24% with histologic evidence of epithelial rather than stromal involution. Prostate sizes were restored within 6 months to pretreatment levels. Only one third of the patients showed clinical improvement and flow rates improved over 15 cm^3/sec in only 3 patients. All patients who were sexually active before the study experienced impotence while taking the medication. These studies suggest that the bulk of the prostate adenoma can be reduced approximately 30% by a variety of agents designed to decrease serum and prostatic androgen levels. Any agent that lowers systemic levels of testosterone is likely to have a negative impact on libido and may also cause associated side effects such as gynecomastia and hot flashes.

The significant side effects and generally inadequate results of the hormonal therapies have contributed to poor acceptance of this treatment. However, the experimental 5-α-reductase inhibitors, in preliminary trials, have shown some promise.[70,71] These agents suppress prostatic DHT levels without affecting plasma testosterone levels. Thus, these agents should not cause erectile dysfunction. Currently trials using finasteride have revealed that prostatic sizes shrink significantly especially in dog models and prostatic DHT levels are reduced by 90% in humans.[73] Most importantly, no significant side effects are reported. The MK-906 (finasteride) Study Group has recently confirmed the reduction in DHT levels to approximately 80% of control values and has shown a 24% to 28% decrease in prostatic volume (in the 1- and 5-mg. dose groups, respectively) after 6 months of treatment.[82,119] Twelve weeks after cessation of treatment, however, the prostatic volumes returned to near pretreatment values. The finasteride study population did show an increase in maximum peak flow rates of nearly 4 ml/sec. The study group revealed no significant improvements in symptoms when compared to those of placebo; however, the authors believed that this may be due to the small population size.[119] The recommended dose of finasteride (Proscar) is 5 mg/day. Relief of

symptoms is of more gradual onset than in some of the other treatment modalities, often requiring several months for initial improvement. Physicians must also be aware that finasteride may lower serum PSA levels up to 40%.[119] Patients on finasteride treatment must have regular follow-up determinations of PSA levels and careful digital rectal examinations so that carcinoma of the prostate will not be missed.

SOCIOECONOMIC CONSIDERATIONS

Throughout much of the world and, most certainly, the United States, people are tending to live longer. A growing number of the population will be over 65, and this group accounts for a large percentage of the health care costs in this country. We will see increasing expenditures for treatment and management of diseases of the elderly in the near future as a result.

The costs for the management of BPH are expected to become a worsening economic burden. As the incidence of BPH increases with age, more men will require medical attention. Lytton[66] showed that 10% of men living to age 80 will eventually undergo surgical intervention and Birkhoff[6] more recently found this number to be 25%. Barry indicated that in 1987 alone 296,000 prostatectomies were performed on men over age 65; only cataract surgery was more common in this age group.[3] This accounted for approximately 70% of the total number of prostatectomies.[44] Holtgrewe[44] reports that the average cost of each prostatectomy in 1987 was approximately $12,000. Thus, the total expense for prostatectomies in the Medicare population was over $3.5 billion, not including the preoperative and postoperative fees, and the expenditures for nonoperative management.

Although prostatectomy, most commonly transurethral prostatectomy, is extremely effective in treating BPH, the rising costs as well as the morbidity and mortality of the procedures have generated an impetus for the development of alternative treatment modalities. Recently, there has been a great increase of information relating to pharmacologic management and less invasive treatments. Many of these are currently under rigorous study and may offer viable altrnatives to surgery. Whether these newer measures will alter the enormous economic burden that BPH incurs is yet to be determined.

PROSTATITIS

Prostatitis is a common diagnosis and an important cause of urinary tract infection in men. Nearly 25% of office visits for genitourinary complaints entail a diagnosis of prostatitis.[75,76] Three basic types exist: acute bacterial, chronic bacterial, and nonbacterial prostatitis. Each of these is a distinct entity, and the proper diagnosis is essential to providing appropriate management.

The organisms that are responsible for bacterial prostatitis are generally the same that cause urinary tract infections. *Escherichia coli* is the most common of these. Other gram-negative bacilli species including *Proteus, Klebsiella,* and *Pseudomonas* are also found. Less often, gram-positive organisms, *Enterobacter* species, cause clinical infection.

Pathogenesis

There are several routes through which the prostate can become infected. Bacteria can traverse the urethra in retrograde fashion and seed the gland. Infected urine can enter the prostate from the bladder through the ducts that empty into the urethra. Direct extension of infection from surrounding tissue or organs into the prostate is possible. This is most likely to originate from the rectum, which is in close proximity posteriorly. The final route of infection is via hematogenous spread. The causative agent(s) of nonbacterial prostatis is not specifically known; therefore, the pathogenesis is also still a mystery.

Symptoms and diagnosis

The onset of symptoms in acute bacterial prostatitis (ABP) is sudden. These often are characterized by fever, chills, perineal and back pain, and irritative voiding complaints (frequency, urgency, dysuria, nocturia). Many patients have obstructive symptoms, and some experience complete urinary retention. The most consistent finding on physical examination is an exquisitely tender prostate gland on rectal palpation. Urinalysis often reveals bacteruria and pyuria, and blood tests show the presence of a leukocytosis. Urine cultures should be obtained in this setting. Prostatic massage and instrumentation of the urinary tract should be avoided if possible to prevent hematogenous spread of the infection.

Chronic bacterial prostatis (CBP) is an uncommon infection. It can be a sequela of an acute infection; however, most patients deny prior history of acute disease. Irritative symptoms, that are commonly associated with CBP are dysuria, frequency, nocturia, and urgency. Pain is generally more vague and can be present in the perineum, back, genitalia, or inguinal areas. Fever and chills are not common. Physical examination (including rectal examination), radiologic studies, and blood tests do not reveal any characteristic abnormal findings. Recurrent urinary tract infections by the same organism are common. Examination of prostatic secretions after prostatic massage (termed expressed prostatic secretions [EPS]) characteristically reveals the presence of more than 15 white cells per high-power field. Lipid-laden macrophages are seen in large numbers.

Nonbacterial prostatis (NBP) is the most common of the three types. Clinically it is similar to CBP except that positive culture results are almost never seen. The EPS contains more than 15 white cells per high-power field; however, lipid-laden macrophages are less likely to be found. The causative organism(s) has not been identified, and attempts to obtain cultures of *Mycoplasma, Chlamydiae, Ureaplasma,* and viruses have all failed. NBP differs from prostatodynia in that the latter shows no evidence of prostatic inflammation.

Prevention and treatment

The introduction of infection into the prostate by various types of instrumentation can be prevented or reduced by strictly adhering to sterile techniques when placing catheters or other instruments in the urinary tract. To obviate these iatrogenic infections, antibiotics are often given before, during, and/or after urologic procedures (see Chapter 57).

Many antibiotics diffuse poorly across the prostatic epithelial barriers to achieve therapeutic levels in the tissue. In the presence of acute inflammation, many of these "barriers" are broken down, allowing for improved penetration of antibiotics into the tissue and secretions of the gland. The most common organisms in the bacterial infections are the gram-negative bacilli. Therapy should be initiated against these organisms until specific sensitivities are available from culture reports. Trimethoprim-sulfamethoxazole combinations are most commonly employed at dosages of trimethoprim 160 mg and sulfamethoxazole 800 mg administered twice daily. More recently the oral quinolones have gained popularity, especially because of their broad spectrum of coverage. Ciprofloxacin 500 mg bid, norfloxacin 400 mg bid, ofloxacin 400 mg bid are effective against most of the usual pathogens. Intravenous aminoglycosides (gentamicin, tobramycin) and ampicillin can be used if oral agents are not appropriate or in cases of severe infection. Treatment should continue for approximately 4 weeks to prevent recurrence and development of chronic infection. Alcohol, caffeine, and medications such as anticholinergics and antidepressants should be avoided if possible because of their effects on the bladder.

In nonbacterial prostatitis cultures show no specific growth and treatment is directed at possible causative agents as listed previously. Minocycline 100 mg bid and erythromycin 500 mg qid for periods of 4 to 6 weeks are frequently effective. Anti-inflammatory medications tend also to alleviate some of the symptoms.

Why some men are susceptible to chronic infections has yet to be discovered. Fair and associates[30] described a prostatic antimicrobial factor, later found to be free zinc,[95] which is deficient in men with CBP. However, oral zinc supplementation does not raise the zinc levels in the prostatic fluid of these men.

Antibiotic penetration into the prostatic tissue and secretions in chronic infection is not similar to the acute situation. Many antibiotics do not achieve therapeutic levels in these patients as they cannot penetrate the epithelial barrier. Trimethoprim-sulfamethoxazole, quinolones, carbenicillin, erythromycin, minocycline, and cephalexin all achieve adequate levels in the prostate. Satisfactory treatment of this chronic infection often requires long courses of antibiotic. Recommended courses range from 4 (ciprofloxacin) to 6 weeks (norfloxacin, ofloxacin). If medical management does not satisfactorily cure the condition, further testing and treatments may be necessary. Prostatic ultrasound may reveal the presence of calcifications that can be infected and nearly impossible to treat with medications. Surgery, either open or transurethral, is often indicated in these situations. Open surgery is more effective because the entire gland can be removed, ensuring the removal of the infected calculi.

Prostate Cancer

Eric A. Klein

In 1990 adenocarcinoma of the prostate became the most common cancer in U.S. males, surpassing in incidence carcinoma of the lung. Estimates are that there will be more than 122,000 new cases of prostate cancer diagnosed in 1990, resulting in more than 32,000 deaths.[112] Despite advances in early detection, staging, and treatment during the last decade, prostate cancer ranks third as a cause of cancer deaths in U.S. males behind cancers of the lung and colon and still accounts for a significant level of morbidity in older males. In view of continued improvements in life expectancy for U.S. males and because the incidence of prostate cancer increases with advancing age, it is likely that the detection and treatment of this cancer will assume increasing importance in the future.

EPIDEMIOLOGY AND RISK FACTORS

Little is known about the biologic origins of prostate cancer. The disparity between clinically evident cancers and the very high incidence of cancer of the prostate observed at autopsy (70% incidence in the ninth decade) remains unexplained. Also unexplained are differences in the incidence and death rates of prostate cancer across geographic and racial boundaries. The incidence of clinically detectable prostate cancer ranges from 0.8 per 100,000 in China to 100.2 per 100,000 blacks in California.[37] Mortality rates for prostate cancer range from 3 per 100,000 in Uruguay, 12 per 100,000 in Germany, 22 per 100,000 in the United States, to 32 per 100,000 in Sweden.[19]

No studies have identified a clear link between prostate cancer and potential causative factors such as diet, sexual activity, venereal disease, smoking, or environmental exposure. Because prostate cancer is usually sensitive to androgen withdrawal, one hypothesis is that high serum testosterone levels are a causative factor. One study has suggested that serum testosterone levels are higher in young blacks than in whites,[101] an intriguing observation in view of the observed higher incidence of prostate cancer in black men (about 1 in 9 lifetime risk) versus white men (1 in 11).

Recent epidemiologic studies have identified a twofold increased risk of prostate cancer in men with an affected first-degree relative and an almost nine-fold risk when both a first- and a second-degree relative are affected.[117] Another clearly associated risk factor is age, with incidence (autopsy and clinical) and mortality rates beginning a steep climb at age 50. The occurrence of benign prostatic hyperplasia (BPH) does not increase the risk of prostate cancer.

SCREENING

Screening for prostate cancer has become a topic of concern because of an increasing incidence of cancer and the availability of sensitive and noninvasive measures such as serum prostatic specific antigen (PSA) and transrectal ultrasonography (TRUS). With reliance on digital rectal examination as the main source of detection, only one half to two thirds of prostate cancers are organ-confined and therefore potentially curable at the time of diagnosis.[51] As a result the mortality rate for prostate cancer has not declined for the last three decades. The rationale for large-scale screening programs has been to detect cancers at an earlier (organ-confined) stage with the hope that earlier treatment will decrease mortality. However, there remains much controversy over who should be screened and which screening tools are best, and some disagreement over whether earlier detection will indeed decrease mortality. Because screening for prostate cancer has not been done on a large scale until recently, and because this tumor has an indolent natural history with survival measurable only at 10 to 15 years (as compared to much shorter intervals for other cancers), there are as yet no reports that demonstrate a beneficial effect on mortality for screening programs. The National Cancer Institute has recently begun a 16-year multicenter randomized trial to evaluate the effect of screening on detection rates and mortality of prostate cancer in the general population to address these issues. A definitive statement on who might benefit from screening must await completion of this and other trials.

Screening tools

There are three tools available for screening for prostate cancer: digital rectal examination (DRE), serum PSA, and TRUS. When used alone, these methods have detection rates of approximately 1.5%, 2.2%, and 2.6%, respectively, with varying degrees of false-negative results, false-positive results, and predictive value (Table 31-1).

One problem with DRE is the infrequency with which it is performed. In a screening program of 433 men over age 40 performed at the Cleveland Clinic in 1989 and 1990, 67% said they had not had a DRE performed in the previous year.[52] Perhaps more alarming was that of the 153 patients who reported having a general physical examination in the previous year, only 56% had had a DRE.

TRUS is limited as an independent screening tool because it is highly operator-dependent, has a significant

Table 31-1. Value of screening tools in detecting prostate cancer*

	Sensitivity (%)	Specificity (%)	Positive Predictive Value(%)	Detection Rate (%)
DRE	69-89	84-98	26-35	1.5
TRUS	36-85	41-79	27-36	2.6
PSA	57-79	59-68	40-49	2.2

*DRE, digital rectal examination; TRUS, transrectal ultrasonography; PSA, serum prostate specific antigen.

Table 31-2. Detection rates of prostate cancer combining DRE and PSA*

	DRE Result	
PSA Level (ng/ml)	Normal (%)	Abnormal (%)
< 4	2.1	11.7
4-10	7.0	42.6
> 10	28.1	76.2

From Cooner WH et al: Prostate cancer detection in a clinical urological practice by ultrasonography, digital rectal examination, and prostate specific antigen, *J Urol* 143:1146, 1990.
*DRE, digital rectal examination; PSA, serum prostate specific antigen.

Recommended screening for prostate cancer

1. All men over the age of 40 have a screening DRE yearly. This is in accordance with American Cancer Society recommendations.
2. Serum PSA level is determined in all men over the age of 50, and in younger men with symptoms suggesting bladder outlet obstruction caused by prostatic enlargement and in those with a family history of prostate cancer.
3. Men with normal DRE findings and PSA level less than 4 ng/ml are followed yearly with repeat DRE and PSA level evaluations.
4. Men with normal DRE results and PSA level of 4 to 10 ng/ml undergo TRUS, with biopsy of any suspicious lesion. If no lesion is seen, random biopsies from the base, middle, apex, and transition zones of both lobes are obtained. The role of PSAD in this setting is currently being evaluated prospectively.
5. Men with an abnormal DRE result or PSA level over 10 ng/ml undergo TRUS and biopsy. If the biopsy result is positive, appropriate treatment is instituted; if the result is negative, DRE and PSA level evaluations are repeated in 6 months; TRUS is again performed if either test result has changed significantly or if the suspicion of cancer remains high.

---

learning curve, is more costly and uncomfortable than either DRE or PSA, and does not detect the 30% of prostate cancers that appear isoechoic rather than hypoechoic. The American Urological Association has recognized the value of TRUS as a diagnostic procedure but has not endorsed its use for screening.

Serum PSA levels are elevated in 20% to 30% of men with BPH; this elevation results in a significant false-positive result overlap in men with organ-confined prostate cancer.[51] This overlap limits the benefit of PSA alone as an independent screening tool. Still, one recent study suggested that of DRE, TRUS, and PSA, serum PSA level was the best individual predictor of the presence of prostate cancer.[20]

There are conflicting reports on whether the addition of TRUS to DRE increases the detection rate of prostate cancer. One study comparing DRE and TRUS in the same population found DRE superior by 5.4% to 4.4%.[94] Both methods have limitations in detecting cancers and each can detect cancers that the other will miss.

There is evidence that the combination of DRE and PSA can increase the detection rate of prostate cancer. In a study of 1807 men with DRE, TRUS, and PSA (using the Hybritech assay), Cooner showed that the rate of detection of prostate cancer in men with abnormal DRE findings was 12% if the PSA was less than 4 ng/ml, 43% if the PSA was 4 to 10 ng/ml, and 76% if PSA was above 10 ng/ml (Table 31-2).[24] In men with normal DRE results the corresponding detection rates were 2%, 7%, and 28%. In patients with normal DRE findings and PSA less than 4 ng/ml, 11 patients had biopsy performed for each cancer detected. The corresponding ratio for PSA level between 4 and 10 ng/ml was 7:1 and for PSA level above 10 ng/ml, 3:1. The cost for detecting a single cancer in this series was $2850, suggesting that it may not be cost-effective to perform biopsy procedures when patients have normal DRE results and PSA levels below 10 ng/ml. Recently, several investigators have suggested using PSA density (PSAD) as a way of defining a subgroup of patients with normal DRE result and PSA level of 4 to 10 ng/ml who are more likely to have cancer.[4,5] PSAD is calculated by dividing serum PSA level by prostatic volume as estimated by TRUS (PSAD = serum PSA level/prostatic volume). PSAD ratios greater than 0.1 to 0.15 have been reported to be associated with a high likelihood of cancer.[5]

Screening guidelines

As mentioned previously, there is much controversy over whether screening for prostate cancer should be limited to patients in urologic practices or applied to the pop-

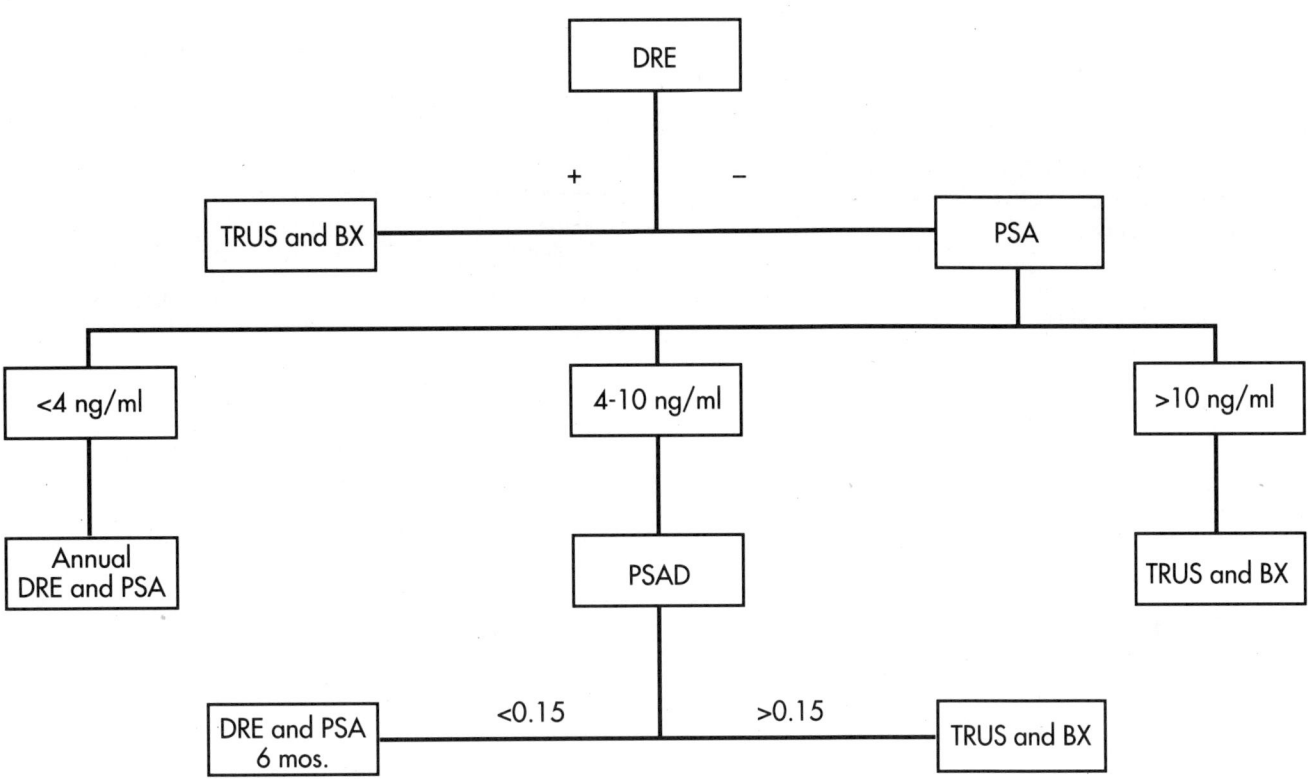

Fig. 31-2. *DRE*, digital rectal examination; *TRUS*, transrectal ultrasound; *BX*, prostate biopsy; *PSA*, prostate specific antigen; *PSAD*, prostate specific antigen density.

ulation at large. On the basis of the foregoing considerations, I use the following guidelines in my (urologic) practice (see the box on p. 646 and Fig. 31-2):

TREATMENT

Treatment of prostate cancer is determined by clinical stage. It is axiomatic that patients with cancers confined to the prostate can be cured, whereas those with extraprostatic spread cannot (Table 31-3).

SUMMARY

Screening for prostate cancer has assumed a prominent role in the arena of preventive medicine because of increasing life expectancy, increasing incidence of this cancer with age, and development of noninvasive screening tools such as PSA and TRUS. Although the increased detection of potentially curable cancers seems likely with screening, no study has yet demonstrated a reduction in mortality by the use of these methods. The precise role of each of the available tools continues to evolve, as does the debate regarding whether screening should be limited to urologic practices or applied to the population at large. The results of large-scale studies currently under way will be needed to answer these questions.

Table 31-3. Staging classification for prostate cancer

Stage	Classification
A	Incidentally discovered, clinically unsuspected cancer found at the time of transurethral prostatectomy and confined to the prostate
	A1 Focal
	A2 Diffuse
B	Palpable cancers confined to the prostatic capsule
	B1 Nodule ≤ 1.5 cm
	B2 Nodule ≥ 1.5 cm or involvement of more than one lobe
C	Palpable cancers that extend beyond the prostatic capsule
	C1 Minimal extension into or through capsule
	C2 Extensive extracapsular tumor or extension into seminal vesicles
D	Metastatic cancer
	D1 Spread to pelvic lymph nodes
	D2 Spread to juxtaregional nodes or distant sites

Histologic classification of testicular neoplasms

Germ cell tumors
    Seminoma
    Embryonal carcinoma
    Choriocarcinoma
    Yolk sac tumor
    Teratoma
    Mixed tumors
Gonadal stromal tumors
    Leydig cell tumors
    Sertoli cell tumors
    Gonadoblastoma
    Mixed tumors
Other tumors
    Epidermoid cyst
    Adenomatoid tumor
    Adrenal rest
    Adenocarcinoma of the rete testis
    Carcinoid

Cancer of the testis

Eric A. Klein

Testis cancer is a rare neoplasm, with an estimated 6100 new cases and 375 deaths in the United States in 1991.[18] The importance of this cancer is not measured by incidence but by the fact that testis cancer is the most common cancer in men between the ages of 20 and 35 and is highly curable even in advanced stages. Compared with other cancers, the psychologic impact of testis cancer is magnified by its occurrence in young and otherwise healthy men, its sexual connotations, and its potential effects on future fertility.

EPIDEMIOLOGY AND RISK FACTORS

More than 90% of testis cancers are germ cell tumors derived from the germinal epithelium of the mature testis (see the box). These can occur in both pure and mixed forms, occur slightly more commonly on the right, and are bilateral in 1% to 2% of patients. Approximately 5% of testis cancers are gonadal stromal tumors, derived from cells that support the generation and maturation of sperm. About 1% of testis tumors are metastatic from another site.

There are three known risk factors for developing testis cancer: age, race, and cryptorchidism (undescended testis). Although testis cancer can occur at any age, there are three peaks of incidence: between ages 20 and 40, above age 60, and from birth to age 10.[99] The histologic characteristics of the primary tumor are closely correlated with age. Seminoma and mixed germ cell tumors are most common in postpubertal men up to age 40, yolk sac tumors and pure teratoma predominate in infants, and men over 50 are most commonly affected by spermatocytic semi-

Table 31-4. Effect of delay in diagnosis on clinical stage

	Percentage of Patients (N = 154)		
Delay	Stage I	Stage II	Stage III
< 30 days	62	30	8
> 30 days	28	33	39

Modified from Wishnow KW et al: Prompt orchiectomy reduces morbidity and mortality from testicular carcinoma, *Br J Urol* 65:629, 1990.

noma, lymphoma, or other secondary tumors. Whites are four times more likely to develop testis cancer than blacks.

Approximately 10% of all testis tumors occur in undescended testes.[68] There is a 3% to 5% chance of cancer's developing in a cryptorchid testis, with the risk proportional to the degree of maldescent. Intra-abdominal testes and dysgenetic testes associated with a chromosomal syndrome (intersex) have the highest risk of malignancy.

Testis cancer has been reported to occur in fathers and sons, twins, and two or more male siblings.[99] However, except for the known forms of intersex, a defined familial inheritance pattern has not been established.

The most common symptom of testis cancer is a discrete mass or enlargement of the testis, which may be painless or painful. Other symptoms include scrotal heaviness; a dull ache in the groin, lower abdomen, or back; or the relatively acute onset of a hydrocele.

SCREENING

The relative rarity of testis cancer makes screening of the general population not cost-effective. There is ample evidence, however, that a delay in diagnosis leads to more advanced clinical stage, higher morbidity, and excess mortality (Table 31-4).[13,131] Both patients and physicians can be the source of delay in establishing a diagnosis of testis cancer. Common reasons for patient delay include misunderstanding of the significance of testicular symptoms, attribution of symptoms to minor testicular trauma, transience of symptoms, and fear of cancer.[13,131] Reasons for physician delay include attribution of symptoms to a benign condition such as infection, epididymitis, or hydrocele and failure to perform a testicular examination.[13,131] These facts and the 90% curability of localized (stage I) and even locoregional (stage II) testis cancer indicate a need to devote resources to education and detection in high-risk groups.

The American Cancer Society recommends a cancer-related history and physical examination every 3 years for men aged 20 to 40 years, including a screen for symptoms related to the testes and a thorough testicular examination.[18] In addition, the National Cancer Institute recommends that physicians instruct patients in testicular self-ex-

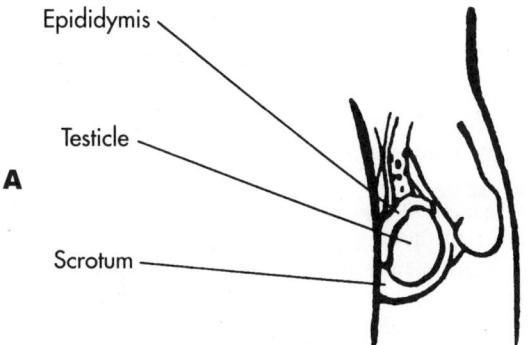

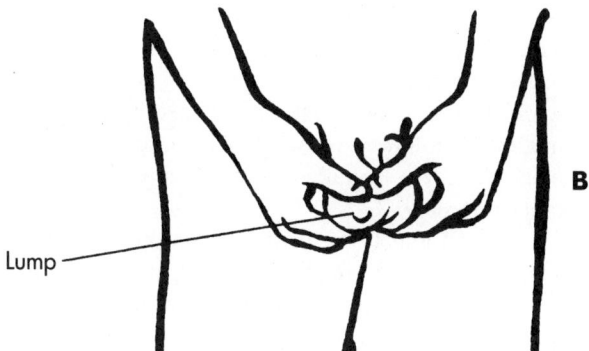

Fig. 31-3. A, Normal anatomy of testis and adjacent structures. Patients should be taught to recognize the epididymis lying posterior to the testis and not confuse it with a tumor. **B,** Technique of testicular palpation by patient. Index and middle fingers are placed behind testis with thumb in front. Palpation is accomplished by rolling testis between the fingers.

amination (TSE) (Fig. 31-3) and that TSE be performed monthly.[122] Patients, particularly those in higher risk groups, should be instructed to perform TSE after a shower when the scrotal skin is relaxed, to search for any abnormalities in the substance of the testis, and to avoid confusing the epididymis with a tumor (Fig. 31-3).

When a testicular tumor is suspected because of symptoms or examination, the diagnosis can be confirmed with a testicular sonogram and measurement of serum human chorionic gonadotropin and alphafetoprotein levels. These studies should not be used as screening tools unless a tumor is suspected.

PREVENTION

Prepubertal patients with cryptorchidism should undergo surgical placement of the testis into the scrotum (orchidopexy) preferably between the ages of 12 and 18 months. Although it remains controversial whether this will lower the risk of malignancy, placement of the testis in the scrotum at an early age is thought to improve fertility and permit easy access for physical examination.[68] Patients with a corrected undescended testis should be taught TSE and examined on a regular basis. In postpubertal males, orchidopexy to move the testis to a palpable position should be performed.[68] Alternatively, because of the diminished fertile potential in an undescended postpubertal testis, orchiectomy may be considered. Orchiectomy should also be performed in a postpubertal male if the testis cannot be moved into a palpable position.

TREATMENT

Treatment of documented testis cancer depends on both histologic characteristics and stage. The sine qua non for diagnosis is inguinal orchiectomy, which provides histologic confirmation, local control of the primary tumor, pathologic stage (T category), and prognostic criteria. Ad-

---

Patient guidelines for testicular self-examination

Perform monthly after warm shower or bath.
Examine each testis with index and middle fingers behind and thumb in front.
Roll testis back and forth between fingers.
Report any abnormalities to your physician immediately.

---

ditional staging studies include serum tumor markers (β-human chorionic gonodotropin [β-HCG] and α-fetoprotein [AFP]) measured both before and after orchiectomy, chest radiograph (CXR), and computed tomographic (CT) scan of the abdomen and pelvis.

Stage I tumors are those histologically confined to the testis with normal postorchiectomy serum markers, CXR, and CT. Stage I pure seminomas can be treated by 30- to 40-Gy external beam irradiation to the retroperitoneum or by observation.[123] Patients with stage I nonseminomatous tumors and those who have mixed histologic findings are treated by nerve-sparing retroperitoneal lymphadenectomy (RPLND). This modification of the standard RPLND can preserve ejaculatory competence in more than 90% of patients.[31] In selected patients with no histologic evidence of lymphatic or vascular invasion in the orchiectomy specimen a wait-and-see "surveillance" approach has been adopted with lower morbidity and overall cure rate approaching that of RPLND.[62] The overall cure rate for stage I tumors is estimated to be 96%.[18]

Stage II tumors are those with radiographic evidence of retroperitoneal metastases up to 5 cm maximum diameter. For stage II seminomas, retroperitoneal irradiation is usually curative. For nonseminomatous tumors, treatment depends on the level of postorchiectomy tumor markers. If the markers are normal, RPLND is performed and if metastatic disease is confirmed patients are generally treated with adjuvant chemotherapy, although observation may be advised if the volume of metastases is small.[90] Stage II nonseminomatous and mixed tumors with elevated postorchiectomy serum markers are treated with systemic chemotherapy followed by surgical resection of any residual metastases. The overall cure rate for stage II tumors is estimated to be 91%.[18]

Stage III tumors are defined as retroperitoneal metastases greater than 5 cm and/or distant metastases (typically lungs, mediastinum, cervical lymph nodes, liver, and bone). All stage III tumors are treated initially with platinum-based chemotherapy followed by resection of residual tumor regardless of histologic findings. The overall cure rate for stage III tumors is estimated to be 54%.[18]

SUMMARY

Testis cancer is a relatively rare but highly curable neoplasm that primarily affects men aged 15 to 40 years. Known risk factors include age, race, and cryptorchidism. Although screening of the general population is not cost-effective, the demonstration that a delay in diagnosis is clearly related to treatment-related morbidity and survival suggests that patient and physician education directed at early recognition is important. It is currently recommended that at-risk patients be taught and perform testicular self-examination monthly and that testicular examination by physicians be part of the routine physical examination of these patients.

Male sexual dysfunction

Drogo K. Montague
Milton M. Lakin

OVERVIEW
Classification of male sexual dysfunction

A classification of disorders of male sexual function is shown in the box. Of disorders of libido, hypoactive sexual desire is quite common, whereas hyperactive sexual desire is seldom a complaint. Erectile dysfunction, a term preferable to impotence, may be either psychogenic, organic, or mixed. Ejaculation is premature if it occurs during foreplay, during intromission, or too soon after intromission. Retarded ejaculation, or inability to reach orgasm, when present usually occurs only during coitus as orgasms are possible either with masturbation or nocturnal seminal emissions. An orgasm with no ejaculate is due to either retrograde ejaculation or failure of seminal emission.

Aging and sexual function in normal men

Sexual function should be possible during a man's entire lifetime if he remains in good health. There are, however, changes in sexual function that occur with aging in normal men.[69] Arousal (erection) is delayed and usually

---

Classification of male sexual dysfunction
Libido
Hypoactive sexual desire
Hyperactive sexual desire
Erection
Psychogenic erectile dysfunction
Organic erectile dysfunction
Mixed organic and psychogenic erectile dysfunction
Ejaculation
Premature ejaculation
Retarded ejaculation
Dry orgasm

---

requires direct genital stimulation. There is a longer interval until orgasm occurs, and orgasm is a shorter event with decreased ejaculate force and volume. After ejaculation there is more rapid detumescence and a longer interval before another erection can be obtained (prolonged refractory period). In a study of 65 healthy married men aged 45 to 74 years, Schiavi et al. found a significant negative relation between age and sexual activity and an increasing prevalence of sexual dysfunction with age. However, no age differences in sexual enjoyment and satisfaction were found.[104]

Commonly held myths

"Normal men lose desire for sex with age."

Loss of sexual desire is not a normal consequence of aging either for men or for women.

"Erection problems are unavoidable with age."

Although some disease processes associated with erectile dysfunction, such as atherosclerosis and type II diabetes mellitus, are frequently seen in aging individuals, men who remain healthy may enjoy sexual activity well into and even beyond the eighth and ninth decades.

"Most sexual problems have psychological causes."

Although psychological factors play a significant role in many sexual dysfunctions, many sexual problems, especially those beginning later in life, are now recognized to have physical causes.

Incidence of male sexual dysfunction

In 300 men with mean age 55 years, Schover et al. reported the following rates of sexual dysfunction: hypoactive sexual desire 11%, premature ejaculation 8%, and erectile dysfunction 21%.[105] Kinsey found a prevalence of erectile dysfunction of 18% by age 60, 27% by age 70, 55% by age 75, and 75% by age 80.[50] Furlow has estimated that there are 10 million men with organic erectile dysfunction in the United States,[33] and 34% of 1180 men in a medical outpatient clinic reported problems with erections.[113]

CAUSES OF MALE SEXUAL DYSFUNCTION
Disorders of libido

Decreased (hypoactive) sexual desire is a common complaint alone or in association with another sexual problem such as erectile dysfunction. The primary determinants of libido are a man's general physical and emotional well-being. Depression and chronic illness (e.g., chronic renal or hepatic disease) have significant deleterious effects on libido. Hypogonadism, primary or secondary, and hyperprolactinemia also decrease libido.[109] Hyperactive sexual desire is a rare complaint.

Disorders of ejaculation

Premature ejaculation is generally regarded as a psychogenic (functional) disorder. Sex therapy techniques are designed to help the man recognize the point of ejaculatory inevitability and to gain control over the ejaculatory demand, and these methods are frequently successful. Retarded ejaculation during coitus when ejaculation is possible at other times is regarded as psychogenic and is more difficult for sex therapists to treat. Retrograde ejaculation commonly occurs after transurethral or open enucleative prostatectomy. Failure of seminal emission occurs after radical prostatectomy when the entire prostate and both seminal vesicles are removed; however, these men can still have orgasms. Aortoiliac surgery and retroperitoneal lymphadenectomy may result in damage to sympathetic nerves and cause either retrograde ejaculation or failure of seminal emission. Diseases associated with autonomic neuropathy such as diabetes mellitus and drugs affecting the autonomic nervous system may also cause dry orgasms.

Disorders of erection

Mechanisms responsible for normal penile flaccid and erect states have recently been described.[63] In the flaccid state corporeal smooth muscle is contracted and spaces between muscle bundles are small. Blood flow into the corpora is low and venous outflow equals arterial inflow; high sympathetic tone maintains the penis in this state. When erections occur the parasympathetic nerves are stimulated and sympathetic tone decreases. The corporeal smooth muscle relaxes and spaces between muscle bundles enlarge. Arterial inflow increases, corporeal spaces fill with blood, and penile expansion (tumescence) occurs. Emissary veins, which course beneath the tunica albuginea and traverse it obliquely, are compressed by the filled corpora, and venous outflow from the corporeal bodies almost ceases. Continued arterial inflow then results in penile rigidity.

Causes of organic erectile dysfunction

Vascular	Postsurgical
Arterial insufficiency	Prostatectomy (simple, radical)
Venous leakage	Cystectomy
Endocrine	Resection of rectum
Hypogonadism	Aortoiliac surgery
Hyperprolactinemia	Pharmacologic (drug classes)*
Diabetes mellitus	Major tranquilizers
Pituitary disease	Minor tranquilizers
Thyroid disease	Antidepressants
Adrenal disease	Antihypertensives
Neurologic disease	Anticholinergics
Trauma	Antihistamines
Spinal cord	Antiandrogens
Pelvic and perineal	Antiparkinsonism drugs
External genitalia	Abused and recreational drugs, tobacco
Peyronie's disease/penile disorders	Pelvic irradiation therapy

*See also box at right.

Drugs implicated in male sexual dysfunction

Drugs decreasing libido	*Drugs affecting erectile capacity*
Antihypertensives	Antihypertensives
Methyldopa	β-Blockers
Clonidine	Thiazide diuretics
Propanolol	Spironolactone
Reserpine	Methyldopa
Recreational	Clonidine
Alcohol	Antipsychotics
Marijuana	Phenothiazines
Methadone	Haloperidol
Psychiatric	Antidepressants
Monoamine oxidase inhibitors	Amitriptyline
Phenothiazines	Doxepin
Amitriptyline	Recreational
Anxiolytic agents— benzodiazepines	Alcohol
	Heroin
Antiandrogens	*Drugs affecting ejaculation*
LHRH agonists	
Estrogens	Antihypertensives
Cimetidine (in very high doses)	Phenoxybenzamine
	Guanethidine
Ketoconazole	Methyldopa
Spironolactone	Antipsychotic
Other drugs	Thioridazine
Antihistamines	Trifluoperazine
Barbituates	Antidepressants
Clofibrate	Amitriptyline
Diphenylhydantoin	Imipramine

Modified from Lakin MM: Diagnostic assessment of disorders of male sexual disfunction. In Montague DK, ed: *Disorders of male sexual function*, Chicago, 1988, Year Book Medical.

Psychogenic or anxiety mediated erectile dysfunction is associated with high sympathetic tone. Organic erectile dysfunction results from many causes as shown in the boxes on p. 651. Whereas psychogenic erectile dysfunction can occur in the absence of significant organic disease, organic erectile dysfunction is invariably associated with some psychogenic elements.

Prostatectomy is a commonly performed procedure in older men, and its effects on sexual function are of particular interest. Simple prostatectomy (transurethral resection, suprapubic or retropubic prostatectomy) is associated with retrograde ejaculation in 50% to 76%, whereas potency (if present preoperatively) is spared in 69% to 95%.[61] In radical prostatectomy using nerve-sparing techniques, 72% maintained potency postoperatively.[127]

EVALUATION OF MALE SEXUAL DYSFUNCTION
Screening

Screening for sexual dysfunction during a routine office visit can be done by asking two simple questions: Are you sexually active? Are you having any problems?

History

A detailed sex history should be obtained;[53] it is important to note how long the problem has been present and whether the chief complaint is a problem with erections, libido, or ejaculation. In general, questions concerning erection problems are intended to help differentiate between organic and psychogenic causes. The sudden onset of an erection problem (in the absence of injury or surgery), variations in erectile quality in different circumstances (coitus, oral stimulation, masturbation, or with different partners), and preservation of morning erections all suggest a psychogenic cause. Conversely, men with organic erectile dysfunction generally notice a gradual onset of the problem, globally poor erections, and absent morning erections. Patients with vascular disease may notice loss of erection with movement such as pelvic thrusting; these men also may rarely notice gluteal claudication. It is very important to ask about premature ejaculation because this results in loss of erections, and men with this disorder frequently present themselves as having an erection problem. Questions regarding libido should try to differentiate between a true lack of desire compared with a decrease in the frequency of sexual activity associated with anxiety over failing. After the sexual history, a complete medical history is obtained, searching in particular for items listed in the boxes that might be expected to contribute to a sexual problem.

Physical examination

The physical examination should place particular emphasis on the man's affect, apparent state of health, and secondary sex characteristics. Gynecomastia if present should be noted. Abdominal masses are potentially impor-

tant and the peripheral pulses, especially in the lower extremities, should be noted. A detailed examination of the external genitalia should be made. At the time of digital rectal examination the anal sphincter tone, bulbocavernosus reflex, and prostate should all be checked. The bulbocavernosus reflex is elicited by squeezing the glans penis; the normal response is a contraction of the anal sphincter against the examiner's finger. The neurologic examination, in addition to the bulbocavernosus reflex, should also include checking saddle and external genital sensation, gait, and lower extremity deep tendon reflexes.

Laboratory tests

A complete blood count (CBC), urinalysis, (SMA) profile, including blood urea nitrogen (BUN), creatinine, and serum electrolyte levels should be obtained. Serum testosterone and serum prolactin level determinations should be made, thyroid blood studies should be ordered, and unless the patient is a known diabetic, a glucose tolerance test should be done.

Psychologic evaluation

We administer two questionnaires: a Dyadic Adjustment Inventory[114] and a Brief Symptom Inventory.[27] If either of these two inventories reveals significant abnormalities, we obtain psychologic consultation with a psychologist who is also a sex therapist. We also obtain psychologic consultation if the history reveals marital problems, chemical dependency, psychiatric disease, personality disorder, a litigious personality, or many unexplained somatic complaints.

Nocturnal penile tumescence studies

If the patient's complaint is erectile dysfunction, we usually obtain a 2 night sleep study to measure nocturnal penile tumescence (NPT). In a man with erectile dysfunction, normal sleep erections suggest that the erectile dysfunction is psychogenic, whereas impaired sleep erections suggest an organic cause. There are some exceptions to this rule, and sleep erections and awake erections cannot always be equated.[49,88]

Specialized diagnostic testing

The evaluation described is sufficient for most patients. Only if a man is a candidate for vascular surgery is more specialized testing necessary. This includes duplex ultrasonographic examination of the penile arteries,[64] infusion pharmacocavernosometry,[85] pharmacocavernosography,[118] and penile arteriography.[26]

PREVENTION

Healthy men should be able to function sexually during their entire life. Maintenance of good physical and emotional health promotes good sexual function throughout life. A low-fat diet, maintenance of ideal body weight, and regular physical exercise would all seem important in this regard specifically in view of preventing atherosclerosis and adult onset diabetes mellitus. The effects of alcohol on sexual function are well known, and avoidance of alcohol abuse is warranted.[106] The adverse effects of smoking on sexual function are less well known but becoming evident.[38,47] Thus in addition to other reasons to avoid smoking, men wishing to preserve normal sexual function should do so. Seat belt use may prevent spinal cord injury and pelvic fracture, both of which are associated with erectile dysfunction.

TREATMENT
Sex therapy

Sex therapy is behavior modification therapy that should be considered as the first line of treatment for men with psychogenic erectile dysfunction or premature ejaculation. Whenever possible the sex therapist treats these problems by working with the couple. Treatment for psychogenic erectile dysfunction may also combine sex therapy and other treatments such as use of vacuum constriction devices or intracavernous injection therapy. In addition to therapy for psychogenic dysfunctions, the sex therapist can provide supportive couple therapy in cases where men are undergoing treatment for organic erectile dysfunction.

Systemic therapy

We find evidence of hypogonadism or hyperprolactinemia in about 1% of the men we evaluate,[67] and these disorders usually respond well to systemic therapy.[109] We do not recommend testosterone replacement in men without evidence of hypogonadism. Yohimbine, an α-adrenergic blocker, has been used for treatment of erectile dysfunction;[89,120] however, we have not found this agent to be helpful. Trazadone, an antidepressant that has been associated with priapism, has been suggested anecdotally as a systemic agent to treat erectile dysfunction.[55]

Vacuum constriction devices

Vacuum constriction devices have achieved widespread popularity in the treatment of erectile dysfunction,[110,124,132] and their use has been associated with few complications.[80] Proper instruction in the use of the device is essential; a nurse clinician provides this service for our patients.

Intracavernous injection therapy

The direct injection of vasoactive drugs into the corpora cavernosa has become a very popular method for treating erectile dysfunction. The initial agent used was papaverine hydrochloride alone or in combination with phentolamine mesylate.[133] We found a significant incidence of fibrosis associated with the use of these agents.[54] More recently prostaglandin E1 has been used for intracavernous injection therapy; initially this drug appears to be associated with a lower incidence of penile fibrosis but a higher incidence of pain after injection.[35] Future research will undoubtedly result in availability of new agents with a lower incidence of prolonged erections, fibrosis, or pain.

Penile vascular procedures

The success of coronary artery bypass surgery has prompted similar attempts to provide penile arterial revascularization.[72] However, during the flaccid state, flow through penile recipient vessels is low, and this can result in bypass graft thrombosis. Success rates with penile arterial revascularization procedures even in carefully selected men have been disappointing. Arterial transluminal angioplasty of the common or internal iliac arteries has resulted in improvement of erectile function; however, this procedure appears applicable to relatively few patients.[125]

Penile venous ligation procedures have been used to increase corporeal outflow resistance in men with erectile dysfunction secondary to venous leakage.[60] In carefully selected patients a return to normal erectile function can be achieved in the majority; however, a recurrence of the erectile dysfunction associated with venous leakage occurs in many patients after 1 year. Transluminal penile venoablation is a relatively new technique; it appears to be both feasible and safe, but future studies are needed to clarify its role in the treatment of venogenic erectile dysfunction.[11]

Penile prosthesis implantation

Treatment of erectile dysfunction by penile prosthesis implantation has continued to improve over the years through the development of better prostheses and improved implantation techniques. New inflatable hydraulic devices, which feel more like tissue and provide control over erections, have a low incidence of mechanical failures.[83] Recently a prosthesis was introduced that on inflation increases both penile girth and penile length.[84]

SUMMARY

Today the man with a sexual dysfunction has a much better chance of obtaining relief than he did only 15 years ago. A better understanding of normal sexual function, improved understanding of disease mechanisms, and new diagnostic techniques usually make it possible to determine the cause of a man's sexual dysfunction. This points the way to effective therapy, and today, in contrast to only a few years ago, a variety of effective treatment options exists (see the box on p. 654).

VASECTOMY

Richard S. Lang

For several years vasectomy has been a common method of contraception in the United States. This minor

Treatment for erectile dysfunction	
Sex therapy	Intracavernous injection therapy
Individual	Papaverine
Couple	Papaverine, phentolamine
Adjunct to other	Prostaglandin E1
therapies	Penile vascular procedures
Systemic therapy	Transluminal arterioplasty
Hypogonadism	Penile arterial revascularization
Hyperprolactinemia	Transluminal venoablation
Vacuum constriction	Penile venous ligation
devices	Penile prosthesis implantation
	Nonhydraulic (rod) prostheses
	Hydraulic, inflatable prostheses

surgical procedure involves cutting or occluding the vas deferens. This is accomplished by ligation, cutting, or clipping the vas deferens followed oftentimes by fascial interposition to prevent spontaneous re-anastomosis. The procedure is done under local anesthesia and is usually accomplished in less than 30 minutes.

The failure rate for vasectomy is generally less than 1 percent.[123a] Failure is due to coitus soon after vasectomy, unrecognized congenital duplication of the vas deferens, ligation of the wrong structure, or spontaneous re-anastomosis.[96a] Sperm concentration and motility decrease by 3 days after vasectomy.[59a] Ideally the absence of sperm should be documented by microscopic analysis of semen. Alternatively, after vasectomy, men are advised to wait 10 to 15 ejaculations or 6 weeks to ensure clearance of sperm from the genital tract.

Complications from vasectomy are generally minor and include scrotal swelling, ecchymosis, and pain, which generally resolve in 1 to 2 weeks. Other complications include hematoma in about 2 percent of cases,[48a] infection, and epididymitis. Increased risk for epididymitis occurs particularly in the first year after vasectomy but also is increased slightly in years thereafter.[68a]

Leakage of sperm at the vasectomy site leads to sperm granuloma formation. This occurs commonly, is usually asymptomatic, but occasionally may cause pain. Microfistula formation within a sperm granuloma is thought to be the method by which spontaneous re-anastomosis may occur.[96a] Vasectomy has no effect on sexual function or satisfaction. Testosterone and hormone function appear not to be changed after vasectomy.[52a]

The long-term effects of vasectomy on mortality have been evaluated in a variety of studies. No increased risk for atherosclerotic heart disease as a result of vasectomy has been demonstrated.[35c,68a,100a] The large study conducted by Massey et al. to evaluate systemic effects of vasectomy particularly related to the formation of antisperm antibodies and immune complexes showed no significant increase for other diseases except epididymitis as described previously.[68a] More recently, the question of prostate cancer risk related to vasectomy has been evaluated. Studies by Giovannucci et al. have suggested an increased risk for development of prostate cancer as a result of vasectomy.[35a,35b] They found a relative risk of about 1.5 to 2.0, with greater risk conferred in those men who had their vasectomy procedure more than 2 decades ago. They postulate mechanisms for explaining the increased risk for prostate cancer as a result of vasectomy, but these remain theoretical. Despite these well-done studies, the risk for prostate cancer in men having undergone vasectomy based on prior studies is not clear, and merits continued investigation.

A common question asked in considering vasectomy is the reversal potential. Reversal of vasectomy is possible, with subsequent pregnancy rates ranging from 30% to 60%.[96a] Reversal is accomplished by microsurgical technique and is dependent on the skill of the surgeon, the technique used for the previous vasectomy, the duration of time elapsed from vasectomy to reversal, the previous amount of vas deferens removed, and the presence of sperm granuloma formation. If a large amount of vas deferens has been removed, reversal is less likely. If reversal is attempted within 10 years of the vasectomy, as many as 90% of men may show normal sperm count, whereas in persons undergoing reversal more than 10 years from time of vasectomy, the same study demonstrated only 35% to have a normal sperm count.[101a] The presence of sperm granuloma at the vasectomy site appears to favor reversibility.[101a]

The decision to undergo vasectomy should include consideration of the factors outlined, as well as the other available methods of contraception and sterilization. Generally, in comparison to tubal sterilization, vasectomy is as effective and as reversible.[96a] The question of prostate cancer risk associated with vasectomy merits further investigation and some consideration in the decision making process. Men having had vasectomy should be screened for prostate cancer after age 50 following the guidelines of the American Cancer Society. Reversal of vasectomy to reduce risk for prostate cancer cannot be recommended at this time based on the data available.

REFERENCES

1. Arrighi HM et al: Symptoms and sign of prostatism as risk factors for prostatectomy, *Prostate* 16:263, 1990.
2. Ball AJ, Feneley RC, Abrams PH: The natural history of untreated "prostatism," *Br J Urol* 53:613, 1981.
3. Barry MS: Epidemiology and natural history of benign prostatic hyperplasia, *Urol Clin North Am* 17(3):495, 1990.
4. Benson MC et al: Use of prostate specific antigen density to enhance predictive value of intermediate levels of serum prostate specific antigen, *J Urol* 147:817, 1992.
5. Benson MC et al: Prostate specific antigen density: means of distinguishing benign prostatic hypertrophy and prosate cancer, *J Urol* 147:815, 1992.

6. Berry SJ et al: The development of human benign prostatic hyperplasia with age, *J Urol* 132:474, 1984.

7. Birkhoff JD: Natural history of benign prostatic hypertrophy. In *Benign prostatic hyperplasia,* New York, 1983, Springer-Verlag.

8. Birkhoff JD et al: Natural history of benign prostatic hypertrophy and acute urinary retention, *Urology* VII(1):48, 1976.

9. Blaivas JG: Multichannel urodynamic studies in men with benign prostatic hyperplasia: indications and interpretation, *Urol Clin North Am* 17(3):543, 1990.

10. Bolton NJ, Lukkarinen O, Vihko R: Concentrations of androgens in human BPH tissues incubated for up to three days, *Prostate* 9:159, 1986.

11. Bookstein JJ, Lurie AL: Transluminal penile veno-ablation for impotence: a progress report, *Cardiovasc Intervent Radiol* 11:253, 1988.

12. Bosch RJLH et al: Treatment of benign prostatic hyperplasia by androgen deprivations: effects on prostatic size and urodynamic parameters, *J Urol* 141:68, 1989.

13. Bosl GJ et al: Impact of delay in diagnosis on clinical stage of testicualr cancer, *Lancet* 2:970, 1981.

14. Caine M: The present role of alpha adrenergic blockers in the treatment of benign prostatic hyperplasia, *J Urol* 136:1, 1986.

15. Caine M: Alpha adrenergic blockers for the treatment of benign prostatic hyperplasia, *Urol Clin North Am* 17(3):641, 1990.

16. Caine M, Perlberg S, Meteyk S: A placebo-controlled double blind study of the effect of phenoxybenzaminc in benign prostatic hypertrophy, *Br J Urol* 50:551, 1978.

17. Caine M, Pfav A, Polbergs: The use of alpha-adrenergic blockers in benign prostatic obstruction, *Br J Urol* 48:255, 1976.

18. *Cancer Facts & Figures - 1991,* Atlanta, 1991, American Cancer Society.

19. Catalona WJ, Scott WW: Carcinoma of the prostate. In Walsh PC et al, editors: *Campbell's urology,* ed 5, Philadelphia, 1986, WB Saunders.

20. Catalona WJ et al: Measurement of prostate-specific antigen in serum as a screening test for prostate cancer, *N Engl J Med* 324:1156, 1991.

21. Chilton LP et al. A critical evaluation of the results of transurethral resection of the prostate, *Br J Urol* 50:542, 1978.

22. Christensen MM et al: Transurethral resection versus transurethral incision of the prostate: a prospective randomized study, *Urol Clinic North Am* 17(3):621, 1990.

23. Coffey DS: The biochemistry and physiology of the prostate and seminal vesicals. In *Campbell's urology,* vol 1, ed 5, Philadelphia, 1986, WB Saunders.

24. Cooner WH et al: Prostate cancer detection in a clinical urological practice by ultrasonography, digital rectal examination, and prostate specific antigen, *J Urol* 143:1146, 1990.

25. Cotran RS, Kumar V, Robbins SL: The male genital system. In *Robbins pathologic basis of disease,* ed 4, Philadelphia, 1989, WB Saunders.

26. Delcour C et al: Penile arteriography: technical improvements, *Int J Impotence Res* 1:43, 1989.

27. Derogatis LR, Melisaratos N: The brief symptom inventory: an introductory report, *Psychological Med* 13:595, 1983.

28. Dowd JB, Smith JJ: Balloon dilatation in the treatment of benign prostatic hyperplasia, *Urol Clin North Am* 17(3):671, 1990.

29. Eckman P: Benign prostatic hyperplasia, epidemiology and risk factors, *Prostate Suppl* 2:23, 1989.

30. Fair WR, Cough J, Wehner N: Prostate antibacterial factor identity and significance, *Urology* 7:169, 1976.

31. Foster R, Donohue J: Nerve sparing retroperitoneal lymphadenectomy, *Urol Clin North Am* 20:117, 1993.

32. Franks LM: Benign nodular hyperplasia of the prostate: review, *Ann R Coll Surg* 14:92, 1954.

33. Furlow WL: Prevalence of impotence in the United States, *Med Aspects Human Sex* 19:13, 1985.

34. Geller J: Pathogenesis and medical treatment of benign prostatic hyperplasia, *Prostate Suppl* 2:95, 1989.

35. Gerber GS, Levine LA: Pharmacological erection program using prostaglandin E1, *J Urol* 146:786, 1991.

35a. Giovannucci E et al: A prospective cohort study of vasectomy and prostate cancer in U.S. men, *JAMA* 269:873-877, 1993.

35b. Giovannucci E et al: A retrospective cohort study of vasectomy and prostate cancer in U.S. men, *JAMA* 269:878-882, 1993.

35c. Giovannucci E et al: A long-term study of mortality in men who have undergone vasectomy, *N Engl J Med* 326:1392-1398, 1992.

36. Gillenwater JY, Grayhack JT, Duckett, editors: *Adult and pediatric urology,* vol 2, ed 2, St. Louis, 1991, Mosby-Year Book.

37. Gittes RF: Carcinoma of the prostate, *N Engl J Med* 324:236, 1991.

38. Glina S et al: Impact of cigarette smoking on papaverine-induced erection, *J Urol* 140:523, 1988.

39. Glynn RJ et al: The development of benign prostatic hyperplasia among volunteers in the normative aging study, *Am J Epidemiol* 121(1):78, 1985.

40. Goldenberg SL et al: Endoscopic ballon dilatation of the prostate— early experience, *J Urol* 144:83, 1990.

41. Guess HA et al: Cumulative prevalence of prostatism matches the autopsy prevalence of benign prostatic hyperplasia, *Prostate* 17:241, 1990.

42. Hald T: Urodynamics in benign prostatic hyperplasia: a survey, *Prostate Suppl* 2:69, 1989.

43. Hargreave TB, Stevenson TP: Potency and prostatectomy, *Br J Urol* 49:683, 1977.

44. Holtgrewe HL: AVA survey of transurethral prostatectomy and the impact of changing medicare reimbursement, *Urol Clinic North Am* 17(3):587, 1990.

45. Isaacs JT, Coffee DS: Etiology and disease process of benign prostatic hyperplasia, *Prostate Suppl* 2:33, 1989.

46. Janknegt RA: Surgical management for BPH: indications, techniques, and results, *Prostate Suppl* 2:79, 1989.

47. Juenemann KP et al: The effect of cigarette smoking on penile erection, *J Urol* 138:438, 1987.

48. Kelly MJ, Roskomp D, Leach GE: Transurethral incision of the prostate: a preoperative and postoperative analysis of symptoms and urodynamic findings, *J Urol* 142:1507, 1989.

48a. Kendrick JS et al: Complications of vasectomies in the United States, *J Fam Pract* 25:245-248, 1987.

49. Kessler WO: Nocturnal penile tumescence, *Urol Clin North Am* 15:81, 1988.

50. Kinsey AC, Pomeroy WB, Martin CE: *Sexual behavior in the human male,* Philadelphia, 1948, WB Saunders.

51. Klein EA: Prostate cancer: current concepts in diagnosis and treatment, *Cleve Clin J Med* 59:383, 1992.

52. Klein EA, Gerlach RW: Prostate examinations are overlooked, *Cleve Clin J Med* 58:51, 1991.

52a. Kobrinsky NL et al: Endocrine effects of vasectomy in man, *Fertil Steril* 27:152-156, 1976.

53. Lakin MM: Diagnostic assessment of disorders of male sexual function. In Montague DK, editor: *Disorders of male sexual function,* Chicago, 1988, Year Book Medical.

54. Lakin MM et al: Intracavernous injection therapy: analysis of results and complications, *J Urol* 143:1138, 1990.

55. Lal S, Rios O, Thavundayil JX: Treatment of impotence with trazodone: a case report, *J Urol* 143:819, 1990.

56. Lepor H: Non-operative management of BPH, *J Urol* 141:1283, 1989.

57. Lepor H: Role of alpha-adrenergic blockers in the treatment of benign prostatic hyperplasia, *Prostate Suppl* 3:75, 1990.

58. Lepor H: Role of long activity alpha-1 blockers in the treatment of benign prostatic hyperplasia, *Urol Clin North Am* 17(3):651, 1990.

59. Lepor H, Knapp-Maloney G, Wozniak-Petrofsky J: The safety and efficacy of terazosin for the treatment of benign prostatic hyperplasia, *Int J Clin Pharmacol Ther Toxicol* 27(8):392, 1989.

59a. Lewis EL, Brazil CK, Overstreet JW: Human sperm in the ejaculate following vasectomy, *Fertil Steril* 42:895-898, 1984.

60. Lewis RW, Puyau FA, Bell DP: Another surgical approach for vasculogenic impotence, *J Urol* 136:1210, 1986.

61. Libman E, Fichten CS: Prostatectomy and sexual function, *Urology* 29:467, 1987.

62. Lowe B: Surveillance for low-stage nonseminomatous germ cell tumors, *Urol Clin North Am* 20:75, 1993.

63. Lue TF, Tanagho EA: Physiology of erection and pharmacological management of impotence, *J Urol* 137:829, 1987.

64. Lue TF et al: Evaluation of arteriogenic impotence with intracorporeal injection of papaverine and the duplex ultrasound scanner, *Semin Urol* 3:43, 1985.

65. Lytton B: Interracial incidence of BPH. In *Benign prostatic hyperplasia,* New York, 1983, Springer-Verlag.

66. Lytton B, Emery JM, Harvard BM: The incidence of benign prostatic obstruction, *J Urol* 99:639, 1968.

67. Maatman TJ, Montague DK, Martin LM: Cost-effective evaluation of impotence, *Urology* 27:132, 1986.

68. Marshall FF, Elder JS: *Cryptorchidism and related anomalies,* New York, 1982, Praeger.

68a. Massey FJ et al: Vasectomy and health. Results from a large cohort study, *JAMA* 252:1023-1029, 1984.

69. Masters WH, Johnson VE: *Human sexual inadequacy,* Boston, 1970, Little, Brown.

70. McConnell JD: Androgen ablation and blockade in the treatment of benign prostatic hyperplasia, *Urol Clin North Am* 17(3):661, 1990.

71. McConnell JD: Medical management of benign prostatic hyperplasia with androgen suppression, *Prostate Suppl* 3:49, 1990.

72. McDougal WS, Jeffery RF: Microscopic penile revascularization, *J Urol* 129:517, 1983.

73. McNeal JE. Normal histology of the prostate, *Am J Surg Pathol* 12:619, 1988.

74. McNeal JE. Pathology of benign prostatic hyperplasia, *Urol Clin North Am* 17(3):427, 1990.

75. Meares EM: Non-specific infections of the genitourinary tract. In *Smith's general urology,* Norwalk, Conn, 1992, Appleton & Lange.

76. Meares EM: Prostatitis and related disorders. In *Campbell's urology,* vol 1, ed 6, Philadelphia, 1986, WB Saunders.

77. Mebust WK: Transurethral prostatectomy, *Urol Clinic North Am* 17(3):575, 1990.

78. Mebust WK et al: Transurethral prostatectomy: immediate and post operative complications—a cooperative study of 13 participating institutions evaluating 3,885 patients, *J Urol* 141:243, 1989.

79. Meghoff HH: Transurethral versus transvesical prostatectomy: clinical, urodynamic, renographic and economic aspects: a randomized study. *Scand J Urol Nephrol* 102(suppl):1, 1987.

80. Meinhardt W et al: Skin necrosis caused by use of negative pressure device for erectile impotence, *J Urol* 144:983, 1990.

81. Melchiar J et al: Transurethral prostatectomy: computerized analysis of 2,223 consecutive cases, *J Urol* 112, 1974.

82. MK-906 Study Group: One year experience in the treatment of benign prostatic hyperplasia with finasteride, *J Androl* 12(6)372, 1992.

83. Montague DK: Experience with the AMS 700CX penile prosthesis, *Int J Impotence Res* 2(suppl 2):457, 1990.

84. Montague DK, Lakin MM: Early experience with the controlled girth and length expanding cylinder of the AMS Ultrex penile prosthesis, *J Urol* 148:1444, 1992.

85. Montague DK et al: Infusion pharmacocavernosometry and nocturnal penile tumescence findings in men with erectile dysfunction, *J Urol* 145:768, 1991.

86. Moore KL: *Clinically oriented anatomy,* ed 2, Baltimore, 1985, Williams & Wilkins.

87. Moore RA: BPH and carcinoma of the prostate: occurrence and experimental production in animals, *Surgery,* 16:152, 1944.

88. Morales A, Condra M, Reid K: Role of nocturnal penile tumescence monitoring in diagnosis of impotence: review, *J Urol* 143:441, 1990.

89. Morales A et al: Is yohimbine effective in the treatment of organic impotence? Results of a controlled trial, *J Urol* 137:1168, 1987.

90. Motzer R, Bosl GJ: Adjuvant chemotherapy for stage II nonseminomatous germ cell tumors, *Urol Clin North Am* 20:111, 1993.

91. Narayan P: Neoplasms of the prostate gland. In *Smith's general urology,* ed 13, Norwalk, Conn, 1992 Appleton & Lange.

92. Orandi A: Transurethral incision of the prostate compared with transurethral resection of the prostate in 132 matching cases, *J Urol* 138:810, 1987.

93. Orandi A: Transurethral resection versus transurethral incision of the prostate, *Urol Clin North Am* 17(3):601, 1990.

94. Palken M et al: Prostate cancer: comparison of digital rectal examination and transrectal ultrasound for screening, *J Urol* 145:86, 1991.

95. Parish RF, Pesinetti EP, Fair RW: Evidence against a zinc binding peptide in pilocarpine-stimulated canine prosatic secretion, *Prostate* 4:189, 1983.

96. Peters CA, Walsh PC: The effect of nafarelin acetate, a luteinizing hormone agonist on benign prostatic hyperplasia, *N Engl J Med* 317:599, 1987.

96a. Peterson HB, Huber DH, Belker AM: Vasectomy: an appraisal for the obstetrician and gynecologist, *Obstet Gynecol* 76:568-572, 1990.

97. Reddy PIC et al: Balloon dilatation of the prostate for benign prostatic hyperplasia, *Urol Clin North Am* 15(3):531, 1988.

98. Reddy PK: Role of balloon dilatation in the treatment of benign prostatic hyperplasia, *Prostate Suppl* 3:39, 1990.

99. Richie JP: Neoplasms of the testis. In Walsh PC et al: *Campbell's urology,* ed 6, Philadelphia, 1992, WB Saunders.

100. Roesch RP et al. Ammonia toxicity resulting from glycine absorption during TURP, *Anaethesiology* 58:577, 1983.

100a. Rosenberg L et al: The risk of myocardial infarction 10 or more years after vasectomy in men under 55 years of age, *Am J Epidemiol* 123:1049-1056, 1986.

101. Ross RK et al: Serum testosterone levels in healthy young black and white men, *J Natl Cancer Inst* 76:45, 1986.

101a. Silber SJ: Vasectomy and vasectomy reversal, *Fertil Steril* 29:125-140, 1978.

102. Rotkin ID; Origins, distribution and risk of benign prostatic hyperplasia. In *Benign prostatic hyperplasia,* New York, 1983, Springer-Verlag.

103. Sapozink et al: Preliminary data reported at the North American Hyperthermia Group Meeting, Seattle, March, 1989

104. Schiavi RC et al: Healthy aging and male sexual function, *Am J Psychol* 147:766, 1990.

105. Schover LR, Evans RB, von Eschenbach AC: Sexual rehabilitation in a cancer center: diagnosis and outcome in 384 cases, *Arch Sex Behav* 16:445, 1987.

106. Schover LR, Jensen SB: *Sexuality and chronic illness: a comprehensive approach,* New York, London, 1988, Guilford Press.

107. Schroeder FH, Blom JHM: Natural history of benign prostatic hyperplasia, *Prostate Suppl* 2:17, 1989.

108. Shapiro E: Embryologic development of the prostate: insights into etiology and treatment of benign prostatic hyperplasia, *Urol Clin North Am* 17(3):487, 1990.

109. Sheeler LR, Lakin MM: Hypogonadism and hyperprolactinemia. In Montague DK, editor: *Disorders of male sexual function,* Chicago, 1988, Year Book Medical.

110. Sidi AA et al: Patient acceptance of and satisfaction with an external negative pressure device for impotence, *J Urol* 144:1154, 1990.

111. Siiteri PK, Wilson JD: Dihydrotestosterone in prostatic hypertrophy: formation and content of DHT in the hypertrophic prostate of man, *J Clin Invest* 49:1737-1745, 1970.

112. Silverberg E, Lubera JA: Cancer statistics, 1989, *CA Cancer J Clin* 39:3, 1989.

113. Slag MF et al: Impotence in medical clinic outpatients, *JAMA* 249:1736, 1983.

114. Spanier GB: Measuring dyadic adjustment: new scales for assessing the quality of marriage and similar dyads, *J Marriage Fam* 38:15, 1976.

115. Spiro LH, Labay G, Lazarus OA: Prostatic infarction: role in acute urinary retention, *Urology* 111(3):345, 1974.

116. Stamey TA: Ultrasound: guided transurethral core biopsies, *Monogr Urol* 10(5):67, 1989.

117. Steinberg GD et al: Family history and the risk of prostate cancer, *Prostate* 17:337, 1990.

118. Stief CG et al: The rationale for pharmacologic cavernosography, *J Urol* 140:1564, 1988.

119. Stoner E, Finasteride Study Group: The clinical effects of a 5-alpha reductase inhibitor, finasteride on benign prostatic hyperplasia, *J Urol* 147:1298, 1992.

120. Susset JG et al: Effect of yohimbine hydrochloride on erectile impotence: a double-blind study, *J Urol* 141:1360, 1989.

121. Tanagho EA: Anatomy of the lower urinary tract. In *Campbell's urology,* vol 2, Ed 5, Philadelphia, 1986, WB Saunders.

122. *Testicular Self-Examination,* NIH publication No 90-2636, 1990.

123. Thomas G: Surveillance for stage I seminoma, *Urol Clin North Am* 20:85, 1993.

123a. Trussell J, Kost K: Contraceptive failure in the United States: a critical review of the literature, *Stud Fam Plann* 18:237-283, 1987.

124. Turner LA et al: Treating erectile dysfunction with external vacuum devices: impact upon sexual, psychological and marital functioning, *J Urol* 144:79, 1990.

125. Valji K, Bookstein JJ: Transluminal angioplasty in the treatment of arteriogenic impotence, *Cardiovasc Intervent Radiol* 11:245, 1988.

126. Vincente J, Salvador J, Chechile G: Spiral urethral prosthesis as an alternative to surgery in high risk patients with benign prostatic hyperplasia: prospective study, *J Urol* 142:509, 1990.

127. Walsh PC: Radical prostatectomy, preservation of sexual function, cancer control, *Urol Clin North Am* 14:663, 1987.

128. Walsh PC, Hutchins GM, Ewing LL: Tissue content of DHT in human prostatic hyperplasia is not supranormal, *J Clin Invest* 72:1772, 1983.

129. Williams PL et al, eds. The reproductive organs of the male. In *Gray's anatomy,* ed 37, New York, 1989, Churchill, Livingstone.

130. Wilson JD: The pathogenesis of benign prostatic hyperplasia, *Am J Med* 68:745, 1980.

131. Wishnow KW et al: Prompt orchiectomy reduces morbidity and mortality from testicular carcinoma, *Br J Urol* 65:629, 1990.

132. Witherington R: Vacuum constriction device for management of erectile impotence, *J Urol* 141:320, 1989.

133. Zorgniotti AW, Lefleur RS: Auto-injection of the corpus cavernosum with a vasoactive drug combination for vasculogenic impotence, *J Urol* 133:39, 1985.

RESOURCES

Prostate Cancer

Prostate Cancer Education Council, c/o Burston–Marstellar, 230 Park Avenue South, New York, NY 10211.

American Cancer Society, 1599 Clifton Road NE, Atlanta, GA 30329.

Testicular Cancer

Office of Cancer Communications, National Cancer Institute, Bethesda, MD 20892.

Cancer Information Service, National Cancer Institute, 1-800-4-CANCER.

American Cancer Society, 1599 Clifton Road NE, Atlanta, GA 30329.

Sexual Dysfunction

Psychologic Inventories

Brief Symptom Inventory, Clinical Psychometric Research, Inc. PO Box 619, Riderwood, MD 21139.

Dyadic Adjustment Inventory, Spanier GB: Measuring dyadic adjustment: new scales for assessing the quality of marriage and similar dyads, *J Marriage and the Family* 38:15-28, 1976.

Support Groups and Information Sources

Impotence Anonymous (IA), 119 S. Ruth St, Maryville, TN 37801-5746.

Recovery of Male Potency (ROMP), c/o Grace Hospital 18700 Meyers Rd. Detroit, MI 48235.

Not For Men Only, c/o Mercy Hospital and Medical Center, Stevenson Expressway at King Drive Chicago, IL 60616.

The Impotence Information Center, P.O. Box 9 Dept. USA Minneapolis, MN 55440.

The American Association of Sex Educators, Counselors and Therapists (AASECT), 11 Dupont Circle, NW, Suite 220 Washington, DC 20036.

Chapter 32

THE GERIATRIC PATIENT

Dennis W. Jahnigen

DEMOGRAPHIC ISSUES

The number of elderly persons in this country has grown rapidly in recent decades. People over 65 years of age now represent almost 12% of the U.S. population, increasing to 17% by 2020. During the last 20 years the absolute size of this group has grown by more than 50%, and the 80- to 90-year-old age group is the fastest growing segment of all. It is estimated that by the year 2000, there will be over 100,000 centenarians in the U.S. Most older people consider themselves to be fairly healthy, with 70% in excellent or good health by self-report.[1] Disability does increase, with almost 50% reporting activity limitations resulting from chronic conditions, with arthritis, hypertension, hearing impairments, and heart conditions leading the list. The need for the physical assistance of another person with one or more basic activities of living reaches 40% for individuals 85 years or older. The use of health care resources by this group is very high for many reasons, including increased prevalence of disability, greater burden of chronic diseases, more medications used, and higher rates of hospitalization and nursing home use. The need for chronic home or institutional services is high. More than half of all older persons will spend some time in a nursing home. Nearly 25% of persons over 80 live in chronic care facilities, with a 145% increase projected by 2020. However, almost twice as many frail elderly persons with equal disabilities and needs live in the community, supported by both formal and informal caregivers.

The average life expectancy at birth in the U.S. is now 78 years. Life expectancy for people who are already very old remains significant (Table 32-1). A woman of 65 today can expect to live another 20 years; a 75-year-old man, nearly 10. Of course, at its best, preventive medicine can only postpone death, not eliminate it (Table 32-2). Even so, preventive health is important in this age group for the same reasons as for younger people[34,57]:

1. To potentially increase the length of life by preventing physical, psychologic, and iatrogenic disorders
2. To prolong the period of independent living
3. To enhance the quality of remaining life, however long

Although aged persons have decreased life expectancy compared with other groups, preventive interventions begun even late in life can show benefits (see box on p. 660).[36]

The scientific basis supporting recommendations for health promotion and disease prevention for elderly persons is limited because, until very recently, there were few specific studies of the elderly. Although there have been a number of recent important investigations, in many areas adequate studies have not yet been done. In particular, mass screening should adhere to established WHO criteria and be linked to a primary care service system. The U.S. Preventive Services Task Force (USPSTF) has produced a set of recommendations for preventive services in adults. For older adults, these cover 34 topic areas.[63,64] These can be used by the primary care physician based on the presence of specific risk factors or overt functional impairment.

Several cohort effects are already influencing the health status of people as they enter their latter years of life. For example, people are arriving at retirement age in better overall health compared with past generations. This is due to improvements in childhood health practices, safer working conditions, and better personal health habits. As an emphasis on life-long health awareness continues, successive generations will make positive lifestyle choices regarding smoking, exercise, and diet that will likely result in higher levels of health at any given age. There is a trend toward assuming increased responsibility for one's own health by the elderly as well as younger groups. The medical consumer movement will make its presence felt

Table 32-1. Average life expectancy

Males	Years of survival	Life expectancy
65	15.1	80.1
70	12.3	82.3
75	9.8	84.8
Females		
65	19.9	84.9
70	16.3	86.3
75	13.0	88.0
85	6.2	91.2

Table 32-2. Gain in life expectancy from eliminating various causes of death

Cause of death	Gain in years if eliminated at birth	Gain in years if eliminated at age 65
All cardiovascular and renal diseases	10.9	10.0
Heart diseases	5.9	4.9
Stroke	1.3	1.2
Cancer	2.3	1.2
Motor vehicle accidents	0.6	0.1
Non-vehicular accidents	0.6	0.1
Influenza and pneumonia	0.5	0.2
Infections	0.2	0.1
Diabetes	0.2	0.2
Tuberculosis	0.1	0.0

From Hazzard WR: Preventive gerontology: strategies for healthy aging, *Post Grad Med* 72:279-287, 1983.

Areas of preventive efforts for older persons

Primary prevention

Infections—influenza, pneumonia, tetanus
Accidents
Adverse drug reactions
Nutrition
Exercise
Alcohol
Smoking

Secondary prevention

Sensory impairment
Hypertension
Cardiovascular disease
Cancer
Osteoporosis
Incontinence
Depression
Dementia

Tertiary prevention

Rehabilitation
Geriatric assessment

---

among aged populations, who will insist on being more involved in all of their physician-recommended decisions.

The effect on overall ability to function independently is the final manifestation of a disease in any individual. Concern over loss of this autonomy frightens older people, often much more than the prospect of death itself. The success of some preventive strategies can be judged according to the extent they reach this goal, as much as by the prevention of a specific disease.

PRIMARY PREVENTION

There are several important illnesses in elderly people for which primary prevention is possible.

Infections

Influenza. Influenza is associated with an excess mortality of about 12,000 people/year, with 89% of these being elderly.[38] Estimates of direct and indirect costs of influenza and its complications range from $1 to $3 billion annually. All persons over the age of 65 are considered at high risk for influenza, with some groups such as those with cardiac or pulmonary diseases or living in nursing homes at even higher risk of morbid events. Nursing home outbreaks have been associated with attack rates of 60% and mortality rates of 30%. Current vaccines are 60% to 80% protective for both occurrence of disease and associated morbidity when the vaccine strain matches the epidemic strain. Unfortunately, only about 20% of this group is vaccinated. Some of this reflects residual fear of the vaccine-associated Guillain-Barré syndrome from 1976.[23] This phenomenon has not recurred since; adverse symptoms (other than a sore arm) from the vaccine have been no higher than with placebo[39] (Table 32-3). All persons over 65 are advised to be vaccinated.[12] Particularly high-risk groups are those with any systemic illness and those residing in nursing homes. The cost/benefit of mass influenza programs is estimated to be about $4000/year of life gained, a bargain compared with many other preventive efforts. Work is underway to improve the antigenicity of influenza vaccine by the use of multiple injections,[17,44] higher doses of vaccine, or the coadministration of thymosin. Because antibody titers decline over 4 to 6 months, the vaccine should be administered in mid-November if possible to protect from late-spring outbreaks.[37] The vaccine requires 4 to 6 weeks for maximum antibody response but can be effective even when given at the time of the first cases in a geographic area.

Amantadine has prophylactic benefits in conjunction

Table 32-3. Symptoms from influenza vaccine

Symptom	Vaccine %	Placebo %
Feverish	5.7	4.2
Cough	6.6	5.1
Coryza	13.2	10.2
Fatigue	8.0	7.7
Malaise	7.2	6.3
Myalgia	4.8	4.2
Headache	6.9	7.6
Nausea	4.5	2.4
Any symptom	27.7	22.9
Sore arm	20.1	4.9
Disability	3.1	3.7

From Margolis KL et al: Frequency of adverse reactions from influenza vaccinations in the elderly, *JAMA* 264:1139, 1990.

with vaccine if given early after exposure. It can also be used for individuals who are allergic to influenza vaccine. Amantadine can ameliorate the course of influenza if given within hours of the onset of symptoms and continued for 4 to 5 days. It can also be used during known outbreaks of influenza A among other household members or nursing home residents. The most common side effects experienced by elderly persons taking amantadine are fatigue, anorexia, depression, insomnia, and nervousness. Because of a potential toxic accumulation of drug in patients with diminished renal function, a dose of 100/mg day is advisable for aged patients.[45,53]

Physicians can play a critical role in helping promote widespread vaccination programs as well as assuring that their own patients are vaccinated. Postcard reminders, well-publicized community-wide programs, and standing orders on hospital discharge or nursing home admission have all been successfully employed.[31]

Pneumococcal pneumonia. Pneumonias are the fourth leading cause of death among elderly persons, with *Streptococcus pneumoniae* (pneumococcus) responsible for 25% of pneumonia deaths. Among the 50,000 cases of bacteremic pneumococcal pneumonia annually, case mortality is almost 50%. A 23-valent vaccine has been shown to be about 70% effective for patients capable of mounting an antibody response.[10] The fact that many vaccination opportunities are missed is evident in one large study of patients hospitalized with pneumonia. Between 60% and 70% had been in the hospital at least once in the prior 5 years.[21,43] The serum antibody titer falls slowly over time, but at present, only one lifetime injection is advised. Studies are being conducted to develop inexpensive assays of individual antibody response to determine whether booster injections are useful. The cost effectiveness of pneumococcal vaccination, using conservative estimates, is $6000 per year of life saved.

The target groups for vaccination are the same as for in-

fluenza. Vaccination is recommended for all persons over 65 years of age. Because the magnitude of antibody response is diminished in many conditions, it is prudent to give the vaccine to healthy elderly if possible rather than waiting until they develop serious illness. Currently physicians are immunizing only one third of their healthy elderly patients and only one half of those at very high risk.

Tetanus. Although rare, tetanus is a preventable illness with a high mortality. Only half of those over 60 years of age have protective levels of antibody. Mass childhood immunization programs and widespread military use of tetanus vaccine have led to tetanus becoming a disease of elderly women, the majority of whom never had primary immunization. For this reason persons who never received primary immunization should receive a series of two tetanus toxoid injections given 1 month apart. A booster is recommended every 10 years.[30]

Accidents

Accidents are the sixth greatest cause of death for older persons.[29] The majority are of three major types: falls, motor vehicle related,[50] and fires or burns.[26] One half of the fatalities are caused by falls, and one fourth are from automobile accidents, followed by thermal injuries. To a young person a fall may be embarrassing, but for an older person it can have serious consequences, with a death rate that is twice as high for people who are 75 to 84 years old as for those 15 to 24 years old. In addition to fatalities, the rate of injury and resulting bed-disability days are three times as high for the older group. There is high morbidity from falls, with 200,000 hip or femur fractures annually. Mortality for people who sustain a hip fracture is nearly 20% in the subsequent 6 months, reflecting the serious associated morbidity. Causes of falls are complex. Factors are both intrinsic (e.g., loss of strength, flexibility, reaction time) and extrinsic (e.g., environmental hazards, slippery or uneven surfaces.[25,32,59] Falling can be an indicator of an underlying acute medical problem or adverse reaction to medication. An office assessment of gait to identify remedial factors as well as a home assessment for safety can eliminate some risks.[3] A simple screening evaluation of gait can identify high-risk individuals[60] (Table 32-4). This test consists of observing sitting balance, rising from a chair, standing balance, stability, and turning 360 degrees. This can be done in an office setting in a few minutes. The home assessment for environmental hazards can be carried out by a visiting nurse, therapist, or family member.

The use of walking aids may be beneficial. Canes can be effective in aiding with balance. The single-prong cane is inexpensive and widely available, but provides minimal support. As with all canes, it should be held on the unaffected or strongest side of the body to decrease the duration of weight bearing by the weaker side. A quadruped cane provides greater support but is somewhat more bulky

Table 32-4. Screening evaluation of balance and gait

Subject is seated in hard armless chair.

Maneuver	Instructions	Maneuver	Instructions
1. Sitting balance • Leans or slides in chair • Steady, safe		10. Able to stand on one leg for 5 seconds • Symptoms or staggering with lateral movement or extension • Marked decreased ROM but without symptoms or staggering • At least moderate ROM and steady	Subject instructed to turn head from side to side as far as possible and look up as far as possible.
2. Arise • Unable without help • Able, but uses arms to help • Able without use of arms	Attempt to get up with arms folded. Subject should fold arms and then get up from the chair. Note the number of attempts.		
3. Attempts to arise • Unable without help • Able, but require more than one attempt • Able to arise with one attempt		11. Back extension (let patient alone) • Refuses to try or no extension or uses walker while doing it • Tries but little extension • Good extension	Patients are instructed to extend backward as far as possible.
4. Immediate standing balance (first 5 seconds) • Unsteady (staggers, moves feet, marked trunk sway) • Steady, but uses walker or cane, or grabs other object for support • Steady without walker, cane, or other support	With arms folded the patient should rise and stand.	12. Reaching up (have subject reach to a high shelf) • Unable or unstable, needs to hold on to steady self • Able to reach up and is stable	Have patient actually take something down from a high shelf.
5. Standing balance • Unsteady Steady, but wide stance (medial heels more than 4 inches apart), or uses cane, walker, or other support • Narrow stance without support	Give patient a chance to gain balance while standing and then instruct him or her to put his or her feet as close as possible.	13. Bending over (place pen on floor and ask subject to pick it up) • Unable or is unsteady • Able and is steady	Self-explanatory.
		14. Sit down • Unsafe (misjudged distance; falls into chair) • Uses chair • Uses arms or not a smooth motion • Safe, smooth motion	Self-explanatory.
6. Nudge (subject at maximum position with feet as close together as possible; examiner pushes lightly on subject's sternum with palm of hand three times). • Begins to fall • Begins to fall, staggers, grabs, but catches self • Steady	Instruct patient to stand with feet as close as possible. Then lightly push for about 2 seconds over the sternum. Do not use sudden jerky motions.	15. Turning • Staggers, unsteady • Discontinuous, but no staggering or uses walker or cane • Steady, continuous	
7. Neck (document exact symptoms) • Symptoms or staggering with lateral movement or extension • Marked decreased range of motion (ROM) but without symptoms or staggering • At least moderate ROM and steady	Subject instructed to turn head from side to side as far as possible and look up as far as possible.	16. Able to pick up walking speed (tell subject to walk as fast as he or she can—a pace at which he or she feels *safe*) • None • Some • Marked	
		17. Is walking aid used appropriately? • No • Yes • Not applicable	
8. Eyes closed • Unsteady • Steady		18. Trunk • Asymmetrical • Symmetrical	
9. Turn 360 degrees • Discontinuous steps • Continuous • Unsteady (grabs, staggers) • Steady	Self-explanatory.		

From Tinetti ME, Ginter SF: Identifying mobility dysfunction in elderly patient: standard neuromuscular examination or direct assessment? *JAMA* 259:1190, 1988.

and cumbersome to move. A "pistol-grip" offers greater strength and comfort. Walkers can also be useful if properly used. The four-post walker is the most common. Patients must lift and move the walker forward. The patient must have reasonable balance, and this type of walker is usually not appropriate for those who tend to fall backward, such as those with Parkinson's disease. Wheeled walkers are easy to push, and the wheels will retract when weight is on the walker, thus preventing it from rolling. Newer versions of three-wheeled walkers with bicycle style handbrakes are also available. These are maneuverable for patients who are cognitively intact. Most walkers can be modified with custom hand grips and forearm supports. Wheelchairs are appropriate for patients who are unable to safely ambulate with one of the other devices. The fitting of walkers and chairs can often be best done by a physiatrist or physical therapist. Participation in a supervised fitness program can improve both strength and flexibility. For high–fall-risk persons living alone, an electronic medical alert device can lead to greatly increased security. These systems are activated when the older person requires help and alerts a local emergency room, which initiates a response by local police or fire department personnel (see Resources at end of this chapter). Table 32-5 displays some of the remediable risk factors for falls.

Driving

Driving holds symbolic as well as practical importance for older persons. The ability to drive is almost synonymous with autonomy for many people. Although older drivers often are conservative and drive fewer miles than younger persons, their overall accident rate is as high as those of teenage drivers, and they have the highest rate of accidents per mile driven of all age groups.[20] Many conditions impair the aged driver, including both normal and disease-related processes.[49] Physicians have an obligation to the community if they believe that a patient's driving represents a hazard; this obligation may override the confidentiality of the doctor-patient relationship. Licensure for driving is a function of individual state laws, which are not uniform. Physicians should be familiar with guidelines for license renewal and reporting obligations for their own state.

Guidelines to help physicians assess the capacity of individual patients to drive are available from the American Medical Association (see Resources at end of this chapter). The decision to restrict a person's driving must be accompanied by help in dealing with the practical problems it may create, such as in shopping and other essential travel. For patients with cognitive impairment who do not recognize their driving hazard, the assistance of the family is essential. In addition to reporting the individual to the appropriate licensing agency, the car can be disabled, allowing the patient to retain the belief that he or she does continue to drive. This approach often will work for patients with Alzheimer's disease.

Table 32-5. Reducing fall risk

Risk factor	Intervention
Vision	Refraction, cataract extraction
Hearing	Audiologic evaluation
Vestibular	Vestibular rehabilitation
Proprioceptive	Physical therapy
Dementia	Supervision, avoid CNS medications
Musculoskeletal	Exercise, gait aids, appropriate medications
Postural hypotension	Avoid specific medications, use compressive stockings
Medication	Cautious use
Environmental	Inspect for hazards
Peripheral neuropathy	Treat specific diseases

Adverse drug reactions

Although the beneficial effects of medications are enormous, side effects associated with their use are common. The risk of such adverse effects increases with age. This is due to the increase in the use of both nonprescription and prescription medications, as well as changes in pharmacokinetics and pharmacodynamics resulting from normal aging and disease. Adverse drug reactions are estimated to cause 10% of all hospitalizations of geriatric patients. The cost of adverse drug reactions is high, estimated at over 3 billion in 1979. Reactions can be the result of excess therapeutic effect; drug-drug, drug-disease, or drug-food interaction; or behavioral factors such as medication misuse or noncompliance. Patients often see multiple physicians, who may be unaware of each other's prescriptions. Patients might use old prescriptions or take a spouse's medications. Many over-the-counter preparations also can cause side effects, and older people (and their physicians) commonly fail to recognize this possibility.

Although side effect profiles are known for many medications, knowledge about their adverse effects when used in combinations of three or more medications are not. For this reason, a safe assumption is that any drug or combination of drugs can cause serious adverse effects in an elderly patient. A decline in mental status, for example, may be due to not only drugs with well-known central nervous system actions, but also digoxin, histamine antagonists, nonsteroidal antiinflammatories, and many over-the-counter agents. Many reactions are preventable by efforts in a primary care setting. Although much of the emphasis in efforts to reduce adverse drug reactions may seem to be on discontinuing medications, the real challenge is simply to use them appropriately. Specific suggestions are shown in the box on p. 664. Perhaps the most important is for the physician to have a very clear idea why the medication is being used and an objective measure of how it is benefiting a specific patient. When it is unclear whether a medication is helping, it should be discontinued. This must be done with appropriate supervision, particularly for medication prescribed for potentially life-threatening conditions.

Reducing adverse drug reactions

Simplify the regimen—reduce both number of preparations and the dose frequency.

Have the patient bring all medications to each office visit.

Discard unneeded medication on the spot.

Have a clear reason and a measurable outcome for every medication used.

Add or delete only one medication per visit.

Consider a "drug holiday"—stopping a medication to determine whether it is helping.

Ask about over-the-counter medications.

When starting one medication, try stopping another.

When possible, keep the total medication number at three or less.

Start therapy with a low dose (one half usual dose if >70, one third if >80).

Educate the patient and family about expected results and side effects.

Ask about alcohol use.

Benefits of exercise for elderly persons

Reduced cardiovascular risk

Reduced body mass and body fat

Increased insulin sensitivity

Decreased resting blood pressure

Improved functional capacity

Improved flexibility

Favorable changes in lipid profile

Better sleep

Increased oxygen uptake

Exercise

The lack of regular exercise by older persons contributes significantly to disability. Less than 10% of this group exercises at least 20 minutes three times weekly.[41] Many of the changes observed in older persons are in fact the result of inactivity, and not of the aging process itself.

Regular exercise has demonstrable benefits for many physiologic functions. Many diseases can be mitigated by exercise, and some studies show increased longevity as well* (see box above and Table 32-6). Primary care physicians can evaluate existing medical conditions, fitness level, and functional ability, and recommend an individualized program. This can be a graded, slowly progressive program with an emphasis on establishing a regular pattern. Many communities have supervised senior exercise programs, which may be useful. A walking or swimming program can lead to significant benefits if it includes

---

*References 9, 11, 22, 35, 42, 55, 56.

Table 32-6. The effect of vigorous exercise on longevity

Age group (years)	Gain in life (years)
35-39	2.51
40-44	2.34
45-49	2.10
50-54	2.11
55-59	2.02
60-64	1.75
65-69	1.35
70-74	0.72
75-79	0.42

From Paffenbarger R: Contributions of epidemiology to exercise science and cardiovascular health, *Med Sci Sports Exerc* 5:426-438, 1985.

sessions at least three times weekly for at least 40 minutes. A target heart rate of only 70% of predicted maximum rate is sufficient to produce measurable benefits.[11,46] This can be obtained accurately with a maximal treadmill or bicycle ergometer test. An alternative approach is to calculate the maximum heart rate (220 minus age equals maximum heart rate) and determine the training heart rate by multiplying by .7. For patients with known disabilities or serious underlying medical illnesses, greater caution is warranted.

Most communities have cardiovascular rehabilitation programs, which may be appropriate. An important theme is that at no age does exercise cease to be beneficial.

Smoking

Cigarettes and other forms of tobacco represent a serious problem among older persons, with 17% of men and 12% of women continuing to smoke.[47] Smoking overall accounts for one of every six deaths in the U.S. Counseling by a physician with strong advice to quit is helpful and can be supplemented through self-help material or referral to smoking cessation programs.[52] It is estimated that a 65-year-old person who quits smoking will gain an average of 4 years of life, justifying a vigorous effort by every physician to promote cessation efforts.

Alcohol use

Alcohol is known to be a problem for about 10% of older persons, with men affected four times as often as women. It is associated with nearly half of all fatal accidents and 30% of suicides in older persons, and has an adverse effect on many medical disorders.[5] Alcoholism is often undetected in older patients because problems observed have alternative explanations. For these reasons, physicians should specifically inquire about drinking habits and counsel patients about health risks associated with the use of alcohol. Screening questionnaires that have been validated for use in elderly populations are available. The

Michigan Alcohol Screening Test (MAST)[15] is very sensitive (100%) and is 90% specific for alcohol abuse. The **CAGE** screening instrument consists of four questions: (1) Have you ever thought you should **C**ut down? (2) Have you ever felt **A**nnoyed by criticism of your drinking? (3) Have you ever felt **G**uilty or bad about your drinking? (4) Have you ever felt the need for an "**E**ye-opener" in the morning? A positive response to even one question should lead to further inquiry.[14] Rehabilitation efforts can be successful for aged alcoholics. Alcoholics Anonymous is a widely available self-help group that can be of assistance.

Nutrition

Diet plays an important role in many of the illnesses elderly people experience. These include coronary artery disease, cancer, osteoporosis, stroke, dental disease, and diabetes. Physicians are advised to counsel their elderly patients to balance caloric intake with activity level and desired body weight. Total dietary fat is recommended to be less than 30% of total calories, with dietary cholesterol to be under 300 mg/day. Avoidance of salt is suggested. Women should be advised to consume at least 1500 mg calcium/day.[16] The average elderly woman's diet does not contain this much calcium, and supplements are often indicated. In spite of widespread use of other vitamin or mineral supplements, there is no evidence that they are beneficial to healthy people who consume an adequate diet (see also Chapter 23, Special Nutritional Needs Through the Life Cycle).

SECONDARY PREVENTION

Secondary prevention screening to detect early disease has utility in several specific conditions that cause disability among elderly persons.

Sensory impairment

Impairment of hearing is one of the most common disabilities that affect older persons. Hearing impairment can lead to social isolation or depression, or aggravate confusional states. Office screening can identify candidates for audiometric assessment and intervention. Hand-held screening devices are available, but formal audiologic evaluations are necessary if impairment is suspected. Amplification and the appropriate use of aids such as telephone amplifiers can restore highly functional hearing. These can be obtained through local telephone service companies.

Visual impairment is also common as a result of several conditions such as cataracts, hypertensive or diabetic retinopathy, macular degeneration, and glaucoma. Some of these conditions have highly effective therapies. Periodic ophthalmologic assessments (every 1 to 2 years) are advisable. Many communities have special services for individuals with impaired vision. These can include access to audiotape books and newspapers and information on low-

---

Treatable causes of cognitive impairment

Drug toxicity
Depression (pseudodementia)
Thyroid disorders
Vitamin B_{12} deficiency
Subdural hematoma
Calcium abnormality
Primary neoplasm
Alzheimer's disease
Vascular dementia
Alcohol induced
Toxic dementia
Neurosyphilis

---

vision aids, such as magnification devices and optical scanners that can actually "read" printed material.

Cognitive impairment

Like many of the conditions previously considered, significant cognitive impairment is a major, underrecognized problem. Recent studies suggest that among community-dwelling persons over 85, up to 47% may have Alzheimers disease, the leading cause of dementia.[19] The societal costs associated with caring for patients with Alzheimer's disease are staggering. With estimates of mean survival from diagnosis at 2.7 years for men and 4.2 for women, the per patient cost of care ranges from $48,544 to $493,277, depending on the age at onset, with a total cost to society of $27.9 to $31.2 billion.[27,61]

Many causes of cognitive problems other than Alzheimer's disease are remediable, particularly those related to medications and depression. Even those with Alzheimer's disease can benefit from careful management of comorbid conditions. Some of the causes of cognitive impairment are shown in the box above. Because of the insidious nature of dementias, it is important to screen for impairment. Several screening scales are available for use in an outpatient setting (see Table 32-7 for example). These can be administered in just a few minutes in an office setting and can identify a baseline level of function. Cognitive functions tested include orientation, registration, memory, calculation, judgment, language, and drawing. This type of screening test may be sufficient if the patient has clear dementia, but for people with very early impairment, more extensive neuropsychological testing may be required. This usually requires several hours of testing under the supervision of a neuropsychologist.

Depression

Depression is both common and underrecognized as a problem in elderly people. Depressive symptoms are reported by 27% of community-living elderly. Older patients in hospitals or nursing homes have a 13% prevalence of

Table 32-7. The Cleveland Clinic Foundation Geriatric Diagnostic Clinic assessment: Folstein mini-mental state

Maximum score	Score	Category
		Orientation
5	____	What is the (year) (season) (date) (day) (month)
5	____	Where are we (state) (county) (town) (hospital) (floor)
		Registration
3	____	Repeat three objects named. Trials.
		Attention and calculation
5	____	Serial 7s
3	____	**Recall**
9	____	**Language**
		Name a pencil and a watch. (2) Repeat the following: "No, ifs, ands, or buts." (1) Follow a three-stage command. (3) Read and obey: "close your eyes." (1) Write a sentence. (1) Copy the following design. (1)
30	____	**Total** ___

From Folstein MF et al: Mini-mental state: a practical method of grading the cognitive state of the patient for the physician, *J Psychiatr Res* 12:189, 1975.

major depression. This is associated with suicide, especially for elderly white males, who have the highest suicide rate of any age, sex, or racial group in the U.S. Clinicians should be alert for signs of depression, such as anhedonia, apathy, weight loss, or early morning awakening. Screening for risk factors such as new sleep disorders, multiple somatic complaints without obvious organic cause, or recent loss or prolonged bereavement should be considered. Diagnosis requires that at least five of the following symptoms be present for at least 2 weeks[8]:

Depressed mood
Loss of interest or pleasure
Significant weight gain or loss
Insomnia or hypersomnia
Psychomotor agitation or retardation
Decreased energy or easy fatigability
Feelings of worthlessness or inappropriate guilt
Decreased ability to think or concentrate
Recurrent thoughts of death or suicide

Coronary artery disease (see also Chapter 41)

Coronary disease is the leading cause of death in the U.S. Its relative importance increases with age, and it causes almost half of all deaths over age 80. Smoking and hypertension are modifiable risk factors that occur among elderly populations.[54] Smoking cessation is discussed in Chapter 16. Blood pressure should be checked at every office visit and at least every 2 years. Hypertension should be diagnosed after several separate readings with diastolic blood pressure greater than 90 mm Hg or systolic blood pressure of greater than 160 mm Hg. Treatment of either systolic or diastolic hypertension in the elderly reduces strokes and congestive heart failure, but so far only treatment of systolic hypertension has led to reduced coronary heart disease deaths.

Cholesterol has been shown to be a risk factor for middle-aged men, but its value as a risk factor for elderly people is controversial. Routine lipid screening is recommended only for elderly patients with other coronary risk factors, such as obesity, smoking, or diabetes (see box on p. 669). If total cholesterol is over 240 mg/dl, or 200 mg/dl for those with two or more risk factors, dietary counseling is recommended. The role, if any, of lipid-lowering agents for elderly persons is uncertain. For patients with known coronary disease or any risk factors shown in the box on p. 669, the USPSTF recommends low-dose aspirin therapy (325 mg every other day). The growing evidence supporting the benefit of this therapy in reducing the risk of myocardial infarction and stroke, coupled with its low cost and minimal side effects, makes this a prudent suggestion.

Cerebrovascular disease (see also Chapter 43)

Stroke causes over 130,000 deaths annually among elderly persons. The morbidity of nonfatal strokes is very severe. Screening for hypertension is an important intervention for primary physicians. There is now strong evidence for the benefit of treatment of both systolic and diastolic hypertension. For patients who have had either a transient ischemic attack or a nondisabling stroke, low-dose aspirin (30 mg/qd) has been shown to reduce subsequent death from vascular causes by 25% to 30%[18] (see also Chapter 43).

Breast cancer (see also Chapter 47)

Breast cancer is the second leading cause of cancer deaths among women. The outcomes of therapy are comparable to those of younger women, and therefore elderly women should be taught and encouraged to perform a monthly breast self-examination (BSE). The percentage of hormonally responsive tumors increases with age, and the therapy for these tumors is well tolerated. Because many older women are unwilling to perform BSE, an annual clinical breast examination is especially important, as is mammography every 1 to 2 years.

Colorectal cancer (see also Chapter 46)

Colon and rectal cancer is the second leading cause of cancer deaths among the elderly. Annually, 110,000 people 65 years of age or older are diagnosed with colorectal

---

Cardiac risk factors

- Male gender
- Diabetes mellitus
- Hypertension
- Smoking
- Strong family history
- HDL cholesterol < 35 mg/dl
- LDL cholesterol > 130 mg/dl
- Severe obesity

From Woolf SH et al: The periodic health examination of older adults, *J Am Geriatr Soc* 38:817-823, 1990.

cancer. Although studies to date demonstrate earlier detection of cancers, they are inconclusive in showing improved mortality. The cost of performing fecal occult blood testing every year and sigmoidoscopy every 2 years is estimated to be $42,000 to $47,000/year of life added. The USPSTF found insufficient evidence to support fecal occult blood testing or sigmoidoscopy for asymptomatic elderly persons. The American Cancer Society recommends an annual rectal examination and testing of stool for occult blood as an appropriate part of a complete examination in elderly persons. Sigmoidoscopy is recommended every 5 years after two negative annual examinations. Although, 20 U.S. medical organizations have endorsed these recommendations, there is not good prospective evidence that this approach is useful in fully asymptomatic populations.[24] Several large-scale studies are underway that may help resolve these questions, but currently clinicians must weigh the individual benefit of such screening against its cost and burden on the patient. The management of colon cancer once detected is highly individualized. Cure is a reasonable goal for many patients, and otherwise good health can justify aggressive surgical intervention (see the section on the role of the primary care physician later in this chapter).

Cervical cancer (see also Chapter 30)

Even though the rate of development of abnormal cervical Pap tests is lower for elderly women, the prevalence of cervical cancer is very significant. More than 7000 elderly women die annually from cervical cancer. Nearly half of the women in this age group have never had a Pap smear. The American Cancer Society recommends that a pelvic examination be performed annually. This permits evaluation for a number of potential problems, including uterine or ovarian enlargement and genitourinary problems such as incontinence. A Pap smear is recommended every 1 to 3 years until the age of 70.

Prostate cancer (see also Chapter 31)

Prostate cancer is the most common cancer among males and has the third highest mortality rate. Among men over 75 years, it is the second leading cause of cancer

deaths. In asymptomatic men, no clinical or laboratory test has been demonstrated to be an effective screening test. At present, a digital prostate examination is the most sensitive test (67% sensitive). Screening for prostate cancer is evolving as tools such as prostate-specific antigen are evaluated.

Skin cancer (see also Chapter 49)

Skin cancer is often completely curable. An annual skin examination is recommended for people with increased sun exposure, prior skin cancers, or strong family history of skin cancer. Premalignant lesions, such as actinic keratoses, can be detected and treated.

Oral cancer (see also Chapter 61)

Both oral and dental problems can contribute to nutritional and other problems for older persons. Inspection of the mouth should be part of a routine examination. In addition to screening for overt malignancies and premalignant lesions such as leukoplakia, one can determine the condition of natural teeth, periodontal tissues, or dentures.

Thyroid disease

Thyroid disease is often subclinical among elderly people. "Classic" findings of either hyperthyroidism or hypothyroidism are often absent. Less than one third of elderly persons with hyperthyroidism display tremor, tachycardia, and sweating. Likewise, patients with hypothyroidism may demonstrate minimal findings. For this reason, serum T-4 is suggested annually for all asymptomatic elderly women. In many laboratories, a sensitive thyroid stimulating hormone (TSH) assay is available at a comparable cost and is adequate to screen for both hyperthyroidism and hypothyroidism. This recommendation is based on the high prevalence of clinically unsuspected hypothyroidism and hyperthyroidism, the relative ease and accuracy of screening, and the availability of effective treatment.

Tuberculosis

Tuberculosis is a decreasing cause of morbidity and mortality in the U.S., but most cases are among aged persons. It is a special problem in nursing homes, where the high prevalence of wasting disease, malnutrition, and close living conditions leads to annual seroconversion rates of 5%. Skin testing should be performed on all frail elderly persons who are losing weight or showing signs of unexplained decline in overall functional level. All patients residing in a nursing home should be tested. A first-step Mantoux test with 5 U of tuberculin derivative is recommended for elderly persons with diabetes, silicosis, long-term steroid use, or chronic lung disease, or who are postgastrectomy, with all nursing home residents receiving a second-step test with 5 U 1 week later if the first is negative. This second step is positive in about 3% of newly admitted residents.

Urine abnormalities

Asymptomatic abnormalities, such as bacteriuria, hematuria, or proteinuria occur often. Dipstick urinalysis is advisable on an annual basis.

Osteoporosis (see also Chapter 30)

Osteoporosis is one of the most important causes of morbidity in elderly women.[4,13,33] One fourth of all women over 60 have evidence of a spinal compression fracture; 15% will have a hip fracture at some time in their lives. Hip fracture itself is associated with a 20% mortality in the following year. Estrogen replacement therapy should be considered in all perimenopausal women, especially if they have a known risk factor (white or Asian, slender build, history of early menopause). The utility of estrogen replacement in women 75 years and older is not established. Weight-bearing exercises and adequate (at least 1500 mg/day) dietary calcium also should be advised for all postmenopausal women. Bone densitometry is not recommended as a routine screening activity.

Incontinence (see also Chapter 30)

Incontinence, or involuntary loss of urine, affects 15% to 30% of community-dwelling elderly persons.[48] It can predispose to skin ulcers, urinary tract infections, and sepsis, and is one of the leading causes of nursing home placement. The costs of care associated with incontinence were over $10 billion in 1987, exceeding the cost of renal dialysis. It is an embarrassing condition, but an older person may accept it as a normal aging change and not seek medical attention as a result. Primary care physicians should ask specifically whether this is a problem for the person. Incontinence is merely a symptom of many underlying disorders of bladder function, many of which can be successfully treated.

Abuse

Physical abuse and neglect of elderly persons is an underrecognized problem. Patients with cognitive or physical impairment may depend entirely on others to meet all of their needs. Caregiver stress or overt hostility can lead to exploitation or abuse similar to that seen in children. Physicians must be alert to circumstances in which abuse may be likely. This includes an obligation, in the case of incompetent patients, to recommend guardianship or similar protection. When abuse is suspected, physicians must take appropriate action to protect the patient. Most communities have adult protective services that have legal authority to assist in abusive circumstances.

TERTIARY PREVENTION

Perhaps the most important type of preventive care for older persons is the identification of symptomatic, treatable disabilities.

Comprehensive geriatric assessment

One of the newer approaches to incorporate all three types of preventive efforts is the comprehensive geriatric assessment.[2,3,40,51] This approach gathers information on the strengths and weaknesses of elderly patients with regard to their physical, psychological, social, and environmental functioning. This information can be obtained in any setting, including hospital, home, nursing home, or outpatient clinic. The data are gathered over one or more visits, usually by a multidisciplinary team of a physician, nurse, and social worker, with other disciplines as needed. Specific evaluation of functional skills related to independence is included (see boxes on pp. 669 and 671). A combined plan of health care is generated that includes diagnostic, treatment, and preventive recommendations, which are prioritized according to the patient's values and wishes. This approach has been shown to lead to more accurate diagnosis, more appropriate use of community services, and reduced use of medications. Studies of the economic effect of assessment programs have reported mixed results.

The use of comprehensive assessment appears to be most useful when linked to an ongoing clinical management program. Assessment can form the basis of recommending a change in living arrangements. Nursing home placement should normally be the last recommendation because so many less restrictive alternatives may be equally effective. The loss of independence in leaving one's own home is often demoralizing, and many older people fear it more than even death. For frail patients, community-based nursing, therapy, or companion services are available. Many communities have day respite or activity programs that provide a temporary relief for stressed caregivers. Planned, temporary nursing home stays of 1 to 2 weeks can be helpful in some settings. Ultimately, permanent nursing home placement should be reserved for circumstances where safety cannot be ensured or needed personal services cannot be arranged in the home.

Role of primary care physician

The older patient's primary physician plays a critical role in educating, advising, and encouraging sound health practices by older patients. As the primary medical decision-maker, this physician is in a position to greatly influence the direction, scope, and magnitude of screening, diagnosis, and treatment decisions.

The following five-step process is one way to emphasize appropriate medical recommendations while demonstrating respect for the individual's values and wishes.[31]

1. Try to determine the person's values. From where does he or she derive enjoyment? How does the person judge the quality of his or her life at present? How does the person see his or her own life? Under what circumstances, if any, would he or she view

life as not worth living? What degree of risk/discomfort/lifestyle change would he or she be willing to undergo for what benefit? Has he or she considered a living will, durable power of attorney, or other advance directive? A few minutes spent in these discussions may prove to be especially valuable in subsequent decision making.

2. Determine the person's objectives. Most aged persons have considered their own mortality. All understand that no amount of preventive care can prevent death. Many seek outcomes other than cure of a condition. These can include preservation of some vital function such as ambulation, symptom relief such as control of incontinence, explanation regarding the significance of a worrisome symptom, advice, help in coping with disability, and even sympathy. The person's particular objectives will largely dictate the extent to which the physician's recommendations will be heeded.

3. Determine the medical facts. What evidence supports a specific recommendation for preventive care for this person? For what conditions should screening be conducted? How does a recommendation for a specific action weigh against disruption of lifestyle? What are the literal risks of the proposed treatments? What are the optimal benefits to be derived?

Physical self-maintenance scale: (activities of daily living or ADL)*

A. Toilet
   1. Cares for self at toilet completely; no incontinence.
   2. Needs to be reminded, or needs help in cleaning self, or has rare (weekly at most) accidents.
   3. Soiling or wetting while asleep, more than once a week.
   4. No control of bowels or bladder.
B. Feeding
   1. Eats without assistance.
   2. Eats with minor assistance at meal times, with help in preparing food or with help in cleaning up after me.
   3. Feeds self with moderate assistance and is untidy.
   4. Requires extensive assistance for all meals.
   5. Does not feed self at all and resists efforts of others to feed him or her.
C. Dressing
   1. Dresses, undresses, and selects clothes from own wardrobe.
   2. Dresses and undresses self, with minor assistance.
   3. Needs moderate assistance in dressing or selection of clothes.
   4. Needs major assistance in dressing but cooperates with efforts of others to help.
   5. Completely unable to dress self and resists effort of others to help.
D. Grooming (neatness, hair, nails, hands, face, clothing)
   1. Always neatly dressed and well-groomed, without assistance.
   2. Grooms self adequately, with occasional minor assistance (e.g., in shaving).
   3. Needs moderate and regular assistance or supervision in grooming.
   4. Needs total grooming care, but can remain well-groomed after help from others.
   5. Actively negates all efforts of others to maintain grooming.
E. Physical ambulation
   1. Goes about grounds or city.
   2. Ambulates within residence or about one block distance.
   3. Ambulates with assistance of (check one): (a) wheelchair (1. gets in and out without help; 2. needs help in getting in and out); (b) railing; (c) cane; or (d) walker.
   4. Sits unsupported in chair or wheelchair, but cannot propel self without help.
   5. Bedridden more than half the time.
F. Bathing
   1. Bathes self (tub, shower, sponge bath) without help.
   2. Bathes self, with help in getting in and out of tub.
   3. Washes face and hands only, but cannot bathe rest of body.
   4. Does not wash self but is cooperative with those who bathe him or her.
   5. Does not try to wash self and resists efforts to keep him or her clean.

From Lawton MP: The functional assessment of elderly people, *J Am Geriatr Soc* 19(6):465, 1971.
*Start by asking the patient to describe her or his ability to perform a given activity (e.g., feeding). Then ask specific questions as needed.

4. Recommend a specific course of action. Educate/ negotiate to arrive at a plan that is acceptable to both patient and physician. A plan that is medically correct but unpalatable to the patient is doomed to failure. For many patients with diminished competence, the family must be involved in all decision making.
5. Establish outcome measures. The plan can be diagnostic, supportive, therapeutic, palliative, or preventive, each having its own measures of success. The specific expected outcomes should be described, such as "prevention of influenza this year," or "helping a person remain in his or her own home longer by implementing the plan developed from a geriatric assessment."

Patients can be encouraged to use one of the available self-administered health-risk appraisals. The Carter Center developed one that is a questionnaire that can be computer scored with an individual risk assessment, life-expectancy calculations, and specific health behavior recommenda-

---

Scale for instrumental activities of daily living (IADL)*

A. Ability to use telephone
   1. Operates telephone on own initiative: looks up and dials numbers, etc.
   2. Dials a few well-known numbers.
   3. Answers telephone but does not dial.
   4. Does not use telephone at all.
B. Shopping
   1. Takes care of all shopping needs independently.
   2. Shops independently for small purchases.
   3. Needs to be accompanied on any shopping trip.
   4. Completely unable to shop.
C. Food preparation
   1. Plans, prepares, and serves adequate meals independently.
   2. Prepares adequate meals if supplied with ingredients.
   3. Heats and serves prepared meals, or prepares meals but does not maintain adequate diet.
   4. Needs to have meals prepared and served.
D. Housekeeping
   1. Maintains house alone or with occasional assistance (e.g., domestic help for heavy work).
   2. Performs light daily tasks such as dishwashing and bedmaking.
   3. Performs light daily tasks but cannot maintain acceptable level of cleanliness.
   4. Needs help with all home maintenance tasks.
   5. Does not participate in any housekeeping tasks.
E. Laundry
   1. Does personal laundry completely.
   2. Launders small items; rinses socks, stockings, etc.
   3. All laundry must be done by others.
F. Mode of transportation
   1. Travels independently on public transportation or drives own car.
   2. Arranges own travel via taxi but does not otherwise use public transportation.
   3. Travels on public transportation when assisted or accompanied by another.
   4. Travel limited to taxi or automobile, with assistance of another.
   5. Does not travel at all.
G. Responsibility for own medication
   1. Is responsible for taking medication in correct dosages at correct time.
   2. Takes responsibility if medication is prepared in advance in separate dosages.
   3. Is not capable of dispensing own medication.
H. Ability to handle finances
   1. Manages financial matters independently (budgets, writes checks, pays rent and bills, goes to bank); collects and keeps track of income.
   2. Manages day-to-day purchases but needs help with banking, major purchases, etc.
   3. Incapable of handling money.

From Lawton MP: The functional assessment of elderly people. *J Am Geriatr Soc* 19(6):465, 1971.
*Start by asking the patient to describe his or her functioning in each category, then complement with specific questions as needed.

tions to achieve optimum survival. The assessment is based on established risk factors for morbidity and mortality for which a health behavior or medical intervention can have a positive effect (see Resources at end of this chapter).

"Rolling physical"

Given the large volume of information and multiple ongoing issues in the care of frail elderly patients, the "rolling" or ongoing physical assessment is preferable to the typical annual physical.[62] Such patients can be seen at 2- to 4-month intervals, at which times current problems can be managed, a portion of a usual comprehensive examination can be performed, and a regular schedule of preventive services can be offered (see Table 32-8). The use of a preventive services checklist as a part of the permanent record can help develop a systematic approach (see Table 32-9).

One area that is not commonly considered in preventive care for older persons but that is associated with enormous unnecessary morbidity is the use of medical care near the end of life. Lack of information about an individual's personal wishes and values often leads to the use of burdensome and expensive medical interventions. The net effect can be to diminish autonomy, increase suffering, and prolong dying. Misapplication of resources also contributes to excessive health care costs with no or minimal benefit. The use of a process, such as the previously described five-step process, is one way to use the benefits of preventive medicine while respecting individual values.

Table 32-8. Regular preventive health care services for elderly patients

Intervention	Frequency
Comprehensive assessment	Initial evaluation
Vaccinations	Flu annually
	Pneumovax once
	Tetanus every 10 years
Functional assessment	ADLs annually
Smoking	Counsel annually
Exercise	Counsel annually
Accident prevention	Annual risk assessment
Medication review	Every visit
Blood pressure	Annually
Rectal examination	Annually
Breast examination	Annually
Mammogram	Annually
Pelvic examination	Every 3 years
Vision assessment	Annually
Hearing assessment	Every 3 years
Cognitive function	Annually
Gait assessment	Annually
Resuscitation decisions	Once, review annually

Table 32-9. Cleveland Clinic Geriatric Health Maintenance Checklist

Pneumovax _____   Name _____

Tetanus _____   Clinic no. _____

Resuscitation _____   Allergies _____

Pharmacy _____

Flu Vaccine					
Folstein					
Mammogram					
Pelvic/Pap					
Physical exam					
Rectal/hemoccult					
Sigmoidoscopy					

Continued.

Table 32-9. Cleveland Clinic Geriatric Health Maintenance Checklist—cont'd

Ambulation	1. Independent device 2. Walks/supervision 3. Walks w/support 4. Bed to chair 5. Bedfast					
Transfer	1. No assistance 2. Equipment only 3. Supervision only 4. Requires transfer w/wo equipment 5. Bedfast					
Bladder control	1. Continent 2. Rarely (once/month) 3. Occasional (once/week) 4. Frequently 5. Total incontinence 6. Catheter/indwelling					
Bowel control	1. Continent 2. Rarely 3. Frequent 4. Total incontinence 5. Ostomy					
Bathing	1. No assistance 2. Supervision only 3. Assistance 4. Bathed (shower/tub) 5. Bathed (bed bath)					
Dressing	1. Dresses self 2. Minor assistance 3. Partial help 4. Has to be dressed					
Feeding	1. No assistance 2. Minor assistance 3. Help in feeding/encouraging 4. Is fed					

I = independent A = requires assistance D = totally dependent				
Telephone				
Shopping				
Food Preparation				
Housekeeping				
Laundry				
Transportation				
Medications				
Finances				

SUMMARY

Preventive services of all types for elderly persons may help prolong life as well as preserve an individually defined quality of life. Much of the success of such measures relies on the belief of the primary care physician in its value, and in his or her knowledge of the most useful interventions. This knowledge, coupled with an accurate assessment of the patient's unique values, can lead to the best use of preventive medicine for elderly people.

REFERENCES

1. *Aging America, trends and projections 1985-86,* U.S. Senate Special Committee on Aging, in conjunction with the American Association of Retired Persons, The Federal Council on the Aging, and the Administration on Aging, Pub 498-116-814, Washington, DC, 1986, Government Printing Office.
2. Applegate WB et al: Impact of a geriatric assessment unit on subsequent health care charges, *Am J Public Health* 81:1302-1306, 1991.
3. Applegate WB et al. A randomized controlled trial of a geriatric assessment and rehabilitation unit in a rehabilitation hospital, *N Engl J Med* 322:1572, 1990.
4. Arden NH et al: The roles of vaccination and amantadine prophylaxis in controlling an outbreak of influenza A (H3N2) in a nursing home, *Arch Intern Med* 148:865-868, 1988.
5. Atkinson RM, editor: *Alcohol and drug abuse in old age,* Washington, DC, 1984, American Psychiatric Press.
6. Beyer WE et al: Antibody induction by influenza vaccines in the elderly: a review of the literature, *Vaccine* 7:385-394, 1989.
7. Blazer DG: Affective disorders in late life. In Busse EW, Blazer DG, editors: *Geriatric psychiatry,* Washington, DC, 1989 American Psychiatry Press.
8. Blazer DG, Hughes DC, and George LK: The epidemiology of depression in an elderly community population, *Gerontologist* 27:281, 1987.
9. Blumenthal JA et al: Effects of exercise training on bone density in older men and women, *J Am Geriatr Soc* 38:1065, 1991.
10. Bolan G et al: Pneumococcal efficacy in selected populations in the United States, *Ann Intern Med* 104:1, 1986.
11. Bruce RA: Exercise, functional aerobic capacity and aging: another viewpoint, *Med Sci Sports Exerc* 16:8, 1984.
12. Centers For Disease Control: Prevention and control of influenza: recommendations of the immunization practices advisory committee (ACIP), *MMWR* 39(RR-7):297-309, 1990.
13. Cummings SR et al: Epidemiology of osteoporosis and osteoporotic fractures, *Epidemiol Rev* 7:178, 1985.
14. Curtis JR et al: Characteristics, diagnosis, and treatment of alcoholism in elderly patients, *J Am Geriatr Soc* 37:310, 1989.
15. Cyr MG, Wertman SA: The effectiveness of routine screening questions in the detection of alcoholism, *JAMA* 259:51, 1988.
16. Department of Health and Human Services: *The surgeon general's report on nutrition and health,* DHHS Publication No (PHS) 88-50210. Washington, DC, 1988, Government Printing Office.
17. Douglas RG: Prophylaxis and treatment of influenza, *N Engl J Med* 322:443-450, 1990.
18. The Dutch TIA Trial Study Group: A comparison of two doses of aspirin (30 mg vs 283 mg a day) in patients after a transient ischemic attack or minor ischemic stroke, *N Engl J Med* 325:1261-1266, 1991.
19. Evans DA et al: Prevalence of Alzheimers disease in a community population of older persons, *JAMA* 262:2551, 1989.
20. Evans L: Older driver involvement in fatal and severe traffic crashes, *J Gerontol* 43:s186-193, 1988.
21. Fedson DS et al: Hospital-based pneumococcal immunization, *JAMA* 264:1117-1122, 1990.
22. Fiatarone M et al: High intensity strength training in nonagenarians, *JAMA* 263:3029, 1990.
23. Fiebach NH, Viscoli CM: Patient acceptance of influenza vaccine, *Am J Med* 91:393-400, 1991.
24. Fleisher DE et al: Detection and surveillance of colorectal cancer, *JAMA* 261:580-584, 1989.
25. Grabiner M, Jahnigen DW: Recovery from stumbles: variable selection and classification efficiency, *J Am Geriatr Soc* 40:910-913, 1992.
26. Gulaid JA, Sacks JJ, and Sattin RW: Deaths from residential fires among older people, United States, 1984, *J Am Geriatr Soc* 37:331-334, 1989.
27. Hay JW, Ernst RL: The economic costs of Alzheimer's disease, *Am J Public Health* 77:1169, 1987.
28. Hazzard WR: Preventive gerontology: strategies for healthy aging, *Postgrad Med* 72:279-287, 1983.
29. Hogue CC: Injury in later life: part 1. Epidemiology, *J Am Geriatr Soc* 30:183-190, 1982.
30. Immunization Practices Advisory Committee, Centers For Disease Control: Diphtheria, tetanus, and pertussis: guidelines for vaccine prophylaxis and other preventive measures, *Ann Intern Med* 95:723, 1981.
31. Jahnigen D, Schrier R: The doctor-patient relationship in geriatric care. In Jahnigen D, Schrier R, editors: *Ethical issues in the care of the elderly,* Philadelphia, 1984, WB Saunders.
32. Jahnigen DW, Grabiner M: Falling in the elderly: biomechanical and neuromotor modeling, *J Am Geriatr Soc* 39:A34, 1991.
33. Jensen GF et al: Epidemiology of postmenopausal spinal and long-bone fractures: a unifying approach to postmenopausal osteoporosis, *Clin Orthop* 166:75, 1982.
34. Kennie DC: Health maintenance of the elderly, *J Am Geriatr Soc* 32:316, 1984.
35. Larson EB, Bruce RA: Health benefits in an aging society, *Arch Intern Med* 147:353-356, 1987.
36. Larson EB: Health promotion and disease prevention in the older adult, *Geriatrics* 43:31-37, 1988.
36a. Lawton MP: The functional assessment of elderly people, *J Am Geriatr Soc* 19(6):465, 1971.
37. Levine MA et al: Characterization of the immune response to trivalent influenza vaccine in elderly men, *J Am Geriatr Soc* 35:609-615, 1987.
38. Lui K, Kendal AP: Impact of influenza epidemics on mortality in the United States from October 1972 to May 1985, *Am J Public Health* 77:712, 1987.
39. Margolis KL et al: Frequency of adverse reactions to influenza vaccine in the elderly: a randomized, placebo-controlled trial, *JAMA* 264:1139, 1990.
40. NIH Consensus Statement: Geriatric assessment methods for clinical decision making, *J Am Geriatr Soc* 35:1071, 1987.
41. Paffenbarger R: Contributions of epidemiology to exercise science and cardiovascular health, *Med Sci Sports Exerc* 5:426-438, 1985.
42. Paffenbarger RS et al: Physical activity, all-cause mortality, and longevity of college alumni, *N Engl J Med* 314:605-613, 1986.
43. Patriarca PA et al: Pneumococcal vaccination practices among private physicians, *Public Health Rep* 97:406, 1982.
44. Peters N et al: Antibody response of an elderly population to a supplemental dose of influenza B vaccine, *J Am Geriatr Soc* 36:594, 1988.
45. Peters NL et al: Treatment of an influenza A outbreak in a teaching nursing home, *J Am Geriatr Soc* 37:210-218, 1989.
46. Posner JD et al: Low to moderate intensity endurance training in healthy older adults: physiological responses after four months, *J Am Geriatr Soc* 40:1-7, 1992.
47. Remington PL et al: Current smoking trends in the United States, *JAMA* 253:2795, 1985.

48. Resnick NM, Yalla SY: Management of urinary incontinence in the elderly, *N Engl J Med* 313:800, 1985.

49. Retchin SM et al: Performance-based measurements among elderly drivers and nondrivers, *J Am Geriatr Soc* 36:813-818, 1988.

50. Reuben DB, Silliman RA, and Traines M: The aging driver, medicine, policy, and ethics, *J Am Geriatr Soc* 36:1135-1142, 1988.

51. Rubenstein LZ et al: Effectiveness of a geriatric evaluation unit: a randomized trial, *N Engl J Med* 31:1664, 1984.

52. Sachs DP: Cigarette smoking: health effects and cessation strategies, *Clin Geriatr Med* 2:337, 1986.

53. Setia V et al: Factors affecting the use of influenza vaccine in the institutionalized elderly, *J Am Geriatr Soc* 33:856, 1985.

54. SHEP Cooperative Research Group: Prevention of stroke by antihypertensive drug treatment in older persons with isolated systolic hypertension, *JAMA* 265:3255-3265, 1991.

55. Shepard RJ: The scientific basis of exercise prescribing for the very old, *J Am Geriatr Soc* 38:62-70, 1990.

56. Siscovic DS, Laporte RE, and Newman JM: The disease-specific benefits and risks of physical activity and exercise, *Public Health Rep* 100:180, 1985.

57. Surgeon General's Workshop: Health promotion and aging, US Department of Health and Human Services, Public Health Service, 1988.

58. Tinetti ME, Ginter SF: Identifying mobility dysfunctions in elderly patients, *JAMA* 259:1190, 1988.

59. Tinetti ME, Speehley M: Prevention of falls among the elderly, *N Engl J Med* 320:1055, 1989.

60. Tinetti ME: Performance oriented assessment of mobility problems in elderly patients, *J Am Geriatr Soc* 34:119, 1986.

61. Weiler PG: The public health impact of Alzheimer's disease, *Am J Public Health* 77:1157, 1987.

62. Wolf-Klein GP et al: Efficacy of routine annual studies in the care of elderly patients, *J Am Geriatr Soc* 33:325-329, 1985.

63. Woolf SH et al: The periodic health examination of older adults: the recommendations of the US Preventive Services Task Force, part 1. Counselling, immunizations, and chemoprophylaxis, *J Am Geriatr Soc* 38:817-823, 1990.

64. Woolf SH et al: The periodic health examination of older adults: the recommendations of the US Preventive Services Task Force, part 2. Screening tests, *J Am Geriatr Soc* 38:933-942, 1990.

RESOURCES

Books

Lavizzo-Mourey R et al: *Practicing prevention for the elderly,* Philadelphia, 1989, Hanley & Belfus.

Bortz WM: *We live too short and die too long,* New York, 1991, Bantam Books.

Self-help guides

Carter Center Health-Risk Appraisal For Older Persons. Information available by writing: Health Risk Appraisal Program, One Copenhill, Atlanta, GA 30307.

Emergency Alert Systems, Emergency Alert, (800) 899-4560.

Doege TC, Engelberg AL, editors: *Medical conditions affecting drivers,* Chicago, Ill, 1986, American Medical Association.

Part VII

RACIAL AND ETHNIC CONSIDERATIONS IN CLINICAL PREVENTION

Chapter 33

SPECIAL HEALTH PROBLEMS OF HISPANICS IN THE UNITED STATES

Tamsen Bassford

This chapter will provide an introduction to health concerns significant for the U.S. Hispanic population. Hispanics comprise the fastest growing ethnic minority population in the United States. Approximately 20 million Hispanics live in the mainland United States, and an additional 3 million live in Puerto Rico. This population is expected to reach 25 million by the year 2000. By the year 2020, the Hispanic population is expected to be the largest ethnic minority group in the United States.[56]

Any consideration of Hispanic health status must take into account the fact that the term *Hispanic* refers to a diverse people, composed of many different groups, each with somewhat different values, traditions, history, and health concerns. Beliefs and practices may vary widely from group to group, and, of course, between individuals within a group. The purpose of this chapter is to increase the health care provider's awareness of certain possibilities when serving the Hispanic patient. It will not obviate each health care provider's need to assess the health concerns, beliefs, and values of the individual Hispanic patients and patient populations they serve.

In the following sections, readers will be introduced to the major sub-populations of Hispanics living in the United States. Major causes of mortality and the prevalence of risk factors for these diseases will be discussed. The impact of social, economic, and cultural factors on the prevalence of disease, and on its prevention and early detection, will be considered. Finally, the cultural milieu and its effect on the patient-health care provider interaction will be examined.

EPIDEMIOLOGY

Two thirds of the Hispanic population live in California, Texas, and New York. Additionally, Florida, Illinois, Arizona, New Jersey, New Mexico, and Colorado have sizeable Hispanic populations. More than 90% of U.S. Hispanics live in urban areas.[56]

Mexican Americans comprise two thirds of the current U.S. Hispanic population. They are also the youngest and fastest growing segment of the population.[56] The bulk of the Mexican American population lives in Texas and the southwestern states. Many Mexican Americans continue to have close ties to Mexico, with frequent visits back to families and friends. In addition, however, much of the current Mexican American population has lived in the United States for generations. Therefore the Mexican American population has a wide range of acculturation and language preference.

The 5.3 million Puerto Ricans living in Puerto Rico and the United States comprise the second largest U.S. Hispanic population.[56] All Puerto Ricans are U.S. citizens, as Puerto Rico is a commonwealth of the United States. Puerto Ricans have a high rate of migration between the mainland and Puerto Rico.[11] Like the Mexican American population, the Puerto Rican population is a mixture of those whose self-identification is primarily with the mainland and those who identify primarily with the island.

Cuban Americans, most of whom live in Florida, make up 5.3% of the Hispanic population.[56] While immigration to the United States from Cuba has occurred since the 1930s, Cubans arriving in the United States since Fidel

Castro's rise to power in 1960 have been considered political refugees by the U.S. government. Because of this, a variety of private charitable and government programs to assist in resettlement have been available to Cuban American immigrants. The 125,000 Cuban immigrants arriving in 1980, however, were not considered refugees, and this group has faced difficulties in resettlement. Because of the political situation, back-and-forth migration or visits by Cuban Americans to Cuba are more restricted than for other groups.

The remaining U.S. Hispanic population includes Central and South Americans. Many Central Americans have fled threatening political situations and have problems specific to refugee populations, including the physical and emotional sequelae of war.

In the broadest sense, a history of using the Spanish language is the unifying factor in the Hispanic population. Even so, a significant segment of the U.S. Hispanic population is English monolingual.

Terminology

It is important to pay attention to data sources when trying to apply information on Hispanic health status to a patient population. Some information may be based on data pooled from small numbers of subjects from many different Hispanic subgroups. This creates a composite picture that may not be applicable to any particular group. Other studies may concentrate on one group of Hispanic Americans in detail, creating information that is accurate for that group but not for other Hispanic groups. In addition, terms used to designate ethnicity have changed over time and may vary from study to study. For example, when using U.S. census data, it is important to be aware of the evolution of census ethnicity designations over time. The U.S. Census Bureau currently uses the term "Hispanic" to refer to persons who self-identify as a member of one of the following five groups: Mexican or Mexican American, Puerto Rican, Cuban or Cuban American, Central or South American, or "Other." Before 1985, Central or South Americans were included in the "Other" category. Before 1970, census information does not note Hispanic ethnicity at all. Self-designation is used to determine ethnicity in other data sources, such as birth certificates, but is not the only method used to make this determination. In some cases, another person will be assigning the ethnic category. Death certificates, for example, are filled out by a coroner or mortician. Other studies of health status use more complex determinations of ethnicity, based on such factors as grandparents' ethnicity. If studies are conducted in certain regions of the country, they may include terminology that reflects country of origin. For example, the majority of Hispanics in the southwest part of the United States are Mexican American, and many studies in that part of the country use that ethnic descriptor.

Finally, chosen self-descriptors vary within the His-

panic population. Some Mexican Americans prefer the terms *Chicano/Chicana*. Some Hispanics prefer the designation *Latino/Latina*, which emphasizes Latin American rather than European origin. All these designations become important when interpreting data on Hispanic health status and applying it to a particular patient population.

Sources of data

The Hispanic Health and Nutrition Examination Survey (HHANES) was performed in 1982-1984 by the National Center for Health Statistics (NCHS). It examined health and dietary practices in three groups of U.S. Hispanics: Mexican Americans of the southwestern United States, Puerto Ricans living in the greater New York City area, and Cuban Americans in Dade County, Fla. This information is some of the most complete health information collected on the Hispanic groups surveyed but is regional, rather than national, data and cannot be over-interpreted to apply to other Hispanics living in the United States.

Birth and death data is also incomplete. The 1989 report of the NCHS estimated mortality among Hispanics based on 18 reporting states. Unfortunately, Florida and New Mexico, both with sizeable Hispanic populations, were not among them. The National Model Birth and Death Certificates program has included Hispanic ethnic identifiers since 1989 and will be an important source of data. As mentioned above, U.S. census data has included some designation of Hispanic ethnicity since 1970.

The 1980 National Health Interview Survey (NHIS)[43] and the 1970 National Health and Nutrition Examination Survey (NHANES) also provide some data. SEER data (the Suveillance, Epidemiology, and End Results Program of the National Cancer Institute) include only Hispanics living in New Mexico and Puerto Rico. For specific disease entities, such as tuberculosis or HIV infection, the Centers for Disease Control has data on prevalence by race and ethnicity. A variety of smaller regional studies examining specific health behaviors or diseases can supplement the data from these larger studies in some instances.

While the top two causes of death are the same for Hispanics and non-Hispanic whites, heart disease and malignant neoplasms (see box) account for two fifths of Hispanic deaths but three fifths of deaths for nonhispanic whites.[41] Homicide and legal intervention, HIV, and perinatal mortality are not in the top ten causes of death for non-Hispanic whites. COPD and allied conditions, and suicide, are in the top ten causes of death for non-Hispanic whites but not for Hispanics (see box on p. 679).

Some of the difference between the two groups is due to differences in age composition. The U.S. Hispanic population is a younger population.[56] As of 1988, 38.7% of Hispanics were under 20 years of age, compared to 29.5% of the U.S. population as a whole. People over 65 years of age made up 12% of the general U.S. population but only 5% of the Hispanic population. Some differences in causes

Causes of death in the U.S. Hispanic population

1. Heart disease
2. Malignant neoplasms
3. Accidents and adverse effects
4. Cerebrovascular disease
5. Homicide and legal intervention
6. Chronic liver disease and cirrhosis
7. Pneumonia and influenza
8. Diabetes mellitus
9. Human immunodeficiency virus infection
10. Perinatal events

From National Center for Health Statistics: *Advance report of final mortality statistics.* In *Monthly Vital Statistics Report,* 38(5) *(suppl).*

of death, such as HIV disease and homicide/legal intervention, persist even within age categories.

SPECIFIC DISEASES
Cardiovascular disease

Heart disease and cerebrovascular accident combined account for a significant percentage of deaths in the Hispanic population.[41] Although some Hispanic groups have a much higher prevalence of known risk factors for cardiovascular disease, cardiovascular mortality in the Hispanic population in general is lower than in the non-Hispanic white population. A 1983 study of Mexican Americans in Los Angeles County demonstrated an age-adjusted mortality rate from heart disease and acute myocardial infarction of 390/100,000, compared with 429/100,000 in the non-Hispanic white population.[10] This is despite the increased prevalence of diabetes mellitus, obesity, and hyperlipidemia in the Mexican American population.[21,28,54,55] Caution must be taken when interpreting regional studies, however. In the Los Angeles County study, for example, mortality from cardiovascular disease in both the Mexican American and non-Hispanic white groups were higher than the 1980 national age-adjusted average of 205/100,000.[14]

Although differences in cardiovascular mortality rates between ethnic groups are important as clues to better understanding the interplay of environmental and genetic factors in the pathogenesis of disease, they are less important for the practitioner caring for Hispanic patients. As in the non-Hispanic white population, Hispanics with known risk factors for cardiovascular disease have a higher mortality rate from heart disease, stroke, and acute myocardial infarction than Hispanics without such risk factors.[8]

Obesity is prevalent for Hispanic women in all groups studied and prevalent among Mexican American and Puerto Rican men.[54,55] Diabetes mellitus, another cardiovascular risk factor known to be associated with obesity, is also present at higher rates in the U.S. Hispanic population than in the general population.[20]

Risk factors appear to cluster. In the San Antonio Heart Study, 40% of Mexican Americans with diabetes also had hyperlipidemia. Only 25% were aware of their diagnosis, and only 10% were being treated.[53] Although the majority of studies examining hypertension have found no excess prevalence, Hispanic men are less likely to have adequately controlled hypertension.[54] Knowledge of preventive strategies for hypertension was found to be low in some studies of Mexican American populations.[1,29] Some studies indicate a lower rate of recreational exercise among Hispanics, suggesting that physical inactivity may be a contributor to the above risk factors.[21,25]

For the practitioner, awareness of and aggressive screening for cardiovascular risk factors is important, but it is only half the picture. An understanding of the effects of socio-economic, cultural, and genetic forces that affect these factors is necessary to more effectively intervene. Such considerations will be discussed in more detail later in this chapter.

Malignant neoplasms

According to SEER data, Hispanics have an overall lower rate of cancer than non-Hispanic whites.[40] Cancer, however, is still the number two cause of death for U.S. Hispanics. The leading cancer diagnoses for women, breast and colorectal, are similar in both Hispanic and non-Hispanic populations, although the incidence for these cancers is lower in Hispanic women.[39] Prostate cancer is more common in Hispanic men than in non-Hispanic white men and is the leading cancer diagnosis in both groups.[40] Hispanics have a higher incidence of pancreatic cancer; cancer of the uterine cervix and the stomach occur at twice the rate among Hispanics as compared to non-Hispanic whites.[39]

Dietary factors may contribute to some of these differences in cancer incidence. The traditional Hispanic diet is higher in fiber and vegetable sources of protein.[22,31] This may be associated with lower rates of colon and breast cancer. With acculturation and an increase in the use of animal sources of protein (and an accompanying rise in fat), disease frequencies among Hispanics become more similar to non-Hispanic whites.[31]

Lack of cancer screening continues to be a major problem for the U.S. Hispanic population.[36] Hispanic women continue to be diagnosed with breast cancer at a later stage of the disease and with a larger tumor size, both associated with poorer outcomes.[50] Hispanic women are less likely to have received mammography or other breast cancer screening services.[26,37,49] Economic barriers to screening are significant in every study examining this problem.

Underutilization of preventive services of all types is found in Hispanic populations and will be discussed in more detail below. In general, Mexican Americans have the lowest utilization rates of U.S. Hispanic groups, and Cuban Americans have the the highest.[36]

Homicide and accidental death

Violent death is a significant cause of death among U.S. Hispanic men. Specific causes vary among Hispanic subgroups. Analysis of death certificate data for Hispanics is problematic due to variable coding of Hispanic ethnicity and possible bias in reporting causes of death. Foreign-born Hispanics are coded by place of birth, so causes of death for this subgroup, while not as generalizable, may be more accurate. Analysis of violent deaths in these nativity groups indicates that age-adjusted rates of death from homicide are higher for Puerto Rican-born men than those of non-Hispanic whites, African Americans, or other Hispanic groups.[52] Accidental death is higher for Mexican-born men than other ethnic subgroups. Both Cuban-born and Puerto Rican-born men have rates of suicide higher than non-Hispanic whites or African Americans. Cuban-born and Mexican-born men have lower homicide mortality than African American men but higher than non-Hispanic whites. Rates of suicide and accidental deaths are lower for foreign-born Hispanic women than for other U.S. women. Mortality rates due to homicide are higher for foreign-born Hispanic women than for non-Hispanic white women but lower than for African-American women.

The factors involved in these rates are complex. Income has been shown to be inversely related to homicide and accidental death rates.[52] This may be through such factors as residence in urban areas with higher rates of violent crime, and delay of emergency treatment for indigent patients. Other factors include substance abuse, risk-taking behaviors, and socio-cultural stressors. High suicide rates among Cuban Americans as compared with other Hispanic subgroups may be related to the political upheaval and loss of access to their homeland that accompanied the migration of this group. Underdiagnosis of depression caused by language or cultural barriers may also play a role.

Tuberculosis

The incidence of tuberculosis in Mexico and Central America is three to ten times greater than in the United States.[45] A higher prevalence of tuberculin reactivity and of active tubercular disease in the U.S. Hispanic population has been demonstrated in numerous regional studies.[45,46] Unlike the non-Hispanic white population, the largest numbers of new tuberculosis cases are occurring in Hispanics under the age of 50 years.[45,47] Although much of the "excess" tuberculosis in the past five years has been attributed to new cases in the HIV-positive population, higher rates of disease have been demonstrated in the Hispanic population for over a decade.[45-47] A screening program directed at the Hispanic community in San Francisco in 1983 and 1984 demonstrated a 37% prevalence of significant tuberculin reactions, almost five times the prevalence of the general urban U.S. population. Although much of this excess prevalence was due to extremely high rates among foreign-born Hispanics, U.S.-born Hispanic children had a prevalence rate of 9%. The prevalence of reactors 5 years of age or less in this study was more than ten times the rate reported for children in this age group in the general population.[45] Most authors recommend routine tuberculosis screening for all Hispanic children and for immigrant Hispanics of all ages.[47]

Diabetes mellitus

Non-insulin dependent diabetes mellitus accounts for the excess diabetes prevalence in the Hispanic population. Twenty-six percent of Puerto Ricans and 24% of Mexican Americans were found to have diabetes in the HHANES data.[19,20] The prevalence of undiagnosed diabetes was higher in all Hispanic groups, 9.6% to 11.8% compared with 6.1% for non-Hispanic whites.[20] Mexican Americans were especially undertreated; 40% of those with diabetes were receiving no treatment for it. Although obese Hispanics are more likely to have diabetes than nonobese Hispanics, the prevalence is greater even when controlled for obesity.[20] A study of Mexican American diabetics in San Antonio found that hyperinsulinemia, a marker for end-organ resistance to insulin, is greater in Mexican American diabetics per degree of central obesity than in non-Hispanic whites.[10] The natural history of the disease also appears to differ. Mexican Americans with diabetes have six times the rate of end-stage renal disease requiring dialysis and three times the rate of retinopathy as their non-Hispanic counterparts.[10] Some of this difference is probably due to poorer control of the disease in the Hispanic population, as discussed previously. However, the fact that Hispanics with more Pima Indian ancestry have a greater prevalence of diabetes, as well as the previously noted differences, strongly suggests the possibility of a genetic component as a causal factor in at least some of these differences.[23]

HIV

The number of AIDS cases is increasing at a greater rate in all ethnic minority populations compared with the general population.[15] The cumulative incidence of AIDS in Hispanics is 2.7 times higher than non-Hispanic whites and slightly less than African Americans.[12] As in the general population, the majority of AIDS cases in adult and adolescent Hispanics are associated with injecting drug use (40%) and men having sex with men (40%). Although a higher proportion of AIDS cases in Hispanics is associated with injecting drug use than in the general population, it should be stressed that 47% of cases among Hispanics are associated with sexual contact.[12]

Although results of the 1988 NHIS indicate that general knowledge about AIDS among Hispanics was equivalent to that in the general population, sources of information about AIDS differed between Hispanic and non-Hispanic populations.[13] Hispanics were less likely to cite written information and more likely to cite radio announcements as sources of information. Hispanic parents were less likely to report having discussed AIDS with their children, and Mexican Americans were less likely to have done so than other Hispanics. Remedying the lack of culturally and linguistically appropriate outreach efforts into Hispanic communities has become a vital priority of Hispanic leadership. The National Coalition of Hispanic Health and Human Services Organizations has developed a national agenda and resource guide for AIDS activism in Hispanic communities (see Resources).

Perinatal mortality

A considerable amount of heterogeneity exists in the Hispanic population with regard to infant mortality. Birth rates of low and very low birth-weight infants, based on 1987 birth and infant death registration from 23 states (comprising greater than 90% of the U.S. Hispanic population) showed that while Puerto Ricans have a higher prevalence of low and very low birthweight infants when compared with the non-Hispanic white population, Mexican Americans and Cuban Americans have rates equivalent to the nonHispanic white population.[38,42] As low birth weight is a major predictor of infant death, it is not surprising that infant mortality rates also conform to this pattern.[27]

This might be expected among Cuban Americans, who have higher socioeconomic status, education, are more likely to be insured, and have higher rates of early prenatal care. Mexican American women, however, are more likely to be living in poverty, least likely to be insured, and most likely to initiate prenatal care in the third trimester or receive none.[42] This suggests that factors in the Mexican American culture are protective against low birth weight, despite factors that are predictive of low birth weight in other segments of the population.[6] Supporting this idea is the finding that Mexican-born women have lower rates of low birth weight than U.S.-born Mexican Americans.[4,51] While lower smoking prevalence among less acculturated Mexican American women accounts for some of this, acculturation increases the relative risk of low birth weight in Mexican American women even when controlled for smoking, age, education, and income.[16,51] Interestingly, educational level had no effect on risk among Mexico-acculturated women but reduced risk among U.S.-acculturated Mexican women.[51] Therefore additional cultural affects must play a role. Among all groups, teen pregnancies had higher low birthweight rates.[4,42]

Although Mexican American women appear to be somewhat "protected" against the deleterious effects of late prenatal care, low birth weight is still higher among Mexican Americans receiving late or no prenatal care than those receiving earlier care.[51] The practitioner would do well to respect and emphasize the traditional dietary, lifestyle and family support factors that reduce low birth weight in Mexican American patients. Programs incorporating these elements may be more successful in reducing the low birth weight rate in higher risk Hispanic groups.

RISK FACTORS
Smoking

Data gathered by the U.S. Census Bureau in its 1989 Current Population Survey indicate that the prevalence of smoking among Hispanics overall is lower than in African American or non-Hispanic white populations and has decreased from 1985 levels[56]; 25.6% of Hispanic males and 13.4% of Hispanic females are current smokers.[32] Among Hispanics, Puerto Rican and Cuban American men who smoke are more likely to report heavy smoking.[11] Both the CPS and HHANES data indicate that smoking incidence is lower for Hispanic women than Hispanic men or non-Hispanic women.[32,33,34,35,36] Puerto Rican women have the highest smoking prevalence at 33.5% and the highest rate of heavy smoking.[24]

Some studies indicate that tobacco use may be a more persistent problem in some segments of the Hispanic population. An estimate of smoking initiation between the ages of 20-24, derived from HHANES data, suggests that decreases in smoking initiation in Mexican American and Cuban American men appear to be lagging behind that of non-Hispanic white men.[17] Smoking initiation in Puerto Rican men appears not to be decreasing at all but remaining constant. Among women, smoking initiation is decreasing in Cuban American and Puerto Rican populations. Mexican American women, who have the lowest smoking prevalence, also show the smallest decrease in smoking initiation, suggesting that smoking may be a larger problem in this population in the future. At least one study indicates a positive association between smoking and acculturation in Mexican American women, although this association does not appear to hold across all Hispanic groups.[33,36]

Both male and female Hispanic adolescents report more smoking than their African American and non-Hispanic white peers.[8,33] As Hispanic smokers are more likely to smoke for social reasons rather than in response to nicotine withdrawal,[11] Hispanic smokers, especially adolescents, may be especially vulnerable to increased advertising directed at ethnic minority communities in the face of a shrinking market. Conversely, they may be more amenable to interventions directed at the community or social network level.

Diet

The traditional Hispanic diet is high in fiber.[22,31] Vegetables, grains, and legumes are used as protein sources. Animal sources of protein, with their accompanying high saturated fat, are less frequent. Puerto Rican diets, for example, have been found to be lower in total calories, cholesterol, and saturated fats, and higher in complex carbohydrates, than the typical U.S. diet.[22,31] Migration to the United States and subsequent acculturation appears to be associated with an increase in reliance on high fat animal products and a decrease in daily fiber.[31] Mexican American diets, in particular, have been found to be higher in their percent of calories as saturated fat, because of use of animal fats for cooking. Mexican Americans also have been found to have lower dietary calcium and vitamins A and C.[5]

Mexican Americans have higher serum triglyceride levels, a higher incidence of diabetes, and higher rates of obesity than non-Hispanic whites.[8,54,55] These are markers of a high-calorie, high-fat diet. Additionally, lower serum high-density lipoprotein levels and higher total serum cholesterol levels have been found in some studies.[21,28,54,55] The relationship of diet to these factors in Mexican Americans is not clear cut. For example, although acculturation appears to be accompanied by a transition from traditional Hispanic diets and an increase in some diseases thought to be associated with the traditional U.S. diet,[31,36] acculturation has also been associated with lower rates of obesity and diabetes in at least one study.

Dietary assessment in Hispanics, whether of a population or of an individual patient, is challenging for several reasons. Currently available USDA data bases are limited to relatively few Hispanic foods.[30] Although data for foods reported in a special study done in Puerto Rico are contained in the current data base, using it for dietary assessment of other Hispanic groups necessitates substituting foods from one Hispanic group for another. As recipes and ingredients vary from group to group, this can result in underassessment or overassessment of certain nutrients. For example, substitution of Puerto Rican recipes for Mexican American will result in an overestimation of salt intake, because of higher use of ham and salt pork in Puerto Rican recipes.[30] Substitutions of non-Hispanic foods or ingredients are also necessary at times, adding further inaccuracy. Data from the NHANES III will be used to improve nutrient data on Mexican American foods in future versions of the USDA data base.

The health practitioner serving Hispanics should be alert to possible problem areas such as total calories, use of saturated fats, and adequacy of fruit and vegetable intake, as well as calcium sources. Adequate dietary assessment may be more time-consuming for both the patient and the practitioner. Recipes and ingredient lists and attention to food preparation technique may be required. Dietary counseling may be strengthened by emphasizing the benefits of traditional Hispanic cooking. The social and family aspects of meals should be respected. When possible, dietary counseling should involve the entire family.

Obesity

Hispanic women are more likely to be obese than non-Hispanic white women and less likely than black women. More than one third of Mexican American, Cuban Ameri-

can, and Puerto Rican women are obese. The age-adjusted prevalence of obesity among Hispanic men living in the United States is 30% for Mexican Americans, 29% for Cuban Americans, and 25% for Puerto Ricans, as compared with 24% for nonHispanic white men and 26% for African American men.[9] While some studies have found that prevalence of obesity decreases with higher socioeconomic status, others have not found such a relationship.[53] Although it is not clear that standards for obesity, generally normed on nonHispanics, are entirely appropriate for Hispanic populations, obesity in Hispanics is a risk factor for both diabetes and cardiovascular disease.

Alcohol

Heavy alcohol abuse is a significant problem for the U.S. Hispanic population. Chronic liver disease and cirrhosis is the sixth most common cause of death for Hispanics. Men, especially younger men, appear to be at highest risk. According to HHANES data, 17% of Mexican American and Puerto Rican men drink heavily (average of one or more ounces of ethanol daily).[36] Cuban American men report somewhat lower rates, with 9% reporting heavy drinking. Hispanic women have low rates of alcohol use.[44] Less than 3% of Hispanic women were classified as heavy drinkers in the HHANES data. The HHANES survey results found a positive association between acculturation and alcohol use, with the effect being most pronounced for women.[36]

Identification of a drinking problem and referral for treatment by a social network or by media messages currently appears to play a bigger role in the Hispanic community than physician referral.[3] There is some indication that Hispanics undergoing alcohol treatment are viewed by treatment personnel as having poorer attitudes, poorer prognosis, and are discharged with less complete aftercare plans than non-Hispanic whites.[3] Outreach and treatment efforts that are linguistically and culturally appropriate are vitally important.

USE OF PREVENTIVE SERVICES

Underutilization of preventive medical examinations of all kinds is prevalent in the U.S. Hispanic population. According to HHANES data, more than 45% of Mexican Americans and more than 30% of Puerto Ricans and Cuban Americans reported not having a complete physical examination in greater than five years.[36] Hispanic men receive fewer screening services than women.[36] Hispanics have low screening rates in every category studied. One fifth of the population has never seen a dentist.[36] Of Mexican American men diagnosed with hypertension in a San Antonio study, 46% were unaware of their disease.[54] Forty percent of Mexican Americans with diabetes are receiving treatment,[20] and two thirds have never had their cholesterol checked. Rates were similar in a study of Puerto Ricans and Dominicans living in New York.[7]

Screening behaviors appear to cluster. Hispanic men

who smoke are less likely to get general medical exams or dental exams, regardless of level of acculturation. Hispanic women with poorer diets are less likely to get PAP smears.[36]

Screening for cancer is also low in the Hispanic population. According to HHANES data, approximately 15% of Hispanic women have never had a Pap smear or have not had one within the past five years.[36] Mammography rates vary from study to study. In a 1987 study, only 25% of older women living in low income housing in Los Angeles had ever received a mammogram.[37] But more than 60% of women living in barrios in Tucson, Arizona, had received at least one mammogram in a 1991 study.[49] There are fewer data on cancer screening in Hispanic men. Taking into account their underscreening in other categories and the low prevalence of colorectal screening in the general population (less than 20% of adults over 50 receiving fecal occult blood testing within the past year, less than 25% ever receiving sigmoidoscopy), it seems safe to assume that rates are low.

As in nonHispanic populations, prevalence of breast and cervical cancer screening is most highly correlated with access to such services and insurance coverage.[26,37] Among insured Hispanic populations, sociodemographic variables such as age, education, and affective reactions toward screening (nervousness, embarrassment) and cues to action play an important role.[26,37,49] As in other screening behaviors, actions cluster. Women who have had a Pap smear are more likely to have had a mammogram.[26,37]

Hispanic women are three times more likely than the general population to have received late or no prenatal care. Cuban American women get the most prenatal care, starting earlier and obtaining more visits.[42] Puerto Rican women have the lowest levels of early prenatal care. Low birth weight infants and infant mortality are inversely related to prenatal care in all U.S. Hispanic groups, although this association is weaker among Mexican American women[42] (see previous section on perinatal mortality).

SOCIO-MEDICO-ECONOMICS
Effects of acculturation

As noted previously, any acculturation process has a variety of effects on health, some positive and some negative. In general, acculturation of the U.S. Hispanic population may be associated with lower rates of obesity and diabetes.[9] It, however, has also been associated with higher infant death rates in some Hispanic populations,[42] and the assumption of other high-risk behaviors, such as smoking,[33,36] alcohol use,[36] and low fiber diets.[31,36] Culture is a factor in the total health environment and is one that must be accounted for and respected in prevention endeavors.

More recently immigrated Hispanics are less "bureaucratically" acculturated and may feel more helpless and overwhelmed when facing serious disease that requires attention from the medical system. Economic status is closely allied to acculturation and has been found to be a more powerful predictor of preventive health activities in many studies.[26,37] However, attention to culture and the acculturation process allows for health care interventions that work with, rather than against, patient beliefs and values.

Sociodemographic variables

Income. Twenty-five percent of Hispanic families live below the U.S. poverty level compared with 10% of non-Hispanic families.[56] Among Hispanics, Cuban Americans are least likely to be living in poverty, with Puerto Ricans being the most likely.[56] Hispanics are less likely to be employed and are more likely to be employed in service, agricultural, or blue-collar jobs.[56] Because of their overrepresentation in low-paying jobs and jobs that do not provide health insurance, Hispanics are least likely to have health insurance coverage. Thirty-eight percent of Mexican Americans, 24% of Puerto Ricans, and 21% of Cuban Americans do not have health insurance.[11] Lack of insurance is a major barrier to use of preventive health services in the Hispanic population.[26,37] Similarly, the economic impact of illness on Hispanic workers is exacerbated by their concentration in jobs without sick leave, parental leave, or disability benefits.

A sizeable number of Hispanics are seasonal farm workers.[11] Basic health information on this population is scanty due to such barriers as migration, undocumented residency, and lack of services.

In this setting of scarce resources, health care, especially preventive services, is often viewed as a luxury rather than a necessity. A conflict is apparent between the medical culture, which may view those patients who seek medical care only when ill as being less interested in preventive health care, and the culture of the poor and underinsured, which views "saving" a medical visit for when really necessary as a wise economic decision. In many practices prevention information is not provided during an acute care visit. Patients may be told to return for health care maintenance, which is not economically feasable, or told nothing at all. This contrasts with the patient perception that the physician would have informed them of any necessary tests (such as mammography). This is especially unfortunate, as referral by a physician has been found to be a strong predictor of use of screening services.[49] This effect is strongest among the poor, those least likely to get such a referral.

Education. Hispanics are less likely to have graduated from high school than other U.S. populations. Sixty percent of Hispanics 25 years of age and older have completed high school, compared with 89% of non-Hispanics. Only 11% have completed 4 years of college or more, compared with 26% of non-Hispanics.[56] English literacy is also low in the Hispanic population in general, a problem compounded by the fact that some groups have low Spanish literacy also. While low educational level has been associated in the Hispanic population with low use of preventive services, it appears that its major effect is socioeconomic. Low educational attainment, then, exerts its major negative effect on health through its association with poverty. Health care providers, however, need to consider literacy levels when planning health education. It should be noted that 12% of the general U.S. population reads below the fourth grade level, making literacy an issue for all healthcare providers.[11]

Aging. The elderly Hispanic population is the fastest growing segment of elderly Americans. It is growing at 3.5 times the rate of older African Americans and at 5 times the rate of older non-Hispanic white Americans.[19] A significant percentage were born in Mexico, many in rural communities. Some effects of aging in the U.S. for this population include a dissonance between traditional values, such as respect for the elderly and familialism, and values based in the U.S. culture, such as an emphasis on youthfulness and personal independence.[48] A language and culture gap may exist between Hispanic elders and their U.S.-born children or grandchildren. The economic impact of aging is greater for Hispanics because of the higher concentration of jobs without retirement benefits.

Values such as familialism, the closeness of extended families and networks of fictive kin, and the participation of grandmothers in child care may help to maintain a useful role for elders in the Hispanic community.[49] Hispanic elderly prefer to live close to relatives and will move rather than be separated.[48] Some studies find that older Hispanics enter nursing homes only after greater degrees of disability than non-Hispanic whites, suggesting an important role for the extended family structure in caretaking.[18]

SPECIAL CONSIDERATIONS IN PHYSICIAN-PATIENT INTERACTION
"Respeto"

Hispanic culture traditionally incorporates respect for people because of their position in the community,[11,48,49] whether by virtue of educational attainment, age, experience, or service. This will affect interactions with Hispanic patients. Many Hispanic patients will hesitate to openly disagree with a physician, question, or even correct misinformation to avoid an indication of lack of *respeto,* or respect. Additionally, Hispanic culture places importance on the quality of *simpatía,* a cultural script promoting pleasant social relationships,[46] which reinforces hesitance to directly question a physician. For the non-Hispanic physician, this can be confusing or frustrating and be interpreted, mistakenly, as obstructive behavior on the part of the patient.

Misunderstanding can be avoided if the practitioner takes care to ask the patient for their input and to leave the door open for new information from the patient. For example, when beginning a new medicine, the practitioner might ask the patient if there is any reason the patient might have trouble taking the medicine. This provides the opportunity for the patient to politely offer the information that a similar medication had to be discontinued because of side effects once before or that the dosing interval would be difficult to maintain while working.

Equally important is the provider's demonstration of *respeto* for patients. Older patients have a wealth of experience and information for which they are accorded respect by their families and communities. Seeking their input with regard to their health care increases the power of any health intervention and strengthens the bond between provider and patient. The opinions and experience of older members of the family will affect how medical information is used by any member of the family. Mothers, grandmothers, and aunts are all important allies in the health care of the family and should be treated as such.

Family

As alluded to previously, the family plays a central role in Hispanic culture and values. The good of the family may be accorded precedence over the good of the individual.[49] Disease, treatment, and preventive activities will be weighed in terms of their effects on the family. Health care–decision making is often a family process. The practitioner must recognize this and respect it to be effective. Often this involves sharing information with the family and extended family. The importance of patient confidentiality cannot be overlooked and the physician must take time to clarify who in the family the patient would like to have access to information. For important decisions, time may need to be taken to convene the entire family.

This process is especially important for preventive interventions. It is clear, for instance, that a sustained dietary change will not be maintained without the support and participation of the entire family. Discussing its importance with the usual cook in the family is not sufficient, as the wishes and opinions of the family will immediately begin to affect the meals. Although for some physicians the "extra" time taken to educate entire families may seem unwieldy, it is actually more effective in terms of effort expended per degree of result.

Community

Allocentrism is an important Hispanic cultural value and emphasizes the needs and perspectives of the group rather than of the individual.[49] Hispanics have been described as having a style that is, relative to Anglos, more interdependent, open to influence from others, empathetic, trusting of members of the group, more willing to sacrifice for group members, and value favorable, respectful, intimate interpersonal relationships. This makes community norms and values significant in the consideration of disease prevention activities among Hispanics. Tobacco and alcohol use among Hispanics appears to have stronger social components[4,11] (see previous section, Risk Factors). Social network and family factors appear to contribute to lower rates of low birth weight among Mexican American mothers,[7] and less use of nursing homes for the care of the elderly.[18] In one study, women receiving more cues from their environment to engage in breast cancer screening, for example, felt more hopeful and powerful about the disease.[49]

Approaches to health care and disease prevention, then, must respect these values. Many projects aimed at increasing desired health behaviors have used community approaches, ranging from community councils to media campaigns stressing family and community responsibility to the use of lay health advisors. Such projects have been targeted at cardiovascular disease prevention, cancer screening, smoking, and maternal child health in such varied settings as low income apartment complexes, urban communities, rural populations, and migrant farm worker communities.

Views on health

The Hispanic view of health is more holistic than traditional Anglo views.[2] The Spanish word for health—*enfermedad*—includes both the concept of disease (physical events within the body) as well as the concept of illness (the events surrounding and affecting disease).[49] The Hispanic patient, then, is more likely to describe an illness not just in terms of physical symptoms but in terms of emotional reactions to those symptoms.[2] A health care provider with a more dichotomous view of health ("in your head" or "in your body") may incorrectly interpret the higher emotional content of the patient's description as an attempt to exaggerate symptom severity or even as malingering. This holistic view of health is an advantage in working with such primary prevention concepts as the impact of life-style on health. Also helpful is the Hispanic concept of illness as an imbalance. This imbalance can either be within an individual or between the individual and the environment.

The concept of conforming to God's will *(estar conforme),*[49] and of some diseases as being *natural causes* can provide a barrier to concepts of secondary prevention (screening). Some authors report the attitude that going to a physician or being tested when healthy is "asking for trouble."[49] Hispanic values of *sacrificio* (sacrifice for one's family) and helping oneself can be used to improve communication around screening issues.

The interpretation of a symptom as an illness may not be made by the patient alone but with input from family and extended family. The ideas a patient presents on probable causes of his/her disease, or its effects, may represent a consensus view. It is important for health care providers to respect this, particularly when new information as to causes or treatments must be presented. The illness doesn't belong solely to the patient, but to the patient's social network (see previous section, Family).

Language

The Spanish language is common to all Hispanic cultures. Spanish is the most commonly spoken second language in the United States today. A wide range of language preference and ability exists, however, in the Hispanic population. Not all Hispanics prefer to speak Spanish or even speak Spanish at all. Practitioners who speak Spanish certainly have an advantage in effective communication with their Spanish speaking patients. Spanish language skills do not have to be flawless to be useful. A practitioner who isn't afraid to use his/her "less than perfect" Spanish will soon find that patients are more willing to use their "less than perfect" English. Even the knowledge of a few courtesy phrases can do much to establish rapport with patients. There are many Spanish language courses available that are tailored to the needs of health care professionals. Hospitals, neighborhood centers, and community colleges are good places to find such training.

Non-Spanish speaking practitioners will need to use interpreters to communicate with their Spanish speaking patients. It is important to use interpreters correctly. The interpreter should not be a family member, friend, or neighbor of the patient. The patient will edit information he/she considers embarrassing if sharing it with a physician means sharing it with an acquaintance. The untrained interpreter also transmits information through the filter of their own perceptions and will add to and modify the physician's words, even deleting at times information or questions they consider embarrassing. When using trained interpreters provided by the health care site, it is important that they notify health care personnel if asked to interpret for an acquaintance so another interpreter can be substituted.

When using an interpreter, the practitioner should introduce the interpreter to the patient and explain that the interpreter will not repeat anything that transpires during the interview. It is important to face the patient and direct all questions and statements directly to the patient, not the interpreter. One thought or sentence should be spoken at a time, allowing an interval for translation. Maintain eye contact with the patient while the interpreter speaks. Look for all the same nonverbal clues for comprehension or discomfort that you would when not using an interpreter. Do not address questions to the interpreter ("Does she have any questions?"). Rather, address them to the patient ("Do you have any questions?").

You may need to work with an interpreter during the physical examination, especially when performing a pelvic or other examination requiring explanation from you or assistance from the patient. Again, emphasizing the interpreter's professional role is important. Interpreters in this role should be the same gender as the patient. It is possible to place an interpreter behind a curtain during the physical examination. Remember to explain to the patient each thing you are about to do and allow time for translation before you start.

Communication style

Practitioners should be aware of an attribute called *personalismo*[11] in their interactions with patients. A warm caring affect is valued greatly by many Hispanic patients. Communication style is as important as language in establishing an effective relationship. Differences in communication style between Hispanic and non-Hispanic cultures may interfere with this process. The distance between two people considered appropriate varies from culture to culture. In general, Hispanic cultures maintain a smaller interperson distance than nonHispanic. Hispanics also often use a more verbally and physically expressive communication style. The style of a health care provider may appear cold and distant with overreliance on medical or scientific language, lack of social inquiries, lack of physical touch, and greater interpersonal distance.

SUMMARY

The U.S. Hispanic population is heterogeneous and fast-growing. Care must be taken not to overgeneralize information gained from a study of one Hispanic subpopulation. Sources of data on U.S. Hispanic health include the 1980 National Health interview survey, the 1970 National Health and Nutrition Examination Survey, the Surveillance Epidemiology and End Result Program of the National Cancer Institute, the CDC, and regional studies.

Cardiovascular disease is a significant source of morbidity and mortality for Hispanics, as it is for non-Hispanic whites. Although overall mortality from heart disease may be the same or lower in U.S. Hispanics, this population has a higher prevalence of risk factors for cardiovascular disease such as diabetes mellitus, obesity, and hyperlipidemia.

Although neoplasia is the second greatest cause of death among Hispanics, as it is in non-Hispanic whites, Hispanics have an overall lower cancer rate. Effective treatment of the above diseases is hindered among the Hispanic population by lower access to health services and underutilization of preventive services.

Violent death, human immunodeficiency virus infection, and perinatal mortality make up a higher proportion of deaths in the Hispanic population than in the non-Hispanic white population. Complex socioeconomic factors contribute to the higher rates of accidental death, suicide, and homicide in various Hispanic subpopulations. Although a higher proportion of AIDS cases in Hispanics is associated with injecting drug use than in the general population, 47% of cases among Hispanics are associated with sexual contact. Higher perinatal mortality rates among Hispanics are associated with a higher prevalence of low birthweight births and delayed access to prenatal care. Mexican American women appear to be somewhat pro-

tected from the deleterious effects of late prenatal care.

Tubercular disease and significant tubercular reactions are more prevalent in the U.S. Hispanic population than the general U.S. urban population. Although extremely high rates among foreign-born Hispanics account for some of this, U.S.-born Hispanic children have a rate of significant tuberculin reactions more than 10 times the rate reported for children in this age group in the general population.

Non-insulin dependent diabetes mellitus is a significant cause of morbidity and mortality in the Hispanic population, affecting nearly a quarter of adult Puerto Ricans and Mexican Americans. Although higher prevalence of obesity in the Hispanic population accounts for some of this, some data suggest the possibility of a genetic component as well.

Barriers to healthcare in the Hispanic population include poverty, unemployment, lack of insurance, and language and cultural barriers. Awareness and sensitivity to cultural themes such as *respeto*, familialism, community, and a holistic approach to health can assist the individual practitioner and in the planning of health care interventions directed at the Hispanic community.

Although the Spanish language is common to all Hispanic cultures, a wide range of language preference exists in the Hispanic population. Spanish fluency is an advantage in effective communication with Spanish-speaking patients. Skilled use of an interpreter and a Spanish-friendly clinic setting can do much, however, to bridge the gap between practitioners and their Spanish-speaking patients.

REFERENCES

1. Ailinger RL: Hypertension knowledge in a Hispanic community, *Nurs Res* 31(3):207-210, 1982.
2. Angel R, Guarnaccia PJ: Mind, body, and culture: somatization among Hispanics, *Soc Sci Med* 28(12):1229-1238, 1989.
3. Babor TF, Mendelson JH: Ethnic/religious differences in the manifestation and treatment of alcoholism, *Ann N Y Acad Sci* 472:46-59, 1986.
4. Balcazar H, Aoyama C, Cai X: Interpretative views on Hispanics' perinatal problems of low birth weight and prenatal care, *Public Health Rep* 106(4):420-426, 1991.
5. Bartholomew AM et al: Food frequency intakes and sociodemographic factors of elderly Mexican Americans and non-Hispanic whites, *J Am Diet Assoc* 90(12):1693-1696, 1990.
6. Becerra JE et al: Infant mortality among Hispanics: a portrait of heterogeneity, *JAMA* 265(2):217-221, 1991.
7. Carrascal A, Rosenberg S: *Hypertension prevalence rates in New York City*. Presented at Conference on Hispanic Health Fare Approaches, Columbia University School of Public Health, 1987.
8. Castro FG, Baezconde-Garbanati L, Beltran H: Risk factors for coronary heart disease in Hispanic populations: a review, *Hispanic J Behav Sci* 7(2):153-175, 1985.
9. Centers for Disease control. Prevalence of overweight for Hispanics—United States, 1982-1984. *MMWR* 38(48):838-842, 1989.
10. Chapman JM, Frerich RR, Maes EF: Cardiovascular diseases in Los Angeles, *Am Heart Assoc GLAA*, 1983.
11. COSSMHO. The National Coalition of Hispanic Health and Human Services Organizations, *Delivering preventive health care to Hispanics: a manual for providers*, 1990.

12. COSSMHO. The National Coalition of Hispanic Health and Human Services Organizations, *AIDS: a guide for Hispanic leadership,* 1989.

13. Dawson DA, Hardy AM: AIDS knowledge and attitudes of Hispanic Americans, U.S. Department of Health and Human Services. *Vital Health Stat,* 166:1-6, 1989.

14. Department of Health and Human Services. Health-United States 1982. (DHHS Publication No. PHS 83-1232. 1983). Hyattsville, MD: Department of Health and Human Services.

15. Department of Health and Human Services. HIV/AIDS Surveillance Report, April 1992: 1-18.

16. Dowling PT, Fisher M: Maternal factors and low birthweight infants: a comparison of Blacks with Mexican-Americans, *J Fam Pract* 25(2):153-158, 1987.

17. Escobedo LG, Reminton PL, Anda RF: Long-term secular trends in initiation of cigarette smoking among Hispanics in the United States, *Public Health Rep* 104(6):583-587, 1989.

18. Espino DV, Burge SK: Comparisons of aged Mexican-American and Non-Hispanic white nursing home residents, *Fam Med* 21:191-194, 1989.

19. Espino DV, Burge SD, Moreno CA: The prevalence of selected chronic diseases among the Mexican-American elderly: data from the 1982-1984 Hispanic health and nutrition examination survey, *J Am Board Fam Pract* 4(4):217-222, 1991.

20. Flegal K et al: Prevalence of diabetes and impaired glucose tolerance in Mexican-Americans, Cubans, Puerto-Ricans, ages 20-74. In *Hispanic Health and Nutrition Examination Survey, 1982-1984. Diabetes Working Group,* National Center for Health Statistics, 1988.

21. Friis R et al: Coronary heart disease mortality and risk among Hispanics and non-Hispanics in Orange County, California, *Public Health Rep* 96:418-422, 1981.

22. Garcia-Palmieri MR et al: Relationship of dietary intake to subsequent coronary heart incidence: The Puerto Rican heart health program, *Am J Clin Nutr* 33:1818-1827, 1980.

23. Gardner L Jr. et al: Prevalence of diabetes in Mexican Americans: relationship to percent of gene pool derived from Native American sources, *Diabetes* 33(1):86-92, 1984.

24. Haynes S et al: Cigarette smoking patterns among Mexican Americans in the Southwest United States, 1982-1984. Paper presented at the 113th Annual Meeting of the American Public Health Association, Washington, DC, Nov. 19, 1985.

25. Hazuda HP et al: Ethnic differences in health knowledge and behavior related to the prevention and treatment of coronary heart disease, The San Antonio Heart Study, *Am J Epidem* 117(6):717-728, 1983.

26. Kirkman-Liff B, Jacobs Kronenfeld J: Access to cancer screening services for women, *Am J Pub Health* 82(5):733-735, 1992.

27. Kleinman JC: Infant mortality among racial/ethnic minority groups, 1983-1984. National Center for Health Statistics. Vol. 39, No. SS-3: pp. 31-38.

28. Kraus JF, Borhani NO, Franti CF: Socioeconomic status, ethnicity and risk of coronary disease, *Am J Epidem* 111:407-414, 1980.

29. Kumanyika S, Savage DD et al: Beliefs about high blood pressure prevention in a survey of Blacks and Hispanics, *Am J Prevent Med* 5(1):21-26, 1989.

30. Loria CM et al: Nutrient data for Mexican-American foods: are current data adequate? *J Am Diet Assoc* 91(8):919-922, 1991.

31. Lowenstein F: Review of the nutritional status of Spanish Americans, Based on published and unpublished reports between 1968 and 1978, National Center for Health Statistics. In *World Rev Nutr Diet* 37:1-37, 1981.

32. Mahaney FX: Lung cancer rates in white males leveling off, *J Natl Cancer Inst* 84(2):83-84, 1992.

33. Marin C, Perez-Stable EJ, Marin BV: Cigarette smoking among San Francisco Hispanics: the role of occulturation and gender, *Am J Pub Health* 79:196-197, 1989.

34. Marcus AC, Crane LA: Smoking behavior among Hispanics: a pre-

liminary report. In Engston PF, Anderson PN, Mortonson LE, editors, *Advances in cancer control: Epidemiology and research,* New York, 1984, Erlan-Liss.

35. Marcus AC et al: Prevalence of cigarette smoking in the United States: from the 1985 current population survey. *J Natl Cancer Inst* 81(6):409-414, 1989.

36. Marks G, Garcia M, Solis JM: Health risk behaviors of Hispanics in the United States: findings from HHANES, 1982-1984, *Am J Pub Health* 80(suppl):20-26, 1990.

37. Marks G et al: Health behavior of elderly Hispanic women: does cultural assimilation make a difference?, *Am J Pub Health* 77(10):1315-1319, 1987.

38. Mendoza FS et al: Selected measures of health status for Mexican-American, Mainland Puerto Rican, and Cuban-American children, *JAMA* 265(2):227-232, 1991.

39. National Cancer Institute. *Cancer Rates and Risks,* ed 3, Publ. No. 85-691, April 1985.

40. National Cancer Institute. *Surveillance, Epidemiology, and End Results Program (SEER),* 1973-1981. Sondik E, et al, Annual Cancer Statistics Review. Public Health Service, Bethesda, Md. 1985.

41. National Center for Health Statistics (NCHS). Advance report of final mortality statistics, 1987. *Monthly Vital Statistics Report* 38, no. 5 (suppl), Public Health Service. 1989.

42. National Center for Health Statistics (NCHS). Advance report of final natality statistics, 1987. *Monthly Vital Statistics Report* 38, no. 3 (suppl), Public Health Service. 1989.

43. National Health Interview Survey. *Smoking data,* National Center for Health Statistics and National Institute on Drug Abuse, 1980.

44. National Institute on Alcohol Abuse and Alcoholism (NIAAA). *National Survey of Alcohol Use.* Rockville, Md, 1979.

45. Perez-Stable EJ et al: Tuberculin skin test reactivity and conversions in United States- and foreign-born Latino children, *Pediatr Infect Dis J* 4(5):476-479, 1985.

46. Perez-Stable E et al: Tuberculin reactivity in United States and foreign-born Latinos: results of a community-based screening program, *Am J Pub Health* 76(6):643-645, 1986.

47. Pust RE: Tuberculosis in the 1990's: resurgence, regimens and resources, *South Med J* 85(6):584-593, 1992.

48. Ruiz RA, Miranda MR: A priority list of research questions on the mental health of Chicano elderly. *Chicano Aging and Mental Health.* U.S. Department of Health and Human Services, National Institute of Mental Health, Rockville, Md.

49. Saint-Germain MA, Longman A: Resignation and resourcefulness: older Hispanic women's responses to breast cancer. In Cayleff SE, Bair B, editors, *Minority women and health: gender and the experience of illness,* Detroit, 1993, Wayne State University Press.

50. Samet JM, Hunt WC, Goodwin JS: Determinants of cancer stage: a population-based study of elderly New Mexicans, *Cancer* 66:1302-1307, 1990.

51. Scribner R, Dwyer JH: Acculturation and low birthweight among Latinos in the Hispanic HANES, *Am J Pub Health* 79:1263-1267, 1989.

52. Shai D, Rosenwaike I: Violent deaths among Mexican-, Puerto-Rican, and Cuban-born migrants in the United States, *Soc Sci Med* (26)2:269-276, 1988.

53. Stern MP, Gaskill SP, Hazuda H: Knowledge attitudes and behavior related to obesity and dieting in Mexican Americans and Anglos: the San Antonio heart study, *Am J Epidemiol* 115:916-928, 1982.

54. Stern MP et al: Cardiovascular risk factors in Mexican Americans in Laredo, Texas. II. Prevalence and control of hypertension, *Am J Epidemiol* 113:556-562, 1981.

55. Stern MP et al: Affluence and cardiovascular risk factors in Mexican Americans and other whites in three Northern California communities, *J Chron Dis* 28:623-636, 1975.

56. U.S. Bureau of the Census. The Hispanic population in the United States: March 1989. *Current Population Reports* (population charac-

teristics), Ser. P-20, No. 444. Washington, DC, May 1990, Government Printing Office.

━━━ RESOURCES ━━━

AIDSFILMS, 50 West 34th Street, Suite 6B6, New York, NY 10001.

American Academy of Family Physicians, 8880 Ward Parkway, Kansas City, MO 64114-2797.

American Association of Retired Persons, 1909 K Street NW, Washington, DC 20049.

American Cancer Society National Office, 1599 Clifton Road, NE, Atlanta, GA 30329.

American Diabetes Association, 1660 Duke Street, Alexandria, VA 22314.

American Red Cross National Headquarters, HIV/AIDS Education Program, 1709 New York Avenue, NW, Suite 208, Washington, DC 20006.

Cancer Information Service, 900 Rockville Pike, BSB, Room 340, Bethesda, MD 20892-4200.

Center for Health Policy Development, Inc., 6905 Alamo Downs Parkway, San Antonio, TX 78238-4519.

Chicano Resource Center, 4801 East Third Street, Los Angeles, CA 90022.

Clearinghouse on Child Abuse and Neglect Information, P.O. Box 1182, Washington, DC 20013.

Coalition for People of Color/AIDS, c/o BIHA Women in Action, 122 West Franklin Avenue, Suite 306, Minneapolis, MN 55404.

COSSMHO, National Coalition of Hispanic Health and Human Services Organizations, 1030 15th Street NW, Suite 1052, Washington, DC 20005.

Environmental Protection Agency, Public Information Center, PM-211B, 401 M Street SW, Washington, DC 20460.

Health Promotion Resource Center, Stanford Center for Research in Disease Prevention, Stanford University School of Medicine, 1000 Welch Road, Palo Alto, CA 94304-1885.

Hispanic AIDS Forum, 121 Avenue of the Americas, Suite 505, New York, NY 10013.

Latino Caucus American Public Health Association, College of Social Work, University of Illinois at Chicago, 4348 MC/309, Chicago, IL 60680.

National AIDS Hotline, P.O. Box 13827, Research Triangle Park, NC 27709.

National AIDS Information Clearinghouse, P.O. Box 6003, Rockville, MD 20850.

National Arthritis and Musculoskeletal and Skin Diseases Information Clearinghouse, Box AMS, 9000 Rockville Pike, Bethesda, MD 20892.

National Asthma Education Program Information Center, 4733 Bethesda Avenue, Suite 530, Bethesda, MD 20814-4820.

National Clearinghouse for Primary Care Information, 8201 Greensboro Drive, Suite 600, McLean, VA 22102.

National Diabetes Information Clearinghouse, Box NDIC, Bethesda, MD 20892.

National High Blood Pressure Education Program Information Center, 4733 Bethesda Avenue, Suite 530, Bethesda, MD 20814.

National Hispanic Council on Aging, 2713 Ontario Road, NW, Washington, DC 20009.

Novela Health Education, P.O. Box 1688, Hollister, CA 95023.

Office of Minority Health Resource Center, P.O. Box 37337, Washington, DC 20013-7337.

Chapter 34

SPECIAL HEALTH PROBLEMS OF AFRICAN AMERICANS

Giesele Robinson Greene

HEALTH CARE DISPARITY

Minority Americans experience poorer health than majority Americans despite tremendous gains in scientific knowledge and technology in the last 100 years. The reasons are not clearly understood, yet minorities—African Americans in particular—have not achieved equity in health status as a result of the medical profession's capacious and expanding ability to diagnose, treat, and cure disease. The inferior health status experienced by African Americans may be attributed to certain specific disease states that are enhanced by individual behavior, adverse health habits, and the social-political-economic environment of the United States.

POPULATION DEFINITION

Precisely racially defining the African-American subset of the United States population is difficult. There is no specific accepted scientific definition of race, particularly in the very heterogeneous American population. Race is not a fixed demographic parameter such as sex and marital status. Definitions may vary with geographic location, social class, and nation of origin. Many African Americans or "Blacks" or "Negroes" are phenotypically indistinguishable from European Caucasians. Racial characterization of population subgroups requires a biogenetic ancestral perspective of the population. Obtaining this information is not practical for the purposes of general health care characterizations of a population subset.[28,30,91,126,133,139]

As discussed in this chapter, the term *African American* or *Black American* is more an ethnic characterization of this American subpopulation, which takes into account anthropologic, social, cultural, and political factors, rather than a racial characterization. Of the three major anthropologic population types (Negroid, Caucasian, and Mongol-

oid), African Americans derive from the Negroid group with significant genetic admixing. The first large numbers of African Americans arrived in colonial America during the early 1600s. By 1860, 90% of the 4.4 million Blacks in America had been born in the United States. Twenty five percent were of Negro, Caucasian, and American Indian descent. Thirteen percent were visibly of mixed Caucasian-Negroid background.[38]

In addition to diverse genetic background, African Americans also share the heritage of ancestry of the North American slave trade.[106,134,160] As the only immigrant minority people entering the United States unwillingly, African Americans during and after slavery experienced the synthesis of powerful, opposing, and diverse cultural forces combining in an unsafe, demeaning, and repressive economic and political environment for Blacks. Brought to the United States in bondage under inhumane conditions, African people carried with them many different languages, religions, tribal cultures, and customs. In forced servitude and used principally as an agricultural labor force, after several generations, a settled working population of African Americans speaking principally English and practicing the Christian faith emerged. The unique form of slavery in North America perpetuated for over three and one half centuries by white racism and the traditional African cultural philosophies and practices that helped structure the Black American adaptation to the environment are the background cultural and political factors socially defining the African-American subpopulation of the United States today. All Black Americans, however, do not claim African ancestry. In the 1980 census, 26.5 million people identified themselves as Black or Negro, whereas only 21 million people related a history of African ancestry. The terms *Black, Black American,* and *African*

American for the purpose of this chapter are used interchangeably and refer to persons in this socially defined non-White population of the United States.

SOCIOECONOMIC CHARACTERISTICS AND HEALTH STATUS

African Americans comprise 12% of the U.S. population of approximately 250 million people counted in the 1990 census. African Americans are the largest minority group in the United States. Although African Americans live in all areas of the country, over 55% are urban dwellers, living in the central metropolitan areas of the United States. These central city areas frequently demonstrate high levels of stress, in part related to impoverished conditions, poor school systems, crowded housing, low socioeconomic status, and exposure to drug culture and street violence.

Slightly more than 82% of Black Americans have completed high school education, as had the general U.S. population in 1988. However, only 15% of Black Americans compared to 28% of the total U.S. population are college graduates. Unemployment among Blacks in 1989 was 11.8%, more than double the unemployment rate of 4.5% for White Americans.[169]

African Americans in the work force are concentrated in blue-collar and service occupations. They are consistently underrepresented in managerial and professional specialty occupations, where they constitute approximately 6% of the work force. African Americans comprise 3% of physicians and hold less than 2% of medical school faculty positions in the United States.[95,180]

Family ties and kinship are extremely important among African-American people and form the base of the individual's support network providing emotional, financial, and social resources. Religion, providing emotional strength, is also a powerful force in the lives of most African Americans. The church is a forum for exchange of ideas and has been both a catalyst and a conduit for social and political change affecting African Americans.[38,78,49,180]

The life expectancy at birth for African-American men and women has lagged behind the total American population average for this entire century. The average life expectancy increased for both Whites and Blacks in the decade of the 1980s although less than expected for Black Americans (see Figure 34-1). Life expectancy has actually decreased for Black male babies born after 1984. The life expectancy for a Black male born in 1990 was 66 years— the same as that of a White male born in 1950. This compares with a life expectancy of 72.6 years for a White male born in 1990. The life expectancy of a Black female born in 1990 was 74.5 years, 5 years less than that of 79.3 years for a White female of similar birth. The overall life expectancy for Black Americans was 69.2 years in 1989, compared to 75.3 years for the total American population.[177,179]

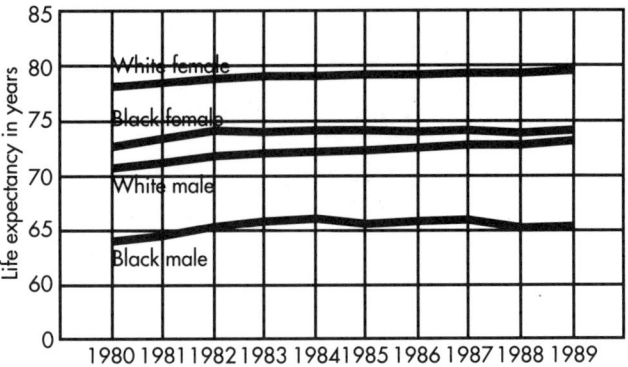

Fig. 34-1. Life expectancy at birth according to race and sex in the United States (1980-1989). (From National Center for Health Statistics: National Health Interview Survey.)

HEALTH PERCEPTIONS

Black Americans have a poorer self-assessed health status than White Americans. Health status self-assessment correlates with actual health status and utilization of health care services and is a predictor of mortality in the elderly.[176,179] In the 1990 National Health Interview Survey, Black Americans were nearly twice as likely as White Americans to assess their health as poor or fair. During the period of 1983 to 1990 the percentage of Black Americans reporting activity incapacitation rendering them unable to carry on their major activities was 80% to 90% higher than for White Americans, as detailed in Figure 34-2.[179] The Black elderly were more likely to assess themselves as sick and disabled than the White elderly. Although the Black elderly aged 65 through 74 have higher mortality rates than the White elderly, Blacks aged 75 and higher have lower mortality with higher rates of poverty and illness.[176]

FOLK BELIEFS

Black American folk beliefs are highly prevalent in the African-American culture, although folk medicine is largely embraced and practiced by African Americans of lower socioeconomic standing. Black-American folk medicine evolved to fill a void in health care access before and after emancipation. This folk medicine is a combination of West Indian Voodoo, elements of African culture, and fragments of Euro-American formal and folk medical beliefs, blended with tenets of Christianity and spiced with magic. Alternate names for Black American folk medicine include Hoodoo, Roots, Rootwork, Mojo, and Spiritualism.[81,162,163]

The system includes beliefs about prevention of sickness; the classification of illness into "natural" or "unnatural" categories; the ranking of healing of folk health care providers according to perceived ability, modes of treatment, and type of illnesses they can cure; and the use of

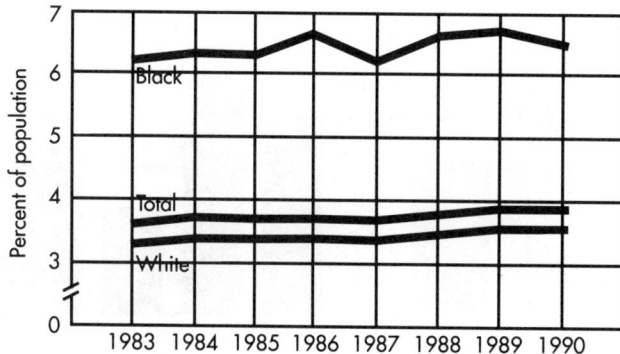

Fig. 34-2. Percentage of people unable to carry on major activity because of chronic conditions according to race in the United States (1983-1990). (From National Center for Health Statistics: National Health Interview Survey.)

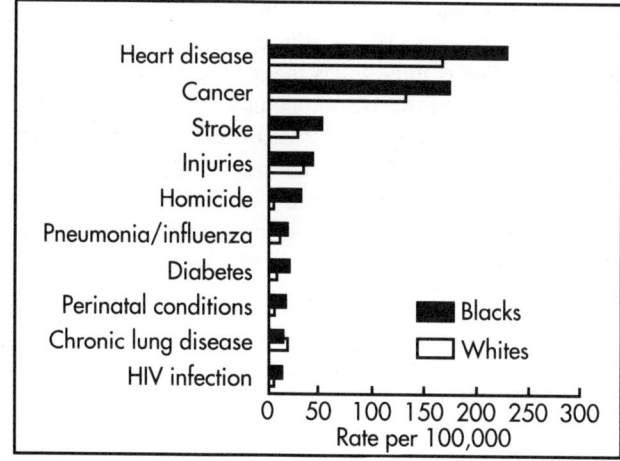

Fig. 34-3. Leading causes of death for blacks compared with whites (1987 age-adjusted rates). (From National Center for Health Statistics.)

home remedies and preventive agents that generally have an herbal basis.

"Natural" illness may result from divine punishment and serve to change behavior in the social network. It results from the effects of improper diet and exposure to cold causing changes in the blood system. There are numerous beliefs about blood and its functions relating to many illnesses and conditions including "high blood" (hypertension), "low blood" (anemia), menstruation, venereal disease, and childbearing.[70,162,163]

"Unnatural" illness is the result of witchcraft and conjuring, in which a "spell"—a hex or a curse—has been placed on the individual. Such illness results from conflict in the social network. It is believed that physicians do not understand and cannot treat an unnatural illness, and that treatment by a medical doctor increases the power of the spell and causes the victim's condition to worsen. Only a folk healer can help him or her. If accepted, the folk medical system is as sensible to the believer as the orthodox medical system is to any physician.[8,44,162,163]

The use of folk practitioners has declined as Blacks have gained access to established medical facilities; however, a glance at the classified ads in any Black-oriented newspaper will provide the reader with a list of active practitioners, attesting to the influence of folk medicine in the African-American community today. Folk beliefs have been understudied as regards the health disparity experienced by African Americans but may be a prominent factor in the poorer health status experienced by them. Delays in diagnosis and treatment may result from late entry into the traditional medical system, particularly if illness is perceived as "unnatural." Failure of the physician to recognize these beliefs and acknowledge and discuss illness from the perspective of the folk believer has serious implications for the acceptance of traditional health care by African Americans who subscribe to folk medicine.

Table 34-1. Ten leading causes of death for black males and females all age groups 1988

Black male		Black female
Heart disease	(1)	Heart disease
Malignant neoplasms	(2)	Malignant neoplasms
Accidental injuries	(3)	Cerebrovascular disease
Homicide*	(4)	Diabetes mellitus
Cerebrovascular disease	(5)	Accidental injuries
HIV disease	(6)	Pneumonia and influenza
Pneumonia and influenza	(7)	Perinatal period
Perinatal period	(8)	Nephritis
Chronic lung disease	(9)	Homicide*
Diabetes mellitus	(10)	Septicemia

Compiled from data from National Center for Health Statistics.
*Number one cause of death in age groups 15 to 34 years.

CAUSES OF MORTALITY AND MORBIDITY: OVERVIEW

The leading causes of death for the Black American population are the same as for the total population, although Black death rates surpass those of Whites in all categories except chronic lung disease. The leading causes of death comparing Black and White Americans are detailed in Figure 34-3.[179]

The 10 leading causes of death specific to Black men and women of all ages are listed in Table 34-1. Heart disease, malignant neoplasms, accidental injuries, homicide, cerebral vascular disease, and human immunodeficiency virus (HIV) disease were the leading six causes of death in the Black male in 1988. Heart disease, malignant neoplasms, cerebral vascular disease, diabetes mellitus, accidental injuries, pneumonia, and influenza were the six leading causes of death for Black females in 1988.[114]

Although Black Americans are represented in all socio-economic groups, 33% of Black Americans live in poverty. This rate is three times that of the White population. Low income or low socioeconomic status impacts all dimensions of health.[177,179,180] Disparities between poor people and those with higher incomes are exemplified by the finding that people with low income have death rates twice those of people with incomes above the poverty level. Low income is a special risk factor for all chronic diseases that rank high on the causes of death for the U.S. population. Poverty affects cancer incidence and survival. The incidence of cancer increases as family income decreases. Low-income patients have lower survival rates for cancer. People with low income are victims of violent crime more often than those with higher income. Poverty is a predisposing factor to injury and death caused by fire, drowning, and suffocation among children. Poverty increases infant mortality rate and is associated with poor pregnancy outcome including prematurity, low birth weight, birth defects, and infant death. Poverty reduces life expectancy by increasing the likelihood of infant death, chronic disease, and traumatic death. Infectious diseases such as tuberculosis and HIV infection are also more prevalent among poor people. Although the disparity in health in most minority populations in the United States is affected by socioeconomic factors, even if socioeconomic effects are set aside, disparities experienced in health by minority population groups are still observed. Differences in health are not totally explained by poverty or other environmental factors.

The 1985 report of the Secretary's Task Force on Black and Minority Health documented the extent of disparity among minority groups in the United States. The Secretary's Task Force reported that Black Americans suffered nearly 60,000 excess deaths per year in the interval 1979 to 1980. "Excess deaths" were defined as the difference between the number of deaths observed in the minority population and the number of deaths that would have been expected if that population had the same age- and gender-specific death rate as the White population. The task force identified six causes of death that accounted for over 80% of the excess deaths in minority populations; in order of negative impact on mortality for Black Americans they were heart disease and stroke, homicides and accidents, cancer, infant mortality, and chemical dependency as measured by deaths caused by cirrhosis of the liver and diabetes mellitus. HIV disease has emerged in the last decade as a major contributor to the health disparity of Black Americans. Sickle cell disease is another longstanding disproportionate cause of morbidity and mortality in African Americans. Although not a cause of mortality among Black Americans, primary open angle glaucoma produces significant morbidity and is the leading cause of blindness in Black Americans.

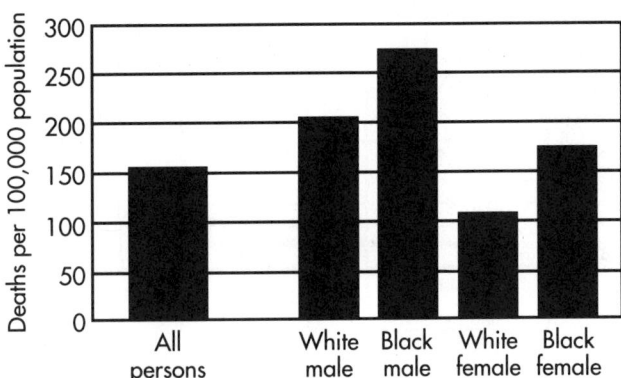

Fig. 34-4. Death rates for heart disease according to sex and race in the United States (1989). (From National Center for Health Statistics: National Vital Statistics System.)

EPIDEMIOLOGY AND PREVENTION OF MAJOR HEALTH PROBLEMS
Heart disease

Diseases of the heart are the leading causes of death in the United States today. Death rates for heart disease in Black males are the highest in the nation (Figure 34-4).[179]

Risk factors for heart disease and stroke in African Americans include the classic cardiovascular risk factors: cigarette smoking, elevated blood pressure, elevated serum cholesterol level, diabetes mellitus, obesity, and physical inactivity. More culturally specific, less well studied risk factors also exist. Socioeconomic factors may influence the multifaceted problem of access to care and the ability to attenuate cardiovascular risk factors when known.[67,156,41,53,144] Knowledge of risk factors and symptoms of heart attack may be less among Black Americans than White Americans.[97,167] A number of studies have linked psychosocial factors and hypertension in Blacks.[18,76,92] Psychosocial stress in African Americans may be a risk factor for cardiovascular mortality.

More than 50% of the deaths caused by heart disease in Blacks were attributed to ischemic heart disease in 1986.[56] At ages 35 through 64 death rates for acute myocardial infarction and chronic ischemic heart disease were higher in Black men than White men. Before age 75, rates of ischemic heart disease were higher in Black women than White women. Chronic ischemic heart disease is more prevalent in Blacks than Whites when compared to acute myocardial infarction. Coronary heart disease is characterized in Blacks as compared to Whites by younger age at onset, higher rates among women, more angina (especially among women), and higher rates of complications associated with hypertensive left ventricular hypertrophy and cardiac function abnormalities. The average Black patient has more severe disease and worse long-term survival rate than Whites.[29,56,97] Blacks have lower rates of invasive di-

Ischemic heart disease and African Americans

Chronic ischemic variety most prevalent
Younger age at onset
More angina, especially in women
Worse disease and shorter survival
More left ventricular function–related abnormalities
More sudden cardiac death

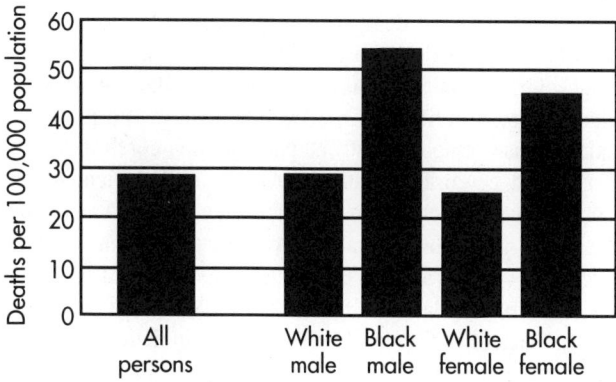

Fig. 34-5. Death rates for stroke according to race and sex in the United States (1989). (From National Center for Health Statistics: National Vital Statistics System.)

agnostic and therapeutic procedures than Whites that are not explained by clinical characteristics of the patient. Coronary artery bypass surgery rates are lower in Blacks than Whites.[51,138] Although understudied, ischemic heart disease is uncommon in many parts of Africa and in Afro-Caribbean people,[2,83,151] raising the question of whether environmental, economic, or social factors increase the rates of disease in the United States. Although most of the coronary artery heart disease data in the literature about Blacks were obtained from studies in the southeastern United States, the studies suggest that coronary heart disease rates increase with urbanization.[2,83] Coronary heart disease in Blacks has higher rates of prevalence, incidence, and mortality in urban than rural areas. The box above summarizes the major clinical differences for ischemic heart disease in African Americans as contrasted with whites. See Chapter 41 for a general discussion of prevention and heart disease.

Death rates for congestive heart failure were higher for Black than White persons in 1981, as were death rates for cardiomyopathy.[185] Gillum[56] examined data from the United States Center for Health Statistics for 1970 to 1982 to determine numbers of deaths and acute care hospital discharges with a diagnosis of cardiomyopathy. Blacks had more deaths and discharges in all age groups. Age adjusted death rates for acute rheumatic fever and rheumatic heart disease combined were slightly lower in Blacks than in Whites in 1982. Hypertensive heart disease causes substantial numbers of deaths; a disproportionate number of these deaths occur in Black persons independent of the effect of hypertension on mortality from ischemic heart disease and cerebral vascular disease.[52,58] In 1985, non-White* males and females experienced hypertensive disease mortality rates at least twice those of White persons of the same sex in all adult groups.[56] The highest mortality rate disparities occurred among adults 35 to 64 years old. Non-White males had mortality rates 7.6 times those of White males in the age group 35 to 44 years, with a de-

clining trend to 2.4 times more mortality in the group 75 to 84 years old. Non-White females experienced mortality rates 12.6 times those of White females in the age group 35 to 44 years; the rate also declined, to 2.6 times more mortality in the age group 75 to 84 years. Non-White men in the south Atlantic region of the United States had the highest death rates for hypertensive disease and hypertensive heart disease in men age 55 to 64 years old. Despite improvement in control of hypertension in the past three decades, Blacks are still highly susceptible to hypertensive cardiac complications particularly in the south Atlantic states.

Sudden cardiac death is more frequent among African Americans than White Americans largely as a result of coronary artery disease.[191] An analysis by Gillum of sudden coronary death in the United States in 1985 included 40 states and demonstrated a greater proportion of ischemic heart deaths occurred out of the hospital or in the emergency department in Blacks than in Whites. Sickle cell trait (AS hemoglobinopathy) is a risk factor for sudden cardiac death and is more common in Blacks. Sudden cardiac death with sickle cell anemia has rarely been reported. Hypertrophic cardiomyopathy is the most common cause of sudden cardiac death among young athletes. Black athletes experience a disproportionate amount of sudden cardiac death due to hypertrophic cardiomyopathy accounting for one third of sudden deaths in athletes younger than 30 years of age.[102]

Stroke

Cerebrovascular disease is the third leading cause of death in the United States. Deaths for the African subpopulation are higher than the Whites for stroke[27,84,179] (Figure 34-5). The incidence, prevalence, and hospitalization rates for stroke are all also higher for Black than White Americans. Stroke death rates have fallen dramatically over the last several decades, diminishing by 66% from

*The non-White classification is used to designate racial groups other than Caucasians and gives a good estimate of rates in Blacks. Blacks accounted for approximately 90% of the U.S. non-White population during the times specified with use of this designation.

88.6 in 1950 to 28 deaths per 100,000 resident population in 1989. Stroke death rates have fallen most strikingly in Black females but remain 66% higher in Black Americans than White Americans. Cerebral hemorrhage is a more frequent cause of death in stroke patients than cerebral thrombosis and cerebral embolism. All three classifications of stroke are more common in Black than White Americans. Cerebral hemorrhage is almost twice as common in Black men and women as in White Americans. This difference is thought to be related to the higher incidence of hypertension, particularly severe hypertension, in Blacks. Blacks experiencing stroke have more hypertension, diabetes mellitus, and small arterial vessel disease than Whites, who have more associated coronary and peripheral vascular disease and hyperlipidemia. In Blacks and Whites, men have more disease than women before the age of 65. Lacunar infarcts have no predilection for race or ethnicity but are related to the incidence of hypertension in the population. Blacks are underrepresented among series of patients who undergo carotid endarterectomy.[138] Recreational use of drugs is a growing risk factor for stroke and cardiac disease among young people.[5,82,87] Cocaine is a prominent drug associated with stroke and cardiac disease and has high use among drugs of abuse in African Americans.[154] (See Chapter 43 for a general discussion of stroke and prevention.)

Hypertension

Hypertension is an underlying risk factor for heart disease and stroke, which figures prominently in the disparate health status of Black Americans. It affects more than 30% of the African-American population. Hypertension is more likely to develop at an early age in Black Americans. Statistically significant racial differences in blood pressure occur after the age of 17 although mean systolic and diastolic blood pressures have been reported to be higher in Black subjects at all ages.[16,71,135,187] Hypertension remains undiagnosed or undercontrolled for longer periods of life in African Americans than in other American population subgroups. *Severe hypertension,* defined as diastolic blood pressure equal to or greater than 115 mm Hg, is five times more common in Black men than White men and seven times more common in Black women than White women. Blood pressure rises more rapidly with advancing age in Blacks and is associated with increased mortality and morbidity rates, especially those for heart disease, stroke, and end-stage renal disease. Cardiac involvement is more prevalent in the Black hypertensive patient and also more severe. Left ventricular hypertrophy is the most prevalent cardiac effect. A higher prevalence of left ventricular hypertrophy is indicated by echocardiography in Blacks than in Whites with similar levels of hypertension. Left ventricular hypertrophy carries a risk for mortality independent of

*References 9,18,63,68,71,142,151,180,187.

Hypertension and African Americans

Younger age at onset
Underdiagnosed and undercontrolled for longer periods of life
More severe hypertension (diastolic blood pressure ≥115 mm Hg)
More rapid progression with age
More left ventricular hypertrophy
More end-stage renal disease
More salt-sensitive disease

---

the risk of hypertension and also is a precursor to left ventricular function abnormalities. Although the rates of strokes have declined significantly over the last four decades, the annual cerebral vascular disease mortality rate remains highest in Blacks. African Americans have a 7.3 times greater risk of development of end-stage renal disease produced by hypertension than Whites. For 50% of Blacks on renal dialysis hypertensive renal disease is the cause of disease, as compared to 18% of dialysis patients in non-Black populations. No proven genetic differences between Black and White hypertensive individuals have been found. Several studies have associated darkness of skin color with level of blood pressure,[37,86,127] but no confirmed studies have associated hypertension and skin color independent of socioeconomic status. Although no evidence indicates unique pathophysiologic mechanisms of blood pressure control in Black Americans as contrasted with White individuals, there are major physiologic differences in blood pressure regulation between Black and Whites. Blacks have more vascular reactivity to stressors, have lower renin levels, respond more slowly to excrete a sodium load, and are more sensitive to the blood pressure elevating effects of increasing dietary sodium intake.[18,63,71,92] Salt sensitive hypertension is much more common in Blacks. The box above summarizes the major clinical differences in hypertension in African Americans versus Whites.

Hypertension control rates among Blacks are unacceptably poor: in 25% of the population hypertension is not controlled. Black men have the highest prevalence rate of any group and also have the poorest control rate. Whereas the rate of hypertension among African Americans is the highest in the world, the rate in West African nations is only about 5% to 20%.[2,63,125] Rates of hypertension grow in prevalence with higher degrees of urbanization,[2,83] raising the question of contribution of nonbiologic factors to the prevalence of hypertension in Black Americans. An NIH funded study is in progress at Loyola University Medical Center, Chicago, Illinois, simultaneously evaluating 11,000 men and women of African origin living in different geographic locations worldwide.[125] The study will

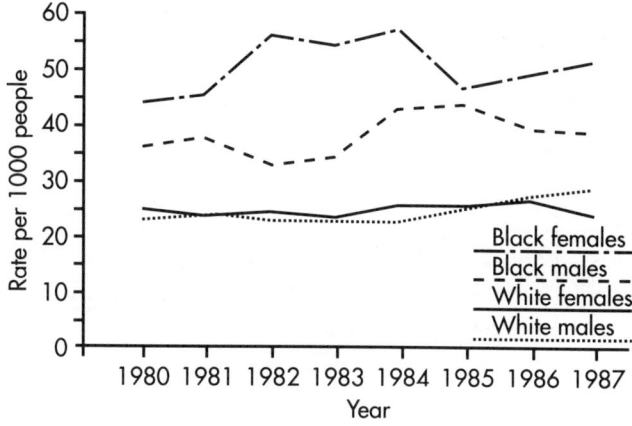

Fig. 34-6. Age-standardized prevalence of diabetes mellitus by race, sex, and year in the United States (1980-1987). (From CDC's National Health Interview Survey for 1980-1987.)

assess the influence of environmental versus biologic factors on the risk of developing high blood pressure and subsequent cardiovascular disease.

Diabetes mellitus

An estimated 6.8 million Americans had diabetes mellitus in 1987.[111] Until 1940, diabetes mellitus was less common in Black Americans than White Americans.[184] In 1989, Black Americans had a 91% higher prevalence of self-reported diabetes mellitus than White Americans.[40] The highest rates of diabetes are found in overweight Black females. As in the majority population, the majority of African-American diabetics have non-insulin-dependent diabetes mellitus, formerly classified as type II diabetes mellitus. At every age and socioeconomic strata, African Americans have a greater prevalence of diabetes and elevated fasting glucose levels.[83] Complications of diabetes (heart disease, stroke, and kidney disease), are more common among Black diabetics than White diabetic individuals. Lower-extremity amputation and blindness are as common in Black diabetic as in White diabetic patients.[25] The National Health Interview Survey 1980–87, a household survey of 120,000 U.S. residents, found the highest rate of diabetes mellitus in African-American adults and highest rates in Black women.[179] As detailed in Figure 34-6, Black women had a prevalence rate twice that of White women (50.9 versus 23.4 per 1000 people) while Black men had a prevalence rate approximately one third higher than White men. From 1980 to 1987 the annual U.S. prevalence of diabetes mellitus increased by 9% from 25.4 to 27.6 per 1000 persons. During the same period the prevalence of diabetes mellitus among Black men increased 16%. Increases among Black women were over 2.6 times the national prevalence increase at 24%.[111] Diabetes and its prevention are discussed in Chapter 60.

Table 34-2. Cancer demographics: African Americans compared to White Americans*

Higher incidence rates	Female breast†
	Cervix uteri
	Larynx
	Lung‡
	Multiple myeloma
	Pancreas
	Prostate
	Stomach
Lower 5-year survival rates	Bladder
	Breast
	Cervix uteri
	Colon and rectum
	Corpus uteri
	Esophagus
	Larynx
	Prostate
Excess mortality	Female breast§
	Esophagus
	Cervix uteri
	Colon and rectum
	Corpus uteri
	Larynx
	Lung‡
	Multiple myeloma
	Pancreas
	Prostate
	Stomach

(Derived from Surveillance, Epidemiology and End Results Program (SEER) 1978-81, 1981-1988.)
*Cancers listed alphabetically.
†Under age 40 only.
‡Primarily men.
§Under age 50-55 only.

Cancer

African Americans have the highest overall age-adjusted rates for cancer incidence and mortality among Americans. Incidence rates were 402.5 per 100,000 for Blacks and 379.1 per 100,000 for Whites in 1987.[4] In the last 30 years, death rates for cancer have risen 17% in White men and 2% in White women. In contrast, death rates have increased 51% in Black men and 10% in Black women. The highest United States mortality rates for all cancers occur among Black men.[4,173,181]

Five-year survival rate for cancer among African-American people is 38% compared to 52% for White Americans.[4,173] Table 34-2 summarizes the disparity related to specific cancers for African Americans. Lung cancer death rates are 45% higher among Black males compared to White males, although death rates for women are approximately equal.[110] The esophageal cancer mortality rate is three times higher in Blacks than nonminorities.[181] Blacks have more than twice the mortality rate of Whites for cervical, uterine, and prostate cancers and for multiple myeloma. The disparity by race for prostate cancer is par-

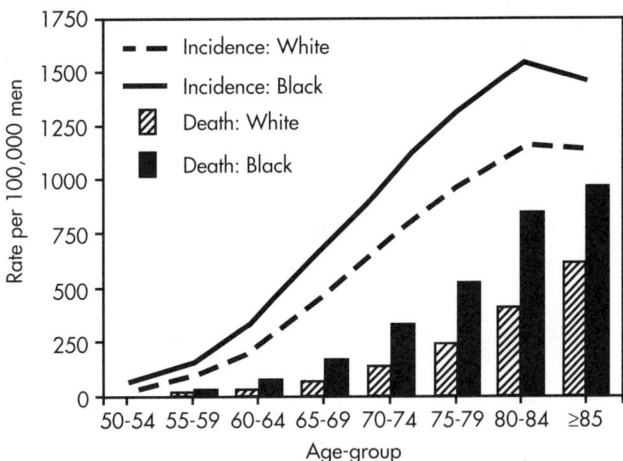

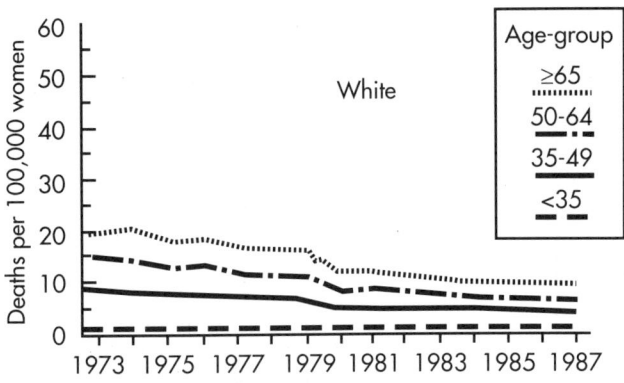

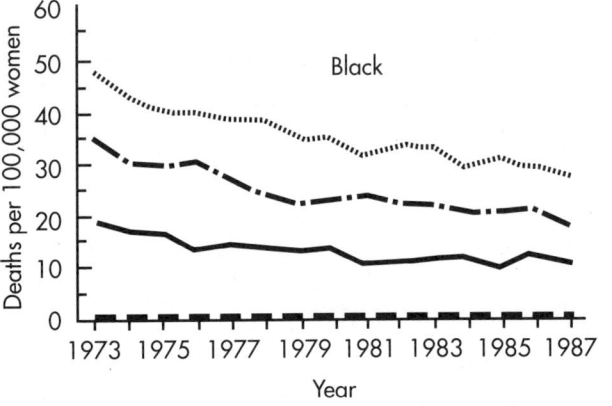

Fig. 34-7. Age-specific prostate cancer incidence and death rates by race in the United States (1984-1988). (From National Cancer Institute: Surveillance, Epidemiology, and End Results program and the CDC's National Center for Health Statistics Multiple Causes of Death Files.)

Fig. 34-8. Cervical cancer mortality rate by age-group and race in the United States (1973-1987). (From National Cancer Institute: Surveillance, Epidemiology and End Results program.)

ticularly pronounced among younger men, aged 50 to 54, among whom the death rate is more than triple that of White men[113] (Figure 34-7). There is an excessive incidence of carcinoma of the breast in African-American women below age 40, and there is excess mortality from carcinoma of the breast in African-American women below age 55.[1,143,174] Death rates for cervical cancer are declining for all women, yet African-American women have a mortality rate 2.6 times that of White women[1,118,143] (Figure 34-8). Although the incidence of colorectal cancer is the same for Black and White Americans at 49 per 100,000, the 5-year survival rate for Blacks is 44% versus 55% for White Americans.[174,186]

Similar risk factors underlie many cancers for which there is increased incidence or excess mortality in Black Americans. Factors in the environment cause the majority of cancers or promote cancer development.[4,74] These include tobacco use, alcohol use, combined alcohol and tobacco use, occupational exposure to carcinogens, dietary practices, nutritional status, and socioeconomic status.

There is a higher prevalence of smoking in Black Americans than in White Americans.[122] Although Blacks accumulate fewer pack-years than Whites,[55] Blacks smoke brands of cigarettes higher in tar and nicotine than Whites.[32] Rates of smoking-related cancers seem to be especially high among Blacks. African Americans appear to be lesser users of smokeless tobacco than nonminorities.[69]

Herd[184] studied and reported no consistent pattern of excessive alcohol consumption nor excessive rate of alcohol problems for Blacks in his 1985 survey of drinking patterns and alcohol problems among U.S. Blacks. The heterogenous pattern and frequency of alcohol consumption among African Americans as a group are comparable to those of the general American population.

Dietary factors account for over one third of all cancer deaths today. This topic has been reviewed more extensively in Section V. There is no evidence that African Americans differ from the general population in susceptibility to dietary and nutritionally related carcinomas.

Occupational exposure as a cause of cancer death may be higher in Blacks than the 4% reported for the general U.S. population. Blacks have a higher rate of assignment to hazardous work sites than Whites. Occupation may account for higher numbers of cancers than previously acknowledged in the African-American population.[181]

African Americans tend to be more pessimistic than nonminorities about the curability of cancer.[181] African Americans are less likely to believe that early detection can make a difference in survival and cure and tend to be more fatalistic in outlook. On average, African Americans are less knowledgeable about cancer warning signs and screening tests.[145] However, this may vary widely, depending on specific cancers.[1] A large number of Black Americans accept common myths regarding the genesis of cancer as fact.[163,181]

Cancer and African Americans

The same risk factors predominate as in the general population: diet, tobacco use, alcohol use, and occupational exposure

Presentation at later stages of disease for diagnosis

Increased mortality rate for most malignancies

Higher incidence at younger ages, especially for breast and cervical cancer in women and lung and prostate cancer in men

Generally less informed about warning signals and available screening modalities for early detection

More pessimistic attitudes regarding early detection

More fatalistic attitude for treatment and cure

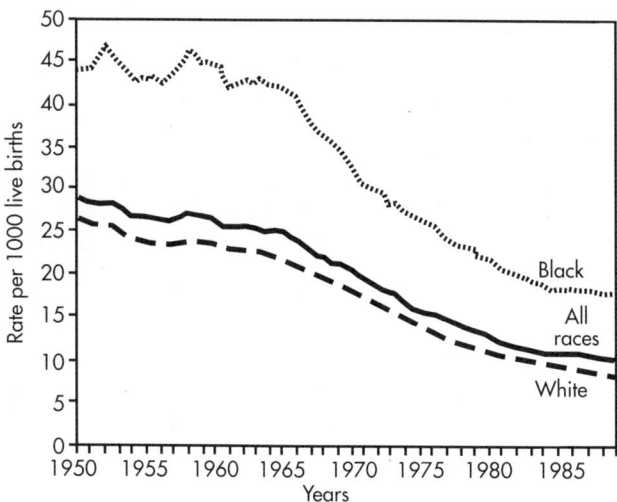

Fig. 34-9. Infant mortality rates by race of child in the United States (1950-1989). Includes Hispanic and non-Hispanic infants. (From National Center for Health Statistics: National Vital Statistics System.)

Black Americans seek cancer diagnosis later than White Americans. This likely affects the increased mortality rate seen in many carcinomas. When diagnosed, Blacks delay longer before accepting definitive treatment.[181]

Historically African Americans have received cancer screening examinations at lower rates than Whites. In recent years, however, screening has increased, especially for breast and cervical cancers in Black women.[1] Mammography and use of clinical breast examinations result in a 30% reduction in mortality rate among women screened. Black women utilize mammography for screening and for current and prior breast problems at rates comparable to those of Whites. The use of the Papanicolaou smear for cervical screening by Black women may exceed that for Whites. Although cervical cancer screening by Papanicolaou smears has never been proved in clinical trials to be efficacious, the marked decline in incidence in mortality rate of cervical cancers since the widespread use of the Papanicolaou smear attests to the efficacy of the test (see Figure 34-8 for death rates for cervical cancer in Whites and Blacks).

The increasing incidence of prostate cancer in both White and Black men may reflect increased screening and enhanced modalities of early detection (prostate specific antigen testing, transrectal ultrasound, in addition to digital rectal examination). Despite increased 5-year survival rate for prostate cancer, death rates have not been significantly reduced. The efficacy of advanced screening for prostate cancer has not been fully evaluated. The box above summarizes major facts regarding cancer in African Americans and Figure 34-7 the incidence of prostate cancer by race.

Culturally specific education is necessary to educate African Americans about cancer-specific screening and to help destroy the cancer-related fatalistic outlook. Given the younger age at onset and worse prognosis despite comparable or better utilization of available screening modalities, cancer screening practices in African Americans may

need to begin at younger ages than those recommended by the American Cancer Society for the general population. The physician should be cognizant of the enhanced risks of cancer in African Americans and the pessimistic attitude of many Black Americans regarding cancer. In addition to screening, follow-up evaluation and treatment of detected abnormalities are essential to reduce morbidity and mortality rates for African Americans. (See Section X for a general discussion of cancer and prevention.)

Infant mortality

Infant mortality is a general indicator of the health status of a nation. The U.S. infant mortality rate declined from 29.2 infant deaths per 1000 live births in 1950 to 9.8 deaths per 1000 live births in 1989, reflecting the general improvement in health status of the U.S. population.[121] Despite this, infant mortality rates (IMRs)* in the United States are among the highest in the industrialized world and many countries report lower rates.[85] Infant mortality rates among Black Americans are the highest of any group in the nation.[182,123] The IMR for Black Americans is twice that of Whites[121] at 18.6 deaths/1000 births compared to 8.1 deaths/1000 births (1989)† and has been so since 1960 (Figure 34-9).

The National Infant Mortality Surveillance project identified low birth weight‡ as the major contributing factor to

*IMR is determined by dividing the number of infant deaths in 1 year (death certificates) by the number of live births in the same year (birth certificates).

†Race-specific IMR is reported by the race of the mother.

‡Low birth weight means less than 2500 grams at birth.

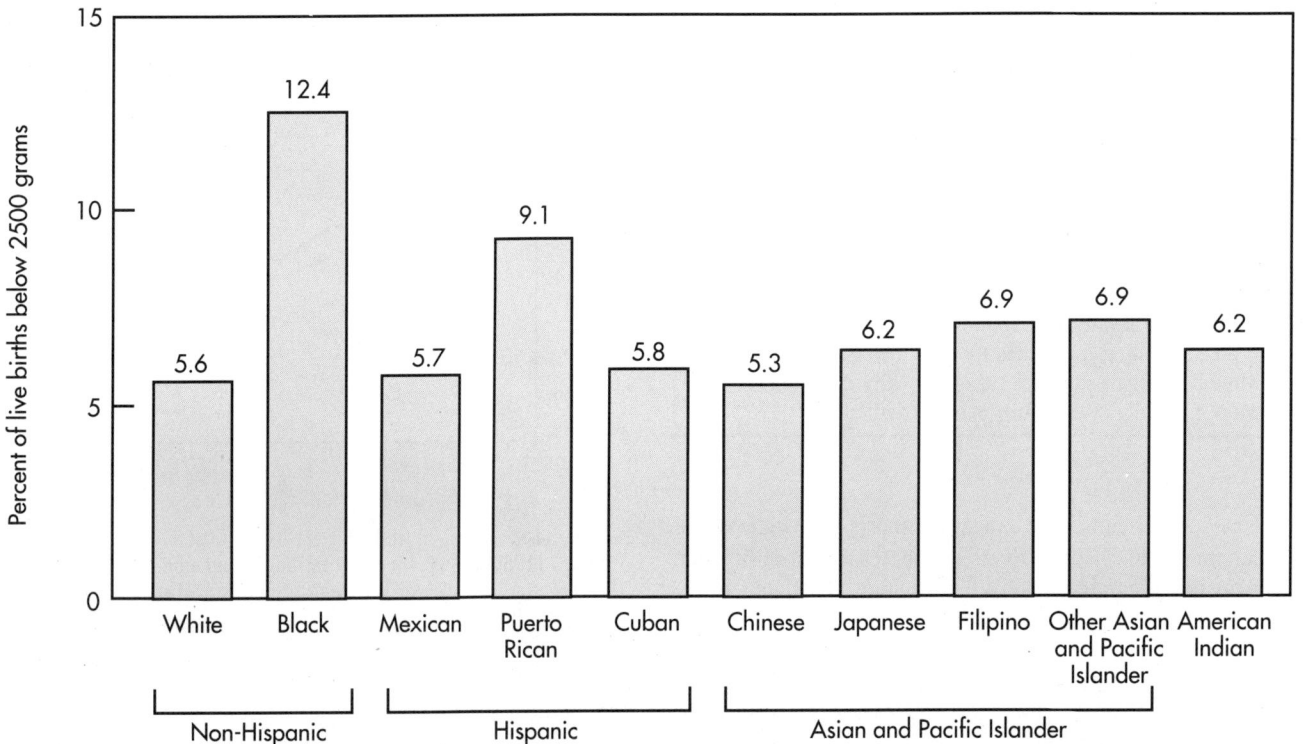

Fig. 34-10. Low birth weight ratios according to race and ethnicity in the United States (1982). (From National Center for Health Statistics.)

high infant mortality rates among Black women.[123] Blacks experience excessive neonatal deaths (0 to 28 days of age) among infants weighing more than 2500 grams and higher postnatal period deaths (28 days to 1 year of age) among infants in all birth weight categories. Except for congenital anomalies,[101] the overall neonatal mortality rate for Black infants is more than twice that of Whites irrespective of causes of death. Black infants are at higher risk of death than Whites from all causes, including preventable illness, in the postnatal period.

Birth weight is the most important predictor of infant survival.[176,182,119,33,123] Low birth weight increases the likelihood of morbidity and mortality before the first birthday. The incidence of low birth weight in Blacks has been double that of Whites for many years by a 2 to 1 ratio, which has remained stable since 1975[85,119,121] (Figure 34-10).

Black mothers are overrepresented in the subgroups of women at enhanced risk of having low birth weight babies.* These risk factors include single marital status, less than 20 years of age, less than 12 years of education, late or absent prenatal care, poor nutritional status, higher rates of unwanted births, higher rates of mistimed pregnancies, weight gain of less than 16 pounds during pregnancy, anemia, and low socioeconomic status with attendant prob-

*References 33,34,43,46,54,85,119,121,123,182.

lems in financing and accessing prenatal and infant health care services. Correspondingly, Black mothers are at high risk for all adverse pregnancy outcomes.

Among Blacks and Whites, smokers have a greater risk of having a low birth weight infant than nonsmokers.[46] The 1985-86 Center for Disease Control Behavioral Risk Factor Surveillance System reported that White pregnant women were more likely to smoke than Black pregnant women and to smoke more cigarettes per day than Black women. Despite this, the difference in risk between smokers and nonsmokers for a low birth weight infant is greater for Black women than White women. The risk increases with age and is greatest in the pregravid underweight Black woman although also elevated in the normal pregravid weight Black woman.

Alcohol, substance abuse, and environmental hazards also affect maternal risk for infant mortality though little ethnic-specific information exists. Heavy alcohol consumption during pregnancy is associated with enhanced risk of fetal alcohol syndrome characterized by malformations and central nervous system dysfunction, including mental and growth retardation. No "safe" amount of alcohol consumption during pregnancy has been quantified, but heavy consumption during early pregnancy is most often associated with development of the fetal alcohol syndrome. Low birth weight and prematurity are the best known ill effects of substance abuse during pregnancy.

The effects of maternal substance abuse caused by drug exposure may be difficult to differentiate from those caused by inadequate nutrition and prenatal care and are difficult to quantify. As many as 10% of babies are born annually to women who have used one or more illicit substances while pregnant.[176] Environmental factors such as viral infections and chemical and radiation exposure affect the fetus directly by disruption of germ cell chromosomes with resultant congenital anomalies. The effect of toxins in the workplace of pregnant women relative to infant mortality outcome is controversial.

Adequate prenatal care of the mother and accessible affordable care for the child after birth are vital components of any planned intervention strategies for the reduction of infant mortality rates in African Americans. Iron supplementation in women with established or marginal anemia assists in achieving measurable reduction in preterm delivery and low birth weight. The reduction of unplanned pregnancies in Black women may substantially reduce the infant mortality rate consistent with findings that infants born less than 2 years after a previous child are at greater risk for low birth weight.[119] Interventions to reduce smoking in pregnant women may achieve major reductions in the number of pregnancies with low birth weight outcome.

HIV disease

African Americans are disproportionately represented in the acquired immunodeficiency syndrome (AIDS) pandemic, comprising 31% of reported cases of AIDS in the United States while totaling only 12% of the U.S. population.[98,116,169,175] Of all children with AIDS, 52% are African American[175] as are 52% of women with AIDS. Death rates for HIV disease are highest in African-American men[161,170,175,179] (Figure 34-11). AIDS transmission occurs in the same manner in the African-American community as in the general population: by intravenous drug use, sexual intercourse, and mother to infant perinatal transmission.

The majority of AIDS cases in all ethnic groups are related to infection through homosexual contact. Minorities more often than Whites report intravenous drug use and heterosexual contact as routes of AIDS transmission. In the United States, 54% of all heterosexual intravenous (IV) drug users with AIDS are African American.[155,175]

The primary mode of HIV transmission in IV drug use is through contaminated needles and syringes. The social setting in which drugs are used is a risk factor for HIV infection as well.[17,154,188] African Americans and Hispanic Americans are more likely than Whites to use IV drugs in group settings where drugs are bought, sold, and injected. These group settings are in clandestine locations believed to be safe from police intervention and are commonly known as "shooting galleries." Although underground operations, likely locations for shooting galleries are inner-city neighborhoods where minorities disproportionately re-

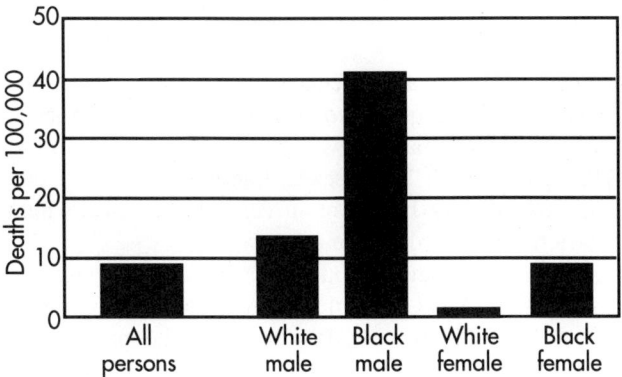

Fig. 34-11. Death rates for human immunodeficiency virus (HIV) infection according to race and sex in the United States (1989). (From National Center for Health Statistics: National Vital Statistics System.)

side. Galleries promote social customs of borrowing and sharing drug paraphernalia ("works") as gestures of goodwill and friendship. "Works" may be rented in galleries and are used and reused by strangers or acquainted individuals. The risk of HIV transmission is highest among IV drug users who share and reuse needles with strangers or acquaintances. This practice is more common among Blacks and Hispanics than White IV drug users.

Cocaine is a favored drug of abuse by African-American IV drug users. Cocaine must be injected frequently to maintain desired effects because of the short half-life of the drug. Frequent injections of drugs increase HIV transmission risk by increasing exposure to needles and syringes.[154]

Intravenous drug use is more often than not daily and habitual. However, periodic IV drug use does occur.[152] Periodic drug users may be less easily identified and may not perceive themselves as IV drug abusers at risk for HIV disease.

Heterosexual contact with IV drug users is a risk factor for HIV disease. Intravenous drug use by women or their sexual partners accounts for much of the growth in the prevalence of HIV disease in women over the last decade. Infected heterosexual IV drug using men or infected bisexual men may transmit HIV to their female partners. Infected pregnant females pass the HIV infection to their offspring in the perinatal period.

Within heterosexual relationships, women of all races generally have less control in the relationship.[22,166] African-American women, who are more likely than White women to be impoverished, underemployed, mothers, and single or divorced,[170] may be more financially, socially, and emotionally dependent in the male-female relationship. Consequently, they may be less insistent on HIV-safe sex practices. More men than women in the United States are HIV-infected. HIV disease is more easily transmitted from men to women, increasing the burden of disease for females. There are no proven effective HIV protective measures that are female controlled.[62,165] Even the female condom requires cooperation of the male partner for correct use, making women quite vulnerable in the AIDS pandemic.[62] Heterosexual transmission of HIV disease is extremely important in communities where both HIV infection and drug use are prevalent.

Homosexual transmission of HIV accounts for 44% of the cases of AIDS in African-American men contrasted with 80% of all cases of AIDS among White men.[175] Despite strong cultural disapproval, nearly 30% of homosexual and bisexual men with AIDS are African American or Hispanic.[11,17,175] There is little information in the literature on the sexual behavior of African-American men. Men who are having sex with women and also engage in sex with other men may not view themselves as bisexual or homosexual, particularly if the male sexual encounter is limited to certain settings such as incarceration.[11,105] The heterosexual identified Black male who is sexually active with other men may have difficulty acknowledging symptoms of HIV disease and a diagnosis of AIDS. He may also be difficult to identify by general demeanor and mannerisms. Denial or poor knowledge may promote the spread of HIV infection in homosexual and bisexual men living in the Black community who are not identified with the larger gay community and are not exposed to AIDS related information. Homosexuality is an understudied phenomenon in the African-American community and must be better understood in order to develop culture-specific treatment interventions.[11,17,105] No race-linked genetic factors account for the higher prevalence of HIV infection in African Americans, nor is there evidence that Black men have a greater preference than White men for anal intercourse, which is the highest-risk sexual practice in HIV transmission.

HIV disease in African Americans is characterized by a short survival time between the diagnosis of AIDS and death.[17,149] A high percentage of patients seek care late in the course of the disease. Many minorities delay health assessment until a symptomatic crises occurs. This reduces opportunities for participation in clinical trials and prophylactic AIDS treatment.

Studies indicate that Black Americans are generally as knowledgeable about HIV transmission and AIDS as the majority population.[10,64] Yet at least two studies of African Americans suggest that knowledge about causes and prevention of HIV disease may not relate to the use of safe sex practices or decrease participation in risky sexual behavior.[79,80] African Americans may be knowledgeable about AIDS but not about who can acquire the disease. Only 3% of Black Americans in the 1990 National Health Interview Survey reported being in any of the high-risk behavior categories associated with HIV transmission, whereas African Americans comprise nearly one third of

all AIDS victims.[64] Blacks may perceive AIDS as a disease of homosexual and White Americans and may not identify themselves as at risk even if participating in risky sexual behavior.

HIV prevention strategies in the African-American community should educate non–drug users to prevent the start of IV drug use and must curtail the use of needle and syringe sharing, where IV drug use is prevalent.[11,17,75,128,151] Strategies for women should improve low self-esteem and impart feelings of control over one's own life. Women must be taught to appreciate their risk of infection and how to change behavior to reduce risk of infection. Risk reduction efforts for African Americans, developed by principally White and homosexual organizations, have been largely ineffective to date. African-American–directed interventions should target at-risk sexual behavior and IV needle sharing rather than targeting at-risk groups, with whom it is not clear that the African-American individual identifies. Physicians can play a large role in identification and education of the high-risk individual patient. Suggested interview questions are listed in the box below. Culturally sensitive education will be necessary to curtail the spread of AIDS in the African American community. AIDS-related broadcast media public service announcements have proved helpful in HIV-related education efforts, and culturally sensitive presenta-

---

HIV risk factor interview questions that avoid high-risk group identification labels

General questions
1. Have you ever used a needle* to give yourself a drug that was not prescribed by a doctor?
2. What drug(s) did you use?
3. How often do you give yourself a shot?
4. Where do you get your needles?
5. Have you ever borrowed a needle someone else has used to give yourself a shot?
6. Have you ever given a needle that you have used to someone else?

Questions for women
1. Do you have more than one sexual partner?
2. Are condoms being used in your sexual relationships?
3. Do you know if your sexual partner(s) has ever given himself an injection (a shot) of drugs not prescribed by a doctor?

Questions for men
1. Do you have more than one sexual partner?
2. Do you routinely use condoms in sexual relationships?
3. Have you ever been in a situation where you had no contact with women for a prolonged period of time? How did you fulfill your sexual needs?
4. Have you ever had a sexual experience with a member of your same sex? Did you have intercourse? Did you use a condom?

*Needle means needle and syringe apparatus.

tions and messages [115] should be encouraged. Research on the sexual attitudes and practices of African Americans is needed to develop culturally specific intervention strategies. (Chapter 56 addresses preventive aspects of HIV infection as well.)

Alcohol and tobacco

All of the major causes of mortality and morbidity for African Americans are enhanced by alcohol use. Alcohol abuse may be the leading health and safety problem in Black America, and alcohol is a legal drug.

Alcohol-related illness has become a problem for African Americans only during the last 100 years.[184] Nineteenth-century Black Americans strongly supported the American temperance movement and were abstinent. Blacks experienced unusually low rates of alcohol-related problems. The 1880 Census reported the lowest rates of alcoholism for the population in Blacks, at 0.7 per 1000 persons. Support for the temperance movement was politically motivated. Temperance was regarded as a means of supporting emancipation and equality efforts. In response to Jim Crow laws and political disfranchisement by the prohibition movement, Black participation in the temperance movement declined in the early twentieth century. Coinciding with this reversal of support for national prohibition was the great northern migration of southern Blacks to the large northern urban centers. By 1930 urban centers had become a focus for heavy-drinking life-styles, which increased and flourished in the wake of repeal. With increasing urbanization and alcoholization of the Black community, rates of alcoholism and alcohol-related illness among Blacks began to rise.

Liver cirrhosis and esophageal cancer are associated with long-term heavy alcohol consumption whether or not the liquor consumption is accompanied by intoxication or other adverse social consequences. Before 1955 age-adjusted rates for liver cirrhosis mortality in non-Whites were lower than rates in the White population. From 1950 to 1973 non-White rates increased 242% while rates among Whites rose only 60%. At all ages the cirrhosis mortality rate for African Americans is nearly twice that of the White population[184] (Figure 34-12). The incidence of esophageal cancer among Blacks is exceptionally high for both men and women as discussed earlier in this chapter. Alcoholic beverage consumption may be the primary etiologic agent in the development of cancer of the esophagus: an estimated 81% of the cancers are attributed to alcohol use.[4,74,181]

Studies of drinking habits in the United States show that Black Americans evidence higher rates of abstention than Whites.[184] Young Black men are less likely to drink than their White counterparts. Frequent heavy alcohol con-

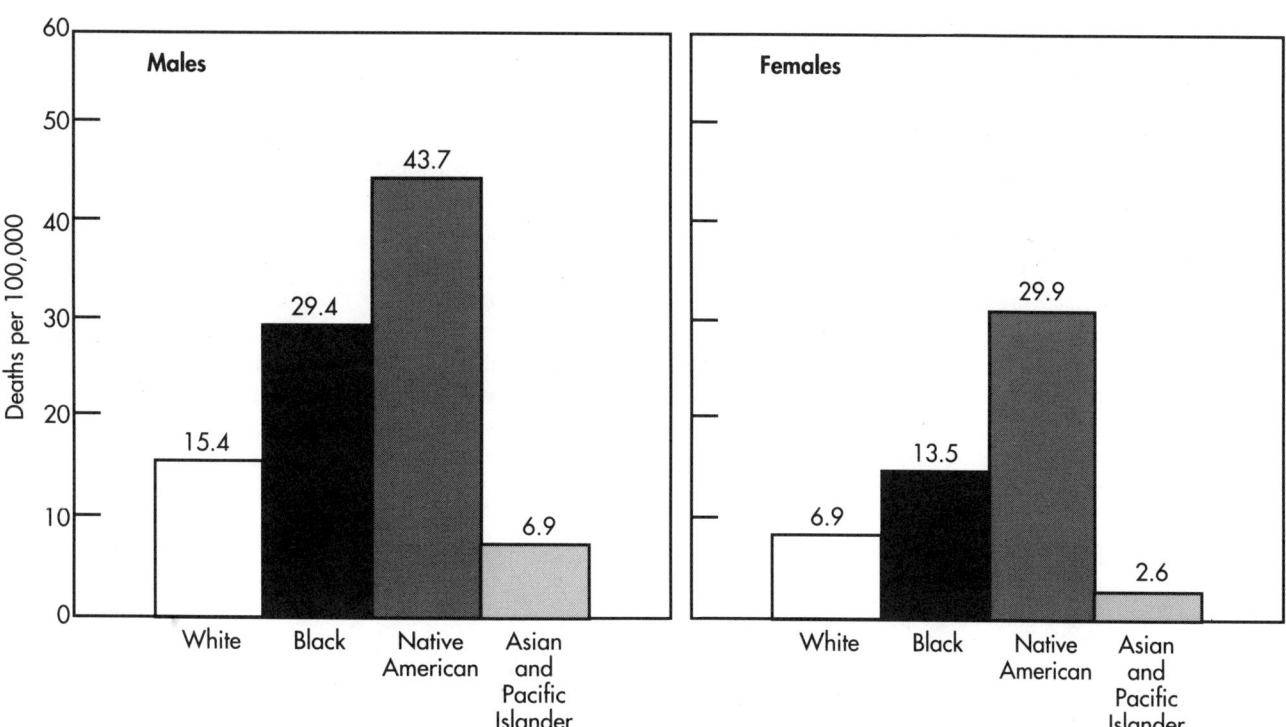

Fig. 34-12. Average annual age-adjusted death rates for chronic liver disease and cirrhosis (1979-1981). Death rates for Hispanics are not available. Death rates for Native Americans and Asian/Pacific Islanders are probably underestimated because of less frequent reporting of these races on death certificates. (From National Center for Health Statistics, Bureau of the Census, and Task Force on Black and Minority Health.)

sumption is more common in men over age 30 in African Americans and may continue as a stable pattern of midlife. White men generally exhibit increased alcohol consumption in youth and decreased alcohol consumption around age 30, when the prevalence of drinking in African Americans begins to rise.

Cigarette smoking is a factor in most causes of excess mortality in Black Americans.[107,184] The prevalence of smoking among Black Americans is the second highest of Americans at 26.2%, exceeded only by that of American Indian and Alaskan Native Americans.[122] African Americans smoke fewer cigarettes than White Americans and begin to smoke at later ages than Whites.[55] Smoking has declined among both Black and White Americans over the last 20 years, and the rate of Black Americans has decreased at a higher rate.[112,122] However, Black Americans have higher relapse rates than nonminorities; thus it is uncertain whether this will improve trends in smoking-related mortality and morbidity.[73,122]

African Americans are strongly encouraged to drink and smoke by the alcoholic beverage and tobacco industries. The young African American is actively pursued. Marketing is specifically targeted at Black youth to decrease rates of abstention and create a new market of consumers.[112,178]

Billboard advertising is highly prevalent in urban Black neighborhoods and uses culturally enticing imagery and messages to encourage drinking and smoking. Many magazines, including Black-oriented magazines, carry a high proportion of alcoholic beverage and tobacco advertisements. The broadcast media also carry a high proportion of alcoholic beverage advertisements. Not surprisingly, media efforts directed at decreasing alcohol and tobacco use are small compared to efforts to curtail other drug use although alcohol and tobacco cause the larger problem. The alcohol and tobacco merchants counter their advertisement campaigns by public affairs campaigns that indebt many African-American organizations to their companies by supporting mainstream African-American community programs. These programs are well funded and enacted in such a way to minimize publicity related to the harmful effects of alcohol and tobacco and maximize appearances of goodwill.[112,178]

Alcohol and tobacco companies target products specifically to entice Black consumers. Malt liquor is an example. Blacks are prime consumers of this beverage, which is sold like beer but has 15% to 50% more alcohol than regular beers.[178] Menthol cigarettes are primarily marketed to African Americans.[32]

Interventions to curtail the use of alcohol and tobacco must begin in young minority youth. High-risk youth should be identified. Risk factors[178] for substance abuse in youth include family history of alcohol or drug abuse, poor parenting, family history of management problems, low value for academic achievement, low value on relationships, parents and friends who are current drug users,

and conducive immediate environment. Risk factors for the environment include large numbers of retail alcohol outlets, weak law enforcement against drug dealing and juvenile crime, and ineffectual community institutions (school, church, recreational facilities). Prevention efforts focused on children will achieve the best primary prevention results. In age-appropriate settings children should be provided factual information about alcohol, tobacco, and drugs; the dangers they pose to health; and how to refuse these substances. Positive recognition should be given to drug-free students.

Prevention efforts should also focus on advertising reform.[112,178] Alcohol and tobacco companies must stop marketing products almost exclusively to Blacks and balance the messages that are given to Black youth in the media. Reform in advertising should focus on avoiding the use of imagery and allowing words and a picture of the product itself; prohibit sponsorship of youth audience directed events (such as sport tournaments) by alcohol and tobacco companies; prohibit alcohol and tobacco advertisement billboards in schools, parks, and other areas where youth congregate; and prohibit advertising in magazines with substantial youth readership. The schools and health care settings can provide tobacco and alcohol abstention programming. This may help reduce the numbers of youth who begin to smoke and drink and will be aided by increased efforts to curtail access to cigarettes by teenagers.[140] (Substance abuse is also discussed in Chapters 15 and 16.)

Violence

Violent behavior leading to intentional injury or death is escalating in the United States and is a major health problem among African Americans.*

The most common risk factors for suicide or for involvement in a homicide as a victim or perpetrator are young age and male sex.[180] White males have the highest death rate for suicide in the United States, followed by that of Black males[61,120,176] (Figure 34-13). The rate of suicide for Black male teenagers, however, has been rising faster than that for other teenagers since 1986 (Figure 34-14). Homicide is the second most common cause of death among persons age 15 to 34 and is exceeded only by deaths from unintentional injury.[114,176] Homicide was the most common cause of death in Black men and women in this age group in 1989[176] (Figure 34-15). Death rates for Black males and Black females for homicide and legal intervention† are the highest of any population group in the United States (Figure 34-16).[114] Other common risk fac-

---

*References 6,88,114,130,147,148,153,176,177,179,180.
†Legal intervention includes death caused by on-duty law enforcement personnel and legal executions. These collectively account for 1.3% of all homicides.

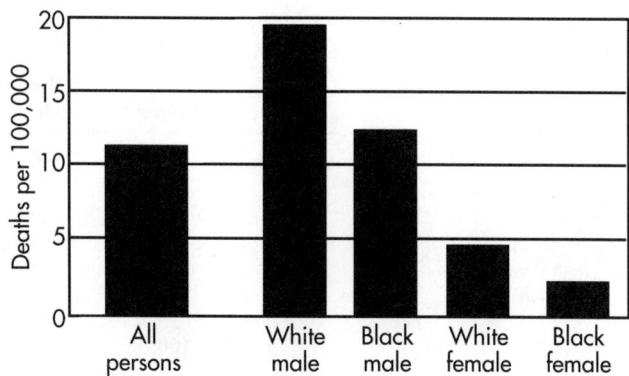

Fig. 34-13. Death rates for suicide according to race and sex in the United States (1989). (From National Center for Health Statistics: National Vital Statistics System.)

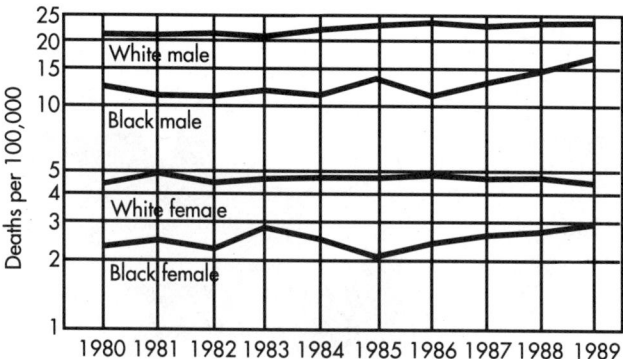

Fig. 34-14. Death rates for suicide among persons 15-24 years of age in the Unites States (1989). (From National Center for Health Statistics: National Vital Statistics System.)

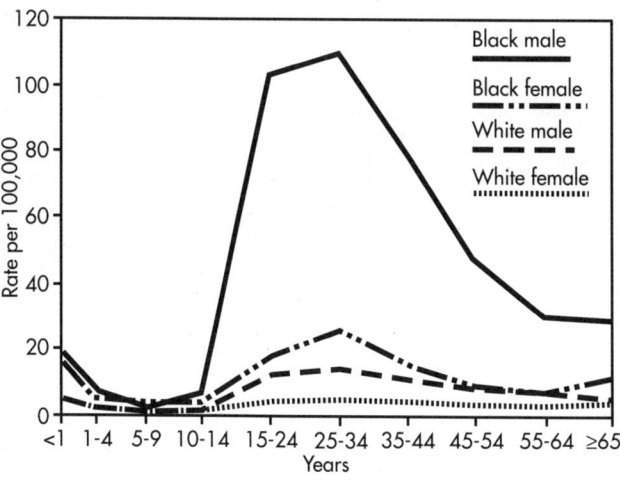

Fig. 34-15. Homicide rates by age-group, race, and sex in the United States (1988). Analyses include black and white races only. (From National Center for Health Statistics Mortality Tapes.)

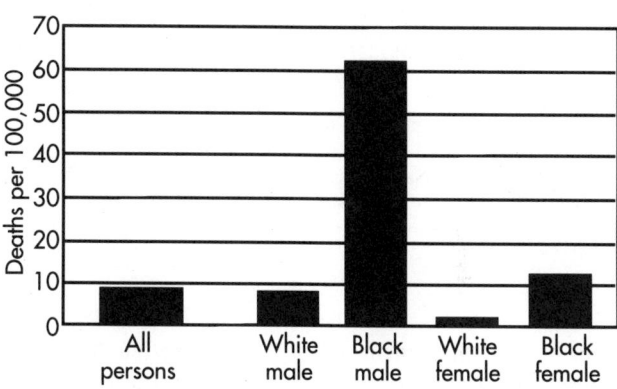

Fig. 34-16. Death rates for homicide and legal intervention according to race and sex in the United States (1989). (From National Center for Health Statistics: National Vital Statistics System.)

tors for violent behavior include urban residence, alcohol or drug use, availability of weapons, and low socioeconomic status. Detailed risk factors for violent behavior are summarized in the box at right.[166,180] Racial differences in homicide rates are significantly attenuated when socioeconomic variables are taken into account.[176]

The most common cause of homicide is conflict.[114] This includes disputes over money, valuables, and lover's triangles; killings of children by babysitters; brawls under the influence of inhibition-lowering drugs and/or alcohol; and other various types of interpersonal arguments. Only 14% of homicides occur in association with another crime[77,114] (Table 34-3). Over 50% of all homicide victims are acquainted with their murderers. Forty-eight percent of Black victims and 43% of White victims are murdered by assailants of the same race.[114]

Nonfatal violence often precedes fatal violence.[166,180,195] Physical fighting is a common form of interpersonal violence and is a precursor to injury and homicide. Physical fighting is greater among males and in minorities.[117]

Risk factors for violent behavior

Male sex
Young age
Urban environment
Poverty
Unemployment
Perceived need for protection
Inhibition-lowering substance use
Preadolescent television exposure
Childhood exposure to violence
Easy access to firearms

Table 34-3. Percentage of homicide victims and circumstance, by race—United States, 1988*

Circumstance	Total	Total white	Total black	Total male	White male	Black male	Total female	White female	Black female
Conflicts*	35.8	34.8	37.0	36.7	36.5	37.0	33.2	30.7	36.9
Drugs	6.5	4.1	9.1	7.7	5.2	10.3	2.7	1.5	4.6
Gangs	2.0	1.7	2.3	2.5	2.2	2.7	0.5	0.3	0.6
Felony	14.0	17.3	10.3	12.9	16.2	9.6	17.3	19.8	13.3
Other	13.1	15.4	10.6	10.6	11.9	9.2	21.0	24.3	16.4
Reverse felony†	3.1	3.5	2.7	4.0	4.8	3.3	0.2	0.2	0.3
Unknown	25.5	23.2	27.9	25.65	23.2	27.9	25.0	23.3	27.9
Total	**100.0**	**100.0**	**100.0**	**100.0**	**100.0**	**100.0**	**100.0**	**100.0**	**100.0**

Data source: Federal Bureau of Investigation—Supplementary Homicide Report. 1988 FBI data do not include Florida or Kentucky.
*Includes the following categories: lovers' triangle, children killed by babysitter, brawl under the influence of alcohol, argument over money, and other arguments.
†Includes the following categories: felon killed by police, felon killed by citizen (both considered justifiable homicide, not murder).

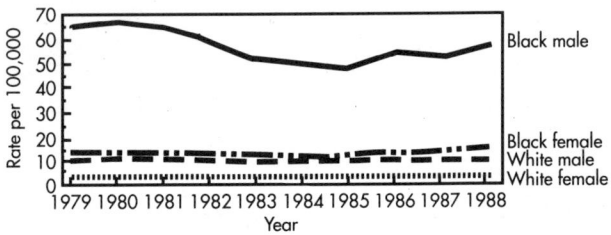

Fig. 34-17. Homicide rate by race and sex of victim in the United States (1979-1988). Analyses include black and white races only. (From National Center for Health Statistics Mortality Tapes.)

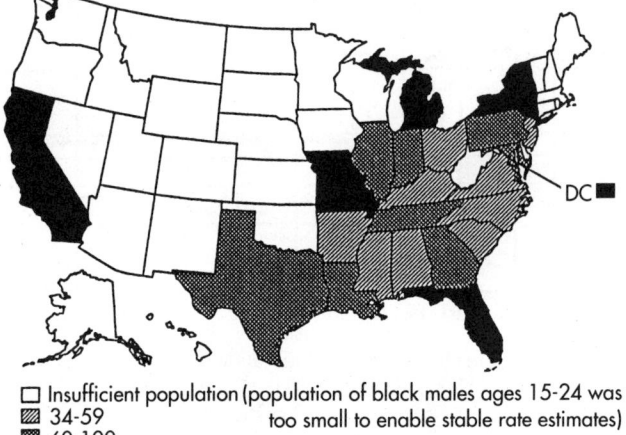

☐ Insufficient population (population of black males ages 15-24 was too small to enable stable rate estimates)
▨ 34-59
▩ 60-100
■ >100

Fig. 34-18. Homicide rates for black males ages 15-24 by state per 100,000 (1987). (From Center for Environmental Health and Injury Control, CDC.)

Homicide rates are highest in the large cities.[48,180] Violent crimes, their victims, and their perpetrators are also most often found in urban environments. The majority of homicide victims are White, although rates of homicide are higher among African Americans. Throughout the last decade, Black males had the highest homicide rate of all Americans, followed by that of Black females (Figure 34-17).

Homicide rates declined in Black males in the early 1980 and have increased sharply since 1984.[114,147] The large difference in homicide rates between Black males and other racial and sexual groups is increasing. Homicide rates for young Black males are 4 to 5 times higher than for young Black females; 5 to 8 times higher than for young White males; and 16 to 22 times higher than for young White females.[147] Certain geographic areas in the United States have the highest homicide rates and have experienced considerable increase in homicide rates[47,48] (Figure 34-18). Five states—New York, Florida, Michigan, Missouri, California, and the District of Columbia—have homicide rates in excess of 100 per 100,000 persons. These areas contained 29% of the young Black male pop-

ulation and total 51% of the death by homicide in this group in 1987.[147]

Firearm-associated homicides are highly prevalent in the United States: 61% of all homicides in 1988 involved the use of a firearm.[48] The rate of firearm homicides parallels the rate of total homicides, and especially among young Black males (Figure 34-19).[147] Fifty-five percent of all Black males murdered in 1988 were killed with a handgun. The rate of homicide by firearms is highest in Black teenage males and is increasing most rapidly in this age group.

Recurrent intentional injuries also disproportionately afflict African Americans.[57,158] These patients are primarily Black males with statistically significant high rates of unemployment but with no significant differences noted in age, sex, educational level, marital status, number of off-

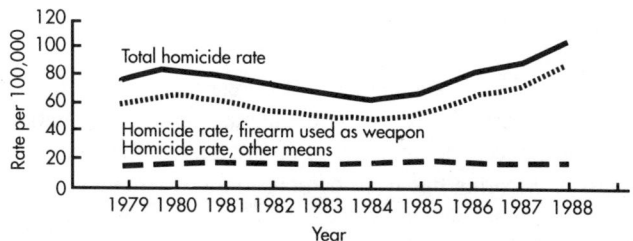

Fig. 34-19. Homicide rates for black males ages 15-24 by use of firearms in the United States (1979-1988). (From National Center for Health Statistics Mortality Tapes.)

Risk factors for domestic violence

Early marriage
More children than wanted
Inadequate child management skills
Disabled children
Physical punishment for disobedient children
Social isolation
Marital conflict
Cohabitation with an elderly demented relative
Male dominance in the household
Substance abuse with drug or alcohol dependence

---

spring, or mechanism of injury. Of the patients in recurrent intentional injury studies 50% to 79% have had one prior episode of assaultive injury, and 31% to 49% two or more prior episodes of assaultive injury. Recurrent intentional injury patients have significantly higher hospital charges than first-time assaulted patients and may have larger financial impact on the health care system.

African Americans are not inherently more violent than other racial groups, yet violent behavior is more likely to result in fatal outcome in the Black community. Although all reasons are not clear, some risk factors are evident. African Americans more often reside in urban metropolitan areas, a prominent risk factor for homicide. African Americans have systematically and historically been excluded from opportunities available to the majority culture and are more commonly in the lower socioeconomic strata of U.S. society.[180,183] Violence is often associated with poverty and lower socioeconomic status. African-American youths are covictimized by poverty and violence in the inner city.[156] They are seen as potential threats to the larger society first and are possibly never seen as victims. Violent behavior can be one possible effect of covictimization, as well as impaired school performance and judgment, vulnerability for substance abuse, and emotional disorders.[39] Potential contributing factors to the increased prevalence of violence in the African-American community, in addition to the general risk factors already mentioned, include immediate access to firearms, often made available through increased drug trafficking in lower socioeconomic areas; poverty; increased exposure to community violence; increased exposure to direct violence (witnessing the violent assault of another person); increased exposure in childhood to direct violence, including the violent injury or death of a parent or first-degree relative; racial discrimination; high rates of unemployment; feelings of powerlessness; low self-esteem; and perceived need for protection.*

Irrespective of race, three factors contribute to the homicide rate and the burden of violence borne by all Amer-

*References 13,39,57,65,124,131,156,180,190.

ican people: domestic violence, television exposure, and easy access to firearms.

Domestic violence or family violence is a major cause of nonfatal injury.[22,42,65] This includes spouse abuse, child abuse, elder abuse, and domestic quarrels. There is usually an identifiable pattern in the family leading to violence although the violent behavior may be spontaneous and impulsive. Identified risk factors for family violence include early marriage; unwanted children; lack of skills in child management; social isolation; premature, handicapped, or mentally retarded children; use of physical punishment in child rearing; expressed marital conflict; presence of a demented elderly relative in the home; male dominance in family decisions; and substance abuse (see the box above).

Long-term childhood exposure to television is a causal factor behind approximately half of the homicides committed in the United States and is a factor in other forms of interpersonal violence regardless of race.[23,24,89] Television exerts its behavior-modifying effect primarily in children (see Chapter 27). The effect of aggression enhancement by television is chronic, extending into later teenage years and adulthood, although exposure after adolescence does not exert additional influence.

Easy access to firearms, particularly handguns, is another risk factor for homicide and accidental firearm injuries in children and adults and a factor in suicide.[26,88,124,150,189] The overall increases in the suicide and homicide rates of the last 20 to 30 years have been attributed to firearm-assisted deaths. Only a small portion of firearm deaths are the result of a crime requiring self-defense,[114] yet the most common stated reason for owning a handgun is protection from crime. Guns present in the home are most often kept loaded. Many homes that have unlocked loaded guns are households with children.[189] Convenient access to firearms, particularly handguns, is a risk factor for violence.

Physicians can assume an important role in the prevention of violence. Primary prevention of violence includes

---

Questions to ask during evaluation for accidental injury

Where and when did the injury occur?

Was the injury caused by another person?

What is the relationship of the person to the victim?

Does the person who inflicted the injury live with the victim?

Was the person who inflicted the injury under the influence of alcohol or other substances when he or she hurt the victim? How often is he or she under the influence?

Has the victim been injured by the person previously?

Was the conflict resolved?

Is there a gun in the home?

---

recognition of risk factors (Box 34-6). Once they are identified, afflicted individuals can be offered counseling or other intervention to prevent primary eruption of violence in the household.

Secondary prevention measures are meant to preclude the recurrence of interpersonal violence. By asking critical questions during the diagnostic interview accompanying treatment for unintentional injury, the medical professional can take an active role in secondary prevention by providing the service of rapid case identification and referral for treatment. Both victims and perpetrators of violence may be identified and referred. Violent behavior may result from treatable illness in the direct domain of the physician such as alcoholism or other substance dependency. Physicians must be trained to elicit a history of violence risk factors much as they are trained to inquire about cardiovascular risk factors (see the box above).

Childhood exposure to television violence is a modifiable risk factor. Physicians and health care facilities can set examples by limiting television viewing in waiting areas to educational videotapes and emphasize the recommendation of the American Academy of Pediatrics that parents limit children's television viewing to 1 to 2 hours per day.[3] Physicians can emphasize the use of time channel locks for working parents to control children's television viewing and can endorse television violence program rating systems for parents to judge how violent a program is without watching it. Physicians should endorse general public education endeavors to teach good television viewing habits (see Chapter 27).

Antiviolence intervention planning should include strategies to prevent firearm injuries. Parents should be assisted to prevent children from having unsupervised access to guns. Efforts to assist families in this regard can be effected in part through public education campaigns. In the privacy of the doctor's office, an inquiry as to whether there is a firearm in the home and storage practices for the firearm may elicit violence risk factors during the routine health interview.

Although immediate access to firearms is a critical element in the high rates of homicide and suicide, limitation of adult access to firearms is controversial. Reducing access to firearms has been demonstrated to reduce firearm-related homicide and suicides.[35,99,132,159] Health, operational, and safety standards exist in all states for motor vehicles, yet firearm ownership and operational safety standards are largely nonexistent.[88,169] Ownership of firearms involves socioeconomic, geographic, victimization, self-protection, racial, cultural, and constitutional issues. Interventions should be developed to evaluate and influence these issues.

Reduction of violent behavior requires drug and alcohol abuse prevention strategies. Physician efforts on the individual patient level to screen for drug and alcohol dependency and make appropriate referrals for treatment will help reduce violent behavior in an unquantifiable manner.

Violence intervention strategies for African Americans must include an understanding of the impact of racism, poverty, environmental violence, childhood violent exposures, childhood media exposures, and socioeconomic status on the African-American individual. Intervention strategies for African Americans should include major programs targeted at children and teenagers in urban centers.* Programs should be developed to screen, identify, refer, and counsel at risk children who exhibit behavioral and emotional disturbances in the public school system. All children should be formally instructed in nonviolent conflict resolution skills.[20] This will erode the cycle of violence through programmatic school structure and educational violence prevention. The traditionally strong Black church environment may also be utilized as a community-based institution through which to effect behavioral change. Physicians can assist by identifying children living in environments at risk for violent behavior and initiating early referral for counseling in the school, church, or appropriate professional center.

Mentoring programs by African-American professionals may assist with role modeling and improving self-esteem in Black minority youth who may not have successful role models in the immediate community.[20,65,95] Mentoring can be linked to programs that address employment and explore other options to violent behavior through self-development.

Interventions are best designed as long-term commitments. Time-abbreviated interventions may evoke feelings of exploitation in minority populations. Interventions should be designed with strong evaluative components so that successful interventions may be duplicated. Interven-

---

*References 20,104,129,146,168,194.

tion strategies should provide linkages among agencies and health professionals to provide a wide range of services and create a comprehensive support system for violence prevention activities. The media can be used to promote and publicize violence prevention service by using culturally appropriate community-based media broadcasts.

Physicians can be advocates for change by one-on-one antiviolence counseling and community leadership supportive of the violence intervention strategies discussed. Medical education institutions must develop curricula to educate future health care providers in violence prevention and intervention strategies. Although the answer to the reduction of violence and its health consequences is not the domain of the doctor alone, physician intervention will be necessary to assist in the control of this public health emergency and curb the rising tide of violence in the United States most disparately afflicting African Americans.

Sickle cell disease

The sickle cell diseases are a group of inherited disorders of abnormal hemoglobin that follow classic mendelian genetic patterns and result in chronic symptomatic sickling hemolytic anemia states in the homozygous (HbSS genotype) or double heterozygous individual (HbSβ thalassemia or HbSC genotypes).

Of African Americans 8% are heterozygous for HbS, known as sickle cell trait. About 0.15% of U.S. Black children are homozygous for HbS and have sickle cell anemia (SCA). Black adults have lower prevalence of SCA because of the decreased life expectancy associated with significant morbidity and mortality as a result of the chronic anemia and recurrent vaso-occlusive episodes that repeatedly damage the lungs, kidney, skeleton, skin, and neurologic system. The prevalence of SC sickle disease among Black adults equals that of SS sickle disease even though the HbC gene frequency is only 25% as common. SC sickle disease is a milder illness; most individuals have an increased morbidity risk but near-normal life expectancy and survive well into adulthood.

The clinical course of sickle cell disease varies greatly. Patient care has improved significantly in the last several decades, though no "cure" has been found. Genetic counseling is the best method for prevention of sickle cell anemia. When both prospective parents are AS heterozygotes, there is a 25% chance of their having a homozygous offspring with sickle cell anemia. Prospective parents should be informed. SS homozygote status may be diagnosed antenatally in the first trimester of pregnancy by analyzing the deoxyribonucleic acid (DNA) in fetal cells obtained by examination of a chorionic villus, giving parents the option of terminating the pregnancy.

All African Americans who do not know their sickle cell status should be screened for sickle cell hemoglobin.

The widely used sickle preparation in which sickled blood cells can be microscopically visualized after the addition of an oxygen-consuming reagent to a drop of blood or solubility testing can be used for screening purposes. Both are inexpensive. Positive screening results should be confirmed by hemoglobin electrophoresis and affected individuals counseled about parenthood.

Primary open angle glaucoma

The term *glaucoma* denotes a group of related disorders associated with elevated intraocular pressure, which may lead to visual field impairment and may progress to blindness.

There are two major categories of glaucoma—open angle glaucoma and angle closure glaucoma. Primary open angle glaucoma (POAG) accounts for over two thirds of all glaucomas. Primary open angle glaucoma describes those open angle glaucoma patients in whom no secondary or developmental abnormality of the iridocorneal angle can be found as the cause. The terms *chronic open angle glaucoma, simple glaucoma,* and *glaucoma simplex* are often used synonymously with *primary open angle glaucoma.* Diagnosis of glaucoma depends on the demonstration of visual field loss in the presence of a funduscopic examination result consistent with glaucomatous anatomic changes. The finding of elevated intraocular pressure increases the likelihood of a diagnosis of glaucoma.

Primary open angle glaucoma is largely an asymptomatic disorder characterized by painless yet progressive loss of vision. Since vision loss occurs first in the periphery and progresses centrally, by the time the patient is symptomatic, extensive damage to the eye has already occurred. Patients who have elevated intraocular pressure (21 mm Hg or higher) but no clinical evidence of glaucomatous damage are described as having ocular hypertension or being "glaucoma suspects."

Primary open angle glaucoma is the third leading cause of blindness in the United States and affects 2% of the U.S. population above the age of 40.[60] It is a leading cause of irreversible blindness worldwide and is the number one cause of irreversible blindness in Black Americans. Prevalence rates of blindness caused by glaucoma are from six to eight times higher in Black than White Americans.[173] By age 70, 1 in 10 Blacks will develop glaucoma, compared to 1 in 50 Whites. The Baltimore Eye Survey, a population-based prevalence survey of 5308 Americans aged 40 and older in East Baltimore, Maryland, established that prevalence rates of glaucoma were four times greater in Blacks than Whites in an urban racially mixed group of Americans consisting of 2395 African Americans and 2913 White Americans from similar socioeconomic backgrounds.[172,173]

Racial differences in glaucoma prevalence are also found in numerous studies from outside the United States

---

Characteristics of glaucoma in African Americans

Younger age of onset of disease
More extensive disease
Greater resistance to medical and surgical treatment
Higher incidence and prevalence of blindness

Risk factors for primary open angle glaucoma

Biologic	**Systemic**
Black race	Hypertension
Increasing age	Diabetes mellitus
Family history	Vascular disease
Increased cup to disc ratio	Prior hypotensive episodes
Myopia	

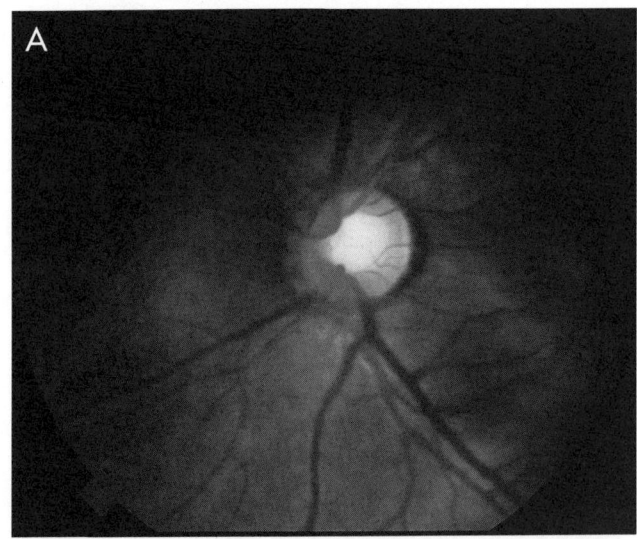

Fig. 34-20. Fundoscopic findings: primary open angle glaucoma. **A,** Fundus demonstrating increased cupping with ratio of 0.4.

Continued

in geographic areas with homogeneous racial populations.[31,141,193] These results are identical to findings in the United States, with higher prevalence rates, younger disease onset, and more resistant treatment patterns among Black African, Black Caribbean, and Black European patients as compared with White European patients. Environmental conditions such as geographic differences in exposure to intense tropical sunlight have been postulated to explain the differences; however, the recent surveys in the United States tend to negate any geographic environmental explanation in favor of a genetic biologic racial predisposition among Blacks.

Not only is primary open angle glaucoma more common in Blacks; it is a much more malignant process that develops earlier and produces greater proportional damage over a shorter period than in non-Black patients with similar intraocular pressure. This suggests a possible genetically enhanced susceptibility to optic nerve damage and development of visual field defects.[12,60,96,100,103]

It is not specifically known why Blacks with glaucoma have a higher incidence of blindness than Whites with glaucoma.[59,66,72] Primary open angle glaucoma is more therapeutically resistant to both medical and surgical treatment in Black patients.[31,60] Some studies have attempted to address this issue and its relationship to glaucoma blindness but results are inconclusive. The box above summarizes characteristics of glaucoma in African Americans.

Additional risk factors for glaucoma include family history and myopia. A family history of glaucoma correlates well with increased risk of disease, although the genetic component of this condition is likely multifactorial. Nearly 50% of all patients with glaucoma have a positive family history. The presence of a positive family history portends a 15- to 20-fold greater risk of development of glaucoma than in the general population.

Myopia ("nearsightedness") is related to primary open angle glaucoma, although the relationship is not entirely understood. This may relate to increased scleral elasticity in myopic individuals, predisposing the patient to greater damage at lower intraocular pressure or to a greater frequency of eye examinations among this group.

Other established risk factors for primary open angle glaucoma include increasing age; systemic hypertension—particularly untreated systolic hypertension; diabetes mellitus; previous hypotensive episodes; ocular hypertension; vascular disease; and increased optic nerve cup to disc ratio. Although the Framingham study[96] reported a higher prevalence of POAG and blindness in males, the Baltimore Eye Study found no significant gender differences. Currently data regarding the possible contribution of diet, exercise, alcohol, and tobacco use and other personal habits to the onset or severity of this disease are poor.[96,164,192,60]

The primary care physician can screen Black Americans to identify those persons at high risk for glaucoma. Specific questions regarding family history of glaucoma and visual loss and personal current visual status should be incorporated into the patient interview. Those identified as having a high-risk history should be referred to an ophthalmologist. Questioning should target the risk factors listed in the second box above.

All patients above age 60 and all Black patients age 40 and older should have a screening examination that includes direct ophthalmoscopic examination of the optic nerve. This is a major screening tool that can be used in the physician's office. Primary care physicians need to become familiar with the suspicious funduscopic appearance of the optic disc suggestive of glaucoma that is characterized by optic cup to disc ratio greater than 0.4 and/or disc asymmetry greater than 0.2 and disc pallor (Figure 34-20).

B

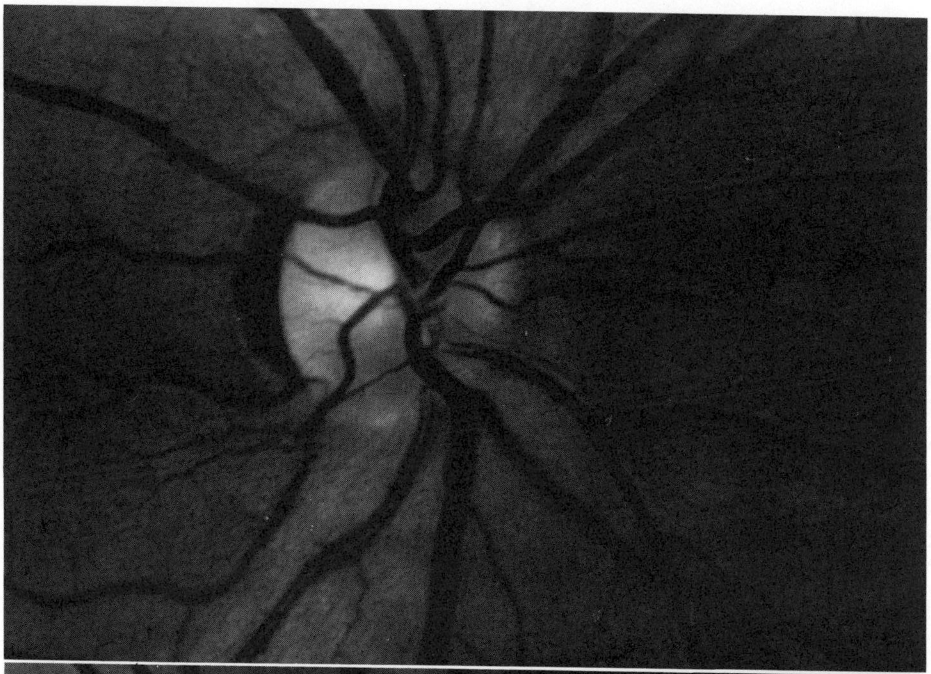

C

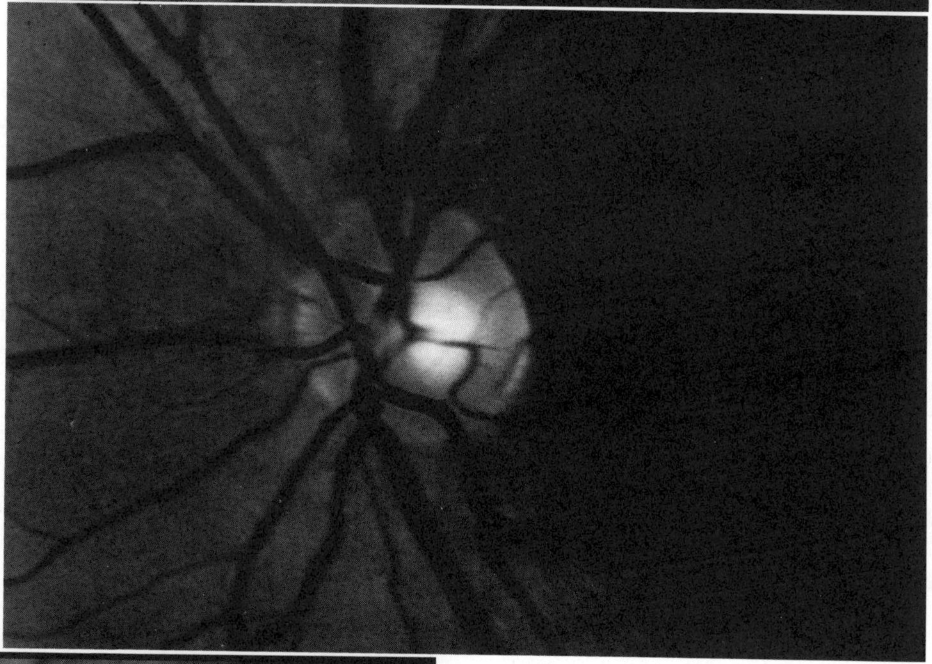

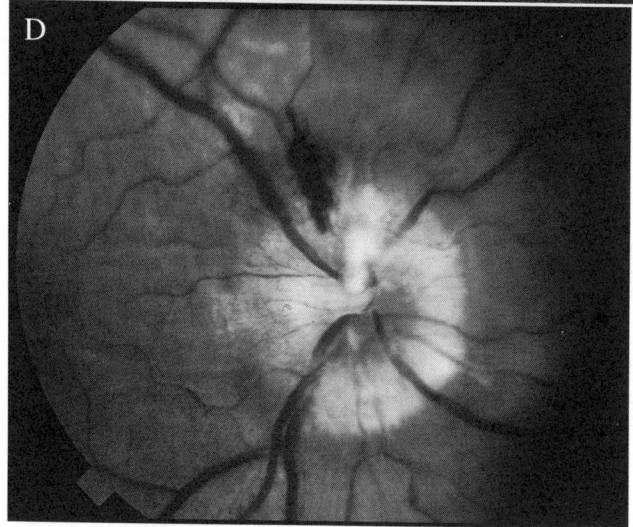

D

Fig. 34-20, cont'd **B & C,** asymmetry of cupping and pallor. Right disc, **B,** shows significantly smaller cup and area of pallor than left disc, **C.** POAG may manifest asymmetric disc to cup ratios. When the eyes differ by more than 0.2, the asymmetry is acquired 98% of the time. The most common cause is POAG. **D,** Disc hemorrhage may be a transient observation in glaucoma. The hemorrhage lasts 4 to 6 weeks and resolves. (**B, C** from Ritch R, Shields B, and Krupin T: *The glaucomas,* St. Louis, 1989, CV Mosby, p 473. **A, D,** courtesy of Dr. Edward Burney, Director of Glaucoma Services, University Hospitals of Cleveland, Cleveland, Ohio.)

Tonometric screening is not sufficiently sensitive as a single screening tool to detect the presence of primary open angle glaucoma, nor is it highly specific. Glaucoma is not always associated with intraocular pressures in excess of 21 mm Hg, nor is it always absent when intraocular pressure measurements are below 21 mm Hg. In the Baltimore Eye Survey[164] roughly one half of subjects with established optic nerve damage would not have been detected by tonometric screening criteria alone. Of the entire population 40 years old or older 7% to 8% have pressures above 21 mm Hg, whereas only 3% have glaucoma.[164] If tonometry alone is used for screening, many more patients will be referred to an ophthalmologist with an elevated intraocular pressure than will ultimately have glaucoma and many with established glaucoma will not be identified. Although intraocular pressure in excess of 21 mm Hg is an independent risk factor for future glaucomatous disease, it is not recommended that primary care physicians make routine tonometric measurements as an exclusive screening modality.

Useful criteria on which to base referral to an ophthalmologist should include a cup to disc ratio greater than 0.4, and disc asymmetry greater than 0.2 with or without a high-risk patient profile. Persons who have several risk factors for this condition also merit referral, as do those with intraocular pressure in excess of 21 mm Hg.

Primary open angle glaucoma is an asymptomatic disease until late in its course. Education of affected and high-risk individuals is critical in order to stress early treatment, early case finding, and compliance with prescribed therapy.

SUMMARY: FOCUS ON PREVENTION

The inferior health status of African Americans is related to low socioeconomic status, adverse personal health habits, ensconced beliefs in folk healing traditions, disease misconceptions, and biologic predisposing factors to some illnesses. Mistrust of the American medical system by African Americans based on historical inequities in care and experimentation[171] and the biased attitudes of many health care professionals in treating Black Americans adversely impacts overall health status as well.[53,36,67,97,157] The health status of Black men is the worst of all segments of the U.S. population. Lagging 30 years behind White men in life expectancy, Black men suffer the highest mortality rates of all people in the United States of cancer, HIV disease, heart disease, hypertension, and the epidemic of violence engulfing the country. Cirrhosis of the liver and stroke are high-mortality-rate diseases also. These excessive casualty rates resulting from multiple disease have caused Black men to become relatively endangered for survival among American people. Black women experience higher than average population rates of hypertension, stroke, angina, and homicide. The highest rates of diabetes mellitus are found among Black women and are related principally to obesity.

While socioeconomic status affects educational level, employment level, access to health care, nutritional status, immune system function, and cancer prevention awareness, attitudes, and practice, the physician can do little to affect the socioeconomic aspect of life of a patient. Nor can biologic health factors be modified.

Prevention strategies must focus on changing adverse health habits and discrediting myths about disease to promote early detection and early treatment of medical illness when interventions are most likely to affect morbidity and prevent fatal outcome. Reduction and cessation of smoking in African Americans reduces the risk of development of cardiovascular disease and cancer and reduces infant mortality rates. Abstinence and moderation in alcohol consumption reduces birth defects contributing to infant mortality and decreases the incidence of esophageal cancer and cirrhosis of the liver. Alcohol abstinence may also improve hypertension control. Aerobic exercise should be encouraged to improve general cardiovascular fitness and to maintain a nonobese body habitus. Efforts to control obesity[19,50,90,92,109,137] are of critical importance for African Americans to assist in decreasing the rising rates of diabetes mellitus. This is best achieved by maintaining a lifestyle that includes regular exercise and caloric intake appropriate to maintain or decrease body weight as necessary. Snacking is a major factor that predisposes to obesity that should be specifically addressed with Black women. Although the intake of sodium in African Americans is comparable to that of the general population, dietary potassium intake is lower in African Americans.[93] The addition of more potassium-rich foods to the diet (such as fresh fruits and vegetables) may improve hypertension control rates and reduce the risk of certain carcinomas by increasing fiber consumption.[93,94,136]

Patient education should be a part of every physician-patient encounter. Conversation with patients should avoid sophisticated medical jargon and be easily understood.

Prevention efforts should specifically target children. Cardiovascular risk factors start early in life,[*] as does risk behavior for cancer.[69] Adverse health habits should be prevented rather than attempting to modify behavior later in life. It is a much easier process to intervene to stop smoking, alcohol and recreational drug use, sedentary life-style, and poor dietary habits before they start. Intervention planning must begin early in the child's social structure and must be culturally as well as economically sensitive. Children learn by example and efforts for interventions in adult populations must continue and expand.

Acknowledgments

I would like to thank Dr. Edward Burney, Director of Glaucoma Services, University Hospitals of Cleveland, for his review of the section on glaucoma and the use of pho-

---

*References 14,15,21,45,108,109,196.

tographs from his private collection. My sincere gratitude is also extended to Karen Spencer, Joanne Billiar, the late Verna Myers, and Darlene Hardiman, all from St. Vincent Charity Hospital, Cleveland, Ohio, for their research, transcription, and hard work on my behalf to complete this chapter.

REFERENCES

1. Ackerman SP et al: Cancer screening behaviors among U.S. women: breast cancer, 1987-1989, and cervical cancer, 1988-1989, *MMWR* 41:SS-2, 1992.
2. Akinkugbe O: Heart disease in Blacks of Africa and the Carribean, *Cardio Clin* 21(3):377-391, 1991.
3. American Academy of Pediatrics, Committee on Communications: Children, adolescents, and television, *Pediatrics* 85:1119-1120, 1990.
4. American Cancer Society: Cancer facts and figures—1992, Atlanta, 1992.
5. Amin M, et al: Acute myocardial infarction and chest pain syndromes after cocaine use, *Am J Cardiol* 66:1434, 1990.
6. Ammirato T. Treating violence as a public health problem. *Urban Med* September 1992.
7. Anderson et al: Hypertension in blacks: psychosocial and biological perspectives, *J Hypertens* 7:161-172, 1989.
8. *Ann Intern Med* 74(5):789-790, 1971 (editorial).
9. Arch Intern Med: The 1988 report of the Joint National Committee on Detection, Evaluation, and Treatment of High Blood Pressure, *Arch Intern Med* 148:1023-1038, 1988.
10. Aruffo JF et al: AIDS knowledge in low-income and minority populations, *Public Health Rep* 106(2):115-119, 1991.
11. Bakeman R et al: The incidence of AIDS among Blacks and Hispanics, *J Natl Med Assoc* 79(9):921-928, 1987.
12. Beck RW et al: Is there a racial difference in physiologic cup size? *Ophthalmology* 92:873-876, 1985.
13. Bell CC, Chance-Hill G: Treatment of violent families, *J Natl Med Assoc* 83:203-208, 1991.
14. Berenson GS et al: Cardiovascular risk factors in children and early prevention of heart disease, *Clin Chem* 34(8B):115-122, 1988.
15. Berenson GS et al: Risk factors in early life as predictors of adult heart disease: the Bogalusa Heart Study, *Am J Med Sci* 141:1989.
16. Berenson GS et al: Pathogenesis of hypertension in black and white children, *Clin Cardiol* 12(4):3-8, 1989.
17. Bing EG et al: Treatment issues for African-Americans and Hispanics with AIDS, *Psychiatr Med* 9(3):455-467, 1991.
18. Blaustein MP, Grim CE: The pathogenesis of hypertension: black-white differences, cardiovascular diseases in Blacks, *Cardiovasc Clin* 21(3):97, 1991.
19. Block G et al: Calories, fat and cholesterol: intake patterns in the U.S. population by race, sex and age. *Am J Public Health* 78(9):1150, 1988.
20. Boruch RF et al: Violence prevention strategies targeted at the general population of minority youth, *Public Health Rep* 106:247-250, 1991.
21. Burke GL et al: Cardiovascular risk factors and their modification in children, *Cardiol Clin* 4:33, 1986.
22. Cascardi M et al: Marital aggression impact, injury, and health correlates for husbands and wives, *Arch Intern Med* 152:1178-1184, 1992.
23. Centerwall BS: Television and violence: the scale of the problem and where to go from here, *JAMA* 267(22):3059-3063, 1992.
24. Centerwall BS: Exposure to television as a risk factor for violence, *Am J Epidemiol* 129:643-652, 1989.
25. Connell FA: Lower extremity amputations among persons with diabetes mellitus—Washington 1988, *MMWR* 40(42):736-750, 1991.
26. Cook PJ et al: Weapons and minority youth violence, *Public Health Rep* 106:254-258, 1991.

27. Cooper ES, Caplan LR: Cerebrovascular disease in hypertensive blacks, cardiovascular diseases in Blacks, *Cardiovasc Clin* 21(3):145, 1991. FA Davis Publisher.
28. Cooper R: A note on the biologic concept of race and its application in epidemiologic research, *Am Heart J* 108:715, 1984.
29. Cooper RS, Ghali JK: Coronary heart disease: black-white differences, *Cardiovasc Clin* 21(3):205, 1991.
30. Cooper RS: Celebrate diversity—or should we? *Ethnicity Disease* 1(1):3-7, 1991.
31. Cowan CL et al: Glaucoma in blacks, *Arch Ophthalmol* 106:738-739, 1988.
32. Cummings KM: Comparison of the cigarette brand preference of adult and teenage smokers—United States, 1989, *MMWR* 41(10):169-176, 1992.
33. David RJ: Did low birth weight among US blacks really increase? *Am J Public Health* 76(4):380-383, 1986.
34. Davis RA: Adolescent pregnancy and infant mortality: isolating the effects of race, *Adolescence* 23:92, 1988.
35. Deutsch SJ, Alt FB: The effect of Massachusetts gun control law on gun related crimes in the city of Boston, *Eval Q* 1:543-568, 1977.
36. Dever J et al: Counseling practices of Primary Care Physicians North Carolina, 1991, *MMWR* 41(31):565-568, 1992.
37. Dressler WW: Social class, skin color, and arterial blood pressure in two societies, *Ethnicity Disease* 1(1):60-77, 1991.
38. DuBois WEB: *Black reconstruction in America 1860-1880*, New York, 1934, Atheneum.
39. Dyson JL: The effect of family violence on children's academic performance and behavior, *J Natl Med Assoc* 82(1):17-22, 1990.
40. Eldridge L et al: Regional variation in diabetes mellitus prevalence—United States, 1988-1989, *MMWR* 39(45):806-820, 1990.
41. Eldridge L et al: Factors related to cholesterol screening and cholesterol level awareness—United States, 1989, *MMWR* 39(37):633-637, 1990.
42. Elsea WR et al: Family and other intimate assaults—Atlanta, 1984. *MMWR* 39(31):525-538, 1990.
43. Emanuel I et al: Poor birth outcomes of American black women: an alternative explanation, *J Public Health Policy* 1989.
44. Engel GL: Sudden and rapid death during psychological stress, folklore or folk wisdom? *Ann Intern Med* 74:771-782, 1971.
45. Enos WF et al: Coronary disease among United States soldiers killed in action in Korea, *JAMA* 152(12):1090-1093, 1953.
46. Fichtner RR et al: Racial/ethnic differences in smoking, other risk factors, and low birth weight among low income pregnant women, *MMWR* 39(SS-3):13-21, 1990.
47. Fingerhut LA et al: Firearm and nonfirearm homicide among persons 15 through 19 years of age: differences by level of urbanization, United States, 1979 through 1989, *JAMA* 267(22):3048-3053, 1992.
48. Fingerhut LA et al: Firearm homicide among black teenage males in metropolitan counties: comparison of death rates in two periods, 1983 through 1985 and 1987 through 1989. *JAMA* 267(22):3054-3058, 1992.
49. Flack JM, Wiist WH: Cardiovascular risk factor prevalence in African-American adult screenees for a church-based cholesterol program: the Northeast Oklahoma City Cholesterol Education Program, *Ethnicity Disease* 1(1):78-90, 1991.
50. Folsom AR et al: Implications of obesity for cardiovascular disease in blacks: the CARDIA and ARIC studies, *Am J Clin Nutr* 53(160):4S-11S, 1991.
51. Ford E et al: Coronary arteriography and coronary bypass survey among whites and other racial groups relative to hospital-based incidence rates for coronary artery disease: findings from NHDS, *Am J Public Health* 79(4):437-440, 1989.
52. Francis CK: Hypertension and cardiac disease in minorities, *Am J Med* 88:(suppl 3B):3S, 1990.
53. Gemson DH: Differences in physician prevention practice patterns for white and minority patients, *J Community Health* 13:1, 1988.

54. Geronimus AT: The effects of race, residence, and prenatal care on the relationship of maternal age to neonatal mortality, *Am J Public Health* 76(12):1416-1421, 1986.

55. Giebel HN: Differences in the age of smoking initiation, *MMWR* 40(44):754, 1991.

56. Gillum RF: Cardiovascular disease in the United States: an epidemiologic overview, *Cardiovasc Clin* 21(3):3, 1991.

57. Goins WA et al: Recurrent intentional injury, *J Natl Med Assoc* 84:431-435, 1992.

58. Gottdiener JS: Hypertensive heart disease in blacks, *Cardiovasc Clin* 21(3):133, 1991.

59. Grant WM, Burke JF: Why do some people go blind from glaucoma? *Am Acad Ophthalmol* 89(9):991-998, 1982.

60. Greenidge KC et al: Glaucoma in the black population: a problem of blindness, *J Natl Med Assoc* 80(12):1305-1309, 1988.

61. Griffith E, Bell CC: Recent trends in suicide and homicide among blacks, *JAMA* 262(16):2265-2269, 1989.

62. Guinan ME: HIV, heterosexual transmission, and women, *JAMA* 268:4520-521, 1992.

63. Hall WD, Saunders E, Shulman N: *Hypertension in blacks: epidemiology, pathophysiology and treatment*, Chicago, 1985, Year Book Medical.

64. Hardy AM et al: AIDS knowledge and attitudes of black americans: United States 1990. Advance Data, Centers for Disease Control, NCHS, no. 206, October 16, 1991.

65. Harrison DD: An anthropologist's view of the roots of violence in the United States, *J Natl Med Assoc* 83:638-642, 1991.

66. Hart WM et al: Multivariate analysis of the risk of glaucomatous visual field loss, *Arch Ophthalmol* 97:1455-1458, 1979.

67. Haywood LJ: Hypertension in minority populations: access to care, *Am J Med* 88(suppl 3B):17S, 1990.

68. Haywood LJ: Hypertension in minority populations. *Am J Med* 88(suppl 3B):3B-17S-3B-20S, 1990.

69. Heath CW et al: Cigarette smoking among youth—United States, 1989, *MMWR* 40(41):713-715, 1991.

70. Heurtin-Roberts S: Health beliefs and compliance with prescribed medication for hypertension among black women—New Orleans, 1985-86, *MMWR* 39(40):701-704, 1990.

71. Hildreth C, Saunders E: Hypertension in blacks: clinical overview, *Cardiovasc Clin* 21(3):85, 1991.

72. Hiller R, Kahn HA: Blindness from glaucoma, *Am J Ophthalmol* 80(1):62-69, 1975.

73. Hoffman A et al: Cigarette smoking and attitudes toward quitting among black patients, *J Natl Med Assoc* 81(4):415-420, 1989.

74. Holleb AI et al: American Cancer Society textbook of clinical oncology, Atlanta, 1991, The American Cancer Society.

75. Hutchinson J: AIDS and racism, *JAMA* 84(6):119-124, 1992.

76. James S: Psychosocial presursors of hypertension: a review of the epidemiologic evidence, *Circulation* 76(suppl I):I-60, 1987.

77. Jason J et al: A comparison of primary and secondary homicides in the United States, *Am J Epidemiol* 117:309-319, 1983.

78. Johnson C: The status of health care among Black Americans: address before the Congress of National Black Churches, *J Natl Med Assoc* 83(2):125-129, 1991.

79. Johnson E et al: Do African-American men and women differ in the knowledge about AIDS, attitudes and condoms, and sexual behaviors? *J Natl Med Assoc* 84(1):49-63, 1992.

80. Johnson RL: Sexual behaviors of African American male college students and the risk of HIV infection, *J Natl Med Assoc* 84(10):864-868, 1992.

81. Jordan WC: Black American folk medicine: minority aging, U.S. Department of Health and Human Services, DHHS Pub No HRS-P-DV 90-4, 1990.

82. Kaku DA et al: Emergence of recreational drug abuse as a major risk factor for stroke in young adults, *Ann Intern Med* 113(11):821-827, 1990.

83. Keil JE, Saunders DE: Urban and rural differences in cardiovascular disease in blacks, *Cardiovasc Clin* 21(3):17, 1991.

84. Kittner SJ et al: Black-white differences in stroke incidence in a national sample, *JAMA* 264(10):1267, 1990.

85. Kleinman JC: Infant mortality among racial/ethnic minority groups, 1983-1984, *MMWR* 39(SS-3):31-39, 1990.

86. Klag M et al: The association of skin color with blood pressure, *Jama* 265(5):599, 1991.

87. Klonoff D, Andrews BT, Obana WG: Stroke associated with cocaine use, *Arch Neurol* 46:989, 1989.

88. Koop CE et al: Violence in America: a public health emergency, *JAMA* 267(22):3075, 1992.

89. Kruttschnitt C et al: Family violence, television viewing habits, and other adolescent experiences related to violent criminal behavior. *Criminology* 24:235-267, 1986.

90. Kumanyaka SK et al: Weight-loss experience of black and white participants in NHLBI-sponsored clinical trials, *Am J Clin Nutr* 53:1631S-1638S, 1991.

91. Kumanyika S, Golden P: Cross-sectional differences in health status in US racial/ethnic minority groups: potential influences of temporal changes, disease, and life-style transitions, *Ethnicity Dis* 1(1):50-59, 1991.

92. Kumanyika S, Adams-Campbell L: Obesity, diet, and psychosocial factors contributing to cardiovascular disease in blacks. *Cardiovasc Clin* 21(3):47, 1991.

93. Langford H et al: Dietary profile of sodium, potassium and calcium in U.S. blacks: Hypertension in Blacks, Chicago, 1985, Yearbook Medical.

94. Lanza E et al: Dietary fiber intake in the U.S. population, *Am J Clin Nutr* 46:790, 1987.

95. Lawrence LE: Driving "Miss Clarabell": to a medical education and beyond. *J Natl Med Assoc* 84:441-446, 1992.

96. Leske MC, Rosenthal J: Epidemiologic aspects of open-angle glaucoma, *Am J Epidemiol* 109(3):250-272, 1979.

97. Lewis CE et al: Risk factors and the natural history of coronary heart disease in blacks. Cardiovascular Disease in Blacks, 21:3:29, 1991. FA Davis Publisher.

98. Lindan CP et al: Underreporting of minority AIDS deaths in San Francisco Bay area, 1985-86, *Public Health Rep* 105(4):400-404, 1990.

99. Loftin C et al: Effects of restrictive licensing of handguns on homicide and suicide in the District of Columbia, *JAMA* 267(22):3017, 1992.

100. Lotufo D et al: Juvenile glaucoma, race, and refraction, *JAMA* 261(2):249-252, 1989.

101. Lynberg MC et al: Contribution of birth defects to infant mortality among racial/ethnic minority groups, United States, 1983, *MMWR* 39(SS-3):1-12, 1990.

102. Maron BJ et al: Sudden death in young athletes, *Circulation* 62:218, 1980.

103. Martin MJ et al: Race and primary open-angle glaucoma, *Am J Ophthalmol* 99:383-387, 1985.

104. Mason J: Reducing youth violence, *JAMA* 267(22):3003-3006, 1992.

105. Mays VM, Jackson JS: AIDS survey methodology with black Americans, *Soc Sci Med* 33(1):47-54, 1991.

106. Mellon J: *Bullwhip days (the slaves remember—an oral history)*, New York, 1988, Avon Books.

107. McGill H Jr: The cardiovascular pathology of smoking, *Am Heart J* 115:250-257, 1988.

108. McNamara JJ et al. Coronary artery disease in combat casualties in Vietnam. *JAMA*, 216(7):1185-1187, 1971.

109. Moore J et al: Participation in school physical education and selected dietary patterns among high school students—United States, 1991, *MMWR* 41(33):597, 1992.

110. Morbidity and Mortality Weekly Report: Trends in lung cancer in-

cidence and mortality—United States, 1980-1987, *MMWR* 39(48): 875-883, 1990.

111. Morbidity and Mortality Weekly Report: Prevalence and incidence of diabetes mellitus—United States 1980-1987, *MMWR* 39(45): 609, 1990.

112. Morbidity and Mortality Weekly Report: Cigarette advertising United States, 1988, *MMWR* 39(16):280, 262, 264, 1990.

113. Morbidity and Mortality Weekly Report: Trends in prostate cancer United States, 1980-1988. *MMWR* 41(23):401-404, 1992.

114. Morbidity and Mortality Weekly Report: CDC surveillance summary, homicide surveillance 1979-1988, *MMWR* 41:SS-3, 1992.

115. Morbidity and Mortality Weekly Report: Assessment of broadcast media airings of AIDS-related public service announcements—United States 1987-1990, *MMWR* 40(31):543-546, 1991.

116. Morbidity and Mortality Weekly Report: The second 100,000 cases of acquired immunodeficiency syndrome—United States, June 1981—December 1991, *MMWR* 41(2):29, 1991.

117. Morbidity and Mortality Weekly Report: Physical fighting among high school students—United States—1990, *MMWR* 41(6):90-94, 1992.

118. Morbidity and Mortality Weekly Report: Black-white differences in cervical cancer mortality—United States, 1980-1987, *MMWR* 39(15):245-248, 1990.

119. Morbidity and Mortality Weekly Report: Low birth weight—United States 1975-1987, *MMWR* 39(9):148, 1990.

120. Morbidity and Mortality Weekly Report: Attempted suicide among high school students—United States, 1990, *MMWR* 40(37):633-634, 1991.

121. Morbidity and Mortality Weekly Report: Infant mortality—United States 1989, *MMWR* 41(5):81, 1992.

122. Morbidity and Mortality Weekly Report: Cigarette smoking among adults—United States, 1990, *MMWR* 41(20):354, 360, 362, 1992.

123. Morbidity and Mortality Weekly Report: Infant mortality among black Americans, *MMWR* 36(1):1-10, 1987.

124. Morbidity and Mortality Weekly Report: Weapon-carrying among high school students—United States, 1990, *MMWR* 40(40):680-684, 1991.

125. National Medical Association News: International study to gauge role of economic, social factors in hypertension among blacks, September/October 1992.

126. National Medical Association News: Federal health statistics seen as marred by inccurate racial and ethnic identification, September/October 1992.

127. Murray R: Skin color and blood pressure, *JAMA* 265(5):639, 1991.

128. Nickens H: AIDS among blacks in the 1990's, *JNMA* 82(4):239-242, 1990.

129. Northrop D et al: Violence prevention strategies targeted towards high-risk minority youth, *Public Health Rep* 106:272-274, 1991.

130. Novello AC, Shosky J et al: From the surgeon general, U.S. Public Health Service, a medical response to violence, *JAMA* 267(22):3007, 1992.

131. Novello AC: Violence is a greater killer of children then disease, *Public Health Rep* 106:231-233, 1991.

132. O'Carroll PW et al: Preventing homicide: an evaluation of the efficacy of a Detroit gun ordinance, *Am J Public Health* 81:576-581, 1991.

133. Osborne NG, Feit MD: The use of race in medical research, JAMA 267(2):275-279, 1992.

134. Palmer C: African slave trade, *National Geographic*182(3):62-91, 1992.

135. Parker FC et al: The association between cardiovascular response tasks and future blood pressure levels in children: Bogalusa Heart Study, *Am Heart J* 5:1174, 1987.

136. Patterson B et al: Food choices and the cancer guidelines, *Am J Public Health* 78(3):282, 1988.

137. Pearson TA et al: Prevention of coronary heart disease in black adults, *Cardiovasc Clin* 21(3):263, 1991. FA Davis Publisher

138. Peniston RL et al: Cardiovascular surgery in blacks, *Cardiovasc Clin* 21(3):321, 1991.

139. Peniston RL, Keita SO: Introduction, *Cardio Clin* 21(3):xxxv-vi, 1991.

140. Pierce JP: Accessibility of cigarettes to youths aged 12-17, United States, 1989, *MMWR* 41(27):485-488, 1992.

141. Poinoosawmy D et al: Glaucoma and race, *Lancet* 1134, 1989.

142. Prineas R, Gillum R: U.S. epidemiology of hypertension in blacks. In Hypertension in Blacks, Chicago, 1985, Yearbook Medical.

143. Qualters JR et al: Breast and cervical cancer surveillance, United States 1973-1987, *MMWR* 41:SS-2, 1992.

144. Rice M: Black health care in America: a political perspective, *J Natl Med Assoc* 83:6, 1991.

145. Robinson RG et al: Cancer awareness among African Americans: a survey assessing race, social status, and occupation, *J Natl Med Assoc* 83(6):491-497, 1991.

146. Roper WL: The prevention of minority youth violence must begin despite risks and imperfect understanding, *Public Health Rep* 106:229-231, 1991.

147. Roper WL et al: Homicide among young black males—United States, 1978-1987, *MMWR* 39:869-872, 1990.

148. Rosenberg ML et al: Let's be clear: violence is a public health problem, *JAMA* 267(22):3071-3072, 1992.

149. Rothenberg R et al: Survival with the acquired immunodeficiency syndrome, *N Engl J Med* 317(21):1297-1302, 1987.

150. Saltzman LE et al: Weapon involvement and injury outcomes in family and intimate assaults, *JAMA* 267(22):3043-3047, 1992.

151. Saunders E: Cardiovascular diseases in blacks, *Cardiovasc Clin* 21:3, 1991.

152. Schilling RF et al: Developing strategies for AIDS prevention research with black and hispanic drug users, *Am J Public Health,* 104(1):2-11, 1989.

153. Schneider D et al: Violence as a public health priority for black Americans, *J Natl Med Assoc* 84(10):843-848, 1992.

154. Schoenbaum E et al: Risk factors for human immunodeficiency virus infection in intravenous drug users, *N Engl J Med* 321(13):874-879, 1989.

155. Selik RM et al: Distribution of AIDS cases by racial/ethnic group and exposure category, United States, June 1, 1981—July 4, 1988, JAMA 261(2):201-205, 1989.

156. Shakoor BH, Chalmers D: Co-victimization of African-American children who witness violence: effects of cognitive, emotional, and behavioral development, *J Natl Med Assoc* 83(3):233-238, 1991.

157. Shulman NB: Economic issues relating to access to medications, *Cardiovasc Dis Blacks* 21(3):75, 1991.

158. Sims DW et al: Urban trauma: a chronic recurrent disease, *J Trauma* 29:940-947, 1984.

159. Sloan JH et al: Handgun regulations, crime, assaults, and homicide: a tale of two cities, *N Engl J Med* 319(3):1256-1262, 1988.

160. Smead H: The Afro-Americans: the peoples of North America, New York, 1989, Chelsea House Publishers.

161. Smith DK: HIV disease as a cause of death for African Americans in 1987 and 1990, *J Natl Med Assoc* 84(6):481-487, 1992.

162. Snow LF: Folk medical beliefs and their implication for care of patients, *Ann Intern Med* 81:82-96, 1974.

163. Snow LF: Traditional health beliefs and practices among lower class black americans, *West J Med* 139(6):820-828, 1983.

164. Sommer A et al: Relationship between intraocular pressure and primary open angle glaucoma among white and black Americans, *Arch Ophthalmol* 109:1090-1095, 1991.

165. Stone KM, Peterson HB: Spermicides, HIV, and the vaginal sponge, *JAMA* 268(4):521-522, 1992.

166. Strauss MA: Domestic violence and homicide antecedents, *Bull NY Acad Med* 62:446-465, 1986.

167. Strogatz D: Use of medical care for chest pain: differences between blacks and whites, *Am J Public Health,* 80(3):290-294, 1990.

168. Sullivan LW: The prevention of violence—a top HHS priority, *Public Health Rep* 106:268-269, 1991.
169. Teret SP et al: The firearm fatality reporting system. *JAMA* 267(22):3073-3074, 1992.
170. The world almanac and book of facts, New York, 1991, Pharos Books.
171. Thomas SB et al. The Tuskegee syphilis study, 1932 to 1972: implications for HIV education and AIDS risk education programs in the black community, *Am J Public Health* 81(11):1498-1505, 1991.
172. Tielsch JM et al: Blindness and visual impairment in an American urban population, *Arch Ophthalmol* 108:286-290, 1990.
173. Tielsch JM et al: Racial variations in the prevalence of primary open-angle glaucoma, *JAMA* 266(3):369-374, 1991.
174. U.S. Department of Health and Human Services. National Cancer Institute: *Cancer among blacks and other minorities: statistical profiles,* 1986.
175. U.S. Department of Health and Human Services: *HIV/AIDS surveillance report,* Center for Disease Control, September 1990.
176. U.S. Department of Health and Human Services: The nation's health: age groups, *Healthy People 2000* 2:9-28, 1990.
177. U.S. Department of Health and Human Services: The nation's health: special populations, *Healthy People 2000* 3:29-42, 1990.
178. U.S. Department of Health and Human Services: Proceedings of a National Conference on Preventing Alcohol and Drug Abuse in Black Communities. Office for Substance Abuse. Pub No (ADM)89-1648, 1990.
179. U.S. Department of Health and Human Services: Health United States and Prevention Profile 1991. National Center for Health Statistics, Pub No (PHS)92-1232, 1992.
180. U.S. Department of Health and Human Services: Report of the Secretary's Task Force on Black and Minority Health. Vol I. Executive summary, August 1985.
181. U.S. Department of Health and Human Services: Report of the Secretary's Task Force on Black and Minority Health. Vol III. Cancer, January 1986.
182. U.S. Department of Health and Human Services: Report of the Secretary's Task Force on Black and Minority Health. Vol VI. Infant mortality and low birth weight, 1986.
183. U.S. Department of Health and Human Services. Institutional racism and community competence. Public Health Service, Alcohol, Drug Abuse, and Mental Health Administration, Center for Minority Group Mental Health Program, Pub No (ADM) 81-907, 1981.
184. U.S. Department of Health and Human Services. Report of the Secretary's Task Force on Black and Minority Health. Vol VII. Chemical dependency and diabetes, 1986.

185. Watkins LO, Williams RA: Cardiomyopathy in blacks, *Cardiovasc Clin* 21(3):279, 1991.
186. Weaver PW et al: Colon cancer in blacks: a disease with a worsening prognosis, *J Natl Med Assoc* 83(2):133-136, 1991.
187. Webber LS et al: Cardiovascular risk factors in hispanic, white, and black children: The Brooks County and Bogalusa Heart Studies, Am J Epidemiology, 133(7):704-714, 1991.
188. Weddington WW: Risk behaviors for HIV transmission among intravenous drug users not in drug treatment, *MMWR* 39(16):273-274, 1990.
189. Weil DS et al: Loaded guns in the home: analysis of a national random survey of gun owners, *JAMA* 267(22):3033-3037, 1992.
190. Widom CS: The cycle of violence, *Science* 244:160-166, 1989.
191. Williams RA: Sudden cardiac death in blacks. Including black athletes, *Cardiovasc Clin* 21(3):297, 1991.
192. Wilson MR et al: A case-control study of risk factors in open angle glaucoma, *Arch Ophthalmol* 105:1066-1071, 1987.
193. Wilson MR: Glaucoma in blacks: where do we go from here? JAMA, 261(2):281-282, 1989.
194. Wilson-Brewer R, Jacklin B: Violence prevention strategies targeted at the general population of minority youth, *Public Health Rep* 106:270-271, 1991.
195. Wishner AR et al: Interpersonal violence-related injuries in an African-American community in Philadelphia, *Am J Public Health,* 81(11):1474-1476, 1991.
196. Zeek P: Juvenile arteriosclerosis, *Arch Pathol* 10:417, 1930.

━━━━━━━━━ **RESOURCES** ━━━━━━━━━

National Medical Association, a national organization of physicians addressing health care needs of the African American community. Contact the Public Relations Department for general information or the Community Health Coalition Project (Formerly NMA—Healthy People 2000), National Medical Association, 1012 10th Street NW, Washington, DC, 20001.

Office of Minority Health Resource Center, US Department of Health and Human Services, A federal government agency dedicated to minority health care, PO Box 37337, Washington, DC, 20013-7337.

Chapter 35

SPECIAL HEALTH PROBLEMS OF EUROPEAN AMERICANS, INCLUDING PEOPLES OF THE MEDITERRANEAN BASIN

Stephen P. Hayden

European, Middle Eastern, and North African countries have citizens of diverse ethnic origins, although the overwhelming majority of people are of the white race. For the purposes of this chapter, some regional groupings were made, on the basis of cultural and historic ties as well as geography. Fig. 35-1 shows the regions of Europe, the Middle East, and North Africa that have been included. North Africa and the Middle East will be considered together as the "Middle East." Although these are times of rapid political change, the epidemiologic studies reported here were performed while the former Soviet Union, Yugoslavia, and Czechoslovakia were still intact, and the map reflects the situation at that time. Fig. 35-2 is a map of the United States showing the largest centers of population of European immigrants, including Italians, Germans, British, Poles, Russians, Irish, Austrians, and Swedes. Tables 35-1 and 35-2 summarize the numbers of immigrants from European countries in the last 3 decades and the distribution of different ethnic groups within the United States.

As in other racial and ethnic groups, the health of the population and its susceptibility to disease depend on both genetic and environmental influences, such as diet; and in the case of immigrants, there are additional changes, brought about by environmental influences in the adoptive country as well as the effects of intermarriage on subsequent generations. The provision of health care and the type and amount of health information available vary greatly among European and Middle Eastern countries. The countries of Western Europe and Israel have in general maintained more complete health records, and there is more information about these populations than about Eastern Europe and other parts of the Middle East. Attitudes toward health care vary among different ethnic groups in the United States. [96] In some countries strong customs and religious convictions have profound effects on certain aspects of medical care, such as circumcision among the Jewish and Muslim communities and abortion in the Republic of Ireland, where it is almost totally banned. Preventive medicine and general concern for health also appear to differ greatly between peoples, and this will tend to affect preventive medicine programs. For instance, these programs have been slower to develop in the United Kingdom than in North America. Where government control of expenditure is strong, such as the U.K., there is little possibility for major initiatives unless supported by central government policy (see Chapter 5).

It is increasingly important to know about the genetic and other diseases and predispositions of the Europeans and their various subgroups, not to mention other population groups of the globe. There are large groups of first- and second-generation people living among us in North America; many patients, with their families, on assignment from their native countries are seen, particularly in

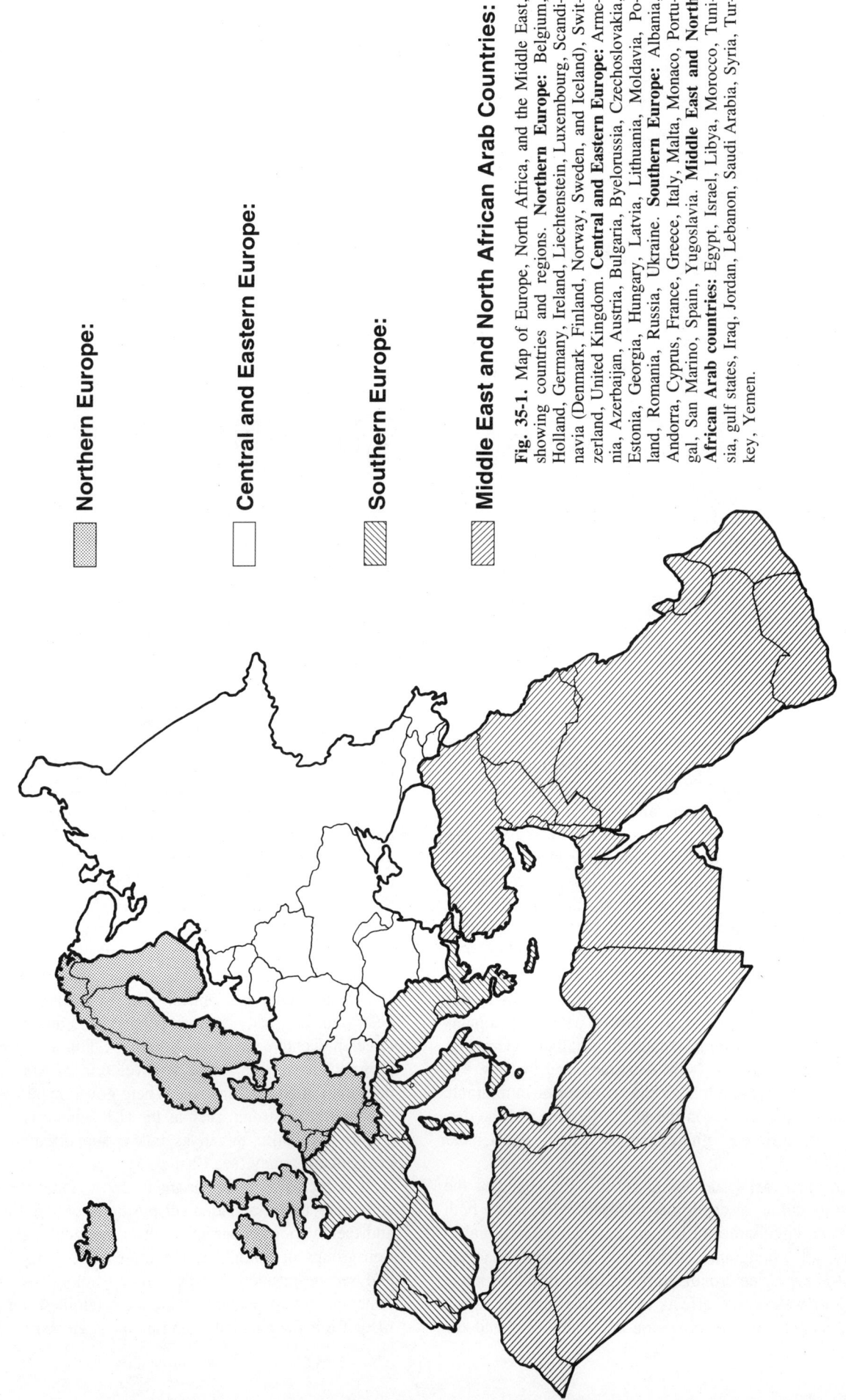

Northern Europe:

Central and Eastern Europe:

Southern Europe:

Middle East and North African Arab Countries:

Fig. 35-1. Map of Europe, North Africa, and the Middle East, showing countries and regions. **Northern Europe:** Belgium, Holland, Germany, Ireland, Liechtenstein, Luxembourg, Scandinavia (Denmark, Finland, Norway, Sweden, and Iceland), Switzerland, United Kingdom. **Central and Eastern Europe:** Armenia, Azerbaijan, Austria, Bulgaria, Byelorussia, Czechoslovakia, Estonia, Georgia, Hungary, Latvia, Lithuania, Moldavia, Poland, Romania, Russia, Ukraine. **Southern Europe:** Albania, Andorra, Cyprus, France, Greece, Italy, Malta, Monaco, Portugal, San Marino, Spain, Yugoslavia. **Middle East and North African Arab countries:** Egypt, Israel, Libya, Morocco, Tunisia, gulf states, Iraq, Jordan, Lebanon, Saudi Arabia, Syria, Turkey, Yemen.

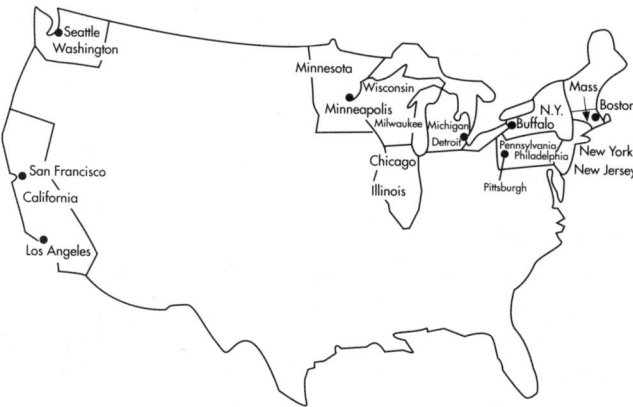

Fig. 35-2. U.S. cities with the highest number of foreign born residents and their children. Numbers are in 1000s.

Italian

New York	1,004
Philadelphia	229
Chicago	197
Boston	192
Newark	139

Russian

New York	513
Los Angeles	129
Philadelphia	120
Chicago	105
Boston	77

German

New York	345
Chicago	225
Philadelphia	100
Milwaukee	90
Detroit	89

Irish

New York	315
Boston	147
Chicago	92
Philadelphia	84
San Francisco	36

British

New York	208
Los Angeles	143
Philadelphia	104
Detroit	95
Chicago	81

Austrian

New York	198
Chicago	57
Pittsburgh	46
Los Angeles	38
Philadelphia	34

Polish

New York	386
Chicago	284
Detroit	160
Philadelphia	88
Buffalo	75

Swedish

Chicago	66
Minneapolis	56
Los Angeles	36
New York	31
Seattle	22

Modified from: Johns SB: *The ethnic almanac,* New York, 1981, Dolphin Books.

Table 35-1. The 10 most populous foreign groups in the United States

Group	Population
Italian	4,240,779
German	3,622,035
Canadian	3,034,556
British	2,465,050
Polish	2,374,244
Mexican	2,339,151
Russian	1,943,195
Irish	1,450,220
Austrian	975,325
Swedish	806,138

From Johns SB: *The ethnic almanac,* Garden City, NY, 1981, Dolphin Books.

Table 35-2. Immigration into the United States from Europe by country of origin, 1951-1985

Country	No. of immigrants
Albania	580
Austria	102,625
Belgium	36,222
Bulgaria	2,689
Czechoslovakia	14,290
Denmark	27,083
Estonia*	497
Finland	13,414
France	134,092
Germany	782,841
Greece	243,574
Hungary	51,529
Ireland	98,154
Italy	553,180
Latvia*	1,195
Lithuania*	1,215
Luxembourg	1,675
Netherlands	99,127
Norway	44,231
Poland	132,711
Portugal	218,764
Romania	30,324
Spain	100,944
Sweden	50,143
Switzerland	48,045
USSR	76,877
United Kingdom	632,833
Yugoslavia	66,919
Other Europe	17,955
TOTAL EUROPE	3,583,728
Israel	111,343
Jordan	59,428
Lebanon	76,939
Turkey	38,295
ALL OF ASIA	3,527,343
TOTAL	5,773,896

*Immigration statistics from these countries partly combined with USSR total.

From *1985 Statistical yearbook of the immigration and naturalization service,* Washington, DC, 1986, Immigration and Naturalization Service.

large clinics and university centers. The transient nature of populations is increasing not only with immigration but also as multinational businesses develop and the world becomes more of a global village. Therefore we must beware of the person from another continent or culture who presents for care and may carry conditions that require different screening or treatment from that of the resident population. For example, the preventive medicine section of the Cleveland Clinic has assumed responsibility for screening Japanese nationals who are on assignment to the United States for cancer of the stomach, which is common in the Japanese population and for which they are regularly screened in their own country.

In this chapter, the following topics will be covered, concentrating on the conditions that are frequent, of major clinical significance, and that show important differences between populations or regional variation within Europe and the Middle East:

- Developmental defects and congenital anomalies
- Disorders of body systems other than cancer
    - Coronary artery
    - Pulmonary and thoracic
    - Gastrointestinal
    - Renal and genitourinary
    - Neurologic and psychiatric
    - Musculoskeletal
    - Endocrine and metabolic
    - Dermatologic
    - Hematologic
- Cancer
- Summary: Screening and counseling guidelines. Infectious diseases will be covered elsewhere in this book and are not included in this chapter.

DEVELOPMENTAL DEFECTS AND CONGENITAL ANOMALIES
Low birth weight

This is defined as 2500 g or less and is linked to infant mortality and developmental disorders. The incidence is 4% in Scandinavia and is as high as 12% in Southern Europe. Risk factors include prematurity (less than 37 weeks' gestation), young maternal age, parity, socioeconomic group, race, maternal height (shorter mothers have increased risk), obstetric disorders, congenital abnormalities, and illegitimate status. Environmental factors include cigarette smoking and nutrition.[38] The countries of Western Europe have generally low perinatal mortality. Prevention of low birth weight can be improved by planning of pregnancy, detection and treatment of hypertension, smoking cessation or prevention, and nutritional and other antenatal care.

Down syndrome

Several articles from Europe, Asia, and South Africa indicate fairly similar rates of 1.02 to 1.4 per 1000 births.

The frequency of Down syndrome (mostly trisomy 21) increases with maternal age. However, the majority of cases are seen in infants of mothers aged less than 35 years, at least in a Scottish survey. Prevention by abortion of fetuses identified by chorionic villus sampling is employed in high-risk pregnancies.*

Neural tube defects

Neural tube defects are the commonest fatal congenital abnormality. Frequency varies considerably; in the U.K. anencephalus occurs at a rate of 1.4 to 3.4 per 1000 live births, compared with 0.3 to 0.4 in Sweden and Finland. In North America rates are intermediate.[38] Migrant studies, such as those in Irish populations, show changes in the rates among immigrants compared with those of the host country over two or three generations.[71] The prevalence rates in the United Kingdom and Ireland are between 24 and 38 per 10,000 pregnancies (including live births, stillbirths, and abortions).[39] Prevention can be achieved by alpha fetoprotein monitoring and fetal ultrasound. These measures appear to be affecting the termination rate of pregnancies with such defects.

In the eastern Black Sea region of Turkey, there was an increase in neural tube defects and anencephaly after the Chernobyl accident.[68] The region downwind of the Chernobyl site must be closely monitored in the future for hazards, such as thyroid cancer. This appears to have extended as far as the Scandinavian peninsula.

Congenital heart disease

The incidence of all congenital heart disease does not differ greatly between populations and is about 1% of live births, but is higher in aborted fetuses and stillborn infants.[51] There have been reports of regional variation; for instance in Czechoslovakia the incidence varied from 0.515% in western Bohemia to 0.958% in Prague.[91] A Finnish study found increased risk with maternal video display terminal use (Odds Ratio [OR] 1.4); alcohol use (OR 2.0); and exposure to dye, lacquer, and paint (OR 2.9); but not with coffee, tea, cola, smoking, or acetylsalicylic acid use.[102]

Pyloric stenosis

It is more common in Northern Europe (2 to 4 per 1000) than other European areas. The rate may be increasing both in Europe and in the United States.[53,66] The male-female ratio is between 3:1 and 6:1.

Congenital dislocation of the hip

Recent publications from the Netherlands, Czechoslovakia, Poland, and Spain have shown rates of dislocation of around 1%, with female preponderance at 3:1 to 6:1. Similar rates are reported from Britain and the United

---

*References 11, 24, 25, 80, 98, 99.

States. When lesser degrees of subluxation and dysplasia are included, the rate is about 4.5%.* Although screening is also carried out in Algeria, it was found that many patients were lost to follow-up.[29]

DISORDERS OF BODY SYSTEMS OTHER THAN CANCER

Coronary artery disease

Striking variations in the rates of coronary artery disease as well as changes in these rates occurred in the period 1969-1978, and these are shown for many countries in Fig. 35-3. In contrast to major reductions in mortality from coronary artery disease in the United States and Australia, albeit from a very high starting point, other countries have shown either a small decrease, or more disturbingly, an increase. Examples are Scotland, Northern Ireland, England, Wales, and the Irish Republic. In general, mortality from coronary artery disease is high among the European countries, but lower in the south, as exemplified by France and Italy.[41] Recent information from the former USSR indicates that age-adjusted mortality increased by 0.7 per 1000 for men and 0.2 per 1000 for women aged 25 to 64 years between 1960-1970 and 1985. All this increase resulted from increased cardiovascular disease mortality, mostly coronary heart disease. This appears to be the result of the high cardiovascular risk profiles of the population.[30]

Pulmonary and thoracic disease

Cystic fibrosis. Several surveys of cystic fibrosis in northern Europe have shown incidence from 1:1857 live births in Northern Ireland[74] to 1:4760 in Denmark.[75] This Danish study estimated that 3% of that population were heterozygotes. In an Australian study, children of Greek and Italian immigrants had an incidence of about 1:3700; the incidence for children of British immigrants was 1:2021.[1] In Brittany, France, there are substantial variations between neighboring districts of 2.9 to 6.0 per 10,000 live births.[32] According to Nazer et al,[72] cystic fibrosis is said to be rare in Saudi Arabia, but these authors described 13 cases and suggested that greater awareness of the disease is needed.

Sarcoidosis. The epidemiology of sarcoidosis was reviewed by James in 1985.[52] In Europe the overall highest prevalence is reported in Scandinavia, Germany, the UK, Ireland, and Hungary, with 25 to 65 per 100,000 population. By contrast, Italy, Yugoslavia, Poland, France, Spain, and Portugal had rates of 0.2 to 11 per 100,000. Data for Arabia are sparse. A study from Kuwait described 20 patients, all with thoracic involvement. Most notable was the rarity of central nervous system and ocular disease, but this may be the effect of selection.[34] In U.S. blacks, the prevalence is about 80 per 100,000.

*References 38, 63, 81, 86, 103, 104.

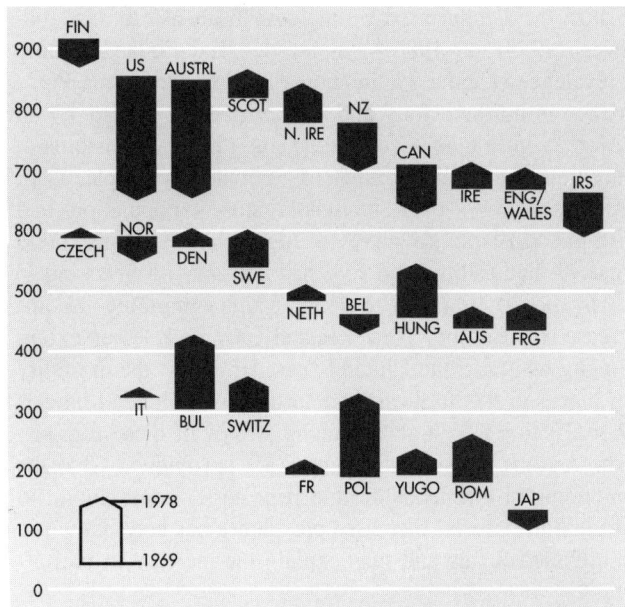

Fig. 35-3. Coronary heart disease motality rates per 100,000 population for men ages 35 to 74 by country (1969 to 1978). Modified from: Friedewald WT: Epidemiology of cardiovascular disease. In *Cecil textbook of medicine,* ed 18, Philadelphia, 1988, WB Saunders.

Familial sarcoidosis has been described in Irish populations,[14,19] with 9.6% of index patients having at least one sibling with sarcoidosis. In London, males and females of British origin have a prevalence of 27 per 100,000. For those of Irish origin, males had a prevalence of 97 and females 213 per 100,000.[52]

The features of sarcoidosis also vary geographically. Erythema nodosum, a feature of this disease, is common in studies from the U.K., occurring in about 30% of cases. In Paris, Geneva, Naples, and New York, erythema nodosum occurred in 6% to 11%. Ocular sarcoidosis varied from 0% to 32% of cases; neurosarcoidosis varied from 0% to 9%.[52] At one time it was suggested that the disease was more frequent in regions with pine forests; further scrutiny has not borne this out in the United States or elsewhere in the world.[27]

Asthma. The prevalence of wheezing and diagnosed asthma has been studied extensively, particularly in northern Europe. The study method has usually been a questionnaire, and some have also used pulmonary function testing. Studies have been done of bronchial responsiveness, showing higher prevalence than asthma, but the significance of these findings is not clear. Several studies with increases in asthma prevalence have shown that these increases seem to be real rather than the result of changing diagnostic patterns. A total review of this literature is outside the scope of this book, and therefore representative studies will be quoted. Prevalence of asthma in South Wales for 12-year-old children rose from 4% to 9%, and history of asthma at any time rose from 6% to 12% between 1973 and 1988.[17] In Sweden and Finland asthma prevalence is about 4% in similar aged children.[13,87] Prevalence in northern Italy and southern France is also 4% to 5%.[21,83] In Prague, Czechoslovakia, a history of asthma at any time was found in 2.3% of a population sample.[105] In Algeria, 1.34% of a household survey population had asthma.[6] In Israel, a survey of high school students found that 9% had asthma and 15% had a history of wheezing.[15]

In the 10 years up to 1986, asthma mortality has increased in Europe, New Zealand, and to a lesser extent among whites in the United States. However, the mortality of blacks in the northeast and north central United States is 7 to 10 times as high as among whites in these regions. The reasons for such differences are not known. Changes in coding or erroneous death certificates are not thought to explain the trends. Increased prevalence has been shown in the United States and may explain the increase in mortality.[84]

Gastrointestinal disease

Peptic ulcer, including gastric ulcer, gastritis, duodenal ulcer, and esophagitis. Information on prevalence and incidence is available for some countries. In Sweden, an autopsy series from Lund, in the south, showed a 5.4% active ulcer rate.[109] In Gothenburg, in the west, the rate of peptic ulcer disease increased with age, the majority occurring in the over-60-year-old population.[92] In Norway, 10.5% prevalence in males and 9.5% prevalence in females were found, with 1% prevalence of asymptomatic ulcer found by endoscopy.[7] There have been changes in the mortality from peptic ulcer in Britain between 1970 and 1985. For gastric ulcer, mortality has fallen except for women aged 65 years or more; for duodenal ulcer, mortality declined for men less than 65 years old but sharply increased for women aged 65 years or more.[9]

Campylobacter pylori was identified in 87% of gastric ulcer and 91% of duodenal ulcer patients in a Swedish study.[42] In Denmark, male bus drivers had twice the frequency of symptoms of ulcer disease (12% vs. 6%) and younger bus drivers had twice the hospital discharge rate for ulcer than the general age-matched male population.[73]

Inflammatory bowel disease

Ulcerative colitis. In northern Europe, the incidence varies from 4.3 per 100,000 population in Stockholm in 1979[69] to 20.3 per 100,000 in the Faroe Islands in 1981-1988.[89] Most reports were between 6 and 13 per 100,000. In the south of Europe, incidence rates were between 0.8 in Catalonia, Spain in 1987[95] and 4.6 in northern France in 1988.[22] In Israel, native-born Jews had the highest incidence. The incidence in all Jews rose from 0.88 to 3.79 in Upper Galilee, being higher in the kibbutz dwellers than others. For Israeli Arabs the incidence was 0.96 per 100,000.[76]

Crohn disease. Rates in northern Europe have risen over the last 20 to 25 years. In recent years, the typical

incidence has been between 4 per 100,000 in Tubingen, Germany[26] and 8.3 per 100,000 in Cardiff, Wales.[90] In southern Europe, the spectrum is between 0.7 per 100,000 in Catalonia and Zagreb[95,106] and 2.7 per 100,000 in Sicily.[23] In Israel, a rate of 3.10 has been reported for 1970-1979,[40] with higher rates for European-American immigrants than those from other areas. Inflammatory bowel disease has a higher frequency among northern Europeans, but it is uncertain how much this is the result of genetic or environmental influences.

Diverticular disease. This condition appears to be a disease of western countries, whereas it is rare in rural Africans.[82] Vegetarian diet also reduces the frequency in western populations.[44]

Celiac disease. Genetic factors have been shown: The presence of HLA B8 is associated with a fivefold to sevenfold relative risk and HLA DR3 with an eightfold to fourteenfold relative risk. The prevalence of celiac disease in European studies varies from 24 to 354 per 100,000. The highest rates are apparently in Austria, Switzerland, Ireland, and Scotland, with low rates in Scandinavia and parts of England.[61] In the United States and Canada the prevalence is 1:3000 to 1:10,000. Celiac disease is rare in blacks and in Japan.[57]

Pancreatitis. The incidence is linked to frequency of cirrhosis and alcohol consumption. Disease is attributed more frequently to alcohol in France (almost 90%) than in the U.K. (less than 5%).[61]

Gallstones. There is a high prevalence in Europe compared with Third-World countries, with prevalence between 30% and 61% in females over the age of 60 years in European studies.[61]

Liver disease: infectious hepatocellular cancer and cirrhosis. The prevalence of liver disease depends on known factors, such as the prevalence of hepatitis B virus infection and alcohol intake. Many cases of cirrhosis in the U.K. are the result of autoimmune liver disease, and cirrhosis is more likely to be attributed to alcohol in some countries.[61] In Trieste, the frequency of cirrhosis was 2.3 times higher in males, corresponding with alcohol intake, whereas hepatitis B infection rates were similar in the sexes.[45] Despite a high alcohol intake, the incidence of cirrhosis on the Island of Lewis, Scotland, is low, suggesting genetics, patterns of drinking, or type of alcohol can play a part in the frequency of alcohol-induced liver disease.[46]

However, autoimmune liver disease may be increasing in frequency or is now identified more accurately in other countries, such as Spain; the reported incidence of 25 per million female population in Spain is similar to that from northern Sweden, with annual incidence in males and females of 13.3 per million, and is greater than in a Canadian study, which found an incidence of 3.26 per million.[12,28,108]

Hemochromatosis is a common genetic disorder leading to liver disease. It is estimated that 10% of the U.S. white population of Northern European ancestry is heterozygous for the hemochromatosis allele. Of all marriages, 1% will be between heterozygotes, and 25% of the offspring will be homozygous. The population frequency of the disease ranges from 3 to 13 per 1000.[36]

Genitourinary disease

Genetic factors. Familial Mediterranean fever (FMF) occurs more frequently among Sephardic Jews, Arabs, and Armenians, probably passed through autosomal recessive inheritance. Renal failure results from amyloidosis.

Recently a gene causing FMF has been mapped to the short arm of chromosome 16.[88] In Israel FMF accounts for 7% of patients requiring dialysis.

One in 10 patients treated for ESRF in Europe, the United States, and Australia has polycystic renal disease.

Inheritance of cystinosis is autosomal recessive; the infantile form, which results in death in the first decade, varies from 1:26,000 in Brittany to 1:326,000 in the rest of France, to 1:150,000 in Switzerland and 1:40,000 in parts of Britain. In parts of Quebec, a high incidence is found, which may result from immigration from Brittany and Normandy. The highest frequency of 1:20,000 is described in North African Jews in Israel.[20]

Drugs and chemicals. In analgesic nephropathy, rates of papillary necrosis vary dramatically, with Australia having a much higher rate of such patients requiring dialysis and transplantation. Of Swiss patients on treatment for renal failure, 18% have drug-induced nephropathy, compared with 1% in the U.K. and 4% in Germany.[20]

Stone disease. Renal stone is a disease of rich nations. Animal protein intake is correlated with renal stone formation. Stones are common in Arabs and Europeans residing in Africa, but blacks seem protected. An increase in the Ruhr district of Germany was secondary to Turkish immigration.[20] My colleagues in preventive medicine, who see many Arabs who travel to the United States for medical examinations, assume that any such patient has a stone, symptomatic or otherwise, because it is so common in their experience.

Bladder stones are more common in North and Central Africa, the Middle East, Iran, Pakistan, Burma, Thailand, and Indonesia. In contrast to renal stone, the incidence is inversely related to protein intake.[20]

Neurologic and psychiatric disease

Multiple sclerosis (MS). Multiple sclerosis is largely a disease of whites. Information from the 1950s gave vari-

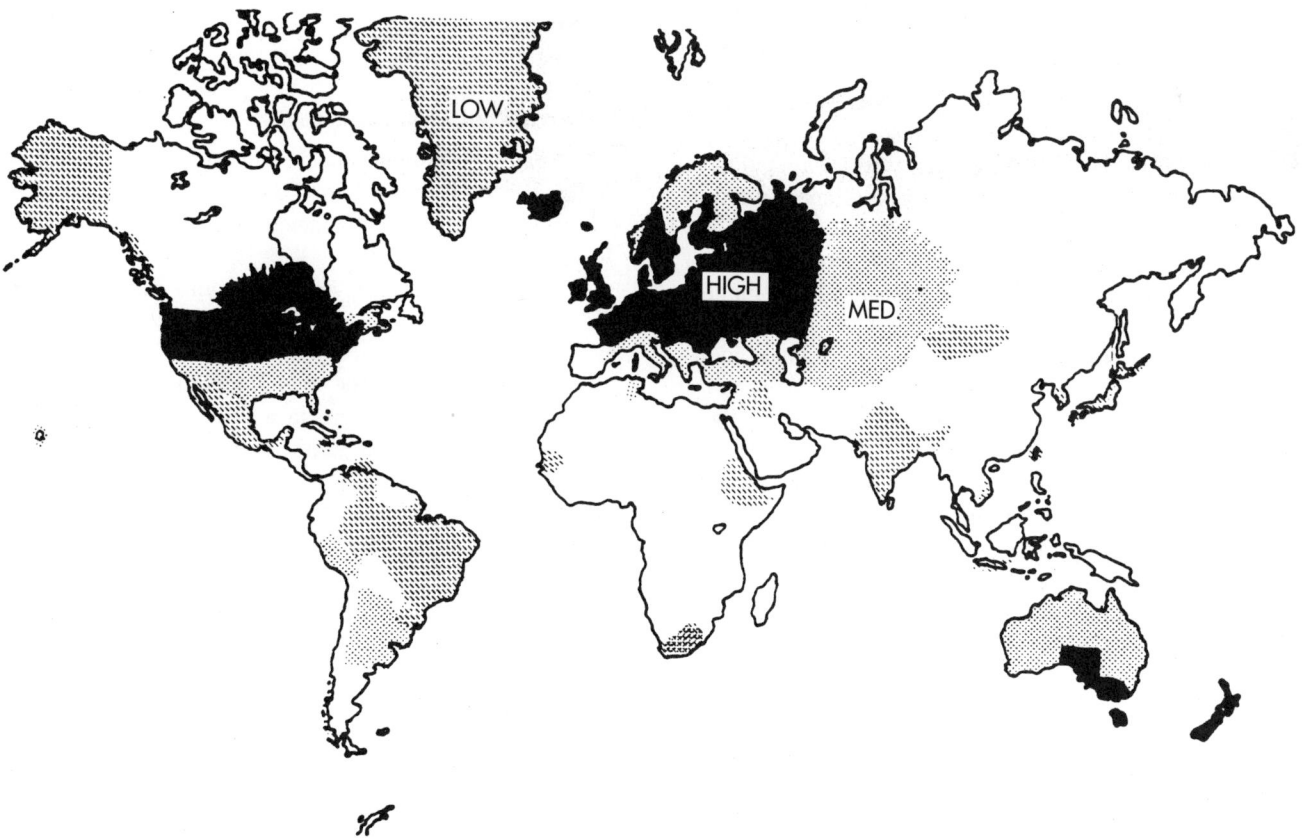

Fig. 35-4. Multiple sclerosis: worldwide distribution as of 1980 according to high *(black)*, medium *(dots)*, and low *(diagonal dashes)* zones of prevalence or frequency. Open areas are without data. South American frequencies are tentative. Modified from Kurtzke JF: *The Oxford textbook of public health*, Oxford, 1984, Oxford University Press.

able death rates from MS, the highest being in Scotland and Ireland (about 3/100,000). Lower rates were generally found in Greece, Italy, Portugal, and northern Scandinavia (about 1/100,000). High prevalence rates exist in Northern and Central Europe, including the former USSR, and the Northern United States and Southern Canada (equal to or greater than 30/100,000 population). The map in Fig. 35-4 illustrates the distribution. Age at migration is important, with those migrating from high-risk to low-risk areas before the age of 15 acquiring the lower risk of their new residence. Whether young immigrants to high-risk areas acquire a greater risk of MS is unclear. Genetic studies including HLA types have shown increased A3, B7, DW2, and DrW2 in Europeans.[60]

Parkinsonism. High death rates are reported in the U.K., Ireland, Belgium, the Netherlands, France, Switzerland, Israel, Uruguay, and New Zealand. Estimated prevalence is 2/1000 white population.[60]

Creutzfeldt-Jakob disease. Jews of Libyan origin have a high frequency, shown to be genetically determined.[59] Zilber et al. found an incidence of 43 per 1 million among Libyan-born Jews, but 0.9 per million in the rest of the population.[113]

Huntington's chorea. Whites have a higher frequency than nonwhites. Other information indicates little variation between Europe, the United States, and Australia.

Musculoskeletal disease

Most rheumatic disorders do not show striking variations in prevalence between populations.

Ankylosing spondylitis. The HLA B27 association in whites is stronger than in black, Japanese, and American Indian populations.

Rheumatoid arthritis. Masi and Medsger[65] report a variable prevalence with the highest (3%) in Finnish whites and the lowest (0.1%) in South African blacks. There is little information about geographic variation in juvenile rheumatoid arthritis.

Systemic lupus erythematosus. Studies in Sweden[65,77] and Finland[50] showed prevalence in hospital and clinic between 2.3 and 39 per 100,000. Jonsson et al.[56] reported a higher incidence in the population aged 55 to 64 and 65 to 74, approximately 7.5 per 100,000 per year. Studies comparing whites with other races have been performed in Hawaii and New Zealand and showed prevalence in whites of 5.8 and 14.6/100,000. Among Polynesians in New Zealand the rate was 50.6/100,000.[48,94]

Systemic sclerosis. The annual incidence of systemic sclerosis does not show major variations between different populations. The rate quoted for a Czechoslovakian district was 7/1,000,000 per year. In the United States rates have varied between 2.3 and 12.[64]

Gout. The frequency is closely related to population serum uric acid levels, which are probably the result of heritable and environmental effects. The annual incidence in Great Britain was 25 to 35/100,000 per year. The prev-

alence in Gothenburg, Sweden was 1.3% in an elderly population. Usually there is a male predominance.[64]

Vasculitis. The most common entity is temporal arteritis. Studies in Denmark and Sweden have shown annual incidence rates in the population over 50 years of age of temporal arteritis and polymyalgia rheumatica of 28.6 to 76.6/100,000. Biopsy-proven temporal arteritis in Scotland was less frequent than in Gothenburg, Sweden (annual incidence 4.2 and 16.8/100,000 over age 50 years).[64]

Behçet's disease. The highest prevalence is found in the Eastern Mediterranean and Japan, where the prevalence is 1:1000. In North America and Western and Northern Europe the disease appears to be fairly rare.[79]

Paget's disease. The epidemiology of Paget's disease has been reviewed[3,4]; Britain has the highest prevalence with 5.4% of the population aged 55 years or more affected. Higher rates were found in Lancashire (in Northwestern England). Lower rates are found in the rest of Europe, with the lowest rates in Sweden and Norway.[33] In Jerusalem 1% of Jews and no Arabs were found to have the disease.[10] The amount of clinically significant disease is much less, estimated at 0.25% of all cases of Paget's disease in a population of 4 million in Germany.[112]

Osteoporosis. Women of Northern European extraction have a higher incidence of osteoporosis.[78] White females, and hence those of European extraction, have a lower bone mineral density of the radius, hip, spine, and back than black women.[62]

Endocrine and metabolic disease

Diabetes. Insulin-dependent diabetes mellitus has a higher incidence in northern Europe and is increasing. It has been estimated that the incidence could double in 20 to 30 years.[8]

Vitamin D deficiency. Reports from France and Algeria indicate that this is a persistent problem, related to socioeconomic, cultural, or religious factors.[43]

Iodine deficiency. The WHO reports that there is a moderate deficiency, severe in a few individuals, in Europe. Subclinical hypothyroidism, goiter, and the consequent mental deficiency, hearing loss, and short stature result.[31]

Phenylketonuria. Screening for iodine deficiency and phenylketonuria (PKU) in the Basque region of Spain was analyzed by Mugarra Bidea and Cabases Hita.[70] The cost per child with mental handicap prevented was estimated at 3300 pesetas. In Greece, G6PD deficiency was added to the PKU screening test at an additional cost of $0.90 per test. This cost was considered justified in high-frequency populations and because the clinical manifestations of the disease are serious.[67]

Dermatologic disease

Nodular cystic acne is 10 times as common among white males aged 15 to 21 years as among black males of the same age. Psoriasis has a high prevalence in Scandinavia and Northern Europe, with up to 4% prevalence in the Faroe Islands. Psoriasis is less frequent in Asia and Africa.[97]

Hematopoietic disease

A number of hereditary diseases are more common in the Mediterranean and Middle East, compared with the rest of Europe. These include sickle cell disease and the thalassemias; glucose 6 phosphate dehydrogenase deficiency; and heavy-chain disease (alpha-chain disease). Pyruvate kinase deficiency is more common with Northern European ancestry.[49] Pernicious anemia has a high prevalence in Scandinavians and other northern Europeans.[2]

CANCER

Information about the incidence of cancer in many countries is available from the World Health Organization publication *Cancer Incidence in Five Continents volume V,* which uses data from certain cancer registries throughout the world.[18] Using this information, a summary of the incidence of major neoplasms is displayed in Table 35-3, comparing the white population of the United States with the population of the European regions. A report from Jensen et al.[54] uses cancer incidence and mortality data from European Community countries to present a recent overview of cancer in the community. Information from some countries in Eastern Europe and Middle Eastern countries is limited because of the lack of registries.

Some generalizations are possible regarding cancer incidence in Europe. In 1986-1988 overall death rates from cancer in males were highest in Hungary, Czechoslovakia, Luxembourg, Belgium, France, Scotland, the Netherlands, and Poland, with rates over 200 per 100,000 population, compared with 163.2 in the United States and 170.6 in Canada. For females, death rates were highest for Denmark, Scotland, Hungary, England, Wales, Ireland, and Czechoslovakia (above 119.9 per 100,000). However, these rates are more comparable to the United States (109.7/100,000) and Canada (111.5/100,000). The most common cancers have similar incidences in Europe and in the United States. In Czechoslovakia, rates of cancer have been increasing, particularly in males, and especially for lung, "other skin," prostate, colon, and rectal cancer. Rates for women also are increasing for breast, "other skin," ovary, and corpus uteri. The incidence of stomach cancer in men and women, cervix in women, and lip in men is declining.[35]

In the former USSR, lung, stomach, breast, and cervical cancer are reported to have the highest incidence and mortality.[111] Stomach and cervical cancer are decreasing; the others increasing.

Lung cancer

Lung cancer is very common in males, and in females it is increasing in several countries. However, several countries in Europe have a large discrepancy between male and lower female deaths from lung cancer, including Belgium, France, Italy, Czechoslovakia, Finland, Germany, Luxembourg, and the former USSR.

Breast cancer

Breast cancer does show some variation, being more common in the northern European countries, compared with many southern and eastern European countries. It has been suggested that vitamin D may play a part in reducing the risk of breast cancer. Gorham et al.[47] also found a statistically significant negative association between sunlight energy striking the ground and breast cancer incidence in the former USSR. Socioeconomic status and breast cancer were positively correlated in this study.

Cancer of the mouth, pharynx, and esophagus

These cancers are greatly increased in areas of France, thought to be the result of smoking and alcohol intake. Pottier et al. reported that poor housing and manual work were strongly associated with the esophageal cancer risk.[85]

Stomach cancer

Death rates in Europe per 100,000 males are highest in the former USSR, Poland, Portugal, and Hungary. In the United States the rate is 5.3 and in Japan 37.9 per 100,000. Fig. 35-5 summarizes recent statistics.[5] Within countries there is variation. In the north of Italy gastric cancer is more frequent than in the south. Lower social class and rural residence were associated with higher rates of gastric cancer. Dietary factors have been implicated.[16] In Montreal, the population of Italian descent had higher rates of stomach cancer than those of other ancestry (mainly French and British).[101] The Republic of San Marino, a small independent country within Italy, has a high incidence of, and mortality from, gastric cancer, with male age-adjusted death rates of 72.3/100,000; 9% of all deaths and 33% of cancer deaths were from this cause in 1969-1983. A screening program of first-degree relatives of San Marinese gastric cancer patients revealed a similar frequency of gastric metaplasia in those living in Detroit (52%) and in San Marino (36%), although whether there is an early environmental cause or a genetic cause is uncertain.[93]

Colon and rectal cancer

These are more common in Central and Northern Europe than in the south. In Austria bowel cancer appears to be a special problem in both sexes, representing 14.8% of all malignancies.[107]

Prostate cancer

In Europe, prostate cancer is most common in Norway and Sweden. The incidence is lower among Asian races.[20] U.S. blacks have a high incidence, whereas Africans do not.

Table 35-3. Cancer incidence in the United States and Europe; age-adjusted incidence per 100,000 population per year

Site	U.S. whites	Northern Europe	Southern Europe	Eastern Europe
Lip, male	1.6-5.3	S	Italy 14.9 Spain 10.7	Hungary 14.0 Romania 13.2 Poland 10.5
Mouth, male	5.4-8.0	Switzerland 14.5	France 14.2-30.8	S
Oropharynx, male	2.7-4.1	S	France 13.1-30.7 Slovenia 10.1	S
Hypopharynx, male	1.9-3.3	Switzerland 14.5	France 11.7-36.3	S
Esophagus, male	3.6-6.2	Switzerland 14.5	France 18.0-54.3	S
Stomach	6.8-12.8	Iceland 34.4	Italy 49.9 Slovenia 41.1 Spain 19.8-38.7	Poland 60.3 Hungary 46.1 Romania 43.3 Czechoslovakia 40.1
Colon	26.3-31	Former Federal Republic of Germany 23.7 Ireland 25.6 Netherlands 23.6 Switzerland 23.7 UK 30.6	France 27.1 Italy 22.7	Czechoslovakia 23.6
Rectum	11.4-19.7	Former Federal Republic of Germany 23.1	S	Hungary 26.3 Czechoslovakia 21.5
Liver	0.7-3.3	Switzerland 12.5	Italy 11.4 France 10.9	Hungary 12.0 Romania 9.8
Gallbladder	1.5-2.7	S	S	Hungary 9.5 Poland 8.5 Czechoslovakia 7.3
Larynx, male	10.0-15.4	S	France 24.4 Italy 30.8 Spain 33.4	Poland 23.3 Czechoslovakia 21.8 Hungary 20.7 Romania 20.4
Lung, bronchus, male	81.1-120.8	UK 120.7 Netherlands 109.4 Switzerland 100.6	Italy 117.0	Czechoslovakia 111.7 Poland 101.9
Lung, bronchus, female	41.5-54.9	S	S	S
Melanoma, skin	8.1-23	Scandanavia 20.4 Switzerland 16.3 Ireland 13.0	S	S
Breast, female	125.8-163.2	S	S	S
Cervix uteri	12.7-17.6	Former German Democratic Republic 51.3 Former Federal Republic of Germany 41.4 Denmark 37.8 UK 36.2 Norway 32.5	France 34.2	Slovakia 53
Corpus uteri	18.4-24.2	S	S	Poland 43.4 Hungary 38.8 Romania 37.9
Ovary	20.2-24.2	S	S	S
Prostate	26.7-34.8	S	S	S
Testis	4.8-7.1	S	S	S
Bladder	22-27.7	Switzerland, Basel 32.3 Denmark 37.8 UK 36.2	Italy 35.6 France 28.6 Spain 28.1	S
Other urinary	11.8-16	S	S	S
Brain	7.4-13.7	S	S	S
Thyroid	3.2-10.69	Iceland 24.4	S	S

From Muir C et al, editors: *Cancer incidence in five continents,* vol 5, Lyon, 1987, International Agency for Research on Cancer.
S, similar to U.S. whites.

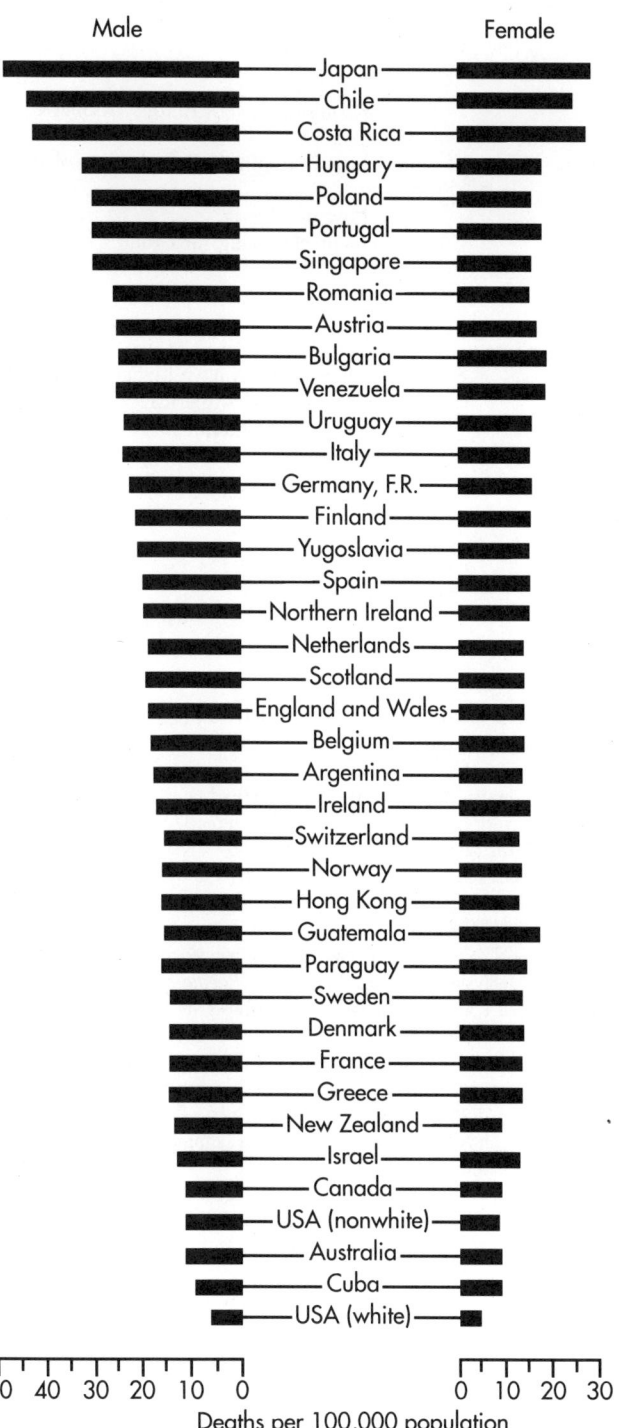

Male   Female

Japan
Chile
Costa Rica
Hungary
Poland
Portugal
Singapore
Romania
Austria
Bulgaria
Venezuela
Uruguay
Italy
Germany, F.R.
Finland
Yugoslavia
Spain
Northern Ireland
Netherlands
Scotland
England and Wales
Belgium
Argentina
Ireland
Switzerland
Norway
Hong Kong
Guatemala
Paraguay
Sweden
Denmark
France
Greece
New Zealand
Israel
Canada
USA (nonwhite)
Australia
Cuba
USA (white)

50 40 30 20 10 0   0 10 20 30
Deaths per 100,000 population

Fig. 35-5. Age-adjusted death rates for malignant neoplasm of the stomach. Modified from Barkin JS: What's new in stomach cancer?, *Pat Care* 26:22, 1992.

Bladder cancer

The European community (EC) statistics do not show any major differences between countries. In the United States it is more common in white than black residents. Schistosomiasis *(S. hematobium)* infection is implicated in bladder cancer, with high rates in Africa and the Middle East, compared with Europe and North America.[20]

Melanoma of the skin

The highest rates are found in the northern countries, particularly Scandinavia. This is probably the result of increased susceptibility in the population and high levels of exposure to available sunlight.

Liver cancer

Greece, Italy, Spain, and France have higher incidence and mortality than the average for the EC in men, and the same is true in women except for France.

Cancer of the cervix uteri

EC countries with a higher-than-average risk included Denmark, the U.K., Germany, Portugal, Italy, and Belgium.

Cancer of the corpus uteri

The highest incidence and mortality were in Luxembourg, Denmark, Italy, and Belgium.

Cancer of the ovary

The highest incidence and mortality were in Denmark, the Netherlands, Germany, Luxembourg, and the U.K.

SUMMARY
Specific screening and counseling guidelines to be attached to a standard health history questionnaire

Among noncancerous conditions considered here, screening and prevention have the greatest scope for coronary artery disease. Several conditions have notable geographic disparities, which can be useful in diagnosis and to increase awareness, because some appear to be relatively uncommon in North America, or largely confined to the population of European or Middle Eastern extraction. Table 35-4 summarizes many of these conditions.

Cancer screening

Stomach cancer screening should be implemented for the highest risk populations, particularly the San Marinese. Italy, Hungary, Poland, Austria, Germany, and Spain have higher-than-average risk, and individuals from these countries may benefit from screening; however, it is not likely that this will be as effective as in Japan, where intensive screening is carried out because of the extremely high rate of gastric cancer.

Head and neck cancer in French and Swiss males is common, and is related to lower socioeconomic class.

Table 35-4. Conditions of high relative frequency in Europe and the Middle East

Condition	Regions of high frequency	Comments
Low birth weight	Southern Europe	
Neural tube defects	Britain and Ireland	
Congenital pyloric stenosis	Northern Europe	
Coronary artery disease	Britain, Ireland, Finland	Rising in Eastern Europe, former USSR
Cystic fibrosis	Britain and Ireland	
Sarcoidosis	Scandinavia, UK, Germany, Hungary, Ireland (familial)	Low in Southern Europe and Poland
Asthma	Britain, Israel	Low in Algeria
Inflammatory bowel disease	Northern Europe	Incidence rising for Crohn's disease
Celiac disease	Ireland, Scotland, Austria, and Switzerland	
Hemochromatosis	Northern Europe	
Familial Mediterranean fever	Sephardic Jews, Arabs, Armenians	
Renal stone	Arabs of North Africa	Richer nations have higher incidence
Multiple sclerosis	Northern Europe	Also in North America
Paget's disease	Britain	Local concentrations
Osteoporosis	Northern Europe	
Diabetes, insulin dependent	Northern Europe	Increasing
Vitamin D deficiency	North Africa and France	
Pernicious anemia	Northern Europe	
Sickle cell, G6PD deficiency, thalassemia	Southern Europe, Middle East	

Special attention to the oral, pharyngeal, and head and neck examination is prudent. There should be a high index of suspicion for esophageal, pharyngeal, and laryngeal cancer among smokers and alcohol users.

Melanoma of the skin in residents of northern Europe and their descendants should be preventable by sun avoidance and use of barriers. Careful examination at intervals and self-examination are clearly wise, as survival is linked to the depth of the tumor. Colon and rectal cancer appear to be more common in the Austrians. In North America there is already considerable awareness of screening for this common cancer in the general population, but more complete screening and careful attention to family history in Austrians may be beneficial. Breast, cervical, testicular, thyroid, prostate, and ovarian cancer screening should probably be carried out according to usual practices in the United States and Canada.

REFERENCES

1. Allan JL, Phelan PD: Incidence of cystic fibrosis in ethnic Italians and Greeks and in Australians of predominantly British origin, *Acta Paediatr Scand* 74:286, 1985.
2. Babior BM: The megaloblastic anemias. In Williams WJ et al, editors: *Hematology,* ed 4, New York, 1990, McGraw Hill.
3. Barker DJ: The epidemiology of Paget's disease of bone, *Br Med Bull* 40:396, 1984.
4. Barker DJ: The epidemiology of Paget's disease, *Metab Bone Dis Relat Res* 3:231, 1981.
5. Barkin JS et al: What's new in stomach cancer, *Pat Care* 26:22, 1992.
6. Belhocine M, Ait-Khaled N: Prevalence of asthma in a region of Algeria, *Bull Int Union Tuberc Lung Dis* 66:91, 1991.
7. Bernersen B et al: Towards a true prevalence of peptic ulcer: the Srreisa gastrointestinal disorder study, *Gut* 31(9):989, 1990 Sep.
8. Bingley PJ, Gale EA: Rising incidence of IDDM in Europe, *Diabetes Care* 12:289, 1989.
9. Bloom BS, Fendrick AM, and Ramsey SD: Changes in peptic ulcer and gastritis/duodenitis in Great Britain, 1970-1985, *J Clin Gastroenterol* 12:100, 1990.
10. Bloom RA et al: Prevalence of Paget's disease of bone in hospital patients in Jerusalem: an epidemiologic study. *Isr J Med Sci* 21:954, 1985.
11. Boo NY et al: Maternal age-specific incidence of Down's syndrome in Malaysian neonates, *J Singapore Paediatr Soc* 31:138, 1989.
12. Borda F et al: Primary biliary cirrhosis in Navarra, *Ann Med Interne* 6:63, 1989.
13. Braback L, Kalvesten L, and Sundstrom G: Prevalence of bronchial asthma among schoolchildren in a Swedish district, *Acta Paediatr Scand* 77:821, 1988.
14. Brennan NJ et al: High prevalence of familial sarcoidosis in an Irish population, *Thorax* 39:14, 1984.
15. Brook U: The prevalence of bronchial asthma among high school pupils in Holon (Israel), *J Trop Pediatr* 37:176, 1991.
16. Buiatti E et al: A case control study of gastric cancer and diet in Italy, *Int J Cancer* 44:611, 1989.
17. Burr ML et al: Changes in asthma prevalence: two surveys 15 years apart, *Arch Dis Child* 64:1452, 1989.
18. *Cancer incidence in five continents,* vol 5, Muir C et al, editors, Lyon, 1987, International Agency for Research on Cancer.
19. Carmichael AJ, Tan CY, and Smith AG: Familial sarcoidosis: high ethnic prevalence, *Acta Derm Venereol* 69:531, 1989.
20. Challah S, Wing AJ: The epidemiology of genito-urinary disease. In Holland WW et al, editors: *The Oxford textbook of public health,* Oxford, 1984, Oxford University Press.
21. Charpin D, Vervloet D, and Charpin J: Epidemiology of asthma in western Europe, *Allergy* 43:481, 1988.
22. Colombel JF et al: Incidence of inflammatory bowel disease in the Nord-Pas-de-Calais region and the Somme area of France in 1988, *Gastroenterol Clin Biol* 14:614, 1990.

23. Cottone M et al: Epidemiology of Crohn's disease in Sicily: a hospital incidence study from 1987 to 1989. "The Sicilian Study Group of Inflammatory Bowel Disease," *Eur J Epidemiol* 7:636, 1991.

24. Cuckle H, Nanchahal K, and Wald N: Birth prevalence of Down's syndrome in England and Wales, *Prenat Diagn* 11:29, 1991.

25. Czeizel E: Some epidemiological characteristics of Down's syndrome in Hungary, *Acta Morphol Hung* 36:63, 1988.

26. Daiss W, Scheurlen M, and Malchow H: Epidemiology of inflammatory bowel disease in the county of Tubingen (West Germany), *Scand J Gastroenterol Suppl* 170:39, 1989.

27. Daniel TM: Sarcoidosis. In Baum GL, Wolinsky E, editors: *Textbook of pulmonary diseases,* ed 3, Boston, 1983, Little Brown.

28. Danielsson A, Boqvist L, and Uddenfeldt P: Epidemiology of primary biliary cirrhosis in a defined rural population in the northern part of Sweden, *Hepatology* 11:458, 1990.

29. Daoud A, Saighi-Bouaouina A: Neonatal diagnosis of hip luxation, *Chir Pediatr* 31:305, 1990.

30. Deev AD, Oganov RG: Trends and determinants of cardiovascular mortality in the Soviet Union, *Int J Epidemiol* 18(3 suppl 1):S137, 1989.

31. Delange F, Burgi H: Iodine deficiency disorders in Europe, *Bull WHO* 67:317, 1989.

32. Demenais F et al: Incidence of cystic fibrosis in Brittany, *Rev Epidemiol Sante Publique* 27:51, 1979.

33. Detheridge FM, Guyer PB, and Barker DJ: European distribution of Paget's disease of bone, *Br Med J* 285:1005, 1982.

34. Diab SM et al: Sarcoidosis in Arabs: the clinical profile of 20 patients and review of the literature, *Sarcoidosis* 8:56, 1991.

35. Dimitrova E et al: Trends and patterns in cancer incidence in Czechoslovakia, 1968-1985, *Neoplasma* 36:245, 1989.

36. Edwards CQ, Griffen LM, and Kushner JP: Southern Blood Symposium: an update on selected aspects of hemochromatosis, *Am J Med Sci* 300:245, 1990.

37. Ekbom A et al: The epidemiology of inflammatory bowel disease: a large, population-based study in Sweden. *Gastroenterology* 100:350, 1991.

38. Elwood JM, Madeley RJ: Developmental defects. In Holland WW et al, editors: *The Oxford textbook of public health,* Oxford, 1984, Oxford University Press.

39. EUROCAT working group: Prevalence of neural tube defects in 20 regions of Europe and the impact of prenatal diagnosis, 1980-1986, *J Epidemiol Comm Health* 45:52, 1991.

40. Fireman Z et al: Epidemiology of Crohn's disease in the Jewish population of central Israel, 1970-1980, *Am J Gastroenterol* 4:255, 1989.

41. Friedwald WT: Epidemiology of cardiovascular disease. In Wyngaarden JB, Smith LH, editors: *Cecil textbook of medicine,* ed 18, Philadelphia, 1988, Saunders.

42. Gad A et al: Campylobacter pylori and gastroduodenal ulcer disease. A prospective study in a Swedish population, *Scand J Gastroenterol Suppl* 167:81, 1989.

43. Garabedian M, Ben-Mekhbi H: Deficiency rickets: the current situation in France and Algeria, *Pediatrie* 44:259, 1989.

44. Gear JSS et al: Symptomatic diverticular disease and intake of dietary fibre, *Lancet* 1:511, 1979.

45. Giarelli L et al: Occurrence of liver cirrhosis among autopsies in Trieste, *IARC Scientific Publications,* Lyon 112:37, 1991.

46. Goodall JA, Bryan C: The low incidence of alcoholic cirrhosis in the islands of Lewis and Harris, *Scott Med J* 33:229, 1988.

47. Gorham ED, Garland FC, and Garland CF: Sunlight and breast cancer incidence in the USSR, *Int J Epidemiol* 19:820, 1990.

48. Hart HH, Grigor RR, and Caughey DE: Ethnic differences in the prevalence of systemic lupus erythematosus, *Ann Rheum Dis* 42:529, 1983.

49. Heath CW, Evatt BL: Haematopoietic diseases. In Holland WW et al, editors: *The Oxford textbook of public health,* Oxford, 1984, Oxford University Press.

50. Helve T: Prevalence and mortality rates of systemic lupus erythematosus and causes of death in SLE patients in Finland, *Scand J Rheumatol* 14:43, 1985.

51. Hoffman JI: Congenital heart disease: incidence and inheritance, *Pediatr Clin North Am* 37:25, 1990.

52. James DG, Williams WJ: Sarcoidosis and other granulomatous disorders. In Smith LH, editor: *Major problems in internal medicine,* vol 24, Philadelphia, 1985, Saunders.

53. Jedd MB et al: Trends in infantile hypertrophic pyloric stenosis in Olmsted County, Minnesota, 1950-1984, *Paediatr Perinat Epidemiol* 2:148, 1988.

54. Jensen OM et al: Cancer in the European community and its member states, *Eur J Cancer* 26:1167, 1990.

55. Johns SB: *The ethnic almanac,* Garden City, NY, 1981, Dolphin Books.

56. Jonsson H et al: Estimating the incidence of systemic lupus erythematosus in a defined population using multiple resources of retrieval, *Br J Rheumatol* 29:185, 1990.

57. Kagonoff MF: Celiac disease. In Yamada T, editor: *Textbook of gastroenterology,* Philadelphia, 1991, Lippincott.

58. Kildebo S et al: The incidence of ulcerative colitis in Northern Norway from 1983 to 1986. The Northern Norwegian Gastroenterology Society, *Scand J Gastroenterol* 25:890, 1990.

59. Korczyn AD: Creuzfeld-Jacob disease among Libyan Jews, *Eur J Epidemiol* 7:490, 1991.

60. Kurtzke JF: Neurological system. In Holland WW et al, editors: *The Oxford textbook of public health,* Oxford, 1984, Oxford University Press.

61. Langman MJS, Logan RFA: Gastrointestinal disease. In Holland WW et al, editors: *The textbook of public health,* Oxford, 1984, Oxford University Press.

62. Liel Y et al: The effects of race and body habitus on bone mineral density of the radius, hip, and spine in premenopausal women, *J Clin Endocrinol Metab* 66:1247, 1988.

63. Martin Sanz AJ et al: Risk factors in 130 children suspected with hip dysplasia; *Ann Esp Pediatr* 35:409, 1991.

64. Masi AT, Medsger TA: Epidemiology of the rheumatic diseases. In McCarthy DJ, editor: *Arthritis and allied conditions,* ed 11, Philadelphia, 1989, Lea and Febiger.

65. Masi AT: Clinical epidemiologic perspective of systemic lupus erythematosus. In: *Epidemiology of the rheumatic diseases. Proceedings of the Fourth International Conference,* National Institutes of Health, New York, 1984, Gower Medical.

66. Mason PF: Increasing infantile hypertrophic pyloric stenosis? Experience in an overseas military hospital, *J R Coll Surg Edinb* 36:293, 1991.

67. Missiou-Tsagaraki S: Screening for glucose-6-phosphate dehydrogenase deficiency as a preventive measure: prevalence among 1,286,000 Greek newborn infants, *J Pediatr* 119:293, 1991.

68. Mocan H et al: Changing incidence of anencephaly in the eastern Black Sea region of Turkey and Chernobyl, *Paediatr Perinat Epidemiol* 4:264, 1990.

69. Monsen U: Inflammatory bowel disease. An epidemiological and genetic study, *Acta Chir Scand Suppl* 559:1, 1990.

70. Mugarra Bidea I, Cabases Hita JM: Cost benefit analysis of the early detection for metabolic diseases in the autonomous basque community, *Gac Sanit* 4:140, 1990.

71. Naggan L, MacMahon B: Ethnic differences in the prevalence of anencephaly and spina bifida in Boston, Massachusets, *N Engl J Med* 227:1119, 1967.

72. Nazer H et al: Cystic fibrosis in Saudi Arabia, *Eur J Pediatr* 148:330, 1989.

73. Netterstrom B, Juel K: Peptic ulcer among urban bus drivers in Denmark, *Scand J Soc Med* 18:97, 1990.

74. Nevin GB, Nevin NC, and Redmond AO: Cystic fibrosis in Northern Ireland, *J Med Genet* 16:122, 1979.

75. Nielsen OH et al: Cystic fibrosis in Denmark 1945 to 1985. An analysis of incidence, mortality and influence of centralized treatment on survival, *Acta Paediatr Scand* 77:836, 1988.

76. Niv Y et al: Incidence and prevalence of ulcerative colitis in the upper Galilee, Northern Israel, 1967-1986, *Am J Gastroenterol* 85:1580, 1990.

77. Nived O, Sturfelt G, and Wollheim F: Systemic lupus erythematosus in an adult population in southern Sweden: incidence, prevalence and validity of ARA revised classification criteria, *Br J Rheumatol* 24:147, 1985.

78. Nordin BEC: International patterns of osteoporosis, *Clin Orthop* 45:17, 1966.

79. O'Duffy JD: Behcet's disease. In Kelley WN et al, editors: *Textbook of rheumatology*, Philadelphia, 1981, Saunders.

80. Op't Hof J, Venter PA, and Louw M: Down's syndrome in South Africa—incidence, maternal age and utilisation of prenatal diagnosis, *S Afr Med J* 79:213, 1991.

81. Padilla Esteban ML et al: Incidence of congenital hip dislocation in 40,243 live births (I), *Ann Esp Pediatr* 33:535, 1990.

82. Painter NS, Burkitt DP: Diverticular disease of the colon. A deficiency disease of western civilisation, *Br Med J* 2:450, 1971.

83. Paoletti P et al: Prevalence of asthma and asthma symptoms in a general population sample of north Italy, *Eur Respir J Suppl* 6:527s, 1989.

84. Pierson WE, Sly RM: Epidemiology and prevention of asthma mortality, *J Respir Dis Suppl* S49, June, 1989.

85. Pottier D et al: Esophageal cancer at the department of Calvados. Geographic and social inequality factors, *Bull Cancer (Paris)* 76:1111, 1989.

86. Poul J, Fait M: Early therapy of congenital hip dislocation and ultrasonic studies of clinically positive cases—results of a prospective epidemiological study in Brunn, *Z Orthop* 129:336, 1991.

87. Poysa L et al: Asthma, allergic rhinitis and atopic eczema in Finnish children and adolescents, *Allergy* 46:161, 1991.

88. Pras E et al: Mapping a gene causing familial Mediterranean fever to the short arm of chromosome 16, *N Engl J Med* 326:1509, 1992.

89. Roin F, Roin J: Inflammatory bowel disease of the Faroe Islands, 1981-1988. A prospective epidemiologic study: primary report, *Scand J Gastroenterol Suppl* 170:44, 1989.

90. Rose JD et al: Cardiff Crohn's disease jubilee: the incidence over 50 years, *Gut* 29:346, 1988.

91. Samanek M et al: Regional differences in the prevalence of congenital heart defects, *Cesk Pediatr* 46:65, 1991.

92. Schoon IM et al: Incidence of peptic ulcer disease in Gothenburg, 1985, *Br Med I* 299:1131, 1989.

93. Schuman BM et al: Gastric cancer in San Marinese and their first degree relatives in San Marino and the United States, *Gastrointest Endosc* 33:224, 1987.

94. Serdula MK, Rhoads GG: Frequency of systemic lupus erythematosus in different ethnic groups in Hawaii, *Arthritis Rheum* 22:328, 1979.

95. Sola Lamoglia R et al: Chronic inflammatory intestinal disease in Catalonia (Barcelona and Gerona), *Rev Esp Enferm Apar Dig* 81:7, 1992.

96. Spector RE: *Cultural diversity in health and disease*, East Norwalk, Conn, 1991, Appleton and Lange.

97. Stern RS: The epidemiology of cutaneous disease. In Fitzpatrick T et al, editors: *Dermatology in general medicine*, ed 3, New York, 1987, McGraw Hill.

98. Stoll C et al: Epidemiology of Down syndrome in 118,265 consecutive births, *Am J Med Genet Suppl* 7:79, 1990.

99. Stone DH, Rosenberg K, and Womersley J: *Paediatr Perinat Epidemiol* 3:278, 1989.

100. Szulc W: The frequency of occurrence of congenital dysplasia of the hip in Poland, *Clin Orthop* (272):100, 1991.

101. Terracini B, Siemiatycki J, and Richardson L: Cancer incidence and risk factors among Montreal residents of Italian origin, *Int J Epidemiol* 19:491, 1990.

102. Tikkanen J et al: Cardiovascular malformations and maternal exposure to video display terminals during pregnancy, *Eur J Epidemiol* 6:61, 1990.

103. Tomas V: Incidence and treatment of congenital dysplasia of the hip joint in the Bardejov District over the 5-year-period 1984-1988, *Acta Chir Orthop Traumatol Cech* 56:502, 1989.

104. Valdivieso Garcia JL et al: Seasonal incidence of congenital hip dislocation. A risk factor, *An Esp Pediatr* 31:567, 1989.

105. Vondra V et al: Epidemiology of bronchial asthma and bronchial hyperreactivity, *Cas Lek Cesk* 129:714, 1990.

106. Vucelic B et al: Ulcerative colitis in Zagreb, Yugoslavia: incidence and prevalence 1980-1989, *Int J Epidemiol* 20:1043, 1991.

107. Weiss W: Colorectal cancer-epidemiologic aspects, *Wien Med Wochenschr* 138:281, 1988.

108. Witt-Sullivan H et al: The demography of primary biliary cirrhosis in Ontario, Canada, *Hepatology* 12:98, 1990.

109. Wroblewski M: Peptic ulcer in geriatric long-term care medicine, *Aging* 1:77, 1989.

110. Zaridze DG, Basieva TH: Incidence of cancer of the lung, stomach, breast and cervix in the USSR: patterns and trends, *Cancer Causes Control* 1:39, 1990.

111. Zaridze DG: Time trends and international geographic variations related to diet and cancer, *Prog Clin Biol Res* 346:21, 1990.

112. Ziegler R et al: Paget's disease of bone in West Germany. Prevalence and distribution, *Clin Orthop* 194:199, 1985.

113. Zilber N, Kahane E, and Abraham M: The Lybian Creutzfeldt-Jakob disease focus in Israel: an epidemiologic evaluation, *Neurology* 41:1385, 1991.

RESOURCES

Holland WW et al, editors: *The Oxford textbook of public health,* Oxford, 1984, Oxford University Press.

Johns SB: *The ethnic almanac,* Garden City, NY, 1981, Dolphin Books.

Thompson MW, McInnes RR, Willard HF: *Genetics in medicine,* ed 5, Philadelphia, 1992, WB Saunders.

World Health Organization publication *Cancer Incidence in Five Continents.*

Chapter 36

SPECIAL HEALTH PROBLEMS
OF NATIVE AMERICANS

David Ray Baines

EPIDEMIOLOGY, BACKGROUND, AND RISK FACTORS

Although Native Americans are the original inhabitants of North America, or the first "Americans," they are the smallest of the minority groups and one of the most diverse. There are more than 500 federally recognized tribes[28] or nations, and each has its own language, traditions, heritage, and culture. The term *Native American* refers to American Indians and Alaska natives. Alaska has three distinct racial aboriginals. These are American Indians (Athebascan, Tlingit, Tsimpsian, and Haida Nations), Eskimos, and Aleuts. Native Hawaiians, although technically Native Americans, are generally considered under the Asian/Pacific Islander group, because they do not have a special trust relationship with the federal government as do the American Indians and Alaska Natives. They do, however, have similar health problems, and much of what is said about American Indians and Alaska Natives can be applied to Native Hawaiians.

There were about 1.7 million American Indians and Alaska Natives in the 1990 census.[15] About one third live on reservations or historic federal trust lands, and about one half live in urban areas.[35] The remainder live on rural nontrust lands (Fig. 36-1).

The Indian Health Service (IHS), an agency of the Public Health Service, provides health care for approximately 60% of this population. The remainder receive care in other federal, state, or county programs, or in the private sector. Although severely handicapped by fiscal concerns, the Indian Health Service has ongoing programs to address all of the preventable causes of death. The IHS is not operational in all eligible locations because of financial and personnel limitations. The IHS also increasingly is utilizing other federal sources, such as the Centers for Disease Control and The National Institutes of Health.[39] Still, there is a tremendous unmet need. Much of the reservation population is scattered over vast territories where it is difficult and expensive to provide care. Travel can be very difficult, and access to care can be very limited.[28]

SOCIOECONOMICS

Native American family income is well below the national average, and 29% of American Indian families live in poverty[28] (compared with 12% for the population as a whole). Unemployment is over twice the national rate and can exceed 70% on many reservations. Only 31% of American Indian adults graduate from high school, only 7% have a college degree,[28] and American Indians have the lowest educational attainment of all the minority groups. The average American Indian family is 4.6 members, which is the largest for any minority or nonminority group.[28]

The Native American population is relatively young. The median age is 9 years younger than the national average (23 compared with 32).[35] This is due to a high birthrate and the fact that 37% of deaths occur before age 45, compared with 12% for the group "U.S. all races."[30]

DEMOGRAPHICS

The 10 leading causes of death for American Indians in reservation states in 1987 are shown in Fig. 36-2.[35] Injuries, liver disease, diabetes, pneumonia/influenza, suicide, and homicide rates are significantly higher than those for nonhispanic whites. Other conditions more prevalent in

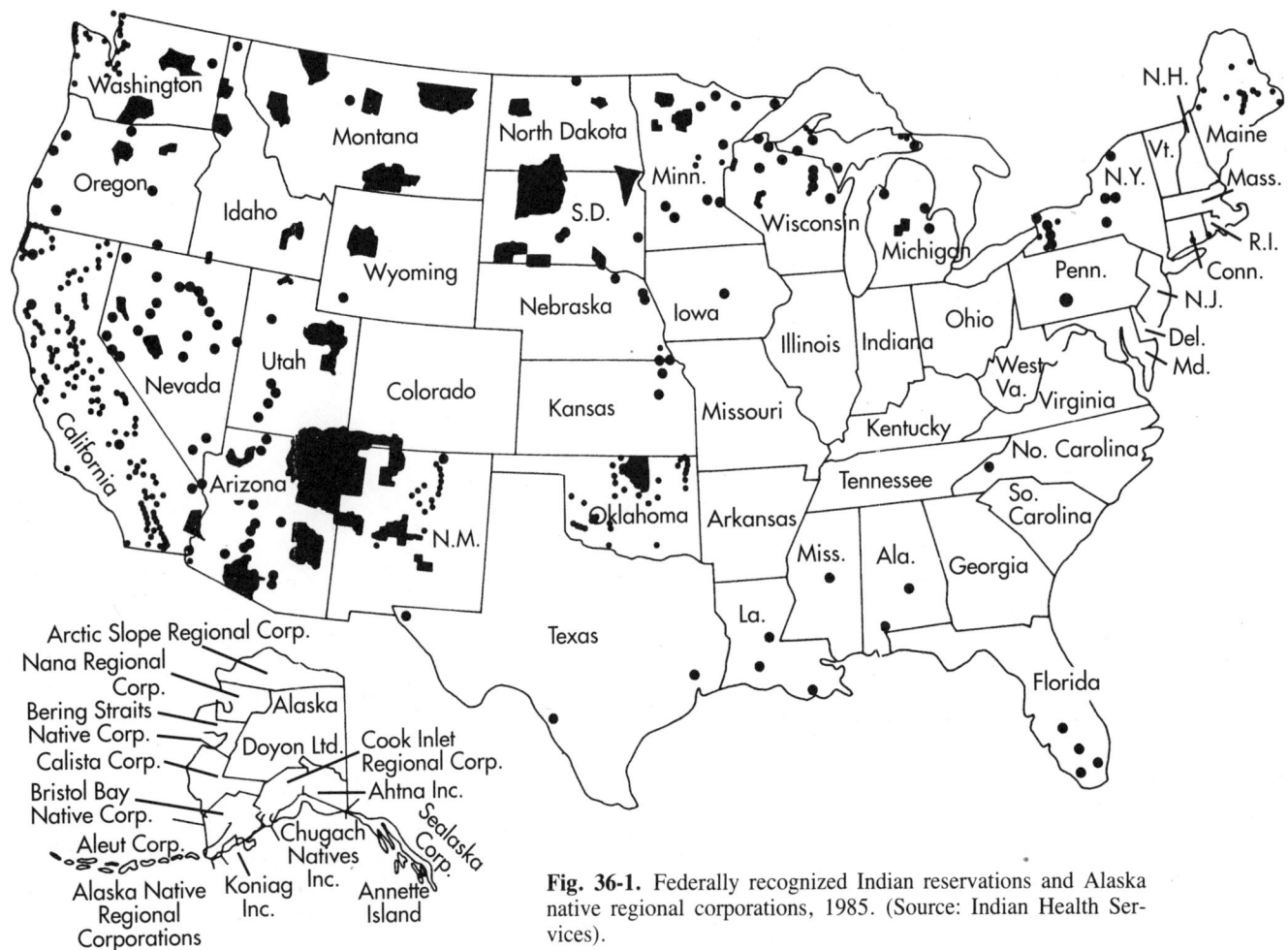

Fig. 36-1. Federally recognized Indian reservations and Alaska native regional corporations, 1985. (Source: Indian Health Services).

American Indians and Alaska Natives include infant mortality, nephritis, septicemia, and tuberculosis (Fig. 36-3). There are regional differences for these problems (Figs. 36-4 and 36-5). These differences have not been broken down by race (e.g., Indian vs. Eskimo), and little effort to determine the etiology of most of these differences has occurred.

Cardiovascular disease is now the leading cause of death in American Indians.[30,36] Early medical literature indicates that ischemic heart disease in this population was rare.[9,19] In 1979 Sieves et al. noted increasing rates of myocardial infarction. As advances were made in other areas such as infant mortality and infectious disease, and as the Native American population aged, heart disease has become the leading cause of mortality. Rates vary from one area to another. The highest rates are seen in the Bemiji (Minnesota) and Aberdeen (South Dakota) areas of the Indian Health Service. Currently a large multicenter study is evaluating cardiovascular disease and risk factors in American Indians.[18] Risk factors such as elevated cholesterol, hypertension, diabetes, smoking, family history, obesity, diet, and level of acculturation are being evaluated. This may identify areas that need to be targeted for intervention.

Cancer is the second leading cause of death, and like cardiovascular disease, the rate is below that for U.S. all races. Lung cancer is noted to be prevalent in the Oklahoma area.[41] Cancer of the gallbladder is more prevalent in the southwest, and an excess mortality from cancer of the liver is noted in Alaska.[5] Cancer of the cervix is noted to be more prominent in Native Americans when compared with U.S. all races.[28] Smoking plays a significant role in lung cancer, and a high incidence of hepatitis B in Alaska Natives is the primary reason that a high incidence of liver cancer is seen. Very low Pap smear rates are a significant reason mortality from cervical cancer is high in Native Americans.

If unintentional and intentional injuries are combined, they become the leading cause of death and the largest cause of years of potential life lost (YPLL).[8,39] Motor vehicle accidents are the most common cause of unintentional injury.[28] Several studies have documented that alcohol was involved in more than 50% of all motor vehicle accidents,[29,38] and detectable blood alcohol levels have

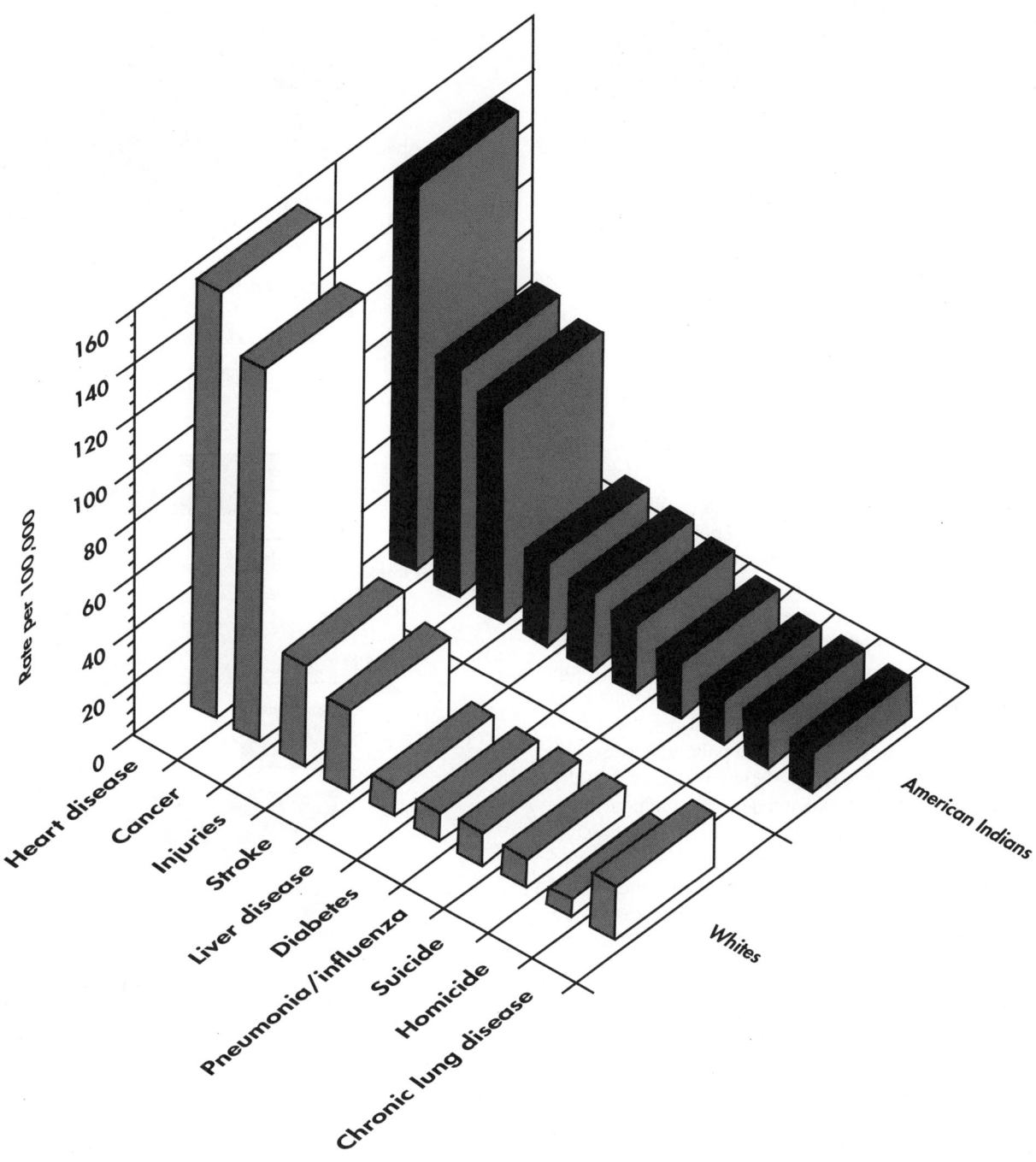

Fig. 36-2. Leading cause of death for American Indians in reservation states compared with whites (1987). (Source: Indian Health Services and National Center for Health Statistics (CDC).)

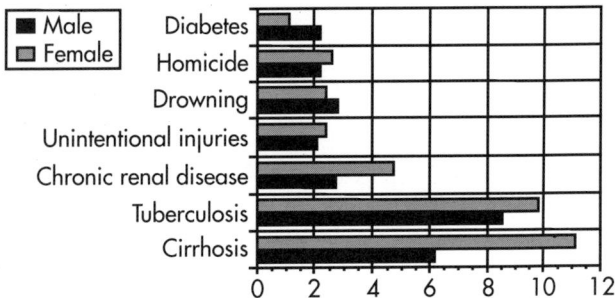

Fig. 36-3. Relative risk of death for American Indians by cause. (Source: Duke University analysis commissioned for the Task Force, 1984.)

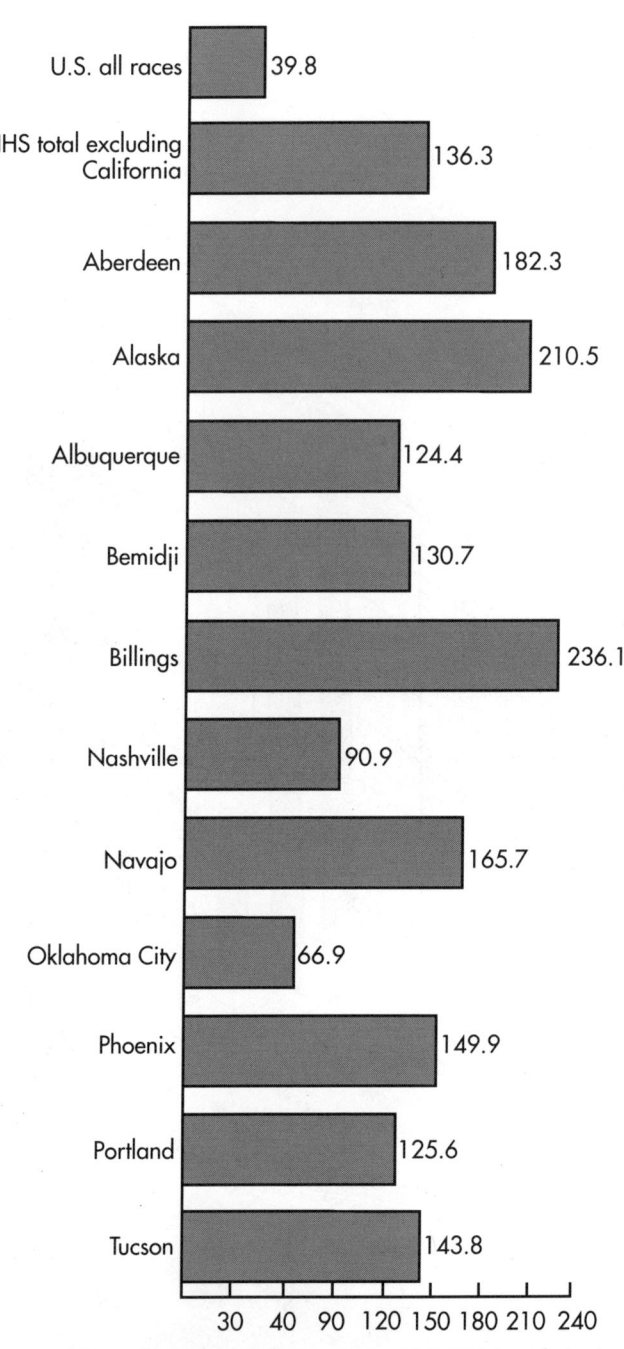

Age-adjusted mortality rate (per 100,000 population)

Fig. 36-4. Age-adjusted death rates for accidents and adverse conditions for American Indians in 11 IHS areas (excluding California) 1980 to 1982. (Source: U.S. Department of Health and Human Services, Public Health Services, Health Resources and Services Administration, Indian Health Service, computer tape supplied to the Office of Technology Assessment, Washington, D.C. 1985.)

been noted in as many as 77% in American Indian victims of motor vehicle accidents.[21] American Indians have the highest mortality rate from unintentional injuries of any group, 3.4 times higher than the U.S.-all-races rate.[30] Homicide is also significantly more prevalent in Native Americans and has been estimated to be 70% greater than the rate for the general population.[28] The suicide rate for Native Americans is 1.7 times the rate for U.S. all races.[26] Suicide is more common in males, and generally a violent method is used (guns and hanging). Tribes with stronger group orientation have lower rates than tribes with more individual orientation, and tribes that are going through rapid cultural changes also have higher rates.[26] The rates were highest in the age group 10 to 24. This age group faces the pressures of moving into adulthood, being a minority, having few economic and educational advantages, and trying to decide between two different pathways (traditional Indian or mainstream) that are polar opposites. Often no good role models exist to show how to successfully meld these two pathways. Role models are commonly persons who have not developed the skills to be a successful, well-adjusted adult and who have many self-destructive behaviors. Profiles of suicide victims indicate they come from unstable families with significant alcohol and drug abuse, where they also acquire these behaviors.[4] Physical and sexual abuse are also more common in those who attempt or complete suicide. A significant number commit suicide while in jail; they are usually intoxicated. Several reservations have instituted programs in which elders stay with them in jail, and there has been a significant drop in the number of suicides in these locations. As in unintentional injuries, alcohol is a significant factor in both homicide and suicide. Transportation and treatment of injury victims costs an estimated $100 million, and the IHS has initiated an injury-prevention program[39] (see Resources at end of this chapter).

Diabetes is becoming more prevalent in all areas of the Indian Health Service, but it is greatest in the Southwest, where more than 40% of the adults of some tribes are afflicted with this disease.[35] Fig. 36-4 shows the wide varia-

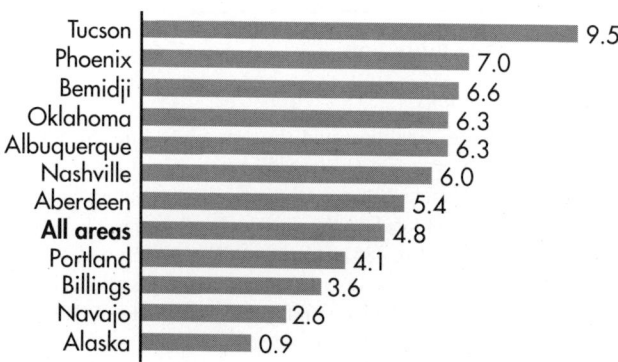

Tucson	9.5
Phoenix	7.0
Bemidji	6.6
Oklahoma	6.3
Albuquerque	6.3
Nashville	6.0
Aberdeen	5.4
All areas	4.8
Portland	4.1
Billings	3.6
Navajo	2.6
Alaska	0.9

Fig. 36-5. Percentage of outpatient visits with diabetes as clinical impression from October 1, 1982, to September 30, 1983. (Data from U.S. Congress Office of Technology and Assessment, Indian Health Care, OTA-H-290, Washington, D.C., 1986, U.S. Government Printing Office.)

tion in prevalence of this disease in Indian country. This is due to increasingly sedentary lifestyles and obesity from high-fat, high-calorie diets.[17,20] Like heart disease, diabetes was also previously rare in Native Americans.

INTERVENTION PROGRAMS AND STRATEGIES

Most of the top 10 causes of death in Native Americans are preventable, and although no estimation of cost savings is known, substantial savings obviously would occur if the rates were brought to a level equivalent to those for nonhispanic whites. Many of these deaths are also attributed to several risk factors:

• Tobacco
• Alcohol abuse
• Obesity
• Low socioeconomic status
• Inadequate access to care

Tobacco

Between 42% and 70% of American Indians use tobacco. It is much more prevalent in the northern midwestern tribes and least prevalent in the Southwest. This compares with a U.S.-all-races rate of 26%.[35] Tobacco use plays a role in cardiovascular disease, lung cancer, chronic lung disease, and susceptibility to pneumonia. Traditionally tobacco was used for ceremonial purposes. Indians believed that tobacco was given to the tribes by the Creator as a sacred substance. It was used to help prayers ascend to the Creator. Indians believed you could not tell a lie when smoking it; thus the peace pipe was used in negotiations. Some traditional Indians believe that it should be used only in ceremonies and that recreational use of tobacco is a misuse. This is why harm comes to those who abuse it. These beliefs could be part of an effective strategy to reduce the incidence of tobacco abuse and thus significantly reduce cardiovascular disease and lung cancer in the Native American population.

Sudden infant death syndrome (SIDS) also has been linked to maternal tobacco use.[24,30,34] Native American neonatal mortality is similar to U.S. all races; however, postnatal mortality is still 1.7 times the rate for whites. SIDS is the leading cause of postnatal mortality,[14,27] (68% of postnatal deaths) and is twice as common in Native Americans as in the general population.[31] Further study is needed to delineate the factors most responsible for this discrepancy while efforts to decrease tobacco abuse continue. A school-based curriculum, starting in grade school, can provide a good base to initiate community prevention efforts. This is a very significant area for intervention, as American Indian/Alaska Native youth have the highest rates of cigarette use.[2]

Alcohol abuse

Alcohol abuse plays a significant role in four of the top 10 causes of death in American Indians (unintentional injuries, liver disease, suicide, and homicide) and also increases infant mortality and morbidity in the form of fetal alcohol syndrome. The mortality rate from alcoholism for American Indians is four times the national average.[32] Native American youth have the highest rate of illicit drug use of all racial groups.[2] A recent study[8] of pedestrian and hypothermia deaths in Native Americans showed 90% of victims were significantly intoxicated. Most deaths occurred off reservations, because alcohol is prohibited on the reservations. Because alcohol could not be obtained on the reservation, individuals had to travel great distances to get alcohol and then travel back to the reservation while intoxicated. Perhaps the concept of a "dry" reservation needs a second look. Traditional Western approaches have been mostly unsuccessful in American Indian populations and have had only limited success in treating alcohol addiction. Programs that integrate traditional native values and community support have been more successful but have not been widely used because of financial and personnel limitations. Additionally, Western medical practitioners have been reluctant to use traditional Indian values and traditions.[3,22,23] Alkali Lake Band in Canada is the model of a community mounting a tremendous response to the alcoholism problem. Their video documentary is being shown to many audiences.[1] The box on p. 734 lists some school- and community-based prevention programs for alcohol and drug addiction.[32] Certainly several communities have been very successful in combating alcoholism. One hopes their efforts will be duplicated, and funding for these programs will increase. The use of family and community support, as well as traditional values, needs to be strongly considered when dealing with alcoholism and drug addiction in Native American patients.

Obesity

No large-scale national study is available to determine prevalence rates for obesity in this population, but 50% to

---

School- and community-based prevention programs for alcohol and drug addiction

Curriculums

Here's Looking at You: Original materials that were produced by the Comprehensive Health Education Foundation, 20832 Pacific Highway South, Seattle, WA 98198-5997, have been revised as "Here's Looking at You 2000" by Roberts, Fitzmahan, and Associates. This complete drug-education curriculum begins in kindergarten and continues through high school. Address: Roberts, Fitzmahan, and Associates, 9131 California Ave. SW, Seattle, WA 98136.

Project CHARLIE: Chemical Abuse Resolution Lies in Education (CHARLIE) is a Storefront/Youth Action drug-prevention program originally funded through the Community Education Training Act. Address: Project CHARLIE, 5701 Normandale Rd, Edina, MN 55424.

BABES: Beginning Alcohol and Addiction Basic Education Studies (BABES) was developed by the National Council on Alcoholism (NCA) in Detroit, in 1978, and is available through any NCA affiliate. Address: NCA, 17330 Northland Park Court, Southfield, MI 48075.

Community programs

TRAILS: Testing Realities and Investigating Life Styles (TRAILS) is a program of alternative activities for youth. Contact: Ms. Nancie Young, Division of Community Services, Department of Health and Social Services, 1 W. Wilson St., P.O. Box 7851, Madison, WI 53707.

Circle of Life: Circle of Life is an annual training seminar in Michigan for Indian and nonIndian service workers. It is sponsored by tribes and financed with federal and state funds.

Children are People: Children are People is a program that deals with sociological-emotional implications of drug abuse. Address: Children are People, Inc., 1599 Selby Ave., St. Paul, MN 55104.

75% of Native American adults are overweight.[6] Obesity affects cardiovascular disease, stroke, and diabetes, three of the top 10 causes of death in Native Americans. Sedentary lifestyles and high-calorie and high-fat diets predispose persons to obesity. Traditional foods are still used by a large number of the reservation population, but they have become a smaller proportion of the diet, being replaced by high-fat, high-sugar, low-nutrient foods. In addition, the number of calories expended by Native Americans has dropped dramatically. Modern conveniences and lifestyle have eliminated many of the physical activities that previously had limited obesity. A number of adolescent and childhood obesity-prevention programs are underway, but some time will be needed to see just how effective they are. Culturally sensitive dietary education programs[37] and a community-wide competitive program[43] have been tried with some success. Both dietary education/counseling and physical activities need to be utilized to maximize chances for success.

Low socioeconomic status

To start, education and job opportunities can provide a stronger base to develop self-esteem. Low self-esteem leads to many psychologic and behavioral problems. Both suicide and homicide have been associated with low socioeconomic status. Infant mortality and unintentional injury in children also have been linked to low socioeconomic status.[25] Providing strong psychologic and social services for those in stressful situations can be beneficial in preventing worsening of the situation. In Native Americans these services should include traditional healers when appropriate.

Inadequate access to care

The Indian Health Service, as well as many rural and inner-city locations where Native Americans reside, often has inadequate health manpower resources. The IHS has had great difficulty in filling many of its primary care positions, and some locations may have only half the number of providers needed to serve the population. The IHS has used physician extenders such as community health representatives, nurse practitioners, pharmacists, and physician assistants to alleviate some of the problem.[16] In addition, a triage method using nurses has been very successful in addressing the burden of an excess patient load. This has led not only to better acute care, but to better preventive care as well.[33] This setup may well prove to be effective in many other settings outside the Indian Health Service.

Overview

The epidemiology program of the Aberdeen area IHS, in conjunction with the Carter Center at Emory University and the Centers for Disease Control, has developed a Health Risk Appraisal (HRA) specific for American Indians[40] (see the box on p. 735). It has a disclosure statement indicating that answering the questionnaire will not in any way jeopardize their receiving health care from the Indian Health Service. The questionnaire includes a section that asks for percentage of American Indian/Alaska Native blood (blood quantum). The questionnaire can be obtained from the Aberdeen IHS (see Resources). The Health Risk Appraisal uses IBM-compatible computers and is useful for screening large numbers of people. Whether it is useful in changing patients' attitudes and life-styles is still uncertain, but it can identify high-risk individuals.

Health risk appraisal for American Indians

1. Your age: _____
2. Your height: _____
3. Your weight: _____
4. Sex: M _____, F _____
5. Have you ever been told that you have diabetes (or sugar diabetes)?
6. Did your mother, father, brothers, or sisters ever have diabetes or sugar diabetes?
7. Are you now taking medicine for high blood pressure?
8. Cigarette smoking:
   How would you describe your cigarette smoking habits?
9. If you smoke cigarettes now:
   How many cigarettes a day do you smoke?
10. If you've quit:
    a. How many years has it been since you smoked cigarettes fairly regularly?
    b. What was the average number of cigarettes you smoked per day?
11. How many cigars do you usually smoke per day?
12. How many pipes of tobacco do you usually smoke per day?
13. How many times per day do you usually use smokeless tobacco (chewing tobacco, snuff pouches, etc.)
14a. In the next year, how many thousands of miles will you travel by car, truck, or van?
14b. In the past year did you ride on a motorcycle, all-terrain vehicle, or snowmobile?
14c. In the next 12 months how many thousands of miles will you travel by motorcycle, all-terrain vehicle, or snowmobile?
15. On a typical day how do you usually travel?
16. How often do you usually buckle your safety belt when traveling by car or truck?
17. On the average, how close to the speed limit do you usually drive?
18. *How many times* in the last month did you drive or ride in a vehicle or boat when the driver had perhaps too much alcohol to drink?
19. *How many drinks* of alcoholic beverages do you have in a typical week? (1 drink = a can or bottle of beer, a small glass of wine, or a shot of hard liquor)

20. *On how many days* in a typical month do you have at least one drink?
21. On the days when you drank any liquor, beer, or wine, about *how many drinks* did you have on the average?
22. How many times during the past month did you have five or more drinks on an occasion?
23. Have you seriously considered suicide?
24. About how long has it been since you had a rectal exam?
25. How often do you get physical exercise, such as running, dancing, bicycling, vigorous walking, or active sports?
26. How often do you brush or floss your teeth?
27. How many cups of caffeinated beverages (e.g., coffee, tea) do you drink per day?
28. Ethnic background: American Indian/Alaska Native
    ☐ Full blood   ☐ ¼-⅞ Blood
    ☐ <¼ blood   ☐ Non-Indian
29. Education: What is the highest grade you completed in school?
30. Employment: What is your employment status?

Questions 31-40: women only

31. At what age did you have your first menstrual period?
32. How old were you when your first child was born?
33. How long has it been since your last breast x-ray (mammogram)?
34. How many women in your natural family (mother and sisters only) have had breast cancer?
35. Have you had a hysterectomy operation?
36. How long has it been since you had a Pap smear for cancer?
37. How often do you examine your breasts for lumps?
38. About how long has it been since you had your breasts examined by a physician or nurse?
39. How many times have you been pregnant? (Include live births, miscarriages, abortions, and stillborns.)
40. Are you now or do you think you might be pregnant?

The box on p. 736 lists objectives proposed for the Indian Health Service regarding preventive health efforts.[31] Many of them are applicable to non-IHS personnel treating Native American patients. It combines community health education, leaders, government agencies, culturally sensitive providers, and involvement of the community. It is somewhat broad in scope but allows for specific adjustments when necessary. The Indian Health Service has done a tremendous job in immunizing much of the population. Immunization has been widely accepted because of the few negative consequences. Contraception is an area that needs more attention. Native Americans have the highest birth rate of any ethnic group. Many women want

to be pregnant or feel that if they do become pregnant, it was meant to be. Many adolescents are ignorant of contraception.[4] Better education, starting at the grade school level and utilizing community members and leaders, will improve this problem. Without community support, there will be little success in reducing unwanted pregnancies.

COUNSELING AND COMPLIANCE

When dealing with Native American patients, one must understand the patient's beliefs regarding health, disease, and healing. This allows for effective communication and a better chance of a positive outcome. Indian patients claim that non-Indian physicians cannot communicate

Summary of objectives proposed for the Indian Health Service

Health status

Lower specific morbidity and mortality rates for the IHS service population.

Awareness

Ensure that the IHS service population has a general knowledge of:
- Stress reduction
- Parenting
- Nutrition
- Sanitation
- Symptoms requiring treatment
- Sources of information and care
- Specific health conditions; for example, diabetes
- Availability of mutual support and self-help for selected conditions, such as alcoholism

Ensure that IHS personnel have:
- Appropriate training and experience
- Knowledge of Indian culture
- Continuing education
- Skills for taking patient histories that detect particular conditions
- Structured treatment protocols
- Self-awareness as role models

Advocate Indian health issues

Risk factors

Collaborate with tribal, other government, and private organizations to encourage healthful behavior, including smoking cessation, diet, exercise, avoidance of substance abuse, injury avoidance, and positive parenting attitudes.

Services

Screen for such conditions as hypertension and diabetes.

Immunize the Indian population against vaccine-preventable diseases.

Ensure universal access to preventive primary care services for Indians, including well-child care, developmental screening, and prenatal care.

Tailor specific programs to Indian culture.

Coordinate regional service delivery with other community health resources.

Surveillance

Establish and continue systems to monitor particular health conditions, including consistent reporting of notifiable diseases.

Conduct periodic health status and health care delivery surveys.

Improve current data gathering.

Track specific health problems, such as diabetes, hypertension, and pregnancy, and events indicating potential health or service delivery problems.

Establish standards for all IHS programs and conduct periodic reviews.

---

well, are difficult to work with, and do not stay long enough to learn about Indian culture and traditions. Physicians complain that Indian patients cannot communicate well, are difficult to work with, and are not motivated enough to care for themselves. This makes for poor doctor-patient relationships. Understanding some of the aspects of Native American culture can help to improve these relationships.

Health in Native American culture is not the absence of disease but rather harmony with oneself (mind, body, and spirit), others, and one's surroundings or environment. When harmony is lost, illness is allowed to enter. Spirituality or religion is inseparable from health. Traditional Indian healers use spiritual means to diagnose and heal. They are viewed as healing from the inside (of the body) because they spiritually correct what was out of harmony. Thereby they treat the cause of illness. Each tribe has its own unique beliefs. Western medicine is viewed as using physical means to diagnose and treat. It is viewed as healing from the outside (of the body), and it treats the symptoms (e.g., headaches, dyspepsia). Both methods are viewed as compatible and are not considered competitive.

They have the same goal—a healthy patient. Through a better understanding one can be more effective and satisfied with encounters with Native American patients.

Both reservation and urban Native Americans utilize traditional healers,[7] and they should be kept in mind as a possible consultant to which to refer Native American patients. Traditional healers are often underutilized and can be a significant resource. Locating one can be a problem if you are not considered a long-term resident in the community. Often the traditional healers are "underground," a position that became necessary for survival as the pressure from religious and legal sources mounted. Traditional healers are also reluctant to work with non-Indians until they get to know them. Having someone in the Indian community to act as a go-between is probably the most effective way to make a referral. In some locations where the physicians and traditional healers have worked in harmony, this may not be necessary. Some hospitals even have areas for the traditional healers to work. Through better understanding, this may become the rule rather than the exception in Indian communities. The Association of American Indian Physicians (see Resources) has an American Indian cross-cultural training workshop that has had good success with medical and nursing students, residents, nurses, and physicians who do or will provide care for Native American patients. The workshop utilizes Indian physicians and traditional healers who discuss traditional Indian beliefs, cultural norms, and specific case histories. (For further information on Indian culture, see Suggested Readings at the end of the chapter.)

REFERENCES

1. Alkali Lake Indian Band, "The Honor of All," video documentary, Issaquah, Wash, 1987, Phil Lucas Productions.
2. Bachman JG: Racial/ethnic differences in smoking, drinking, and illicit drug use among American high school seniors, 1976-89, *Am J Public Health* 81:372-377, 1991.
3. Blum K: Peyote, a potential ethniopharmacologic agent for alcoholism and other drug dependencies: possible biochemical rationale, *Clin Toxicol* 11(4):459-472, 1977.
4. Blum RW: American Indian-Alaska Native youth health, *JAMA* 267:1637-1644, 1992.
5. Boss LP: Cancers of the gallbladder and biliary tract in Alaska Natives, *J Nat Cancer Institute* 69(5):1005-1007, 1982.
6. Donato K: *Obesity in minority populations,* unpublished background paper prepared for the National Heart, Lung and Blood Institute's Ad Hoc Committee on Minority Populations, April, 1990.
7. Fuchs M: Use of traditional Indian medicine among urban Native Americans, *Med Care* 13(11):915-927, 1975.
8. Gallaher MM: Pedestrian and hypothermia deaths among Native Americans in New Mexico, *JAMA* 267:1345-1348, 1992.
9. Gilbert J: Absence of coronary thrombosis in Navajo Indians, *Calif Med,* 82:114-115, 1955.
10. Gohdes DM: Diabetes in American Indians: a growing problem, *Diabetes Care* 9:609-613, 1986.
11. *Healthy People 2000: national health promotion and disease prevention objectives,* Washington, DC, 1990, US Department of Health and Human Services.
12. Hill G: San Francisco Bay Area American Indian needs assessment, Personal communication of unpublished paper, 1985.
13. Hill G: Klamath Tribe needs assessment, Chiloquim, Ore, 1986, Klamath Tribe, personal communication.
14. Honsifeld LS: Native American postneonatal mortality, *Pediatrics* 80(4):575-578, 1987.
15. *Indian Health Service: Injuries among American Indians and Alaska Natives, 1990,* Washington, DC, 1990, US Department of Health and Human Services.
16. Johnson KG: Strategies for prevention using allied health professionals, *Prev Med* 6:386-390, 1977.
17. Knowler WC: Diabetes incidence in Pima Indians: contributions of obesity and parental diabetes, *Am J Epidemiol* 113(2):144-156, 1981.
18. Kumanyika SK, Savage DD: *Ischemic heart disease risk factors among American Indians and Alaska Natives,* vol 1, Commissioned unpublished paper for the Task Force on Black and Minority Health, Department of Health and Human Services, 1985.
19. Kunitz SJ: *Disease change and the role of medicine. The Navajo experience,* Berkeley, Calif, 1983, University of California Press.
20. Lillioja S: Obesity and insulin resistance: lesson learned from the Pima Indians, *Diabetes Metab Rev* 4(5):517-540, 1988.
21. Mahoney MC: Fatal motor vehicle traffic accidents among Native Americans, *Am J Prev Med* 7(2):112-116, 1991.
22. Marum L: Rural community organizing and development strategies in Alaska Native villages, *Arcumpolar Health* 47(1):354-356, 1988.
23. May PA: Alcohol and drug misuse prevention programs for American Indians: needs and opportunities, *J Stud Alcohol* 47(3):187-195, 1986.
24. Malloy MH: The association of maternal smoking with age and cause of infant deaths, *Am J Epidemiol* 128(1):46-55, 1988.
25. May PA: The health status of Indian children: problems and prevention in early life, *American Indian and Alaska Native mental health research,* monograph no 1.
26. May PA: Suicide among American Indian youth: a look at the issues, *Child Today* July, August 1987.
27. Nakamura RM: Excess infant mortality in an American Indian population, 1940-1990, *JAMA* 266(16):2244-2248, 1991.
28. National Center for Health Statistics: Health, United States, 1990, Hyattsville, Md, 1991, Public Health Service.
29. National Highway Traffic Safety Administration, US Department of Transportation: *National Accident Sampling System, 1984,* Report DPT HS, Washington, DC NHTSA, 1985.
30. *Report of the Secretary's Task Force on Black Minority Health,* executive summary, Washington, DC, 1985, US Department of Health and Human Service, US Government Printing Office.
31. Rhodes ER: The Indian burden of illness and future health interventions, *Public Health Rep* 102(4):361-368, 1987.
32. Rhodes ER: The Indian health service approach to alcoholism among American Indians and Alaska Natives, *Public Health Rep* 103(6):621-627, 1988.
33. Shorr G: *Improving outpatient care with concurrent visit planning: a case for industrial strength triage,* unpublished draft, IHS, Division of Health Systems Development, personal communication from Thomas Welty, MD, MPH.
34. Shannon DC: SIDS and near SIDS, *N Engl J Med* 306(16):959-965, 1982.
35. Sievers ML: Diseases of North American Indians. In Rothchild H, Chapman C, editors: *Biocultural aspects of disease,* New York, Academic Press.
36. Sievers ML: Increasing rate of acute myocardial infarction in Southwestern American Indians *Ariz Med* 36:739-742, 1979.
37. Stegmayer P: Designing a diabetes nutrition education program for a Native American Community, *Diabetes Educator* 12(1):64-66, 1987.
38. US Congress, Office of Technology Assessment: *Indian health care,* OTA-H-290, Washington, DC, 1986, US Government Printing Office.
39. Waller JP: Injury: conceptual shifts and preventive implications, *Ann Rev Public Health* 8:21-49, 1987.
40. Welty TK: Indian specific health risk appraisal being developed, *IHS Primary Care* Provider 13(7):1, 1988.
41. Welty TK: The Strong Heart Study: a study of cardiovascular disease and its risk factors in American Indians, *IHS Provider* 17(2):32-33, 1992.
42. West KM: Diabetes in American Indians and other native populations of the New World, *Diabetes* 23(10):841-855, 1974.
43. Wilson R: A low cost competitive approach to weight reduction in a Native American community, *Int J Obesity* 13:731-738, 1989.
44. Young TJ: Poverty, suicide and homicide among Native Americans, *Psychol Rep* 67:1153-1154, 1990.

Suggested readings

1. Aitken LP: *Two cultures meet: pathways for American Indians to medicine,* Garrett Park, Md, 1990, Garrett Park Press.
2. Camazine SM: *Traditional and Western health care among the Zuni Indians of New Mexico,* vol 14, Social Science Medicine.
3. Coulehan JL: Navajo Indian medicine: implications for healing, *J Fam Pract* 10(1):55-61, 1980.
4. Halfe LB: The circle: death and dying from a native perspective, *J Palliat Care* 13(11):915-927, 1975.
5. Hammarschlag CA: *The dancing healers, a doctor's journey of healing with native Americans,* San Francisco, 1988, Harper Row.
6. Kunitz SJ: Traditional Navajo health beliefs and practices. In *Disease change and the role of medicine, The Navajo experience,* Berkeley, Calif, 1983, University of California Press.

◼◼◼ RESOURCES ◼◼◼

Welty, Thomas K., MD MPH, Epidemiologies, Aberdeen Area IHS, Strong Heart Study, 3200 Canyon Lake Drive, Rapid City, SD 57702.

Kauley, Matthew, executive director, Association of American Indian Physicians, 10015 S. Pennsylvania Ave, Oklahoma City, OK 73159.

Smith, Richard J., manager, Injury Prevention Program, Parklawn 5A 39, 5600 Fishers Lane, Rockville, MD 20857.

Chapter 37

SPECIAL HEALTH PROBLEMS OF ASIANS AND PACIFIC ISLANDERS

Arthur Chen, Peter Ng, Peter Sam, Don Ng, Denise Abe, Rosalinda Ott, Wally Lim, Sue Chan, Winston Wong

OVERVIEW

Until recently, health problems of the U.S. Asian and Pacific Islander (API) population have gone largely unnoticed nationally. Asians have long been portrayed as America's high-achieving "model minority" and as a community without problems. They have been noticed culturally with prominent displays in our major cities where "Chinatowns" are common. Meanwhile "Little Saigons," "Koreatowns," "Little Tokyos," and "Manilatowns" are also growing in number. Hawaii is still known to the U.S. public only as a vacation paradise where exotic tropical Pacific Island culture abounds. However, the 1980 and 1990 census revealed astounding growth, which has notably had an impact on our nation's cultural and political landscape. A rapid influx of API immigrants and refugees while still grieving their losses, faced challenges of adjusting to a totally different culture. In the process, a variety of social problems began to emerge, including health problems, most notably tuberculosis, hepatitis B, depression, and thalassemia. The community itself began speaking out about the need to explore and address the multitude of problems confronting them. Policy makers and the general public are now beginning to respond.

This chapter draws on the experience of the co-authors, all primary care physicians serving API communities. Distinctions are made periodically between "Asians" and "Pacific Islanders." The acronym API will refer to "Asians and Pacific Islanders" as an entire group.

Diverse nationalities and cultures

API represent the fastest growing minority group in the United States.[119] Approximately 40,000 to 50,000 refugees arrive from Asia annually (340,000 total 1989 Asian immigrant and refugee admissions).[146] Between 1980 and 1990 this population increased 108% from 3.5 million to 7.3 million persons.Currently API comprise 2.9% of the total U.S. population.[165]

API represent over 25 distinct ethnic groups. Major groupings identified by the 1990 Census include Chinese, Filipino, Japanese, Asian Indian, Korean, Vietnamese, Hawaiian, Guamanian, and Samoan. Other groups include Cambodian, Hmong, Laotian, Thai, Bangladeshi, Burmese, Indonesian, Malaysian, Okinawan, Pakistani, Sri Lankan, as well as Pacific Islander groups including Tongan, Tahitian, Northern Mariana Islander, Palauan, and Fijian. The various nationalities each have their own languages and unique cultural beliefs and practices. Up to 50% of the U.S. API community use languages other than English in their household, with corresponding low rates of English fluency.[47] The language barrier limits their access to preventive health information and primary care services.

Despite the perception that API are recent newcomers to North American shores, they encompass fourth- and fifth-generation Americans as well as newly arrived immigrants. The earliest Asian immigrants to America arrived in the early portion of the nineteenth century. This historical root continues today, with the settlement of thousands of Southeast Asian refugees. On the other hand, indigenous Pacific Islander populations predated any formal relationships with the United States.

Distinctions should be made between immigrant or refugee API and those that are American born. Recent arrivals tend to be low income, less educated, and uninsured, with little or no English fluency.[24,47,109] The language barrier may limit access to health services and compromise ability to lead a healthy life-style. These access barriers may explain the excess mortality rates seen among foreign born Chinese, Filipino and Japanese Americans.[175]

Although the media has often portrayed API as a homogeneous community,[11,29,80] their socioeconomic status displays a bipolar characteristic.[96,99] Whereas portions of the API community clearly demonstrate well-established educational achievements and family income, equally prominent segments are disenfranchised families that fall below the poverty level. According to the 1990 census, for example, API earn the highest median annual household income ($38,450). However, 12.2% of this same population live below the federally defined poverty level, in contrast to 10.7% for whites. API tend to have larger families, which results in a lower per capita income.[120] These grouped figures under the broad "API" category also mask the tremendous variation in incomes of specific API ethnic subgroups.

EPIDEMIOLOGY

Cerebrovascular, cardiovascular disease, and risk factors

Data are limited because the National Center for Health Statistics does not routinely report the leading causes of death for API ethnic subgroups. In 1988, heart disease and cerebrovascular disease ranked first and third, respectively, for all API.[58] A 1980 ethnic breakdown showed similar rankings for Chinese, Japanese, and Filipinos and the general U.S. population.[175] However, stroke, rather than coronary heart disease, is the major cause of mortality in both China and Japan.[88,143] Sixty-one percent of Southeast Asian patients at a California community health facility had at least one of four risk factors (hypertension, hypercholesterolemia, smoking, and obesity).[5]

Hypertension. Prevalence of hypertension ranges from 18.1%[147] to 39% among Bostonian elderly Chinese,[24,26] 14%[147] to 24.7%[2,56] among Japanese, and 19.9%[2] to 26.6%[147] among Filipinos. These figures contrast with 15% to 17% prevalence seen in California's 1990 general population.[58] Southeast Asians (Vietnamese, Laotian, Cambodians, Hmong) have a prevalence of hypertension between 10% to 41%.[5,25,109] This marked difference is likely due to different methodology and time periods of each study. The 1990 Hawaiian Behavioral Risk Factor Survey (BRFS) reported that Hawaiians had a prevalence of hypertension of 22.4% in contrast to whites (15.8%).

Awareness of hypertension in API is poor, with only 46% of hypertensives aware of their condition.[147] In one Ohio study, 94% had no knowledge of what hypertension was.[25] The level of knowledge regarding consequences and treatment of hypertension is quite varied, with the Japanese being most knowledgeable and Southeast Asians the least. Control of hypertension is likewise poorer than the average population, even among Japanese and Filipinos.[147]

Cholesterol and triglycerides. The 1990 Centers for Disease Control (CDC) survey conducted in Hawaii and California revealed higher rates of hypercholesterolemia among most API subgroups as compared to the general population. For example in Hawaii, prevalence of hypercholesterolemia among Japanese was 43.7%, among Filipino 41.6%, among Hawaiians (22.5%), and among whites 31.9%.[56] California Vietnamese men (38%) and women (32%) and Oakland Chinese men (41%) and women (38%) had higher prevalence than the general male (29%) and female (28%) population.[24,109] Additionally, the percentage of Chinese (70%), Filipino (63%), Vietnamese (56%), and Hawaiians (52%) who never had a blood cholesterol check was high in contrast to their white (41% in Hawaii) and general population (38% in California) counterparts. Among the Oakland Chinese, 60% lacked knowledge of the association between high cholesterol levels and heart disease. This lack of knowledge was mainly evident among Chinese not fluent in English and rose to 70% among those with low incomes (less than $10,000 annually) and less than high school education. The general impression is that with immigration to the United States, dietary shifts lead to higher cholesterol levels. Cholesterol levels have been documented to be higher among Japanese Americans living in Hawaii compared with their counterparts in Japan.[131] Similar comparisons between China and western nations indicated lower total cholesterol levels in China, although HDL levels differed less significantly.[81] This trend, however, has not been consistently substantiated for all API subgroups. For example, total cholesterol, LDL and HDL levels, in 346 elderly Chinese in Boston were similar to those in China.[26]

Smoking. The 1985 and 1987 National Health Interview Survey reported API age-adjusted smoking prevalence for men (25%) and women (12%) as less than non-Hispanic white men (31%) and women (29%).[58] Due to intense local and national "smoke free" campaigns, these rates have been declining rapidly for the general population, but less so for the API community, as evidenced by API men maintaining almost the same prevalence (24.3%) in 1990. Furthermore, closer examination of 1990 API male subgroups reveals even higher rates for Vietnamese (35%)[109] and Chinese (28%).[24] Hawaii's 1991 BRFS, showed male smoking rates for Hawaiians (30.4%) Filipinos (28.7%), Koreans (39.4%), and Japanese (18%) in contrast to whites (26.2%).[56] A 1985 study reported that 72% of male Lao refugees were smokers.[135] These same

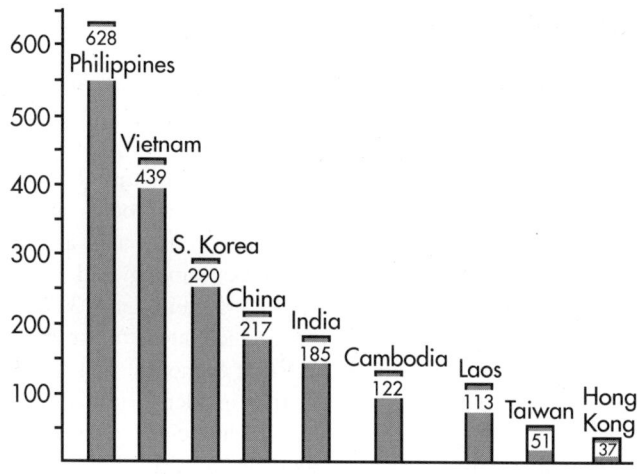

Fig. 37-1. 1987 Tuberculosis in the United States: Breakdown by Asian country of origin. (Modified from tuberculosis statistics in the United States, 1987, US Department of Health and Human Services, CDC, Atlanta, 1989.)

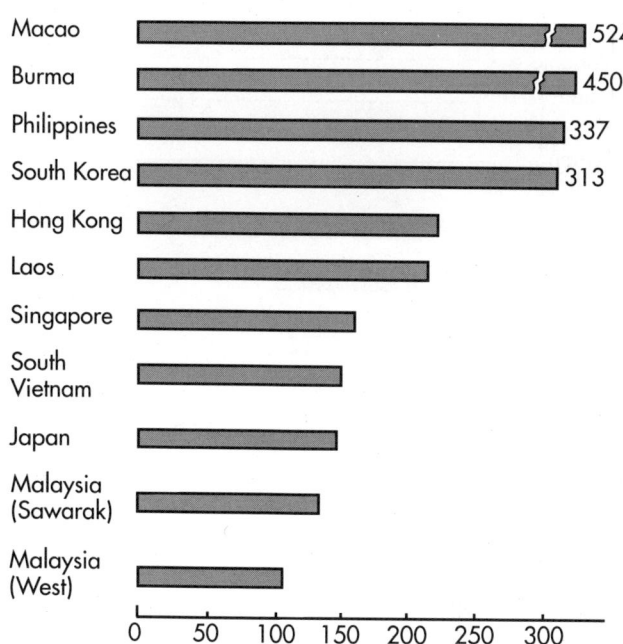

Fig. 37-2. New tuberculosis cases reported (per 100,000) 1971 in Asia. (Modified from Bulla A: *WHO statistics report* 39:2-38, 1977.)

studies suggest that with the exception of Hawaiians (27.9%) and Koreans (30.5%), smoking among API women (<1% to 12.6%) tends not to exceed rates of their white counterparts (18.3% to 19.6%).

The higher prevalence seen among most API men is most likely related to patterns seen in their native countries. In China, one study reported that 61% of men over age 15 were smokers.[176] Similar trends have been reported for men from Japan (61%), Korea (75%),[49] and the Philippines (47%).[129]

Diabetes mellitus. In 1980, diabetes was the eighth leading cause of death for Chinese and the seventh leading cause for Japanese, Filipinos, and whites.[175] One study found that 13.3% of elderly Chinese women and 12.5% of elderly Chinese men in Boston had a history of diabetes.[26] Another study showed elevated fasting blood glucoses in 9.6% to 20.8% of API subgroups with the highest rates among Japanese (20.8%), Filipino (16.1%), and Chinese (15.9%) men.[86] The differences among subgroups did not reach statistical significance, but contrasted with the 12% prevalence of diabetes among U.S. non-Hispanic whites aged 45 to 74.[58] A 1985 rural study found that 17% to 23% of Hawaiians aged 40 to 59 had diabetes.[31] Micronesians from Nauru have a 30% prevalence.[3] The prevalence of other Pacific Islander groups, including Polynesians, Melanesians, and Fijians, is less than 12%.[154,181,182]

Infectious disease

Tuberculosis. The 1991 overall incidence rate for tuberculosis (TB) was 10.3/100,000. By contrast API had the highest 1985 TB incidence (49.6/100,000), which was 8.7 times the 1985 rate for U.S. whites (5.7/100,000).[163] These cases accounted for 2530 of 22,201 total cases. Ap-

proximately 93.6% of those affected were foreign born, with the largest contingent coming from Southeast Asia and the Philippines. Southeast Asian refugees from Kampuchea, Laos, and Vietnam have the highest TB rates. They rose from 231/100,000 in 1980 to 310/100,000 in 1985.

In 1987 these trends continued, with 2332 TB cases among API. The greatest number were from the Philippines, South Vietnam, South Korea, and China (Fig. 37-1).[164]

Among all Asian subgroups 1126 (44.5%) of reported 1985 TB cases occurred in patients younger than 35 years. The geographic distribution of patients was California 45.6%, Hawaii 6.9%, New York 6.5%, Texas 5.7%, and Illinois 5.3%. In San Francisco, where API comprised 29% of the 1990 population, they accounted for 48.6% of the TB cases in 1989.[136,137] Existing international data sets indicate patterns consistent with US findings (Figs. 37-2 and 37-3).[14]

TB is still a major public health problem in many of these areas today. Data on extrapulmonary TB in API populations are limited. Immigrants from India may contract intestinal TB secondary to *Mycobacterium bovis*.[4]

Hepatitis B. From 8% to 22% of Chinese, Korean, Filipino, Southeast Asian, and Pacific Islander populations may be chronic carriers of the hepatitis B (HB) virus.[39,46,55,149,160] In contrast, the U.S. general population carrier rate is 0.2% to 0.9%.[110] One study showed a lower prevalence of chronic HB carriers among US-born Asians

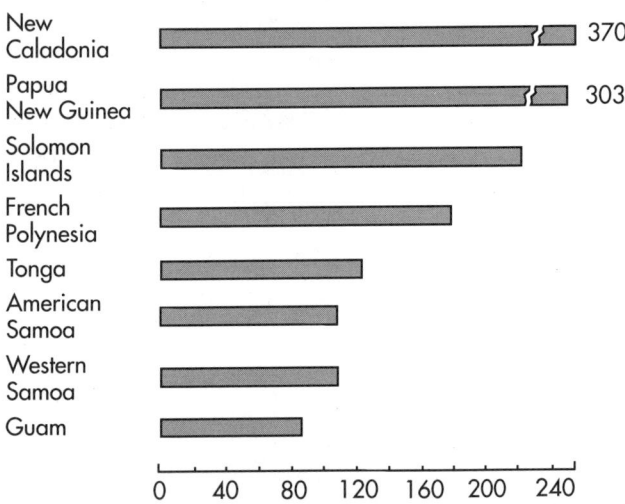

Fig. 37-3. New tuberculosis cases reported (per 100,000) 1971 in the Pacific Islands. (Modified from Bulla A: *WHO statistics Report,* 39:2-38, 1977.)

compared with foreign born of the same ethnicity.[149] Because estimates show that more than 25% of chronic HB carriers develop chronic active hepatitis and die of cirrhosis or hepatocellular cancer,[6,7] API are at higher risk for these complications.

Parasitism. Up to 50% of Asian immigrants and refugees continue to carry some type of parasite long after they have arrived in the United States. Most are helminthic intestinal parasites, which are relatively benign and not easily transmitted to others.[19,77,90,152] Examples include *Trichuris* (whipworm), *Ascaris* (roundworm), *Necator* (hookworm), and *Strongyloides*. Some of these organisms may persist in the gastrointestinal (GI) tract for up to 6 years. Common protozoans include *Giardia lamblia* and *Entamoeba histolytica*. These organisms pose a different public health risk because they tend to cause symptoms and are transmitted by the fecal-oral route. The liver fluke, *Clonorchis sinensis* or *Opisthorchis vivierri* is associated with cholangiocarcinoma and recurrent pyogenic cholangitis.[18] It has been found to persist in the Chinese from the Chinatown area of Manhattan for as long as 50 years.[78]

Other parasites are much less common, but worthy of attention. Immigrants from Southeast Asia and southern China may carry malaria to the United States. The majority organism is *Plasmodium vivax* with the remainder being *P. falciparum*.[15,52] Patients from Southeast Asia and the Philippines may harbor *Schistosoma japonicum* for 47 years or longer. Disease may still occur after a prolonged latent period.[105] At least four outbreaks of trichinosis involving Southeast Asians have occurred over the past 15 years. Southeast Asians accounted for 60 of 1260 trichinosis cases (4.8%) reported to the CDC from 1975 to 1984.[148] In 1990, an outbreak affected 90 Southeast Asians who ate uncooked pork sausage.[22] Finally, *Para-*

gonimus (lung fluke) occurs and may cause clinical symptoms similar to tuberculosis.

HIV. The number of reported AIDS cases among Asians and Pacific Islanders in the United States as of October 1991 was 1235.[61] Nationwide statistics for AIDS and HIV seroconvertors are difficult to obtain, as not all local tracking systems identify API or their subgroups separately. California includes ethnic subgroups and as of March 1991 reported 469 AIDS cases among API men (92%), women (7%) and children (1%).[75] Filipinos (37%), Chinese (18%) and Japanese (15%) accounted for the majority of cases. The Thai, Hawaiians, Samoans, and Guamanians had the highest cumulative incidence for AIDS. Similar to the general population, homosexual/bisexual men comprise the greatest proportion of API AIDS cases (78%). Transfusion with HIV infected blood (8%) ranked second in contrast to the general population (1%). Additionally, API intravenous drug abusers (7.9%) constituted a smaller proportion of AIDS cases compared to 14% for non-API. Among API female AIDS cases, the largest group (41%) were heterosexual. Intravenous drug abuse, which ranks first as an exposure category for women from other racial groups, is much less prevalent among API female AIDS cases.

It is difficult to obtain AIDS data from Asian countries. However, the epidemic is growing rapidly in Southeast Asia, especially in Thailand.[107a] This increase poses risks to epidemiologic trends among API. Although the immigration policy of HIV testing will screen out those with the virus, those with false-negative results will be missed. In addition, many immigrants/refugees eventually return to their homeland to visit friends and relatives, and are at risk should they have intercourse with prostitutes or infected partners. Upon return to the United States, they may become the vector of transmission of HIV as well as other sexually transmitted diseases in their communities.

Measles. In 1990, 12,500 cases of measles (one half the national total) were reported in the state of California, the highest in over 25 years. Over 2500 patients in the state were hospitalized, the majority being less than 5 years of age. In that same year in California over 50 people died from measles and related complications. Approximately one half were API (specifically Hmong and Samoan). The API deaths were in preschool-aged children and young adults.[162]

Genetic disorders

Important genetic disorders in this population include thalassemia and glucose-6-phosphate dehydrogenase (G6PD) deficiency. These disorders are discussed in the Clinical Strategies section.

Lactose intolerance. Low lactose digestion capacity or lactase deficiency is found in 75% to 100% of Chinese, Japanese, Koreans, Thai, and Vietnamese.[43] Studies of Chinese children receiving physiologic doses of lactose

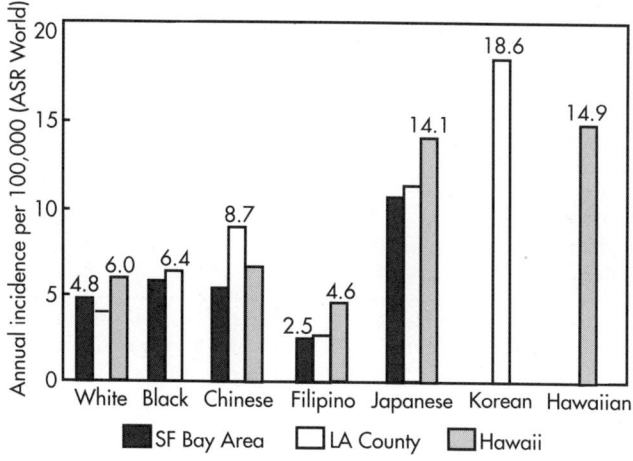

Fig. 37-4. Stomach cancer in females in 1978-1982 in the San Francisco Bay area, Los Angeles County, and Hawaii. (From Muir C et al: WHO IARC Sci Pub 88: Cancer Incidence in Five Countries, Vol V, Lyon, 1987.)

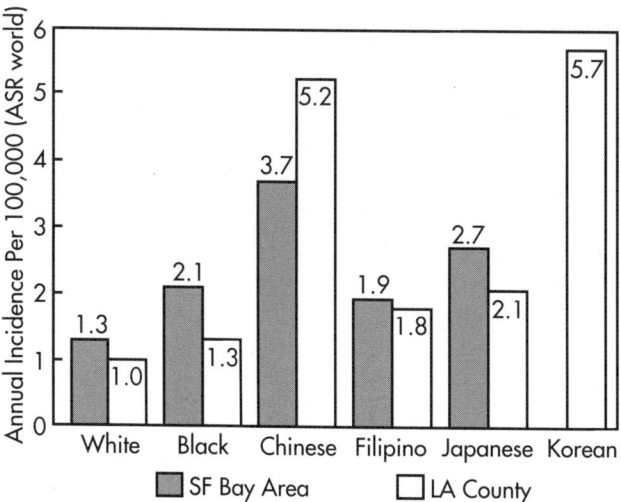

Fig. 37-5. Annual incidence of liver cancer per 100,000 among various groups of women in the San Francisco Bay area and Los Angeles County. (From Muir C et al: WHO:IARC Sci Pub 88: Cancer Incidence in Five Countries, Vol V, Lyon, 1987.)

(0.5g/kg) demonstrated that all 3-year-olds were able to digest lactose. By 4 to 6 years of age, lactose malabsorption was detected in 12% to 14%, by 7 years it was detected in 43%, and by 13 to 14 years it was detected in 74%.[158]

Cancer

In 1988, cancer ranked second among the leading causes of death for both API and the general population.[58] Incidence for specific cancers varies widely among API subgroups. Data sets on these populations are limited to narrow geographic samples, but they reveal patterns of high incidence for some cancers.

Women. Average annual age-adjusted incidence rates between 1983 and 1988 were compiled for Chinese, Japanese, and Filipino Americans in the San Francisco Bay Area.[17] Breast, lung, colon, and cervical cancer were the most common types among women from these groups as well as among whites. Invasive cervical cancer incidence was highest however among Filipinos (15.1 per 100,000) and Chinese (11.3 per 100,000). Similarly, 1978 to 1982 data including Hawaii, Los Angeles, and San Francisco demonstrated high rates for both Korean (17.5 per 100,000) and Hawaiian women (12.3 per 100,000).[116,168] Hawaiian women also demonstrated the highest breast cancer incidence (93.9 per 100,000) in the world. Maori women living in New Zealand had the highest rates of female lung cancer (68.1 per 100,000). By 1988 stomach cancer ranked fourth among Japanese women (21.6 per 100,000) and occurred at four times the rate of white women (5.4 per 100,000). These findings confirm data showing Japan to have the highest rates in the world for both sexes. Earlier findings revealed that Hawaiian, Filipino, and Chinese women also had a high incidence of stomach cancer (Fig. 37-4). By 1988, Chinese women contracted liver cancer more than five times as often as

whites. Earlier data show similar trends among Korean, Filipino, and Japanese women (Fig. 37-5).

Nasopharyngeal carcinoma (NPC) is a rare cancer in most world populations. It is remarkably concentrated among Chinese from the Guongdong province of southern China where incidence may exceed 30 per 100,000. Carryover has been documented among Chinese in Los Angeles and San Francisco.[13,177] Chinese, Filipino, and Korean female incidence exceeded their white and African American counterparts in these regions.

The incidence for thyroid cancer among many API females is two to three that of US whites and African Americans. This higher rate is especially noted for Filipinos and Hawaiians.[116,168]

Polynesian women from New Zealand have the highest incidence in the world for myeloid leukemia among women.[116,168]

Men. Lung, prostate, and colon cancer were the most common among white, African American, and API male subgroups. Hawaiian men (82.8 per 100,000) had a higher lung cancer incidence than whites (66.2 per 100,000) in Hawaii.[116] Polynesians and Maori men living in New Zealand had even higher rates (91.8 and 101.3 per 100,000, respectively). Currently, Japanese men have the highest incidence of rectal cancer in the San Francisco Bay Area. Male cancer trends parallel those of API women in most respects. Stomach cancer incidence among Japanese men was 2.7 times the rate of whites in San Francisco. (Table 37-1) From 1978 to 1982, Los Angeles Korean men showed the highest rates (44.8 per 100,000). Hawaiian men (31.2 per 100,000) had similarly high incidence.

Chinese men in San Francisco contract liver cancer 8.6 times more often than whites and nearly five times the rate

Table 37-1. 1983-1988 Male stomach cancer incidence (per 100,000), San Francisco Bay area

	Rate per 100,000
Chinese	20.5
Filipino	13.0
Japanese	33.8
White	12.4
African American	18.7

From cancer incidence data collected by the Northern California Cancer Center under contract N01-CN-05224 with the Division of Cancer Prevention and Control, National Cancer Institute, and under subcontract 050C-8708 with the California Public Health Foundation.

Table 37-2. 1983-1988 Male liver cancer incidence (per 100,000), San Francisco Bay area

	Rate per 100,000
Chinese	30.2
Filipino	15.7
Japanese	2.3
White	3.5
African American	6.1

From cancer incidence data collected by the Northern California Cancer Center under contract N01-CN-05224 with the Division of Cancer Prevention and Control, National Cancer Institute, and under subcontract 050C-8708 with the California Public Health Foundation.

Table 37-3. 1978-1982 Male thyroid cancer incidence (per 100,000), Hawaii

	Rate per 100,000
Chinese	8.8
Filipino	6.1
Japanese	5.3
Hawaiian	5.9
White	2.3

From Muir C et al: WHO:IARC Sci Pub 88: Cancer Incidence in Five Continents, Vol V, Lyon, 1987; and Whelan S, Parkin D, Masuyer E: Patterns of cancer in five continents, WHO:IARC Sci Pub 102: Lyon, 1990.

of African Americans (Table 37-2). Koreans (15.8 per 100,000) from Los Angeles, Hawaiians (7.3 per 100,000), and Polynesians from New Zealand (26.6 per 100,000) all showed relatively high incidence.

The incidence of NPC among Chinese men (30.0 per 100,000) from Hong Kong is the highest in the world. Rates among San Francisco Bay Area and Los Angeles Chinese men between 1978 and 1982 ranged from 9.9 to 14.8 per 100,000 in contrast to their white (0.6 to 0.7 per 100,000) and African American (1.0 to 1.1 per 100,000) counterparts.[13,177] Filipino (3.6 to 4.3 per 100,000), Japanese (0 to 1.4 per 100,000) and Korean (1.2 per 100,000) men also demonstrated comparatively high rates as well as Vietnamese in Los Angeles County.[133]

In Hawaii, thyroid cancer among Chinese men occurred 3.8 times more often than among whites. Other API subgroups also showed relatively higher incidence (Table 37-3).

Among men, the incidence per 100,000 for myeloid leukemia was higher for Chinese in Hawaii (5.2), Filipinos (6.1) in Los Angeles, Hawaiians (6.3), New Zealand Maori (6.1) and Polynesians (5.1) than for U.S. whites (4.7) and African Americans (4.7). Finally, Korean men in Los Angeles County displayed high rates of pancreatic cancer per 100,000 (16.4) compared with their white (8.1) and African American (11.0) counterparts.[116,168]

Major knowledge and screening barriers. According to the 1990 CDC BRFS carried out in Hawaii and California, API subgroups demonstrate low rates of cancer screening (Table 37-4).

The Chinese women surveyed were less likely to know the purpose of a Pap smear if they were either of low income, not fluent in English, less educated, or illiterate in their native language. Similar patterns exist for selected cancer screening measures among Vietnamese in California.

Nutrition, obesity, and exercise

Nutrition. Nutrition practices among API are best considered in the context of cultural beliefs and practices (see

Cultural Practices). However, some important western generalizations can be made.

The diets of API share many similarities. The main source of calories is rice, with relative less intake of animal fats and higher consumption of vegetables, fruits, and fish. The chief source of calcium is soybean curd, fish (sardines), and leafy green vegetables. Intake of dairy products is limited due to lactose intolerance.

Salt intake is common with sources being soy sauce, salted/pickled vegetables, fish sauce, and fermented bean curd.[128,151] A survey of various provinces in China measured 24-hour urinary sodium excretion and determined higher salt intake equivalent to 14.9 g/day while the World Health Organization recommends 3 to 5 g/day. They also identified a urinary sodium/potassium ratio of 10.76, which was over five times that seen in the United States.[180] Nutritional data taken on Southeast Asian pregnant women seen in a Southern California teaching hospital clinic revealed higher sodium intake and few differences between ethnic subgroups. Exceptions included the Cambodians who ate less fat, riboflavin, vitamin D, and calcium than the Vietnamese.[117] Of Chinese subgroups in California, the Taiwanese used the most oil in their cooking.[170] In a San Francisco survey, 46 Chinese women 50

Table 37-4. Women surveyed by 1990 BRFS in Oakland (Chinese) and statewide (Vietnamese and general population)[24,109]

Screening examination	Chinese		Vietnamese		California	
	%	95% CI*	%	95% CI*	%	95% CI*
Never had Pap smear†	45	(37-53)	53	(49-58)	6	(4-7)
Never had mammogram‡	68	(59-77)	48	(41-55)	27	(23-30)
Never had clinical breast exam (BE)‡	—	—	47	(42-51)	11	(9-14)
Never did self-BE‡	75	(66-83)	—	—	9	(7-11)

*Confidence interval.
†Women aged ≥18 years.
‡Women aged ≥40 years.

years and older had high daily cholesterol intakes of 576 mg.[26,81,169] Southeast Asian women showed decreased fat intake compared to other races in Southern California.[117]

Obesity. In Hawaii in 1990, Native Hawaiians had the highest percentage of obesity.[56] Obesity is also thought to be higher in Chinese Americans,[2] although perhaps not among the elderly Chinese.[26] Obesity has been documented to increase in a stepwise fashion with the lowest rates among Japanese men living in Japan, higher rates among those in Hawaii, and the highest rates among those in California.[127] The incidence of coronary heart disease among these cohorts of Japanese men increased in a similar manner from Japan to California.[132] Obesity among Filipinos is higher in the United States compared with the Philippine Islands.

Exercise. Studies documenting the activity level of Asians are scant. Immigrants from Asia, especially those from rural areas, have led physically active lives. In the United States, these immigrants view exercise as a luxury, not as an important aspect of maintaining good health. The 1990 Hawaiian BRFS identified sedentary life-styles (no physical activity or physical activity less than three times per week or less than 20 minutes per occasion) in Hawaiians (60.2%), Filipinos (71%), and Japanese (67.8%) as compared with whites (54.1%).[56] A slightly higher percentage of women were sedentary. Of 1009 Vietnamese adults in a 1990 California survey, a large proportion of men (40%) and women (50%) pursued no physical activity outside of work during the preceding month in contrast to the state's overall population (men 24% and women 28%).[109]

Mental health

The characteristic mental health problems of Asian immigrants and refugees are strongly influenced by circumstances that motivated them to leave their native countries and their expectations for starting a new life in the United States. These disorders include intrusive and frightening thoughts, sleep disturbances, anxiety, depression (over 50% of adults in one Vietnamese refugee community[95]), somatization, posttraumatic stress disorder (PTSD), and

psychosis. Problems of substance abuse, domestic violence, compulsive gambling, and suicide are on the rise. Immigrants, while being spared the often extreme hardships of the refugee experience, also disproportionately experience mental health problems.[64] However, these problems may be masked by negative cultural attitudes toward mental illness that prevent many Asians from seeking out care.

Refugees, in their often precipitous decision to leave their country of origin and seek asylum, frequently leave behind loved ones, a familiar system of providing food and shelter, and the sense of a predictable future. The refugees may bring with them both the physical and psychologic scars of torture, malnutrition, a disintegrating social structure, and memories of atrocities inflicted by war on their family and friends. The dangers of the escape often end in a protracted confinement in a crowded refugee camp. This disorienting episode is followed by transplantation into an alien environment and culture, which takes its toll on the adaptive skills of the hardiest survivors.

The profound sense of personal distress from these stressors may begin at the time the individual contemplates flight, but may need to be suppressed to qualify for acceptance by a host country. This potential legal barrier to entry into a host country compounds a frequent cultural barrier to mental health care in many Asian countries. Many Southeast Asians believe that mental illness results from retribution for a previous lifetime's wrongdoing, from a spell cast by a jealous rival, or from being haunted by an unhappy ghost. The resulting shame to one's family may prevent one from openly acknowledging that a problem exists.[64] In short, upon arrival in the United States where culture shock and major adjustment awaits them, refugees have yet to fully grieve their immense losses. This problem has a profound impact on their mental health problems.

Disillusionment over the realities of making a new life in the host country replaces romanticized dreams and high expectations.[32] Other influences include marital status,[114] isolation from others of the same community, ability to learn the host country's language, and degree of racism encountered. Lack of gainful employment and separation from traditional family support networks are two powerful stress factors, especially for refugees.[64] Marital conflict (sometimes resulting in domestic violence) and intergenerational conflict become increasingly common among these groups as ancestral gender roles become blurred by the need for two incomes, and strict intergenerational traditions conflict with host country norms.

Models of psychologic adjustment of refugees and immigrants identify the period of maximal risk for depression or other psychiatric disorder as 10 to 18 months after arrival in the host country.[8,134] When psychologic stressors overwhelm the coping mechanisms of the individual, somatization of depression may often be the mode of presentation to the health care system.[94,167] In this case, primary care providers are usually the first line of contact with the western treatment system. Multiple visits are often required to establish the diagnosis. In one study, 95% of Vietnamese refugees diagnosed with depression had initially presented with physical complaints.[95] Common presenting symptoms include chronic headache, intermittent abdominal pain, both upper and lower back pain, and multiple joint pains.[94]

Post Traumatic Stress Disorder as defined by the American Psychiatric Association (DSM III R), denotes "a psychologically distressing event that is generally outside the range of usual human experience." The characteristic symptoms involve reexperiencing the traumatic event often leading to detachment from the external world, painful and intrusive flashbacks, recurrent nightmares, and the loss of ability to find enjoyment in life. After a triggering stressor (e.g., news report about country of origin or letter from family member) occurs in the affected individual's life, symptoms of hyperalertness, sleep difficulties, decreased concentration and/or impaired memory may develop.[84] One study of young Khmer survivors of the Pol Pot regime concluded that 50% suffered from PTSD.[85]

CULTURAL (HEALTH) PRACTICES THAT INFLUENCE CARE

API culture and folk health beliefs contrast significantly with Western values and medical models. Yet their influence depends on the individual's educational level, socioeconomic status, familiarity with Western health care systems, level of acculturation, influence of religion and family, and health status.

A Southeast Asian refugee from the hills of Laos may have a shamanistic belief system. A peasant from a rural agricultural village may incorporate herbal remedies. A foreign graduate student may have access to Western health care. A third-generation Asian American infant may receive both routine well-child checkups and immunizations as well as traditional folk medicine from an immigrant grandmother who is the primary caretaker while both parents work. This combination using both traditional and western systems occurs frequently even within tight-knit and exclusive ethnic communities such as the Chinatowns in major US cities.[60]

Yin-Yang and balance

Chinese Taoist philosophy is at the root of most traditional Asian medical theories and incorporates the concept of Yin and Yang also known as the hot-cold theory.[28,37,67,79,145] Filipinos call their principle of balance *Tim-bang*.[1] Yin is cold, dark, female, negative, sour; Yang is hot, light, male, positive, sweet. Most body organs are also labeled as either Yin (heart, lungs, spleen, liver and kidneys) or Yang (gallbladder, stomach, small intestine, large intestine, bladder, and triple burner [best understood as the functional relationship between the organs that regulate water]). Qi or Ch'i (energy), blood (which also has aspects of Qi), Jing (essence), Shen (spirit), and fluids comprise the five "fundamental substances" that flow through body pathways (meridians). Illness and disease are interpreted as a state of imbalance in the Yin and Yang.

Causes of illness. Illness is generated by factors in one of three categories—environment, emotion, and way of life. The factors are never seen as separate from the illness. The environmental factor of illness include the "six pernicious influences"—wind, cold, heat or fire, dampness, dryness and summer heat. The "seven emotions" include joy, anger, sadness, grief, pensiveness, fear, and fright. The category of "way of life" includes diet, sexual activity, physical activity, and miscellaneous factors.[79]

Diagnostic techniques. To distinguish among patterns of disharmony, the Chinese traditional healers use the "four examinations": inspection (appearance, facial color, tongue, secretions, and excretions), listening and smelling, asking, and touching (pulse taking and abdominal palpation).[67] The pulse is taken from 12 different positions along the radial pulse of both wrists. Each position is closely linked with the meridians and internal organs. Combining the four examinations enables the traditional practitioner to visualize a matrix of signs that relate to the fundamental substances, the pernicious influences, body organs, emotions, and the patient's way of life. The astute clinician can thereby perceive a total body landscape of harmony and disharmony that transcends purely physical categories of description—the excesses and deficiencies, the cold and hot, the Yin and the Yang.[79]

Nutrition. The practical application of this interwoven culture, philosophy, and traditional belief system is best understood by examining nutrition beliefs and practices. Nutrition is an important element in health and illness. It is useful for prevention and recovery. Foods are also classified as Yin (cold) or Yang (hot); hot-cold is not related to temperature of the food. A balance between the Yin and Yang is the basis for a balanced diet. Foods also have different flavors (pungent, sour, salty, sweet, bitter, and bland), energies (cold, cool, warm, hot, and neutral), movements (inside, outside, upper, and lower), and organic action (in reference to the internal organs), as well as many common actions (arrest bleeding, promote digestion, relieve pain, tone up the spleen, etc.).[102]

The knowledge of hot and cold foods is passed down in the family by tradition and practice and heavily influences meal patterns. Intake of food should be a balance of the two forces; cold foods need to be eaten to balance hot foods. Examples of cold and hot foods can be seen in the accompanying box. Lu[102] has developed a chart of y-scores by which foods and body types, diseases, moods, and four seasons may be classified into Yin ($-$) and Yang ($+$); a score of 0 is neutral. Watermelon has a y-score of -2 (Yin), beef has a y-score of $+2$ (Yang), and bean cake is neutral with a y-score of 0. The chart includes almost 200 foods.

The choice of foods will depend on the individual's health at the moment. Yin conditions require the consumption of more Yang foods. Yang conditions require Yin foods. In addition, the nature of food may change after cooking. Hot ingredients such as pepper and ginger increase the hotness of meat. Boiling for a long time makes a cold food hotter (more Yang). Other cultural beliefs such as "Bo" or "enriching" foods (meat, poultry, seafood, and eggs) are used to deal with imbalances that occur with recent illness, after giving birth, or after surgery. These foods must be used sparingly, however, or they in turn will cause an imbalance. Another belief is that intake of animal organs will help the same human organ function; i.e., eating pork brain will improve brain function.

This classification of food can be both beneficial and harmful. Chinese babies are breast-fed because neither cows' milk nor goats' milk is acceptable.[145] However, infants are allowed only neutral foods, which excludes most fruits and vegetables.[45,98]

TRADITIONAL TREATMENTS
Traditional treatment techniques

Traditional and folk treatments include acupuncture, acupressure, skin scraping (coin-rubbing), spinal pinch-pull, cupping (heating the inside of a cup and then placing it on the skin; the resulting vacuum opens up skin pores and causes the cup to attach to the skin), and moxibustion (use of heat by burning a powdered mixture). These various techniques involve points on the skin surface that are linked with meridians of internal organs. Theoretically, they either stimulate or withdraw the activity of fundamental substances traveling along the meridians, thereby relieving congestion and allowing for regulation of blood and energy. This technique helps restore balance to organ function and states of mind.

Herbal medicine

When nutrition and other measures fail, herbal remedies are used as the next step. This practice is an ancient tradition in Chinese medicine, but it is also used by tribal peoples such as the Mien, H'mong, Khmer, Lao, Vietnam-

---

> **Yin (cold) and Yang (hot) conditions and foods**[16,41,115,170]
>
> Cold conditions—anemia, chills, colds and flu, diarrhea, frequent urination, miscarriage, muscle cramps, poor appetite, weakness, cancer, weight loss
>
> Hot conditions—blurry vision, dry cough, fever, constipation, infection, hypertension, pimples, rashes
>
> Cold foods—most fruit and fruit juices, rice cooking water, spinach, cabbage, other green leafy vegetables, mung beans and sprouts, seaweed, water, Chinese herbal medicine
>
> Hot foods—Alcohol, red and black beans, cereal, coffee, fat and oil, some fruits (ripe mango, papaya, tangerines, watermelon), ginger, ice, chicken, meat, poultry, nuts, black pepper, spices, chili beans, Western medicines, sugar, vitamins and iron pills

---

ese,[115] and some Filipinos.[108] Herbal shops are found in many urban centers with large Asian populations. China is developing a body of medical knowledge that combines the best of both worlds—traditional and Western. Research on the pharmacology of herbal medicines is underway. Physicians, paramedical trainees, and other health care professionals receive basic courses on treating patients with herbs, acupuncture, and Western medicines.[51] One published guide, *A barefoot doctor's manual*, contains a listing of over 500 herbal medicines. For example both *Coptis* and *Scutellena* inhibit the growth of *Streptococcus* bacteria.[141] *Coptis* is one Chinese herbal remedy listed in addition to penicillin for the treatment of acute tonsillitis.[156] Digitalis and reserpine are well-known pharmaceuticals derived from plants. Unfortunately, the collection and processing of herbs are not controlled, which may yield contaminated final products.[123] There have been several reports of heavy metal poisoning, agranulocytosis, and other adverse reactions to such herbal remedies.[34,93,130,144,161]

Patients boil herbs in the prescribed amount of water for the designated time to achieve proper concentrations of broth. Usually, a single dose of the correct herb is sufficient. In contrast, Western medicines are given in many pills over a period of time.

BARRIERS TO PREVENTION
Traditional health practices

Recent arrivals are more likely to rely on folk medicine and traditional/religious healers as a first resort. Even after visiting a Western practitioner, they may continue to use two methods of care simultaneously. The slightest dissatisfaction with Western care may reinforce reliance primarily on traditional care. This reaction limits opportunities for primary and secondary prevention. Cultural taboos about mental illness also prevent many API refugees and immigrants from actively pursuing western services.

Other barriers to preventive and ongoing care include blood drawing, surgery, and the hospital.[145] Blood is seen as a nonrenewable vital life and energy source for the body. Its loss is considered deleterious to one's health. According to traditional Chinese medicine practice, a good clinician should be able to make a diagnosis, based on history and examination alone.[145] Hence, many patients abhor routine blood draws to monitor their cholesterol, glucose, potassium, hemoglobin, or coagulation status. Surgery may involve mutilation of the body; Confucius taught that the body must be revered and kept whole and sound. Understandably, some people will refuse any operation, including biopsy to detect problems early.[82,145] Hospitals are thought to be a place to die, where surgery is performed, where a person's spirit may get lost, or where the right food to prevent illness will not be served. It is a place where there is no translator[16] and where you will not be understood even with translators because you are different culturally.

Communication

Language barriers undermine preventive health practices by immigrants in several ways. The non-English-speaking or illiterate immigrant does not benefit from current mainstream U.S. media campaigns that emphasize health promotion and disease prevention. Overcoming this knowledge gap is of paramount importance given the multitude of barriers this population already faces in obtaining preventive services. Standardized CDC surveys conducted in Hawaii and California reveal major knowledge deficits and access problems among API regarding cardiovascular risk factor control and cancer screening.[24,56,109] Lack of English fluency has been associated with less likelihood for Vietnamese men to obtain stool occult blood tests; for Chinese to obtain serum cholesterol screening, and for Chinese to recognize the influence of cholesterol on heart disease.[24,109] This problem is further complicated by a high rate of illiteracy among some ethnic subgroups (e.g., Mien people from Laos). Even if an individual is motivated by acute symptoms, public transportation imposes a formidable obstacle to a non-English speaker.

Not knowing whether a hospital or doctor's office has sufficient multilingual/multicultural staffing can be an added deterrent for even the most health-conscious individuals. The frightening experience of venturing into a health facility without adequate translation capacity undermines efforts to convince API immigrants and refugees to make future follow-up visits. Without skilled interpretors or multilingual and multicultural professionals on site, vital preventive education and counseling for genetic disease (thalassemia), AIDS and HIV testing, cholesterol reduction, and cancer prevention will fail to reach API communities.

Cultural insensitivity

Most public health institutions and primary care providers lack knowledge about the epidemiology, history, cultural background, and barriers facing immigrant and refugee populations in accessing health services. Cultural insensitivity occurs when little or no action (individual or institutional) is taken to address both the knowledge gaps and the critical health access issues. For example, lack of awareness about somatization, depression, PTSD, and other common mental disorders in this population will cause unnecessary delay in arriving at an accurate diagnosis. Inadequate multilingual and multicultural staffing of major health institutions will send a negative message to new arrivals and make preventive follow-up an impossible task. At the community voluntary level, Chinese seniors may continue with traditional daily exercises such as Tai Chi or Chi Kung. However, lack of organized groups and facilities may restrict participation.

Socioeconomic barriers

Financial barriers are ever present, mainly among recent arrivals who tend to be low income, work long hours, and have minimal or no benefits such as sick leave, health insurance, or health promotion programs. Consequently, unless symptoms occur, most individuals are reluctant to lose valuable work time or to pay doctor fees for preventive checkups or any other beneficial programs (e.g., smoking cessation workshops). In Oakland Chinatown, 23% of uninsured Chinese over age 40 never had their blood pressure checked in contrast to only 6% among insured Chinese.[24] Vietnamese women were less likely to have had a breast examination if they had no health insurance. Failure to have a mammogram was associated with below poverty level income.[109] Even with a common understanding of the benefits from childhood immunizations, the costs are obstacles to full compliance with immunization recommendations.[71]

Less educated and illiterate subgroups exist among API, particularly in groups at the lowest income level and among those with communication or language barriers. Young immigrant and refugee children are often cared for by elderly family members who are less familiar with Western traditions and more likely to adhere strongly to traditional cultural beliefs. This type of care can result in several barriers to prevention. For example in San Francisco young Chinese children may not get adequate exercise because immigrant caretakers may be uncomfortable with their external environment and be fearful of venturing outside. School-aged children are expected to do their class work as a first priority to the exclusion of afternoon physical activities.

Lack of health data

A relatively small population size and the perception of a "model minority" without problems have limited efforts to assess API health status. Until recently, most national survey instruments were not conducted in any Asian languages. Race coding has often lumped API into one category or as "other," combining them with Native Americans and Hispanics. That approximately one half of the 1990 California deaths from measles occurred only among Samoans and Hmong underscores the importance of data collection that monitors all API subgroups. Consequently, many API preventable health risks and health care needs are poorly understood.[128]

SCREENING AND COUNSELING GUIDELINES SPECIFIC FOR API
Transcultural strategies

Bridging cultural gaps requires provider initiative toward becoming knowledgeable about the patient's culture and health beliefs. Interpreters and patients themselves can offer a great deal of information. An open and flexible attitude can build trust and help overcome even the most profound cultural differences between practitioner and patient. Familiarity with both major and unique diseases that afflict the particular community will enhance early detection capability. Community workshops, videos, and opportunities for continuing medical opportunities are available (see Resources).

Berlin[9] provides a model and mnemonic for dealing with increasingly diverse patient populations: LEARN

L   *Listen* with sympathy and understanding to the patient's perception of the problem
E   *Explain* your perceptions of the problem
A   *Acknowledge* and discuss the differences and similarities
R   *Recommend* treatment
N   *Negotiate* agreement

Linkages between social services, community groups, churches, or ongoing orientation classes for new arrivals can facilitate their adjustment to a new society. They may also provide a rich information resource for the practitioner. National organizations also provide a wealth of resources including health education pamphlets, posters, and videos in several API languages.

Skilled multilingual and multicultural interpreters are essential to communicate effectively across both language and cultural barriers. They assist the health care provider in establishing a respectful and trusting environment in which to introduce a new client to the western medical/mental health system.[83] In areas where the monolingual API population is sizable, a commitment should be made to ensure adequate translation capacity in all major health facilities. Family members and friends can be helpful. However, the practitioner will be compromised in handling confidentiality issues that arise unpredictably, particularly true in mental health settings. Putsch[125] provides some excellent guidelines in using medical interpreters.

The following excerpt is from a videotape summary handout:[65]

How To Use Interpreters' Services

1. Learn and use a few phases of greeting and introduction in the patient's native language.
2. Identify, for the interpreter, a seating arrangement that facilitates eye contact between the patient and you.
3. Ask the interpreter to use the first person "I" (refraining from using "He/she says. . .").
4. Use the second person "you" to address the patient (for example, "Are you married?" instead of "Ask her if she's married").
5. Identify, for the interpreter, the interpreting method to be used. Explain it, if necessary.
6. Direct the interpreter not to give advice, offer comments, or make assumptions. This helps you to maintain control of the interview and guides the interpreter in defining his/her role.
7. Verify mutual understanding of the information exchanged, asking the interpreter to translate back your questions/instructions and using specific questions to check the patient's comprehension.
8. Stay with the patient until the interview has been completed.
9. Become acquainted with relevant aspects of your patient's culture.
10. Refine your general communications skills as well as your expertise as an interviewer.
11. Define the roles of a health care interpreter. Promote those most useful to you.
12. Study the status of health care interpretations in your area. Identify available resources.
13. Establish a communication partnership with your interpreter.

It is also important to ascertain the individual's level of education and exposure to western culture, and to assess the extent to which the cultural gap needs to be addressed. Concepts of disease and treatment vary widely among groups. For example the Mien use folk medicine and religious shamanism to treat illness, whereas many Chinese, Japanese, Koreans, and Vietnamese believe in the concepts of traditional Chinese medicine and acupuncture. The least educated will require basic education about concepts such as germ theory and infectious disease transmission. Educated individuals from cosmopolitan cities tend to use western medicine or a combination of western and traditional Chinese medicine. Those with little or no exposure to western medicine will find its concepts totally foreign and yet may believe that because it is so sophisticated anything can be cured. Even within one ethnic group diversity exists. Knowledge and education levels vary tremendously from the frankly illiterate rural villager who relies solely on folk remedies and traditional Chinese medicine to the well-educated person totally familiar with western medicine techniques.

Individual patients also use traditional practices to different degrees. A study of Boston Chinatown residents found diverse use of medical care as well as different attitudes about medical beliefs. Utilization patterns and beliefs varied also based on sex. The study concluded that ethnic groups cannot be viewed as homogeneous and uniform. Individual members have different sets of attitudes, values, beliefs, and behaviors.[60]

Many API, especially Chinese, go to a traditional herbalist for ailments more often than to a western practitioner. Personal attacks on herbal medicine in these situations are best avoided. Some herbal treatments have been proven effective in treating mild hypertension.[171] If the practitioner acknowledges the potential effectiveness of these remedies, patients will readily mention their current use, thereby offering an opportunity to avoid mixing unknown herbs with western prescriptions during treatment initiation. Clinicians can also explain how western medicine differs from folk remedies to achieve better understanding and compliance.

Coin rubbing (Cao Gio) on the skin surface is common among the Vietnamese and the Khmer for treatment of fever, chills, and headaches.[115] It usually leaves bruises on the chest and back. Several cases of pseudobattering in Vietnamese children have been reported.[10,48,101,173] Herbal mixtures are burned (moxibustion) over the skin surface causing first-, second-, and third-degree burns. These may be misinterpreted as cigarette burns on an infant or young child. It is important, therefore, to distinguish this cultural health custom from a true case of child abuse.

Convincing the patient about the importance of test or examination results requires time and patience, but can enhance compliance. When drawing blood, reassuring the patient that blood production is ongoing is helpful.

Many API regard western medicine as being very powerful and worry about long-term adverse affects. This attitude becomes a self-fulfilling prophecy if they experience even minor side effects from medications. Therefore, in prescribing medications, low doses with gradual increases, low side-effect profiles, and convenient dosing are helpful in improving compliance.

Clinical strategies

In considering preventive intervention in API, specific recommendations help to supplement standard preventive health practices. These following suggestions are organized by age group or condition.

Prenatal care. Traditional Chinese high-iron, high-calcium, low-sugar diets should be encouraged. Patients may avoid iron due to the belief that it may harden the bones and make delivery difficult. Pregnancy and delivery, with its accompanying blood loss, are considered a Yin condition.[16] High sugar intakes are common and in late pregnancy, eggs scrambled with rock sugar are commonly used to "clean the system and lubricate the passage."[112] Milk and dairy products are not part of the standard Asian diet. Alternative sources (tofu, green leafy vegetables) can provide adequate calcium.

Prenatal screening procedures are often incomprehensible to healthy traditionally minded immigrants whose prenatal experiences were satisfactory without advanced technology. Glucose tolerance testing, with its multiple blood draws, nonstress testing, ultrasonography, and amniocentesis, are seen as "meddlesome, dangerous, unnecessary, and frightening." Noncompliance is common.[112]

In the prenatal period screening should take place for tuberculosis, hepatitis B, parasitism, and thallassemia. In general, however, only active TB, symptomatic parasitism, and *Ascaris* infections should be treated during the prenatal period. HB carriers should have all family members screened and vaccinated as needed. Their newborn should also receive one dose of hepatitis B immune globulin in addition to the HB vaccine. Partners of thalassemia-trait mothers should be screened and receive appropriate counseling and management.

Support for traditional postpartum care beliefs and presentation of alternatives such as sponge baths and hot water hair washing are often beneficial. Some emphasize the importance of perineum and breast care.[16] The traditional postpartum recovery period requires decreasing the Yin energy forces or cold air in the body. The body pores are believed to remain open for a month after delivery during which time cold air can enter the body. The new mother is advised against going outdoors or taking a shower or even washing her hair during this time. Southeast Asian mothers are permitted to take hot baths and steam baths, but only after the second postpartum day.[90]

The classical Chinese postpartum diet is high in hot foods (Yang) and hot drinks. A popular soup consists of pig's feet or knuckles, sweet black vinegar, black beans, ginger, and hard-boiled eggs.[28] These foods are said to help get rid of gas; assist in the involution of the uterus; and provide calcium, protein and minerals. Another dish consists of rice wine, chicken, lichen, and ginger (*gai jow* "chicken whiskey"). Because the alcohol in the rice wine may cause bleeding, eating this dish should be postponed for at least 2 weeks. The new mother should also be encouraged to supplement her diet with other culturally acceptable foods as well as nutritious foods such as eggs, meat, and liver.[16]

Care should be taken to review the benefits of breast feeding. "Resistance to breast-feeding reflects a cultural identification of breast-feeding with a primitive or agrarian past and a perceived adaptation to modern, urbanized and western life-style. . . . additional educational reinforcement for breast-feeding during the critical early puerperal period" is needed.[112] Southeast Asian mothers do not breast feed until their milk has come because of the belief that their vital heat and fluids would be further depleted.[91]

Pediatric Issues. Asian children, whether born in Asia or in the United States, frequently have poor dental care. Dental caries and orthodontic problems range from 18% in children ages 0 to 4 to 42% in those between 5 and 14.[57] Prolonged bottle use with consequent nursing bottle caries is common. Nursing bottle caries beginning as early as 16 months, with eventual erosion down to the gumline, is not rare. Aggressive prevention of nursing bottle caries may involve asking the child to "surrender" the bottle to the physician. Molar caries from excessive sweets is also common.

Excessive whole milk from the bottle, often to the exclusion of other foods, often leads to iron deficiency and severe constipation. Fresh meats, fish, and poultry should be recommended over preserved salted fish. Because eggs are at a premium in Asia and are inexpensive in the United States egg intake among children may be excessive.

Although excessive whole milk and infant formula intake with the bottle is common, excessive and prolonged breast feeding may also occur. Prolonged breast-feeding is seen more often in Southeast Asians; these mothers tend to have many children. Calcium drain with respect to the prevention of osteoporosis should be addressed.

Overt lead poisoning is rare, but given the near universal use of ceramics from Asia, even among second- and third-generation Asian-Americans, subclinical low-dose chronic exposure may be common (see Plates 1 and 2 between p.16 and p.17).

Although the FDA has entered into a Memorandum of Understanding with the People's Republic of China to ensure that no ceramic ware manufactured in China with an unsafe quantity of leachable lead or cadmium be imported into the United States, much of the older ceramic ware is still in use.

Parents should be warned not to place acid foods (e.g., juice, vinegar) in ceramic ware from Asia. Simple to use, relatively inexpensive FDA-approved testing kits are available (see Resources).

Southeast Asians may additionally make use of traditional medications that contain high concentrations of lead, arsenic, and mercury, although parents may often not admit to such items.

Teaching parents and grandparents about first aid for burns should be a routine part of primary care during the well-child visit. Hot water burns are fairly common in young children, who sometimes require hospitalization. Parents or grandparents are often not aware of simple first aid measures of immediate cold water flushing and may instead use traditional methods such as application of toothpaste, soy sauce, and ointments.

Mothballs are frequently used to protect clothing. If the mothballs are made from naphthalene, their use poses a hemolytic anemic threat if ingested, or inhaled.[166] Children with and without G6PD deficiency may have hemoly-

sis on exposure to naphthalene. Both p-dichlorobenzene and naphthalene mothballs are commonly sold in Asian markets. Primary care providers should discourage Asian parents from using mothballs, especially those made of naphthalene.

Medications common around the house include *Bai Hua Yao* (White Flower Oil) and/or *Hung Hua Yao* (Red Flower Oil). These medications can be bought from Asian markets. Like the western ointment Ben-Gay, these medications contain methyl salicylate or wintergreen oil and are used externally to treat muscle and joint pain. Because of the extremely high concentrations of methyl salicylate (often 40% to 70%), parents should be cautioned to keep them out of reach of children.

In Hong Kong[174] and among Asian children in San Francisco,[138] *Salmonella* and *Campylobacter* are the two most common bacterial causes of diarrhea. *Salmonella* is also the most common bacterial cause of diarrhea in Singapore.[126] In Hong Kong and San Francisco, a great number of these cases occur in the very young; in Hong Kong, most of the *Salmonella* cases occur in children less than 2 years of age; a similar pattern is seen in San Francisco.

The preparation of chicken may be a major contributing factor for the high incidence of *Salmonella* and *Campylobacter* infections. Chicken is inexpensive and easily obtained in Asian markets. The high frequency of such infections during the first year among Chinese may be related to the custom of preparing a wine with chicken specialty to strengthen the mother after giving birth. Great quantities of this dish are prepared, as it is served to all the friends and relatives when they come to visit. In San Francisco, high population density, the use of shared kitchens, visiting grandparents, and relatives unfamiliar with use of the western kitchen may also contribute to the high incidence of these infections.

Prenatal, postnatal, and pediatric primary care should repeat the need for handwashing and the proper cleaning of kitchen utensils and cutting boards. Providers should obtain stool cultures in Asian children with diarrhea, especially those less than 1 year old who account for a large number of persons with this infection.[138]

Among the preventive health modalities Asian immigrants confront after arrival, immunizations are one of the more familiar and accepted. Incomplete immunizations at age 2 years are not uncommon, however, despite statistics that may indicate a higher rate of full immunization in Asian children at 2 years of age as compared to other children.[72] Documentation of the type and number of immunizations received in the home country is frequently difficult as records are unavailable. Relying on the memory of parents or the individual is unreliable. Many school districts will only acknowledge immunizations from other countries when exact dates are supplied. Asking parents to write to relatives overseas to get records is often helpful; however, these records may be misleading. Three vaccines ending with "B" (Japanese B, HB, and *Haemophilus influenza* B) often causes confusion. Japanese B encephalitis vaccines are routinely given in Hong Kong, China, Taiwan, Japan, and Korea. Before 1985, China gave monovalent and bivalent oral polio vaccines. These vaccines were often given 1 to 2 months apart. Credit should be given for only one vaccination ([type 1 monovalent] + [type 2+3 bivalent]). This approach has often caused confusion when staff has credited the child with two trivalent polio vaccinations. Fortunately, trivalent polio vaccines have been administered since then. It is always helpful to copy the original vaccination record and keep it in the patient's chart. Without reliable records, children need to begin a complete battery of immunizations.

Special attention should be paid to the history of adverse reactions to vaccines so as to take necessary precautions. Immigrants may not be knowledgeable about changes in recommendations for childhood immunizations. Therefore, reviewing and updating immunizations are necessary, especially in the older school-aged child whose immunizations are "complete" and who rarely returns for health care visits.

To treat fever and pain after immunizations, parents need careful instructions on acetaminophen use. Parents should be cautioned about the different concentrations of various preparations. Language barriers have caused mix-ups between infant drop bottles (80 mg/0.8 ml) and elixirs (160 mg/5ml).

Grandparents should be involved in the discussion of child-care problems (dental, nutritional, safety, psychologic) in Asian families. Children often spend most of the day with grandparents while both parents are working. On the other hand, the provider must assess each family individually. In some cases one might openly support the parent who seeks to become independent and progressive in the face of more traditional and resistant grandparents. The influence of grandparents can be very strong.

Mental health. The practitioner should thoroughly document the patient's journey to the current residence. This social history should include the client's life-style and family unit before any upheaval, flight experience from country of origin, description of life within the refugee camp, immigration experience, and description of settlement and adjustment in the country of permanent residence. From this database, a health provider can anticipate some of the predictable stressors of resettlement. These stressors can include issues around war trauma and grieving losses, physical safety, adequate housing, ability to use the transportation system, finding culturally familiar foods, learning to access emergency medical care, and social and cultural isolation.

A complete psychiatric evaluation may be warranted. This evaluation can be enhanced by the use of Kinzie's Vietnamese Depression Scale (based on DSM III criteria).[83] The potential for suicide should be considered in any patient who finds little hope for the future of their chil-

dren or family.[32] In many Asian cultures the individual is often considered less important than the family. Symptomatic treatment is useful and appreciated by many who are truly suffering. Antidepressant medications can be extremely helpful, not only in major depression but in PTSD patients.[32,64] A supportive, stable comprehensive health care environment is one model that patients seem to appreciate. A support group and/or individual psychotherapy, used in tandem with the primary medical visits, is perceived to address the total health of the individual; these opportunities rely on a holistic belief in which many immigrant and refugee patients can find comfort. The patient may have already resorted to home remedies, traditional healers, and spiritual leaders. Treatment plans are often facilitated by cooperation between the various treatment modalities the patient has chosen.

SPECIFIC DISEASES
Thalassemia

Thalassemia is a genetic disorder affecting the synthesis of the globin chain (alpha or beta) of the hemoglobin molecule. It occurs with high frequency in a broad tropical belt that extends from the Mediterranean basin through the Middle East and Southeast Asia. Due to Asian immigration, previously rare occurrences of hydrops fetalis (alpha thal homozygous) with maternal complications (preeclampsia and placental retention) are now more frequent in U.S. hospitals serving large Asian populations.[53,155] These hydrops fetalis cases occur mainly among Asian ethnicities because this expression does not exist among patients of Mediterranean extraction. Homozygous beta thalassemia (and beta/HgbE) results in severe transfusion-dependent anemia, a condition that parallels the clinical course of sickle cell anemia. Consequently, thalassemia is viewed as the most important genetic disorder among Asians in the United States.

Practically all types of thalassemia and its related disorders are found in Southeast Asia. Prevalence of thalassemia trait, both in native countries and among Asian immigrants, is displayed in Table 37-5.

Alpha thalassemia. There are four alpha genes located in two closely linked sets of chromosome 16. The alpha thalassemia syndromes are caused by deletions, in varying degree, of these genes.

Silent Carriers involve a single gene deletion and appear clinically and hematologically normal. **Alpha thalassemia trait** involves deletion of two alpha genes resulting in mild anemia with microcytosis, mean corpuscular volume (MCV) < 80. Diagnosis is by exclusion, i.e., low MCV in the absence of iron deficiency anemia and with normal hemoglobin A2 levels on hemoglobin electrophoresis. Family studies support the diagnosis.

Hemoglobin H disease results from deletion of three alpha genes and leads to chronic hemolytic anemia, microcytosis, marked hypochromia, anisocytosis, poikilocyto-

Table 37-5. Prevalence of thalassemia trait

	Alpha	Beta	E
China[179]	4-15%	1-1.5%	—
Taiwan[30]	1.4%	—	—
Thailand	20-30%	5-10%	35-50%
Laos	44%	—	35-50%
Cambodia	—	—	35-50%
Burma	10.5%	—	>10%
Vietnam, Malaysia, Indonesia, Philippines	—	—	2-5%
U.S. Studies			
Chinese[140]	4.9%	3.5%	0.05%
Samoan	1.9%	—	—
Filipino	6.4%	0.7%	—
Laotian	7.5%	—	15%
Mien	12%	6.1%	—
Boston			
1970s Chinese[27]	9%	4.8%	—
1990 Chinese/Southeast Asians[122]	5%	3.6%	0.45%
California[70]			
Vietnamese	8%	8%	<1%
Cambodia	12%	3%	36%
Laos	14%	3%	28%
Filipino (newborn)[97]	5.4%	—	—
Hawaii*	25%	7.2%	7.3%

*Referral Center.

sis, and the presence of hemoglobin inclusions in the peripheral blood. **Fetal hydrops syndrome** involves deletion of all four alpha genes except in rare cases. It is not compatible with life. Affected fetuses suffer from severe anemia, progressive heart failure, and edema leading to stillbirth or death immediately after birth. Pregnant women carrying affected fetuses have a high risk for obstetric complications such as toxemia of pregnancy.

Beta thalassemia. The beta gene is located on chromosome 11. Three syndromes may result. **Beta thalassemia trait** occurs in persons with a single beta thalassemia gene, and is clinically benign with mild hematologic findings of low MCV, low hemoglobin and hematocrit, and normal iron levels. **Thalassemia intermedia** presents with moderately severe hemolytic anemia. This anemia may result in chronic icterus, jaundice, and splenomegaly. Pneumococcal vaccination is advised in these persons. In **thalassemia major** (Cooley's anemia) homozygosity results in severe hemolytic anemia, which requires regular transfusion to sustain life. Most patients manifest symptoms in the first year of life. Repeated transfusions cause iron overload requiring chelation on a regular basis.

Hemoglobin (Hb) E is a beta-chain variant and is a hallmark of thalassemia in Asia, where it is common. **Hb E trait** results from heterozygosity of the Hb E gene. The Hb level on Hb electrophoresis is between 30% and 40%. This condition is clinically and hematologically benign. **Hb EE disease** represents homozygous state for the E gene. Patients are clinically and hematologically benign with low MCV and mild anemia.

Hb E/beta thalassemia represents double heterozygosity of Hb E and beta thalassemia and results in severe clinical manifestations similar to Cooley's anemia. **Hb E/alpha thalassemia** is the double heterozygosity of Hb E and the alpha gene. This combination is also generally benign.

Hgb E is identified differently depending on the electrophoresis technique used. Verify your local laboratory's technique to ensure accurate interpretation of results.

Alpha/beta thalassemia. This occurs when an alpha trait is combined with a beta trait and the characteristic Hb A2 elevation is not found. There is a balanced globin synthesis resulting in less red blood cell pathology and the MCV is usually normal.

Clinical strategies for thalassemia

Fig. 37-6 depicts a strategy for thalassemia screening in the API population.

The common practice of doing only a hematocrit or hemoglobin for anemia screening often does not identify patients with low MCV and possible diagnosis of thalassemia. A complete blood count (CBC) should be obtained on the first visit, especially with prenatal patients. In the case of Cambodians, Laotians, or Thais it is advisable to do a CBC and hemoglobin electrophoresis on the same visit. This technique will identify persons with hemoglobin E

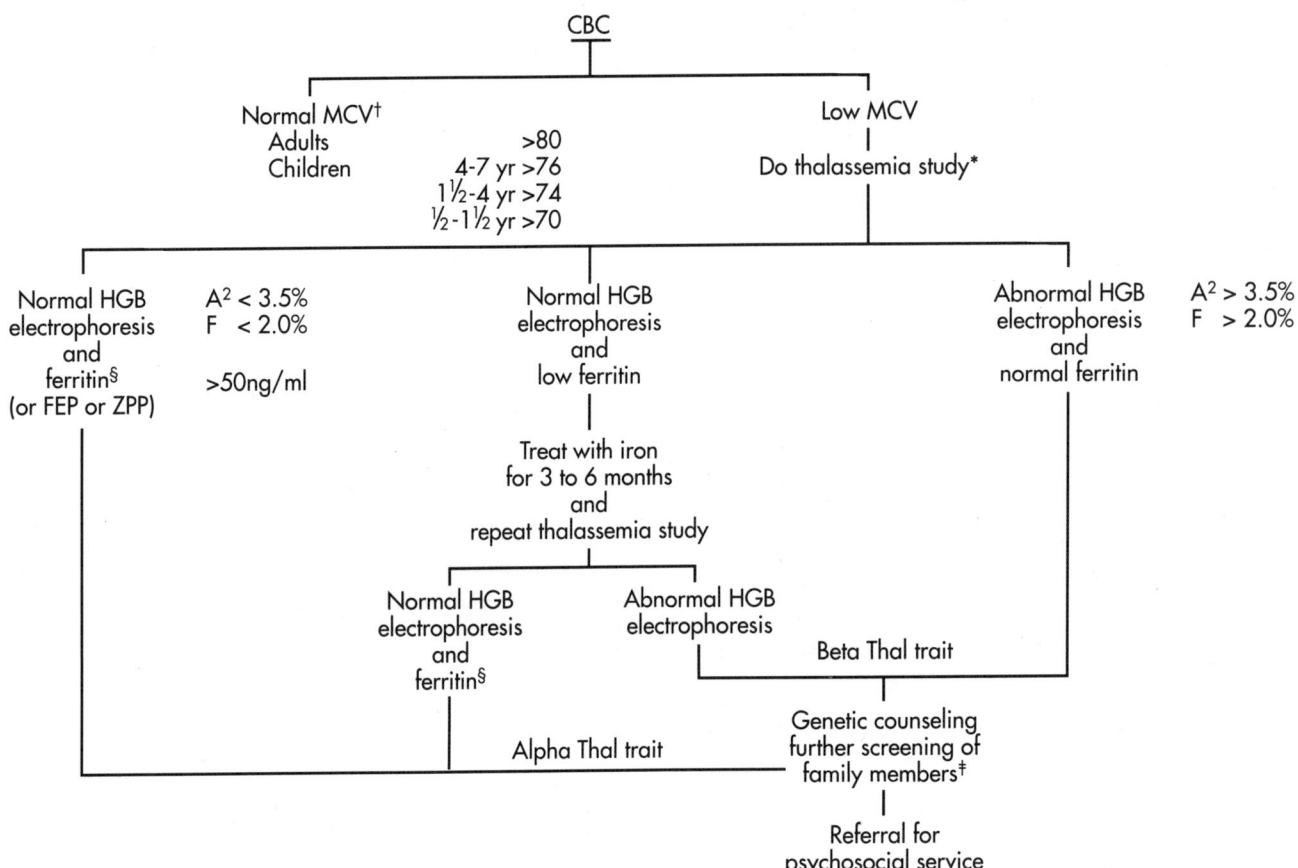

Fig. 37-6. Thalassemia Screening Protocol.

*Thalassemia Study includes ferritin, Hgb H prep and Hgb electrophoresis. Children under 6 years of age will also have FEP and lead screening.

†Because of the possibility of missing the Hgb E carriers among Southeast Asians, especially Cambodians, Laotians and Thais, Hgb electrophoresis is recommended even when MCV is normal.

‡Husband/mates of prenatal patients who are identified to have thal trait should have work-up. If found to have the same trait, provide genetic counseling and offer prenatal diagnosis—chorionic villus sampling or amniocentesis.

§Microcytosis with normal ferritin, consider alpha thalassemia trait in spite of normal Hgb electrophoresis. Provide genetic counseling and perform family study.

trait, which is more prevalent among this population some of whom will have normal MCVs.

Iron deficiency anemia is also a common finding among the newly arrived refugee/immigrant population. Therefore, it is important to obtain free erythrocyte protoporphyrin (FEP) or serum ferritin or serum iron and total iron binding capacity (TIBC) levels for proper diagnosis. These studies will also prevent a misdiagnosis of iron deficiency and risks of iron overload therapy. The Hb A2 in beta thalassemia trait may be depressed in the presence of iron deficiency anemia, and the Hb H in alpha thalassemia trait and the intraerythrocytic inclusion bodies may not be expressed. Treatment with iron, therefore, is required, followed by a repeat hemoglobin electrophoresis. Therapeutic trial of iron is acceptable before definitive studies have been conducted.

Timing of testing is important. In the newborn, Hgb Bart's is detectable but disappears by 3 to 6 months. Hb E is also detectable. Retrograde parental screening can identify carrier/carrier couples. In the pediatric age group, identification avoids misdiagnosis and unnecessary iron therapy of low MCVs.

In the premarital/child-bearing age, early identification allows carrier/carrier couples to have thoughtful family planning, which may include not having children, adoption, and prenatal diagnosis. The disadvantage is that this is an emotionally charged time. Unfortunate labeling of an identified trait carrier can create problems with future in-laws. In Asian cultures, because marrying a person that is less than perfect is not acceptable, being a trait carrier may become a stigma. When a patient is diagnosed in the prenatal period as a carrier, it is essential to screen the partner as soon as possible to identify at-risk couples. At-risk couples should be offered genetic counseling and prenatal diagnosis options.

Genetic counseling and education are urgent for at-risk couples identified through prenatal care. The deliberations around prenatal diagnostic procedures and possible termination of pregnancy may be extremely delicate, for in many Southeast Asian patients, babies are viewed as gifts from God and the delivery is not to be interfered with. An inherited disease is interpreted as possible punishment for bad behavior in a previous life. For newborn, childhood, and premarital screening, the same considerations apply, although the circumstances are less urgent. Many genetic terms are nonexistent in the Asian languages, making translations very challenging. Models for Chinese, Korean, Vietnamese, and Laotian exist (see Resources).

G6PD clinical issues

G6PD deficiency is an important genetic disease in the Asian population; G6PD is rare in whites except in those of Mediterranean extraction.[168a] In Japan and Korea, the deficiency is rare with a prevalence of about 0.5% and 0.1%, respectively.[122b] Among Southern Chinese, Hakka Chinese, and overseas Chinese men, the prevalence of G6PD deficiency is about 5%. Among Chinese and Taiwanese, there are 11 G6PD variants.[122a] In Thailand the prevalence is 9% to 15% with 17 known G6PD variants. In south Vietnam, G6PD deficiency occurs in 1% to 4% of persons. In Laos and Cambodia, the prevalence is about 12% to 15%.

Because this condition is more prevalent in this population the practitioner should act to avoid precipitation of hemolytic episodes, which may occur in G6PD deficient patients. Therefore, caution should be exercised against the use of naphthalene moth balls and fava beans, both of which may be found in the Asian home. Fava beans are sold in Asian markets; most commonly they are dried and cooked, and are rarely fresh. Wong et al.[172] described a 2½-year-old Chinese-Burmese boy who developed hemolysis after eating fava beans. Du[36] described 11 such cases in China. Fava beans have been grown in China for many centuries. Additionally, G6PD status should be determined before use of primaquine for malaria therapy. G6PD deficiency should also be considered in API newborns with hyperbilirubinemia, as G6PD deficiency has been associated with increased incidence of severe neonatal hyperbilirubinemia in Chinese infants in both Taiwan[103] and Singapore.[12]

Cardiovascular disease

Health education is the key need in preventing cardiovascular disease in this population. As described earlier, APIs have major knowledge deficits about the risks of hypertension, smoking, cholesterol, and obesity. Educational materials on these issues are available in several Asian languages (see Resources). Video health "commercials," calendars with health tips and reminders and classes may be helpful strategies to educate communities with sizable API populations.[25]

Tuberculosis

In contrast to the U.S. general population, TB occurs in younger Asian Pacific Americans. Over half of the foreign-born immigrant patients arrive in the United States before the age of 35 years. The timing of screening is critically important because in 1985 approximately 50% of the foreign-born API TB cases developed within the first 2 years in the United States.[163] Therefore, screening, treatment, and prophylaxis should ideally be initiated before immigration. Alternatively, tuberculin skin testing along with aggressive follow-up should occur immediately upon arrival in the United States.

In most cases, prior Bacille-Calmette-Guerin (BCG) vaccination may be disregarded as a potential cause of a positive tuberculin skin test. BCG vaccine was originally derived from a strain of *Mycobacterium bovis,* which was attenuated through years of serial passage in culture.[104] Currently several BCG vaccines are available. API patients with positive tuberculin skin tests (PPDs) will often give a history of one or more BCG vaccinations. Because TB is so prevalent in Asian countries, TB exposure is highly likely, even with a negative history of known contact. Initial infection with TB may be completely asymptomatic and may not manifest as disease until years later. There is also doubt about the permanence of BCG-induced tuberculin hypersensitivity. The protection they provide has varied from 0 to 80%.[40] We have seen patients with a history of BCG develop TB.

Because one can never be sure that a positive PPD is secondary solely to the BCG the chance for exposure is high and BCG is not 100% protective, we favor single-drug prophylactic therapy with isoniazid in this setting. Adults with negative PPDs should be retested within approximately 2 to 3 weeks. Adults previously exposed to TB may lose their tuberculin sensitivity as they get older.[157] Any older adult with a negative PPD should have another repeated within a few weeks to confirm the initial reaction. A positive reaction indicates renewed (booster phenomenon) tuberculin sensitivity. The initial PPD, although negative, serves to boost the immune system's memory. A follow-up positive PPD confirms this phenomenon. This approach helps to avoid future misdiagnoses as a "recent convertor."

The prevalence of isoniazid (INH) resistance among

cases of active TB in Southeast Asian refugees ranges from 4% to 25%.[35,100,118] For documented cases of active tuberculosis, treatment with rifampin, ethambutol, and pyrazinamide is recommended until sensitivities can be identified. Prophylaxis of household or close contacts of INH-resistant cases is less clear. Rifampin alone has been used but without conclusive effectiveness.[100]

Because Asians tend to be rapid INH acetylators, they respond better to more frequent drug dosing. In a study of 682 Asians from Taiwan, Hong Kong, and Singapore, approximately 80% were rapid INH acetylators. Acetylator status was of little consequence in TB treatment regimens given daily or twice per week. In treatment regimens given once per week however, treatment is less effective in rapid acetylators than in slow acetylators,[38] so this dosing schedule should be avoided in Asians.

The clinician should also be aware that other endemic organisms and conditions may mimic TB among APIs. These conditions include meloidosis *(Pseudomonas pseudomallei)*, which is endemic in areas of Southeast Asia, Malaysia, the Philippines and Guam,[4] and *Paragonimus* (lung fluke), a fresh water parasite found in shellfish from Southeast Asia, China, Japan, Korea, Taiwan, and the Philippines.[76]

Hepatitis B

High API HB carrier rates and the availability of HB vaccine make screening essential to prevent transmission and limit morbidity and mortality secondary to chronic active hepatitis, cirrhosis, and hepatoma. Particular attention should be directed toward screening API prenatal patients to interrupt perinatal transmission. Since 1988, the CDC Advisory Committee on Immunization Practices (ACIP) in consultation with the American College of Obstetricians and Gynecologists and the American Academy of Pediatrics has recommended HBsAg screening for all prenatal patients.[124] Once an HB carrier has been identified, all household members should be screened and unprotected members immunized.[21] Child-to-child transmission has been an important vector among Southeast Asian refugees.[44] Special attention should also be directed toward immunizing all newborns of HB carrier mothers until universal HB immunization is fully implemented.

Parasites

Three purged stool specimens for ova and parasites should be obtained on all API immigrants and refugees at least once after arrival. The majority of infected patients may be asymptomatic. Follow-up stool specimens should be collected at least 3 weeks after completion of antiparasitic therapy. Repeat screening is necessary if patients make return visits to their country of origin. Additionally, the CDC recommends that in areas with large populations of Southeast Asians, health education programs directed at preventing trichinosis should be considered.[107]

AIDS and HIV

Cultural beliefs and misinformation. The threat of HIV spread in this community is great due to numerous factors: (1) low level of education among many immigrants/refugees, (2) unfamiliarity with the concepts and practices of western medicine, (3) cultural taboos about open discussion of sexual matters and terminal illness, (4) fear of ostracization, and (5) the growing spread of HIV in Southeast Asia.

There is an attitude within Asian communities that AIDS is a disease of non-Asians and they will not contract the disease if sexual activities are limited to their own people.[89] Yet some persons continue to surreptitiously engage the services of non-Asian prostitutes. Some Asian communities are generally aware of AIDS but are misinformed about the modes of transmission.[50,74,75] Open discussion of sex and sexuality does not occur and is discouraged. Homosexuality and bisexuality are not accepted, and those thought to have such preferences are stigmatized and/or ostracized, thus creating problems in identifying persons at risk. Discussion of terminal illnesses and death is strongly discouraged, as it is felt to ruin any chances or hope for recovery.

Educating API patients about HIV is best conducted by community organizations familiar with both the language and culture of the API subgroup. Health education materials, including pamphlets and videos, are available (see Resources). As with the general population, the process of education will be time consuming. For APIs breaking through cultural beliefs and misconceptions will be even more difficult.

Cancer

Due to language, cultural, and financial barriers, API lack information and knowledge about the benefits of regular screening. These same barriers limit their access to primary care services. Consequently, many API have higher rates of invasive cervical cancer at the time of diagnosis.[17] Health education and aggressive screening will be essential for primary care practitioners to impact poor screening rates for this population. Materials in several Asian languages are available from the American Cancer Society and the National Cancer Institute.

Special attention should be given to education about screening and avoidable risk factors for less common cancers including stomach, liver, thyroid, nasopharyngeal, and myeloid leukemia as these cancers occur with higher frequency among various API subgroups than among their white counterparts.

All chronic HB carriers should be screened at least annually for elevated liver function tests and serum alpha feto protein (AFP) levels. The AFP tumor marker will rise in approximately 85% of patients but may miss up to 30% of patients that develop hepatoma.[87,92,153] Therefore, patients with negative AFP and elevated liver function tests should pursue further screening with abdominal ultrasound. Early detection is essential, as nonsurgical cures are being developed for small tumors.

Currently, there are no standardized cost-effective measures to screen for NPC. NPC is associated with the consumption of salted fish (a Cantonese preparation) early in life.[62] Various nitrosamines have been detected in salted fish, some being known nasal and paranasal carcinogens.[68,69] The Epstein-Barr virus (EBV) has also been associated with NPC.[33] Measuring a titer of IgA against the EBV viral capsid antigen (IgA/VCA) at a level ≥1:10 may be the first indication of subclinical NPC.[63] This test is sensitive and has been used successfully for large-scale early screening in China.[178] A more specific test measures titers of IgA against the EBV diffuse type of "early antigens" (IgA/EA-D). In the multistep progression toward malignancy, IgA-EA develops after the rise in IgA/VCA titers. Combined use of IgA/VCA with IgA/EA-D can be effective in the detection of early NPC.[33]

Our current impression suggests that ingestion of salted fish is still common, especially among poorer members of the Cantonese Chinese community, the elderly, and young children cared for by grandparents. Salted fish and rice have traditionally been the cheapest foods of the Southern Chinese.[62] These are peasant foods, and are a reflection of the difficult times of the past. Many of the grandparents remember those times. Caution against ingestion of salted fish should be part of the primary care of all Chinese children and adults.

Adult immunizations

Adult Asian immigrants tend to think that immunizations are for infants and children. As the recent resurgence in measles has shown, a substantial number of deaths and serious illness now resulting from vaccine-preventable diseases occur in older adolescents and adults. Seven vaccine-preventable diseases—influenza, pneumococcal disease, HB, rubella, measles, tetanus, and diphtheria—still often cause fatal illness.[20] Yearly influenza vaccines and a pneumococcal vaccine are achievable standards in most elderly Asian immigrants. Ongoing education, mass immunization efforts coordinated with local health departments, senior centers, churches, and other community organizations have yielded impressive numbers of elderly who receive vaccinations.

Nutrition and exercise

Nutrition may be enhanced in persons of these groups by obtaining a diet history, exploring use of specific foods and food myths, providing alternative healthy nutritional choices, and using published guides.[41] A brochure by the San Francisco Chapter of the American Heart Association "Eat Heart Smart—Chinese Style" incorporates traditional dietary practices in its recommendations. Encouraging culturally acceptable foods and classifying foods by function (e.g., high calcium foods are "good" for the bones) will allow for nutritional recommendations to fit into patient's traditional framework. Exercise levels may be enhanced by suggesting specific activities such as walking, use of exercise facilities, or specific exercise equipment. Available video tapes demonstrate forms of traditional exercise such as Tai Chi or Chi Goong (see Resources).

HEALTH DATA

Much of the difficulty in presenting objective information on each ethnic subgroup stems from inadequacies in our national data collections systems. Measures must be taken to accurately identify and report health status indicators on all API ethnic subgroups. High-risk groups include recent arrivals who are less educated, low income, uninsured, and not fluent in English. Reporting the health status of these subgroups is essential in developing planning strategies to address the health needs of this new American community.

CONCLUSION

The multipicity of API national backgrounds coincides with differential morbidity and mortality trends.[58] When combined with several languages, cultural beliefs and practices, and different levels of acculturation, plus a variation in socioeconomic status, it becomes impossible to view API as a homogeneous group.

Our health care system is duly challenged to provide quality care to non-English speaking API. Primary care practitioners, individually and collectively, can initiate efforts to bridge cultural gaps, thereby expanding our capacity to serve a more diverse population. Special attention to recent-arrival, high-risk API subgroups will help the overall effort to achieve our nation's Year 2000 health objectives.[59]

REFERENCES

1. Anderson JN: Health & illness in Pilipino immigrants, *West J Med* 139(6):811-819, 1983.
2. Angel A, Armstrong MA, Klatsky AL: Blood pressure among Asian-Americans living in northern California, *Am J Cardiol* 64:237-240, 1989.
3. Balkau B, King ZP, Raper R: Factors associated with the development of diabetes in the Micronesian population of Nauru, *Am J Epidemiol* 122:594-605, 1985.
4. Barrett-Connor E: Latent and chronic infections imported from Southeast Asia, *JAMA* 239:1901-1906, 1978.
5. Bates SR, Hill L, Barrett-Connor E: Cardiovascular disease risk factors in an Indochinese population, *Am J Prev Med* 5(1):15-20, 1989.
6. Beasley RP: Hepatitis B virus as the etiologic agent in hepatocellular carcinoma—epidemiologic considerations, *Hepatology* 2(Suppl): 21-26, 1982.
7. Beasley RP et al: Hepatocellular carcinoma and hepatitis B virus: a prospective study of 22,707 men in Taiwan, *Lancet* 2:1129-1133, 1981.
8. Beiser M: Influences of time, ethnicity and attachment on depression in Southeast Asian refugees, *Am J Psychiatry* 145:46-51, 1988.

9. Berlin E Ann, Fowkes WC: A teaching framework for cross-cultural health care—applications in family practice, *West J Med* 139(6):934-938, 1983.

10. Beware: Vietnamese coin rubbing, *Ann Emerg Med* 17(4):384, 1988.

11. Brand D et al: Those Asian American whiz kids, *Time Magazine* August 31, 1987, pp 42-51.

12. Brown W, Boon WH: Hyperbilirubinemia and kernicterus in glucose-6-phosphate dehydrogenase-deficient infants in Singapore, *Pediatrics* 41:1055-1061, 1968.

13. Buell P: The effect of migration on the risk of nasopharyngeal cancer among Chinese, *Cancer Res* 34:1189-1194, 1972.

14. Bulla A: Global review of tuberculosis morbidity and mortality in the world, *WHO Statistics Report* 39:2-38, 1977.

15. *Calif Morbidity #43*, Malaria and Hong Kong, California Health Services.

15a. Henderson A: Endemic Malaria in Hong Kong (letter), *Lancet* 8497(i):1324, 1986.

16. Campbell T, Chang B: Health care of the Chinese in America, *Nursing Outlook* 21:245-249, 1973. Reprinted in Spradley BW: *Contemporary community nursing*, Boston, 1975, Little Brown.

17. Cancer incidence data collected by the Northern California Cancer Center under contract N01-CN-05224 with the Division of Cancer Prevention and Control, National Cancer Institute, and under subcontract 050C-8708 with the California Public Health Foundation.

18. Case Records of the Massachusetts General Hospital: Case 33-1990, *N Engl J Med* 323:467-475, 1990.

19. Catanzaro A, Moser RJ: Health status of refugees from Vietnam, Laos and Cambodia, *JAMA* 247:1303-1308, 1982.

20. CDC: An introduction to adult immunization in the U.S., 1986-631-008/45636, 1986, US Government Printing Office.

21. CDC: Protection against viral hepatitis: recommendations of the ACIP, *MMWR* 39:1-26, 1990.

22. CDC: Trichinella spiralis infection—United States, 1990. *MMWR* 40:57-60, 1991.

23. CDC: Malaria surveillance annual summary 1987, Issued Nov. 1988.

24. Chen A et al: Chinese behavioral risk factor survey 1990, *MMWR* 41(16):266-270, 1992.

25. Chen MS et al: Promoting heart health for Southeast Asians: a database for planning interventions, *Public Health Rep* 106(3):304-309, 1991.

26. Choi ESK et al: The prevalence of cardiovascular risk factors among elderly Chinese Americans, *Arch Intern Med* 150:413-418, 1990.

27. Choi ESK, Necheles TF: Thalassemia among Chinese Bostonians: usefulness of the hemoglobin H preparation, *Arch Intern Med* 143:1713-1715, 1983.

28. Chow E: Cultural health traditions: Asian perspectives. In Branch MF, Paxton PP: *Providing safe nursing care for ethnic people of color*, New York, 1976, Appleton-Century-Crofts.

29. Chua-Eoan HG, Brown S, Hull T: Strangers in paradise, *Time Magazine* April 9, 1990, pp 32-35.

30. Crocker AC, editor: Thalassemia in Southeast Asian refugees: public health planning aspects, Irvine, Calif., 1984, Developmental Evaluation Clinic, Children's Hospital, Boston.

31. Curb JD et al: Cardiovascular risk factor levels in ethnic Hawaiians, *Am J Public Health* 81:164-167, 1991.

32. De Lay P, Fause S: Depression in Southeast Asian refugees, *Am Fam Physician* 36:179-184, 1987.

33. de-The G, Zeng Y: Population screening for EBV markers: toward improvement of nasopharyngeal carcinoma control. In Epstein MA, Achong, editors: *The Epstein Barr virus: recent advances*, New York, 1986, Wiley-Medical.

34. Dolan G et al: Lead poisoning due to Asian ethnic treatment for impotence, *J Royal Soc Med* 84(10):630-631, 1991.

35. Drug resistance among Indochinese refugees, *MMWR* 28:385-398, 1979.

36. Du SD: Favism in West China, *Chin Med J* 70:17-26, 1952.

37. Eisenberg D: *Encounters with Qi: exploring Chinese medicine*, New York, 1985, WW Norton.

38. Ellard GA: Variations between individuals and populations in the acetylation of isoniazid and its significance for the treatment of pulmonary tuberculosis, *Clin Pharm Ther* 19:610, 1976.

39. Engebretsen B, Knight A, Shah R: Hepatitis B in Southeast Asian refugees in Iowa, *Iowa Med* 74:105-108, 1984.

40. Fine PEM: The BCG story: lessons from the past and implications for the future, *Rev Infect Dis* 11:S353-S359, 1989.

41. Fishman C et al: Background information and counseling tips for working with Indochinese WIC clients 1987. California Department of Health Services, Maternal and Child Unit.

42. Reference deleted in proofs.

43. Flatz G: The genetic polymorphism of intestinal lactase activity in adult humans. In Scriver C et al, editors: *The metabolic basis of inherited disease*, ed 6, New York, 1989, McGraw-Hill.

44. Franks AL et al: Hepatitis B virus infection among children born in the US to Southeast Asian refugees, *N Engl J Med* 321(19):1301-1305, 1989.

45. Freimer N et al: Cultural variation—nutritional and clinical implications, *West J Med* 139(6):928-933, 1983.

46. Friede A et al: Transmission of Hepatitis B virus from adopted Asian children to their American families, *Am J Public Health* 78(1):26-29, 1988.

47. Gardner RW, Bryant R, Smith PC: Asian Americans: growth, change and diversity, *Pop Bull* 40(4):28, 1985.

48. Gellis SS, Feingold M: Pseudobattering in Vietnamese children, *Am J Dis Child* 130:857, 1976.

49. Goldstein C: Drags to riches, *Far Eastern Econ Rev* 29:62-63,1990.

50. Gorrez L, Araneta MRG: AIDS knowledge, beliefs and behaviors in a household survey of Filipinos in San Francisco, 1990, San Francisco Department of Public Health, AIDS Surveillance Office.

51. Griggs B: *Green pharmacy: a history of herbal medicine*, New York, 1981, Viking Press.

52. Guerrero IC, Chin W, Collins W: A survey of malaria in Indochinese refugees arriving in the United States, 1980, *Am J Trop Med Hyg* 31:897-901, 1982.

53. Guy G et al: Thalassemia hydrops fetalis: clinical and ultrasonographic considerations, *Am J Obstet Gynecol* 153:500-504, 1984.

54. Hall SC, Kehoe EL: Prolonged survival of *Schistosoma japonicum*, *Calif Med* 113:75-77, 1970.

55. Hann HWL et al: Prevention of hepatitis B and primary liver cancer in Asian populations in the United States. Proceedings from "The Next Decade," 1986 Conference on Refugee Health Care Issues and Management. State of Wisconsin, 1986, pp 95-109.

56. Hawaii's Health Risk Behaviors 1991 (unpublished): Health Promotion and Education Office, Hawaii State Dept of Health.

57. Health Screening of resettled Indochinese refugees—Washington, DC, Utah. *MMWR* 29(1):4-11, 1980.

58. Health United States 1990, National Center for Health Statistics, US Public Health Service, USDHHS, 1991:80-82. DHHS Pub. No. (PHS) 91-1232.

59. Healthy People 2000: National Health Promotion and Disease Prevention Objectives. US Public Health Service, 1990. DHHS Pub. No. (DHS) 91-50213.

60. Hessler RM et al: Intraethnic diversity: health care of the Chinese-Americans, *Human Organization* 34(3)348-363, 1975; Reprinted in Logan MH, Hunt EE Jr: *Health and the human condition: perspectives on medical anthropology*, North Scituate, Mass, 1978, Duxbury Press.

61. HIV/AIDS Surveillance Report, November 1991, Atlanta, U.S. Public Health Service.

62. Ho JHC: Genetic and clinical study of nasopharyngeal carcinoma. In Nakahara W et al, editors: *Recent advances in human tumor virology and immunology*, Tokyo, 1971, University of Tokyo Press.

63. Ho, WJM: Personal communication, July 1985.

64. Holtman WH, Bornemann TH: *Mental health of immigrants and refugees*, Hogg Foundation for Mental Health, 1990.

65. How to use interpreters' services (videotape): Produced by Meister J, Tucson Ariz, Area Health Education Center, Arizona Rural Health Office, 1987.

66. Hsia YE: Comprehensive hereditary anemia program for Hawaii, Honolulu, Maternal and Child Health Project, 1990.

67. Hsu H-Y, Peacher WG. *Chinese herb medicine & therapy*, rev ed, Los Angeles, 1982, Oriental Healing Arts Institute.

68. Reference deleted in galleys.

69. Huang D et al: Volatile nitrosamines in salt-preserved fish before and after cooking, *Food Cosmet Toxicol* 19:167-171, 1981.

70. Hurst D et al: Anemia and hemoglobinopathies in Southeast Asian refugee children, *J Pediatr* 102:692-697, 1983.

71. Immunizations in the United States, *Pediatrics,* 86(suppl):1064-1066,1990.

72. Immunization Update, Immunization Unit, California Department of Health Services, 8/7/91.

73. Ja DY, Kitano KJ, Ebata A: Report on a survey of AIDS knowledge, attitudes and behaviors in San Francisco's Chinese communities, executive summary, May 23, 1990, Asian American Recovery Services, 300 Fourth Street, San Francisco, CA 94107.

74. Reference deleted in proofs.

75. Jew S: AIDS among California Asian and Pacific Islander Subgroups, *Calif HIV/AIDS Update,* 4(9):90-98, 1991.

76. Johnson RJ, Johnson JR: Paragonimus in Indochinese refugees, *Am Rev Respir Dis* 128:534-538, 1983.

77. Judson FN et al: Health status of Southeast Asian refugees, *West J Med* 141:183-188, 1984.

78. Kammerer WS et al: Clonorchiasis in New York City Chinese, *Trop Doct* 7:105-106, 1977.

79. Kaptchuk TJ: *The web that has no weaver: understanding Chinese medicine,* New York, 1983, Congdon & Weed.

80. Kasindorf M et al: Asian Americans: a model minority, *Newsweek Magazine* December 6, 1982, pp 39-51.

81. Kersteloot H et al: Serum lipids in the People's Republic of China, *Arteriosclerosis,* 5(5):427-433, 1985.

82. Kim SS. Ethnic elders and American health care: a physician's perspective, *West J Med* 139(6):885-891, 1983.

83. Kinzie JD: Evaluation and psychotherapy of Indochinese refugee patients, *Am J Psychother* 35:251-261, 1981.

84. Kinzie JD, Fleck J: Psychotherapy with severely traumatized refugees, *Am J Psychother* 41:82-94, 1987.

85. Kinzie JD et al: The psychiatric effects of massive trauma on Cambodian children, Part I. The children, *J Am Acad Child Psychiatry* 215:370-376, 1986.

86. Klatsky AL, Armstrong MA: Cardiovascular risk factors among Asian Americans living in northern California, *Am J Public Health* 81(11):1423-1428, 1991.

87. Kobayashi K et al: Screening methods for early detection of hepatocellular carcinoma, *Hepatology* 5:1100-1105, 1985.

88. Komachi Y, Tanaka H: A collaborative study of stroke incidence in Japan: 1975-1979, *Stroke* 15(1):28-36, 1984.

89. Lee DA, Fong K: HIV/AIDS and the Asian and Pacific Islander community, SIECUS Report, February/March 1990.

90. Lee M et al: Intestinal parasitic infections in immigrants from China and Southeast Asia. San Francisco, 1986. Proceedings of the Third Conference on Health Problems Related to the Chinese in America.

91. Lee RV et al: Southeast Asian folklore about pregnancy and parturition. *Obstet Gynecol* 71(4):643-645, 1988.

92. Lehmann FG: Early detection of hepatoma: prospective study in liver cirrhosis using passive hemagglutination and radioimmunoassay, *Ann NY Acad Sci* 259:196, 1975.

93. Lightfoote J et al: Lead intoxication in an adult by Chinese herbal medication, *JAMA* 238:1539, 1978.

94. Lin EH, Carter W, Kleinman A: An exploration of somatization among Asian refugees and immigrants in primary care, *Am J Public Health* 75:1080-1084, 1985.

95. Lin EH, Ihle LJ, Tazuma L: Depression among Vietnamese refugees in a primary care clinic, *Am J Med* 78:41-44, 1985.

96. Lin-Fu JS: Population characteristics and health care needs of Asian Pacific Americans, *Public Health Rep* 103(1):18-27, 1988.

97. Lin-Fu JS: Thalassemia screening among Asian Pacific Americans. In Asian American Health Forum, San Francisco, 1990, Asian specific protocols.

98. Ling S, King J, Leung V: Diet, growth and cultural food habits in Chinese-American infants. *Am J Chin Med* 2:125-132, 1975.

99. Liu WT, Yu ESH: Asian/Pacific American elderly: mortality differentials, health status and use of health services, *J Appl Gerontol* 4(1):35-64, 1985.

100. Livengood JR et al: INH-resistant tuberculosis—a community outbreak and report of a rifampin prophylaxis failure, *JAMA* 253:2847-2849, 1985.

101. Longmire AW, Broom LA: Vietnamese coin rubbing, *Ann Emerg Med* 16(5):602, 1987.

102. Lu HC: *Chinese system of food cures: prevention and remedies,* New York, 1986, Sterling Publishing.

103. Lu TC, Wei H, Blackwell R: Increase incidence of severe hyperbilirubinemia among newborn Chinese infants with G-6-P-D deficiency, *Pediatrics* 37:994-998, 1966.

104. Luelmo F: BCG vaccination, *Am Rev Respir Dis* 125:3 (part 2)70, 1982.

105. Markel S, LoVerde P, Britt E: Prolonged latent schistosomiasis, *JAMA* 240:1746-1747, 1978.

106. Markell EK, Voge M, John DT: *Medical parasitology,* ed 6, Philadelphia, 1986, WB Saunders.

107. McAuley JB, Michelson MK, Schantz PM: Trichinosis surveillance, United States, 1987-90. *MMWR* 40:(No.SS-3) 35-42, 1991.

107a. McDermott J: Asia—epicenter of the AIDS epidemic, *Washington Post,* Sunday, June 23, 1991.

108. McKenzie JL, Chrisman NJ: Healing, herbs, gods and magic: folk health beliefs among Filipino-Americans, *Nurs Outlook* 25(5):326-329, 1977.

109. McPhee SJ et al: Behavioral risk factor survey of Vietnamese—California, 1991. *MMWR* 41(5):69-72, 1992.

110. McQuillan GM et al: Seroepidemiology of hepatitis B virus infection in the United States: 1976 to 1980, *Am J Med* 87(3A):5S-10S, 1989.

111. Miller LH: Transfusion malaria and immigrant blood donors, *J Infect Dis* 133:727, 1976.

112. Minkler DH: The role of a community-based satellite clinic in the perinatal care of non-English speaking immigrants, *West J Med* 139(6):349-354, 1983.

113. Lettau LA et al: Locally acquired neuro-cysticercosis: North Carolina, Massachusetts and South Carolina, 1989-1991, *MMWR* 41(1):1-4, 1992.

114. Mollica R, Syshak G, Lavelle J: The psychosocial impact of war trauma and torture on southeast Asian refugees, *Am J Psychiatry* 144:12:1567-1572, 1987.

115. Muecke MA: In search of healers—Southeast Asian refugees in the American health care system, *West J Med* 139(6):835-840, 1983.

116. Muir C et al: WHO:IARC Sci Pub 88: Cancer Incidence in Five Continents, Vol V, Lyon 1987.

117. Newman V et al: Nutrient intake of low-income southeast Asian pregnant women, *J Am Diet Assoc* 91(7):793-799, 1991.

118. Nolan CM et al: Active tuberculosis after INH chemoprophylaxis of Southeast Asian refugees, *Am Rev Respir Dis* 133:431-436, 1986.

119. O'Hare W: Asian Americans—the fastest growing minority, *Am Demogr* 26-31, Oct.,1990.

120. O'Hare WP, Felt JC: Asian Americans: America's fastest growing minority group, *Population Trends and Public Policy,* 19:7, 1991.

121. McDermott J: Asia—epicenter of the AIDS epidemic, Office of AIDS, California Dept of Health Services, *The Washington Post,* Sunday, June 23, 1991.

122. Ott RJ, Wu N: Proceedings of thalassemia and Southeast Asians in New England, Region I Conference, Needham, Mass, 1990.

122a. Panich V: Glucose-6-phosphate dehydrogenase deficiency: genetic heterogeneity in Asia. In Weatherall D et al, editors: *Advances in red cell biology,* New York, 1982, Raven Press.

122b. Panich V: Glucose-6-phosphate dehydrogenase deficiency: Part 2: tropical Asia, *Clin Hematol* 10:800-813, 1981.

123. Pizer H: *Guide to the new medicine: what works, what doesn't,* New York, 1982, William Morrow.

124. Immunization Practices Advisory Committee (ACIP): Hepatitis B: a comprehensive strategy for eliminating transmission in the U.S. through universal vaccination, *MMWR* 40(RR 13): 1-16, 1991.

125. Putsch RW III: Cross-cultural communication: the special case of interpreters in health care, *JAMA* 254(23):3344-3348, 1985.

126. Quak SH: Gastrointestinal infections in Singapore children, *Ann Acad Med* (Singapore) 20:265-268, 1991.

127. Reed, D, Yano K: Epidemiological studies of hypertension among elderly Japanese and Japanese Americans, *Asia-Pacific J Public Health* 1(2):49-56, 1987.

128. Report of the Secretary's Task Force on Black and Minority Health: Executive Summary, USDHHS, 1986, vol I, Washington, DC, 1986, US Govt. Printing Office.

129. Research & Development, Lung Center of the Philippines: National smoking prevalence survey, *Phillippine J Intern Med* 27:133-156, 1989.

130. Ries C, Sahud M: Agranulocytosis caused by Chinese herbal medicines, *JAMA* 231:352, 1975.

131. Robertson TL, Kato H: Epidemiologic studies of coronary heart disease and stroke in Japanese men living in Japan, Hawaii and California: incidence of myocardial infarction and death from coronary heart disease, *Am J Cardiol* 39:239-243, 1977.

132. Robertson TL et al: Epidemiologic studies of coronary heart disease and stroke in Japanese men living in Japan, Hawaii and California: coronary heart disease risk factors in Japan and Hawaii, *Am J Cardiol* 39:244-249, 1977.

133. Ross R et al: Cancer patterns among Vietnamese immigrants in Los Angeles County, *Br J Cancer* 64:185-186, 1991.

134. Rumbaut R: Mental health and the refugee experience: a comparative study of Southeast Asian refugees. In Owan TC, editor: *Southeast Asian mental health: treatment, prevention, services, training and research,* Rockville, Md, 1985, USDHHS.

135. Rumbaut RG: IHARP: smoking and drinking prevalence data, San Diego, 1986, San Diego State University.

136. *San Francisco Epidemiologic Bulletin* 5:31-33, 1989.

137. *San Francisco Epidemiologic Bulletin* 6:19-20, 1990.

138. *San Francisco Epidemiological Bulletin* 7:27-29, 1991.

139. Schwartz I et al: Glucose-6-phosphate dehydrogenase deficiency in Southeast Asian refugees entering the United States, *Am J Trop Med Hyg* 33:182-184, 1984.

140. Screening of Asian and Pacific Islander Prenatal Patients in Community Health Centers From 1988-1991 (unpublished data). Association of Asian Pacific Community Health Organizations, Oakland, Calif.

141. Shanghai First Medical Hospital: *Clinical handbook of antimicrobial medicines (Ling-chuang kang-jun yao-wu shou-ce).* Shanghai, 1977, People's Press.

142. Shaw PK et al: Malaria surveillance in the United States, *J Infect Dis* 133:95-101, 1976.

143. Shi F et al: Stroke in the People's Republic of China, *Stroke* 20(11):1581-1585, 1989.

144. Siao, GW-T: Officials warn of dangers of some herbal medicines, *Asian Week* 10(28):17, 1989.

145. Spector RE: *Cultural diversity in health and illness,* ed 2, New York, 1985, Appleton-Century-Crofts.

146. *Statistical Year Book of Immigration & Naturalization Services,* 1990, U.S. Goverment Printing Office.

147. Stavig GR, Igra A, Leonard A: Hypertension and related health issues among Asians and Pacific Islanders in California, *Public Health Rep* 103(1):28-37, 1988.

148. Stehr-Green K, Schantz P: Trichinosis in Southeast Asian refugees in the United States, *Am J Public Health* 76:1238-1239, 1986.

149. Stevens CE et al: Perinatal hepatitis B virus transmission in the United States. Prevention by passive-active immunization, *JAMA* 253:1740-1745, 1985.

150. Stevenson CS: Oil of wintergreen (methyl salicylate) poisoning. Report of three cases, one with autopsy, and a review of the literature, *Am J Med Sci* 193:772-788, 1937.

151. Story M, Harry LJ: Food habits and dietary changes of Southeast Asian refugee families living in the United States, *J Am Diet Assoc* 89(6):800-803, 1989.

152. Safran D et al: Survey of Intestinal Parasites—Illinois: *MMWR* 28(29):346-347, 1979.

153. Tatsuta M et al: Value of serum alpha-fetoprotein and ferritin in the diagnosis of hepatocellular carcinoma, *Oncology* 43:306-310, 1986.

154. Taylor RJ et al: The prevalence of diabetes mellitus in a traditional-living Polynesian population: the Wallis Island survey, *Diabetes Care* 6:334-340, 1983.

155. Reference deleted in galleys.

156. The Revolutionary Health Committee of Hunan Province: *A barefoot doctor's manual,* Rev, enlarged ed, Seattle, 1977, Cloudburst Press.

157. Thompson N et al: The booster phenomenon in serial tuberculin testing, *Am Rev Respir Dis* 119:587-597, 1979.

158. Ting CW, Hwang B, Wu TC: Developmental changes of lactose malabsorption in normal Chinese children: a study using breath hydrogen test with a physiologic dose of lactose, *J Pediatr Gastroenterol Nutr* 7:848-851, 1988.

159. Todisco V, Lamour J, Finberg L: Hemolysis from exposure to naphthalene mothballs (letter), *N Engl J Med* 325:1660, 1991.

160. Tong MJ: Screening for hepatitis B virus in pregnant Asian Pacific women and immunoprophylaxis of newborns. Asian Specific Protocols: 3-6, 1990. Asian American Health Forum, Inc, San Francisco, CA.

161. Toxic reactions to plant products sold in health food stores. *The Medical Letter,* 21(7):29-31, 1977.

162. Trends in pediatric immunization in California, Immunization Unit, State of California of Health Services, 1991.

163. Tuberculosis among Asian/Pacific Islanders—US, 1985, *MMWR* 36:331-334, 1987.

164. Tuberculosis statistics in the United States, 1987, Atlanta, 1989, USDHHS Technical Information Service, CDC,

165. US Bureau of the Census Statistical Abstract of the United States, ed 110, Washington, DC, 1990.

166. Valaes T, Doxiadis SA, Fessas P: Acute hemolysis due to naphthalene inhalation, *J Pediatr* 63:904-915, 1963.

167. Westermeyer J et al: Somatization among refugees: an epidemiologic study, *Psychosomatics* 30:34-43, 1989.

168. Whelan S, Parkin D, Masuyer E: Patterns of cancer in five continents, WHO:IARC Sci Pub 102: Lyon, 1990.

168a. Wintrobe MM, et al: *Clinical hematology,* Philadelphia, 1981, Lea and Febiger.

169. Wong C: Nutritional status of Chinese at a community fair, 1987 (unpublished). Health Center #4, San Francisco Dept of Public Health, San Francisco.

170. Wong C: Nutritional needs of Chinese. California Dietetic Association Annual Meeting 1988. Health Center #4, San Francisco Department of Public Health, San Francisco.

171. Wong ND et al: A comparison of Chinese traditional and western medical approaches for the treatment of mild hypertension, *Yale J Biol Med* 64:79-87, 1991.

172. Wong W, Powars D, Williams W: 'Yewdow'-induced anemia, *West J Med* 151:459-460, 1989.

173. Yeatman GW et al: Pseudobattering in Vietnamese children, *Pediatrics* 58(4):616-618, 1976.

174. Yeung CP: Acute infantile gastroenteritis in Hong Kong. In Eeckels RE, Ransome-Kuti O, Kroonenborg CC, editors: *Child health in the tropics,* Boston, 1985, Nijhotff.

175. Yu ESH et al: Asian-White mortality differentials: are there excess deaths? In *Task force on black and minority health,* vol II, Washington DC: DHHS, 1985.

176. Yu JJ et al: A comparison of smoking patterns in the People's Republic of China With the United States, *JAMA* 264(12):1575-1579, 1990.

177. Yu M et al: Nasopharyngeal carcinoma in Chinese—salted fish or inhaled smoke? *Prev Med* 10:15-24, 1981.

178. Zeng Y et al: Serological mass survey for early detection of nasopharyngeal carcinoma in Wuzhou City, Chine, *Int J Cancer* 29:139-141, 1982.

179. Zeng YT, Huang SZ: Disorders of hemoglobin in China, *J Med Gen* 24:578-583, 1987.

180. Zhao-Guang-Sheng, Chai Shang-da: An epidemiological study on the correlation of urinary sodium and potassium excretion to blood pressure in China. In Lovenberg W, Yamori Y, editors: *Nutritional prevention of cardiovascular disease,* Orlando, 1984, Academic Press.

181. Zimmet P et al: Prevalence of diabetes and impaired glucose tolerance in the biracial (Melanesian and Indian) population of Fiji: a rural-urban comparison, *Am J Epidemiol* 118:673-688, 1983.

182. Zimmet P, Taylor R, Whitehouse S: Prevalence rates of impaired glucose intolerance and diabetes in various Pacific populations according to the new WHO criteria, *WHO Bulletin* 60:279-282, 1982.

RESOURCES

National organizations—health issues and advocacy

Association of Asian Pacific Community Health Organizations (AAPCHO), 1212 Broadway #730, Oakland, CA 94612.

Asian American Health Forum, 116 New Montgomery St #531, San Francisco, CA 94105.

Oriental Healing Arts Institute, 1945 Palo Verde Ave., Suite 208, Long Beach, CA, 90815.

Community Health Centers—primary care and health education

Asian Health Services, 310 8th Street #200, Oakland, CA 94607.

Asian Pacific Health Care Venture, 300 W. Sunset Blvd., Los Angeles, CA 90012.

Chinatown Health Clinic, 89 Baxter Street, New York, NY 10013.

International District Community Health Center, 416 Maynard South, Seattle, WA 98104.

Kokua Kalihi Valley Health Center, 1846 Gulick Avenue, Honolulu, HI 96819.

North East Medical Services, 1520 Stockton Street, San Francisco, CA 94133.

South Cove Community Health Center, 885 Washington Street, Boston, MA 02111.

Waianae Coast Comprehensive Health Center, 86-260 Farrington Hwy, Waianae, HI 96792 .

Hawaii Department of Health, Food and Drug Branch, 591 Ala Moana Blvd., Honolulu, HI 96813. For brochures on lead-containing dishware.

Videotapes

How to use interpreters' services. 20 minutes, with facilitator's guide. Division of Biomedical Communication, University of Arizona Health Sciences Center, Tucson, AZ, 85724.

Tai Chi for Health, by Terry Dunn, 1-800-937-0234 (Catalog #937).

The bilingual medical interview I and II. Includes discussion guide. Boston Area Health Education Center, Videos, Boston City Hospital, 818 Harrison Ave., Boston MA 02118.

Miscellaneous

American Foundation of Traditional Chinese Medicine, 1280 Columbus Ave., Suite 302, San Francisco, CA 94133.

Lead Testing Kits available from Leadcheck 1-800-262-LEAD (Framingham, Mass) or Frandon Enterprises 1-800-359-9000 (Seattle, Wash).

National Research Center on Asian American Mental Health, Department of Psychology, UCLA, 405 Hilgard Ave., Los Angeles, CA, 90024-1563.

Oriental Healing Arts Institute, 1945 Palo Verde Ave. Suite 208, Long Beach, CA 90815.

Southeast Asian Genetics Program (SEAGEP), Dept. of Pediatrics, Route 81, Bldg 29A, UC Irvine Medical Center, 101 The City Drive, Orange, CA 92668.

Vietnamese Community Health Promotion Project, UC San Francisco, Div General Internal Med, 44 Montgomery Street, #2862, San Francisco, CA 94104.

Part VIII

GENETICS

Chapter 38

INTEGRATION OF GENETIC INFORMATION INTO PREVENTIVE CARE

Ronald T. Acton
Richard Bamberg
Jeffrey M. Roseman

In recent years there has been considerable increase in knowledge regarding the role genes play in the etiology of various disease states. This increase in knowledge has mainly been due to the development of recombinant DNA technology, which has provided the tools to more easily identify genes involved in disease states. Of approximately 4000 diseases for which genetic factors are involved in their etiology, the genes for 700 have been mapped to a specific chromosome.[44,127] An estimated 300 of these genes have been cloned and sequenced. In many instances these data have provided insight into the etiology of a given disease and/or the ability to predict predisposition to or diagnose the disease. In fact, for several diseases it is possible to predict in utero or shortly after birth the risk of an individual developing the disease.

Genetic tests currently can predict carrier status of several diseases for which there are no known cures.[32,71] However, this information can be utilized to make reproductive and other decisions. Fortunately, for many of the diseases that can be predicted there is the possibility to intervene and prevent early onset or lessen severity. For the multifactorial diseases there is the possibility to prevent the disease entirely. These possibilities currently provide exciting opportunities for the clinician interested in preventive medicine. Future advances will provide the means to correct genetic disorders. This knowledge is only beginning to be used in prevention strategies. This avalanche of genetic information will require an understanding of genetics by the medical as well as lay communities, availability of personnel trained in medical genetics, strategies for assessing genetic risk of adult-onset disorders, and integration of this information into preventive measures.[78]

This chapter will suggest approaches that might help practicing physicians incorporate current genetic knowledge into the evaluation of their patients. This chapter will not attempt to deal with all the more prevalent genetic disorders. We have selected for discussion familial disorders that usually begin to appear from adolescence on, where genetic or laboratory testing is available to refine risk estimates, to aid in early diagnosis, and, where intervention measures are available, to reduce either risk of onset or severity. This is designed to give the physician interested in preventive medicine the basics on which they can integrate into their practice additional genetic information as it becomes available.

OVERVIEW OF GENETICS
Traditional genetics

Traditionally, investigators studying abnormal genes as causes of disease used methods to evaluate gene products. High levels of metabolic products in plasma or urine, the failure to detect enzyme activity, or the presence of enzymes or other proteins that migrated differently during electrophoresis were all clues that abnormal genes were related to the disease state. These protein polymorphisms (i.e., of at least two detectable forms, both occurring in greater than 1% of the population) were called *genetic markers*. One of the first genetic markers found to be related to disease states was the ABO blood group antigens.[4] This marker was found to differentiate risk for gastric ulcers. Individuals with blood type O had increased risk for ulcers. Since that time many other genetic markers have been identified.

Heretofore some of the more useful genetic markers for categorizing individuals by disease risk have been the human leukocyte antigens (HLA).[2,198] These are antigens present on the surface of white blood cells and other tissues. They are important as determinants of acceptance or rejection of transplanted tissues or organs. Different forms (or alleles) of these HLA markers have identified persons at high risk for ankylosing spondylitis,[128] insulin-dependent diabetes,[134,151,156] and narcolepsy,[208] among many other diseases.[2,198] Although traditional genetic markers still are useful for studying certain diseases, the "new" genetics as defined by use of recombinant DNA technology have opened the door to additional possibilities.

The "new" genetics

The essential features of recombinant DNA technology are as follows[138]:

* DNA from cells can be highly purified.
* The purified DNA can be cleaved at specific nucleotide sequences by use of restriction endonucleases.
* A number of vectors such as plasmids and bacteriophages are found in *Escherichia coli* into which the cleaved fragments of DNA of interest can be inserted. The DNA fragments from an individual with a given disease, for example, can be joined with the DNA of a plasmid or bacteriophage by use of DNA ligase.
* The human DNA-vector artificial recombinant can be used to transform to *E. coli*. The bacteria can be grown, thus replicating the recombinant and generating large quantities.
* The bacteria can be propagated under conditions whereby clones derived from a single bacterium that contain a single recombinant (or in other words, a specific fragment of human DNA) can be selected.
* The human DNA fragment of choice can be purified from the vector DNA fragment.
* The purified human DNA fragment can be used as a probe to identify similar copies of the DNA in individuals other than the one from whom the material was cloned. This provides the ability to look for polymorphisms at the nucleotide sequence level that may be different in individuals with a given disease compared with healthy controls. Variants within DNA can be assessed by several methods.[32]

The now classical method of assessing variants is Southern blot analysis[185] (Fig. 38-1). In this analysis, one purifies genomic DNA. The DNA is cleaved by restriction endonucleases, and the cleaved fragments separated by electrophoresis through an agarose gel. The cleaved DNA fragments will separate based on their size, with the larger fragments remaining at the top of the gel and the smaller ones migrating toward the positive pole of the electrical field. The separated DNA fragments are transferred to a membrane of nitrocellulose or nylon. Variation within the nucleotide sequence can be detected by use of cloned DNA (i.e., probe), that has been tagged with a radioactive molecule. This probe will seek out complementary sequences of DNA with which to hybridize. The membrane with the radioactive probe attached is placed against an x-ray film to capture an image of the DNA fragments. The resulting autoradiograph reveals the fragments of DNA to which the probe hybridized.

This analysis is designed to determine whether individuals with a given disease have a different sequence (i.e., variant), in the area recognized by the restriction endonuclease. This variant is termed a *restriction fragment length polymorphism (RFLP)*.[20] One might observe that individuals with a given disease have a smaller or larger fragment than a normal individual. This RFLP may in fact be an abnormal gene involved in the etiology of a given disease or linked to the actual predisposing gene. The Southern blot and RFLP analysis are currently being used to search for genes involved in the etiology of a disease, or, if the gene has been located, as a test to determine risk of developing the disease.

An example of an RFLP analysis is illustrated in Fig. 38-2. The DNA from a normal individual and from patients with hypertriglyceridemia was evaluated with regard to polymorphisms within the apolipoprotein A1-C3-A4 gene complex.[154] As can be seen, all individuals possess a 5.7kb fragment. Lane 1 contains the DNA from a normal individual who has 5.7kb and 4.2kb DNA fragments generated by cleavage with the restriction endonuclease SstI. This individual is homozygous (S1/S1) for the 4.2kb fragment. However, individuals with hypertriglyceridemia have been observed to possess a different SstI cleavage site, which leads to the generation of a 3.2kb fragment. This can result in individuals (lane 2 of Fig. 38-1) who are heterozygous (S1/S2) in that they possess both the 4.2kb and the 3.2kb fragments, or homozygous (S2/S2) if they possess only the 3.2kb fragment (lane 3). The frequency of the S2 allele (3.2kb fragment) has been observed increased fivefold in white hypertriglyceridemic subjects.[154]

Another approach to assessing whether there are variants at the DNA level is to actually determine the nucleotide sequence of cloned DNA from diseased individuals for comparison with healthy individuals. Several techniques are available to accomplish this analysis.[32] In fact, one need not sequence entire genes because techniques are available to look at discrete segments.

In summary, recombinant DNA technology allows one to look for variation within the nucleotide sequence of entire genes or discrete segments. Using the appropriate statistical techniques, one can ask whether certain variants

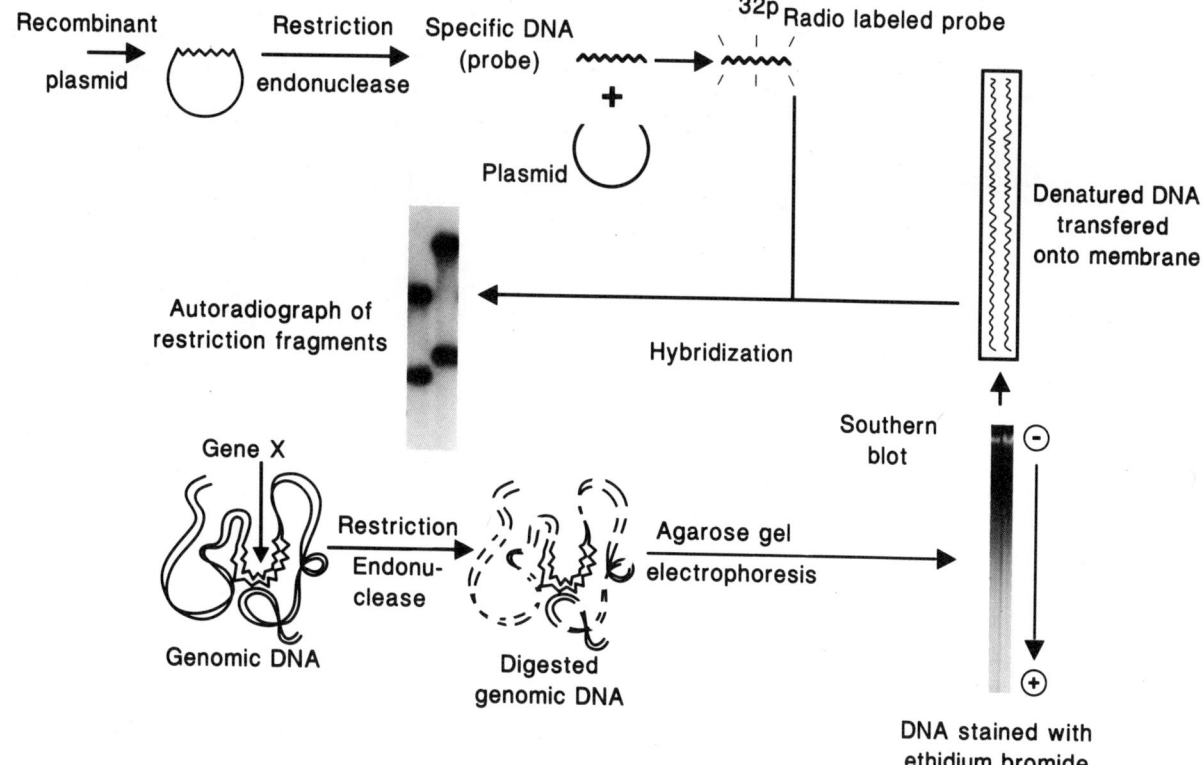

Fig. 38-1. Schematic illustrating the steps involved in a Southern blot analysis.

are associated or linked with the disease state. Once a DNA mutation has been determined to be related to a disease state, several laboratory methodologies can be used to detect these variants, which form the basis for diagnostic testing. The ability to determine genetic variation at the nucleotide sequence level has by and large not changed any of the fundamental principles of genetics. However, the techniques are more powerful because they give the ability to deduce from variants within the nucleotide sequence the molecular basis for disease states. For the practicing physician, understanding the details of the technology is less important than knowing how this information can be used for presymptomatic diagnosis and to select preventive interventions. We will now turn to a discussion of approaches for using genetic information in preventive medicine.

OBTAINING GENETIC INFORMATION

A concern for the busy practicing physician might be how best to obtain genetic information. Physicians may obtain genetic information during the taking of a medical history. To fully evaluate a person's genetic risk of disease and to determine the laboratory or screening test that could further refine the risk estimate or aid in the diagnosis of a disease, the physician needs detailed information. Thus a more structured approach should be used to obtain genetic

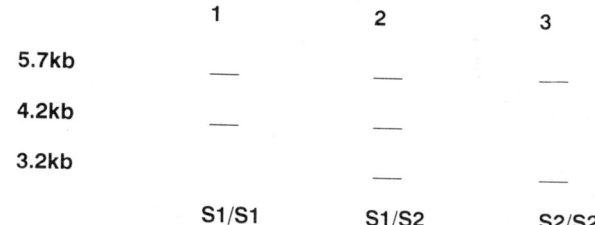

Fig. 38-2. Diagrammatical representation of an autoradiograph of DNA from a normal individual and individuals with hypertriglyceridemia. The DNA was cleaved with the restriction endonuclease Sst-1, electrophoresed through agarose, Southern blotted to a membrane, and hybridized with a ^{32}P-labeled probe that detects nucleotide sequences within the apolipoprotein A1-C3-A4 gene complex.

information. In this section we will discuss variables that must be considered when obtaining genetic information. In Chapter 39 we will discuss approaches that can make the process more efficient.

Family history of disease

There are a number of recognized familial disorders. Table 38-1 is a selection of diseases and an estimate of the relative risk associated with having a positive family history for the specific disease. These are diseases that often

Table 38-1. The association of positive family history with disease

Disease	Estimated relative risk*	Reference
Alcoholism	2-20	50,102,131,162,166,171
Breast cancer	2-10	28,39,82,84,107,173,192,201
Colorectal carcinoma/adenomatous polyposis	2-8	21,27,30,67,93,116-120,164
Coronary heart disease	2-25	3,26,70,79,85
Diabetes: IDDM	7-18	55,103
NIDDM	3-16	5,37
IGT	2-3	33
Emphysema	2	24,219
Glaucoma	3-4	122,163,216
Hemochromatosis	2-6	53,54,108
Hypercholesterolemia	24-499	64,133,174
Hypertension	2-4	3,206,210,214
Lung cancer	2-5	126,141,167,175,176,199,218
Manic depression	2-3	92,222,109
Marfan syndrome	↑	34,123,144
Melanoma	3-148	46,52,56,77,101,160
Obesity	4-25	22,76,110,184,190
Osteoporosis	↑	42,182,202
Ovarian cancer	3-69	100,115,146,170
Polycystic kidney disease (AD)	199	63,96
Prostate cancer	2-11	129,186,187

*Relative risks are estimated from studies referenced. The range represents the difference observed in the various studies. If the appropriate data were not available to estimate familial relative risks based on FHD, increased risk is indicated by ↑ .

do not become clinically apparent until adolescence on. With the exception of the autosomal dominant disorders (e.g., Marfan syndrome,[153] polycystic kidney disease,[63,96] and familial hypercholesterolemia[133]) they represent multifactorial diseases. Life-style and environmental factors also appear to play a role in clinical expression of many of these disorders.[97] Thus a positive family history of disease (FHD) can be due to shared environment and/or shared genes. However, for some of these diseases (e.g., coronary heart disease), FHD appears to be an independent predictor of risk. Lastly, as will be discussed, once risk of disease based on FHD is apparent, there are genetic and other laboratory tests that can be used to refine one's risk or screening tests that may lead to early diagnosis. Using these diseases as examples, we will suggest approaches for obtaining information on one's risk for familial disorders.

Obtaining a family history of disease

The first step in obtaining genetic information on a subject is to obtain a detailed FHD. Traditionally, the physician has collected FHD information as part of the history and physical to help sort out the differential diagnosis for the presence of disease. However, FHD has usually not been collected to target those patients who might benefit from additional laboratory or screening tests or interventions to prevent the disease from occurring. In fact, evidence suggests FHD information often is not obtained or is inaccurate. A review of the clinic charts of 200 cancer patients revealed that 62% of these charts lacked FHD of cancer information.[114] Subsequent interviews revealed that

17% of these patients had two or more first-degree relatives affected by cancer. A negative FHD of cancer was recorded in 21% of the patients. The FHD of cancer information was correct for 79% of these patients.

Henry Lynch, a leader in the field of cancer genetics, has said, "The family history is one of the most powerful methods for identification of cancer risk and provides useful guidelines for surveillance and management. Paradoxically, the cancer family history is one of the most neglected portions of the medical workup of cancer-affected individuals."[116] We add that for most adult-onset disorders, a family history is neglected during the medical history. The American Medical Association (AMA) recently recognized that knowledge of one's FHD could lead to earlier detection and treatment for many diseases. Thus one of the AMA's 1992 "New Year's Resolutions for a Healthier America" is to write a family health history.[7] It has become apparent that FHD information can be used to more effectively target populations for additional screening and/or diagnostic tests that can predict disease or detect onset of disease in its earlier stages. To enhance the utility of a FHD, detailed and accurate information must be obtained. Thus the physician should be aware of variables that may affect conclusions drawn from FHD information.

Variables affecting the quality of family history of disease

Information collected. Several factors must be considered when collecting FHD data (see the box on p. 769). The genetic nature and severity of the disorder will clearly

FHD data collection

Genetic nature of disorder
Type of disorder
Educational level of subjects
Method of data collection
Site of data collection
Confirmation of data

Variables affecting FHD risk estimates

Correct diagnosis
Race/ethnic background
Sex
Age at onset of disease
Relationship of family member affected
Number of relatives affected
Consanguinity
FHD risk not static

influence the patient's knowledge as well as the accuracy of information collected. The patient is more likely to be aware of the more common diseases. Another consideration when assessing an FHD is whether the disorders for which information is desired are single-gene defects or multifactorial. The patient may be more aware of the genetics of a single-gene type disorder than of a more complex disease.

The quality of the information collected also is related to the educational level and socioeconomic status of the subjects being assessed. Moreover, educational level should be considered when deciding whether to obtain FHD information by a self-administered questionnaire or through an interviewer. The setting for FHD data collection also should be considered. One is more likely to obtain detailed information and increase accuracy if the subject can consult with parents, grandparents, or other relatives. Again, depending on the educational level of the subject, the information obtained may need to be checked by an interviewer. One also must consider that certain diseases in an FHD must be confirmed by contacting other members of the family or by obtaining medical records. There are ethical issues that should be considered before attempting the latter. These issues will be discussed later in this chapter. Contacting family members and obtaining medical records should be the responsibility of the subject on whom an FHD is being obtained. In addition to the factors that influence the quality of data collected, the physician should be aware of variables that can affect the assessment of an FHD risk.

Variables affecting FHD risk estimates

As can be seen in the box above right, a number of variables can affect one's FHD risk. It is imperative that the disease occurring in family members be diagnosed correctly. The incidence of various diseases differs among the races and ethnic groups. This is well established for some of the pediatric disorders, such as cystic fibrosis with an incidence of 1/600 to 1/2000 among American whites, compared with 1/17,000 in African Americans. An example of a disease that varies in incidence among ethnic groups is beta thalassemia, which affects 1/800 to 1/2500 individuals of Greek and Italian descent living within the

United States, compared with U.S. whites of Norwegian ancestry, in whom the disorder rarely occurs.

Obviously, the sex of the patient is important in assessing risk. With the exception of the sex-specific diseases, such as cervical cancer in women and prostate cancer in men, there are diseases such as coronary heart disease (CHD), in which the incidence is greater in males than in females. The age of onset of disease, sex, degree of relationship to family member affected, number of relatives affected, and presence of consanguinity within the family are all important variables to consider. Lastly, FHD is not a static variable; it changes over time as more family members enter and transit the period of risk.

To illustrate the effect of these variables on risk, we have chosen a family from our early-onset CHD study. The pedigree of this family is shown in Fig. 38-3. The proband (II-5) is a white male who presented at age 46 with chest pains. He was found by coronary angiography to have 100% occlusion of the left anterior descending coronary artery, and he underwent successful angioplasty. This individual smoked and had a positive family history of CHD and diabetes. His mother had developed non–insulin-dependent diabetes mellitus (NIDDM) at age 34 and presented at age 64 with chest pains. Coronary angiography revealed 99% occlusion of the left anterior descending artery and 40% occlusion of the right coronary artery. She underwent three coronary artery bypass grafts. Her father had died of a heart attack in his early 60s. Approximately 6 months after the proband presented, an older brother (II-3) presented with chest pains. He also had hypertension and smoked. He was found by coronary angiography to have 60% occlusion of the left anterior descending artery, and the right coronary artery was occluded proximally. He underwent three coronary artery bypass grafts. Within the same year the proband's oldest brother (II-1) had a myocardial infarction while undergoing coronary angiography and underwent four coronary artery bypass grafts. He was a nonsmoker. The father (I-1) of these three brothers smoked most of his life and died at age 73 of adenocarcinoma of the right lung.

Now let us consider the risk of CHD to individual III-2, that is, the son of the proband's middle brother (II-3). If

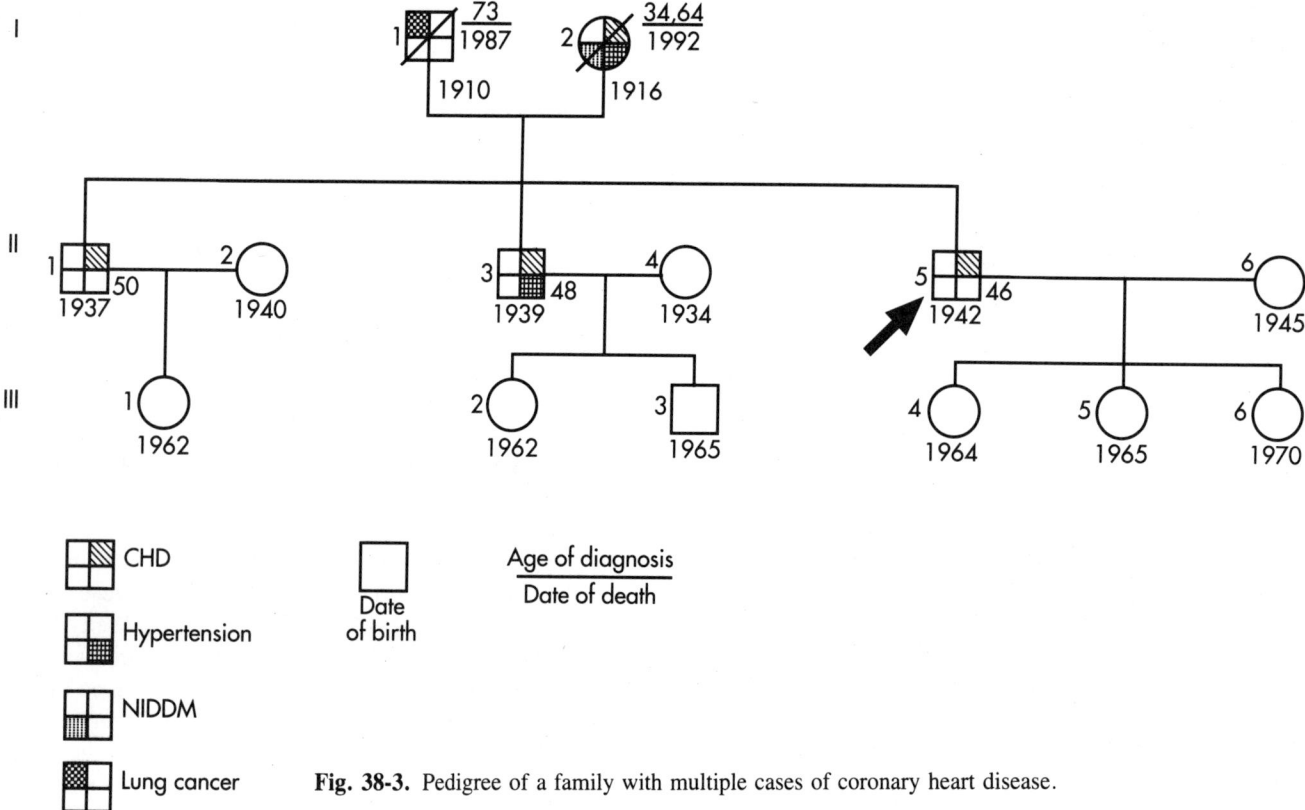

CHD

Hypertension

NIDDM

Lung cancer

Date of birth

Age of diagnosis
Date of death

Fig. 38-3. Pedigree of a family with multiple cases of coronary heart disease.

Table 38-2. CHD risk as a function of age and paternal relative affected

Age of male subject	Relative affected	Age at onset	Relative risk estimate[3,85]
18	0	—	—
20	Grandmother	64	2.9
21	Uncle 5	46	5.9
22	Father	48	12.7
22	Uncle 1	50	↑

this individual's FHD had been assessed at age 18, the only known affected member would have been his paternal grandmother's father. Because the great-grandfather presented with CHD after the age of 55, this would present a minimal risk for the 18-year-old male (Table 38-2). The paternal grandmother presented with CHD when individual II-3 was age 20, thus he would now have a threefold risk of developing CHD. At age 21 this individual's relative risk would be raised to six because his uncle (II-5) had presented with CHD. At age 22 the individual's relative risk for developing CHD would be approximately 13 because his father had presented and he now had two first-degree relatives with CHD below the age of 55. In addi-

tion, within that same year his oldest paternal uncle presented, which would of course increase risk of CHD further.

After his father developed CHD, the 22-year-old male was referred to a physician. He had few life-style risk factors because he did not smoke and was not overweight. He said that as a salesman he was under a lot of stress and did not have much time for exercise. The evaluation of this individual's lipid and lipoprotein values revealed a total cholesterol of 188 and total triglycerides of 147. However, his LDL/HDL ratio was 3.63, which placed him in a moderate-risk category. Therefore his physician advised a low-cholesterol diet and regular exercise, started him on 20 mg daily of Lovostatin, and recommended a follow-up visit in 3 months.

The pedigree of this family demonstrates the need for a physician to periodically update the FHD information. The presentation of CHD in this family also illustrates how age of onset and relative affected influence the risk estimate. Moreover, the physician should assess and consider other risk factors. Some have suggested that additional weight be placed on a positive FHD of CHD and that interventions be more aggressive if the subject being evaluated shares other risk factors with the affected relative(s).[180]

Another disease in which a number of variables also influence the risk estimate is breast cancer. As shown in Table 38-3, a woman's relative risk estimate for breast cancer is influenced by whether the female family member affected is a first- or second-degree relative, whether a mother or sister, age of onset of disease in the relative, menopausal status of the affected relative, laterality of the breast cancer, and age of delivery of first child. Currently, FHD of breast cancer is the best genetic indicator of risk. Genes have been identified that appear to be involved in the etiology of breast cancer.[48,69,183] Thus one can anticipate in the future using a genetic test to presymptomatically determine those women at risk for the disease.

As just these two diseases show, obtaining the best FHD risk estimate for disease requires one to obtain detailed information.

Quality of family history of disease information

As has already been discussed, the quality of FHD information will vary according to the disease. With most of the diseases listed in Table 38-1, the patient probably will know whether the disease occurred in an immediate family member. FH information will not be useful for all diseases. For example, we have observed that information obtained on family history of arthritis is not very good. We suspect that the reason for this is that everyone has heard their parents or grandparents complain about stiffness or aching of a joint. The basis for these complaints could be rheumatoid arthritis or osteoarthritis, two entirely different disorders with perhaps different genes playing a role in their etiology.

Patients also are often confused about the specific type of diabetes affecting a relative. Patients usually know if they have a relative affected with diabetes. However, when questioned as to whether the affected relative has insulin-dependent (type 1) or non–insulin-dependent (type 2) diabetes, the patient is often not sure. Even if the patient says that the family member is taking insulin, one cannot be certain that the family member has insulin-dependent diabetes (IDDM), because many people with non–insulin-dependent diabetes (NIDDM) are treated with insulin to better control their blood glucose levels. When assessing the patient's risk of diabetes, one must determine the type of diabetes, because there are specific genetic and biologic markers that can be used to determine risk of IDDM. Moreover, genetic factors play a stronger role in NIDDM than in IDDM as emphasized by the fact that concordance in identical twins is greater than 90% for NIDDM compared with about 50% for IDDM.[37,106]

In a study to assess the accuracy of FHD of diabetes information, Hispanic and non-Hispanic white patients and controls were interviewed at clinic visits.[91] Their family members also were questioned. There was complete agreement between the information given by the proband regarding diabetic status and answers given by family members who were interviewed by telephone.

Another study has shown that FHD information re-

Table 38-3. Variables affecting family history of breast cancer risk estimates

Variable	Relative risk
Family member affected	
First-degree relative	2.1
Mother	1.9
Sister	2.3
Second-degree relative	1.3
Age at diagnosis/relative affected	
<45/First-degree	2.0
<45/Mother	1.7
<45/Sister	6.9
>60/First-degree	1.9
>60/Mother	2.1
>60/Sister	2.3
Laterality status/relative affected	
Unilateral/first-degree	2.0
Unilateral/mother	1.9
Unilateral/sister	2.3
Bilateral/first-degree	2.9
Bilateral/mother	1.9
Bilateral/sister	4.7
Menopause status/relative affected	
Premenopausal/first-degree	2.1
Premenopausal/mother	1.6
Premenopausal/sister	4.4
Natural menopausal/first-degree	2.0
Natural menopausal/mother	1.9
Natural menopausal/sister	2.1
Age at first full-term birth/relative affected	
<20/First-degree	2.3
<20/Mother	1.8
<20/Sister	3.1
≥30/First-degree	3.4
≥30/Mother	2.7
≥30/Sister	3.9

Modified from Byrne C et al: Heterogeneity of the effect of family history on breast cancer risk, *Epidemiology* 2:276, 1991.

ported by cancer patients is quite good.[111] In this study, of 121 probands who contacted a cancer-prevention clinic, 216 cases of cancer were reported in 180 first-degree relatives. Medical records were obtained to validate these reports. It was found in 83% of the cases that the primary cancer site had been correctly identified by the proband in the first-degree relative. The reported site was accurately identified in 67% of second-degree and 60% of third-degree relatives. The incidence of false positives was only 5%.

There are two approaches for obtaining FHD information for familial psychiatric disorders such as schizophrenia, depression, bipolar illness, and panic disorder. The family-study method involves direct interviewing of as many relatives as possible using a standard psychiatric diagnostic instrument. The family-history method obtains FHD information through interviews with the proband or a relative. A number of investigators have sought to deter-

Table 38-4. Familial diseases for which follow-up measures are available

Disease	Life-style/environmental risk factors	Genetic test*	Reference
Alcoholism	+	R	19,40,45,58
Breast cancer	+	R	36,48,69,83,84,192,203,213
Colorectal cancer/adenomatous polyposis	+	A	11,27,30,62,65,67,98,120,150,165,179
Coronary heart disease	+	A,R	26,59,79,112
Diabetes:			
Insulin dependent	±	A	103,220
Non-insulin dependent	+	R	135,149
IGT	+	R	33,135
Emphysema	+	A	23,80,137,219
Glaucoma	+	N/A	122,163,216
Hemochromatosis	+	A	53,54,108
Hypercholesterolemia	+	A	112,174
Hypertension	+	R	112,214
Lung cancer	+	R	18,31,75,178
Manic depression	±	R	217
Marfan syndrome	−	R	34,51,104,123,125,153
Melanoma	+	R	14,46,52,56,77,121,160,178
Obesity	+	R	22,43,110
Osteoporosis	+	N/A	42,182,202
Ovarian cancer	+	N/A	107,115
Polycystic kidney disease (AD)	+	A	16,63,73
Prostate cancer	+	N/A	129,169,186,187

*NA, not available; R, research stage; A, available

+, risk factors identified; ± risk factors may be involved in etiology of disease; − risk factors not identified.

mine the utility of the family-history method. One study observed that this method underestimates the prevalence of affective illness in psychiatric disorders in family members of the proband, while overestimating the age of onset of illness in the relative.[130] The probands reported affective illness more accurately in their spouses and parents than in their siblings and children. Another study suggested that the family-study method was likely to be more accurate than the family-history method in that the latter leads to significant underreporting, but it can be improved by the use of diagnostic criteria.[8,9] Including criteria for diagnosing 12 psychiatric disorders was found to increase sensitivity, but there is still underreporting by the family-history method.[8]

Others have compared the family-history method with the direct-interview method for detecting psychiatric disorders in relatives of patients. The specificity of the family-history method was observed to range from 93% to 99%, based on the relationship of the informant.[196] However, the sensitivity was low. The spouses and offspring were shown to provide more accurate information than parents and siblings. When the information was obtained from multiple individuals, the sensitivity was improved, but there was no effect on specificity. It also has been shown that the family-history method for detecting major depression and general anxiety disorder in relatives reveals the psychiatric history of the person being interviewed as well as the relative.[94] These problems may be reduced when

multiple informants are used to obtain the history. Others have shown that the specificity of the family-history method for obtaining information on depression in relatives is high, but the sensitivity is influenced by subject and illness characteristics.[142] The sensitivity was found to be higher for females than males and higher for probands than first-degree relatives and spouses. In the psychiatric community as a whole, the family-history method is thought to be a useful instrument for diagnosing affective disorders. In addition, the use of the family history method has been extended to include the personality disorders.[155] A standardized family-history method also apparently can identify dependent personality disorder in relatives of probands.

In summary, for many of the diseases listed in Table 38-1 there are data supporting the validity of FHD information obtained. Formal studies have not been conducted to determine how good FHD information is for identifying the presence of all the disorders in relatives of the proband. However, most of the diseases are readily recognized by a lay person and are similar to the other diseases for which information is available. In Chapter 39 we will discuss the type of instruments that should be considered for obtaining FHD information, as well as studies supporting the validity of this approach. In Chapter 40 we will discuss how genetic information may increase patient compliance with the recommended preventive interventions. We suggest that FHD information for many disorders is

Table 38-5. Follow-up screening of individuals with positive family history

Disease	Screening tests	Reference
Alcoholism	Cage questionnaire	157
Breast cancer	Breast exam, mammogram	157
Colorectal cancer/polyposis	Fecal occult blood, colonoscopy	27,67,68,120,150,157
Coronary heart disease	Non-fasting blood cholesterol, LDL-C, Lp(a), blood pressure	157,158
Diabetes:		
Insulin dependent	HLA, islet cell and insulin autoantibodies	66,220,143
Non-insulin dependent	Fasting plasma glucose	136,157
Glaucoma	Interocular pressure	157
Hemochromatosis	HLA, iron stores	53,108
Hypertension	Measure blood pressure	157,194
Hypercholesterolemia	Non-fasting blood cholesterol, LDL-C	157,158
Manic depression	Questionnaire	157
Marfan syndrome	Phenotype, opthalmologic evaluation, echocardiogram	34,44,153
Melanoma	Skin exam	45,157
Obesity	Height and weight measurement	157
Osteoporosis	Measure bone, mineral content	157
Ovarian cancer	Ultrasound	115,157
Polycystic kidney disease	Genetic test, ultrasound	16
Prostate cancer	Digital rectal exam, transrectal ultrasound, PSA	47,157,169

useful to assess a patient's risk. Moreover, we feel this information can be used to identify high-risk patients who should be targeted for additional genetic and/or laboratory testing and preventive interventions. These uses will now be discussed.

USING FAMILY HISTORY OF DISEASE INFORMATION

Several strategies have been proposed for using genetics to predict or diagnose diseases. There are two major schools of thought regarding the best strategy to influence the course of a common disease in a population:

1. Direct risk-factor screening of and preventive interventions for the entire population
2. Stratification of the population by risk and screening intervention strategies directed toward those at high risk

Taking CHD as an example, some think that the risk factors of everyone in the population should be assessed, but others think that one should evaluate only those who are at high risk.[139,140]

The cost of risk-factor screening for a given disease often dictates which of the approaches will be taken. For many of the familial disorders, there is evidence that FHD screening is an efficient and cost-effective approach for identifying high-risk individuals who should receive additional genetic and/or laboratory testing to either refine their risk or diagnose the disease and to whom preventive measures should be targeted.* Table 38-4 provides a selection of familial diseases for which follow-up measures are available. For many of these diseases, life-style and/or environmental factors also predispose one to the disease. Moreover, there are recognized preventive measures that, if practiced by the subject, could reduce risk of disease developing, delay onset of disease, or reduce severity. In addition, for many of these diseases genetic tests could be used to presymptomatically assess one's risk of developing the disorder. For most of the diseases listed, research is being conducted to identify the gene(s) involved in the etiology. Although patients cannot change their genetic risk of disease, they should be encouraged to reduce their lifestyle/environmental risk factors. The physician should target those individuals with a high genetic risk and aggressively apply preventive or therapeutic measures.

Strategies for using FHD information to stratify the use of genetic and/or laboratory tests to predict risk of disease will be discussed in the next chapter.

Table 38-5 is a summary of screening tests recommended for individuals who have a positive FHD of the diseases listed. For many of the diseases listed, FHD information can help determine the age at which an individual should receive clinical interventions and how often the screening test should be performed.

Because a gene involved in the etiology of some colon cancers has been identified, these disorders have been chosen to illustrate how genetic information can be used to stratify screening tests to detect disease earlier. As shown in the box on p. 774, FHD information and the results of an RFLP genetic test are variables that are considered in defining the hereditary nature of colon cancer as well as the type of screening tests and age at which they are utilized.[27,67,120,150]

Insulin-dependent diabetes mellitus (IDDM) provides

*References 90, 121, 123, 124, 188, 204, 212, 215.

Recommendations for screening subjects with positive family history of colon cancer

I. Familial adenomatous polyposis
   Offsprings of affected parent at 50% risk.
   1. If one or more affected relatives available offer genetic testing:
      A. If subject positive begin flexible proctosigmoidoscopy at age 10-12 years, repeat yearly until 40 years of age and then every 3 years.
      B. If subject negative perform flexible proctosigmoidoscopy at age 10-12 years, repeat every 3 years until age 35 years.
   2. In the absence of available affected relatives for genetic testing follow screening recommendations in 1.A.

II. Hereditary non-polyposis colorectal cancer
   Family members of affected individuals should have yearly fecal occult blood testing and full colonoscopy every 2 years beginning at age 25 or at an age 5 years younger than age of family member at diagnosis of colorectal cancer.

III. Sporadic colorectal cancer
   1. One first-degree relative affected.
      A manual digital rectal exam and fecal occult blood test. Beginning at 35-40 years of age proctosigmoidoscopy every 3-5 years.
   2. Two first-degree relatives affected.
      Same as in 1 except begin colonoscopy at 35-40 years of age or at an age 5 years younger than the age of the youngest affected relative at diagnosis, whichever is the youngest age.
   3. Three or more affected relatives.
      Screen as for hereditary non-polyposis. Suspect an inherited colon cancer syndrome.
   4. First-degree relative diagnosed with colon cancer at age younger than 30 years. Suspect inherited colon cancer syndromes.

Modified from Burt RW: Familial Screening, *J Gastro Hepat* 6:548, 1991; and Peterson GM et al: Screening guidelines and premorbid diagnosis of familial adenomatous polyposis using linkage, *Gastroenterology* 100:1658, 1991.

another example of how information derived from genetic and other laboratory testing might be used to predict the risk of an individual developing the disorder and to determine whether pathological events have begun. IDDM or type 1 diabetes is characterized by a dependency on injected insulin to prevent hyperglycemia, ketosis, and subsequent death.[136] Although the peak incidence of this disease is in adolescence, onset can occur at any age.[103] The disease was originally thought to be characterized by a sudden onset, but we now know that the disease may smolder for several years before clinical presentation.[86] IDDM is regarded as an autoimmune disorder because insulitis is a hallmark of the disease, and it subsequently re-

sults in destruction of the pancreatic beta cells.[55] Circulating serum pancreatic islet cell autoantibodies and insulin autoantibodies are present in subjects several years before the development of hypoglycemia and insulin dependency and suggest that the pancreatic beta cells are being destroyed.[66] These autoantibodies provide serologic markers that can be used to predict those individuals at high risk of developing IDDM.[193] IDDM appears to be a multifactorial disease in that environmental factors such as viruses or chemicals may act to initiate the disease process in a genetically predisposed host. The fact that even in monozygotic twins the concordance rate is 50% or less suggests that environmental etiologic factors are involved in IDDM.[106]

A number of retrospective and prospective population and family studies have provided data that can be used to estimate one's risk of developing IDDM based on the knowledge of presence or absence of specific risk factors. Table 38-6 summarizes the genetic and immunological tests that can be used to predict one's risk of developing this disease. As can be seen, the lifetime risk of the disease in the U.S. white population is about 2 per 1000.[103] The genetic markers HLA-DR3 and HLA-DR4, which are located within the major histocompatibility complex (MHC) on the short arm of chromosome 6, have been shown to be strongly associated with IDDM in population studies of several racial and ethnic groups.[134,151,156,191] The fact that an individual who possesses both DR3 and DR4 is at greater than the additive risk compared with their risk if only one of these genetic markers is possessed, suggests that there are two genes for IDDM susceptibility, one each associated with DR3 and DR4. While DR3 and DR4 can reveal risk of IDDM for the population as a whole, their predictive value is not very high because the frequency of these genetic markers in North American whites is 23% and 28%, respectively. In addition, the cost of the test may be prohibitive for many. Thus DR3 and DR4 are currently not useful for population screening. More recently even greater risk differentials have been noted by comparing the risk of those with and without certain subtypes of DQw3.[201]

If the patient has a positive FHD of IDDM, the risk depends on the number of first-degree relatives affected and whether the affected relative is a sibling, child, or parent.[197] The risk could be from 20 to 100 per 1000. The risk of developing IDDM in an individual who has an affected sib can be further refined by use of HLA typing data. For example, the risk of an individual with an affected sib is 50 per 1000, but if that person has no HLA identity to the affected sib, the risk is only 7 per 1000. If a sibling is haploidentical to the affected sib, that is, both sibs share one identical HLA haplotype, the unaffected sib's risk is 86 per 1000. When a sibling is HLA identical, that is, he or she shares both HLA haplotypes with the affected sib, that person's risk is 157 per 1000. Thus HLA

Table 38-6. Lifetime risk estimates for insulin-dependent diabetes mellitus in whites based on presence of specific risk factors

Risk variable	Estimated lifetime risk per 1000*
Population overall	2
HLA-DR3$^+$	5
HLA-DR4$^+$	20
HLA-DR3/4$^+$	58
Family history of IDDM (FHD)	20-100
FHD$^+$ + HLA − DQB3-2	100
Children of IDDM	49
Any sibling of affected sib	50
Sibling non-HLA identical to affected sib	7
Sibling haploidentical to affected sib	86
Sibling HLA-identical to affected sib	157
FHD$^+$ islet-cell autoantibody positive	423
FHD$^+$ insulin autoantibody positive	84

*References 12,13,55,66,86,103,134,143,151,156,191,193,197,201.

typing of individuals with an affected sib helps to refine their actual risk of developing IDDM.

Pancreatic islet cell and insulin autoantibodies can be used to determine whether the autoimmune process has begun.* Individuals who have a positive FHD as well as serum pancreatic islet cell autoantibodies have a risk of 423 per 1000 of developing IDDM, compared with 84 per 1000 in individuals who have a positive FHD and insulin autoantibodies. Individuals who have both types of autoantibodies have a greater likelihood of impaired insulin secretion than those with islet cell autoantibodies alone.[13] Metabolic testing, such as first-phase insulin secretion at 1 and 3 minutes after intravenous administration of glucose, can be used to monitor the progression toward insulin dependency in high-risk individuals. Thus it is now possible not only to predict the individuals at high risk for developing IDDM, but also to identify those with subclinical disease and follow their clinical progression to an active disease state.[35]

Unfortunately, a cure for IDDM does not exist at present. Randomized trials of immunosuppressive therapy indicate that some patients can be brought into remission for variable lengths of time, but the efficacy and safety of this approach remain to be determined.[15,57,189] Although an effective intervention does not exist, there are several reasons one might want to screen for IDDM. First, mothers of IDDM children are usually very anxious to know whether their children are at risk or the risk to other children they may choose to have. Second, a nationwide survey has revealed that the frequency of coma in new-onset cases of IDDM is greater than 10%.[89] The death rate

*References 12, 55, 66, 86, 143, 193.

among subjects presenting with coma was 3%, compared with 0.1% in noncoma patients. Because the early stages of the pathologic process can be detected, the health care provider can keep a close eye on those developing disease and prevent coma. Third, if high-risk subjects are identified, they would be the group to target for intervention, should it become available.

The U.S. Preventive Services Task Force has also recommended using FHD information as well as other risk factors to decide on the type of screening tests and when they should be administered for CHD, hypercholesterolemia, breast cancer, colorectal cancer, depression, diabetes, and skin cancer.[157] Other groups such as the National Heart, Lung, and Blood Institute, American Heart Association, American Diabetes Association, National Cancer Institute, and American Cancer Society emphasize FHD as a risk factor and recommend considering this variable along with other risk factors in their screening recommendations.

For many of the diseases listed, the agencies do not agree on the type of screening test to be used or frequency at which the test should be administered. For example, there is a debate about whether occult blood screening is a cost-effective method of detecting colorectal cancer.[6] It has been argued that although occult blood testing is not a perfect approach to detecting colon cancer and adenomas, there is no cost-effective alternative test.[99] Therefore, it has been stated that this practice need not be changed.[99] There is also a debate about the age at which one should conduct a cholesterol test on a child and whether all children should be screened as opposed to only those with a positive FHD of CHD or hypercholesterolemia.[49,87]

There will continue to be debate about the age to begin screening and type of test that should be administered to individuals at risk for various diseases. However, one can be more liberal in recommendations if the screening test does not place the individual at risk or is not very costly. For example, screening for cholesterol or blood sugar level, administering a questionnaire, or paying close attention to certain organ systems, such as the skin exam for cancer, carry little risk for the patient and are not expensive procedures compared with other medical tests. The process would require the physician or office personnel to spend time explaining to the patient genetic risk factors and recommending that certain lifestyle/environmental risk factors be modified to reduce the patient's overall risk. Unfortunately, the cost of providing cognitive genetic services currently may not be totally reimbursed.[17] Some of the issues surrounding genetic testing and counseling will be discussed in the next two sections of this chapter.

Genetic counseling

Having obtained FHD information on a patient, the physician now must analyze and determine how best to use the information. The physician must make decisions about ordering genetic or other laboratory tests, choosing the ap-

---

Process of genetic counseling

Obtain and confirm FHD
Accurate diagnosis
Construct a pedigree
Assess risk
Discern educational level of patient and whom in family to
    inform of results
Informing the patient or family members
Preventive measures or treatment
Follow-up

---

propriate preventive interventions, and informing the patient of risks for developing a given disease. Many physicians do not feel comfortable in providing genetic counseling for their patients. Thus they may wish to refer their patient to a medical geneticist or a genetic counselor. Because the physician usually has a rapport with the patient and has history, physical, and laboratory information in hand, at least for many of the disorders listed in Table 38-1, it may be more effective and efficient if they counseled their patient. We recommend that, for any complicated genetic disorder or one that may require a reproductive decision on the part of a patient, the patient be referred to a medical geneticist or counselor. Therefore we will provide suggestions for conducting limited genetic counseling.

The box above lists the steps involved in the process of genetic counseling.[74,132] As previously discussed, the first step is to obtain accurate FHD information. An essential component of the family history is accurate diagnosis of any disease that appears in the family. To accomplish this the patient may be required, often with help from the physician, to obtain status of disease, medical records, or death certificates on family members.[145] In fact, it has been recommended "that medical records be sought in any situation where family history will influence management."[111]

A pedigree should be constructed containing all relevant information and should be part of the patient's medical record. The physician or office personnel can draw the pedigree or use one of the many personal computer programs that are now available (see Resources at end of this chapter). The pedigree is useful in that the counsellee can visualize the family history and correct any mistakes that may have crept into the written history. Moreover, it helps communicate to the counsellee the disease for which the counsellee or his or her family members are at risk. Lastly, it is used by the physician to assess the risk of disease for the counsellee and his or her family members.

The next step is to inform the counsellee as well as relevant family members of their risk of disease. This is done after discerning who should be involved and their level of

knowledge. The available options for refinement of the risk estimate, screening tests for detecting disease, preventive measures, or treatment should also be explained. Genetic counseling should be nondirective. That is, the physician or counselor provides the patient with information so that the patient or his or her guardian can make an informed decision. However, whether nondirective counseling is appropriate or possible in every situation has been questioned.[38,132] Others have suggested that "clinicians counseling patients with or at high risk for genetic cancers should be directive and urge implementation of the medical options most conducive to preserving a patient's health."[145] The physician can certainly be more directive when recommending a preventive measure that has little risk, such as quitting smoking, a change of diet, exercise, or a screening test for fecal occult blood.

The importance of follow-up to ensure that the patient and/or family members are adhering to the preventive recommendations, have obtained genetic or screening tests that may have been ordered, or where indicated have seen the appropriate health care provider or self-help group(s) to which they were referred cannot be overemphasized. The physician should realize that the patient may feel guilty about the possibility of possessing a deleterious gene that has been or can be passed to the patient's offspring and may need appropriate help to cope with this burden.[81,95,105] Moreover, the patient may deny the risk or suffer psychologic distress that may prevent the patient from following preventive recommendations or keeping appointments for screening tests. These issues are discussed in more detail in Chapter 40.

Some elements of this counseling process are outside the scope of the normal physician-patient relationship. Normally, the physician is dealing with a patient who has presented with a problem or for a routine examination. The process of assessing a patient's risk for a familial disorder requires that family members be involved at a minimum to provide information about their health status or to authorize release of medical records.

Another issue is determining who has the responsibility of informing family members that they may be at risk for a given disease and need to be evaluated. Take as an example the family whose pedigree is illustrated in Fig. 38-3. When the proband II-5 was diagnosed as having CHD, his brothers (II-1 and II-3) as well as nieces and nephews should have been informed of the need to have their cholesterol measured. The problem in routine medical practice is that the appropriate family members of a patient presenting with a familial disorder may not be informed. This lack of information on the part of family members may influence whether their own physician is alerted to their risk and recommends the appropriate preventive interventions. For example, the report from the National Institutes of Health Consensus Development Conference recommends that in adults with borderline high levels of cholesterol

(200 to 239 mg/dl), other risk factors such as "family history of premature CHD, definitive myocardial infarction or sudden death before age 55 years in a parent or sibling" be considered when selecting appropriate follow-up measures.[158] If the patient with a 235 mg/dl cholesterol is unaware of his or her family history of CHD, the physician would most likely not be as aggressive in prescribing preventive interventions. Thus physicians should inform their patients who have been diagnosed with a familial disorder of the need to alert their relatives.

For patients with certain diseases, self-help groups or disease registries may provide assistance to family members.

Identifying and counseling the individual with a familial disorder does require extra effort by the physician and his or her office personnel. However, this effort may produce dividends in the form of early detection and/or prevention of disease. Moreover, if the physician fails to identify a person's genetic risk, he or she may be legally and ethically liable.

PHYSICIAN RESPONSIBILITIES: ETHICAL AND LEGAL ISSUES OF GENETIC TESTING

The ability to predict through genetic testing risk of diseases that occur later in life raises several ethical and legal issues.[74,78,95,105,161] These issues are somewhat different from those related to a reproductive decision. An individual's rights regarding reproductive options are legally protected.[147,177] A health care provider who fails to inform prospective parents of genetic risks and testing options or who fails to provide proper counseling could be found to have violated their rights. This could result in a suit brought either by the parents for a wrongful birth or by a defective child for wrongful life. Wrongful birth and/or life lawsuits have resulted from alleged failure of health care providers to consider a patient's positive FHD or misinterpreting an FHD.[177] Most of the lawsuits dealing with alleged negligence in offering genetic testing and counseling have heretofore mainly involved reproductive decisions.

The physician should be aware of the ethical concerns created by genetic risk information. Many of these problems are related to the effect of this knowledge on the individual for whom the risk assessment has been conducted, as well as the family, health care provider, employer, and others. Knowledge of genetic risk may increase anxiety, expose an individual to discrimination, affect employment opportunities, and unnecessarily influence decision-making. Some studies regarding attitudes toward predictive genetic testing suggest that each genetic disease will have its own related issues and burden.[209] Even in high-risk families, such as those with the Li-Fraumeni syndrome, there is question about what one would do with a young child who has a p53 mutation but is cancer-free. F.P. Li said that in his group "there was a moratorium on testing presymptomatically until many issues had been resolved."[1]

International standards for access to genetic test results were urged in a 1991 conference sponsored by the NIH. "In the Netherlands, the government's health council approved a resolution in 1990 stating that access by insurance companies to previously existing genetic information should be 'restricted rather than prohibited.'[159] This resolution insures 'that the individual's right to privacy is protected, since insurance companies cannot require genetic testing as a condition of coverage, nor mandate disclosure of genetic test results previously obtained as long as the individual seeks to purchase only enough insurance to provide for adequate economic security. In turn. . .access to genetic testing is not impeded. The policy also protects the interests of insurance companies, by helping to counter the effects of so-called adverse selection, in which individuals who discover through testing that they are at risk for developing a disease, subsequently purchase more insurance without disclosing the test result to their insurer."

There are additional issues that one should consider concerning the patient's rights and health care provider's responsibility regarding diseases that often do not appear until adolescence or later in life. The health care provider has a responsibility to obtain an FHD, advise the patient of the genetic risk, suggest further genetic or laboratory screening tests that could refine the risk estimate, and offer preventive interventions.[147,148] Failure of the health care provider to perform these duties or even failure to suggest life-style changes that could lower a patient's risk could result in malpractice lawsuits. A study conducted by the Physician Insurers of America found that delay in diagnosing breast cancer had become a major reason for malpractice lawsuits.[25] As part of the study, 273 cases of breast cancer where indemnity payments were made to the claimants were reviewed. A delay in diagnosis caused by the physician was alleged in 269 of these cases. Several reasons were found for these delays in diagnosis of breast cancer. Failure to obtain or be influenced by the physical history or conduct the appropriate screening test were cited as frequent reasons for delays. In 37% of the cases an FHD of breast cancer was unknown or not recorded. In the remaining 172 patients, 53% had a positive FHD of breast cancer. One of several recommendations to physicians for reducing malpractice lawsuits was, "take a complete family history."

From a legal standpoint medical negligence can be due to acts of omission, which include failure to take an FHD (which one could argue should be part of the physical history), failure to identify and inform the patient of his or her genetic risks, and failure to recommend appropriate screening tests or preventive interventions.[113] This may also include a duty to recontact a patient who is known to be at risk and inform him or her of new genetic testing and preventive interventions. For example, a person might be found to have a positive FHD for a given genetic disorder for which there are no genetic tests available to refine the risk, no screening tests for early diagnosis, or no known preventive interventions. At issue is whether, in the event that the defective gene responsible for the disorder is cloned, a diagnostic test is developed, and preventive interventions become available, the physician has a legal responsibility to recontact the patient and inform him or her of these possibilities. The physician is thought to have a legal responsibility to inform individuals who are still their patients of these new findings.[10] Whether this responsibility also extends to individuals who are no longer patients is not clear. In addition, new information may suggest a different interpretation of previous genetic test results. Here again, the legal responsibilities of the physician are not clear because there are no legal precedents.

Another issue concerns the responsibility of the physician to inform the patient's relatives of their genetic risks. As discussed by Lynch, the physician's responsibility to inform relatives of a genetic risk before developing a disease may be akin to informing them of their risk for a communicable disease.[113] There is a legal precedent for informing household members of their risk for the latter. The physician should encourage the patient to inform his or her relatives who are at risk. However, if the physician is the informant in this situation, there is the issue of potentially violating the right to privacy of both the patient and the relative. The President's Commission for the Study of Ethical Problems in Medicine and Biomedical and Behavioral Research has recommended guidelines for disclosure.[10] However, if a relative could potentially be at great risk for a genetic disorder that could be prevented or the severity of which could be reduced by early diagnosis, the physician might have a legal right to inform the relative of the potential risk and advise him or her to see a health care provider. Whether the physician has a legal duty to inform the relative is unclear because legal precedents are lacking. Many think that the patient known to have a familial disorder has an ethical responsibility to inform relatives of their potential risk. The health care provider could help the patient who wishes to inform relatives. However, the notification of at-risk relatives by health care professionals could be a financial burden that is not reimbursable by existing third-party carriers.[17]

There are additional issues surrounding genetic screening of which the physician should be aware. These will be mentioned only briefly because they have been the subject of much discussion, and there is no consensus about how one should address several of these issues. One very germane issue is the need to retain medical records of deceased family members if these records could be useful to the physician trying to sort out the FHD for a given individual.[195] These records may contain clues about the presence of a disorder in a family member that was not diagnosed previously. There also is the issue of whether to store DNA from elderly individual family members. For example, consider a 55-year-old woman confined to a nursing home because of Alzheimer's disease whose children wish to obtain and store her DNA to be able to determine their risk once the gene(s) for the disorder have been isolated and a diagnostic test perfected. Reference laboratories are available that have the capability of storing DNA, but several issues surround this practice, such as the children's right to obtain the DNA, who has the right to use the DNA, and the concern for confidentiality.[10]

There has been much debate over the use of genetic screening to determine fitness for employment and approval to buy insurance. Currently genetic testing information does not appear to be misused in these areas. A recent report by the Office of Technology Assessment reported that companies over the past few years have actually decreased their use of genetic screening tests.[60] Health and life insurers do not seem to be rushing to use the technology. However, guidelines and legislation are needed that will govern the use of the information obtained for these purposes.

Lastly, the physician should be aware that the patient might suffer psychologic consequences by learning that he or she has a risk of developing a debilitating disorder.[212] These problems surfaced at the advent of testing for Huntington's disease, which stresses the need for pretest and posttest counseling of the subject desiring these genetic tests. The physician should be aware that the patient may need psychologic counseling after learning that he or she may be at risk for a certain disease or his or her children may be at risk.

The age at which genetic testing should be conducted also is at issue. For late-onset disorders, where the child has not reached an age at which intervention is appropriate, there is no justification for genetic testing. Some have suggested that testing of children under any other circumstance should be delayed until official debate has occurred and guidelines have been established.[72]

SUMMARY

The taking of a detailed FHD should be a routine part of the medical examination. If the appropriate information has been obtained, one can estimate a patient's relative risk for several diseases. This information can be used to alert the physician to the need to conduct additional genetic and other screening tests to aid in early diagnosis of the disorder or to predict subsequent risk of onset of disease. The information should help identify high-risk patients and alert the physician to begin preventive interventions to reduce the likelihood of the patient developing the disease or to reduce severity should the disease occur. The physician has an ethical and legal responsibility to obtain FHD information, conduct the appropriate screening tests, and institute preventive interventions. The patient should be informed of available tests for refining risk and counseled about the need to inform family members who might also be at risk for developing the disease. Several issues must be resolved to fully realize the promise of molecular genetics. However, the physician interested in preventive medicine currently has powerful tools at his or her disposal. Wise use of these tools will significantly advance disease prevention in the future.

Acknowledgments

The authors thank Dr. Bracie Watson for reviewing the manuscript and Celestine Hicks and Teri Jacob for preparing the manuscript.

This study was supported by grants No. DK32767 from the National Institute of Diabetes and Digestive and Kidney Disease and No. NS26795 from the National Institute of Neurological Disorders and Stroke.

REFERENCES

1. Abnormal genes, prevalent diseases, *Lancet* 337:1538, 1991.
2. Acton RT: Relationship of genes within the major histocompatibility complex to disease states. In Tardif GN, MacQueen M, editors: *SEOPF HLA technical reference manual,* Richmond, 1992, Southeastern Organ Procurement Foundation.
3. Acton RT et al: Use of self-administered family history of disease instruments to predict individuals at risk for cardiovascular diseases, hypertension and diabetes, *Am J Hum Genet* 45:A275, 1989.
4. Aird I et al: The relationship between cancer of the stomach and the ABO blood group, *Br Med J* 1:799, 1953.
5. Alcolado JC, Alcolado R: Importance of maternal history of noninsulin dependent diabetic patients, *Br Med J* 302:1178, 1991.
6. Allison JE et al: Hemoccult screening in detecting colorectal neoplasm: sensitivity, specificity, and predictive value, *Ann Intern Med* 112:328, 1990.
7. American Medical Association: *New Year's resolution for a healthier America,* Chicago, 1991, The Association
8. Andreasen NC et al: The family history method using diagnostic criteria. Reliability and validity, *Arch Gen Psychiatry* 34:1229, 1977.
9. Andreasen NC et al: The family history approach to diagnosis. How useful is it? *Arch Gen Psychiatry* 43:421, 1986.
10. Andrews LB: Legal aspects of genetic information, *Yale J Biol Med* 64:29, 1991.
11. Anton-Culver H: Smoking and other risk factors associated with the stage and age of diagnosis of colon and rectum cancers, *Cancer Detect Prev* 15:345, 1991.
12. Arslanian SA et al: Correlates of insulin antibodies in newly diagnosed children with insulin-dependent diabetes before insulin therapy, *Diabetes* 34:926, 1985.
13. Atkinson MA et al: Are insulin autoantibodies markers for insulin-dependent diabetes mellitus? *Diabetes* 35:894, 1986.
14. Bale SJ et al: Mapping the gene for hereditary cutaneous malignant melanoma-dysplastic nevus to chromosome 1p, *N Engl J Med* 320:1367, 1989.
15. Bell DSH et al: Futility of predicting onset of type 1 diabetes mellitus, *Diabetes Care* 10:788, 1987.
16. Bennett WM et al: Polycystic kidney disease: II. Diagnosis and management, *Hosp Pract* 27(4):61-64, 69-72, 1992.
17. Bernhardt BA, Pyeritz RE: The economics of clinical genetics services. III. Cognitive genetics services are not self-supporting, *Am J Hum Genet* 44:288, 1989.
18. Birrer MJ, Minna JD: Genetic changes in the pathogenesis of lung cancer, *Ann Rev Med* 40:305, 1989.
19. Blum K et al: Allelic association of human dopamine D₂ receptor gene in alcoholism, *JAMA* 263:2055, 1990.
20. Botstein D et al: Construction of a genetic linkage map in man using restriction fragment length polymorphism, *Am J Hum Genet* 32:314, 1980.
21. Bonelli L et al: Family history of colorectal cancer as a risk factor for benign and malignant tumours of the large bowel. A case-control study, *Int J Cancer* 41:513, 1988.
22. Bouchard C: Genetic factors in obesity, *Med Clin North Am* 73:67, 1989.
23. Brantly ML et al: Clinical features and history of the destructive lung disease associated with alpha-1 antitrypsin deficiency of adults with pulmonary symtoms, *Am Rev Respir* 138:327, 1988.
24. Bruce RM et al: Collaborative study to assess risk of lung disease in Pi MZ phenotype subjects, *Am Rev Respir Dis* 130:386, 1984.
25. Brylawski R: Delay in cancer diagnosis now leads in malpractice $$$, *Oncol Times* September 1, 1990.
26. Burke GL et al: Relation of risk factor levels in young adulthood to parental history of disease, the CARDIA study, *Circulation* 84:1176, 1991.
27. Burt RW: Familial screening, *J Gastro Hepat* 6:548, 1991.
28. Byrne C et al: Heterogeneity of the effect of family history on breast cancer risk, *Epidemiology* 2:276, 1991.
29. Reference deleted in galleys.
30. Cannon-Albright LA et al: Common inheritance of susceptibility to colonic adenomatous polyps and associated colorectal cancers, *N Engl J Med* 319:533, 1988.
31. Caporaso NE et al: Lung cancer and the debrisoquine metabolic phenotype, *J Natl Cancer Inst* 82:1264, 1990.
32. Caskey CT: Disease diagnosis by recombinant DNA methods, *Science* 236:1223, 1987.
33. Cederholm J, Wilbell L: Impaired glucose tolerance: influence by environmental and hereditary factors, *Diabetes Metab* 17:295, 1991.
34. Chan K-L et al: Marfan syndrome diagnosed in patients 32 years of age or older, *Mayo Clin Proc* 62:589, 1987.
35. Chase HP et al: Diagnosis of pre-type 1 diabetes, *J Pediatr* III:807, 1987.
36. Chen LC et al: Loss of heterozygosity on the short arm of chromosome 17 is associated with high proliferative capacity and DNA aneuploidy in primary human breast cancer, *Proc Natl Acad Sci* 88:3847, 1991.
37. Cheta D et al: A study on the types of diabetes mellitus in first degree relatives of diabetic patients, *Diabetes Metab* 16:11, 1990.
38. Clarke A: Is non-directive genetic counselling possible? *Lancet* 338:998, 1991.
39. Claus E et al: Age at onset as an indicator of familial risk of breast cancer, *Am J Epidemiol* 131:961, 1990.
40. Cloninger CR: D2 dopamine receptor gene is associated but not linked with alcoholism, *JAMA* 266:1833, 1991.
41. Committee on Nutrition: Indications for cholesterol testing in children, *Pediatrics* 83:141, 1989.
42. Coralli CH et al: Osteoporosis: significance, risk factors and treatment, *Nurse Pract* 11:16, 1986.
43. Council on Scientific Affairs: Treatment of obesity in adults, *JAMA* 260:2547, 1988.
44. Cooper DN, Schmidtke J: Molecular genetic approaches to the analysis and diagnosis of human inherited disease: an overview, *Ann Med* 24:29, 1992.
45. Comings DE et al: The dopamine D₂ receptor locus as a modifying gene in neuropsychiatric disorders, *JAMA* 266:1793, 1991.
46. Cruthcher WA, Cohen PJ: Dysplastic nevi and malignant melanoma, *Am Fam Physician* 42:372, 1990.
47. Culkin DJ et al: Evaluation of a new tumor marker for localized prostate cancer, *Prostate* 20:117, 1992.
48. Davidoff AM et al: Genetic basis for p53 overexpression in human breast cancer, *Proc Natl Acad Sci* 88:5006, 1991.
49. Davidson DM et al: Family history fails to detect the majority of

children with high capillary blood total cholesterol, *J Sch Health* 61:75, 1991.

50. Devor EJ, Cloninger CR: Genetics of alcoholism, *Ann Rev Genet* 23:19, 1989.

51. Dietz HC et al: Marfan syndrome caused by a recurrent de novo missense mutation in the fibrillin gene, *Nature* 352:337, 1991.

52. Duggleby WF et al: A genetic analysis of melanoma-polygenic inheritance as a threshold trait, *Am J Epidemiol* 114:63, 1981.

53. Edwards CQ et al: Hereditary hemochromatosis: contributions of genetic analyses, *Prog Hematol* 12:43, 1981.

54. Edwards CQ et al: Prevalence of hemochromatosis among 11,065 presumably healthy blood donors, *N Engl J Med* 318:1355, 1988.

55. Eisenbarth GS: Type I diabetes: clinical implications of autoimmunity, *Hosp Pract* 15:167, 1987.

56. English DR, Armstrong BK: Identifying people at high risk of cutaneous malignant melanoma: results from a case-control study in Western Australia, *Br Med J* 296:1285, 1988.

57. Feutren G et al: Cyclosporin increases the rate and length of remissions in insulin-dependent diabetes of recent onset (results of a multicenter double-blinded trial), *Lancet* 2:119, 1986.

58. Gelernter J et al: No association between an allele at the D_2 dopamine receptor gene (DRD2) and alcoholism, *JAMA* 266:1801, 1991.

59. Gemson DH et al: A public health model for cardiovascular risk reduction, *Arch Intern Med* 150:985, 1990.

60. *Genetic monitoring and screening in the workplace,* Congress of the United States Office of Technology Assessment, OTA-BH-455 Washington, DC, 1990, Government Printing Office.

61. Gershon ES, Guroff JJ: Information from relatives, *Arch Gen Psychiatry* 41:173, 1984.

62. Giovannucci E et al: Relationship of diet to risk of colorectal adenoma in men, *J Natl Cancer Inst* 84:91, 1992.

63. Grantham JJ: Polycystic kidney disease: I. Etiology and pathogenesis, *Hosp Pract* 15:51, 1992.

64. Griffin TC et al: Family history evaluation as a predictive screen for childhood hypercholesterolemia, *Pediatrics* 84:365, 1989.

65. Groden J et al: Identification and characterization of the familial adenomatous polyposis coli gene, *Cell* 66:589, 1991.

66. Groop LC et al: Islet cell antibodies identify latent type I diabetes in patients aged 35-75 years at diagnosis, *Diabetes* 35:237, 1986.

67. Grossman S, Milos ML: Colonoscopic screening of persons with suspected risk factors for colon cancer, *Gastroenterology* 94:395, 1988.

68. Gyr K, Meir R: Preventive colonoscopy. In Weber W, Coffer UT, and Dürig M, editors: *Hereditary cancer and preventive surgery,* Basel, Switzerland, 1990, Karger.

69. Hall JM et al: Linkage of early-onset familial breast cancer to chromosome 17q21, *Science* 250:1684, 1990.

70. Hamsten A, Faire U: Risk factors for coronary artery disease in families of young men with myocardial infarction, *Am J Cardiol* 59:14, 1987.

71. Handelin B: Genetic analysis of inherited disease, *Diagn Clin Test* 27:31, 1989.

72. Harper PS, Clarke A: Should we test children for "adult" genetic diseases? *Lancet* 335:1205, 1990.

73. Harris PC et al: Rapid genetic analysis of families with polycystic kidney disease 1 by means of microsatellite marker, *Lancet* 338:1484, 1991.

74. Harris R: Genetic counseling and the new genetics, *TIG* 4:52, 1988.

75. Heim M, Meyer UA: Genotyping of poor metabolisers of debrisoquine by allele-specific PCR amplification, *Lancet* 336:529, 1990.

76. Heller R et al: Family resemblances in height and relative weight in the Framingham heart study, *Int J Obesity* 8:399, 1984.

77. Holman CDJ, Armstrong BK: Pigmentary traits, ethnic origin, be-

nign nevi, and family history as risk factors for cutaneous malignant melanoma, *J Natl Cancer Inst* 72:257, 1984.

78. Holtzman NA: Recombinant DNA technology, genetic tests and public policy, *Am J Hum Genet* 42:624, 1988.

79. Hopkins PN, Williams RR: Human genetics and coronary heart disease: a public perspective, *Ann Rev Nutr* 9:303, 1989.

80. Horne SL, et al: Pulmonary function in Pi M and MZ grainworkers, *Chest* 89:795, 1986.

81. Hoskins IA: Genetic counseling for cancer patients and their families, *Oncology* 3:84, 1989.

82. Houlston RS et al: Family history and risk of breast cancer, *J Med Genet* 29:154, 1992.

83. Howe GR et al: Dietary factors and risk of breast cancer: combined analysis of 12 case-control studies, *J Natl Cancer Inst* 82:561, 1990.

84. Hsieh CC et al: Age at menarche, age at menopause, height and obesity as risk factors for breast cancer: associations and interactions in an international case-control study, *Int J Cancer* 46:796, 1990.

85. Hunt SS et al: A comparison of positive family history definitions for defining risk of future disease, *J Chron Dis* 39:809, 1986.

86. Irvine WJ, Gray RS, and McCallum CJ: Pancreatic islet-cell antibody as a marker for asymptomatic and latent diabetes and prediabetes, *Lancet* 2:1097, 1976.

87. Jacobson MS et al: The pediatrician's role in atherosclerosis prevention, *J Pediatr* 112:836, 1988.

88. Janus ED, Phillips NT, and Carrell RW: Smoking, lung function and antitrypsin deficiency, *Lancet* 1:152, 1985.

89. Japan and Pittsburg Childhood Diabetes Research Groups: Coma at the onset of young insulin-dependent diabetes in Japan, *Diabetes* 34:1241, 1985.

90. Jarvinen HJ: Epidemiology of familial adenomatous polyposis in Finland: impact of family screening on the colorectal cancer rate and survival, *Gut* 33:357, 1992.

91. Kahn LB et al: Accuracy of reported family history of diabetes mellitus. Results from San Luis Valley Diabetes Study, *Diabetes Care* 13:796, 1990.

92. Kay DWK: Assessment of familial risks in the functional psychoses and their application in genetic counseling, *Br J Psychiatry* 135:385, 1978.

93. Kee F et al: Histologic characteristics and outcome of familial nonpolyposis colorectal carcinoma, *Scand J Gastroenterol* 26:419, 1991.

94. Kendler KS et al: The family history method: whose psychiatric history is measured? *Am J Psychiatry* 148:1501, 1991.

95. Kessler S: Psychological aspects of genetic counseling: VI. A critical review of the literature dealing with education and reproduction, *Am J Med Genet* 34:340, 1989.

96. Kimberling WJ et al: The genetics of cystic diseases of the kidney, *Semin Nephrol* 11:596, 1991.

97. Kingston HM: Genetics of common disorders, *Br Med J* 298:949, 1989.

98. Kinzler KW et al: Identification of a gene located at chromosome 5q21 that is mutated in colorectal cancers, *Science* 251:1366, 1991.

99. Knight KK et al: Occult blood screening for colorectal cancer, *JAMA* 261:587, 1989.

100. Koch M, Gaedke H, and Jenkins H: Family history of ovarian cancer patients: a case-control study, *Int J of Epidemiol* 18:782, 1989.

101. Kopf AW et al: Familial malignant melanoma, *JAMA* 256:1915, 1986.

102. Kosten TR et al: Gender differences in the specificity of alcoholism transmission among the relatives of opioid addicts, *J Nerv Ment Dis* 179:392, 1991.

103. LaPorte RE, Cruickshanks KJ: Incidence and risk factors for insulin-dependent diabetes. In National Diabetes Data Group: *Diabetes in America,* NIH Publication No. 85-1468, 1985.

104. Lee B et al: Linkage of Marfan syndrome and a phenotypically related disorder to two different fibrillin genes, *Nature* 352:330, 1991.

105. Lerman C et al: Cancer risk notification: psychosocial and ethical implications, *J Clin Oncol* 9:1275, 1991.

106. Leslie RDG, Pyke DA: Genetics of diabetes. In Alberti KGMM, Krall LP, editors: *The diabetes annual,* New York, 1985, Elsevier Science Publishers.

107. Li FP: Familial cancer syndromes and clusters, *Curr Probl Cancer,* 14(2):73-114, 1990.

108. Lin HJ et al: Disease risk estimates from marker association data: application to individuals at risk for hemochromatosis, *Clin Genet* 27:127, 1985.

109. Loehlin JC et al: Human behavior genetics, *Ann Rev Psychol* 39:101, 1988.

110. Longini IM et al: Genetic and environmental sources of familial aggregation of body mass in Tecumseh, Michigan, *Hum Biol* 56:733, 1984.

111. Love RR et al: The accuracy of patient reports of a family history of cancer, *J Chron Dis* 38:289, 1985.

112. Luis A, Rotter J, and Sparkes R, editors: *Molecular genetics of coronary heart disease and stroke. Monogram human genetics,* Basel, Switzerland, 1992, Karger.

113. Lynch PM, Lynch HT: Genetics: a link to malpractice? *J Legal Med* 4(5):10-16, 1976.

114. Lynch HT et al: Family history in an oncology clinic, *JAMA* 242:1268, 1979.

115. Lynch HT et al: Surveillance and management of patients at high genetic risk for ovarian carcinoma, *Obstet Gynecol* 59:589, 1982.

116. Lynch HT et al: Hereditary nonpolyposis colorectal cancer. Lynch syndromes I and II, *Gastroenterol Clin North Am* 17:679, 1988.

117. Lynch HT et al: Genetic epidemiology of colon cancer. In Lynch HT, Hirayama T, editors: *Genetic epidemiology of cancer,* Boca Raton, Fla, 1989, CRC Press.

118. Lynch HT et al: Genetic diagnosis of Lynch syndrome II in an extended colorectal cancer-prone family, *Cancer* 66:2233, 1990.

119. Lynch HT et al: Hereditary colorectal cancer, *Semin Oncol* 18:337, 1991.

120. MacDonald F et al: Predictive diagnosis of familial adenomatous polyposis with linked DNA markers: population based study, *Br Med J* 304:869, 1992.

121. Masri GD et al: Screening and surveillance of patients at high risk for malignant melanoma result in detection of earlier disease, *J Am Acad Dermatol* 22:1042, 1990.

122. Margolis KL, Rich EC: Open-angle glaucoma, *Prim Care* 16:197, 1989.

123. Marsalese DL et al: Mafan's syndrome: natural history and long-term follow-up of cardiovascular involvement, *J Am Coll Cardiol* 14:442, 1989.

124. Marshall CJ et al: Cytologic identification of clinically occult proliferation breast disease in women with a family history of breast cancer, *Am J Clin Pathol* 95:157, 1991.

125. Maslen CL et al: Partial sequence of a candidate gene for the Marfan syndrome, *Nature* 352:334, 1991.

126. McDuffie HH: Clustering of cancer in families of patients with primary lung cancer, *J Clin Epidemiol* 44:69, 1991.

127. McKusick VA: Human genetic disorders, *J NIH Res* 3:143, 1991.

128. McDaniel DO et al: Association of 9.2-kilobase *PVU* II class I major histocompatibility complex restriction fragment length polymorphism with ankylosing spondylitis, *Arthritis Rheum* 30:894, 1987.

129. Meikle AW et al: Familial factors affecting prostatic cancer risk and plasma sex-steroid levels, *Prostate* 6:121, 1985.

130. Mendlewicz J et al: Accuracy of the family history method in affective illness, *Arch Gen Psychiatry* 32:309, 1975.

131. Merikangas KR: The genetic epidemiology of alcoholism, *Psychol Med* 20:11, 1990.

132. Muller H: Genetic counselling and cancer. In Weber W, Laffer UT, and Durig M, editors: *Hereditary cancer and preventive surgery,* Basel, Switzerland, 1990, Karger.

133. Motulsky AG: Genetic aspects of familial hypercholesterolemia and its diagnosis, *Arteriosclerosis Suppl I* 9:1, 1989.

134. Murphy CC et al: Population genetic analyses of insulin dependent diabetes mellitus using HLA allele frequencies, *Clin Genet* 23:405, 1983.

135. Mykkanen L et al: Prevalence of diabetes and impaired glucose tolerance in elderly subjects and their association with obesity and family history of diabetes, *Diabetes Care* 13:1099, 1990.

136. National Diabetes Data Group: Classification of diagnosis of diabetes mellitus and other categories of glucose intolerance, *Diabetes* 28:1039, 1979.

137. Nukiwa T et al: Evaluation of "at risk" alpha 1-antitrypsin genotype SZ with synthetic oligonucleotide gene probes, *J Clin Invest* 77:528, 1986.

138. Old RW, Primrose SB: *Principles of gene manipulation,* ed 4, Oxford, England, 1989, Blackwell Scientific Publications.

139. Oliver MF: Strategies of preventing and screening for coronary heart disease, *Br Heart J* 54:1, 1985.

140. Olson RE: Mass intervention vs screening and selective intervention for the prevention of coronary heart disease, *JAMA* 255:2204, 1986.

141. Ooi WL et al: Increased familial risk for lung cancer, *J Natl Cancer Inst* 76:217, 1986.

142. Orvaschel H et al: Comparison of the family history method of direct interview, *J Affective Disord* 4:49, 1982.

143. Palmer JP et al: Insulin antibodies in insulin-dependent diabetics before insulin treatment, *Science* 222:1337, 1983.

144. Pan CW et al: Echocardiographic study of cardiac abnormalities in families of patients with Marfan's syndrome, *J Am Coll Cardiol* 6:1016, 1985.

145. Parry DM et al: Strategies for controlling cancer through genetics, *Cancer Res* 47:6814, 1987.

146. Parazzini F et al: Family history of reproductive cancers and ovarian cancer risk: an Italian case-control study, *Am J Epidemiol* 135:35, 1992.

147. Pelias MZ: Duty to disclose in medical genetics: a legal perspective, *Am J Med Genet* 39:347, 1991.

148. Pelias MZ: Torts of wrongful birth and wrongful life: a review, *Am J Med Genet* 25:71, 1986.

149. Permutt MA: Use of DNA polymorphisms for genetic analysis of non-insulin dependent diabetes mellitus, *Bailliere's Clin Endocrinol Metab* 5(3):495-526, 1991.

150. Peterson GM et al: Screening guidelines and premorbid diagnosis of familial adenomatous polyposis using linkage, *Gastroenterology* 100:1658, 1991.

151. Pittman WB et al: HLA-A, -B, and -DR associations in type I diabetes mellitus with onset after age forty, *Diabetes* 31:122, 1982.

152. Powledge TM: Ethical and legal implication of genetic testing: a synthesis. In: *The genome, Ethics and the law,* Washington, DC, 1992 American Association for the Advancement of Science.

153. Pyeritz RE: The Marfan syndrome, *Am Fam Physician* 34:83, 1986.

154. Rees A et al: DNA polymorphism adjacent to human apoprotein A-1 gene: relation to hypertriglyceridaemia, *Lancet* 1:444, 1983.

155. Reich J: Using the family history method to distinguish relatives of patients with dependent personality disorder from relatives of controls, *Psychiatry Res* 39:227, 1991.

156. Reitnauer PJ et al: HLA association with insulin-dependent diabetes mellitus in a sample of the American black population, *Tissue Antigens* 17:286, 1981.

157. Report of the U.S. Prevention Services Task Force: *Guide to clinical preventive service,* Baltimore, 1989, Williams & Wilkins.

158. Report of the Expert Panel on Detection: Evaluation and treatment

of high blood cholesterol in adults, NIH Publication No. 89-2925, 1989.

159. Research policy. International standards for access to genetic test results urged at conference sponsored by NIH, *The Blue Sheet* 2:1, 1991.

160. Rhodes AR et al: Risk factors for cutaneous melanoma, *JAMA* 258:3146, 1987.

161. Robertson JA: Legal issues in genetic testing. In *The genome, ethics and the law,* Washington, DC, 1992 American Association for the Advancement of Science.

162. Rogosch F et al: Personality variables as mediators and moderators of family history risk for alcoholism: conceptual and methodological issues, *J Stud Alcohol* 51:310, 1990.

163. Rosenthal AR, Perkins ES: Family studies in glaucoma, *Br J Ophthalmol* 69:664, 1985.

164. Rozen P et al: Family history of colorectal cancer as a marker of potential malignancy within a screening program, *Cancer* 60:248, 1987.

165. Rustgi AK, Podolsky DK: The molecular basis of colon cancer, *Ann Rev Med* 43:61, 1992.

166. Rybakowski J, Ziolkowski M: Clinical and biochemical heterogeneity of alcoholism: the role of family history and alexithymia, *Drug Alcohol Depend* 27:73, 1990.

167. Samet JM et al: Personal and family history of respiratory disease and lung cancer risk, *Am Rev Respir Dis* 134:466, 1986.

168. Sarfarazi M et al: A linkage map of 10 loci flanking the Marfan syndrome locus on 15q: results of an international consortium study, *J Med Genet* 29:75, 1992.

169. Scardino PT: Early detection of prostate cancer, *Urologic Clin North Am* 16:635, 1989.

170. Schildkraut JM, Thompson WD: Familial ovarian cancer: a population-based case-control study, *Am J Epidemiol* 128:456, 1988.

171. Schuckit MA: Genetics and the risk for alcoholism, *JAMA* 254:2614, 1985.

172. Schumacher MC et al: Major gene effect for insulin levels in familial NIDDM pedigree, *Diabetes* 41:416, 1992.

173. Schwartz AG et al: Family risk index as a measure of familial heterogeneity of cancer risk. A population based study in metropolitian Detroit, *Am J Epidemiol* 128:524, 1988.

174. Scientific Steering Committee on behalf of the Simon Broome Register Group: Risk of fatal coronary heart disease in familial hypercholesterolaemia, *Br Med J* 303:893, 1991.

175. Sellers TA et al: Increased familial risk for non-lung cancer among relatives of lung cancer patients, *Am J Epidemiol* 126:237, 1987.

176. Sellers TA et al: Evidence for mendelian inheritance in the pathogenesis of lung cancer, *J Natl Cancer Inst* 82:1272, 1990.

177. Shaw MW: Editorial comment: avoiding wrongful birth and wrongful life suits, *Am J Med Genet* 25:81, 1986.

178. Shields PG et al: Molecular epidemiology and the genetics of environmental cancer, *JAMA* 266:681, 1991.

179. Shike M et al: Primary prevention of colorectal cancer, *Bull WHO* 68:377, 1990.

180. Singer F: Risk factors for coronary artery diseases: taking the family history, *Am Heart J* 121:947, 1991.

181. Skolnick MH et al: Inheritance of proliferative breast disease in breast cancer kindreds, *Science* 250:1715, 1990.

182. Smith DM et al: Genetic factors in determining bone mass, *J Clin Invest* 52:2800, 1973.

183. Sommer SS et al: Pattern of p53 gene mutations in breast cancer of women of the midwestern United States, *J Natl Cancer Inst* 84:246, 1992.

184. Sørensen TI et al: Genetics of obesity in adult adoptees and their biological siblings, *Br Med J* 298:87, 1989.

185. Southern EM: Detection of specific sequences among DNA fragments separated by gel electrophoresis, *J Mol Biol* 98:503, 1975.

186. Spitz MR et al: Familial patterns of prostate cancer: a case-control analysis, *J Urol* 146:1305, 1991.

187. Steinberg GD et al: Family history and the risk of prostate cancer, *Prostate* 17:337, 1990.

188. Stevenson GW et al: Single-visit screening and treatment of first-degree relatives, *Dis Colon Rectum* 34:1120, 1991.

189. Stiller CR et al: Effects of cyclosporin immunosuppression in insulin-dependent diabetes mellitus of recent onset, *Science* 223:1362, 1984.

190. Stunkard AJ et al: An adoption study on human obesity, *N Engl J Med* 314:193, 1986.

191. Svejgaard A et al: Insulin-dependent diabetes mellitus. In Terasaki PI, editor: *Histocompatibility testing 1980,* Los Angeles, 1980, UCLA Tissue Typing Laboratory.

192. Taplin SH et al: Revisions in the risk based breast cancer screening program at group health cooperative, *Cancer* 66:812, 1990.

193. Tarn AC et al: Predicting insulin-dependent diabetes, *Lancet* 1:845, 1988.

194. *The 1988 Report of the Joint National Committee on Detection, Evaluation and Treatment of High Blood Pressure,* NIH Publication No. 88, Washington, DC, 1988, NIH.

195. The retention of medical records in relation to genetic disease. Report of the Clinical Genetics Committee of the Royal College of Physicians, *J Royal Coll Phys London* 25:291, 1991.

196. Thompson WD et al: An evaluation of the family history method for ascertaining psychiatric disorders, *Arch Gen Psychiatry* 39:53, 1982.

197. Tillil H, Kobberling J: Age-corrected empirical genetic risk estimates for first-degree relatives of IDDM patients, *Diabetes* 36:93, 1987.

198. Tiwari JI, Terasaki PI: *HLA and disease associations,* New York, 1985, Springer-Verlag.

199. Tokubata GK, Lilienfeld AM: Familial aggregation of lung cancer in human, *J Natl Cancer Inst* 30:289, 1963.

200. Trucco M: To be or not to be ASP 57, that is the question, *Diabetes Care* 15:705, 1992.

201. Tulinius H et al: Epidemiology of breast cancer in families in Iceland, *J Med Genet* 29:158, 1992.

202. Tylavsky FA et al: Familial resemblance of radial bone mass between premenopausal mothers and their college-age daughters, *Calc Tissue Int* 45:265, 1989.

203. Varley JM et al: Loss of chromosome 17p13 sequences and mutation of p53 in human breast carcinomas, *Oncogene* 6:413, 1991.

204. Vasen HFA et al: Screening of hereditary non-polyposis colorectal cancer: a study of 22 kindred in the Netherlands, *Am J Med* 86:278, 1989.

205. Vogel VG: High-risk populations as targets for breast cancer prevention trials, *Prev Med* 20:86, 1991.

206. Volpe M et al: Abnormal hormonal and renal responses to saline load in hypertensive patients with parental history of cardiovascular accidents, *Circulation* 84:92, 1991.

207. Wagener DK et al: The Pittsburg study of insulin-dependent diabetes mellitus. Risk for diabetes among relatives of IDDM, *Diabetes* 31:136, 1982.

208. Watson B et al: Genetic epidemiology of narcolepsy, *Am J Hum Genet* 49:(suppl)486, 1991.

209. Watson B et al: Neurofibromatosis 1: attitude toward predictive testing, *J Hum Genet,* in press, 1992.

210. Watt GCM: Design and interpretation of studies comparing individuals with and without a family history of high blood pressure, *J Hypertension* 4:1, 1986.

211. Weber W et al: Familial cancer: consequences for the oncological practice, *Cancer Detect Prev* 9:455, 1986.

212. Wexler NS: Disease gene identification: ethical considerations, *Hosp Pract* 15:145, 1991.

213. Willett W: The search for the causes of breast and colon cancer, *Nature* 338:389, 1989.

214. Williams RR et al: Are there interactions and relations between ge-

netic and environmental factors predisposing to high blood pressure? *Hypertension* 18(suppl)I:29, 1991.

215. Williams RR et al: Evidence that men with familial hypercholesterolemia can avoid early coronary death, *JAMA* 255:219, 1986.

216. Wilson MR et al: A case-control study of risk factors in open angle glaucoma, *Arch Ophthalmol* 105:1066, 1987.

217. Winokur G: A familial ("genetic") methodology for determining valid types of affective illnesses, *Pharmacopsychiatry* 25:14, 1992.

218. Wu AH et al: Personal and family history of lung disease as risk factors for adenocarcinoma of the lung, *Cancer Res* 48:7279, 1988.

219. Wu MC, Eriksson S: Lung function, smoking and survival in severe alpha-antitrypsin deficiency, PiZZ, *J Clin Epidemiol* 41:1157, 1988.

220. Ziegler AG et al: Predicting type 1 diabetes, *Diabetes Care* 13:762, 1990.

221. Zimmerman M et al: The reliability of the family history method for psychiatric diagnoses, *Arch Gen Psychiatry* 45:320, 1988.

222. Zimmerman M, Coryell W: The validity of a self-report questionnaire for diagnosing major depressive disorder, *Arch Gen Psychiatry* 45:738, 1988.

RESOURCES

Health care provider

Berini RT, Kahn E, editors: *Clinical genetics handbook,* New Jersey, 1987, Medical Economics.

Go RCP: FTREE. Pedigree Drawing Program for P.C. Department of Epidemiology, 720 So. 20th St, Birmingham, AL 35294.

Mamelka PM, Dyke B, and MacCluer JW: Pedigree/Draw for the Apple Macintosh, Population Genetics Laboratory, Department of Genetics, Southwest Foundation for Biomedical Research, San Antonio, TX 78284.

Gelehiter TD, Collins FS: *Principles of medical genetics,* Baltimore, 1990, Williams & Wilkins.

Genetic applications: a health perspective, Lawrence, Kan, 1988, Learner Managed Designs. Book and instructional software program employs a seven-step tutorial model for a study of genetic applications in health care.

Lay persons

Gormley MV: *Family diseases. Are you at risk?* Baltimore, 1989, Genealogical Publishing.

Ince S: *Genetic counseling,* New York, 1987, March of Dimes Birth Defects Foundation.

Pierce BA: *The family genetic sourcebook,* New York, 1990, John Wiley & Sons.

Milunsky A: *Choices not chances. An essential guide to your heredity and health,* Boston, 1989, Little, Brown.

Milunsky A: *Heredity and your family health,* Baltimore, 1992, The Johns Hopkins University Press.

Chapter 39

HEALTH AND GENETIC RISK ASSESSMENT INSTRUMENTS

Jeffrey M. Roseman
Ronald T. Acton
Richard Bamberg

WHAT IS A HEALTH RISK ASSESSMENT?
Overview

In the last half of the twentieth century in the United States, prevention efforts have focused on heart disease, the various types of cancer, stroke, diabetes, and now injuries and AIDS. One of the preventive approaches to these diseases is to identify and provide preventive information to those at high risk, and one of the tools that has been developed for this purpose is the health risk assessment (HRA), or health risk appraisal, or health hazard appraisal (HHA), as it has been variously called.* The HRA is an organized approach to collect the individual's pattern of risk factors (usually through a questionnaire), to estimate the individual's risk of a disease(s) or other health outcome(s) using this pattern (usually with a computer), to present the estimate to assist the individual and the physician to put risks in perspective, to make risk-specific recommendations, and to establish priorities for risk reduction and screening.

The origin of the HRA is traced to Dr. Lewis Robbins, an early investigator in the Framingham Prospective Study, which identified risk factors for cardiovascular disease. This experience suggested that a physician could adopt a more prospective orientation by noting a patient's health hazards. During the late 1950s, while chief of the Cancer-Control Program of the U.S. Public Health Service, he proposed that cancer "control should preferably begin with the identification, appraisal, and reduction of cancer precursors."[44] To this end he directed that race-sex-age specific statistical tables be developed to provide estimates of the risk of death of the 12 leading causes over the next 10 years.[39] These tables became the basis of the first HRAs, which were tested by Dr. John Hanlon at the Department of Preventive Medicine of Temple University in 1959 and a few years later by the Department of Preventive Medicine and Community Health of the George Washington University School of Medicine.

The availability of HRAs lead to the birth of a new preventive medicine discipline, prospective medicine. The term *prospective medicine* was first used in 1962 and has been attributed to both Cecilia Conrath of the Cancer Control Program and Dr. William DeMaria of the School of Medicine of Duke University.[44] The focus of prospective medicine, Dr. DeMaria said, is "the identification of the individual's changing risks of disease. . . ." It complements "the art of medical care with a scientific method which reduces long-term health risks."[44] In 1968, Drs. Sadusk and Robbins proposed in *The Journal of the Ameri-*

---

*For convenience, we will use HRA throughout this chapter unless quoting someone else. Our apologies to those who use the other terminologies. We will use HRAs as the plural. Also, we will call those attributes useful in sorting persons by their risk, *risk indicators,* and the specific categories of the risk indicators associated with high risk, *risk factors.* For example, blood pressure is a risk indicator for stroke; high blood pressure is a risk factor for stroke. It should be noted that the use of the term *risk factor* in this chapter arises out of an epidemiologic context, where, for example, high cholesterol is described as a risk factor for coronary artery disease. In the terminology of the HRAs, *risk factor* has been used as the term for the multiplier weight used in calculating risk. We will not use this latter definition unless specifically identified.

can Medical Association, "the use of a health hazard appraisal as a method of outlining a preventive medicine program in comprehensive health care by the physician."[76] They suggested that the "concept is applicable to the three hazards of premature death; those of potential (asymptomatic) importance from a statistical basis, those of early (incipient) disease, and those of fully developed (overt) disease." The charge of the physician, they argued, was to "promote useful life expectancy."[76]

The first book about the HRA, *How to Practice Prospective Medicine,* was written by Drs. Robbins and Jack Hall in 1970 and published by Methodist Hospital in Indianapolis where much of the early development of the HRA took place.[71] The utilization of HRAs has expanded rapidly since that time. In the mid 1970s the Centers for Disease Control developed their own HRA, which was widely utilized. In 1974, The Society for Prospective Medicine was formed with a primary focus on HRAs. By 1987 it was estimated that between 5 million and 15 million people had completed an HRA.

The explosion in studies of genetic markers (see Chapter 38) has made it possible to include them directly in an HRA for physicians. Before discussing their use specifically, however, we will describe the HRA and its usefulness more thoroughly.

Description

Predicted outcome(s). The central element in the design of the HRA is the outcome (also called *event, consequence*) to be predicted. The outcomes on which Robbins and Hall focused represented 36 different causes of death.[44] HRAs need not focus only on leading causes of death. They have been used with less common causes of death, morbidities, dysfunctions, disabilities, and side effects. The choice of outcome depends in part on the characteristics of the individual for whom the HRA is intended. Although most HRAs have been designed for adults, they also have been designed specifically for elderly, children, adolescents, pregnant or fertile women, and occupational and diseased groups. Depending on the group of interest, HRAs have focused on such diverse outcomes as depression, alcoholism, medication problems, nursing home admission, pregnancy, and having a low-birth-weight child. An HRA for industry might be concerned with risk of a particular problem such as chronic back pain or lung disease or estimated employee's health care utilization cost. The increasing focus on less common causes of death and morbidities opens more possibilities for use of the HRA by the physician. Specific uncommon diseases and other outcomes, for which it would not be cost-effective to estimate risk and/or counsel at a work site or health fair, might be feasible in a physician's office.

Some argue that no outcome is appropriate in an HRA unless there is at least one risk indicator that is useful in risk sorting and, as a result of its use, some risk-modifying

or screening intervention is possible. Nevertheless, Robbins and Hall in the first HRA gave risk estimates for causes of death such as leukemia and aleukemia, which did not use risk indicators other than age, race, and sex to derive; for those, population average risk was used.[44] In some cases, it may be useful simply to know the risk, for example, to put various outcomes in perspective.

Risk indicators. Once the outcome(s) has been chosen, the particular risk indicators must be chosen. The literature has discussed the criterion(a) by which a risk factor is included. These criteria include the sensitivity, specificity, prevalence, and whether it is causal and/or modifiable.

Risk indicators used in HRAs vary considerably in scope and number. The original HRA of Robbins and Hall had 35 different risk indicators.[71] In addition to standard demographic risk indicators (e.g., age, race, sex, education), many HRAs have asked about medical history, behaviors (e.g., exercise level, diet, smoking and alcohol history), driving habits (e.g., miles per year, seat belt use), exposure to violence (e.g., carrying a weapon), participation in screening programs (e.g., recency of stool test for occult blood, breast self-examination and Pap smear), psychiatric symptoms (e.g., depression), stress, social support, and family history of disease.

Multiple questions or pieces of data are often necessary to discern a particular risk indicator (e.g., the information from multiple questions is necessary to determine whether a person has a type A personality). Some HRAs have included extensive questionnaires about medical history, stress, nutrition, behavioral type and attitudes, occupational exposures, home safety risks, and, as will be discussed later, family history. Sometimes, these additional risk indicators are not used in the computation of risk, but directly as the basis for risk reduction recommendations. Most HRAs collect information on risk factors through questions and, therefore, include very few physiologic measures—usually only height, weight, blood pressure, pulse, and serum cholesterol—because most people don't know or remember other measures. There is no a priori reason why some of these or other risk indicators cannot be obtained more validly from charts or laboratory or other test results, especially when an HRA is conducted in a physician's office. Some HRAs do include other physiologic risk indicators such as electrocardiographic (ECG) results, exercise tolerance tests, oxygen consumption,[63] and genetic markers.[73]

When designing an HRA, a tension often exists between the benefit of adding a particular risk indicator and the detriment of increasing the length of the HRA. Some of the short HRAs do not include risk indicators for which there is not strong evidence for causation and for intervention that can reduce the risk. From the perspective of the physician, it may make sense to include risk indicators that are good predictors, even without evidence that they are causal.

In the original proposal by Sadusk and Robbins, the physician took the risk indicator information from the patient in a face-to-face interview.[76] Currently interviews have been conducted by nonprofessionals or have been self-administered. Self-administration may be a problem where illiteracy is prevalent. In some situations the answers are recorded directly on paper, sometimes on optically scanable forms. In other cases, data are entered directly into a computer, through the use of a keyboard, mouse, or touchscreen. In the physician's office, a secretary or clerk can enter the data or, where feasible, the patient can directly enter the data. One study examined the effectiveness of the equipment in the administration of the HRA and found that a mouse interface did not appear to be as effective as a keyboard or touchscreen for the elderly.[29]

Risk estimation. In the context of the HRA, "risk" is the probability that an individual will develop a particular outcome in some defined period of time. The defined period of time can be a number of years (e.g., the risk of dying of a heart attack in the next 10 years) or a lifetime (e.g., the lifetime risk of developing breast cancer). Risk for the individual is estimated by applying the results of groups or families with similar characteristics. The estimates of an individual's risk of disease come from epidemiologic or genetic studies.

The basic idea of the risk estimation for an HRA is simple. A risk indicator(s) is connected with an outcome by algorithms, formulae, or tables generated from studies that provide an estimate of the risk. A risk indicator may be connected to more than one disease, and a disease could be connected with many different risk indicators. For example, cigarette smoking status could be involved in the computation of the estimated risks of heart disease, lung cancer, emphysema, etc. (in this case it is called a "cross-cutting risk"); coronary heart disease, could be connected with age, race, sex, cigarette smoking status, blood pressure, diabetes, and, cholesterol level, HDL/LDL ratio, personality type, and family history of heart disease among many others.

Two major types of epidemiologic studies have been useful in measuring risk: the prospective/longitudinal/cohort study and the case-control study. Of the two, the prospective study is the most useful in obtaining an estimate of the absolute risk. In this type of study, a group of outcome-free individuals are assessed for a variety of potential risk indicators and are then followed over time to see which ones develop the outcome in some particular time frame. The estimated absolute risk for those with the factor(s) measured from such a study is simply the number of people with the factor(s) who develop the disease in that time period divided by the total number of people with the factor(s). By dividing the absolute risk of those with the factor by the absolute risk of those without the factor, a relative risk can be estimated. In many of the HRAs, the relative risk is estimated by dividing by the population average risk, rather than by dividing by the risk of those without the factors.

Prospective studies are good for estimating risks of common outcomes, but they are less useful for rare outcomes because unless one has a large sample to follow, few cases of the outcome would be likely to occur. Because testing and following a large sample for a long time are expensive, not many large prospective studies have been conducted.

In the case-control study, cases (those with the outcome) are selected and then compared with controls (those without the outcome). The odds of cases having the risk factor are compared with the odds of controls having the risk factor. This approach provides an estimate of the relative risk. If the population prevalence of the risk factor and the incidence of the disease (average risk) are also known, through a series of mathematical manipulations, one can estimate the absolute risk of disease for those with the risk factor.

Certain types of family studies are also useful for providing risk estimates. Family studies provide estimates of recurrence risk (the probability that with age, an unaffected individual will become affected, given that another specific family member is affected) and risks estimated from segregation and linkage models.

Many algorithms have been used to predict risk. The original HRA of Robbins and Hall used a formula by which the age-sex-race absolute risk is multiplied by a weight that is used to quantify the relative deviation of those with the particular risk factor (which they called *prognostic characteristic*) to the average of those of the same age, race, and sex.[71] This technique is different from that used for relative risk, which is relative to those at lowest risk.

The population average absolute risk tables (Geller tables) used in the HRA of Robbins and Hall were based on U.S. vital statistics.[39] In other countries, different mortality data have been used. Canadian HRA used Canadian mortality statistics.[21] Because of regional differences in "average risk," several investigators have suggested the use of regional data.[39,53] If, however, regional differences are accounted for by the differences in prevalence of the risk factors, using the risk multiplier tables unchanged would lead to inaccurate risk estimates.[21]

Often no single study involves all the risk factors reported to have predictive value. Decisions must be made as to whether to include the additional variables and, if so, how they should be combined. In their original HRA, Robbins and Hall used a "credit-debit" method, which multiplies risk multipliers below 1.0 and adds those over 1.0 (after subtracting 1.0) to obtain a composite risk multiplier.[71] With the increasing numbers of epidemiologic studies reporting results in a multivariable format, such as multiple logistic or Cox regression models, recent HRAs have begun to use such models. These models can directly estimate absolute risk. Early HRAs assumed that all risk factors were independent, which is problematic when risk factors share variance. Today interaction among risk factors can be estimated directly from multivariate methods, which include interaction terms. There is no a priori reason why any algorithm or type of calculation that can be performed on a computer cannot be used in an HRA.

Some HRA software uses a branching approach to risk calculation. Different methods may be used depending on rules of risk indicator status and/or the availability of data. For example, a different calculation could be used depending on whether the subject is a male or female. Or, if a data value is missing, a risk estimation method that does not use the missing indicator can be selected. (Other HRAs substitute the population average value for a missing value).

Today, the risk estimates are often calculated by computer; however, some HRAs including the original HRA developed by Robbins and Hall used hand calculation.[71] Problems have been reported with self-scoring. In a field trial among randomly selected adults, Smith et al.[85] report: "Mathematical errors made by respondents completing self-scored instruments . . . decrease the accuracy of HRA risk estimates."[85]

Output. Results vary among HRAs, both with respect to the information provided and the presentation format. The information provided may include an estimate of the patient's risk (absolute, relative, or both), an estimate of what risk reduction might be achieved with risk factor modification, educational messages about the disease and/or risk factor, a recommendation for risk reduction and/or screening, and information about where to locate help in achieving risk reduction or disease screening. It has been argued that absolute rates are not meaningful for many people without a risk against which to compare it,[41] so many HRAs provide the age-race-sex average risk for comparison. Relative risks alone cannot be compared across diseases and can give false assurance to an individual somewhat below average for a relatively common outcome. Absolute risk estimates are necessary to provide a relative ranking among the outcomes. Estimation of "achievable" risk is achieved by calculating the patient's risk, substituting their modifiable high-risk behaviors with low-risk behaviors.

Whether there is an advantage to numerical estimates compared with semiquantitative estimates such as high, average, or low has not been demonstrated. The former can be seen as having scientific validity; the latter is easier to understand. Even if numerical estimates are provided, there is disagreement as to how precise they should be (how many significant digits? should a range be given?) given the scientific uncertainty of the estimate.

Because of the perceived need to provide the patient with an overall measure of risk, some HRAs have calculated a *risk age*, which is also called *health age* or *assessed age*. The risk age is the age with the sex-race average risk closest to the subject's calculated risk. Life expectancy has also been predicted in some HRAs.

All HRA outputs are designed to assist the subject in understanding and remembering the results. The differences in HRA outputs reflect the purpose for which the HRA was designed and the program context. HRA outputs can be written, verbal, or both and by mail, computer, phone, or in person. Those administered and returned by mail may rely on extensive output, including an explanation of the output itself. Others, designed to be interpreted by a health care provider, may be more concise (some only a single page). A written output alone may be insufficient; HRA interpretation by a physician or other health care provider may be necessary. Outputs can be organized by disease, by risk indicator, or both. Many HRAs display the risk in graphic forms, such as bar charts, speedometers, thermometers, etc. The risk reduction recommendations used in the HRAs are usually based on studies showing that these recommendations are effective in reducing risk. Some of the recommendations, however, are not based on demonstrated effective interventions and are controversial. Some outputs provide information about where to seek assistance with the risk reduction and screening recommendations including agencies, programs, and literature. Some HRAs permit programming of local addresses and phone numbers. Most include a disclaimer with respect to the validity of the risk estimate and an assurance of confidentiality. Some HRAs provide two different outputs: one for the patient, which is simple and easy to read, and another for the physician, which may contain more detailed information.

HRA software programs may provide the capability to generate group summary reports. This option permits the physician or organization to examine the prevalences of the health behaviors. HRA software programs may also allow for the export of the group data to other software programs such as statistical and graphics packages.

USES OF THE HRA

Many factors have led to the widespread use of the HRA, including its simplicity, adaptability, and ease of administration. HRAs have been administered in a variety of settings including schools, work sites, health fairs, churches, and even grocery stores by TV, magazines and newspapers, mail, and telephone. It can be modified for use in a variety of situations and patients generally like it. HRAs have been used by individuals, health departments, insurance companies, HMOs and PPOs, employers, community and voluntary organizations, fitness and nutrition centers, educators, government agencies, nurses, dentists, health educators and genetic counselors, as well as physicians. The application of HRAs to large groups is feasible and relatively inexpensive. One very important factor has been the development of the computer. Only a computer could store all the risk tables, make the calculations, and provide such a nice looking output in a reasonable period of time. The questionnaires, computers, computer software, and other parts of a wellness program can be packaged, which has attracted commercial firms.

In addition HRAs have uses other than to assist the individual in risk reduction. They have been used to evaluate educational interventions,[94,95] to collect population profiles,[14,26] to train medical students,[32] and to develop a database for future research and health planning.[81]

Perhaps the most important reason for the increased use of the HRAs has been the change in the focus of the medical system. Along with the increasing prevalence of chronic diseases has been a shift toward prevention. As the cost of medical care has skyrocketed, ways to reduce costs have attracted more attention. Because the HRA is a low-cost way of identifying individuals at risk and for promoting healthful behaviors, HRAs have begun to play an increasing role in modern medicine. In addition to identifying high-risk persons for targeting disease prevention and control efforts, the HRA can be used for the following reasons:

- To stimulate interest and increase participation in health promotion/disease prevention programs
- To structure the interaction between the patient and the provider; to facilitate the discussion of potentially emotional or embarrassing issues and the range of preventive activities; to more efficiently use provider time
- To establish priorities regarding various health behaviors; to help to focus those that are easy to reduce and those that promise great benefit
- To provide additional impetus for an individual to change behaviors that put them at increased risk
- To keep track of the patient's risk factors over time

Although physicians have not been the primary users of HRA, the HRA is becoming an ever more important tool for the physician involved in preventive care.* The use of the HRA in clinical medicine offers some special circumstances not present in many of the situations in which HRAs are typically used. Among these circumstances are the following:

- Increased motivation to spend considerable time filling out the forms and a willingness to provide more personal information
- An opportunity to collect more sophisticated and valid laboratory and test measures that can be used as risk indicators
- A physician's office in which subjects are likely to be fasting, if requested. (Many of the laboratory values used in the epidemiologic studies from which the risk

*References 20, 21, 30, 34, 47, 63, 65.

estimate algorithms are derived are based on fasting levels.)
- An opportunity to use a sequential approach (to output information to recommend collecting additional risk indicator information that might be useful in further refining the risk estimates)
- An interest in risk estimates of morbidities and rare causes of death; an interest in persons who are already ill, not just the well
- The special saliency of the recommendation by a physician for risk factor modification
- An opportunity to educate health care providers about the current state of knowledge about risk indicators and risk-reduction and screening recommendations
- A need to make the input and output compatible with the particular preferences and biases of the clinician
- A place where the participation of the minority and/or disadvantaged persons might be increased[12,19]

CRITICISMS OF THE HRA

The HRA has raised a number of criticisms, problems, and questions, which can be divided into three types: questions about the validity of the risk estimate, concerns about which output should be presented, and questions about effectiveness. The last concern will be addressed in the next section. Regarding validity of the risk estimate, problems could arise with respect to the following:

- Data collection errors and omissions
- Differences between the risk factor as measured in the HRA and in the epidemiologic study from which it was derived
- Lack of generalizability of the risk estimate from the studies from which it is derived
- Inaccuracies in the original study on which the algorithm is based
- Data processing

The subject may provide inaccurate risk factor information because of ignorance, inadvertently, or deliberately. Subjects could misread or misinterpret the questions. In areas with low literacy rates, it may be necessary to consider interview rather than self-administration.

Some studies demonstrate problems with test-retest reliability of the subject's responses. Others have reported considerable variation in intrasubject response in test-retest studies. Sacks et al.[75] found that only 15% of a sample of adults had HRAs without a single difference between the two responses and an average of 1.6 contradictions per person. Best and Milsum[13] reported an average of 1.5 changes in 6 months and stated "such a degree of unreliability creates major problems for the Health Risk Appraisals." Most evaluations, however, have not reported such high difference rates.[19,36,62,68] Alexy found high correlations except for systolic blood pressure and HDL. Smith et al.[84] found that self-reported "cigarette smoking and relative weight were generally accurate, but correlations between physiological measurements and scores for blood pressure, cholesterol, and physical activity were always lower than .51." The low correlation with the physiologic measurements suggests that an HRA using data collected in a physician's office would be more accurate. Overall, it seems that lack of reliability is not a critical issue for HRA risk estimation.

It has been suggested that individuals will modify the validity of their responses to meet a "need to look good in front of others."[24,82] Sieber-Martin[80] tested the reliability by comparing the HRA questionnaire and personal interview responses concerning tobacco, alcohol, and drugs in young men and found those who were more often unreliable were trying to make a socially desirable impression. Killeen[57] found that a higher score on the Social Desirability Scale was associated with nonuse of tobacco and alcohol. This result could reflect a need to be socially acceptable either by not engaging in these behaviors or by giving socially desirable answers. As evidence against this theory, Best and Milsum[13] found as many errors in questions about unchangeable risk factors and those related to lifestyle.

Another concern is the selection of the information to measure the risk factor. Ideally, the risk factor would be assessed in exactly the same way as in the epidemiologic research, which was the basis for its use in risk estimation in the HRA. Practically, however, this approach is often not possible. Information collected by subject recall may not be a valid measure of the risk factor used in the studies. For example, subjects' recall of their blood pressure levels when they were last checked is not as accurate as the blood pressure measures taken from the current record. Again, this problem may be less likely with an HRA administered in a physician's office.

Problems may occur with respect to the studies on which the risk estimates are based. The estimates are subject to the deficiencies of the epidemiologic studies on which they were based. Many HRAs use as the "average risk" data from the U.S. National Center of Health Statistics. These statistics depend on the accuracy of the cause of death stated on the death certificate. There may also be errors in the accuracy of the population size estimates used in the denominator.

It is often necessary to generalize beyond the conditions of the study sample. Epidemiologic data for blacks, Hispanics, and other minority populations are sparse. Although the same characteristics that are related to risk in whites also often increase risk in other racial and ethnic groups, the risk multiplier may differ. Studies are also often similarly restricted with respect to age and socioeconomic status.

Frequently, more than one study examines the relationship between a particular risk factor and a disease. For example, many studies have quantified the relationship between number of cigarettes smoked and risk of lung cancer, and there are many longitudinal studies of the risk of coronary heart disease given a particular level of cholesterol in the blood. Most HRAs, however, base their risk estimates on the results of a single study. For example, many use the relationship between cholesterol and heart disease risk from the Framingham Heart Disease Study alone. By combining the results of many studies, the risk estimate would be influenced less by the characteristics of the participants in a particular study, whose representativeness may be uncertain. However, meta-analysis, a formal approach to combining the results across studies, is in its infancy. Another problem with the validity of the risk estimates is that they are based on empirical data, which by its nature is already out of date; and changes over time can be substantial.[89]

A number of studies have examined the validity of HRA risk estimates. The predictive ability of the algorithms of various HRAs has been evaluated by comparing their results with the results of prospective studies. For the most part, the tendency is to overestimate the risk severalfold, although there have been strong correlations between the predicted and empirical results.[28,35,83,85,96] These findings do not obviate the efficacy of the HRA as a prevention tool; they do, however, suggest the necessity for careful evaluation of the accuracy of the estimated risks.

There is also question as to the reversibility of the risk. How good an estimate is the "achievable" risk? How rapidly does the risk of someone with a risk factor return to the risk of those without the risk factor after the individual has modified the behavior? For example, the risk of heart disease declines much more rapidly than the risk of cancer in an ex-smoker.

Some debate has involved the clinical utility of risk factor data for disease prediction. Baron,[10] using a mathematical approach, concluded that even a risk factor with high relative risk may not be effective when used clinically. Although one study found that not even multivariate algorithms provide useful predictive power,[91] several studies have demonstrated that combinations such as used in the HRA are useful.[69,93]

It has been argued that HRAs do not provide any information not already known by subjects.[25] There is evidence from a primary care rural practice, however, that people do not perceive their risk of even common diseases such as coronary heart disease (CHD) correctly. They found a discrepancy between perceived and actual risk for CHD. "Smoking was not recognized as a risk factor for heart disease among smokers."[66]

One of the major concerns with the HRA is the complexity of the output. Many individuals do not understand the concepts of probability or risk. Again, this may be more of a problem in areas of low literacy or education. This problem is minimized when the physician or other health care provider reviews the results with the subject. A study of the perception of risk found that an HRA focused only on heart disease risk was more effective in changing perceived heart disease risk than an HRA that addressed many causes of death.[7] This result might imply that focusing on a specific disease may be more effective, but the study provided no feedback to help the patient focus attention.

The usefulness of the risk-based approach has been questioned with adolescents and the elderly. For the adolescent, the most likely causes of death in the next 10 years are not those most likely to kill them over their lifetime. Moreover, risk of death is often minimized by adolescents. For the elderly, the risks might be seen as so high and life expectancy so short that they are discouraging and depressing. However, Roseman et al.[74] found both physicians and elderly lay persons were very interested to know the risks of dying in the next year of heart disease, stroke, senility, cancer, diabetes, falling, as well as the risk of severe depression, entering a nursing home, expected medical expenses, and the proportion of the rest of life being healthy. One study found "that older users found the HRA was significantly more useful and reported significantly more intent to change behavior."[29]

Are there counterproductive side effects? Could HRAs reinforce less than optimal levels of risk factors for those in the "average" category? Possible negative effects, such as anxiety, depression, hypochondriasis, unnecessary medical expenses, and confusion, can result from health promotion programs, including those using HRAs. Patients may be uncomfortable in discussing one or more risk factors, which may dampen the effectiveness of the entire message. An approach based on risk of dying may be less conducive to learning than a more positive approach. One study found no difference in anxiety scores between groups that received HRA feedback and a group that did not.[60] Otherwise, possible risks of the HRA have received little attention; nonetheless, negative consequences appear to be minor and uncommon.

EVIDENCE FOR THE EFFECTIVENESS OF THE HRA

The value of HRAs in a prevention program is only beginning to be examined. Many reviewers have remarked on the complexity, difficulty, and challenge of evaluating approaches that rely solely on the provision of health information.[15,22,42,55] Few studies have demonstrated any efficacy of HRAs and no studies have reported long-term effects. Many uncontrolled studies[*] have supported the effectiveness of the HRA, but not all of them.[45] The scientific validity of these studies has been limited by methodologic problems such as volunteer bias, lack of reliable

---

*References 1, 8, 11, 18, 28, 37, 51, 59, 61, 72.

and valid measures, secular change in the population, and lack of a control group.[92] Of the randomized control studies of the HRA, several found no impact on health-related behaviors[19,45,86]; however, others found behavior improvement in HRA groups as compared to the control group.[54,60] One study reported that a group given an HRA and risk reduction education had a significantly lower mortality risk 1 year later than a group given an HRA alone, or neither.[87] It should be noted, however, that HRAs were designed to aid the physician and not by themselves to reduce risk.

The next two sections discuss how an HRA, including detailed family history of disease and genetic markers, can aid the physician.

USE OF FAMILY HISTORY OF DISEASE IN HRAS
Family history of disease

Traditionally, family history of disease (FHD) information has been collected by the physician as part of the history to help with the differential diagnosis. FHD is being increasingly used in preventive medicine to target more effectively risk reductions and screening/diagnostic tests that can detect onset of disease in its earliest stages (see Chapter 38). Although for many of the familial diseases FHD appears to be an independent predictor of risk, most widely used HRAs obtain little FHD information.

Collection of FHD information

Several factors must be considered in the design of an FHD data collection form:

- Whether the disorder for which information is desired is a single gene defect or multifactorial
- Whether the target population is pediatric, adolescent, adult, or elderly
- Educational level and socioeconomic status of the target population
- Setting in which the data will be collected, e.g., home, clinic
- Whether the FHD information will be confirmed by contacting other members of the family
- Access of relatives to medical care and diagnosis
- Adoptive or estranged status of patient from relatives
- Whether the data will be collected by means of a trained interviewer or by a self-administered interview form

Because the age at onset of disease, sex, relationship of family member affected, and number of relatives affected must be known to assign risk for many diseases, the FHD data collection form also must be designed to collect this information. For example some HRAs ask, "How many women in your natural family (mother and sisters only) have had breast cancer?" This question does not consider age of the subject's relatives at onset, potentially informative second-degree relatives, and whether the disease was unilateral or bilateral. With this additional information, a more precise risk estimate can be obtained. Whether the number and degree of the person's affected relatives offer important additional risk information to that gained when one simply asked "Does anyone in your family have this disease?" depends on the disease. The risk estimate usually increases more than linearly as the number of affected persons increases and when first-degree as opposed to second-degree relatives are affected. FHD information must be updated periodically over an individual's life span because risk information changes with age. As detailed in Chapter 39, FHD is not static; it changes over time as more family members enter the period of risk.

An optically scannable questionnaire has been suggested as a more efficient and economic means of obtaining and entering FHD information into a computer.[98] A self-administered questionnaire works well with subjects who have at least completed high school. Having the opportunity to fill out the questionnaire at home without a strict time constraint may give the subject more time to check disease statuses with relatives.[98] Currently, no data are available to determine if the best information is obtained when the questionnaire is mailed to the subject's home before the subject comes to the clinic or when the subject takes the questionnaire home to complete. Subjects with less education often will need to have the questionnaire checked or administered by a trained interviewer. Albano et al.[5] found that providing subjects with a family history of cancer questionnaire for completion before their visit and reviewing the questionnaire by a nurse interviewer from a cost-efficient approach yields reliable data.[5]

Williams et al.[98] described the use of "health family trees" as "a tool for finding and helping young family members of coronary and cancer prone pedigrees in Texas and Utah." The form was "a large fold-out chart, the size of a road map (2 ft by 3 ft)", with a box of questions for each relative with the boxes arranged in the form of a pedigree. Among the questions asked about the student's family members were whether the person was a blood relative, whether they lived in the state, whether they were living or dead, what of a list of diseases they had (heart attack, angina pectoris, coronary bypass surgery, stroke, high blood pressure, high blood cholesterol, diabetes, and breast, lung, and colon or other cancer) and if dead, cause of death. It also asked about a number of behaviors such as smoking, alcohol, and exercise.[98] The authors reported the feasibility and utility of this family medical history, demonstrating that they were able to collect and process over 24,000 family trees, representing 68% of the enrolled "students" in 37 high schools in 14 urban and rural communities in Texas and Utah between 1980 and 1986. The estimated cost to identify each unaffected high-risk person was less than $10.

Validity of patient-reported family history of disease information

Most studies of the validity of a well-designed, self-administered FHD suggest that it is generally sensitive for detecting affected family members. Acton et al.[4] assessed the validity of the self-administered FHD instrument in identifying family members with cardiovascular disease (CD), hypertension (HT) and diabetes (DM) and found it to be generally good. The population consisted of white men 50 years of age or less who were referred with presumptive CD for coronary angiography and age-, race-, and sex-matched controls from the same geographic region. All subjects were asked to complete a detailed FHD questionnaire, which also requested the addresses and telephone numbers of all first-degree relatives as well as grandparents, aunts, and uncles. Relatives of cases and controls 20 years of age and older were sent an interview form designed to assess their personal health status. The sensitivity and specificity of the FHD self-administered instrument for detecting MI, HT, and DM were determined. The sensitivity of detecting MI, HT, and DM in relatives of cases was found to be 79%, 70%, and 89%, respectively and 67%, 58% and 83%, respectively, in controls. The specificity was 99%, 97%, and 99% in relatives of cases for MI, HT, and DM, respectively and 98%, 95%, and 99%, respectively, in controls. Hunt et al.[52] have shown that a health family tree completed by high school students with the help of their parents yielded a sensitivity and specificity of identifying CD comparable to our observations.[52] Instruments also are available for assessing psychiatric illnesses with good sensitivity and specificity for identifying these diseases in relatives (see Chapter 38).

Not all studies, however, have reported such good results. Napier et al.[67] compared family histories obtained from participants in the Tecumseh Community Health Study with information obtained directly from the relative or death certificate and found many false-negative and false-positive results, "but the major feature of such histories was gross underreporting" of the diseases among the living, from 57% unreported heart disease to 65% to 75% for hypertension, stroke, and diabetes to more than 90% for kidney, stomach, and thyroid. The accuracy of information about death was much better, with over 70% agreement for heart disease, cancer, and trauma.[67]

Family history information is not equally valid for all diseases. A case in point is rheumatoid arthritis (RA). When the family members of probands who were identified as having RA were further evaluated by reviewing their medical records or physician examination, only approximately 50% were confirmed as actually having the disease.[40] It will be essential to validate an FHD instrument for various populations and diseases and make changes as required to obtain reliable information.

Risk estimation

The use of FHD from epidemiologic studies in the estimation of risk is usually the same as for any other risk indicator; however, it is important to discriminate between the covariance of FHD and and other known risk factors for the disease. Family study estimates of recurrence risk can also be used. The recurrence risk is the likelihood that another family member will develop the disease after one member of the family has already developed the disease.

FHD output

Our approach has been to generate two outputs. One output is designed to inform the subject of risk for a given disease based on the data provided that preventive measures are suggested. A pedigree is provided as reported by the subject. Subjects often are delighted at having received the pedigree. It is one positive outcome of the experience from their perspective. A disclaimer statement is also included.

The other output is directed to the physician who ordered the assessment or to whom the patient requested that the assessment be sent. This output includes all or some of the following items, as indicated:

- A copy of the patient's pedigree
- A brief synopsis on the genetics of the disease(s)
- The patient's disease risk estimates
- The availability of genetic and/or other tests that could be ordered, which might refine the risk of disease
- Preventive measures that might reduce either the risk or severity of disease or delay its onset
- Other family members that should be tested
- Screening tests that might lead to earlier detection of the disease
- References and other sources of information for the physician

Usefulness of HRA with FHD information

A positive FHD can be used either to alert the physician to the need for further testing or, if obtained by the physician, to indicate the need for more aggressive and/or more frequent screening. An FHD may suggest that a particular screening test(s) be used earlier in life for those with a family history. For example, a family history of early onset coronary heart disease or of hyperlipidemia may indicate cholesterol screening at an earlier age.[97] Although a mammogram is recommended for all women beginning at age 50, "for the special category of women at high risk because of FHD premenopausally diagnosed breast cancer in first-degree relatives, it may be prudent to begin regular clinical breast examinations and mammography at an earlier age, e.g. age 35."[33] Earlier sigmoidoscopic screening is recommended for individuals with first-degree relatives affected with colorectal cancer, familial polyposis coli or cancer family syndrome.[16] Even when no good screening

test is available, it is possible to make preventive recommendations that could reduce the risk of developing the disease. Those with a positive FHD for emphysema or lung cancer should be advised about the risks of smoking, while persons with a first-degree relative affected with melanoma who have a high-risk complexion would be especially advised to use sun screens and avoid long exposure to the sun.

As detailed in Chapter 40, we and others have observed that genetic risk information motivates subjects to comply with suggested preventive measures. One's family genetic and medical history has a particular saliency with respect to most other risk factors. Family history personalizes the risk for some people. Siblings of colon cancer patients or subjects with first-degree relatives affected are more likely to participate in colon cancer screenings than those without an affected relative.[64,77] Parents with a positive FHD of cardiovascular disease were reported more likely to allow their children to be screened for hypercholesterolemia than parents lacking an FHD.[43] Moran et al.[66] found that "a positive family history of heart disease was the only risk factor that significantly affected risk perception among the patients enrolled in the study." Other data suggest that in a person with a positive family history for CHD, the presence of life-style risk factors such as smoking magnifies their overall risk for developing the disorder.[50] Thus an FHD can be used to identify individuals at high risk for certain diseases who are more likely to submit to additional screening tests and follow the recommended preventive measures. In addition, in some situations involving the entire high-risk family in a health promotion program provides the opportunity for them to act synergistically to change health risk behaviors. For example, they might all agree to modify their diet, thereby easing the transition for any single individual.

Patients seem to find an FHD useful. Evans et al.[31] used an interactive computer program to assess the familial cancer risk of breast and colon cancer. The vast majority (87% of 620 persons) found the assessment had "value"; 96% would recommend the interview to others. It is also anticipated that the physician, when provided the appropriate information, will be stimulated to apply more aggressively preventive or therapeutic measures in those with an FHD.

USE OF GENETIC MARKERS IN HRAS

As described in Chapter 38, genetic markers are also useful for risk sorting; and, with advances in recombinant DNA technology, new genetic markers are continuously being identified. Many of these markers might be useful in an HRA for physicians. As discussed by Khoury et al.,[58] however, the relationship between marker and disease prevalence influences marker sensitivity and positive predictive value (PPV) and affects its usefulness. A rare genetic marker, even with a high relative risk and a common disease, has only low sensitivity (many false-negative re-sults) and a common marker and rare disease, a low PPV (many false-positive results). Once an individual is noted to have a family history of specific diseases, however, ge-netic markers and other laboratory test results that would not necessarily be cost-efficient or would generate too many false-positive results when applied to the general population would be acceptable when applied only to this select group. It is also important in selecting a genetic marker to consider cost, co-variance and reliability of the test, and the presence of risk-modifying recommendations.

The risk estimates on which the use of genetic markers in an HRA is based can arise from both genetic and epide-miologic studies. In epidemiologic studies, genetic mark-ers are used as are other risk indicators. In case-control studies, the association is estimated by comparing the pro-portion of those with the disease who possess the particu-lar allele with the proportion in those without the disease. Case-control studies can be conducted with genetic mark-ers without worrying about the antecedent-consequent questions that always surround this particular study design. Unlike other biologic markers that might have changed as the result of disease rather than be the cause of it, genetic markers are not affected in this way.

Multiple genetic markers can also be used to estimate the degree of individual genetic admixture. This technique would be useful in diseases where the causal and linked genes are not known, but where the risk of the disease is related to the degree of admixture. For example, insulin-dependent diabetes mellitus (IDDM) is more likely to oc-cur in African Americans with more white admixture.[70] With genetic markers, linkage studies can yield estimates of risk. These linkage studies determine the likelihood that the disease gene is linked (close on the same chromosome) to a particular genetic marker. To make this prediction, at least two other affected individuals in the family must be evaluated.

Genetic markers can make the following contributions to the HRA:

- A significant contribution to the estimation of risk.
- Additional impetus for behavioral change in those who are at increased genetic risk. (Persons might be more likely to quit smoking if they were told that their genetic susceptibility makes them 100 times more likely to get emphysema if they smoke. Knowl-edge of genetic susceptibility for melanoma might be a stronger motivation to control sun exposure. It should be noted that the stimulatory effect of this knowledge may be important, even if the biologic marker is not an independent risk indicator.)
- Different screening recommendations for those known to be genetically susceptible to that disease. (For example, those with genetic susceptibility to breast cancer or colorectal cancer probably should be

screened more frequently and earlier in life than those without genetic susceptibility.)
- Information that might be useful in career selection and sports participation. (Men with HLA-B27 and a family history of ankylosing spondylitis are at very high risk for developing ankylosing spondylitis. Knowledge of this risk might be helpful in avoiding jobs that require heavy lifting.)
- Reduce unnecessary anxiety. (Absence of a high-risk genetic marker may suggest that an individual is not at increased risk for a particular disease, even though they have a strong family history).

In applying a health risk assessment using genetic risk indicators, it is necessary to consider the ethical concerns of inclusion in an HRA. These concerns are the same as described in Chapter 39 with respect to their general use. Many of these problems are related to the effect of their knowledge on the individual for whom the risk assessment has been conducted, as well as the family, health care pro-vider, employer, etc. Knowledge of genetic risk may in-crease anxiety, expose an individual to discrimination, af-fect employment opportunities, and unnecessarily influ-ence decision making.

Part of the attractiveness of HRAs has been their low cost. It might be asked if the inclusion of genetic risk fac-tors makes the HRA more expensive. The present cost of screening for RFLPs (restriction fragment length polymor-phisms) are about the same as the cost for a lipid and li-poprotein profile. The advantage is that genetic testing would have to be performed only once in a lifetime. Un-like results of most medical tests, these results do not change over time. Therefore, the cost is amortized over many years. Genetic tests will become less and less expen-sive because as technology advances, the price drops. In addition, recommendations for particular tests can be se-quenced so that the specificity of each test is maximized while the costs are minimized. For example, in the first se-ries of questions a family history may be obtained. Only if family history of certain diseases is present would a partic-ular marker test be recommended. For example, a person who gives a family history of ankylosing spondylitis would be told that presence or absence of HLA-B27 would be very useful in more precisely quantifying risk. This per-son might then reconsider the value of obtaining the HLA test.

In addition, genetic marker information usefulness ex-tends beyond the health risk assessment itself; therefore, the cost can be amortized over other possible uses such as the following:

- Differential diagnosis (The presence of HLA-B27 is useful to evaluate and diagnose ankylosing spondyli-tis[79]; DR2 and DQw1 is useful to evaluate and diag-nose narcolepsy.[49])

- Prognosis (HLA-A2 is associated with prolonged survival with acute lymphocytic leukemia.)[46]
- Selecting appropriate therapy (Persons with rheumatoid arthritis and HLA-DR3 are more likely to suffer side effects of gold therapy.)[9]
- Identifying those appropriate for selective intervention when gene therapy becomes available

For all these reasons, assessing risk of disease using genetic risk indicator information has the potential (when used with care) for making an important contribution to the health risk assessment. Genetic risk indicators should become more and more important as more sensitive and specific markers are discovered and their costs are reduced.

FUTURE OF HRAS

Using an HRA will increasingly become the standard of good preventive care. The HRA of the future will be used for diseased as well as healthy persons, will be longer and more complex, will allow sequential data entry, will predict many more outcomes, will use many more physiologic risk indicators, and will have an output that educates not only the patient but also the physician.

HRAs already make risk predictions for persons who are not entirely healthy. Many HRAs use hypertension and diabetes as risk indicators. An HRA for use by a physician could include many more disease states as risk predictors, because the physician would have access to valid disease information that would be important factors in refining risk estimates. For example, although it may not be cost-effective to ask about rare diseases such as xeroderma pigmentosa in a survey of the general population, it might be useful for physicians to have the ability to include it as a risk indicator in their HRAs, as it is useful in refining the risk of skin cancer for those who suffer from it and possibly for heterozygous carriers. This approach will be facilitated by the conceptual similarities between the HRA and outcome evaluation methodology, which looks at predictors of outcome in those already diseased. This examination of the prognosis for patients in hospital settings is developing quickly. Already the APACHE III (Acute Physiology, Age, and Chronic Health Evaluation) system for estimating the probability of a patient's death in the intensive care unit or hospital and estimating length of stay uses 27 pieces of data in its searches. This program will become part of routine care.

Many current HRAs are designed for brevity. They anticipate a short contact time with the subject. We see a use in preventive medicine of longer HRAs focusing on less common causes of death and morbidity. We envision physicians focusing more on prevention, using more detailed family history, nutrition, and chemical exposure questionnaires. Patients are more likely to be willing to spend more time filling out the HRA in the doctor-patient setting than

perhaps in other circumstances where HRAs are used. This approach would all be enhanced by adequate reimbursement for the time spent in counseling by the physician.

We have tended to view the interpretation and effectuation of the results of the HRA as an ongoing process, but the data collection has evolved into a single encounter. There is no reason for this constraint in the physician's office where the patients are seen many times. There is little obstacle to performing sequential tests where multiple encounters naturally occur between the testee and the tester. There may be many laboratory tests that might not be cost-effective for routine screening, but would be cost-effective when used after a routine screening that identified the individual as benefiting from the additional test to further refine the risk estimate. A detailed family history is a first step in a sequential approach to an HRA using genetic markers because it can identify persons for whom genetic tests would be most useful.

Genetic markers are useful to identify many diseases, especially when there is a gene-environment interaction. It has already been reported among smokers that lung cancer is associated with the ability to metabolize debrisoquine by oxidation,[17] and bladder cancer from arylamine chemicals is increased in those who are slow acetylators.[43] Oncogene screening will be useful in cancer-prone families. It will also be possible to identify persons at high risk for sequelae of infectious diseases when they are infected. With most infectious diseases, persons are at differential risk for developing symptoms or a particular sequela because of their genetic constitution. For example, enteric infections are more likely to lead to seronegative spondyloarthropathies in HLA B27-positive persons. Genetic markers may be useful in determining those who are HIV-1 infected who will most rapidly develop AIDS.

We are in the growth phase of the curve of the number of genetic markers over time. It is difficult to keep up with all the new ones. With the Genome Project to map the entire human genome, vast numbers of potential genetic markers will be identified in the near future. The costs will keep decreasing. Many of the activities are already automated and the valuable restriction enzymes mass produced. There are plans to obtain DNA samples in large numbers. "The Armed Forces Institute of Pathology plans a data bank of the nearly two million active members of the military, designed to help identify soldiers killed in war or accidents."[56] Entrepreneurs are recommending its use in hospitals as a better way of identification. The DNA analyses will also make possible linkage analyses, which will be extremely useful in identifying genes that modify the risk considerably within specific families. By combining improved storage techniques, use of smaller quantities of sample, computers, better access to more accurate diagnoses, and increasing interest in genealogy, family linkage studies of disease risk will be easier.

The newly discovered technique of amplifying the DNA

How to choose an HRA

The following questions should be addressed when selecting an HRA:

1. What are the risk factors? The physician may wish to use an HRA that reflects his or her own opinion as to which risk factors are important. Does it collect the data in an appropriate and sufficient detail for the purpose for which it will be used? Is it easy for most patients to use? What are the quality-control procedures to protect against input errors?
2. Is the HRA computer scored? Does it use state-of-the-art formulae and algorithms?
3. Are its outputs useful in terms of content and readability for the patient population for whom it is intended? Considerations include the age and education level of patients and applicability of the specific HRA. It is important that physicians test the HRA themselves to evaluate its ease of use and its ability to identify obvious input errors. Does it provide quantitative results, qualitative results, or both? Are risk-reduction and screening recommendations appropriately compatible with the best available information as to how to reduce the risk? If not, can they be easily updated? Can it be modified to include recommendations specific for the community in which the physician resides?
4. How will the HRA be linked to other health care and health promotion activities? What is its usefulness to the physician as a focus for counseling and its cost-benefit?
5. Are there protections for privacy and confidentiality?
6. Is the software vendor likely to remain in business for the foreseeable future? Are they committed to updating the HRA as new epidemiologic studies and genetic markers become available and new risk-reduction recommendations are made? Are they willing to orient the physician to its use and accessible if questions arise?[27]

Guidelines for the appropriate use of HRA

All HRA programs should provide the following:

1. Established instructions for assuring the informed consent for the participant
2. Written statement of the objectives of the program and limitations
3. Evidence of a scientific base for the risk appraisal instruments
4. Evidence that appropriate risk reduction resources are available to participants
5. Demonstration of staff's capability to organize and conduct risk appraisal/risk reduction programs in accordance with stated objectives
6. Evidence that participants receive the results of their appraisal in a form they can comprehend, including recommendations to consult an appropriate health provider when needed
7. Mechanisms to protect the confidentiality of the data on individual participants
8. Evidence of efforts to evaluate the program periodically in relation to objectives[88]

using the polymerase chain reaction (PCR) has markedly decreased the amount of sample necessary for evaluation. Perhaps blood will not be necessary at all. Hair roots, urine, and mouth scrapings have also been successfully used as DNA sources. For DNA techniques, preservation is less of a concern due to its stability.

There are also rapidly developing techniques for measuring other physiologic risk indicators: antibodies, immune function, minerals, hormones, steroids, etc., which may also be useful in prospective medicine. For example, significant associations between specific autoantibodies and the occurrence of early onset coronary artery disease and gestational diabetes mellitus have been reported, which may be important risk indicators.[2,3] Chemical exposures could be assessed either directly, through their metabolites, or through their effects such as thymine dimers or DNA adducts. The levels may be useful in predicting risk. One way molecular biology might revolutionize pro-

spective medicine would be to discover a reliable and valid measure of biologic age as opposed to the current use of chronologic age. We all know people aged 60 who look 90 and those 90 who look 60. Age is already such a central measure in prospective medicine. Imagine what an improvement in risk prediction might accrue if we had a good measure of biologic age. With the increasing emphasis on aging research, including research into the basic molecular mechanisms of aging, it is likely that one will be available in the future.

The lack of good epidemiologic and genetic studies has been one drawback to the development of the use of genetic markers in prospective medicine. To get the best estimate of risk of occurrence of a particular disease, it is necessary to combine the marker information with other risk indicator information for the occurrence of that disease. For example, a child with a family history of IDDM with DR3,4 is at greater risk to develop IDDM than a child with DR3,4 and no positive family history. In almost all cases where genetic marker studies have been conducted, they have not been combined with the other risk indicators to get a risk estimate based on all the known risk indicators taken together. Studies will need to collect both the genetic and standard risk factors to develop the appropriate multivariable logistic regression models of risk. Many large prospective studies of healthy populations such as the Coronary Artery Disease in Young Adults Study of studies diseased persons have stored DNA for future analysis.

Statistical advances are likely to occur, particularly with respect to the nonindependent models. In addition, further development of meta-analysis will permit a more quantitative approach to combining studies.

Software will allow for individualizing the choices of risk indicators, risk estimates, and output messages. For example, some clinicians may wish to include fasting insulin as a predictor of heart disease, whereas others may think the data are insufficient at present to include it. There is disagreement about what levels of cholesterol or body weight to recommend, whether HDL and personality type should be included, how to utilize dietary information, and other issues. How the physician stands on these controversies may influence choice of cutpoint and output. Some providers may wish to use the mammography recommendations in the *Guide to Clinical Preventive Services*,[33] whereas others may prefer those of the American Cancer Society. An HRA for clinical medicine must allow the flexibility of conforming to the beliefs of the individual clinician.

Because of the multiplicity of and rapid increase in risk indicators, physicians will have trouble keeping up with the everchanging literature in this area. HRA might play an important part in continuing education of the physician. Frequently, updated software will let the physician know what markers are available and appropriate to use. Feedback from the HRA to the physician will describe the risk indicators, the meaning of the risk estimates, and what tests to order to better estimate risk and make recommendations.

It is our view that genetic risk indicators will become increasingly important in prospective medicine. Their numbers will rapidly increase. They will be more useful in sorting individuals with respect to risk. They will become easier to obtain and less expensive. Many of them are fixed at conception so they only need to be measured once, thus amortizing their cost over a lifetime, and in the future, over many other uses. For some currently interview-obtained risk factors, they will offer a more reliable and valid assessment. Their growing usefulness will be moderated by ethical concerns and the lack of good epidemiologic studies to evaluate their utility, particularly in situations where environmental interactions are important. Each one will need to be evaluated on its own cost-benefit merits and together with other known risk factors (see boxes).

REFERENCES

1. Acquista VW et al: Home-based health risk appraisal and screening program, *J Comm Health* 13:43-52, 1988.
2. Acton R et al: Immunogenetic and AI/CIII polymorphisms are risk factors for early onset coronary heart disease, Berlin, West Germany, 1986, 7th International Congress of Human Genetics, 750.
3. Acton R et al: The association of autoantibodies with gestational diabetes (GDM) in a sample of black women, *Diabetes Suppl* 208a, 1988.
4. Acton R, Go R, Roseman J: Strategies for the utilization of genetic information to target preventive interventions, *Proceedings of the 25th Annual Meeting of the Society of Prospective Medicine*, Indianapolis, Indiana, 1989, Society of Prospective Medicine, pp 88-100.
5. Albano WA et al: Familial cancer in an oncology clinic, *Cancer* 47:2113-2118, 1981.
6. Alexy BJ: Health risk appraisal: reliability demonstrated. In Miller LA, editor: *Proceedings of the 20th Annual Meeting of the Society of Prospective Medicine*, Bethesda, 1984, Society of Prospective Medicine Publishers.
7. Avis NE, Smith KW, McKinlay JB: Accuracy of perceptions of heart attack risk: what influences perceptions and can they be changed, *Am J Public Health* 79:1608-1612, 1989.
8. Bamberg R et al: The effect of risk assessment in conjunction with health promotion education on compliance with preventive behaviors, *J Allied Health* 18:271-280, 1989.
9. Barger B et al: DR antigens and gold therapy in whites with rheumatoid arthritis, *Arthritis Rheum* 27:601-605, 1984.
10. Baron JA: The clinical utility of risk factor data, *J Clin Epidemiol* 42:1013-1020, 1989.
11. Bartlett E et al: Health hazard appraisal in a family practice center: an exploratory study, *J Community Health* 9:135-144, 1983.
12. Berkanovic E: Behavioral science and prevention, *Prev Med* 5:92-105, 1976.
13. Best JA, Milsum JH: Health hazard appraisal and the evaluation of lifestyle change programs. In Ross CM, editor: *Proceedings of the Thirteenth Annual Meeting of the Society of Prospective Medicine*, Bethesda, 1977, Health and Education Resources.
14. Bosworth K: The health hazard appraisal as a survey instrument for a population profile. In *Proceedings of the 16th Meeting of the Society of Prospective Medicine*, Bethesda, 1980, Society of Prospective Medicine.
15. Breslow L: A policy assessment of preventive health practice, *Prev Med* 6:242-251, 1977.
16. Burt RW: Familial screening, *J Gastroenterol Hepatol* 6:548-551, 1991.
17. Caporaso N et al: Lung cancer risk, occupational exposure, and the debrisoquine metabolic phenotype, *Cancer Res* 49:3675-3679, 1989.
18. Chenowith D: The effects of a health risk appraisal with personalized conferences on the health age of university undergrads. In *Proceedings of the 16th Annual Meeting of the Society of Prospective Medicine*, Bethesda, 1981, Society of Prospective Medicine.
19. Cioffi JP: The effect of health status feedback on health beliefs. In Ross CM, editor: *Proceedings of the Fifteenth Annual Meeting of the Society of Prospective Medicine*, Bethesda, 1979, Health and Education Resources.
20. Clendenin JG et al: Prospective medicine. How four practitioners are using HHA, *Patient Care* 20-61, 1974.
21. Colburn HN, Baker PM: Health hazard appraisal—a possible tool in health protection and promotion, *Can J Public Health* 64:490-492, 1973.
22. Cohen CI, Cohen EJ: Health education: panacea, pernicious or pointless? *N Engl J Med* 13:718-720, 1978.
23. Coronary Prevention Group: Risk assessment in the prevention of coronary heart disease: a policy statement, *Br Med J Gen Pract* 40:467-699, 1990.
24. Crowne D, Marlow D: *The approval motive*, New York, 1964, John Wiley.
25. Crumrine JL: Health risk appraisals, *J Occup Med* 27:786, 1985.
26. Current Trends. Health risk appraisal—United States, *MMWR* 30:133-135, 1981.
27. DeFriese GH, Fielding JE: Health risk appraisal in the 1990s: opportunities, challenges, and expectations, *Annu Rev Public Health* 11:401-18, 1990.
28. Dunton S, Rasmussen W: Comparative data on risk reduction, 1975-1977. In *Proceedings of the 13th Annual Meeting of the Society of Prospective Medicine*. Bethesda, 1977, Health and Education Resources.
29. Ellis LBM, Joo H-Y, Gross CR: Use of a computer-based health risk appraisal by older adults, *J Fam Pract* 33:390-394, 1991.

30. Emory ML et al: Prospective medicine. The case for doing health hazard appraisals, *Patient Care* 8:110-118, 1974.

31. Evans S et al: Computer-based expert system for cancer risk analysis for breast and colon cancer. In *Proceedings of the American Society of Clinical Oncology,* Philadelphia, 1990, W.B. Saunders.

32. Fenger TA: The role of prospective medicine in medical education. In *Proceedings of the 14th Annual Meeting on Prospective Medicine and Health Hazard Appraisal,* Bethesda, 1978, Health and Education Resources.

33. Fisher M, Eckhart C: *Guide to clinical preventive services,* Baltimore, 1989, William & Wilkins.

34. Fletcher DJ, Smith GL: Health-risk appraisal: helping patients predict and prevent health problems, *Postgrad Med* 80:69-82, 1986.

35. Foxman B, Edington DW: The accuracy of health risk appraisal in predicting mortality, *Am J Public Health* 77:971-974, 1987.

36. Fullerton J: Health hazard appraisal: its limitations and new directions for risk assessment. In Ross CM, editor: *Proceedings of the Thirteenth Annual Meeting of the Society of Prospective Medicine,* 1977, Health and Education Resources.

37. Fultz FG: Effects of an experimental personal health education course and HHA on selected college students in Illinois. In *Proceedings of the 13th Annual Meeting of the Society of Prospective Medicine,* Bethesda, 1977, Health and Education Resources.

38. Gazmararian JA et al: Comparing the predictive accuracy of health risk appraisal: the Centers for Disease Control versus Carter Center Program, *Am J Public Health* 81:1296-1301, 1991.

39. Geller H, Steele F: Updating tables of probability of dying within next ten years. In *Proceedings of the Thirteenth Annual Meeting of the Society of Prospective Medicine,* Bethesda, 1978, The Society of Prospective Medicine.

40. Go R et al: Analyses of HLA linkage in white families with multiple cases of seropositive rheumatoid arthritis, *Arthritis Rheum* 30:1115-1123, 1987.

41. Goetz A, McTyre R: Health risk appraisal: some methodological considerations, *Nurs Res* 30:307-313, 1981.

42. Green LW: Determining the impact and effectiveness of health education as it relates to federal policy, *Health Educ Monogr* 6:28-66, 1978.

43. Griffin TC et al: Family history evaluation as a predictive screen for childhood hypercholesterolemia, *Pediatrics* 84:365-373, 1989.

44. Hall JH, Zwemer JD: *Prospective medicine,* Indianapolis, 1979, Methodist Hospital of Indiana.

45. Hancock JR et al: Patient compliance with health hazard appraisal recommendations, Annual Conference of the Canadian Public Health Association, Vancouver, 1977.

46. Harris R, Lowler S, Oliver R: The HLA system in active leukemia and Hodgkin's disease, *Br Med Bull* 34:301-304, 1982.

47. Health Hazard appraisal, dovetailing HHAs into practice routine. *Patient Care* 8:120-140, 1974.

48. Hein D: Genetic polymorphism and cancer susceptibility: evidence concerning acetyltransferases and cancer of the urinary bladder, *Bioassays* 9:6, 1988.

49. Honda Y, Juji T: *HLA in narcolepsy,* Berlin, 1988, Springer-Verlag.

50. Hopkins PN, Williams RR, Hunt SC: Magnified risks from cigarette smoking for coronary prone families in Utah, *West J Med* 141:192-202, 1984.

51. Hsu DHS, Milsum JH: Implementation of health hazard appraisal and its impediments, *Can J Public Health* 69:227-232, 1978.

52. Hunt SC, Williams RR, Barlow GK: A comparison of positive family history definitions for defining risk of future disease, *J Chronic Dis* 39:809-821, 1986.

53. Imrey PB, Williams B: Statistical hazards of health hazard appraisal. In *Proceedings of the Thirteenth Annual Meeting of the Society of Prospective Medicine,* Bethesda, 1978, The Society.

54. Johns RE: Health hazard appraisal—a useful tool in health education? *Proceedings of the 12th Annual Meeting of the Society of Prospective Medicine,* 1976, Health Education and Resources.

55. Kasl SV: Cardiovascular risk reduction in a community setting: some comments, *J Consult Clin Psychol* 48:143-149, 1980.

56. Keehn J: The long arm of the gene, *American Way* March 16, 1992, pp 36-40.

57. Killeen ML: What is health risk appraisal telling us? *West J Nurs Res* 11:614-620, 1989.

58. Khoury MJ, Newill CA, Chase GA: Epidemiologic evaluation of screening for risk factors: application to genetic screening, *Am J Public Health* 75:1204-1208, 1985.

59. LaDou J, Sherwood JN, Hughes L: Health hazard appraisal in patient counseling, *West J Med* 122:177-180, 1975.

60. Lauzon RRJ: A randomized controlled trial on the ability of health hazard appraisal to stimulate appropriate risk-reduction behavior, Unpublished doctoral dissertation, Eugene, Ore, 1977, University of Oregon.

61. Leppick HB, DeGrassi A: Changes in risk behavior: a two year follow-up study. In *Proceedings of the 13th Annual Meeting of the Society of Prospective Medicine,* Bethesda, 1977, Health and Education Resources.

62. Logie AR, Madirazza JA, Webster IW: Patient evaluation of a computerised questionnaire, *Comput Biomed Res* 9:169-176, 1976.

63. Lowe WP, Correll W: Lifestyle change: a delegated model in private practice. In *Proceedings of the 25th Annual Meeting of the Society of Prospective Medicine.* Bethesda, 1989, Health and Education Resources.

64. Macrae FA et al: The Ballarat General Practitioner Research Group, Predicting colon cancer screening behavior from health benefits, *Preventive Medicine* 13:115-126, 1984.

65. McCoy JJ, Sinacore JM: Health hazard appraisal. Its application as data base information and first attempt at measuring its clinical efficacy, *Ill Med J* 149:41-42, 1976.

66. Moran MT et al: Coronary heart disease risk assessment, *Am J Prev Med* 5:330-336, 1989.

67. Napier JA, Metzner MA, Johnson BC: Limitations of morbidity and mortality data obtained from family histories—a report from the Tecumseh Community Health Study, *Am J Public Health* 62:30-35, 1972.

68. Pecoraro RE, Inui TS, Chen MS: Validity and reliability of a self-administered health history questionnaire, *Public Health Rep* 94:231-238, 1979.

69. Pryor DB et al: Estimating the likelihood of significant coronary artery disease, *Am J Med* 75:771-780, 1983.

70. Reitnauer PJ et al: Evidence for genetic admixture as a determinant in the occurrence of insulin-dependent diabetes mellitus in U.S. blacks, *Diabetes* 31:532-537, 1982.

71. Robbins LC, Hall JH: *How to practice prospective medicine,* Indianapolis, 1970, Methodist Hospital of Indiana.

72. Rodnick JE: Health behavior changes associated with health hazard appraisal counseling in an occupational setting, *Prev Med* 11:583-94, 1982.

73. Roseman J et al: A computerized system to assess risk of disease-specific morbidity and mortality utilizing immunogenetic marker information. In *Proceedings of the 23rd Annual meeting of the Society of Prospective Medicine,* Indianapolis, 1990, Society of Prospective Medicine, 205-212.

74. Roseman J et al: The development and validation of a health risk assessment for the elderly. In *Proceedings of the 23rd and 24th Annual Meeting of the Society of Prospective Medicine, Healthier People, New Trends in Health Risk Assessment and Health Promotion,* Bethesda, 1990, Society of Prospective Medicine.

75. Sacks JJ, Krushat WM, Newman J: Reliability of the health hazard appraisal, *Am J Public Health* 70:730-732, 1980.

76. Sadusk JF, Robbins LC: Proposal for health-hazard appraisal in comprehensive health care, *JAMA* 203:1108-1112, 1968.

77. Sandler RS et al: Participation of high-risk subjects in colon cancer screening, *Cancer* 63:2211-2215, 1989.

78. Schoenbach VJ: Appraising health risk appraisal, *Am J Public Health* 77:409-411, 1987.

79. Schlosstein L et al: High association of HLA antigen W27 with ankylosing spondylitis, *N Engl J Med* 288:704-706, 1973.

80. Sieber-Martin A: The reliability of statements about one's self in questionnaires, *J Exp Social Psychol* 26:157-167, 1979.

81. Siegel LP: Utilization of the health risk appraisal for a needs assessment, *Am J Public Health* 77:1228, 1987.

82. Smith D: Correcting of social desirability response sets in opinion-attitude survey research, *Public Opin Q* 31:87-94, 1967.

83. Smith KW, McKinlay SM, Thorington BD: The validity of health risk appraisal instruments for assessing coronary heart disease risk, *Am J Public Health* 77:419-424, 1987.

84. Smith KW, McKinlay SM, McKinlay JB: The reliability of health risk appraisals: a field trial of four instruments, *Am J Public Health* 79:1603-1607, 1989.

85. Smith KW, McKinlay SM, McKinlay JB: The validity of health risk appraisals for coronary heart disease: results from a randomized field trial, *Am J Public Health* 81:466-470, 1991.

86. Smith WA, Ekdahl SS, Henley CE: Use of health hazard appraisal in counseling for reduction of risk factors, *J Am Osteopath Assoc* 85:809-814, 1985.

87. Spilman MA et al: Effects of a corporate health promotion program, *J Occup Med* 28:285-289, 1986.

88. Peterson KW, Hilles SB, editors: *SPM Directory of Health Risk Appraisals,* Charlottesville, VA, 1992, Occupational Health Strategies, Inc.

89. Stallones RA: The rise and fall of ischemic heart disease, *Sci Am* 243:53-59, 1980.

90. Stange KC et al: Demographic and health characteristics of participants and nonparticipants in a work site health-promotion program, *J Occup Med* 33:474-478, 1991.

91. Vlietstra RE et al: Risk factors and angiographic coronary artery disease: a report from the Coronary Artery Surgery Study (CASS), *Circulation* 62:254-261, 1980.

92. Wagner EH et al: An assessment of health hazard/health risk appraisal, *Am J Public Health* 72:347-352, 1982.

93. Wasson JH et al: Clinical prediction rules. Applications and methodological standards, *N Engl J Med* 313:793-799, 1985.

94. Wheeler RJ: Factors of well-being and health promotion. In *Proceedings of the 17th Annual Meeting of the Society of Prospective Medicine,* Bethesda, 1981, Society of Prospective Medicine.

95. Wilbur CS: Live for life: an epidemiological evaluation of comprehensive health promotion program. In *Proceedings of the 17th Annual Meeting of the Society of Prospective Medicine,* Bethesda, 1981, Society of Prospective Medicine.

96. Wiley JA: Preventive risk factors do predict life events. In *Prospective Medicine and Health Hazard Appraisal, State for the Art: Proceedings of the 16th Annual Meeting of the Society of Prospective Medicine,* Bethesda, 1981, Society of Prospective Medicine.

97. Williams RR et al: Evidence that men with familial hypercholesterolemia can avoid early coronary death, *JAMA* 255:219-224, 1986.

98. Williams RR et al: Health family trees: a tool for finding and helping young family members of coronary and cancer prone pedigrees in Texas and Utah, *Am J Public Health* 78:1283-1286, 1988.

RESOURCES

HealthFinder on Health Risk Appraisal, Office of Disease Prevention and Health Promotion of the U.S. Department of Health and Human Services. List of HRAs and how to order them.

Peterson KW, Hilles SB, editors: *SPM directory of health risk appraisals,* The Society of Prospective Medicine, Charlottesville, Va, 1992, Occupational Health Strategies. Contains a section on the HRA, its uses, implementation strategies, validity and reliability, Guidelines of the Society of Prospective Medicine for Health Risk Appraisal Users; and descriptions and comparisons of 29 different HRAs. There will be updates once a year. The directory can be ordered from the Society of Prospective Medicine, 6220 Lawrence Drive, Indianapolis, IN 46226.

Chapter 40

HEALTH AND GENETICS RISK IMPACT ON PREVENTIVE BEHAVIORS

Richard Bamberg
Ronald T. Acton
Jeffrey M. Roseman

The assessment of an individual's risk to disease and illness based on health and genetic factors has come of age only within the past decade. Previously little was understood about the association of life-style and biochemical parameters in relation to risk for disease. For genetically based diseases, virtually no reliable diagnostic procedures were available, and effective interventions to improve the course of the disease were not known.

Today risk factors associated with common diseases such as diet for coronary heart disease and smoking for lung cancer are now well established. In addition, procedures such as restriction fragment length polymorphisms are available to detect genetic markers for certain diseases and preventive measures can be recommended to improve the course of some diseases in patients. Therefore, assessing a patient's health and genetic risk becomes a realistic component to include in the routine practice of preventive medicine.

HEALTH BELIEF MODEL AND PREVENTIVE BEHAVIOR
Health belief model in concept

The health belief model, which was developed in the early 1950s, was conceptualized to explain the lack of acceptance of preventive measures (e.g., vaccines) and established screening tests for the early detection of asymptomatic diseases of a widespread nature.[29] During this time, the US Public Health Service was largely oriented toward preventing, not treating, diseases. The lack of public participation in early screening tests and vaccines for relatively common diseases such as tuberculosis, cervical cancer, rheumatic fever, polio, influenza, dental caries, and venereal diseases was of concern, particularly, in light of the fact that most of these measures were offered either free or at a reduced rate to the public.[49] A group of social psychologists attempted to explain these behaviors by the health belief model.[29]

The health belief model indicates that a person's attitude, and thus their overt behavior with respect to a particular disease process or entity, is a combination of several factors that can be positive or negative in facilitating their compliance with preventive behaviors or therapeutic/treatment interventions. These factors are all highly individual in their assessment by a particular person.

Perceived susceptibility. Persons vary widely in the degree to which they feel they are personally susceptible to a disease or condition. Their beliefs about the validity of their personal diagnosis, the reliability of diagnostic criteria for the disease or condition, and the prevalence of the disease can increase or decrease their perceived susceptibility.[29,49] Life-style risk factors, family history, and presence of genetic markers and their beliefs about the validity of these factors as predisposing conditions for the disease also can affect their perceived susceptibility.[9] For example, persons vary widely in their perceived susceptibility to injury or accidents as reflected in the fluctuating and inconsistent use of seat belts by many drivers and passengers as well as the overall low usage rate by motorists in general. Other models to predict health behavior such as the theory of reasoned action and the protection motivation theory also include perceived susceptibility (sometimes referred to as risk or vulnerability) as a possible motivating factor.[6]

Perceived seriousness. Persons also vary as to their reactions to the level of discomfort they perceive concerning contracting a given disease or condition or leaving it untreated. Individuals' perceptions of their endurance and acceptance of pain, disability, and death as well as limitations in family life, work capacity, and social relationships vary. An individual's perception relative to these aspects can increase or decrease their perceived seriousness of the disease or condition.[29,49] Many persons diminish the discomfort and potential disability of cancer and other diseases and do not comply with established preventive behaviors for cancer or deny early warning signs when present.

Perceived benefits and barriers (efficacy). Once a sufficient level of perceived susceptibility and seriousness has motivated individuals to pursue a course of action in intervening in the disease process or condition, they will analyze the pros and cons of intervention. They will compare the potential benefits of treatment/intervention methods (e.g., drugs, technologies, nutrition) in ameliorating the disease versus potential barriers or side effects (e.g., iatrogenic effects, pain, nausea, expense, inconvenience, time). Based on their perception of the balance between perceived benefits and barriers, a particular course of action will be pursued. The action may be very direct and medically relevant such as a treatment regimen. Or, the action may be more psychologically overt to pacify momentary feelings of guilt such as the espoused commitment to quit smoking even though a smoking cessation program, formal or informal, is never begun.[29,49]

Cues to action. Even though perceived susceptibility and seriousness provide the motivation for action and the perceived benefits and barriers indicate a specific course of action, the health belief model theorizes that a final factor,—cue to action,—is the trigger to initiate the selected intervention. Such triggers may be physical manifestations of the disease or condition such as pain, disfigurement, or symptoms or external cues such as mass media communications, reactions/caring from family members and significant others, similar illness of a family member or friend, or reminder postcards from health care providers.[29,49]

Preventive behavior in relation to the health belief model

The association of personal characteristics with the use of preventive behaviors and detection services, although the socioeconomic reasons are not completely understood, reveal the generalization that such services are used more frequently by younger or middle-aged people, by women, by persons with relatively higher incomes and higher lev-

els of education, and by whites.[50] Persons who delay or forego such behaviors and services are more likely to be older, of less education, and male.[5]

The health belief model factors have been investigated in relation to several variables including acceptance of vaccines and screening tests, reduction of risk-factor behaviors, compliance with therapeutic interventions and regimens, and physician office and clinic use. A study of 122 predominantly black and Portuguese-American senior citizens[2] as well as a second study of 500 senior citizens in Tompkins County, New York[51] found that perceived susceptibility and efficacy were statistically significant in distinguishing subjects who had received the swine flu inoculation from those who had not. In Oakland County, Michigan, perceived susceptibility, severity, and efficacy all produced a statistically positive significant correlation with obtaining the swine flu vaccination for 286 adults.[20] A study of 241 patients over the age of 65 years and with high-risk complications for influenza (e.g., diabetes, bronchopulmonary disease), half of whom received a reminder postcard from their physician, found that the inoculation rate for those receiving the reminder was twice that of those not receiving the postcard and that perceived susceptibility, severity, and efficacy significantly correlated with obtaining the vaccine.[35]

A study by Hochbaum[26] of 1200 adults, all of whom accepted the benefits of chest radiography in the early detection of tuberculosis, found that 64% of individuals who perceived a personal susceptibility to the disease voluntarily obtained this screening test, whereas only 29% of those without perceived personal susceptibility had a chest radiograph.[50] Regarding perceived susceptibility, severity, and efficacy, a study of 77 individuals in a prepaid dental care plan found that 78% of persons scoring high on all three factors (n=18) had obtained preventive dental check-ups or prophylaxis in the absence of symptoms, whereas 66% of persons scoring high on two factors (n=38) and 61% of persons scoring high on only one factor (n=18) had obtained such dental care. Of the three persons scoring low on all three factors, none had obtained prophylactic dental care.[31] A study of 207 American women found a significant correlation between perceived susceptibility and benefits and the preventive practice of breast self-examination,[21] and a second study of 640 Canadian women found perceived benefits as well as social support system and associated level of comfort (i.e., practice not being distasteful) to be significantly correlated with the practice of breast self-examination.[45]

Some studies have examined the relationship between the health belief model factors and behaviors to reduce known risk factors for given diseases or conditions as well as physician office and clinic visits. A study of 30 adults who had undergone coronary artery bypass operations found only perceived barriers to be statistically significant in its relation to exercise compliance.[58] A study of 120 outpatients receiving care in a municipal teaching hospital found that ex-smokers were significantly more likely to score high on both perceived susceptibility and severity than moderate smokers (10 or less cigarettes per day) and heavy smokers (greater than 10 cigarettes smoked per day).[62] Perceived susceptibility and barriers were significantly correlated with obtaining preventive medical checkups relative to heart disease, stroke, high blood pressure, and lung cancer in a study of 781 adults in Washtenaw County, Michigan.[52]

A study of 769 Los Angeles County adults with various symptoms found perceived susceptibility significantly positively associated with the use of physician services for symptoms in general, whereas perceived efficacy and severity were more strongly correlated with physician visits based on symptom-specific analysis.[15] Interviews of a random sample of 250 low-income mothers of children enrolled in the Children and Youth Program of a teaching hospital found perceived susceptibility and severity positively related to visits for acute illness but negatively associated to well-child visits. In this same study, perceived benefits were positively associated to well-child visits and negatively related to visits for acute illness.[12]

Other studies have investigated the relationship between the health belief model factors and compliance with therapeutic regimens. A study of 50 obese adults with non-insulin-dependent diabetic mellitus (NIDDM) found a positive association between perceived severity and compliance with weight loss and blood glucose control.[3] A second study of 50 adults with NIDDM, treated as outpatients by a Veterans Administration Medical Center, found significant positive correlations between perceived susceptibility and dietary compliance, benefits and exercise compliance, and barriers and medication compliance.[25] Perceived benefits were found to correlate positively with taking phosphate-binding medication and perceived barriers correlated positively with potassium intake restriction and weight gain control in a study of 116 renal disease patients on outpatient hemodialysis.[21] Results from studies concerning antihypertensive regimen compliance and health belief model factors have produced conflicting and inconclusive results.[29]

The increasing availability of specific blood tests to detect genetic markers for various diseases has led to a concern about the relationship of such genetic risk information and the health belief model factors. One study examined the differences between 500 participants and 386 nonparticipants of a screening program for Tay-Sachs disease, all of whom were Jewish. A significantly greater number of participants than nonparticipants had a high level of perceived susceptibility. But perceived severity was inversely related to participation in that those with lower levels of perceived severity were more likely to participate in genetic screening. It seems from these findings, that a mini-mum low level of perceived severity is necessary to motivate participation in genetic screening, particularly as related to future family planning, whereas participants who perceived Tay-Sachs disease as being severe felt that knowledge of being a carrier of the Tay-Sachs gene could be disruptive to family planning and thus did not participate in the screening program.[13,29]

A study of 732 Massachusetts adults aged 25 to 65 years found that death of a parent due to coronary heart disease had the highest correlation coefficient with perceived risk of heart attack, indicating that persons may weigh family history heavily in their perceived susceptibility to cardiovascular diseases.[6] Another study of 883 patients (mean age 61 years) visiting two primary care, rural practices in western Maryland found the only risk factor that significantly increased a patient's perceived risk for coronary heart disease was family history.[42] With regard to breast cancer, a study of 501 Texas women found a significantly greater percentage of women with a family history for the disease to consider their perceived risk moderate or great as compared to those without a family history (79% versus 54%).[60]

HEALTH RISK ASSESSMENT AND PREVENTIVE BEHAVIOR
Health risk assessment instruments

Health risk assessment (HRA), also called health hazard appraisal (HHA), is a technique that has gained considerable use and undergone investigation over the past decade as a way to motivate individuals to make positive changes in their health-related behaviors. HRAs and HHAs provide a person with individual mortality and/or morbidity estimates for the usually 10 to 12 major causes of death and illness for persons of that age and sex. Estimates are based on the person's responses to questions concerning lifestyle, nutrition, medical history, and participation in screening tests and physician visits, which are used to determine the status on known risk factors for the 10 to 12 diseases and conditions.[7,46,61]

Family history of diseases is frequently included in HRAs/HHAs. Physiologic parameters such as blood pressure, total blood cholesterol level, and blood glucose level are included as a part of some HRAs/HHs in determining the individual's mortality and/or morbidity estimates.[27,46,61] Some innovative researchers and developers have included testing for specific genetic markers such as human lymphocyte antigens (HLA) and restriction fragment length polymorphisms (RFLP) as well as biologic assays such as islet-cell antibodies and alpha-1 antitrypsin to determine an individual's mortality and/or morbidity values.[1,17,32,47,63] Adults have been the target audience of most HRAs/HHAs, although a few instruments have been pursued for the needs of special populations such as children, the elderly, and college students.[46,61] The administration of most HRAs/HHAs involve a follow-up counseling session with the patient to explain the individual's assessment/printout.

Preventive behavior in relation to health risk assessment

Studies have been undertaken with a variety of populations to determine the effect of HRAs/HHAs in motivating individuals to comply with preventive health behaviors. The results have been mixed but encouraging (see Chapter 63).

A study of 107 California-based NASA employees found the net risk age reduced by a statistically significant 1.4 years due to health behavior changes after administration of an HHA.[34] In a study of 69 family practice adult patients administered HHAs and recommended to pursue health-related behavioral changes, 41% began a program of vigorous exercise, 28% stopped smoking cigarettes, 20% limited their alcohol consumption, 24% reduced their driving mileage to less than 10,000 miles per year, 33% underwent a rectal examination, and 75% of the women had begun breast self-examination.[10] Among 49 allied health professionals, those subjects receiving HRA, health promotion education and sessions (e.g., exercise training), and peer support had greater improvement in treadmill capacity, capacity for sit-ups per minute, sit-and-reach capacity in inches, and greater reductions in total blood cholesterol level and cholesterol/high density lipoprotein ratio as compared to a control group.[39]

Some studies have investigated the use of HRA/HHA specifically with the college student population, as such persons are in a formative stage and tend to develop lifelong health-related behaviors. These studies have examined the impact on preventive health behavior of HRAs/HHAs alone as well combined with feedback.

As part of a general health education course for Central Michigan University students, 61% of the students reported that they had improved on health-related behaviors or risk factors including weight reduction, attendance at stress reduction education, pursuit of exercise programs, reduction of alcohol consumption, and increased use of seat belts, after HRA administration.[14] A study of 234 undergraduates in a general health education class at Pennsylvania State University reported improvements in behavior for persons receiving HRA as compared to a control group only for factors and behaviors specifically mentioned and evaluated through the HRA.[19] A study of 345 entering freshmen at Virginia Commonwealth University, Richmond, Virginia reported statistically significant differences in preventive behaviors related to cigarette smoking when comparing persons receiving only HRA and those receiving HRA and feedback counseling. Twenty-six percent of those in the group receiving feedback stopped smoking as compared to 6% in the group not receiving feedback after HRA administration; 59% of those in the feedback group as compared to 19% of the no-feedback

group who could not quit smoking had reduced their consumption by more than six cigarettes per day.[18]

A comprehensive study of 55 adult employees of an electric cooperative in rural Alabama provided encouraging results related to behavior change after HRA administration. The employees were administered three HRAs, including one that incorporated family history for diseases/conditions prevalent in the general public (i.e., heart attack, stroke, hypertension, and diabetes), a detailed nutritional assessment, and a type A personality assessment, along with measurements of weight, pulse, blood pressure, and total blood cholesterol level. Each subject received individualized recommendations for behavioral change to reduce the risk to disease and disability based on their status on the associated risk factors and medical screenings. Health promotion educational programs were also made available, including weight reduction, smoking cessation, gun safety, hypertension prevention, exercising, healthy eating, and stress management with follow-up administration of all three HRAs as well as the medical tests conducted 1 year later.

Statistically significant improvements were found in limiting saturated fat in the diet, in taking less than 200 calories and 300 mg of cholesterol daily, reducing daily intake of sodium and percent of calories from fat, walking 1 continuous mile or climbing 10 flights of stairs daily, doing at least 20 minutes of vigorous exercise at least once per week, participating in less vigorous forms of recreation (e.g., bowling, golfing) at least once per week, and having an examination of the rectum or colon. Of the 10 women in the study, 60% of those who had not done so the previous year, underwent a physician breast examination, and 50% of those not receiving PAP smears the previous year did so after HRA administration. Subjects also improved in the areas of eating a balanced breakfast daily and having a pulse rate lower than 70 beats per minute, with 20% of the subjects changing from noncompliance to compliance for these two health-related factors.[7]

Overall, from the findings of studies of the impact of HRA/HHA on preventive health behavior, it appears that HRA/HHA usually provides a cue or trigger to action for behavioral changes that would eventually take place anyway, although at a slower rate. The HRA/HHA may simply provide the added feedback to place a person beyond the needed motivational threshold to engage in preventive behaviors, practices, and life-styles. It also appears that when HRAs/HHAs focus more on morbidity than mortality estimates, they may be better able to motivate persons to comply with positive life-styles and preventive behaviors. An emphasis on mortality alone could actually demotivate an individual by prompting a fatalistic attitude.[11] The vast majority of HRA research is limited by the reliance on self-reports of compliance with recommended behaviors or changes in health-related behaviors.

GENETIC RISK INFORMATION AND PREVENTIVE BEHAVIOR

Genetic risk information regarding diseases and conditions is usually related to an individual's family history or status on a specific genetic marker test. As illustrated in the preceding chapter of this section, a person's risk is known to be increased if the individual has a family history, particularly in first-degree relatives, for some prevalent diseases such as coronary heart disease and myocardial infarction, as well as several cancers including breast, colon, and lung.* Specific genetic markers have been found for a number of diseases including the chromosomal abnormalities in Down, Turner's, Edward's, Klinefelter's, and Patau's syndromes; the S2 RFLP flanking the apolipoprotein A1-C3-A4 gene complex in hypertriglyceridemia; and the human lymphocyte antigen (HLA) associations of DR4 with rheumatoid arthritis, B27 with ankylosing spondylitis and Reiter's disease, DR3 with celiac disease, DR2 with narcolepsy and Goodpasture's syndrome, and B37 with lung cancer. Some biologic assays also have been found to offer promise as markers for certain diseases such as the alpha-1-antitrypsin deficiency associated with chronic obstructive pulmonary disease.†

Studies of the impact of genetic risk information, alone or in conjunction with health risk assessment, have been limited and produced varying results. A study of 92 Welsh patients with Huntington's chorea and their spouses reported that 56% of the total subjects but 40% of those who were already parents would be in favor of taking a predictive test to determine if they carried the gene for this disease.[59] A comparison of 141 individuals diagnosed with polycystic kidney disease (PKD) and 137 at-risk relatives of PKD patients found that 97% of the at-risk individuals would undergo gene testing. More than 88% of both groups in the PKD study would favor gene testing for their children, whereas 50% of PKD patients and 65% of at-risk relatives would submit to prenatal testing for future children.[55]

In a study comparing 159 siblings of newly diagnosed colorectal cancer patients and 194 control subjects, 52% of those with a family history in first-degree relatives for this disease participated in a fecal occult blood screening test and only 38% of those without such a family history participated; the difference was statistically significant.[53] A similar comparison of siblings of patients diagnosed with colorectal cancer and a control group found higher participation in the fecal occult blood screening test by those with a family history than those without (60% vs 47%), although only 20% of compliant subjects with a family history for colorectal cancer cited this risk-increasing factor

as the reason for their participation.[16] When 69 freshmen college students with a family history for cardiovascular disease (CVD) were compared to 154 such students without a family history for CVD, students with this history were more likely to be smokers themselves and to have parents who smoked and were less likely to exercise and to have had a blood cholesterol test.[57]

One comprehensive study examined the effect of genetic risk information in conjunction with HRA on preventive, health-related behaviors. All 82 healthy, adult subjects participating in the study were provided eight recommendations to reduce their risk for coronary heart disease (CHD) and lung cancer (LC) including not smoking, exercising aerobically, limiting alcohol intake, losing weight if overweight, eating baked or broiled fish weekly, reducing cholesterol and saturated fat intake, having blood cholesterol level rechecked within the next 3 months if greater than 200 mg/dl or asking their personal physician when to be rechecked if below 200, and staying calm when under stress or pressure. All subjects received individual printouts from a general HRA, a detailed nutritional HRA, and a type A personality assessment with explanatory information as well as results from weight, blood pressure, and total blood cholesterol measurements. Subjects with a family history of parents or siblings with either disease or who had the S2 RFLP (a genetic risk factor for CHD) or the HLA-B37 (a genetic risk factor for LC) (i.e., the treatment group) were told that they should comply with the suggested recommendations due to their increased genetic risk for the disease(s). Subjects without any genetic risk factor (i.e., the control group) were told that because of the prevalence of CHD and LC in the general public, all persons should comply with the suggested preventive behaviors.

Compliance before receiving their assessments and preventive behavior recommendations was similar for the treatment and control groups. Based on self-report, there was an at least 18% higher compliance rate and an at least four times greater likelihood of performing the behavior when comparing the treatment and control groups for the preventive behaviors of having blood cholesterol level rechecked, seeking advice from the physician or a registered dietitian for weight loss for those overweight, and limiting fat and cholesterol intake for those with a blood cholesterol value below 200. When those subjects with a blood cholesterol level above 200 were analyzed as a subgroup, the treatment group had a statistically significant higher compliance rate than the control group for having blood cholesterol level rechecked.[8]

INTERVENTION STATEMENTS AS A PART OF HEALTH AND GENETIC RISK FEEDBACK TO PROMOTE PREVENTIVE BEHAVIOR

Health and genetic risk information can be conveyed to patients in several ways. It is advisable to include the ge-

---

*References 4, 22, 36, 43, 54, 63.
†References 17, 24, 27, 32, 33, 38.

netic risk assessment in a larger, general health risk assessment as part of the patient's health promotion. This approach allows one to identify life-style and environmental risk factors, which can be modified, as opposed to genetic factors, which cannot. The assessments can be made on individual patients or with groups such as in industry or business. The patient should be told that the feedback is only as reliable as the honesty of the responses, as the analyses for risk factor status are based on self-report of behaviors, sometimes in conjunction with limited physiologic measures (e.g., blood pressure, weight, and blood cholesterol level) and genetic marker analyses.

Some patients will be reluctant to reflect accurately behavior in areas that may carry social ramifications such as alcohol consumption, particularly if the health and genetic risk assessment is being administered as part of a group such as at the employment site. In addition, patients may be reluctant to participate in genetic marker screening due to the social consequences, although this problem is more prominent in screenings for diseases that are psychologic (e.g., Huntington's disease) or widespread (e.g., CHD) as opposed to those with a purely physical and less common symptomology (e.g., cystic fibrosis).

The feedback from genetic and health risk assessments can be provided in a variety of methods. For patients comfortable with high technology and who learn better through visual, interactive formats, results could be conveyed through computer-based programs. This will not be the preferred mode for the majority of patients and, realistically, should not take the place of the provider-patient contact. However the information is conveyed, it should stress that the patient's control over positive health outcomes is the most effective way to produce preventive behavior.[37] As many individuals underestimate their risk for common diseases, especially cardiovascular diseases,[44] and high anxiety can sometimes reduce compliance with preventive and screening behaviors,[30,56] results that convey both the patient's current risk level and the reduced risk through behavior modification will be particularly beneficial in promoting preventive behavior and positive life-style modifications.

The provider could convey the patient's results in a group format, although this approach is generally not as effective as individual contact and should be attempted only in those instances where the size of the group provides no other logistically feasible method of feedback. Genetic risk information should never be conveyed in a group format.

Overall, initial explanation by the physician in an individual session followed by detailed risk assessment counseling by a qualified health promotion practitioner (e.g., medical geneticist, genetic counselor, health educator, or nurse) is the preferred method of feedback in the routine practice of preventive medicine. Telephone or written reminders by a nurse may help patients keep follow-up counseling appointments, particularly for younger patients and those with less education and relatively few health problems.[40,41] If the results are conveyed without any follow-up counseling, the patient may not develop the necessary skills and attitudes to effect successful behavior change and may be left without reinforcers of healthy life-style modification.[28]

A method to approach facilitating the clinical management of patients with genetic risk factors such as family history, specific genetic markers, or abnormal values of biologic measures known to be associated with an increased prevalence of a specific disease or condition, is to use educational materials that may promote preventive behaviors. Such health education materials can be referred to as intervention statements.

The Immunogenetics Program at the University of Alabama at Birmingham has developed more than 20 intervention statements for specific diseases and conditions with known genetic risk factors and for which certain behavior modifications related to nutritional intake, life-style practices, and medical screenings can reduce an individual's chances of contracting the illness. The intervention statements were developed for use in health promotion education in conjunction with health risk assessment that incorporated genetic risk measures. Each intervention statement was developed based on a review of the literature pertinent to the specific disease or condition and content validated by physician specialists.[48]

Through a counseling session and/or written educational materials, the patient could be informed of the specific genetic marker (or family history) that increases the risk for a disease or condition. This information should be placed in context to promote perceived susceptibility by indicating the relative risk associated with the marker, or how much greater the occurrence of the disease/condition is in persons with the genetic risk factor as compared to persons without the factor (e.g., three times, 4.5 times, 28 times etc).

Specific relative risk values vary by race. Prevalence or incidence figures could be included in the written materials unless they are at levels so low that they would probably decrease an individual's perceived susceptibility and thus negatively affect preventive behavior. The patient should understand that his or her genetic status makes it more important to practice preventive behaviors and adopt positive life-styles than for persons who do not possess the genetic risk factor(s).

It is advisable to target the educational materials for a general, nonmedical population by using concise, direct, and simple language. This goal can be challenging when explaining medical conditions, risk factors, biologic parameters, and medical screening tests. The intervention statements can be written in a narrative format or in a "bullet" format with emphasizing punctuation (e.g., exclamation points).

Some suggested intervention statements for specific diseases are presented as the remainder of this chapter. Each disease has a genetic risk factor associated with it such as a specific molecular marker or family history (see Chapter 38 for genetic risk factor information). Use of the intervention statements should be accompanied by a counseling session between the physician and patient to put the individual's case into perspective based on the physician's total knowledge and assessment of the patient.

Coronary heart disease

The intervention statement in a narrative, paragraph format is as follows (also see Chapter 41):

Coronary heart disease (CHD) is the most common cause of death in the United States. CHD includes a long period without symptoms during which time fat deposits on the walls of coronary arteries (atherosclerosis). CHD is then detected by a clinical event including myocardial infarction (MI or "heart attack"), angina pectoris (chest pain), or sudden death from a massive heart attack. About 200 per 100,000 Americans die from CHD each year.

Some factors have been found to increase your risk for developing CHD. As you are genetically at risk for CHD, you should make an effort to reduce any of the other risk factors you have. Persons who smoke are at greater risk. If you do not smoke, it is best to never start. If you do smoke, it is best to QUIT! You can contact your doctor or local health department to find out about smoking cessation (quit smoking) programs in your area. Your local chapter of the American Heart Association, American Lung Association, or American Cancer Society may also offer such programs.

Being obese (overweight) increases your chances of getting CHD. You should not let your weight increase 20% more than your recommended weight. Proper calorie intake based on your level of activity is essential for weight control. Doing aerobic exercise (swimming, biking, or brisk walking) for at least 20 minutes three to four times a week can help control your weight, improve your overall health, and help prevent CHD. Strenuous isometric and calisthenic exercise is not advised for anyone who already has a heart condition. Ask your doctor about the recommended weight for your height and body frame as well as the needed diet and amount and type of exercise to keep your weight at the recommended level and to remain healthy. It is always best to check with your doctor before beginning any diet or exercise program.

High blood cholesterol as well as triglyceride levels can increase your chances of developing CHD. Cholesterol and triglyceride levels are measured from a blood sample and expressed in a weight per volume unit called milligrams per deciliter (mg/dl). It is best to keep your cholesterol level at less than 200 mg/dl and your triglyceride level at less than 250 mg/dl. The lower your cholesterol and triglyceride levels, the lower your risk for CHD. A fat-modified diet can help reduce and maintain your cholesterol and triglyceride levels. It is best if fat makes up no more than 30% of your total calories. This goal can be achieved by eating less fat, by using polyunsaturated and nonsaturated fat products (i.e., skim milk or low-fat milk, vegetable margarine and oils) *instead of* saturated fat products (i.e., whole milk, butter, solid cooking lards, and shortenings), by using poultry and fish and avoiding red meats and organ meats such as liver and kidney, and by using egg substitutes and no egg yolks. You can replace calories lost through eating less fat by increasing by no more than 50% your intake of complex carbohydrates (i.e., fruits, vegetables, whole-grain breads, and cereals). It is also best to eat less refined sugars as in table sugar, baked goods, candy, and other sweets.

Research has demonstrated that low-density lipoprotein (LDL) is the most harmful type of cholesterol, whereas high-density lipoprotein (HDL) actually improves health. You may want to ask your doctor about the need for periodic assessment of cholesterol, LDL, HDL, and triglyceride blood levels, as well as any needed dietary changes. Since having low thyroid hormone (hypothyroidism) can increase cholesterol and triglyceride blood levels, ask your doctor about the need for T3 and T4 blood tests if your cholesterol and triglyceride levels are high. You may wish to consult a registered dietitian or nutritionist to help determine an appropriate diet. The American Heart Association and American Dietetic Association can also give you detailed guides. Be sure to read carefully the labels for contents of the products you cook with and the foods you eat.

Some research suggests that eating baked or broiled fish three or more times per week can reduce the chances of developing CHD. Dark fleshy fish such as anchovy, capelin, carp, dogfish, herring, mackerel, salmon, sardines, scad, sturgeon, lake trout, tuna, whitefish, and sablefish are the most protective. Fish oil supplements in the form of capsules or tablets are not advised unless you are taking them under the supervision of a physician.

Excessive alcohol intake can increase your chances of developing CHD. It is best to have no more than 2 oz of alcohol per day. Some research suggests that moderate intake on a weekly, not daily, basis may reduce your risk for CHD. If you feel you may have an excessive drinking problem, you can contact your doctor or local health department for treatment programs in your area as well as your local chapter of Alcoholics Anonymous.

An electrocardiogram (ECG) is a graph of the electrical actions of the heart. An ECG can tell when the heart is not functioning as it should. An exercise or stress ECG sometimes gives more useful information than a resting ECG. You may want to ask your doctor about the possible need for a periodic ECG.

Persons who are very hostile, impatient, uptight, aggressive, and compulsive; who easily get angry and irritated; and who are always in a hurry have an increased chance of developing clinical complications from CHD. If you are this type of person, which is called type A personality, you should make an effort to stay calm, relaxed, and easygoing. In your daily life, avoiding situations and persons, as much as possible, that you know make you feel angry and hostile can help. When you have to wait in line, try to go to the shortest line. Travel as much as possible at times other than rush hour. Setting aside a certain amount of time each day to relax by doing deep breathing exercises, pleasure reading, or hobbies can help. When you feel yourself getting angry, count to at least 10 and take deep breaths. Remind yourself that getting angry is not going to change or help the situation. Simply, you should try to stay calm and relaxed when you feel tense, irritated, under pressure or stressed. You may wish to ask your doctor about a type A personality test and any behavioral changes you need to make.

The same preventive behavior information could also be communicated in a more direct format as follows:

Coronary heart disease (CHD) is the most common cause of death in the United States. The major form of coronary heart disease includes a long period without symptoms during which fat deposits on the walls of coronary arteries (atherosclerosis). CHD is then detected by a clinical event including myocardial infarction (MI or "heart attack"), angina pectoris (chest pain), or sudden death from a massive heart attack. About 200 per 100,000 Americans die from CHD each year.

Some factors have been found to increase your risk for getting CHD. Because you are genetically at increased risk for CHD, you should take the following are actions to decrease your risk of developing CHD.

Do not smoke!

Smoking cigarettes increases your risk for CHD. If you quit smoking, your risk decreases. If you do not smoke, it is best to never start. If you do smoke, it is best to QUIT! You can contact your doctor or local health department to find out about smoking cessation (stop smoking) programs in your area. Or, you can contact your local chapter of the American Heart Association, the American Cancer Society, or the American Lung Association as these groups offer stop smoking programs (see Chapter 16).

Exercise regularly!

Leading a highly sedentary (inactive) life-style increases your risk for CHD. Doing some form of aerobic exercise, which increases your heart rate, (for example, swimming, brisk walking or biking) for a least 20 minutes three to four times per week can decrease your risk (see Chapter 18).

Do not drink excessively!

Excessive alcohol intake increases your chances of developing CHD. It is best to have no more than one mixed drink or shot of liquor, bottle of beer, or glass of wine per day. If you feel you may have an excessive drinking problem, you can contact your doctor or local health department to find out about treatment programs in your area. Or, you can contact your local chapter of Alcoholics Anonymous (see Chapter 15).

Lose weight if you are overweight!

Being overweight increases your chances for CHD. Dieting (eating less) and exercising regularly can help you lose weight. You should check with your doctor (or a registered dietitian or nutritionist) about your recommended weight and ways for you to lose weight if you are overweight (see Part V).

Reduce your intake of cholesterol and saturated fat!

The less cholesterol and saturated fat you eat, the less chance you have of developing CHD. There are many ways you can reduce cholesterol and saturated fat in your diet. Eat as little fat as possible. Eating low-cholesterol and low-saturated-fat foods instead of high-cholesterol and high-saturated-fat foods helps. High-cholesterol foods include eggs and organ meats such as liver and kidney. High-saturated-fat foods include whole milk and whole-milk products, butter, products with coconut oil or palm oil, ice cream, and meat fat. Foods high in both cholesterol and saturated fat include solid cooking lards and shortenings, salad dressings, pork, and red meats such as beef. Low-cholesterol and low-saturated-fat foods, which are better for you, include egg substitutes, skim or low-fat milk, poultry and fish, margarine, vegetable oils, and vinegar as a salad dressing. Baked or broiled foods are preferable to fried foods. Contact your local chapter of the American Heart Association for detailed guidelines for reducing your intake of cholesterol and saturated fat (see Part V).

Have your blood cholesterol level checked periodically!

Cholesterol levels are measured from a blood sample and expressed in a weight per volume unit called milligrams per deciliter (mg/dl). You should keep your cholesterol level at less than 200 mg/dl to decrease your chances of developing CHD. Therefore, it is important to know your blood cholesterol level and to have it rechecked periodically. If it is greater than 200 mg/dl, it is even more important to reduce cholesterol and saturated fat in your diet as much as possible and to have your blood level rechecked by your doctor within the next 3 months. Even if your cholesterol is below 200 mg/dl, it is still good to reduce cholesterol and saturated fat in your diet as much as possible and to ask your doctor when and how often you should have your blood level rechecked. See your doctor today about having your blood cholesterol levels (total, LDL, and HDL) checked!

Eat baked or broiled fish!

Eating baked or broiled fish two to three times per week may decrease your chances of developing CHD. Dark fleshy fish such as anchovy, capelin, carp, dogfish, herring, mackerel, salmon, sardines, sturgeon, lake trout, tuna, whitefish, and sablefish are the best to eat. Fish oil supplements in the form of capsules or tablets should be taken only after asking your doctor (see Part V).

Stay calm and relaxed!

Persons who are impatient, uptight, aggressive, compulsive; who easily get angry and irritated; and who are always in a hurry are at increased risk for CHD. Persons who have these kinds of behavior are called type A personalities. Type A persons need to make an effort to stay calm and relaxed whenever they feel tense, irritated, under pressure, or stressed to decrease the risk of developing CHD. Even if you are not a type A person, you should still make an effort to stay calm and relaxed whenever you feel tense, irritated, under pressure, or stressed. See your doctor about taking a type A personality test (see Chapter 12).

Non-insulin-dependent diabetes mellitus

The intervention statement is as follows:

The body's cells need sugar (in the form of glucose) to make energy. The sugar is taken to the cells by the bloodstream. In diabetes mellitus the glucose stays in the bloodstream in high levels. If the glucose in the blood gets very high, some of it will be given off in the urine. If the blood sugar is not controlled, it can lead to serious problems such as coma, infection, heart disease, kidney disease, foot ailments, and blindness.

There are two major types of diabetes mellitus: type I or insulin-dependent diabetes mellitus (IDDM) and type II or non-insu-lin-dependent diabetes mellitus (NIDDM). Type I used to be called juvenile-onset diabetes; type II used to be called adult-onset or maturity-onset diabetes. IDDM generally has an early onset, usually before age 20; NIDDM occurs more often in persons over age 40. Both can occur at any age. About 1 person per 400 has IDDM; 3 out of 100 persons have NIDDM.

Because you are genetically at increased risk for type II diabetes mellitus, it is particularly important to know the warning signs for this disease: extreme hunger, a gain or loss of weight, frequent urination, thirst, nausea, drowsiness (being sleepy most of the time), weakness, fatigue (being tired most of the time), blurred vision; itching, tingling or numbness of hands and feet; and slow healing of cuts and scratches. If you notice any of the warning signs, see your doctor. As with any condition, early detection of diabetes mellitus gives a better chance of control and less chance of disability due to complications.

You may want to undergo certain medical screening tests periodically, as changes in these tests over time can give an early warning that you are developing diabetes mellitus. These tests include the oral glucose tolerance test, fasting glucose, 2-hour postprandial glucose, and urine glucose. Ask your doctor about the need to undergo these tests periodically.

Type II diabetes occurs more often in obese (overweight) persons, particularly in persons whose excess weight is above the waist. It is important to maintain weight at not greater than 20% above your recommended level. Proper calorie intake based on your level of activity is essential for weight control. Diets high in fiber (fruits, vegetables, whole-grain breads and cereals, nuts, seeds, bran) and low in sugar (table sugar, baked goods, candy, sweets) are helpful in controlling weight and preventing the development of type II diabetes. Proper exercise can also help control your weight. Doing aerobic exercise (swimming, biking, or brisk walking) for at least 20 minutes three or four times a week can help control your weight, improve your overall physical health, and help the body move sugar from the bloodstream into the cells. Ask your doctor about the recommended weight for your height and body frame as well as the needed diet and amount and type of exercise to keep your weight at the recommended level and to prevent the onset of type II diabetes mellitus. It is always best to check with your doctor before beginning any diet or exercise program.

Higher than normal cholesterol and triglyceride levels in the blood have also been found to be related to type II diabetes mellitus. It is best if fat makes up no more than 30% of your total calories. Fat that is less saturated and more polyunsaturated can help reduce cholesterol and triglyceride levels. Diets low in whole milk, butter, egg yolks, red meats, and organ meats (i.e., liver and kidney) can help reduce cholesterol and triglyceride levels. Low-fat or skim milk, margarine, egg substitutes, fish, and poultry can be used in place of these foods. It has also been found that high insulin levels in the blood occur before the onset of type II diabetes. Ask your doctor about the need for periodic tests for cholesterol, triglyceride, and insulin blood levels. Since having low thyroid hormone (hypothyroidism) can also increase your cholesterol and triglyceride blood levels, you may want to ask your doctor about the need for T3 or T4 blood tests if your cholesterol and triglyceride levels are high (see Chapter 60).

Chronic obstructive pulmonary disease

The intervention statement is as follows:

Chronic obstructive pulmonary disease (COPD) affects the lungs. Because of obstructions in the airways, a person with COPD has increased difficulty breathing.

Persons who smoke have a greater risk of developing COPD. Since you are genetically at increased risk of developing COPD, you should not smoke. If you do not smoke, it is best to never start. If you do smoke, QUIT! You can contact your doctor or local health department to find out about smoking cessation (stop smoking) programs in your area. Or, you can contact your local chapter of the American Heart Association, the American Cancer Society, or the American Lung Association as these groups offer stop smoking programs.

Evidence suggests that being in environments heavy in dust or smoke can increase your chance of developing COPD. If you work in an occupation or industry that is dust or smoke laden (e.g., farming, steel, textiles, etc.), check with your supervisor to be sure you are using all necessary clothing and equipment to reduce your exposure to dust and smoke (see Chapter 55).

Lung cancer

The intervention statement is as follows:

Lung cancer is basically an uncontrolled growth of abnormal cells in the lungs. It is a leading cause of death in the United States. About 50 per 100,000 people die from lung cancer each year. The following is an action you should take to decrease your risk of getting lung cancer since you are genetically at increased risk.

At least 80% of lung cancer cases can be directly linked to smoking cigarettes. If you quit smoking, your risk decreases. If you do not smoke, it is best to never start. If you do smoke, it is best to QUIT! You can contact your doctor or local health department to find out about smoking cessation (stop smoking) programs in your area. Or, you can contact your local chapter of the American Heart Association, the American Cancer Society, or the American Lung Association, as these groups offer stop smoking programs (see Chapter 48).

Breast cancer

The intervention statement is as follows:

Breast cancer is basically an uncontrolled growth of abnormal cells in the breasts. Breast cancer is the leading cancer in women. About 85 per 100,000 women get breast cancer each year.

Some factors have been found to increase the chances of getting breast cancer. If you do develop the disease, early detection offers the best chances for survival and reduced disability and disfigurement. Since you are genetically at increased risk of developing breast cancer, reduce your risk as much as possible and practice screening methods for early detection.

Lumps in the breast can be detected by doing a breast self-examination (BSE). You should do this at least once per month on both breasts. The BSE should be performed 2 to 3 days after your period ends, or on the same day each month if you no longer have periods. The warning sign of breast cancer is any change in size, shape, appearance, or feel of your breast, both on the surface and underneath, including any lump, thickening, swelling, puckering, dimpling, redness or irritation, whitish scale, or discharge. Contact your doctor or local chapter of the American Cancer Society for detailed instructions on how to do a breast self-examination. And see your doctor immediately if you detect any change!

See your doctor yearly for a routine preventive examination of your breasts. Ask your doctor about the need for a mammogram or thermogram, which are medical tests that can detect lumps in the breast at an early stage before they can be felt by touch. You should ask your doctor when you should begin these important tests and how often you should have them.

Evidence suggests that excessive fat intake and alcohol consumption can increase your chances of developing breast cancer. Limit fat to less than 30% of your total calorie intake by trimming excess fat from meat, avoiding fried foods, using polyunsaturated and nonsaturated fat products (i.e., skim milk or low-fat milk, vegetable margarine and oils) *instead of* saturated fat products (i.e., whole milk, butter, solid cooking lards and shortenings), and substituting vegetables, whole grains, and fruits for meats. Contact your doctor or local chapter of the American Heart Association to get detailed guides for a fat-modified diet. Limit your alcohol intake to less than three drinks or 6 oz of alcohol per week. If you feel you may have an excessive drinking problem, contact your doctor, health department, or local chapter of Alcoholics Anonymous (see Chapter 47).

Colon cancer

The intervention statement is as follows:

Cancer is basically an uncontrolled growth of abnormal cells. Colon cancer is a cancer of the end part of the large intestine (colon), an organ that aids in digesting the food you eat. About 35 per 100,000 people get colon cancer each year.

Some factors have been found to increase the risk of getting colon cancer. Since you are genetically at increased risk of getting colon cancer, it is important that you do everything you can to reduce your risk.

Diets low in fiber may increase your chances of developing colon cancer. You should include a source of fiber in your diet every day such as whole grains, fruits, and vegetables. You can also substitute whole flour in any recipe calling for refined flour. Contact your doctor or local chapter of the American Lung Association to get detailed guides about how to increase fiber in your diet.

Diets high in fat may increase your chances of getting colon cancer. You should limit your intake of fat to no more than 30% of your total calorie intake by trimming excess fat from meat, avoiding fried foods, using polyunsaturated and nonsaturated fat products (i.e., skim milk or low-fat milk, vegetable margarine and oils) *instead of* saturated fat products (i.e., whole milk, butter, solid cooking lards and shortenings), and substituting vegetables, whole grains, and fruits for meats. Contact your doctor or local chapter of the American Heart Association to get detailed guides for a fat-modified diet.

Excessive alcohol intake, especially beer, may increase your chances of developing colon cancer. Limit your intake of alcohol to no more than three drinks or beers or 6 oz of alcohol per week. If you feel you may have an excessive drinking problem,

contact your doctor, health department, or local chapter of Alcoholics Anonymous.

People with a sedentary or inactive life-style have an increased chance of developing colon cancer. Aerobic exercise (e.g., brisk walking, biking, or swimming) for 20 minutes three to four times per week provides an active life-style. Always contact your doctor before beginning any exercise program.

Certain medical tests can give an early warning that colon cancer is developing. These tests are the digital rectal exam stool test and proctosigmoidoscopy. You should see your doctor yearly for these tests. Ask your doctor when and how often you should undergo these important tests.

The warning signs of colon cancer include alternating constipation and diarrhea, stomach cramps, painful bowel movements (stools), blood in the stool, or unexplained weight loss. See you doctor if you notice any of the warning signs. Remember, early detection offers the best chances for survival and decreased disability.

Note: For additional specific information on clinical management of patients as related to health and genetic risk, refer to the information provided in Chapters 38 and 39, and Chapter 46 regarding colorectal cancer screening.

SUMMARY

Genetic assessment in combination with an overall health risk assessment can provide a valuable tool for physicians to incorporate a preventive focus to their practices. Knowing an individual's genetic and other health risks can identify specific life-style, environmental, and nutritional factors, which can be modified and for which the physician and patient can jointly establish a behavior modification plan. By knowing the patient's risk factors that can be positively altered, the physician can provide realistic and effective preventive counseling. Genetic and health risk assessment together can provide a more complete profile of a patient's risk status and potential risk reductions than either component could do alone and should be an integral and routine part of any preventive medicine practice. The information provided in the three chapters in this section offer practical guidelines, applications, and examples of ways to incorporate genetic and health risk assessment along with preventive feedback and counseling into a medical practice.

REFERENCES

1. Acton RT et al: Utilization of genetic and other laboratory test results to predict and reduce the risk of disease. In *Proceedings of the 23rd and 24th annual meetings of the Society of Prospective Medicine,* Indianapolis, 1990, Society of Prospective Medicine.
2. Aho WR: Participation of senior citizens in the swine flu inoculation program: an analysis of health belief model variables in preventive health behavior, *J Gerontol* 34:201-208, 1979.
3. Alogna M: Perception of severity of disease and health locus of control in compliant and noncompliant diabetic patients, *Diabetes Care* 3:533-534, 1980.
4. Anderson DE: Genetic study of breast cancer: identification of a high risk group, *Cancer* 34:1090-1097, 1974.
5. Antonovsky A, Hartman H: Delay in the detection of cancer: a review of the literature, *Health Educ Monogr* 2:98-128, 1974.

6. Avis NE, Smith KW, McKinlay JB: Accuracy of perceptions of heart attack risk: what influences perceptions and can they be changed? *Am J Public Health* 79(12):1608-1612, 1989.

7. Bamberg R et al: The effect of risk assessment in conjunction with health promotion education on compliance with preventive behaviors, *J Allied Health* 18:271-280, 1989.

8. Bamberg R et al: The effect of genetic risk information and health risk assessment on compliance with preventive behaviors, *Health Educ* 21(2):26-32, 1990.

9. Bamberg R et al: Genetic risk information as an impetus to health related behavioral change. In *Proceedings of the 23rd and 24th annual meetings of the Society of Prospective Medicine,* Indianapolis, 1990, Society of Prospective Medicine.

10. Bartlett EE et al: Health hazard appraisal in a family practice center: an exploratory study, *J Community Health* 9:135-144, 1983.

11. Becker MH, Janz NK: On the effectiveness and utility of health hazard/health risk appraisal in clinical and nonclinical settings: behavioral science perspectives on health hazard/health risk appraisal, *Health Serv Res* 22:546-547, 1987.

12. Becker MH et al: Mothers' health beliefs and children's clinic visits: a prospective study, *J Community Health* 3:125-135, 1977.

13. Becker MH et al: Some influences on public participation in a genetic screening program, *J Community Health* 1:3-14, 1975.

14. Bensley LB: Health risk appraisals in teaching health education in colleges and universities, *Health Educ* 12(6):31-33, 1981.

15. Berkanovic E, Telesky C, Reeder S: Structural and social psychological factors in the decision to seek medical care for symptoms, *Med Care* 19:693-709, 1981.

16. Blalock SJ et al: Risk perceptions and participation in colorectal cancer screening, *Health Psychol* 9(6):792-806, 1990.

17. Caskey CT: Disease diagnosis by recombinant DNA methods, *Science* 236:1223-1229, 1987.

18. Chan CW, Witherspoon JM: Health risk appraisal modifies cigarette smoking behavior among college students, *J Gen Intern Med* 3:555-559, 1988.

19. Cottrell RR, Pierre RW: Behavioral outcomes associated with HRA use in a college level health education course utilizing a lifestyle theme, *Health Educ* 14(7):29-33, 1983.

20. Cummings KM et al: Psychosocial determinants of immunization behavior in a swine influenza campaign, *Med Care* 17:639-649, 1979.

21. Cummings KM et al: Psychosocial factors affecting adherence to medical regimens in a group of hemodialysis patients, *Med Care* 20:567-579, 1982.

22. Friedlander Y, Karak JD, Stein Y: Family history of myocardial infarction as an independent risk factor for coronary heart disease, *Br Heart J* 53:382-387, 1985.

23. Hallal JC: The relationship of health beliefs, health locus of control, and self-concept to the practice of breast self-examination in adult women, *Nurs Res* 31:137-142, 1982.

24. Harris R: Genetic counseling and the new genetics, *Trends Genet* 4(2):52-56, 1988.

25. Harris R et al: Relationship between the health belief model and compliance as a basis for intervention in diabetes mellitus, *Pediatr Adolesc Endocrinol* 10:123-132, 1982.

26. Hochbaum GM: Public participation in medical screening programs: a sociopsychological study, Washington, DC, 1958, US Public Health Service, US Government Printing Office (PHS Publ No 572).

27. Hunt SC, Williams RR, Barlow GK: A comparison of positive family history definitions for defining risk of future disease, *J Chron Dis* 39:809-821, 1986.

28. Hyner GC, Melby CL: Health risk appraisals: use and misuse, *Fam Community Health* 7(4):13-25, 1985.

29. Janz NK, Becker MH: The health belief model: a decade later, *Health Educ Q* 11:1-47, 1984.

30. Kash KM et al: Psychological distress and surveillance behaviors of women with a family history of breast cancer, *J Natl Cancer Inst* 84(1):25-30, 1992.

31. Kegeles SS: Some motives for seeking preventive dental care, *J Am Dent Assoc* 67:90-98, 1963.

32. Khoury MJ, Newill CA, Chase GA: Epidemiologic evaluation of screening for risk factors: application to genetic screening, *Am J Public Health* 75:1204-1208, 1985.

33. Kolata G: Reducing risk: a change of heart? *Science* 231:669-670, 1986.

34. LaDou J, Sherwood JN, Hughes L: Health hazard appraisal in patient counseling, *West J Med* 122:177-180, 1975.

35. Larson EB et al: The relationship of health beliefs and a postcard reminder to influenza vaccination, *J Fam Pract* 8:1207-1211, 1979.

36. Leo ten kate L et al: Familial aggregation of coronary heart disease and its relation to known genetic risk factors, *Am J Cardiol* 50:945-953, 1982.

37. Lermin C, Rimer BK, Engstrom PF: Cancer risk notification: psychosocial and ethical implications, *J Clin Oncol* 9(7):1275-1282, 1991.

38. Lewin R: DNA fingerprints in health and disease, *Science* 233:521-522, 1986.

39. Maki D et al: Health promotion and allied health professionals: considerations for program design, *J Allied Health* 17:231-241, 1988.

40. Manfredi C, Lacey L, Warnecke R: Results of an intervention to improve compliance with referrals for evaluation of suspected malignancies at neighborhood public health centers, *Am J Public Health* 80:85-87, 1990.

41. Michielutte R et al: Noncompliance in screening follow-up among family planning clinic patients with cervical dysplasia, *Prev Med* 14:248-258, 1985.

42. Moran MT et al: Coronary heart disease risk assessment, *Am J Prev Med* 5(6):330-336, 1989.

43. Muller H, Weber W, Kuttapa T, editors: *Familial cancer,* New York, 1985, Karger.

44. Niknian M et al: A comparison of perceived and objective CVD risk in a general population, *Am J Public Health* 79:1653-1654, 1989.

45. Norman RMG, Tudiver F: Predictors of breast self-examination among family practice patients, *J Fam Pract* 22:149-153, 1986.

46. Robbins LC, Hall JC: Prospective medicine. In Rakel RE, Conn HF, Johnson TW, editors: *Family practice,* Philadelphia, 1978, WB Saunders.

47. Roseman JM et al: A computerized system to assess risk of disease-specific morbidity and mortality utilizing immunogenetic marker information. In *Proceedings of the 23rd and 24th annual meetings of the Society of Prospective Medicine,* Indianapolis, 1990, Society of Prospective Medicine.

48. Roseman JM et al: The risk of morbidity and mortality assessment (ROMMA): a health risk assessment utilizing genetic markers. In *Proceedings of the 23rd and 24th annual meetings of the Society of Prospective Medicine,* Indianapolis, 1990, Society of Prospective Medicine.

49. Rosenstock IM: Historical origins of the health belief model, *Health Educ Monogr* 2:328-333, 1974.

50. Rosenstock IM: The health belief model and preventive health behavior, *Health Educ Monogr* 2:355-361, 1974.

51. Rundall TG, Wheeler JRC: Factors associated with utilization of the swine flu vaccination program among senior citizens, *Med Care* 17:191-200, 1979.

52. Rundall TG, Wheeler JRC: The effect of income on use of preventive care: an evaluation of alternative explanations, *J Health Soc Behav* 20:397-406, 1979.

53. Sandler RS et al: Participation of high-risk subjects in colon cancer screening, *Cancer* 63:2211-2215, 1989.

54. Sattin RW et al: Family history and the risk of breast cancer, *JAMA* 253:1908-1913, 1985.

55. Sujansky E et al: Attitudes of at-risk and affected individuals regarding presymptomatic testing for autosomal dominant polycystic kidney disease, *Am J Med Genet* 35:510-515, 1990.

56. Stoate HG: Can health screening damage your health? *J R Coll Gen Pract* 39:193-195, 1989.
57. Tamragouri RN et al: Cardiovascular risk factors and health knowledge among freshmen college students with a family history of cardiovascular disease, *Coll Health* 34:267-270, 1986.
58. Tirrell BE, Hart LK: The relationship of health beliefs and knowledge to exercise compliance in patients after coronary bypass, *Heart Lung* 9:487-493, 1980.
59. Tyler A, Harper PS: Attitudes of subjects at risk and their relatives towards genetic counseling in Huntington's chorea, *J Med Genet* 20:179-188, 1983.
60. Vogel VG et al: Mammographic screening of women with increased risk of breast cancer, *Cancer* 66(7):1613-1620, 1990.
61. Vogt TM: Risk assessment and health hazard appraisal, *Annu Rev Public Health* 2:31-47, 1981.
62. Weinberger M et al: Health beliefs and smoking behavior, *Am J Public Health* 71:1253-1255, 1981.
63. Zylke JW: Once identified, will high-risk families make life-style changes, lower coronary disease rate? *JAMA* 258:433, 1987.

RESOURCES

Organizations that may be helpful in providing health promotion educational materials for preventive behavior or assistance in the development of such communications, as well as contacts for employment of health education professionals include the following:

Association for the Advancement of Health Education, American Alliance for Health, Physical Education, Recreation, and Dance, 1900 Association Drive, Reston, VA 22091.

Society for Public Health Education, American Public Health Association, 2001 Addison St., Suite 220, Berkeley, CA 94704.

Society of Prospective Medicine, PO Box 55110, Indianapolis, IN 46205.

Office of Disease Prevention and Health Promotion, Public Health Service, Department of Health and Human Service, 330 C Street SW, Room 2132, Washington, DC 20201.

National Commission for Health Education Credentialing, Inc, 475 Riverside Drive, Room 740, New York, NY 10115.

American Heart Association, 7272 Greenville Avenue, Dallas, TX 75231.

American Cancer Society, 1599 Clifton Road NE, Atlanta, GA 30329.

American Lung Association, 1740 Broadway, New York, NY 10019.

American Dietetics Association, 216 West Jackson Blvd, Chicago, IL 60606.

Part IX

PREVENTION IN CARDIOVASCULAR DISEASE

Chapter 41

CORONARY ARTERY DISEASE

Michael Cressman

Coronary artery disease has been and continues to be the number one cause of death in the United States. During the past several years, mortality caused by this disease has been substantially reduced. This decline has occurred among men, women, whites, and blacks and is due both to improved therapy for myocardial infarction and to modification of known risk factors for coronary artery disease. An enormous volume of information that describes efforts to identify and/or modify these risk factors has been published in the medical literature. Risk factors for coronary artery disease include cigarette smoking, elevated blood cholesterol level, hypertension, diabetes, obesity, and sedentary life-style. Modification of several of these factors is covered in other chapters: smoking and smoking cessation in Chapter 16, diabetes in Chapter 60, control of obesity in Chapters 22 and 26, and improvement of physical conditioning in Chapter 19. This chapter primarily focuses on approaches to hypertension and hypercholesterolemia in the prevention of coronary artery disease. Population-based and patient-based methods of coronary heart disease prevention have been developed during the last 10 years and represent complementary strategies that seek to identify and/or modify risk factors for premature atherosclerosis in the entire population of adults and to bring high-risk subsets of adults to the attention of physicians. These two approaches share the same ultimate goals and use similar methods as intermediate steps to achieve the long-term goal of further reducing morbidity and mortality attributable to this disease. The U.S. government has been an active participant in population-based health promotion efforts that are designed to reduce blood pressure and blood cholesterol levels of the entire adult population. Two examples of health promotion programs that utilize population-based approaches are the National High Blood Pressure Education Program and the National Cholesterol Education Program. The former program has been in progress for more than two decades'; the latter effort was initiated

approximately 10 years ago. Examining the prevalence of cardiovascular deaths that occurred in men and women in the United States in 1988 (Fig. 41-1) makes it obvious that continued efforts to reduce the risk of cardiovascular disease are necessary. It should be recognized that more men and women die of a cardiovascular event each year than of malignancy, accidental death, and acquired immunodeficiency syndrome (AIDS), even when these three noncardiovascular causes of death are combined. (Fig. 41-2).

An important component of both of these programs is related to population-based methods to identify individuals with hypertension or hypercholesterolemia. These "diseases" have been the most extensively scrutinized "modifiable risk factors" for premature coronary heart disease studied to date.[33,36,43,45,50] As an operational concept, the population-based and patient-based approaches to prevention of coronary heart disease merge when measurements of blood pressure or blood cholesterol levels are performed in community-based screening programs. The fact that screened individuals are (or should be) advised to consult their physician if an elevated blood pressure or blood cholesterol level is identified on a screening measurement is the most obvious example of this merger. Another example of overlap of the population-based and patient-based approaches is that management of hypertension or hypercholesterolemia incorporates education in a process designed to promote long-term changes in life-style, including changes in diet and the level of physical activity. It is probably safe to say that introduction of a "life-style change prescription" as the sole method to treat hypertension and/or hypercholesterolemia takes more time than most physicians in clinical practice have to dedicate to this process. The physician may, in fact, provide a better service to his or her patients by spending a few minutes strongly endorsing the need to make life-style changes and provide a list of names and locations of a qualified registered dietitian and health education programs in the com-

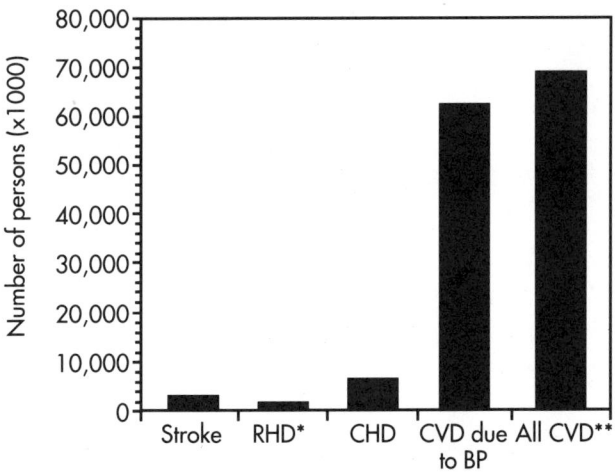

Fig. 41-1. Estimated prevalence of major cardiovascular diseases, United States, 1989 estimates. *, rheumatic heart disease, **, sum of the individual estimates exceeds 69,080,000 since many people have more than one cardiovascular disorder. *CHD*, Coronary heart disease; *CVD*, cardiovascular disease.

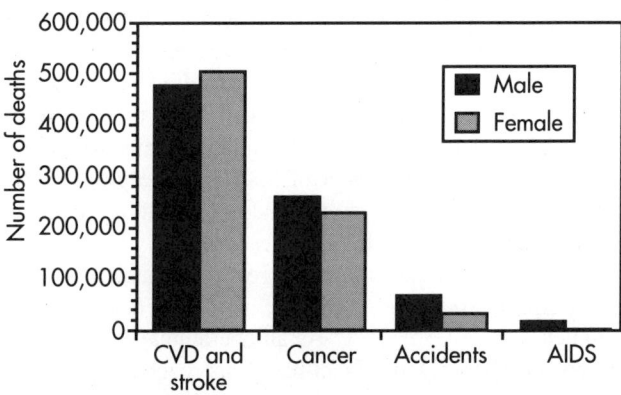

Fig. 41-2. Deaths due to cardiovascular disease, cancer, accidents, and AIDS: men and women in the United States, 1988. *CVD*, cardiovascular disease.

munity that address dietary issues and the need to make major changes in life-style. Another approach that can be useful is for the physician to use a member or members of his or her office staff as a resource for similar information. If the latter approach is utilized, it is usually advisable to address issues related to the quality and realistic goals of efforts such as dietary counseling when the dietary program can represent a successful form of treatment.

This preamble to the current chapter is provided for two interrelated reasons. The first is the author's opinion that the information in the previous paragraph may be useful advice that can immediately be put into practice in most geographic areas and physicians' clinical care routines. This is particularly true in the current era of heightened public interest in these programs. There are obviously situations that require very different levels of direct physician involvement in life-style modification approaches to risk factor modification just as there is considerable variability in the ways different physicians approach other health care problems. The other reason is related to the emphasis on drug treatment of hypertension and hypercholesterolemia in the current chapter. Every effort to prevent repetition of topics covered in other sections of this text has been made in this discussion of prevention of coronary artery disease (CAD). It is also important to note that most of the following discussion is actually a review of two important approaches to prevention of coronary heart disease (CHD) events that probably represent strategies that prevent or delay the development or reduce the progression of CAD. Abundant data are now consistent with the concept that although not ideal, secondary prevention of CHD not only is possible but may be the most cost-effective preventive effort that a physician is capable of providing.

THE TREADMILL STRESS TEST AS A MODEL OF COST-EFFECTIVENESS IN PREVENTION OF CORONARY HEART DISEASE

Beginning a discussion of treatment strategies used to prevent coronary heart disease by reducing blood pressure or blood cholesterol levels with a topic such as exercise testing may appear unusual but is useful to illustrate several concepts. This is particularly true with respect to introduction of cost-effectiveness as a factor to consider in areas of activity that range from screening (to detect individuals who may have high blood pressure or hypercholesterolemia) to selection of a specific form of antihypertensive and/or cholesterol-lowering drug treatment. The following review of the cost-effectiveness of exercise testing as a "screening" test to detect asymptomatic individuals with severe obstructive coronary artery disease[42] emphasizes the following points:

1. Reasonable precision and accuracy of the method used to screen are requirements that must be met before any realistic hope of obtaining useful information from a screening program can be justified.
2. A subset of the general population that has a very low risk for development of coronary heart disease during the next 10 years represents a portion of the population not ideal for a cost-effective risk factor modification strategy that involves the use of expensive tests or expensive drugs.
3. Individuals with established coronary artery disease, irrespective of the presence of symptoms, have a high risk for sustaining coronary heart disease events during a relatively brief period. They are probably the best candidates for application of risk modification strategies that involve expensive diagnostic procedures and/or drugs.

Sox and co-workers published an analysis of the cost-effectiveness of treadmill exercise testing as a screening procedure to detect asymptomatic individuals with severe

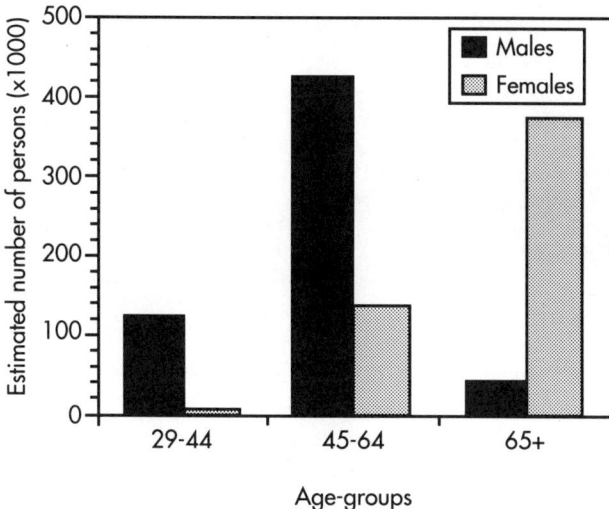

Fig. 41-3. Estimated annual number of Americans experiencing heart attack. Note that the number of men or women who are less than 45 years of age who have a heart attack each year is very small, particularly for women. However, the number of women is much higher than the number of men who have a myocardial infarction in the over 65 age-group.

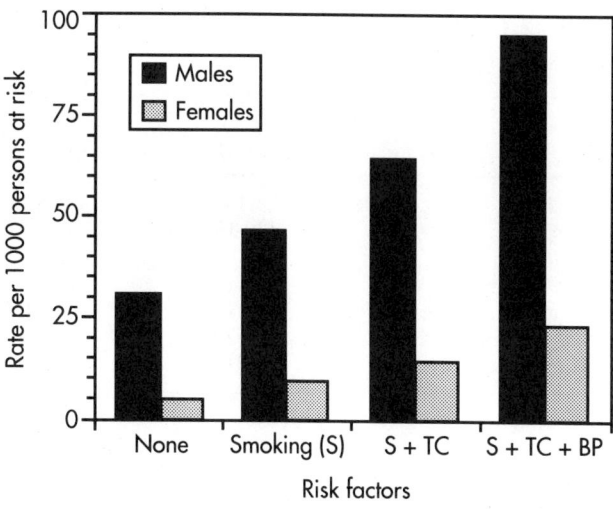

Fig. 41-4. Danger of heart attack within 8 years by risk factors present. Note that the 8-year risk of CHD was higher in men with no risk factors than it was in women who were smokers and had hypertension and hypercholesterolemia. *S,* smoking; *TC,* hypercholesterolemia; *BP,* hypertension; *CHD,* coronary heart disease.

but asymptomatic coronary artery disease.[42] In this model, the exercise test is theoretically used for a group of asymptomatic individuals with the assumption that surgical treatment is available and effectuve as a method to prolong life in a selected group of screenees ultimately found to have severe coronary artery disease. A statistical model was used to assess the cost and projected number of years of life saved (cost per year of life saved) as an index of cost-effectiveness. This type of estimate requires (1) a reasonable estimate of the prevalence of the disease of interest (in this case, severe but asymptomatic coronary disease in the general population), (2) published information about the performance of exercise testing (cost, risk of adverse events, sensitivity, and specificity of the testing procedure), and (3) costs and risks associated with the evaluation of individuals who ultimately had a false-positive exercise test result, such as the cost of performing thallium stress tests to prove that an exercise test yields a false-positive finding. Finally, the cost of treating any complications that occurred throughout the screening and subsequent evaluation procedures was included in the estimated costs of treating surgical complications in individuals undergoing coronary bypass surgery.

It was estimated that performing routine stress testing in asymptomatic 60-year-old men would ultimately cost $24,600 per person screened to gain an additional year of life in the 60-year-old men screened. In contrast, the cost estimate was $216,496 to achieve a 1-year estimated prolongation of life for asymptomatic 40-year-old women. A substantial proportion of the difference in cost is related to the fact that 60-year-old men, as a group, have a higher prevalence of coronary artery disease than 40-year-old

women. By analogy, a similar difference in cost and number of lives saved would result from lowering blood cholesterol levels from 250 mg/dl to 200 mg/dl, because in many more 60-year-old men than 40-year-old women coronary artery disease develops in a period of 5-10 years (Fig. 41-3). As suggested in Figure 41-3, the major increment in the incidence of myocardial infarction occurs 20 years later in women than in men, although the risk increases substantially for 29- to 44-year-old versus 45- to 64-year-old women or men. However, the difference in the number of heart attacks that occur during the 15- to 20-year period in the "early versus later" years of a middle-aged person's life is much greater in men because the prevalence of CHD is much higher in men than in women during that period. Interestingly, the opposite effect is observed when age increases into the "elderly" range. In this phase of life, many more women experience a heart attack annually than men. However, there are individuals within the subsets of 40-year-old women and 60-year-old men who have substantial differences in prognosis even though both individuals may be 40-year-old women or 60-year-old men. For example, a 40-year-old woman who smokes, has high blood pressure, and has inherited a condition such as heterozygous familial hypercholesterolemia is probably a better candidate for having a myocardial infarction during the next 10 years than the average 60-year-old man in the general population. As seen in Fig. 41-4, the presence of multiple risk factors for CHD markedly increases CHD risk in women or men. Unfortunately, it is very easy to lose sight of the fact that blood pressure or blood cholesterol levels per se are usually much less important from the standpoint of overall coronary heart disease risk than the

Table 41-1. Classification of blood pressure for adults age 18 years and older

	Systolic (mm Hg)	Diastolic (mm Hg)
Normal	<130	<85
High normal	130-139	85-89
Hypertension		
Stage 1 (mild)	140-159	90-99
Stage 2 (moderate)	160-179	100-109
Stage 3 (severe)	180-209	110-119
Stage 4 (very severe)	≥210	≥120

Table 41-2. Classification of total blood cholesterol and LDL-C levels in adults

Desirable blood cholesterol (mg/dl)	<200
Borderline-high blood cholesterol (mg/dl)	200-239
High blood cholesterol (mg/dl)	≥240
Desirable LDL-C level (mg/dl)	<130
Borderline-high risk LDL-C (mg/dl)	130-159
High risk LDL-C (mg/dl)	≥160

clinical conditions that accompany the hypertensive or hypercholesterolemic state.

Sox used an estimate to consider the costs and benefits associated with reducing diastolic blood pressure levels from 110 to 90 mm Hg in middle-aged men or women with assumptions similar to the ones made in his exercise test cost-benefit analysis. His estimate suggested that it would cost approximately $16,300 to produce a 1-year addition of life to hypertensive 60-year-old men by using antihypertensive therapy, which approximates the estimated cost of performing stress tests in asymptomatic men to detect a correctable coronary artery lesion. In regard to the use of stress testing, the following recommendations were given and appear to be appropriate:

1. Exercise testing is not recommended as a routine screening procedure in adults with no evidence of coronary heart disease.
2. An asymptomatic person who has already had a negative exercise electrocardiogram (ECG) result has an excellent prognosis and does not require further testing.
3. If exercise testing is to be used to screen high-risk patients for coronary artery disease, performing thallium scintigraphy is a reasonable method to detect individuals with a "false"-positive exercise test finding. We generally recommend coronary arteriography only if the results of both noninvasive tests are abnormal. This approach detects most patients who have serious coronary artery disease and is considerably more cost-effective than an exercise ECG alone.

DEFINITIONS OF HYPERTENSION AND HYPERCHOLESTEROLEMIA

Recognizing the theoretic problems associated with the use of a specific level of blood pressure or blood cholesterol to define hypertension or hypercholesterolemia, there have been no justifiable alternative proposals to replace the use of systolic blood pressure, diastolic blood pressure, or serum cholesterol concentration as parameters to define

systolic hypertension, diastolic hypertension, or hypercholesterolemia, respectively. Table 41-1 summarizes the recently recommended classification of blood pressure from the fifth Joint National Committee (JNC) for detection, evaluation, and treatment of hypertension.[39] Using these definitions, the average of several systolic blood pressure levels of 160 to 179 mm Hg or diastolic blood pressure (DBP) of 100 to 109 mm Hg is a criterion for "stage 2" hypertension. A patient with a blood pressure of 164/88 (formerly defined as isolated systolic hypertension) would have stage 2 hypertension since the highest stage of the systolic/diastolic blood pressure is used in the classification system.

The necessity of using several measurements of blood pressure or blood cholesterol cannot be overemphasized to prevent misclassification of individuals identified as "hypertensive" or "hypercholesterolemic" at a single screening examination. Results of repeat measurements of these and other tests tend to be lower when initial values are high, and higher when the initial levels are lower than the average value (regression toward the mean). However, treatment decisions in patients with hypercholesterolemia are based on estimated concentrations of low density lipoprotein-cholesterol (LDL-C) levels, which are measured if the average of two total cholesterol levels is elevated.[38] Decisions about the use of pharmacologic treatment of hypercholesterolemia are based on the number of risk factors present (Table 41-2 and the box on p. 817). Analysis of LDL-C levels is generally performed by estimating LDL-C levels by means of measurements of fasting total cholesterol (TC), triglyceride (TG), and HDL-C concentrations with the formula LDL-C = TC-(TG/5 + HDL-C). These factors are considered in subsequent discussions of screening, confirmation, evaluation, and treatment of hypercholesterolemia.

SCREENING FOR HYPERTENSION AND HYPERCHOLESTEROLEMIA

Hypertension and hypercholesterolemia are largely asymptomatic conditions that may be present but not identified or may be present transiently in normotensive individuals who are evaluated for symptomatic medial conditions. Large-scale population-based screening programs have been particularly useful for detection of hypertensive

---

Coronary heart disease (CHD) risk factors

Definite cardiovascular disease including the history of a surgical or nonsurgical revascularization procedure
Family history of premature CHD (in a first-degree relative less than 55 years of age)
Hypertension
Cigarette smoking
Severe obesity (greater than 30% above ideal body weight)
Diabetes mellitus
Male gender
Low HDL cholesterol (less than 35 mg/dl)
Increased LDL cholesterol (greater than 159 mg/dl)

Laboratory evaluation of patients with hypertension or hypercholesterolemia

- Complete blood count
- Urinalysis (at least dipstick for protein, glucose, blood)
- Serum chemistry profile including serum creatinine, potassium, glucose, and uric acid levels
- Serum cholesterol (total and HDL-C) levels, preferably combined with a fasting serum triglyceride level
- Alkaline phosphatase levels and a thyroid stimulating hormone level for patients with hypercholesterolemia
- Electrocardiogram

---

individuals and more recently have been used to identify patients with hypercholesterolemia. "Screening" for hypercholesterolemia requires acquisition of a blood sample, reasonably precise and accurate assays for total cholesterol measurements, and availability of adequate resources to evaluate and possibly treat individuals who have hypercholesterolemia. If all of these criteria cannot be met, a screening program should probably not be performed. Considerable progress has been made during the last few years because of the availability of relatively inexpensive automated devices that are capable of providing fairly precise and reliable total cholesterol measurements when recommendations of the manufacturers of these devices are followed. High-quality community screening programs are therefore theoretically attractive as an alternative to office-based cholesterol testing.

DIAGNOSIS AND EVALUATION OF HYPERTENSION

Because blood pressure (BP) levels fluctuate considerably in certain individuals, the diagnosis of hypertension requires repeated BP measurements. BP should initially be measured in both arms, and the arm with the higher BP should be used to obtain follow-up measurements.[39] At least two measurements should be obtained at each visit; both levels or the average value should be recorded. Additional measurements should be obtained if the first two systolic or diastolic readings differ by more than 5 mm Hg. Classification of hypertension is based on the average level obtained on at least two separate visits. If hypertension is confirmed, a hypertensive evaluation should assess the patient's general health, evaluate hypertensive target organs, determine overall cardiovascular risk status, and rule out secondary causes of high BP. This evaluation requires a careful history and physical examination and a few laboratory tests. Treatment should generally not be initiated until the entire evaluation is completed. An exception to this general rule is when hypertension is severe or cardiovascular compromise seems imminent. It is usu-

ally not necessary to discontinue medications during the evaluation, but the history of medication use and results of treatment should be recorded. The patient should be informed about the level of BP and the results of the hypertensive evaluation in a timely fashion.

History

When a patient is evaluated for hypertension, the history should begin with a discussion of previous BP measurements. BP usually rises slowly in patients with essential hypertension (EH); an abrupt rise provides a clue to the presence of a secondary cause of high BP. EH is usually detected between ages 35 and 55, although it is the most common cause of adolescent hypertension. It is useful to know whether there is a family history of hypertension or premature cardiovascular disease. Hypertension is quite common in the general population, particularly in family members of patients with EH. The absence of a family history of hypertension in a young patient with moderate or severe hypertension may also be a clue to the presence of a secondary cause of high BP. In addition, a family history of polycystic kidney disease or other hereditary forms of renal parenchymal disease, medullary carcinoma of the thyroid, hyperparathyroidism, or pheochromocytoma may provide a clue to the presence of an inherited secondary cause of high BP.

It is well known that mild to moderate EH does not in itself cause symptoms. Symptoms in patients with EH are usually due to an unrelated illness or complications of hypertension. In contrast, patients with pheochromocytoma generally have symptoms such as headaches, sweating, or palpitations associated with high BP. Severe headaches should raise the suspicion of an intracranial mass lesion, particularly if unilateral papilledema is noted on physical examination. Muscle weakness is a prominent feature in patients with Cushing's syndrome, hypothyroidism, hyperthyroidism, and primary hyperaldosteronism. Polyuria and nocturia develop in patients with poorly controlled diabetes mellitus or chronic renal failure. Other historic clues to the presence of chronic renal disease include a history of previous renal disorders, such as "nephritis," recurrent urinary tract infections, hematuria, or renal calculus formation.

A careful history of medication use should also be elicited. This includes the response to antihypertensive medications that have previously been used as well as a history of ingestion of drugs that may secondarily cause high BP. For example, excessive use of a variety of analgesics may lead to chronic interstitial renal disease and hypertension. Nonsteroidal anti-inflammatory drugs may blunt the antihypertensive response to diuretics and other antihypertensive drugs. Heavy alcohol consumption is associated with an increased prevalence of hypertension. The prevalence begins to increase when three or more alcoholic beverages are consumed daily. Oral contraceptives, particularly those with a high progesterone content, may also increase BP. Discontinuation of oral contraceptives is reasonable if their use is thought to contribute to hypertension and an alternative form of contraception is acceptable to the patient. BP may not return to normal levels for several weeks even if the oral contraceptive caused the hypertension. Use of cold remedies or "diet pills" containing sympathomimetic drugs or amphetamines can induce hypertension in certain individuals. Heavy use of or withdrawal from amphetamines, cocaine, or narcotics should also be considered, particularly when tachycardia, sweating, or irritability is a prominent symptom. Similar symptoms and signs may occur after abrupt withdrawal from clonidine or other centrally acting sympatholytic agents. A pheochromocytomalike syndrome can develop when patients receiving monoamine oxidase (MAO) inhibitors ingest food with a high tyramine content.

The presence of associated disorders in the patient or family members may influence the approach to the hypertensive evaluation or plan of treatment. A strong family history of premature CHD (definite CHD in a first-degree relative before age 55) raises the possibility of a serious genetic form of hyperlipoproteinemia, such as familial heterozygous hypercholesterolemia or the familial combined hyperlipidemia syndrome. The patient may also be aware of a personal or family history of elevated blood glucose or blood lipid level. A useful way to approach the family history from the standpoint of risk factors for coronary heart disease is to ask (1) whether either of the patient's parents or grandparents died before the age of 55 or (2) if either of these groups of first-degree relatives had a heart attack before the age of approximately 55 years. If the answer to either one of these questions is yes, it is prudent to ask whether the death occurred in a smoker versus nonsmoker and if other health problems were known to exist. The presence of high blood pressure or elevated blood cholesterol levels in the patient's siblings and/or children is other information that is useful if a familial disorder of blood pressure regulation or lipid metabolism is suspected by other aspects of the history or physical examination.

This is particularly true in patients with hypercholesterolemia, as described later in the chapter. The recording of symptoms referable to the target organs of hypertension (central nervous system, eyes, heart, kidneys, peripheral vasculature) or a history of other medical conditions should be elicited because depression, migraine headache, bronchial asthma, Raynaud's phenomenon, "brittle" diabetes, or supraventricular tachyarrhythmias may ultimately influence the choice of drugs.

Physical examination

The physical examination supplements the historical evaluation and provides additional information about the degree of hypertensive target organ involvement. It may provide evidence suggesting a secondary cause of high BP. A diagnosis of Cushing's disease is suggested by the presence of moon facies and truncal (as opposed to generalized) obesity. Diffuse hyperpigmentation of the skin in a patient with rapidly developing muscle weakness and/or hypokalemia suggests an ectopic adrenocorticotrophic hormone (ACTH) syndrome, which is often accompanied by hypertension. Café au-lait spots, which are seen in neurofibromatosis, suggest the possibility of pheochromocytoma (which occurs in about 1% of patients with neurofibromatosis) in a symptomatic hypertensive patient. In patients with neurofibromatosis, renovascular hypertension can also develop if a neurofibroma impairs blood flow to the kidney. Finally, hypertension occurs in approximately 40% of patients with acromegaly, but unfortunately the clinical manifestations of acromegaly can be quite subtle and escape detection for many years.

A careful funduscopic examination should be performed, particularly in individuals with symptoms or signs referable to the central nervous system. This includes an evaluation for retinal arteriolar spasm, sclerosis of these vessels, flame-shaped hemorrhages, or cotton-wool exudates that are characteristic of severe hypertension. When severe retinal arteriolar vasospasm is associated with bilateral papilledema, a diagnosis of malignant hypertension can be made. This finding should prompt urgent evaluation and treatment even if the patient has minimal symptoms. In this setting, a secondary cause of hypertension, renovascular hypertension, should be considered. Significant retinal arteriolar spasm in patients with minimal arteriolar sclerosis suggests recent onset of hypertension. Careful auscultation of the carotid arteries at the angle of the jaw should always be performed. Although there is continued controversy about the approach to management of patients with asymptomatic carotid bruits, radiographic evaluation should be strongly considered in patients with long, high-pitched systolic carotid bruits and those with systolic/diastolic carotid bruits. This is particularly true if the patient has suffered from a previous stroke or transient ischemic attacks. The thyroid gland should be carefully palpated because detection of thyroid gland enlargement may point to the presence of hypothyroidism, which can cause a secondary form of high BP or hypercholesterolemia.

Distention of the internal jugular veins and the presence of rales in the lung bases may be found in patients with right- or left-sided heart failure, respectively. Careful auscultation of the heart with the bell of the stethoscope may reveal a third heart sound (S_3) in a patient with heart failure. Left ventricular dilatation of hypertrophy is suggested when the point of maximal impulse is diffuse or displaced inferolaterally. A fourth heart sound (S_4) indicates reduced compliance of the left ventricle, which is common in diastolic hypertension. The abdominal examination should include careful palpation and measurement of the size of the abdominal aorta. An abdominal aortic aneurysm should be suspected when a pulsatile mass is noted in the midline between the xiphoid process and umbilicus. Palpation of bilateral renal masses should raise the suspicion of polycystic kidney disease. Occasionally, a hydronephrotic kidney may be palpated. Auscultation deep within the epigastrium may reveal a systolic/diastolic bruit that is suggestive of severe stenosis of the renal artery. Systolic abdominal bruits are quite common in older individuals but usually arise from the mesenteric vessels. The femoral, popliteal, dorsalis pedis, and posterior tibial pulses should also be examined. Delayed and diminished femoral pulses suggest the possibility of coarctation of the aorta, particularly in young patients with intermittent claudication. Palpation of the popliteal pulse should be performed to detect popliteal artery aneurysms. Absence or asymmetry of the popliteal, posterior tibial, or dorsalis pedis pulses points to the presence of atherosclerosis and may be the only sign of atherosclerosis in middle-aged or older individuals. There are very few differences in this general approach to clinical evaluation of patients with hypertension or hypercholesterolemia since the goal of these examinations is to assess status of the target organ systems of hypertensive and/or atherosclerotic cardiovascular disease.

Laboratory investigation

An extensive laboratory evaluation is generally not required in a hypertensive patient, but certain simple and relatively inexpensive tests should be performed before treatment is initiated[39] (see box on p. 817). These tests are used to determine the severity of vascular disease, detect secondary causes of hypertension, assess overall coronary risk status, and provide baseline values that can be used to judge adverse biochemical effects of treatment (Table 42-4). The minimal evaluation should include a urinalysis, complete blood count, and determination of serum potassium, creatinine, glucose, uric acid and total cholesterol levels (if prior level is unknown). Serum triglyceride and high-density lipoprotein (HDL)-cholesterol levels should be performed with the total cholesterol level if a prior TC value was above 240 mg/dl. If a diagnosis of hypertension has already been confirmed, it is reasonable to obtain fasting TC, TG, and HDL-C levels at the first visit of a patient who has had an elevated blood cholesterol level in the past. An automated battery of blood chemistry tests is often used and may be more cost-effective than obtaining separate blood tests. Fasting samples are preferable for measurement of glucose and lipids levels. Although accurate total and HDL-cholesterol levels do not require a 12- to 14-hour fast, calculation of low-density lipoprotein (LDL)-cholesterol levels requires fasting to estimate very-low-density lipoprotein (VLDL) cholesterol from triglyceride levels.[38] As previously stated, this estimate is used to calculate LDL-cholesterol (when triglyceride levels are less than 400 mg/dl [4.52 mmol/L]) according to the formula[12]

$$LDL\text{-}C = total\ cholesterol - (triglyceride/5 + HDL\ cholesterol)$$

Finally, the electrocardiogram (ECG) may show evidence of left ventricular hypertrophy or previous myocardial infarction. It is of note that over 25% of myocardial infarctions were discovered only through the appearance of new ECG abnormalities during biennial ECG examinations in the Framingham study.[6,31] Thus the ECG can provide important prognostic information and influence the choice of drug treatment in patients with hypertension or hypercholesterolemia.

MANAGEMENT OF HYPERTENSION

After the initial history and physical examination have been performed and the appropriate laboratory evaluations obtained and reviewed, the patient should be scheduled for another visit to repeat BP readings, review results of the evaluation, and outline a treatment plan and its goals. Patients should be made aware that treatment of hypertension is designed to prevent the development of hypertensive complications, such as stroke, myocardial infarction, and heart failure, and usually requires continuous lifelong therapy. It should also be clearly stated that the patient cannot judge his or her BP level by "the way he feels." This common misconception is a frequent cause of erratic use of antihypertensive medications and inadequate BP control. As previously stated, most patients with hypertension have no symptoms and may be reluctant to make dietary or other life-style changes or use drugs, particularly if the drugs are expensive or cause bothersome side effects. A number of methods have been used in an attempt to improve adherence to antihypertensive treatment regimens. It is important for the patient to understand the risks of hypertension and potential benefits of treatment, in order to take an active role in the management of his or her health care. Home BP monitoring is one excellent method to provide positive reinforcement, enhance adherence to treatment, and reduce costs associated with prevention of cardiovascular disease. The specific type of blood pressure measuring device or a specific manufacturer of the device is much less important than assurance of accurate calibration.[39] A convenient way to check calibration of the home BP device is to compare it to the monitoring device in the physician's office. BP levels with both should be within 5 mm Hg of each other. Obviously, the physician or nurse and the "gold standard" BP measurement (the office BP level) have to be accurate.

Nonpharmacologic treatment of hypertension

Clinical trials in which the benefits of reducing BP have been demonstrated employed pharmacologic approaches to treatment, usually with diuretic-based antihypertensive drug therapy. However, there are legitimate concerns about the potential hazards of long-term diuretic therapy in the treatment of hypertension. For this and several other reasons, an adequate trial of life-style modification, or, on occasion, addition of oral calcium supplements as nonpharmacologic methods of treatment should be considered before drug treatment is initiated.[8] This is particularly true in patients with mild uncomplicated hypertension who have hypercholesterolemia, diabetes mellitus, and/or obesity. Patients treated with nonpharmacologic therapy should be followed as closely as individuals receiving drugs and BP should be monitored by the patient or physician (or both) periodically to assure that goal BP levels have been achieved. Unfortunately, patients frequently cancel physician visits scheduled for routine health maintenance, placing the physician in a difficult situation as a provider of preventive care. Again, patients must be made aware of their responsibilities as active participants in these long-term treatment programs.

In general, it is usually appropriate for a physician to recommend that a hypertensive (or normotensive) patient increase his or her level of exercise, attempt to lose weight, avoid obvious sources of salt in the diet (i.e., adding salt at the table, eating potato chips instead of unsalted celery for a snack), reduce the use of alcohol to one or two drinks per day, and stop smoking altogether (see the box above right).[8,10,35,39,47] It is also appropriate for a physician to warn patients with severe hypertension, known coronary artery disease, malnutrition, and/or alcoholism that initiating a vigorous exercise program, going on a rigid diet, and beginning a program of mental feedback or transcendental meditation while ignoring advice about pharmacologic treatment of hypertension probably has a better chance of ending the patient's life rather than prolonging it. Patients may not be aware that many of the statements made in the nonmedical press are merely opinions about issues that have not been addressed in a carefully conducted scientific trial. It may be useful to point out that guidelines for treatment of hypertension and hypercholesterolemia have been based on information from a very large number of controlled clinical trials. On occasion, it may be helpful to keep a copy of these guidelines in the office and use the document as a resource for patient edu-

---

Nonpharmacologic therapy in the hypertensive patient

Lose weight if overweight

Limit alcohol intake to no more than 1 ounce of ethanol/day (24 ounces of beer, 8 ounces of wine, or 2 ounces of 100 proof whiskey)

Exercise (aerobic) regularly.

Reduce sodium intake to less than 100 mmol/day (<2.3 g of sodium or <6 g of sodium chloride).

Interventions of limited or unproven efficacy
  Stress management
  Potassium (pill) supplementation
  Fish oil (pill) supplementation
  Calcium (pill) supplementation
  Magnesium (pill) supplementation
  Macronutrient alteration
  Fiber supplementation

Stop smoking and reduce dietary saturated fat and cholesterol intake for overall cardiovascular health. Reducing fat intake also helps reduce calories, which is important for control of weight and type II diabetes.

From National High Blood Pressure Education Program Working Group Report on Primary Prevention of Hypertension, *Arch Intern Med* 153:186-208, 1993. Copyright 1993, American Medical Association.

---

cation. The initial pages of the Fifth Report of the Joint National Committee on Detection, Evaluation, and Treatment of High Blood Pressure (JNC V) and National Cholesterol Education Program documents describe their purpose and how they were developed.[39,47]

A physician can use printed material that deals with dietary treatment of hypertension to endorse the concept that dietary treatment is important and give the patient some direction about how to go about changing his or her lifestyle. County or state medical societies frequently have information available for this specific purpose and may have lists of addresses or phone numbers of resources in the community that provide these services. Face-to-face interview and instruction of patients with problems that require long-term dietary management are probably more likely to succeed if a registered dietitian assists in this effort. The physician can write a "dietary prescription," for example, transmitting specific instructions for a specific level of sodium restriction (4 g sodium/day or a 2-g level of restriction if indicated for other reasons). A desirable level of weight loss or saturated fat restriction can be specified. Thus, a reasonable dietary prescription for a hypertensive patient with hypercholesterolemia could read "4 g sodium, 10% saturated fat diet to achieve a 10 pound weight loss." Registered dietitians usually develop a dietary plan that is appropriate for the specific needs of the patient. Patients often view this approach as an indication that dietary treatment is, in fact, part of the treatment process. I find it useful to rely on information that the nutritionists provide after their assessment in deciding when the patient should return to the outpatient department to monitor the response to dietary treatment. I find it difficult to predict whether a patient will or will not follow the nutritionist's advice, particularly when weight loss is one of the goals of dietary treatment. Our nutritionists feel that a large number of patients think they know much more about their diet than they actually know, and often make mistakes reading labels about sodium versus salt content, total fat versus saturated fat, and content per serving versus per unit weight of food.

Data from controlled clinical trials warrant a recommendation to include sodium restriction, weight loss, and alcohol restriction as a nutritional method to treat hypertension. Smoking cessation and avoidance of large doses of caffeine on a chronic basis are more likely to be beneficial than harmful to a hypertensive patient's long-term health. If a postmenopausal woman is going to begin a course of low-dose estrogen with or without progesterone, oral calcium supplementation should probably be added to the regimen for its effect on bone mineralization. Oral calcium also may lower blood pressure as an added benefit. Potassium or magnesium supplement should be added to the diet of an overweight, diuretic-treated hypertensive individual.

Pharmacologic therapy of hypertension (Table 41-3)

The 1988 report of the Joint National Committee report included a recommendation for use of either thiazide-type diuretics, β-blockers, angiotensin-converting enzyme (ACE) inhibitors, or calcium channel blockers (CCBs) as initial agents for treatment of patients with high BP.[47] Until recently, the thiazide-type diuretics and β-adrenergic receptor blockers were generally used as the first step in drug treatment for the majority of patients with hypertension. They were usually included in the blinded blood pressure regimens in controlled clinical trials that demonstrated reduction in the incidence of stroke, congestive heart failure, and other pressure-related complications of hypertension. A large number of drugs with various pharmacologic properties have been developed and marketed during the last 10 years for the treatment of hypertension. Since hypertension is a heterogeneous pathophysiologic condition, it is useful to become familiar with one or two agents in each of the major drug classes (diuretics, β-blockers, calcium channel blockers, etc). Individual differences exist in the pharmacologic properties of drugs within a specific pharmacologic class, but in most situations these differences are not important clinically. Although the diuretic-based stepped-care approach to management of hypertension remains useful, the availability of newer antihypertensive agents permits considerable room for individualization of treatment. An obvious concern about the thiazide-type diuretics and β-blockers that is particularly applicable to the discussion of prevention of cor-

onary heart disease is the issue of lipoprotein abnormalities that can occur with these agents.*

Diuretics. Diuretics have been used in treatment of hypertension for three decades and are still recommended as first step pharmacologic agents.[39] Diuretics are inexpensive, convenient to administer, well tolerated, and unquestionably effective in reducing BP for prolonged periods. Diuretics are particularly useful in treatment of blacks, older individuals, patients with chronic renal disease, or individuals with chronic congestive heart failure. The 1988 JNC report included recommendations for a reduced diuretic dose range of 12.5 to 50 mg of hydrochlorothiazide per day (or equivalent).[47] This dose reduction was prompted largely by concerns about the metabolic complications of diuretics, which are dose-related. On the basis of clinical studies, a drop in serum potassium level of about 0.4 mEq/L (0.4 mmol/L) or 0.6 mEq/L (0.6 mmol/L) can be expected with 25-mg and 50-mg hydrochlorothiazide doses, respectively. When serum potassium levels fall to below 3.0 mEq/L (3.0 mmol/L) in a patient receiving a low dose of a thiazide diuretic, a diagnosis of primary hyperaldosteronism should be considered.

Serum cholesterol levels may increase during short-term thiazide administration but frequently return to baseline levels after the first few weeks or months of treatment.[48] Administration of a diet low in saturated fat and cholesterol abolishes the initial increase in total and LDL cholesterol associated with diuretic administration.[20] However, in the MRFIT study, the reduction in serum cholesterol associated with the low-saturated fat and low-cholesterol diet was blunted in men receiving diuretic therapy for over 5 years compared to that in those not receiving diuretics.[30,34] Thiazide diuretics can also impair glucose tolerance. Certain studies suggest that hypokalemia underlies this hyperglycemic tendency, but a few studies have shown that potassium replacement does not correct thiazide-induced carbohydrate intolerance. Hyperglycemia occurs much less frequently than hypokalemia and is most likely to develop in patients whose carbohydrate metabolism is not truly normal before treatment. Diuretics cause renal magnesium wasting and produce hypomagnesemia. This may contribute to the presumed arrhythmogenic effect of diuretics. The combined effect of hypokalemia and hypomagnesemia may enhance the arrhythmogenic effect of digitalis. Symptomatic side effects associated with diuretic use occur much less frequently than the biochemical changes previously described. In the placebo-controlled Medical Research Council (MRC) trial comparing bendroflumethiazide and propranolol, impotence (12.8 per 1000 patient years), and gout (12.6 per 1000 patient years) accounted for the majority of treatment withdrawals caused by symptomatic side effects in men receiving diuretics.[30] In women, nausea, dizziness, headache, lethargy, and gout

*References 1, 19, 20, 24, 44, 46, 49.

Table 41-3. Antihypertensive agents

Type of drug	Usual dosage range (total mg/day)*	Frequency (per day)	Comments
Initial antihypertensive agents			
Diuretics			
Thiazides and related agents			
Bendroflumethiazide	2.5-5	Once	Possible situations for decreased antihypertensive effects
Benzthiazide	12.5-50	Once	• Cholestyramine and colestipol decrease absorption of thiazides.
Chlorothiazide	125-500	Twice	• NSAIDs (including aspirin and over-the-counter ibuprofen) may antagonize diuretic effectiveness.
Chlorthalidone	12.5-25	Once	Effects of diuretics on other drugs
Cyclothiazide	1.0-2	Once	• Diuretics can raise serum lithium levels and increase toxicity by enhancing proximal tubular reabsorption of lithium.
Hydrochlorothiazide	12.5-50	Once	• Diuretics may make it more difficult to control dyslipidemia and diabetes.
Hydroflumethiazide	12.5-50	Once	For thiazide and loop diuretics, lower doses and dietary counseling should be used to prevent metabolic changes.
Indapamide	2.5-5	Once	More effective antihypertensive than loop diuretics except in patients with serum creatinine level ≥221 μmol/L (2.5 mg/dl).
Methyclothiazide	2.5-5	Once	Hydrochlorothiazide or chlorthalidone is generally preferred; both were used in most clinical trials.
Metolazone	0.5-5	Once	
Polythiazide	1.0-4	Once	
Quinethazone	25.0-100	Once	
Trichlormethiazide	1.0-4	Once	
Loop diuretics			
Bumetanide	0.5-5	Twice	Higher doses of loop diuretics may be needed for patients with renal impairment or congestive heart failure.
Ethacrynic acid	25.0-100	Twice	Ethacrynic acid is the only alternative for patients with allergy to thiazide and sulfur-containing diuretics.
Furosemide	20.0-320	Twice	
Potassium sparing			
Amiloride	5-10	Once or twice	Weak diuretics. Used mainly in combination with other diuretics to prevent or reverse hypokalemia resulting from other diuretics.
Spironolactone	25-100	Twice or thrice	Avoid when serum creatinine level ≥221 μmol/L (2.5 mg/dl).
Triamterene	50-100	Twice	May cause hyperkalemia, which may be exaggerated when combined with ACE inhibitors or potassium supplements.
Adrenergic inhibitors			
β-blockers			
Atenolol	25-100†	Once	Possible situations for decreased antihypertensive effects
Betaxolol	5-40	Once	• NSAIDs may decrease the effects of β-blockers.
Metoprolol	50-200	Once or twice	• Rifampin, smoking, and phenobarbital decrease serum levels of agents primarily metabolized by the liver as a result of enzyme induction.
Metoprolol (long-acting)	50-200	Once	Effects of β-blockers on other drugs • Combinations of diltiazem or verapamil with β-blockers may have additive SA and AV node depressant effects and may also promote negative inotropic effects on the failing myocardium.
Nadolol	20-240†	Once	• Combination of β-blockers and reserpine may cause marked bradycardia and syncope. • β-Blockers may increase serum levels of theophylline, lidocaine, and chlorpromazine through reduced hepatic clearance.
Propranolol	40-240	Twice	• Nonselective β-blockers prolong insulin-induced hypoglycemia and promote rebound hypertension through unopposed α stimulation. All β-Blockers mask the adrenergically mediated symptoms of hypoglycemia and have the potential to aggravate diabetes.

Drug	Dosage range (mg/day)*	Frequency	Comments
Propranolol (long-acting)	60-240	Once	• β-Blockers may make it more difficult to control dyslipidemia. • Phenylpropanolamine (which can be obtained over-the-counter in cold and diet preparations), pseudophedrine, ephedrine, and epinephrine can cause elevations in blood pressure through unopposed α-receptor-induced vasoconstriction. Selective agents also inhibit β₂-receptors in higher doses; e.g., all may aggravate asthma.
Timolol	20-40	Twice	
β-Blockers with ISA			No clear advantage for agents with ISA except in those with bradycardia who must receive a β-blocker; they produce fewer or no metabolic side effects.
Acebutolol	20-1200†	Twice	
Bisoprolol	2-10†	Once	
Carteolol	20-80†	Once	
Penbutolol	10-60†	Once	
Pindolol		Twice	
α-β-Blocker			Possibly more effective in blacks than other β-blockers. May cause postural effects, and titration should be based on standing blood pressure.
Labetalol	200-1200	Twice	
α₁-Receptor blockers			Possible situations for increased antihypertensive effects • Concomitant antihypertensive drug therapy (especially diuretics) may increase chance of postural hypotension. All may cause postural effects, and titration should be based on standing blood pressure.
Doxazosin	2.0-15	Once	
Prazosin	2.0-20	Twice or thrice	
Terazosin	1.0-20	Once	
Ace inhibitors			Possible situations for decreased antihypertensive effects • NSAIDs (including aspirin and over-the-counter ibuprofen) may decrease blood pressure control. • Antacids may decrease the bioavailability of ACE inhibitors. Possible situations for increased antihypertensive effects • Diuretics may lead to excessive hypotensive effects (hypovolemia). Effect of ACE inhibitors on other drugs • Hyperkalemia may occur with potassium supplements, potassium-sparing agents, and NSAIDs. • ACE inhibitors may increase serum lithium levels Diuretic doses should be reduced or discontinued before starting ACE inhibitors whenever possible to prevent excessive hypotension. Reduce dose of those drugs marked † in patients with serum creatinine level >221 μmol/L (2.5 mg/dl). May cause hyperkalemia in patients with renal impairment or in those receiving potassium-sparing agents. Can cause acute renal failure in patients with severe bilateral renal artery stenosis or severe stenosis in an artery to a solitary kidney.
Benazepril	10.0-40†	Once or twice	
Captopril	12.5-150†	Twice	
Cilazapril	2.5-5.0	Once or twice	
Enalapril	2.5-40†	Once or twice	
Fosinopril	10.0-40	Once or twice	
Lisinopril	5.0-40†	Once or twice	
Perindopril	1.0-16†	Once or twice	
Quinapril	5.0-80†	Once or twice	
Ramipril	1.25-20†	Once or twice	
Spirapril	12.5-50	Once or twice	
Calcium antagonists			Possible situations for decreased antihypertensive effects • Serum levels and antihypertensive effects of calcium antagonists may be diminished by interactions of rifampin-verapamil; carbamazepine-diltiazem and verapamil; phenobarbital and phenytoin-verapamil. Possible situations for increased antihypertensive effects • Cimetidine may increase pharmacologic effects of all calcium antagonists through inhibition of hepatic metabolizing enzymes resulting in increased serum levels.
Diltiazem	90-360	Thrice	
Diltiazem (sustained release)	120-360	Twice	

*The lower dose indicated is the preferred initial dose, and the higher dose is the maximum daily dose. Most agents require 2 to 4 weeks for complete efficacy, and more frequent dosage adjustments are not advised except for severe hypertension. The dosage range may differ slightly from the recommended dosage in *Physicians' Desk Reference* or package insert.

NSAID, nonsteroidal antiinflammatory drug; ACE, angiotensin-converting enzyme; SA, sinoatrial; AV, atrioventricular; ISA, intrinsic sympathomimetic activity.

†Indicates drugs that are excreted by the kidney and require dosage reduction in renal impairment.

Continued.

Table 41-3. Antihypertensive agents—cont'd

Type of drug	Usual dosage range (total mg/day)*	Frequency (per day)	Comments
Calcium antagonists—cont'd			
Diltiazem (extended release)	180-360	Once	Effects of calcium antagonists on other drugs
			• Digoxin and carbamazepine serum levels and toxicity may be increased by verapamil and possibly by diltiazem.
Verapamil	80-480	Twice	• Serum levels of prazosin, quinidine, and theophylline may be increased by verapamil.
Verapamil (long acting)	120-480	Once or twice	• Serum levels of cyclosporine may be increased by diltiazem and verapamil. Cyclosporine dose may need to be decreased.
			These agents also block the slow channels in the heart and may reduce sinus rate and produce heart block.
Dihydropyridines			
Amlodipine	2.5-10	Once	Dihydropyridines are more potent peripheral vasodilators than diltiazem and verapamil and may cause more dizziness, headache, flushing, peripheral edema, and tachycardia.
Felodipine	5-20	Twice	
Isradipine	2.5-10	Twice	
Nicardipine	60-120	Thrice	
Nifedipine	30-120	Thrice	
Nifedipine (GITS)	30-90	Once	
Supplemental antihypertensive agents			
Centrally acting α₂-agonists			
Clonidine	0.1-1.2	Twice	Possible situations for decreased antihypertensive effects
			• Tricyclic antidepressants may decrease the effects of centrally acting and peripheral norepinephrine depleters.
Clonidine TTS (patch)†	0.1-0.3	Once *weekly*	• Sympathomimetics including over-the-counter cold and diet preparations, amphetamines, phenothiazines, and cocaine may interfere with the antihypertensive effects of guanethidine and guanadrel.
Guanabenz	4-64	Twice	• The severity of clonidine withdrawal reaction can be increased by β-blockers.
Guanfacine	1-3	Once	• Monoamine oxidase inhibitors may prevent degradation and metabolism of norepinephrine released by tyramine-containing foods and may cause hypertension. They may also cause hypertensive reactions when combined with reserpine or guanethidine.
Methyldopa	250-2000	Twice	Clonidine patch is replaced once a week. None of these agents should be withdrawn abruptly. Avoid in nonadherent patients.
Peripherally acting adrenergic neuron antagonists			
Guanadrel	10-75	Twice	May cause serious orthostatic and exercise-induced hypotension.
Guanethidine	10-100	Once	
Rauwolfia alkaloids			
Rauwolfia root	50-200	Once	
Reserpine	0.05‡-0.25	Once	
Direct vasodilators			
Hydralazine	50-300	Twice to four times	Hydralazine is subject of phenotypicly determined metabolism (acetylation). For both agents: should treat concomitantly with a diuretic and a β-blocker because of fluid retention and reflex tachycardia.
Minoxidil	2.5-80	Once or twice	

†Weekly patch is 1, 2, 3 equivalent to 0.1-0.3 mg per day.
‡0.1 mg dose may be given every other day to achieve this dosage.

were the only symptomatic side effects that required treatment withdrawal more frequently in bendroflumethiazide- than placebo-treated patients.

As a general recommendation, it is reasonable to institute diuretic treatment in patients with mild hypertension at a daily dose of 12.5 to 25.0 mg of hydrochlorothiazide or equivalent. This is particularly true if the patient is elderly and has no clinical evidence of ischemic heart disease. The physician should recognize that elderly individuals may be at greater risk for the arrhythmogenic effects of the thiazides because of the high prevalence of organic heart disease in this population. However, data from the Systolic Hypertension in the Elderly Program and HDFP data do not indicate that the risk is excessive.[17] Dose titrations should proceed at monthly intervals with a maximal dose of 50 mg of hydrochlorothiazide per day (or equivalent). Serum potassium levels should be monitored when the maintenance dose of the thiazide diuretic is reached or even sooner in patients at risk for diuretic-associated arrhythmias (patients receiving digitalis or those with known organic heart disease). Potassium supplements or potassium-sparing diuretics should be given to patients with cardiac disease if hypokalemia (serum potassium <3.5 mEq/L [3.5 mmol/L]) develops.

The potassium-sparing diuretics (amiloride, spironolactone, and triamterene) are usually given in combination with a thiazide-type diuretic when used as antihypertensive agents (Table 41-3). Some physicians advocate routine use of these combinations, but it should be recognized that (1) in many patients given low doses of thiazides hypokalemia does not develop, (2) thiazide/potassium-sparing drugs do not always prevent hypokalemia, and (3) potassium-sparing agents can cause hyperkalemia. Thus, use of a thiazide/potassium-sparing combination does not eliminate the need to monitor serum potassium levels but increases the cost of therapy. However, it is reasonable to initiate therapy with a potassium-sparing diuretic alone or use a thiazide/potassium-sparing combination in individuals with preexisting cardiac disease, particularly if digitalis has been prescribed. Hyperkalemia is the most serious side effect of use of the potassium-sparing drugs and is most likely to occur in patients with severe chronic renal failure, diabetes mellitus, or the syndrome of hyporeninemic hypoaldosteronism. Concomitant administration of nonsteroidal antiinflammatory drugs, ACE inhibitors, and potassium supplements also increases the risk of hyperkalemia. As a general rule, potassium-sparing diuretics should not be administered with ACE inhibitors (which blunt diuretic-induced hypokalemia) or potassium supplements unless hypokalemia persists despite administration of the potassium-sparing agent.

The loop diuretics (e.g., bumetanide, ethacrynic acid, furosemide) are not generally used for treatment of hypertension except in the presence of chronic renal insufficiency or a concomitant edematous state (cirrhosis, congestive heart failure, nephrotic syndrome). The short duration of action of the loop diuretics requires at least twice-daily administration. Combined administration of thiazide-type and loop diuretics may be quite helpful in patients with refractory edema or those in whom resistant hypertension appears to be due to inadequate volume control. However, hypovolemia and electrolyte abnormalities may develop rapidly when this combination is used. Most of the metabolic complications previously described for the thiazides also occur with loop diuretics, although the long-term carbohydrate and lipid changes are less precisely defined. It should be recognized that the flat relationship between dose and antihypertensive effect of the thiazides previously discussed does not apply to use of loop diuretics. This is particularly true in azotemic patients with hypertension. For this reason, recommended dose ranges are quite wide for the loop diuretics. If hypertriglyceridemia and/or hypercholesterolemia is present in a patient receiving a diuretic, it seems reasonable to discontinue the diuretic and either (1) monitor the patient during a trial of nonpharmacologic treatment; (2) repeat the blood test that suggested the metabolic problem, particularly if the problem was a mild, isolated elevation of serum triglyceride level; or (3) substitute a nondiuretic for the diuretic antihypertensive agent. It should be recognized that a previous serum triglyceride level of 200 mg/dl could be 100 mg/dl on a repeat test with no change in the patient's metabolic state.

β-Adrenergic receptor antagonists. The efficacy of monotherapy with β-blockers in long-term treatment of hypertension has been convincingly demonstrated, and the 1984 JNC report first recommended β-blockers as first-step agents.[38] β-Blockers are useful in treating various conditions that may coexist with hypertension, such as supraventricular tachyarrhythmias, hypertrophic cardiomyopathy, angina pectoris, essential tremor, and migraine headache. Several β-blockers have been shown to reduce the incidence of reinfarction and sudden death after a myocardial infarction. It is generally assumed that β-blockers induce metabolic changes less frequently than diuretics. However, changes in carbohydrate and lipid metabolism may occur. A greater increase in fasting blood glucose level occurred during 1 year of propranolol compared to hydrochlorothiazide treatment in a large published Veterans Administration study.[48] Triglyceride levels also increase by as much as 25% during treatment with β-blockers alone or in combination with diuretics.[30] Total cholesterol levels do not usually change, but HDL-cholesterol may be reduced. The prognostic effects of these changes in hypertensive patients treated with β-blockers are not known but again are of theoretic concern. The reduction in HDL cholesterol level is particularly bothersome from the standpoint of risk factor analysis for coronary artery disease.[17] Interestingly, β-blockers with intrinsic sympathomimetic activity do not appear to induce lipid abnormalities.[1]

β-Blockers usually reduce BP by decreasing cardiac output. This effect or the reduced β-adrenergic receptor sensitivity in elderly persons may contribute to the age-related difference in antihypertensive efficacy (young patients respond better than older patients) noted with these drugs. Some of the side effects associated with treatment, such as reduced exercise tolerance, coldness of extremities, or Raynaud's phenomenon, reflect the hemodynamic effects of β-blockade. The overall frequency of symptomatic side effects is quite similar for β-blockers and diuretics, but the pattern of the adverse effects is quite different. Central nervous system side effects (fatigue, lethargy, depression, insomnia, hallucinations), dyspnea, bronchospasm, Raynaud's phenomenon, and coldness of extremities occur more frequently during β-blocker than diuretic treatment. Gout and impotence occur less frequently with β-blockers than diuretics. The reported incidence of side effects depends to some extent on the type of β-blocker used. Although any β-blocker can cause central nervous system effects, such effects may occur less frequently with hydrophilic (e.g., acebutolol, atenolol, nadolol) than lipophilic β-blockers. In addition, β_1-selective adrenergic blockers affect small airway flow to a lesser extent than those that are noncardioselective, but it should be recognized that β_1-selectivity is often lost with the high doses used to treat hypertension, and β-blockers should generally be avoided in bronchospastic lung disease. Probably the major advantage of cardioselective β-blockers is that they do not prolong insulin-induced hypoglycemia to as great an extent as noncardioselective agents. β-Blockers with intrinsic sympathomimetic activity reduce resting heart rate to a lesser extent than those that do not possess this property. Furthermore, the incidence of Raynaud's phenomenon and coldness of extremities is probably lower with β-blockers that have intrinsic sympathomimetic activity.

The prophylactic effect of postinfarction β-blockade has been demonstrated in normotensive and hypertensive patients who have sustained a myocardial infarction. Furthermore, postmyocardial infarction patients who do not have contraindications to β-blockade tolerated the relatively high β-blocker doses used in clinical trials quite well. There is no consensus about the optimal time to initiate (that is, in the first few hours versus first few days) β-blocker treatment after a myocardial infarction, but continuing the treatment for a 2- to 3-year period seems reasonable on the basis of the results of the Beta Blocker Heart Attack Trial (using propranolol) and the Norwegian Multicenter Trial (using timolol). The threshold β-blocker dose required to achieve long-term prophylaxis is also not known; the studies mentioned used relatively large daily doses (200 mg of metoprolol, 180 to 240 mg of propranolol, 20 mg of timolol). The efficacy of β-blockers that have intrinsic sympathomimetic properties has not been shown in the setting of postmyocardial infarction prophylaxis.

β-Blockers are quite useful as initial therapy for hypertension in young patients, particularly those with evidence of hyperkinetic circulation (resting tachycardia, wide pulse pressure, systolic flow murmurs, hyperdynamic precordium, labile BP, episodic palpitations, sweating or flushing). Whites as a group tend to respond better than blacks, but a significant percentage of blacks respond. β-Blocker monotherapy is particularly useful in hypertensive patients with angina pectoris, hypertrophic cardiomyopathy, or supraventricular tachyarrhythmias. The incidence of reinfarction and sudden death after a myocardial infarction is reduced when appropriately selected patients are treated with certain β-blockers. A useful rule in clinical practice is never to stop β-blocker treatment abruptly since a withdrawal syndrome can develop and lead to tachycardia, myocardial ischemia, or unstable angina, particularly in patients with underlying, but clinically silent, coronary artery disease.

Angiotensin-converting enzyme inhibitors. ACE inhibitors have been increasingly used for treatment of hypertension and chronic congestive heart failure. These agents reduce conversion of angiotensin I to the potent vasoconstrictor angiotensin II (A II). As a result of decreased production of A II, aldosterone secretion is also reduced. Systemic vascular resistance falls and transient accumulation of sodium occurs. However, this sodium-retaining state is short-lived. The magnitude of the BP-lowering response to an ACE inhibitor is related to the degree of activation of the renin-angiotensin system. Salt restriction or diuretic administration activates the renin-angiotensin system and increases responsiveness to these drugs. In addition, renal hypoperfusion, which occurs in patients with chronic heart failure or renal artery obstruction, is typically accompanied by increased renal secretion of renin, high plasma renin levels, and angiotensin II-mediated vasoconstriction. The acute antihypertensive response to ACE inhibition correlates with pretreatment levels of plasma renin activity, but the strength of this association is diminished during chronic treatment. In fact, patients with "high," "normal," or "low" levels of plasma renin activity may respond to chronic ACE inhibitor therapy. As a group, young hypertensive patients have higher levels of plasma renin activity than older individuals, and white hypertensive patients have higher levels than blacks. This may explain the enhanced efficacy of ACE inhibitors in young and/or white hypertensive patients. The racial difference in response is abolished when patients receive simultaneous diuretic treatment. In addition, ACE inhibitors blunt the hypokalemic response to diuretics.

ACE inhibitors are particularly useful in treatment of patients with renovascular hypertension. However, acute renal failure has been noted in patients with severe stenosis of an artery to a solitary kidney and those with severe bilateral renal artery stenosis. In these conditions, it is thought that removal of the postglomerular effect of angiotensin II (that is, constriction of the efferent arteriole) decreases transglomerular hydraulic pressure and reduces the glomerular ultrafiltration rate. This effect of ACE inhibitors may be beneficial in patients with renal parenchymal disease. Reducing the angiotensin II–mediated glomerular "hyperfiltration" that occurs in remaining functional nephrons in patients with renal parenchymal disease is thought to reduce progressive damage to remaining glomeruli and slow the progression of chronic renal failure. Captopril and enalapril have been the agents used in controlled clinical trials of patients with diabetic or other causes of chronic renal parenchymal disease. It is not clear whether reduced progression of renal disease is a generic property of ACE inhibitors or whether structural differences in ACE inhibitors (presence or absence of a sulfhydryl group) produce differences in their renal protective effects. Clinicians should recognize, however, that patients with severe azotemia are at risk for developing hyperkalemia during ACE inhibitor treatment. Hypotension can occur when ACE inhibitors are given to patients who are dehydrated or receiving diuretics, and treatment should be initiated cautiously in these settings. It is prudent to discontinue diuretics for several days if an ACE inhibitor is added to a diuretic treatment regimen. Chronic nonproductive cough, rash, and agesusia (loss of taste) are probably the most common adverse effects; central nervous system effects and sexual dysfunction are uncommon. Occasionally, angiodema of the face, mouth, or larynx has been described and may be life-threatening. ACE inhibitors should not be used during pregnancy.

Thus, ACE inhibitors are useful as monotherapy for patients with mild to moderate EH but are particularly useful in combination with low-dose thiazide-type diuretics. Patients with unilateral renal artery disease, chronic renal parenchymal disease, or chronic heart failure are logical candidates for ACE inhibitor treatment, but careful monitoring for adverse effects, such as hypotension, azotemia, or hyperkalemia, is required. The potential benefit of reduced progression of chronic renal failure must be weighed against the role of hyperkalemia and/or increased azotemia in patients with chronic renal failure. In general, patients with mild hyperkalemia or severe azotemia (serum creatinine level >8 mg/dl) have a high risk of complications during ACE inhibitor treatment. It is prudent to avoid ACE inhibitors with longer durations of action in patients with any severe underlying health problem (renal failure, liver disease, heart failure) since prolonged hypotension and/or hyperkalemia is more likely when they are used. There has been an increasing interest in the use of ACE inhibitors early in the course of acute myocardial infarction, particularly when evidence of left ventricular dysfunction develops.[37] There is no consensus about the indications for use of ACE inhibitors in this setting.

Calcium entry blockers. All of the calcium channel blockers reduce BP through vasodilation. Nifedipine is the most potent vasodilator and does not have significant cardiac electrophysiologic effects. For this reason, reflex tachycardia can be a problem when this agent or another agent in the dihydropyridine class is used alone or in combination with a diuretic to treat hypertensive patients. In contrast, verapamil reduces atrioventricular nodal conduction and produces little change or slight reduction in heart rate. Although some studies suggest that the efficacy of the calcium channel blockers is greater in blacks and older individuals (who tend to have low-renin hypertension), these associations have not been universally observed. The calcium channel blockers have been used as monotherapy or in combination with diuretics, β-blockers, and ACE inhibitors. In patients receiving nifedipine, β-blockers are particularly useful to prevent reflex tachycardia. However, there is some concern about the combined use of β-blockers and diltiazem or verapamil because of the potential for profound bradycardia when β-blockers are administered with these calcium channel blockers.

Calcium channel blockers are particularly useful in patients with high BP and angina pectoris, especially when absolute or relative contraindications to β-blocker treatment are present. However, bradyarrhythmias may occur with diltiazem or verapamil in patients with underlying cardiac conduction defects. In addition, verapamil and, possibly, diltiazem may reduce cardiac output and aggravate symptoms in patients with congestive heart failure. The protective effect of postinfarction β-blocker treatment is more clearly established when compared to the available evidence of a postinfarction benefit of calcium channel blocker. Experimental evidence of an antiatherosclerotic effect of certain channel blockers has been found, but the clinical relevance of these findings is currently unknown. The development of an effective "delivery system" for nifedipine has provided a substantial improvement in the clinical utility of this agent, which has proved to be a versatile antihypertensive agent.

Other antihypertensive agents

α-Blockers. Prazosin, terazosin, and doxazosin are selective α_1 antagonists that have been used alone or in combination with diuretics and other antihypertensive agents (Table 41-3). These agents reduce both preload and afterload and are effective in the treatment of congestive heart failure. The α_1-receptor blockers do not induce hyperglycemia, hypertriglyceridemia, hypercholesterolemia, hypokalemia, or hyperuricemia. In fact, a reduction in serum triglyceride and LDL-C level and an increase in HDL level have been shown in several studies. However, the effects are small and are not sufficient to justify the use of these agents for the specific purpose of lowering blood lipid levels. The most important side effect of the α_1-blockers is orthostatic hypotension. This is most likely to occur after the first dose and is most hazardous in elderly patients. Chronic orthostatic hypotension can be a problem, particularly in elderly individuals, those receiving diuretics, and those with autonomic neuropathy (such as diabetic patients) or severe lower extremity venous varicosities.

α- and β-Receptor antagonists. Labetalol was the first α-/β-blocker approved for treatment of hypertension and is a combined nonselective β-blocker and selective α_1-antagonist. It is available for oral and intravenous administration and is useful in treatment of all grades of severity of hypertension. This drug reduces BP by reducing peripheral vascular resistance (a manifestation of α_1-receptor blockade); heart rate and cardiac output do not change substantially because of the simultaneous β-blockade. Side effects and contraindications to labetalol are similar to those described for β-blockers; orthostatic hypotension can also be a problem because of the drug's α_1-blocking property. Raynaud's phenomenon and coldness of extremities occur much less frequently with this drug than with other β-blockers, and serum cholesterol and triglyceride levels do not change during labetalol monotherapy. Interestingly, labetalol monotherapy appears to be more effective than propranolol therapy in black patients and, possibly, elderly individuals. Despite the fact that labetalol tends to reduce afterload, it should be used with great caution, if at all, in cases of congestive heart failure. An initial 50- to 100-mg bedtime dose is reasonable in elderly individuals to minimize possible orthostatic hypotension. Maintenance doses generally range from 200 to 800 mg/day (given on a twice-daily basis), but doses as high as 2400 mg/day have been used.

Centrally acting sympatholytic agents. Clonidine, guanabenz, guanfacine,[27] and methyldopa are α_2-receptor agonists that lower BP mainly by reducing sympathetic efferent flow. These agents are effective as monotherapy but are usually given in combination with a diuretic. Diuretics reduce dose requirements of the centrally acting drugs; this effect undoubtedly reduces the frequency of lethargy, fatigue, and dry mouth that is commonly associated with these agents. The centrally acting agents usually do not induce important metabolic side effects. Methyldopa treatment has been shown to prevent left ventricular hypertrophy in rats with spontaneous hypertension and reverse left ventricular hypertrophy in hypertensive humans. This may be a property of all of the centrally acting sympatholytic agents, but the most convincing clinical evidence has been obtained with methyldopa. Therefore, monotherapy with methyldopa should be considered in a hypertensive patient with ECG or echocardiographic evidence of left ventricular hypertrophy. This is particularly true if cost is a major concern since generic preparations of methyldopa are available and should reduce the cost of drug treatment per se by 50% or more when compared to the cost of nongeneric preparations of most antihypertensive drugs. Epidemiologic evidence and data from treatment trials clearly demonstrate the adverse effect of left ventricular hypertrophy on cardiovascular mortality, and measures to prevent or reverse hypertrophy would appear to be reasonable.

However, a benefit of reducing left ventricular mass per se in reducing mortality has not been to date demonstrated.

Peripheral adrenergic antagonists. Reserpine, guanethidine, and guanadrel lower BP primarily through reduction in catecholamine availability in adrenergic synapses rather than via adrenergic receptor blockade. Reserpine is the least expensive nondiuretic antihypertensive agent and is effective and fairly well tolerated when used in low doses (0.1 to 0.2 mg/day) with a diuretic. Depression and other central nervous system side effects that were quite common when higher doses of reserpine were used occur much less frequently at low doses. Guanethidine and guanadrel do not usually cause central nervous system side effects unless orthostatic hypotension occurs, but diarrhea, impotence, and orthostatic hypotension (especially in the morning) can be problems. Guanadrel has a much shorter duration of action than guanethidine, therefore causing such side effects less frequently. Guanethidine can be given once daily, whereas guanadrel requires twice-daily administration. Tricyclic antidepressants and indirect acting sympathomimetics (ephedrine, phenylpropranolamine) can reverse the antihypertensive effects of guanethidine and guanadrel. Diuretics enhance their efficacy and prevent the fluid retention that can lead to pseudotolerance or edema when these agents are used alone. It is prudent to avoid guanethidine or guanadrel in patients with congestive heart failure because reduction of adrenergic support to the heart can aggravate heart failure. Even the newer agents in this class are more likely to cause bothersome side effects and have prompted united application of these agents as monotherapy for hypertensive drug therapy. The use of these drugs in a regimen for treatment of individuals with resistant hypertension is an appropriate clinical application of these agents. It is advisable to consider the issues reviewed in Table 41-3 before a diagnosis of truly drug resistant hypertension is applied.

Direct vasodilators. Hydralazine and minoxidil are the only available direct vasodilators approved for chronic treatment of hypertension. These agents are almost always used in combination with diuretics and adrenergic inhibitors to prevent vasodilator-induced fluid retention and reflex tachycardia. Minoxidil is a highly potent vasodilator, and loop diuretics are usually required to prevent edema. Hydralazine has been used as an afterload-reducing agent in patients with congestive heart failure. Although minoxidil is a more potent vasodilator, it is less useful in these patients because fluid retention and pleural and pericardial effusions are associated with its use. Minoxidil is generally reserved for treatment of patients with resistant hypertension. Hirsutism limits its use in women. Hydralazine may be useful as monotherapy or in combination with a diuretic in elderly hypertensive patients, particularly those with ischemic heart failure (ISH). In many of these individuals reflex tachycardia does not develop with vasodilators because of reduced baroreceptor sensitivity. However, low doses of hydralazine (10 mg twice daily) should be initiated because reflex tachycardia can occur and may induce myocardial ischemia. It is prudent to avoid use of hydralazine in patients with connective tissue disease because of the risk of hydralazine-induced autoantibody formation.

Goal setting in antihypertensive drug treatment

It is very easy to lose sight of the fact that hypertension is treated to prevent clinical events that are either directly caused by high blood pressure (pressure-related complications) or associated with complications of advanced atherosclerosis. In the former situation, the risks associated with moderate to severe hypertension are reduced substantially even if blood pressure is reduced to high normal levels chronically. In fact, overzealous acute reduction of blood pressure (i.e., administration of sublingual nifedipine to an asymptomatic patient with no evidence of target organ involvement and a BP of 210/120 mm Hg) may do more harm than good. In contrast, administration of an antihypertensive agent that alters carbohydrate or lipid metabolism for a period of years may increase the risk of development of symptomatic atherosclerotic cardiovascular disease even if excellent BP control is achieved. The critical issue is that there are no data from controlled clinical trials that provide convincing evidence to support the suggestions that are stated or implied in advertisements that mention "adverse metabolic complications or the risks of diuretics and/or β-blockers." The observation of borderline elevations of blood glucose, triglyceride, and/or cholesterol level after initiation of a diuretic does not necessarily mean that (1) the diuretic has caused the blood test abnormalities (they may be identical if the drug is stopped), (2) the risk for heart attack is increased, or (3) the results of the tests will be the same if they are repeated. The physician can use the observation of hypertriglyceridemia as a reason to reinforce the need for more exercise, weight loss, or other therapeutic maneuvers that contribute no additional cost and have the potential to produce additional BP-lowering effects, triglyceride-lowering effects, and other beneficial health effects that are unrelated to blood pressure or blood lipid levels. Reinforcement or further restriction of the dietary methods previously mentioned should also be considered if an inadequate blood pressure–lowering response to drug therapy is observed (see the box at right). It is not clear how much blood pressure lowering is sufficient or what the "J-curve" phenomenon noted in epidemiologic studies or certain controlled clinical trials of antihypertensive treatment actually means in terms of choosing a goal for long-term antihypertensive drug treatment.[9] The J-curve phenomenon represents the finding of higher mortality rate in individuals with the lowest blood pressure levels (for example, the lowest decile [10th percentile] of the distribution of BP values in the general population). A similar phenomenon has been reported in studies of the serum cholesterol–cardiovascular risk relationship.

Considerations when blood pressure response is inadequate

Nonadherence to therapy, which may be related to
  Cost of medication
  Unclear instructions or nonwritten instructions to the patient
  Inadequate or no patient education about diet or adherence to drugs
  Lack of patient involvement in the treatment plan
Clinical cues
  Patient complaint about high cost
  Lack of knowledge of names of drugs or when they are taken
  Patient failure to take medications to physician's office on repeated request
  Patient gains weight
  Patient cancels appointments, etc.
Drug-related causes
  Doses too low or reduced absorption in patients receiving a bile acid sequestrant*
  Inappropriate combinations (e.g., two centrally acting adrenergic inhibitors)
  Drug interactions
    Sympathomimetics
    Antidepressants
    Adrenal steroids
    Nonsteroidal antiinflammatory drugs
    Nasal decongestants
    Oral contraceptives
    Licorice-containing substances (e.g., chewing tobacco)
    Cocaine
    Cyclosporine
    Erythropoietin
Associated conditions
  Increasing obesity
  Alcohol intake more than 1 ounce of ethanol a day
  Renal insufficiency
  Renovascular hypertension
  Other secondary causes of hypertension
Volume Overload
  Inadequate diuretic therapy
  Excess sodium intake
  Fluid retention from reduction of blood pressure
  Progressive renal damage

---

*Particularly true of diuretics.

DIAGNOSIS AND EVALUATION OF HYPERCHOLESTEROLEMIA

One difference in the approach to evaluation and treatment of hypertension and hypercholesterolemia relates to the potential value of family history of high blood pressure or high blood lipid levels from a practical and a mechanistic standpoint.[16,21,22,25,26,41] A patient often knows something about the history of hypertension in a parent, sibling, or child, but much less often is aware of similar information about blood lipid levels. In addition to knowledge about the family history of these risk factors, information about history of cardiovascular events may be helpful. Although hypertension and hypercholesterolemia are both risk factors for cardiovascular diseases, the diseases that they lead to are somewhat different. For example, severe hypertension is a relatively common cause of hypertensive intracerebral hemorrhage. Severe hypercholesterolemia may be associated with a higher risk of stroke in general, but the excessive number of strokes would not be expected to be of the "hemorrhagic" variety.[41] Severe hypertension is a common cause of hypertensive left ventricular hypertrophy and/or failure and "hypertensive nephrosclerosis." The latter condition accounts for a major percentage of the population of African American patients with end-stage renal disease in the United States. Severe hypercholesterolemia does not cause left ventricular hypertrophy and is rarely accompanied by left ventricular failure in the absence of large vessel obstruction in the coronary arteries or ischemic infarction of left ventricular segments. There are, however, very difficult problems that arise during attempts to assign a hypertensive or atherosclerotic cause to an event that occurred in a family member (or even a patient) who experienced a clinical event that was considered cardiovascular in origin.

As previously stated, the currently recommended definitions of hypertension or hypercholesterolemia approximate the 75th percentile (upper quartile) of the population distribution of BP or serum TC levels in the adult population of the United States. When a BP or blood cholesterol level exceeding these levels is discovered in a community-based screening program, the intent is to confirm or not confirm the screening level in the medical practice setting. The subsequent evaluation of hypercholesterolemia in adults involves assessment of the general health status of the patient and determination of low-density-lipoprotein-cholesterol levels. The recommended classification of total cholesterol and LDL-cholesterol levels has been described (Table 41-2). The previous discussion of aspects of the history, physical examination, and laboratory assessment of the patient with hypertension is applicable to the evaluation of patients with hypercholesterolemia.

A simplified approach to the genotypic classification of "atherogenic dyslipidemias" divides hypercholesterolemia into two types: classic "familial" hypercholesterolemia (FH) and "nonfamilial" hypercholesterolemia. This classification is simple but ignores the fact that many patients with nonfamilial hypercholesterolemia probably have a range of genetic defects that contribute to the elevated blood cholesterol level. Other investigators have used the term "primary moderate" or "polygenic" hypercholesterolemia to describe these conditions. It is felt that genetic as well as environmental factors (e.g., diets high in saturated fats and cholesterol) contribute to the elevation in blood cholesterol levels observed in these individuals. In con-

trast, patients with heterozygous FH have approximately a 50% reduction in functional apoB-LDL receptors caused by the presence of a single-site mutation in the gene that encodes for synthesis of the apoB-LDL receptor.[16] Clinically, heterozygous FH is characterized by an autosomal dominant pattern of inheritance, severe hypercholesterolemia (total blood cholesterol blood levels typically above 350 mg/dl), tendinous xanthomas (see Fig. 41-5), and a very high incidence of premature CHD in patients and their first-degree relatives. It occurs in approximately 1 in 500 persons in the population. Another disorder, the "familial combined" hyperlipidemia syndrome is more common but is currently classified as a syndrome rather than a specific disease.[21] These individuals usually have mild to moderate elevations of serum cholesterol and/or triglyceride level, a fairly strong family history of premature coronary heart disease and/or lipid abnormalities in about 50% of their first-degree relatives. An increasing body of evidence also suggests involvement of a lipoprotein called lipoprotein (a) or "Lp(a)" in a familial disorder of lipoprotein metabolism. This disorder may account for 20% to 40% of what are now called "risk factor–negative" premature myocardial infarctions.[14] Individuals with high Lp(a) levels may not have high levels of either total cholesterol or triglyceride values (see the following discussion).

NCEP guidelines

Case finding versus screening. Serum total cholesterol level should be measured in all adults over age 20 at least once every 5 years; this measurement may be made in the nonfasting state.[38] Levels below 200 mg/dl are classified as "desirable blood cholesterol," levels of 200 to 239 mg/dl represent a "borderline-high blood cholesterol level" and levels exceeding 240 mg/dL are considered to be "high blood cholesterol level." The cutoff point that defines high blood cholesterol (240 mg/dl) is a value above which risk of CHD rises steeply; it corresponds approximately to the 75th percentile for adults in the U.S. population. The cutoff points currently recommended (in the first set of published NCEP guidelines) are uniform for adult men and women of all ages. Patients with desirable blood cholesterol levels (<200 mg/dl) should be given general dietary and risk reduction education materials and advised to have another serum cholesterol test within 5 years irrespective of where the blood test was obtained. Patients with cholesterol levels 200 mg/dl or greater should have the value confirmed by a repeat test; the average of the two test results is then used to guide subsequent decisions. Patients with a high blood cholesterol level (≥240 mg/dl) should undergo lipoprotein analysis, as should those with borderline-high blood cholesterol (200 to 239 mg/dl), who are at high risk because they have definite CHD or two other CHD risk factors (see Table 41-2). Individuals with confirmed borderline-high blood cholesterol levels who do not have CHD or two other risk factors need no further evaluation or active medical therapy; they should be given the dietary information designed for the general population and reevaluated after 1 year. There may be a place for measurement of HDL-C levels in community-based screening programs in the future, but improved precision and accuracy of HDL-C levels obtained on portable serum chemistry analyzers are required.

Evaluation. Once someone is identified as requiring lipoprotein analysis, the focus of attention should shift from total cholesterol to LDL-cholesterol level. The ultimate objective of case finding or screening is to identify individuals with elevated LDL-cholesterol levels. Similarly, the specific goal of treatment is to lower LDL-cholesterol levels. Hence, the level of LDL-cholesterol serves as the key index for clinical decision making about cholesterol-lowering therapy. As previously stated, lipoprotein analysis involves measurement of the fasting levels of total cholesterol, total triglyceride, and HDL-cholesterol.[51] LDL-cholesterol is calculated as follows:

LDL-cholesterol (LDL-C) =
 total cholesterol − (HDL-cholesterol [HDL-C] + triglyceride/5)

Levels of LDL-cholesterol of 160 mg/dl or greater are classified as "high-risk LDL-cholesterol," and those 130 to 159 mg/dl as "borderline-high-risk LDL-cholesterol." Patients with high-risk LDL-cholesterol levels and those with borderline-high-risk LDL-cholesterol levels who have definite CHD or two other risk factors (one of which can be male sex) should have a complete clinical evaluation and then begin cholesterol-lowering treatment. The clinical evaluation should include a complete history, physical examination, and basic laboratory tests. The most useful laboratory tests to be included in the evaluation of patients with hypercholesterolemia or other lipoprotein abnormalities are (1) fasting blood glucose, (2) thyroid-stimulating hormone, (3) alkaline phosphatase, (4) serum creatinine, (5) serum albumin level determinations, and (6) urinalysis. Most of the secondary dyslipoproteinemias are detected with these relatively inexpensive tests. Hypothyroidism, diabetes mellitus, and liver or renal disease should be excluded with these tests. The patient's total coronary risk and clinical status, as well as age and gender, should be considered in developing a cholesterol-lowering treatment program.

Genetic dyslipidemias associated with atherosclerosis

Familial hypercholesterolemia (FH). This is the prototype of a genetic dyslipidemia that is due to a single gene defect that results in failure to produce functionally active cell-surface receptors that normally bind and internalize the apoprotein B in LDL particles. The heterozygous form of familial hypercholesterolemia is present in approximately 0.2% of the U.S. population. The disease is transmitted as an autosomal dominant trait. Individuals who inherit one normal and one abnormal gene (heterozy-

gote) have only one half the normal number of LDL receptors and a twofold to threefold increase in circulating LDL-C level (usually in the 250 to 400 mg/dl range). Patients with the rare homozygous form of the disease have no functioning LDL receptors; massive hypercholesterolemia, accelerated atherosclerosis, and death occur during the first to third decades. Combined cardiac and liver transplantation has been used to treat these unfortunate patients. Although LDL receptor assays in fibroblasts and peripheral blood lymphocytes could probably be used to confirm the presence of an LDL receptor defect in patients with heterozygous familial hypercholesterolemia, results of these tests are usually not necessary to establish the diagnosis. These patients usually have at least two of the following triad of clues to the presence of heterozygous FH: (1) tendinous xanthomas (see Fig. 41-5), (2) LDL-C levels greater than 250 mg/dl, and (3) a family history of severe hypercholesterolemia and/or premature CHD in approximately 50% of the patient's first-degree relatives. It is important to screen relatives of patients with familial hypercholesterolemia for lipid abnormalities. The elevation in LDL-C level is apparent at birth (and should be two to three times the level of a normal neonate). In adults adequate treatment to lower LDL-C levels below approximately 200 mg/dl rarely occurs in the absence of lipid altering drug treatment.

Familial combined hyperlipidemia. Goldstein et al. proposed the designation familial combined hyperlipidemia (FCHL) to characterize families exhibiting multiple lipoprotein phenotypes (IIa, IIb, IV, and occasionally V) and premature CHD.[16] These investigators originally suggested that an autosomal dominant mode of inheritance was present in this syndrome as it is in familial hypercholesterolemia. Unfortunately, there is no unique marker for this syndrome, thus impairing the ability precisely to determine its prevalence or mode of inheritance. The diagnosis depends on finding elevated levels of total cholesterol, LDL-C, and/or triglycerides in affected patients and approximately 50% of their first-degree relatives. Multiple lipoprotein phenotypes are often observed in a single patient. In addition to the abnormalities of lipoprotein concentration, the composition of lipoproteins is often abnormal. Ten percent of patients less than 60 years old with myocardial infarction have FCHL.

Lipoprotein particles that are contained in the LDL ultracentrifugation range vary in size, density, and chemical composition. Patients with FCHL tend to have a higher percentage. The concentration of apoB in whole plasma is almost always increased, but the LDL-C level may be normal. Several lines of evidence suggest that there is an increased synthetic rate of hepatic apoB-containing lipoproteins. This could lead to simultaneous overproduction of LDL. However, the fractional catabolic rate of LDL tends to be high, so that LDL levels, and particularly LDL-C levels, may not increase. Thus in patients with FCHL,

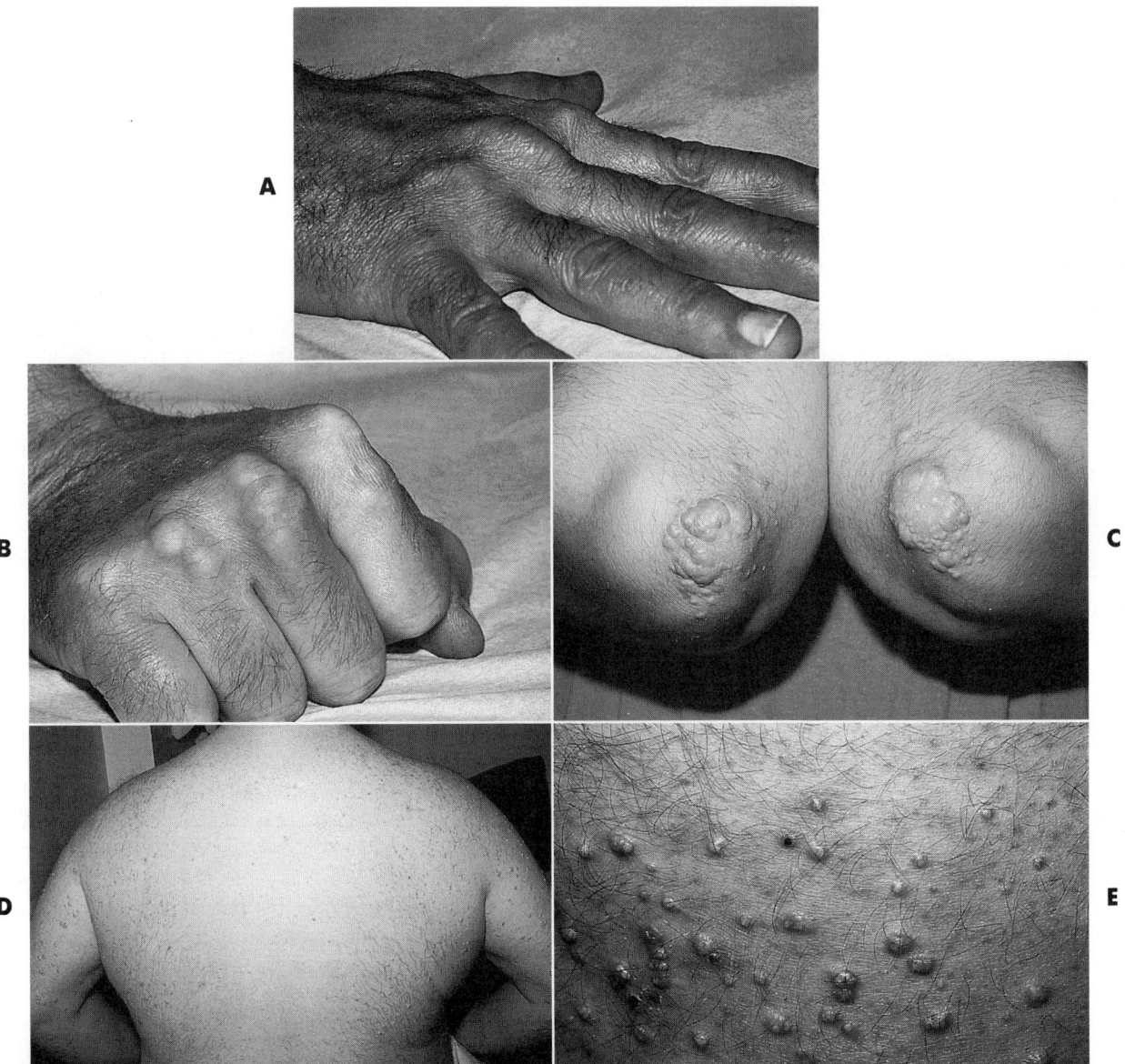

Fig. 41-5. Tendinous xanthomas, which are virtually diagnostic of heterozygous familial hyper-cholesterolemia in adults, may be present on extensor tendons of the hands, elbows, or "Achilles tendons." They are less prominent when the fingers are extended *(A)* than flexed *(B)*. Tendinous xanthomas do not involve the skin overlying these lesions. Patients with familial hypercholester-olemia may also have lesions that are cutaneous, due to lipid deposition and most commonly are observed on the skin overlying the elbows or knees *(C)*. These lesions, which are tuberous xan-thomas, also occur in patients with familial dysbetalipoproteinemia. These individuals do not de-velop tendinous xanthomas but occasionally have an "eruption" of cutaneous xanthomas. Severe hypertriglyceridemia is invariably present and accompanied by fasting hyperchylomicronemia. These lesions are more likely to occur in patients with an underlying phenotype V hyperlipopro-teinemia *(D and E)*. A dorsal rather than ventral location is also more comon in patients with eruptive xanthomas. The lesions usually have an erythematous base and a yellowish central core. They are frequently present in clusters of individual lesions that are 0.5 to 1.5 cm in diameter. Poorly controlled diabetes mellitus and hypothyroidism should be considered in patients who have eruptive xanthomas.

overproduction of apoB-containing lipoproteins, many of which are small, dense, and possibly highly atherogenic, appears to occur. A high percentage of these patients are overweight and may have an excellent response to weight loss. Nicotinic acid and gemfibrozil are particularly useful agents in hypertriglyceridemia patients with FCHL syndrome. However, LDL-C values may paradoxically increase during treatment with these agents. This is particularly true with gemfibrozil. When this occurs, addition of a bile-acid sequestrant is appropriate but may not be tolerated due to the gastrointestinal side effects of the bile acid sequestrants. One of the HMG-CoA reductase inhibitors could be substituted for the bile-acid sequestrant or be administered alone. The latter approach may be safer because of the increased risk of myositis when an HMG-CoA reductase inhibitor is added to gemfibrozil and niacin.[25]

Lipoprotein(a). Lipoprotein(a), or Lp(a), is an atherogenic lipoprotein structurally related to LDL. The lipid compositions of Lp(a) and LDL are similar, and both of these cholesterol-rich lipoproteins contain apoB. The presence of a glycoprotein, apo(a), that is covalently bound to apoB in the Lp(a) lipoprotein accounts for the distinct immunologic properties of Lp(a) when compared to LDL. Apo(a) may be responsible for the markedly reduced binding of Lp(a) by the hepatic LDL receptor. Lp(a) apparently is synthesized by the liver, but its route of catabolism is not known. Serum Lp(a) metabolism does not appear to be related to metabolism of other lipoproteins, and Lp(a) levels do not correlate with other lipoprotein levels.

Lp(a) levels are primarily under genetic control, with different Lp(a) glycoprotein phenotypes related to serum Lp(a) concentrations. The Lp(a) glycoprotein phenotypes associated with the highest Lp(a) levels are relatively uncommon in the population so that the frequency of distribution of Lp(a) levels is highly skewed, with higher frequencies of low Lp(a) values. This skewed distribution of Lp(a) levels has been observed in all Caucasian populations studied. Clinical laboratories do not routinely measure serum Lp(a) levels at this time, but it may be useful to include Lp(a) measurements in the evaluation of patients with significant atherosclerosis and no conventional cardiovascular risk factors. Commercially available "sandwich" enzyme linked immunosorbent assays (ELISA) methods to quantitate Lp(a) levels have been introduced but standardization of these assays has proved extraordinarily difficult.[54]

Secondary dyslipidemias

Obesity is commonly associated with a "clustering" of hypercholesterolemia, hypertriglyceridemia, and low HDL-C levels.[22,26] Hypertriglyceridemia and low HDL-C level are particularly common in individuals with hyperinsulinemia or glucose intolerance and, when detected, should prompt a careful assessment of glucose metabolism. Weight reduction may alleviate the lipid disorder, re-

duce fasting blood glucose levels, correct hyperinsulinemia, and decrease blood pressure. Upper body (android) obesity is of particular importance from the standpoint of coronary heart disease risk. Android obesity with a waist/hip ratio greater than 0.85 is associated with increased cardiovascular risk. Alcohol consumption contributes to obesity and may adversely affect lipoprotein metabolism, leading to elevations in triglyceride and VLDL levels even in the absence of obesity. Alcohol also may contribute to the development of hypertension and may further impair glucose tolerance.

CHD mortality rate is two to four times higher in diabetic than in nondiabetic individuals and is the main cause of death in patients with non–insulin dependent diabetes mellitus (NIDDM) or insulin-dependent diabetes mellitus (IDDM). Even mild abnormalities of glucose metabolism seem to be associated with an increased risk of CHD. Hypertriglyceridemia seems to be more common than an isolated elevation of LDL-C levels in diabetics. There is controversy regarding the role of high plasma triglyceride levels (the most common lipid abnormality in patients with diabetes) and CHD in general. The low HDL-C levels frequently observed in hypertriglyceridemic patients may contribute to or account for the increased risk. Structural alterations in VLDL and LDLs also occur and may cause certain subclasses of these lipoproteins to be particularly atherogenic in diabetics or nondiabetics. For example, hypertriglyceridemia may be a marker for the presence of increased levels of VLDL remnants or small, dense LDLs. Massive hypertriglyceridemia and chylomicronemia with eruptive xanthomas (Fig. 41-5, A-E), lipemia, retinalis, and chronic abdominal pain or pancreatitis occur in hypertriglyceridemic patients with poorly controlled diabetes mellitus. In treating the dyslipidemia of diabetes, achievement of ideal body weight and control of blood sugar with diet, oral hypoglycemics, and/or insulin often correct the underlying lipid disturbance. Lipid-lowering drug therapy should be used when good diabetic control alone is not effective in achieving "desirable" LDL-C levels.

In patients with hypothyroidism, TC, VLDL-C, and LDL-C levels may all be increased. The association of elevated cholesterol levels with hypothyroidism has been recognized for many years and has been used as an aid to the diagnosis of hypothyroidism in the past. In patients with "subclinical hypothyroidism" (elevated thyroid-stimulating hormone levels with normal thyroxine levels) hypercholesterolemia may also develop. Treatment of hypothyroidism with thyroid replacement usually improves or corrects the underlying abnormality. If a paradoxic elevation in LDL-C levels occurs after initiation of treatment with a bile acid sequestrant in a patient on thyroid replacement therapy consider the possibility that the bile acid sequestrant is binding the thyroid hormone supplement, thereby reducing absorption of the hormone and leading to a hypothyroid state.

A variety of abnormalities of lipoprotein concentration and/or composition occur in patients with chronic renal failure. Hypertriglyceridemia and low HDL-C level are the most frequently observed abnormalities. It is not certain that the abnormalities in lipoprotein metabolism contribute to the development or progression of atherosclerosis in patients with renal disease. Marked hypertriglyceridemia and/or hypercholesterolemia frequently occurs in patients with the nephrotic syndrome. Overproduction of apoB-containing lipoproteins by the liver apparently is the major cause of these abnormalities. There is also considerable controversy about the role of the dyslipoproteinemia of nephrotic syndrome in the development of atherosclerosis.

Physical manifestations of hyperlipidemias

During the physical examination several ocular and cutaneous abnormalities may suggest the presence of an abnormality of lipoprotein metabolism or suggest a specific genotypic or phenotypic dyslipidemic state. Xanthomas (yellow to gray plaques) on the eyelids and periorbital skin and corneal arcus (a light gray pigment deposition in the periphery of the cornea) are seen with increased frequency with aging and may be associated with presence of hypercholesterolemia. The presence of xanthomas and corneal arcus appears to be associated with an increased risk of developing ischemic heart disease in men less than 49 years of age. The clinical findings of xanthomas or corneal arcus, especially in younger patients, should serve as a reminder to assess lipid status and other cardiovascular risk factors. Lipemia retinalis, which is a salmon or creamy coloration of the retinal blood vessels, occurs with marked elevation of triglycerides to greater than 2500 mg/dl. These patients usually have fasting hyperchylomicronemia and phenotype V dyslipoproteinemia.

Cutaneous markers occur for lipoprotein disorders associated with the genetic forms of dyslipidemia and with the acquired disorders of triglyceride-rich lipoprotein metabolism (see Fig. 41-5). Deposition of lipids, lipoproteins, and their remnants in tissues close to the surface of the body causes xanthomas of various types. Recognition of these physical findings should lead to a complete lipoprotein evaluation and may allow the physician to recognize specific disease states. The type of skin lesion frequently correlates with the type of lipid or lipoprotein abnormality that is present. Eruptive xanthomas are reddish yellow, 1- to 4-mm dermal papules that are somewhat acniform in appearance. They are most commonly located on the extensor surface of the hands, arms, knees, and buttocks. When they first appear, they can be puritic and somewhat tender. In contrast, tendinous xanthomas are rarely puritic and rarely tender. Eruptive xanthomas usually occur in people with a secondary cause of hypercholesterolemia who have fasting hyperchylomicronemia. When a patient has a fasting blood serum triglyceride level that exceeds 1500 mg/dl, chylomicron remnants are nearly always present. Hyperchylomicronemia in adults is almost always associated with what was formerly called a phenotype V lipid abnormality. Phenotype V refers to the presence of chylomicrons in fasting blood in conditions of elevated concentrations of very-low-density lipoproteins. Whenever eruptive xanthomas are identified, it is imperative to rule out the presence of uncontrolled diabetes or untreated hypothyroidism. There are types of xanthomas that have some characteristics of the hard, firm tendinous xanthoma and some characteristics of an eruptive xanthoma. They are often called tuberoeruptive or tuberous xanthomas. They usually occur on the elbows, knees, and buttocks and less commonly in other areas. These patients almost always have high serum triglyceride levels and high LDL values, at least when the LDL is calculated by the formulas that are now generally used in clinical practice.

When a physician encounters a patient with formerly normal blood cholesterol and triglyceride levels who suddenly has serum cholesterol and triglyceride values in the 300 to 400 mg/dl range, a diagnosis of "familial dysbetalipoproteinemia" or phenotype III dyslipoproteinemia should be entertained. If a pure appearing tendinous xanthoma with no other overlying skin changes is present, the patient probably has heterozygous familial hypercholesterolemia and high triglyceride level. In contrast, if the hand is examined and found to contain yellow to orange appearing discoloration in the creases in the palms and fingers, the patient probably has what are called palmar crease xanthomas. These are associated with familial dysbetalipoproteinemia or phenotype III dyslipoproteinemia. In general, a patient who is less than 50 years of age with relatively severe hypercholesterolemia and hypertriglyceridemia and a history of coronary heart disease probably has heterozygous familial hypercholesterolemia. The reason for this is that heterozygous FH is inherited, has a very high degree of penetrance, and the appearance of the lipid abnormality occurs at an early stage in life. In contrast, in patients with "familial dysbetalipoproteinemia," who may also have severe hypercholesterolemia and hypertriglyceridemia, lipid problems usually do not develop until later in life or until another condition such as diabetes mellitus or hypothyroidism occurs. The other conditions that can cause a secondary form of hypercholesterolemia have dyslipidemic states that have an uncertain relationship to the risk of development of CHD. These conditions include obstructive liver disease, chronic renal insufficiency, and nephrotic syndrome. It is certainly true that patients with chronic renal disease have a high incidence of subsequent cardiovascular disease, but the role of lipids and lipoproteins in this process is still under investigation.

Drug treatment of hypercholesterolemia (Table 41-4)

Bile acid sequestrants. Cholestyramine and colestipol selectively lower LDL-C levels by increasing the clearance of LDL. These agents bind bile acids in the gut; this leads

Table 41-4. Drug treatment of hypercholesterolemia

Type of drug	Usual dosage range (total/day)	Frequency (per day)	Comments
Bile acid sequestrants			Anticipated side effects
Cholestyramine	8-24 g	2-3 Times*	Bloating
Colestipol	10-30 g	2-3 Times*	Midepigastric fullness or pain
			Constipation (may be decreased by adding 3-4 g psyllium to each dose of resin)
			Tolerance increased by slow upward dose titration
			Avoidance of high doses
			Possible binding of other agents including antihypertensive agents; in general, give other drugs at least 1 hour before or 4 hours after resin
			Avoid with serum triglyceride levels >400 mg/dl unless gemfibrozil or niacin is also given
Nicotinic acid	1000-6000 mg	2-3 Times	Anticipated side effects
			Flushing—especially with regular crystalline niacin preparations; usually diminishes with time, administration with food, and/or addition of low-dose aspirin
			Gastrointestinal distress/dyspepsia—probably more common with slow release preparations and may represent early symptoms of chemical hepatitis
			May cause itching, headache, insomnia, recurrence of gout, unmasking of glucose intolerance, or diabetes mellitus; may cause toxic amblyopia, acanthosis nigricans, dry skin, or myositis (particularly when combined with an HMG CoA reductase inhibitor)
Gemfibrozil	1200 mg	2 Times	Most potent and consistently effective triglyceride-lowering agent, tends to increase HDL-C level and reduce LDL-C level by 10%-20%; seems to be more effective in reduced primary CHD risk in hypertriglyceridemic patients with high LDL-C/HDL-C ratios than predicted by its LDL-C lowering effect
HMG CoA reductase			Capable of lowering LDL-C by 35%-45% in high percentage of patients
inhibitors	20-80 mg	1 Time	Side effects infrequent, liver enzyme elevations frequently occur but are
Lovastatin	10-40 mg	1 Time	of questionable significance, liver function testing still recommended
Pravastatin	5-40 mg	1 Time	but of questionable usefulness (except for medicolegal reasons)
Simvastatin			Mainly lowers LDL-C level; modest elevation of HDL-C level and reduction of serum triglyceride level also occur
			Do not cause cataracts; most feared side effect is myositis, which is rare except when used with niacin, gemfibrozil, cyclosporine, or possibly erythromycin
			Most cost-effective use may be in high-risk patients, addition of low-dose resin therapy may be particularly effective.
Probucol	1000 mg	2 Times	Lowers HDL-C levels—the effect of this property on risk is unknown
			Has antioxidant properties—theoretically beneficial but clinically untested
			Avoid in patients with prolonged Q-T interval

*May be given as a single dose at bedtime (1-2 scoops or packets). Daytime doses should be given before meals. HMG CoA, Hydroxy methylglutaryl coenzyme A.

to increased conversion of hepatic cholesterol to bile acids and reduction of intercellular cholesterol in the liver. Stimulation of LDL receptor synthesis, leading to enhanced clearance of LDL from the blood, occurs. The bile acid binding resins can produce bothersome gastrointestinal side effects (bloating, abdominal pain, and constipation), but because they are not absorbed, serious systemic side effects are infrequent. Constipation can be a major problem for older adults, particularly if other drugs are being taken that cause constipation. Gastrointestinal side effects can be minimized by mixing the resin with a pulpy noncarbonated beverage, increasing fluid and dietary fiber intake,

and increasing the dose slowly. The bile acid sequestrants should be administered with meals or before bedtime.

Because bile acid sequestrants may increase triglyceride levels, they should be avoided by patients with triglyceride levels above 500 mg/dl. Bile acid binding resins may reduce the absorption of several drugs; therefore, other drugs should be administered at least 1 hour before or several hours after the ingestion of the resins. Cholestyramine is available in 4-g packets and bulk containers; colestipol is available in 5-g packets and bulk containers. The bulk containers are less expensive than the individual packets. The dosage of cholestyramine ranges from 4 to 24 g/day;

that of colestipol from 5 to 30 g/day. It may be helpful to add a psyllium preparation to the resin to reduce constipation. The bile acid sequestrants are a good choice for initial treatment in patients who are greatly concerned about serious side effects of medications. Because of their safety profile, these drugs are favored for young patients who may require treatment for decades. Cholestyramine and gemfibrozil are the only lipid-lowering drugs that have been shown to reduce the incidence of fatal and nonfatal coronary heart disease in hypercholesterolemic adults.[11,32] The bile acid sequestrants have also been included in most of the angiographic studies subsequently described.[29] The use of a single bedtime dose of one to two scoops or packets of colestipol or cholestyramine frequently achieves 10% to 20% reduction in LDL-C level and is much more acceptable than higher doses of these agents.

Nicotinic acid. Nicotinic acid has been used for more than three decades to treat patients with lipoprotein abnormalities.[25] Nicotinic acid reduces TC, TG, and LDL-C levels and increases HDL-C levels. Although cutaneous and gastrointestinal side effects may occur, nicotinic acid is a good first choice drug for most hypercholesterolemic patients. Exceptions include those with poorly controlled diabetes, peptic ulcer disease, chronic liver disease, and recurrent gouty arthritis. Cutaneous flushing is common with nicotinic acid, particularly early in the course of therapy. To reduce this effect, the patient can increase the dose slowly, take the drug with meals, or precede the dose with aspirin. A slow release preparation may also be helpful in this regard. Several over-the-counter slow-release niacin preparations are available and are relatively inexpensive (i.e., a 2000-mg dosage regimen should cost about $10 a month). The regular release formulations are even less expensive. Although slow-release nicotinic acid helps prevent flushing, these preparations cause a higher incidence of hepatitis than regular-release forms.[28] It is prudent to measure fasting blood glucose and liver transaminase levels before and after 6 to 12 weeks of niacin treatment. Nicotinic acid can also cause acanthosis nigricans, toxic amblyopia, or myositis, but these complications are uncommon.

Nicotinic acid is, in certain respects, the "thiazide diuretic" of the lipid-lowering drugs. In our lipid management clinic, we have found the use of printed instructions describing methods to reduce the flushing that occurs early in the course of niacin treatment to be very helpful. We provide a toll-free phone number for the manufacturer of a niacin preparation. Niacin can be ordered from the manufacturer by the patient, and the drug sent directly to the patient at a cost of about $5 per month for a niacin dose of 1000 mg twice daily. We generally encourage selection of regular niacin tablets because of the concerns about slow-release-niacin-induced hepatitis. The key points to cover in a set of instructions are that flushing is a normal response to niacin and is not an allergy; that administration of a

small dose of aspirin may reduce the flushing induced by niacin and is probably a reasonable recommendation for prevention of coronary heart disease because of its controlled clinical trials; that niacin should be taken with meals; and that ingestion of hot beverages should be avoided at the time of niacin administration. We suggest an initial dose of 100 mg twice a day and instruct the patients to add 100 mg to the previous niacin dose at intervals of every 3 days. We generally limit the total daily dose of niacin to approximately 1600 mg/day in women and 2000 mg/day in men in part because of the smaller body mass in women.

Niacin can impair glucose tolerance in people who are "prediabetic" or inadequately controlled diabetics. Whether hyperinsulinemia has an adverse effect on coronary heart disease risk is unclear; however, hyperinsulinemia is clearly a common component of clinical syndromes characterized by the "clustering phenomenon." This clustering frequently includes hypertension, hyperinsulinemia, glucose intolerance, and male pattern obesity. Postmenopausal women appear to be a high-risk subset of adults for development of glucose intolerance, hypertriglyceridemia, and/or hypertension. The perimenopausal period is frequently accompanied by flushing, which may be more likely to occur in women who are receiving niacin. In contrast, middle-aged men with a history of documented coronary artery disease are usually excellent candidates for niacin treatment. A survival benefit appeared to follow administration of niacin treatment in the Coronary Drug Project, which was used in combination with a bile acid sequestrant in the Familial Atherosclerosis Treatment Study (FATS).[4] Niacin was also combined with colestipol in the Cholesterol-Lowering Atherosclerosis Study (CLAS), reported by Blackenhorn and coworkers.[3] The FATS and CLAS studies have convincingly demonstrated that patients with coronary artery disease and hypercholesterolemia frequently have demonstrable progression of atherosclerosis during as brief a period as 2 years. In addition, data from the CLAS Study using colestipol and nicotinic acid and data from the FATS study that evaluated either a bile acid sequestrant and niacin or a bile acid sequestrant and lovastatin provide very convincing evidence that aggressive cholesterol-lowering treatment slows progression of established coronary artery disease. There is also some evidence of atherosclerotic regression, but this aspect of these studies has probably been overemphasized. It is important to point out that the degree of regression found in these trials is extremely small and has generally been in the 10% range, a range that is barely detectable by visual inspection. Thus, patients who strongly desire initiation of lipid-altering treatment as a means to avoid a surgical procedure must be aware that regression of atherosclerosis during cholesterol-lowering treatment is probably the exception rather than the rule. All of the available evidence suggests that the ability to delay progression of atherosclerosis has some relation to the extent of cholesterol-lowering treatment. Although precise estimates of the goal of therapy cannot be stated with certainty at this time, it seems reasonable to attempt to reduce the LDL/HDL-C ratio to less than 3 and perhaps even to less than 2 in the subset of hypercholesterolemic patients with established coronary artery disease.

Fibric acid derivatives. Clofibrate and gemfibrozil are the only fibric acid derivatives that have been used to any great extent in the United States. Clofibrate is used infrequently because of concerns about long-term toxicity that emerged from several previous clinical trials. In contrast, gemfibrozil was shown to be effective and safe in the Helsinki Heart Study.[11] The fibric acid derivatives have several effects on lipoprotein metabolism. They increase cholesterol excretion into the bile, probably accounting for the lithogenic effect of these drugs. They also stimulate lipoprotein lipase activity, which increases the fractional catabolic rate of triglyceride-rich lipoproteins. Gemfibrozil is a potent triglyceride-lowering agent, reducing triglyceride levels by approximately 40%. The fibric acid derivatives and nicotinic acid are the most effective drugs in the management of patients with phenotype V hyperlipoproteinemia (characterized by fasting chylomicronemia and elevated VLDL-C levels). In the Helsinki Heart Study, total cholesterol and LDL-C levels were reduced by approximately 10% while HDL-C levels were increased 10%.[11] The LDL-C reducing efficacy of these drugs is lower in patients with hypertriglyceridemia, and a paradoxic increase in LDL-C levels is not unusual in these patients. However, participants with phenotype IIB hyperlipidemia had the greatest gemfibrozil association coronary risk reflection in the Helsinki Heart Study.[11] A subset analysis of participants with serum triglyceride levels above 200 mg/dl and LDL-C/HDL-C ratios above 5 appeared to have a 70% reduction in coronary heart disease risk.

Gastrointestinal disturbances resulting from gemfibrozil occur in 5% to 10% of patients and are most common early in treatment. Serious toxicity from gemfibrozil is unusual, but this agent and clofibrate should not be used in patients with cholelithiasis. Routine monitoring of blood chemical levels for evidence of systemic toxicity is not required. Gemfibrozil is available in 600-mg tablets; the usual dose is 600 mg twice daily. Gemfibrozil is a convenient agent to use, and although the current cost of treatment is fairly high (approximately $70 to $80 per month), it is usually is not prohibitive. The fact that gemfibrozil was shown to be effective in the Helsinki Heart Study should not be trivialized since the trial had a scientifically valid design, specific objectives, and the same goals as lipid-altering treatment.

HMG-CoA reductase inhibitors. Lovastatin, pravastatin, and simvastatin are the three currently available HMG-CoA reductase inhibitors. These agents reduce activity of HMG-CoA reductase, which is the rate-limiting enzyme in endogenous cholesterol synthesis. Reduction of intracellular cholesterol synthesis in the liver leads to depletion of intracellular cholesterol concentration, stimulation of LDL receptor synthesis, and increased clearance of LDL from the circulation. The production of apoprotein B–containing lipoproteins may also be reduced. These agents reduce LDL-C levels by up to 40% to 50%,[40] and produce a modest reduction in triglyceride levels and slight increase in HDL-C levels. Side effects of the HMG-CoA reductase inhibitors are uncommon. Gastrointestinal complaints develop in about 5% of patients and usually occur early in treatment. Elevated liver transaminase levels occur in less than 2% of patients. It is not clear whether the newer agents cause hepatic dysfunction more or less often than lovastatin. In fact, there is more convincing evidence that a 20-mg daily dose of lovastatin does not cause persistent elevation of liver transaminase levels more frequently than placebo does. It is not clear whether the elevation of liver transaminase levels that occurs during treatment with lovastatin or other HMG-CoA reductase inhibitors actually represents an effect of these agents, a response to reducing cholesterol levels per se, or the patient's recent use of alcohol or other potential hepatotoxins. Although studies in dogs and early clinical trials with lovastatin suggested that this drug causes cataracts, clinical trial data do not support this effect. Diffuse muscle pain and marked elevation in (CPK) levels occur in approximately 0.5% of patients treated with lovastatin alone. The incidence of myositis is increased three- to five-fold in patients receiving nicotinic acid or gemfibrozil in combination with lovastatin. The incidence of rhabdomyolysis in patients receiving the combination of lovastatin, gemfibrozil, and cyclosporine may be as high as 30%.

The usual dose ranges for lovastatin, pravastatin, and simvastatin are 20 to 80 mg/day, 10 to 40 mg/day, and 5 to 40 mg/day, respectively. There may be subtle differences in the side effect profiles of these three approved HMG-CoA reductase inhibitors, but they are probably not substantial. One difference is that there have been no reported cases of rhabdomyolysis with the combination of either gemfibrozil or nicotinic acid plus pravastatin. However, caution should still be exercised when consideration is given to the use of any HMG-CoA reductase inhibitor/gemfibrozil or nicotinic acid regimen. The most easily definable indication for an HMG-CoA reductase inhibitor is in the management of familial hypercholesterolemia. Because of the LDL cholesterol values in affected individuals, 50% reductions of LDL-C concentration are required to achieve adequate LDL-C values. In addition, an increasingly strong case can be made for the use of an HMG-CoA reductase inhibitor alone or in combination with a bile acid sequestrant in individuals with established coronary artery disease.[4] There is no evidence that the combination of an HMG-CoA reductase inhibitor and a bile acid resin is any better than the combination of a bile acid binding resin and nicotinic acid, but the former regimen is almost certainly easier to tolerate.

The most significant difficulty in assigning the cost-effectiveness potential of lipid-altering treatment with an HMG-CoA reductase inhibitor occurs when individuals have only a small or mild increase in risk of premature coronary artery disease. A good way to illustrate this point is to examine the estimated number of heart attacks that actually occur in individuals with a different risk status (Figure 41-4). The risk of experiencing a heart attack in women below the age of 45 is so small that it would be almost impossible to reduce this risk by lowering blood cholesterol levels. This is certainly true when considering women as a group but does not exclude the possibility that a woman with heterozygous familial hypercholesterolemia who is a smoker and has high blood pressure would benefit from cholesterol-lowering treatment. However, as a group, low-risk individuals are not ideal candidates for aggressive treatment of hypercholesterolemia with expensive drugs. It is instead the high-risk individuals who probably have the best chance of achieving cost-effective reduction of coronary risk through interventions that include pharmacologic lipid-lowering intervention. One should consider the use of HMG-CoA reductase inhibitors with respect to age as well as presence of several risk factors for coronary disease (Figures 41-3 and 41-4). Considering these general guidelines may be more appropriate than defining specific subsets of the population who should or should not receive a specific cholesterol-lowering or any other pharmacologic agent.

Probucol and other potential lipid-altering agents. It may be reasonable to consider probucol in a category of agents that includes vitamins C and E, since both probucol and these vitamins probably represent orally active lipid-altering agents that are lipoprotein antioxidants.[23] There is convincing evidence in experimental models of atherosclerosis that oxidized lipoproteins cause several toxic effects. These effects include cytoxicity to endothelial cells and migration and proliferation of smooth muscle cells and other cellular components of the atherosclerotic lesion. It is difficult to ascribe a precise place for probucol or any of the antioxidants in a lipid-lowering treatment algorithm, but they are certainly not first-step agents.[25] Studies currently in progress may give more convincing evidence for a beneficial effect of probucol or another antioxidant in the treatment of atherosclerosis in humans, but presently there is not sufficient information to justify any specific recommendations.

Other agents that have been proposed as useful in preventing coronary heart disease in certain subsets of the population include estrogen administered to postmenopausal women,[7] fish oil supplements,[18] and triglyceride-lowering agents in general.[41] The preventive effect of triglyceride-lowering therapy is useful to consider within the context of a "hypercoagulable state." It should be recognized that there is considerable evidence that hemostatic factors have some relation to the paradoxic difference in the risk of stroke and coronary heart disease.[15] It is possible that the use of fish oil as a triglyceride-lowering agent could reduce the risk of stroke or myocardial infarction through an antiplatelet effect. There is evidence that postprandial hyperlipemia (which is largely due to elevated levels of serum triglyceride levels) is in fact a situation that induces hypercoagulability, at least in certain individuals. There is a considerable amount of information that needs to be learned about the therapeutic use of antithrombotic/antiplatelet agents in the preventive therapy of patients with risk factors for coronary heart disease. It is interesting to recall that the markedly beneficial effect of low-dose aspirin initially reported from the Physicians' Health Study[53] was subsequently found to be offset by an increased risk of hemorrhagic stroke in physicians randomized to the low-dose aspirin group. It is not difficult to imagine the dangers that could occur if individuals ingested over-the-counter fish oil supplements and used aspirin to prevent heart attack while neglecting to control hypertension. Poor control of hypertension during antiplatelet or antithrombotic treatment could result in an increased risk for stroke. Information about these kinds of agents can be difficult to interpret, yet early media release and widespread dissemination of data can lead to premature application to the general population. Recognizing the uncertainty of aspirin's effectiveness in specific subsets of the population, recommending the use of 80 mg per day or 160 mg every other day appears reasonable as a preventive intervention for most individuals, if no contraindication to aspirin exists. The risk/benefit ratio for aspirin probably favors its use in males compared to premenopausal women because of the comparatively increased risk for myocardial infarction in males. Aspirin use needs to be individualized in females.

SUMMARY

There seems to be considerably less danger in recommending that efforts continue in areas such as encouragement of health promotion in children.[45] We should continue to encourage physicians to utilize the "coronary risk profile" carefully to assess and detect risk factors for coronary disease.[2] We need to continue to scrutinize the advantages and disadvantages of performing cholesterol screenings in the community[5] and not relax our efforts to utilize nonpharmacologic approaches to the control of high blood pressure. The possibility that blood pressure can be reduced to too low a level is certainly a reality, particularly in the acute setting. However, whether or not there is any real danger in careful utilization of a stepped care approach to antihypertensive drug treatment because of pharmacologic reduction of elevated blood pressure levels is still highly debatable. There is still much to be learned about the potential costs and effectiveness of lowering cholesterol levels in the elderly.[13] However, older individuals have a much higher risk of development of acute coronary heart disease events and thus have a greater potential benefit from cholesterol-lowering therapy that would occur in a much briefer period than in younger individuals. In fact, there is so little information that use of the newer cholesterol-lowering agents causes significant toxicity that the cost-effectiveness issue probably has more relevance to the cost of drugs and the effectiveness of lowering risk than it does to the induction of a new risk imposed by drug treatment per se. There will probably never be another 2 year period that will see such a soaring increase in the use of cholesterol-lowering treatment as there was in the late 1980s.[52] However, the experience gained during this time places us on a different area of the learning curve and certainly provides some potential for physicians to consider the possibility that the favorable trends in reduction of coronary heart disease in the United States will continue.

REFERENCES

1. Ames RP: The effects of antihypertensive drugs on serum lipids and lipoproteins. II. Non-diuretic drugs, *Drugs* 32:335-357, 1986.
2. Anderson KM et al: An updated coronary risk profile: a statement for health professionals, *Circulation* 83(1):356-362, 1991.
3. Blankenhorn DH et al: Beneficial effects of combined colestipol-niacin therapy on atherosclerosis and coronary venous bypass grafts, *JAMA* 257:3233-3240, 1987.
4. Brown G et al: Regression of coronary artery disease as a result of intensive lipid-lowering therapy in men with high levels of apolipoprotein B, *N Engl J Med* 323:1289-1298, 1990.
5. Bush TL et al: Screening for total cholesterol: do the National Cholesterol Education Program's recommendations detect individuals at high risk of coronary heart disease? *Circulation* 83:1287-1293, 1991.
6. Castelli WP, Anderson K: A population at risk: prevalence of high cholesterol levels in hypertensive patients in the Framingham study, *Am J Med* 80:23-32, 1986.
7. Crook D et al: Comparison of transdermal and oral estrogen-progestin replacement therapy: effects on serum lipids and lipoproteins, *Am J Obstet Gynecol* 166:950-955, 1992.
8. Final Report of the Subcommittee on Nonpharmacological Therapy of the 1984 Joint National Committee on Detection, Evaluation, and Treatment of High Blood Pressure: Nonpharmacological approaches to the control of high blood pressure, *Hypertension* 8:444-467, 1986.
9. Fletcher AE, Bulpitt CJ: How far should blood pressure be lowered? *Curr Concepts* 326(4):251-254, 1992.
10. Fletcher GF et al: Benefits and recommendations for physical activity programs for all Americans: a statement for health professionals by the Committee on Exercise and Cardiac Rehabilitation of the Council on Clinical Cardiology, American Heart Association, *Circulation* 86(1):340-344, 1992.
11. Frick MH et al: Helsinki Heart Study: primary-prevention trial with gemfibrozil in middle-aged men with dyslipidemia, *N Engl J Med* 317:1237-1245, 1987.
12. Friedewald WT, Levy RI, Fredrickson DS: Estimation of the concentration of low density lipoprotein cholesterol in plasma, without use of the preparative ultracentrifuge, *Clin Chem* 18:499-502, 1972.
13. Garber AM et al: Costs and health consequences of cholesterol screening for asymptomatic older Americans, *Arch Intern Med* 151:1089-1095, 1991.
14. Genest J Jr et al: Prevalence of lipoprotein(a) [Lp(a)] excess in coronary artery disease, *Am J Cardiol* 67:1039-1045, 1991.
15. Gliksman M, Wilson A: Are hemostatic factors responsible for the paradoxical risk factors for coronary heart disease and stroke? *Stroke* 23:607-610, 1992.
16. Goldstein JL, Schrott HG, Hazzard WR: Hyperlipidemia in coronary heart disease. II. Genetic analysis of lipid levels in 176 families and delineation of a new inherited disorder combined hyperlipidemia, *J Clin Invest* 52:1544-1568, 1973.
17. Gordon DJ et al: High-density lipoprotein cholesterol and cardiovascular disease: four prospective American studies, *Circulation* 79:8-15, 1989.
18. Gorlin R: The biological actions and potential clinical significance of dietary omega-3 fatty acids, *Arch Intern Med* 148:2043-2048, 1988.
19. Greenberg G, Brennan PJ, Miall WE: Effects of diuretic and beta-blocker therapy in the Medical Research Council Trial, *Am J Med* 76:45-51, 1984.
20. Grimm RH Jr, Leon AS, Hunninghake DB: Effects of thiazide diuretics on plasma lipids and lipoproteins in mildly hypertensive patients: A double-blind controlled trial, *Ann Intern Med* 94:7-11, 1981.
21. Grundy SM, Chait A, Brunzell JD: Familial combined hyperlipidemia workshop, *Arteriosclerosis* 7:203-207, 1987.
22. Haffner SM et al: Clustering of cardiovascular risk factors in confirmed prehypertensive individuals, *Hypertension* 20:38-45, 1992.
23. Harats D et al: Effect of vitamin C and E supplementation on susceptibility of plasma lipoproteins to peroxidation induced by acute smoking, *Atherosclerosis* 85:47-54, 1990.
24. Helgeland A: The impact on serum lipids of combinations of diuretics and β-blockers and of β-blockers alone, *J Cardiovasc Pharmacol* 6:S474-S476, 1984.
25. Hoeg JM, Gregg RE, Brewer HB Jr: An approach to the management of hypercholesterolemia, *JAMA* 255:512-521, 1986.
26. Hubert HB et al: Life-style correlates of risk factor change in young adults: an eight-year study of coronary heart disease risk factors in the Framingham offspring, *Am J Epidemiol* 125:812-831, 1987.
27. Kiechel JR: Pharmacokinetics and metabolism of guanfacine in man: a review, *Br J Clin Pharmacol* 10:25S-32S, 1980.
28. Knopp RH et al: Contrasting effects of unmodified and time-released forms of niacin on lipoproteins in hyperlipidemic subjects: clues to mechanism of action of niacin, *Metabolism* 34:642-647, 1985.
29. LaRosa JC: Cholesterol-lowering as a treatment for established coronary heart disease, *Circulation* 85(3):1229-1235, 1992.
30. Lasser NL et al: Effects of antihypertensive therapy on plasma lipids and lipoproteins in the multiple risk factor intervention trial, *Am J Med* 76:52-66, 1984.
31. Levy D et al: Stratifying the patient at risk from coronary disease: new insights from the Framingham Heart Study, *Am Heart J* 119:712-717, 1990.
32. Lipid Research Clinic's Program: The Lipid Research Clinic's Coronary Primary Prevention Trial results. I. Reduction in the incidence of coronary heart disease, *JAMA* 251:351-364, 1984.
33. Martin MJ et al: Serum cholesterol, blood pressure, and mortality: implications from a cohort of 361,662 men, *Lancet* 2:933-936, 1986.
34. Multiple Risk Factor Intervention Trial Research Group: Multiple risk factor intervention trial: risk factor changes and mortality results, *JAMA* 248:1465-1477, 1982.
35. National High Blood Pressure Education Program. The 1984 Report of the Joint National Committee on Detection, Evaluation, and Treatment of High Blood Pressure: (U.S. Department of Health and Human Services, National Heart, Lung, and Blood Institute), NIH Publication No 84-1088, June 1984. (The entire report was published originally in *Arch Intern Med* 144:1984, and in *J Am Osteopat Assoc* 83:1984.)
36. Neaton JD, Wentworth D: Serum cholesterol, blood pressure, cigarette smoking, and death from coronary heart disease, *Arch Intern Med* 152:56-64, 1992.
37. Pfeffer MA et al: Effect of captopril on mortality and morbidity in patients with left ventricular dysfunction after myocardial infarction, *N Engl J Med* 327:669-677, 1992.
38. Report of the National Cholesterol Education Program Expert Panel

on Detection, Evaluation, and Treatment of High Blood Cholesterol in Adults, *Arch Intern Med* 148:36-80, 1988.

39. Report of the Joint National Committee on Detection, Evaluation and Treatment of High Blood Pressure: The fifth report of the joint national committee on detection, evaluation, and treatment of high blood pressure, (JNC V) *Arch Intern Med* 153:154-183, 1993.

40. Shear CL et al: Expanded clinical evaluation of lovastatin (EXCEL) study results: effect of patient characteristics on lovastatin-induced changes in plasma concentrations of lipids and lipoproteins, *Circulation* 85:1293-1303, 1992.

41. Simpson HCR et al: Hypertriglycerideaemia and hypercoagulability, *Lancet* 786-789, 1983.

42. Sox HC Jr, Littenberg B, Garber AM: The role of exercise testing in screening for coronary artery disease, *Ann Intern Med* 110:456-469, 1989.

43. Stamler R et al: Higher blood pressure in adults with less education: some explanations from INTERSALT, *Circulation* 19(3):237-241, 1992.

44. Stamler J, Wentworth D, Neaton JD: Prevalence and prognostic significance of hypercholesterolemia in men with hypertension: prospective data on the primary screenees of the Multiple Risk Factor Intervention Trial, *Am J Med* 80:33-36, 1986.

45. Strong WB et al: Integrated cardiovascular health promotion in childhood: a statement for health professionals from the subcommittee on atherosclerosis and hypertension in childhood of the council on cardiovascular disease in the young, American Heart Association, *Circulation* 85(4):1638-1650, 1992.

46. Tanaka N et al: Effect of chronic administration of propranolol on lipoprotein composition, *Metabolism* 25:1071-1075, 1976.

47. The 1988 Report of the Joint National Committee on Detection, Evaluation and Treatment of High Blood Pressure, *Arch Intern Med* 148:1023-1038, 1988.

48. Veterans Administration Cooperative Study Group on Antihypertensive Agents: Comparison of propranolol and hydrochlorothiazide for the initial treatment of hypertension. II. Results of long-term therapy, *JAMA* 248:2004-2011, 1982.

49. Weinberger MH: Antihypertensive therapy and lipids: evidence, mechanisms, and implications, *Arch Intern Med* 145:1102-1105, 1985.

50. Williams RR, Hunt SC, Hopkins PN: Familial dyslipidemic hypertension: evidence from 58 Utah families for a syndrome present in approximately 12% of patients with essential hypertension, *JAMA* 259:3579-3586, 1988.

51. Wilson PWF, Abbott RD, Castelli WP: High density lipoprotein cholesterol and mortality: The Framingham Heart Study, *Arteriosclerosis* 8:737-741, 1988.

52. Wysowski DK, Kennedy DL, Gross TP: Prescribed use of cholesterol-lowering drugs in the United States, 1978 through 1988, *JAMA* 263(16):2185-2188, 1990.

53. Young FE, Nightingale SL, Temple RA: The preliminary report of the findings of the aspirin component of the ongoing Physicians' Health Study, *JAMA* 259(21):3158-3160, 1988.

54. Yeo KHJ et al: A competitive ELISA for lipoprotein(a), *Clinica Chimica Acta* 205:213-222, 1992.

RESOURCES

Fletcher GF et al: Benefits and recommendations for physical activity programs for all Americans: a statement for health professionals by the Committee on Exercise and Cardiac Rehabilitation of the Council on Clinical Cardiology, American Heart Association, *Circulation* 86:340-344, 1992.

Gifford RW Jr et al: Office evaluation of hypertension: a statement for health professionals by a writing group of the council for high blood pressure research, American Heart Association, *Circulation* 79:721-731, 1989.

Joint National Committee on Detection, Evaluation, and Treatment of High Blood Pressure: The fifth report of the Joint National Committee on Detection, Evaluation, and Treatment of High Blood Pressure (JNC V), *Arch Intern Med* 153:154-183, 1993.

National High Blood Pressure Education Program working group report on primary prevention of hypertension, *Arch Intern Med* 153:186-208, 1993.

Stone EJ, Van Citters RL, Pearson TA, editors: *Preventive cardiology: perspectives in physical education,* New York, 1990, Oxford University Press. (Published as a supplement of *Am J Prev Med*).

Report from the Laboratory Standardization Panel of the National Cholesterol Education Program on Blood Cholesterol Measurement in Clinical Laboratories in the United States. NIH Publication No 88-2928, January 1988.

Report of the National Cholesterol Education Program on Community Guide to Cholesterol Resources. NIH Publication No 88-2927, February 1988.

Report of the National Cholesterol Education Program on Highlights of the Report of the Expert Panel on Blood Cholesterol Levels in Children and Adolescents. NIH Publication No 91-2731, September 1991.

Report of the National Cholesterol Education Program Expert Panel on Population Strategies for Blood Cholesterol Reduction: executive summary, *Arch Intern Med* 151:1071-1084, 1991.

Strong WB et al: Integrated cardiovascular health promotion in childhood: a statement for health professionals from the subcommittee on atherosclerosis and hypertension in childhood of the council on cardiovascular disease in the young, American Heart Association, *Circulation* 85:1638-1650, 1992.

Chapter 42

OTHER CARDIAC CONDITIONS

Loretta R. Isada
Donald A. Underwood

RHEUMATIC FEVER
Definition

Acute rheumatic fever (ARF) is characterized by non-suppurative inflammatory lesions affecting the heart, joints, central nervous system, and subcutaneous tissues. The disease is a delayed sequela of upper respiratory infection with group A beta-hemolytic streptococci. The exact mechanisms mediating the development of rheumatic fever remain elusive; ARF is variable in its manifestations, and the diagnosis is primarily clinical.[4,8,57]

Epidemiology

Factors such as latitude, altitude, age, and crowding affect the incidence of streptococcal disease severity. Certain data suggest that the severity of streptococcal upper respiratory tract infections (based on clinical, bacteriologic, and immunologic criteria) influences the likelihood of subsequent ARF. Nevertheless, up to one third of the cases of rheumatic fever can occur after asymptomatic streptococcal upper respiratory tract infections.[8,57]

Rheumatic fever occurs most commonly in school-aged children. There is no sex predilection for the disease, although certain clinical manifestations occur more frequently in girls (i.e., mitral stenosis, and Syndenham's chorea, when the latter occurs post puberty). Crowding also affects the incidence of ARF in untreated cases of streptococcal pharyngitis. In endemic infections, such as open populations of school children, the attack rate is approximately 0.5%. It appears, however, that with increased antistreptolysin O titers as a marker of greater immunogenicity, the attack rates in such open populations can reach up to 1%. In addition, in crowded situations such as military bases, attack rates can escalate to as high as 3%.[8,57,87]

There is general agreement that the incidence of ARF in the United States has markedly diminished, although exactly why this is so is not clear. Physicians and epidemiologists point to a host of factors including improved living standards, easier access to medical care, widespread antibiotic use, and fewer "rheumatogenic" serotypes of *Streptococcus*.[57,59,91] Crowding and associated socioeconomic status seem to affect the incidence of rheumatic fever, which is especially noteworthy in third world countries.[1,91] However, the 1980s have seen several outbreaks of rheumatic fever in middle class neighborhoods. In many of these outbreaks, bacteriology revealed colonies of highly mucoid streptococci. Other clear predisposing factors were not found.[92]

Persons who have suffered an initial attack of rheumatic fever are at increased risk for recurrence of the disease with another episode of streptococcal pharyngitis. Rate of recurrence of the disease is highest in the first year after the initial episode of ARF and can be as great as 50%. Thereafter, there is a decline in the rate of recurrence with subsequent infections, until 4 to 5 years after the initial attack, at which point recurrence of the disease with streptococcal pharyngitis remains about 10%.[8,56,57]

Rheumatic fever is no longer the significant health problem that it once was in the United States. Most young physicians today have never seen a case of acute rheumatic fever. Nevertheless, the primary care physician of young children should keep the diagnosis in mind, especially when dealing with indigent populations or young immigrants of third world countries.[1,57,59,87,91]

Clinical presentation

The diagnosis of ARF is based on clinical presentation. Because the manifestations of ARF are variable, in 1944, Jones established a set of criteria for guidance in its diagnosis. These criteria were subsequently modified and revised by the American Heart Association.[21] They were proposed to assist not only in diagnosis, but to minimize overdiagnosis. With the realization that single laboratory test or clinical sign or symptom is in itself pathognomonic for rheumatic fever, the Jones criteria divides certain clinical and laboratory findings into major and minor categories based on their diagnostic significance. Major manifestations are arthritis, carditis, chorea, subcutaneous nodules, and erythema marginatum. Minor criteria for rheumatic fever include previous history of rheumatic fever, arthralgia, fever, acute phase reactants in the blood (elevated white blood cell [WBC] count, elevated sedimentation rate, elevated C-reactive protein), and prolongation of the P-R interval on the electrocardiogram (ECG).[8,21,57]

The latent period between an episode of pharyngitis and the onset of rheumatic fever varies between 1 and 5 weeks, with an average onset of 19 days. There is no difference in this latent period between initial and recurrent attacks. Most attacks begin with episodes of polyarthritis (approximately 75% of cases). Polyarthritis is almost always migratory, manifesting with heat, swelling, erythema, tenderness, and limitation of motion of two or more joints. Knees, ankles, elbows, and wrists are most often involved.[8,21,57,87]

Carditis, which occurs in 40% to 50% of patients, is the most disabling manifestation of ARF in terms of its potential for acute and chronic morbidity and mortality. Cardiac involvement is frequently a pancarditis involving endocardium, myocardium, and pericardium; but is often asymptomatic. Cardiac involvement, if not associated with pericarditis or congestive heart failure, can go unnoticed; or it can be brought to attention by a previously unheard murmur in the face of other symptoms that bring the individual to the attention of a physician.

Cardiac involvement in ARF usually is seen within the first 3 weeks of onset. Clinical signs and symptoms at presentation include congestive heart failure (5% to 10%), pericarditis (5% to 10%), and new or changing murmurs (85%). Pericardial effusion and cardiac dilation can also be seen. The murmurs associated with ARF are high-pitched, apical, holosystolic; low-pitched, apical, mid-diastolic (Carey Coombs); and apical high-pitched, decrescendo, diastolic. Murmurs of mitral stenosis and aortic stenosis are associated with chronic rheumatic fever and are not heard in the acute phase of the disease. Delayed arteriovenous conduction occurs in up to 75% of patients with ARF. The most common conduction abnormality is the prolongation of the P-R interval, but it is not diagnostic of rheumatic carditis.[8,57]

Chorea occurs in about 15% of patients with ARF; nodules and erythema marginatum are rarest of all, occurring in 10% of cases. Chorea, otherwise known as "St Vitus' dance" is characterized by emotional lability, muscular weakness, and uncoordinated purposeless movements. Such involuntary movements are most notable in the hands, feet, and face and tend to subside with rest and sedation. Syndenham's chorea can occur with a significant latent period (1 to 6 months) and has a variable duration (1 week to 2 years, averaging 8 to 15 weeks). The latent period is long enough to allow the acute phase reactants and antibody titers to return sometimes to normal at the time that the patient manifests the neurologic disorder.[21,57]

Subcutaneous nodules most often occur with severe carditis and present weeks after the onset of cardiac involvement. They are round, firm, painless lesions located over bony surfaces and tendons, particularly extensors of fingers, toes, and flexors of wrists and ankles. Such lesions can be seen in rheumatoid arthritis and systemic lupus erythematosus; they are not pathognomonic for ARF. Nodules are evanescent and usually last a week or two, but sometimes are seen only for several days, which can then distinguish them from those seen with rheumatoid arthritis.[8,21,57]

Erythema marginatum can be seen with ARF, but like subcutaneous nodules is not pathognomonic of the disease, as it may be seen with *Staphylococcus* sepsis, glomerulonephritis, and drug reactions. The rash is described as serpiginous; like a "smoke ring"; and is not indurated, raised, pruritic, or painful. It is seen on the trunk and proximal extremities, sparing the face, and may occur intermittently for weeks. Presence of the rash does not necessarily indicate recrudescence of the disease.[4,21,57]

Prevention of attacks of rheumatic fever may be primary and secondary. Primary prevention of first attacks is managed by recognition and treatment of upper respiratory infections with group A beta-hemolytic streptococcus. Common symptoms of initial streptococcus infection include swelling of the anterior cervical lymph node chain, sore throat, tonsilar exudate, and scarlitiniform rash. These symptoms are nonspecific, and additional testing may be needed to assist in making the proper diagnosis.[4,21,91]

Diagnostic testing

Throat cultures are valuable in establishing a diagnosis of strep throat, but cannot distinguish the carrier state from actual infection. A negative culture, however, is quite helpful in allowing the physician to withhold antibiotic therapy reliably in the majority of patients. Rapid antigen detection tests have also been used, with results available in minutes as opposed to the 1- or 2-day lag time for throat culture results. Unfortunately, although the test is fairly specific, it is not as highly sensitive and, therefore, a negative test should still be followed by a throat culture.[4,21,57,87,91]

Streptococcal antibody testing has no value in immediate diagnosis of streptococcal infections acutely. Antibody tests such as antistreptolysin-O (ASO) and antideoxyribonuclease B (anti-DNase B) are helpful only in confirming recent infections. Most throat infections are of viral etiology. Only one fourth to one third of children complaining of sore throat will have positive cultures for group A beta-hemolytic streptococcus. Approximately one half of children with positive cultures will have significant antibody titers. It is believed that most of the children with low immunologic response are simply carriers of streptococci.[57,87,91]

Prophylaxis—primary and secondary

Patients with a history of rheumatic carditis should receive long-term antibiotic treatment. Prophylaxis of rheumatic fever should continue into adulthood, and possibly for life in such patients. In patients with a known history of rheumatic fever without cardiac involvement, prophylaxis should continue until the patient is in his or her 20s, and 5 years have elapsed since the last attack.[8,21,57,87,91] Patients with evidence of rheumatic valvular disease who have undergone prosthetic valve involvement should also be continued on long-term prophylaxis, as well as receive

short-term antibiotics before certain invasive procedures (see Endocarditis).

Some difficulties remain with regard to treatment failures, chronic carriers of streptococcus, and family contacts. Reports have been made that 5% to 30% of treated patients harbor streptococcus after a full course of antibiotics, with oral regimens less effective than intramuscular therapy. Causes of failure are numerous and include noncompliance with treatment, reinfection, or true treatment failures. The cost-benefit rate of a repeat throat culture to pick up such failures after a full course of medical treatment, however, is not sufficient in the United States to warrant routine reculture. In high-risk circumstances, such as persistent or recurrent symptoms of streptococcal infection, or in patients with a known history of rheumatic fever, repeat cultures become much more important. If reculture is undertaken, only a single course of retreatment is necessary for positive cultures. It is generally accepted that the presence or persistence of weakly positive throat

Table 42-1. Antibiotics in rheumatic fever

Primary prevention (for the treatment of group A beta-hemolytic streptococcus)

Drug	Dose/Route	Duration	Comments
Penicillin V	125-250 mg TID or QID orally	10 days	Same dose adults and children Associated with fewer allergic reactions than parenteral Compliance problems
Erythromycin estolate	20-40 mg/kg BID to QID orally	10 days	Used for penicillin allergic patients Compliance problems
Benzathine penicillin*	<27kg=600,000 u intramuscularly >27kg=1.2 million u intramuscularly	1 dose	Allergic reactions more frequent Discomfort at injection site

*Procaine penicillin is associated with less discomfort at the injection site, but efficacy is not certain in adults.

Secondary Prevention (for the treatment of patients who have suffered rheumatic fever, and prevention of further attacks)

Category	Drug	Dose/Route	Duration
ARF without carditis	Sulfadiazine	<27 kg=500 mg daily orally >27 kg= 1 gm daily orally	Until young adulthood or 5 years years since last episode of ARF
	Penicillin V	125-250 mg daily orally	Same
	Erythromycin estolate	250 mg daily orally	Same
	Benzathine penicillin	1.2 million u intramuscularly every 4 weeks	Same May be best for those at greatest risk of another attack of ARF (school teachers, adults with young children, army recruits)
ARF with carditis	Same prophylaxis as patients without carditis; however, prophylaxis should continue for lifetime		

From Braunwald E, editor: Specific arrhythmias. In *Heart disease,* ed 3, Philadelphia, 1988, WB Saunders.
Dajani AS et al: Prevention of rheumatic fever, *Am Heart Assoc* 78(4):1082-1086, 1988.
Mandell GL, Douglas RG, Bennett JE, editors: Nonsuppurative poststreptococcal sequelae:rheumatic fever and glomerulonephritis. In *Principles and practice of infectious diseases,* ed 2, New York, 1990, Churchill Livingstone.
Shulman ST et al: *Circulation,* 70(6):1118A-1127A, 1987

cultures in asymptomatic individuals usually identifies the chronic carrier state. Carriers of streptococcus do not appear to be at increased risk for the development of rheumatic fever, nor do they appear to pose a threat to patients with a known history of rheumatic fever.[21,57,59,87,91]

The issue of management of family contacts poses another question. Asymptomatic household contacts of patients with streptococcus pharyngitis do not need treatment. However, streptococcal acquisition rates have been found to be as high as 25% in family contacts. In households with a rheumatic individual, the risk is high enough to warrant testing even for asymptomatic individuals.[21,87]

The treatment schedule for streptococcal upper respiratory infections should be initiated as soon as the definitive diagnosis is made. Penicillin is the treatment of choice and is effective in the prevention of rheumatic fever, even if started several days after the onset of illness. Penicillin may be administered orally or intramuscularly. If oral therapy is used, a full 10 days of treatment is necessary. Although this route is associated with fewer allergic reactions, patient compliance may be a problem. Penicillin V, 125 to 250 mg three to four times daily for 10 days, is the standard oral regimen. The dose of penicillin is the same for adults and children. For patients allergic to penicillin, erythromycin may be used. Erythromycin estolate can be given in a dose of 20 to 40 mg/kg/day in two to four divided doses, or erythromycin ethyl succinate can be given in a dose of 40 mg/kg/day in two to four divided doses a day. Oral treatment should be continued for 10 days regardless of drug choice[8,21,57,87] (Table 42-1).

When considering the intramuscular route, benzathine penicillin G is preferred. The recommended dose of penicillin G is 600,000 units intramuscularly for patients less than 27 kg, and 1.2 million units for patients over 27 kg. Procaine penicillin mixtures are associated with less discomfort at the injection site, but the efficacy of penicillin combinations is not certain for adults. It should be noted that tetracyclines and sulfonamides are not adequate treatment for cases of acute streptococcal pharyngitis.[21,57,87]

Secondary prevention of ARF is accomplished with long-term continuous antibiotic prophylaxis. Oral agents are considered more appropriate for patients at a lower risk of rheumatic recurrence. Some physicians prefer to place a patient on oral prophylaxis until the patient has reached young adulthood and has remained free of rheumatic attacks for 5 years. Sulfadiazine can be used in a dose of 0.5 g daily in patients less than 27 kg, and 1 g in patients weighing over 27 kg. Side effects are not common, although leukopenia has been reported. Penicillin can be used as well, in a dose of 125 to 250 mg daily by mouth. In the rare instance that a patient is allergic to both penicillin and sulfa, erythromycin may be used in a dose of 250 mg daily[8,21,57,87] (see Table 42-1).

Intramuscular benzathine penicillin is the other method of secondary prevention of rheumatic fever. The injection is given every four weeks in a dose of 1.2 million units, and is often the preferred approach to avoid recurrent rheumatic fever. Many physicians believe that this is the best method for those patients at high risk of contracting rheumatic fever. Adults with a high risk of exposure to streptococcal infection include the parents of small children, teachers, health care workers, and people living in crowded conditions[21,57,87,91] (see Table 42-1).

ENDOCARDITIS
Definition

One important aspect of caring for patients with heart disease is the question of endocarditis prophylaxis—which patients should receive it, for what procedures, and for how long. For patient and physician alike, prophylaxis against endocarditis should be easy to administer, low in cost, effective, and selective. To this end, multiple recommendations have been made to guide clinicians.[11,22,34,84] Perhaps the best known set of guidelines is that of the American Heart Association (AHA), most recently updated and published in 1990. The AHA is careful to state that their recommendations are a general set of guide rules, and "not meant to replace the physician's clinical judgment in individual cases."[22]

Approaches for the prevention of bacterial endocarditis are based on indirect information. There have been no adequate controlled clinical trials in humans with regard to antimicrobial prophylaxis of bacterial endocarditis; therefore, conclusive proof of the efficacy of antibiotic prophylaxis is not available. Current concepts and recommendations are based on animal models, in vitro studies, pharmacokinetics, microbiologic data (such as virulence of a specific organism and most likely source of infection), and other clinical experience.[22,34,42,43] In the preantibiotic era, the disease was almost uniformly fatal, and today endocarditis still carries a mortality of 10% to 20%.[87] For this reason, it seems justified to use antibiotic prophylaxis in the hope that a significant fraction of cases of endocarditis can be prevented.[9]

Infective endocarditis is defined as infection of the endocardial surface of the heart, with microorganisms physically present in the lesion. Multiple etiologic factors are believed to play a role in the pathogenesis of infective endocarditis. The surface of the heart must be altered in some way to produce a site for fibrin and platelet deposition. Transient bacteremia and turbulent blood flow are also well-recognized contributors in the development of the disease. Prediction of the sites of bacterial deposition and vegetation formation can be made based on the pattern of disturbed blood flow.[9]

The prevention of bacterial endocarditis involves several fairly specific observations/considerations. First, certain invasive procedures appear to be more commonly associated with bacteremias causing endocarditis. Second, certain hosts are at a greater risk for the development of endocarditis associated with transient bacteremia. Finally, certain bacteria appear to be responsible for a majority of the cases of endocarditis, and these organisms seem to have fairly predictable antibiotic sensitivities.[9,53,56]

Transient bacteremia is the primary event in the development of infective endocarditis. Common sources of organisms include the oral cavity, gastrointestinal (GI) tract, respiratory tract, and genitourinary (GU) tract. Manipulation at any one of these sites can allow the intrusion of bacteria into the bloodstream, thus creating the potential for deposition and proliferation of organisms on cardiac valves.[26,38]

Risk factors

The recognized patient populations at risk for endocarditis include those with prosthetic valves, hypertrophic cardiomyopathy, a known previous history of endocarditis, rheumatic and other acquired valvular disease, most congenital abnormalities, and surgically created systemic pulmonary shunts[6,42,61] (Table 42-2). Patients with mitral valve prolapse are a special population, for which some controversy exists, and will be discussed separately.

A fairly new and growing population of patients are those who have undergone valvular repair procedures including bioprosthetic or pericardial rings and sliding annuloplasties.[5,16,20,97] Currently, not enough data are available on the actual risk of infection in such patients. As the number of individuals undergoing valvular repair increase in number, a better understanding of relative risk of endocarditis should develop. Until then, endocarditis prophylaxis remains the clinical decision of the individual physician caring for the patient.

Bacterial endocarditis is associated with a host of predisposing conditions. Illicit drug use and prolonged use of intravascular catheters have contributed to the rising number of cases of right-sided endocarditis. Cirrhotics, burn victims, patients with underlying neoplasms, and other immunosuppressed hosts all appear to have an increased likelihood of developing endocarditis when compared with the general population of hospitalized patients. The existence of such conditions should raise the physician's awareness of the possibility of endocarditis.[9,56]

It is not possible to predict with certainty which patients will develop or which procedures will cause endocarditis.* The exact risk of endocarditis in specific cardiac lesions is unknown. Transient bacteremias not related to procedures are responsible for a large number of cases of endocarditis and appear to be related to simple daily activities. For example, chewing and tooth brushing can cause transient bacteremia, and significant gingival disease can increase the frequency and intensity of such events. The best prevention against these events is maintenance of good oral hygiene. In addition, simple measures such as the gingival

*References 22, 26, 34, 42, 68, 88, 90.

Table 42-2. Cardiac conditions and endocarditis antibiotic prophylaxis*

Prophylaxis recommended	Prophylaxis not necessary
1. Prosthetic cardiac valves	1. Secundum atrial septal defect (ASD)
2. History of endocarditis in any patient	2. Surgical repair of ASD, ventricular septal defect, patent ductus arteriosus, without residual beyond 6 months
3. Most congenital malformations	
4. Rheumatic/acquired valve disease	3. Previous coronary bypass
5. Hypertrophic cardiomyopathy	4. MVP without regurgitation
6. Mitral valve prolapse (MVP) with regurgitation	5. Physiologic murmurs
	6. Previous Kawasaki disease without valve dysfunction
	7. Rheumatic fever, without valve disease
	8. Pacemakers, defibrillators

From American Heart Association and Dajani AS et al: Prevention of bacterial endocarditis, *JAMA* 264(22):2919-2922, 1990.
*This table is a general set of guidelines and is not all inclusive.

application of chlorhexidine solution can reduce bacteremia associated with dental manipulation.[11,43]

Incidence and epidemiology

The incidence of infective endocarditis has been reported to be approximately 1 in 1000 hospital admissions. With the arrival of the antibiotic era, the mean age of patients presenting with infective endocarditis has steadily increased. Slightly over half the cases of endocarditis occur in the 30- to 60-year-old age group, and approximately one fourth of these patients are less than 30 years old. Those patients over age 60 account for a little less than 25% of all cases. In patients under the age of 35, more cases of endocarditis occur in women; however, the overall male/female ratio shows a male preponderance, which can be as great as 3:1.[9,56]

As the mean age of patients has changed, so too has the spectrum of the underlying lesions that predispose to the disease. In the early 1900s, rheumatic heart disease was undisputedly the most common predisposing condition in patients with endocarditis, accounting for approximately 80% of recognized underlying cardiac abnormalities. Congenital heart disease accounted for most other reported incidents at that time. Today, cases of native valve endocarditis show a much different distribution of predisposing lesions, including degenerative valvular disease (20% to 25%), mitral valve prolapse (25% to 30%), congenital heart disease (10% to 15%), and rheumatic disease (5% to 10%). It is estimated that nearly 50% of endocarditis cases have no clear underlying cardiac abnormality.[9,42,61]

Infection of the heart valves occurs in the following frequency, from most common valve involved to least: mitral, aortic, tricuspid, and pulmonic. Left-sided lesions are by far the most common. Right-sided endocarditis is reported in about 5% to 10% of cases. Clinical presentation is vastly different in left- versus right-sided endocarditis. Manifestations of the disease also depend on whether the infection is acute or subacute.[9,56]

The differentiation between acute and subacute forms of the disease is based on the organism responsible for the infection. Such a distinction seems legitimate, as duration of the course, complications, and mortality differ greatly between the two groups, despite appropriate intervention. It is apparent, however, that in a number of patients, the clinical presentation does not relate to the responsible pathogen, and patients in whom the course may change from one category to another.[56]

Procedures and prophylaxis

The incubation period between the procedure thought to be the inciting event and the onset of symptoms of endocarditis has been reported to be about 2 weeks in half the cases. Nearly 80% of the patients manifest symptoms within 5 weeks of the event.[31,38] Dental procedures contribute the majority of precipitating events, and *Streptococcus viridans* is the most common organism involved (Table 42-3). Antibiotic prophylaxis is recommended for all dental procedures that are likely to produce gingival trauma. Edentulous patients are not immune from endocarditis and may develop bacteremia from ill-fitting dentures; therefore, periodic dental examinations are appropriate. Simple readjustment of orthodontic appliances do not usually require prophylaxis.[22,84,88]

Other procedures involving the upper respiratory tract, such as tonsillectomy and adenoidectomy, and bronchoscopy with a rigid bronchoscope can produce a bacteremia similar to that seen with dental manipulation (see Table 42-3). The standard prophylactic regimen for dental and upper respiratory procedures for patients at risk is amoxicillin, 3 g before the procedure and 1.5 g 6 hours after the procedure. Penicillin and ampicillin are effective against *Streptococcus* in vitro, but the absorption of amoxicillin is better and the serum levels are sustained longer. Erythromycin or clindamycin can be used in patients allergic to penicillin. Tetracyclines and sulfonamides do not provide adequate prophylaxis[22,56] (see box).

For patients in whom oral administration of antibiotic prophylaxis is not possible, the parenteral route is used. In such cases, ampicillin, 2 g, can be used intravenously 30 minutes before the procedure, with a postprocedure dose of 1 g given 6 hours later. Clindamycin can be used in penicillin-sensitive patients, with 300 mg administered intravenously 30 minutes before the procedure and half the dose 6 hours later. In high-risk patients, gentamicin can be added to the ampicillin regimen at a dose of 1.5 mg/kg (maximum dose of 80 mg) before the procedure. A postprocedure dose of gentamicin is not necessary, but can be

---

Recommended prophylactic regimens*

1. Dental, oral, upper respiratory tract
   a. Standard: amoxicillin 3.0 g orally before procedure; repeat 1.5 g 6 hours after first dose
   b. Penicillin allergic: erythromycin ethylsuccinate 800 mg, or erythromycin stearate 1 g orally 2 hours before procedure, half the dose to be repeated 6 hours after the initial dose; or clindamycin 300 mg orally 1 hour before procedure and 150 mg 6 hours after the initial dose
   c. Patients unable to take oral medication: intravenous (IV) or intramuscular (IM) administration of 2.0 g ampicillin, ½ hour before procedure; repeat IV or IM ampicillin 1 g 6 hours after the initial dose
   d. Penicillin-allergic patients unable to take oral medications: clindamycin 300 mg IV ½ hour before procedure; repeat clindamycin 150 mg IV 6 hours after the initial dose
   e. High-risk patients, not candidates for standard regimen: ampicillin 2.0 g IV or IM, plus gentamicin 1.5 mg/kg (not to exceed 80 mg) ½ hour before procedure; amoxicillin 1.5 g orally 6 hours after the initial dose, or repetition of the parenteral regimen 8 hours after the initial dose
   f. Penicillin-allergic patients considered high risk: vancomycin 1 g IV over 1 hour before procedure, repeated dose not needed
2. GU/GI tract
   a. Standard: ampicillin 2.0 g IV or IM, plus gentamicin 1.5 mg/kg (not to exceed 80 mg) ½ hour before procedure; followed by amoxicillin 1.5 g orally 6 hours after the initial dose—alternatively, the parenteral regimen may be repeated 8 hours after the initial dose
   b. Penicillin allergic: vancomycin 1 g IV over 1 hour, plus gentamicin 1.5 mg/kg IM or IV (not to exceed 80 mg) 1 hour before the procedure; regimen may be repeated 8 hours after the initial dose
   c. Alternate regimen for the low-risk patient: amoxicillin 3.0 g orally 1 hour before procedure; repeat half the dose 6 hours after the initial administration

From American Heart Association and Dajani AS et al: Prevention of bacterial endocarditis, *JAMA,* 264:2919-2922, 1990.
*This information represents a general set of guidelines and is not all inclusive.

---

repeated 8 hours after the initial dose. Vancomycin is the alternative regimen of choice for high-risk patients who are allergic to penicillin and is given as a single dose of 1 g 1 hour before the procedure over a 1-hour period. (Faster infusion rates can cause unpleasant cutaneous reactions.) The AHA advises that individuals at high risk for endocarditis (patients with prosthetic valves, previous history of endocarditis, or with systemic-pulmonary shunts) be strongly considered for the parenteral route whenever possible[6,13,22,42] (see box, above).

Table 42-3. Procedures and endocarditis antibiotic prophylaxis*

Prophylaxis recommended	Prophylaxis not necessary
1. Dental procedures associated with trauma, i.e., professional cleaning	1. Dental procedures without significant trauma, i.e., adjusting orthodontic appliances
2. Tonsillectomy/adenoidectomy	2. Flexible bronchoscopy with or without biopsy
3. Rigid bronchoscopy	3. Injection of local oral anesthetic
4. Esophageal sclerotherapy/dilation	4. Tympanostomy tube insertion
5. Gallbladder surgery	5. Endotracheal intubation
6. Cystoscopy	6. Shedding of primary teeth
7. Urinary tract catheterization/surgery in the presence of infection	7. Cardiac catheterization
8. Prostate surgery	8. GI endoscopy
9. Incision and drainage of infected tissue	9. Cesarean section
10. Vaginal hysterectomy	10. Uncomplicated vaginal delivery, insertion/removal of intrauterine devices
11. Vaginal delivery in the presence of infection	

From Am Heart Association and Dajani AS et al: Prevention of bacterial endocarditis, *JAMA* 264(22):2919-2922, 1990.
*This table is a general set of guidelines and is not all inclusive.

The GU and GI tracts also provide sources of bacteria, which can potentially cause endocarditis (see Table 42-3). The GU tract is second only to the oral cavity as a potential source of bacteremia, and the rate of bacteremia can rise significantly in the presence of urinary tract infection. Some procedures known to cause transient bacteremia associated with the GU and GI tracts include sclerotherapy of esophageal varices, esophageal dilation, cholecystectomy, cystoscopy, prostate surgery, vaginal hysterectomy, and incision and drainage of infected tissues (see Table 42-3). *Streptococcus faecalis* is the most frequent offending organism in such cases. Gram-negative bacillary bacteremia is not unusual after GU or GI procedures; however, gram-negative bacilli rarely cause endocarditis. Therefore, antibiotic prophylaxis is directed against enterococci.[22,42,56,63]

The antibiotic regimen for low-risk patients undergoing GI or GU procedures is oral amoxicillin, in the same dose as that given for dental procedures. The standard high-risk prophylactic regimen is ampicillin and gentamicin, given intravenously, in the same doses and dosing intervals as stated for upper respiratory tract procedures in high-risk patients. A combination of vancomycin and gentamicin can be used in the penicillin-sensitive individual[9,22,42,56] (see box on p. 846).

It should be noted that regimens used in the secondary prophylaxis of rheumatic fever recurrences are inadequate for the prevention of bacterial endocarditis. Patients on penicillin for secondary prevention of rheumatic fever may be colonized with *Streptococcus viridans,* which has developed some penicillin resistance. In such cases, the practitioner may consider erythromycin or clindamycin as an alternative for endocarditis prophylaxis.[8,9,22,56]

There have been many arguments against the routine use of antibiotics for the prophylaxis of endocarditis. Most of these arguments are based on factors such as the relative risk of an allergic or other adverse reaction to the antimicrobial agent, the inability to predict with accuracy which patients will develop endocarditis and with which procedures, the fact that daily events create more episodes of bacteremia than isolated invasive procedures, and the fact that prophylaxis itself cannot be 100% effective (it is believed that theoretically less than 10% of cases can be reliably prevented).*

Failed prophylaxis

Some cases of apparent prophylactic failures have been reported. In 1983, 52 cases were submitted to a national registry established by the AHA.[31] The questions addressed included the following: (1) Did failures occur when antibiotics were given as prophylaxis? (2) Which organisms were most commonly involved when antibiotics failed and what were their specific sensitivities? (3) What were the underlying cardiac lesions and did the regimens actually provide adequate prophylaxis. The paper concluded that failures in the prevention of endocarditis are not rare, but the exact incidence cannot be determined. In addition, in vitro sensitivities did not always correlate with in vivo success of the prophylactic regimen. The registry also found that mitral valve prolapse was a common underlying cardiac lesion. Finally, antibiotic prophylaxis was not always received according to the recommended standards of the AHA or other well-known authorities such as the British Society for Antimicrobial Prophylaxis.[26,31,38,43,53]

In essence, the recommendations of the AHA are a simple and applicable set of guidelines targeted at high- and moderate-risk patients and represent the ideal standard of care in the United States. Low-risk lesions and low-risk patients need not be given routine chemoprophylaxis. There is no reliable way to measure the outcome of patients prospectively with regard to administration of antibiotic prophylaxis. However, the cost-benefit analysis of those patients with increased risk for endocarditis would suggest that antibiotic prophylaxis may be the best way to avoid a prolonged hospital stay, long-term antibiotic administration, and potentially valve replacement.

MITRAL VALVE PROLAPSE
Definition

Prolapse is defined as "the slipping or displacement of an organ or part of an organ from its normal position

*References 34, 38, 43, 68, 84, 90.

through an opening or into a cavity."[93] Mitral valve prolapse (MVP) is defined by the superior and posterior displacement of the leaflets of the mitral valve in relation to the mitral annulus. This displacement may be due to structural enlargement or abnormal distensibility of the mitral valve itself and is evidenced by the detection of certain abnormal auscultatory, angiographic, and/or echocardiographic findings.[8,27,28,71]

Epidemiology

MVP is the most prevalent cardiac abnormality known, and with the current advances in cardiac imaging, has been recognized in 2.5% to 5% of the general population. There are primary and secondary causes of mitral valve prolapse. Primary MVP, more commonly encountered by physicians, is identified as valvular-ventricular disproportion associated with an abnormality of connective tissue that is either inherent or in response to injury at sites of minor normal anatomic variations in the architecture of the mitral valve apparatus (including chordae tendinae and leaflets).* Secondary causes of MVP include Marfan syndrome, Ehler-Danlos syndrome types I and II, and conditions in which the left ventricular size is reduced relative to that of the mitral valve (i.e., anorexia nervosa and ostium secundum atrial septal defects). Normalization of the size of the left ventricle (for example by repair of an ostium secundum atrial septal defect, or return to normal body weight in anorexia nervosa) has resulted in the disappearance of MVP. Conversely, such conditions as significant aortic insufficiency may mask MVP due to increased left ventricular volume. In clinical practice, the secondary causes of MVP are quite rare.

Diagnosis

The diagnosis of MVP and its severity may be established by a variety of methods. Clinically, it is important to identify which patients or subset of patients are at risk for cardiac complications based on such a diagnosis. An enormous amount of literature has addressed the potential complications, phenotypic associations, and existence of what has been considered the "MVP syndrome." Auscultatory diagnostic criteria include mid to late systolic clicks and a late systolic murmur. Midsystolic clicks that shift their timing with respect to the first and second heart sounds in response to various maneuvers are the most widely used diagnostic criteria. These maneuvers alter the relationship between the mitral valve and left ventricular size. For example, sitting and standing move the click closer to the first heart sound and prolong the systolic murmur. Squatting increases the ventricular size, moves the click closer to the second heart sound, and shortens the murmur.[8,27,28,29]

Unfortunately, auscultatory manifestations can be variable. Fluctuation of the murmur and click can require repeated examinations to determine whether a patient may intermittently have evidence of prolapse and mitral regurgitation. Identification of patients with regurgitant lesions becomes important with respect to prevention of potential complications. Therefore, it has become increasingly common to find patients with so-called "silent" MVP, which is detected by a method other than auscultation.[27,32,49,67,83]

Echocardiography has contributed greatly to the diagnosis and evaluation of the severity of MVP. M-mode and two-dimensional cardiac imaging have both been used to identify patients with MVP, although the use of two-dimensional imaging has probably become the most popular method. With the use of various imaging positions and planes, two-dimensional echocardiography is ideally suited to record the range of motion of the mitral valve leaflets, the point of leaflet coaptation, left atrial size, and other structural abnormalities, such as chordal rupture. With the aid of color imaging and Doppler echocardiography, the direction and severity of regurgitant jets can also be assessed.*

MVP may also be diagnosed during cardiac catheterization. Contrast angiography initially played an important role in the identification of patients with prolapse of the mitral valve; however, this procedure may not be as accurate as newer noninvasive methods. Difficulty in differentiating mild prolapse from normal findings, high interobserver variability, and a limited number of imaging planes contribute to some of the difficulties with diagnosis using this technique.[29,32]

Associated conditions—the "MVP syndrome"

Significant attention has been directed at a collection of symptoms thought to be associated with MVP, the so-called "MVP syndrome." Interestingly, the high prevalence of symptoms in subjects with MVP in several clinical series did not correlate with the prevalence of symptoms in subjects with MVP in population-based studies and studies of healthy volunteers. Such discrepancies were attributed to selection bias. Controlled studies have not been able to demonstrate an increased prevalence of chest pain, dyspnea, panic attacks, anxiety disorders, or ECG abnormalities in patients with MVP compared with normal persons.[27,29,32,49]

Some studies have taken advantage of the apparent autosomal dominant inheritance pattern (with variable penetrance) of MVP and have studied the first-degree relatives of patients identified with MVP. These studies provided the opportunity to compare affected and unaffected relatives of patients with MVP. Such investigations revealed a strong association between echocardiographic and auscul-

*References 27, 28, 30, 49, 78, 83.

*References 27, 29, 30, 48, 67, 77.

Table 42-4. Mitral valve prolapse and endocarditis prophylaxis

Lesion	Prophylaxis	Comments/References
MVP and audible murmur or click	Highly recommended	Recommended by the AHA[14]
MVP and mitral regurgitation by echo, but **no** murmur	Probably recommended	Large randomized clinical trials not available[20,31,32,44]
MVP in men	Variably recommended	Some evidence suggests greater risk in men[10,11,13,19,32]
MVP in patients over age 45	Variably recommended	Some evidence suggests greater risk in older patients[10,11,13,19,32]

tatory features of MVP when comparing affected relatives to control groups. In addition, significant associations were observed between MVP and thoracic bony abnormalities, low body weight (<90% of ideal), low systolic blood pressure, and palpitations. With these studies, the spectrum of clinical features associated with MVP appears narrower than initially thought. There was no clear evidence that chest discomfort, anxiety disorders, panic attacks, ECG abnormalities, or dyspnea were associated with MVP.[27,29,30,83]

Estimates of the prevalence of MVP may vary depending on the population studied, the method of diagnosis, and specific criteria used for diagnosis. In addition, prevalence seems to be affected by gender and age. In general, MVP is twice as common in women as men. The prevalence (or at least the recognition) of MVP appears to increase through childhood and peaks in early adulthood. Thereafter, the prevalence of MVP declines slowly. Multiple studies, including the Framingham Study, indicate that the prevalence of MVP remains fairly constant in men, at about 2% to 4%. In women, however, prevalence of MVP varies greatly with age and can be found in up to 17% of women in the 20 to 29 age group, whereas in women over 80 years of age, the prevalence drops markedly to less than 2%.[8,27-30,37]

Evidence from clinical studies suggests that MVP is a genetic disorder and that the trait is inherited in an autosomal dominant pattern with variable penetrance. Such data may account for the variable severity of MVP among patients. In addition, this finding also raises the question as to whether racial differences may affect the prevalence of MVP. Currently, there is no clear evidence of detectable differences in the prevalence of MVP between races when the same diagnostic criteria are used.[37,49]

Morbidity and mortality

The most important issue in dealing with MVP, both for the patient and the physician, is the potential for increased morbidity and/or mortality. With increasing research into this problem, it is clear that not all individuals have an equal risk for complications. It is also apparent that MVP has different degrees of severity. Identifying

which patients are at risk and which method of follow-up, prophylaxis, and intervention should be used is the greatest challenge.

Many investigators note an increased risk ranging from three to eight times for endocarditis in patients with MVP when compared to the general population.[19,23,51,60] Certain studies have shown a gradual trend away from underlying rheumatic heart disease in patients presenting with endocarditis and have found that up to 29% of patients with underlying cardiac abnormalities presenting with endocarditis had MVP.[61] Factors such as male gender, age greater than 45 years, and a history of preexisting murmur were found to be independent risk factors in patients with MVP and endocarditis.* The majority of cases of endocarditis appeared to be associated with dental manipulation. Major complications occurred in up to one third of these patients, including valve replacements and death.[32,94]

Decisions concerning antibiotic prophylaxis for patients with MVP require knowledge about the risk of infective endocarditis, the consequences of infection, and the risks/benefits of prophylaxis itself. The AHA recommends prophylaxis for patients with MVP and evidence of systolic murmur[21]; however, the murmur of mitral regurgitation associated with MVP may not always be detectable.[29,49,52,77] Thus the clinician may be presented with a difficult dilemma: whether to provide prophylaxis for a specific patient with MVP. The recommendations of the AHA with regard to antibiotic prophylaxis for infective endocarditis do state that decisions in individual cases must be made by the physician caring for the patient, as it would be virtually impossible to envision every scenario in which antibiotic prophylaxis might be required. Suffice it to say that antibiotic prophylaxis is highly advisable in those patients with MVP who have evidence of mitral regurgitation and may be more strongly indicated in men and in patients over 45 years[18,19,21,28,52] (Table 42-4).

Another proposed complication of MVP deals with malignant arrhythmias. Rare cases of sudden death have been associated with MVP. Sudden cardiac death is natural death due to cardiac causes, which occurs in individuals

*References 10, 11, 15, 19, 24, 32, 38, 45.

with or without known underlying disease, but in whom death was unexpected. Cardiac arrest is an associated term relating to abrupt cessation of pump function, which may be reversible with prompt intervention. (Some clinicians use these terms interchangeably, but many authorities prefer to maintain a distinction.)[16,28,29]

The strongest evidence for an association between sudden death and MVP has been from autopsy studies and from the evaluation of patients who have survived sudden death, in which MVP was the only demonstrable abnormality. These observations, however, do not clearly prove cause and effect. Referral and selection bias, lack of definitive autopsy data, and inconstant documentation all contribute to difficulty in accurately assessing the incidence of serious arrhythmias with MVP. The strength of association between sudden death and MVP in patients without mitral regurgitation is not well documented. In patients with significant regurgitation, however, sudden death appears to be a definite risk and has been estimated to be 50 to 100 times greater in this subset of patients than in the population of patients with MVP as a whole.[32,46,71]

The prevalence of arrhythmias is difficult to estimate in patients with MVP. Several studies have yielded a variety of results, with atrial premature complexes recorded in 35% to 90% of patients, atrial tachycardias found in 3% to 32% of patients, premature ventricular complexes noted in 58% to 89%, and complex ventricular arrhythmias reported in 43% to 56% of patients. Definitions of ventricular arrhythmias have not been uniform among studies and again selection bias adds to the difficulty in interpreting these results. With the present information available, it seems that in patients with MVP and significant mitral regurgitation, both the risk of sudden death and the prevalence of ventricular arrhythmias are greater than in the general population of patients with prolapse.[46,71]

The vast majority of patients with MVP require no treatment for arrhythmias. Unfortunately, there is no clear data on management of patients who have MVP and mitral regurgitation with regard to antiarrhythmic therapy. In symptomatic patients, treatment may be necessary to alleviate discomfort; however, there is no evidence that symptomatic palpitations are a marker for more serious rhythm disturbances. Ambulatory monitoring may be helpful in these patients to evaluate which patients may be having significant ventricular arrhythmias. In mildly symptomatic patients with supraventricular arrhythmias, reductions in nicotine, caffeine, and alcohol may be sufficient to relieve symptoms. On the other hand, patients with syncope or presyncope and evidence of ventricular ectopy require therapy. The role of electrophysiologic testing, antiarrhythmic drug therapy, mitral valve surgery, and other interventions must be individualized. At this point, there are no adequate controlled prospective studies with sufficient numbers to yield definitive answers in these cases.[32,46,60,67]

An additional complication of MVP may be an in-creased risk for cerebrovascular accidents (CVA). Neurologic ischemic events are believed to be caused by fibrin-platelet emboli forming on the roughened surface of an abnormal mitral valve. Estimates of MVP prevalence in young patients with stroke vary markedly from 2% to 40%; however, a causal relationship has not been clearly established. Data are conflicting with regard to the relationship of MVP with cerebral vascular ischemic events, and many studies have failed to find any association. The risk of stroke with primary MVP is low, and prophylactic treatment with antiplatelet agents or anticoagulants is not warranted. When a neurologic event occurs in the face of MVP, recurrence seems infrequent. Nevertheless, in the face of MVP and recent CVA, a thorough investigation into causes other than mitral valvular disease should be initiated. If there is no other definable cause for cerebral ischemia, then a trial of antiplatelet agents is considered the first course of action. In the event of repeated episodes of ischemia on antiplatelet therapy, consideration should be given to anticoagulation with warfarin.[32,60,67,71,96]

Hemodynamically, significant mitral regurgitation requiring surgical intervention is yet another complication of MVP. Progressive myxomatous changes with gradual chordal attenuation and chordal rupture are responsible for an increase in mitral regurgitation. This complication appears to be more frequent in men, patients older than 45, and those who lack the low systolic blood pressure and asthenic body habitus that is usually associated with MVP. Some investigators have calculated that the lifetime risk for needing mitral valve surgery is approximately 1.5% for women, and 4% for men with MVP.[94] When surgical intervention is required, establishing degenerative myxomatous disease of the mitral valve has important significance with regard to whether a valve can be repaired or must be replaced.[5,16,20] Optimal timing of surgical intervention for mitral regurgitation with regard to left ventricular function must also be considered.

With the advent of new cardiac imaging techniques, recognition of MVP has become more common. From available data, it is obvious that there are gradations of severity of disease. Diagnosis of MVP should be based on objective evidence by auscultation or clearly defined by an established laboratory technique. The subset of patients with MVP associated with mitral regurgitation seems to be at greatest risk of serious complications. These patients require close follow-up, with repeat examination to assess any changes in mitral regurgitation, and are also candidates for antibiotic prophylaxis.

The difficulty arises with those patients in whom prolapse is documented, with little or no regurgitation. In young women in whom the disorder seems to be especially prevalent and the risk fairly low, there is genuine concern that labeling a patient with a diagnosis of MVP may have significant detrimental effects on the patient's psychologic and emotional state. Adding to the problem in these patients are financial issues such as insurability and cost of follow-up. Most authorities in the field suggest that reassurance is appropriate in these cases, and limited follow-up is necessary.[29,30,51,52,60] Annual examination is probably sufficient (with or without the addition of cardiac imaging), and more often if symptoms should arise. Due to the heterogeneity of the disorder, blanket recommendations are difficult to make, and much of the evaluation and treatment of these patients remains highly individualized.

COMMON CARDIAC RHYTHM DISTURBANCES AND SUBSTANCES THAT AFFECT THE HEART
Definition

Arrhythmia or dysrhythmia are terms often used interchangeably to describe a disturbance in the heart's normal sinus rhythm. Factors that can affect heart rhythm include mechanical, electrical, and chemical influences. Common arrythmias and their precipitating causes will be discussed in brief particularly where preventive intervention can be most helpful. Perhaps most difficult for both the physician and patient is the fact that rhythm disturbances are not entirely predictable, although there are some clinical situations in which arrythmias are distinctly more frequent.

Clinical presentation/evaluation

Patients with rhythm disturbances present in a variety of ways. Such patients may seek the advice of a physician for complaints of syncope, presyncope, palpitations, shortness of breath, chest pain, or even heart failure.[15,25,50,65,81] A variety of tests are available for the evaluation of patients with rhythm disturbances. The most frequently used tests are the 12-lead ECG, exercise stress testing, and Holter monitoring (both continuous, and event recorders).[62,66,70] Additional tests such as the tilt table examination and invasive electrophysiologic evaluation are also useful in selected cases.* In general, the more malignant and life-threatening the arrythmia, the more invasive the testing becomes. The approach to a patient with a rhythm problem is to document and define the arrythmia, determine and eliminate its cause (if possible), and consider the consequences of the arrhythmia itself as well as the potential complications of antiarrhythmic treatment.

Common precipitating factors

Rhythm disturbances can be precipitated by a number of factors including electrolyte imbalance (most notably potassium, magnesium, and calcium), acidosis or alkalosis, myocardial ischemia, hypoxemia, drugs, and environmental toxins.[12,33,73,85] In addition, many common disease states such as general infection, thyroid disease, and anemia can aggravate or even precipitate rhythm disturbances.[17,44,80,82,89]

*References 3, 7, 39, 41, 54, 64.

Rhythm disturbances

One of the most common causes of an irregular pulse is premature beats. Premature complexes can occur from any area of the heart, but are most commonly ventricular in origin. Normal patients can have all types of premature beats; however, these irregularities, or ectopics, occur more often with advancing age and underlying heart disease.[36,74] The significance and urgency for treatment relates to the type and frequency of ectopy, the patient's symptoms, the presence of any underlying disease state, and the potential for morbidity and mortality related to the specific rhythm disturbance.

Premature atrial contractions (PACs) can occur in a variety of clinical situations, such as in general infection or myocardial ischemia. Other factors such as tension, caffeine, alcohol, and tobacco can also cause PACs. PACs can precede the onset of sustained atrial (or less commonly ventricular) arrhythmias. However, isolated PACs require no specific treatment and may resolve completely if an offending agent such as alcohol or caffeine can be eliminated. In symptomatic patients, or when PACs precipitate sustained tachycardias, even after correction of aggravating problems (ischemia, infection, psychologic stressors, etc.), pharmacologic agents such as digoxin, beta-blockers, or verapamil may be tried. If these agents are unsuccessful, a trial of Ia antiarrhythmics (quinidine, procainamide, disopyramide) may be warranted. It should be noted that with **any** antiarrhythmic agent, side effects, including worsening of the initial arrhythmia or precipitation of a new and more malignant rhythm disturbance, can occur.[14,15,47,72] The physician must be especially wary of drug interactions in patients on multiple medications who require antiarrhythmic therapy.

Atrial fibrillation (AF) is an extremely common rhythm disturbance seen in a wide variety of clinical settings such as myocardial infarction/ischemia, valvular heart disease, chronic obstructive lung disease, pulmonary embolism, thyroid disease, and after open heart surgery patients. This arrhythmia consists of disorganized atrial depolarizations without effective atrial contraction and an irregular (and usually rapid) ventricular response.[15,47]

AF can be intermittent or chronic. Chronic AF is more commonly associated with underlying heart disease than is intermittent AF. When treating new onset AF, or AF of uncertain duration, it is important to detect possible underlying precipitants such as thyrotoxicosis, pericardial disease, myocardial infarction, or pulmonary emboli. History and physical examination are extremely important in pointing to possible etiologies for the irregular rhythm, and laboratory tests such as ECG, oxygen saturation/arterial blood gas, thyroid function tests, electrolytes, and cardiac enzymes are helpful.

The patient's clinical picture and hemodynamic status dictates initial therapy. With sudden decompensation or hemodynamic compromise, DC cardioversion is the treatment of choice. In hemodynamically stable patients, slowing of the ventricular response with digoxin, beta-blockers, or verapamil can be accomplished. Digoxin works slowly to decrease rate, so used alone it is not effective in immediate relief of tachycardia. Doses of beta-blockers or verapamil are often used to decrease rate quickly, especially when given intravenously, but these agents may precipitate hypotension and can have deleterious negative inotropic effects. Ia antiarrhythmics can also be used to convert AF to normal sinus rhythm, keeping in mind that drug interactions can and do occur, most notably with quinidine and digoxin (the former raising the levels of the latter). A general rule to keep in mind is that when initiating quinidine therapy, digoxin dose should be decreased by one half. Drug levels, clinical response, and signs of toxicity can then be monitored.[10,15,47,58,72]

In patients with chronic AF, change in ventricular response rate may be due to changes in underlying disease status. Questions with regard to anticoagulation and cardioversion are somewhat complicated and depend on the clinical situation.[55,86,95] Extensive information on embolic risk, anticoagulation, and cardioversion continues to be collected and is the subject of ongoing clinical trails (see also Chapter 43).

When there is a rapid atrial mechanism and the rhythm is regular, usually at a rate of 150 to 200 beats/min, the diagnosis of paroxysmal supraventricular tachycardia (SVT) may be considered. The term *paroxysmal* indicates a tachycardia of sudden onset that can change from normal sinus rhythm in one beat. The term *nonparoxysmal* refers to a tachycardia that is gradual in onset and termination and can often be found in patients with enhanced automaticity as the underlying mechanism.

The two basic mechanisms involved in SVT are reentry and enhanced automaticity. For example, when an atrial tachycardia is due to reentry, the arrhythmia may be initiated with a PAC. Vagal maneuvers can terminate tachycardia due to a reentrant pathway. In contrast, when tachycardia is due to enhanced automaticity, the arrhythmia is usually not initiated by a premature complex. There may also be a "warming-up" phenomenon in tachycardia due to enhanced automaticity, that is, a gradual onset of increasing heart rate. The response to carotid sinus massage and other vagal maneuvers in patients with tachycardia due to enhanced automaticity is transient, if at all.[10,15,47,58] Automatic atrial tachycardias can occur in all age groups and may be related to a variety of factors, including myocardial infarction, chronic lung disease, metabolic derangements, and acute alcohol intoxication. Digitalis intoxication should always be considered in patients who present with atrial tachycardia, especially patients with atrial tachycardia *with block* or *paroxysmal* atrial tachycardia. In patients not on digoxin, atrial tachycardia can be treated with this medication and the Ia antiarrhythmics. In patients who are currently on digoxin, the medication itself should

be suspected as the precipitating cause of the rhythm disturbance and should be discontinued. In addition, correction of electrolyte imbalance may bring the arrhythmia under control.[12,58,72,73]

Chaotic or multifocal atrial tachycardia may be regular or irregular, with a rate between 100 to 130 beats/min and has at least three demonstrable P wave morphologies. This rhythm disturbance is most often associated with patients who have underlying lung disorders and is often refractory to digoxin. Treatment is usually targeted at treating the underlying cause of the arrhythmia, such as an acute exacerbation of chronic obstructive pulmonary disease, repletion of potassium and magnesium, and occasionally the administration of verapamil. Beta-blockers are usually avoided in such cases, as a significant number of patients with multifocal atrial tachycardia have underlying lung disease with a bronchospastic component that could be aggravated by beta-blockers.[10,47]

Premature ventricular contractions (PVCs) are characterized by the early occurrence of a QRS complex, which is abnormal in shape and usually exceeds the duration of the dominant QRS pattern (most often QRS duration of a PVC = 120 msec). PVCs can often be confused with supraventricular premature beats. Usually, but not always, a fully compensatory pause follows a PVC because the retrograde impulse produced by the ventricular impulse collides with the antegrade impulse originating from the sinus node. Generally, the R-R interval produced by the sinus initiated QRS complexes on either side of the PVC equals two times the normal R-R interval.[15,47]

PVCs increase in frequency with age.[36,74] Patients may be asymptomatic or may feel palpitations or an uncomfortable awareness of the postextrasystolic beat (most often felt in the neck or chest). Runs of PVCs, or ventricular tachycardia, can result in hypotension, angina, shortness of breath, and/or syncope. A variety of stimuli can provoke ventricular ectopy similar to those that contribute to atrial rhythm disturbances.[50,72,81]

The importance of ventricular ectopy is mainly related to the clinical setting. Isolated PVCs in a young individual may require no treatment, and simple reassurance may suffice. Frequent PVCs in a young individual could relate to mechanical trauma (motor vehicle accident and myocardial contusion), psychologic stresses and stimulation (so-called "hyperbeta state"), chemical inducers (caffeine, alcohol, cocaine), or unrecognized structural abnormalities of the heart (congenital heart disease, right ventricular arrhythmogenic dysplasia). On the other hand, older persons with PVCs are more likely to have known or suspected underlying heart disease. Myocardial infarction/ischemia, left ventricular dysfunction (cardiomyopathy), and side effects of medications are some of the many causes of ventricular ectopy more common in the older patient.[10,15,47]

Treatment of ventricular arrhythmias is extremely complex and relates to etiology, degree of left ventricular dysfunction, and the presence of underlying disease in other organ systems (liver, lung, kidney) among other considerations. The Cardiac Arrhythmia Suppression Trial (CAST) underscored the importance of the proarrhythmic effects of certain antiarrhythmic drugs, specifically the type Ic antiarrhythmics.[14,75,79]

Because there is no simple set of recommendations for antiarrhythmic therapy for ventricular ectopy, patient treatment must be highly individualized. The subspecialty of cardiac electrophysiology deals with such dilemmas, and knowledge in this area is expanding dramatically. When dealing with the patient who has highly complex and malignant rhythm disturbances, it may be best to request the assistance of an expert, as much of the evaluation and treatment of cardiac arrhythmias requires in-hospital monitoring and specialized testing.

CARDIAC MURMURS: WHO TO EVALUATE?

A common problem encountered by the physician in daily practice is the presence of a new or previously undiscovered heart murmur. The question may then arise as to whether this murmur is benign or the manifestation of a more serious underlying cardiac problem. The dilemma may then become whether the presenting murmur requires further evaluation. In many cases, patients go on to further evaluation, often with echocardiography.

Echocardiographic imaging

Advances in cardiac ultrasound imaging make this modality an attractive, noninvasive method for evaluating patients with a variety of cardiac conditions, including patients with different types of heart murmurs. With two-dimensional echocardiography, the valves and chambers can be viewed with relative clarity, and with the addition of Doppler echocardiography and color-flow imaging, an enormous amount of information can be obtained on a patient in a matter of minutes.[35,69]

The most commonly used (and least invasive) echocardiographic study is the transthoracic examination, which entails taking pictures from a number of different locations on the patient's chest with an ultrasound imaging transducer. Other types of echocardiographic examinations that may be required in certain clinical settings include stress echocardiography (exercise and pharmacologic), transesophageal echocardiography (on the conscious sedated patient, or in the operating room), and epicardial echocardiographic imaging (operating room technique).

Patient selection

When evaluating the patient with a heart murmur, history and physical examination provide the most valuable information to the physician regarding the need for further evaluation. Heart murmurs are so common that evaluation of every patient presenting with a cardiac murmur would clearly not be cost-effective. In cases of young, asympto-

matic patients presenting with a murmur on routine physical examination, the yield of an echocardiographic examination is extremely low. One possible exception is the young patient with unsuspected hypertrophic obstructive cardiomyopathy. In such cases, however, additional clues to the diagnosis may be provided by the changes in the murmur with provocative maneuvers, family history of the condition, and an ECG showing ventricular hypertrophy. Provocative maneuvers that decrease blood flow to the left ventricle increase the obstruction and make the murmur louder.

In most cases of young asymptomatic patients presenting with a murmur, echocardiography is not necessary because trivial or mild age-related valvular regurgitation is common in normal subjects. For example, mitral regurgitation can be detected in up to nearly 40% of normal subjects under the age of 50; tricuspid regurgitation can be found in nearly 60% of normal patients under the age of 50; pulmonic and aortic insufficiency are much less prevalent, but can also be found in the normal patient. Prevalence of valvular regurgitation as well as the potential for underlying heart disease increases in patients over the age of 50, and it is generally in this age group that the physician must make a decision on further evaluation of a cardiac murmur.[76] When the physical examination suggests valvular stenosis or regurgitation of uncertain severity, es-

---

Use of cardiac ultrasound

Generally accepted uses of the echocardiographic examination

Native and prosthetic valve disease
Endocarditis
Cardiac masses (tumors, thrombi, vegetations)
Pericardial effusion/tamponade
Pericardial disease (MRI, if available, may be more useful)
Constrictive/restrictive disease
Left ventricular function (global and segmental)
Cardiomyopathies (i.e., hypertrophic, dilated)
Complications of acute myocardial infarction (i.e., ischemic ventricular septal defect or aneurysm)
Pulmonary hypertension
Congenital heart disease
Precardiac/lung transplantation
Stroke in patients <45 years old or with known heart disease

Echocardiography generally not useful

Chronic coronary artery disease
Pulmonary embolism
Stroke in patients >45 years old or with known cerebrovascular disease

Feigenbaum H: *Echocardiography,* ed 4, Philadelphia, 1986, Lea & Febiger.

pecially in the symptomatic or older patient, echocardiography can be a valuable tool. In patients with known underlying valvular disease or left ventricular dysfunction, echocardiography is clearly a useful, reproducible, noninvasive method for evaluating severity and/or progression of disease. Furthermore, the use of echocardiography may obviate the need for additional invasive testing such as cardiac catheterization.[2,40,45,69]

Who then are the patients that may benefit most from an echocardiographic examination? Perhaps the patients who can benefit the most are those in whom the physical examination and symptoms do not correlate, causing uncertainty as to diagnosis. The older patient who is a poor historian, has vague symptoms and who presents with a new or previously undiscovered systolic murmur is also a good candidate.[69]

Other uses of echocardiography

Echocardiographic examination is appropriate in a number of different clinical situations other than the evaluation of cardiac murmurs. Echocardiography can be used not only in the evaluation of valvular heart disease (both native and prosthetic), but also in the evaluation of primary myocardial disease, pericardial disease, cardiac masses, aortic pathology, and in selected cases as an adjunct in the evaluation of ischemic heart disease (see accompanying box).[35] Certain modalities are more useful in particular clinical situations when evaluating the cardiac patient; and in many situations, echocardiography may be inappropriate or supplanted by a better test. For example, cardiac catheterization is a better method to determine the severity and extent of coronary disease, and magnetic resonance imaging (MRI) is more appropriate to evaluate pericardial tumors.

In summary, echocardiography is a valuable test in the evaluation of the cardiac patient. Careful selection of patients who should undergo this test may be based on history and physical examination in most cases. In less common situations, where the physician may be unable to obtain a clear assessment of the patient's cardiac status due to a confusing clinical picture (especially in the older patient), echocardiography may be a helpful screening tool.

REFERENCES

1. Agarwal BL: Rheumatic heart disease unabated in developing countries, *Lancet* 2:910-911, 1981.
2. Akasata T et al: Age-related valvular regurgitation: a study by pulsed Doppler echocardiography, *Circulation* 76:262-265, 1987.
3. Akhtar M et al: Role of cardiac electrophysiologic studies in patients with unexplained recurrent syncope, *PACE Pacing Clin Electrophysiol* 6:192-201, 1983.
4. American Heart Association: Jones criteria (revised) for guidance in the diagnosis of rheumatic fever, *Circulation* 69:204A-208A, 1984.
5. Arrigo L et al: Mitral valve repair: results and the decision-making process in reconstruction, *J Thorac Cardiovasc Surg* 99:622-630, 1990.
6. Bayer AS, Nelson RJ, Slama TG: Current concepts in prevention of prosthetic valve endocarditis, *Chest* 97(5):1203-1206, 1990.
7. Benditt PG et al: Prevention of recurrent sudden cardiac arrest: role of provocative electropharmacologic testing, *J Am Coll Cardiol* 2:418-425, 1983.
8. Braunwald E, editor: Valvular heart disease. In *Heart disease*, ed 3, Philadelphia, 1988, WB Saunders.
9. Braunwald E, editor: Infective endocarditis. In *Heart disease*, ed 3, Philadelphia, 1988, WB Saunders.
10. Braunwald E, editor: Specific arrhythmias. In *Heart disease*, ed 3, Philadelphia, 1988, WB Saunders.
11. British Society for Antimicrobial Chemotherapy: Antibiotic prophylaxis of infective endocarditis, *Lancet* 335:88-89, 1990.
12. Burawicz B: Is hypomagnesemia or magnesium deficiency arrhythmogenic? *J Am Coll Cardiol* 14:1098-1096, 1989.
13. Calderwood SB et al: Risk factors for the development of prosthetic valve endocarditis, *Circulation* 72(1):31-37, 1985.
14. CAST investigators: Preliminary report: effect of encainide and flecainide on mortality in a randomized trial of arrhythmia suppression after myocardial infarction, *N Engl J Med* 321:406-412, 1989.
15. Chatterjee K et al, editors: Syncope. In *Cardiology*, vol 1, Philadelphia, 1991, JB Lippincott.
16. Carpentier A: Cardiac valve surgery—the "French correction," *J Thorac Cardiovasc Surg* 86:323-337, 1983.
17. Ceremuzynski L: Hormonal and metabolic reactions evoked by acute myocardial infarction, *Circ Res* 48:767-772, 1981.
18. Cheng TO: Should antibiotic prophylaxis be recommended for all patients with mitral valve prolapse? *Am J Cardiol* 68:564, 1991.
19. Clemens JD et al: A controlled evaluation of the risk of bacterial endocarditis in persons with mitral valve prolapse, *N Engl J Med* 307:776-781, 1982.
20. Cosgrove DM, Stewart WJ: Mitral valvuloplasty, *Curr Probl Cardiol:* 14:359-415, 1989.
21. Dajani AS et al: Prevention of rheumatic fever: a statement for health professionals by the Committee on Rheumatic Fever, Endocarditis, and Kawasaki Disease of the Council on Cardiovascular Disease in the Young, the American Heart Association, *Circulation* 78(4):1082-1086, 1988.
22. Dajani AS et al: Prevention of bacterial endocarditis, *JAMA* 264(12):2919-2922, 1990.
23. Danchin N et al: Mitral valve prolapse with systolic murmur, a true risk factor for infective endocarditis. A case controlled study, abstract, *Circulation* (suppl II)78(4):210, 1988.
24. Danchin N et al: Mitral valve prolapse as a risk factor for infective endocarditis, *Lancet* 1:743-745, 1989.
25. Day SC et al: Evaluation and outcome of room emergency patients with transient loss of consciousness, *Am J Med* 73:15-22, 1982.
26. De Geest et al: Dental health, prophylactic antibiotic measures and infective endocarditis: an analysis of the knowledge of susceptible patients, *Acta Cardiol* 45(6):441-453, 1990.
27. Devereux RB et al: Relation between clinical features of the mitral valve prolapse syndrome and echocardiographically documented mitral valve prolapse, *J Am Coll Cardiol* 8:763-772, 1986.
28. Devereux RB et al: Complications of mitral valve prolapse. Disproportionate occurrence in men and older patients, *Am J Med* 81(5):751-758, 1986.
29. Devereux RB et al: Diagnosis and classification of severity of mitral valve prolapse: methodologic, biologic, and prognostic considerations, *Am Heart J* 113(5):1265-1280, 1987.
30. Devereux RB, Kramer-Fox R, Kligfield P: Mitral valve prolapse: causes, manifestations, and management, *Ann Intern Med* 111(4):305-317, 1989.
31. Durack DT, Kaplan EL, Bisno AL: Apparent failures of endocarditis prophylaxis. Analysis of 52 cases submitted to a national registry, *JAMA* 250(17):2318-2322, 1983.
32. Duren DR, Becker AE, Dunning AJ: Long-term follow-up of idiopathic mitral valve prolapse in 300 patients: a prospective study, *J Am Coll Cardiol* 11:42-47, 1988.

33. Emerman CL, Delvin C, Connors AF: Risk of toxicity in patients with elevated theophylline levels, *Ann Emerg Med* 19:643-648, 1990.

34. Farber BF: Prophylaxis of endocarditis. Comparison of new regimens, *Am J Med* 82:529-531, 1987.

35. Feigenbaum H: *Echocardiography*, Philadelphia, ed 4, Philadelphia, 1986, Lea & Febiger.

36. Fleg JL, Kennedy HL: Cardiac arrhythmias in a healthy elderly population: detection by 24-hour ambulatory electrocardiography, *Chest* 81:302-307, 1982.

37. Hickey AJ, Wilken DE: Age and the clinical profile of idiopathic mitral valve prolapse, *Br Heart J* 55:582-586, 1986.

38. Imperiale TF, Horwitz RI: Does prophylaxis prevent postdental infective endocarditis? A controlled evaluation of protective efficacy, *Am J Med* 88:131-136, 1990.

39. Jaeger FJ et al: Vasovagal syncope: diagnostic role of head-up tilt test in patients with positive ocular compression test, *PACE Pacing Clin Electrophysiol* 13:1416-1423, 1990.

40. Jaffe WM et al: Clinical evaluation versus Doppler echocardiography in the quantitative assessment of valvular heart disease, *Circulation* 78:267-275, 1988.

41. Josephson ME et al: Electrophysiologic and hemodynamic studies in patients resuscitated from cardiac arrest, *Am J Cardiol* 46:948-962, 1980.

42. Kaye D: Prophylaxis for endocarditis: an update, *Ann Intern Med* 104(3):419-423, 1986.

43. Kaye D, Abrutyn E: Prevention of bacterial endocarditis: 1991, *Ann Intern Med* 114:803-804, 1991.

44. Kimura K et al: Cardiac arrhythmias in hemodialysis patients, *Nephron* 53:201-207, 1989.

45. Klein AK et al: Age-related prevalence of valvular regurgitation in normal subjects: a comprehensive color flow examination of 118 volunteers, *J Am Soc Echocardiogr* 2:54-63, 1990.

46. Kligfield P et al: Arrhythmias and sudden death in mitral valve prolapse, *Am Heart J* 113(5):1298-1307, 1987.

47. Kloner RA, editor: Diagnosis and management of cardiac arrhythmias. In *The guide to cardiology*, ed 2, New York, 1990, Le Jacq Communications, Inc.

48. Levine RA et al: Reconsideration of echocardiographic standards for mitral valve prolapse: lack of association between leaflet displacement isolated to the apical four chamber view and independent echocardiographic evidence of abnormality, *J Am Coll Cardiol* 11:1011-1019, 1988.

49. Levy D, Savage D: Prevalence and clinical features of mitral valve prolapse, *Am Heart J* 113(5):1281-1290, 1987.

50. Librach G et al: The initial manifestations of acute myocardial infarction, *Geriatrics* 31:41-46, 1976.

51. MacMahon SW et al: Risk of infective endocarditis in mitral valve prolapse with and without precordial systolic murmurs, *Am J Cardiol* 58:105-108, 1986.

52. MacMahon SW et al: Mitral valve prolapse and infective endocarditis, *Am Heart J* 113(5):1291-1297, 1987.

53. Madlon-Kay DJ: Endocarditis prophylaxis in a primary care clinic, *J Fam Pract* 32(50):504-507, 1991.

54. Maloney JD et al: Malignant vasovagal syncope: prolonged asystole provoked by head-up tilt, *Cleve Clin J Med* 55:542-548, 1988.

55. Mancini GBJ, Goldberger AL: Cardioversion of atrial fibrillation: consideration of embolization, anticoagulation, prophylactic pacemaker, and long-term success, *Am Heart J* 104:617-624, 1982.

56. Mandell GL, Douglas RG, Bennett JE, editors: Cardiovascular infections. In *Principles and practice of infectious diseases,* ed 2, New York, 1990, Churchill Livingstone.

57. Mandell GL, Douglas RG, Bennett JE, editors: Nonsuppurative poststreptococcal sequelae: rheumatic fever and glomerulonephritis. In *Principles and practice of infectious diseases,* ed 2, New York, 1990, Churchill and Livingstone.

58. Margolis B, DeSilva RA, Lown B: Episodic drug treatment in the management of paroxysmal arrhythmias, *Am J Cardiol* 45:621-626, 1980.

59. Markowitz M: The decline of rheumatic fever: role of medical intervention, *J Pediatr* 106(4):545-550, 1985.

60. Marks AR et al: Identification of high-risk and low-risk subgroups of patients with mitral valve prolapse, *N Engl J Med* 320:1031-1036, 1989.

61. McKinsey DS, Ratts TE, Bisno AL: Underlying cardiac lesions in adults with infective endocarditis, *Am J Med* 82:681-688, 1987.

62. McManus BM et al: Exercise and sudden death, *Curr Probl Cardiol* 6:10, 1981.

63. Meyer GW: Endocarditis prophylaxis and gastrointestinal procedures, *Am J Gastroenterol* 84:1492-1493, 1989.

64. Morady F et al: Long-term follow-up of patients with recurrent unexplained syncope evaluated by electrophysiological testing, *J Am Coll Cardiol* 2:1053-1062, 1983.

65. Morady F et al: Clinical symptoms in patients with sustained ventricular tachycardia, *West J Med* 142:341-347, 1985.

66. Nikolic G, Bishop RL, Singh JB: Sudden death recorded during Holter monitoring, *Circulation* 6:218-226, 1982.

67. Nishimura RA et al: Echocardiographically documented mitral valve prolapse. Long-term follow-up of 237 patients, *N Engl J Med* 313:1035-1039, 1985.

68. Oakley CM: Controversies in the prophylaxis of infective endocarditis: a cardiological view, *J Antimicrob Chemother* 20(suppl A):99-104, 1987.

69. O'Rourke RA: Value of Doppler echocardiography for quantifying valvular stenosis or regurgitation, *Circulation* 78:483-485, 1988.

70. Panadis IP, Morganroth J: Sudden death in hospitalized patients: cardiac rhythm disturbances detected by ambulatory electrocardiographic monitoring, *J Am Coll Cardiol* 2:798-803, 1983.

71. Perloff JF, Child JS: Clinical and epidemiologic issues in mitral valve prolapse: overview and perspective, *Am Heart J* 113:1324-1332, 1987.

72. Podrid PJ: Aggravation of arrhythmia: a complication of antiarrhythmic drug therapy, *Eur Heart J* 10(suppl E):66-72, 1989.

73. Podrid PJ: Potassium and ventricular arrhythmias. *Am J Cardiol* 65:33E-44E, 1990.

74. Pomerance A: Cardiac pathology in the elderly. In Noble RJ, Rothbaum, editors: *Geriatric cardiology, cardiovascular clinics,* Philadelphia, 1981, FA Davis.

75. Pratt CM: Introduction: the aftermath of CAST—a reconsideration of traditional concepts, *Am J Cardiol* 65:1B-2B, 1990.

76. Rahko PS: Prevalence of regurgitant murmurs in patients with valvular regurgitation detected by Doppler echocardiography, *Ann Intern Med* 111(6):466-472, 1989.

77. Rahko PS: Antibiotic prophylaxis and regurgitant murmurs, *Ann Intern Med* 112:148-149, 1990.

78. Ranganathan N et al: Morphology of the human mitral valve. II. The valve leaflets, *Circulation* 41:459-467, 1970.

79. Roberts WC: Sudden cardiac death: a diversity of causes with focus on atherosclerotic coronary artery disease, *Am J Cardiol* 65:13B-19B, 1990.

80. Rokas S et al: Proarrhythmic effects of reactive hypoglycemia, *PACE Pacing Clin Electrophysiol* 15:373-376, 1992.

81. Roy D et al: Clinical characteristics and long-term follow-up of 119 survivors of cardiac arrest: relation to inducibility at electrophysiologic testing, *Am J Cardiol* 52:969-978, 1983.

82. Rubin DA et al: Prospective evaluation of heart block complicating early Lyme disease, *PACE Pacing Clin Electrophysiol* 15:252-255, 1992.

83. Savage DD et al: Mitral valve prolapse in the general population. I. Epidemiologic features: The Framingham Study, *Am Heart J* 106(3):571-581, 1983.

84. Shanson DC: Antibiotic prophylaxis of infective endocarditis in the

United Kingdom and Europe, *J Antimicrob Ther* 20(suppl A):119-131, 1987.

85. Sheps DS et al: Production of arrhythmias by elevated carboxyhemoglobin in patients with coronary artery disease, *Ann Intern Med* 113:343-351, 1990.

86. Sherman DG et al: Thromboembolism in patients with atrial fibrillation, *Arch Neurol* 41:708-711, 1984.

87. Shulman ST et al: Prevention of rheumatic fever. A statement for health professionals by the Committee on Rheumatic Fever and Infective Endocarditis of the Council on Cardiovascular Disease in the Young, *Circulation* 70(6):1118A-1127A, 1987.

88. Shulman ST: Prevention of infective endocarditis: the view from the United States, *J Antimicrob Ther* 20(suppl A):111-118, 1987.

89. Skelton CL: The heart and hyperthyroidism, *N Engl J Med* 307:1206-1214, 1982.

90. Steinberg W: Antibiotic prophylaxis for gastrointestinal procedures: the case against antibiotics, *Am J Gastroenterol* 85(8):1043, 1990.

91. Stollerman GH: Global changes in Group A streptococcal diseases and strategies for their prevention, *Adv Intern Med* 27:373-406, 1982.

92. Veasy LG et al: Resurgence of acute rheumatic fever in the intermountain area of the United States, *N Engl J Med* 316(8):421-427, 1987.

93. *Webster's ninth collegiate dictionary,* Springfield, 1983, Merriam-Webster.

94. Wilcken DEL, Hickey AJ: Lifetime risk for patients with mitral valve prolapse of developing severe valve regurgitation requiring surgery, *Circulation* 78:10-14, 1988.

95. Wolf PA et al: Duration of atrial fibrillation and imminence of stroke: the Framingham study, *Stroke* 14:664-671, 1983.

96. Wolf PA, Sila CA: Cerebral ischemia with mitral valve prolapse, *Am Heart J* 113(5):1308-1315, 1987.

97. Yacoub M et al: Surgical treatment of mitral regurgitation caused by floppy mitral valves: repair versus replacement, *Circulation* 64(suppl II):210-216, 1981.

RESOURCES

American Dental Association, 211 East Chicago Avenue, Chicago, Illinois 60611. Provides pamphlets on conditions, including procedures and prophylaxis for endocarditis.

American Heart Association, National Center, 7320 Greenville Avenue, Dallas, Texas 75231. Provides pamphlets on medication, exercise, diet and other preventive measures.

Centers for Disease Control, 1600 Clifton Road NE, Atlanta, Georgia 30333. Contact to report the incidence of rheumatic fever.

North American Society of Pacing and Electrophysiology, 377 Elliott Street, Newton Upper Falls, Massachusetts 02164. Provides pamphlets on testing methods and conditions and information on electrophysiologic procedures and underlying conditions that require such evaluation.

Chapter 43

STROKE

Cathy Sila

Stroke is a generic term representing a group of cerebrovascular disorders in which part of the brain is "transiently or permanently affected by ischemia or hemorrhage and/or in which one or more blood vessels of the brain are primarily affected by a pathological process."[57] The clinical entities included are transient ischemic attack, cerebral infarction, intracerebral hemorrhage, and subarachnoid hemorrhage.

In the 1970s, epidemiologists recognized a decline in stroke mortality. The rate of decline in cerebrovascular mortality was 1%/year in the 1950s and accelerated to 5%/year in the mid 1970s. The decline in cerebrovascular mortality was greater than the decline for cardiovascular disease in general and was circumstantially linked to improvements in identification and management of hypertension.[25]

In 1971 the Council on Cerebrovascular Disease of the American Heart Association issued a special subcommittee report that, although dogmatic statements were premature, transient ischemic attacks, cerebral infarction, hypertension, cardiac abnormalities, other consequences of atherosclerosis, and diabetes mellitus were major risk factors for stroke.[37] By focusing attention on risk factors, they hoped that a better understanding of pathophysiologic mechanisms of stroke would emerge and lead to the development of specific therapeutic interventions.

Population studies from Framingham, Massachusetts and Rochester, Minnesota continue to improve understanding of the frequency and relative importance of risk factors. In 1984 the subcommittee published an updated review that divided risk factors into groups according to the strength of their association with stroke and their ability to be modified (see the box at right).

The identification of risk factors in populations at risk provides a framework for individual patient management.[70] Within this framework, however, other specific preventive therapies require an understanding of the underlying pathophysiologic mechanism of stroke. In population studies, cerebral infarction accounts for 85% of all strokes, with 60% related to atherothrombosis and/or thromboembolism from the cervico-cephalic vessels and 40% to cardioembolism.[54] Therefore the majority of preventive strategies have been targeted to these types of stroke.

PRIMARY PREVENTION OF STROKE

Although stroke is clinically and etiologically heterogeneous, for most cases, and specifically for cases of cerebral infarction, the event itself is the culmination of a series of pathological processes that began decades before. Despite the advances in our understanding of the basic pathophysiology of cerebral ischemia, applications of pharmacologic manipulation of acute cerebral ischemia, and increased attention to rehabilitative efforts for stroke victims, the results of these efforts remain disappointing. The most significant effect on stroke will come from *primary prevention* of the processes that lead to a stroke in at-risk individuals before the development of symptoms. Failure of primary prevention is heralded by the develop-

---

Risk factors for stroke

Hypertension
Transient ischemic attacks
Prior cerebral infarction
Cardiovascular disease
Atrial fibrillation
Hyperlipidemia
Cigarette smoking
Diabetes mellitus
Sickle cell disease
Advancing age

Table 43-1. Cardiac risk factors for stroke

Risk factor	Increased risk
Rheumatic mitral stenosis	
With atrial fibrillation	18× Increase
Without atrial fibrillation	3-6× Increase
Nonvalvular atrial fibrillation	5.8%/year
Acute myocardial infarction	
Overall	3%/First month
With mural thrombus	20%/First month
Prosthetic heart valves, anticoagulated	
Mitral position	4%/year
Aortic position	2%/year
Left ventricular hypertrophy (EKG or CXR)	4× increase
With coronary artery disease or congestive heart failure	Additional 2× increase
Cardiac mortality for patients with asymptomatic bruit, TIA, prior stroke	5%/year

ment of symptoms, most commonly transient ischemic attacks and cerebral infarction. For high-risk individuals, alternative strategies for *secondary prevention* of stroke recurrence are necessary.

Hypertension

Hypertension is the single most important predisposing factor for stroke. The risk of stroke is directly related to the magnitude of elevation of both the systolic and diastolic blood pressure for both sexes and all age groups. Improvements in the identification and management of hypertension were circumstantially linked with the observed decline in stroke mortality. The efficacy of hypertension management as a strategy for stroke prevention has been confirmed by a series of controlled clinical trials performed over the last 30 years. In the 1960s, the efficacy of blood pressure reduction in stroke prevention was first demonstrated for severe and moderately severe diastolic hypertension (115 to 130 mm Hg).[67] Subsequently, efficacy in treating mild diastolic hypertension (90 to 109 mm Hg) was demonstrated in both placebo-controlled and treatment-vs.-usual-care trials.[34,39] Most recently, the value of treating isolated systolic hypertension (systolic >160 mm Hg and diastolic <90 mm Hg) was demonstrated in 4736 people over the age of 60 in a randomized double-blind placebo-control trial.[56] Fatal and nonfatal stroke, the primary endpoint, was reduced by 36%, which is consistent with the overall 42% reduction in stroke demonstrated by the previous hypertension treatment trials. Moreover, because of the significant number of individuals over the age of 80 who were enrolled in the trial, this is the first demonstration of a treatment benefit for any form of hypertension in individuals 80 years of age or older.

Cardiac disease

Cardiac diseases, including coronary heart disease, congestive heart failure, evidence of left ventricular hypertrophy, and cardiac dysrrhythmias, notably atrial fibrillation, double the risk of stroke determined by the level of blood pressure. (Table 43-1). This powerful statistical relationship is attributable to a number of mechanisms. Atherothrombotic and thromboembolic stroke share the same risk factors as coronary artery disease, the major contributor to overall cardiovascular disease. In turn, cardiogenic embolism accounts for approximately 15% of all ischemic strokes.[15] Although many types of cardiac disease have been linked with cerebral embolism (see Table 43-1), the major causes include:

- Nonvalvular atrial fibrillation
- Acute myocardial infarction
- Ventricular aneurysm
- Rheumatic heart disease
- Prosthetic cardiac valves

Atrial fibrillation. Atrial fibrillation in the setting of rheumatic mitral valve disease has long been recognized as a high-risk subgroup for stroke and systemic embolism. Chronic atrial fibrillation in the absence of rheumatic heart disease was subsequently suspected as an independent risk factor when a fivefold increased risk of stroke persisted after adjustment for other risk variables.[71] The incidence of nonvalvular atrial fibrillation increases with advancing age from 6.7% for ages 50 to 59 to 36.2% for ages 80 to 89.[69] More than a third of ischemic strokes occurring in the elderly are in the setting of atrial fibrillation. One third of patients with atrial fibrillation will experience a stroke sometime during their lifetime, and two thirds of these have clinical characteristics suggesting cardioembolism. In a series of hospitalized patients with an initial stroke associated with atrial fibrillation, the dysrhythmia was known to be present before the stroke in 76%. In this subgroup, 71% had a poor outcome with a significantly disabling deficit or death. In addition to the significant risk of clinical symptoms of stroke, "silent" cerebral infarcts were present on computed tomography in more than a third of patients.[50] Within the last 3 years, four prospective randomized clinical trials (Table 43-2) addressing primary prevention of stroke and systemic embolism with chronic anticoagulant or antiplatelet therapy in patients with nonvalvular atrial fibrillation were published.*

In the four trials, 3135 patients were followed from 15 to 27 months. Treatment consisted of placebo, aspirin at dosages at 75 mg or 325 mg per day, and warfarin with a protime ratio ranging from 1.2 to 1.9 times the control value, but standardized for differences in reagent by an international normalized ratio. The primary endpoints were thromboembolic complications of cerebral infarction and

*References 2, 11, 17, 49, 60, 61

Table 43-2. Stroke prevention in nonvalvular atrial fibrillation

Study	Thromboembolic risk: Cerebral infarction and systemic embolism			Treatment risk: Warfarin complications		Treatment			
	Control	Aspirin (risk reduction)	Warfarin (risk reduction)	ICH	Major hemorrhage	Control	Aspirin	Warfarin (INR)	Protime ratio
AFASAK[49]	5.5%/yr	4.7%/yr (15%)	2.2%/yr (58%)	1	0.8%/yr	Placebo	75 mg/day	2.4-4.2	1.5-1.9
SPAF[60,61]	6.3%/yr	3.6%/yr (42%)		1	1.5%/yr	Placebo	325 mg/day	1.5-5.0	1.3-1.8
(Group I, II)									
(Group I)	7.4%/yr		2.3%/yr (67%)						
BAATAF[11]	3.0%/yr		0.4%/yr (86%)	1	0.8%/yr	None/Aspirin		1.5-2.7	1.2-1.5
CAFA[17]	4.6%/yr		3.0%/yr (35%)	1	2.5%/yr	Placebo	—	2.0-3.0	1.3-1.5
Aggregate	5.8%/yr	(34%)	2.6%/yr (63%)	0.3%/yr					

From Peterson P et al: The Copenhagen AFASAK study, *Lancet* I:175-179, 1989.

systemic embolism and treatment complications of intracranial hemorrhage, major hemorrhage (bleeding requiring hospitalization, transfusion, or surgery), and minor bleeding. Exclusion criteria typically included significant bleeding history including intracranial hemorrhage, predisposition to trauma, inability to provide adequate follow-up, uncontrolled hypertension, alcohol abuse, or a requirement for anticoagulant therapy. In the Copenhagen AFASAK trial, 60% of the cerebral infarcts occurred at times of inadequate anticoagulation, and one third of the patients dropped out because of the inconvenience of monthly monitoring.[49]

The Stroke Prevention in Atrial Fibrillation (SPAF) study consisted of group I patients randomized to receive placebo, aspirin 325 mg per day, or warfarin, and group II of warfarin-ineligible patients. The study was prematurely interrupted when active treatment (aspirin or warfarin) was found to be significantly superior to placebo within group I patients.[60,61] Insufficient endpoints occurred at the time of interruption to assess the relative value of aspirin vs. warfarin, and the SPAF II study continues to address this question.

The Boston Area Anticoagulation Trial for Atrial Fibrillation (BAATAF) randomized patients to anticoagulation or usual care in an unblinded fashion.[11] The discretionary use of aspirin was carefully monitored and 8 of 13 endpoints in the control group occurred in patients taking aspirin of at least 325 mg per day.

Aggregate data indicates that chronic anticoagulation reduces stroke risk 63% from 5.8% per year to 2.6% per year; the reduction increases to an impressive 83% when target anticoagulation is achieved.

Complications of anticoagulant treatment included intracerebral hemorrhage at a rate of 0.3%/year. Major hemorrhage occurred in 1.5%/year regardless of treatment, but minor bleeding was three times more frequent in anticoagulated patients.

These studies clearly document the efficacy and safety of chronic low-level anticoagulation in a heterogeneous population of eligible patients with nonvalvular atrial fibrillation. Data are insufficient to assess the relative value of aspirin vs warfarin, and subgroup analyses suggest that the effect of aspirin may not be uniform across all variables. Metaanalysis of the completed trials should help in identify high- and low-risk subgroups, although many high-risk (recent embolic event, acute myocardial infarction, significant congestive heart failure, or cardiomyopathy) and low-risk (lone atrial fibrillation) patients were largely excluded. The prospective trials were able to show that left atrial size was not a reliable predictor of stroke risk, but insufficient data are available to assess other echocardiographic variables, and transesophageal echocardiography was not employed.

Acute myocardial infarction. Of patients suffering acute myocardial infarction, 3% suffer an ischemic stroke within the first month, most within the first 2 weeks. The majority occur in patients with large transmural anteroseptal myocardial infarctions associated with a dyskinetic segment. When mural thrombus can be identified, the risk increases to approximately 20%. Aggregated data from three randomized controlled clinical trials involving a total of 3562 patients showed that three months of warfarin anticoagulation to prolong the protime to 1.3 to 1.5 times control (INR 2.0 to 3.0) reduced the risk of stroke by 59%.[19,43,66] To prevent cardioembolic stroke, short-term warfarin anticoagulation is recommended for acute anterior transmural myocardial infarction and should be continued long term if complicated by atrial fibrillation, systemic embolism, or persistent left ventricular dysfunction.[51]

Valvular heart disease. Rheumatic mitral stenosis in association with atrial fibrillation increases the risk of stroke by eighteenfold, which is three to seven times the rate with mitral stenosis alone. On the basis of nonrandomized studies with historical controls, the evidence was sufficiently convincing that long-term anticoagulant therapy has been recommended for all patients with rheumatic mitral valve disease and paroxysmal or chronic atrial fibrillation.[38] Even in the absence of atrial fibrillation, there are probably subgroups that are at sufficiently increased risk to warrant chronic anticoagulant therapy as well, such as those associated with enlargement of the left atrium greater than 5.5 centimeters. Recently, 3 months of anticoagulation before balloon valvuloplasty of the mitral valve has also been recommended to reduce the embolic risk of the procedure.[47]

Thromboembolism continues to be one of the most serious and feared complications of prosthetic heart valves, occurring with such frequency as to warrant chronic anticoagulant therapy. Many of the technical valve modifications have been designed to reduce thromboembolic potential and permit sufficient protection with lower-dose anticoagulation or antiplatelet therapy. Therefore treatment recommendations are based on the type of prosthetic valve employed. The overall rate of embolism for anticoagulated patients with mechanical valves averages 4%/year for mitral valve replacements and 2%/year for aortic valve replacements. Dipyridamole in combination with warfarin has also been shown to further reduce thromboembolic risk. Current recommendations for mechanical prosthetic heart valves include long-term anticoagulation (protime ratio 1.5 to 2 times control, INR 3.0 to 4.5). Patients who fail or require lower-dose warfarin therapy should receive dipyridamole 400 mg/day as well. Bioprosthetic valves have been associated with an increased frequency of thromboembolic events, largely within the first 3 months after operation. The long-term risk of thromboembolic complications with bioprosthetic valves is low and can often be attributed to associated atrial fibrillation, left atrial enlargement, or thrombus. For patients with bioprosthetic heart valves, low-dose anticoagulant therapy (protime ratio 1.3 to 1.5 times control, INR 2.0 to 3.0) should be employed for the first 3 months after mitral valve replacement, is optional for aortic valve replacement associated with a normal sinus rhythm, and should be continued in those patients whose bioprosthetic valves are complicated by atrial fibrillation, left atrial thrombus, or a history of systemic embolism.[59] Long-term antithrombotic therapy with aspirin, 325 mg per day, is optional but typically used.

Impaired cardiac function. Subclinical cardiac dysfunction as evidenced by left ventricular hypertrophy on electrocardiogram or chest x-ray measures the effect of hypertension, and this evidence of end-organ involvement produces more than fourfold risk of cerebral infarction, even when adjusted for age and level of blood pressure. Additional clinical evidence of impaired cardiac function, including coronary artery disease and congestive heart failure, further doubles the stroke risk. Epidemiologic studies have demonstrated much stronger associations with coronary artery disease than with stroke for certain risk factors such as genetic predisposition, hyperlipidemia, smoking, and diabetes mellitus. The risk of cardiovascular complications increases with an increasing number of risk factors and increasing levels of any single risk factor. (See Chapter 41 for the prevention of cardiovascular disease.)

Coronary heart disease is the major cause of death among stroke survivors as well as patients with transient ischemic attacks or asymptomatic carotid bruits at a rate of 5%/year. The cardiac events are catastrophic in two thirds, with 15% to 25% presenting with sudden death, 40% with acute myocardial infarction, and 35% with angina. In a heterogeneous group of patients with cerebrovascular disease, 40% have severe coronary artery disease as determined by stress radionucleid ventriculography or cardiac catheterization, but 86% of patients have angiographic evidence of coronary artery disease.[31,53] The neurologic presentation does not predict the severity of coronary artery disease.

Asymptomatic carotid artery disease

Cervical bruits occur with increasing frequency with age in 7% to 10% of those over the age of 65. However, cervical bruits correlate poorly with the degree of underlying carotid artery stenosis, are a poor indicator of the risk of an ipsilateral cerebral infarction, and essentially are a marker of generalized atherosclerosis. The most important independent predictors of carotid artery stenosis are duration of cigarette smoking, hypertension, diabetes mellitus, and systolic blood pressure at the time of examination.[35]

Longitudinal data from noninvasive vascular laboratories have provided insight on the risk associated with asymptomatic carotid stenosis. In a heterogeneous group of patients with an asymptomatic bruit studied with duplex carotid ultrasound, transient ischemic attacks and cerebral infarction occurred at a rate of 4%/year; however, the annual rate of an unheralded ipsilateral infarct was only 1.3%.[52] Subsequent prospective cohort studies determined that stroke incidence increases with the degree of carotid stenosis, with a break in the risk at approximately 75% stenosis.[16] The annual overall stroke rate associated with a carotid stenosis of less than 75% was 1.3%/yr, which increased to 3.3%/yr as the stenosis progressed to greater than 75%. However, even in the higher-risk group, the rate of ipsilateral cerebral infarction was 2.5%/yr, but the combined risk of myocardial ischemia and vascular death was 9.9%/yr.[48] As a marker for generalized atherosclerosis, asymptomatic carotid artery disease is a better indicator for myocardial infarction and vascular death than stroke.

Antiplatelet therapy for primary prophylaxis of myocardial events has been demonstrated to be effective.[58] Although aspirin has not been shown to alter cerebrovascular events in asymptomatic individuals, the number of patients studied has been too small to specifically address this is-

Table 43-3. Carotid endarterectomy trials

	Diagnostic criteria	Medical therapy	
		Specific risk factor education	Antiplatelet therapy
Asymptomatic carotid disease			
CASANOVA[14]	50%-90%	−	ASA 300 mg tid + dipyridamole 75 mg tid
VA #167[64]	>50%	−	ASA 650 mg bid
ACAS[6]	>60%	+	ASA 325 mg qd
Symptomatic carotid disease			
VA #309[42]	>50%	−	ASA 325 mg qd
NASCET[45,46]	>30%	+	ASA 650 mg bid
ECST[23]	Physician discretion	Local center discretion	Local center discretion

From Howard VJ et al: Comparison of multicenter study designs for investigation of carotid endarterectomy efficacy, *Stroke* 23:583-593, 1992.

sue. A randomized study of the value of antiplatelet therapy in patients with asymptomatic cervical bruits is now underway with completion planned in May, 1994.[7]

Carotid endarterectomy has been considered a prophylactic procedure for patients judged to be at high risk for stroke, and various degrees of carotid artery stenosis have been included in this high-risk category. The 1980s witnessed a flurry of emotionally charged publications regarding carotid endarterectomy. Perhaps the most powerful was the Rand report on the appropriateness of carotid endarterectomy, stating that a third of procedures are done inappropriately and another third for questionable indications.[44] In this wake, a series of multicenter prospective randomized clinical trials have organized to address whether carotid endarterectomy provides additional benefit over best medical therapy. Three prospective, multicenter, randomized trials have been designed to determine the safety and effectiveness of carotid endarterectomy for asymptomatic carotid atherosclerosis[33] (Table 43-3). The Carotid Artery Stenosis with Asymptomatic Narrowing: Operation Versus Aspirin (CASANOVA) study randomized 410 patients with 50% to 90% asymptomatic internal carotid artery stenosis, excluding those patients with a recent myocardial infarction or other severe medical disease. There was no statistical difference in the number of neurological deficits and deaths between the two groups. However, because greater than 90% stenosis was excluded from the study, no conclusion could be offered about this subgroup.[14] The Veteran's Administration's Asymptomatic Carotid Stenosis Trial (VA #167) randomized 444 patients with greater than 50% internal carotid artery stenosis. Preliminary analysis has shown that coronary artery disease has been the prime determinant of operative mortality, and the follow-up of the two cohorts continues.[64] The Asymptomatic Carotid Atherosclerosis Study (ACAS) plans to randomize 750 patients with greater than 60% in-

ternal carotid artery stenosis.[6] Patient acquisition began in early 1988 and randomization continues.

Until further data are available, management of risk factors associated with asymptomatic carotid artery stenosis is indicated. The role of surgery awaits the results of all the randomized surgical trials, but in the interim, there is no evidence to support carotid endarterectomy for asymptomatic patients with less than 90% internal carotid stenosis. Patients with asymptomatic stenosis greater than 90% continue to be managed on a case-by-case basis, which should take into account the annual ipsilateral stroke rate of approximately 2.5%, the number of patient years at risk for complications, the surgical risk, and the risk of non-neurologic complications, such as cardiovascular morbidity and mortality.

Lipids

Lipids and lipoprotein abnormalities have strong associations with coronary atherosclerosis; however, their relationship to stroke is poorly established and inconsistent. In fact, total serum cholesterol in individuals over 65 is inversely related to stroke incidence, which is primarily determined by the negative association of low-density lipoprotein cholesterol with stroke in women.[72] A review of more than 20 studies suggests that a relationship between lipid abnormalities and cerebrovascular atherosclerosis does exist, but the significance may be blurred by the heterogeneity of indicators used to define cerebrovascular disease and the small sample size of the studies.[62] Plaque regression in a serial ultrasound study of seven patients with heterozygous hypercholesterolemia treated with heparin-induced extracorporeal LDL precipitation has recently been reported, analogous to its effects on coronary artery plaques. Although coronary events have been reduced with this therapy, the results in cerebrovascular complications are not established.[30]

In the absence of further scientific data, the rationale for management of hyperlipidemia is its relationship to coronary artery disease.

Diabetes mellitus

Although diabetes mellitus is an independent risk factor for cerebral infarction, it correlates strongly with hypertension and has a stronger association for women than men. The greater relative risks appear to be a fourfold increase in intermittent claudication and cardiovascular complications in women at a rate equal to their male counterparts. When adjusted for hypertension and diabetes, obesity is no longer an independent risk factor for stroke.[72]

Although diabetic control has not been clearly shown to influence the risk of stroke, hyperglycemia at the onset of cerebral infarction has been suggested to increase infarct size by supporting anaerobic glycolysis and lactate production, which accentuates secondary ischemic damage.

Red blood cell disorders

Sickle cell anemia is the most common hemoglobinopathy, and 10% to 15% of patients have cerebrovascular complications representing a threefold to fourfold increase. These are more common in patients with severe disease and sickle crisis, when tissue hypoxia and acidosis result in polymerization, stasis, and vascular occlusion.[28]

An elevated hematocrit has been linked in epidemiologic studies to increased stroke risk. Hematocrit is one of the major determinants of viscosity, with maximal oxygen-carrying capacity occurring between 33% and 35%. When adjusted for blood pressure and cigarette smoking, elevated hematocrit loses statistical significance.

Genetic factors

Atherosclerosis is thought to be a complex genetic disorder caused by multiple gene interactions with variable phenotypic expression and influenced by environmental factors. Studies have demonstrated a strong genetic component, with an approximate tenfold increased risk of myocardial infarction in the presence of a first-degree relative with premature coronary artery disease. Although a few families have been described with a similar type of premature cerebrovascular disease, the role of genetic factors for most patients is difficult to determine, largely because of the heterogeneous etiology and clinical manifestations of stroke. Some forms of amyloid angiopathy, certain coagulopathies, and some metabolic disorders associated with stroke are inherited, and hypertension and diabetes may also have a genetic basis.[3] Homogeneous cerebrovascular conditions, such as cavernous malformations, 10% to 15% of all saccular intracranial aneurysms, and intracranial aneurysms associated with polycystic kidney disease, Ehlers-Danlos type IV, and Marfan's syndrome have been more amenable to genetic analysis.

Alcohol and tobacco

Alcohol consumption has been linked with stroke in epidemiologic studies. However, hypertension, cigarette smoking, and paroxysmal atrial fibrillation with alcoholic cardiomyopathy are confounding associated factors, making the role of alcohol as an independent risk factor unclear.[27]

SECONDARY PREVENTION OF STROKE

The failure of primary preventive measures and the progression of disease is heralded by the development of cerebral or retinal ischemia, as manifest by transient ischemic attacks, transient monocular blindness (amaurosis fugax), or cerebral or retinal infarction. Patients with transient ischemic attacks (TIA) form a high-risk subgroup with a significantly higher prevalence of hypertension, ischemic heart disease, diabetes, cigarette smoking, and prior stroke than the general population. In the absence of associated risk factors, data suggest that a TIA may not be an independent risk factor but rather identifies patients at increased risk from a combination of comorbid conditions.[32]

Transient ischemic attacks resolve within 24 hours by definition, but the majority last less than 15 minutes. The usefulness of this clinical definition has been questioned, as correlation with neuroimaging (computed tomography or magnetic resonance imaging) has demonstrated that 25% of patients clinically diagnosed with a transient ischemic attack actually have a cerebral infarction.[63] Because the brevity of the event and the absence of objective neurological abnormalities result in interobserver variability from 40% to 70%, TIAs are usually not included as an endpoint event subject to statistical analysis, and most studies use combinations of transient and persistent ischemic events as qualifying inclusion criteria.

As determined by natural history studies and the placebo groups of treatment trials,[8,10,18,40] the annual risk for stroke in persons with prior transient ischemic attack or minor stroke is 4% to 12% per year and risk of death is 10% to 17% per year, of which two thirds are vascular deaths.

Although these are overall statistics, the group identified by transient ischemic attacks and minor stroke is heterogeneous. Although the ipsilateral infarct rate is associated with the degree of underlying carotid stenosis, the overall outcome is largely influenced by vascular mortality, myocardial infarction, and strokes of other mechanisms. For example, the fate of 45 symptomatic patients with greater than 75% carotid stenosis was followed when their surgical risk precluded endarterectomy.[8] Although 10% had an ipsilateral cerebral infarct within the first year and the annual rate subsequently dropped to 2.4%, one third of the strokes were lacunar infarcts probably unrelated to the carotid stenosis. The cumulative death and

Table 43-4. Recent antiplatelet trials in stroke prevention

Study	Patients	Treatment		Endpoint	Risk reduction*	Comments
Antiplatelet Trialists' Collaboration[5]	metaanalysis >29,000	ASA 300-1300 mg/day	Placebo	Stroke, MI, vascular death	25%	No difference between ASA doses
SALT[55]	1360: 33% TIA, 67% stroke	ASA 75 mg/day	Placebo	Stroke, death	18%	Both men and women
Dutch[20]	3131: 32% TIA, 68% stroke	ASA 30 mg/day	ASA 283 mg/day	Stroke, MI, vascular death	NS	No difference between ASA doses
TASS[29]	3069: 50% TIA, 35% stroke, 15% >1 type	Ticlopidine 250 mg bid	ASA 650 mg bid	All stroke	19%	But 47% in the first year, both men and women
CATS[26]	1072: all stroke, 26% lacunar	Ticlopidine 250 mg bid	Placebo	Stroke, MI, vascular death	23%	Both men and women

*Intent-to-treat analysis

stroke rate was 24% within the first 2 years and claimed half the patients during a 6-year follow-up.

The majority of clinical trials for stroke prevention have been for the secondary prevention of patients with ischemic symptoms. Major therapies include antiplatelet therapy, anticoagulant therapy, and carotid endarterectomy.

Antiplatelet therapy

Aspirin has become the standard preventive therapy for patients at risk for stroke, although controversy continues regarding efficacy and optimum dosage. The major statistical support for antiplatelet therapy is derived from a metaanalysis of 31 randomized trials of more than 29,000 patients receiving antiplatelet therapy for TIA, stroke, unstable angina, and myocardial infarction (Table 43-4). With a combined endpoint of nonfatal stroke, myocardial infarction, or vascular death, a 25% risk reduction was demonstrated with antiplatelet therapy, typically aspirin at a dosage of 1000 to 1300 mg per day. Addressing specifically cerebrovascular trials, the reduction of nonfatal stroke was 22%.[5] The data also suggest that the major effect of aspirin is in the reduction of minor, not major, strokes.

The UK-TIA trial was the single cerebrovascular trial included in the metaanalysis that used lower aspirin doses, randomizing patients to either 300 mg daily or 600 mg twice daily. Although the combined endpoint of stroke, myocardial infarction, and vascular death was reduced by 22%, the 7.7% reduction of disabling stroke and vascular death was not significant. There was no difference in endpoints between the two dosage levels, but the rate of gastrointestinal side effects was significantly lower in the low-dose group.[65]

In the metaanalysis, this trial was combined with two cardiac trials of low-dose aspirin, and these were com-

pared with the 15 trials using doses of 900 to 1300 mg/day. This subgroup analysis suggested that the studies using 300 to 325 mg of aspirin per day yielded results that were comparable with those obtained by 900 to 1300 mg/day.[5] The next year the World Health Organization concluded that the optimum dose of aspirin remains uncertain, but given the available data, for patients who are unable to tolerate 1300 mg of aspirin per day, 325 mg/day may be as effective and the gastrointestinal side effects are less.[68] At the International Conference on Cerebrovascular Disease and Stroke in 1991, a show of hands indicated that nearly all the physicians present used 325 mg/day routinely in their practice.

The European Stroke Prevention Study (ESPS), which followed 2500 patients for 2 years yet took 11 years to publish, compared a regimen of aspirin 330 mg and dipyridamole 75 mg combined in a single capsule administered three times a day with a regimen of placebo. The 35% reduction in stroke and vascular death and 38% reduction in fatal and nonfatal stroke was the highest obtained in any antiplatelet trial, although the relative benefit of the two drugs could not be assessed.[22] This antiplatelet combination failed to regenerate enthusiasm because a concurrent trial published 7 years before failed to demonstrate any additional benefit of dipyridamole over aspirin alone.

The Dutch TIA trial used a water-soluble carbaspirin calcium preparation and demonstrated no statistically significant difference in the frequency of stroke, myocardial infarction, or vascular death between 30 mg/day and 283 mg/day groups, although major bleeding complications were slightly fewer and minor bleeding was significantly less in the low-dose group.[20] In the SALT trial, aspirin 75 mg reduced the risk of stroke and vascular death by a significant 17%. The 16% reduction in fatal and nonfatal stroke, however, was not significant, perhaps because fatal hemorrhagic stroke occurred in six patients in the aspirin group and not in the placebo group.[55] Although an increased frequency of hemorrhagic stroke has been noted before, this trend has never attained statistical significance.[58]

Ticlopidine is a novel antiplatelet agent that has demonstrated efficacy in secondary prevention of vascular events after transient ischemic attack and a completed stroke. The Ticlopidine Aspirin Stroke Study (TASS) compared ticlopidine 250 mg twice daily with aspirin 650 mg twice daily in patients with TIAs or minor strokes.[29] Ticlopidine reduced the overall risk of fatal or nonfatal stroke by 19% over aspirin, but within the first, highest-risk year of treatment, the risk reduction was 48%. In the Canadian-American Ticlopidine Study (CATS) of patients with a completed stroke, ticlopidine 250 mg/day reduced recurrent stroke by 34% and the combined risk of stroke, myocardial infarction, or vascular death by 30%.[26] These studies included sufficient women to prove efficacy for both sexes. Serious adverse reactions were present in 2% of both groups, with gastrointestinal bleeding being the major aspirin-induced effect. Significant neutropenia (absolute neutrophil count [ANC] less than 450) occurred in ticlopidine-treated patients almost exclusively within the first 3 months of therapy.

As a result of these studies, ticlopidine was released as an alternative treatment for transient ischemic attacks in aspirin-intolerant patients. During the first 3 months of treatment, the complete blood counts should be monitored every 2 weeks and ticlopidine discontinued if the absolute neutrophil count drops below 1200.

Anticoagulant therapy

The only placebo-controlled trials of warfarin in the prevention of recurrent stroke date back more than 30 years, with fewer than 200 patients investigated. A recent metaanalysis was unable to find evidence for benefit in stroke prevention; however, the sample sizes were small and may reflect a type II error of missing a beneficial effect.[36] Until the recent atrial fibrillation trials, the complication rates of warfarin therapy were thought to outweigh any potential benefit in all but extreme situations where medical therapy had failed. In view of the acceptable risk of low-dose anticoagulant therapy, the Warfarin Aspirin Recurrent Stroke Study (WARSS) trial has begun to compare low-dose anticoagulant therapy with aspirin 325 mg/day and is expected to be completed in 1998.

Carotid endarterectomy

Three prospective, multicenter, randomized trials have been designed to determine safety and efficacy of carotid endarterectomy for symptomatic internal carotid artery stenosis. Although randomization began about the same time as the asymptomatic carotid stenosis trials, a rapid acquisition of statistical significance has allowed results to be published for some subgroups.

The Veteran's Administration Symptomatic Carotid Stenosis Trial (VA #309) randomized only 3.8% of 5000 patients screened with 50% to 99% internal carotid stenosis and failed to demonstrate a significant reduction in the endpoints of stroke and death between 7% and 8% in the medical and surgical treatment arms respectively.[42] Only by adding crescendo TIAs to the combined endpoint could the trial demonstrate a benefit for surgery for patients with greater than 50% carotid stenosis, which was even more impressive in the presence of greater than 70% stenosis.

The North American Symptomatic Carotid Endarterectomy Trial (NASCET) randomized patients with symptomatic 30% to 99% carotid stenosis and prematurely terminated the greater-than-70% subgroup because of a statistically significant benefit for surgical treatment.[45,46] Carotid endarterectomy reduced the rate of ipsilateral stroke from 26% to 9% and major ipsilateral stroke from 13.1% to 2.5% at 2 years. This was accomplished at the lowest perioperative stroke morbidity and mortality rate of 5%, which included major stroke and death of 2% and a mortality of more than 1% alone. During this 30-day period, approximately 3% of the medical group had a similar 3% stroke morbidity or mortality rate. Secondary analyses have determined that finer divisions in stenosis from 70% to 99% also correlate with the degree of relative risk. The study of the subgroup of 30% to 69% stenosis has not yet been concluded.

The European Carotid Surgery Trial (ECST) allowed individual physicians to randomize 2500 patients for whom there was "substantial uncertainty" about which treatment they should receive.[23] This unique and inexpensive statistical method allowed for a heterogeneous group based on individual practice bias and included subgroups of less than 30%, 30% to 69%, and 70% to 99% stenosis. For patients with severe symptomatic 70% to 99% carotid stenosis, the benefits of surgery outweighed the 30-day stroke and death rate of 7.5%. The highest-risk period for severe or fatal stroke alone appeared to be the first year after randomization, and surgery reduced ipsilateral stroke from 16.8% to 2.8% over 3 years. Too few strokes occurred within the less-than-30% stenosis subgroup to justify the risk of surgery, and the 30% to 69% subgroup continues to be studied.

SOCIO-MEDICO-ECONOMICS

Cerebrovascular disease exerts a tremendous influence on medical resources and social productivity. Stroke is the third leading cause of death in the United States, after cardiovascular disease and cancer. In 1981, more than 164,000 Americans died from stroke and there were 1.87 million stroke survivors, 70% of whom had some limitation of vocational capacity.[4] Approximately 400,000 patients are discharged from hospitals with either an initial or recurrent stroke, which accounts for more than half of the hospitalizations for acute neurologic disease.

The incidence of stroke more than doubles with each

decade over the age of 55.[21] Stroke currently is the most prevalent neurological public health problem, and its effect will be felt especially by the growing proportion of elderly people. Over the last 4 decades, the proportion of cerebral infarctions occurring in the over-65 population has increased by 14%, and this age group accounts for approximately 80% of cerebral infarctions in a community study.[13] Most of the stroke prevention and therapy trials have focused on the younger patients because of age restrictions in the protocols, and this will have an increasing effect on recruitment in treatment trials as perhaps 50% of patients would be ineligible because of age.[13]

The economic effect of these statistics is formidable. In 1976 the estimated annual direct cost of health care was $2.3 billion, and in 1988 this had increased to $83.7 billion.[1] Hospitalization for a severely disabling but nonfatal stroke can average $20,000, and subsequent inpatient rehabilitation for an average 25-day stay an additional $21,000.

The pharmacologic cost of prevention can include $5 to $20/year for aspirin, $250/year for warfarin, and $1200/year for ticlopidine. Additional costs of prevention include identification of risk factors, education, and nonpharmacologic and pharmacologic management of hypertension, diabetes mellitus, hyperlipidemia, and cigarette smoking, all of which have beneficial effects on other comorbid conditions.

Within 3 decades of its introduction, carotid endarterectomy became one of the most frequently performed vascular procedures in the United States. The number of procedures increased from 15,000 in 1971 to more than 82,000 in 1982 and was predicted to reach 125,000 by 1987. However, instead of reaching this predicted figure, the rate declined by 22%, largely because of publications questioning the efficacy of the procedure in stroke prevention. To resolve these questions, six multicenter prospective clinical trials were organized to address whether carotid endarterectomy provided an additional benefit over best medical therapy for asymptomatic and symptomatic carotid stenosis. Unfortunately, the swing in public opinion has seriously reduced recruitment in some of the clinical trials, which delays the scientific results. However, if the multicenter studies confirm the Rand prediction that one third of the procedures are indicated, the estimated savings of 83,750 endarterectomies at an average cost of $13,000 would pay for the roughly $50 million budget of the four U.S. carotid endarterectomy trials within 3 weeks.

SCREENING

For the majority of patients, appropriate screening consists of a thorough history and physical guided by our knowledge of predisposing risk factors. Auscultation for cervical bruits should be a part of the general physical examination in the fashion that palpating peripheral pulses and listening for fourth heart sounds gives information about the severity of end-organ damage and directs the aggressiveness of patient management required to prevent further complications. Although cervical bruits may originate from the internal, external, or common carotid artery or be transmitted from the subclavian artery or the heart, bruits that are maximal at the angle of the mandible are more likely to originate from the carotid artery itself. A bruit that extends into diastole is highly suggestive of a severe stenosis. Bruits that seem to disappear and reappear, depend on patient position (sitting or supine), or can be obliterated with light neck pressure are often transmitted from the venous system and are of no clinical significance. However, a cervical bruit is a nonspecific and insensitive indicator of ipsilateral significant internal carotid artery (ICA) stenosis. For patients without symptoms of cerebral or retinal ischemia, further screening tests for ICA stenosis remain an option, pending the results of the carotid endarterectomy trials. Until the trials are completed, our cerebrovascular group believes that carotid endarterectomy for asymptomatic carotid stenosis should be reserved for young, otherwise healthy individuals with a low surgical risk who have 90% or greater carotid stenosis.

Once patients have become symptomatic with retinal or cerebral ischemia, the evaluation is designed to identify the mechanism to provide a rational basis for subsequent treatment. Depending on the circumstance, a wide variety of testing may be required, ranging from noninvasive vascular techniques to cerebral angiography, electrocardiogram to specialized echocardiography, and simple blood tests to complex batteries of coagulation factors. In the presence of clear carotid distribution symptoms, if the patient is considered a surgical candidate, one may proceed directly to carotid angiography or screen for the presence of greater-than-70% or less-than-30% carotid stenosis, for which clear surgical guidelines exist.[24] Carotid artery screening can be performed with duplex or doppler ultrasonography.

Duplex carotid ultrasonography combines a b-mode anatomic image with a doppler assessment of blood flow. This is the preferred noninvasive study (85% sensitive, 90% specific). High-grade stenoses with low flow can be mistaken for occlusion, requiring angiographic confirmation. The usual cost is $200 to $400. Doppler ultrasound alone (70% sensitive, 95% specific) is an alternative screening modality at a reduced cost and can be used when duplex ultrasonography is not available.

Magnetic resonance angiography (MRA) is an emerging technology with the advantage of providing a vascular image in less than 10 minutes of additional data acquisition. Preliminary reports indicate a 95% sensitivity of and specificity for detecting a 70% carotid bifurcation stenosis.[41] The major limitations are that approximately 25% of patients are unable to tolerate the procedure because of claustrophobia and that MRA is contraindicated in certain patients with implanted metal including pacemakers, defibrillators, and certain aneurysm clips. Although a cost has not yet been determined, magnetic resonance imaging ranges from $1000 to $2000. Carotid angiography is the reference diagnostic test for carotid artery disease and is usually required before carotid endarterectomy. Serious complications occur in less than 2%. The procedure usually requires hospitalization, although intraarterial digital subtraction techniques employ smaller catheters and less contrast material and may be conducted on an outpatient basis. The cost ranges from $1000 to $3000.[24]

SUMMARY

Stroke is the third leading cause of death and the most prevalent neurological public health problem in the United States. Cerebral infarction accounts for 85% of all strokes, with most caused by atherothrombosis and thromboembolism from the cervico-cephalic vessels and cardioembolism.

Prevention efforts are directed toward identification and management of risk factors in presymptomatic individuals as well as specific pharmacologic and surgical management of patients symptomatic with cerebral or retinal ischemia.

Despite advances in acute stroke management and rehabilitation, prevention remains the best course.

REFERENCES

1. Adelman SM: The national survey of stroke. Economic impact, *Stroke* 12(suppl I):1-69, 1981.
2. Albers GW et al: Stroke prevention in nonvalvular atrial fibrillation; a review of prospective randomized trials, *Ann Neurol* 30:511-518, 1991.
3. Alberts MJ: Genetic aspects of cerebrovascular disease, *Stroke* 22:276-280, 1991.
4. American Heart Association: *Heart facts 1984,* Dallas, 1984, the Association.
5. Antiplatelet Trialists' Collaboration: Secondary prevention of vascular disease by prolonged antiplatelet treatment, *Br Med J* 296:320-331, 1988.
6. The Asymptomatic Carotid Atherosclerosis Study Group: Study design for randomized prospective trial of carotid endarterectomy for asymptomatic atherosclerosis, *Stroke* 20:844-849, 1989.
7. The Asymptomatic Cervical Bruit Study Group: Natural history and effectiveness of aspirin in asymptomatic patients with cervical bruits, *Arch Neurol* 48:683-686, 1991.
8. Bogouslavsky J, Despland PA, and Regli F: Prognosis of high risk patients with non-operative symptomatic extracranial carotid tight stenosis, *Stroke* 14:108-111, 1988.
9. Reference deleted in galleys.
10. Bogousslavsky J, Regli F: Prognosis of symptomatic intracranial obstruction of internal carotid artery, *Eur Neurol* 22:351-358, 1983.
11. The Boston Area Anticoagulation Trial for Atrial Fibrillation Investigators: The effect of low-dose warfarin on the risk of stroke in patients with non-rheumatic atrial fibrillation, *N Engl J Med* 323:1505-1511, 1990.
12. Bousser MG et al: "AICLA" controlled trial of aspirin and dipyridamole in the secondary prevention of atherothrombotic cerebral ischemia, *Stroke* 14:5-14, 1983.
13. Broderick J et al: Incidence rates of stroke in the eighties: the end of the decline in stroke? *Stroke* 20:577-582, 1989.
14. The CASANOVA Study Group: Carotid surgery versus medical therapy in asymptomatic carotid stenosis, *Stroke* 22:1229-1235, 1991.
15. Cerebral Embolism Task Force: Cardiogenic brain embolism, *Arch Neurol* 43:71-84, 1986.
16. Chambers BR, Norris JW: Outcome in patients with asymptomatic neck bruits, *N Engl J Med* 315:860-865, 1986.
17. Connally SJ et al: Canadian atrial fibrillation anticoagulation (CAFA) study, *J Am Coll Cardiol* 18:349-355, 1991.
18. Craig DR et al: Intracranial internal carotid artery stenosis, *Stroke* 13:825-828, 1982.
19. Drapkin A, Mersky C: Anticoagulant therapy after acute myocardial infarction: relation of therapeutic benefit to patient's age, sex, and severity of infarction, *JAMA* 222:541-549, 1972.
20. The Dutch TIA Trial Study Group: A comparison of two doses of aspirin (30 mg vs. 283 mg a day) in patients after a transient ischemic attack or minor ischemic stroke, *N Engl J Med* 325:1261-1266, 1991.
21. Dyken ML et al: Risk factors in stroke: a statement for physicians by the subcommittee on risk factors and stroke of the stroke council, *Stroke* 15:1105-1109, 1984.
22. ESPS Group: European stroke prevention study, *Stroke* 21:1122-1130, 1990.
23. European Carotid Surgery Trialists Collaborative Group: MRC European carotid surgery trial: interim results for symptomatic patients with severe (70-99%) or with mild (0-29%) carotid stenosis, *Lancet* 337:1235-1243, 1991.
24. Feussner JR, Matchar DB: Where and how to study the carotid arteries, *Ann Intern Med* 109:805-818, 1988.
25. Garraway WM et al: The declining incidence of stroke, *N Engl J Med* 300:449-452, 1979.
26. Gent M et al: The Canadian American ticlopidine study (CATS) in thromboembolic stroke, *Lancet* 1:1215-1220, 1989.
27. Gorelick PB: Alcohol and stroke, *Stroke* 18:268-270, 1987.
28. Grotta JC et al: Red blood cell disorders and stroke, *Stroke* 17:811-817, 1986.
29. Hass WK et al: A randomized trial comparing ticlopidine hydrochloride with aspirin for the prevention of stroke in high-risk patients, *N Engl J Med* 321:501-507, 1989.
30. Hennerici M, Kleophas W, and Gries FA: Regression of carotid plaques during low density lipoprotein cholesterol elimination, *Stroke* 22:989-992, 1991.
31. Hertzer NR et al: Coronary angiography in 506 patients with extracranial cerebrovascular disease, *Arch Intern Med* 145:849-852, 1985.
32. Howard G et al: Reevaluation for transient ischemic attacks as a risk factor for early mortality, *Stroke* 22:582-585, 1991.
33. Howard VJ et al: Comparison of multicenter study designs for investigation of carotid endarterectomy efficacy, *Stroke* 23:583-593, 1992.
34. Hypertension Detection and Follow-up Program Cooperative Group: The effect of treatment on mortality in "mild" hypertension, *N Engl J Med* 307:976-980, 1982.
35. Ingall TJ et al: Predictors of intracranial carotid artery atherosclerosis, *Arch Neurol* 48:687-691, 1991.
36. Jones S: Anticoagulant therapy in cerebrovascular disease: review and meta-analysis, *Stroke* 19:1043-1048, 1988.
37. Kannel WB et al: Risk factors in stroke due to cerebral infarction, *Stroke* 2:423-428, 1971.
38. Levin HJ, Panker SG, and Salzman EW: Antithrombotic therapy in valvular heart disease, *Chest* 95(suppl):98S-106S, 1989.
39. Management Committee: The Australian therapeutic trial in mild hypertension, *Lancet* I:1261-1267, 1980.
40. Marzewski DJ et al: Intracranial internal carotid artery stenosis: long-term progress, *Stroke* 13:821-824, 1982.
41. Masaryk AM et al: 3DFT MR angiography of the carotid bifurcation: potential and limitations as a screening examination, *Radiology* 179:797-804, 1991.
42. Mayberg MR, Wilson SE, and Yatsu F: Carotid endarterectomy and

prevention of cerebral ischemia in symptomatic carotid stenosis, *J Am Med Assoc* 266:3289-3294, 1991.

43. Medical Research Council: Assessment of short-term anticoagulant administration after myocardial infarction, *Br Med J* 1:335-342, 1969.

44. Merrick NJ et al: The appropriateness of carotid endarterectomy, *N Engl J Med* 318:721-727, 1988.

45. NASCET Investigators: Clinical alert: benefit of carotid endarterectomy for patients with high-grade stenosis of the internal carotid artery, *Stroke* 22:816-817, 1991.

46. NASCET Steering Committee: North American symptomatic carotid endarterectomy trial. Methods, patient characteristics, and progress, *Stroke* 22:711-720, 1991.

47. Nishimura RA, Holmes DR, and Ruder GS: Percutaneous balloon valvuloplasty, *Mayo Clin Proc* 65:198-220, 1990.

48. Norris JW et al: Vascular risks of asymptomatic carotid stenosis, *Stroke* 22:1485-1490, 1991.

49. Peterson P et al: Placebo-controlled, randomized trial of warfarin and aspirin for prevention of thromboembolic complications in chronic atrial fibrillation: the Copenhagen AFASAK study, *Lancet* I:175-179, 1989.

50. Peterson P et al: Silent cerebral infarction in atrial fibrillation, *Stroke* 18:1098-1100, 1987.

51. Resnekov L et al: Antithrombotic agents in coronary artery disease, *Chest* 95(suppl):52S-72S, 1989.

52. Roederer GO et al: The natural history of carotid arterial disease in asymptomatic patients with cervical bruits, *Stroke* 15:605-613, 1984.

53. Rokey R et al: Coronary artery disease in patients with cerebrovascular disease: a prospective study, *Ann Neurol* 16:50-53, 1984.

54. Sacco RL et al: Infarction of undetermined cause: the NINCDS stroke data bank, *Ann Neurol* 25:382-390, 1989.

55. The SALT Collaborative Group: Swedish aspirin low-dose trial (SALT) of 75 mg aspirin as secondary prophylaxis after cerebrovascular ischaemic events, *Lancet* 338:1345-1349, 1991.

56. SHEP Cooperative Research Group: Prevention of stroke by antihypertensive drug treatment in older persons with isolated systolic hypertension, *JAMA* 265:3255-3264, 1991.

57. Special Report From the National Institute of Neurological Disorders and Stroke: Classification of cerebrovascular diseases III, *Stroke* 21:637-676, 1990.

58. Steering Committee of the Physicians' Health Study Research Group: Final report on the aspirin component of the ongoing physicians' health study, *N Engl J Med* 321:129-135, 1989.

59. Stein PD, Kantrowitz A: Antithrombotic therapy in mechanical and bioprosthetic heart valves and saphenous vein bypass grafts, *Chest* 95(suppl):107S-117S, 1989.

60. The Stroke Prevention in Atrial Fibrillation Investigators: Preliminary report of the stroke prevention in atrial fibrillation study, *N Engl J Med* 322:863-868, 1990.

61. The Stroke Prevention in Atrial Fibrillation Investigators: The stroke prevention in atrial fibrillation study: final results, *Circulation* 84:527-539, 1991.

62. Tell GS, Crouse JR, and Furberg CD: Relation between blood lipids, lipoproteins, and cerebrovascular atherosclerosis, *Stroke* 19:423-430, 1988.

63. Toole JF: The Willis lecture: transient ischemic attacks, scientific method, and new realities, *Stroke* 22:99-104, 1991.

64. Towne JB, Weiss DG, and Hobson RW II: First phase report of cooperative Veterans Administration asymptomatic carotid stenosis study: operative morbidity and mortality, *J Vasc Surg* 11:252-259, 1990.

65. UK-TIA Study Group: United Kingdom transient ischaemic attack (UK-TIA) aspirin trial: interim results, *Br Med J* 296:316-320, 1988.

66. Veteran's Administration Cooperative Study: Anticoagulants in acute myocardial infarction: results of a cooperative trail, *JAMA* 225:724-729, 1973.

67. Veteran's Administration Cooperative Study Group on Antihypertensive Agents: Effects of treatment on morbidity in hypertension. 1. Results in patients with diastolic blood pressures averaging 115 through 129 mm Hg, *JAMA* 202:116-122, 1967.

68. WHO Report, *Stroke* 20:1407-1431, 1989.

69. Wolf PA, Abbott RD, and Kannel WB: Atrial fibrillation: a major contributor to stroke in the elderly, The Framingham Study, *Arch Intern Med* 147:1561-1564, 1987.

70. Wolf PA et al: Probability of stroke: a risk profile from the Framingham study, *Stroke* 22:312-318, 1992.

71. Wolf PA et al: Epidemiologic assessment of chronic atrial fibrillation and the risk of stroke: the Framingham study, *Neurology* 28:973-977, 1978.

72. Wolf PA, Kannel WB, and Verter J: Current status of risk factors for stroke, *Neurol Clin North Am* 1:317-343, 1983.

RESOURCES

American Heart Association, 7320 Greenville Ave, Dallas, TX 75231, and local affiliate chapters (see local white pages), publish a wide variety of multimedia educational materials in English and Spanish for health professionals and the public and sponsor a speakers bureau.

National Stroke Association, 330 E Hampden Ave, Suite 240, Englewood, CO 80110-2622 and local chapters. Nonprofit organization publishes multimedia educational materials for health professionals and the public.

Chapter 44

PERIPHERAL VASCULAR DISEASE

Jeffrey W. Olin

ARTERIOSCLEROSIS OBLITERANS

Atherosclerosis of the aorta and lower extremity arteries [arteriosclerosis obliterans (ASO)] may cause intermittent claudication, ischemic rest pain, and limb-threatening ischemia. The exact incidence of ASO in the general population is not known. In the Framingham Study, the incidence of intermittent claudication and coronary heart disease increased with age. The average annual rate of intermittent claudication without coronary heart disease was 19/10,000 for men and 10/10,000 for women. If coronary heart disease was present, the average annual rate was 156/10,000 for men and 98/10,000 for women. The onset of disease in women lags behind men by approximately 10 years.[32] Dormandy et al.[12] reported that 1.5% of men under 49 years old and 5% of men over 50 years old developed intermittent claudication during their lifetime. It should be noted, however, that the incidence of asymptomatic arterial disease is much higher. Only approximately 25% of patients progressed to the point of requiring reconstructive surgery and less than 5% required a major amputation.

Intermittent claudication, even if mild, may indicate underlying diffuse atherosclerosis. When compared with a general population of comparable age, men with ASO have a mortality rate two to three times higher after 5 years. Most patients die from either myocardial infarction or stroke. The mortality rate for patients with ASO is approximately 30% at 5 years, 50% at 10 years, and 70% at 15 years. There is an average decline in life expectancy of about 10 years in patients with ASO.[5] These data emphasize that atherosclerosis is a systemic disease. To make a significant impact on morbidity and mortality, atherosclerosis should not only be treated at the location causing symptoms but screening should be undertaken to identify disease in other areas such as the coronary and cerebrovascular circulation.

Risk factors for ASO

The same risk factors that are important in coronary heart disease are also important in peripheral arterial diseases. These risk factors include age and sex, hypertension, diabetes, elevated total and low-density lipoprotein (LDL) cholesterol, decreased high-density lipoprotein (HDL) cholesterol, smoking, obesity, sedentary life-style, family history of vascular disease, and genetic factors. Other factors have been identified recently such as altered platelet function, abnormal levels of fibrinogen and fibrinolytic activity, hyperinsulinemia, and endothelial cell function.

Cigarette smoking. Cigarette smoking is the most important risk factor for the development of ASO. In the classic review by Juergens et al.,[26] only 2.5% of 520 male patients with arteriosclerosis obliterans were nonsmokers.[26] Amputation occurred in 11.4% of those patients who continued to smoke, whereas none of the patients who stopped smoking required amputation during a 10-year follow-up. In an 18-year follow-up study from Framingham, smoking correlated more closely with the development of intermittent claudication than any other risk factor for atherosclerosis.[30] Cigarette smoking doubled the risk for intermittent claudication in both men and women, and this risk increased in proportion to the number of cigarettes smoked per day.

Jonason and Bergstrom[25] have shown that patients who

Table 44-1. Cessation of smoking in patients with intermittent claudication

	Smokers n = 304 (89%)	Ex-smokers n = 39 (11%)	
Rest Pain	16%	0	$P < 0.05$
Myocardial infarction	53%	11%	$P < 0.05$
Cardiac death	43%	6%	$P < 0.05$
10-year survival	43%	82%	$P < 0.05$

Modified from Jonason T, Bergstrom R: Cessation of smoking in patients with intermittent claudication, *Acta Med Scand* 221:253-60, 1987.

discontinue cigarette smoking had less rest pain, less myocardial infarctions after 10 years, fewer cardiac deaths, and greater 10-year survival (Table 44-1). Using multivariate Cox regression analysis, the association between smoking and infarction ($P < 0.05$) and cardiac death ($P < 0.05$) was significant. The study study concluded that discontinuing cigarette smoking was of the utmost importance in patients with intermittent claudication. Unfortunately, only 11% of patients were able to stop smoking for at least 1 year.

In another report, 124 limbs of patients with intermittent claudication were studied over a 10-month period.[46] Forty-one patients continued to smoke, and 15 patients discontinued cigarette smoking at the initiation of the study. Resting ankle systolic pressures *decreased* in smokers' limbs by a mean of 10.2 mm Hg ($P < 0.001$) and *increased* in those patients who stopped smoking by a mean of 8.7 mm Hg (not statistically significant). The patients who discontinued smoking also noted an increase in exercise tolerance.

If patients with diabetes mellitus are excluded, nonsmokers comprise only 1% of all patients with intermittent claudication. The risk of claudication is nine times greater for smokers than for nonsmokers. Evidence also suggests that cigarette smoking significantly contributes to aortic and femoral popliteal graft failure.[38]

It has been estimated that cigarette smoking is directly related to 325,000 to 350,000 deaths annually in the United States. In 1965 approximately 40% of American adults smoked cigarettes. The prevalence decreased to 29% by 1987. However, the number of women smokers is increasing. Abstinence from smoking may reduce the risk of death from coronary disease by 50% after 2 years of cessation, with a further reduction in risk to that of nonsmokers after 20 years of cessation.[29]

The exact method by which cigarette smoking accelerates atherosclerosis is unknown. Smoking has been implicated as a factor in altering platelet function, directly injuring endothelial cells, causing proliferation of arterial smooth muscle cells, and altering circulatory neurophar-

macology. It also lowers HDL cholesterol. In addition, cigarette smoking increases carboxyhemoglobin levels in the blood, thereby decreasing the oxygen-carrying capacity of the red blood cell. It stimulates the sympathetic nervous system and increases heart rate, blood pressure, stroke volume, and cardiac output. Many of these mechanisms may play a significant role in the development of atherosclerosis.[9,34]

Cigarette smoking has been accepted as a recognized medical disorder described as tobacco dependency disorder. It is defined as the "inability to discontinue cigarette smoking despite awareness of its medical consequences." Physicians should strongly recommend the cessation of smoking to all patients, not only those with clinically significant vascular disease (see Chapter 16).

Diabetes mellitus. Diabetes mellitus is a significant risk factor for the development of ASO. The Framingham Study has clearly demonstrated that glucose intolerance, even when mild, is associated with an increased risk of ASO.[31] The relative risk of ASO in patients with glycosuria is 3.5% among men and 8.6% among women. When diabetes mellitus or impaired glucose tolerance is present, the incidence of ASO is equal in men and women. Patients with diabetes and ASO often demonstrate multisegment disease, which is more severe and extensive than seen in patients without diabetes. Patients with diabetes mellitus have a higher incidence of below knee (tibial-peroneal) disease, a similar incidence of femoropopliteal disease, and a lower incidence of aortoiliac occlusive disease than their nondiabetic counterparts.

Most studies in nondiabetic persons support the conclusion that limb loss rarely occurs in patients with intermittent claudication (approximately 1.4% per year). Patients with diabetes mellitus, however, account for 50% to 80% of all amputations, although they compose only 5% of the general population.

Patients with type II diabetes mellitus often have significant clinical atherosclerosis when their diabetes is first diagnosed. Haffner et al.[19] demonstrated that patients who eventually developed diabetes had a higher body mass index and central fat distribution, increased levels of triglycerides, total and LDL cholesterol and decreased levels of HDL cholesterol, increased systolic and diastolic blood pressure, increased fasting and 2-hour glucose and increased fasting insulin levels compared to those patients who remained nondiabetic over an 8-year follow up period. Using multivariate analysis, they showed that most of these risk factors could be abolished by adjusting for fasting insulin levels. Thus hyperinsulinemia may cause perturbations in other cardiovascular risk factors (i.e., lipids, blood pressure). Even before patients who eventually become diabetic exhibit clinical diabetes, their blood vessels are exposed to a milieu, which is favorable to the development of accelerated atherosclerosis.

Hypertension

The Framingham Study[31] has also shown that hypertension imposed a threefold increased risk of intermittent claudication during a 26-year follow-up. No reports published to date demonstrate that aggressive treatment of hypertension alters the clinical course of lower extremity occlusive disease. Nevertheless, control of hypertension is considered to be important to one's overall cardiovascular health (see Chapters 41 and 43).

Lipids. An abnormality in blood lipids is also a potent adverse cardiovascular risk factor. Increased total and LDL cholesterol and decreased HDL cholesterol are strongly associated with coronary and peripheral vascular disease. Effective treatment of blood lipids has been shown to decrease the incidence of myocardial infarction and other cardiac deaths. Multiple studies have demonstrated that regression of atherosclerosis in the coronary circulation is possible. The details of these studies are discussed in Chapter 41.

The data on lipids in peripheral vascular disease are not as extensive as that for coronary heart disease. However, the Lipid Research Clinics Program Prevalence Study[44] showed that men with intermittent claudication had a lower high-density lipoprotein cholesterol (35.6 vs 46.4 mg/dl) and a higher mean triglyceride level than those patients without claudication. In this study, the total and LDL cholesterol were no different in the groups with and without claudication. In a recent series of 125 consecutive patients with intermittent claudication, 87% of patients had one or more abnormalities in the lipid profile.[41] The mean values for total cholesterol were 238 ± 60 mg/dl, triglycerides 241 ± 224 mg/dl, HDl cholesterol 38 ± 13 mg/dl, and low density lipoprotein cholesterol 153 ± 45 mg/dl. Nearly half of the patients in this series had a low HDL cholesterol. However, 28% of patients had a total cholesterol <200 mg/dl and 32% of patients had an LDL cholesterol <130 mg/dl. This study underscores the limitations of the National Cholesterol Education Program guidelines, as some patients would be improperly characterized as having "desirable" values if only the total or LDL cholesterol was used to decide on treatment options. Therefore, the entire lipid profile should be examined and treatment should be initiated based on all of the lipoprotein fractions.

Two older studies have demonstrated that regression of femoral atherosclerosis is possible with aggressive treatment of lipid abnormalities.[2,13] These reports, however, did not use quantitative computerized angiography, which many of the more recent coronary regression studies have used. Although the lipids were not controlled nearly as well as in these early reports, lack of progression and regression of atherosclerosis still occurred. Blankenhorn et al.[3] recently reported the 2-year therapy effect on femoral atherosclerosis in the Cholesterol Lowering Atherosclerosis Study (CLAS), a randomized-controlled, computer-estimated angiographic study comparing patients on diet and placebo to patients on diet, colestipol, and niacin therapy. The effects on lipid lowering was impressive in the actively treated group. There was significantly more regression and lack of progression of femoral atherosclerosis in the drug-treated group compared to the placebo group. For more details on regression of atherosclerosis see Chapter 41.

Association with coronary artery disease

It has long been known from the Framingham Study that the risk of coronary artery disease in patients with peripheral atherosclerosis is 2.4 times greater in men and 1.4 times greater in women than in age- and sex-matched control subjects.[11] As previously stated, there is an overall decline in life expectancy of approximately 10 years in patients with ASO, and most of this mortality is due to cardiovascular deaths.

Hertzer et al.[20] evaluated 1000 consecutive patients with a diagnosis of peripheral arterial disease with coronary angiography. The primary vascular diagnosis was abdominal aortic aneurysm in 263 patients, cerebrovascular disease in 295 patients, and lower extremity ischemia in 381 patients. Two hundred fifty-one patients (25%) had severe, surgically correctable coronary artery disease while 58 patients (6%) had severe, inoperable coronary artery disease. Only 85 patients (8%) had completely normal coronary arteries. This high incidence of significant coronary disease has been confirmed in other studies from our institution and others. Because of the likelihood of coronary disease in patients with atherosclerosis elsewhere, we currently screen all patients for the presence of coronary disease and surgically correct significant coronary disease before performing many peripheral vascular operations.

Patients with intermittent claudication who are not candidates for operative intervention because their symptoms are mild are also screened for the presence of coronary and carotid artery disease. This approach seems prudent, as only 25% of patients with intermittent claudication live 15 years or longer. Most of these deaths are cardiovascular in nature. Intermittent claudication is merely a marker for atherosclerosis elsewhere.

If patients cannot walk on a standard treadmill, we screen with either a dobutamine echocardiogram, a rubidium 82 positron emission tomography myocardial perfusion study, or an arm ergometer stress thallium examination. If significant ischemia is detected, a cardiac catheterization would then be performed and the appropriate course taken based on the results of the cardiac catheterization.

Signs and symptoms of lower extremity ASO

The primary symptom of lower extremity occlusive disease is intermittent claudication. Often, the onset is insidious and goes unrecognized for many years. Older patients may attribute these symptoms to arthritis or aging. The

Table 44-2. Differentiating true claudication from pseudoclaudication

	Intermittent claudication	**Pseudoclaudication**
Character of discomfort	Cramping, tightness, tiredness	Same or tingling, weakness, clumsiness
Location of discomfort	Buttock, hip, thigh, calf, foot	Same
Exercise induced	Yes	Yes or no
Distance to claudication	Same each time	Variable
Occurs with standing	No	Yes
Relief	Stop walking	Often must sit or change body positions

From Krajewski LP, Olin JW: Atherosclerosis of the aorta and lower extremity arteries. In Young JR et al, editors: *Peripheral vascular diseases,* St Louis, 1991, Mosby–Year Book.

classic description of intermittent claudication is an aching sensation associated with walking. Most commonly, the discomfort occurs in a muscle group distal to the area of arterial obstruction. Therefore, if the superficial femoral artery is occluded, patients exhibit calf claudication. If the disease is in the aortoiliac segment, the claudication is in the buttock, hip, or thigh region. Rarely, one may experience claudication of the foot alone. This is most common in nonatherosclerotic disease such as thromboangiitis obliterans. If multilevel occlusive disease is present, the most distant muscle group is affected first followed by more proximal muscle groups if the patient continues to walk.

Most patients can provide an accurate description of the walking distance before claudication occurs. If the speed of walking is increased or if the patient walks up an incline or grade, the claudication will be experienced sooner. A classic description of intermittent claudication is discomfort in the leg when walking, which rapidly (2 to 5 minutes) disappears when one stops and stands still. Generally, the patient does not have to sit down to get relief. True claudication must be differentiated from pseudoclaudication (i.e., neurogenic claudication from lumbar canal stenosis or degenerative disc disease). This differentiation can usually be made on the basis of the history and physical examination alone (Table 44-2).

In addition to a careful history, palpation of the arterial pulses at the femoral, popliteal, posterior tibial, and dorsalis pedis areas is one of the most important clinical diagnostic maneuvers. Although most patients with significant ASO demonstrate a decrease in the arterial pulsation, some may have normal arterial pulses at rest. It is important, therefore, to perform pulse volume recordings and Doppler blood pressures at rest and then have the patient walk on a treadmill until symptoms are reproduced. Pulse volume recordings and Doppler blood pressures should be repeated after exercise. When arterial obstruction is present, the pressures in the ankles decrease after exercise because exercise increases the metabolic demands of the muscles. Because there is arterial obstruction, however, oxygen can only be delivered at a fixed rate. In an attempt to compensate, more blood is shunted into the collateral vessels

---

Conservative treatment of patients with ASO of the lower extremities

1. Discontinue smoking tobacco in all forms
2. Engage in a regular walking program
3. Foot care
4. Trial of pentoxifylline
5. Aspirin
6. Put bed in vascular position (reverse Trendelenburg) for patients with rest pain or ischemic ulcers that will not heal

---

proximal to the obstruction and the capacitance vessels distal to the obstruction dilate. Therefore, less blood is delivered to a dilated segment of the distal vasculature and the pressure decreases.[33]

Many patients with diabetes have highly calcified blood vessels and if only arterial pressures are obtained in the lower extremities, one may be under the false assumption that the circulation is actually better than it is, as the systolic blood pressure will be falsely high because of the calcification (pseudohypertension). Therefore it is especially important to perform pulse volume recordings in these patients.

Prevention and treatment

Medical therapy is advocated for the majority of patients with ASO (see accompanying box). The usual indications for surgical or interventional therapy include patients who develop limb-threatening ischemia with ischemic rest pain and/or tissue necrosis or patients with lifestyle disabling claudication.

The most important aspect in the treatment of lower extremity ASO is to encourage the patient to completely discontinue smoking cigarettes or tobacco in any form. This step is the single most important measure that may prevent the progression of atherosclerosis and reduce the risk of amputation. Quick and Cotton[46] demonstrated that patients who stopped smoking successfully improved treadmill

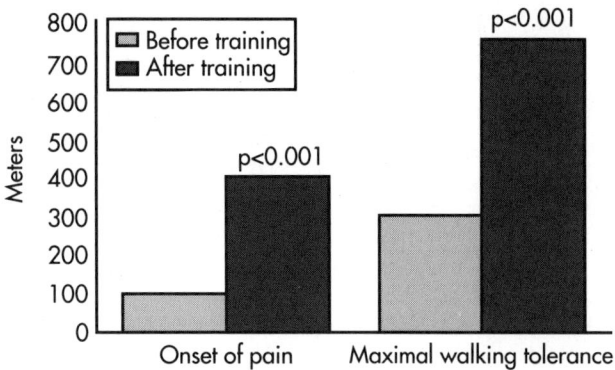

Fig. 44-1. Walking tolerance in patients with intermittent claudication (n=129) before and after 4 to 6 months of physical training. (From Elkroth R et al: Physical training of patients with intermittent claudication: indications, methods and results, *Surgery* 84:640, 1978.)

walking distance compared to those who continued to smoke. Every effort should be made to assist patients to stop smoking completely (see Chapter 16).

Exercise rehabilitation is an effective method of increasing walking distance in patients with peripheral arterial disease.[21,47] The first randomized controlled trial of exercise training in patients with lower extremity ASO demonstrated a significant improvement in treadmill walking ability in patients who engaged in a regular exercise program.[35] Since then numerous reports have demonstrated the efficacy of such an exercise program. Most studies show an increase in treadmill exercise time and a decrease in claudication pain after several months of exercise (Fig. 44-1).[14] This result underscores the importance of an exercise program on the functional capacity of the patient.

Hiatt and Regensteiner[21] summarized the results of 26 trials of exercise conditioning. The improvement in claudication pain averaged 134% (range 44% to 290%). Peak walking time increased an average of 96% (range 25% to 183%). Thus a significant training effect occurs in patients who engage in an exercise program. These patients not only demonstrate an improvement in pain-free walking time, but also in peak exercise performance and oxygen consumption. Along with discontinuing cigarette smoking, an exercise program is an extremely important aspect in the treatment of patients with peripheral arterial occlusive disease. Yet many physicians proceed directly to medications (which often are not helpful) and fail to thoroughly instruct their patients on proper exercise training.

The exact reason for improvement in exercise tolerance in patients with peripheral arterial disease is unclear. There may be adaptions in peripheral blood flow or the distribution of flow, changes in muscle metabolism (training effect), or changes in pain threshold. Others have suggested that exercise may decrease whole blood and plasma vis-

cosity and improve abnormal hemorheology in patients with ASO. It also has been suggested that an exercise training program may increase collateral blood flow to the ischemic limb; however, this theory has never been definitively proven.

Several different techniques can be used when instructing a patient on an exercise program. We prefer to have the patient exercise for approximately 45 minutes daily, usually at one time. The patient is instructed to walk at a pace fast enough to bring on the intermittent claudication at approximately ½ block. When the claudication begins, the patient is instructed to continue walking for a short time and then stop, stand still, and wait until the pain or discomfort disappears. The patient is then instructed to walk again until the onset of claudication and this pattern repeated for 45 minutes. The patient will usually note an improvement in walking distance in a short time. When this improvement occurs, the patient is instructed to increase the pace of walking so as always to bring on the claudication at approximately ½ block. See Chapter 19 for further details on a structured exercise program.

In summary, a structured exercise program may increase pain-free walking, distance, and time, and may preclude the need for future vascular reconstruction or nonsurgical intervention.

Although there is no convincing evidence to support the use of vasodilating agents in the treatment of peripheral arterial occlusive disease, their use continues to be popular among primary care physicians. Direct-acting vasodilators have provided no objective evidence of benefit in patients with ASO.[6] Other agents such as ketanserin and L-carnitine have been used; however, their effectiveness has not been clearly demonstrated. Preliminary studies suggest that iloprost, a prostacyclin analog, may be effective in patients with ischemic ulcers and ischemic rest pain.

The most commonly used agent in the treatment of ASO in recent years has been pentoxifylline (Trental). A multicenter, prospective, randomized study in the United States has demonstrated its effectiveness in patients with mild to moderate intermittent claudication (Table 44-3).[45] Pentoxifylline does not affect the natural history of the arterial disease. It is reported to act by reducing blood viscosity and enhancing oxygen delivery to the tissue of the affected limb. The dose of pentoxifylline is 400 mg three times a day; it should be taken with meals, as its major side effect is gastrointestinal intolerance. Only approximately 20% of patients who take pentoxifylline will subjectively note improvement.

Pentoxifylline should be administered after patients have been thoroughly instructed on discontinuing cigarette smoking and placed on a structured exercise program. If they have not gained the amount of improvement that they had wished or if they are unwilling or unable to participate in an exercise program, then a 2-month trial of pentoxifylline is warranted. The most common mistake is initially

Table 44-3. Pentoxifylline in ASO

	Initial claudicating distance (meters)		Actual claudicating distance (meters)	
	Pentoxifylline (n = 42)	Placebo (n = 40)	Pentoxifylline (n = 42)	Placebo (n = 40)
Baseline	111	117	172	181
Week 24	195	180	268	250
Percent increase	59	36	38	25

Modified from Porter JM et al: Pentoxifylline efficacy in the treatment of intermittent claudication: multicenter controlled double-blind trial with objective assessment of chronic occlusive arterial disease patients, *Am Heart J* 104:66, 1982.

Patient instructions for the care of the diabetic foot

1. Do not smoke.
2. Inspect the feet daily for blisters, cuts, and scratches. The use of a mirror can aid in seeing the bottom of the feet. Always check between the toes.
3. Wash feet daily. Dry carefully, especially between the toes.
4. Avoid extremes of temperatures. Test water with hand or elbow before bathing.
5. If feet feel cold at night, wear socks. Do not apply hot water bottles or heating pads. Do not soak feet in hot water.
6. Do not walk on hot surfaces such as sandy beaches, or on the cement around swimming pools.
7. Do not walk barefoot.
8. Do not use chemical agents for the removal of corns and calluses. Do not use corn plasters. Do not use strong antiseptic solutions on your feet.
9. Do not use adhesive tape on the feet.
10. Inspect the inside of shoes daily for foreign objects, nail points, torn linings, and rough areas.
11. If your vision is impaired, have a family member inspect feet daily, trim nails, and buff down calluses.
12. For dry feet, use a very thin coat of a lubricating oil or cream. Apply this after bathing and drying the feet. Do not put the oil or cream between the toes. Consult your physician for detailed instructions.
13. Wear properly fitting stockings. Do not wear mended stockings. Avoid stockings with seams. Change stockings daily.
14. Do not wear garters.
15. Shoes should be comfortable at time of purchase. Do not depend on them to stretch out. Shoes should be made of leather. Running or special walking shoes may be worn after checking with your physician.
16. Do not wear shoes without stockings.
17. Do not wear sandals with thongs between the toes.
18. Take special precautions in winter. Wear wool socks and protective foot gear, such as fleece-lined boots.
19. Cut nails straight across.
20. Do not cut corns and calluses: Follow instructions from your physician or podiatrist.
21. See your physician regularly and be sure that your feet are examined at each visit.
22. Notify your physician or podiatrist at once if you develop a blister or sore on your feet.
23. Be sure to inform your podiatrist that you have diabetes.

Adapted from Levin ME: The diabetic foot: pathophysiology, evaluation and treatment. In Levin ME, O'Neal LW, editors: *The diabetic foot,* ed 4, St Louis, 1988, Mosby–Year Book.

---

starting the patient on this medication, as the patient then mistakenly believes that the medicine is affecting the natural history of the disease.

Aspirin has been shown to be effective in preventing myocardial infarction and stroke. Until recently there was no convincing evidence that aspirin limited the progression of peripheral arterial disease. However, Goldhaber et al.[18] demonstrated that low-dose aspirin (325 mg every other day) reduced the subsequent occurrence of peripheral arterial surgery in healthy men (relative risk 0.54, $P = 0.03$).[18] Because many patients with ASO have coexisting coronary heart disease and carotid artery disease and because aspirin may help patients with ASO directly, one as-

pirin daily should be advocated if there are no contraindications.

Foot care is extremely important in preventing amputations, especially in patients with diabetes. These patients account for only 5% of the general population but 50% to 80% of all amputations. In those patients undergoing one amputation, 42% will have an amputation of the remaining leg in 1 to 3 years and 56% in 3 to 5 years. The overall life expectancy after an amputation in a patient with diabetes is significantly reduced.[36] More than 50,000 major diabetic amputations were reported in 1985. With special foot care programs, amputation rates can be cut by 50% to 83% (see accompanying box). The most important aspect in the care of the diabetic foot or the foot of the patient with peripheral arterial occlusive disease is prevention. Once injury to the foot occurs, limb-threatening ischemia or infection may occur resulting in amputation.

In addition to the other treatment modalities mentioned, an overall program of cardiovascular risk factor modification should be undertaken (see Chapter 41).

VENOUS DISEASE
Deep venous thrombosis

Rationale for prophylaxis. Venous thromboembolic disease is one of the most common causes of death in the hospitalized setting. Estimates have suggested that pulmonary embolism is associated with 300,000 to 600,000 hospital admissions each year in the United States, and between 50,000 and 100,000 patients die from a pulmonary embolism each year.[10,39] In all likelihood, these statistics are an underestimation of the frequency of this diagnosis, as many patients with deep venous thrombosis and pulmonary embolism have not been diagnosed.

Risk factors associated with deep venous thrombosis include advancing age, major surgery, trauma, malignancy, immobilization, myocardial infarction, congestive heart failure, stroke, previous venous thromboembolic disease, obesity, and pregnancy or the use of oral contraceptive agents.

Pulmonary embolism arises from venous thrombosis in the legs 90% of the time. Most often the thrombi originate in the calf veins. In 20% of the cases, calf vein thrombosis extends to the popliteal veins, resulting in a 50% chance of embolization to the pulmonary vasculature. If one waits for clear-cut physical signs of deep venous thrombosis, approximately 50% of patients will not be correctly diagnosed, as they will have a normal physical examination. Ninety-five percent of patients with *calf* deep venous thrombosis have a completely normal physical examination. Most often, the only abnormality is pain in the calf or thigh. The classic findings of a swollen leg, dilated superficial veins, suffusion, or a palpable cord are often not present. Homan's sign is nonspecific because it can be positive when there is muscular strain and soreness.

Venous thrombosis is extremely common in hospitalized patients when some form of screening measure is undertaken (Table 44-4). In patients undergoing total knee replacement, there is an 84% incidence of lower extremity deep venous thrombosis. For any given surgical procedure, the risk is substantial and increases as the age of the patient increases. For example, there is a 20% incidence of deep venous thrombosis in patients with a myocardial infarction between the ages of 50 and 60, whereas the incidence is 40% for patients between the ages of 60 to 70 and close to 60% for those nearing 80 years of age.

Although prophylaxis of deep venous thrombosis is effective, it is clearly underused. In a recent study, 2017 pa-

Table 44-4. Hospitalized patients screened for venous thrombosis (VT) with routine leg scanning or venography

Diagnostic category	Screening test(s)	VT (%)
Trauma		
Hip fracture	Venogram	40-49
Tibial fracture	Venogram	45
Multiple injuries	Venogram	35
Elective surgery		
General abdominal	Leg scan/venogram	3-51
Splenectomy	Leg scan	6
Thoracic	Leg scan	20-45
Gynecologic	Leg scan	7-45
Prostatectomy (open)	Leg scan	29-51
Prostatectomy (closed)	Leg scan	7-10
Aortofemoral	Leg scan/venogram	4-43
Neurosurgery	Leg scan	29-43
Meniscectomy	Venogram	8
Knee surgery	Venogram	17-57
Knee replacement	Venogram	84
Hip replacement	Venogram	30-65

From Hirsh J: Prophylaxis of deep vein thrombosis: current techniques. In Bergan JI, Yao JST, editors: *Venous disorders,* Philadelphia, 1991, WB Saunders.

tients with multiple risk factors for venous thromboembolism were evaluated.[1] Prophylaxis for venous thromboembolism was received by 32% of these high-risk patients. Prophylaxis use in the 16 hospitals in the study ranged from 9% to 56%. Prophylaxis use was much higher in teaching hospitals than in nonteaching hospitals (44% vs 19%, P <0.001). The study concluded that prophylaxis for venous thromboembolism is underused, particularly in nonteaching hospitals.

Routine screening for deep venous thrombosis with impedance plethysmography or duplex scanning is effective for identifying proximal venous thromboembolic disease. However, routine screening should not and does not replace primary prophylaxis.

Methods of prophylaxis. Low-dose heparin regimens prevent thrombosis by enhancing antithrombin III and by inhibiting activated factor X (Xa). Factor Xa is important in the conversion of prothrombin to thrombin. The most commonly used regimen is minidose heparin (5000 Units subcutaneously every 12 hours). For surgical prophylaxis, the heparin should be administered 2 hours before the operation and every 12 hours thereafter. For some high-risk patients, the frequency of administration can be increased to every 8 hours.

Low-dose heparin administration is effective in most general surgical patients and in medical patients who need prophylaxis. Some physicians have the unfounded fear that minidose heparin will increase bleeding, but this problem has not occurred.[23,24] In some situations such as patients undergoing neurologic or eye surgery, however, heparin

---

Prophylaxis for deep venous thrombosis and pulmonary embolism

Underlying condition or operation	*Prophylaxis*
Abdominal or thoracic surgery	Low-dose heparin: 5000 units subcutaneously every 12 hours (begin 2 hours before surgery)*
Eye or neurosurgery	Pneumatic compression stockings
Open prostatectomy	Pneumatic compression stockings
Orthopedic surgery (total hip or knee replacement)	Pneumatic compression stockings
	or
	Adjusted dose subcutaneous heparin every 8 hours to prolong the aPTT† 1-3 seconds
	or
	Low-dose warfarin
Medical patients (e.g., stroke, myocardial infarction, congestive heart failure)	Low-dose heparin (5000 units subcutaneously every 12 hours)*
Hemorrhagic stroke	Pneumatic compression stockings

*In the high-risk patient, may give heparin every 8 hours *and* use pneumatic compression stockings.
†aPTT, activated partial thromboplastin time.

---

should not be administered even in low doses. Administration of minidose heparin is also not effective in patients undergoing orthopedic surgery or open prostatectomy.

Pneumatic compression stockings have gained an increased amount of popularity in the last several years. They reduce venous stasis and enhance blood flow in the legs.[48] It has been suggested that intermittent pneumatic compression increases the body's fibrinolytic activity, thus further preventing venous thrombosis. Pneumatic compression stockings are an ideal choice in patients who are not candidates for receiving minidose heparin, such as patients undergoing neurosurgery, eye surgery, open prostatectomy, and total joint replacements.

Some investigators combine low-dose heparin with pneumatic compression stockings in the high-risk patient.[49] Other approaches include low-molecular-weight heparin, oral low-dose warfarin,[16] and adjusted-dose heparin.[37] Bleeding complications with oral anticoagulants in patients undergoing hip surgery are about twice that in a control population. Hirsh[22] performed a pooled analysis of seven studies comprised of 505 patients in the oral anticoagulant group and 505 patients in the control group: 20% of those receiving oral warfarin developed bleeding compared to 9.7% in the control group.[22]

A common approach to prophylaxis for deep venous thrombosis and pulmonary embolism is shown in the box.[22,23,39] About 4000 to 8000 postoperative deaths could be prevented each year if routine prophylactic measures were undertaken in general surgical patients.[17]

Kakkar et al.[27] studied over 4000 patients undergoing elective general surgery. Fatal pulmonary embolism occurred in 2 of 2045 patients in the low-dose heparin group compared to 16 of 2076 patients in the control group

($P < .005$). Clagett and Reisch[8] reviewed 49 studies using low-dose heparin (5000 Units subcutaneously every 12 hours) and mididose heparin (5000 units subcutaneously every 8 hours) in preventing deep venous thrombosis.[8] The incidence was 11.8% when heparin was given every 12 hours and 7.5% when given every 8 hours, compared to an average incidence of approximately 30% in the general surgical patient not receiving prophylaxis.

Two recent studies have suggested that low-molecular-weight heparin may produce a lower incidence of venous thrombosis than standard heparin, with no difference in bleeding manifestations.[15,28] Further data will be required to confirm these conclusions.

The most difficult area in prophylaxis for venous thrombosis is in total hip and total knee replacements. In the patient not receiving prophylaxis, the incidence of deep vein thrombosis is extraordinarily high, approaching 80% for total knee replacement and 50% to 60% in total hip replacement. The easiest method of prophylaxis is to use pneumatic compression stockings. Even with this modality, 15% to 20% of patients will develop deep venous thrombosis. Low-dose warfarin is also associated with a 20% incidence of deep venous thrombosis.[16]

In our experience (unpublished data), adjusted dose subcutaneous heparin may be slightly more effective than pneumatic compression stockings; however, this technique is cumbersome. Subcutaneous heparin is administered every 8 hours in an attempt to prolong the activated partial thromboplastin time 1 to 3 seconds (aPTT = 31 to 35 seconds). Even with this method, the incidence of deep venous thrombosis is approximately 15%.

In a recently completed study at our institution using low-molecular-weight heparin, the incidence of deep venous thrombosis was approximately 10% in patients undergoing total hip and knee replacement (unpublished data). This rate is similar to the 12% rate from the pooled data reported by Hirsh.[22]

Aspirin, dextran, and low-dose heparin have uniformly been ineffective in the prevention of deep venous thrombosis in patients undergoing hip or knee replacement. In patients undergoing total joint replacement, our approach has been to screen every patient 5 days after surgery with a venogram. If duplex ultrasound examination is used to screen for deep venous thrombosis, it is important to remember that calf thrombi may not be detected.

In summary, physicians do not use prophylaxis as often as they should despite the effectiveness of this approach in preventing deep venous thrombosis and pulmonary embolism.

Varicose veins

Varicose veins are extremely common in the United States. It has been estimated that primary varicose veins may occur (to some degree) in up to 50% of the adult female population. Primary varicose veins are thought to be genetically based, but the specific genetic abnormality is not known. In some unknown way there is an inherited structural weakness in the vein wall. Between 40% and 80% of patients with varicose veins have a family history of varicose veins. Age, female sex, parity, race, and occupation, (i.e., prolonged standing) may all contribute to the development of varicose veins. Other factors such as weight, height, and alcohol are less clearly associated with their development.[4]

Secondary varicose veins are caused by increased venous pressure such as postthrombotic changes, pregnancy, or venous obstruction in the pelvis and congenital abnormalities such as the Klippel-Trenaunay syndrome.

Varicose veins may cause symptoms of aching, swelling, heaviness, cramps, and itching. Patients may be concerned that varicose veins represent a serious problem with the circulation. Once they are reassured many live a normal life without disabling symptoms. In patients with varicose veins who have leg pain, the pain is not always due to the varicose veins. Their symptoms may be due to peripheral arterial disease, muscular leg pain, degenerative joint disease, lumbar canal stenosis, lumbar disc disease, edematous states of other etiologies, or obesity. It is important to identify these other causes, as intervention for the varicose veins may not relieve these symptoms.

Indications for intervention in patients with varicose veins include the following: recurrent superficial thrombophlebitis in the varicose veins, bleeding from the varicose veins, chronic pain, and aching or heaviness in the area of the varicose veins. Many patients simply want therapy for cosmetic reasons.

Several modalities are useful in managing patients with varicose veins. The first is the use of graduated compression stockings. Support stockings can be administered with varying degrees of compression. They compress the veins so that they do not dilate when the patient is standing, thus eliminating many of the symptoms of heaviness and aching. Stockings are extremely useful in patients who have to stand for prolonged periods of time or whose symptoms of varicose veins exacerbate during portions of the menstrual cycle. In addition, compression stockings are the mainstay in the treatment of chronic venous insufficiency.

The second option is sclerotherapy. This technique involves directly injecting the vein with a hypertonic saline solution. Sclerotherapy has become extremely popular and is used to treat patients with varicose veins or small spider veins when the patient is concerned about the cosmetic appearance. Sclerotherapy obliterates the vein by causing an inflammatory reaction inside of the vein. Some patients need to come back for repeated injections because the small spider veins continue to form. Generally, this technique is safe and effective. It is performed in the outpatient setting and requires 15 to 30 minutes for a series of injections. The patient then either wears a mild compression stocking or wraps the leg in Ace bandages for several days until the acute inflammation disappears. If the hypertonic saline is injected outside of the vein, staining may occur on the skin.

The third intervention is surgical (vein stripping). We reserve venous stripping for those patients who have large varicose veins. Most other patients can be successfully treated with sclerotherapy. Venous stripping is a useful modality when there is reflux at the saphenofemoral level or saphenopopliteal level or when there are large clusters of varicosities. Surgical intervention is particularly useful when there are large varicosities high in the thigh or in the region of the groin.[4]

MISCELLANEOUS VASCULAR CONDITIONS

Prevention is the best form of treatment of most vascular diseases. Some diseases would cease to exist (thromboangiitis obliterans [TAO]) and others would be less bothersome (Raynaud's phenomenon) with proper prevention.

Thromboangiitis obliterans (Buerger's disease)

TAO is a nonatherosclerotic inflammatory condition of the small arteries, veins, and nerves. There has never been a reported case of TAO in a patient who does not smoke (usually cigarette smoking). It is associated with distal extremity ischemia and ischemic ulcerations of the lower and/or upper extremities. Forty percent of patients have concomitant superficial thrombophlebitis. Amputation may occur in a large percentage of patients who continue to smoke. The only treatment for TAO is discontinuation of tobacco use permanently and completely. If a patient stops smoking at a time when there is not irreversible critical ischemia of the limb, amputation will usually not be necessary.[42]

Raynaud's disease or phenomenon

Raynaud's disease or phenomenon is a vasospastic disease usually brought on by exposure to the cold or emotional stimuli. The classic presentation of Raynaud's is a tricolor response which consists of: pallor due to arterial vasospasm, cyanosis due to capillary venous congestion, and rubor due to reactive hyperemia.

Raynaud's *disease* has no underlying secondary cause. It most commonly occurs in women and is bilateral. Ischemic ulcerations do not occur in Raynaud's disease and the overall prognosis is favorable. Before labeling a patient as having Raynaud's *disease,* the patient should be followed for at least 2 years and a careful search should be made for a secondary cause.

Raynaud's *phenomenon* is said to occur when there is a known cause of the vasospasm. These causes are numerous and include drugs (beta-adrenergic receptors, ergotamines, methylsurgide, vinblastine, bleomycin, bromocriptine, clonidine, imipramine, amphetamines, cyclosporin, withdrawal from nitroglycerin exposure, and oral contraceptives). Other secondary causes include scleroderma, systemic lupus erythematosus, Sjögren's syndrome, polymyositis, dermatomyositis, and mixed connective tissue disease. There are multiple occupational causes such as the use of vibratory tools, pneumatic hammers, and chain saws and chronic pounding of the hypothenar eminence known as hypothenar hammer syndrome. Thoracic outlet syndrome, vasculitis (including TAO), and multiple other less common diseases may be associated with Raynaud's phenomenon.[7]

The treatment of Raynaud's phenomenon is mainly conservative. If there is a known secondary cause, it should be treated. If patients smoke cigarettes, they should stop. It is helpful to keep the hands and feet as warm as possible. Mittens are generally better than gloves. The patient should be told to keep the entire body warm, as chilling of any part of the body can precipitate an attack. Multiple foot- and hand-warming devices (either battery-operated or chemical) may be helpful in some patients. If conservative therapy is not helpful, nifedipine is often useful in preventing vasospasm. Nifedipine is a calcium-channel blocking agent and may be given by several methods. A patient may take 10 to 20 mg orally ½ to 1 hour before going out into the cold. This regimen often prevents an attack. A patient who experiences more frequent attacks can be started on nifedipine XL 30 to 90 mg a day. Other calcium-channel blocking agents have also been shown to be beneficial. Other drugs that have been used include reserpine, prazosin, and other alpha₁-blocking agents. Sympathectomy has been used in some patients and has a short-term success rate of 50% to 60%; however, vasospastic attacks often recur after 6 months to several years.

Chronic pernio

Chronic pernio is another cold-induced vasospastic disease. Why one patient exposed to cold develops Raynaud's phenomenon and another pernio is unknown. These diseases appear to be a continuum, with Raynaud's phenomenon representing an acute and readily reversible vasospasm and pernio representing more prolonged vasospasm with more chronic changes.[40] Pernio may develop soon after exposure to the cold. There may be single or multiple erythematous purple-, brown-, or yellow-appearing lesions generally affecting the toes and the dorsum of the feet. The fingers, nose, ears, and thighs have also been involved. These ulcerations may be shallow and may have a hemorrhagic base. Generally, the peripheral pulses are normal. Chronic pernio occurs when repeated exposure to cold results in the persistence of the lesion with subsequent scarring and atrophy.

Pernio usually is not difficult to diagnose. The patient develops the previously described ulcerations, which first appear in the fall or winter and disappear each spring. This seasonal variation is characteristic of chronic pernio.

As in all cold-induced vascular disorders, prevention is the best form of treatment. Again, nifedipine is the drug of choice in this condition.

Frostbite

Frostbite is another condition that is entirely preventable. It is defined as a state of actual freezing of the tissue resulting from exposure to the cold.[40] Prevention is achieved by wearing several thin layers of loose clothing. The first layer should be a water-resistant material (i.e., polypropylene) and the outer layer should be waterproof material. Warm, loose footwear should be worn. When one is exposed to the cold for a prolonged time, careful inspection of the feet should be undertaken. The skin should be kept well oiled, as this greatly protects the skin from low temperature. Mittens should be worn on the hands. Facial hair growth increases the likelihood of frostbite on the face because of moisture collecting on the mustache or beard.

SUMMARY

Most vascular diseases are entirely preventable. Lifestyle modification such as discontinuing smoking, achieving ideal body weight, following a diet high in fiber and low in cholesterol and saturated fat, and following a regular exercise program will go a long way to prevent the development or progression of the most common form of vascular disease, arteriosclerosis. Although advances in surgical and nonsurgical interventional techniques are occurring at a rapid rate, clearly prevention is the best form of therapy.

In addition, venous thromboembolic disease can be effectively prevented by using appropriate prophylactic measures in high-risk patients.

REFERENCES

1. Anderson FA et al: Physician practices in prevention of venous thromboembolism, *Ann Intern Med* 115:591, 1991.
2. Barndt R et al: Regression and progression of early femoral atherosclerosis in treated hyperlipoproteinemic patients, *Ann Intern Med* 86:139, 1977.
3. Blankenhorn DH et al: Effects of Colestipol-Niacin therapy on human femoral atherosclerosis, *Circulation* 83:438, 1991.
4. Browse NL, Burnand KG, Thomas ML: Varicose veins. In *Diseases of the veins. Pathology, diagnosis and treatment*, London 1988, Edward Arnold.
5. Coffman JD: Intermittent claudication: not so benign, *Am Heart J* 112:1127, 1986.
6. Coffman JD: Vasodilator drugs and peripheral vascular disease, *N Engl J Med* 300:713, 1979.
7. Coffman JD: Vasospastic diseases. In Young JR, Graor RA, Olin JW, Bartholomew JR, editors: *Peripheral vascular disease* St Louis 1991, Mosby–Year Book.
8. Clagett GP, Reisch JS: Prevention of venous thromboembolism in general surgical patients, *Ann Surg* 208:227, 1988.
9. Couch NP: On the arterial consequences of smoking, *J Vasc Surg* 3:807, 1986.
10. Dalen JE, Alper JS: Natural history of pulmonary embolism, *Prog Cardiovasc Dis* 17:259, 1975.
11. Dawber TR, Moore FE, Mann GV: Measuring the risk of coronary heart disease in adult population groups. II. Coronary heart disease in the Framingham Study, *Am J Public Health* 47:4, 1957.
12. Dormandy J et al: Fate of the patient with chronic leg ischaemia, *J Cardiovasc Surg* 30:50, 1989.
13. Duffield RGM et al: Treatment of hyperlipidaemia retards progression of symptomatic femoral atherosclerosis. A randomized control trial, *Lancet* 2:639, 1983.
14. Ekroth R et al: Physical training of patients with intermittent claudication: Indications, methods, and results, *Surgery* 84:640, 1978.
15. European Fraxiparin Study Group. Comparison of a low molecular weight heparin and unfractionated heparin for the prevention of deep vein thrombosis in patients undergoing abdominal surgery, *Br J Surg* 75:1058, 1988.
16. Francis CW et al: Two step warfarin therapy: prevention of postoperative venous thrombosis without excessive bleeding, *JAMA* 249:374, 1983.
17. Frantantoni J, Wessler S: *Prophylactic therapy of deep vein thrombosis and pulmonary embolism*. Department of Health, Education and Welfare Publication (NIH) 76-866, Washington DC, 1975, United States Government Printing Office.
18. Goldhaber SZ et al: Low dose aspirin and peripheral arterial surgery in the physicians health study, *Lancet* 340:143, 1992.
19. Haffner SM, Stern MP, Hucuda HP: Cardiovascular risk factors in confirmed prediabetic individuals. Does the clock for coronary heart disease start ticking before the onset of diabetes? *JAMA* 263:2893, 1990.
20. Hertzer NR et al: Coronary artery disease in peripheral vascular patients. A classification of 1,000 coronary angiograms and results of surgical management, *Ann Surg* 199:223, 1984.
21. Hiatt WR, Regensteiner JG: Exercise rehabilitation in the treatment of patients with peripheral arterial disease, *J Vasc Med Biol* 2:163, 1990.
22. Hirsh J: Prophylaxis of deep vein thrombosis: current techniques, In Bergan JJ, Yao JST, editors: *Venous Disorders*, Philadelphia, 1991, WB Saunders.
23. Hull FD, Raskob GE, Hirsh J: Prophylaxis of venous thromboembolism. An overview, *Chest* 89(suppl):374S, 1986.
24. International multicenter trial. Prevention of fatal post-operative pulmonary embolism by low doses of heparin, *Lancet* 2:45, 1975.
25. Jonason T, Bergstrom R: Cessation of smoking in patients with intermittent claudication, *Acta Med Scand* 221:253, 1987.
26. Juergens JL, Barker NW, Hines EA: Arteriosclerosis obliterans: review of 520 cases with special reference to pathogenic and prognostic factors, *Circulation* 21:188, 1960.
27. Kakkar VV, Corrigan TP, Fossard DP: Prevention of fatal postoperative pulmonary embolism by low doses of heparin, *Lancet* 2:45, 1975.
28. Kakkar VV, Murray WJG: Efficacy and safety of low molecular weight heparin (CY 216) in preventing postoperative venous thromboembolism. A cooperative study, *Br J Surg* 72:786, 1985.
29. Kannel WB: Update on the role of cigarette smoking and coronary heart disease, *Am Heart J* 101:319, 1981.
30. Kannel WB, McGee D, Gordon T: A general cardiovascular risk profile: the Framingham Study, *Am J Cardiol* 38:4, 1976.
31. Kannel WB, McGee DL: Update on some epidemiologic features of intermittent claudication: the Framingham Study, *J Am Geriatr Soc* 33:13, 1985.
32. Kannel WB, Skinner JJ Jr, Schwartz MJ: Intermittent claudication. incidence in the Framingham Study, *Circulation* 41:875, 1970.
33. Krajewski LP, Olin JW: Atherosclerosis of the aorta and lower extremities. In Young JR, Graor RA, Olin JW, Bartholomew JR, editors: *Peripheral vascular diseases,* St Louis, 1991, Mosby–Year Book.
34. Krupski WC: The peripheral vascular consequences of smoking, *Ann Vasc Surg* 5:291, 1991.
35. Larsen O, Lassen N: Effective daily muscular exercise in patients with intermittent claudication, *Lancet* 2:1093, 1966.
36. Levin ME: Diabetic foot lesions. In Young JR, Graor RA, Olin JW, Bartholomew JR, editors: *Peripheral vascular disease,* St Louis, 1991, Mosby–Year Book.
37. Leyvraz PF, Richard J, Bachmann F: Adjusted vs. fixed dose subcutaneous heparin in the prevention of deep vein thrombosis after total hip replacement, *N Engl J Med* 309:154, 1983.
38. Myers KA et al: The effect of smoking on the late patency of arterial reconstruction in the legs, *Br J Surg* 65:267, 1978.
39. National Institutes of Health Consensus Development Conference Statement: Prevention of venous thrombosis and pulmonary embolism, *JAMA* 256:744, 1986.
40. Olin JW, Arrabi W: Vascular diseases related to extremes in environmental temperature. In Young JR, Graor RA, Olin JW, Bartholomew Jr, editors: *Peripheral vascular disease,* St Louis, 1991, Mosby–Year Book.
41. Olin JW et al: Lipid and lipoprotein abnormalities in patients with lower extremity arteriosclerosis obliterans, *Cleve Clin J Med* 59:491, 1992.
42. Olin JW et al: The changing clinical spectrum of thromboangiitis obliterans, *Circulation* 82(suppl:IV-3), 1990.
43. Pollin W: The role of the addictive process as a key step in causation of all tobacco related diseases, *JAMA* 252:2874, 1984.
44. Pomrehn P, Duncan B, Weissfeld L: The association of dyslipoproteinemia with symptoms and signs of peripheral vascular disease. The Lipid Research Clinics Program Prevalence Study, *Circulation* 73(suppl I):1-100, 1986.

45. Porter JM et al: Pentoxifylline efficacy in the treatment of intermittent claudication: multicenter controlled double-blind trial with objective assessment of chronic occlusive arterial disease patients, *Am Heart J* 104:66, 1982.

46. Quick CRG, Cotton LT: The measured effect of stopping smoking on intermittent claudication, *Br J Surg* 69(suppl):S-24, 1982.

47. Radack K, Wyderski RJ: Conservative management of intermittent claudication, *Ann Intern Med* 113:135, 1990.

48. Turpie ACG et al: Prevention of deep vein thrombosis in potential neurosurgical patients: a randomized trial comparing graduated compression stockings alone or graduated compression stockings plus intermittent pneumatic compression with control, *Arch Intern Med* 149:679, 1989.

49. Wile-Jorgensen O et al: Prophylaxis of thromboembolism following emergency abdominal surgery, *Thromb Haemost* 62:128, 1989.

━━━━━━━━━━ **RESOURCES** ━━━━━━━━━━

American Diabetes Association, 1660 Duke Street, Alexandria Va. 22314. Provides monthly magazine *Diabetes Forecast* and other periodicals helpful in patients with diabetes and peripheral vascular disease.

American Heart Association, National Center, 7320 Greenville Avenue, Dallas Texas 75231. Provides information and periodicals on heart and vascular disease.

Part X

CANCER PREVENTION

Chapter 45

PRINCIPLES OF CANCER PREVENTION

Robert Gerlach

Cancer is one of the major causes of death in the United States. For American women, cancer is the leading cause of death. For all individuals across the United States under age 54, cancer is the number one cause of death. Should current trends persist, cancer will be for the general U.S. population the leading cause of death by the start of the twenty-first century.

Important aspects of cancer are addressed in earlier chapters of this book. Two leading contributing factors in the etiology of cancer, smoking and diet, affect a variety of diseases in addition to cancer. Considerations regarding "Smoking and smoking cessation" appear in Chapters 16 and 48, and "Nutrition, disease, and prevention" are discussed in Chapter 24. For many cancers, preventive interventions often are integrated into more general health care services. For this reason, cancer prevention is addressed in this book in the Chapter 30 discussion of "The adult female" and the Chapter 31 coverage of "The adult male."

Cancer is not one disease but rather a family of diseases, sharing the trait of uncontrolled proliferation of cells that spread through local invasion and distant metastasis. The natural history of these diseases varies dramatically by site of origin in the body, posing a wide variety of potential approaches to cancer prevention. Because of this diversity, the Section X discussion of cancer prevention includes four chapters that address specifically common cancers amenable today to preventive interventions. Detailed information follows on "Colorectal cancer screening" (Chapter 46), "Breast cancer" (Chapter 47), "Lung cancer" (Chapter 48), and "Skin cancer and protection of the skin" (Chapter 49).

This discussion of principles of cancer prevention begins with an overview of the epidemiology of the disease. Unavoidable risk factors, such as family history of dis-

ease, are noted for reference in identifying high-risk patients. Voluntary patient behaviors or lifestyle choices that raise cancer risk are discussed early in this chapter, because patients themselves have the opportunity to reduce their chances of developing the disease. Major examples of such risk-reduction behaviors include abstinence from tobacco, moderation in the use of alcohol, compliance with dietary recommendations, and regular exercise. In some cases, exposure to factors that contribute to cancer risk can be reduced but not eliminated, or patients with a documented history of exposure can be monitored more frequently to improve the chances for early detection of disease. Examples of such "environmental" exposures include hormones, viruses, ultraviolet light, workplace, and radiation. Patients also may present with premalignant conditions or lesions, placing them in a high-risk population that warrants increased surveillance.

After the discussion of cancer risk, this chapter will outline social, medical, and economic factors in the delivery of health care services that influence the provision of cancer prevention services. These considerations include efforts of the National Cancer Institute to promote cancer prevention, insurance coverage, training of health providers, integration of services into general periodic medical exams, interpretation of diagnostic tests, and effect on quality of life.

For many common cancers, disease prevention is not feasible. Early detection of disease, however, can improve greatly the opportunities for effective treatment. Examples include major diseases such as breast and colon cancer. For this reason, this chapter will address the rationale for screening asymptomatic patients, expected outcomes of these interventions, the effectiveness of screening programs, appropriate follow-up, therapeutic interventions for high-risk patients, and counseling interventions to improve patient compliance with recommendations.

EPIDEMIOLOGY OF CANCER

Cancer is rising in the relative ranking of major diseases primarily because of a substantial decline since 1950 in heart disease mortality. Given that cancer risk increases with age, the aging of the American population also has contributed to the increase in the cancer death rate. Actually, cancer mortality rates for Americans under the age of 55 have decreased during the period 1950 to 1985. If lung cancer, a preventable disease, is excluded from consideration, the cancer mortality for all age groups under the age of 85 years has declined during this period. And more recently, for the period 1973 to 1985, overall cancer mortality rates, including lung cancer, have decreased. Dramatic improvements in cancer survival, however, have occurred only in select types of cancer in the United States, including cancer of the stomach, cancer of the cervix, and Hodgkin's disease.[8] Unfortunately, over the past 30 years survival rates for patients with cancers common in the United States have not improved significantly. In general, the majority of the leading cancers remain resistant to currently available therapies. Completely effective technology to control cancer does not exist today.

Cancer incidence for all sites combined has increased approximately 36% over the past 36 years.[10] The combination of an increase in the incidence of cancer and limited advances in treatment of some tumors has fueled growing interest in preventive interventions. For example, the variance in cancer mortality rates across counties throughout the United States is substantial. When ranked by cancer mortality rate, counties in the tenth decile actually have less than 71% of the national average. In specific diseases, for reports on the period 1950 to 1969, this variation represented cancer mortality rates for breast cancer in women of 13.4 (compared to the national average of 25.5), and lung cancer rates for men of 17.5 (compared to the national average of 38.0), per 100,000 residents.[6]

Cancer epidemiology is affected by a variety of social and economic factors that are interrelated, and the actual contribution of individual factors is difficult to isolate. Socioeconomic status may alter host factors, such as nutritional status and/or resistance to disease, that can change an individual's risk of developing cancer and the prognosis for responding to treatment. Socioeconomic status, however, also is linked closely to an individual's level of education and subsequent employment, thus introducing consideration of environmental factors. Differences in representation in the work force can result in variation in the history of exposure to occupational carcinogens. For example, studies in the steel and rubber industries have noted that African-Americans are overrepresented in work sites with greater exposure to hazardous toxins and carcinogens.

In addition to influencing host and environmental factors, socioeconomic status may alter access to trained health professionals and health facilities. Regardless of the interdependency of these considerations, it is clear that the risk of cancer varies between segments of the U.S. population. Studies consistently confirm, for example, that Mormons and Seventh-Day Adventists have cancer incidence and mortality rates substantially lower than the overall white U.S. population. For Mormons, the incidence of cancers of the lung, larynx, oral cavity, esophagus, and bladder is reported as 55% lower, and mortality from colorectal cancer is 75% lower.[6] On the other hand, the cancer death rate for African-Americans remains 27% higher than for whites.[5] Special target groups, therefore, for cancer prevention efforts include low-income, ethnic minority, and medically underserved subpopulations.

GENETICS AND CANCER

Identifying populations at high risk, or specific high-risk individuals within target subpopulations, remains a challenge. Reliance on self-reporting is not effective, and the high cost of mass screening of broad populations for individuals at elevated risk often lacks a positive yield sufficient to justify the commitment. In many instances, family physicians may play a significant role in identifying individuals particularly susceptible to cancer. For example, a patient's personal medical history may document factors (e.g., prior breast or skin biopsies for histological results) that justify continuing surveillance, or the record of family history of disease (e.g., first-degree relative with premenopausal and/or bilateral breast cancer) may warrant more intensive follow-up with the individual. Clinical reports of findings also historically have played a key role in triggering studies and new insights into the epidemiology of cancer, including the first observations of scrotal cancer in chimney sweeps, lung cancer in coal miners, and bladder cancer in dye workers. More recently, reports of the effect of transcultural migration on cancer incidence and mortality rates have provided leads for further research on the effect of lifestyle on cancer risk. Descriptive epidemiology, even in the absence of conclusive evidence of causal mechanisms, therefore plays an important role in advancing our understanding of populations at elevated risk of cancer.

Advances in genetic research offer new capabilities and great promise for identifying high-risk individuals. Although exposure to carcinogens may remain difficult to document, and variation in susceptibility to carcinogens remains likely, genetic observations such as chromosomal abnormalities, DNA adducts, micronuclei, oncogene activation, and sister chromatid exchange offer new approaches for case identification. In many cases, these genetic alterations involve gross, visible chromosomal changes that readily can be observed. Today, a deletion in chromosome 13 may reveal loss of a gene critical to suppression of retinoblastoma.[11] In some cases, such as a second major suppressor gene (p53), genetic alterations are associated with a variety of cancers rather than a specific disease. In other instances, including p53, a specific genetic change is known to require additional cytogenetic abnormalities to result in manifestation of the disease. Some cancers that are preceded by a series of premalignant changes, such as colorectal cancer, have revealed that individual genetic alterations are associated with progression between these stages of cancer development. Beyond their relevance to cancer prevention or early detection, some genetic rearrangements now are utilized to classify more precisely the cancer diagnosis, as in the cases of B and T cell lymphomas and in chronic myelogenous leukemia (CML). Genetic observations also can contribute to the formulation of treatment recommendations, serving as predictors of more aggressive tumors in breast or ovarian cancer (erbB-2 amplification) and neuroblastoma (N-myc amplification).[1]

Chromosomal confirmation of the role of genetic factors in the development of cancer dates to observation in 1960 of the association of the Philadelphia chromosome in CML. Technical advances eventually led to the ability to demonstrate the reciprocal translocation between the long arms of chromosome 9 and chromosome 22. The field has advanced rapidly, with translocations identified in approximately 3% of all tumors and definition of over 100 recurrent translocations. The realization that particular genes lie at translocation breakpoints, and confirmation that these rearranged genes contribute directly to the new phenotype, now is the model for the study of translocations in tumors.

PERSONAL CHOICES AND CANCER RISK

One major reason for the growing public attention to cancer prevention is the emerging evidence that the way people live can affect their chances of getting cancer. The most obvious case has been the dramatic increases in lung cancer rates after adoption in the early part of this century of cigarette smoking by men and women. Although large international variations in cancer could be consistent with either lifestyle or environmental factors, migrant studies tend to confirm the significance of diet in disease rates. The major causes of cancer (i.e., tobacco, alcohol, diet, ultraviolet light), then, are associated with voluntary lifestyle choices and not involuntary environmental exposures. Public concern regarding environmental pollution fails to recognize appropriately that individuals have the opportunity to alter significantly their personal risk of developing cancer.

Smoking

The causal link between smoking and cancer is firmly established, and primary prevention strategies are available to reduce smoking prevalence. Former Surgeon General Dr. C. Everett Koop simply labeled smoking "the chief, single, avoidable cause of death in our society and the most important public health issue of our time."[5] Cigarettes are far and away the most important cause of tobacco-related cancer, but other forms of tobacco, notably chewing tobacco and snuff, are well-established carcinogens. Smoking is estimated to be responsible for 30% (135,000 annually) of American cancer deaths and 430,000 deaths each year from cancer, heart disease, and chronic obstructive lung disease.[12]

Alcohol and diet

Most dietary recommendations regarding cancer include an admonition to avoid consumption of alcohol in excess. Alcohol consumption has independent effect as well as synergistic effects with tobacco. Risk of liver cancer is known to increase with the use of excessive amounts of alcohol, and the chances of cancers of the mouth, throat, larynx, and esophagus also increase, particularly in combination with smoking. Spirits, beer, and wine appear to produce an equivalent effect on cancer risk, suggesting that alcohol content rather than type of beverage is the risk determinant. In a rat model, alcohol stimulates rectal cell proliferation, providing a possible mechanism for an observed association with large bowel cancer.

There is substantial agreement that the major cancers of the gastrointestinal tract (i.e., stomach, colon, and rectum) are related causally to certain dietary factors. In the United States, 10 cancer sites account for more than 73% of all cancer deaths (i.e., lung, colon and rectum, breast, prostate, pancreas, leukemia, stomach, ovary, bladder, and liver). Most of these, including cancers of the alimentary tract and hormonally influenced cancer, are considered to be influenced by diet. Doll and Peto have estimated that 35% of cancer deaths may be related to dietary components, and that 150,000 lives could be saved annually through dietary changes.[6] The NCI estimates that 30,000 American lives could be saved in the year 2000 if Americans would modify their dietary habits.

The mechanism by which diet influences carcinogenesis is complex and remains under investigation. In the case of breast cancer, for example, studies continue to attempt to separate the effects of caloric intake, type of fat, fat ratios, and caloric expenditure. In general, both the NCI and the American Cancer Society have issued public dietary recommendations encouraging people to eat a variety of foods that are high in fiber, low in fat, and low enough in calories so that regular exercise will keep an individual trim. It is estimated specifically that a reduction in fat intake to 25% of total calories and an increase in daily dietary fiber to 20 to 30 g could result in an 8% reduction in total cancer mortality.[6] Such a reduction in total fat intake and the approximate doubling of current dietary fiber intake of the average American will require major modifications of deeply ingrained eating habits.[5] For this reason, emphasis has been placed on promotion of general principles of diet and nutrition, to include the following:

- Eat a variety of foods, including fruits, whole-grain breads and cereals, lean meats, poultry and fish, dry peas, and beans.
- Maintain a desirable, healthy weight.
- Avoid too much fat, saturated fat, and cholesterol.
- Eat foods with adequate starch and fiber, including vegetables, fruits, and grains.
- Use sugar and salt only in moderation.
- Use alcoholic beverages only in moderation.

These principles provide guidance in efforts to modify current dietary habits and promote the goals of weight control, fat reduction, and increased fiber.

Chemoprevention

In contrast to attempts to make major restrictions on the typical American diet, one very promising line of cancer prevention research is the practice of adding items to the diet that reduce cancer risk. Chemoprevention involves administering specified amounts of distinct natural and synthetic chemicals to prevent, halt, or reverse carcinogenesis. Chemoprevention research focuses on identification of compounds that demonstrate cancer-inhibiting effects, selecting promising candidate inhibitors for efficacy and safety screening, and eventually applying these approaches to human interventions. Potential agents include phenolic antioxidants, retinoids, prostaglandin inhibitors, indoles, dehydroepiandrosterone analogs, and pharmaceuticals. These natural compounds, their analogs, and synthetic agents need to demonstrate initial efficacy and then undergo pharmacological and toxicological studies similar to pharmaceuticals. In addition to studies in general populations, chemoprevention trials are focusing on use in high-risk subpopulations, for preventing precancerous lesions from progressing to malignancy, and for prevention of second primaries.

Particular attention is being directed at the relationship between cancer and dietary vitamin A, β-carotene, and vitamin C. These and other substances may function as antioxidants that prevent the formation of nitrosamines and mutagens in the dietary tract. Most retrospective studies confirm that vitamin A may afford protection against cancers of the esophagus, larynx, lung, and other epithelial tissues. The best source of vitamin A appears to be fresh foods (not vitamin pills) with β-carotene, including carrots, peaches, apricots, squash, and broccoli. Studies are under way currently in persons with asbestosis to test the combined protective effect of β-carotene and vitamin A. Prospective studies consistently have found that patients who develop cancer, especially lung and other smoking-related cancers, have lower levels of serum β-carotene than

healthy controls, although conclusions are confounded by the tendency of smokers to consume less β-carotene than nonsmokers. The NCI has initiated a randomized trial to study the effect of isoretinoin in reducing the incidence of basal cell carcinoma, and a joint U.S.-Finnish study is investigating the effectiveness of β-carotene and α-tocopherol in lowering lung cancer risk in smokers.

Much less data are available on the relationship between lung cancer and other micronutrients such as vitamin C and vitamin E, but case-control studies suggest that they can serve as antioxidants and have a protective effect against cancers of the esophagus, larynx, oral cavity, and stomach. Good sources of natural vitamin C include fruits (grapefruit, cantaloupe, oranges, strawberries) and vegetables (red and green peppers, broccoli, and tomatoes). Other dietary substances of interest include vitamin B_{12} and folic acid, which may prevent the progression of precancerous lesions, and selenium, a trace element that has shown possible anticancer effects in animal models and geographic correlation studies. Interest in chemoprevention extends to regions of the world with unusually high incidence of cancers with potential for dietary intervention, as in the case of studies in China currently to test the efficacy of vitamin and mineral supplements in reducing the incidence of esophageal cancer.

Exercise

In addition to diet, regular exercise appears to contribute to reduced risk of cancer. The association of physical activity with lowered colon cancer incidence is believed based on reduced transit time and, as in the case of dietary fiber, decreased colonic mucosal exposure to animal fat. For hormonally-regulated cancer, regular exercise may have important protective effects on breast, endometrial, and ovarian cancer because of the resulting delay in the onset of regular ovulatory cycles.

Sun exposure

After smoking and diet, solar radiation may play the next largest role in worldwide incidence of cancer. Exposure to the sun is considered a factor in the onset of cancer in perhaps as many as 20% of all cases, primarily because of its major association with skin cancer. These considerations are discussed in Chapter 49, dedicated to "Skin cancer and protection of the skin."

OTHER FACTORS IN CANCER RISK
Environment

Research on carcinogenesis has demonstrated that most human cancer in some way is associated with environmental factors. Genetic research, rather than minimizing the role of environmental agents, has demonstrated that carcinogenic exposures may be genotoxic for DNA, may increase cell proliferation, or both. The International Agency for Research on Cancer and other cancer research organizations periodically publish lists of human carcinogens. These lists typically focus on individual chemicals for which epidemiological evidence is accompanied by sufficient experimental evidence to establish causation beyond a reasonable doubt. With regard to cancer risk attributable to environmental agents, the most pervasive factors appear to be diet (up to 35% of all cancers) and tobacco (30% of cancers).

Research also has suggested that most cancers may involve a "web" of causation factors. Synergistic effects are well established in specific cases, such as the interaction of asbestos and tobacco in lung cancer and the combined influence of smoking and alcohol for oral-pharyngeal cancers. The interplay of biologic and physicochemical factors has been suspected in cases such as hepatocellular carcinoma (hepatitis B virus and aflatoxin) and nasopharyngeal carcinoma (Epstein-Barr virus and salted fish). Genetic research, rather than forwarding the theory of a single-hit explanation for cancer, also has confirmed the relevance of models proposing a series of carcinogenic events. Multistep carcinogenesis can be rationalized by a series of definable genetic changes that are accumulated successively in the genome of the evolving cancer cell. Studies in colon carcinoma suggest many alterations result from somatic mutations. Carcinogenesis often appears to involve both the activation of oncogenes and the inactivation of suppressor genes.

Hormones

Hormones are known to have a critical role in cancer etiology and prevention. In the 1970s, evidence arose of a miniepidemic of vaginal cancer in the daughters of women who took diethylstibesterol during pregnancy. Hormonal influences on cancers of the female (Chapter 30) and male (Chapter 31) genital tracts are discussed in detail elsewhere. Differences in premenopausal steroid hormone levels, in average age at menarche, and in weight are sufficient to explain why breast cancer incidence in the United States is four- to sixfold greater than in Japan. In general, attempts to modulate relevant hormone effects should be pursued. A better understanding of the determinants of adult hormone levels is necessary, however, before primary prevention of these cancers through alteration in lifestyle is feasible.

Viruses

Virus infections are associated with 15% of cancers in the world. Hepatocellular carcinoma and cancer of the cervix account for about 80% of virus-linked cancer to date. Several different mechanisms may be involved in the overall contribution of viruses to development of human tumors. Viruses may act indirectly, by inducing immunosuppression or by modifying the host cell genome without persistence of viral DNA. Directly, viruses may induce oncoproteins or alter the expression of host cell proteins at the site of viral DNA integration. The papilloma virus, Epstein-Barr virus, and hepatitis B virus appear to act through modification of host genes or production of viral oncoproteins. HIV infection results in immunosuppression that increases the risk of Kaposi sarcoma and B cell lymphomas. In most cases virus infections per se are not sufficient to induce cancer. The requirement for additional modifications after viral infection in cancer development is suggested by observation of long latency periods, a low number of infected individuals who eventually develop the particular type of cancer, and known carcinogenic interactions with chemical or physical factors. Nevertheless, Epstein-Barr virus (EBV), hepatitis B virus, several types of papillomaviruses, and HTLV-I and possibly -II (human T cell leukemia-lymphoma virus) are linked to specific malignancies. The strongest evidence for a direct cause-and-effect relationship between a putative cancer virus and a human cancer is hepatitis B virus and hepatocellular carcinoma. Beasley's cohort study in Taiwanese civil servants found a relative risk close to 100 for liver cancer in hepatitis B carriers.[11] EBV, in conjunction with an immunodeficiency state, appears to be an opportunistic viral carcinogen that is effective in causing Burkitt's and other high-grade lymphomas. There is evidence that human papillomavirus is related causally to cervical cancer, having demonstrated capacity to bind and inactivate two major suppressor genes. Women with earlier intercourse and with more sexual partners are known to be at higher risk of cervical cancer, and viral infections of the cervix and vagina are associated with cervical cancer. The recent increased incidence of certain types of lymphomas in younger age groups can be attributed to the increasing prevalence of human immunodeficiency virus (HIV) infection, an established cause of these cancers. There is strong epidemiological evidence to support a causal relationship between human T cell lymphotropic virus type I and certain T cell lymphomas. Other types of microorganisms may play a role in human carcinogenesis. Infection with *Helicobacter pylori* recently has been implicated in stomach cancer etiology.[7] Identification of the role and mechanism by which virus contributes to human cancer provides new leads for the use of vaccines to control cancer. In Africa and Asia, attempts are underway to control liver cancer through hepatitis B vaccination programs. Development of an effective HIV vaccine is a major public health priority, given the likelihood of a growing epidemic of HIV-associated lymphomas and Kaposi's sarcoma.

Occupation

Workplace exposures are estimated to be responsible for perhaps 4% to 8% of U.S. cancer deaths. Although relatively small, this risk represents a clearly defined opportunity for cancer control through workplace regulations and protective practices that ensure safe environments for workers. The single most important known occupational carcinogen is asbestos. Asbestos-related lung cancer and mesothelioma peaked during the mid-to-late 1980s as a result of extensive occupational exposure in shipyards during World War II. As in the case of other factors, occupational exposures to asbestos fibers, environmental smoke, and/or radon have a synergistic role in the elevated risk of smoking-related lung cancer.

Iatrogenic

Although iatrogenic causes of cancer (i.e., chemotherapeutic agents, diagnostic or therapeutic radiation) represent a small portion of the total cancer burden, these cases are largely preventable. Health professionals must monitor exposures that are potentially carcinogenic. As the number of available pharmaceuticals and the degree of diagnostic x-ray exposure grow, additional etiological associations are inevitable. Ionizing radiation is known to cause leukemias and some solid tumors, such as thyroid, breast, and salivary gland. These relationships were established after exposures to relatively high-dose radiation. During the middle of this century, radiation was used in many settings in the treatment of adolescent acne, and these individuals subsequently required periodic physical examination of the thyroid as adults to detect early onset of radiation-induced disease. In the United States, medical x-rays represent 80% of exposure to man-made sources of ionizing radiation. It is agreed generally that the risk of chronic myelogenous leukemia increases with a history of exposure to diagnostic x-rays to the trunk, with risk rising in correlation to increasing x-ray dose to active bone marrow. Data to date support a similar relationship in acute myelogenous leukemia. It is estimated that in the United States perhaps 16% of all leukemias are caused by diagnostic radiation. Exposure to dental x-rays, particularly in the use of early generation equipment that involved much higher exposures, may have contributed to a real increase in CNS tumor incidence.

Physical and mechanical trauma

There also are numerous examples of an association between specific tumors and physical or mechanical irritation or trauma. Gallstones are present in some 80% of patients with gallbladder cancer. Head trauma is known to have the potential to lead to development of intracranial meningiomas. Asbestos fibers lodged in the lung can induce lung cancer or mesothelioma. Asbestos exposure is no longer a major public health problem in the United States because of strategies put in place over the past 20 years for reduced use and better handling. Asbestos exposure, however, still is of considerable clinical importance because of the long latency period (greater than 20 years), for its carcinogenic effects, and because of its potentiation of the cancer-causing effects of smoking.

Precancerous conditions

For some cancers, detectable precancerous conditions are well defined that are known to, or likely to, progress to malignancy. Identification of these conditions can permit preventive interventions or heightened surveillance to detect early the onset of cancer. Colonic polyps are associated with colon cancer. Individuals with familial polyposis, characterized by the early onset of numerous polyps in the colon, warrant counseling and close monitoring. Approximately 10% of melanomas develop in families with distinctive development of dysplastic nevi. As noted earlier, molecular epidemiology studies are achieving sufficient sensitivity to provide the opportunity to define biomarkers that may identify high-risk populations and monitor the progression of precancerous conditions. Many current studies are aimed at confirming the prognostic value of these sentinel developments.

PROVIDING CANCER PREVENTION

The previous considerations have focused on ability to identify opportunities for cancer prevention. Social, medical, and economic factors, however, influence the actual availability and provision of appropriate interventions. One major constraint on adoption of cancer prevention services in community practice is limited third-party payor coverage for services to asymptomatic patients. In some cases services simply can be incorporated into routine medical care (e.g., physical examination of the breast, digital rectal examination); in other cases the detection technique has relatively little incremental cost (e.g., Pap smears). Other cancer detection technologies, however, entail significant cost (e.g., mammography, sigmoidoscopy), and reimbursement for screening of individuals without symptoms is not routinely available. Health insurance plans based on prepayment mechanisms, such as health maintenance organizations, have more incentive to cover services that, through early detection of disease, can reduce the eventual costs for treatment and continuing care. In general, however, substantial research is necessary to demonstrate the sensitivity, specificity, and cost effectiveness of preventive services.

CANCER PREVENTION RESEARCH

Cancer prevention research recently has received significant endorsement and support from the National Cancer Institute. Mortality rates are only one dimension in the measurement of public health concerns. In the effort to reduce the effect of cancer on the community, the term "cancer control" has been defined formally as

. . . the reduction of cancer incidence, morbidity and mortality through an orderly sequence from research on interventions and their impact in defined populations to the broad, systematic application of the research results.[4]

The National Cancer Act of 1971 noted that cancer control efforts include new research and the promotion of the community use of known methods.[4]

Increased knowledge regarding the natural history of cancer has revealed a variety of stages for potential cancer prevention interventions. Research on colorectal cancer has exemplified our new understanding of the chain of events preceding clinical manifestation of the disease. The term *primary prevention* typically refers to avoidance of factors that can trigger or initiate the cascade of events leading to cancer. Primary prevention of cancer is feasible when causative factors can be identified and removed. The most readily apparent examples of primary prevention are avoidance of exposure to initiators present in tobacco, diet, or occupational and nonoccupational environments. In the best of situations, however, primary prevention efforts are slow and inefficient, and in many cases their potential efficacy is impeded by the need to rely on self-regulation and individual changes in behavior. *Secondary prevention* interventions may serve as antipromoters after initiation of the cancerous process. For example, studies in rats have indicated that the major benefit of a low-fat diet in inhibiting mammary tumors occurred after (rather than before) exposure to a carcinogen. Similarly, fat is known to stimulate the release of bile acids, which bacteria convert into chemicals known to act as co-carcinogens contributing to changes in the intestinal walls. Finally, *tertiary prevention* refers to factors that can inhibit progression of disease to full malignancy.

Until recently two approaches, the elimination of carcinogenic agents and the early detection of precancerous lesions, dominated the field of cancer prevention and control research. While these efforts continue to be important, prevention strategies today include a number of new approaches. Many of the new interventions support the initiative of individuals to reduce their risk of cancer. Some new strategies reinforce behavioral initiatives, such as smoking cessation, dietary modification or avoidance of excessive sun exposure. These approaches vary in intensity from self-help interventions to individual or group counseling. In addition to behavioral reinforcements, biological aids can complement or supplement the initiative of motivated individuals. Leading examples include the use of chemopreventive agents for protection from aerodigestive tract cancers and the use of nicotine substitutes in smoking cessation programs.

As research and technological advances trigger new, promising leads for future cancer control interventions, it remains important to test rigorously the efficacy and effect of these potential advances. The NCI Division of Cancer Prevention and Control, most recently under the direction of Dr. Peter Greenwald, has developed a five-phase model of cancer control research that assists in evaluating the extent to which a new concept has been tested for theoretical and practical merit.[4] These five phases are: (1) hypothesis development, (2) methods development, (3) controlled intervention trials, (4) defined population studies, and (5) demonstration and implementation studies.

In the earliest phase of hypothesis development, researchers may review data from laboratory, epidemiological, and clinical studies to formulate a testable cancer control intervention hypothesis. In the second phase of methods development, studies establish an intervention design and investigate instruments capable of testing the postulated hypothesis. Considerations addressed in this methodological research include participant compliance rates, validity of data collection instruments, sensitivity and specificity of indicators, cost-effectiveness of the intervention, and risks to participants. With a reasonable hypothesis and a valid study design, the third phase of cancer control research involves a controlled intervention trial to test the efficacy of an intervention in a select group of individuals. The aim of such trials is to establish clearly the effect of the intervention in a controlled setting. For prevention research, clinical trials provide valuable information about the ability of study subjects to participate in a lifestyle change such as a dietary modification over a long period of time. After efficacy is established, the relevance of the observations to a general target population is tested in the fourth phase by defined population studies that involve applying the intervention to a large, distinct, well-characterized population. In the fifth and final phase of cancer control research, an intervention is applied to the community at large to measure public health effect. The intent is to confirm a reduction in risk factors or cancer rates that alters cancer mortality.

Rigorous attention to research design and methodology is particularly critical for studies addressing preventive interventions. Initial study design must incorporate consideration of incidence rates in the target population, ability to define risk status, study recruitment efforts, necessary sample sizes, and compliance issues. Ability to monitor behavioral, as well as pharmacological, interventions may depend on the availability of biomarkers and epidemiological risk factors. Analysis of outcomes can be compromised seriously by unpredictable developments during the study, lack of compliance, and lag time in effect of the intervention.

The long period of latency associated with carcinogenesis has made it difficult to identify etiological factors. Interventions usually target an individual subject, but that person concurrently is affected by a number of variables external to the intervention (e.g., family, social contacts, health care services, school, worksite, mass media, legislation) that may change over time and compromise a controlled study environment.

One common concern in prevention research is establishment of a "true incidence" rate. Disease incidence generally increases after implementation of techniques for early detection of a condition. Additional persons diagnosed in that time period increase the previously reported incidence rates. If the true incidence of disease in the population remains unchanged, however, then the increased incidence of cases detected earlier because of the intervention will be offset in later periods by decreased incidence in the period in which they would have been reported if undetected by the intervention. When cancers are detected earlier than otherwise expected, survival calculated from the time of diagnosis will appear to be increased even though the true effects of treatment may not extend the actual life expectancy. This potential phenomenon is termed *lead-time bias.*

Given the variability in the natural history of the disease, researchers also have recognized that persons with relatively slow-growing tumors are likely to be overrepresented in cases detected by screening interventions compared with individuals with fast-growing tumors because the window for subclinical detection is wider. Because persons with slow-growing tumors by definition have longer survival times, the survival times for disease detected by screening are likely to be longer even if early detection of disease has no beneficial effect on treatment. Researchers refer to this additional bias as *length-time bias.*

The most recognizable and least controversial criterion for confirming efficacy of a proposed intervention is the randomized trial. Advantages of clinical trials are that their prospective nature and experimental designs provide a specificity and ability to separate out potential confounding factors not otherwise possible in epidemiological studies. Although randomized trials are particularly useful for determining the efficacy of preventive measures, ethical considerations dictate that they rarely will be appropriate to evaluate harmful exposures. Many known effective cancer control measures never have been subject to the rigor of confirmation by a randomized trial, for good reason. The Surgeon General's report on smoking and cancer was not based on randomized trials. Similarly, in the case of Pap smears, no trial has ever been carried out. In prevention studies, where the probability of an observed event is far lower than the likelihood of disease recurrence or death in a cancer patient target population, the number of people required for study and control arms rises rapidly. Studies in lung cancer prevention may require 30,000 enrollees, and rarer diseases such as testicular cancer would require 7 million study participants. In these instances, clinical trials are technically feasible but not practical.

In general, given the time and resources required for large-scale human prevention trials, they must be limited to situations where there is a clear potential for human effect. Prevention trials are not feasible when (1) the "true incidence" of disease is very low, (2) the time of hazardous exposure is very distant from onset of observable effect (e.g., childhood diet), and (3) the effect of the intervention requires a long period until an observable payback.

In the absence of rigid adherence to a requirement for randomized trials, other principles must be developed to permit reliance on a series of observations. These principles include the consistency of the observation across studies, the strength or magnitude of the observed difference, the specificity of the hypothesis and the number of independent variables, the immediacy of the response, and the mechanistic and biologic plausibility of the observed association. Fortunately, research technology has developed a number of new data analysis methodologies, such as the Mantel-Haenszel procedure and multivariate techniques, to interpret epidemiological studies.

Compliance issues are particularly critical to interpretation of prevention trials. In general, difficulties may be encountered in sustaining maximal compliance of healthy subjects on altered regimens for long periods of time to prevent disease onset. Some regimens, however, such as chemopreventive agents, may have toxicities and biological effects on other organ systems that adversely affect health and intent to comply.

Regardless of the strength of compliance, length of study inherently introduces additional research concerns as the period of susceptibility to unanticipated complicating factors is extended. Endpoints in a study may vary, including time to death, progression of disease, onset of disease, or change in a biological marker. Reliance on a definitive event such as death raises the concerns associated with long time periods between intervention and effect. These complexities reinforce the need for shorter-term trials using intermediate marker endpoints. Intermediate endpoints, however, require validation as appropriate proxy variables for eventual end-results. In some cases, the applicability of experimental animal studies to humans can be demonstrated, establishing a model system with significantly shorter time relationships between intervention and outcome.

Interpretation of the results of prevention trials often is compromised by difficulty in quantification or scaling of variables to detect changes over time. Examples include detection of changes in behavior or lifestyle, the correlation of biological measurements to such changes, and the sensitivity of quality-of-life measures to interpret the effect of any changes.

Given the need for preventive interventions and the constraints on research initiatives, great effort has been made to define priorities for prevention demonstration and implementation. These priorities are based on three fundamental requirements for cancer control research: the need for human trials to evaluate an intervention, the need for strong laboratory and/or epidemiological evidence to justify such trials, and the need for flexibility in designing the flow of basic and applied research. Within this framework, laboratory and epidemiological research results are unequivocal regarding smoking cessation. In diet modification and nutrition, the data are sufficient to justify human trials of the relationship between fat intake and breast cancer. Additional basic studies of other dietary components are required to define further their role in human cancer. For chemoprevention, the convergent evidence is adequate to warrant human trials of a number of naturally occurring substances and several synthetic agents. For promising leads, priority should be given to cancers with the greatest mortality rates, to cancers for which substantial risk has been associated with common exposures, and to cancers for which control strategies already are available.

REDUCING CANCER MORTALITY RATES

In the 1980s the National Cancer Institute proposed as a goal for the year 2000 a reduction in the cancer mortality rate of 25% to 50% from 1980 levels, which appears feasible through full and rapid application of existing knowledge.[6] In general, this improvement depends on a reduction in tobacco smoking by 50% from 1980 levels, adoption of a prudent low-fat and high-fiber diet, and compliance with recommended cancer screening guidelines. To maximize the effect of public health efforts on the community, priority is placed on advancements in cancers causing the greatest morbidity and mortality, cancers for which substantial risk is associated with common exposures, and cancers for which effective actions are available. Programs to decrease the percentage of adults who smoke, and to decrease the percentage of fat and increase the percentage of fiber in the American diet, have been accompanied by wide-scale research projects on antismoking and chemoprevention interventions. Other lifestyle factors and environmental or occupational exposures associated with cancer at this time have more limited bases of scientific information and understanding to utilize in developing interventions. With regard to early detection, emphasis has been placed on increasing the percentage of women in compliance with recommended guidelines on screening for breast and cervical cancer.

A recent study by McPhie and Bird concluded that physician forgetfulness is the major reason patients fall outside the recommended guidelines for cancer screenings. Physicians may not recognize the true magnitude of their contribution to noncompliance, because the same study observed that physicians tend to overestimate their actual performance of screening tests.[9] Other than Pap smears, cancer screening tests consistently are underutilized by the majority of physicians. These professionals likely are aware of basic risk factors, but their actions do not reflect the magnitude of cancer risk associated with specific factors or the interaction of factors. Unfortunately, training of health professionals in cancer prevention remains largely indirect or outside the mainstream of academic curriculum. Professional education must better recognize that health practitioner knowledge, attitude, and behavior are critical to furthering the goal of cancer prevention.

Responsibilities of the health professional should begin with disseminating information on cancer prevention and counseling patients on preventive steps. Where time is a concern, allied health professionals should be utilized to complement the physical exam. The essential cancer prevention messages to convey to the patient population can be summarized as:

- Stop cigarette smoking.
- Avoid excessive alcohol consumption.
- Keep exposure to the sun at a minimum.
- Maintain desirable weight.
- Cut high-fat, salt-cured, smoked, and nitrite-cured foods from your diet.
- Eat more vegetables in the cabbage family, foods high in fiber, and foods with vitamins A and C.

Eliciting a complete occupational and medical history also can identify those patients who warrant more extensive examination and follow-up. Any report of tobacco dependence should be treated as a primary medical problem, resulting in instruction in the risks of tobacco and cessation methods. Even in the absence of symptoms, the complete medical check-up should, where applicable, include examination of the skin, mouth, lymph nodes, breasts, cervix, pelvis, testicles, rectum, and prostate.

Health professionals committed to cancer prevention must take on the additional responsibility of monitoring follow-up actions resulting from initial observations. Cases should be considered open until the outcome of referrals for mammography, Pap tests, stool blood tests, sigmoidoscopy, prostate specific antigen (PSA) blood work, or skin biopsies are known. In some instances, such as suspicious mammograms or elevated PSA, physicians will need to consult with patients regarding the issues of risk, invasive follow-up, and quality of life in determining the appropriate level of additional surveillance necessary.

Most of the progress that has been made in the early detection of cancer has come from the premise that most cancers begin with a few cells and that, as the cancers increase in size, the potential for metastasis to regional lymph nodes becomes greater. For most cancers, detection and treatment in the early stage does afford a much greater chance of patient survival than detection and treatment at later stages of the disease. Screening is an attempt to detect in a population a group of individuals with higher probability of having a particular disease. The efficiency of screening is increased by targeting the population using factors known to associate with higher risk, such as sex, age, race, or occupation. To be effective, both health care professionals and the lay population must have knowledge of appropriate examinations. Correct performance of tests must accompany knowledge, and positive findings must lead to appropriate referral for treatment.

Today, effective screening procedures are well established that can reduce greatly mortality from breast and cervical cancers. In the short run, early-detection programs may lead to substantial increases in cancer incidence without correspondingly large changes in mortality rates, which may currently be the case in prostate and breast cancer. Much of the recent increase in breast cancer incidence reflects the detection of early-stage disease resulting from increased utilization of mammography. The recent increase in the incidence of brain and other central nervous system tumors may be explained largely by the increased availability of computerized tomography to detect previously "silent" tumors. In the long run, if screening leads to earlier diagnosis and more effective treatment of otherwise fatal cancers, mortality rates will decline.

Recommendations regarding effective prevention and early detection interventions are based on (1) the identification of a human carcinogenic exposure that can be used to identify high-risk individuals, (2) the availability of biomarkers to serve as intermediate endpoints to document effect of the intervention, and (3) compliance of individuals with recommendations for behavioral changes. With regard to cancer screening, the variety of methods include reliance on self-examination, health surveys and risk factor assessments, physician examination, and mass public screening. The National Cancer Institute has disseminated a set of early detection working guidelines addressing breast, cervical, endometrial, colorectal, testicular, prostate, oral cavity, and skin cancers. Three relatively visible and/or palpable sites of cancer lend themselves to self-examination and warrant patient instruction in and encouragement of periodic assessment: the breast, the testes, and the skin. NCI recommendations for early cancer detection in the physician's office include examinations of the colon and rectum, skin, oral cavity, and prostate, fecal occult blood testing, and sigmoidoscopy for patients of specific sex and age groups. NCI estimates that adoption of these practices could result in a 25% decrease in current U.S. cancer mortality rates.

In 1985, NCI limited recommendations for mass screening to cancer of the breast and cervix. Mass screening interventions were expected to contribute only 3% to the desired 50% decrease in overall cancer mortality. The NCI made no recommendations for screening of several major cancers, including lung, pancreas, and ovary.

Chemoprevention is the use of specific chemicals for the purpose of reducing the occurrence of cancer before it becomes clinically manifest.[3] In 1991, for example, one study reported that colon cancer death rates among people who took more than 16 aspirin tablets per month was 40% lower than among people who did not report taking aspirin.[2] Research currently is focusing on ways to improve methods for selecting promising chemopreventive agents and developing new analogs to known chemopreventive agents. Given the difficulties cited previously in cancer

prevention research in the asymptomatic population, many preliminary chemoprevention studies are conducted in cancer patients or individuals at high risk for the disease. The study endpoint in these investigations may be development of second primaries, disease recurrence, or progression of known conditions. One current active area of interest is the potential for retinoids to improve the prognosis of patients with a history of head and neck cancer. Some agents with known therapeutic efficacy may have additional potential for cancer prevention. A current example is a national study to determine the long-term effect of tamoxifen on women at elevated risk of breast cancer based on an assessment of personal and family history of disease.

In addition to developing tools to prevent cancer, adoption of cancer prevention strategies in the community requires conveying information and creating a setting that promotes acceptance of these positive behaviors. Efforts are needed that focus on transmitting knowledge and facilitating modification of current lifestyle practices. Some themes may reinforce positive behaviors, such as diet and exercise. Other messages may advocate avoidance of cancer-associated habits, such as tobacco cessation and avoidance of sunburn. Lay education can play a critical role at many different junctures in the implementation of risk-reduction practices. Information that helps shape beliefs or attitudes regarding cancer can predispose individuals to preventive strategies. Attitude may represent a key factor in the decision of an individual to abstain from smoking, perform breast self-examination, or maintain a recommended program of Pap smears. School-based interventions, from elementary to high school curricula, can be an effective channel for educating young people in cancer-related habits and lifetime risk. Knowledge of prevention and detection interventions can enable individuals to initiate, adopt, or change behavior. Most physicians agree that publicizing warning signs of cancer will lead a segment of the population to seek earlier medical help, whereas a lack of knowledge can reduce cancer survival by contributing to delay in seeking diagnosis and treatment. The American Cancer Society has been very effective in conveying information on early signs of cancer through their "CAUTION" campaign regarding seven warning signs of cancer:

- **C** hange in bowel or bladder habits
- **A** sore that does not heal
- **U** nusual bleeding or discharge
- **T** hickening or lump in breast or elsewhere
- **I** ndigestion or difficulty in swallowing
- **O** bvious change in a mole or wart
- **N** agging cough or hoarseness

Demonstration of and exposure to cancer prevention services can reinforce the desire to maintain positive practices. Efforts in the workplace may address general themes, such as diet modification or weight control, or target specific cancers for worksite education and early detection programs (e.g., lung, breast, cervical, or colon cancer). Recently, the National Cancer Institute and the FDA have focused on consumer education in the marketplace, through shelf- and item-labeling, in-store promotional materials, and public advertising of health messages. Given the persisting differential in cancer mortality across population subgroups (e.g., African-Americans, the elderly), educational campaigns aimed at altering attitudes, knowledge, and behavior need to be targeted to messages and settings specific to these audiences.

Health professionals' knowledge, attitudes, and behavior are critical to furthering the goal of cancer prevention. Patients generally are very willing to comply with a physician's advice regarding cancer prevention. Therefore we must do a better job of educating physicians in cancer risk assessment and prevention. Increasing the role of physicians as change agents for cancer prevention and control requires the development and promotion of consistent and simple recommendations for professionals to implement in their usual office practices. In 1987, the NCI approved *Working Guidelines for Early Cancer Detection*. The word *guideline* was used instead of recommendation because the physician, knowing the entire history and clinical setting of his or her patient, might correctly choose to advise a patient differently. In general, patients should be educated by their primary care physician in good health principles that contribute to cancer prevention, such as abstinence from smoking, avoidance of severe sunburn, and avoidance of dietary and other factors that predispose to cancer.

Dentists, during routine oral examinations, can educate patients about the effects of oral cancer associated with tobacco. Qualified dietitians and nutritionists also can effectively complement the physician's and dentist's efforts when the focus is diet. Health professionals also should share their commitment to health promotion, such as advocacy of abstinence from tobacco, with other professions (e.g., teachers, coaches, public figures) whom young people emulate as role models.

REFERENCES

1. Aaronson SA: Growth factors and cancer, *Science* 254:1146-1153, 1991.
2. *The Cancer Letter* 18:3, 1992. (Editor Boyd J, Cancer Letter, Inc., Washington, D.C.)
3. Department of Health and Human Services: *Healthy People 2000: national health promotion and disease prevention objectives,* US Department of Health and Human Services, Boston, Mass, Jones and Bartlett Publishers, 1992.
4. Greenwald P, Cullen JW: The scientific approach to cancer control, *CA Cancer J Clin* 34:328-332, 1984.
5. Greenwald P, Cullen JW, and McKenna JW: Cancer prevention and control: from research through applications, *J Natl Cancer Inst* 79:389-400, 1987.
6. Greenwald P, Sondik ET, editors: *Cancer control objectives for the nation: 1985-2000,* NCI Monograph 2:3-74, 1986.
7. Henderson BE, Ross RK, and Pike MC: Toward the primary prevention of cancer, *Science* 254:1131-1138, 1991.
8. Koshland DE Jr: Cancer research: prevention and therapy, *Science* 254:1089, 1991.
9. McPhee SJ, Bird JA: Implementation of cancer preventive guidelines in clinical practice, *J Gen Intern Med* (suppl) 3:5116-5122, 1990.
10. National Cancer Institute: *Annual cancer statistics review including cancer trends 1950-1985,* National Institutes of Health, NIH Publication No 88-2789. Bethesda, Md, 1988.
11. Pelayo C: The new era of cancer epidemiology, *Cancer Epidem, Biomark Prev* 1:5-11, 1991.
12. Orleans CT: American Society of Preventive Oncology Position Statement on Tobacco and Nicotine, *Cancer Epidemiology, Biomarkers, and Prevention* 1:255-256, 1991.

RESOURCES

American Cancer Society, 1599 Clifton Road NE, Atlanta GA 30329. (Offers information and educational materials on cancer related topics.)

National Cancer Institute. (Provides free publications, cancer information service, and computerized up-to-date data access.) (800) 4-CANCER or (800) 422-6237.

Cancer Prevention and Early Detection. (A patient booklet by Gambosi JR and Kennedy JM outlining checkup guidelines and cancer warning signs.) Available from: Cleveland Clinic Cancer Center, 9500 Euclid Ave., Cleveland OH 44195-5232.

Chapter 46

COLORECTAL CANCER SCREENING

Jacques Van Dam
Goren Hellers
Michael V. Sivak, Jr.

Colorectal cancer is one of the most common cancers in the industrialized world and the incidence is increasing. There has been no substantial improvement in the outcome after surgical therapy for colorectal carcinoma in the past 30 to 40 years.[17,73] The results for chemotherapy are equally disappointing. Less than one third of patients with colon cancer will survive 5 years.[17,109] Because the disease is often asymptomatic in its early stages, a diagnosis is often not reached until the disease is widespread. Survival is closely related to the stage at time of surgery. Eddy et al[34] developed a mathematical model for estimating the likelihood of survival based on tumor stage and found that patients with Dukes' A or B tumors have an 80% chance of 5-year survival.[34] Survival falls dramatically with increasing tumor stage. Early detection, therefore, should play a critically important role in improving survival. Colorectal cancer screening should be a paradigm for preventing other cancers by mass screening. Before a screening program is initiated however, a number of requirements have to be fulfilled. The requirements were formulated in a World Health Organization (WHO) report published in 1968 (see box on p. 896).[119]

POLYPS

A polyp is a grossly visible protrusion from a mucosal surface. Polyps may be sessile (attached across a broad, flat base with no stalk), semisessile (attached across a broad base by a very short stalk), or pedunculated (attached across a narrow base by a long stalk). Five major types of polypoid lesions occur in the colon: juvenile polyps (hamartomatous epithelial retentions), Peutz-Jeghers polyps (hamartomas), hyperplastic polyps, adenomatous polyps, and mixed hyperplastic-adenomatous polyps. Of these, the adenomatous polyp is the most important precursor for colorectal cancer.[38]

Histologically, polyps may be divided into two categories: neoplastic and nonneoplastic. Adenomatous polyps are benign neoplastic polyps, which may be further classified as either tubular or villous. A tubular adenoma is defined as a polyp composed of straight or branched tubules of adenomatous (dysplatic) epithelium within a qualitatively normal lamina propria. A villous component is defined as adjacent crypts or folia of adenomatous (dysplastic) epithelium, which without branching, are elongated to a minimum of twice the length of a normal crypt.[84] The larger the adenoma, the more likely a villous component. The prevalence of adenomas is not precisely known, but based on autopsy studies it may be 30% or more in the over-40 population of the United States and northwestern Europe.

Substantial evidence suggests that most, if not all, colorectal cancers arise from preexisting adenomas or neoplastic polyps.[39,78] Although only 1% of benign adenomas undergo malignant transformation, the high incidence of colonic adenomas in the Western population places a large number of people at risk. Over two thirds of Americans over the age of 65 years have a colonic polyp.[98] Adenomatous polyps require removal because they have a 2.7% to 9.4% chance of containing invasive carcinoma.[26]

The chance of a benign polyp undergoing malignant

Requirements for mass screening (WHO)*

The disease should be a major health problem for the individual and the population.

Effective treatment for the disease should be available.

The natural history of the disease should be well known, as should its development from a latent to a symptomatic stage.

The latent asymptomatic stage of the disease should be detectable.

There should be an appropriate screening method available.

Adequate resources should be available for screening.

The definition between treatable patients and healthy individuals should be defined.

Early treatment should positively affect disease outcome.

Case-finding should be continuous and not a one-time event.

---

*Wilson JML and Jungner C: *Principles and practices of screening for disease,* Public Health Paper No. 34, Geneva, 1968, World Health Organization.

transformation depends on its histologic type, size, and the number of polyps found at initial colonoscopy. A villous adenoma is more likely to contain cancer than is the more common tubular adenoma. As the size of a polyp increases, so does its malignant potential. Cancer develops in 1% of polyps less than 1 cm in diameter, in 10% of polyps between 1 and 2 cm in diameter, and in 50% of polyps larger than 2 cm.[37] It is estimated that one third of tubular adenomas and one half of villous adenomas larger than 2 cm in diameter will contain cancer.[78] The number of adenomatous polyps discovered at colonoscopy may also predict the risk of colon cancer. In a retrospective analysis of over 3800 patients who underwent colonoscopy over a 10-year period, 4% of patients with adenomas discovered at their initial colonoscopy had multiple (more than five) adenomatous polyps.[104] Of the patients with multiple adenomas, 20% to 30% had invasive cancer at the time of their index colonoscopy.[104] Preliminary results from the National Polyp Study demonstrate a similar association between multiple adenomatous polyps and high-grade dysplasia.[84] Patients with multiple adenomas are more likely to have at least one adenoma with high-grade dysplasia (13.8%) than are patients with single adenomas (7.3%).

Unlike adenomatous polyps, hyperplastic polyps are nonneoplastic and develop from a focal abnormality in cell replication, resulting in an expansion of the proliferative zone of the glandular crypt. Although the proliferative zone is expanded, the cells lining the individual crypts differentiate and mature in a truly hyperplastic process, as opposed to the neoplastic proliferation seen in adenomas.[38] Hyperplastic polyps are generally small (<0.5 cm diameter), sessile, sharply marginated mucosal elevations composed of parallel crypts aligned perpendicular to the mus-

cularis mucosae. Hyperplastic polyps are not generally considered premalignant lesions.[78] Classically, they were not regarded as an indicator of synchronous malignant or premalignant colonic lesions until Achkar and Carey[2] reported that 29% of patients who had hyperplastic polyps in the distal 35 cm of the colorectum had more proximal adenomatous polyps. The incidence of more proximal colonic adenomatous polyps, therefore, may be nearly as prevalent in patients with distal hyperplastic polyps (29%) as it is in patients found to have distal adenomatous polyps (33%). Continued investigation in this area demonstrates data both supporting and refuting an association between distal hyperplastic polyps and proximal adenomas.

Supporting the work of Achkar and Carey, Deal et al.[27] demonstrated that both distal hyperplastic and adenomatous polyps are markers for proximal adenomas and, therefore, require full colonoscopic examination. Blue et al.,[18] in a prospective analysis, also found proximal adenomas in 28% of patients with hyperplastic rectosigmoid polyps. Ansher et al.[11] demonstrated that the prevalence rate for an adenomatous polyp in patients without a hyperplastic polyp is 15% but 49% among patients with a hyperplastic polyp.

Refuting the work of Achkar and Carey, Provenzale et al.[90] found that patients with distal hyperplastic polyps were as likely to have proximal adenomas (32%) as patients without distal hyperplastic polyps (23%) and, therefore, could not justify a full colonoscopy in patients found to have hyperplastic polyps on flexible sigmoidoscopy. Similarly, preliminary reports from the National Polyp Study refute the assertion that distal hyperplastic polyps are a marker for more proximal adenomatous polyps.[121] Of 300 patients discovered to have hyperplastic polyps, 51% had one or more associated adenomatous polyps and 49% had no association with adenomatous polyps. The preliminary data generated by the National Polyp Study, therefore, do not demonstrate a relationship between hyperplastic polyps and adenomatous polyps.[121] Similarly, when 482 asymptomatic patients with negative fecal occult blood tests were screened using colonoscopy, the incidence of adenomas in the colon proximal to the sigmoid-descending junction in subjects with hyperplastic polyps distal to that point was 18% and not significantly different from the incidence of proximal adenomas in subjects with no distal hyperplastic polyps (15%).[97] Despite a number of editorials supporting both sides of the argument and a number of ongoing prospective studies, there is currently no consensus regarding the management of hyperplastic polyps discovered on flexible sigmoidoscopy.[3,24,48]

METHODS FOR SCREENING

Because the vast majority of persons screened for colorectal cancer will never get the disease, the screening test must meet certain basic criteria. A strategy for effective screening must include all adults over the age of 40 years,

Table 46-1. Diet for hemoccult testing
(Diet should be followed for 48 hours before testing and then throughout the test period)

Food	Allowed	Avoid
Animal products	Well-cooked pork Well-cooked poultry Well-cooked fish	Beef Lamb Processed lunch meat
Fruit	Any cooked fruit	Raw fruit, especially melon and citrus
Vegetables	Any cooked vegetable	Raw vegetables, turnips, radishes, and horseradish
Grains	Any high fiber foods including popcorn, bran, whole grain bread	None
Alcohol	In moderation	
Over the counter medication	None	Vitamins and minerals, especially vitamin C and Iron Aspirin, aspirin substitute, corticosteroids anticoagulants

(From Grossman MI et al: Fecal blood loss produced by oral and intravenous administration of various salicylates, *Gastroenterology,* 40(3):383, 1961; Johnson FC: Gastrointestinal consequences of treatment with drugs in elderly patients, *J Amer Ger Soc* 30(11):s52; 1982; Macrae FA et al: Optimal dietary conditions for Hemoccult testing, *Gastroenterology* 82(5):899; 1982.)

with special consideration given to patients at increased risk. The ideal screening test for colorectal cancer should be sensitive (few false-negative results) and specific (few false-positive results), simple to perform (for both the patient and physician), and cost-effective. Furthermore, the test should be able to detect the cancer, or precancerous lesions, at a treatable stage (see box at right).

Rectal palpation

The digital rectal examination is an "old" method used not only for detecting rectal carcinoma, but also for detecting prostatic carcinoma. The test is obviously inexpensive when used in conjunction with other tests as part of an overall general health plan. No studies support the value of rectal palpation for the detection of rectal carcinoma. Thus the frequency of false-negative tests is unknown.

Chemical tests

The guaiac test was developed during the 1800s and was used by Boas in 1901 to detect occult gastric bleeding.[19] Other reagents, such as benzidine and ortholidine have also been used, but are too sensitive for clinical use.[53] Guaiac is by far the most common method used for fecal occult blood testing in clinical practice today. The rationale for the test is that hemoglobin contains a pseudoperoxidase activity that oxidizes guaiac, turning it blue. False-positive tests, therefore, occur in the presence of dietary animal hemoglobin. Vegetables containing the enzyme peroxidase also produce false-positive tests. An additional source of error is the microscopic bleeding that may follow salicylate intake. The guaiac test was first developed as a screening test for widespread use in clinical practice by Greegor.[44] The test is customarily performed in triplicate on three consecutive stools. Two samples are taken from each stool. A complete test, therefore, is com-

Screening tests
Rectal examination
Fecal occult blood testing
Immunologic testing
Endoscopic examination
Rigid sigmoidoscopy
Flexible sigmoidoscopy
Colonoscopy
Radiologic examination
Barium enema x-ray
Enzymatic assay/tissue-specific enzymatic analysis
Carcinoembryonic antigen
Ornithine decarboxylase/tyrosine kinase*
Optical/laser analysis
Laser-induced fluorescence spectroscopy*

*Experimental.

prised of six samples and is considered positive if at least one sample is positive. Initial evaluations of the fecal occult blood test demonstrated a high frequency of false-positives results due to the interference by meat and/or peroxidase-containing vegetables. Dietary restrictions now accompany the test (see Table 46-1). Patients are instructed to consume fiber-rich foods and avoid meat and peroxidase-containing food for 3 days.

The ability of the test to detect cancer or polyps depends on the degree to which these lesions are bleeding.[51] Cr-labeling techniques have demonstrated that normal individuals bleed approximately 1 ml/day.[52] Most patients with cancer bleed approximately 20 to 30 ml/day.[110] The diagnostic "window" for the fecal occult blood test is directed toward these values. Bleeding from polyps is more varied and irregular. The sensitivity of the guaiac test in patients with known colorectal cancer is 65% to 90%.[4] The positive predictive value for cancer screening in the population however, varies considerably (0 to 16%).[108]

Other chemical tests that have been performed on stool specimens to predict colorectal cancer include fecal lysozyme and other fecal proteins. High levels of fecal lysozyme have been reported in the stool of patients with colorectal cancer; however, when measured in the stool of patients with colorectal cancer and compared with normal healthy subjects, no statistically significant differences were detected.[31] Molecular biologic techniques including sodium dodecyl sulfate-polyacrylamide gel electrophoresis (SDS-PAGE) and protein immunoblotting have been used to identify fecal proteins that may be useful in detecting early colorectal cancer.[32] Early results from such high-powered laboratory techniques have been equivocal thus far.

Immunologic tests

Most currently employed chemical tests for occult fecal blood use hemoglobin peroxidase activity as an indicator. Most tests are guaiac-based. Drawbacks in chemical testing techniques have lead to the development of more specific immunologically based tests. The first method thoroughly evaluated was designed in Great Britain.[113] The test used gel diffusion methodology and was based on fluorescein-labeled rabbit antihuman hemoglobin. In vitro studies proved the test to be high accurate; however, due to the extended time to analyze the results (24 hours), the test was not suitable for population screening.

Recently, a novel test (Hemolex, Orion Diagnostica, Esbo, Finland) has been introduced. It is more "user friendly" and does not require specially trained personnel. The test is a latex agglutination test and includes a latex reagent consisting of polystyrene beads coated with antibodies directed against human hemoglobin.[112] The reagent agglutinates when hemoglobin is present in the specimen dilution vial to free the hemoglobin from the fecal material. In a recent study, this immunologic test was compared to three guaiac-based chemical tests.[112] The Hemolex test proved to be slightly more sensitive than the guaiac-based tests. Hemolex required 0.6 ml blood/100 g stool to demonstrate the presence of blood. The guaiac-based tests required 1 to 4 ml blood/100 g stool to demonstrate the presence of blood. Hemolex was also found to be less sensitive to bleeding in the upper gastrointestinal tract than the guaiac-based tests, but more sensitive for bleeding in the lower tract. Hemolex, therefore, appears to be more specific than the guaiac-based tests, but is limited because it is cumbersome to use and may be unsuitable for home testing. Another immunologically-based test used to overcome the disadvantages of chemical testing is the immunologic determination of both fecal hemoglobin and transferrin levels. The simultaneous detection of fecal hemoglobin and transferrin levels improves the accuracy of screening and can be performed in patients without dietary restriction.[76] A more simple immunologic test (InTime, Eureka Medical, Stockholm, Sweden) has been developed and is currently undergoing clinical trial. If successful and as simple to use as guaiac-based tests, InTime may be an immunologic test suitable for mass screening. At present, it is available in Sweden and has been used for this purpose.

Molecular genetic alterations in colorectal cancer

Colorectal cancer does not appear to result from a single abnormal gene; rather, multiple genetic mutations may be required. Altered total nuclear DNA content is frequently associated with colorectal carcinoma; however, the mechanisms producing aneuploidy remain unknown. DNA aneuploidy, as measured by flow cytometry, is associated with a poor prognosis. Another genetic alteration is the loss of a set of chromosomal segments, which can be observed by cytogenetics or by investigating loss of alleles. When compared with diploid carcinomas, aneuploid tumors are associated with some of the genetic alterations of colorectal carcinomas, (a greater mean allelic loss; i.e. the fraction of evaluable nonacrocentric autosomal arms with deletions), but may not be a reliable indicator of metastatic potential.[85] However, specific allelic losses, such as the loss of 17p alleles, appear to be a marker for tumor aggressiveness, and may help select those patients for whom adjuvant chemotherapy may be useful.[65] The molecular genetic mechanisms underlying the evolution of colorectal neoplasia should continue to be determined and will have profound implications in colorectal cancer screening.[5]

Rigid sigmoidoscopy

The use of sigmoidoscopy as a screening tool is based largely on the results of a study by Gilbertsen and Nelms[43] who reported a lower than expected incidence of rectal carcinoma in patients who underwent sigmoidoscopic examination and polypectomy. Although the rigid sigmoidoscope is being replaced by the flexible model in most practices, there continue to be reports documenting the clinical utility of the rigid instruments. One limitation of the rigid scope is diminished patient acceptance of the procedure, which may be uncomfortable at the hands of less experienced physicians. The major limitation of the rigid instrument, however, is that a high percentage of lesions are beyond the reach of this instrument and, therefore, are not discovered on examination. The rigid scope will detect only one third to one sixth of the lesions detectable by the flexible sigmoidoscope. The 65 cm flexible sigmoidoscope detects about twice as many cancers and six times as many adenomas as does the rigid sigmoidoscope.[123]

Flexible sigmoidoscopy

Commercially available sigmoidoscopes vary in length from 30 to 77 cm, although the 60 to 65 cm instruments are the most frequently used. Controversy continues regarding the optimum length of flexible sigmoidoscopes.[95] When used for colorectal cancer screening, the 60 cm flexible sigmoidoscope will detect cancer in approximately 0.2% and adenomas in approximately 11% of average risk subjects.[72,125] Using the 35 cm flexible sigmoidoscope, the yield of adenoma detection falls to approximately 80% of the adenomas detected using the 60 cm instrument.[30] Achkar[1] notes, however, that the difference in detection rates between the 35 and 60 cm sigmoidoscopes does not justify the use of the longer instrument. The use of sigmoidoscopes longer than 60 cm, or even colonoscopes for screening sigmoidoscopy, does not result in a proportionally greater yield of detected neoplasms. Schuman et al.[103] performed screening sigmoidoscopy in 64 patients using a 130 cm instrument and did not report an improved yield of polyp detection. Similarly, Rex et al.[95] performed screening sigmoidoscopy in 500 patients using the 168 cm colonoscope and detected adenomas in 12% of subjects, similar to the 11% detection rate with the 60 cm instrument.[95] On the other hand, Lieberman and Smith studied the screening sensitivity of the 60 cm sigmoidoscope in asymptomatic men over the age of 50 years and found it to be relatively insensitive for detecting colonic adenomas or cancers (sensitivity, 44%).[67] In addition, Foutch et al.[40] used both a 60 cm flexible sigmoidoscope, and then a colonoscope to screen asymptomatic men over the age of 50 and found that 20% of patients screened with the sigmoidoscope, and found to have no adenomas and therefore no indication for full colonscopy, had adenomas detected in the proximal colon by colonoscopy.[40] However, it remains to be determined if the 20% miss rate for colonic adenomas (for those with normal sigmoidoscopic examinations) has a significant impact in population screening.

Considerable debate continues regarding the proper management of polyps discovered on screening proctosigmoidoscopy. The most expedient approach is to remove all polyps by snare or electrocautery biopsy technique; however, the risk of explosion in an inadequately prepared rectosigmoid is considered by many to be a contraindication to polypectomy. The discovery of large polyps on screening proctosigmoidoscopy requires a full colonoscopy to examine the colon for additional polyps and to remove polyps discovered on proctosigmoidoscopy. Patients with rectosigmoid polyps larger than 5 mm have a higher rate of additional proximal adenomas (44%) than patients with smaller (<5 mm diameter) rectosigmoid polyps (24%).[18] Therefore, the size of the rectosigmoid polyp, rather than its histology, is a better predictor for the presence of additional proximal adenomas. The management of smaller polyps found on screening proctosigmoidoscopy is the subject of current prospective analysis. However, all polyps should be removed, as neither polyp size nor endoscopic appearance adequately predicts the histologic nature of the polyp.[2,18,82,99]

Colonoscopy

A complete examination of the large bowel is indicated in patients with either a positive screening test, or symptoms referable to the colorectum. Barium enema x-ray examinations and colonoscopy are the two tests currently used to examine the entire colon, and both tests are also used in periodic surveillance of high-risk individuals. There are no unbiased, controlled studies comparing barium enema and colonoscopy in the diagnosis of cancer,[21] but both methods appear to be at least 85% sensitive for detecting colonic tumors.[74,91] The entire colon can be examined in over 90% of cases. The risk of perforation for colonoscopy and barium enema x-ray is 0.2% and 0.02%, respectively.[21] Colonoscopy is more accurate for detecting smaller lesions and has the added advantage of allowing for biopsy specimens or resecting polyps. Colonoscopy will miss approximately 9% of polyps less than 1 cm in diameter, whereas barium enema x-ray may miss as many as 41%.[37]

Colonoscopy as a screening examination for asymptomatic individuals is currently being evaluated despite its apparent impracticality. In one study of 210 asymptomatic, average-risk persons, aged 50 to 70 years with negative fecal occult blood tests, 25% of subjects had adenomas and two had cancer.[96] Stratifying the results of the study for age, all of the adenomas >1 cm and both cancers were discovered in subjects older than 60 years. Screening colonoscopy, therefore, was judged to have a high yield for detection of neoplasms in asymptomatic, average-risk persons with negative fecal occult blood tests who were older than 60 years. Currently, however, neither colonoscopy nor barium enema x-ray is used for screening asymptomatic, average-risk individuals because neither is practical nor cost-effective.

Newer screening methods used in association with endoscopy for colorectal carcinoma involve chromoscopy, specialized assays for colorectal biopsy specimens, or the combined use of endoscopy and laser-induced fluorescence spectroscopy. Chromoscopy, or the use of dyes during colonoscopy, increase fine mucosal detail. Indigo carmine dye is often used as a colonic dye because it is poorly absorbed by colonic epithelium. When given before polyethyleneglycol electrolyte lavage, indigo carmine dye highlights irregularities in the mucosal architecture by pooling in mucosal grooves and interstices and defining minute endoscopic lesions that might be overlooked by conventional endoscopic methods.[75]

Specialized assays of colonic biopsies obtained at the time of colonoscopy may be useful in detecting colonic neoplasia. The enzyme ornithine decarboxylase (ODC) is the rate-limiting step in the polyamine biosynthetic pathway and has been shown to correlate with proliferative activity and neoplasia in colonic mucosa. Tyrosine kinase (TK) is also associated with proliferation, differentiation, and transformation of colonic tissue. Arlow et al.[13] evaluated the variable enzyme (ODC and TK) activity in the rectal mucosal biopsy specimens from occult blood positive subjects with no prior history of colonic polyps, undergoing colonoscopy. They demonstrated that TK activity is increased in patients who have either hyperplastic or adenomatous polyps, whereas ODC activity is increased in the rectal mucosa of subjects who have adenomatous polyps or adenomatous polyps in combination with hyperplastic polyps. Thus the variable activity of specific proliferative enzymes may be used to predict those subjects in whom the colonic mucosa is predisposed to either hyperplastic or neoplastic polyp formation. If further studies confirm these results, then analysis of enzyme activity in rectal mucosa may become an important adjunct to future colorectal screening strategies.

The use of optical spectroscopy for tissue diagnosis is a new approach in medical diagnostics. Optical properties of tissue such as absorption and fluorescence may yield valuable diagnostic information regarding tissue composition and pathology.[14,114] Low power laser illumination can induce endogenous tissue fluorescence (autofluorescence) with spectral characteristics that reflect the physicochemical composition of the tissue. Single optical fibers of small caliber (400 μm diameter) may be used in conjunction with endoscopic techniques to both transmit ultraviolet radiation from the laser to the tissue and to transmit the fluorescence emitted by the tissue to the spectral analyzer at endoscopy.

Preliminary reports evaluating this new optical technique have demonstrated a high degree of accuracy in differentiating adenomatous polyps from hyperplastic polyps and normal colonic mucosa.[25,55,102] Furthermore, laser-induced spectroscopy obtained from normal-appearing rectosigmoid mucosa can distinguish normal patients from those with a history of adenoma formation.[41] Thus endoscopic spectral analysis of rectosigmoid mucosa may become an important future method for detecting, and thereby screening, patients at increased risk for developing colon adenomas and carcinomas.

SCREENING

The incidence of colorectal cancer deaths is generally closely related to a nation's economic development, with developed countries having a higher incidence than developing countries. The incidence of colorectal cancer death in Western Europe, Canada, the United States, and Australia ranges from 20 to 32 per 100,000 population; the rate in Thailand and Honduras ranges from 0.2 to 3.8 per 100,000.[107] It is probably not industrialization per se that increases the risk for colorectal cancer, but rather the adoption of Western dietary habits.[77]

Colorectal cancer is the second most common form of cancer in the United States (after lung cancer), with the second highest mortality rate.[9] Approximately 150,000 new cases of colorectal cancer are diagnosed yearly, and

the disease claims 61,000 lives annually.[9] The three United States policy-making organizations—the National Cancer Institute, the American Cancer Society, and the American College of Physicians—endorse similar strategies for screening persons over the age of 50: annual fecal occult blood tests and sigmoidoscopy every 3 to 5 years.[94] On the other hand, the United States Preventive Task Force states that "there is insufficient evidence to recommend for or against fecal occult blood testing or sigmoidoscopy as effective screening tests for colorectal cancer in asymptomatic persons. There are also inadequate grounds for discontinuing this form of screening where it is currently practiced or for withholding it from persons who request it. It may be clinically prudent to offer screening to persons 50 years and older with known risk factors for colorectal cancer."[124] In other countries with similarly high incidences of colorectal cancer, such as Canada, Great Britain, and Germany, screening recommendations also vary, probably due to the lack of direct evidence indicating that screening reduces mortality from colorectal carcinoma.[94]

Who should be screened?

Approximately 5% of men and 6% of women born in the United States develop colon cancer during their lifetime.[111] Of all the risk factors for colorectal cancer, the most important is age. Beginning at age 40 years, both men and women are at an increased risk for developing colorectal cancer (see box below). The risk doubles with each decade after 50 years, peaking at age 70.[36,122] Johnson et al.[54] used colonoscopy to investigate the prevalence of colonic neoplasia in asymptomatic individuals with only an age-related risk. In patients over the age of 50 years (51 to 82 years), 24% were found to have adenomatous polyps (27% men; 14% women), of which 66% were proximal to the rectosigmoid junction. A linear association between age and the prevalence of colonic neoplasia was not demonstrated; however, the study documented a high prevalence of colonic neoplasia in patients with only an age-related risk.[56]

Other principal risk factors for colorectal cancer include a family history of colorectal cancer, familial polyposis

---

Risk factors for colorectal cancer

Age over 50 years
Familial polyposis coli
Gardner's syndrome
Family cancer syndrome
Adenomatous polyps
Family history of colorectal cancer
Long-standing inflammatory bowel disease
Previous colorectal cancer
Personal history of endometrial, ovarian, or breast cancer

coli, or family cancer syndrome; a personal history of endometrial, ovarian, or breast cancer; and a history of long-standing ulcerative colitis, adenomatous polyps, or previous colorectal cancer.[124] The majority of patients who develop colorectal cancer, however, have no such recognizable risk factors. With regard to asymptomatic patients with no identifiable risk factors for developing colorectal carcinoma, opinions vary with regard to screening, and some suggest that no colorectal screening is justified in such individuals at the present time.[93]

Patients who have one cancer resected from the colon are at an increased risk of subsequent cancer of the large bowel,[22] as well as an increased risk of having cancer in extracolonic sites.[117] Therefore, patients who have a history of resected colorectal carcinoma constitute a group that requires increased surveillance. Colonoscopy remains unsurpassed for the routine postoperative examination of the colon and anastomosis after colonic resection for colorectal carcinoma[115]; however, routine endoscopy should not be the sole method of follow-up, as the incidence of intraluminal recurrence is small and may initially be detected by other means, such as an elevated carcinoembryonic antigen.[15,87] For the first 5 years after resection of a cancer of the colon or rectum, the patient should be studied frequently for recurrence. If there is no recurrence after 5 years, cure is probable, but the risk of a new colorectal cancer remains high.[81] The chance of having two or more distinct colonic sites for colorectal cancer (synchronous tumors) is approximately 4%.[118] For unclear reasons, women with a history of either breast or genital cancer have a risk of developing colorectal cancer that is at least 1.5 times greater than the general population.[37]

Colonoscopic surveillance is recommended for all persons having had a colonic adenoma. This recommendation is based on the assumption that such individuals are at an increased risk for having additional asymptomatic colorectal neoplasms.[60,120] But what is the risk of subsequent colon cancer in individuals in whom a small adenoma has been removed? The degree of this risk has important implications for surveillance after adenoma removal.[92] Grossman and Milos[45] prospectively evaluated the use of colonoscopy as a method of surveillance in asymptomatic patients with a history of colonic neoplasms ranging from small tubular adenomas to invasive cancers. They demonstrated that persons whose only risk factor is a single, small (<1.0 cm), tubular adenoma and no first-degree relative with colorectal carcinoma may not be at increased risk for developing colonic neoplasms. If confirmed by additional studies, these results may permit current screening guidelines to be modified to recommend techniques less invasive and costly than colonoscopy.[45]

Controversy continues regarding the risk of colorectal carcinoma in persons who have a first-degree relative with colorectal cancer. Some authorities, having noted that the risk of colorectal cancer may be increased 2.5 times in persons with such a family history have recommended that the usual surveillance program begin 10 years earlier[81] or that screening colonoscopy should be performed.[51] Guillem et al.[47] performed screening colonoscopy in 48 asymptomatic individuals whose only risk was one or more first-degree relatives with colorectal carcinoma and reported a striking increase in the prevalence of adenomas (46%) in men over the age of 50 years. Other investigators have questioned the degree of cancer risk in these patients and argue that colonoscopy would not be cost-effective in this group.[34]

Grossman and Milos[45] performed initial screening colonoscopy in 154 asymptomatic individuals whose only suspected risk factor was one or two first-degree relatives with colorectal cancer. The overall prevalence of colonic neoplasia was not greater in the study group than might be expected in the general population. The authors suggested that colonoscopy is not an appropriate first step in screening persons with affected first-degree relatives.[45]

Polyp syndromes are a heterogeneous group of gastrointestinal disorders that place its subjects at an increased risk for colorectal cancer. Familial adenomatous polyposis is a rare disease inherited as an autosomal dominant trait. The disease is characterized by the development of hundreds or thousands of colonic polyps by adolescence or early adult life. The genetic defect responsible for familial adenomatous polyposis resides at a locus called APC (adenomatous polyposis coli), which has been localized to the long arm of human chromosome 5. Patients with familial adenomatous polyposis may remain asymptomatic until the polyps undergo malignant transformation. Analysis of chromosome 5 may improve the accuracy of the presymptomatic diagnosis of patients with familial polyposis.[86] Examination of lymphocyte metaphases in peripheral blood lymphocyte cultures may also be useful in identifying individuals predisposed to colon cancer who do not have familial adenomatous polyposis.[88] The incidence of colorectal cancer in patients with familial adenomatous polyposis is virtually 100% by the fifth decade.

Gardner's syndrome is a variant of familial adenomatous polyposis associated with numerous extracolonic manifestations such as retinal lesions, abnormalities in the teeth and osteomas of the jaw, desmoid tumors, and papillary thyroid carcinoma. Patients with Gardner's syndrome are also at an increased risk for colorectal cancer and, therefore, are advised to undergo prophylactic proctocolectomy. Patients with familial adenomatous polyposis and Gardner's syndrome carry the additional risk for neoplasms elsewhere in the gastrointestinal tract, including the liver and especially the duodenal periampullary area. These patients' risk for ampullary cancer is approximately 100 times greater than that of the general population, and their ratio of stomach cancers to other upper gastrointestinal cancers is much lower than that of the general population.[28] Many authors recommend upper gastrointestinal endoscopy, specifically inspection of the papilla with a side-viewing instrument, and biopsy as surveillance for these individuals.[8,28,57]

Certain rare families without hereditary polyp syndromes appear to manifest a strong genetic predisposition to colorectal cancer.[59] Lynch et al.[69] have described kindreds with a high incidence of colonic malignancies.[69] Hereditary nonpolyposis colorectal cancer is at least seven to eight times more common than familial adenomatous polyposis.[61] This syndrome, referred to as the family cancer syndrome or hereditary site-specific colon cancer, is characterized by predominantly right-sided malignancies. Many authorities suggest, therefore, that colonoscopy be the primary screening modality in these high-risk individuals.[61,69] Individuals in families with hereditary nonpolyposis colorectal cancer should have colonoscopy every 2 years beginning at age 25, or at an age 5 years younger than the age of the earliest colon cancer diagnosis in the family, whichever comes first.[20] After age 35 years, colonoscopic examination should be performed annually.

Inflammatory bowel disease, both ulcerative colitis and Crohn's disease, increase the risk for colorectal cancer. For ulcerative colitis, the risk is related to the extent and the duration of the disease. The incidence of carcinoma appears to be directly proportional to the extent of colonic involvement by colitis. When the entire colon is involved (pancolitis), the incidence of colorectal carcinoma after 20 years ranges from 13% to 24%. When ulcerative colitis is limited to the rectosigmoid, the incidence of carcinoma is less than 1%.[16] The risk for colorectal carcinoma begins to increase after 10 years of chronic disease. The incidence of cancer over the first 10 years is 2% to 3%; however, after 10 years the incidence increases dramatically to approximately 2% per year.[29] Specifically, the risk of cancer is 2.5% at 20 years, 4% at 25 years, 7% at 30 years, 13% at 35 years, and 20% at 40 years.[62,64] Age at diagnosis is a strong, independent risk factor for colorectal carcinoma and requires close surveillance.[35] Other risk factors such as chronic symptoms and a severe first attack have been cited as significant; however, convincing data regarding these risks are lacking.

Virtually all patients who develop colorectal carcinoma have dysplasia, and virtually all have high-grade dysplasia or a mass lesion. Thus screening for dysplasia in ulcerative colitis should improve cancer-related survival by advancing the diagnosis of cancer to a more favorable pathologic stage or by identifying patients at high risk for developing colorectal carcinoma.[63,68,83] In a historical cohort study, Lashner et al.[63] demonstrated that a program of annual screening for carcinoma/dysplasia in patients with ulcerative colitis improved survival and delayed colectomy.

Similarly, Nugent et al.[83] evaluated the utility of a biopsy surveillance program in patients with long-standing (>8 years) ulcerative colitis. They concluded that a biopsy program can be an effective aid in helping control the risk

of carcinoma in patients with long-standing ulcerative colitis, that the short-term risk of carcinoma for patients with negative biopsy results is low, and that colectomy for risk of carcinoma can be deferred in this group.[83] At present, however, there are no well-established data on the optimal manner of surveillance for patients with ulcerative colitis.

Many gastroenterologists perform surveillance colonoscopy with biopsy at 10 cm intervals throughout the colon in such high-risk patients; however, the optimal number of biopsies, the optimal time to begin surveillance, and the interval for colonoscopic surveillance remains controversial. Some practitioners begin surveillance in the fifth year from the diagnosis of disease, others in the seventh or eighth year. Scheduling screening tests using patient-specific hazard rates to minimize the delay in the diagnosis of cancer reduces the number of colonoscopies, associated costs, and morbidity.[62] It is not possible from the current limited data to make recommendations regarding the optimal interval for colonoscopic surveillance. There is no evidence that a program of annual surveillance will not fail to detect premalignant lesions, although many practitioners perform yearly surveillance colonoscopy in these high-risk patients. It seems clear, however, that if dysplasia persists, progresses, or is associated with any suspicious gross lesion or stricture, colectomy should be considered. Attempts to identify a specific histochemical or immunohistochemical marker to reliably detect mucosal dysplasia in ulcerative colitis have been largely unsuccessful.[7]

Patients with Crohn's colitis, although not at the same degree of increased risk for colorectal cancer as patients with ulcerative colitis, have a higher incidence for colorectal cancer, estimated to be approximately 20 times greater than the general population.[116] As with ulcerative colitis, the extent and duration of Crohn's disease appear to be risk factors. The risk for colon cancer in patients with Crohn's disease is particularly increased if loops of bowel are obstructed or by-passed.[101] Although extremely rare, carcinoma of the ileum occurs about 300 times more often in patients with Crohn's disease than in the general population.[106] The precise role for surveillance in patients with Crohn's disease is controversial. In contrast to patients with ulcerative colitis, patients with Crohn's disease limited to the small intestine would derive little benefit from colonoscopic surveillance. Patients with Crohn's disease involving the colon (Crohn's colitis), however, may require periodic surveillance with biopsy. Dysplasia in association with Crohn's disease has been described; however, its significance in this setting remains largely unknown.[89]

RESOURCES

Of the many principles underlying screening, the principle that cost should not outweigh benefit is one of the most difficult to assess. The cost of mass colorectal screening has been estimated for a variety of settings. The initial cost of a program of mass screening using fecal occult blood tests (FOBT) would include advertising, mailing, cost of the guaiac cards, testing of returned samples, and notification of patients with abnormal results.[77] The cost of colonoscopic examination for colorectal carcinoma in those subjects with a positive screening test has also been investigated. Moore and LaMont[77] have estimated that colonoscopy, polypectomy, and ancillary administrative and laboratory tests would cost $1500 per patient (1984 dollars).[77] About 3.5% of patients will have a positive result from an initial fecal occult blood test screening, leading to 350 diagnostic evaluations per 10,000 population. The total cost of $525,000 would adjust to a cost of $52.25 per patient screened.

In 1987, the American insurance companies Blue Cross and Blue Shield investigated the costs of a screening program based on the recommendations of the American Cancer Society,[10] which included annual FOBT and flexible sigmoidoscopy every 3 to 5 years after negative findings from two consecutive annual examinations in persons more than 50 years of age. The cost of a number of screening tests were averaged from among 12 insurance plans in diverse regions of the country. The "usual, customary and reasonable fee" in 1987 for these tests are as follows: FOBT $5 to $7; flexible sigmoidoscopy $97 to $203; and air contrast barium enema examination, $110 to $210 (Table 46-2). The average fees were $11, $160 and $162, respectively. Adding a nominal administrative charge of 10% brought the annual insurance premium for this screening strategy to more than $1.1 billion.[24]

Ransohoff et al.[94] estimated the costs for screening Americans over the age of 50 years (60 million) as follows: fecal occult blood tests $300 million (60 million FOBT at $5 each); plus $900 million for the subsequent 1.8 million complete colonic evaluations required, given a 3% rate of positive screening tests (at $500 per evaluation); for a total cost of $1.2 billion per year. And this figure does not take into account the considerable costs for flexible sigmoidoscopy.

The cost of using colonoscopy as a screening test in asymptomatic individuals has also been evaluated. Neugut and Forde[80] compared the estimated cost of screening colonoscopy to the amount saved by early detection of cancer. The charge for the procedure in New York City in 1988 was $600,[80] whereas the average charge for colonoscopy in major cities outside New York in the mid 1980s averaged $450.[71] After including the ancillary and administrative costs, as well as the cost of surgery for the estimated two persons per thousand screened who will suffer a bowel perforation, the cost per individual if screened at 7-year intervals starting at age 40 (approximately five colonoscopies per individual) would be $2800 or $2.8 million per 1000 persons. If colonoscopy reduced colon cancer mortality by half (saving an estimated 15 lives per 1000 adults) and eliminated the cost of terminal hospital care for these patients, the savings would amount to

Table 46-2. Costs for recommended screening tests

Test	Fee (U.S. $)
Fecal occult blood tests	$ 5[33,34]
	$ 5-7[23]
Rigid sigmoidoscopy	$ 70[33,34]
Flexible sigmoidoscopy	
Length not specified	$ 97-203[23]
35 cm	$100[33,34]
60 cm	$135[33,34]
Colonoscopy	$500[33,34]
	$600[80]
	$450[71]
Air contrast	
Barium enema x-ray	$200[33,34]
	$110-210[23]

$25,000 per patient.[80] Thus screening would yield a savings of $375,000 per 1000 patients screened, at a cost of $2.8 million. Lieberman and Smith[66] addressed a similar question in a prospective evaluation of the cost-effectiveness of screening colonoscopy in asymptomatic individuals as compared to the current practice using 60 cm flexible sigmoidoscopy. The authors similarly concluded that the costs of screening colonoscopy would have to be reduced before this procedure could provide a cost-effective means for reducing colon cancer mortality, compared to the current screening recommendations.

Periodic surveillance has been recommended after the removal of colonic adenomatous polyps, and a 1-year follow-up colonoscopy is recommended after adenomatous polypectomy to ensure that the colon has been "cleared" of neoplastic growths. Ransohoff et al.[94] assessed the cost-effectiveness of these current recommendations using data from the medical literature in a simulation model.[94] Assuming a 50-year-old man's cumulative risk for colon cancer is 2.5% after the removal of a single adenoma, and assuming 100% effectiveness of colonoscopic surveillance every 3 years, one death from colorectal cancer could be prevented by performing 283 colonoscopies at a cost of $82,000. If colonoscopic surveillance every 3 years was 50% effective and the cumulative risk for colorectal cancer in a 50-year-old man was only 1.25% (a more likely scenario), then 1131 colonoscopies would be required to prevent one death from colorectal cancer, at a cost of $331,000. According to this simulation model, therefore, colonoscopic surveillance programs for persons whose risk for death from colorectal carcinoma is low, such as persons with a single small adenoma, may be excessively costly.[94]

A mathematical model was used to estimate the cost-effectiveness of colorectal cancer screening strategies for people at high risk by virtue of a first-degree relative with colorectal cancer.[35] The costs (1986 US dollars) for the

Table 46-3. Five-year survival based on Dukes' classification of colorectal cancer

Stage	Description	5-Year survival
A	Tumor confined to bowel mucosa	80%
B_1	Invasion of muscularis; serosa clean	65%
B_2	Serosal invasion (complete bowel wall involvement)	50%
C_1	Stage B_1 and lymph node involvement	40%
C_2	Stage B_2 and lymph node involvement	10%
D	Distant metastases	<5%

From Bruckstein AH: Update on colorectal cancer: risk factors, diagnosis, and treatment, *Postgrad Med* 86(3):83-92, 1989.

testing in this study were as follows: FOBT, $5; rigid sigmoidoscopy, $70; 35 cm flexible sigmoidoscopy, $100; 60 cm flexible sigmoidoscopy, $135; air-contrast barium enema x-ray, $200; colonoscopy, $500. Mathematical models are not without substantial error; however, either colonoscopy or barium enema x-ray at 3- to 5-year intervals, in conjunction with yearly fecal occult blood testing, were expected to reduce mortality due to colorectal cancer by 85% in this high-risk population. Furthermore, although both barium enema and colonoscopy appeared to be effective in reducing mortality, the lower cost of barium enema x-ray made it a more cost-effective strategy.

Rozen and Ron also evaluated the cost-effectiveness of various screening strategies for family members of colorectal cancer patients.[100] They found that screening asymptomatic adults by colonoscopy is fourfold more cost-effective if the subjects have two or more first-degree relatives with colorectal carcinoma. Screening families with only one affected relative by flexible sigmoidoscopy, together with fecal occult blood testing, is otherwise a more economic strategy. No published controlled trials have evaluated colorectal cancer screening strategies for high-risk populations.

It is not possible, however, to estimate the exact cost of colorectal cancer screening for large populations. Nor is it possible to estimate accurately the benefits of screening on purely financial criteria. Screening costs must be balanced against the costs for diagnosing and treating those in the population who go unscreened, as well as the intangible benefits of reduced mortality, including reduced agony and other family benefits. Currently, the cost of an annual mammogram is comparable to that of a screening colonoscopy every 5 years. When public health policy required the development of mammography as a breast cancer screening tool, the costs of mammography were substantially reduced.[79] It is conceivable that a similar reduction of costs may occur if colonoscopy is found to be a useful screening tool.

EARLY TREATMENT

The overall mortality rate for colorectal cancer approaches 60%. The detection of early lesions, such as cancer confined to the colon without regional or distant metastases and without lymph node involvement, results in a mortality rate of 20% or less.[37,122] Dukes' staging is as follows (Table 46-3): Stage A, cancer limited to the colonic mucosa; stage B, cancer that penetrates the muscularis mucosa with or without an intact serosa (B_1 and B_2, respectively); stage C, cancer with regional lymph node involvement; and stage D, evidence of distant metastatic disease. The 5-year survival rate is approximately 80% in stage A, 50% to 65% in stage B, 10% to 40% in stage C, and less than 5% in stage D.[37] Eddy (1990) calculated that screening persons from 50 to 75 years of age should decrease the chance of a person dying from colorectal cancer by 10% to 75%, depending on the choice and frequency of tests.[33]

No randomized, prospective studies are yet available that demonstrate a reduction in cancer mortality as a direct result of colorectal cancer screening. In one case-controlled study, the use of screening by rigid sigmoidoscopy in patients who died from cancer of the colon or rectum was compared with sigmoidoscopic screening in control subjects matched for age and gender.[105] Only 8.8% of the case subjects had undergone screening by sigmoidoscopy in the 10 years preceding their death from colorectal cancer, as compared with 24.2% of the controls. Screening by sigmoidoscopy was therefore shown to reduce mortality from cancer of the rectum and distal colon.[105] Two major American studies have been published,[42,120] but neither was population-based and, therefore, are unlikely to provide reliable mortality data. Three major European population-based studies have been published. In the Danish study, 60,000 individuals were selected from the population and randomized to either a screening group, or a control group, which was not screened.[58] Compliance was 67%. The positive predictive value for screening was 17% for cancer and 41% for adenomatous polyps. In the group that underwent screening, 51% of the cancers detected were Dukes' A, compared to only 2% in the control group. No mortality data are yet available.

The designs of the other two European population-based studies were similar to the Danish study. The compliance in the Gothenberg study was 66%. As in the Danish study, this study was able to detect cancer at an earlier stage in the screened group than in the control group.[56] In the Nottingham study, 120,000 individuals were randomized to either a screening group, or a control group.[49] Fifty-four percent of the cancers detected in the screened group were Dukes' A as compared to 8% in the control group. Mortality data are not yet available.

The early surgical treatment of patients with familial polyposis coli remains controversial. When left untreated, virtually all patients with familial polyposis develop colorectal carcinoma. Complete excision of the colon and rectum is the only certain method of preventing colorectal cancer in these individuals. However, patients with polyposis coli have few, if any, symptoms and may be reluctant to undergo total proctocolectomy and permanent ileostomy. Mucosal proctocolectomy with ileoanal anastomosis is gaining acceptance as an alternative surgical treatment for ulcerative colitis, which allows removal of the diseased mucosa without loss of continence. Mucosal proctocolectomy with ileoanal anastomosis is also becoming a surgical alternative in patients with polyposis coli and is equally or better tolerated than in patients with ulcerative colitis.[50]

As for the outcome for the surgical treatment of colorectal cancer in the elderly, it appears to be independent of the patient's age. The number of elderly (>80 years of age) is rapidly rising in our population. In a retrospective analysis of surgery for colorectal carcinoma, the 5-year survival—taking into account the tumor site, tumor stage, and type of operation—was not significantly different from the 5-year survival of younger patients with colorectal carcinoma.[12] (See Chapter 38 for gene identification of some colon cancers)

REFERENCES

1. Achkar E: Screening patients for colorectal cancer, *Pract Gastroenterol* 13(1):37-42, 1989.
2. Achkar E, Carey W: Small polyps found during fiberoptic sigmoidoscopy in asymptomatic patients, *Ann Intern Med* 109:880-883, 1988.
3. Achord JL: Hyperplastic colon polyps do not predict adenomas, *Gastroenterology* 100:1142-1143, 1991.
4. Adlercreutz H, Partanen P, Virkola P, et al: Five guaiac-based tests for occult blood in faeces compared in vitro and in vivo, *Scand J Clin Lab Invest* 44:519-528, 1984.
5. Ahlquist DA et al: Hemo Quant, a new quantitative assay for fecal hemoglobin, *Ann Intern Med* 101:297-302, 1984.
6. Ahlquist DA, Thibodeau SN: Will molecular genetic markers help predict the clinical behavior of colorectal neoplasia? *Gastroenterology* 102:1419-1421, 1992.
7. Ahnen DJ et al: Search for a specific marker of mucosal dysplasia in chronic ulcerative colitis, *Gastroenterology* 93:1346-1355, 1987.
8. Alexander JR, Andrews JM, Buchi KN: High prevalence of adenomatous polyps of the duodenal papilla in familial adenomatous polyposis, *Dig Dis Sci* 34(2):167-170, 1989.
9. American Cancer Society: Cancer Statistics, 1989, *CA Cancer J Clin* 39:3-20, 1989.
10. American Cancer Society: Cancer of the colon and rectum, *CA Cancer J Clin* 30:208-215, 1980.
11. Ansher AF et al: Hyperplastic colonic polyps as a marker for adenomatous colonic polyps, *Am J Gastroenterol* 84(2):113-117, 1989.
12. Agarwal N et al: Outcomes of surgery for colorectal cancer in patients age 80 years and older, *Am J Gastroenterol* 85(9):1096-1101, 1990.
13. Arlow FL et al: Differential activation of ornithine decarboxylase and tyrosine kinase in the rectal mucosa of patients with hyperplastic and adenomatous polyps, *Gastroenterology* 100:1528-1532, 1991.
14. Baraga JJ, Feld MS, Rava RP: Rapid near-infrared Raman spectroscopy of human tissue with a spectograph and CCD detector, *Applied Spectroscopy* 46(2):187-190, 1992.
15. Barkin JS et al: Value of a routine follow-up endoscopy program

16. Bayless TM, Yardley JH: Cancer in inflammatory bowel disease. In DeCosse JJ, Sherlock P, editors: *Gastrointestinal cancer,* The Hague, 1981, Martinus, Nijhoff.
17. Berge T et al: Carcinoma of the colon and rectum in a defined population, *Acta Chir Scand* 438(suppl):1-86, 1973.
18. Blue MG et al: Hyperplastic polyps seen at sigmoidoscopy are markers for additional adenomas seen at colonoscopy, *Gastroenterology* 100:564-655, 1991.
19. Boas I: Uber occulte Magenblutungen, *Dtsch Med Wochenschr* 27:315-317, 1901.
20. Bond JH: Are the guidelines changing for the screening of colon cancer? *ASGE Postgraduate Course Syllabus* 315-321, 1991.
21. Bond JH: Screening for colorectal cancer: need for controlled trials, *Ann Intern Med* 113(5):338-340, 1990.
22. Bussey HJR, Wallace MH: Metachronous carcinoma of the large intestine and intestinal polyps, *Proc R Soc Med* 60:208-210, 1967.
23. Clayman CB: Mass screening for colorectal cancer: are we ready? *JAMA* 261(4):609, 1989.
24. Cohen ME, Barkin JS: Small polyps found during fiberoptic sigmoidoscopy (editorial), *Gastrointest Endosc* 35(6):591, 1989.
25. Cothren RM et al: Gastrointestinal tissue diagnosis by laser-induced fluorescence spectroscopy at endoscopy, *Gastrointest Endsosc* 36(2):105-111, 1990.
26. Cranley JP et al: When is endoscopic polypectomy adequate therapy for colonic polyps containing invasive carcinoma? *Gastroenterology* 91:419-427, 1986.
27. Deal SE et al: Screening sigmoidoscopy for colonic neoplasms: hyperplastic polyps (HP) require further evaluation and 30cm flexible sigmoidoscopy (FS) is inadequate, abstract, *Gastrointest Endosc* 37(2):261, 1991.
28. DeCosse JJ: Clinical studies of familial adenomatous polyposis, *Resid Staff Physician* 36(2):32-35, 1990.
29. Devroede GJ et al: Cancer risk and life expectancy of children with ulcerative colitis, *N Engl J Med* 285:17-21, 1971.
30. Dubrow R, Kim CS, Eldred A: Fecal lysozyme: an unreliable marker for colorectal cancer, *Am J Gastroenterol* 87(5):617-621, 1992.
31. Dubow RA et al: Short (35cm) versus long (60cm) flexible sigmoidoscopy: a comparison of findings and tolerance in asymptomatic screening for colorectal neoplasia, *Gastrointest Endosc* 31:305-308, 1985.
32. Dubrow R, Yannielli L: Fecal protein markers of colorectal cancer, *Am J Gastroenterol* 87(7):854-858, 1992.
33. Eddy DM: Screening for colorectal cancer, *Ann Intern Med* 113:373-384, 1990.
34. Eddy DM et al: Screening for colorectal cancer in a high-risk population, *Gastroenterology* 92:682-692, 1987.
35. Ekbom A et al: Ulcerative colitis and colorectal cancer: a population-based study, *N Engl J Med* 323:1288-1233, 1990.
36. Fath RB, Winawer SJ: Early diagnosis of colorectal cancer, *Annu Rev Med* 34:501-517, 1983.
37. Fedotin MS, Ginsberg BW: Practical considerations in screening for colorectal cancer, *Mod Med* 56:127-135, 1988.
38. Fenoglio-Preiser CM, Hutter RVP: Colorectal polyps: pathologic diagnosis and clinical significance, *CA Cancer J Clin* 35(6):322-344, 1985.
39. Fleischer DE et al: Detection and surveillance of colorectal cancer, *JAMA* 261(4):580-585, 1989.
40. Foutch PG et al: Flexible sigmoidoscopy may be ineffective for secondary prevention of colorectal cancer in asymptomatic, average-risk men, *Dig Dis Sci* 36(7):924-928, 1991.
41. Gardner DA et al: Tissue fluorescence spectroscopy as a means of identifying increased risk for colon adenomas and carcinomas, *Am J Gastroenterol* 86:1353a, 1991.

42. Gilbertsen VA et al: The early detection of colorectal cancer. A preliminary report of the results of the occult blood study, *Cancer* 45:2899-2901, 1980.

43. Gilbertsen VA, Nelms JM: The prevention of invasive cancer of the rectum, *Cancer* 41:1137-1139, 1978.

44. Greegor DH: Diagnosis of large bowel cancer in the asymptomatic patient, *JAMA* 201:943-945, 1967.

45. Grossman S, Milos ML: Colonoscopic screening of persons with suspected risk factors for colon cancer: I. Family history, *Gastroenterology* 94:395-400, 1988.

46. Guidelines for cancer related check-ups, recommendations and rationale, *Cancer* 30:208-230, 1980.

47. Guillem JG et al: Colonic neoplasms in asymptomatic first-degree relatives of colon cancer patients, *Am J Gastroenterol* 83(3):271-273, 1988.

48. Hacker JF: Adenoma markers or busy work? (editorial), *Am J Gastroenterol* 86(6):784-785, 1991.

49. Hardcastle JD et al: Faecal occult blood screening for colorectal cancer in the general population. Results of a controlled trial, *Cancer* 58:397-403, 1986.

50. Heimann TM, Gelernt I, Salky B: Familial polyposis coli: results of mucosal proctocolectomy with ileoanal anastomosis, *Dis Colon Rectum* 30:424-427, 1987.

51. Herrera L, Hanna S, Petrelli N: Screening endoscopy in patients with family history positive (FH+) for colorectal neoplasia (CRN), abstract, *Gastrointest Endosc* 36(2):211, 1990.

52. Herzog P et al: Faecal blood loss in patients with colonic polyps: a comparison of measurements with 51Cr-labelled erythrocytes and with the Haemocult test, *Gastroenterology* 83:957-962, 1982.

53. Irons GV, Kirschner JB: Routine chemical test of the stool for blood: an evaluation, *Am J Med Sci* 249:247-260, 1965.

54. Johnson DA et al: A prospective study of the prevalence of colonic neoplasms in asymptomatic patients with an age-related risk, *Am J Gastroenterol* 85(8):969-974, 1990.

55. Kapadia CR et al: Laser-induced fluorescence spectroscopy of human colonic mucosa: detection of adenomatous transformation, *Gastroenterology* 99:150-157, 1990.

56. Kewenter J, Bjorck S, Haglind E: Screening and rescreening for colorectal cancer: a controlled trial of fecal occult blood testing in 27,700 subjects, *Cancer* 62:645-651, 1988.

57. Kotzampassi K et al: Duodenal polyposis in Gardner's syndrome: the significance of endoscopic surveillance, *Am J Gastroenterol* 85(11):1541-1542, 1990.

58. Kronberg O et al: Initial mass screening for colorectal cancer with fecal occult blood test: a prospective randomized study at Funen in Denmark, *Scand J Gastroenterol* 22:278-286, 1987.

59. Kussin SZ, Lipkin M, Winower SJ: Inherited colon cancer: clinical implications, *Am J Gastroenterol* 72:448-457, 1979.

60. Lambert R et al: The management of patients with colorectal adenomas, *CA Cancer J Clin* 34:167-76, 1984.

61. Lanspa SJ, Lynch HT, Smyrk TC: Colorectal adenomas in the Lynch syndromes: results of a colonoscopy screening program, *Gastroenterology* 98:1117-1122, 1990.

62. Lashner BA, Hanauer SB, Silverstein MD: Optimal timing of colonoscopy to screen for cancer in ulcerative colitis, *Ann Intern Med* 108:274-278, 1988.

63. Lashner BA, Kane SV, Hanauer SB: Colon cancer surveillance in chronic ulcerative colitis: historical cohort study, *Am J Gastroenterol* 85(9):1083-1087, 1990.

64. Lashner BA, Silverstein MD, Hanauer SB: Hazard rates for dysplasia and cancer in ulcerative colitis: results from a surveillance program, *Dig Dis Sci* 34(10):1536-1541, 1989.

65. Laurent-Puig P et al: Survival and acquired genetic alterations in colorectal cancer, *Gastroenterology* 102:1136-1141, 1992.

66. Lieberman DA, Smith FW: Screening for colon malignancy with colonoscopy, *Am J Gastroenterol* 86(8):946-951, 1991.

67. Lieberman D, Smith F: Cost effectiveness of screening colonoscopy in asymptomatic individuals, *Gastrointest Endosc* 36(2):209-210, 1990.

68. Lofberg R et al: Colonoscopic surveillance in long-standing total ulcerative colitis: a 15-year follow-up study, *Gastroenterology* 99:1021-1031, 1990.

69. Lynch HT et al: Natural history of colorectal cancer in hereditary nonpolyposis colorectal cancer (Lynch syndromes I and II), *Dis Colon Rectum* 31:429-444, 1988.

70. Mason JO: *Healthy people 2000: National health promotion and disease prevention objectives.* Public Health Service, Department of Health and Human Services, Washington, DC, 1991, US Government Printing Office.

71. McGill DB: The president and the power of the colonoscope, *Mayo Clin Proc* 60:886-889, 1985.

72. Meyer CT, McBride W, Goldblatt RS: Clinical experience with flexible sigmoidoscopy in asymptomatic and symptomatic patients, *J Biol Med* 53:345-352, 1980.

73. Miller AB: Trends in cancer mortality and epidemiology, *Cancer* 51:2413-2418, 1983.

74. Miller RE: Detection of colon carcinoma and the barium enema, *JAMA* 230:1195-1198, 1974.

75. Mitooka H et al: Chromoscopy of the colon using indigo carmine dye with electrolyte lavage solution, *Gastrointest Endosc* 38(3):373-374, 1992.

76. Miyoshi H et al: Immunological determination of fecal hemoglobin and transferrin levels: a comparison with other fecal occult blood tests, *Am J Gastroenterol* 87(1):67-73, 1992.

77. Moore JRL, LaMont JT: Colorectal cancer: risk factors and screening strategies, *Arch Intern Med* 144:1819-1823, 1984.

78. Muto T, Bussey HJR, Morson BC: The evolution of cancer of the colon and rectum, *Cancer* 36:2251-2270, 1975.

79. Neugut AI: Screening for colorectal cancer, *Ann Intern Med* 113(11):899-900, 1990.

80. Neugut AI, Forde KA: Screening colonoscopy: has the time come? *Am J Gastroenterol* 83(3):295-297, 1988.

81. Norfleet RG: Early detection of colorectal neoplasms: methods for screening and surveillance, *Postgrad Med* 79(6):121-124, 1986.

82. Norfleet RG, Ryan ME, Wyman JB: Adenomatous and hyperplastic polyps cannot be reliably distinguished by their appearance through the fiberoptic sigmoidoscope, *Dig Dis Sci* 33(9):1175-1177, 1988.

83. Nugent FW, Haggitt RC, Gilpin PA: Cancer surveillance in ulcerative colitis, *Gastroenterology* 100:1241-1248, 1991.

84. O'Brien MJ et al: The national polyp study: patient and polyp characteristics associated with high-grade dysplasia in colorectal adenomas, *Gastroenterology* 98:371-379, 1990.

85. Offerhaus GJA et al: The relationship of DNA aneuploidy to molecular genetic alterations in colorectal carcinoma, *Gastroenterology* 102:1612-1619, 1992.

86. Olschwang S et al: Genetic characterization of the APC locus involved in familial adenomatous polyposis, *Gastroenterology* 101:154-160, 1991.

87. Ovaska J et al: Follow-up of patients operated on for colorectal carcinoma, *Am J Surg* 159:593-596, 1990.

88. Pathak S et al: Identification of colon cancer-predisposed individuals: a cytogenetic analysis, *Am J Gastroenterol* 86(6):679-684, 1991.

89. Petras RE, Mir-Madjlessi SH, Farmer RG: Crohn's disease and intestinal carcinoma: a report of 11 cases with emphasis on associated epithelial dysplasia, *Gastroenterology* 93:1307-1314, 1987.

90. Provenzale D et al: Risk for colon adenomas in patients with rectosigmoid hyperplastic polyps, *Ann Intern Med* 113:760-763, 1990.

91. Rankin GB: Indications, contraindications, and complications of colonoscopy. In Sivak MV, editor: *Gastroenterologic endoscopy*, Philadelphia, 1987, WB Saunders.

92. Ransohoff DF, Lang CA: Small adenomas detected during fecal occult blood test screening for colorectal cancer: the impact of serendipity, *JAMA* 264(1):76-78, 1990.

93. Ransohoff DF, Lang CA, Kuo HS: Colonoscopic surveillance after polypectomy: considerations of cost effectiveness, *Ann Intern Med* 114:177-182, 1991.

94. Ransohoff DF, Lang CA: Screening for colorectal carcinoma, *New Eng J Med* 325(1):37-41, 1991.

95. Rex DK et al: Performing screening flexible sigmoidoscopy using colonoscopes: experience in 500 subjects, *Gastrointest Endosc* 36:486-488, 1990.

96. Rex DK et al: Screening colonoscopy in asymptomatic average-risk persons with negative fecal occult blood tests, *Gastroenterology* 100:64-67, 1991.

97. Rex DK et al: Distal colonic polyps do not predict proximal adenomas in average-risk subjects, *Gastroenterology* 102:317-319, 1992.

98. Rickert RR et al: Adenomatous lesion of the large bowel: an autopsy survey, *Cancer* 43:1847-1857, 1979.

99. Rokkas T, Karameris A: The significance of small colonic polyps found at flexible sigmoidoscopy, *Gastrointest Endosc* 36(6):635, 1990.

100. Rozen P, Ron E: A cost analysis of screening methodology for family members of colorectal cancer patients, *Am J Gastroenterol* 84(12):1548-1551, 1989.

101. Sales DJ, Kirsner JB: The prognosis of inflammatory bowel disease, *Arch Intern Med* 143(2):294-299, 1983.

102. Schomaker KT et al: Ultraviolet laser-induced fluorescence of colonic polyps, *Gastroenterology* 102:1155-1160, 1992.

103. Schuman BM, McKay MD, Griffin JW: The use of the 130cm colonoscope for screening flexible sigmoidoscopy, *Gastrointest Endosc* 34:459-460, 1988.

104. Schuman BM, Simsek H, Lyons RC: The association of multiple colonic adenomatous polyps with cancer of the colon, *Am J Gastroenterol* 85(7):846-849, 1990.

105. Selby JV et al: A case-control study of screening sigmoidoscopy and mortality from colorectal cancer, *New Engl J Med* 326(10):653-657, 1992.

106. Sherlock P: Cancer surveillance in inflammatory bowel disease, *Postgrad Med* 74(6):191-204, 1983.

107. Silverberg E: Estimated cancer deaths by sex for all sites, *CA Cancer J Clin* 33:9-25, 1983.

108. Simon JB: Occult blood screening for colorectal carcinoma: a critical review, *Gastroenterology* 88:820-837, 1985.

109. Stower MJ, Hardcastle JD: Five year survival of 1115 patients with colorectal cancer, *Eur J Clin Oncol* 11:119, 1985.

110. Stroehlein JR et al: Haemoccult detection of faecal occult blood quantified by radioimmunoassay, *Dig Dis* 21:841-899, 1976.

111. Sugarbaker PH, MacDonald JS, Querllson LL: Colorectal cancer. In DeVita VT Jr, Hellman S, Rosenberg SA, editors: *Cancer: principles and practice of oncology,* New York, 1982, JB Lippincott.

112. Vaananen P, Tenhunen R: Rapid immunological detection of fecal occult blood by use of a latex-agglutination test, *Clin Chem* 34:1763-1766, 1988.

113. Vellacott KD, Baldwin RW, Hardcastle JD: An immunofluorescent test for fecal occult blood, *Lancet* 1:18-19, 1981.

114. Verbunt RJAM et al: Characterization of ultraviolet laser-induced autofluorescence of ceroid deposits and other structures in atherosclerotic plaques as a potential for laser angiosurgery, *Am Heart Journal* 123(1):208-216, 1992.

115. Weber CA et al: Routine colonoscopy in the management of colorectal carcinoma, *Am J Surg* 152:87-92, 1986.

116. Weedon DD et al: Crohn's disease and cancer, *N Engl J Med* 289:1099-1103, 1973.

117. Weir JA: Colorectal cancer: metachronous and other associated neoplasms, *Dis Colon Rectum* 18:4-5, 1975.

118. Welch JP: Multiple colorectal tumors: an appraisal of natural history and therapeutic options, *Am J Surg* 142:274-280, 1981.

119. Wilson JML, Jungner C: *Principles and practices of screening for disease,* Public Health Paper No. 34, Geneva, 1968, World Health Organization.

120. Winawer SJ: Detection and diagnosis of colorectal cancer, *Cancer* 51:2519-2524, 1983.

121. Winawer SJ et al: The national polyp study: colorectal adenomas and hyperplastic polyps, abstract, *Gastroenterology* 94:499, 1988.

122. Winawer SJ, Miller PG, Sherlock P: Risk and screening for colorectal cancer, *Adv Intern Med* 35:33-48, 1984.

123. Winnan G et al: Superiority of the flexible to the rigid sigmoidoscope in routine proctosigmoidoscopy, *N Engl J Med* 302(18):1011-1012, 1980.

124. Woolf SH, Kamerow DB, Mickalide AD: *Guide to clinical preventive services: an assessment of the effectiveness of 169 interventions.* Report of the US Preventive Services Task Force. Baltimore, 1990, William & Wilkins.

125. Yarborough GW, Waisbren BA: The benefits of systematic fiberoptic flexible sigmoidoscopy, *Arch Intern Med* 145:95-96, 1985.

Chapter 47

BREAST CANCER

Andres Bhatia
G. Thomas Budd

EPIDEMIOLOGY AND RISK FACTORS

The United States has one of the highest rates of breast cancer in the world. Estimates suggest that the U.S. incidence of breast cancer in 1991 was 175,000, and that 44,500 deaths occurred from this disease.[1] Breast cancer had been the leading cause of cancer death in women, but was recently surpassed by lung malignancies. The U.S. incidence of breast cancer has increased by about 3% per year, from 84.8 cases per 100,000 in 1980 to 111.9 cases in 1987.[1]

One out of four women with cancer has breast cancer, with 18% of all cancer deaths being secondary to breast cancer. As in most cancers, the survival rate correlates directly with the stage of the disease at diagnosis. The 5-year survival rate of all stages of breast cancer is approximately 75%. In localized disease (negative lymph nodes, negative skin or muscle invasion, and a lesion less than 3 cm in diameter), the 5-year survival is 91%; with regional disease, 5-year survival is 69%. In metastatic disease, 5-year survival decreases to 18%; and, at this stage, the disease is generally considered to be incurable. Unlike some malignancies, breast cancer can recur at any time after diagnosis. This tendency for continuing relapse reduces the significance of 5-year survival data. Although the incidence of breast cancer is increasing, the mortality has remained about the same, perhaps reflecting earlier detection and improved management.

The information available on clinical risk factors, so far, accounts for only 20% of all breast cancer cases in younger patients and less than 30% in older patients.[62] This section addresses relative risk factors, comparing incidence of breast cancer or death from breast cancer among people with a particular risk factor to that of people without that risk factor. In contrast, absolute risk factor is the rate of occurrence of cancer or mortality from cancer in the general population.

We usually refer to patients as being at high risk of developing breast cancer if relative risk is greater than 4.0 (i.e., the chance of getting breast cancer is four times higher than in the general population). A moderate relative risk factor is between 2.0 and 4.0 and low risk is considered to be 1.1 to 1.9.

Among high-risk factor groups are 5 independent risks (see box on p. 909). The greatest risk for developing breast cancer is being a woman older than 65 years old.[55] The second highest risk is personal history of prior breast cancer, in situ or invasive. The risk in this situation is an annual incidence of .5 to 1.0 per year.[22] A third high-risk factor is a strong family history; two or more relatives of the proband (index case) with history of premenopausal and/or bilateral breast cancer. Having one first-degree relative (sister or mother) with breast cancer carries a lower relative risk factor of between 2 to 3.[47] In fact, this seems to be the case only if the first-degree relative is younger than 60 years old.[51] The risk of a family member developing breast cancer can only be inferred by family history, as no biologic or genetic marker has been identified.[62]

Calculations using pedigrees containing affected first-degree relatives (mother/daughter, sister/sister) who were diagnosed premenopausally, in which at least one member had bilateral disease, yield a lifetime risk of 50%, suggesting an autosomal dominant gene transmission in mendelian genetics. The Li-Fraumeni syndrome, identified in 1969,[31] can be used as a model to study the genetics of cancer. This multiple, primary cancer syndrome (soft tissue and osteosarcomas, breast and brain cancer, leukemia, adrenocortical tumor) is associated with an inherited mutation in the p53 gene of chromosome 17.[39,30] The p53 gene is among the first tumor suppressor genes to be identified. If the p53 gene product, a suppressor protein, is deleted or abnormal, the growth of a cell may become unregulated, leading to transformation.

The fourth high-risk factor is history of a breast biopsy showing a proliferative lesion with atypia. Past data have tended to group all benign breast diseases together as fibrocystic disease. Fibrocystic disease of the breast, however, can be divided into the following categories: (1) nonproliferative benign breast diseases (fibroadenoma cyst, ductal ectasia, apocrine metaplasia, and myohyperplasia), which are not associated with increased risk[32]; (2) epithelial hyperplasia, which carries an increased relative risk of 1.5; and (3) atypical hyperplasia, which yields an increased relative risk of more than 4.[10,32,44] Finally, women born in North America and northern Europe have a relative risk of more than 4.[17,46,49] This has been confirmed by studies showing first generation of immigrants to the United States from low-risk areas acquiring increased risk.[17]

A history of a first-degree relative having breast cancer increases the risk twofold to threefold.[47] Obesity, especially in the older population, seems to increase risk of breast cancer moderately.[9,36] First full-term pregnancy after age 30 and nulliparity also confer a relative risk of about 2.[36,37,45] Most studies show a decreased risk of breast cancer if a woman attains pregnancy before age 20.[47] Relative risk in these women is less than 1.0. A personal history of ovarian or endometrial carcinoma has been associated with a moderate risk of developing breast cancer.[10,19]

Prior history of radiation to the thorax has consistently been found to increase moderately the risk of developing breast cancer.[27] This factor has been observed in Japanese atomic bomb survivors,[64] radiation for postpartum mastitis,[23] multiple x-rays for management of scoliosis in girls,[24] thymus irradiation during infancy,[21] fluoroscopies for management of artificial pneumothorax as treatment of tuberculosis,[25] and radiation for Hodgkin's disease.[4] The sensitivity to radiation seems to be higher in persons under 20 years of age receiving radiation. The latency period peaks around 20 years later. Neither chest x-rays nor mammograms have been shown to increase the risk of breast cancer. Mammographic parenchymal patterns DNY (dysplasia) and P2 (prominent duct pattern), the densest parenchymal pattern, are also associated with a twofold to threefold increase in risk for subsequent development of breast cancers.[52]

Relative risks lower than 2.0 and more than 1.0 are considered low risk. These risk factors include heavy alcohol consumption, menarche before age of 12 years, and menopause after age of 55 years. Several studies have associated moderately heavy alcohol consumption and risk

---

Breast cancer risk factors

High (relative risk >4)

- Age >65 years
- Prior invasive or in situ breast cancer
- Family history of 2 or more relatives with premenopausal and/or bilateral breast cancer
- Atypical hyperplasia on prior breast biopsy
- Having been born in North America or Northern Europe

Moderate (relative risk 2-4)

- Family history of first-degree relative with breast cancer
- Obesity
- Age at first full-term pregnancy of greater than 30 years
- Nulliparity
- History of prior ovarian or endometrial cancer
- Prior radiation to the thorax
- Mammographic pattern of dysplasia and prominent ductal tissue

Low (relative risk 1-2)

- Alcohol consumption
- Early menarche
- Late menopause

---

of breast cancer,[34] whereas others have found no relationship.[30,31] Meta-analysis estimated that 13% of breast cancers in the United States are attributable to alcohol intake.[34] One daily drink (liquor, beer, wine) was associated with a relative risk of 1.4, and two drinks a day almost double any earlier risk.[20] However, there are other socioeconomic variables operative that makes the analysis of these data difficult. The association, however, between alcohol and breast cancer seems to start with low alcohol consumption levels. Therefore if the risk of developing breast cancer is to be reduced significantly through reduction of alcohol intake, nearly total abstinence would be required.[35]

Both early menarche and late menopause increase risk for breast cancer slightly.[28] The risk increases by 12% for every year that a person is younger than the mean at the time of menarche, but is reduced by 6% for every year earlier than the mean at the time of menopause.[40] Thus it seems that the less time that a woman is ovulatory the less the chance of developing breast cancer.

The use of oral contraceptives, especially long-term, has been reported by some to increase the risk of breast cancer[61]; however, other studies do not support this finding.[50] A recent analysis[54] suggests that long-term oral contraceptive use promotes earlier clinical manifestations of breast cancers in some women but has no impact on their lifetime risk of disease. Conjugated estrogen replacement at doses less than or equal to 0.625 mg/day does not increase the risk of breast cancer, even among women with a history of benign disease of the breast, as reported by a recent meta-analysis.[11]

Finally, a number of factors at one time or another have been implicated as high-risk factors for breast cancer, but their importance has not been confirmed. Some of these are high-fat diet, consistency of cerumen, cigarette smoking, emotional stress, viruses (oncornavirus, B virus), Rauwolfia alkaloids, and methylxanthines.[15] The relative importance of each as a risk factor for breast cancer may be further delineated in future studies. Nonetheless, prudence would indicate counseling women to eliminate tobacco use and to follow a low-fat diet to be appropriate as possibly reducing risk for breast cancer while at the same time reducing risk for other problems.

BREAST EXAMINATION

The female breast resides between the second and the sixth ribs, and between the sternal edge and the mid-axillary line. About two thirds of the breast is superficial to the pectoralis major muscle; one third is superior to the serratus anterior muscle. For descriptive purposes, the breast can be divided into four quadrants. Most, but not all, of the lymphatic drainage of the breast drains into the central axillary lymph nodes located around the chest wall high in the axilla and mid-way between the anterior and the posterior axillary folds.

Most authorities recommend breast physical examination by a physician every 3 years between the ages of 20 and 40 years and annually thereafter. So far, this seems to be the most powerful tool in detecting early breast cancer.[38] The best time to examine the female breast is 1 week after menstruation. The breast should be examined systematically. For inspection, the patient should be in the sitting position, disrobed to the waist with her arms at her side. Note the following: appearance of the skin (color, thickening, prominent pores), size and shape of each breast, contour of the breast (looking for masses, flattening or dimpling). Look for an inverted nipple (may be normal, especially if chronic), discharges, ulcerations, or rashes. To reveal dimpling or retraction otherwise not seen, have the patient raise her arms over her head and press her hands against her hips. If the patient has large or pendulous breasts, more information may be gained by having the patient lean forward while standing (may use a chair for support).

The female breast should be palpated while the patient is in the supine position. A small pillow behind the ipsilateral shoulder may help spread the breast tissue more evenly. Using a rotary motion against the chest wall, compress the tissue gently with the fingers flat on the breast. Tissue consistency may vary from more nodular and fibrous in a premenopausal female to soft and fatty in a postmenopausal woman. Upon palpation, feel for nodules or masses and describe their location, size, shape, consistency, tenderness and mobility, or fixation to underlying skin, pectoralis muscle, or ribs. To palpate the axilla for lymph nodes most clinicians recommend having the patient in the sitting position, although sometimes a supine position may be used.[3,7]

BREAST SELF-EXAMINATION

About 70% to 80% of breast cancers are discovered by women themselves. Although it is not clear that breast self-examination (BSE) increases the chances of earlier detection of breast cancer, it is easy to teach and perform. Some retrospective trials of BSE do report an increase in earlier detection and survival rates.[13,14]

A patient should be instructed to be aware of signs that may represent early breast cancer, such as a lump or a thickening in the breast, change in breast shape, or discharges from the nipple. In the premenopausal female, the breasts should be examined about 7 days after menses, starting at age 20 years. Postmenopausal women should perform BSE on the first day of each month. The NIH (National Institutes of Health) has published guidelines for women who want to practice BSE (NIH publication no. 88-2409). Patients should realize that 80% of lumps are benign, as some women are "afraid of finding something bad". In addition, any abnormality found in the breast or axilla should be reported to the physicians immediately. Fig. 47-1 is provided as an introduction to BSE and can be copied and given to patients.

MAMMOGRAPHY SCREENING

Breast cancer is one of the few malignancies for which the value of screening has been demonstrated in prospective, randomized trials. These trials are important, as a number of inherent biases reduce the value of alternative trial designs. The first of these biases is lead time bias. The survival after detection of a clinically inapparent malignancy will necessarily be longer than the survival after clinical diagnosis of the same tumor, even if death is not delayed by earlier detection. This difference results because the date of detection is moved forward, so that the time between detection and death is greater in the tumor detected by screening. Furthermore, rapidly proliferating tumors, with an attendingly poor prognosis, are more likely to become clinically detectable between screening tests than are more slowly growing tumors. Slowly progressing tumors are more likely to remain subclinical during the time between screening tests and to be detected by screening. This tendency of screening to detect more slowly growing tumors with a good prognosis is called length time bias. In addition, a screened population is likely to differ from an unscreened population because of referral bias. That is, patients participating in screening programs may be more likely to have a family history of breast cancer or, on the other hand, a greater degree of

BREAST SELF-EXAMINATION (BSE)

Here is one way to do BSE:

1. Stand before a mirror. Inspect both breasts for anything unusual, such as any discharge from the nipples or puckering, dimpling, or scaling of the skin.

The next two steps are designed to emphasize any changes in the shape or contour of your breasts. As you do them, you should be able to feel your chest muscles tighten.

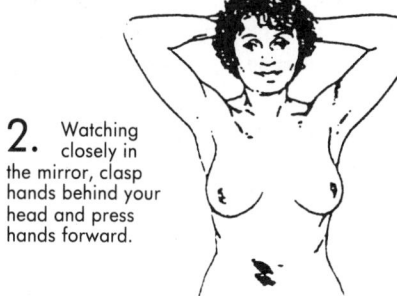

2. Watching closely in the mirror, clasp hands behind your head and press hands forward.

3. Next, press hands firmly on hips and bow slightly toward the mirror as you pull your shoulders and elbows forward.

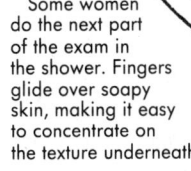

Some women do the next part of the exam in the shower. Fingers glide over soapy skin, making it easy to concentrate on the texture underneath.

4. Raise your left arm. Use three or four fingers of your right hand to explore your left breast firmly, carefully, and thoroughly. Beginning at the outer edge, press the flat part of your fingers in small circles, moving the circles slowly around the breast. Gradually work toward the nipple. Be sure to cover the entire breast. Pay special attention to the area between the breast and the armpit, including the armpit itself. Feel for any unusual lump or mass under the skin.

5. Gently squeeze the nipple and look for a discharge. (If you have any discharge during the month, see your doctor.) Repeat the exam on your right breast.

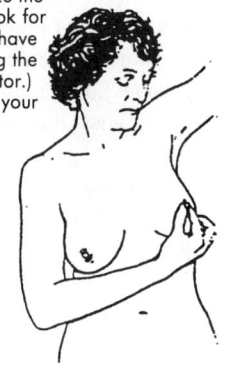

6. Repeat steps 4 and 5 lying down. Lie flat on your back with your left arm over your head and a pillow or folded towel under your left shoulder. This position flattens the breast and makes it easier to examine. Use the same circular motion described earlier. Repeat on your right breast.

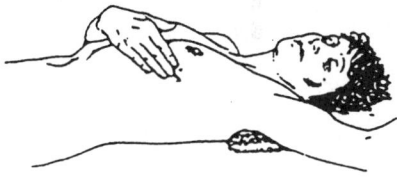

Warning signs   (Do not always mean cancer; eight out of ten lumps are not cancer.)

1. A lump of thickening in the breast
2. A change in breast shape
3. Discharge from the nipple

Remember, you know your body better than anybody else. Therefore, you can probably detect subtle changes earlier, **but you need to look.**

Fig. 47-1. Breast self-examination. (Modified from U.S. Department of Health and Human Services, National Institutes of Health, NIH 88:2409, revised March, 1988.)

health awareness than patients not participating in a screening program.

Because most of these biases inherently confer a more favorable prognosis to tumors detected by screening programs, the true value of screening can only be determined by trials randomizing subjects to either routine care or screening. The value of the policy of screening can then be determined by observing the cancer-specific mortality in the two groups. Several such trials have been performed. In three, the value of screening mammography, with or without professional examination or SBE, was demonstrated by a reduction in the number of deaths due to breast cancer in the screened groups.

The first such study was performed by the Health Insurance Program of New York, termed the HIP study. It was performed in a population of approximately 62,000 women aged 40 to 64 years who were members of a comprehensive, prepaid group health plan. Patient entry occurred between December 1963 and June 1966. Women were randomized to standard care or were offered a total of four annual examinations, consisting of physical examination and mammography.[59] Compliance with the initial screening examination was 65%, and 88% of these women had at least one subsequent examination.

Ten years after entry in the trial, the group of patients randomized to receive screening had a 30% reduction in mortality due to breast cancer, as compared to the control group. The initial reports of this study concluded that screening was of particular value in women between 50 and 59 but that screening was not helpful in women between 40 and 49.[59] This conclusion was made even though patients in the younger age group who were screened had a lower mortality rate (not statistically significant) than those who were not screened. The conclusion was made, however, because the advantage observed for women in the younger age group seemed to be due to differences in cases diagnosed when these women had entered their 50s.

More recent analyses of the HIP study have led to the conclusion that screening is probably of value in women in their 40s.[58] The HIP study, using mammographic technology now outdated, nevertheless stands as a landmark screening study, for a significant decrease in deaths due to breast cancer was found in the group of women randomly assigned to screening.

Subsequent trials have generally supported the conclusions reached by the HIP investigators. These confirmatory trials are summarized here. The Swedish two-county study was begun in 1977 by the Swedish Board of Health and Welfare to determine the effectiveness of single-view mammography. The results of this trial were reported in 1985.[63] A total of 162,981 women 40 years of age or older were randomized in socioeconomically stratified blocks to receive either routine care or to be offered screening mammography every 24 to 33 months, depending on age. Although compliance was poor in women over age 74, 89% of women between 40 and 74 complied with the first screening test, and 83% complied with the second screen.

A 31% reduction in mortality was noted in the screened group ($P = 0.013$). This difference in mortality was due to a divergence in the mortality rates first noted 4 years after randomization and persisting thereafter. The overall difference in breast cancer mortality was due to a difference observed in the patients aged 50 to 74, but the confidence interval for patients aged 40 to 50 was wide and the death rate was low in this group, so that further follow-up will be necessary for these younger women.

As of December 31, 1984, the incidence of invasive cancer was 13.7/1000 in the screened group and 10.5/1000 in the control group. The incidence of stage II and of axillary node-positive breast cancer was slightly higher in the unscreened group, and the incidence of stage I cancer was greater in the screened group. Interestingly, ductal carcinoma in situ was detected in 1.3/1000 of the screened women but only 0.4/1000 of the unscreened women. The implications of this ability to detect preinvasive breast cancer are not known, but it is clear that with widening use of screening mammography, preinvasive breast cancer is becoming a more common clinical problem.

The Malmo mammographic screening trial began in 1976.[2] Based upon a population registry in Malmo, Sweden, all women over the age of 45 were identified; half the

women in each 1-year cohort were randomized to a screening program consisting of mammography every 18 to 24 months (21,088 women) and half were not (21,195 women). Attendance rate at the initial screening session was 74%. This rate dropped slightly to 70% for subsequent screening sessions. At a mean duration of follow-up of 8.8 years, 588 women in the screened group and 447 in the control group had developed breast cancer. After 8.8 years of follow-up, 94 patients in the screened group and 99 in the study group had died of breast cancer. Thus an overall reduction in mortality due to breast cancer was not observed. A 20% reduction in breast cancer mortality was observed, however, in women 55 years and older. If it is assumed that the effects of screening are delayed and only the deaths occurring 6 years or more after screening are considered, a 30% reduction in mortality due to breast cancer was observed, suggesting that further follow-up of this patient group may result in a significant overall reduction.

The U.K. Trial of Early Detection of Breast Cancer was performed between 1979 and 1981.[65] This trial was not a randomized study, but a comparison of breast cancer detection and mortality rates between eight districts offering different screening services. The services compared were no special services, BSE, and biannual mammography with physical examination.

The initial acceptance rate among women offered screening services varied from 30% to 53% for BSE and 60% to 72% for mammography. In the districts offered screening mammography and physical examination, the rate of diagnosis of breast cancer was 2.57/1000 woman yrs. compared to 1.70/1000 woman years in the control district. The rate for in situ cancer was five times higher and the rate for invasive cancer was 1.4 times higher in the screening districts. The diagnosis rate in the districts utilizing BSE was 1.95/1000 woman yrs.

When breast cancer mortality was analyzed in the various districts, a statistically insignificant reduction in breast cancer mortality was noted in the districts offered screening mammography as compared to the control districts (relative risk = 0.86, 95% confidence interval [CI] 0.69 to 1.08, $P = 0.23$). When the mortality figures were adjusted for geographic differences in breast cancer mortality based on population statistics during the period before the study, the relative risk reduction in the screened districts was 0.80, but this difference remained statistically insignificant. Although the observed differences may reach statistical significance after further follow-up, this study demonstrates the weakness of nonrandomized trials and the importance of a high participation rate if a screening policy is to be evaluated adequately.

EXPECTED OUTCOME OF SCREENING

As noted previously, the incidence of breast cancer is higher in screened than in nonscreened populations due to the detection of subclinical disease. Thus with wider application of screening mammography, an increase in the overall incidence of breast cancer would be expected. This trend seems to be occurring. Although other factors may be involved in the rising incidence of breast cancer, such as the aging of the population, the expanding use of mammography is probably responsible for much of the observed increase.[29,56] For example, it has been estimated that mammography has been responsible for approximately 75% of the increased incidence noted in Wisconsin in the 1980s.[29] Screening studies have shown that the incidence of breast cancer rises rapidly in the screened population, as subclinical tumors are detected in the initial, prevalence screen. If patients continue to undergo screening, the incidence rate in the screened population declines after the initial screen to a rate roughly equivalent to that in the general, unscreened population.[56] When screening is applied to an increasingly larger group of women, the incidence rate for breast cancer should increase. This rate of increase should eventually decline as the use of mammography stabilizes. Some of the detected tumors might never become clinically manifest, accounting for some increase in the overall rate of breast cancer.

Despite this anticipated rise in the incidence of breast cancer attributable to screening, the rate of death due to breast cancer is expected to decline. This favorable effect would be expected to be delayed compared to the initial effects on the incidence rates, based on the results of the randomized trials performed to date.

THERAPEUTIC INTERVENTIONS

Because tumors detected by screening tend to be of a lower stage than tumors detected by other methods, breast-conserving therapy is more likely to be possible in tumors detected by screening. Whereas the most aggressive systemic treatments are generally used in patients with high-risk operable breast cancer, adjuvant hormonal and chemotherapies have been shown to have effects on the clinical course of node-negative breast cancer.[12] Some very early stage tumors, however, are associated with recurrence risks too low to justify systemic therapy; screening may result in an increase in the diagnosis of such good-prognosis tumors. Thus, although screening may not decrease the proportion of patients who receive adjunctive therapy, the intensity of such therapy may be reduced. It is important to note that the screening studies discussed earlier were performed when adjuvant therapy was not routinely given; therefore, the effects of early detection on cancer-specific mortality may be different now that such therapy has been shown to be of value.

Another approach to the problem of early breast cancer is to intervene before the diagnosis of breast cancer is made in the hopes of reducing the risk that breast cancer will develop. Intervention could be guided by consideration of the risk factors discussed earlier. Such trials designed to reduce the incidence of breast cancer are now being performed. This primary intervention approach must be considered experimental until these studies are completed.

For some time, some women at particularly high risk have undergone bilateral prophylactic mastectomy. This procedure substantially (but not completely) reduces the chance that a woman will develop breast cancer, but there is no clear consensus with regard to which patients should undergo this procedure, except in women who are psychologically crippled by the fear of developing breast cancer. Obviously, prophylactic mastectomy will never become sufficiently widespread to have a significant impact on the epidemiology of the disease. Three major approaches to primary intervention are now being investigated: (1) alteration in the hormonal milieu in patients at risk to develop breast cancer, (2) dietary changes, and (3) the administration of retinoids.

Tamoxifen is being studied as a chemopreventative agent in several large clinical trials, including a U.S. trial being performed by the National Surgical Adjuvant Breast and Bowel Project. The rationale for these studies is the effectiveness of tamoxifen at every stage of the established disease, the activity of tamoxifen in the reduction of carcinogen-induced rodent mammary tumors,[41] and the reduction of contralateral breast cancers reported in women receiving tamoxifen as adjuvant therapy after local treatment of breast cancer. In a compilation of trials randomizing women to receive or not receive tamoxifen after local therapy for operable breast cancer, patients receiving tamoxifen reduced the rate at which breast cancer developed in the contralateral breast by 40%.[12]

At the University of California at Los Angeles, ovarian suppression with a gonadotropin-releasing hormone superagonist is being investigated.[41] Women entering this trial are also being given low doses of estrogen in an attempt to reduce the adverse effects of ovarian suppression on blood lipids and bone mineralization. Assessment of the usefulness of these approaches and determination of the constellation of risk factors that should be considered when selecting a woman for treatment with a chemopreventative agent must await completion and analysis of these ambitious trials.

Considerable epidemiologic evidence implicates dietary fat as a risk factor for the development of breast cancer.[15,33] Preclinical studies have suggested that dietary fat affects the rate of development of breast cancer in a rodent model system.[6] Because women who reported that they received fewer than 30% of their dietary calories from fat did not have a reduced mortality rate from breast cancer,[66] it is thought that any dietary intervention trial should use a target of 20% of total calories from fat. The large trial that would be required to adequately test the effectiveness of such a substantial change in life-style has hampered the activation of a primary dietary intervention study, but pilot studies have suggested that such a trial is feasible.[43]

Retinoids have been demonstrated to reduce the risk of second primary tumors in patients with treated head and neck cancers.[24] In Sprague-Dawley rats, treatment with the retinoid 4-hydroxy phenyl retinamide (4-HPR, Fenretinide) reduces the number of mammary carcinomas developing after treatment with the carcinogen MNU.[48] In this activity, 4-HPR and tamoxifen have additive or superadditive effects.[48] A trial comparing 4-HPR with placebo in women with a history of node-negative breast cancer is being performed in Milan, Italy. This trial is designed to determine whether 4-HPR reduces the risk of developing contralateral breast cancer in women with a history of node-negative breast cancer.[8] Clinical trials of the combination of 4-HPR and tamoxifen are also being performed.[5]

These chemoprevention trials are important in a disease such as breast cancer, which constitutes a major public health problem. Large prospective trials may help determine which patients are at particular risk to develop mammary carcinoma and who might benefit from primary intervention.

SOCIOMEDICOECONOMICS

Various estimates of the cost-effectiveness of breast cancer screening have been made. These estimates vary widely, depending on the assumptions made in the mathematical models used. Estimates of the cost of screening vary, depending on the number of views assumed to be needed, the frequency of screening, and the estimates of expenditures for equipment and personnel. Other so-called induced costs, such as follow-up mammograms or biopsy procedures and treatment, must be considered. The estimates of the costs of therapy according to stage of disease are variable and will change as practice patterns evolve. Subtracted from these screening costs would be the costs of palliative and terminal care saved by the reduction in breast cancer mortality associated with screening. Estimates of the number of years of life saved by screening can be made, based on the clinical trials described earlier. These estimates can then be used to calculate the number of dollars expended per year of life saved.

Although cost-effectiveness estimates of breast cancer screening vary widely, the estimates available suggest that breast cancer screening is a cost-effective public health strategy.[42] The cost per year of life saved by breast cancer screening has been estimated between $3800 and $126,000, with most estimates being in the $20,000 to $50,000 range for women between 50 and 65 years.[42] This amount compares favorably to the estimated costs of $7300/life year for coronary artery by-pass grafting for a left main coronary artery lesion, $32,600/life year for treatment of mild hypertension, or $225,000 per life year for liver transplantation.[42]

The maximal cost-effectiveness of breast cancer screening is likely to be in women between 50 and 70, as the

Table 47-1. Recommended breast cancer screening program ACS, ACR, NCI

Age	Frequency Clinical breast exam	Frequency Mammography
>20	Monthly BSE	
20-35	Every 3 years	
35-39	Every 3 years	Once as "baseline"
40-49	Annually	Every 1-2 years, depending on risk
≥50	Annually	Annually

Adapted from American Cancer Society: *Cancer facts and figures—1993*, Atlanta, American Cancer Society, 1993.

effectiveness of screening is clear in this age group, the incidence of breast cancer is significant, and competing causes of mortality may be less important than in older age groups. For an individual patient, the utility of screening will depend on her individual risk for developing breast cancer and the severity of other medical conditions likely to result in mortality. From a public health perspective, an expansion of screening efforts to include larger numbers of women in the group most likely to benefit is more important than extending screening to groups less likely to benefit, such as younger women. For this reason, further studies of the benefits of screening in different populations of women are needed.

GENERAL SCREENING RECOMMENDATIONS

In the United States, the American Cancer Society (ACS), the American College of Radiologists (ACR), and the National Cancer Institute (NCI) agree in general with the screening guidelines listed in Table 47-1; these recommendations are appropriate for general use. The United States Preventive Services Task Force (USPSTF) of the U.S. Department of Health and Human Services has recommended a slightly different schedule of breast screening. The USPSTF recommends annual clinical (physical) breast examinations for all women 40 and older; mammography is recommended at 1- to 2-year intervals for women of between 50 and 75 years.[57] They further recommend regular screening examinations, and mammography at a younger age (e.g., 35 years) for women with a family history of premenopausal breast cancer in first-degree relatives. In most other Western countries, mammography is recommended every 2 to 3 years, based on randomized trials that demonstrate a benefit to screening at these longer intervals.[57]

SUMMARY

Breast cancer is a common disease among Western women. The benefits of screening have been demonstrated in controlled and uncontrolled clinical trials. Further research is needed to quantify these benefits so that rational public health policy can be formulated. Clinical trials of interventions hypothesized to reduce the risk of developing breast cancer are underway. The identification of risk groups likely to benefit from such interventions and quantitation of the costs of such efforts will be important if these trials are to be applied to women in general.

REFERENCES

1. American Cancer Society: *Cancer facts and figures—1991*, Atlanta, American Cancer Society, 1991.
2. Andersson I et al: Mammographic screening and mortality from breast cancer: the Malmo mammographic screening trial, *Br Med J* 297:943-948, 1988.
3. Bates B: *A guide to physical examination*, ed 3, 1983, JB Lippincott.
4. Yahalom J et al: Breast cancer in patients irradicated for Hodgkin's disease: a clinical and pathologic analysis of 45 events in 37 patients, *J Clin Oncol* 10(11):1674-1681, 1992.
5. Cobleigh MA et al: Phase I Trial of tamoxifen with or without fenretinide, an analogue of vitamin A in patients with metastatic breast cancer, *Breast Cancer Res Treat* (abstract 65), 19:173, 1991.
6. Cohen LA et al: Effect of varying proportions of dietary fat on the development of NMU-induced rat mammary tumors, *Anticancer Res* 6:215-218, 1986.
7. DeGowin EL, DeGowin RL: The female breast. In *A guide to physical examination*, ed 4 New York, 1981 Macmillan.
8. De Palo G et al: Human breast cancer trial with fenretinide (4-HPR), abstract, *Eur J Cancer* 27 (supplement 2):S40, 1991.
9. DeWaard F: A prospective study of breast cancer risk in post-menopausal women, *Cancer* 14:153-160, 1974.
10. Dupond WD, Page PL: Breast cancer risk associated with proliferative disease, age at first birth, and a family history of breast cancer, *Am J Epidemiol* 125:769-779, 1987.
11. Dupont WD, Page DL: Therapy and breast cancer, *Arch Intern Med* 151:67-72, 1991.
12. Early Breast Cancer Trialists' Collaborative Group: Systemic treatment of early breast cancer by hormonal, cytotoxic, or immune therapy: 133 randomized trials involving 31,000 recurrences and 24,000 deaths among 75,000 women, *Lancet* 339:1-15, 71-85, 1992.
13. Foster RS, Costanza MC: Breast self-examination practices and breast cancer survival, *Cancer* 53:999-1005, 1984.
14. Foster RS et al: Breast self-examination practices and breast cancer stage, *N Engl J Med* 299:265-270, 1978.
15. Gardner J et al: Management of high risk group. In Harris J et al: *Breast diseases*, ed 2, Philadelphia, 1991, JB Lippincott.
16. Greenwald P et al: Estimated effect of breast self-examination and routine physician examinations on breast cancer mortality, *N Engl J Med* 299:271-273, 1978.
17. Haeszel W: Cancer mortality among the foreign born in the US, *J Natnl Cancer Inst* 26:37-137, 1968.
18. Harris RE, Wynder EL: Breast cancer and alcohol consumption: a study in weak associations, *JAMA* 259:2867-2871, 1988.
19. Harvey EB et al: Second cancer following cancer of the breast in Connecticut, 1935-1982, *NCI Monographs* 68:99-112, 1985.
20. Henderson IC: What can a woman do about her risk of dying of breast cancer? *Curr Probl Cancer* 144:161-230, 1990.
21. Hidreth NG et al: The risk of breast cancer after irradiation of the thymus in infancy, *N Engl J Med* 321:1281-1284, 1989.
22. Hishup TG et al: Second primary cancer of breast, incidence and risk factors, *Br J Cancer* 49:79-85, 1984.
23. Hoffman DA et al: Breast cancer in women with scoliosis exposed to multiple diagnostic x-rays, *J Natnl Cancer Inst* 81:1307-1312, 1989.
24. Hong WK et al: Prevention of second primary tumors with isotretinoin in squamous-cell carcinoma of the head and neck, *N Engl J Med* 323:795-801, 1990.
25. Hrubec Z et al: Breast cancer after multiple chest fluoroscopics: second follow-up of Massachusetts women with tuberculosis, *Cancer Res* 49:229-234, 1989.
26. Huguley CM, Brown RL: The value of breast self-examination, *Cancer* 47:989-995, 1981.
27. Kelsey J: Epidemiology of breast cancer, *Epidemiol Rev* 12:231-232, 1990.
28. Kvale G et al: Menstrual factors and breast cancer risk, *Cancer* 62:1625-1631, 1988.
29. Lantz PM, Remington PL, Newcomb PA: Mammography screening and increased incidence of breast cancer in Wisconsin, *J Natl Cancer Inst* 83:1540-1546, 1991.
30. Levine AJ: The p53 tumor suppressor gene, *Nature* 35:453-56, 1991.
31. Li FP, Fraumeni JF: Soft-tissue sarcomas, breast cancer and other neoplasms, *Ann Intern Med* 71:747, 1969.
32. London SJ, et al: Benign breast disease and breast cancer risk, *JAMA* 267:941-44, 1992.
33. Longcope C: Relationships of estrogen to breast cancer of diet to breast cancer, and of diet to estradiol metabolism, *J Natl Cancer Inst* 82:896-897, 1990.
34. Longnecker MP et al: A meta-analysis of alcohol consumption in relation to risk of breast cancer, *JAMA* 260:652-656, 1988.
35. Lowenfels AB, Zevola S: Alcohol and breast cancer: an overview, *Alcohol Clin Exp Res* 13:109-111, 1989.
36. Lubin F et al: Overweight and changes in weight through adult life in breast cancer etiology, *Am J Epidemiol* 122:579-588, 1985.
37. Lubin JH et al: Risk factors for breast cancer in women in northern Alberta, Canada, as related to age at diagnosis, *J Natnl Cancer Inst* 68:211-217, 1982.
38. Mahoney LJ: Annual clinical examination, *N Engl J Med* 301(6):315-316, 1979.
39. Malkin D, Li FP, Fraumeni JF: Germ line p53 mutation in familial syndrome of breast cancer, sarcoma, and other neoplasms, *Science* 250:1233, 1990.
40. Moolgavkar SH et al: Two stage model for carcinogenesis: epidemiology of breast cancer in females, *J Natnl Cancer Inst* 65:559-569, 1980.
41. McCormick DL, Moon RL: Retinoid-tamoxifen interaction in mammary cancer chemoprevention, *Carcinogenesis* 7:193-196, 1986.
42. Mushlin AI, Fintor L: Is screening for breast cancer cost-effective? *Cancer* 69 (supplement 7), 1962-1967, 1992.
43. News: Women's health trial on trial, *J Natl Cancer Inst* 83:321-323, 1991.
44. Page PL et al: Atypical hyperproliferative lesions of the female breast. A long-term follow-up study, *Cancer* 55:2698-2708, 1985.
45. Pathak DR: Parity and breast cancer risk, *Int J Cancer* 37:21-25, 1986.
46. Petrakis NL: Breast. In Schottenfeld D, editor: *Cancer, epidemiology, and prevention*, Philadelphia, 1982, WB Saunders.
47. Phillips RI et al: Familial breast cancer, *Postgrad Med J* 64:847-49, 1988.
48. Ratko TA, Detrisac CJ, Dinger NM, et al: Chemopreventive efficacy of combined retinoid and tamoxifen treatment following surgical excision of a primary mammary cancer in female rats, *Cancer Res* 49:4472-4476, 1989.
49. Robbins GF et al: Studies of Japanese migrants. Mortality from cancer and other diseases among Japanese in US, *J Natnl Cancer Inst* 40:43-68, 1968.
50. Romicu I et al: Prospective study of oral contraceptives use and risk of breast cancer in women, *J Natnl Cancer Inst* 81:1313-1321, 1989.
51. Roseman DL: A positive family history of breast cancer. Does its effect diminish with age? *Arch Intern Med* 150(1):191-194, 1990.
52. Saflas AF: Mammographic parenchymal patterns and breast cancer risk, *Epidemiol Res* 9:146-174, 1989.
53. Schatzkin A et al: Is alcohol consumption related to breast cancer?

Results from the Fremingham Heart Study, *J Natnl Cancer Inst* 81:31-35, 1989.

54. Schlesselman JJ: Oral contraceptives and breast cancer, *Am J Obstet Gynecol* 163:1379-1387, 1990.

55. Seidman H et al: Surveillance, epidemiology, and end results (SEER). Breast cancer, current trends in diagnosis and treatment, *Cancer* 34:186, 1985.

56. Shapiro S: More on screening and breast cancer incidence, *J Natl Cancer Inst* 83:1522-1523, 1991.

57. Shapiro S: Periodic breast cancer screening in seven foreign countries, *Cancer* 69 (Supplement 7):1919-1924, 1992.

58. Shapiro S et al: Selection, follow-up, and analysis in the health insurance plan study: a randomized trial with breast cancer screening, *Natl Cancer Inst Monogr* 67:65-75, 1985.

59. Shapiro S et al: Ten to fourteen-year effect of screening on breast cancer mortality, *J Natl Cancer Inst* 69:349-355, 1982.

60. Shore PE et al: Breast cancer among women given x-ray therapy for acute post partum mastitis, *Natl Cancer Inst* 77:689-696, 1986.

61. Stadel BV et al: Oral contraceptives and breast cancer, *Lancet* 1:1257-1258, 1989.

62. Stoll BA: Quantifying the risk of breast cancer, *Eur J Surg Oncol* 17:36-41, 1991.

63. Tabar L et al: Reduction in mortality from breast cancer after screening with mammography, *Lancet* 8433:829-832, 1985.

64. Takunga M et al: Breast cancer in Japanese atomic bomb survivors, *Lancet* 2:924, 1982.

65. UK Trial of Early Detection of Breast Cancer Group: First results on mortality reduction in the UK trial of early detection of breast cancer, *Lancet* 2:411-416, 1988.

66. Willet WC et al: Dietary fat and the risk of breast cancer, *N Engl J Med* 316:22-28, 1987.

━━━━━━━━━━ **RESOURCES** ━━━━━━━━━━

National Headquarters: American Cancer Society, Inc, 1599 Clifton Road, N.E., Atlanta, GA 30329-4251.

National Cancer Institute, c/o National Institute of Health, Bethesda, MD 20892.

Chapter 48

LUNG CANCER

Richard S. Lang

Lung cancer is the leading cause of cancer death among men and women in the United States. This is a sobering fact considering that the major cause of this disease has long been known and is avoidable—smoking. The American Cancer Society estimates the 1993 incidence of lung cancer to be 17% of all cancers in men and 12% in women. They further estimate lung cancer to account for 34% of all cancer deaths in men and 22% in women in 1993.[10] Approximately 170,000 new cases of lung cancer will be diagnosed in the United States in 1993 (100,000 in men and 70,000 in women), and 149,000 lung cancer deaths will occur (93,000 in men and 56,000 in women).[10]

Lung cancer is divided into types categorized by the predominant cell type of the tumor. These include small-cell carcinoma and non–small-cell carcinoma types. Non–small-cell carcinoma is further subdivided into squamous or epidermoid carcinoma, adenocarcinoma, and large-cell carcinoma. Other types of lung cancer include alveolar cell, metastatic, and mixed types. In this discussion lung cancer will be considered as a single disease, recognizing that the clinical aspects and behavior of the various types may differ.

Lung cancer has a relatively long period between exposure and disease. This latency period thereby represents an opportunity for intervention to prevent the disease. Lung cancer is often diagnosed in a relatively late stage, with only 18% of cases found to be localized at time of diagnosis. Symptoms and signs of lung cancer include cough, hemoptysis, dyspnea, wheezing, chest pain, and hoarseness. The disease may present as a postobstructive pneumonia or as one of a variety of paraneoplastic syndromes. The 5-year survival rates for lung cancer have been relatively poor (see Table 48-1).

Although the 5-year survival rate for lung cancer has improved with time, the current rates are still considered

Table 48-1. 5-Year survival rates for lung cancer by race, 1983-1987

Stage	White	Black
Localized	46%	40%
Regional	13%	11%
Distant	1%	1%
All stages	13%	11%

From Boring CC, Squires TS, and Tong T: Cancer statistics, 1993, *CA Cancer J Clin* 43:7-26, 1993.

to be among the worst prognoses of the major cancers. Efforts at primary prevention therefore are crucial to reducing this important cause of mortality in the United States and throughout the world.

EPIDEMIOLOGY

Lung cancer death rates have climbed in men since the 1940s and in women since the 1960s. The age-adjusted lung cancer death rate for men has risen from about 15 per 100,000 in 1945 to 40 per 100,000 in 1965 to about 73 per 100,000 in 1985. In women, the rate has increased from about 7 per 100,000 in 1965 to approximately 29 per 100,000 in 1985.[10] These trends, however, have not been the same for all age groups (see Figs. 48-1 and 48-2). In men, lung cancer death rates are increasing only in the older age groups. In women, the only age where rates are not increasing is the 35 to 44 age group.[32] Much of these trends is related to smoking habits (see risk factors section later in this chapter). Among smokers, lung cancer may have surpassed coronary artery disease as the number one cause of death.[76]

Lung cancer is a worldwide problem. Table 48-2 de-

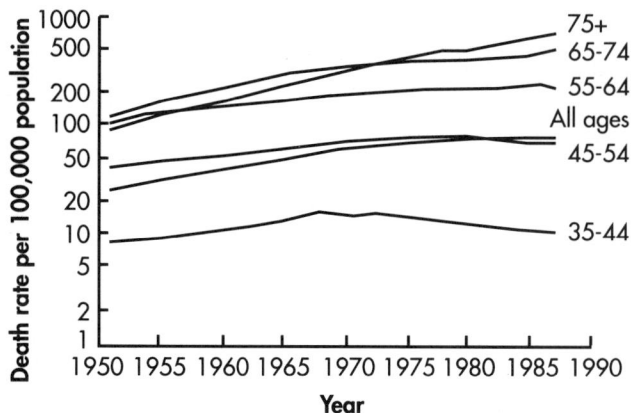

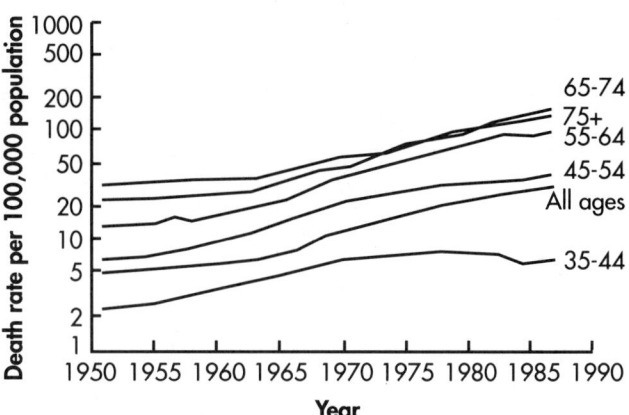

Fig. 48-1. Male lung cancer death rates, United States, 1950 to 1987. Standardized on the age distribution of the population of the United States, 1970. (From Garfinkel L, Silverberg E: Lung cancer and smoking trends in the United States over the past 25 years, *CA Cancer J Clin* 41:137-145, 1991.)

Fig. 48-2. Female lung cancer death rates, United States, 1950 to 1987. Standardized on the age distribution of the population of the United States, 1970. (From Garfinkel L, Silverberg E: Lung cancer and smoking trends in the United States over the past 25 years, *CA Cancer J Clin* 41:137-145, 1991.)

Table 48-2. Lung cancer age-adjusted death rates per 100,000 population for selected countries 1986-1988

World Rank	Male		Female	
1	Belgium	77.2	Scotland	27.1
2	Scotland	75.5	Hong Kong	25.0
3	Netherlands	75.5	Iceland	23.1
4	Czechoslovakia	74.5	United States	22.7
5	Hungary	73.3	Denmark	22.5
6	Luxembourg	71.8	England and Wales	20.1
7	Poland	67.5	Canada	19.5
8	Former USSR	61.0	Singapore	18.3
9	England and Wales	60.9	Ireland	17.7
10	Italy	58.8	Northern Ireland	17.5
11	Hong Kong	57.3	New Zealand	15.7
12	United States	56.9	China	15.1
13	Canada	56.5	Cuba	14.3
14	Uruguay	55.4	Hungary	13.2
15	Singapore	54.7	Australia	11.9

From Boring CC, Squires TS, and Tong T: Cancer statistics, 1993, *CA Cancer J Clin* 43:7-26, 1993.

picts countries around the world with the highest lung cancer death rates in men and women. By the year 2000, deaths related to lung cancer will increase worldwide to 2 million.[15] This worldwide lung cancer problem is related to tobacco consumption. Smoking rates vary throughout the world. In a 1987 European survey, the percentage of smokers in populations varied from 33% in Ireland, Italy, and Portugal to 43% in Greece, 44% in the Netherlands, and 46% in Denmark.[39] Daily consumption of cigarettes for the population in Europe was highest for Greece, Switzerland, Yugoslavia, Hungary, and Poland.[39] Cigarette consumption in the Third World is a major problem, and smoking rates are rapidly increasing. Tobacco consumption can help to predict lung cancer mortality rates for a given country. Tobacco consumption data suggest that

lung cancer mortality rates will likely increase in most European countries and Japan until the year 2000, and that a lung cancer epidemic is likely to occur in Asia in the 21st century.[65]

Lung cancer rates have been generally higher in men than in women, reflecting to a degree the higher smoking rates historically for men compared with women both in the United States and worldwide. This difference in lung cancer rates between the sexes is not fully explained, however, by differing smoking habits. The association of smoking and lung cancer for women is less impressive than in men. Additionally, adenocarcinoma is the predominant lung cancer cell type in women, whereas squamous cell has been the most common type in men.[63] The reason for these differences appears to involve a variety of factors. Horwitz et al. suggest women may have some genetic predisposition or susceptibility for lung cancer. They hypothesize that an environmental (smoking)– genetic (family history) relationship may exist for lung cancer in women.[42] By 1986, lung cancer became the leading cause of cancer death in women. The lung cancer increase in women smokers has been dramatic and is depicted in Table 48-3. These changes in relative risk reflect the higher smoking rates in women over the interval and the earlier age that women began smoking in the more recent time periods.[33]

Smoking rates differ among races, educational groups, and socioeconomic classes. Because lung cancer is so closely tied to cigarette consumption, lung cancer rates differ among these groups as well. Lung cancer is a particular problem in black males, who are 50% more likely than white males to develop lung cancer. Black men are also more likely to smoke, and to use cigarettes higher in tar and nicotine.[21] Smoking rates for black women are more similar to those in white women. Smoking is more common in persons with less than a high school education.[32] Lung cancer mortality rate increases with the level of urbanization, suggesting that air pollution plays some role in risk for lung cancer.

Table 48-3. Relative risk for lung cancer mortality for smokers compared with nonsmokers over time, by sex

Sex	1965-1968	1969-1972	1982-1986
Female	2.9	4.5	10.8
Male	9.3	9.6	17.4

From Garfinkel L, Silverberg E: Lung cancer and smoking trends in the United States over the past 25 years, *CA Cancer J Clin* 41:137-145, 1991.

RISK FACTORS
Smoking

Cigarette smoking is beyond a doubt the major cause of lung cancer. About 91% of lung cancer in men and 77% in women is attributable to cigarette smoking.[59] Smokers have up to 25 times the risk of developing lung cancer as do nonsmokers, depending on number of cigarettes smoked, age when smoking began, and degree of inhalation. Table 48-4 reflects relative risk for lung cancer stratified by sex, number of cigarettes smoked daily, and length of time since smoking cessation. The risk of lung cancer in relation to smoking increases with the number of cigarettes smoked. Risk decreases significantly after stopping smoking, particularly after 5 years or more of cessation.[76] A study in Japan showed lung cancer risk in exsmokers after 5 years of smoking cessation to be half that of persons continuing to smoke.[78] Studies have shown that quitting smoking even intermittently can reduce lung cancer risk.[8] Generally, smokers, regardless of number of packs smoked per day, are 10 times more likely to die of lung cancer than are nonsmokers. The association of lung cancer and smoking is greatest when smoking is at least one pack per day for 10 years. There are no "safe" levels of smoking, nor such thing as a "safe" cigarette. All cigarettes, including those with "low" tar and nicotine, carry risk for lung cancer. One study has suggested the use of a "cumulative tar exposure index from smoking" as a measure of relative risk for development of lung cancer.[93] They were able to demonstrate a near linear dose response for lung cancer risk in relation to cumulative exposure to tar. This index considers the tar content of the brand of cigarette smoked, the number of cigarettes smoked per day, and the number of years each brand was smoked. This demonstrates what would seem intuitive, that the longer a person smokes, the higher the tar content of the

Table 48-4. Effect of quitting smoking on lung cancer risk among male and female former smokers, by length of time off cigarettes and number of cigarettes smoked daily

	Relative risk			
	Males		Females	
	1-20 cigarettes/day	≥21 cigarettes/day	1-19 cigarettes/day	≥20 cigarettes/day
Current smokers	18.8	26.9	7.3	16.3
Former smokers, yr since stopped				
<1	26.7	50.7	7.9	34.3
1-2	22.4	33.2	9.1	19.5
3-5	16.5	20.9	2.9	14.6
6-10	8.7	15.0	1.0	9.1
11-15	6.0	12.6	1.5	5.9
≥16	3.1	5.5	1.4	2.6

From Shopland DR, Eyre HJ, and Pechacek TF: Smoking attributable cancer mortality in 1991: Is lung cancer now the leading cause of death among smokers in the United States? *J Natl Cancer Inst* 83:1142-1148, 1991.

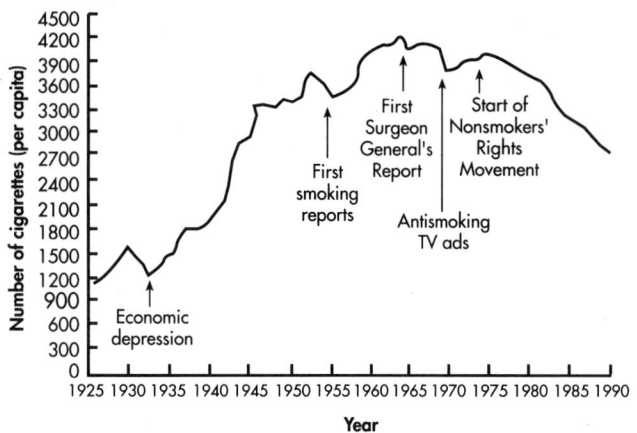

Fig. 48-3. Cigarette consumption per capita, age 18 and older, United States, 1925 to 1989. (From Garfinkel L, Silverberg E: Lung cancer and smoking trends in the United States over the past 25 years, *CA Cancer J Clin* 41:137-145, 1991.)

Table 48-5. Cigarette production and consumption in the United States and exports 1985-1989

Year	Production (billions)	Exports Number (billions)	Exports Percent
1985	665.3	58.9	8.9
1986	658.0	64.3	9.8
1987	689.4	100.2	14.5
1988	694.5	118.5	17.1
1989	677.2	141.8	20.9

Excerpted in part from Garfinkel L, Silverberg E: Lung cancer and smoking trends in the United States over the past 25 years, *CA Cancer J Clin* 41:137-145, 1991.

cigarette smoked, and the greater the number of cigarettes smoked, the greater the lifetime risk for lung cancer. Pipe and cigar smoking carry less risk for lung cancer but still more risk than in nonsmokers.[51] Risk in Denmark and the Netherlands, where deeper inhalation is common in pipe and cigar smokers, is closer to the risk in cigarette smokers.[87] Smokeless tobacco (chewing tobacco and snuff) do not appear to be a risk factor for lung cancer, but are carcinogens for the upper aerodigestive tract.

The number of cigarettes smoked per capita in the United States has gradually decreased since the first Surgeon General's report in the 1960s (see Fig. 48-3). However, the export of tobacco by the United States has increased in recent years (see Table 48-5). Exports have particularly increased to Third World countries, where legislative controls and other measures, which have limited tobacco use in the United States and in other industrialized countries, appear inadequate.[53] Selling higher tar cigarettes, advertising on television, and selling cigarettes without health warnings are all practiced in Third World countries.[53] As smoking consumption in the United States continues to decline, one hopes attention will be focused also on worldwide smoking consumption and the resultant serious threat to the world's health.

In recent years "sidestream" smoke as a risk factor for development of lung cancer in persons who have never themselves smoked has become an issue. If heavy smokers of more than two packs per day have lung cancer mortality rates 15 to 25 times greater than nonsmokers,[59] what is the risk for persons exposed to sidestream smoke who themselves do not smoke? If we extrapolate from the concept and data of cumulative tar exposure we would conclude that the greater the dose of sidestream smoke and the higher the tar content of that smoke, the higher the risk for lung cancer. Beginning in about 1981 and since, a body of data has accumulated to suggest that sidestream or environmental tobacco smoke does in fact increase risk for lung cancer in a nonsmoking spouse.* A population-based case control study found 17% of lung cancers among nonsmokers to be attributable to high levels of exposure to cigarette smoke during childhood and adolescence in the home.[45] A multicenter case control study showed an increased relative risk for lung cancer, particularly adenocarcinoma in spouses of smokers, with a greater risk in the spouses of the heaviest smokers.[26] A recent population-based case control study confirms these findings.[12] An autopsy study found an increase in "epithelial, possibly precancerous lesions" in the spouses of smokers.[85] The lifetime increased relative risk for development of lung cancer from exposure to sidestream smoke in a spouse of a heavy smoker approximates 1.5 to 2.

Eliminating cigarette smoking from our environment is the obvious key to reducing lung cancer mortality. Even if this were to occur, the number of persons already exposed to significant tobacco smoke makes lung cancer a significant public health problem for years to come. Smoking cessation is addressed in Chapter 16. Progress has been made in reducing the percentage of adult smokers. Much progress still is needed, particularly considering that more than 100,000 youths 12 years and under are habitual smokers.[59] All primary care physicians, including and especially pediatricians and family practitioners, need to make it a priority of patient care to counsel patients about smoking cessation and the reasons for not beginning to smoke. One hopes that tobacco-control strategies to promote smoking cessation that focus on the environmental influences rather than the individual also will reduce tobacco use.[13]

Radon

Radon is considered the second leading cause of lung cancer. This ranking is a result of studies in the uranium mining industry, where ionizing radiation has been shown

*References 40, 44, 47, 71, 81, 86.

to cause lung cancer.[90] The combination of radon exposure and cigarette smoking appears to act synergistically in causing risk for lung cancer.[5] Radon is a naturally occurring radioactive gas resulting from the natural breakdown of uranium. Many soils contain varying amounts of uranium. Radon gas is found in rock and soil but also in well water. Radon gas is odorless and colorless. Outside, radon is diluted in the air to low concentrations that are thought to pose no significant health problem. However, in enclosed spaces such as the home, radon can accumulate to significant levels. Radon decay products attach to the surface of aerosols and dust in the air and are inhaled and trapped in the lungs. Alpha particle emissions from the radon can damage the cells of the airways, leading to lung cancer.[68] Many epidemiologic studies of uranium and other underground miners show an increase in lung cancer mortality from exposure to radon and its decay products. Risk for lung cancer depends on the level and duration of exposure, age of the individual, time since initiation of exposure, and personal use of tobacco.[4] The combination of smoking with radon exposure appears to cause a synergistic effect for development of lung cancer. The combined risk when both of these factors are present is greater than the sum of the individual risks from smoking and radon exposure alone.[68] Radon gas can enter homes via cracks in concrete slabs, blocks, and mortar joints; through open tops of block walls; via exposed soil such as in a sump; through loose-fitting pipe penetrations; and through floor draining.[4] The EPA has established standards for radon exposure levels in homes at 4 picocuries (pCi)/liter (L). Canadian home standards are set at 20 pCi/L. Saccomanno's extrapolations from studies of uranium miners also suggest that standards be liberalized to 20 pCi/L.[67] The majority of homes in the United States contain an average concentration of 1 to 2 pCi/L.[37] Some studies have suggested that children may be more sensitive to radon than adults. This difference is postulated to be a result of their higher respiration rate and their more rapidly dividing cells.[4] Control or minimization of radon exposure is achieved by testing the home for radon levels. Reasonably priced and accurate radon measurement kits are available (see Chapter 64 and Resources section of this chapter). Radon measurements should be taken in the home, particularly in geographic areas where radon levels are known to be high. Currently, the EPA standard of 4 pCi/L should be followed.

Asbestos

Asbestos has long been recognized as a risk factor for lung cancer. Asbestos includes a variety of fibrous hydrated silicate materials. Asbestos minerals are divided into amphiboles, which include amosite, crocidolite, anthophyllite, and tremolite; and serpentines, which include chrysotile. The vast majority of asbestos used in the United States is of the chrysotile type. Asbestos exposure has been implicated in causing asbestosis, mesothelioma, laryngeal cancer, gastrointestinal tract cancers, and lung

---

> **Partial list of occupations involving potential asbestos exposure**
>
> Insulation workers
> Asbestos textile workers
> Shipyard workers
> Railroad yard workers
> Construction workers
> Sheet metal workers
> Automobile brake repair workers
> Electricians
> Plumbers
> Carpenters

cancer. Among heavily exposed asbestos workers, 20% of all deaths are from lung cancer.[73] Although the time from exposure to asbestos and development of lung cancer is long (20 years or more), exposure as a risk for lung cancer can be short.[72] All forms of asbestos are capable of causing lung cancer.

Asbestos exposure is encountered in a variety of occupations (see the box above). Asbestos exposure conveys about a 1.5 to 4-fold increase in development of lung cancer in a nonsmoker depending on the occupational group.[19] Like radon, asbestos exposure appears to act synergistically with smoking to increase risk for lung cancer. In persons smoking less than one pack per day and exposed to asbestos, lung cancer risk is found to be 50 times greater than in unexposed nonsmokers. In heavier smokers, the risk is as much as 90 times greater.[36] Chemoprevention studies using beta carotene and retinol are being conducted with persons previously exposed to asbestos in an attempt to reduce lung cancer risk.[60] The risk for lung cancer from long-term exposure to low levels of asbestos such as is found in schools, commercial buildings, and homes is controversial. The risk to children and office workers in these situations is not known. The risk to persons likely to have higher exposure in these buildings, such as maintenance workers, may be greater.

Other occupational exposures

Other occupational exposures have been recognized as risk factors for lung cancer. These include arsenic, chloromethyl ethers, chromium, polycyclic aromatic compounds, nickel, and vinyl chloride.[18,19,30] Arsenic is encountered in smelting operations, particularly of copper and lead, in the pharmaceutical manufacturing industry, and in the manufacture and application of pesticides and herbicides. Arsenic is thought to act synergistically with smoking to cause lung cancer.[64] Chloromethyl ethers are encountered in the production of organic chemicals. Their importance as industrial lung carcinogens has been reduced by industrial hygiene containment in closed processing systems.[19] Although chromium metal and its alloys such as stainless steel are relatively nontoxic, exposure to the hexavalent chromium compounds has been shown to increase risk for lung cancer.[11] These compounds are encountered in chromate production, pigment production, chromium plating, chromium alloy production, and other industrial processes.[19] The polycyclic aromatic compounds are found in coke production, aluminum production, iron and steel founding, and combustion processes of organic materials. Roofing and paving are other occupations that involve polycyclic aromatic compound exposure. Substances containing these compounds include coal tar, coal pitch, diesel exhaust, and soot. Exposure to these substances appears to increase risk for lung cancer.[19] Increased risk for lung cancer has also been found in nickel mining, smelting, and refining workers.[19] Metallic nickel exposure is not thought to be associated with increased risk for lung cancer,[20] whereas nickel compounds, such as nickel oxide and nickel subsulfide, appear to be carcinogenic.[19] Vinyl chloride exposure is known to cause angiosarcoma of the liver. The association of vinyl chloride with lung cancer is less strongly supported.[19] Vinyl chloride is encountered in the plastics and rubber industry. Other compounds suspected to be carcinogenic to the lung in humans are beryllium, cadmium, and acrylonitrile.[18,19] Mustard gas used for chemical warfare during World War I and manufactured but not used in World War II also has been shown to cause lung cancer.[18]

Lung cancer risk is increased in many and varied occupations. Determining that a person has increased risk for lung cancer on the basis of the person's present or past occupation depends on the probability the person was exposed to a lung carcinogen, the degree of the actual exposure, and the presence of additional risk factors for lung cancer, particularly smoking. The primary prevention of lung cancer in persons engaged in occupations associated with known lung carcinogens should include education of the individual about personal protection when in the workplace (see Chapter 62, Industrial Hygiene and Safety in the Workplace) and about smoking cessation and avoidance (see Chapter 16, Smoking and Smoking Cessation).

Chronic obstructive lung disease

Cigarette smoking causes both chronic obstructive lung disease and lung cancer. The presence of chronic obstructive lung disease in a smoker confers a higher risk for future development of lung cancer than if airways obstruction were not present.[22,77,83] Poor clearance of carcinogens resulting from the airways obstruction has been postulated as a possible mechanism for this association.[83] A twofold increased risk for lung cancer in persons with physician-diagnosed chronic bronchitis and emphysema was found by Samet et al.[69] The presence of giant bullous changes of the lungs in smokers confers a higher risk for lung cancer than in smokers without bullous disease.[34] Conversely, there appears to be an inverse relationship between allergic disease and lung cancer.[17,89] Persons with chronic asthma

appear to develop less lung cancer than would be expected.[28]

Previous lung cancer or head and neck cancer

A previous primary cancer of the lung, or of the head and neck to which smoking has contributed, confers a markedly increased risk for a later second primary lung cancer. Lung cancer study group data estimate that persons with a previously resected early-stage lung cancer have a likelihood of developing a second lung cancer at a rate of 1% to 2% per year.[52] Patients with cured early-stage head and neck cancer develop a second primary aerodigestive tract cancer at a rate of about 3% to 4% per year, of which half will be a primary lung cancer.[38,75] Persons in these high-risk groups are now being evaluated for appropriate intensified screening and chemopreventive intervention.

Other factors

Diet has been considered in relation to risk for developing lung cancer. Smokers with an increased intake of foods high in fat, animal protein, or cured meats are at increased risk for developing lung cancer.[35,92] Conversely, high intake of fruits and vegetables has been demonstrated to have a protective effect against lung cancer in high-risk populations.[16,29] Studies suggest that beta carotene, the provitamin found in spinach, leafy green vegetables, broccoli, squash, carrots, and other fruits and vegetables that is converted in the body to vitamin A, may be protective against lung cancer.[27] Retinol, found in dairy products and liver, appears to show a similar protective effect. Several studies are underway to evaluate the chemopreventive effects of beta carotene and compounds related to retinol. Studies have also suggested that vitamin E and vitamin C may be protective against lung cancer in nonsmokers,[48] but these studies have been somewhat inconsistent. Whether these vitamins will prove effective as chemopreventive agents or whether other constituents in the food that contain these nutrients prove to be protective is yet to be determined. A role for alcohol in the development of lung cancer has been suggested but not definitively proven.[7,16] Therefore the physician is prudent to recommend a diet high in fruits and vegetables, emphasizing vitamins A and C and beta carotene, and accompanied by low alcohol intake, especially to persons at high risk for developing lung cancer.

Studies also show a trend for higher incidence of lung cancer for smokers and nonsmokers as body mass index (weight/height^2) decreases. The thinner the person, the greater the risk for lung cancer.[46,49] Whether this association is due to leanness itself or to an associated effect of leanness is not known.

Lung cancer is generally not considered to be a genetic disease. However, family studies and case control studies have shown a component of family risk for lung cancer that is not explained by smoking or other environmental exposures. A genetic component for lung cancer risk has thereby been suspected. A relative risk of about 2.4 for relatives of persons having had lung cancer has been observed.[62] Some have suggested a genetic susceptibility for lung cancer that is then effected by smoking or other carcinogen exposure, leading to lung cancer.[42,74] Whether this ecogenetic hypothesis proves to be true, and if true, what the precise mechanism of inheritance susceptibility is, are under investigation.

SCREENING
Background

Until recently, two methods of screening for lung cancer were available, chest radiography and sputum cytology. A large multicenter study sponsored by the National Cancer Institute in the late 1970s and early 1980s was undertaken. The study, known as the National Cancer Institute Cooperative Early Lung Cancer Detection Program, was conducted at Johns Hopkins Hospital, Memorial Sloan-Kettering Cancer Center, and the Mayo Clinic. More than 30,000 men aged 45 years and older who smoked at least one pack of cigarettes per day were enrolled and followed. Persons were screened with combinations of chest x-rays and sputum cytology. Prevalence studies from this project showed screening could detect lung cancer early. Overall mortality from lung cancer, however, was the same in the screened and the non-screened control populations.[9,23,24,31,58] This reflected lead time bias: despite identifying persons with lung cancer at an earlier stage of their disease, screening did not detect the cancer early enough to reduce cancer-related mortality. In the screening aspect of the program that then followed, the Mayo arm of the study showed chest radiography to be better than sputum cytology for detection of early lung cancer, although sputum cytology was effective in detecting early squamous-cell cancer. Neither sputum cytology nor chest radiography was of value in the early detection of small-cell carcinoma.[91]

Despite showing a significantly increased lung cancer detection, resectability of lesions, and survivorship in the study group compared with the controls, death rates from lung cancer and from all causes were almost the same in both the study and control groups.[25] They concluded that "these results do not justify recommending large scale radiographic and cytologic screening for lung cancer, nor did they prove that selective case finding effort in 'high risk' patients is without value."[70] The Johns Hopkins group showed no benefit from the addition of sputum cytology to annual radiographic screening and concluded that mass screening for lung cancer could also not be recommended based on the findings.[82] Taken together, the groups appeared to agree that screening for lung cancer should not be offered to the general population.[54] The value of the chest x-ray to screen high-risk individuals who consult a physician, however, was not clear.[54]

Citing these large studies as well as earlier studies, the American Cancer Society concluded that early detection using a combination of chest x-rays and sputum cytology did not have a beneficial effect on lung cancer mortality even in high-risk patients and therefore recommended in their guidelines that no tests for the early detection of cancer of the lung be undertaken. They urged a focus instead on primary prevention: smoking cessation and encouragement of nonsmokers to avoid beginning smoking.[3] Similarly, the U.S. Preventive Services Task Force in its review concluded that evidence does not show that screening programs reduce mortality from lung cancer but does show that the cost of routine population testing is substantial (estimated at as much as $1.5 billion annually in the United States)[43] and that unnecessary expense and morbidity results from false-positive testing.[6] The task force also recommended that no screening be done and that attention instead focus on reducing cigarette smoking.[88] Whereas population or community-based screening should not be done, and chest radiography and sputum cytology evaluation are not advocated for general screening, this author believes that the individual patient documented to be at high risk from smoking history, occupational exposure, presence of chronic obstructive lung disease, or other risk factors who presents for a cancer-related examination should undergo chest x-ray and sputum cytology.

Present and future directions

Since the completion of these large studies, attention has shifted to detecting early precursor lesions rather than looking for early lung cancer. To understand the concept of precursor screening and detection, a hypothetical model for the natural history of lung carcinogenesis should be considered: normal cells are exposed to carcinogens; cancer is initiated; a promotion phase then takes place, leading to a stage of invasion and metastasis.[57] The ideal goal for screening and early detection would be to identify the problem and intervene before the stage of development of metastatic competence. To this end, current research is attempting to identify both intermediate markers for lung cancer in the promotion phase and chemopreventive agents that can affect the process and prevent the development of the invasive stage of the cancer.

Lung cancer cells acquire a number of genetic lesions, such as activation of dominant oncogenes and inactivation of tumor suppressor genes. Detection of these genetic lesions to focus early diagnosis and chemoprevention is a prospect. Similarly, a search for growth factors is proceeding, with the goal being identification of persons before clinically detectable disease occurs.[1,2] Lung cancer cells produce a variety of peptide hormones that stimulate their growth. Those identified so far include gastrin-releasing peptide, transferrin, and insulin-like growth factor. Antagonists to one or more of these growth factors might be developed as intervention agents in individuals at high risk

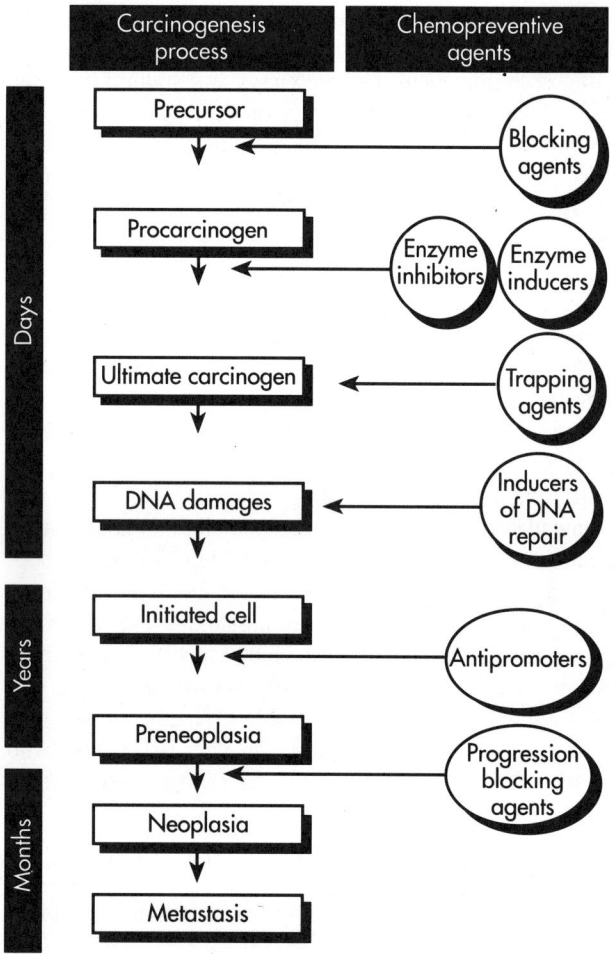

Fig. 48-4. Chemopreventive agents of carcinogenesis. (From Castonguay A: Methods and strategies in lung cancer control, *Cancer Res* [suppl] 52:2641S-2651S, 1992.)

for lung cancer.[56] Carcinoembryonic antigen (CEA) has been found to be increased in serum of persons with resectable lung cancer, and levels also correlate with increasing stage. Unfortunately, CEA is also found to be elevated in persons without lung cancer who are heavy smokers, as well as in a variety of other diseases.[80] Currently there is no proven serologic markers that should be utilized in practice to screen for early lung cancer.

An exciting prospect in the detection of clinical lung cancer is analysis of sputum by application of monoclonal antibodies. Tockman et al. used two lung-cancer–associated monoclonal antibodies to stain banked sputum specimens acquired in the course of the Johns Hopkins arm of the National Cancer Institute–sponsored lung cancer early detection trial. By this method they were able to identify abnormalities in the sputa of confirmed lung cancer patients 2 years before the clinical appearance of lung cancer with a sensitivity and specificity of approximately 90%.[84] Several monoclonal antibodies are now being investigated and applied to sputum cytology.

At the same time, based on the finding that dysplasia of the bronchial epithelium can improve after smoking cessation,[66] research is proceeding to identify immunologic and physiologic indicators of bronchial irritation and damage.[55]

Inherent in the success of a lung cancer early detection program is the ability to intervene in persons found to be positive. For this purpose, chemoprevention trials are underway to identify substances to be used in high-risk individuals. These trials are designed to evaluate the effectiveness of the agent, and as important, the frequency and intensity of the side effects. Fig. 48-4 outlines the concept of chemopreventive agents acting in the carcinogenesis process. Hong et al., using 13 cis-retinoic acid in a randomized control trial, were able to show a statistically significant reduction in the rate of second new cancers in patients with previously resected head and neck cancer.[41] Retinoic acid is one of the retinoid compounds, which are a group of naturally occurring or synthetic derivatives of vitamin A. Dietary sources of vitamin A are listed in Chapter 22, Nutritional Guidelines for Diet and Health. In addition to the retinoids, another substance being utilized as a chemopreventive agent for lung cancer in current studies is beta carotene. This provitamin is converted by the liver to vitamin A. Foods containing beta carotene are listed in Chapter 22. Retinol is thought to act through promotion of cellular differentiation, whereas carotenoids seem to act by their antioxidant capacity for trapping free radicals.[14,79] Until the effectiveness and toxicity of these agents are known, their clinical use, even in patients with high risk for lung cancer, is not currently justified.

In the future we will likely see identification of tools and methods for identifying patients with preclinical disease. These may include a variety of methods for analyzing shed bronchial cells,[57] fluorescence imaging to identify dysplastic lesions using differences in tissue autofluorescence,[50] or even breath analysis for biomarkers.[61] As these methods are developed, chemopreventive agents stratified for degree of risk can be applied to patients either systemically or endobronchially to reverse or slow the carcinogenic process.

SUMMARY

Despite the fact that the major cause of lung cancer is well known and avoidable, this disease remains and will continue for many years to be a major health problem throughout the world. Lung cancer cannot be discussed without reemphasizing the need to eliminate smoking for all individuals. The physician's role as counselor, role model, and advocate within the community at large for stopping smoking cannot be emphasized enough. Primary prevention of lung cancer is the key to making any inroads into this fatal disease. In addition to addressing smoking cessation and smoking prevention with individual patients, particularly those who are young, when smoking most often begins, physicians should encourage radon detection in homes, personal protection in occupational settings that involve lung carcinogens, and diets low in fat and high in vegetables and fruits. Whether chemopreventive agents for lung cancer will prove to be beneficial and generalizable to the public is yet to be determined.

What then can we do for the millions of people who carry increased risk for lung cancer based on present or past smoking habit, past asbestos exposure, other occupational carcinogen exposure, presence of chronic obstructive lung disease, previous radiation to the lungs from occupation or medical therapy, or previous cancer of the lung or head and neck? Most important, anyone in these high-risk categories should be counseled strongly about the need to stop smoking permanently. These people should be offered periodic chest x-ray and sputum cytology analysis when presenting for cancer-related check-ups. Hopefully, effective and safe chemopreventive therapy, whether oral or endobrachial, for people who are at highest risk or who have preclinical disease will be developed.

REFERENCES

1. Aguayo SM et al: Increased levels of bombesin-like peptides in the lower respiratory tracts of asymptomatic cigarette smokers, *J Clin Invest* 84:1105-1113, 1989.
2. Aguayo SM et al: Urinary levels of bombesin-like peptides in asymptomatic cigarette smokers: a potential risk marker for smoking-related disease, *Cancer Res* (suppl) 52:2727S-2731S, 1992.
3. American Cancer Society: Cancer of the lung, *CA Cancer J Clin* 30:199-207, 1980.
4. American Medical Association: *The health threat with the simple solution—radon—a physician's guide,* American Medical Association, Chicago, Ill, 1990.
5. Archer VE, Gillam JD, and Wagoner JK: Respiratory disease mortality among uranium miners, *Ann NY Acad Sci* 271:280-293, 1976.
6. Bailar JC: Screening for lung cancer: where are we now? *Am Rev Respir Dis* 130:541-542, 1984.
7. Bandera EV et al: Alcohol consumption and lung cancer in white males, *Cancer Causes and Control* 3:361-369, 1992.
8. Becher H et al: Smoking cessation and non smoking intervals: effect of different smoking patterns on lung cancer risk, *Cancer Causes and Control* 2:381-387, 1991.
9. Berlin NI et al: The National Cancer Institute cooperative early lung cancer detection program: results of the initial screen (prevalence): introduction, *Am Rev Respir Dis* 130:545-549, 1984.
10. Boring CC, Squires TS, and Tong T: Cancer statistics, 1993, *CA Cancer J Clin* 43:7-26, 1993.
11. Braver ER, Infante P, and Chu K: An analysis of lung cancer risk from exposure to hexavalent chromium, *Teratogenesis, Carcinogenesis Mutagenesis* 5:365-378, 1985.
12. Brownson RC et al: Passive smoking in lung cancer in non smoking women, *Am J Public Health* 82:1525-1530, 1992.
13. Burns DM: Positive evidence on effectiveness of selected smoking prevention programs in the United States, *J Nat Cancer Inst Monogr* 12:17-20, 1992.
14. Burton GW, Ingold KU: B-carotene: an unusual type of antioxidant, *Science* 224:569-573, 1984.
15. Castonguay A: Methods and strategies in lung cancer control, *Cancer Res* (suppl) 52:2641S-2651S, 1992.
16. Chow WH et al: A cohort study of tobacco use, diet, occupation, and lung cancer mortality, *Cancer Causes and Control* 3:247-254, 1992.
17. Cockroft DW et al: Is there a negative correlation between malignancy and respiratory atopy? *Ann Allergy* 43:345-347, 1979.
18. Cone JE: Occupational lung cancer, *Occup Med* 2:273-295, 1987.
19. Coultas DB, Samet JM: Occupational lung cancer, *Clin Chest Med* 13:341-354, 1992.
20. Cox JE et al: Mortality of nickel workers: experience of men working with metallic nickel, *Br J Ind Med* 38:235-239, 1989.
21. Cullen JW: The National Cancer Institute's Smoking, Tobacco, and Cancer Program, *Chest* (suppl) 96:95-135, 1989.
22. Davis AL: Bronchogenic carcinoma in chronic obstructive pulmonary disease, *JAMA* 235:621-622, 1976.
23. Flehinger BJ et al: Early lung cancer detection: results of the initial (prevalence) radiologic and cytologic screening in the Memorial Sloan-Kettering study, *Am Rev Respir Dis* 130:555-560, 1984.
24. Fontana RS et al: Early lung cancer detection: results of the initial (prevalence) radiologic and cytologic screening in the Mayo Clinic study, *Am Rev Respir Dis* 130:561-565, 1984.
25. Fontana RS et al: Lung cancer screening: the Mayo program, *J Occup Med* 28(8):746-750, 1986.
26. Fontham ET et al: Lung cancer in non smoking women: a multi center case-control study, *Cancer Epidemiol Biomark Prev* 1:35-43, 1991.
27. Fontham ET: Protective dietary factors and lung cancer, *Int J Epidemiol* (suppl) 19:532-542, 1990.
28. Ford RM: Primary lung cancer and asthma, *Ann Allergy* 40:240-242, 1979.
29. Forman MR et al: The effect of dietary intake of fruits and vegetables on the odds ratio of lung cancer among Yunnan tin miners, *Int J Epidemiol* 21:437-441, 1992.
30. Frank AL: Occupational cancers of the respiratory tract, *Occup Med Revs* 2:71-83, 1987.
31. Frost JK et al: Early lung cancer detection: results of the initial (prevalence) radiologic and cytologic screening in the Johns Hopkins study, *Am Rev Respir Dis* 130:549-554, 1984.
32. Garfinkel L, Silverberg E: Lung cancer and smoking trends in the United States over the past 25 years, *CA Cancer J Clin* 41:137-145, 1991.
33. Garfinkel L, Stellman SD: Smoking and lung cancer in women: findings in a prospective study, *Cancer Res* 48:6951-6955, 1988.
34. Goldstein MJ et al: Bronchogenic carcinoma and giant bullous disease, *Am Rev Respir Dis* 97:1062-1070, 1968.
35. Goodman MT et al: High-fat foods and the risk of lung cancer, *Epidemiology* 3:288-299, 1992.
36. Hammond EC, Selikoff IJ, and Seidman H: Asbestos exposure, cigarette smoking and death rates, *Ann NY Acad Sci* 330:473-490, 1979.
37. Harley NH, Harley JH: Potential lung cancer risk from indoor radon exposure, *CA Cancer J Clin* 40:265-275, 1990.
38. Heyne KE, Lippman SM, and Hong WK: Chemoprevention in head and neck cancer, *Hematol Oncol Clin North Am* 5:783-795, 1991.
39. Hill C: Trends in tobacco use in Europe, *J Nat Cancer Inst Monogr* 12:21-24, 1992.
40. Hirayama T: Non-smoking wives of heavy smokers have a higher risk of lung cancer: a study from Japan, *Br Med J* 282:183-185, 1981.
41. Hong WK et al: Prevention of second primary tumors in squamous cell carcinoma of the head and neck with 13-cis retinoic acid, *N Engl J Med* 323:795-801, 1990.
42. Horwitz RI et al: An ecogenetic hypothesis for lung cancer in women, *Arch Intern Med* 148:2609-2612, 1988.
43. Hubbel FA et al: The impact of routine admission chest x-ray films on patient care, *N Engl J Med* 312:209-213, 1985.
44. Humble CG, Samet JM, and Pathak DR: Marriage to a smoker and lung cancer risk, *Am J Public Health* 77:598-602, 1987.
45. Janerich DT et al: Lung cancer and exposure to tobacco smoke in the household, *N Engl J Med* 323:632-636, 1990.

46. Kabat GC, Wynder EL: Body mass index and lung cancer risk, *Am J Epidemiol* 135:769-774, 1992.

47. Kabat GC, Wynder EL: Lung cancer in nonsmokers, *Cancer* 53:1214-1221, 1984.

48. Knekt P et al: Dietary anti-oxidants and the risk of lung cancer, *Am J Epidemiol* 134:471-479, 1991.

49. Knekt P et al: Leaness and lung-cancer risk, *Int J Cancer* 49:208-213, 1991.

50. Lam S: Detection of dysplasia and carcinoma in situ by fluorescence imaging, *Lung Cancer Res Quart* 2:4-6, 1992.

51. Lubin JH, Richter BS, and Blott WJ: Lung cancer risk with cigar and pipe use, *J Natl Cancer Inst* 73:377-381, 1984.

52. Lung Cancer Study Group: Cancer recurrence after resection: T1 NO Non-small cell lung cancer, *Ann Thorac Surg* 49:242-247, 1990.

53. Mackay J: U.S. tobacco export to third world: third world war, *J Natl Cancer Inst Monogr* 12:25-28, 1992.

54. Miller AB: Screening—summary, *Chest* (suppl) 89:325S-326S, 1986.

55. Mittman C, Roby TJ: Current status of sputum cytology in the detection of lung cancer, *Primary Care Cancer* 11:15-20, 1991.

56. Mulshine JL et al: Lung cancer: rational strategies for early detection and intervention, *Oncology* 5:25-32, 1991.

57. Mulshine JL, Tockman MS, and Smart CR: Consideration in the development of lung cancer screening tools, *J Nat Cancer Inst* 81:900-906, 1989.

58. The National Cancer Institute cooperative early lung cancer detection program. Summary and conclusions, *Am Rev Respir Dis* 130:565-567, 1984.

59. National Cancer Institute Monograph: *Cancer control objectives for the nation: 1985-2000,* Greenwald P, Sondik EJ, editors, US Department of Health and Human Services, Public Health Service, National Institutes of Health, Bethesda, Md, 1986.

60. Omenn GS et al: CARET, the beta carotene and retinol efficacy trial to prevent lung cancer in asbestos-exposed workers and in smokers, *Anti-cancer Drugs* 2(1):79-86, 1991.

61. O'Neill HJ et al: A computerized classification technique for screening for the presence of breath biomarkers in lung cancer, *Clin Chem* 34(8):1613-1618, 1988.

62. Ooi WL et al: Increased familial risk for lung cancer, *J Natl Cancer Inst* 76:217-222, 1986.

63. Osann KE: Lung cancer in women: the importance of smoking, family history of cancer, and medical history of respiratory disease, *Cancer Res* 51:4893-4897, 1991.

64. Pershagen G et al: On the interaction between arsenic exposure and smoking and its relationship to lung cancer, *Scand J Work Environ Health* 7:302, 1981.

65. Pierce JP et al: Trends in cigarette smoking in the United States: projections to the year 2000, *JAMA* 261:61-65, 1989.

66. Roby TJ, Schumann GB: Reversibility of lung injury following smoking cessation, *Acta Cytol* 33:715-716, 1989.

67. Saccomanno G: Lung cancer and radon in uranium miners, *Lung Cancer Res Quart* 1:7-8, 1991.

68. Samet JM: Radon and lung cancer: how great is the risk? *J Respir Dis* 10(7):73-86, 1989.

69. Samet JM et al: Personal and family history of respiratory disease and lung cancer risk, *Am Rev Respir Dis* 134:466-470, 1986.

70. Sanderson DR: Lung cancer screening—the Mayo study, *Chest* (suppl) 89:324S, 1986.

71. Sandler DP, Wilcox AJ, and Everson RB: Cumulative effects of lifetime passive smoking on cancer risk, *Lancet* 1:312-314, 1985.

72. Seidman H, Selikoff IJ, and Hammond EC: Short-term asbestos work exposure and long-term observation, *Ann NY Acad Sci* 330:61-89, 1979.

73. Selikoff IJ, Hammond EC, and Seidman H: Mortality experience of insulation workers in the United States and Canada 1943-1976, *Ann NY Acad Sci* 330:91-116, 1979.

74. Sellers TA et al: Lung cancer detection and prevention: evidence for an interaction between smoking and genetic predisposition, *Cancer Res* 52(suppl)9:2694S-2697S, 1992.

75. Shons AR, McQuarrie DG: Multiple primary epidermoid carcinomas of the upper aerodigestive tract, *Arch Surg* 120:1007-1009, 1985.

76. Shopland DR, Eyre HJ, and Pechacek TF: Smoking—attributable cancer mortality in 1991: is lung cancer now the leading cause of death among smokers in the United States? *J Natl Cancer Inst* 83:1142-1148, 1991.

77. Skillrud DM, Offord KP, and Miller RD: Higher risk of lung cancer in chronic obstructive lung disease, *Ann Intern Med* 105:503-507, 1986.

78. Sobue T et al: Lung cancer risk among ex-smokers, *Jpn J Cancer Res* 82(3):273-279, 1991.

79. Sporn MB, Roberts AB: Role of retinoids in differentiation and carcinogenesis, *Cancer Res* 43:3034-3040, 1983.

80. Stevens DP, Mackay IR: Increased carcinoembryonic antigen in heavy cigarette smokers, *Lancet* ii:1238, 1973.

81. Stockwell HG et al: Environmental tobacco smoke and lung cancer risk in non smoking women, *J Nat Cancer Inst* 84:1417-1422, 1992.

82. Tockman MS: Survival and mortality from lung cancer in a screen population—the Johns Hopkins study, *Chest* (suppl) 89:324S-325S, 1986.

83. Tockman MS et al: Airways obstruction and the risk for lung cancer, *Ann Intern Med* 106(4):512-518, 1987.

84. Tockman MS et al: Sensitive and specific monoclonal antibody recognition of human lung cancer antigen on preserved sputum cells: a new approach to early lung cancer detection, *J Clin Oncol* 6(11):1685-1693, 1988.

85. Trichopoulos D et al: Active and passive smoking and pathological indicators of lung cancer risk in an autopsy study, *JAMA* 268:1697-1701, 1992.

86. Trichopoulos D et al: Lung cancer and passive smoking, *Int J Cancer* 27:1-4, 1981.

87. US Department of Health and Human Services: The health consequences of smoking: cancer. A report of the surgeon general, US Public Health Service, Rockville, Md, 1982.

88. US Preventive Services Task Force: *Guide to clinical preventive services: an assessment of the effectiveness of 169 interventions,* Baltimore, 1989, Williams and Wilkins.

89. Vena JE et al: Allergy-related diseases and cancer: an inverse association, *Am J Epidemiol* 12:66-74, 1985.

90. Wagoner JK et al: Radiation as the cause of lung cancer among uranium miners, *N Engl J Med* 273:181-188, 1965.

91. Woolner LB et al: Mayo Lung Project: evaluation of lung cancer screening through December 1979, *Mayo Clin Proc* 56(9):544-555, 1981.

92. Wynder EL, Taioli E, and Fujita Y: Ecologic study of lung cancer risk factors in the US and Japan with special reference to smoking and diet, *Jpn J Cancer Res* 83:418-423, 1992.

93. Zang EA, Winder EL: Cumulative tar exposure, a new index for estimating lung cancer risk among cigarette smokers, *Cancer* 70:69-76, 1992.

■■■■■ **RESOURCES** ■■■■■

National Cancer Institute. (800) 422-6237. (Provides guidelines to help health care professionals counsel smokers about quitting and other information related to lung cancer.)

American Cancer Society. (800) ACS-2345. (Provides a variety of pamphlets and educational materials regarding lung cancer. State and local branches can be found in local telephone directories.)

Lung Cancer Research Quarterly (provides information about research on lung cancer etiology, diagnosis, and treatment) published by the Lung Cancer Institute of Colorado, 1905 Sherman St, Suite 803, Denver, CO 80202.

EPA Radon Hotline. (800) SOS-RADO. (Provides information on radon and radon test kits.)

(See also related resources listed in Chapter 16, Smoking Cessation.)

Chapter 49

SKIN CANCER AND PROTECTION OF THE SKIN

Kristin Thorisdottir
Jacob W.E. Dijkstra
Kenneth J. Tomecki

SKIN CANCER

Skin cancer is the most common type of malignancy, with a 30% to 40% prevalency. Approximately 600,000 U.S. citizens develop a skin cancer, either basal or squamous cell type, every year, and another 32,000 to 35,000 develop a melanoma.[3,39] Epidemiological data support a causal role for sun exposure in the development of basal cell (see Plate 3 after page 16) and squamous cell carcinomas (see Plate 4 after page 16). These typically occur on sun-exposed areas of fair-skinned people after chronic (years) sun exposure.[15,17] Each 1% increase in ultraviolet B exposure increases the lifetime risk of nonmelanoma skin cancer by about 2%.[11] Other contributing factors include occupational exposure to chemicals such as coal tar, pitch, creosote, arsenic, or radium.[14]

Sun exposure also contributes to the formation of melanoma, a potentially lethal form of skin cancer (see Plate 5 after page 16). Melanoma is 10 times more common in white people than in blacks and has an incidence higher in equatorial areas than in more temperate climates.[33,36,38] Known risk factors for melanoma include:

- Intense, blistering sunburns at an early age
- Giant congenital nevi
- Family history of melanoma (parent, children, or siblings)
- Dysplastic/atypical nevi

Although melanoma generally affects white adults, persons of other skin types may develop this disease in such areas as the soles of the feet, under the nails, or in the mouth. Rigel et al. have identified six independent risk factors for development of malignant melanoma[13]:

1. Family history of malignant melanoma in a first-degree relative
2. Presence of blond or red hair
3. Presence of marked freckling of the upper back
4. History of three or more blistering sunburns before the age of 20
5. History of 3 or more years of working at an outdoor summer job as a teenager
6. Presence of actinic keratoses

They have found that people with one or two of these risk factors have an increased risk of three and a half times that of the general population. Those with three or more of these factors have an increased risk of about 20 times that of the general population for developing malignant melanoma.[13]

Melanoma skin cancer accounts for about 73% of deaths caused by skin diseases. Since 1973 the incidence rate of melanoma has increased about 4% per year.[3]

Characteristics of sunlight. Solar energy is a form of electromagnetic energy involving high-speed photons. The solar spectrum at sea level includes wavelengths of 290 to 3000 nm. Shorter wavelengths of ultraviolet (UV) solar rays (less than 400 nm) penetrate the skin more than longer wavelengths of visible light (400 to 700 nm) and infrared rays (greater than 700 nm). Of the solar radiation reaching the earth, 6% is UV radiation. Ozone, a three-atom molecule of oxygen present in the atmosphere, absorbs most UV radiation.[16,18] The continued decrease of the ozone layer will lead to decreased natural protection from UV radiation.[50]

Ultraviolet radiation is composed of ultraviolet A (UVA) rays (320 to 400 nm), also called black or invisible light; ultraviolet B (UVB) rays (290 to 320 nm), the sunburn spectrum; and ultraviolet C (UVC) rays (200 to 290 nm). UVC does not reach the earth's surface but is usually present in artificial light sources such as sunlamps. Although UVB radiation constitutes less than 0.5% of terrestrial sunlight, it is responsible for most of the acute and chronic actinic damage to normal skin.[15] Its relative and absolute intensity is directly related to time and location; it is greater in summer than in winter, at noon than in the early morning or late afternoon, in places close to the equator than in temperate zones, and at higher altitude than at sea level.[15,29] The likelihood of sunburn varies accordingly.

During the summer months with the sun at its zenith, solar radiation at sea level is: UVB rays, 0.5%; UVA rays, 6.3%; visible light, 48.9%; and infrared light, 46.3%. UVA rays represent 90% to 92% of the total amount of UV light (UVL) and potentiate the burning action of UVB rays.[15] Although the dose required for UVA-induced skin reactions is significantly higher than the dose for UVB reactions (300 to 1000 times greater), UVA rays directly contribute to both acute and chronic skin damage and play a distinctive role in the production of cutaneous erythema, increased melanogenesis and proliferation of melanocytes, cutaneous carcinogenesis, drug-induced photosensitizing reactions of the skin, photoaging and elastosis, and changes in immune functions in the skin.[22,24,52] UVA radiation may also produce corneal burns, cataracts, and retinal damage,[7,32,42,46] and may contribute to malignant melanoma.[6]

Adverse effects of sun exposure

Acute effects. Acute adverse effects of sun exposure include delayed erythema or sunburn reaction, photosensitivity or phototoxic reactions, and alteration of immune responses. Erythema (redness), the most apparent component of the sunburn reaction, includes damage to cell membranes and DNA, and suppression or induction of many cytokines and inflammatory mediators.[15] Erythema occurs within 2 to 6 hours after sun exposure, and the maximal erythema occurs within 15 to 24 hours.[29]

Shorter UVB wavelengths produce erythema more significantly than longer UVB or UVA wavelengths. Under experimental conditions, UVA rays alone can evoke a sunburn reaction, but the amount of energy to produce erythema in a fair-skinned person is approximately 1000 times the UVB amount of energy and equivalent to 20 to 30 hours of continous UVB sun exposure.[15,29]

Photosensitivity is a general term commonly used for an abnormal cutaneous reaction to sun exposure; examples include the photosensitivity of lupus erythematosus and por-

phyria, a reaction to endogenous photosensitization by one or more porphyrin compounds in the skin.[29] Polymorphous light eruption (PMLE) is the most common abnormal response to sunlight and affects 12% to 16% of the population, usually women. Termed *sun poisoning* or *sun allergy* by many affected patients, it is an acquired idiopathic response, classically occurring after the first intense exposure to springtime sun. PMLE exhibits pruritic plaques, papules, or papulovesicles that typically appear within 2 days after sun exposure; skin disease may not appear on habitually exposed areas such as the face or forearms, but will appear on the arms, chest, and thighs. History typically suggests the correct diagnosis, with skin disease resulting after exposure to intense sunlight (e.g., a vacation in the Caribbean) but possibly not appearing at home in northern latitudes, even during the summer.[40] The action spectrum for PMLE is in UVB and UVA range or both.[10,41]

Phototoxic reactions produce an exaggerated sunburn (i.e., more severe sunburn than expected from the length of sun exposure) after ingestion of or contact with a photosensitizer. Such reactions are not immunologically mediated and theoretically can occur in any individual exposed to sufficient doses of light and chemical. The most common drugs capable of producing phototoxic reactions are thiazides, phenothiazines, tetracyclines, sulfonylureas, sulfonamides, psoralens, nalidixic acid, and coal tars.[4,15] Topical phototoxicity follows cutaneous contact with a plant containing a furocoumarin compound; limes, parsley, celery, bishop's weed, and figs are classical offenders.[4]

UVL alters immune responses in both normal and diseased skin. Ultraviolet radiation suppresses cell-mediated immunity. Exposure of skin to UV light will sometimes lead to immunologic tolerance to contact allergens placed there, so the severity of allergic contact dermatitis can be diminished by prior exposure of the skin to UV radiation.[3] Reduced immunoreactivity is probably responsible for the therapeutic effects of sun exposure and photochemotherapy in patients with a variety of skin diseases, including psoriasis, atopic eczema, and even certain photodermatoses.[15]

Chronic effects. Chronic adverse effects of sun exposure include the induction of precancerous (solar/actinic keratoses) lesions (see Plate 6 after page 16), skin cancers, both nonmelanoma and possibly melanoma, photoaging, premature aging of the lens of the eye, and cataract formation.

Photoaging refers to cutaneous changes that arise from chronic repeated sun exposure rather than simply to passage of time alone.[15] Often labeled "premature aging," photoaging is distinct from chronologic or intrinsic aging seen in sun-protected skin.[27,28] Characteristic signs of photoaging include fine and coarse wrinkling; mottled pigmentation; yellowed, redundant, leathery skin, often with telangiectasia; and a variety of benign, premalignant, and malignant changes.[27]

Chronically irradiated skin is metabolically hyperactive, with epidermal hyperplasia and neoplasia, increased production of elastic fibers, accelerated breakdown and synthesis of collagen, and inflammation. In contrast, protected aged skin exhibits negligible or slow, gradual decline in many of these factors.[27] Animal studies have shown that UVB rays are responsible for the destruction of dermal connective tissue seen in photoaged skin, and that UVA and infrared radiation, which penetrate the skin more deeply than UVB, contribute significantly to photoaging, causing alterations in elastic tissue or elastosis.[23,25,27,28,48]

PREVENTIVE MEASURES
Skin typing

Skin susceptibility to UV radiation varies primarily with the amount of melanin in the skin and the amount of melanin produced by UV exposure.[16]

Skin types are divided into six types based on personal history of sunburning (degree of erythema) and suntanning (the ability to tan) after the first 45 to 60 minutes of exposure to midday sun in the summer[16,42] (see Table 49-1). Knowledge of skin type helps physicians and patients to estimate the relative risk for development of acute and chronic changes related to sun exposure.[42] Skin types I and II particularly and also skin type III require the greatest care in protection from the sun. More frequent application of sun screens and protective clothing are indicated in people of these skin types.

Sunscreens

Sunscreens are topical preparations that reduce the deleterious effects of UV radiation by absorption, reflection, or scattering.[51] The use of sunscreen is an effective way to prevent photoaging and skin cancer.[8] Animal studies have shown that sunscreens inhibit UV-induced tumors.[54] Their regular use during the first 18 years of life has been estimated to reduce the lifetime incidence of nonmelanoma skin cancers by 78%.[49]

Clothes are the simplest and perhaps most practical form of photoprotection. Window glass is a useful photoprotectant and blocks virtually all UVB rays and at least half of all UVA energy, especially the shorter and biologically more active wavelengths.[15]

Sunscreens are available as either oral or topical preparations. Topical sunscreens are either chemical or physical formulations. Chemical sunscreens contain two major ingredients, the UV-attenuating agent that absorbs, scatters, or reflects the rays, and a vehicle to carry the agent, such as an oil, cream, or gel.[16] Desirable characteristics of these preparations include ease of application, ability to form a uniform, protective layer over the exposed areas, noncomedogenicity (resistance to form acne-like lesions), and resistance to removal by perspiration or water activities.[16] The sunscreen should also be nonirritating, nonsensitizing, stable to UV radiation, nonstaining, nonmutagenic, and noncarcinogenic.[42]

Table 49-1. Classification of sun-reactive skin types

Skin type	Sun sensitivity	Pigmentary response
I	Very sensitive, always burn easily	Little or no tan (Irish, Scots, freckled red-heads)
II	Very sensitive, always burn	Minimal tan (blue-eyed, fair-skinned whites)
III	Sensitive, burn moderately	Tan gradually (light brown average whites with dark hair and eyes)
IV	Moderately sensitive, burn minimal	Tan easily (brown whites with Mediterranean ancestry)
V	Minimally sensitive, rarely burn	Tan darkly (dark brown, Hispanics, Orientals, Indians)
VI	Insensitive, never burn	Deeply pigmented (blacks)

From Pathak MA: Sunscreens and their use in the preventive treatment of sunlight-induced skin damage, *J Dermatol Surg Oncol* 13:739-750, 1987; and Norris PW, Hawk JLM: Polymorphic light eruption, *Photodermatol Photoimmunol Photomed* 7:186, 1990.

The majority of sunscreens marketed today are excellent UVB (290 to 320 nm) absorbers and appropriate for preventing sunburn and skin cancer.[1] Newer formulations provide a higher degree of protection through a combination of UV absorbers.[16]

The most commonly available sunscreens contain paraaminobenzoic acid (PABA), PABA esters, benzophenones, cinnamates, salicylates, and anthranilates, all of which absorb predominantly within the UVB range.[42] Butylmethoxydibenzoylmethane, available commercially since 1989, is a UVA-absorbing chemical, but a poor UVB absorber, used in combination with UV absorbers in broad-spectrum sunscreens, which absorb UVA and UVB radiation and are particularly useful for people with photosensitivity disorders. Because of their UVA-absorbing ability, these sunscreens help to retard photoaging.

The sun protective factor (SPF) indicates the degree of protection provided by the sunscreen. The SPF is defined as the ratio of the amount of sun exposure required to produce a minimal erythema reaction, called minimal erythema dose (MED), through a sunscreen film to the amount of exposure required to produce the same erythema without any sunscreen application.[12]

$$SPF = \frac{MED \text{ of sunscreen-protected skin}}{MED \text{ of nonprotected skin}}$$

Sunscreens with an SPF of 15 or more filter more than 92% of the UV radiation responsible for erythema (UVB), and this makes sunburn unlikely in most users. Newer preparations with SPF of 20 to 40 may be unnecessary except for those exquisitely sensitive to the sun. From sunrise to sunset, even in an equatorial region, it is difficult for an average fair-skinned individual to receive UV radiation exceeding 15 MED.[42] During the summer months, sunscreens with SPF of 15 are adequate for average daily exposure. At present there is no standardized testing system for topical agents that offer protection against long-wave UV radiation.

"Water-resistant" and "waterproof" sunscreens remain effective and continue to exert photoprotective properties after water activities/sports for periods of 40 minutes for "water-resistant" screens and 80 minutes for "waterproof" products.[12] Such products are ideal for people who sunbathe for long periods or indulge in physical or athletic activities at the beach or in general outdoor sports activities that cause sweating.[42]

The use of potent UVB sunscreens allows individuals to expose their skin to quantities of UVA radiation that would not normally be possible without UVB protection (protection for sunburning). The ideal sunscreen should protect from UVB rays and deeper-penetrating UVA rays.

Physical sunscreens are usually opaque (colored) formulations, particulate in nature; when applied to the skin, they primarily reflect and scatter UV and visible radiation. Physical sunscreens do not selectively absorb UV radiation but rather scatter and reflect all light. Some of these formulations adhere well to the skin and do not easily wash off with perspiration or water (water sports).[42] Physical sunscreens include zinc oxide, titanium dioxide, talc, kaolin, ferric chloride, starch, magnesium silicate or oxide, and ichthammol. These sunscreens, often white or colored, are often cosmetically unacceptable and can be messy to use. Nonetheless, they are essential for those individuals who are unusually sensitive to UV and visible radiation.

Outdoor workers (lifeguards, farmers, road constructors, sailors, etc.) with fair skin should use opaque sunscreens on selected areas of the body, such as the bridge of the nose, helix of the ears, back of the neck, shoulders, and lips. Those with melasma should also use opaque sunscreens. Melasma is a blotchy hyperpigmentation occurring on the forehead, cheeks, and upper lip, often seen in women, and often brought about by pregnancy, use of oral contraceptives, or use of other hormones. UV light may penetrate melasma-type skin.

The American Academy of Dermatology offers seven recommendations regarding sunscreen use[2,16]:

1. Apply the sunscreen to the face, ears, neck, chest, back, abdomen, upper and lower legs, arms, hands, and feet each morning before dressing. It is best applied 45 minutes before going outside.
2. Use sunscreens from May through September. Reapplication once or twice a day is recommended if the person remains outside. Reapplication every 2 hours while in the sun is a good general rule.
3. Develop a regular habit of daily sunscreen application. Encourage children to get in the habit of applying the sunscreen before they go outside, as sun damage is cumulative over a lifetime. Infants and young children should have the sunscreen applied by their parents.
4. The midday sun is the most intense. Try to limit sun exposure between 10:30 AM and 3 PM, when the sun is most intense.
5. Sunscreen should be used each time a person goes outdoors, even if it is only for a brief trip to the grocery store or the office. A sunscreen should also be applied on cloudy days, as the burning rays can penetrate the cloud cover.
6. Makeup may be applied over sunscreens.
7. Proper clothing and a hat also offer good sun protection and should be used in conjunction with a sunscreen.

Tighter weaves of clothing, preferably colored, tend to filter radiation, thus fewer rays penetrate the skin. The use of hats and umbrellas or parasols helps to minimize the effect of radiation on the face and scalp. Water, snow, and sand may reflect sunlight onto the skin and increase chances of sunburning. Risk for sunburn also is greater at high altitudes. The thinner atmosphere at high altitudes absorbs less UV rays, thereby causing greater UV exposure. Tanning booths should also be avoided, as the UV light emitted may cause sunburn, skin cancer, and premature skin aging.

Sun screen should be applied to the face even when wearing a hat. Men should apply sun screen to any bald scalp areas. Lip screens should be used to prevent cancer of the lips. If irritation of the skin occurs with a given sun screen, a change to another brand is often all that is needed. Reactions to sunscreen may include contact sensitivity, photosensitivity, and delayed hypersensitivity or photoallergic reactions.[42]

People with known allergic hypersensitivity to benzocaine, procaine, hair dyes, sulfonamides, or thiazides should avoid PABA- or PABA-ester–containing sunscreens to avoid allergic reactions.[42] Severe skin reactions to sunscreens should be referred to a dermatologist.

Systemic photoprotectants

Systemic photoprotectants would be desirable because of their ease of use; unfortunately, such agents have had limited success.

Oral sunscreens are antioxidants that have the ability to prevent oxidative damage to cells. Because oxidation reactions are important in various stages of carcinogenesis, these agents interfere with carcinogenesis, blocking the damaging effect of the carcinogen on cells.[54] UV radiation generates free radicals; antioxidants act as scavengers of free radicals and thereby minimize UV-radiation–induced biochemical changes in skin.[42] Unfortunately, PABA, antihistamines, aspirin, indomethacin, corticosteroids, and vitamins A, C, and E (antioxidants) have all failed to provide useful sunburn protection for normal human skin.[43]

Oral sunscreens are novel and promising photoprotectants, especially in the prevention of skin photoaging and dermatoheliosis, where photoprotection is necessary daily and the chronic effects of solar radiation on dermal components (collagen, elastin, etc.) must be minimal. Three systemic agents have limited efficacy for photosensitivity disorders: certain psoralens (for PMLE)[21] beta-carotene (for porphyria)[37] and antimalarials (for PMLE, systemic lupus erythematosus, and possibly porphyria).[9,47] Beneficial effects may be immunologically mediated as well as simply photoprotective.

Retinoids

Retinoids are a family of agents that include preformed vitamin A (retinol) and its isomers, vitamin A derivatives (retinal, retinoic acid), and synthetic analogues. Vitamin A is essential for normal growth and differentiation of epithelial tissue and bone, vision, and reproduction.[34] The use of retinoids as chemopreventive agents is based on data from patients and animals with vitamin A deficiency, which yields squamous metaplasia, a common occurrence in epithelium as it undergoes malignant transformation. Vitamin A administration rapidly reverses the metaplasia of the deficiency state.[8]

Individuals with risk factors such as xeroderma pigmentosum or nevoid basal cell carcinoma syndrome, a history of severely sun-damaged skin, exposure to arsenic, or radiation exposure can develop many basal cell carcinomas in a lifetime. They may benefit from chemopreventive treatment with retinoids, given in high doses and continued long term.[34,44] Topical tretinoin can also produce complete regression of actinic keratoses and certain premalignant skin lesions.[8,45] Retinoids are capable of repairing photodamaged skin, previously thought to be an irreversible change. Observations in mice and humans have shown that damaged connective tissue can repair itself, but only when complemented by photoprotection in the future.[28] Retinoids can stimulate wound healing by enhancing collagen deposition in granulation tissue[31] and by inhibiting collagenase in certain model systems.[28]

The use of topical retinoic acid (e.g., Retin A) can help to repair the dermis, characterized by broad regions of new collagen deposited subepidermally. The amount and depth of repair depend on the duration of treatment and the concentration/dose of retinoid. Retinoic acid will not reverse severe photoaging but can help to efface fine wrinkles and minimize deeper ones.[26-28]

Skin cancer screening

The incidence of skin cancer continues to increase at an alarming rate. The current incidence for malignant melanoma, for example, is 1 in 105 in 1992. Approximately 20 years ago, public skin cancer screening programs began to appear in the United States. The goals have included early

---

Skin self-examination

- Perform monthly after a bath or shower.
- Use a full-length and hand mirror.
- Note any moles, blemishes or birthmarks, from the top of your head to your toes.
- Note changes in color, size, or shape of these or any sore that does not heal.
- Follow these steps:
    1. Examine your body front and back in the mirror; then examine both sides with your arms raised.
    2. With your elbows bent, check your forearms, upper arms, and palms carefully.
    3. Examine the back of your legs and feet (sit if it's more comfortable); check the soles and spaces between your toes.
    4. Check the back of your scalp and neck using both mirrors; part your hair or use a blow dryer to give you a closer look.

If you find any changes in size, color, or shape of any previously noted mole or other skin markings, or if you develop a sore that does not heal, see your physician.

---

detection of cutaneous malignancies and public education in the harmful effects of excessive sun exposure, the clinical characteristics of skin cancer, and the need for prompt intervention.[5] Initially these programs were organized on a local level,[35,53] but since 1985 they have been sponsored nationwide by the American Academy of Dermatology (AAD). Since 1985, more than 260,000 Americans have been screened for melanoma/skin cancer in the annual efforts sponsored by the AAD.[30] A community education and screening program like this seems to be an effective method of informing the public about the importance of this health problem and of identifying affected individuals.[19]

The importance of public education and awareness about sun protection and early identification and treatment of skin cancers cannot be overemphasized. Regular self-examination is the best way to become familiar with the many moles and spots on the skin. The Cleveland Clinic department of dermatology uses the information in the box above as a handout to explain self-examination.

Special attention should be paid to the size, shape, edge, and color of skin moles. A simple way to remember the features that make a mole suspicious for malignancy is to think of A-B-C-D, for Asymmetry, Border (irregularity), Color (nonuniformity of pigmentation), and Diameter (greater than 6 mm) (see Fig. 49-1 and Plate 5 after page 16). With malignant melanoma, early detection and treatment can improve prognosis. Periodic self-examination may be taught, and is especially important to individuals of highest risk. A partial list of risk factors is outlined in the box on p. 934. People with many moles are best screened by a dermatologist. Patients with few moles

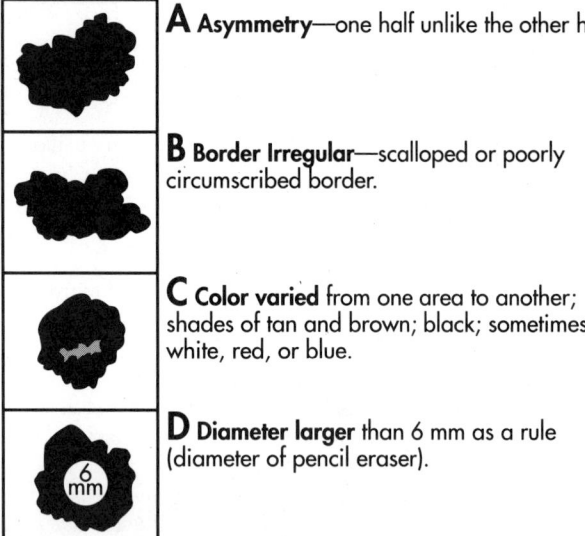

A Asymmetry—one half unlike the other half.

B Border Irregular—scalloped or poorly circumscribed border.

C Color varied from one area to another; shades of tan and brown; black; sometimes white, red, or blue.

D Diameter larger than 6 mm as a rule (diameter of pencil eraser).

Fig. 49-1. The ABCDs of examining moles or pigmented spots. (From American Academy of Dermatology: *Sunscreens*, Evanston, Ill, 1987, The Academy.)

Risk factors for melanoma

1. Family history of malignant melanoma
2. Blond or red hair
3. Marked freckling on the back
4. History of frequent sunburns before age 20
5. Blue, green, or grey eyes
6. Inability to tan
7. Personal history of nonmelanoma skin cancers
8. Sensitivity to the sun
9. Personal history of melanoma
10. Large numbers of moles, particularly those that are atypical or dysplastic
11. History of outdoor summer jobs in the teenage years
12. Living near the equator

From Friedman RJ et al: The continued importance of early detection of malignant melanoma, *CA Cancer J Clin* 41:201-226, 1991.

may be instructed in self-examination. Self-examination brochures may be obtained from the American Academy of Dermatology (see Resources section at the end of this chapter). Photographing questionable moles can often assist the practitioner in the following of that lesion.

SUMMARY

Sunlight is a beneficial source of energy that few people can avoid. It promotes the synthesis of previtamin D_3, used in bone metabolism, and stimulates the production of melanin as a form of photoprotection for the skin.[14,20,42]

Sun exposure can produce acute and chronic adverse effects of medical importance. Acute, short-term effects include sunburn, photoallergic and phototoxic reactions, altered immunoreactivity, and a variety of photosensitivity disorders. Chronic, long-term effects include photoaging (dermatoheliosis or actinic elastosis), precancerous changes (solar/actinic keratoses), and photocarcinogenesis (basal and squamous cell carcinomas and melanomas).

Cutaneous photoprotection represents preventive measures against the acute and chronic effects of the sun on the skin.[15]

REFERENCES

1. Algra RJ, Knox JM: Topical photoprotective agents, *Int J Dermatol* 17:628-633, 1978.
2. American Academy of Dermatology: *Sunscreens,* Evanston, Ill, 1987, American Academy of Dermatology.
3. American Cancer Society: *Cancer facts and figures—1992,* Atlanta, 1992, American Cancer Society.
4. Bernhard JD et al: Abnormal responses to ultraviolet radiation. In Fitzpatrick TB et al, editors: *Dermatology in general medicine,* ed 3, New York, 1987, McGraw-Hill.
5. Bolognia JL, Berwick M, and Fine JA: Complete follow-up and evaluation of skin cancer screening in Connecticut, *J Am Acad Dermatol* 23:1098-1105, 1990.
6. Brodthagen H: Malignant melanoma caused by UVA suntan bed? *Acta Derm Venereol* (Stockh) 62:404-408, 1982.
7. Council on Scientific Affairs: Harmful effects of ultraviolet light radiation, *JAMA* 262:380-384, 1989.
8. Deleo VA: Prevention of skin cancer, *J Dermatol Surg Oncol* 14:902-906, 1988.
9. Dubois EL: Antimalarials in the management of discoid and systemic lupus erythematosus, *Semin Arthritis Rheum* 8:33-51, 1978.
10. Epstein JH: Polymorphous light eruption, *Dermatol Clin* 4:243-251, 1986.
11. Fears TR, Scotto J: Estimating increases in skin cancer morbidity due to increases in ultraviolet radiation exposure, *Cancer Invest* 1:119-126, 1983.
12. Federal Register: Sunscreen drug products for over-the-counter human drugs: proposed safety, effectiveness, and labelling conditions, 43(166):38206-38269, 1978, Washington, DC, DHEW, Food and Drug Administration.
13. Friedman RJ et al: The continued importance of early detection of malignant melanoma, *CA Cancer J Clin* 41:201-226, 1991.
14. Giese AC: The sun, myths, and worship. In *Living with our sun's ultraviolet rays,* New York, 1976, Plenum.
15. Gilcrest BA: Actinic injury, *Annu Rev Med* 41:199-210, 1990.
16. Gilmore GD: Sunscreens: a review of the skin cancer protection value and educational opportunities, *J Sch Health* 59(5):210-213, 1989.
17. Green AES, Hedinger RA: Models relating ultraviolet light and nonmelanoma skin cancer incidence, *Photochem Photobiol* 28:283-291, 1978.
18. Groves GA: Sunburn and its prevention, *Aust J Dermatol* 21:115-138, 1980.
19. Hazen PG: Skin cancer awareness programs: success of a statewide program of education and screening in Ohio, *Ohio Med* June: 449-451, 1989.
20. Holick MK: The photobiology of vitamin D and its consequences for humans, *Ann NY Acad Sci* 453:1-13, 1985.
21. Jansen CT, Karvonen J, and Malmiharju T: PUVA therapy for polymorphous light eruptions: comparison of systemic methoxsalen and topical trioxsalen regimens and evaluation of local protective mechanisms, *Acta Derm Venereol* (Stockh) 62:317-320, 1982.
22. Kaidbey KH, Kligman AM: The acute effects of longwave ultraviolet radiation on human skin, *J Invest Dermatol* 72:252-256, 1979.
23. Kligman AM: Early destructive effects of sunlight on human skin, *JAMA* 210:2377-2380, 1969.

24. Kligman LH, Akin FJ, and Kligman AM: Contributions of UVA and UVB to connective tissue damage in hairless mice, *J Invest Dermatol* 84:272-276, 1985.

25. Kligman LH, Akin FJ, and Kligman AM: Prevention of ultraviolet damage to the dermis of hairless mice by sunscreens, *J Invest Dermatol* 78:181-189, 1982.

26. Kligman LH, Kligman AM: The nature of photoaging: its prevention and repair, *Photodermatol* 3:215-227, 1986.

27. Kligman LH: Photoaging: manifestations, prevention, and treatment, *Clin Geriatr Med* 5:235-251, 1989.

28. Kligman LH: Preventing, delaying, and repairing photoaged skin, *Cutis* 41:419-421, 1988.

29. Kochevar IE, Pathak MA, and Parrish JA: Photophysics, photochemistry, and photobiology. In Fitzpatrick TB et al, editors: *Dermatology in general medicine,* New York, 1987, McGraw-Hill.

30. Koh HK et al: Who is being screened for melanoma/skin cancer? Characteristics of persons screened in Massachusetts, *J Am Acad Dermatol* 24(2):271-277, 1991.

31. Lee KH, Tong TG: Mechanism of action of retinyl compounds on wound healing: effect of active retinyl derivatives on granuloma formation, *J Pharm Sci* 59:1195-1197, 1970.

32. Lerman S: Effects of sunlight on the eye. In Ben Hur E, Rosenthal I, editors: *Photomedicine,* Boca Raton, Fla, 1987, CRC Press.

33. Lew RA et al: Sun exposure and melanoma skin cancer, *J Dermatol Surg Oncol* 9:981-986, 1983.

34. Loescher LJ, Meyskens FL Jr: Chemoprevention of human skin cancers, *Semin Oncol Nurs* 7:45-52, 1991.

35. Lynch H, Lynch J, and Kraft C: A new approach to cancer screening and education, *Geriatrics* 28:152-157, 1973.

36. Magnus K: Incidence of malignant melanoma of the skin in five nordic countries: significance of solar radiation, *Int J Cancer* 20:477, 1970.

37. Mathews-Roth MM et al: Beta carotene therapy for erythropoietic protoporphyria and other photosensitivity diseases, *Arch Dermatol* 113:1229-1232, 1977.

38. Moshovitz M, Modan B: Role of sun exposure in the aetiology of malignant melanoma: epidemiologic inference, *J Natl Cancer Inst* 51:777, 1973.

39. National Cancer Institute: Nonmelanoma skin cancers, basal and squamous cell carcinomas: research report, NIH Publication No. 88-2977, Bethesda, Md, 1988, US Department of Health and Human Services, Public Health Services, National Institutes of Health.

40. Norris PW, Hawk JLM: Polymorphic light eruption, *Photodermatol Photoimmunol Photomed* 7:186, 1990.

41. Ortel B et al: Polymorphous light eruption: action spectrum and photoprotection, *J Am Acad Dermatol* 14:748-753, 1986.

42. Pathak MA: Sunscreens and their use in the preventive treatment of sunlight-induced skin damage, *J Dermatol Surg Oncol* 13:739-750, 1987.

43. Pathak MA: Sunscreens: topical and systemic approaches for protection of human skin against harmful effects of solar radiation, *J Am Acad Dermatol* 7:285-312, 1982.

44. Peck GL et al: Treatment and prevention of basal cell carcinoma with oral isotretinoin, *J Am Acad Dermatol* 19:176-185, 1988.

45. Peck GL: Topical tretinoin in actinic keratoses and basal cell carcinoma, *J Am Acad Dermatol* 15:829-835, 1986.

46. Pitts DG: Threat of ultraviolet light radiation to the eye—how to protect against it, *J Am Optom Assoc* 52:949-957, 1981.

47. Sams WM Jr: Chloroquine: its use in photosensitive eruptions, *Int J Dermatol* 15:99-111, 1976.

48. Smith JH Jr et al: Alterations in human dermal connective tissue with age and chronic sun damage, *J Invest Dermatol* 39:347-350, 1982.

49. Stern RS, Weistein MC, and Baker SG: Risk reduction for nonmelanoma skin cancer with childhood sunscreen use, *Arch Dermatol* 122:537-545, 1986.

50. Stolarski RS: The Antarctic ozone hole, *Sci Am* 258:30-36, 1988.

51. Taylor CR et al: Photoaging/photodamage and photoprotection, *J Am Acad Dermatol* 22:1-15, 1990.

52. Urbach F, Gange RW: *The biological effects of UVA radiation,* New York, 1986, Praeger.

53. Weary PE: A two-year experience with a series of rural skin and oral cancer detection clinics, *JAMA* 217:1862-1863, 1971.

54. Wolf HC et al: Sunscreens for delay of ultraviolet induction of skin tumors, *J Am Acad Dermatol* 7:194-202, 1982.

RESOURCES

The American Academy of Dermatology, 1567 Maple Ave., Evanston, IL 60201; provides brochures and other educational materials.

Office of Cancer Communications, National Cancer Institute, Bethesda, MD 20892. Provides information service and educational materials.

The Skin Cancer Foundation, P.O. Box 561, New York, NY 10156. Provides educational posters, audiovisual aids, brochures, newsletters, and other educational material including:

- *Skin cancer: preventable and curable,* an audiovisual presentation
- *Dysplastic nevi and malignant melanoma, a patient's guide*
- *The ABCD's of moles and melanomas*
- *The 1990 Skin Cancer Foundation Journal*
- *The melanoma letter*

Part XI

SPECIFIC CLINICAL PROBLEMS OF COMMON CONCERN

Chapter 50

GASTROINTESTINAL DISORDERS

David Pietz

This chapter discusses the more common gastrointestinal (GI) pathologic entities, stressing prevention or at least early recognition that allows for the eradication, improvement, or prevention of the progression of a condition together with intelligent follow-up care. It presents information on the underlying disease mechanism, epidemiology, patient and socioeconomic factors, and preventive therapy where applicable. A thorough discussion with the patient of findings; explanation of the disease, expected course, and options to consider; and counseling all lead to a good patient-physician relationship and encourage inclusion of the patient in treatment decisions, management, and compliance in the medical program.

Surveillance indications for the GI tract, with the exception of colorectal cancer and polyps as well as hemoccult studies, which are discussed elsewhere (see Chapter 46), are given. An exception is surveillance of chronic ulcerative colitis for malignancy. Human immunodeficiency virus (HIV) and acquired immunodeficiency syndrome (AIDS) are discussed elsewhere (see Chapter 56).

ESOPHAGUS
Gastroesophageal reflux disease

Hiatus hernia associated with gastroesophageal reflux and gastroesophageal reflux disease (GERD) without a coexistent hiatus hernia are among the most common conditions that the primary care physician encounters in office practice. They are also conditions in which preventive medicine truly has a place, for the prevention of not only the symptoms but the complications that may be the sequelae of chronic reflux and can be of considerable magnitude in terms of disease, disability, and a constellation of secondary symptoms. To prevent the primary symptoms and the sequelae the physician should fully understand the

functional anatomy and physiology of GERD and appreciate the presenting symptoms that are primary to the condition (e.g., heartburn) and secondary (e.g., asthma and hoarseness) to its effects. The anatomy, physiology, and pathophysiology of GERD and the diseases in which it may occur are therefore reviewed in some detail so that the reader may better employ prevention in this common disorder.

Antireflux barrier. The lower esophageal sphincter (LES) and the crural diaphragm have been recognized as the primary anatomic structures contributing to the antireflux barrier. The phrenoesophageal ligament, acute angle of His (the junction of the tubular esophagus and the sacular stomach), and location of the LES may contribute.[39] The LES is 2.5 to 3.5 cm in length, the terminal portions of the esophagus are normally located at the hiatus of the diaphragm.

The intraluminal pressure at the esophagogastric junction determines the strength of the reflux barrier and varies by 10 to 20 mm Hg although at times it may be higher (e.g., from a usual pressure of 15 to 35 mm Hg to 80 mm Hg) as a result of gastric contractions.

A pressure gradient between the stomach and esophagus promotes gastroesophageal reflux, which is offset by pressure at the esophagogastric junction. The pressure in the stomach results from contractions of gastric musculature and transmission of intraabdominal pressure. The esophageal pressure is related to contraction of the LES and intrathoracic pressure. The negative intrathoracic and intraesophageal pressures promote gastroesophageal reflux. During inspiration the esophageal pressure becomes negative and gastric pressure becomes positive, favoring reflux. These effects are offset by an increase of the LES pressure aided by contraction of the diaphragm. A readily available and rapid mechanism is required to counteract the sudden increased intragastric pressure during coughing, straining, and so on.[39]

Pathophysiology of gastroesophageal reflux. LES dysfunction plays a predominant role in causing reflux. In the past it was considered secondary to a chronically weak sphincter that lacked the capacity to oppose forces promoting reflux. In the majority of cases, however, an absent LES pressure results from an intermittent transient abrupt LES relaxation (TLESR), which lasts 5 to 30 seconds, occurring without preceding swallows; otherwise an intervening LES pressure is normal.[28] In asymptomatic persons about 35% of TLESRs occur with reflux versus 65% of GERD.

Gastric distention provokes TLESRs, which may be caused by a vagovagal reflux resulting from stimulation of the mechanical receptors of the gastric wall. In healthy individuals two major factors control the occurrence of TLESRs: (1) they do not occur during sleep, and (2) there is a significant suppression of TLESRs and belching while the person is in the supine position. Approximately 50% of patients with peptic esophagitis have a delay in gastric emptying as well as probable impairment of suppression of TLESRs in response to gastric distention when they are supine. The mean basal LES pressure was decreased only in patients with severe esophagitis, 30% of whom had a basal LES pressure less than 10 mm Hg.[28]

The LES is also supported by the diaphragmatic crus, as well as by its position within the abdominal cavity. Hiatus hernia and obesity may cause a loss of these mechanisms with effects noticed particularly during straining. Reflux occurring during straining is often seen when the basal LES pressure is low (that is, less than 5 mm Hg), usually in the presence of a hiatus hernia and prevalent in GERD.

Fifty percent to 60% of hiatus hernia patients have esophagitis; 94% of esophagitis patients have hiatus hernia. The hernia impairs the LES function particularly during straining. When the LES is displaced from the abdomen into the chest, mechanical defects cause a loss of the pressure effect of the diaphragmatic curve on the LES segment. Particularly with large hernias or impaired phrenoesophageal ligament, the LES segment moves from the normal position with abdominal pressure, thereby decreasing sphincter pressure and causing reflux.[28]

Esophageal motor activity and acid clearance. Esophageal injury is determined on the basis of duration of acid exposure and caustic potency of reflux contents. GERD occurs when aggressive forces (acid reflux) dominate defensive forces, namely, esophageal acid clearance and mucosal resistance.[32] Patients with reflux esophagitis are likely to have more reflux events and prolongation of each exposure. The duration of exposure of the esophageal mucosa is termed the *esophageal clearance time.* The esophageal volume clearance occurs almost immediately

after acid exposure; this differs from acid clearance.

Swallowed saliva rather than subsequent peristalic contractions result in acid clearance. Essentially all the volume is cleared by esophageal peristalsis, leaving only a slight residual that has an acid pH until neutralized by swallowed saliva. Approximately 7 ml of saliva is required to neutralize 1 ml of 0.1 N HCl; 50% of this neutralizing capacity is attributed to salivary bicarbonate.[32]

Saliva output ceases during sleep, thereby affecting acid clearance should reflux occur during sleep or acid clearance not be completed before sleep.

The return of the pH of the esophageal mucosa occurs progressively with each swallow. The esophageal volume clearance is usually completed by one to two peristalic contractions in the normal individual. When volume clearance is impaired, acid clearance time is markedly prolonged because of the minimal neutralizing capacity of saliva.

Instances of delayed clearance are related to failed propagated peristalsis. An upright position or elevation of the head of the bed improves impaired volume clearance. Peristaltic dysfunction significantly increases with progression of esophagitis. Reflux causes injury, prolonging acid clearance, which, in turn, causes greater injury. Hiatus hernia patients have delayed acid clearance as a result of rereflux from the sac during swallowing, present with or without esophagitis.[32]

Poor esophageal volume clearance and reduced salivary neutralizing capacity impair restoration of esophageal pH. In young active subjects acid perfusion results in an esophagosalivary reflux that increases the salivary rate two to three times and may explain the symptom of water brash observed in some patients with reflux disease. The effect on neutralizing acid, however, is probably minimal because of latency of 20 to 30 minutes. This reflex is absent in GERD. Cigarette smokers demonstrate prolonged esophageal acid clearance times because of low salivation. Cigarette smoking adversely affects GERD by causing a 50% increase in acid clearance time compared to that of nonsmokers; the salivary titratable base content of the smokers is 60% that of the nonsmoker. This effect persists 6 hours after cessation of smoking.[32]

Gastric emptying in gastroesophageal reflux. Gastroesophageal reflux is more common after meals and is related to volume of gastric contents.[38] The volume depends on quantity of food and saliva swallowed, amount of gastric secretions, duodenal gastric reflux, and gastric emptying.

Patients who have GER usually have normal gastric acidity. Bile acid induced antral gastritis causes antral hypomotility, increasing reflux of bile acids and other alkaline secretions. Fifty-seven percent of GERD patients have solid food retention and delayed gastric emptying of solids but not liquids. Symptoms of nausea, vomiting, fullness, epigastric distress, and postprandial satiety occur in 25%

of reflux patients and suggest delayed gastric emptying. Smoking and high-fat meals decrease LES pressure and slow gastric emptying. Other foods such as chocolate and a high-fiber diet cause these changes, as do drugs such as anticholinergics, nitrates, theophyllines, α-blockers, calcium channel blockers, levodopa, and narcotics. Prostaglandins, β-antagonists, estrogen, and progesterone likewise decrease LES pressure and delay gastric emptying.[38]

The prokinetic agent metoclopramide increases LES pressure and amplitude of esophageal contractions and stimulates GI smooth muscle, increasing gastric emptying and improving small bowel transit. It tends to coordinate gastric, pyloric, and duodenal motor activity, facilitating forward peristalsis. These effects result in significant reduction in daytime and nighttime heartburn, and regurgitation, and decrease the need for antacids. A fairly high percentage of patients, however, cannot tolerate metoclopramide.[38]

Esophageal mucosal resistance. Esophageal mucosal resistance is important in esophagitis as physiologically it serves as a mucosal barrier maintaining an effective separation between mucosa and lumen.[24]

The primary agent for esophageal injury is acid, but pepsin, bile salts, pancreatic enzymes, and hypertonic meal contents may likewise cause injury. The esophageal mucosa is a nonkeratinized squamous epithelium, approximately 25 to 30 layers thick. A few submucosal glands are present in the distal and proximal esophagus. The barrier retarding diffusion of noxious contents seems to exist primarily as tight intercellular junctions in the first few cell layers of the stratum corneum.

Mucosal resistance depends on the resistance to ionic movement at the intercellular and cellular levels. The esophageal mucosa is considered tight and resistant to significant hydrogen ion diffusion; this resistance is not maintained, however, in the presence of bile salts or pepsin.[24]

Epithelial barrier effectiveness is maintained by an electrochemical gradient across the mucosa. Active mucosal to serosal absorption of sodium relies on the integrity of both cellular and paracellular pathways. Should there be an excess entry of H^+ ions, sodium absorption is impaired. The cells in the stratum spinosum become "ballooned" and necrotic. The basal lateral membrane becomes exposed to the H^+ ion, causing an inactivation of Na^+-K^+- adenosine triphosphatase (ATPase).

The presence of bile acids in the reflux may cause H^+ ion absorption. Bile salts, more hydrophobic and lipid soluble, permeate membranes more readily. The H^+ ion also appears to facilitate bile salt entry.[23]

Pepsin at a low pH, for example pH 2, can cause disruption of the mucosal barrier associated with accelerated H^+ ion influx. Trypsin may cause similar problems although at pH 5 to 8, which is its optimal activity range.

Hyperosmolar foods including coffee, orange juice, and tomato juice, independent of acidity, cause heartburn in acid sensitive patients (positive Bernstein test result). These liquids do not affect esophageal motor activity but do modify permeability.[23]

Medical and surgical conditions that may cause GERD. In addition to the factors listed certain medical and surgical conditions may also cause GERD. These include scleroderma, pregnancy, Zollinger-Ellison syndrome, and after gastric surgery.[13]

Scleroderma. Esophageal disease has been reported in 70% to 90% of patients with scleroderma, usually accompanied by Raynaud's phenomenon. There is relative sparing of the skeletal muscle but smooth muscle peristalsis is severely impaired. LES pressure is decreased and may be undetectable in 30% to 50% of patients. Symptoms of GERD may be the initial presenting feature of scleroderma because of severe reflux related to LES incompetency in conjunction with poor esophageal clearance. Progressive dysphagia with weight loss may occur with secondary stricture. Idiopathic GERD may have an incidence of 10% stricture compared to 48% in patients with scleroderma. Patients may have recurrent pulmonary infections, a cough at night, wheezing, and morning hoarseness suggestive of occult aspiration. The severity of GERD seems to correspond to the severity of the pulmonary disease. Seventy-five percent have a Barrett's esophagus and adenocarcinoma of the esophagus may appear. Odynophagia may occur and often is a manifestation of *Candida* associated esophagitis.[13]

Gastroesophageal reflux disease in pregnancy. In about 30% to 50% of pregnant women GERD is severe in the third trimester, although it can begin in the first trimester. This is common when eating large meals and assuming the recumbent position and usually represents no significant health risk. Symptoms are attributed to increased intraabdominal pressure, loss of the intraabdominal LES segment, alteration of anatomic structures surrounding the LES, hiatus hernia formation, and delayed gastric emptying. LES pressure is reduced but returns to normal levels after delivery. Reduction in LES pressure relates closely to changes in estrogen and progesterone levels during pregnancy. Endoscopy has demonstrated esophagitis in 40 of 43 pregnant women with reflux symptoms.[13]

Life-style changes of eating smaller meals, avoiding spicy and fatty foods, maintaining an upright position, elevating the head of the bed, and avoiding smoking are advised. Antacids or sucralfate can be used; metoclopramide use in the third trimester demonstrates a significant increase in LES pressure and complete relief of symptoms in most patients. H_2-receptor blockers are considered probably safe late in pregnancy although not frequently prescribed.[13]

Zollinger-Ellison syndrome. GERD in the Zollinger-Ellison syndrome is more difficult to treat because of high gastric acidity. In many of these patients esophageal lesions fail to heal with H_2-receptor blockers and require omeprazole therapy, lowering the gastric acid output to less than 10 mEq/hr. Seventy-three percent of cases of esophagitis resolved.[13] A larger dose of H_2-receptor antagonists or more likely omeprazole therapy is usually required.

Gastroesophageal reflux after gastric surgery. Alkaline esophagitis frequently follows surgical procedures for decreasing gastric acidity.[13] Bile reflux gastritis has an estimated incidence of 20% in these patients. All patients having alkaline reflux esophagitis have bile gastritis although the opposite is not true. Increased mucosal influx of hydrogen ions is an indication of mucosal damage and varies directly with the bile salt concentration and duration of exposure.

Often surgery such as vagotomy promotes GER by blocking the normal elevated LES pressure resulting from abdominal compression. In a study of 32 patients before and after vagotomy, in 9 patients GER occurred preoperatively whereas 24 patients had reflux, which frequently was severe, postoperatively. Modification of the angle of His may contribute to this. Decreasing gastrin by antrectomy may lower LES pressure. Patients with alkaline reflux disease are likely to have heartburn, dysphagia, regurgitation, and water brash. A higher incidence of vomiting, severe regurgitation, and resulting pulmonary complications occurs in patients having alkaline reflux from previous gastric surgery (63.5%) compared to those undergoing antireflux surgery for acid reflux disease (37%).[13]

The observation of bile in the stomach or esophagus is not diagnostic of alkaline gastritis and esophagitis; endoscopic and histologic characteristics cannot be used to distinguish acid from alkaline reflux disease.[99] Nuclear medicine bilary scan may help distinguish these patients from those with acid reflux disease. One may also undertake prolonged esophageal pH monitoring: that is, a diagnosis of alkaline reflux may be made by pH greater than 7.[13]

Therapeutically metoclopramide may be used to increase LES and gastric emptying. More success has been derived from surgery, particularly the Roux-en-Y diversion. In the intact stomach Nissen fundoplication combined with gastroplasty may be successful.[13]

Barrett's esophagus. Barrett's esophagus is the replacement of stratified squamous epithelium of the distal esophagus by abnormal columnar epithelium, which may be congenital. The proliferation of columnar mucosa and reepithelization of squamous mucosa of the distal esophagus through the process of metaplasia suggest that the condition may be acquired rather than congenital.[48] Esophageal cancer in Barrett's esophagus is 30 to 50 times the expected incidence. The white/black ratio is 10:1; the male/female ratio, 5:1.[37] Heavy cigarette smoking and alcohol abuse are practiced by up to 85% and 16% of patients, respectively. Most patients have heartburn and regurgitation. Complications of GERD are esophageal ulcer, stricture, bleeding, deficiency anemia, dysplasia, and adenocarcinoma. Cancer incidence is reported as 4.8% to 15%.[48]

The usual GERD management is advocated; often omeprazole therapy is required, rather than use of H_2-antagonist blockers. Esophageal dilation, fundoplication, and possibly vagotomy may be required when response is poor.

If the initial endoscopy result is negative for dysplasia, it should be repeated at least twice. For low-grade dysplasia endoscopy every 3 to 6 months with ongoing medical management is advised. For high-grade dysplasia repeat endoscopy in 2 weeks is recommended; if high-grade dysplasia or intramucosal carcinoma is found, consider esophageal resection.[37]

Symptoms of GERD

Throat symptoms

Globus. A sensation of a lump in the throat may be related to the esophagus in the form of either dysmotility of the esophagus or gastroesophageal reflux.[22,41] Depression, hysteria, and stress are not considered likely causes, and the term "hystericus" should be avoided. Upper esophageal sphincter abnormalities have not been demonstrated.

Water brash. Hypersalivation, or water brash, may be produced by acid reflux into the distal esophagus resulting in reflux hypersalivation. This may induce swallowing, peristalsis, and increased acid clearance.[65]

Hoarseness. It has been estimated that 25% of patients with GERD have head and neck symptoms alone. Hoarseness is uncommon but can result from acid reflux into the hypopharynx resulting in erythema of the arytenoids, pharynx, and/or posterior portion of the true vocal cords. GERD may bathe the pharynx and the larynx, especially at night when the patient is supine.[65]

Chest symptoms. Heartburn is the most common symptom of GERD, occurring in more than 50% of patients. It is most common after meals but can occur during sleep, bending over, and exercise.

Regurgitation is the effortless return of gastric acid into the pharynx. The absence of nausea, retching, and abdominal contractions indicates that this is not vomiting.[65]

Dysphagia, a sensation of delayed passage of food from the mouth into the stomach, is a common complaint. Chronic esophagitis of the distal esophagus may slowly result in scarring and stricture(s). Dysphagia initially is noted with solid foods. Patients with Barrett's mucosa may have severe GERD but little heartburn because of lack of acid sensitivity of the Barrett's mucosa. Dysphagia with or without GERD may be related to Schatzki's ring, present in 5% of the general population. Esophageal dysmotility and dysphagia may also result from reflux associated esophageal spasm. Odynophagia is a rather infrequent symptom of GER but when present suggests severe esophagitis or presence of an esophageal ulcer. Superimposed esophageal candidiasis in the presence of severe motor dysfunction may cause odynophagia.[65]

The esophagus may cause chest pain; this is related

more to GERD than esophageal dysmotility. Manometric events and episodes of chest pain may correlate poorly.

Chest pain of anginal type may also be a presenting symptom of esophageal disorders, and when the patient exhibits an atypical pattern this suspicion must be reserved and addressed in diagnostic studies,[8] not only of the heart (e.g., stress testing, catheterization) but also of the esophagus. One is often frustrated in trying to make a precise definition of the cause and is left with a "best guess." The studies per se, having relieved the patient's mind, often are therapeutic. When a preventable esophageal cause (e.g., GERD) is identified, appropriate prevention recommendations produce great psychological and symptomatic relief to the patient. It is interesting that hypersensitivity to esophageal distention may cause chest pain and may be noted during catheterization within the right atrium—a response not seen in patients with coronary heart disease.[26]

Pulmonary symptoms. Pulmonary symptoms such as chronic asthma, bronchitis, bronchiectasis, aspiration pneumonia, atelectasis, hemoptysis, and pulmonary fibrosis may be associated with GERD.[65] According to Sontag 81.8% of asthmatics studied had GER.[60] It is uncertain whether reflux causes asthma or vice versa.[1] The link between asthma and GERD may not be apparent because *the reflux often is silent and unrecognized.* Possible causal relationships are that GERD could be a stimulant of a vagal reflex or a source of aspiration, and that asthma may develop first with wheezing and coughing sufficient to induce reflux. Reflux has been estimated to be an aggravating factor in at least 5% to 15% of asthmatics. It has been estimated that 20% of asthmatics with reflux are sensitive to its acid content. Clinical features suggesting the possibility of GERD as the cause of asthma include symptoms, middle-age onset of asthma, negative history of allergy.[65]

"Gastric" symptoms. GERD may have associated symptoms of bloating, early satiety, belching, and nausea. The cause of these symptoms may be related to antral gastritis with delayed gastric emptying.[65]

Miscellaneous symptoms. GERD patients may have acute or chronic gastrointestinal blood loss. Hematemesis and melena are uncommon but may result from a discrete esophageal ulcer or from a hiatus hernia causing linear erosions of the stomach. Occasionally hiccups may be associated with GERD although not caused by it.

Medical management and prevention of reflux. Sontag in his description of medical management of reflux esophagitis uses the term *gastroesophageal reflux disease* (GERD) to refer to any symptom or esophageal mucosal damage that results from reflux of gastric acid into the esophagus.[60] Others use the term *gastroesophageal reflux* in those cases where there is no esophageal mucosal damage. The "Castell iceberg" is commonly used to demonstrate that most GERD patients have only mild or sporadic symptoms, not requiring medical assistance; this is the iceberg submerged in water. The next group, which is small,

represents those patients who have troublesome or persistent symptoms without complications. These "office refluxers" are in contrast to "hospital refluxers," who represent the very tip of the iceberg and have complications.[51]

Management and prevention include:

- A 6 inch elevation of the head of the bed, decreasing acid clearance time though having little effect on reflux
- Avoidance of smoking and use of alcohol and drugs that promote reflux (e.g., theophylline, calcium channel blockers, anticholinergics, and progesterone)
- Use of antacids (Gaviscon®), prokinetic drugs as metoclopramide, H_2-receptor antagonists, or omeprazole
- Eating modifications, including losing weight, if the patient is obese, as loss of only 10 to 15 pounds may significantly relieve symptoms; eating small, frequent low-fat meals slowly and decreasing fluid intake at meals
- Avoiding carbonated beverages
- Avoiding meals and snacks within 2 hours of sleeping
- Decreasing intake of chocolate, fats, and carminatives, which may impair LES function
- Avoiding citrus juices, tomato products, and coffee because of esophageal irritation.[51]

Summary of prevention in esophageal conditions or GERD. A detailed description of the mechanisms of gastroesophageal reflux has been presented to promote a better understanding of the disease as well as its therapy. The antireflux barrier consists of LES, crural diaphragm, and phrenoesophageal ligaments. The pressure gradient between the stomach and esophagus that tends to cause gastroesophageal reflux is offset by pressure at the esophagogastric junction, which serves as a barrier.

Transient abrupt LES relaxation (TLESR) causing a sudden absence of LES pressure appears to be a greater factor in causing reflux than a chronically low LES pressure. GERD patients may have delayed gastric emptying as well as impairment of suppression of TLESRs.

Esophageal injury is proportional to the length of time that the mucosa is acidified; swallowing of saliva rather than subsequent peristalic contractions results in acid clearance, although peristalsis is important for esophageal volume clearance. Delayed clearance may be related to failed propagated peristalsis. Hiatus hernia patients may have delayed acid clearance as a result of rereflux from the sac during swallowing. Cigarette smokers have decreased salivary titrable base and delayed acid clearance time.

There may be delayed gastric emptying in reflux patients, which may be helped by the prokinetic agent metoclopramide.

Esophageal mucosal resistance serves as a mucosal barrier protecting the mucosa from the luminal contents. It prevents hydrogen ion diffusion; however, in the presence of bile salts or pepsin the barrier is not maintained.

Therapy includes changes in life-style, such as eating smaller, more frequent meals and avoiding fats, alcohol, smoking, and medications that promote reflux. H_2-receptor blockers and metoclopramide may be needed. The vast majority of patients with GER have only mild symptoms and often need only antacids.

Drug-induced esophagitis

Esophagitis, when drug induced, is a condition preventable by selection of alternative treatment, proper timing, and manner of taking medication. At times when alternative medication cannot be used secondary prevention of the condition through the use of H_2-receptor blockers is necessary.

Drug induced esophagitis has been an underdiagnosed entity recognized only since 1970 as esophageal injury produced by local caustic effects of drugs.[17] One hundred and seventy-five drugs that may cause the condition have been collected from the literature; the most commonly demonstrated to cause esophagitis are tetracycline; doxycyline; emepronium bromide, which has been used in England for bladder spasms; slow released potassium chloride; quinidine; aspirin and nonsteroidal antiinflammatory drugs (NSAIDs), which represent 149 of the 175 listed.

In a clinical trial of health volunteers taking NSAIDs esophagitis was diagnosed in 15.7% to 20%. Of patients with esophageal strictures 31% used NSAIDs compared to 14% of controls.[17]

The acidity or alkalinity of a drug is a major factor in its causative action; for example, tetracycline, doxycycline, and ferrous sulfate dissolved in water form solutions with pH below 3. NSAIDs' inhibition of cyclooxygense affects the biosynthesis of prostaglandins. These drugs are also relatively acidic.

Barium sulfate tablets similar in size to aspirin tablets showed a 5-minute delay or longer in 57 of 98 patients undergoing barium swallow studies for gastrointestinal symptoms.[17]

The studies indicate that medications should be taken only when sitting or standing along with an adequate amount of liquid to wash the drugs down. Ulcerogenic drugs should be given only as liquids in patients with dysphagia or known obstructive conditions in the esophagus.[17]

Cancer of the esophagus

Esophageal cancer varies considerably in different geographic regions.[61] In the United States it is relatively uncommon, consisting of about 1% of all malignancies, whereas the incidence is exceptionally high in areas of South Africa, northern China, parts of Iran, and areas of the former Soviet Russia. Gender incidence is also highly variable; in the United States it is threefold higher in men. The development of esophageal cancer is multifactorial. Alcoholism and cigarette smoking appear very significant in the United States but not in Moslem Iran. Esophageal cancer is frequently associated with other malignancies

particularly of the head and neck. About one third of the esophageal malignancies are adenocarcinoma derived from Barrett's esophagus. The risk of developing esophageal cancer is increased 30 to 40 times in patients who have Barrett's esophagus.[61] Prevention of this cancer in the United States is therefore largely a case of smoking cessation and moderate use of alcohol, especially in the patient with esophageal symptoms.

STOMACH AND DUODENUM
Peptic ulcer disease

Peptic ulcer disease in terms of prevention can be likened to coronary artery disease. In the latter primary prevention results from assumption of a healthy life-style: abstinence from tobacco, abstinence or moderation in alcohol use, proper diet, and avoidance or amelioration of stress by modifying one's environment (opting for a job with fewer stressors) or behavior. Virtually the same points apply to ulcer prevention. In addition the recurrence of the condition, or secondary prevention, is the cardiologist's responsibility after bypass surgery. The physician, having "cured" the ulcer, assumes the task of preventing recurrences. Just as one must know the causes of atherosclerosis one must understand the pathophysiology of ulcer disease. As is the case with hiatus hernia and GERD this is a very common problem for the office practitioner and has increased with the use of NSAIDs and age of the patient population. This entity is addressed in some depth because it is common and "preventable." Emphasis on prevention is "cost effective" in managing health care cost.

Peptic ulcer disease in the past 50 years. The overall incidence of peptic ulcer disease grew continuously through the first half of the twentieth century, reached a peak in 1950, and since has declined.[18] This decline began before the introduction of cimetidine in 1978. There was a significant decline (43%) in hospital admissions for duodenal ulcer (DU) disease but not gastric ulcer (GU) during the period 1970 to 1978. Reduced hospitalization, doctor visits, and mortality of peptic ulcer disease (PUD) may also be explained by greater use of endoscopy, recognizing closely related entities such as gastritis, erosions, and nonulcer dyspepsia. Revised criteria for hospital admission and improved general medical care may also have decreased mortality without a change in incidence or severity of ulcer disease. Since 1980 there has been a 100% increase in hospitalizations for bleeding GU, considered to be primarily caused by greater use of NSAIDs.[20]

Elective operations for PUD have decreased 30% to 45% since the introduction of H_2-receptor antagonists. At the Mayo Clinic there was an incidence of 49 operations per 100,000 circa 1960 compared to 6 in 1981 to 1985.[20]

It has been established that the age of patients requiring emergency surgery is increasing again, probably as a result of use of NSAIDs. The age of patients with peptic ulcers is also increasing. Hospitalization for bleeding GU is increasing; for DU it is decreasing. Primary prevention is possible through use of drugs other than NSAIDs or their judicious use (see Esophagitis/GERD).

Control of acid secretion. Understanding peptic ulcer disease requires knowledge of gastroduodenal protection and healing of peptic ulcers as well as acid secretion.

The secretion of acid is controlled by neural, hormonal, and paracrine mechanisms.[54] Histamine, gastrin, and acetylcholine stimulate acid secretion by acting on specific receptors on the parietal cell. Acetylcholine and gastrin stimulate the parietal cell output of acid by increasing the level of cytosolic calcium in the parietal cell. They also have a direct effect on histamine stores, causing release of histamine. Histamine attaching to the histamine receptor of the parietal cell increases the level of cyclic adenosine monophosphate (cAMP). The neural, hormonal, and paracrine mechanisms converge on and modulate the activity of H^+K^+-ATPase, the gastric proton pump located on the luminal surface of the parietal cell that produces the hydrochloric acid.

Acid secretion is regulated by cholinergic neurons that cause direct stimulation of the parietal cell and indirect stimulation by decreasing somatostatin secretion, which eliminates the inhibitory effect on the parietal cell. Increased formation of acid from the stomach stimulates the somatostatin cells, resulting in decreased acid output.[54]

Gastrin is released from the antrum on ingestion of a meal and represents the main, although not the exclusive, variable in the regulation of acid secretion. Stimuli, whether central or peripheral, converge on intramural neurons that regulate gastrin secretion directly or indirectly via somatostatin cells.

There is also a central regulation of gastric acid secretion in that thought, sight, smell, and taste of food, via the vagus, influence gastric acid secretion. Sham feeding produces a similar response. In dogs truncal vagotomy permanently abolishes the acid response to cephalic stimuli. The inhibitory effects of somatostatin and prostaglandin E on acid secretion are mediated by receptors inhibiting adenylate cyclase activity in the parietal cell.[54]

Growth factors and peptic ulceration. The gastrointestinal mucosa, having marked proliferative capabilities, is affected by nongastrointestinal hormones, such as growth hormone and thyroxin, and by gut hormonal peptides, particularly epidermal growth factor (EGF), gastrin, and somatostatin.[34] Prostaglandins contribute significantly as a cytoprotective agent. Certain food products, aspirin, ethanol, bile cells, hyperosmolar NaCl, or stress may cause extensive injury in the surface epithelium with loss of continuity and basal membrane. The mucosal barrier becomes damaged, through a loss or decrease of surface mucous gel and the anatomic integrity of the surface epithelium. Its extraordinary rapidity of restoration of surface epithelium after injury (restitution) consists of migration of viable cells adjacent to the area to cover the denuded basal

membrane. This process may begin within 5 minutes after injury, for example, in a rat's stomach exposed to ethanol in which 90% of the mucosa is reepithelized within 1 hour.[34]

Acute and chronic peptic ulcers are considered to represent an imbalance between aggressive factors and mucosal defensive factors. Stimulation of lateral growth of undifferentiated epithelium concurrent with the removal of necrotic tissue is important in the healing process. EGF stimulates the growth of these cells and is present in saliva. In animals when the salivary glands have been removed, delayed healing in both DU and GU results. Salivary content of EGF has been found to be significantly lower in GU and DU patients than in healthy subjects. Similarly smoking suppresses EGF in saliva as well as delaying ulcer healing. Growth hormone, gastrin, and growth hormone releasing factor (GRF) facilitate ulcer healing.[34]

Experimental gastric and duodenal ulcers. Studying ulcers from the time of onset to further progression in animals has given added important information in the study of ulcers. Motility abnormalities, cytoprotective mechanisms, abnormal acid emptying, and a "misplaced mix of duodenal bicarbonate and acid" are found to play important roles in PUD.[63]

Gastric ulcer. Prostaglandins at a dose lower than needed to reduce gastric acid secretion were shown to protect GU and DU from effects of concentrated ethanol and indomethacin. This action, termed "cytoprotection," served to *prevent* acute hemorrhagic erosions. The essential part of mucosal protection was the functional maintenance of mucosal blood flow. The status of the microcirculation determined the extent of vascular damage. Rapid restitution of cell migration occurs after superficial injury, whereas regeneration requires cell division or proliferation to fill deeper defects in the mucosa. Sulfhydryls and prostaglandins are able to minimize or *prevent* endothelial injury and maintain blood flow in subepithelial capillaries in this situation. If the damage is deep cell proliferation or regeneration involving epithelial cells, fibroblasts, and angiogenesis is required to repair the injury.[63]

Motility changes contribute to the pathogenesis of both GU and DU. Muscle spasm in the stomach tends to cause congestive hypoxia and congestion, which may lead to hemorrhagic injury. Relieving this spasm by administration of papaverine or related drugs may tend to *prevent* this. High-amplitude gastric contractions of prolonged duration cause gastric mucosal lesions.

Duodenal ulcer. The pathogenesis of a DU seems to be multifactorial; this includes factors of increased acid and pepsin output, decreased bicarbonate secretion, and rapid gastric emptying of acid and pepsin. Aggressive factors (manifested as acid and pepsin) and duodenal, pancreatic, and biliary bicarbonate (the defensive forces) need to be transported into the proximal duodenum, which is regulated by gastroduodenal motility. Normally this neutralization of acid occurs in the proximal duodenum with mixing of acid and bicarbonate produced by Brunner's glands and pancreas. In ulcer disease the locus of neutralization may shift distally; acidity in the proximal duodenum is increased (referred to as a "displaced mix"). Rapid gastric emptying of fluids is observed in most patients with uncomplicated DU. DU alters the normal myoelectric migrating complex (MMC), decreasing frequency of the duodenal slow waves. Hence a DU may occur even in the presence of decreased acid output if duodenal dysmotility leads to disturbed acid neutralization. Bicarbonate secretion was found to be decreased before the development of DU resulting from decreased submucosal Brunner's gland secretion.[63]

Treatment and prevention of peptic ulcer disease. In considering therapy and especially prevention, the epidemiology of PU has to be considered particularly in treatment of the older age groups.[63]

The annual incidence (new cases) is estimated to be about 2 to 3/1000; the 1-year prevalence (number of cases at a specific time) is about 17/1000 and the lifetime prevalence is approximately 5% to 10%. Hospitalizations for bleeding remains approximately the same at 30 to 40/100,000, although the number of surgeries, hospitalizations, and deaths has decreased. The incidence of PUD complications appears proportional to advancing age. About 80% of ulcer deaths occur in individuals above ages 65; the average mortality of complicated ulcers in the elderly is about 30%. The average age for death from PUD has increased from 65 to 70 years. Mortality for GU is higher than that for DU.[47]

Decreased mucosal defense is illustrated by the cigarette smoker who takes a maintenance level of 300 mg ranitidine. The smoker's recurrence rate for DU for this dose is comparable to the nonsmoker taking 150 mg.[35]

Healing ulcers by decreasing gastric acidity theoretically aims to restore the balance between the intragastric acidity (aggressive factors) and mucosal defenses.[20]

Most DU patients have increased basal acid secretion throughout the day and night as well as a prolonged secretory response to food. H_2-receptor antagonists, however, demonstrate that suppression of nocturnal gastric acidity without suppression of daytime acidity is sufficient for healing. Increasing acid suppression merely accelerates healing so that moderate acid suppression has resulted in healing at 4 to 8 weeks compared to that produced by more potent suppression at 2 to 4 weeks.[20]

GU has demonstrated no definite mathematical relationship between healing rates and degree of acid suppression. Extending duration of treatment was found to be more effective than increasing H_2-receptor antagonist dose for healing GU. Healing rates of greater than 90% are common at 8 weeks for DU, whereas similar rates require 10 to 12 weeks for GU. Some elect to treat GU for 8 weeks, checking at this time endoscopically or radiographically

for malignancy, when about 80% of ulcers will be healed. Eight to twelve week treatment is advocated in the elderly and smokers because unhealed GUs are more likely to result in symptomatic recurrences and increase of morbidity and mortality in the elderly.[20]

Half of the healing dose of H_2-receptor antagonists given at bedtime resulted in DU recurrence at an annual rate of about 25% to 30% compared with 70% in placebo treated patients.[20]

Options for managing DU recurrence include intermittent full-dose treatment, chronic maintenance treatment with low doses of H_2-receptor antagonists, and treatment for symptoms only. Patients who continue to smoke, are elderly, or have had ulcer complications should have continuous maintenance therapy for at least 1 to 2 years.[20]

The safety of the newer H_2-receptor antagonists appears similar to that indicated by the many studies performed on cimetidine though fewer studies of H_2-receptor antagonists have been conducted. Cimetidine is considered a very safe drug: frequency of side effects is about 4.4%. Gastrointestinal (GI) symptoms, particularly diarrhea (1%) and nausea and vomiting (0.8%), are the most frequent adverse reactions. Oral and intravenous (IV) cimetidine on occasion may cause minimal confusion, drowsiness, and headache. There has been no objective evidence that the incidence of central nervous system (CNS) reaction is higher with cimetidine than with the other H_2-receptor antagonists. The antiandrogen effects of cimetidine, gynecomastia and impotence, have been rare and occur primarily with the use of high doses for prolonged periods as given for the Zollinger-Ellison syndrome. There was no evidence of higher incidence of sexual dysfunction when using ordinary doses as compared to that of control subjects.[20]

Cimetidine binds reversibly to the hepatic cytochrome P-450 microsomal enzyme system and hence has the potential to elevate blood levels of phenytoin, theophylline, and warfarin. The prothrombin time ratio increased very minimally during administration of cimetidine, then stabilized in 8 days. Elevation of the theophylline level was not considered a problem, and there was no significant difference between the effects of cimetidine and ranitidine. For added safety the blood levels should be monitored for toxicity.

Related gastric disorders

Nonsteroidal antiinflammatory drugs. As was noted in the discussion of GERD, ulcers may be prevented by use of alternate therapy in the treatment of various diseases, or by dosage and timing change of medications associated with PUD and patient selection or concomitant therapy.

There has been a substantial increase in peptic ulcer perforation, hemorrhage, and mortality especially in elderly women caused primarily by increased use of NSAIDs. The American Rheumatism Association Medical

Information System [ARAMIS] reports that NSAID users over age 60 are 2.5 times more likely to have a major complication compared to users below this age. They estimate 2600 excess deaths and 20,000 hospitalizations per year relating to rheumatoid arthritis alone. The Committee on Safety of Medicines estimates that 75% of bleeding and perforations and 90% of mortality attributed to use of NSAIDs occur in individuals over the age of 60.[31]

The elderly female is especially susceptible related in part to higher incidence of gastric ulcers. The dose of NSAIDs is often excessive when considering the weight of the individual, the increased half-life of many of the NSAIDs, and larger doses used for anti-inflammatory properties being unnecessary when used solely for analgesia.[1]

The incidence of gastric ulcers in elderly patients was much higher in women taking NSAIDs (25%) compared to 8% in male users and 7% in NSAID abstainers $p < 0.001$. Hemorrhage was as common in the NSAID aspirin-users (45%) compared with standard dose NSAIDs without aspirin (39%) even though 86% were taking 300 mg of aspirin or less per day.[3]

Gastric mucosal damage from NSAIDs is considered primarily from suppression of systemic and gastroduodenal prostaglandin synthesis. Acid secretion is depressed by prostaglandin binding to parietal cell receptors causing inhibition of adenylate cyclase and decreased release of histamine from the mucosa. Prostaglandins increase mucosal defense mechanisms by synthesis of gastroduodenal mucous and bicarbonate, increased mucosal blood flow, and regeneration of mucosa. Maximal damage from NSAIDs occurs as erosions, mucosal hemorrhages, gastritis, and ulcers primarily in the antrum and prepyloric areas.[31]

Regarding prophylaxis and treatment of NSAID gastropathy [perhaps toxicity], additional factors must be considered:

1. Prevalence and follow-up data suggest that almost 100% of NSAID users will have had ulcers.
2. The majority of these ulcers subside, perhaps reoccur, are superficial, and cause few or no symptoms.
3. ARAMIS study on rheumatoid arthritis patients suggests that serious complications occur in about one per thousand patient—drug years—per year incidence of 0.1%.
4. In elderly individuals taking NSAIDs, 76% of gastric ulcers and 27% of duodenal ulcers are likely to be asymptomatic before hemorrhage or perforation making it more difficult to decide which patients should be treated to prevent these catastrophies.
5. Serious complications are more common in the elderly female.[3,31]

Misoprostol 100-200 ug q.i.d. given with NSAIDs resulted in less than two percent ulcer occurrence using the higher dose compared to 22% without misoprostol. H2-re- ceptor antagonists are of little value for NSAID GU but probably worthwhile for NSAID DU. It appears unreasonable to give misoprostol to all patients taking NSAIDs, including those taking one aspirin per day to prevent the one patient in a thousand or less from developing severe symptoms and subjecting these patients to possible diarrhea.[31]

Selection of high-risk patients who cannot be managed off NSAIDs should be considered for misoprostol treatment. These include the elderly especially elderly women, who have had recent or past episodes of peptic ulcer disease, hemorrhage, and large ulcers. NSAIDs may control the pain and the stiffness of elderly patients incapacitated by musculoskeletal disease making it difficult to stop medication. At times, acetaminophen, propoxyphene, or salsalate may be substituted for NSAIDs. Attempts should be made to stop NSAIDs or at least use a lower dose, an analgesic dose when possible. Physical therapy may be helpful. In rheumatoid arthritis, 10 mg/d of Prednisone may be tried. Smoking and alcohol intake should be discontinued. NSAID drug holiday should be tried periodically. When NSAIDs are necessary, the suggestion has been given to try to stop misoprostol in 3 months as studies on aspirin and indomethacin suggest mucosal adaptation to continued ingestion. Seventy percent of NSAID complications are thought to occur during the first few months of therapy. If symptoms develop when taking NSAIDs suggesting a possible ulcer, endoscopy should be considered. There does not appear to be any significant difference in the various NSAIDs causing complications although less potent drugs have been advised.[3,31]

Stress ulcers. "Stress ulcers are defined as acute gastric and duodenal mucosal lesions occurring in critically ill patients. These may be multiple small mucosal defects or single ulcers and occur mainly after multiple trauma, burns, sepsis, or after major surgery."[52] Stress ulcers commonly are complicated by bleeding and perforation.

The lesions develop when there is a back diffusion of acid into the mucosa; this commonly occurs when there is decreased blood flow. A drop of pH below 6.7 to 6.5 in the lamina propria causes mucosal ulcerations. The mucosa is protected by bicarbonate, which creates an alkaline microenvironment in the mucosa as well as below a necrotic layer of cells referred to as "mucoid cap." Overlying this is mucous gel, which serves as a further barrier against hydrogen ions and pepsin entering the mucosa. The bicarbonate facilitates rapid restitution and migration of cells into the ulcer defect.[52]

Two factors have contributed to a marked improvement in therapy and prevention: the routine prophylaxis with an H_2-receptor blocker and antacids and a better understanding of the pathophysiology. Treatment concentrates on antacids to maintain a pH above 4, suppression of acid secretion with H_2-receptor antagonist, and maintenance of all body functions. Prostaglandins and sucralfate have not been effective, even though NSAIDs increase permeability of H^+ ions and inhibit prostaglandin synthesis.

Intraluminal buffering plays an important role in acid neutralization in the duodenum and is achieved by bicarbonate flux from bile and pancreatic secretion. This buffering is facilitated by acid's coming in contact with the proximal duodenum, which in turn causes an increase in pancreatic and biliary bicarbonate secretion.[52]

***Helicobacter pylori* infections.** Serologic tests in a study in Switzerland showed that a large proportion of healthy people (49%) had antibodies (anti-Hp [ELISA]) against *Helicobacter pylori*, whereas only 34% had active infection (13_C-urea breath test). Theoretically those who remained infected or were reinfected had a defect in the gastric mucosa that made it susceptible to *H. pylori* colonization and in turn vulnerable to acid attack.[47]

Patchett supports the contention that eradication of *H. pylori* from the gastric antrum favorably and significantly alters the natural history of peptic ulcer disease. At least 90% of all DUs and a large majority of GUs are associated with antral *H. pylori* infection. Of 100 patients 51 had DU with *H. pylori;* initially the DU responded to therapy and the *H. pylori* was eradicated by bismuth and antibiotics. In 33 patients test results remained negative for *H. pylori* and DU at 1 year while 18 became *H. pylori* positive and of these 12 had recurrent peptic disease (DU, 5; duodenitis, 7). A treatment program for active *H. pylori* could be considered for frequent recurrent DU.[45]

Nonulcer dyspepsia—functional dyspepsia. Functional dyspepsia is a common clinical syndrome consisting of episodic or persistent abdominal symptoms often related to eating. This is interpreted as arising from the stomach but with no apparent organic or anatomic abnormality present.[9] The patient often experiences upper abdominal pain or discomfort, nausea or vomiting, postprandial fullness, early satiety, anorexia, and bloating.

Although symptomatically similar to GERD and PUD this condition, diagnosed by the exclusion of the aforementioned, should be differentiated in the physician's mind as it does not lend itself to prevention readily if at all; hence preventive therapy is unlikely to be successful.

Excessive acid production, *H. pylori*, somatization disorder, and environmental factors such as diet, smoking, or alcohol use do not contribute significantly to this condition. Abnormal gastrointestinal motility may play a role, warranting a trial of prokinetic agents. There may also be a greater perception of gut function.

These patients appear to have a high negative perception of major life events, which may contribute to the pathogenesis of nonulcer dyspepsia. The number of daily "hassles" representing minor events and nuances of life is probably not different from that of controls. The effect of events is to disrupt social relationships and activities that represent the pattern of daily stress. A trial of fluoxetine hydrochloride or trazodone hydrochloride may help.[9]

Summary of peptic ulcer disease

PUD reached a peak in 1950 and has declined since. This decline began before the introduction of cimetidine. Since 1980 there has been a 100% increase in hospitalizations for bleeding gastric ulcers considered to be related to NSAIDs. The mechanisms of ulcer formation of gastric ulcers, stress ulcers, and NSAID ulcers are similar, representing primarily a loss of mucosal defense. "Cytoprotection" provided by prostaglandins plays an instrumental role in these three ulcers. The mechanism for developing DU primarily concerns acid and pepsin output; modifications of bicarbonate secretion and acid delivery to the duodenal bulb probably also contribute significantly.

The discussion of experimental gastric and duodenal ulcers is intended to facilitate understanding of these two entities. Therapy and prevention of DUs and GUs and their differences have been discussed, including delay in healing from smoking, which may require larger doses of H_2-receptor antagonists.

GASTRIC CARCINOMA

Surveillance programs for premalignant and early malignant lesions by interval gastroscopy for upper gastrointestinal x-rays can be recommended in geographic areas with high incidence such as Japan and China, where preventive screening programs are carried out.[37] Japan's age-adjusted mortality for gastric carcinoma was found to be the greatest in the world in 1960 and has remained so. This led to a mass survey for gastric cancer in 1960.[27] This surveillance has progressively increased in number, having a governmental goal of an annual examination rate of 30% of those at risk, age 40 years and older. In 1978-1979 the incidence per 100,000 was 50 males and 25 females, which compares to the lowest rate in the world, that is, the United States having a male and female rate of about 5 per 100,000.[27]

Photoflurographic air contrast studies using seven views were standardized in 1984 for asymptomatic persons and scheduled every 1 to 2 years. Thirteen percent required full-size films, endoscopy with/without biopsy, and follow-up.

Studies in a localized screening area during 1960 to 1986 in Japan of all gastric carcinomas revealed an increase of percentage of early cancers (limited to mucosa and submucosa) from 13.8% in 1960 to 1964 to 62.1% in 1985 to 1986. The average annual detection rate, however, remained about the same (0.18 to 0.20%).[27] However, age-adjusted studies demonstrated a decreased incidence from 1960 to 1980, with a fall of mortality rate to 31% in males and 20.8% in females. Likewise, the risk of dying from cancer of the stomach among screened cases was 50% of those detected by other means.

There has been a marked decrease in incidence and mortality of gastric carcinoma in Western countries, and perhaps there may be a trend in Japan because of modifications of diet. In Japan there appears to be a general agreement that a double-prong approach, consisting of prevention (dietary modification and incidence reduction) and early detection and reduction of mortality, should be used. Mass screening has been advised only for Japan, but screening for specific high-risk groups should be strongly advised. An example of this is the very common incidence of gastric cancer in the mountainous regions of Italy.

Surveillance is also recommended for gastric epithelial dysplasia, adenomatous polyps of the stomach, and adenomatous polyposis, the latter because of a 40% incidence of polyps in the duodenum and stomach.[37] Gastric ulcer is evaluated for malignancy usually by its endoscopic and x-ray appearance and biopsies (6-8) when possible around its margin. Recommendations vary considerably because of cost of follow-up, but endoscopy is usually favored at least for part of the follow-up study. Establishing complete healing is essential, and after this occurs, follow-up studies are usually not done.

LIVER
Hepatitis

Epidemiology. "The acute and chronic consequences of hepatitis B virus [HBV] infection are major health problems in the United States. The reported incidence of acute hepatitis B increased 37% from 1979 to 1989, and an estimated 200,000 to 300,000 new infections occurred annually during the period 1980-1991. The estimated 1 to 1.25 million persons with chronic HBV infection in the United States are potentially infectious to others. In addition, many chronically infected persons are at risk of long-term sequelae, such as chronic liver disease and primary hepatocellular carcinoma; each year approximately 4000 to 5000 of these persons die from chronic liver disease."[40]

Hepatitis markers. Acute Hepatitis A [HAV] is diagnosed by IgM anti-HAV, whereas past infection is diagnosed by IgG anti-HAV. HAV is a rare cause of fulminant hepatitis but does not progress to chronic liver disease and there are no chronic carriers.

Diagnosis of acute Hepatitis B [HBV] is diagnosed by IgM anti-HBc and usually the presence of serum HBsAg. Rarely, this latter marker is not positive early. Recovery is characterized serologically by the presence of IgG anti-HBc, anti-HBs, and at times anti-HBe. Acute hepatitis A, B, or C may be relatively asymptomatic and illness and diagnosis missed. The marker for Hepatitis C is not very precise and may be delayed for several weeks or months. During early, acute HBV, markers of high HBV replication, HBeAG, and HBV DNA may be present. In chronic HBV (symptoms for more than 6 months) HBsAg remains positive, while replicative markers may persist.

The diagnosis of delta Hepatitis (HDV) is diagnosed by anti-HD and occurs either at the time of acute HBV or in the presence of chronic HBV. More severe sequelae of HBV (fulminant hepatitis, chronic active hepatitis, and cirrhosis) may be associated with HBV.

Vaccination. The most recent preventive recommendations regarding active and passive immunization for hepatitis B virus are listed in the *Morbidity and Mortality Weekly Report (MMWR)* published November 22, 1991, issued by the Center for Disease Control.[40] The detailed report can be obtained from Superintendent of Documents, U.S. Government Printing Office, Washington, D.C. 20402-9325, (202-783-3238).

Various factors negatively influence antibody response to Hepatitis B vaccine, including increasing age over 50, injection into the buttock, obesity, improper storage of vaccine (freezing) and cases of immunosuppression that include end-stage renal disease, chemotherapy, positive HIV status, and alcoholic liver disease.[40,46]

Patients who have had hepatitis B vaccine have a positive anti-HBs, whereas persons with resolved HBV infections have both anti-HBs and anti-HBc. In patients with resolved HBV infections serologic evidence of only one positive test often indicates poor immunity.[46]

Drug-induced liver disease. Drug-induced liver disease (DILD) is thought to represent 2% to 5% of hospital admissions for jaundice in the United States and 10% to 43% of hospital cases of "acute hepatitis" abroad. More than 600 drugs have been incriminated.[36] Their avoidance or circumspect use constitutes prevention of this malady.

Traditional symptoms of hypersensitivity such as fever, rash, and eosinophilia act through drug allergy mechanisms. Examples include chlorpromazine, dapsone, phenytoin, sulfonamides, erythromycin, estolate, and halothane.

Acute DILD is of the cytotoxic (hepatocellar necrosis, steatosis), cholestatic, mixed cytotoxic-cholestatic, granulomatous, and vascular types. Hepatic necrosis may suggest acute viral hepatitis. Serum glutamic-oxaloacetic transaminase (SGOT) and serum glutamic-pyruvic transaminase (SGPT) levels may be elevated 10 to 100 times. The most important clinical aspect is that this may develop into fulminant hepatic failure, which carries a case fatality rate of up to 50%.[36]

Chronic DILD includes chronic necroinflammatory disease, chronic steatosis, pseudoalcoholic liver disease, chronic cholestasis, granulomatous disease, vascular injury, cirrhosis, and noncirrhotic portal hypertension. There are two major categories of hepatotoxins in acute drug-induced liver injury: intrinsic and idiosyncratic. Intrinsic (true or predictable) hepatotoxins are agents that lead to a high incidence of hepatic injury in exposed individuals. Idiosyncratic (nonpredictable) hepatotoxins have a latent period, which is variable and longer than that seen with intrinsic hepatotoxins (hours to days).[36]

Genetic and other factors modify susceptibility to idiosyncratic injury. These include polymorphic differences in drug metabolism, cytochrome P-450 isoenzymes, and their respective genes and the effects of alcohol on drug toxicity. At least 10 distinct P-450 gene families have been identified; families I, II, and III are clinically important in terms of drug metabolism and potential hepatotoxicity.

Isolated liver enzyme elevations in the asymptomatic patient. The frequent use of the automated laboratory tests (discussed in Chapter 7) may result in elevation of results of one or two enzyme tests, often referred to as liver function tests, in asymptomatic patients.[33] This has been evaluated by Kaplan for patients for whom only the elevated enzyme test result was abnormal. These tests include alkaline phosphatase, alanine aminotransferase (ALT; SGPT), aspartate aminotransferace (AST; SGOT), and γ-glutamyl transpeptidase (GGT).

The normal range includes two standard deviations of the mean, or 95%. Five percent of healthy patients, however, may have values outside this range. Isoenzyme studies to differentiate between bone and liver disease are often difficult to interpret. GGT is not elevated in bone disorders and usually is elevated in liver disease although occasionally it is normal in early liver dysfunction.[33]

AST/ALT is used to diagnose alcoholic liver disease; this ratio above 2-3 and ALT less than 300 suggest alcoholic liver disease; a ratio above 3 is considered highly suggestive. ALT is usually not higher than 200 and AST above 300 in alcoholic liver disease. The abnormal ratio is maintained even though there are marked elevations from concomitant heart failure or viral hepatitis.[33]

Skeletal and cardiac muscle damage may cause elevation of both AST and ALT, primarily of AST; elevated ALT may occur with secondary liver dysfunction. Vigorous exercise such as jogging may cause a transient elevation of both values.

GGT may be elevated in patients taking barbiturates and dilantin or consuming large quantities of alcohol. One has to be cautious about overinterpreting GGT elevation as being indicative of surreptitious alcohol intake.[33]

Alcoholic liver disease

Alcoholic liver disease is primarily preventable, of course, by abstinence. Secondary prevention of further damage, or primary prevention by very early diagnosis, depends on aggressive intervention where abstinence is a problem to the patient and on long-term follow-up observation.

Three major patterns have been associated with chronic alcohol consumption: alcoholic steatosis (alcoholic fatty liver), alcoholic steatonecrosis (alcoholic hepatitis), and alcoholic cirrhosis.[14]

Most people who drink alcohol do not develop these lesions although at times even modest drinkers may do so. The incidence of serious liver disease increases in men who consume more than 80 g (equivalent to a six-pack of beer) of alcohol per day and in men and women who consume more than 20 g of alcohol per day for 10 years.

The metabolism of ethanol occurs primarily in the liver and involves oxidation of ethanol. It may be associated with several toxic consequences considered to be the major route through which alcoholic liver disease is produced. The principal route in nonalcoholic subjects involves three hepatic enzyme systems. The primary systems two cytosolic enzymes, alcohol dehydrogenase (ADH) and aldehyde dehydrogenase, which form acetaldehyde, acetate, and reducing equivalents. In chronic alcoholic subjects cytosolic metabolism of ethanol is supplemented by a third enzyme system, the microsomal oxidizing enzymes (MOES). In the presence of oxygen and the reduced form of nicotinamide-adenine dinucleotide phosphate (NADPH) MOES oxidizes ethanol to acetaldehyde, NADP, and water.[14]

Acetaldehyde is a highly reactive substance with numerous toxic and metabolic effects. Because MOES require oxygen, they may cause an insufficient oxygen supply, producing injury in the centrilobular area.

In alcoholic hepatitis histologic features are increased fat, presence of Mallory's bodies, acute inflammation, and centrilobular fibrosis.

An extrahepatic consequence of ethanol metabolism is malnutrition, associated with decreased food intake, impaired assimilation, and storage. Recent evidence has shown that ethanol is also metabolized extrahepatically, namely, through ADH activity in the stomach. Women have significantly less of this activity, suggesting that the same amount of ethanol produces higher alcohol levels, perhaps explaining an apparent increased susceptibility to alcoholic liver disease. Chronic alcohol consumption has also been demonstrated to decrease gastric ADH activity in both sexes so that a given oral amount produccs higher blood levels in the habitual drinker.[14]

In alcoholic liver disease as in many other types of liver injury the height of the liver enzyme level elevations correlates poorly with the severity of the clinical manifestations and histopathologic injury. The AST (SGOT) level is disproportionally more elevated than the ALT (SGPT) level; 80% of patients have an AST/ALT ratio of 2 or more. The mortality of patients with acute alcohol liver injury ranges from between 0% and 50% and seems to be determined by three variables: the severity of the acute alcohol induced injury, the presence or absence of cirrhosis, and the continuance of alcohol ingestion.

Abstinence is considered extremely important as most patients (especially males) with acute alcoholic hepatitis improve clinically with abstinence and resumption of a nutritious diet during the acute management. The variable tolerance to alcohol is demonstrated in epidemiologic surveys reporting cirrhosis in fewer than 20% of males consuming an average of 160 g (two six-packs of beer) of ethanol daily for more than 10 years. An additional 40% had potentially precirrhotic lesions but the remaining 40% to 50% had no histologic evidence of hepatic necrosis or fibrosis. Encephalopathy, peripheral edema, ascites, hypoalbuminemia, hyperbilirubinemia, anemia, and hypoprothrombinemia are factors that correlate with an increased risk of death after 1 month of acute illness. Alcohol abstinence and a good nutritious diet without limiting protein and given as frequent feedings including a late evening meal have been advocated. Decreased hepatic glycogen reserves demonstrate that these patients cope poorly with even brief episodes of fasting. Adjunctive treatments such as androgens, D-penicillamine, colchicine, and prophyliouracil appear to be of no value for acute alcoholic hepatitis or chronic alcoholic liver disease.[14]

Primary biliary cirrhosis and primary hemochromatosis

For many years symptoms may be absent or very mild and hence diagnosis and awareness of illness not forthcoming. Blood tests for primary biliary cirrhosis and hemochromatosis may, however, yield positive and diagnostic results.[59,62] There may be a mild hepatomegaly and slight elevation of transaminase and alkaline phosphatase as well as some weakness, lethargy, and abdominal discomfort. The diagnosis is first made by considering the possibility of hemochromatosis and therefore ordering appropriate tests. An elevated serum iron level, usually greater than 200 μg/dl (n = 80-120); serum ferritin level of 200 to 5000 (n = 10-200 ng/ml); or transferrin saturation (serum iron divided by total iron binding capacity) of 50% to 100% (n = 25-50) suggests the diagnosis. Early the arthralgias, loss of libido or potency, and a bluish discoloration of the skin may not be apparent. It is important to make an early diagnosis as *prevention* of significant iron stores by repeated phlebotomy will *prevent* complications of cirrhosis, liver cancer, severe heart disease, diabetes, and possibly arthropathy and loss of libido.[62]

Early the diagnosis of primary biliary cirrhosis may also be overlooked and be first suggested by finding a high alkaline phosphatase level. The patient may remain asymptomatic for as long as a decade. Early there may be no physical findings. A finding of a high alkaline phosphatase level with pruritus in a middle-aged woman 35 to 60 years old should suggest the possibility of primary biliary cirrhosis. A positive antimitochondrial antibody (AMA) finding, which is detectable in 90% to 95% of cases and is uncommon in other disorders, is diagnostic. As in hemochromatosis a liver biopsy should be obtained.[59]

Hepatocellular carcinoma

Hepatocellular carcinoma (HCC) is a preventable late result of not picking up occult early liver disease. In the United States 50% of hepatocellular carcinoma has underlying cirrhosis. Less than 5% of patients with long-standing cirrhosis may eventually develop HCC.[57] Luk does not advise a regular surveillance program for patients with cirrhosis.[37] A major risk factor for the development of HCC is chronic HBV infection. The HBV DNA becomes inte-

grated into the tumor genomic DNA (See the section on screening for occult HBV).[57]

GALLSTONES

For many years physicians advocated cholecystectomy for the prevention of cancer of the gallbladder, pancreatitis, and cholecystitis with or without duct obstruction. This was in essence preventive advice. This position has been reversed.

There are approximately 20 million cases of gallstones in the United States and about 1 million new patients yearly. Approximately 500,000 cholecystectomies are performed yearly at a cost around $1 billion.[53] Gallstone related symptoms and complications are among the most common causes of hospital admission of gastroenterologic disorders. Several studies evaluating silent gallstones for incidence of subsequent symptoms and complications have been performed.[49] A silent gallstone was defined as one that does not cause biliary pain or biliary complications such as acute cholecystitis. Such symptoms as flatulence, belching, and fatty food intolerance were not considered as representing gallbladder disease. "Life-table analysis demonstrates the accumulative probability of developing biliary pain from silent stones to be 10% at 5 years, 15% at 10 years and 18% at 15 and 20 years."[49] This demonstrates a decrease in yearly risk of developing pain with the passage of time. On the other hand of those patients who became symptomatic over the previous year 69% developed gallbladder pain in the next 2 years and 6% required cholecystectomy. The risk of acute cholecystitis with pancreatitis appears to be about 3% per year. The incidence of gallbladder cancer in patients with gallstones is listed as anywhere from 0.09% to 1%. Surgery is not advised for silent gallstones.[49]

About 25% of obese patients who lose weight rapidly (e.g., 20 kg in 2 to 4 months) develop gallstones. A study indicates that this is *preventable* by use of ursodeoxycholic acid.[53]

PANCREAS
Pancreatitis

About 90% of chronic and calcific pancreatitis in the United States is caused by alcohol, whereas in some European countries idiopathic and miscellaneous causes predominate.[4] Chronic alcoholism is often defined in terms of consumption of 80 g of alcohol daily (equivalent to a six-pack of beer) for 10 years. The consumption of at least 50 g of alcohol/day has been considered to be required to cause alcohol-induced pancreatitis. This quantity may be less in susceptible individuals—those who have dietary, genetic, or metabolic predisposition as well as hyperlipidemia and hypercalcemia. In these individuals pancreatitis may develop with as little as 20 g/day: that is, a half bottle of wine or two to three jiggers of hard liquor. The quantity and not the type of alcohol seems important. Prevention in this disease is therefore usually prevention of alcoholism per se.

Chronic alcoholic pancreatitis versus idiopathic pancreatitis. Hayakawa et al. compared the features of chronic alcoholic pancreatitis (n = 88) with those of idiopathic pancreatitis (n = 67).[24] The 155 patients who had a known 3-year course were examined again 5 years later. At the time of diagnosis significant differences included severe pain (59% versus 33%), pancreatitic calcification (63% versus 31%), and overt diabetes (48% versus 17%); the higher values represented alcoholic pancreatitis.

The rate of abstinence was higher in groups with pain relief and the cumulative 5-year mortality rate was higher in alcoholic than idiopathic pancreatitis (26% versus 10%). Results suggested that a more favorable course of the disease can be accomplished by abstinence from alcohol.

Pancreatitis secondary to severe hypertriglyceridemia. One type of pancreatitis is certainly subject to prevention: pancreatitis associated with hypertriglyceridemia, which can be reversed.

Patients with pancreatitis commonly have elevated triglyceride levels that predate onset of the disease. Acute pancreatitis does not appear unless the triglyceride level reaches 1000 to 2000 mg/dl; there is a preexisting abnormality in lipid metabolism, whether or not the patient ingests alcohol. Lipoprotein electrophoresis shows that type V is the most common pattern and hyperchylomicronemia a key element.[64]

Other conditions that may be associated with marked elevated triglyceride levels include pregnancy, estrogen therapy, use of β-blockers, and vitamin A therapy. Pancreatitis (from all causes) in pregnancy may have a mortality rate as high as 20%, most commonly as a result of cholelithiasis, but hypertriglyceridemia has to be considered. Women using oral contraceptives in whom severe hypertriglyceridemia develops often have prompt and marked hypertriglyceridemia and abdominal pain after starting oral contraceptives. The estrogen of the oral contraceptive induces hypertriglyceridemia. Hyperlipidemia is often present in other family members and patients may have obesity and impaired glucose tolerance. The pattern may simulate gallbladder colic, and many of these patients have had a previous laparotomy for presumed cholecystitis.[64]

Hyperchylomicronemia may or may not occur. The clinical picture may suggest acute pancreatitis, often not very severe and having a normal ultrasound computed tomography (CT) scan result. About 50% of these patients with abdominal pain have normal serum amylase and lipase levels. Occasionally there may be a mild asymptomatic hypertriglyceridemia that develops into gross hyperchylomicronemia caused by use of drugs such as estrogens, vitamin A, β-blockers, and thiazides.

Managing an attack of pancreatitis with marked hypertriglyceridemia involves initially decreasing the triglyceride level to below 500 mg/dl to alleviate abdominal pain.

Hypolipidemic therapy consisting of diet, gemfibrozil, clofibrate, nicotinic acid, or a combination is used to lower the triglyceride level. Feedback inhibition of pancreatic secretion to suppress nausea and abdominal pain may be accomplished by administering pancreatic extracts. After several weeks to months of levels below 500 mg/dl the pancreatic enzymes are stopped.[64]

Summary of pancreatitis. The diagnosis of pancreatitis can usually be made when a patient has abdominal pain and an elevated serum amylase level over three times the upper limit of normal. Other conditions also may cause amylase elevation. Amylase is composed of salivary isoamylase and pancreatic isoamylase. Pancreatitis does not necessarily indicate that pancreatic isoamylase is the predominant fraction. The two isoamylases may be differentiated by using lectin, which is a relatively specific inhibitor of salivary isoamylase.

Alcohol accounts for about 90% of chronic and calcific pancreatitis in the United States. Alcohol-induced pancreatitis usually entails a history of consumption of 50 g or more of alcohol/day times 10 years. Dietary, genetic, and metabolic features may affect the individual's susceptibility; however, abstinence or minimal use constitutes prevention.

Chronic alcoholic pancreatitis was compared to idiopathic pancreatitis and found to be the more serious disease. Abstinence from alcohol is an important factor affecting the progression of pancreatitis.

Pancreatitis associated with hypertriglyceridemia occurs at levels reaching 1000 to 2000 mg/dl. Pregnancy, estrogen therapy, β-blockers, and vitamin A therapy may precipitate pancreatitis. The pattern may simulate gallbladder colic, and many of these patients will have had a previous laparotomy for presumed cholecystitis. Using hypolipidemic agents plus diet to lower the triglycerides below 500 mg/dl usually alleviates the abdominal pain. Feedback inhibition of pancreatic secretion by pancreatic extracts is also used.

Carcinoma of the pancreas

There are 24,000 new cases of cancer of the pancreas and 20,000 cancer-related deaths annually in the United States. It is the fourth cause of cancer death in men and fifth in women. The mean age of onset is the seventh and eighth decades and there is a 2:1 male incidence.[11]

Cigarette smoking is considered a definite risk: the two pack/day smoker has twice the incidence of pancreatic cancer of the nonsmoker.[11] Those former smokers who had quit for 10 years had an incidence similar to that of lifelong nonsmokers.[7]

The vast majority of lesions are unresectable and surgery is used in only about 15% of the total number of cases presented. Most patients are deceased by 6 months and the 5-year survival is under 2%. In one study patients having all gross malignant disease removed plus adjuvant radiation and chemotherapy had a 20 month survival.[7]

Prevention (if this is possible) lies in tobacco abstinence.

COLON AND SMALL INTESTINE
Irritable bowel syndrome

Epidemiology. The irritable bowel syndrome (IBS) is probably *the most common of all GI disorders.* Surveys show that 7% to 15% of the population have symptoms without seeking medical care.[59] Some suggest that as many as 30% of the population will have symptoms at one time or another. IBS has a 3:1 female/male incidence and a 5:1 white/black incidence. Age prevalence is from 45 to 64 years. Most do not require hospitalization (at least not those patients released with a diagnosis of IBS), *but absenteeism from work attributed to IBS is second to absence caused by the common cold.*[55]

Diagnosis. The Manning criteria have been used to identify patients. These include abdominal pain relieved by defecation, more frequent and looser stools with the onset of pain, and bloating.[55] These criteria have been modified as follows[15]:

Symptoms are described as continuous or recurrent for at least three months and include: (1) abdominal pain or discomfort relieved with defecation or associated with a change in the frequency or consistency of stool; and (2) an irregular or varying pattern of defecation at least 25% of the time having three or more of the following: (a) altered stool frequency; (b) altered stool form [hard or loose/watery stool]; (c) altered stool passage [straining or urgency, feeling of incomplete evacuation]; (d) passage of mucosa; (e) bloating or feeling of abdominal distention.

The whole problem of IBS is described well by Heaton et al., who evaluated three groups of women 20 to 44 years of age, having 26 hospital patients with IBS, 27 women who had recurrent colonic pain but had not consulted a doctor (noncomplainers), and 27 healthy control women.[25] Control women previously considered as asymptomatic did list abdominal pain and bloating, but these were considerably more severe in IBS. In patients defecation was more frequent and more erratic in timing and stool form, interpreted as rapid fluctuations in intestinal transit time; urgency was four times that of the control group; straining to finish defecation was nine times the control rate and often accompanied by feelings of incomplete evacuation. This combination could lead to an erroneous diagnosis of constipation. IBS patients would commonly have straining even though the stools were normal. Noncomplainers were intermediate but more closely approximated the control group. The authors concluded that IBS patients had justified complaints and that their bowel function was definitely abnormal.

Psychological considerations in IBS. Several studies indicate that the psychiatric pathology of the IBS patient contributes significantly to a frequent seeking of medical care. Noncomplainers having similar GI complaints show little neuroticism and do not seek medical care for these symptoms. Psychometric test results were abnormal in 80% of IBS patients and psychiatric interview findings were considered abnormal in 100%. In 50% of patients stress aggravated symptoms or precipitated their initial onset. In these patients, avoidance of stress or its treatment may be preventive (see Chapter 12). IBS patients show a much greater propensity to report multiple complaints, have more surgical procedures, and overuse medical services.[69] These features are considered learned behavior from parents' response to symptoms and a result of the modeling demonstrated when they themselves are ill.[69] The sick role is often increased by the parent's giving the child toys, gifts, or ice cream while he or she is ill.[69] Stress does influence the course and possibly the onset of IBS but this association has been overestimated.

IBS symptoms

Constipation. Constipation is one of the most common office GI complaints, perhaps accounting for 2.5 million medical visits per year in the United States. Most patients can be successfully managed and this complaint prevented with relatively simple measures as constipation is a symptom and not a disease. It is important for the patient to define the complaint precisely and for the physician to identify possible causative factors.[68] Diagnostic criteria for functional constipation include two or more of the following present for at least 3 months, once organic abnormality has been excluded: "(1) straining more than 25% of the time; (2) hard stools for more than 25% of the time; (3) two or fewer bowel movements per week; and (4) incomplete evacuation more than 25% of the time." In general functional constipation is considered as separate from IBS if there is no alternating bowel pattern.[15]

Certain historical factors are associated with a greater risk for constipation (see the box below).

A colonic transit study should be considered if defecation is infrequent; that is, fewer than two per week for at

---

Risk factors for constipation

- Demographic status of older patients, decreased education, female sex, and nonwhite race
- Chronic illness
- Medications, e.g., opiates, psychotropics, anticonvulsants, anticholinergics, and bile acid binders
- Psychological status, e.g., depression and psychological stress
- Low-fiber diet
- Low activity level
- Medical diagnosis, e.g., diabetes, hypothyroidism, porphyrea, hyperparathyroidism, and pseudoobstruction

(From Drossman DA, Thompson WG: Management of irritable bowel syndrome and idiopathic constipation, *Am Gastroenteral Assoc,* annual postgraduate course, 1991.)

least 6 months. These patients often have palpable stool in the sigmoid area. The study is performed by using two different radiopaque markers given on consecutive days while the patient has a high-fiber diet and obtaining films at 48-hour intervals.[68] The passage of at least 80% of the markers 5 days after ingestion indicates normal transit.[15] About a third of the patients with infrequent defecation exhibit normal colonic transit and over 90% of these exhibit psychological distress with high scores for anxiety, depression, and somatization.[68] The remaining patients have slow colonic transit, which can be divided into three subgroups: "(1) the most common is colonic inertia in which transit is delayed in the proximal colon; (2) hind gut dysfunction in which transit is delayed in the left and rectosigmoid colons; (3) outlet dysfunction having stagnation in the rectum only."[68] The latter is common in children and the elderly and suggests anorectal dysfunction. The majority of constipated patients with slow transit have normal psychological profiles. Colonic inertia involves the entire enteric nervous system or smooth muscle, has persistent symptoms, and responds poorly to therapy. Where there are outlet obstruction and defecatory straining are present, anorectal manometry and defecography are used to evaluate the patient's problem. Inappropriate contraction of the external anal sphincter and puborectalis muscle during attempted expulsion may be demonstrated. Biofeedback may be completely successful, more so in children than adults.[68]

Therapy for constipation focuses around increasing the fiber in the diet, for example, up to 30 g/day of indigestible bran, fruits, or vegetables or use of soluble fiber bulk laxatives (e.g., psyllium products). This improves gut transit, stool frequency, and stool consistency and decreases intracolonic pressure, thereby reducing pain. Fiber increases the stool weight by binding intraluminal water, by stimulating bacterial growth, and by altering nondigestible characteristics of its chemical structure. This also results in more rapid transit. Hydrophilic properties of fiber can be overcome in the presence of dehydration. Therefore quantities of fluids sufficient to maintain hydration are needed. However, supplemental fiber may further impair contractile force in the dilated impacted colon. Initially laxatives or enemas are used to empty the colon intermittently to prevent overdistention.[50]

Drossman's advice on exercise and other life-style improvements, although not specific for IBS, encourages the patient to take some responsibility for his or her own health maintenance.[15] I heartily agree with this approach and believe it can be successful when there is a good patient-physician relationship including an adequate testing and instruction. Reviewing all of the findings as well as explaining the mechanisms of the pain and symptoms with the patient are essential. Where possible showing the patients the roentgenograms can facilitate this instruction.

The program I have followed for many years, which seems to be quite successful, includes the following:

- Stopping active, stimulant laxatives, when possible
- Increasing fiber content
- Stressing the importance of exercise, especially before breakfast, because exercise decreases transit time and theoretically may help relieve constipation[46]
- Eating a breakfast that has at least a moderate amount of fiber
- Drinking hot diluted orange juice (4 ounces of orange juice and 4 ounces of hot water mixed) on arising in the morning
- Using the urge for defecation even though it may be mild
- Sitting on the toilet for 15 minutes after breakfast reading, without emphasis on attempting to have a bowel movement
- Using a glycerin suppository in the morning if there is no bowel movement in 1 or 2 days and then if unsuccessful, having a small tap water enema
- Adding prunes or prune juice to breakfast if needed.

The program is less effective for delayed colon transit.

Diarrhea—IBS. Tenesmus in patients with chronic diarrhea is directly related to liquidity of stool, which may improve with the use of psyllium. Psyllium swells in water, forming a stiff mucilage and thereby increasing the firmness of stools and reducing stool frequency in people with diarrhea.[19] Side effects may include distention, flatulence, and intestinal obstruction.

Loperamide has morphinelike effects on gut motility without morphine's behavioral influence. It reduces frequency and improves stool consistency, urgency, and incontinence. The dose should not exceed 8 mg/day and works best when given 1 hour before meals.

Bloating. Certain foods may increase IBS symptoms. Caffeine in coffee, tea, cola, chocolate, and cocoa causes excessive intestinal secretion at a dosage of 60 to 150 mg (150 mg equals 1 cup of weak coffee) and may be a factor in diarrhea in patients with inadequate colonic reabsorption. Fat increases sigmoid contraction and IBS should be considered when LLQ (left lower quadrant) pain or splenic flexure syndrome occurs after a fatty meal.[5]

Lactase deficiency is inherited as a recessive trait and is common in most of the world's population. Half of individuals note symptoms with one or two glasses of milk; 60% are aware of milk intolerance. Postweaning decrease in lactase activity is the most common cause; symptoms usually appear in the late teens in the United States. Fructose malabsorption (gas, diarrhea) is to be suspected with such foods as apple purée and pear juice. Sorbitol (sugar alcohol) intolerance should be considered when there are increased symptoms from sugar-free gums, mints, apple juice, or pear juice.[5]

Patients' complaints of "too much gas" may refer to excessive eructation, bloating, and abdominal pain all attributed to too much gas in the gut or excessive passage of flatus.[6]

Ninety-nine percent of intestinal gas represents the five gases N_2, O_2, CO_2, H_2, and CH_4. These occur from swallowed air, production from within the gut, and diffusion from the blood into the gut lumen.[6]

Gas is produced in the gut when acid reacts with bicarbonate to release CO_2, or by intestinal bacteria. One milliequivalent (mEq) of acid with bicarbonate produces 22.4 ml of CO_2. The stomach normally secretes about 30 mEq of H^+ in response to a meal. Additional acid is released from ingested lipid, which is digested to fatty acids by pancreatic lipase; this releases about 100 mEq of fatty acids from 30 g of fat ingested in a fairly hearty meal. Theoretically 200 mEq of acid may be released and if completely neutralized may represent a liberation of about 3000 ml of CO_2.[6]

The major source of H_2 production in the gut is from the ingestion of carbohydrates poorly digested and hence malabsorbed in the small intestine. The massive quantities of gas produced after ingestion of beans are generated by stachyose and raffinose, which cannot be digested and are passed unabsorbed through the small bowel. These are fermented by colon bacteria with a direct release of H_2 and CO_2. Intestinal gases are highly soluble and diffuse rapidly between lumen and blood depending on the partial pressure gradient.[6]

Eructation may be influenced by posture, so that reclining supine causes a fluid layer to form over the gastroesophageal (GE) junction preventing belching.

The gastric gas bubble is largely N_2 and O_2 as it results from swallowed air rather than from production within the lumen. Chronic eructation does not remove gas from the stomach; rather the subject precedes each belch with a relaxation of the upper esophageal sphincter at the same time as a negative pressure is produced in the chest, thereby sucking air into the esophagus. This is almost immediately eructated, little reaching the stomach. The gas in the stomach of the chronic belcher is not helped by the use of anticholinergics, antacids, or simethicone. Using rapid infusion of argon into the duodenum and then studying volume and composition reveal that the intestines of the normal individual and IBS patient contain about 200 ml of gas. The intestinal gas remains normal in composition and volume and does not cause bloating and cramping. The primary abnormality appears to be a motility disorder that causes these patients to experience pain when their guts are distended by volumes of gas that are tolerated by normal subjects. Disorderly transit of gas through the gut together with increased sensitivity to bowel distention cause the symptoms.[6]

Passage of excessive flatus is related to gas production

and not air swallowing. The only feasible method to reduce flatus production is to consume a diet that reduces the quantity of carbohydrate reaching the colon: namely, a legume-free, low-wheat diet, and a lactose-free diet when indicated. High gas producers include beans, cabbage, and brussels sprouts; bread, pasta, and other wheat products; apples, pears, peaches, and prunes; and corn, oats, potatoes, and processed bran. Low gas producers include white rice, bananas, citrus fruits, grapes, hard cheese, meat, eggs, peanut butter, noncarbonated sugar-containing beverages, saccharin, and unprocessed bran.[6] Prevention of this often embarrassing problem is, therefore, largely dietary.

Anticholinergics are of limited value in combatting abdominal cramping. Lying down and using a heating pad may help relieve severe cramping. Metoclopramide used may be tried to stimulate motility.

Abdominal pain. An abdominal pain entity that should be distinguished from IBS is "chronic intractable abdominal pain" or chronic undiagnosed abdominal pain.[17] This pain primarily reflects a somatization or hypochondriasis, is vague, and does not specifically relate to defecation or any other physiological processes, thereby differing from IBS. Diagnosis depends on whether it has been present for more than 6 months, is unresponsive to treatment, limits physical and social activities, and is unresponsive to medication. The pain is often present for years and described as "the worse ever," and the patient demands that the physician "do something now." Particularly the multiple complaints are described as metaphors, for example, as "tormenting," "agonizing," or a sensation of being "seared by hot coals." The patient often does not exhibit clinical features associated with acute abdominal pain and hence the physician interprets the pain as not real. The syndrome may be precipitated by a recent stress. The patient often has inadequate coping strategies or bad childhood experiences and may seek secondary gain through drugs, disability, or litigation.[16]

The pain should be accepted as real, narcotics and benzodiazepines should be avoided, and the goal should be reset to achieve improvement in function despite the pain rather than complete relief of pain. NSAIDs, aspirin, and tricyclic antidepressants such as imipramine, amitriptyline, and doxepin, which stimulate serotonin, may be helpful for depression as well as having an independent analgesic effect through action on the descending inhibitory pain control system. The physician should avoid implying that the condition is imagined, as this is counterproductive. Indicate that other medical disciplines, including psychiatric consultation, may be useful, to achieve maximal benefit.

Therapy—emphasis on physician-patient relationship. Developing a good physician-patient relationship is essential to the successful treatment of IBS and its prevention of recurrence. It may determine why 30% to 90% of

IBS patients respond to "placebo."[15] A history should be obtained through a nondirective patient centered interview; it should be nonjudgmental and determine the patient's understanding of the illness and his or her concerns. Establishing why the patient is being seen at this time can give insight about his or her personal concerns as well as environmental stresses.[15] Patient satisfaction and symptom improvement are likely to occur if the patient gains a realistic understanding of the disease and the factors contributing to its exacerbation. The physician should emphasize that both physiologic and psychological factors interact to produce the symptoms and that the disorder is not solely organic or psychological. It is a very real disorder in which the intestine is oversensitive to a variety of stimuli and motility response is exaggerated. It is best for the physician to state recommendations firmly and involve the patient in the treatment ("Let me suggest a few types of treatment for you to consider").[15] The patient should be assured that further studies or treatment will be done when clinically indicated. There should be continuing care through brief, regular appointments with the physician, which may be as infrequent as one to two times per year. This reinforces the physician's commitment to the patient and helps minimize "doctor shopping." Reassurance of the absence of more serious disease is important.[15]

Summary of irritable bowel syndrome. IBS is a common entity having a threefold greater incidence among females than males and fivefold greater incidence among whites than blacks. Its symptoms include abdominal pain relieved by bowel movements, more frequent and looser stools with the onset of pain, and abdominal distention or bloating. IBS patients are differentiated from individuals who have similar symptoms but do not consult a doctor. Symptoms may be quite severe such as more frequent defecation, erratic and marked variability of stool form, urgency, and often feelings of incomplete evacuation.

IBS patients report multiple somatic complaints, have more surgical procedures, overutilize medical services, and have increased somatization or hypochondriasis. Noncomplainers with gastrointestinal symptoms do not demonstrate these traits and are much closer to control subjects in personality traits than to patients. A good patient-physician relationship includes an adequate evaluation, education and instruction, and periodic return visits to minimize doctor shopping and possible harmful alternative treatments, such as colonic lavage, and does a lot to prevent recurrent symptoms. The physician should avoid unduly accommodating with the patient's behavioral style (e.g., ordering tests to reassure and assuming full responsibility in the care) as these are countertherapeutic.[16] Insoluble or soluble fiber is frequently prescribed and may need to be continued even when symptoms are absent. Diet, symptomatic management as described for constipation, and use of a heating pad as needed for cramping with or without anticholinergics are advised.

Diverticulitis

Diverticulosis is the condition of having diverticula in the colon and is asymptomatic and unknown to the patient unless it is discovered in an incidental sigmoidoscopy, colonoscopy, or during barium enema given for other reasons. Diverticulitis is the inflammation of one or more of these "tics" precipitated by plugging of their ostia, for example, by cellulose, with consequent bacterial proliferation in the obstructed "tic."

Indirect evidence (discussed later) suggests that this is a disease of civilization (and hence preventable), if one may apply that term, or at least industrialized society where bulk and fiber are low in the diet. If so, it is preventable or modified by the adoption of high-fiber diets in childhood, when dietary habits and preferences largely are formed, and their continuation into adulthood.

The experience of many physicians is that diverticulitis may be prevented (or at least the number of attacks decreased) by appropriate dietary habits.

The subject is addressed here in that it has preventive aspects, and as with subjects addressed in the balance of this chapter it is exceedingly common in office practice.

In Western countries where the fiber content of the diet is low, approximately 50% of the population will have diverticulosis by the ninth decade. About 35% of individuals with diverticulosis observed for 20 years developed diverticulitis. One third to one half of patients with acute diverticulitis have recurrent attacks. Diverticulosis is limited to the sigmoid colon in 66%, and in one study of 350 patients having diverticulitis requiring surgery, the diverticulitis occurred in the sigmoid in 94%.[66]

The diverticulum is composed only of mucosa and submucosa, which may facilitate obstruction at its narrowed neck. Bacteria plus continued mucosal secretion may result in distention, apical inflammation, and finally apical micro-perforation. The peridiverticulitis may remain confined or lead to a macro-perforation developing an abscess. This may be small or large. If it is large, it may be associated with a tender mass and frequently sepsis. Recurrent episodes may cause segmental narrowing with or without obstruction.

There is a relative contraindication for colonoscopy and single-contrast or double-contrast barium enema studies during an acute attack of diverticulitis. A barium enema without preparation is performed during the acute attack only if management would be significantly modified by the x-ray finding. Computerized tomography [CT] is advised as the initial procedure by several authors. Shrier, however, reports in his surgical group that 90% of contrast enemas and 69% of CT exams reported either diverticulitis or findings compatible with diverticulitis. He reports no complications resulting from his barium studies or other studies. If a perforation is considered, a water-soluble contrast agent is usually used. Barium studies or a colonoscopy a few weeks after the acute diverticulitis, using an adequate preparation, may be used to confirm the clinical impression and rule out underlying neoplasm.[58]

DIVERTICULITIS

Burkitt and others, basing their opinions on African studies of Blacks 20 to 30 years ago, became strong proponents for increasing fiber content in Western industrialized countries. This was advised because of the low fiber intake and high incidence of diverticular disease in the West.[21,56] I can clearly recall listening to a lecture about twenty years ago given by Burkitt, who described the extreme rarity of colon diverticulosis and diverticulitis, hemorrhoids, appendicitis, and colon cancer in Africa. He states that the stools would be huge, and the diet often times contained about 60 to 80 grams of fiber although low in fat. The fiber intake in the West is about 17 grams, although an intake of 30 grams is desired. The diet of the West was progressively getting worse because of increased refining of carbohydrates and further lowering of fiber content. As urbanization increased, refined sugars and flours becamed preferred, and fresh fruits and vegetables, decreased in popularity because of expense.[56] Increased fiber does increase stool weight, stool frequency, softness of the stool (can cause diarrhea), and may shorten transient time. "Roughage" does not irritate the gut but rather becomes "softage" when it becomes moist. The increased stool volume lowers colonic pressure by decreasing "segmentation" that is formed by intrahaustral contraction rings that may occlude the lumen causing high pressure in these isolated compartments and transmitted also to the diverticula contained therein.[56]

The results of studies on fiber in diverticulitis are varied, ranging from having little value except for constipation and others showing definite improvement.[21,56] Hyland demonstrated that 91%, for example, remained symptom free for 5 to 7 years, attributed to following a 38-gram fiber diet. The 100 subjects were hospitalized with symptomatic diverticular disease, with 25 receiving surgery initially followed by a high-fiber diet. Among the 25 patients who did not comply, there was a 20% complication rate. This series was compared to four studies between 1966 to 1970 before the use of high-fiber diet and the percent of those being symptom free varied from 38% to 64%. Value of high fiber is also supported by a much lower incidence of diverticula among vegeterians compared with nonvegetarians in the same English community,[42] which suggests that adopting a high-fiber diet will postpone diverticular development.

On the other hand, metabolic studies show that a high-fiber vegetable diet increases fecal loss of calcium, magnesium, and zinc that might lead to malnutrition, especially if intake is marginal. The author believes that there is no proven net long-term benefits demonstrated as yet and so suggests the physician make his or her own decision.[42]

This problem of fiber is further complicated by the difficulty of determining an accurate analysis of fiber in the unprocessed food and in turn the amount that is consumed.[21] This makes the evaluation of fiber more difficult.

To attain a high-fiber diet, one should aim for an increase of 10 grams of crude fiber, emphasizing whole grain breads and cereals, fresh fruits, and fresh vegetables. Bran 20 grams (2 T) equals 8.8 gm and may be sprinkled on a salad. Psyllium products as a packet or rounded teaspoon contains 3.4 grams. One final note about diet refers to the ingestion of seeds as in berries, grapes, popcorn hulls, and so on as a possible concern in causing diverticulitis. There has been no information found to substantiate this as being a risk factor, though many years ago these restrictions, as well as a bland diet, were advised.

Acknowledgment

The author is indebted to Jane Thompson for preparation of the manuscript and to Pat Niblick for library assistance.

REFERENCES

1. Alexander W: Gastroesophageal reflux: an unrecognized link to asthma, *Modern Medicine* 59:14, 1991.
2. Alpers DH: Dietary management and vitamin-mineral replacement therapy. In Sleisenger MH, Fordtran JS, editors: *Gastrointestinal disease: pathophysiology diagnosis, management,* ed 4, Philadelphia, 1989, W.B. Saunders.
3. Ballary SV, Isaacs P, Hee FI: Upper gastrointestinal lesions in elderly patients from NSAIDS, *Am J Gastroenterol* 86:961, 1991.
4. Banks S: The clinical features of alcohol and drug induced pancreatitis, *Am Coll of Gastroenterol,* Annual postgraduate course 1984.
5. Bayless TE: Dietary causes of gastrointestinal symptoms, *Am Coll Gastroenterol,* Annual postgraduate course 215, 1990.
6. Bond JH: Intestinal gas, *Am Coll Gastroenterol,* Annual postgraduate course 255, 1990.
7. Brennan MF: Surgical management of pancreatic and biliary tract cancer, *Am Gastroenterol Assoc,* Annual postgraduate course 111, 1990.
8. Browning TH: Diagnosis of chest pain of esophageal origin: a guideline of the patient care committee of the American Gastroenterological Association, *Dig Dis Sci* 35:289, 1990.
9. Camilleri M: Functional dyspepsia, *Am Coll Gastroenterol,* Annual postgraduate course 83, 1990.
10. Carter KJ, Schaffer HA, Ritchie WP: Early gastric cancer, *Ann Surg* 199:604, 1984.
11. Cello J: Carcinoma of the pancreas. In Sleisenger MH, Fordtran JS, editors: *Gastrointestinal disease: pathophysiology, diagnosis, management,* ed 4, Philadelphia, 1989, WB Saunders.
12. Davis GR: Neoplasms of the stomach. In Sleisenger MH, Fordtran JS, editors: *Gastrointestinal disease: pathophysiology, diagnosis, management,* ed 4, Philadelphia, 1989, WB Saunders.
13. Day JP, Richter JE: Medical and surgical conditions predisposing to gastroesophageal reflux disease, *Gastroenterol Clin North Am* 19(3):587, 1990.
14. Diehl AM: Update on alcoholic hepatitis, *Am Coll Gastroenterol,* Annual postgraduate course 577, 1991.
15. Drossman DA, Thompson WG: Management of irritable bowel syndrome and idiopathic constipation, *Am Gastroenterol Assoc,* Annual postgraduate course 1991.
16. Drossman DA: The patient with chronic undiagnosed abdominal pain, *Hosp Pract* 21:22, 1986.

17. Eng J, Sabanathan S: Drug-induced esophagitis, *Am J Gastroenterol* 80:1127, 1991.

18. Fine SN, Dannenberg AJ, Zakim D: The impact of medical therapy on peptic ulcer disease. In Zakim D, Dannenberg AJ, editors: *Peptic ulcer disease and other related disorders,* Armonk, New York, 1991, Academic Research Associates.

19. Fordtran JS: Symptomatic therapy of diarrhea, *Am Gastroenterol Assoc,* Annual postgraduate course 1991.

20. Freston JW: Overview of medical therapy of peptic ulcer disease, *Gastroenterol Clin North Am* 19(1):121, 1990.

21. Friedman G: Nutritional therapy for irritable bowel syndrome, *Gastroenterol Clin North Am* 18(3):519, 1989.

22. Gaynor EB: Otolaryngologic manifestations of gastroesophageal reflux, *Am J Gastroenterol* 86:801, 1991.

23. Goldstein JL et al: Esophageal mucosal resistance, *Gastroenterol Clin North Am* 19(3):587, 1990.

24. Hayakawa T et al: Chronic alcoholism and evolution of pain and prognosis in chronic pancreatitis, *Dig Dis Sci* 35:33, 1989.

25. Heaton KW, Ghosh S, Braddon FE: How bad are the symptoms and bowel dysfunction of patients with the irritable bowel syndrome? A prospective controlled study with emphasis on stool form, *Gut* 32:73, 1991.

26. Hewson EG, Dalton CB, Richter JE: Comparison of esophageal manometry, provocative testing, and ambulatory monitoring in patients with unexplained chest pain, *Dig Dis Sci* 35:302, 1990.

27. Hisamichi S: Screening for gastric cancer, *World J Gastroenterol* 13:31, 1989.

28. Holloway RH, Dent J: Pathophysiology of gastroesophageal reflux, *Gastroenterol Clin North Am* 19(3):517, 1990.

29. Hunt RH: The role of colonoscopy in diverticular disease, *Am Coll Gastroenterol,* Annual postgraduate course 601, 1989.

30. Hyland JMP, Taylor I: Does a high fiber diet prevent the complications of diverticular disease? *British J Surg* 67:77, 1980.

31. Jones MP, Schubert ML, Smith JL: Prophylaxis in elderly women taking NSAIDS, *Am J Gastroenterol* 86:264, 1991.

32. Kahnlas PJ: Esophageal motor activity and acid clearance, *Gastroenterol Clin North Am* 19(3):537, 1991.

33. Kaplan MM: Elevated liver enzymes in the asymptomatic patient, *Am Coll Gastroenterol,* Annual postgraduate course 33, 1988.

34. Konturek SJ: Role of growth factors in gastroduodenal protection and healing of peptic ulcers, *Gastroenterol Clin North Am* 19(1):41, 1990.

35. Lee FI, Hardman M, Jaderberg ME: Maintenance treatment of duodenal ulceration and ranitidine: 300 mg. at night is better than 150 mg. in cigarette smokers, *Gut* 32:151, 1991.

36. Lewis JH: Drug-induced liver disease, *Am Coll Gastroenterol,* Annual postgraduate course 595, 1991.

37. Luk GD: Cancer surveillance for premalignant GI disorders, *Am Coll Gastroenterol,* Annual postgraduate course 423, 1990.

38. McCallum RW: Gastric emptying in gastroesophageal reflux and the therapeutic role of prokinetic agents, *Gastroenterol Clin North Am* 19(3):551, 1990.

39. Mittal RK: Current concepts of the antireflux barrier, *Gastroenterol Clinic North Am* 19(3):501, 1990.

40. *Morbidity and Mortality Weekly Report* 40:No. RR-13, Hepatitis B virus, 1991.

41. Moser G et al: High incidence of esophageal motor disorder in consecutive patients with globus sensation, *Gastroenterology* 101:1512, 1991.

42. Naitove A, Almy TP: Diverticular disease of the colon. In Sleisenger MN, Fordtran JS, editors: *Gastrointestinal disease: pathophysiology, diagnosis, management,* ed 4, Philadelphia, 1989, W.B. Saunders.

43. Oettle' GJ: Effect of moderate exercise on bowel habit, *Gut,* 32:941, 1991.

44. Orstein MH et al: Are fiber supplements really necessary in divertic-

ular disease of the colon? A controlled clinical trial, *British Med J* 282:1353, 1981.

45. Patchett S et al: Helicobacter pylori and duodenal ulcer recurrences, *Am J Gastroenterol* 87:24, 1992.

46. Perrillo RP: Hepatitis B vaccine: Issues of importance for the practicing physician, *Am Gastroenterol Assoc,* Annual postgraduate course 247, 1989.

47. Peterson WL: Bleeding peptic ulcer, *Gastroenterol Clin North Am* 19(1):155, 1990.

48. Polepalle SC, McCollum RW: Barrett's esophagus, *Gastroenterol Clin North Am* 19(3):733, 1990.

49. Ranschoff DF: Natural history of gallstones, *Am Gastroenterol Assoc,* Annual postgraduate course 1988.

50. Reynolds JC: The management of chronic constipation, *Am Coll Gastroenterol,* Annual postgraduate course 27, 1988.

51. Richter JE: New insights into the diagnosis and treatment of gastroesophageal reflux disease, *Am Coll Gastroenterol,* Annual postgraduate course 1991.

52. Schiessel R, Feil W, Wenzl E: Mechanisms of stress ulceration and implications for treatment, *Gastroenterol Clin North Am* 19(1):101, 1991.

53. Schoenfield LJ: Medical treatment of gallstones, *Am Coll Gastroenterol,* Annual postgraduate course 451, 1991.

54. Schubert ML, Shamburek RD: Control of acid secretion, *Gastroenterol Clin North Am* 19(1):1, 1990.

55. Schuster MM: Diagnostic evaluation of the irritable bowel syndrome, *Gastroenterol Clin North Am* 20(2):269, 1991.

56. Shackelford R, Zuidema G, editors: Diverticular disease. In *Surgery of the alimentary tract,* ed 2, Philadelphia, 1982, W.B. Saunders.

57. Shorey J: Evaluation of mass lesions in the liver. In Sleisenger MH, Fordtran JS, editors: *Gastrointestinal disease: pathophysiology, diagnosis, management,* ed 4, Philadelphia, 1989, W.B. Saunders.

58. Shrier D, Skucas J, Weiss S: Diverticulitis: an evaluation by computed tomography and contrast edema, *Am J Gastroenterol* 86:1466, 1991.

59. Simon JB: Sclerosing cholangitis and primary biliary cirrhosis, *Am Coll Gastroenterol,* Annual postgraduate course 1987.

60. Sontag SJ: Medical management of reflux esophagitis, *Gastroenterol Clin North Am* 19(3):683, 1990.

61. Spechler SJ: Cancer of the esophagus: a gastroenterologists' prospective, *Am Gastroenterol Assoc,* Annual postgraduate course 106, 1989.

62. Sterrlieb I: Hemochromotasis, *Am Coll Gastroenterol,* Annual postgraduate course 1987.

63. Szabo S, Vottay P: Experimental gastric and duodenal ulcers, *Gastroenterol Clin North Am* 19(1):67, 1990.

64. Toskes PT: Hyperlipemic pancreatitis, *Gastroenterol Clin North Am* 19(4):783, 1990.

65. Traube MI: The spectrum of the symptoms and presentations of gastroesophageal reflux disease, *Gastroenterol Clin North Am* 19(3):609, 1990.

66. Van Ness M, Peller C: Acute diverticulitis: diagnosis and management, *Hosp Pract* 26:83, 1991.

67. Venu RP et al: Idiopathic recurrent pancreatitis, an approach to diagnosis and treatment, *Dig Dis Sci* 35:56, 1989.

68. Wall A: Evaluation and therapy of intractable constipation, *Am Coll Gastroenterol,* Annual postgraduate course 303, 1990.

69. Whitehead WE, Crowell MD: Psychologic considerations in the irritable bowel syndrome, *Gastroenterol Clin North Am* 20(2):249, 1991.

*Several of the Annual Postgraduate Course syllabi are not numbered consecutively, so no page numbers are listed. The syllabi are not listed by publisher or volume. AGA National Office, 6900 Grove Road, Thorofare, NJ 08086-9447; ACG, 4900 B South 31st Street, Arlington, VA 22206-1656.

Chapter 51

THE UROLOGIC SYSTEM

Protection of the kidney and nephrolithiasis

Phillip M. Hall

PREVENTION OF PROGRESSION OF RENAL DISEASES

Currently more than 100,000 patients with end-stage renal disease are enrolled in the Medicare program in the United States.[34] The cost for such care exceeds $2 billion and seems to be rising. This huge cost, together with the high mortality and morbidity rates of end-stage renal disease, supports the need for effective preventive therapy. The cause of most renal diseases is not known or is only incompletely understood. Thus specific treatments are not possible.

Until 10 or 15 years ago it was believed that most renal diseases that progressed did so as a result of an ongoing insult by the original injurious process. Such renal conditions as recurring infection in pyelonephritis, immune complex deposition disease, immunologic injury in glomerulonephritis, uncontrolled hypertension with arterial nephrosclerosis, and the cyst formation and enlargement in polycystic renal diseases are all examples in which a progressive, ongoing injury is occurring.

However, in many renal diseases evidence of ongoing injurious processes is lacking, yet renal excretory function worsens and end-stage renal failure ensues. Examples include vesicoureteral reflux, in which renal failure often progresses despite correction of the anatomic abnormality.[43]

The current wave of interest in prevention of renal disease derives primarily from experience with animal models of progressive renal failure. In rats removal of significant portions of the renal tissue (⅚ nephrectomy) is associated with the development of proteinuria and progressive loss of renal function despite the absence of any actual ongoing injurious insult.[36] In these models of renal failure it has

been shown that dietary protein restriction, control of systemic hypertension, treatment with angiotensin-converting enzyme (ACE) inhibitors and calcium channel blockers, and control of plasma lipids have proved effective in retarding the rate of progression.[32,42,64,74] In this animal model of progressive renal failure the removal of a significant number of functioning nephrons is thought to set in motion a deleterious process in the remaining nephrons, which eventually results in their becoming sclerotic and destroyed. The mechanism for this deleterious process includes glomerular hyperfiltration, in part mediated by increased levels of angiotensin II; glomerular hypertrophy mediated by various growth factors; glomerular injury mediated by systemic hypertension; glomerular hypermetabolism produced by increased work load per glomerulus and nephron; and lipid deposition or injury in the glomerular tuft.[45] The variety of demonstrated mechanisms of injury illustrate that progressive renal failure in this rat model does not apparently have a single final common pathway. From these animal studies several clinical strategies that may be beneficial in preventing progressive renal failure can be described.

Control of systemic hypertension lessens morbidity and mortality caused by stroke, renal failure, and congestive heart failure. Since hypertension is present in 60% to 80% of patients with renal parenchymal disease, its treatment becomes important for prevention of both stroke and heart failure morbidity and progressive renal failure.[10] In patients with diabetic nephropathy Mogensen et al.[65] and Parving et al.[71] have shown that excellent blood pressure control slowed the rate of progression of renal failure. Preliminary data from the pilot phase of a study to test the efficacy of dietary protein restriction on progression of renal

959

disease show a weak but significantly positive correlation between rate of progression and mean arterial pressure.[44] Although a variety of antihypertensive agents may be effective in lowering systemic blood pressure, ACE inhibitors and calcium channel blockers may be preferred because they retard progressive renal failure in animals with subtotal nephrectomy.

Dietary protein restriction is also effective at reducing the rate of progression of renal failure in animals. In the past several years more than 15 uncontrolled studies in humans have tested the effect of dietary protein restriction on progression of renal disease. In these studies dietary protein intake from 0.3 to 0.8 g/kg/day was prescribed. The rate of progression in renal failure was assessed by measuring the change in creatinine clearance or the slope of the relationship between 1/serum creatinine concentration and time. Generally the results of these studies support the belief that dietary protein restriction retards progression. The major flaws in these studies are that they were not controlled and that the indicators used to assess renal function were serum creatinine concentration measurements, which are known to be inaccurate estimates of renal function in advanced renal failure. Further, other factors such as systemic hypertension that in themselves may increase the rate of progression were not examined or controlled. More recently two randomized prospective studies of patients with nondiabetic renal disease have shown that dietary protein restriction to 0.4 to 0.6 g/kg was associated with reduced rate of progression of renal failure.[38,53] In patients with diabetic nephropathy dietary protein restriction has been shown to retard progression of renal disease.[23,98]

In view of the foregoing studies it seems reasonable to recommend a modest dietary protein restriction in the range of 0.4 to 0.6 g/kg/day for diabetic and nondiabetic patients with progressive renal disease. Such dietary protein intervention requires the help of trained dietitians in counseling and providing follow-up care of patients. More severe degrees of dietary protein restriction are more hazardous because they may result in dietary deficiencies of essential amino acids or other minerals or vitamins.

As noted previously, administration of ACE inhibitors prevents progressive renal failure in animals with subtotal nephrectomy. Likewise, ACE inhibitors are known to reduce the occurrence of diabetic renal disease in animals with diabetes experimentally induced by islet cell destruction. In 1985 Taguma and colleagues[89] reported that captopril reduced urinary protein excretion in human patients with diabetic renal disease and azotemia. Mathiesen et al. have shown that ACE inhibitors postpone the develop of overt diabetic nephropathy in normotensive insulin-dependent diabetics.[59] The protective effect seems to occur in the presence or absence of systemic hypertension. Thus in diabetics with or without hypertension, ACE inhibitors are recommended both to postpone overt diabetic nephropathy and to retard its progression when present.

Finally although not of proven benefit in humans, it does appear that control of hyperlipidemia is associated with prevention of progression of renal disease in animals. Since hyperlipidemia control is of known benefit to the prevention of human atherosclerotic disease, it seems entirely sensible to prescribe lipid-lowering diet and/or pharmacotherapy in patients with renal disease who have significant hyperlipidemia. Studies to show the benefit of such intervention in human progressive renal disease remain unreported.

MEASUREMENT OF NORMAL KIDNEY FUNCTION

The most feared consequence of renal diseases is the progressive loss of excretory function leading to symptomatic or end-stage renal failure. Thus the clinical measurement of renal function is an important element in diagnosing and monitoring various renal diseases. In an adult, significant renal disease is unlikely if the urinalysis result, including microscopic examination of the centrifuged urine sediment, is normal and the plasma creatinine concentration (P_{Cr}) is less than 0.9 mg/dl. This latter statement needs some qualification as follows.

The measurement of P_{Cr} is a practical method of estimating renal excretory function. The concentration of creatinine in the plasma is the result of creatinine production by the body muscle mass and the rate of renal excretion. Since muscle mass (thus creatinine production) varies little over time in the same individual, renal excretion is the predominant determinant of P_{Cr}.

Interpretation of the P_{Cr} requires consideration of the following: individuals who are older, female, and of small body size have a smaller muscle mass resulting in less daily creatinine production and lower P_{Cr} concentration for any level of renal function; individuals who are young, male, and of large body size have a larger muscle mass with consequent greater creatinine production and higher P_{Cr}. A review of Table 51-1 reveals that normal kidney function (glomerular filtration rate [GFR] of 100%) is reflected by P_{Cr} 0.6 to 1.2 mg/dl in women and by P_{Cr} 0.7 to 1.6 mg/dl in men.[78] The range in P_{Cr} levels is due to individual variation in creatinine production and not to variation in the analytic method of P_{Cr}.

From these considerations it is apparent that in a small or elderly person a P_{Cr} of 1.0 mg/dl may represent a 30% to 50% decline in renal excretory function. Such analysis of P_{Cr} is necessary in assessing and monitoring renal function. In such individuals a measurement of GFR by either creatinine clearance or, more accurately, ^{131}I iothalamate isotopic clearance may be important to establish the relationship between P_{Cr} and GFR.[39] Such additional measurements of GFR are especially important in following renal function in disease states progressing slowly over years or in individuals whose illness leads to progressive loss in muscle mass.

Table 51-1. Relationship between iothalamate GFR and serum creatinine levels according to age and gender*

		Mean measured serum creatinine values ± 2 SD (mg/dl)					
Age (years)		15-30		40-50		60-70	
	Sex	M	F	M	F	M	F
GFR	Number	297	334	297	256	388	255
10		6.6 ± 4.6	5.4 ± 3.2	5.8 ± 3.9	4.7 ± 2.5	4.6 ± 3.5	5.1 ± 3.2
25		3.0 ± 1.3	2.6 ± 1.9	3.0 ± 1.6	2.4 ± 1.2	2.6 ± 1.7	2.2 ± 1.5
50		1.8 ± 0.9	1.4 ± 0.6	1.7 ± 0.7	1.4 ± 0.5	1.6 ± 0.6	1.3 ± 0.5
100		1.2 ± 0.4	0.9 ± 0.3	1.2 ± 0.4	0.9 ± 0.3	1.1 ± 0.4	0.9 ± 0.3

From Jacobson HR, Striker GE, Klahr S: *Principles and practice of nephrology,* Philadelphia, 1991, BC Becker
*Serum creatinine values done on SMA (Technicon). GFR values in units of ml/min/1.73 m^2.

In general a doubling of P_{Cr} value is equivalent to a 50% reduction in GFR. Table 51-1 shows that a doubling of P_{Cr} is often equivalent to more than a 50% reduction in renal function. Such information should be helpful in estimating initial as well as serial renal function.

SCREENING FOR RENAL DISEASE

The best screening tests to detect important nonmalignant renal disease are the dipstick for urinary protein concentration, microscopic examination of the sediment, and plasma creatinine. If all of these tests have normal results, significant renal disease is not present—with one exception. The exception is polycystic kidney disease (PKD), which is present long before azotemia or an abnormal urinalysis result occurs. Screening for polycystic renal disease is best done by obtaining family history data and performing computer tomographic (CT) or ultrasound evaluation of the kidney. If the latter tests show more than five simple cysts in both kidneys, PKD is likely.

Unfortunately a random urinalysis result in an asymptomatic child or adult can be abnormal for hematuria and proteinuria and yet not indicate any significant genitourinary disease. Several large studies have determined that asymptomatic microhematuria is associated with definite significant disease in only 0% to 2% of cases in adults.[3,15,24,30,66,67] Asymptomatic proteinuria in healthy adults is associated with significant disease in only 0% to 1.4% of patients. In children proteinuria is even less likely to be an indicator of clinically significant disease.[2,15,52,93] These observations suggest that routine screening of urine for protein and blood in asymptomatic healthy adults is not warranted.

RENAL NEPHROLITHIASIS
Stone formation

The formation of a stone within the urinary tract is not a specific disorder but may result as a complication of many disorders. The incidence of nephrolithiasis is variously re-ported as 0.36 to 20.8/10,000 population.[85] Translating this into prevalence means that about 12% of men and 5% of women have one episode of renal colic by age 70 years. Individuals with their first stone event have a recurrence of 14% at 1 year, 35% at 5 years, and 52% at 10 years.[92] Because nephrolithiasis is common and responsible for patient discomfort, hospitalization, loss of work time, and medical expense, prevention is a worthy goal.

Stones forming in the urinary tract are composed of crystals and matrix skeleton. Seventy to eighty percent of stones contain calcium, as either calcium oxalate monohydrate or dihydrate, or calcium phosphate, or both. Struvites, or magnesium ammonium phosphate stones, are formed in the presence of chronic urinary infection and occur in 15% of patients. Uric acid stones occur in 10% of cases and cystine stones are found in less than 1% of cases.

Physicochemical factors including type of solute, ion strength, pH, and state of saturation are important causes of stones. At a clinical level these physicochemical factors are difficult to measure. Therefore in the clinical evaluation of risk factors favoring stone formation one usually assesses urine volume; daily solute excretion of calcium, oxalate, urate, cystine, and citrate; urine pH; and presence of bacterial infection of the urine. A complete 24-hour urine collection obtained when the patient is on his or her usual diet easily identifies patients with low urine volume, the most frequent risk factor. Other risk factors, including hypercalciuria, hyperoxaluria, hyperuricosuria, hypocitric aciduria, cystinuria, and disturbances of urine pH, can also be identified (Table 51-2).

Daily urine volume of less than 1200 ml is frequent in stone formers. The most important and least expensive intervention is to encourage the oral intake of water to achieve daily urine volumes of greater than 2000 ml. Eight to ten 8-ounce glasses of fluid per day including fluid at bedtime (to lessen nocturnal urinary concentrations) should be advised for all patients.

Table 51-2. Renal stone disease

Condition	Treatment*
Calcium stones	
Idiopathic hypercalciuria	Thiazides
Idiopathic hyperuricosuria	Allopurinol
	Low purine diet
Idiopathic hyperoxaluria	Low oxalate diet
Idiopathic hypocitraturia	Potassium citrate
Hyperparathyroidism	Parathyroidectomy
Enteric hyperoxaluria	Low oxalate diet
	Potassium citrate
Uric acid stones	Low purine diet
	Allopurinol
	Alkalinization of urine
Struvite stones	Control/prevent infection
	Stone removal
Cystine stones	Alkalinization of urine
	Penicillamine
	Captopril

*In all patients 8-12 glasses of water/day is necessary to reduce solute concentration.

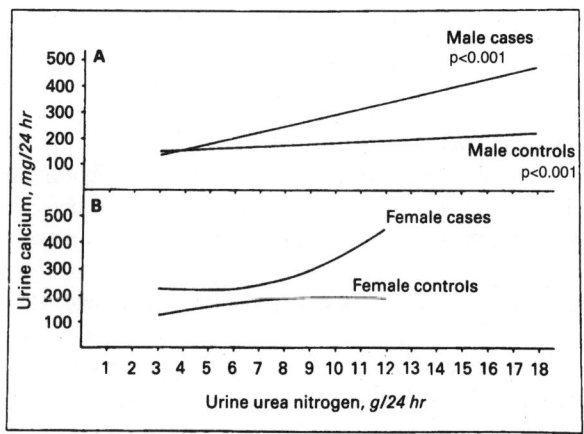

Fig. 51-1. Urinary calcium excretion (mg/24 hr) and urinary urea nitrogen excretion (g/24 hr), an index of dietary protein ingestion, are plotted for male *(upper panel)* and female *(lower panel)* subjects in a large epidemiologic study of risk factors for calcium nephrolithiasis. (From Wasserstein AG et al: Case-control study of risk factors for idiopathic calcium nephrolithiasis, *Mineral Electrolyte Metab* 13:85, 1987.)

Hypercalciuria and other predisposing conditions

Hypercalciuria is defined as the excretion of more than 300 mg calcium/day in men and more than 250 mg calcium/day in women. Approximately 50% of patients with calcium stones have hypercalciuria. At least two dietary factors—protein and sodium—may play a role in hypercalciuria. For several decades studies have supported the finding that upper tract calcium renal lithiasis is more common in affluent societies wherein dietary protein intake is

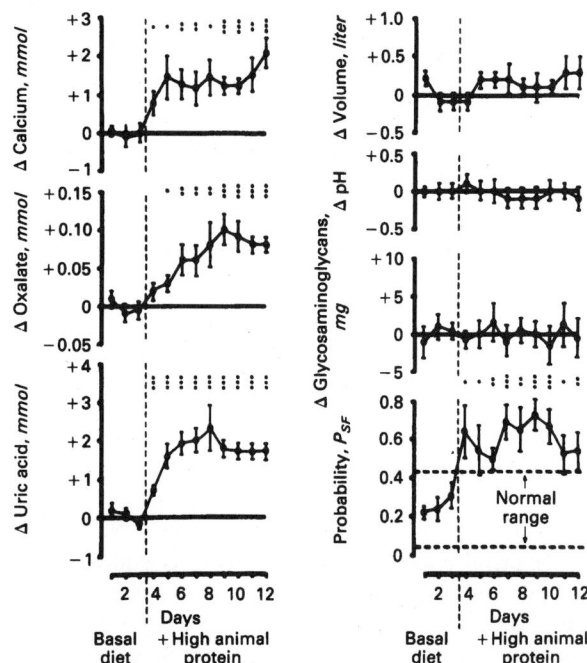

Fig. 51-2. Effects of a short-term increase of dietary animal protein (34 g/24 hr above basal) in six normal male subjects on various urinary constituents. "Probability" score *(lower right)* refers to a derived index of the risk of stone formation based on urinary constituents. (From Robertson WG et al: The effect of high animal protein intake on the risk of calcium stone formation in the urinary tract, *Clin Sci* 57:285, 1979.)

high.[4] In these same societies the calcium stone frequency declines during times of national calamity, such as war, when dietary protein is limited.[77] Further, vegetarians have a significantly lower rate of calcium lithiasis than nonvegetarians.[76] Studies by Wasserstein et al. have shown a strong correlation between calcium excretion and urinary urea excretion in calcium stone formers (Fig. 51-1).[94] Short-term feeding of high dietary protein to male calcium stone formers is associated with an increased excretion of calcium oxalate and uric acid (Fig. 51-2).[75] Together these observations clearly support a relationship among high dietary protein intake, hypercalciuria, and calcium lithiasis in patients prone to stones. The mechanism whereby dietary protein intake leads to hypercalciuria is unproved; it may be (1) increased GFR, (2) reduced tubular calcium reabsorption, or (3) increased net renal acid excretion induced by protein stimulated increases in endogenous acid production.[50]

Ingestion of high dietary protein intake also is associated with hyperuricosuria, which is a risk factor for calcium nephrolithiasis. It seems that uric acid in the urine can absorb glutamic acid crystals (also found in urine), which in turn promote calcium oxalate crystal growth.[81]

Kleeman[46] showed that maneuvers that increase urinary sodium excretion also increase urinary calcium excretion.

The only way to ensure a sustained increased urinary sodium excretion is to ensure a sustained increase in sodium intake. Thus high dietary sodium intake is a risk factor for hypercalciuria. Wasserstein has shown that patients who have calcium nephrolithiasis have a more significant hypercalciuric response to high dietary sodium intake than who do not.[94] The exact mechanism for this relationship is not proved. The close relationship between calcium handling and sodium handling by the kidney points to the proximal tubule and Henle's loop as sites of decreased calcium reabsorption in states of high sodium intake.

General advice regarding dietary factors in renal lithiasis should include modest restrictions in dietary animal protein and no addition of salt to foods (less than 4 g NaCl). Previous studies have shown that a patient who salts food before tasting is usually ingesting more than 31 g of salt daily.[88] Such high salt intake not only causes hypercalciuria but may override the hypocalciuric effect of thiazide diuretics that may be prescribed to treat hypercalciuric renal lithiasis.

The hypercalciuria in renal stone formers not only is enhanced by dietary protein and sodium intake but also results from hyperabsorption of intestinal calcium.[70] Though not certain the mechanism seems to be enhanced gastrointestinal absorption of calcium caused by mildly increased levels of 1,25 vitamin D.[11] Ideally such patients will respond to dietary calcium restriction or to agents that bind intestinal calcium (cellulose phosphate). However, neither of these corrects the metabolic derangement and both pose the risk of negative calcium balance with accompanying skeletal calcium loss.

Therefore, if dietary protein and sodium restriction coupled with high fluid intake do not control calcium stone formation, thiazide diuretics (not loop diuretics) are the preferred intervention. Thiazide diuretics reduce urinary calcium excretion and calcium stone frequency.[20,96] Two caveats are to be considered in this treatment regimen: First, patients given thiazides for hypercalciuria should be instructed to observe a modest sodium restriction since high sodium intake promotes increased urinary sodium and calcium excretion, thus reducing the benefit of the thiazides. Second, thiazides may produce hypokalemia, which in turn reduces urinary citrate excretion. Citrate is a naturally occurring urinary crystal inhibitor, and its reduction in the urine may cause enhanced stone formation.

Hyperoxaluria (greater than 40 mg/day) rarely occurs as an inherited disorder. Most often it is found in patients with enhanced intestinal absorption of oxalate caused by ileal disease.[95] This disturbance may be encountered in patients with inflammatory bowel disease, gastric or small bowel resection, or jejunal ileal bypass. Two factors are responsible for enhanced oxalate absorption: (1) bile salts and fatty acids reaching the lower intestine increase the bowel permeability for oxalate, and (2) fat malabsorption allows more intestinal fat to bind calcium leaving more free oxalate available for intestinal absorption.[21] In such patients low urine volume caused by enhanced gastrointestinal fluid losses, low urinary magnesium produced by magnesium malabsorption, and hypocitraturia resulting from hypokalciuria and metabolic acidosis all contribute to the tendency to calcium oxalate stone disease. Generally enteric hyperoxaluric stone disease only occurs in patients with sufficient mucosa to hyperabsorb the entering oxalate-laden small bowel effluent.

Hyperuricosuria seems to be a predisposing factor in 10% of calcium stone patients. This is thought to be due either to dietary overindulgence of purine-rich foods or to uric acid overproduction. The hyperuricosuria enhances calcium stone disease by the urinary uric acid's forming the crystal nucleus, causing calcium oxalate crystals to grow, or by making the urine supersaturated, so that calcium oxalate more readily precipitates. Dietary purine restriction is the preferred treatment. This would include elimination of meat extracts, herring, organ meats, and sardines and maintaining fat intake at a moderate level. Further restriction in meat, poultry, fish, and legumes, and elimination of beer, wine, and ale may be helpful.[16] Studies have shown also that allopurinol is both effective and safe in reducing hyperuricosuria and reducing calcium oxalate stone frequency.[22]

Uric acid stones, which are radiolucent, are most likely to occur in individuals who have persistently acid urine (pH < 5.0), wherein the uric acid is least soluble, or have hyperuricosuria caused by purine overproduction, as seen in myeloproliferative disorders. Prevention includes hydration, administration of allopurinol (100 to 300 mg/day) to reduce uric acid production, and use of sodium bicarbonate or potassium citrate to alkalinize the urine to pH > 6.0 and thus enhance urinary uric acid solubility. Alkalinization of the urine provides the safest and most effective means of dissolving formed uric acid stones and of preventing urate stone formation. The patient should be instructed to measure the pH of the urine two to three times daily, using pH paper (provided with an accompanying color chart).

Struvite stones are formed in the presence of persistent urinary tract infection with urea-splitting bacteria. Since these stones only form in the presence and as a result of bacterial infection, their prevention requires eradication of the infection. Careful examination of struvite stones reveals viable bacteria in the stone matrix; therefore, removal of the infected stones is also important in eventually eradicating the infectious agents and the stone disease. Chronic urinary infection is more frequent in individuals with abnormal urinary tract anatomy or disordered urinary bladder emptying. Thus complete evaluation of a patient with struvite stones should include urodynamics and voiding cystourethrogram. Surgical removal is less often required now that percutaneous pyelolithotomy and extracorporeal shock wave lithotripsy are readily available.

Cystinuria is an inborn error of metabolism characterized by a disturbance in renal and intestinal transport of dicarboxylic acid, cystine, ornithine, arginine, and lysine. Cystine stones are caused by increased urinary cystine excretion and low solubility of cystine in urine. Treatment or prevention consists of two major interventions besides encouraging high fluid intake to produce dilute urine and reduce the cystine concentration to less than 30 mg/l. Alkalinization of urine to raise pH to greater than 7.5 increases the solubility of cystine twofold. Penicillamine and more recently captopril are both known to enhance solubility of cystine by changing it to a mixed disulfide. Penicillamine is poorly tolerated because of gastrointestinal side effects and is potentially dangerous because of its tendency to induce nephrotic syndrome, dermatitis, and pancytopenia. A recent small study of nine patients with cystinuria showed that captopril (chemical structure similar to penicillamine) 75 to 100 mg/day reduced urinary cystine excretion by 20% to 70% and was not associated with any serious side effects.[87]

GENETIC RENAL DISEASES

The two most common genetic renal diseases are autosomal dominant polycystic kidney disease (ADPKD) and Alport's syndrome. ADPKD accounts for a significant proportion (10% to 12%) of patients who reach end-stage renal disease.[27] About 1 in 500 to 1 in 1000 individuals are affected resulting in about 6000 new cases each year. The disease is caused by an abnormal gene on the short arm of chromosome 16 (PKD1 gene) in about 90% of cases. In most, the gene produces clinical expression (cysts in the kidney) of the disease, though not all patients develop severe or end-stage renal failure. In 75% of cases the family history is consistent with a dominant mode of inheritance. A recent study of 580 subjects with ADPKD found that 71% of subjects at age 50, 53% at age 58, and 23% at age 70 were alive without end-stage renal disease.[25]

The clinical diagnosis is made by finding multiple cysts (usually more than five per kidney) by ultrasound or CT with contrast. Liver and pancreas cysts, hypertension, and nonspecific abdominal pain are found in more than 50% of individuals. Since the disease is frequently silent until later in life, effective genetic counseling regarding childbearing is difficult. The renal failure, when it occurs, is usually slowly progressive over many years. Microscopic and gross hematuria, renal stones, and urinary infection are more common in patients with ADPKD.

Since there is no known treatment for the disease, the use of deoxyribonucleic acid (DNA) probes for diagnosis can only be recommended when a patient with a family history of ADPKD wants to know whether the disease is present. Analysis by Gabow et al. has shown that the following factors are associated with worse mean renal function at any age in persons with ADPKD: PKD1 genes, younger age at diagnosis, male gender, hypertension, increased left ventricular mass, hepatic cysts in women, three or more pregnancies, gross hematuria, and urinary tract infections in men.[25] Therefore, control of hypertension, prompt treatment of urinary infections, and counseling regarding multiple pregnancies are important in reducing the rate of renal failure. It appears that searching for cerebral aneurysms, known to occur more frequently in ADPKD, should be done only in individuals with a family history of ADPKD and cerebral hemorrhage or known ruptured aneurysms.[51]

Alport's syndrome (AS) may not be one disorder, but several closely similar inherited renal disorders. To date gene markers for the disease are not known. Generally AS is considered to be an X-linked dominant trait, but about 18% of new cases are due to mutations. A metabolic defect in type IV collagen is thought to be responsible for the eye lens membrane, glomerular basement membrane, and possibly the cochlear membrane disorder of AS.[7]

Gross and/or microscopic hematuria and sensorineural hearing loss are usually present before azotemia is significant. Anterior lenticonus is characteristic but only occurs in 15% of cases. Thirty to forty percent of patients develop nephrotic syndrome. Azotemia advances to renal failure in the second to fourth decades of life in men. It is uncommon for women to develop azotemia, but microhematuria may be seen in women. The renal biopsy is suggestive of the disorder when it shows thinning and splitting of the glomerular basement membrane. However, such histologic features are also seen in benign familial hematuria.[29] There is no known treatment to alter the course of the disease. Genetic counseling should be done before childbearing when possible.

PREVENTION OF DRUG-INDUCED RENAL DISEASE

An increasing number of drugs are known to cause renal injury or renal failure (Table 51-3). The first principle in the prevention of drug-induced nephrotoxicity is to avoid the drug exposure. Since many of these drugs are of significant benefit to patients with various illnesses, and since not all patients are equally vulnerable to the nephrotoxicity, their avoidance is not always warranted. Rather, the clinician must be particularly circumspect in prescribing potentially nephrotoxic drugs for patients who may be predisposed to the adverse renal effect.

A number of factors are known to increase the likelihood of drug-induced nephrotoxicity (see box on p. 965). Any clinical state associated with a decrease in "effective" (congestive heart failure [CHF], nephrotic syndrome, cirrhosis) or actual (diarrhea, vomiting, diuretics) circulating plasma volume produces conditions within the kidneys that render them more susceptible to nephrotoxicity.[6] The decrease in actual or effective circulatory volume is accompanied by stimulation of the sympathetic nervous system in order to restore or sustain the systemic blood pressure.

Table 51-3. Drugs associated with interstitial nephritis

Strong association	Probable association	Weak association
Acute		
Methicillin	Carbenicillin	Phenytoin
Penicillin	Cephalosporins	Tetracycline
Nonsteroidal antiinflam-	Oxacillin	Probenecid
matory drugs	Ampicillin	Captopril
Cimetidine	Sulfonamides	Allopurinol
Cephalothin	Rifampin	Erythromycin
Leukocyte interferon	Thiazides	Chloramphenicol
	Furosemide	Clofibrate
	Phenindione	
Chronic		
Analgesic abuse	Lithium	
Cyclosporine		
Nitrosoureas		

Modified from Adler SG, Cohen AH, Border WA: Hypersensitivity phenomena and the kidney: role of drugs and environmental agents, *Am J Kidney Dis* 5:75-97, 1985.

Factors that increase likelihood of drug-induced nephrotoxicity

- Advanced age
- Prior renal disease or azotemia
- Conditions known to decrease renal perfusion
  Cirrhosis
  CHF
  Nephrotic syndrome
  Extracellular volume depletion (GI losses, excessive use of diuretics)
- Prolonged therapy with nephrotoxic agent
- Concurrent use of several nephrotoxins
- High doses or too frequent dosing

This stimulation not only restores systemic pressure but also results in stimulation of renin-angiotensin and of prostaglandin activity. The former stimulates glomerular efferent arteriolar constriction, and the latter produces glomerular afferent arteriolar relaxation. The effect of these events is to raise or maintain intraglomerular hydrostatic pressure and thereby to maintain or protect glomerular filtration in the face of ineffective circulating volume. These hemodynamic changes also result in sluggish flow of concentrated urine containing small amounts of sodium.

In such a state of renal compensation with low urine flow rate use of any drug that would interfere with these compensatory mechanisms (drugs whose nephrotoxicity is partially related to their concentration in tubular fluid because of low urine flow rate) quickly results in further decline in GFR. For example, nonsteroidal antiinflammatory drugs (NSAIDs), given in the presence of conditions that reduce renal perfusion, produce excessive falls in GFR because of inhibition of prostaglandin-mediated afferent arteriolar vasodilation. ACE inhibitors given to patients with decreased renal perfusion reduce GFR through inhibition of A II-mediated efferent arteriolar constriction. Radiocontrast agents that cause initial renal vasodilation followed by prolonged renal vasoconstriction further compromise any clinical situation in which maintenance of GFR depends on the combination of afferent vasodilation and efferent vasoconstriction.

Many drugs that are directly nephrotoxic to the kidney are also primarily excreted by the kidney. Agents that are not toxic in low concentrations may become so in higher concentrations. The renal tubules represent an extensive epithelial surface area and the means for toxic agents to be concentrated within the tubular lumina. Thus many nephrotoxins not only cause azotemia but also produce disor-

ders of renal electrolyte, glucose, or hydrogen ion homeostasis (i.e., renal tubular acidosis, glucosuria, Fanconi's syndrome, hypokalemia, hypomagnesemia).

As indicated previously, prevention of drug nephrotoxicity can be quite successful if one avoids potentially nephrotoxic drugs in patients who are particularly predisposed to the adverse effect. When such potentially nephrotoxic agents must be given one should attempt to do so with the least risk. This should include (1) correcting any predisposing condition of impaired renal perfusion, (2) discontinuing any other potentially nephrotoxic drug, (3) using the lowest dose of drug consistent with the purpose, (4) inducing a high urine flow rate during the period of nephrotoxic drug exposure. This latter can usually be attainted by oral or intravenous (IV) fluid administration. Some however would also combine mannitol with IV fluids to maximize urine flow rate during the period of toxin exposure (i.e., immediately before, during, and 8 hours after radiocontrast administration). Finally because NSAIDs are readily available across the counter, careful history is required to detect those patients who are taking these agents to avoid exposure to another potential nephrotoxin, which is medically required.

Cancers of the kidney and bladder

Eric A. Klein

TUMORS OF THE KIDNEY
Renal cell carcinoma

Adenocarcinoma of the kidney (renal cell carcinoma, RCC) accounts for approximately 3% of adult malignancies and is the third most common urologic tumor after cancers of the prostate and bladder. Approximately 90% of renal parenchymal tumors are adenocarcinomas, with a peak incidence in the sixth and seventh decades and a 1.6:1 male to female preponderance.[12] In 1992 there were an estimated 26,500 new cases of renal cancer in the United States, with 10,700 deaths.[12] For unknown reasons there has been an approximately 30% increase in the age-adjusted death rate for renal tumors in the 30-year period from 1958 to 1988. Most patients with tumors confined to the kidney can be cured by surgical resection, and the number incidentally discovered low-stage RCC amenable to partial or total nephrectomy appears to be increasing.[49] Unfortunately, more than one half of the new cases each year include regionally advanced or metastatic disease and are rarely curable.[47]

The cause of renal adenocarcinoma is unknown. RCC occurs more frequently in urban environments. Both environmental and occupational causes have been hypothesized, emphasizing the role of renal proximal tubular cells, which excrete toxic agents and metabolites as potential targets for environmental carcinogens. Animal studies have supported a role for estrogen in causation, but these theories have not been borne out in clinical practice.[8]

Renal cell carcinoma occurs in both sporadic and familial forms, with sporadic cancers accounting for more than 95% of RCC. Two syndromes of familial RCC have been described. The most common familial syndrome is von Hippel-Lindau (VHL) disease, a neurocutaneous disorder associated with a high incidence of multifocal and bilateral RCC.[48] The other syndrome is in families with constitutional chromosomal translocations involving chromosome 3.[17] Recent molecular genetic analysis of patients with sporadic or familial RCC has implicated a gene or genes on the short arm chromosome 3 as playing a central role in the development of these tumors.[26]

Clinical presentation. Renal cell carcinoma may present with nonspecific manifestations or remain clinically silent until late in the course of the disease. The classic presentation of pain, hematuria, and palpable abdominal mass occurs in only about one fifth of patients and typically indicates the presence of advanced disease. Common constitutional symptoms include fever, weight loss, fatigue, and anorexia. Significant physical findings are often absent in low-stage or incidentally discovered tumors. In more advanced stages physical findings may include cachexia, flank or abdominal mass, hypertension, tachycardia caused by either intra-tumoral arteriovenous shunting or anemia, and occasionally palpably enlarged cervical or supraclavicular lymph nodes. The presence of a varicocele, especially one of acute onset, suggests a tumor thrombus in the renal vein or inferior vena cava.

Common laboratory findings include gross or microscopic hematuria, elevated red blood cell sedimentation rate, and hypochromic anemia; erythrocytosis is seen less commonly. Hypercalcemia occurs in 3% to 15% and is caused by either extensive bone metastases or ectopic production of parathyroid-like hormones by the tumor. Severe hypercalcemia may result in mental obtundation. Two syndromes of reversible, nonmetastatic hepatic dysfunction are occasionally seen with RCC. Stauffer's syndrome is characterized by hypoalbuminemia, prolonged prothrombin time, and elevated serum alkaline phosphatase, bilirubin, and serum glutamic oxaloacetic transaminase (SGOT).[31] Budd-Chiari syndrome due to obstruction of the hepatic veins by a tumor thrombus in the inferior vena cava causes hepatomegaly, ascities, and mild abnormalities in serum liver enzymes. Both types of hepatic dysfunction usually resolve with resection of the tumor.

Patients with VHL disease typically present as young adults with dizziness, ataxia, signs of increased intracranial pressure, or visual disturbances because of tumors of the cerebellum and retina. Renal lesions in VHL may take the form of cysts, adenomas, angiomas, or renal cell carcinomas. About 60% of affected individuals will have cysts, 15% adenomas, 7% angiomas, and almost half will be affected by renal cell carcinomas (RCC).[48] The carcinomas are by the far the most important of the renal lesions and account for a significant degree of morbidity and mortality in VHL. Although these renal tumors can have any of the signs or symptoms described for sporadic RCC, they are often asymptomatic, clinically occult, and are detected only upon radiographic screening of the kidneys. There are several important differences in the nature of the renal cancers encountered in VHL and the sporadic RCC that occurs in the general population. The first is that the RCC of VHL is often unsuspected because it frequently arises in the wall of an otherwise benign appearing cyst. Current radiographic techniques are inadequate in distinguishing between benign simple cysts and those that contain cancer in VHL, and the distinction is usually made only at the time of surgical excision. The second important difference is the age of onset. The RCC of patients with VHL is typically found at a much earlier age (usually in the 20s to 40s) than in sporadic RCC (40s to 60s), with about 40% of patients with VHL under the age of 35 at the time of diagnosis. The final difference is the propensity of RCC in VHL to be both multifocal and bilateral. The reported incidence of bilateral RCC in VHL is as high as 75%, in contrast to the 2% incidence in sporadic RCC.[48]

Risk factors. The association of risk factors for the development of sporadic RCC has been less systematically studied and is more poorly defined than for other tumors of the upper urinary tract. Smoking appears to be the single most important factor, accounting for about 25% of tumors.[60] Other life-style factors that carry an increased risk include obesity and abuse of phenacetin-containing analgesics, particularly in women.[54,97] Occupational exposure to cadmium, asbestos, gasoline, and leather tanning agents have also been associated with an increased risk of RCC.[56,58,61]

Patients on long-term dialysis because of renal failure are also at increased risk of developing renal adenocarcinoma. This risk is time-dependent and is closely associated with the development of acquired renal cystic disease. Acquired cysts occur in 35% to 50% of patients on dialysis for 3 or more years and may occur in those treated with either chronic ambulatory peritoneal dialysis (CAPD) or hemodialysis.[5,28] Histologically the cysts are characterized by papillary hyperplasia of cyst endothelium that appears to be a precursor to frank RCC. The risk of developing RCC in this population is 5% to 7%.[55]

Patients with VHL disease carry a 50% risk of developing RCC.[5] Because VHL is transmitted as an autosomal dominant, 50% of siblings, 50% of offspring, and one parent of an affected individual would be expected to have VHL and therefore also be at risk for RCC. Rarely will an individual with no affected family members (sporadic VHL) be identified.

Screening and prevention. Screening the general population for renal cell carcinoma commands interest because of several recent reports of an increasing incidence of incidentally discovered RCC (from about 10% in the 1970s to 40% in the late 1980s) during abdominal sonography or computed tomography (CT) scans performed for unrelated reasons.[49,91] Generally, incidentally discovered tumors are smaller, of lower stage, and occur in patients with better performance status than those discovered in symptomatic patients; therefore patients have an improved survival following nephrectomy.[90,91] Screening of the general population, however, appears to be limited by the low sensitivity and specificity of available tools to detect RCC. For example, routine urinalysis detected only 8% of 74 incidental RCC in one study.[91] Furthermore, the results of large-scale prospective screening studies using abdominal ultrasonography have shown a detection rate of only 0.028 to 0.13%.[80,90] In one report of 355 renal masses detected by abdominal ultrasonography in 41,364 asymptomatic patients, renal cell carcinoma was histologically proven in only 19 (0.04%), and no RCC were detected in 1667 patients with microscopic hematuria (Table 51-4).[90] Of the 355 asymptomatic patients with renal masses, all required abdominal CT scans and some required renal arteriography for definitive diagnosis, while three underwent nephrectomy for what proved to be benign problems.

Asymptomatic patients treated with any form of dialysis should be screened yearly for the development of renal cysts and tumors by renal ultrasonography. Lesions that are indeterminate or suspicious by ultrasound imaging should be further evaluated by computed tomography. Solid lesions should be assumed to be cancers and be treated by nephrectomy.

Because the number and location of lesions in VHL are variable, all potentially affected organ systems upon suspicion of diagnosis should be screened for involvement by appropriate physical or radiographic examination. Attention to the central nervous system is particularly important because the principal cause of death is cerebellar tumors. Because the renal lesions of VHL are typically asymptomatic and the incidence of renal cancer is high, the kidneys should be visualized. All patients suspected of VHL should undergo renal ultrasonography or a CT scan as part of the evaluation. Siblings and first-degree relatives of af-

Table 51-4. Incidence of renal cell carcinomas (RCC) in a population screened prospectively with abdominal ultrasonography

Patient group	No.	No. with renal mass (%)	No. with RCC (%)
Asymptomatic	41,364	355 (0.86)	19 (0.04)
Microscopic hematuria	1,667	39 (2.30)	0 (0.00)
Symptomatic*	2,874	75 (2.60)	16 (0.56)
Routine physical	21,818	56 (0.26)	—
Any symptoms	24,087	413 (1.71)	—
Total	45,905	469 (1.02)	35 (0.08)

From Tosaka A et al: Incidence and properties of renal masses and asymptomatic renal cell carcinoma detected by abdominal ultrasonography, *J Urol* 144:1097, 1990.
*Symptoms related to urinary tract.

fected patients should also be screened for renal and CNS involvement because of the autosomal dominant nature of hereditary transmission. Affected individuals who have yet to bear children should be advised of the risk of transmission to offspring. If renal lesions are demonstrated, surgical exploration is indicated to rule out the presence of RCC.

Screening therefore for renal cell carcinoma is indicated for high risk populations, which includes persons on long-term dialysis and patients with a personal or familial history of VHL. Screening of the general population is not cost effective with currently available tools. The prevention of renal cell carcinoma is directed to the avoidance of smoking, possible occupational carcinogens, and phenacitin-containing analgesics.

Tumors of the renal pelvis and ureter

Tumors of the renal pelvis and ureter (the upper urinary tract) account for only 5% of all renal tumors. Detailed demographic statistics on the incidence, prevalence, and outcome of treatment for these tumors are lacking because these tumors are rare and are not considered separately from other renal tumors in most cancer databases.[12]

Transitional cell carcinoma (TCC) accounts for more than 90% of upper urinary tract tumors, with a peak age incidence of 50 to 70 years. The occurrence of a TCC of the upper urinary tract carries a high risk of concomitant or subsequent development of TCC of the bladder, which occurs in as many as 40% of patients. In contrast, the risk of developing bilateral upper urinary TCC is low, with a reported incidence of only 2% to 4%.

Squamous cell carcinoma, adenocarcinoma, mesenchymal tumors, and metastases account for about 10% of renal pelvic tumors. These tumors do not carry the same risk of subsequent bladder cancers or bilaterality as TCC.

Clinical presentation. Most upper tract TCC present with painless hematuria but may be associated with flank pain caused by ureteral obstruction or the passage of clots. Approximately 15% are found incidentally during evalua-

Table 51-5. Relative risks for development of transitional cell carcinoma (TCC) of the upper urinary tract

Factor	Relative risk (odds ratio)	Reference
Analgesic abuse	2.4 to 4.2	57, 86
Coffee consumption	1.0 to 1.3	79
Industrial exposure		
Health care	0.4	40
Office work	1.0	40
Metal industries	1.4	40
Rubber industry	1.6	40
Paint manufacture	1.8	40
Leather and tanning	2.2	40
Chemical, coke, and coal industries	4.0	40
Tobacco		
Never smoked	1.0	40, 62
Cigars only	1.3	40
Pipe only	2.2	40
Cigarettes only	2.6 to 3.1	40, 62
Mixed, including cigarettes	3.8	40
Mixed, excluding cigarettes	6.5	40

Table 51-6. Dose- and time-related effects of tobacco use on the risks for development of transitional cell carcinoma (TCC) of the upper urinary tract

Factor	Relative risk (odds ratio)
Pack-years of smoking	
None	1.0
1-20	2.0
21-38	3.3
39-59	3.8
≥60	6.2
Depth of inhalation	
never/slight	1.0
deep	3.4
Filtration	
unfiltered cigarettes	1.0
filtered cigarettes	0.5
Years of cessation	
Current smoker	1.0
<10	0.9
10-24	0.3
≥25	0.3

Data from Jensen OM et al: The Copenhagen case-control study of renal pelvis and ureter cancer: role of smoking and occupational exposures, *Int J Cancer* 41:557, 1988.

tion for other conditions. Occasionally irritative bladder symptoms due to infection or associated bladder tumors may occur. Systemic symptoms are rare in the absence of advanced disease. Physical findings are usually absent, although a flank mass caused by a tumor or hydronephrosis is occasionally seen. Except for hematuria, laboratory findings are typically normal.

Risk factors. The major risk factor for TCC of the renal pelvis and ureter is smoking. Several studies have demonstrated that tobacco use alone accounts for 40% to 70% of all TCC of the upper tract, with a clear dose-related effect.[9,40,62,79] In a widely quoted Danish study, cigarette smoking was shown to be responsible for more than half of the observed tumors, with a relative risk of 2.6 compared with nonsmokers.[40] The addition of cigar and/or pipe smoking, the depth of inhalation, and smoking frequency all increased the relative risk of tumor development, whereas using filtered cigarettes and smoking cessation appeared to decrease the risk (Tables 51-5 and 51-6). Other studies have corroborated these findings.[9,62,79] These studies suggest that tobacco-derived carcinogens that are excreted in the urine act as inducers or promoters of urothelial carcinogenesis.

A higher risk for upper tract TCC (up to 4 to 5 times control) has also been reported for some occupational exposures, including the chemical, petrochemical, plastics, coal, coke, and asphalt industries (Table 51-5).[14,40]

Studies that have linked a higher risk of renal pelvic TCC and coffee consumption are difficult to interpret be-

cause coffee drinkers are often smokers as well. However, when smoking is controlled for, some studies have suggested a modest increase in risk (1.3 vs. control) associated with heavy coffee consumption.[79]

Residents of the Balkan states (Bulgaria, Rumania, Greece, and the former Yugoslavia) are at risk for developing an interstitial nephritis called Balkan nephropathy that predisposes to the development of renal pelvic TCC.[72,73] In contrast to sporadic TCC, these tumors account for up to 40% of all renal tumors in these countries, are more frequently bilateral (about 10% of cases), and behave less aggressively. The pathophysiology of tumor development in this syndrome is not understood.

Analgesic abuse accounts for up to 15% to 20% of renal pelvic TCC. Chronic use of oral phenacetin-containing analgesics increases the risk of renal pelvic TCC by 2.4 to 4.2 times normal, and up to 70% of abusers will develop TCC.[41,79,86] More than half of the patients with this form of TCC have reported consumption of at least 5 kg of phenacetin-containing drugs at the time of diagnosis.[57] Although the exact pathophysiology of tumor development in this setting is unknown, chronic analgesic exposure induces sclerosis of subepithelial capillaries. Cessation of drug use does not appear to alter the risk of later tumor development.[86]

Other factors that have been suggested to increase the risk of renal pelvic TCC include bacterial and viral infection, and exposure to cyclophosphamide.[9] Although cyclophosphamide does appear to increase the risk of bladder cancer, a clear association with tumors of the renal pelvis has not been shown for any of these agents. Chronic irritation of the upper urinary tract has been associated with squamous cell carcinoma, with more than half of these patients having a history of renal calculi.[40]

There are no known familial syndromes or genetic predispositions to tumors of the renal pelvis or ureter.

Screening and prevention. There are no generally accepted guidelines for screening the general population or populations at higher risk for the presence of TCC of the upper urinary tract. This reflects both the relative rarity of these tumors and the lack of noninvasive screening tests that have high sensitivity and specificity. In Tosaka's prospective study of renal ultrasonography in 45,905 Japanese, no tumors of the upper urinary tract were discovered in asymptomatic patients (N = 41,364) and only 3 were found in 2874 patients with urinary symptoms, an incidence of only 0.10% in the symptomatic group.[90] These observations, coupled with the high prevalence of smoking in the United States, makes even screening of smokers unlikely to be cost effective despite their 2.6-fold increased risk of tumor development.

The presence of an upper tract TCC should be considered in any patient with hematuria (gross or microscopic) or a positive urinary cytology. Given the high incidence of upper tract tumors in patients with Balkan nephropathy or analgesic abuse, clinical prudence suggests that these patients should be screened by urinalysis, urine cytology, and intravenous urography to exclude the presence of an asymptomatic tumor. Treatment for TCC of the upper urinary tract is usually surgical.

Patients with a history of upper tract TCC should undergo surveillance cystoscopy of the bladder to monitor for the development of TCC of the bladder, which may occur concurrently or subsequently. Cystoscopy should be performed at the time of initial diagnosis and at 3- to 4-month intervals for the following two years. Frequency of cystoscopy after the first two years depends upon the number and grade of bladder tumors observed.

Avoidance of smoking is the single most important factor in the prevention of upper tract TCC, and the data suggest that cessation of smoking lowers the risk for an established smoker within 10 years (Table 51-6). In contrast, cessation of analgesic abuse does not appear to lower the risk of tumor development, and it is not known if avoidance of acute or chronic industrial exposure will modify the risks of tumor development.

TUMORS OF THE BLADDER

Cancer of the bladder is the second most frequent urologic cancer, with an estimated 51,600 new cases and 9500 deaths in 1992.[12] Transitional cell carcinoma accounts for 90% of all bladder cancers, with squamous cell carcinomas, adenocarcinomas, metastatic cancers, and other histologies occurring rarely. Males are more frequently affected than females by a 3:1 ratio, and whites are more affected than blacks by 30% to 50%. The incidence of bladder cancer appears to be increasing in men and decreasing in women since the 1940s, although 30-year mortality rates show a decline in disease-specific deaths for both groups.[12,68] The incidence of bladder cancer rises steadily beginning at age 30 and peaks late in life, with more than one half of cases occurring after age 70.[84]

TCC of the bladder occurs in two forms, superficial and muscle invasive. Superficial tumors arise from the urothelial lining of the bladder and account for 70% of bladder tumors. Depending upon the size, number, grade, degree of mucosal invasion, and frequency of recurrence, superficial TCC are generally treated by transurethral resection and intravesical chemotherapy or immunotherapy. Most superficial tumors behave in a nonaggressive fashion, exhibit little tendency to invade the underlying bladder muscle, and are rarely the cause of patient death. However, approximately 10% to 15% of these tumors ultimately manifest progression to muscle invasion and require more aggressive therapy. Presently the ability to distinguish between the less and more aggressive forms of superficial TCC is limited.

Muscle-invasive bladder cancers show a marked tendency for local progression, invasion into surrounding organs, and lymphatic and hematogenous metastases. Even if treated early by radical cystectomy with or without systemic chemotherapy, long-term survival is approximately 50%.[12] Although most invasive bladder cancers are invasive at the time of presentation, approximately 10% to 15% arise from tumors that present initially as superficial TCC.

Clinical presentation. The most common clinical presentation of superficial or muscle-invasive bladder cancers is painless hematuria, which occurs in the majority of patients. Both types of tumors can be associated with bladder irritability manifested by urinary frequency, urgency, and dysuria, a symptom complex that is also typical of diffuse carcinoma in situ. In locally advanced disease, patients may have flank pain caused by ureteral obstruction or a pelvic mass. With metastases, systemic signs such as anorexia, weight loss, or abdominal or bone pain may occur.

Risk factors. As for TCC of the upper urinary tract, smoking is the greatest risk factor for TCC of the bladder. Compared with nonsmokers, cigarette smokers carry a 2- to 3-fold lifetime increased risk of developing bladder cancer.[68] The risk appears to be dose-related, with higher risks associated with smoking frequency and depth of inhalation (Table 51-7).[19,69] In contrast to studies on upper tract TCC, there is mixed data regarding the effects of duration of smoking, pipe smoking, beneficial effects of smoking cessation, and benefits of filtered versus unfiltered cigarettes in bladder cancer.[68,69] However, cigar smoking does not appear to increase the risk of bladder cancer.[37,68]

Table 51-7. Tobacco-related risks for the development of transitional cell carcinoma of the bladder

| | Relative risk | | | | | |
| | United States | | United Kingdom | | Japan | |
Factor	Males	Females	Males	Females	Males	Females
Nonsmoker	1.0	1.0	1.0	1.0	1.0	1.0
Ex-smoker	1.5	3.4	1.8	0.7	1.0	—
<1 pack/day	1.4	4.3	1.9	2.1	1.6	4.4
1 pack/day	3.2	—	3.2	—	2.1	—
≥1 pack/day	—	6.2	—	2.2	—	4.2
≥2 packs/day	4.7	—	—	—	2.8	—
All smokers	1.9	4.2	2.2	1.3	1.7	4.3

Modified from Morrison A, et al: Advances in the etiology of bladder cancer, *Urol Clin North Amer* 11:557, 1984.

Occupational exposure has also been associated with an increased risk of bladder cancer. Workers in the dyestuffs industry since 1895 have been known to have an increased incidence of bladder cancer, caused by exposure to highly carcinogen aromatic amines such as benzidine and 2-napthylamine.[13] Other industries reported to be associated with smaller but still increased risks of bladder cancer include rubber manufacturing and processing, and the leather, metal, paint, and textile manufacturing.[68]

Several reports have examined the relationship of coffee consumption with bladder cancer.[18,33,63] The results of these studies have been inconsistent in establishing a clear link between coffee and bladder TCC. Some of these studies have incompletely controlled for the effects of smoking.

The observations that the artificial sweeteners saccharin and cyclamate produce bladder cancers in laboratory rats have not been borne out in several large-scale human studies.[35,68] Most studies have also not established an increased risk of bladder cancer with the use of hair dyes and consumption of any dietary factors.[68]

Squamous cell carcinoma of the bladder is seen in high frequency in areas such as Egypt where bladder infection with *Schistosoma hematobium* is endemic, but is rare in the United States. Squamous cancers are occasionally seen in patients with chronic bladder irritation due to long-standing untreated bladder stones or long-term treatment with indwelling Foley catheters or suprapubic tubes. These tumors are invariably associated with multiple, recurrent urinary tract infections and inadequate urologic care over a period of many years.

Screening and prevention. Screening programs for bladder cancer are attractive because of the relative ease and convenience with which patients can provide urine samples for repeated testing as well as a plethora of reliable screening tests, including urinalysis dipsticks, standard urine cytology, DNA ploidy analysis by flow cytometry, quantitative fluorescent image analysis, and immuno-

histochemistry for TCC-related cell surface antigens. However, several factors mitigate the potential success of a wide-spread screening program. These include a long latency period in tumor development, a relatively low prevalence of bladder TCC, and a small potential for affecting patient mortality rates because most of the aggressive tumors present with muscle invasion at the time of diagnosis and can be cured only 50% of the time. A State-of-the-Art Conference on Bladder Cancer Screening called in 1977 by the National Institute for Occupational Safety and Health concluded that "there was a lack of good evidence on which to base a recommendation of screening for bladder cancer."[82] Based on numerous epidemiologic investigations that helped define groups at high risk for developing bladder cancer, a second conference was convened in 1989. The emphasis of this conference was to define what screening tests should be applied to high-risk groups, although again the consensus was that screening even high-risk populations remains investigational.[83] Thus beyond urinalysis advocated by some in an adult physical examination, a recommendation for the routine screening for bladder cancer of the general population or within the context of an individual medical practice by other means cannot be justified at present.

TCC of the bladder should be ruled out in any patient with microscopic or gross hematuria or with otherwise unexplained irritative urinary symptoms. A minimum evaluation for these patients includes microscopic urine examination, urine culture, urine cytology, intravenous urography or ultrasonography of the kidneys and bladder, and cystoscopy.

Avoidance of smoking is the single most important factor in preventing bladder cancer, although there is inconclusive data on the beneficial effect of cessation in long-term smokers. Avoiding occupational exposure to known carcinogens is also important in prevention. Patients managed with long-term indwelling bladder catheters should have the catheters changed every 6 to 8 weeks to prevent encrustation and be monitored for the development and treatment of bladder infections and stones.

REFERENCES

1. Adler SG, Cohen AH, Border WA: Hypersensitivity phenomena and the kidney: role of drugs and environmental agents, *Am J Kidney Dis* 5:75-97, 1985.
2. Alwall N, Lohi A: A population study on renal and urinary tract diseases, *Acta Med Scand* 194:525, 1973.
3. Alwall N, Lohi A: A population study on renal and urinary tract diseases, *Acta Med Scand* 194:529, 1973.
4. Anderson DA: Environmental factors in the etiology of urolithiasis. In Cifuentes-Delatte A, Rapado A, Hodgkinson A, editors: *Urinary calculi,* Basel, 1973, Karger.
5. Babiarz JW et al: The association of acquired cystic disease with renal cell carcinoma in patients on chronic ambulatory peritoneal dialysis. Abstract, North Central Section, American Urological Association Meeting, October 1992.
6. Badr KF, Ichikawa I: Prerenal failure: a deleterious shift from renal compensation to decompensation, *N Engl J Med* 319:623, 1988.
7. Barker DF et al: Identification of mutations in the COL4A5 collagen gene in Alport syndrome, *Science* 248:1224, 1990.
8. Bloom HJG et al: Hormone dependent tumors of the kidney, *Br J Cancer* 17:611, 1963.
9. Booth CM, Cameron KM, Pugh RCB: Urothelial carcinoma of the kidney and ureter, *Brit J Urol* 52:530, 1980.
10. Brazy PC, Stead WW, Fitzwilliam JF: Progression of renal insufficiency: role of blood pressure, *Kidney Int* 35:670, 1989.
11. Broadus AE et al: Evidence for disordered control of 1,25 dihydroxyvitamin D production in absorptive hypercalcuria, *N Engl J Med* 311:73, 1984.
12. *Cancer Facts & Figures—1992*. American Cancer Society, 1992.
13. Case RAM et al: Tumors of the urinary bladder in workmen engaged in the manufacture and use of certain dyestuff intermediates in the British chemical industry, *Brit J Ind Med* 11:75, 1954.
14. Catalona WJ: Urothelial tumors of the renal pelvis and ureter. In Walsh PC, Retik AB, Stamey TA, Vaughan ED, editors: *Campbell's Urology,* ed 6, Philadelphia, 1992, WB Saunders.
15. Chen BTM et al: Comparative studies of asymptomatic proteinuria and hematuria, *Arch Intern Med* 134:901, 1974.
16. Cleveland Clinic Foundation: *Diet manual: Key to nutritional care,* 1986.
17. Cohen AJ et al: Hereditary renal cell carcinoma associated with a chromosomal translocation, *New Engl J Med* 301:592, 1979.
18. Cole P: Coffee drinking and cancer of the lower urinary tract, *Lancet* 1:1335, 1971.
19. Cole P et al: Smoking and cancer of the lower urinary tract, *New Engl J Med* 284:129, 1971.
20. Costanzo LS, Windhager EE: Calcium and sodium transport by the distal convoluted tubule of the rat, *Am J Physiol* 235:F492, 1978.
21. Dobbins JW, Binder HJ: Effect of bile salts and fatty acids on the colonic absorption of oxalate, *Gastroenterology* 70:1096, 1976.
22. Ettinger B et al: Randomized trial of allopurinol in the prevention of calcium oxalate calculi, *N Engl J Med* 315:1386, 1986.
23. Evanoff GV et al: The effect of dietary protein restriction on the progression of diabetic nephropathy, *Arch Intern Med* 147:492, 1987.
24. Froom P, Ribak J, Benbassat J: Significance of microhaematuria in young adults, *Br Med J* 288:20, 1984.
25. Gabow PA et al: Factors affecting the progression of renal disease in autosomal-dominant polycystic kidney disease, *Kidney Int* 41:1311, 1992.
26. Gnarra JR et al: Molecular studies of sporadic and familial renal cell carcinoma. In: Klein EA, Bukowski R, Finke J, editors, *The Immunobiology of Renal Cell Carcinoma,* New York, 1993, Marcel Dekker.
27. Grantham JJ: Acquired cystic kidney disease, *Kidney Int* 40:143, 1991.
28. Grantham JJ, Levine E: Acquired cystic disease: replacing one kidney disease with another, *Kidney Int* 28:99, 1985.
29. Gretz N et al: Aport's syndrome as a cause of renal failure in Europe, *Pediatr Nephrol* 1:411, 1987.
30. Guidicelli P et al: Étude critique des hématuries microscopiques par examens de dépistage, *Ann Med Intern* 135:557, 1984.
31. Hanash KA: The nonmetastatic hepatic dysfunction syndrome associated with renal cell carcinoma (hypernephroma): Stauffer's syndrome, *Prog Clin Biol Res* 100:301, 1982.
32. Harris DC et al: Verapamil protects against progression of experimental chronic renal failure, *Kidney Int* 31:41, 1987.
33. Hartge P et al: Coffee drinking and risk of bladder cancer, *J Natl Cancer Inst* 70:1021, 1983.
34. HCFA patient statistics, *Nephrology News Issues* August, 1987.
35. Hoover R, Strasser PH: Artifical sweetners and human bladder cancer, *Lancet* 1:837, 1980.
36. Hostetter TH et al: Hyperfiltration in remnant nephrons: a potentially adverse response to renal ablation, *Am J Physiol* 241:F85, 1981.
37. Howe GR et al: Tobacco use, occupation, coffee, various nutrients, and bladder cancer, *J Natl Cancer Inst* 64:701, 1980.
38. Ihle BU et al: The effect of protein restriction on the progression of renal insufficiency, *N Engl J Med* 321:1773, 1989.
39. Israelit AH et al: Measurement of glomerular filtration rate utilizing a single subcutaneous injection of 125-iothalamate, *Kidney Int* 4:346, 1973.
40. Jensen OM et al: The Copenhagen case-control study of renal pelvis and ureter cancer: role of smoking and occupational exposures, *Int J Cancer* 41:557, 1988.
41. Johansson S, Wahlqvist L: A prognostic study of urothelial renal pelvic tumors, *Cancer* 43:2525, 1979.
42. Kasiske BL et al: Pharmacologic treatment of hyperlipidemia reduces glomerular injury in rat 5/6 nephrectomy model of chronic renal failure, *Circ Res* 62:367, 1988.
43. Kincaid-Smith P: Reflux nephropathy, *Br Med J* 286:2002, 1983.
44. Klahr S: The modification of diet in renal disease study, *N Engl J Med* 320:864, 1989.
45. Klahr S, Schreiner G, Ichikawa I: The progression of renal disease, *N Engl J Med* 318:1657, 1988.
46. Kleeman CR et al: Effect of variation in sodium intake on calcium excretion in normal humans, *Proc Soc Exp Biol Med* 115:29, 1964.
47. Klein EA: The challenge of advanced renal cell carcinoma. In Klein EA, Bukowski R, Finke J, editors: *The Immunobiology of Renal Cell Carcinoma,* New York, 1993, Marcel Dekker.
48. Klein EA, Novick AC: Urologic manifestations of von Hippel-Lindau disease, *AUA Update Series* 9:258, 1990.
49. Konnak JW, Grossman HB: Renal cell carcinoma as an incidental finding, *J Urol* 134:1094, 1985.
50. Lemann J Jr et al: The importance of renal net acid excretion as a determinant of fasting urinary calcium excretion, *Kidney Int* 29:743, 1986.
51. Levey AS, Pauker SG, Kassirer JP: Occult intracranial aneurysms in polycystic kidney disease, *N Engl J Med* 308:986, 1983.
52. Levitt JI: The prognostic significance of proteinuria in young college students, *Ann Intern Med* 66:685, 1967.
53. Locatelli F et al: Prospective, randomized, multicenter trial of effect of protein restriction on progression of chronic renal insufficiency, *Lancet* 337:1299, 1991.
54. Lornoy W et al: Renal cell carcinoma, a new complication of analgesic nephropathy, *Lancet* 1:1271, 1986.
55. MacDougall ML et al: Renal adenocarcinoma and acquired renal cystic disease in chronic hemodialysis patients, *Amer J Kidney Dis* 9:166, 1987.
56. Maclure M: Asbestos and kidney cancer, *Environ Res* 42:353, 1987.
57. Mahoney JF et al: Analgesic abuse, renal parenchymal disease, and carcinoma of the kidney or ureter, *Aust New Zeal J Med* 7:463, 1977.

58. Malker HR et al: Kidney cancer among leather workers, *Lancet* 1:56, 1984.

59. Mathiesen ER et al: Efficacy of captopril in postponing nephropathy in normotensive insulin dependent diabetic patients with microalbuminuria, *Br Med J* 303:81, 1991.

60. McLaughlin JK et al: A population-based case-control study of renal cell carcinoma, *J Natl Cancer Inst* 72:275, 1984.

61. McLaughlin JK et al: Petroleum-related employment and renal cell cancer, *J Occup Med* 27:672, 1985.

62. McLaughlin JK et al: Cigarette smoking and cancers of the renal pelvis and ureter, *Cancer Res* 52:254, 1992.

63. Mettlin C, Graham S: Dietary risk factors in human bladder cancer, *Amer J Epidemiol* 110:255, 1979.

64. Meyer TW et al: Converting enzyme inhibitor therapy limits progressive glomerular injury in rats with reduced renal mass, *J Clin Invest* 76:612, 1985.

65. Mogensen CE: Long-term antihypertensive treatment (over six years) inhibiting the progression of diabetic nephropathy, *Acta Endocrinol* 242:31, 1981.

66. Mohr DN, Offord KP, Melton LJ: Isolated asymptomatic microhematuria: a cross-sectional analysis of test-positive and test-negative patients, *J Gen Intern Med* 2:318, 1987.

67. Mohr DN et al: Asymptomatic microhematuria and urologic disease, *JAMA* 256:224, 1986.

68. Morrison A: Advances in the etiology of bladder cancer, *Urol Clin North Amer* 11:557, 1984.

69. Morrison AS et al: An international study of smoking and bladder cancer, *J Urol* 131:650, 1984.

70. Pak CYC et al: Gastrointestinal calcium absorption in nephrolithiasis, *J Clin Endocrinol Metab* 35:261, 1972.

71. Parving H-H et al: Effect of antihypertensive treatment of kidney function in diabetic nephropathy, *Br Med J* 294:1443, 1987.

72. Petkovic SD: Epidemiology and treatment of renal pelvic and ureteral tumors, *J Urol* 114:858, 1975.

73. Radovanovic Z et al: Family history of cancer among cases of upper urothelial tumors in a Balkan nephropathy area, *J Cancer Res Clin Oncol* 110:181, 1985.

74. Raij L et al: Therapeutic implications of hypertension-induced glomerular injury: comparison of enalapril and a combination of hydralazine, reserpine and hydrochlorothiazide in an experimental model, *Am J Med* 79:37, 1985.

75. Robertson WG et al: The effect of high animal protein intake on the risk of calcium stone formation in the urinary tract, *Clin Sci* 57:285, 1979.

76. Robertson WG et al: Should recurrent calcium oxalate stone formers eat less animal protein? In Smith LH, Robertson WG, Finlayson B, editors: *Urolithiasis: clinical and basic research,* New York, 1981, Plenum.

77. Robertson WG, Peacock M, Hodgkinson A: Dietary changes and the incidence of urinary calculi in the UK between 1958 and 1976, *J Chronic Dis* 32:469, 1979.

78. Rolin H, Hall P: Evaluation of glomerular filtration rate and renal plasma flow. In Jacobson H, Striker G, Klahr S, eds. *The principles and practice of nephrology,* Philadelphia, 1991, BC Decker.

79. Ross RK et al: Analgesics, cigarette smoking, and other risk factors for cancer of the renal pelvis and ureter, *Cancer Res* 49:1045, 1989.

80. Saita H et al: Mass screening of kidneys in 10,914 patients by ultrasound, *J Urol* 49:1035, 1987.

81. Sarig S: The hyperuricosuric calcium oxalate stone former, *Mineral Electrolyte Metab* 13:251, 1987.

82. Schulte PA: Screening for bladder cancer in high-risk groups: delineation of the problem, *J Occupat Med* 32:789, 1990.

83. Schulte P et al: Final discussion: where do we go from here? *J Occupat Med* 32:936, 1990.

84. Smart CR: Bladder cancer survival statistics, *J Occupat Med* 32:926, 1990.

85. Smith LH: The medical aspects of urolithiasis: an overview, *J Urol* 141:707, 1989.

86. Steffens J, Nagel R: Tumors of the renal pelvis and ureter: observations in 170 patients, *Br J Urol* 61:277, 1988.

87. Streem SB, Hall PM: Effect of captopril on urinary cystine excretion in homozygous cystinuria, *J Urol* 142:1522, 1990.

88. Swaye PS, Gifford RW Jr, Berrettoni JN: Dietary salt and essential hypertension, *Am J Cardiol* 29:33, 1972.

89. Taguma Y et al: Effect of captopril on heavy proteinuria in azotemic diabetics, *N Engl J Med* 313:1617, 1985.

90. Tosaka A et al: Incidence and properties of renal masses and asymptomatic renal cell carcinoma detected by abdominal ultrasonography, *J Urol* 144:1097, 1990.

91. Tsukamoto T et al: Clinical analysis of incidentally found renal cell carcinomas, *Eur Urol* 19:109, 1991.

92. Uribarri J, Oh MS, Carroll HJ: The first kidney stone, *Ann Intern Med* 111:1006, 1989.

93. von Bonsdorff M et al: Prevalence and causes of proteinuria in 20-year-old Finnish men, *Scand J Urol Nephrol* 15:285, 1981.

94. Wasserstein AG et al: Case-control study of risk factors for idiopathic calcium nephrolithiasis, *Mineral Electrolyte Metab* 13:85, 1987.

95. Williams HE: Oxalic acid and the hyperoxaluric syndromes, *Kidney Int* 13:410, 1978.

96. Yendt ER, Cohanim M: Prevention of calcium stones with thiazides, *Kidney Int* 13:397, 1978.

97. Yu MC et al: Cigarette smoking, obesity, diuretic use, and coffee consumption as risk factors for renal cell carcinoma, *J Natl Cancer Inst* 72:275, 1984.

98. Zeller K et al: Effect of restricting dietary protein on the progression of renal failure in patients with insulin-dependent diabetes mellitus, *N Engl J Med* 324:78, 1991.

RESOURCES

American Cancer Society, 1599 Clifton Road NE, Atlanta, GA 30329.

National Kidney Foundation, 30 East 33rd Street, Suite 1100, New York, NY 10016. Provides a variety of booklets, resource manuals, public information, and audio visual materials.

National Kidney and Urology Disease Information Clearinghouse (NKUDIC), P.O. Box NKUDIC, 9000 Rockville Pike, Bethesda, Md 20892. Provides resource, referral, and educational information.

Chapter 52

MUSCULOSKELETAL AND NEUROLOGIC DISORDERS

Daniel J. Mazanec

Musculoskeletal and neurologic disorders represent an enormous problem in occupational medicine today. Nationally, cumulative trauma disorders, of which carpal tunnel syndrome represents more than one third of cases, account for 48% of recorded occupational disease conditions.[10] Nonarticular rheumatic complaints ranging from shoulder periarthritis to DeQuervain's tenosynovitis and plantar fasciitis account for significant morbidity in the working and nonworking populations as well. Back pain is second only to upper respiratory infection as a reason for days lost in the workplace.[55] These conditions are of particular concern as they affect individuals in their most vigorous and productive years. Unfortunately, medical diagnosis and management is complicated by frequent associated litigation or compensation-related issues. Osteoarthritis represents the most common arthropathy affecting the U.S. population. As the mean age of the U.S. population rises, this age-related disorder will confront medical practitioners with increasing frequency.

The etiology or pathogenesis of these musculoskeletal and neurologic disorders is varied and in many cases not completely understood. Preventive strategies are therefore empirical in some cases. For certain conditions such as osteoarthritis, modifiable risk factors have been identified and can be incorporated into preventive management.

CUMULATIVE TRAUMA DISORDER
Overview

Cumulative trauma disorders (CTDs) encompass an array of musculoskeletal syndromes and nerve entrapments sharing a common pathogenesis: repetitive microtrauma with resultant tissue injury, inflammation, and, in some cases, ultimately, fibrosis. Overuse syndromes in competitive and recreational athletes share a similar mecha-

nism.[85,46] CTDs account for approximately 50% of occupational illnesses reported in the United States in recent years.[10] Approximately 60% of cases of CTDs reported occur in persons in assembly/production jobs and machine operators. In the upper extremity, cumulative trauma most commonly results in either nerve entrapment or tendinitis (see the box on p. 974).

Occupations requiring the repetitive application of high force at high frequency are associated with greatest risk of hand-wrist CTDs.[97] Use of vibratory tools in a variety of occupations increases risk of CTD, particularly if added to a highly repetitive, high force hand and/or wrist motion.[83,87] Repeated or prolonged direct pressure over an affected area will also contribute to these syndromes.

Carpal tunnel syndrome (CTS)

Definition. The carpal tunnel is bounded by the carpal bones on three sides and the transverse carpal ligament on the volar surface of the wrist (Fig. 52-1). In addition to the median nerve, nine flexor tendons course through the tunnel into the hand. The median nerve supplies the motor fibers innervating the thenar eminence and sensory fibers to the radial aspect of the thumb, second, third, and one half of the fourth digit. Carpal tunnel syndrome (CTS) refers to symptoms related to compression of the median nerve in the tunnel. Symptoms may be sensory or motor. The classical history is one of nocturnal pain and paresthesias in the distribution of the median nerve, often awakening the patient in the early morning hours. Similar symptoms may occur while driving, reading the newspaper, or when using the hands in fine motor activities (e.g., sewing or knitting).

Etiology and epidemiology. Carpal tunnel syndrome may occur as a primary disorder related to cumulative

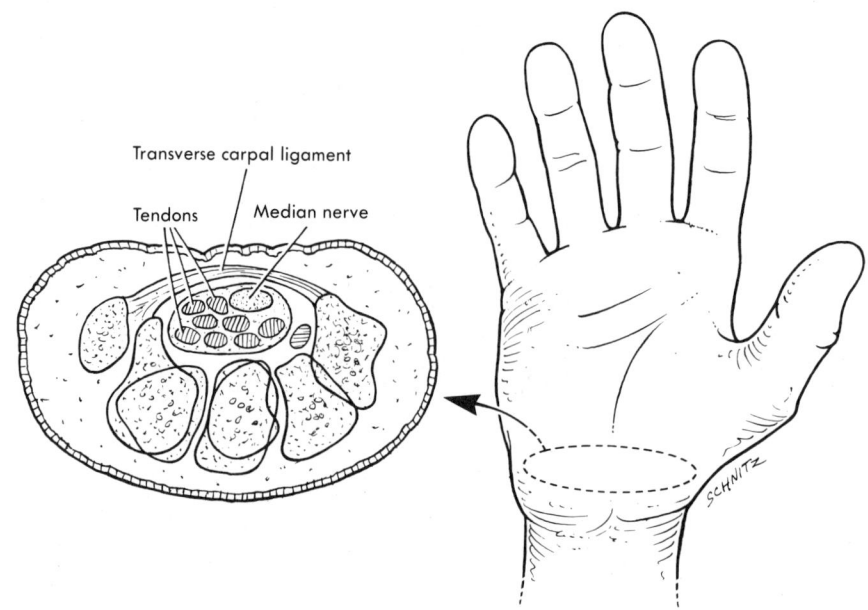

Fig. 52-1. Cross-sectional anatomy of the carpal tunnel illustrating its anatomic boundaries. (From Fess EE, Philips CA: *Hand splinting: principles and methods,* St. Louis, 1987, Mosby, 1987. Courtesy Gary Schnitz.)

Cumulative trauma disorders

Upper extremity

Shoulder periarthritis
Epicondylitis
Tendinitis (DeQuervain's)
Hand-arm vibration syndrome (HAVS)
Carpal tunnel syndrome

Lower extremity

Tendinitis
Plantar fasciitis

Carpal tunnel syndrome secondary causes

Arthritis
   osteoarthritis
   inflammatory arthropathy (i.e., rheumatoid arthritis, systemic lupus erythematous, etc.)
Calcium pyrophosphate dihydrate disease (pseudogout)
Pregnancy
Endocrine
   diabetes
   hypothyroidism
   acromegaly
Amyloidosis (multiple myeloma)

---

trauma or as a secondary condition related to another, often systematic illness (see box above, right). In addition, controversy exists regarding the role of pyridoxine deficiency in producing the syndrome. Recent evidence suggests pyridoxine deficiency results in peripheral neuropathy rather than actual carpal tunnel syndrome, despite evidence suggesting therapeutic benefit of the vitamin.[11,96] Occupations associated with increased risk of carpal tunnel syndrome require repetitive wrist movements as well as, in some cases, use of vibratory tools.[14] The role of repetitive flexion-extension movements in the pathogenesis of carpal tunnel syndrome is underlined by histopathologic studies that confirm maximum "stress" changes—increased subsynovial and connective tissue thickness as well as arterio-

lar and venular hypertrophy—at the flexor crease of the wrist.[3] Magnetic resonance imaging studies have demonstrated significant reduction in cross-sectional carpal canal area in flexion as compared with extension.[98] Studies comparing cross-sectional carpal tunnel area in patients and controls fail to demonstrate significant differences, however.[69,106,111]

Middle-aged women are at greatest risk for CTS.[49] In a study of hourly aircraft factory workers, a history of gynecologic surgery, particularly hysterectomy with bilateral oophorectomy was strongly associated with the condition.[14] The role of hormonal factors in the genesis of the syndrome is not understood but is also suggested by the association of oral contraceptive use with CTS.[91] Another factor in female predisposition for the syndrome may be a smaller carpal canal cross-sectional area in women than men.[20]

Screening and diagnosis. Diagnosis of carpal tunnel syndrome is suggested by the symptoms described earlier and the presence of Tinels and Phalen's signs. Tinels sign is "positive" when light tapping over the volar flexor crease of the wrist reproduces symptoms—pain or paresthesias—in the distribution of the median nerve. Phalens' sign is present when full flexion of the wrists with the hands suspended downward for 60 seconds produces similar symptoms. Phalen's sign is the more sensitive of the two tests (71% versus 44%), but Tinel's may be more specific (94% versus 80%).[37] Thenar atrophy is a late finding. Electrodiagnostic testing has been viewed as the "gold standard" for the diagnosis of CTS, but as many as 27% of patients with CTS have negative studies.[101] Abnormal digital vibrotactile sensation as assessed by vibrometry may be more sensitive than electrodiagnostic studies in the early diagnosis of CTS and is noninvasive and painless.[63] It is clearly superior to two-point discrimination testing, which has up to a 60% false negative rate.[21]

The role of screening tests—symptom questionnaires, physical examinations, vibrometry—for early detection of CTS in high-risk individuals in occupations discussed above has not been well studied.

Individuals with CTS, who do not work in a high-risk occupation, should be screened for secondary causes such as hypothyroidism, myeloma, diabetes, inflammatory arthropathy, acromegaly, osteoarthritis, or benign tumors.[96] Other conditions that may mimic CTS should be considered when symptoms are atypical and the diagnosis is not confirmed by vibrometry or electrodiagnostic studies. In this circumstance, cervical radiculopathy, thoracic outlet syndrome, and peripheral neuropathy should be considered as diagnostic possibilities.[87]

Approach to prevention and treatment. Prevention of CTS begins with recognition of the role of repetitive flexion and extension movements in the pathogenesis and analysis of occupational situations posing greatest risk to the worker. Modification of the work station may be appropriate.

Conservative (nonsurgical) therapy of CTS includes splinting of the wrist in the neutral position, anti-inflammatory drug therapy, and local corticosteroid injection and is effective in up to 65% of patients followed up to 3 years.[72] A specific exercise regimen (see box above) may be useful in rehabilitation as well. Treatment of other underlying medical conditions such as hypothyroidism or rheumatoid arthritis is often successful in relieving symptoms of nerve compression. Following recovery, analysis of the job site and modification of the workplace or work task as mentioned earlier should be considered. For patients failing conservative measures, surgical decompression should be performed. Surgical treatment may be the

---

Carpal tunnel syndrome preventive strategies

- Avoid strain to the wrist, especially in extremes of motion and force. Try to use the larger, stronger joints of the arm (elbow, shoulder) to tighten a vise or jar lid, or in turning a wrench. When driving, try to hold the wrist in a neutral position, not a prolonged, flexed, or extended position.
- Avoid jolting or vibratory motions or activities, such as hammering, stapling, or using a jackhammer.
- Avoid weight bearing on the hands with the wrists in extremes of motion. Avoid getting on your hands and knees, which puts pressure on the wrists in an extended position. Use a long-handled mop for the floors, or sit on the floor and move the sponge around with the wrist held in a neutral position, using more movements with the shoulder. Evaluate the daily movements that involve your wrist. You may be able to add more do's and don'ts to the list.
- Don't staple papers using palm of hand.
- Don't use a hammer.
- Don't apply force with a wrench or vice holding wrist in bent position.
- Don't use wide range of wrist motion while dusting.
- Don't use wrist motion while brushing hair or using curling iron.
- Don't drive for long periods of time with wrists held in extreme flexion or extension.
- Do use long-handled mop or sit on floor and keep wrist in neutral position.
- Do keep wrists straight and use shoulder motions instead.
- Do keep wrists straight and use compensatory movements with shoulder and elbows.

---

therapy of first choice when thenar atrophy is present or weakness of the thenar eminence is identified.

Hand-arm vibration syndrome (HAVS)

Hand-arm vibration syndrome is characterized by Raynaud's-like vasospastic digital symptoms ("white finger"), sensory and motor disturbances (paresthesias, numbness) and rheumatic findings including muscle fatigue, tendinitis, bone cyst formation and avascular necrosis (Kienbock disease).[84] This syndrome results from prolonged use of vibrating tools including compressed air tools, power hammers, chain saws, drills and grinders.[87] The condition is probably a result of cumulative vibratory injury to the neural tissue and microvasculature.

A number of strategies have been recommended to prevent the development of hand-arm vibration syndrome.[84] These include recognition of the hazard by vibration measurement and attempted reduction of vibratory transmission either at the source or by the use of antivibration gloves and antivibration pads on tools and saws. Development of alternative work methods or at least rotation of

---

Lateral epicondylitis rehabilitation exercises

These progressive exercises require only a few minutes a day and a set of dumbbells that can be increased 1 pound at a time from 3 to 6 pounds. Each of the four steps is increasingly difficult. You may move up to the next step only after mastering the preceding step.

Step 1: Grip firmly a 3-pound dumbbell in the playing-arm hand and then place the forearm, palm down, on a firm surface of books or cushions, with the wrist positioned at the edge so that the hand gripping the dumbbell hangs free. Then bend the wrist upward and toward the thumb as far as possible. Hold this position for 5 seconds, then return to the starting position and rest for 3 seconds. Repeat this 10 times, gradually increasing to 15 times.

Step 2: Hold the dumbbell as in Step 1 but with the palm up, and bend the wrist upward toward the ceiling as far as possible. Hold this position for 5 seconds, then return to starting position and rest for 3 seconds. Repeat 10 times and build up to 15 times.

Step 3: Holding the dumbbell as in Step 1, with the palm down, rotate the wrist straight upward toward the ceiling as far as possible, hold this position for 5 seconds before returning to the starting position and resting for 3 seconds. Repeat 10 times and increase to 15 times.

Step 4: Beginning with palm down, rotate the forearm 180 degrees, bring the palm upward and the dumbbell to horizontal. This motion should take 5 seconds. Repeat 10 times building up to 15 times.

Step 5: Hold the 3-pound dumbbell palm down and rotate toward the ceiling. Perform this routine 8 times quickly with no rest between repetitions. Do 3 sets of 8 repetitions with no more than 1 minute rest between sets. Gradually increase the weight until you can comfortably do 3 sets with 15 repetitions per set using an 8-pound dumbbell.

---

work tasks that require use of vibratory tools is recommended. Reduction of the "tightness" of the grip on the tool if consistent with safe work practices may reduce the risk of development of the condition. Early recognition of the signs and symptoms of HAVS with prompt removal from vibration exposure should reduce the likelihood of irreversible neural and microvascular damage.

Lateral epicondylitis

Particularly in the upper extremity, tendinitis as a result of repeated microtrauma with resultant inflammation and degeneration is common. Lateral epicondylitis (tennis elbow) refers to a painful condition resulting from inflammatory changes in the subtendinous space at the point of insertion on the lateral epicondyle of the forearm, wrist, and finger extensors.[39] Most cases are seen not in tennis players but in individuals who typically repetitively pronate and supinate the forearm with the wrist extended, such as construction workers using screwdrivers. The diagnosis is made by identifying the presence of discrete, exquisite tenderness over the lateral epicondyle at the point of soft tissue insertion. The elbow joint itself is normal to examination. Resisted wrist extension frequently produces pain at the epicondyle site. Typically, the patient's dominant side is affected.

Prevention rests on identification of the activity that precipitated the symptoms. As noted above, construction workers or electricians are particularly prone to the problem, but anyone engaged in repetitive pronation and supination of the forearm, particularly with wrist extension, is at risk, including gardeners, dentists, and politicians.[68]

Modification of the task or substitution of power equipment (power screwdriver) may be effective in preventing the condition. A "tennis elbow band" is a 2 to 4 cm wide elastic strap worn 1 to 2 cm distal to the epicondyle in the upper forearm. It has been proposed that the band, by changing the nature of the tension in the forearm muscles and tendons at the attachment point on the lateral epicondyle, may prevent or at least reduce the likelihood of degeneration or inflammation at that site.

Treatment of lateral epicondylitis may begin with a short course of a nonsteroidal antiinflammatory drug, but in many cases local corticosteroid injection is required and is usually successful. Surgical therapy is rarely indicated. Referral to a sports medicine physical therapist for instruction in an exercise-based rehabilitation program may be helpful, particularly if the individual will be required to continue the activity that precipitated the symptoms[27] (see box above).

DeQuervain's tenosynovitis

DeQuervain's tenosynovitis is another upper extremity disorder frequently related to repetitive overuse. The tendons of the abductor pollicis longus and the extensor pollicis brevis course through the distal forearm relatively superficially and angulate shortly at the radial styloid before insertion on the thumb. Repetitive manual tasks requiring grasping with the thumb and movement of the hand in a radial direction may result in inflammation of the tendon at the radius. Commonly, pain is localized to this area and aggravated by thumb flexion. In addition to local tenderness, the diagnosis is suggested by painful response to the

Finkelstein test. In this maneuver, the thumb is placed in the palm and clasped by the fingers with subsequent ulnar deviation of the wrist, eliciting increased pain.[105]

Prevention of forms of tendinitis such as DeQuervain's has not been well studied. Theoretically, the principles that apply to prevention of other cumulative trauma disorders, including identification of the repetitive activity responsible for the condition and avoidance of the offending activity by job modification or at least rotation of the task in the workplace, may reduce the likelihood of development of DeQuervain's disease. Treatment of DeQuervain's tenosynovitis includes a short course of oral nonsteroidal antiinflammatory drugs, immobilization with a splint (the splint should extend to the thumb tip), and corticosteroid injection if required.[51] In resistant cases or when resumption of normal activity including the repetitive movement that triggered the inflammation results in prompt recurrence of symptoms, surgical removal of the tendon sheath at the radius results in permanent resolution of the problem.

Plantar fasciitis or the painful heel syndrome

The clinical syndrome of plantar fasciitis, one of the most common causes of foot pain, is characterized by pain and tenderness over the plantar aspect of the foot often focused at the heel, typically worse on arising in the morning or after prolonged sitting. The condition, which is most common in people between 40 and 60 years of age and occurs with equal frequency in both sexes, is associated with obesity in more than one third of patients and pes planus in almost 25%.[36] In this same series, 16% of the patients were found to have an underlying and associated systemic illness including rheumatoid arthritis, gouty arthritis, and ankylosing spondylitis. The condition is also believed to result from prolonged standing or jumping and is more common in dancers.[95]

The diagnosis of plantar fasciitis is a clinical one, relying on the demonstration of point tenderness at the insertion of the plantar fascia on the medial process of the tuberosity of the calcaneus and extending distally along the longitudinal bands of the plantar fascia. Radiographic examination demonstrates calcaneal spurs in almost 60% of patients with the clinical syndrome of plantar fasciitis. It is likely that these spurs represent a consequence of plantar inflammation rather than a primary etiology of the syndrome. The presence of bilateral fasciitis in association with articular involvement elsewhere should suggest the possibility of an underlying systemic inflammatory condition such as rheumatoid arthritis or seronegative spondyloarthropathy. Prevention strategies for plantar fasciitis include treatment of obesity and pes planus. Particularly in individuals with pes planus who are required to stand for long periods of time, support of the plantar arch with arch-supporting shoes or arch supports including custom-fit inserts (orthotics) may reduce the likelihood of the syndrome.

Treatment of plantar fasciitis includes correction of any associated structural foot deformity such as pes planus noted above, nonsteroidal antiinflammatory agents, and local corticosteroid injection. The approach is effective in more than 70% of patients. Surgery is rarely required, but if it is necessary it is usually successful.[60] As the presence of a calcaneal spur is a consequence of the plantar inflammation rather than the primary cause, surgery to remove a heel spur, particularly in asymptomatic individuals, is not indicated. Once symptoms have resolved, patients should be advised to wear properly supportive shoes at all times in an effort to prevent recurrence.

THE PAINFUL SHOULDER

Shoulder pain represents a common musculoskeletal symptom, often attributed to injury in the industrial setting where it ranks second to low back pain in frequency.[41] Though "shoulder pain" can originate from the glenohumeral joint itself, or from referred sites, i.e., diaphragmatic irritation or cervical radiculopathy, more commonly the periarticular structures or rotator cuff are the source of the pain (Fig. 52-2, A, B).

The supraspinatus tendon and the tendon of the biceps muscle are most vulnerable to trauma or impingement between the head of the humerus and the coracoacromial arch. When the arm is raised to the position in which most upper extremity functions are performed, with the hand in front of the shoulder, the supraspinatus passes under the anterior edge of the acromion and the acromioclavicular joint.[78] Repetitive activities with the arm raised above the head result in the so-called "impingement syndrome" characterized by anterolateral shoulder pain, often with a painful arc at 60 degrees to 75 degrees of abduction.[96] Diagnosis is confirmed by the presence of a positive impingement sign. This is demonstrated with the examiner behind the patient, using one hand to prevent scapular rotation while the other hand raises the arm in forced forward elevation.[78] This produces pain that can be alleviated by injection of local anesthetic beneath the anterior acromial process (Fig. 52-2, B). Radiographic evidence of the impingement syndrome, characteristically a subacromial spur, is found in more than 20% of patients.[17]

Individuals at risk for the impingement syndrome include workers engaging in repetitive activities with the arm above shoulder level, such as overhead assemblers, carpenters, painters, or welders. Athletic pursuits, including swimming, baseball, tennis, and golf, may also be associated with the development of impingement symptoms.

The subdeltoid or subacromial bursa is the most important and dominant bursa in the shoulder region, located between the deltoid muscle and the capsule extending under the acromion and the coracoacromial ligament.[59] Inflam-

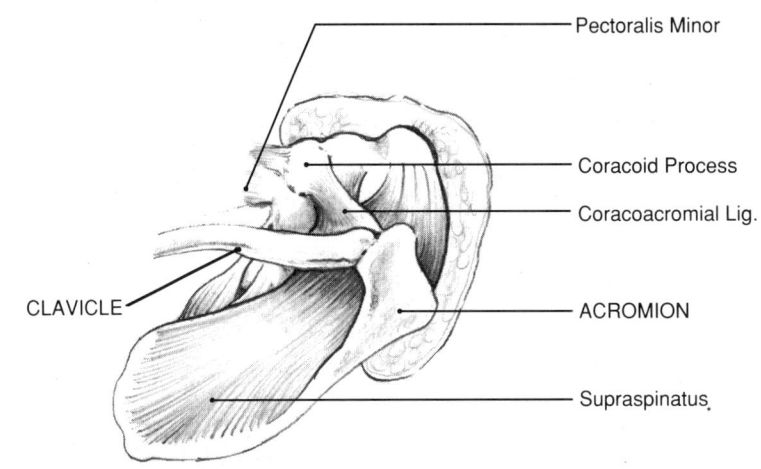

Pectoralis Minor

Coracoid Process

Coracoacromial Lig.

CLAVICLE

ACROMION

Supraspinatus

SUPERIOR

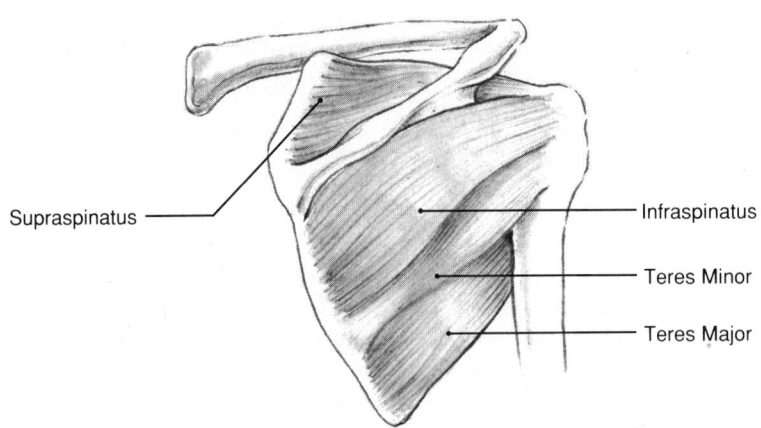

Supraspinatus

Infraspinatus

Teres Minor

Teres Major

POSTERIOR

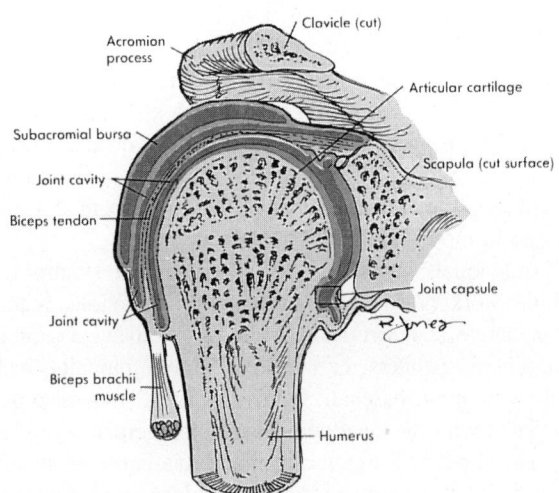

Acromion process

Clavicle (cut)

Articular cartilage

Subacromial bursa

Joint cavity

Biceps tendon

Scapula (cut surface)

Joint cavity

Joint capsule

Biceps brachii muscle

Humerus

Fig. 52-2. A, Long head of the biceps tendon and components of the rotator cuff (musculotendinous cuff derived from the subscapularis, supraspinatus, infraspinatus and teres minor muscles, which cover the glenohumeral joint before inserting on the humeral head). (From Reckling FW, Reckling JB, Mohn MP: *Orthopaedic anatomy and surgical approaches,* St. Louis, 1990, Mosby.) **B,** Shoulder joint. Frontal section of right shoulder. (From Seeley RR, Stephens TD, Tate P: *Anatomy and physiology,* St. Louis, 1989, Times Mirror/Mosby College.)

mation of the bursa related to rotator cuff trauma or degenerative change is common and produces local pain and tenderness extending distally to the insertion of the deltoid at the junction between the upper and middle third of the arm. Rotator cuff tear is a surprisingly common complication of shoulder periarthritis.[62] Tears typically occur in the supraspinatus tendon and may be partial or complete. In the younger patient, such tears are occasionally posttraumatic, but in an older patient the tears result from the degenerative changes described earlier. Though acute tear is dramatic with severe pain and inability to maintain arm abduction beyond 90 degrees, the more common presenting symptoms feature resistant "periarthritis," i.e., a painful shoulder unresponsive to usual conservative management. In such a patient, arthrography may demonstrate partial or complete tear.[56]

Bilateral severe rotator cuff tear with marked glenohumeral degenerative change has recently been described in older, predominantly female patients. This condition has been referred to as "cuff tear arthropathy," or Milwaukee

shoulder syndrome.[44,76] The difference in terminology relates to differing thoughts on pathogenesis. Cuff tear arthropathy presumes the primary event is massive tear of the rotator cuff, whereas Milwaukee shoulder syndrome implicates basic calcium phosphate (BCP) crystalline induced inflammation with resultant dissolution of the rotator cuff and subsequent glenohumeral joint degeneration as the pathogenetic mechanism. Clearly there is overlap as a number of patients with Milwaukee shoulder syndrome describe a history of joint injury or overuse. On the other hand, patients with Milwaukee shoulder syndrome have an increased incidence of polyarticular involvement, particularly of the knees, suggesting a systemic rather than a local traumatic etiology in at least some cases.[44]

Prevention of rotator cuff inflammation, including impingement syndrome, bicipital tendinitis, bursitis, and even rotator cuff tear, involves identification of activities, occupational or athletic, which expose the vulnerable aspects of the rotator cuff to degenerative change and inflammation. If possible, assessment of the job task by an

Shoulder range of motion exercise

A

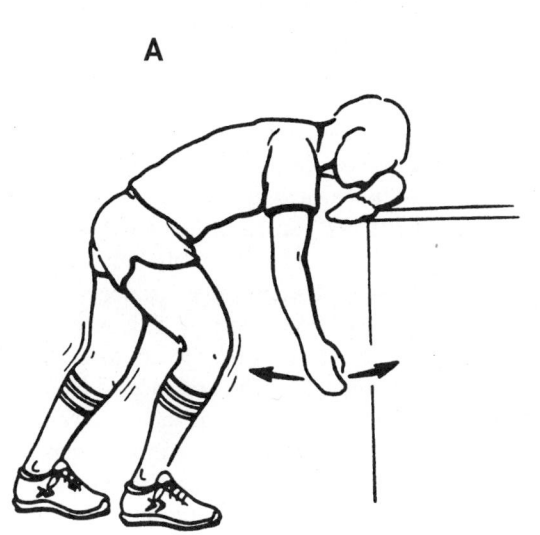

Pendulum exercise

Bending over at waist, circle entire arm, palm facing forward. Then circle entire arm counter-clockwise, palm facing backward.

B

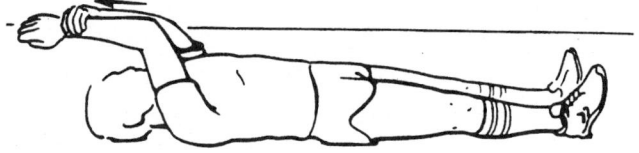

Assisted forearm elevation

Holding involved arm at wrist, assist arm overhead, keeping elbow as straight as possible. Uninvolved arm should provide most of the support to carry out the motion, both up and lowering arm down again.

Fig. 52-3. A, Pendulum exercise. Bending over at waist, circle entire arm palm facing forward. Then circle entire arm counter-clockwise, palm facing backward. **B,** Assisted forearm elevation. Holding involved arm at wrist, assist arm overhead, keeping elbow as straight as possible. Uninvolved arm should provide most of the support to carry out the motion, both up and lowering arm down again.

occupational therapist, with job modification to reduce the work required with overhead arm use, or at least to rotate such tasks with other jobs that don't require such a posture, should be considered. Avoidance of sports activities that require repetitive shoulder use should be recommended. Training programs, including isokinetic exercise strengthening, may particularly benefit athletes.[48]

Early management of shoulder periarthritis, a term used to encompass bicipital tendinitis, subdeltoid bursitis, or supraspinatus tendinitis, i.e., rotator cuff inflammation, includes avoidance of activities that aggravate symptoms, particularly overhead occupational or sports-related movements. Early treatment with nonsteroidal antiinflammatory agents in conjunction with physical therapy modalities may be successful.[16,40] However, for severe symptoms or symptoms resistant to NSAID therapy alone, local corticosteroid/anesthetic injection is usually effective.[90] Range of motion exercises are important in an effort to avoid the complication of adhesive capsulitis (Fig. 52-3). Initially, these exercises may be passive or use the opposite arm to assist in mobilization of the affected extremity. If loss of mobility is apparent at the initial evaluation, referral to a physical therapist for an aggressive, carefully supervised exercise regimen is appropriate.

Individuals with chronic shoulder pain determined to be related to a torn rotator cuff may respond to the same program outlined above.[106] However, in acute situations, or in patients with pain refractory to more conservative measures, surgical therapy effectively relieves pain and improves function.[86] Treatment of cuff tear arthropathy (Milwaukee shoulder syndrome) is more complicated, requiring a resurfacing total shoulder joint replacement with rotator cuff reconstruction and special rehabilitation.[76]

OSTEOARTHRITIS
Epidemiology and risk factors

Osteoarthritis (degenerative joint disease) is the most common arthropathy affecting the U.S. population. In particular, from the standpoint of preventive medicine, osteoarthritis of the *knee* represents a major cause of chronic disability in the United States.[9] Fortunately, though the etiology of osteoarthritis is not entirely understood, much information is available regarding risk factors for the development of knee osteoarthritis that permit some reasonable guidelines for preventive strategies (see the box above).

The prevalence of knee osteoarthritis has been estimated using radiographic techniques as well as by assessment of symptomatic disease. Radiographically, knee osteoarthritis is nearly two times more common in women and increases with increasing age, reaching a prevalence in the U.S. population of 19.5% to 25% in women by age 65.[19,29] Approximately one third of patients with radiographic knee osteoarthritis experience symptoms.[19,29] These same surveys suggest that black women may be

Risk factors for osteoarthritis of the knee
Well established
Obesity
Trauma
Possible
Anatomic variance
Knee valgus or varus
Leg length discrepancy
Questionable
Recreational—jogging/running

more susceptible than white women and prevalence rates plateau at approximately 80 years of age.

The most well-studied risk factor for knee osteoarthritis is obesity. Obesity at a young age is indeed predictive of increased risk of osteoarthritis in later years.[28] Risk of osteoarthritis of the knee is increased in obese symptomatic and asymptomatic individuals suggesting that obesity is etiologic rather than consequential in the development of osteoarthritis.[18] The association of obesity with osteoarthritis of the hips is relatively weak and demonstrated in white and nonwhite men only.[47]

Long-term heavy physical activity, occupational or otherwise, and joint trauma, particularly in the knee, are associated with increased risk of osteoarthritis.[57] Workers engaged in heavy material handling (e.g., dock workers) may be at increased risk for osteoarthritis of the weight-bearing joints as well as the spine.[82] On the other hand, recreational weight-bearing exercise such as jogging or running does not appear to be associated with increased risk of osteoarthritis in the knee. This appears to be true even in marathon class runners.[81] The presence of biomechanical abnormality or anatomical variance, however, may increase the risk of premature osteoarthritis even in moderate runners.[66] Such anatomic variances include knee valgus or varus deformity, leg length discrepancy, or mild hip dysplasia.[58]

Whether or not runners are at increased risk of osteoarthritis of the hip, even with normal biomechanics, remains controversial. A recent study suggests that high intensity high mileage running may, in fact, predispose individuals to premature osteoarthritis of the hip.[64]

Possible associations of other athletic activity with osteoarthritis have been recently reviewed.[80] For athletic activities other than running, the association of a specific sport and osteoarthritis in a particular joint is questionable at best.

Recently, in certain families a specific genetic association coding for a type II pro-collagen has been associated with generalized osteoarthritis.[1] Whether or not similar genetic associations underlie osteoarthritis in most patients remains unclear.

Prevention

Though the pathogenesis of osteoarthritis is incompletely understood, strategies to prevent or slow its development are available. Based on the previous discussion, maintenance of reasonable body weight and avoidance of obesity, particularly at a young age, are associated with reduced risk of knee osteoarthritis and reduced likelihood of significant disability. Modest weight reduction (approximately 10 pounds over 10 years) may reduce the risk of symptomatic knee osteoarthritis in women by more than 50%.[30] Avoidance of obesity as a preventive strategy, however, applies primarily to osteoarthritis of the knee and not to other sites, with the exception perhaps of the hip.

Repetitive trauma at other articular sites has been associated with the development of degenerative (osteoarthritic) changes. In the occupational setting, workplace design and rotation of job tasks are reasonable but untested strategies for reduction of osteoarthritic risk. Instability of the joint (i.e., excess, abnormal joint motion) is associated with accelerated degenerative change. For example, unrecognized rotator cuff tear with abnormal glenohumeral motion may result in "cuff tear arthropathy," a condition of severe, almost Charcot-like, degenerative joint disease at that site.[76] A similar situation may occur in a knee rendered unstable by significant meniscal or cruciate injury. Early recognition of articular instability and prompt repair may reduce the likelihood of secondary osteoarthritis in these situations.

Other biochemical abnormalities should be corrected, if possible, in individuals participating in weight-bearing athletic activities. For example, leg length discrepancy should be managed by a heel lift. Individuals in whom the biomechanical abnormality cannot be conservatively corrected should be encouraged to engage in nonweight-bearing exercise such as swimming or bicycling.

LOW BACK PAIN
Epidemiology and risk factors

Back pain represents a major health problem for society because of its frequency and its cost. The lifetime prevalence of low back pain is between 60% and 90%.[33] With the first episode typically occurring before age 40, the impact on workers in their most productive and vigorous years is significant. In the United States, impairments of the back and spine are the chronic conditions that most often result in limitation of activity in individuals younger than 45 years of age.[55] Low back injury accounts for 20% to 25% of all worker's compensation claims but a disproportionately high percentage of costs.[100,112]

The clinical problem of low back pain is compounded by the fact that in only 10% to 20% of cases can a specific anatomic etiology be defined.[74] Fewer than 1% of individuals with acute low back pain experience true nerve root compression, i.e., sciatica.[33] An array of physical findings and radiographic abnormalities have been found to be as common in individuals without back pain as in those with symptoms. Leg length discrepancy, increased lumbosacral angle, spondylolisthesis, transitional lumbosacral vertebrae, single disc space narrowing, Schmorl's nodes, disc space calcification, mild to moderate scoliosis, and spina bifida occulta are findings of doubtful clinical significance.[75,89] Magnetic resonance imaging and computed tomography are quite sensitive (80% to 90%) in detection of herniated lumbar discs.[70] In asymptomatic individuals, however, abnormalities are found in nearly 50% of scans—most commonly herniated discs, facet degeneration, or spinal stenosis (lateral and central)—indicating that careful clinical correlation is crucial to proper use of imaging studies.[109] In essence, most acute low back pain is attributed to a myofascial origin, i.e., "lumbosacral strain or sprain."

Fortunately, for most patients, acute low back pain resolves spontaneously. Fifty percent of back-injured workers recover sufficiently to return to work within 30 days and 90% return within three months.[2] The high cost of back pain is accounted for by the remaining minority of cases—about 10%—that are responsible for 90% of dollar cost.[100] Nonmechanical "serious" inflammatory causes of low back pain, the identification of which affects immediate therapy—malignancy, infection, spondylitis—are uncommon, found in .1% to 1.0% of unselected patients with back pain.[65] Clinical clues are usually present in such cases permitting more aggressive investigation and detection.

Many risk factors have been associated with low back pain, not all related to one's occupation (see the box below). Cigarette smokers are at increased risk for low back pain.[34] Increased cough with increased intradiscal pressure, smoking-related life-style factors, or even nicotine-

---

Risk factors for low back pain

Occupation

Truck drivers
Material handlers
Nurses

Life-style

Cigarette smoking
Poor fitness

Psychosocial

Job dissatisfaction
Depression
Previous back injury

induced vertebral blood flow reduction have been suggested as possible explanations for the association. Increased level of fitness and cardiovascular conditioning is associated with concomitant decrease in risk for back injury as demonstrated in fire-fighters.[12]

Certain occupations are clearly associated with greater risk for back pain. The three occupations with the highest rates of compensable back injuries are truck drivers, material handlers, and nurses.[54] These occupations share a common characteristic—frequent demand for heavy lifting, at times when bending and twisting. For nurses, the association of lifting requirement with back problems may explain the increased risk of back injuries in LPNs versus RNs or supervisory personnel.[45,102] In addition to lifting, vibratory exposure as in the use of jackhammers or machine tools may increase risk of back pain.[34] The vibration exposure in prolonged driving may compound the risk for truck drivers who load and unload heavy objects and then ride for lengthy periods in their vehicles.

Purely biomechanical factors are not the whole story, however, in assessment of risk for reported back injury. Psychologic factors, particularly job satisfaction and enjoyment, may strongly influence whether a worker will report an episode of back pain.[7] In jobs often without requirements for repeated heavy lifting, subjects who "hardly ever" enjoyed their job tasks were 2.5 times more likely to report a back injury than subjects who "almost always" enjoyed their work. A previous report of a back injury strongly increases the risk of subsequent back pain.[7,102] Whether this factor has a physical basis or is related to recognized or unrecognized psychosocial issues is not clear.

Compensation related issues

The costs of low back pain in the workplace are enormous. Estimates vary, but total costs—direct medical expenses, disability payments, and lost earnings and indirect costs—exceed 30 billion dollars per year in the United States.[104] Two percent of the entire U.S. work force sustains a compensable back injury each year.[8] In Ohio in 1990, the average days lost from work per back injury numbered 16.5.[79] Low back injury presently accounts for 20% to 25% of all worker's compensation claims. Approximately 10% of claims account for 80% of total costs caused by back injury.[100]

The current worker's compensation system, which requires employers to assume the expenses of a work-related job injury irrespective of fault, creates economic disincentives to recovery that may affect the success of medical or surgical therapy. These economic disincentives are magnified in individuals who have a higher degree of personal unhappiness and job dissatisfaction, with greater "secondary gain." Clearly, workers injured on the job recover more slowly from back pain. Railway workers with "lumbosacral sprain" incurred on the job missed 14.9 months of work compared to those with similar nonwork-related

symptoms who missed only 3.6 months.[92] The level of benefits affects the duration of back-related work loss. The greater the financial compensation, the greater the time the individual is off work.[104] Outcome of surgical therapy for lumbar disc disease is adversely affected by the presence of compensation issues as well. Surgically treated compensation patients are less likely to have complete relief of sciatic pain and less likely to be working 1 year after surgery than noncompensation patients similarly treated.[50] Certainly not all of this difference is necessarily related to compensation issues alone. The injured worker may well be in an occupation demanding heavy lifting to which he or she cannot return postoperatively. Second and subsequent surgical procedures in compensation patients have even more dismal outcome; only 40% of second procedures are "successful" in such patients.[103] Clearly, very careful patient selection for such procedures is mandatory.

Prevention and screening

In approximately 85% of cases, the specific etiology of an episode of low back pain is unclear.[107] Furthermore, probably as a result of current compensation laws, in the workplace back pain is commonly and at times inaccurately blamed on "injury."[42] Despite these considerations, the enormous cost of back-related symptoms has driven efforts aimed at prevention. Life-style modifications such as avoiding cigarette smoking and improving cardiovascular fitness have been associated with reduced risk of back pain and injury.[12,34]

Preemployment radiography. Preemployment screening has been used to attempt to identify prospective employees at increased risk for back pain. Several studies have addressed the value of preemployment spine radiographs in predicting risk of back pain with generally similar conclusions. Frequently commented on radiographic findings including transitional vertebrae, Schmorl's nodes, disc vacuum phenomenon, spina bifida occulta, scoliosis, loss of lumbar lordosis, and spondylolysis are observed as frequently in asymptomatic as well as symptomatic individuals.[35,38] The only two radiographic findings consistently reported increased in symptomatic individuals are spondylolisthesis and degenerative disc disease, particularly at the L4-5 level.[6,35,38,88] In younger employees, the maximum detection rate of clinically important radiographic findings with preemployment screening has been estimated at 10%.[88] In older individuals, the increasing prevalence of degenerative disc disease increases the likelihood of detection, but even in these individuals the positive predictive value of radiographic degenerative disc disease for back pain has been estimated at only 55% to 65%.[38] Clearly disk degeneration is a frequent finding in asymptomatic individuals. Based on these considerations, preemployment radiographic screening is not indicated.

Muscle strength testing. The conclusion that most acute low back pain is myofascial in origin, e.g., lumbosacral strain, raises the possibility of muscle strength testing as a screening tool to identify individuals at increased risk of back injury. In fact, earlier studies suggested that risk of back injury is increased when job lifting requirements exceed preemployment isometric strength assessment in work simulation.[15] A more recent study in industrial workers performing a variety of manual tasks found isometric lifting strength ineffective in identifying individuals at risk for back problems.[4] This study, however, did not address the possibility of mismatch between isometric lift strength and job demands as a predictor of back injury. Isokinetic lifting strength was not found to correlate with development of low back pain or injury in nursing personnel in a recent two-year prospective trial.[73] Preemployment strength testing—isometric or isokinetic—is clearly of little value when lifting requirements vary as widely as in the nursing profession. Mismatch of strength and lifting requirement cannot be assessed in this situation.

Preventive strategies. In addition to careful selection of workers in a preemployment screening process, prevention of back injury has been attempted by good training in proper lifting techniques. Unfortunately, there is little data that this information reduces the incidence of job-related back symptoms. The frequency of back "injuries" is not reduced in workers provided with lifting training in comparison with those who are not formally trained.[99]

Job modification to fit the worker—ergonomics—may offer effective prevention of back pain in those occupations in which lifting tasks are predictable and modifiable, unlike nursing as noted earlier.[99] Perhaps an even more effective means of preventing back "injury" is recognizing workers at high risk for reporting back symptoms as job "injury" on the basis of dissatisfaction with supervisors, perception of mistreatment by the employer, or even unhappy personal lives. This relatively recently described set of "risk factors" for back pain may explain the failure of prior preventive efforts, which focused primarily on physical variables such as muscle strength and radiographic abnormalities.[7]

Evaluation and treatment

Proper early management of acute low back pain is a critical factor in reducing the likelihood of chronic symptoms and disability. Recognizing the self-limited nature of most low back pain and the lack of a specific anatomic etiology in the majority of cases, diagnostic studies should be reserved for carefully selected patients only, particularly within the first month of symptoms. Treatment of most episodes of low back pain without sciatica should emphasize limited rest with early resumption of physical activity, accompanied by appropriate patient education and active exercise-oriented physical therapy in some cases. The importance of early return to work or "working through the pain," when appropriate, in reducing the risk of prolonged work absence cannot be overemphasized. Early recognition and treatment of individuals not progressing as expected may permit early intervention with more compre-

---

> **Selective criteria for X-ray use in acute low back pain**
>
> 1. Age more than 50 years
> 2. Significant trauma
> 3. Neuromotor deficits
> 4. Unexplained weight loss
> 5. Suspicion of ankylosing spondylitis
> 6. Drug or alcohol abuse
> 7. History of cancer
> 8. Use of corticosteroids
> 9. Temperature $\geq 100°$ F (37.8° C)
> 10. Recent visit for same problem and not improved
> 11. Patients seeking compensation for back pain

From Deyo RA: Early diagnostic evaluation of low back pain, *J Gen Inter Med* 1:328-338, 1986.

hensive rehabilitative services including assessment of psychosocial issues. An employer willing to provide opportunities for lighter duties, part-time work, and on the job rehabilitation is critical in limiting risk of prolonged work absence and, ultimately, permanent disability.

Diagnostic studies. Beyond careful history and physical examination, initial diagnostic studies in the patient with acute low back pain are directed by two considerations: the favorable natural history of the condition in most individuals and the low likelihood of serious, "urgent" causes mandating immediate identification and therapy.[65] In the majority of patients with acute low back pain, lumbar spine radiographs are not indicated. Ninety percent of patients with back "injury" return to work within 3 months.[2] The most common systemic disease responsible for back pain, cancer, is found in less than 1% of patients presenting with low back pain in a primary care setting.[23] Lumbar spine x-ray films are found to be normal or reveal "incidental findings" unrelated to the primary symptom in almost 80% of patients in whom they are ordered.[93] Oblique and spot lateral views provide additional information not present on routine views in less than 3% of cases, while nearly doubling x-ray exposure and cost.[94] Criteria for selective use of lumbar spine x-ray examination in acute low back pain cases at the first visit have been proposed[26] (see the box above). These criteria are intended for patients at the time of initial evaluation, within 1 month of onset of symptoms. Radiographic evaluation of patients with symptoms of greater duration, who have been unresponsive to usual therapy, should be individualized. Application of these criteria in a primary care setting resulted in a three-fold increase in yield of explanatory x-ray findings in patients with indications for radiography.[24] Indications for x-rays were present in all patients in whom malignancy was identified and in 13 of 14 patients with fractures, suggesting a high degree of sensitivity. Others have estimated the sensitivity of plain lumbosacral radiography for malignancy at 65% to 70% and for osteomyelitis at almost 90%.[61] Whether application of these guidelines in routine clinical practice will result in cost savings is unclear.[32] Patient expectation may affect physician ordering of radiographic studies as well. Patients given a diagnostic label, even if inappropriate from a medical standpoint, on the basis of an x-ray film study, may be more satisfied with their medical care and less likely to pursue care elsewhere.[53] This concern may be addressed by a proactive patient education program at the time of the first visit.[29]

Computed tomography (CT) scanning and magnetic resonance imaging (MRI) are appropriate studies in only a small fraction of patients with acute (less than 1-month duration) nonsciatic low back pain. CT or MRI is indicated in patients in whom spinal infection or malignancy is suspected clinically or on the basis of plain lumbosacral x-ray examinations. Both techniques are extremely sensitive (greater than 95%) for detection of abnormality in these situations and have reasonable specificity (approximately 80% to 90%).[71] For the vast majority of patients with acute low back pain, however, CT scanning or MRI is not indicated. Most patients have pain of myofascial origin for which scanning has no diagnostic value. Furthermore, the clinical significance of "abnormal" findings on CT scan or MRI is doubtful in most such patients. Regardless of age, 35% of CT scans in asymptomatic individuals are "abnormal," with findings of herniated disc, facet degeneration, and stenosis most commonly reported.[108] The frequency of "abnormal" findings in asymptomatic individuals increases with age. Clearly, attaching clinical significance to these findings in symptomatic individuals is difficult and risks inappropriate diagnostic labelling and unnecessary therapy including surgery.

An important, though often overlooked, element of the evaluation in selected patients is assessment of psychosocial barriers to recovery. As already described, issues related to job satisfaction, personal happiness, and compensation strongly influence the reporting of back pain as work-related and the speed of recovery.[7,104] Investigation of these issues in selected patients may avoid unnecessary interventions, including expensive and often repeated imaging studies and even surgical therapy. One avoided operation offsets the expense of 10 neuropsychologic evaluations.[13]

Rest in low back pain. Proper treatment of the patient with acute, nonsciatic low back pain may begin with a brief period of bed rest, but prolonged inactivity is inadvisable and may prolong disability. Comparison of two recommendations for bed rest, e.g., 2 days versus 7 days, in 203 patients with back pain demonstrated no difference in outcome other than the patients in whom 7 days rest was suggested missed 45% more work days.[25] Patients should be encouraged to gradually resume normal activities—including work—as soon as possible (see the box on p. 985). A cooperative employer offering "light duty" for a limited period with the employee's early return to work assists considerably in facilitating recovery and reducing the risk of long-term disability. Employees off work for approximately 6 months may only have a 50% chance of ever again returning to productive employment.[67]

Other conservative therapy. An array of "conservative" therapies are often employed in the management of patients with back pain. Examples of such measures include corsets, TENS units, traction, manipulation, ultrasound, electrical stimulation, epidural steroid injections, and medications of various categories. Though claims of significant benefit have been made for all of these modalities, in general benefits are short-lived and good clinical studies are few.[22,33] The assessment of the value of any of these therapies is difficult in a condition with a very favorable prognosis for full functional recovery in most patients regardless of treatment. Perhaps the most effective approach in terms of early return to full activity including work involves patient education and encouragement of active exercise by a physical therapist. A similar approach can be developed in a group setting or so-called "back school."[31,43] The back school approach emphasizes group instruction in spinal anatomy and physiology, body mechanics, psychiatric aspects of chronic pain, and methods of acute and chronic pain reduction, including exercise. Group interaction is encouraged. Patients are encouraged to assume responsibility for their own health status. Goals include return to full activity and reduction of future pain episodes. A comparison of physical therapy, back school, and "placebo" in 217 auto plant workers reporting work-related back pain suggested back school and physical therapy were equally effective and superior to placebo in reducing pain.[5] Absence from work during the initial episode was least in the back school group. However, time lost from work during the following year as a result of recurrence was the same in all groups.

Medical monitor/managed care. The use of an independent "medical monitor" to reduce days lost from work, unnecessary surgery, and compensation costs in industrial low back pain appears promising.[110] Using an algorithm for "appropriate" medical care of the back-injured patient, a physician uninvolved in the actual care of the individual reviewed the patient's progress on a regular basis (active group) or if the worker missed an expected return to work date (passive group). All patients for whom surgery was suggested were seen and imaging studies reviewed. If the monitor felt inappropriate physical or medical therapy was suggested, the treating physician was contacted. This medical surveillance approach resulted in marked decrease in low back patients (up to 44%), days lost from work (up to 60%), and low back surgery (up to 88%). Similar managed care approaches to occupational back injury using case management and practice guidelines or clinical algorithms are presently under investigation.

Recommendations for management of acute low back pain—patient instructions

Instructions—when in acute low back pain

The key to recovery from acute low back pain is maintaining the hollow or lordosis. When one loses the hollow in the back, it prolongs the recovery phase. It must be remembered that it is essential for the next 10 to 20 days that one retains the hollow in the back.

Sitting

- When in acute pain, one should sit as little as possible and then only for short periods of time (10 to 15 minutes)
- At all times, one must sit with a lordosis. One must place a supportive roll (sheet) in the small of the back. One must have a roll for the car as well as for use at home.
- One should sit in a high back chair with arms or use your lumbar roll. Sitting on a soft couch or chair will tend to make one round the back and lose the lordosis.
- Move to the front of the seat when rising from sitting. Stand up by straightening the legs. Avoid bending forward at the waist. Immediately do 10 standing backbends.
- **Remember**—poor sitting postures are certain to keep one in pain or make it worse.

Driving a car

- When driving, make sure to use the lumbar roll, as well as making sure that the seat is close enough to the steering wheel to maintain the lordosis.

Bending forward

- When in acute pain, one should avoid activities that require bending forward or stooping as you will be forced to lose the lordosis.
- **Remember**—keep the back straight and bend at the knees and hips to pick up any object off the floor or any surface lower than waist level.

Lifting

- When in acute pain, one should avoid lifting altogether.
- If this is not possible, one should at least not lift objects that are awkward or heavier than 30 pounds.
- One must use the correct lifting technique. The back must remain upright, and one must not bend forward. Stand close to the load, have a firm footing and wide stance; bend the knees and keep the back straight. Lift by straightening the knees and hips in a steady, fluid motion; come to a complete, upright position, and then one can walk with this object to where it needs to go.
- **Remember**—do not twist when coming to the upright position. Always move the feet.

Lying

- A good firm support is usually desirable when lying. If the bed is sagging, slats or plywood supports between mattress and the base will firm it. One can also place the mattress on the floor, a simple but temporary solution.
- One may be more comfortable at night when using a supportive roll. A rolled sheet or towel wound around your waist, tied down in front, is usually satisfactory.
- If one has always been on a soft surface, then going to a hard surface may lead to more pain.
- At times, one will find that the above positions cannot be maintained. Therefore, one should lie in the most comfortable position. However, do not get in a position where the lordosis can be lost, such as on the side, drawing knees to the chest.
- When rising from lying, one must retain the lordosis. Turn on the side, draw both knees up and drop the feet over the edge of the bed. Sit up by pushing up with the hands and avoid bending forward at the waist.

Coughing and sneezing

- When in acute pain, one must try to stand up, bend backward, and increase the lordosis while coughing and sneezing.

Remember

- **At all times,** one must retain the lordosis. If one slouches, one will have discomfort and healing time will increase.

SUMMARY

The musculoskeletal and neurologic syndromes reviewed in this chapter are extremely common and affect all segments of the adult U.S. population. Whereas medical management and diagnosis itself may be extremely costly, the costs incurred by disability are even greater, particularly as many of the disorders reviewed affect men and women in their prime working years. The preventive principles suggested in this chapter on the basis of a sound understanding of the likely pathogenesis of the various disorders are a reasonable approach to reduction of the significant medical, social, and economic impact of these conditions.

REFERENCES

1. Ala-Kokko L et al: Single base mutation in type II pro-collagen gene (COL2A1) as a cause of primary osteoarthritis associated with a mild chondrodysplasia, *Proc Natl Acad Sci USA,* 87:6565-6568, 1990.
2. Andersson GJB, Svensson HO, Oden A: The intensity of work recovery in low back pain, *Spine* 8:880-884, 1983.
3. Armstrong TJ et al: Some histological changes in carpal tunnel contents and their biomechanical implications, *Jour Occup Med* 26:197-201, 1984.

4. Battié MC et al: Isometric lifting strength as a predictor of industrial back pain reports, *Spine* 14:851-856, 1989.

5. Bergquist-Ullman M, Larsson U: Acute low back pain in industry, *Acta Ortho Scand* 170 (suppl):73, 1977.

6. Biering-Sorensen F et al: The relation of spinal X-ray to low back pain and physical activity among 60-year-old men and women, *Spine* 14:851-856, 1989.

7. Bigos SJ et al: A prospective study of work perceptions and psychsocial factors affecting the report of back injury, *Spine* 16:1-6, 1991.

8. Bond MB: Low back injuries in industry, *Industrial Med Surg* 39:204-208, 1970.

9. Brandt KD, Schumacher HR: Osteoarthritis and crystal deposition diseases, *Curr Opin Rheumatol* 4:543-545, 1992.

10. Bureau of Occupational Health: *Occupational Health Issues in Ohio,* Number 8, Nov. 1991.

11. Byers CM et al: Pyridoxine metabolism in carpal tunnel syndrome with and without peripheral neuropathy, *Arch Phys Med Rehabil* 65:712-716, 1984.

12. Cady LD et al: Strength and fitness and subsequent back injuries in firefighters, *Jour Occup Med* 21:269-272, 1979.

13. Camp PE: Invasive procedures for treating herniated discs: clinical and cost considerations, *Occup Med* 3:75-90, 1988.

14. Cannon LJ, Bernacki EJ, Walter SD: Personal and occupational factors associated with carpal tunnel syndrome, *Jour Occup Med* 23:255-258, 1981.

15. Chaffin D, Herin G, Keyserling W: Pre-employment strength testing: an updated position, *J Occup Med* 20:403-408, 1978.

16. Cogan L: Medical management of the painful shoulder, *Bulletin of Rheu Disease* 32:54-58, 1982.

17. Cone RO, Resnick D, Danzig L: Shoulder impingement syndrome: radiographic evaluation, *Radiology* 150:29-33, 1984.

18. Davis MA, Ettinger WH, Neuhaus JM: Obesity in osteoarthritis of the knee: evidence from the National Health and Nutrition Examination Survey (NHANES I), *Semin Arthritis Rheum* 20:34-41, 1990.

19. Davis MA, Ettinger WH, Neuhaus JM: Sex differences in osteoarthritis of the knee (OAK): the role of obesity, *Arthritis Rheum* 29:S16, 1986.

20. Dekel S et al: Idiopathic carpal tunnel syndrome caused by carpal stenosis, *British Med Jour* : 280(6227):1297-1299, 1980.

21. Dellon AL: Clinical use of vibratory stimuli to evaluate peripheral nerve injury and compression neuropathy, *Plast Reconstruct Surg* 65:466-476, 1980.

22. Deyo RA: Conservative therapy for low back pain. Distinguishing useful from useless therapy, *JAMA* 250:1057-1062, 1983.

23. Deyo RA, Diehl AK: Cancer as a cause of back pain: frequency, clinical presentation, and diagnostic strategies, *J Gen Intern Med* 3:230-238, 1988.

24. Deyo RA, Diehl AK: Lumbar spine films in primary care. Current use and effects of selective ordering criteria, *Gen Intern Med* 1:20-25, 1986.

25. Deyo RA, Diehl AK, Rosenthal M: How many days for acute low back pain? A randomized clinical trial, *New Engl J Med* 315:1064-1070, 1986.

26. Deyo RA, Diehl AK, Rosenthal M: Reducing roentgenography use. Can patient expectations be altered? *Arch Intern Med* 147:141-145, 1987.

27. Deyo RA: Early diagnostic evaluation of low back pain, *J Gen Inter Med* 1:328-338, 1986.

28. Duncan BF: Rehabilitation of tennis elbow syndrome, *Contemp Orthopaedics* 7:61-65, 1983.

29. Felson DT: The epidemiology of knee osteoarthritis: results from the Framingham Study, *Semin Arthritis Rheum* 20:42-50, 1990.

30. Felson DT et al: Weight loss reduces the risk for symptomatic knee osteoarthritis in women. The Framingham Study, *Ann Intern Med* 116:535-539, 1992.

31. Fisk JR, Dimonte P, Courington SM: Back schools. Past, present, and future. *Clin Ortho Rel Res* 179:18-23, 1983.

32. Frazier LM et al: Selective criteria may increase lumbosacral spine roentgenogram use in acute low back pain, *Arch Intern Med* 149:47-50, 1989.

33. Frymoyer JW: Back pain and sciatica, *N Engl J Med* 318:291-300, 1988.

34. Frymoyer JW et al: Risk factors in low back pain, *J Bone Joint Surg* 65A:213-218, 1983.

35. Frymoyer JW et al: Spine radiographs in patients with low back pain, *J Bone Joint Surg* 66A:1048-1055, 1984.

36. Furey JG: Plantar fasciitis, the painful heel syndrome, *J Bone Joint Surg* 57AL:672-673, 1975.

37. Gellman H et al: Carpal tunnel syndrome: an evaluation of the provocative diagnostic tests, *J Bone Joint Surg* 68A:735-737, 1986.

38. Gibson ES: The value of preplacement screening radiography of the low back, *Occup Med St* 3:91-107, 1988.

39. Goldie I: Epicondylitis lateralis humeri (epicondylalgia or tennis elbow): a pathogenitical study, *Acta Ortho Scand* 339(suppl):1, 1964.

40. Guerin BK, Burnstein SL: Conservative therapy of acute painful shoulder, *Orthop Rev* 11:29-37, 1982.

41. Hadler NM: Industrial rheumatology: clinical investigations into the influence of the pattern of usage on the pattern or regional musculoskeletal disease, *Arthritis Rheum* 20:1019-1025, 1977.

42. Hadler NM: Legal ramifications of the medical definition of back disease, *Ann Inter Med* 89:992-999, 1978.

43. Hall H, Iceton JA: Back school: an overview with specific reference to Canadian back education units, *Clin Orthop Rel Res* 179:10-17, 1983.

44. Halverson PB, Carrera G, McCarty DJ: Milwaukee Shoulder Syndrome: 15 additional cases and a description of contributing factors, *Arch Intern Med* 150:677-682, 1990.

45. Harber P et al: Occupational low back pain in hospital nurses, *J Occup Med* 27:518-524, 1985.

46. Hartz AJ et al: The association of obesity with joint pain and osteoarthritis in the HANES data, *J Chronic Disease* 39(4):311-319, 1986.

47. Hawkins RJ, Kennedy JC: Impingement syndrome in athletes, *Am J Sports Med,* 8:151-158, 1980.

48. Herring SA, Nilson KL: Introduction to overuse injuries, *Clin Sports Med* 6:225-239, 1987.

49. Howard FM: Controversies in nerve entrapment syndromes in the forearm and wrist. *Orthop Clin North Am* 17:375-381, 1986.

50. Hudgins WR: Compensation and success of lumbar disc surgery, *Tex Med* 70:62-65, 1974.

51. Janecki CJ: Extraarticular steroid injection for hand and wrist disorders, *Postgrad Med* 68:178-181, 1980.

52. Reference deleted in proofs.

53. Kaplan DM et al: Low back pain and x-ray films of the lumbar spine: a prospective study in primary care, *South Med J* 79:811-814, 1986.

54. Kelsey JL, Golden AL: Occupational and workplace factors associated with low back pain, *Occup Med* 3:7-16, 1988.

55. Kelsey JL, Pastides H, Bisbee GE Jr: *Musculoskeletal disorders: their frequency of occurrence and their impact on the population of the United States,* New York, 1978, Neale Watson Academic Publications.

56. Kerwein G, Rosenberg B, Snee WR: Aids in the differential diagnosis of the painful shoulder syndrome, *Clin Orthop* 20:11-20, 1961.

57. Kohatsu ND, Schurman DJ: Risk factors for the development of osteoarthrosis of the knee, *Clin Orthop* 261:242-246. 1990.

58. Lang N: Exercise in osteoarthritis, *Bull Rheum Dis* 41(4):5-7, 1991.

59. Larsson L, Baum J: *Bull Rheum Dis* 36(1):1-8, 1986.

60. Lester KD, Buchanan W Jr: Surgical treatment of plantar fasciitis, *Clin Orthop Rel Res* 186:202-204, 1984.

61. Liang M, Komaroff AL: Roentgenograms in primary care patients with acute low back pain: a cost-effectiveness analysis, *Arch Intern Med* 142:1108-1112, 1982.

62. Lie S, Mast WA: Subacromial bursography, *Radiology* 144:626-630, 1982.

63. Lundborg G et al: Digital vibrogram: a new diagnostic tool for sensory testing in compression neuropathy, *J Hand Surg* 11A:693-699, 1986.

64. Marti B, Knobloch M, Tschopp A: Is excessive running predictive of degenerative hip disease? Controlled study of former athletes, *Brit Med J* 299:91-93, 1989.

65. Mazanec DJ: Low back pain syndrome. In Panzer RJ, Black ER, Griner PF (editors) *Diagnostic strategies for common medical problems,* Philadelphia, 1991, American College of Physicians.

66. McDermott FP: Osteoarthritis in runners with knee pain, *Brit J Sports Med* 17:84-87, 1983.

67. McGill C: Industrial back problems: a control program, *J Occup Med* 10:174-178, 1968.

68. Medical Letter: Management of tennis elbow, *Medical Letter* 9:33-36, 1977.

69. Merhar GL et al: High-resolution computed tomography of the wrist in patients with carpal tunnel syndrome, *Skeletal Radiol* 15:549-552, 1986.

70. Modic MT et al: Lumbar herniated disk diseases and canal stenosis: prospective evaluation by surface coil MR, CT, and myelography, *Amer J Nucl Rad* 7:709, 1986.

71. Modic MT et al: Magnetic resonance imaging of musculoskeletal infections, *Rad Clin North Am* 24:247-258, 1986.

72. Moore L, Bernat J, Taylor T: Carpal tunnel syndrome: a conservative management program, *Arthritis Rheu* 26 (suppl):S33, 1983.

73. Mostardi RA et al: Isokinetic lifting strength and occupational injury, *Spine* 17:189-193, 1992.

74. Nachemson AL: Advances in low back pain, *Clin Orthop* 200:266-278, 1985.

75. Nachemson AL: The lumbar spine—an orthopedic challenge, *Spine* 1:59-70, 1976.

76. Neer CS, Craig EV, Fukuda H: Cuff-tear arthropathy, *J Bone Joint Surg* 65A:1232-1244, 1983.

77. Reference deleted in proofs.

78. Neer CS: Impingement lesions, *Clin Orthop* 173:70-77, 1983.

79. Occupational Health and Safety Research Section, Ohio Bureau of Workman's Compensation, *Ohio Back 1990 Injury/Illness Statistics,* 1990.

80. Panush RS, Brown DG: Exercise in arthritis, *Sports Med* 4:54-64, 1987.

81. Panush RS et al: Is running associated with degenerative joint disease? *JAMA* 255:1152-1154, 1986.

82. Partridge REH, Duthie JJR: Rheumatism in dockers and civil servants: a comparison of heavy manual and sedentary workers, *Ann Rheum Dis,* 27:559-567, 1968.

83. Pelmear PL, Taylor W: Hand-arm vibration syndrome: clinical evaluation and prevention, *J Occup Med* 33:1144-1149, 1991.

84. Reference deleted in proofs.

85. Pitner MA: Pathophysiology of overuse injuries in the hand and wrist, *Hand Clin* 6:355-364, 1990.

86. Post M, Silver R, Singh M: Rotator cuff tear: diagnosis and treatment, *Clin Orth* 173:78-91, 1983.

87. Rempel DM, Harrison RJ, Barnhart S: Work-related cumulative trauma disorders of the upper extremity, *JAMA* 267:838-842, 1992.

88. Rowe ML: Are routine spine films on workers in industry cost- or risk-benefit effective? *J Occup Med* 24:41-43, 1982.

89. Rowe M: Low back pain in industry—a position paper, *J Occup Med* 11:161-169, 1969.

90. Roy S, Oldham R: Management of painful shoulder, *Lancet* 1:1322-1324, 1979.

91. Sabour M, Fadel H: The carpal tunnel syndrome: a new complication ascribed to the pill, *Am J Gynec* 107:1265-1267, 1970.

92. Sander RA, Meyers JE: The relationship of disability to compensation status in railroad workers, *Spine* 11:141-143, 1986.

93. Scavone JG, Latshaw RF, Rohrer GV: Use of lumbar spine films: statistical evaluation at a university teaching hospital, *JAMA* 246:1105-1108, 1981.

94. Scavone JG, Latshaw RF, Weidner WA: AP and lateral radiographs: an adequate lumbar spine examination, *Am J Roentgenol* 136:715-717, 1981.

95. Sheon RP, Moskowitz RW, Goldberg VM: *Soft tissue rheumatic pain—recognition, management, prevention,* ed 2, Philadelphia, 1987, Lea & Febiger.

96. Reference deleted in proofs.

97. Silverstein BA, Fine LJ, Armstrong TJ: Hand wrist cumulative trauma disorders in industry, *Br J Ind Med* 43:779-784, 1986.

98. Skie M et al: Carpal tunnel changes and median nerve compression during wrist flexion and extension seen by magnetic resonance imaging, *J Hand Surg* 15A:934-939, 1990.

99. Snook SH, Campanelli RA, Hart JW: A study of three preventive approaches to low back injury, *J Occup Med* 20:478-481, 1978.

100. Spengler DM et al: Back injuries in industry: a retrospective study. I. Overview and cost analysis, *Spine* 11:241-245, 1986.

101. Stevens JC: The electrodiagnosis of carpal tunnel syndrome, *Muscle Nerve* 10:99-113, 1987.

102. Venning PJ, Walter SD, Stitt LW: Personal and job-related factors as determinants of incidence of back injuries among nursing personnel, *J Occup Med* 29:820-825, 1987.

103. Waddell G et al: Failed lumbar disc surgery and repeat surgery following industrial injuries, *J Bone Joint Surg* 61A:201-207, 1979.

104. Walsh NE, Dumitru D: The influence of compensation on recovery from low back pain, *Occup Med* 3:109-121, 1988.

105. Watson FM: Non-arthritic inflammatory problems of the hand and wrist, *Emerg Med Clin North Am* 3:275-282, 1985.

106. Weiss JJ: Intra-articular steroids in the treatment of rotator cuff tear: reappraisal by arthrography, *Arch Phys Med Rehabil* 62:555-557, 1981.

107. White AA, Gordon SL: Synopsis: workshop on idiopathic low back pain, *Spine* 7:141-149, 1982.

108. Wiesel SW et al: A study of computer-assisted tomography. I. The incidence of positive CAT scans in an asymptomatic group of patients, *Spine* 9:549-551, 1984.

109. Reference deleted in proofs.

110. Wiesel SW, Feffer HL, Rothman RH: Industrial low-back pain: a prospective evaluation of a standardized diagnostic and treatment protocol, *Spine* 9:199-203, 1984.

111. Winn FJ, Habes DJ: Carpal tunnel area as a risk factor for carpal tunnel syndrome, *Muscle Nerve* 13:254-258, 1990.

112. Worral JD, Appel D: The impact of worker's compensation benefits on low back claims. In Hadler NM (editor): *Clinical concepts in regional musculoskeletal illness,* Orlando, 1987, Grune and Stratton.

━━━━━━━━━━ **RESOURCES** ━━━━━━━━━━

Osteoarthritis

The Arthritis Foundation, P.O. Box 19000, Atlanta, GA 30326. Provides information and materials related to osteoarthritis and many other rheumatic disorders.

American Physical Therapy Association, Inc., 1111 North Fairfax Street, Alexandria, VA 22314-9902. Provides information for patients related to the role of physical therapy in the management of musculoskeletal disorders.

Chapter 53

HEADACHE

Glen D. Solomon

EPIDEMIOLOGY OF HEADACHE

Headache is the seventh most common presenting complaint for ambulatory care encounters in the United States. The problem of headache generates 18.3 million outpatient physician visits in the United States per year.[23] In spite of the enormous scope of the headache problem until recently little had been known about the prevalence of this common disorder. Most data about headache sufferers had been obtained from specialized headache clinics, whereas little was known about the majority of headache sufferers—those who did not consult physicians about their headaches.[23]

The advent of sophisticated epidemiologic methods and the widespread acceptance of the International Headache Society (IHS) criteria[20] (see box on p. 989) for the diagnosis of headache disorders stimulated a new understanding of the epidemiology of headache in the early 1990s. Four key studies,[23,25,30,38] each using a different method, definition of migraine, and population group, were performed in the late 1980s and early 1990s to detail the prevalence of headache disorders. Each of these studies is reviewed in detail.

Prevalence of headache

In order to determine the overall prevalence of headache in the general population Rasmussen and colleagues[30] examined 740 persons randomly chosen to constitute a representative sample of the population of Copenhagen, Denmark. The group was 25 to 64 years old and was representative of the Danish population as regards sex and age distribution and marital status. Subjects underwent a structured interview, examination by a neurologist, and laboratory evaluation. Headache disorders were classified according to the IHS criteria[20] (see box p. 989). This indepth evaluation offered the highest likelihood of differentiating among headache disorders and recognizing tension-type headache and migraine; however, the size of the population studied was, of necessity, limited.

The investigators reported a lifetime prevalence of headache of 96%, which was significantly higher among women (99%) than among men (93%). Only one case of cluster headache was found in this group. Men aged 55 to 64 years had the lowest lifetime and last-year prevalence of headache. Headache at the time of examination (point prevalence rate) was twice as common in women as in men (see Table 53-1).

The overall lifetime prevalence of migraine was 16%, 25% among women and 8% among men. A migraine occurring during the last month was reported by 4% of patients. The male/female ratio was about 1:3. There were no significant differences in migraine prevalence rates according to age.

Of migraine sufferers 15% had migraine 8 to 14 days/yr and 9% had it more than 14 days/yr. Of migraine patients 85% reported severe pain intensity.

The lifetime prevalence of tension-type headache was 78%, 88% among women and 69% among men. Of the subjects 48% had had a tension-type headache in the previous month. The male/female ratio was about 4:5. Men aged 55 to 64 had the lowest lifetime prevalence of tension-type headache. Among women there was a significant decrease in prevalence of tension-type headache with increasing age.

Of tension-type headache sufferers 23% had headache 8 to 14 days/year and 36% had it several times per month. Chronic tension-type headache (tension-type headache occuring $\geq$ 180 days/yr) was noted by 3% of the population. Only 1% of tension-type headache patients reported severe pain intensity; moderate pain was noted by 58% and mild pain by 41%.

International Headache Society diagnostic criteria

Migraine without aura

A. At least 5 attacks fulfilling B-D
B. Headache lasting 4-72 hours
C. At least 2 of the following characteristics:
    1. Unilateral location
    2. Pulsating quality
    3. Moderate or severe intensity
    4. Aggravation by walking stairs or similar routine physical activity
D. During headache at least 1 of the following:
    1. Nausea and/or vomiting
    2. Photophobia and phonophobia

Chronic tension-type headache

A. Average headache frequency ≥ 15 days/month for ≥ 6 months fulfilling criteria B-D
B. At least 2 of the following pain characteristics:
    1. Pressing/tightening quality
    2. Mild or moderate severity
    3. Bilateral location
    4. No aggravation by walking stairs or similar routine physical activity

C. Both of the following:
    1. No vomiting
    2. No more than 1 of the following: Nausea, photophobia, or phonophobia

Cluster headache

A. At least 5 attacks fulfilling B-D
B. Severe unilateral orbital, supraorbital, and/or temporal pain lasting 15 to 180 minutes untreated
C. Headache associated with at least one of the following signs, which have to be present on the pain side:
    1. Conjunctival injection
    2. Lacrimation
    3. Nasal congestion
    4. Rhinorrhea
    5. Forehead and facial sweating
    6. Miosis
    7. Ptosis
    8. Eyelid edema
D. Frequency of attacks: from 1 every other day to 8 per day

From Headache classification committee of the International Headache Society: Classification and diagnostic criteria for headache disorders, cranial neuralgias, and facial pain, *Cephalagia* 8(supp 7):1-96, 1988.

Table 53-1. Prevalence of headache by type of headache (% population)

	All headache	Migraine	Tension-type	Cluster
Last month	67	4-5.2	48	
Last year		4.1-10	74	
Lifetime	93-96	11.6-16	78	1

Table 53-2. Prevalence of headache by gender (% population)

	Linet et al.	Stewart et al.	Rasmussen et al.
Lifetime headache			
Total population	93		96
Males	90		93
Females	95		99
Last month headache			
Total population	67		
Males	57		
Females	76		
Lifetime migraine			
Total population	11.6	16	
Males		5.7	8
Females		17.6	25
Last month migraine			
Total population	5.2		4
Males	3		2
Females	7.4		6

Data from Linet MS et al: *JAMA* 261:2211-2216, 1989; Stewart WF et al: *JAMA* 267:64-69, 1992; Rasmussen BK et al: *J Clin Epidemiol* 44:1147-1157, 1991.

Headache prevalence in young adults

To assess the prevalence of headache in young adults and their use of medical care Linet and her associates[23] performed a population-based telephone interview study of 10,169 young adults (12 to 29 years) in Washington County, Maryland. This study was able to evaluate a community population sample and obtain specific data on medical consultation and medication use. This method did not allow for the diagnosis of specific types of headache.

More than 90% of males and 95% of females had a history of headache during their lifetime. Of males 57.1% and of females 76.5% reported that their most recent headache occurred within the previous 4 weeks. Only 9% of males and 5% of females had no headache during the previous year.

Of males 6.1% and of females 14% noted four or more headaches in the preceding month. Migraine headache (defined in this study as headache with nausea/vomiting and a visual prodrome, unilateral headache with a visual pro-

drome, or unilateral headache with nausea/vomiting) within the previous month was reported by 3% of males and 7.4% of females (Table 53-2).

Headaches caused significant disability. Almost 8% of males and 14% of females reported missing work or school. Disability was greatest for women aged 24 to 29 years. In addition, women described headaches that were more severe and longer than those of men.

In spite of the disabling nature of their headaches 85% of male and 72% of female headache sufferers never consulted a physician for a headache-related problem. Family practioners, internists, and ophthalmologists were the physicians most commonly consulted; neurologists were consulted by only 5% of headache sufferers.

The most common nonprescription drugs used for headache were acetaminophen (Tylenol, Tylenol Extra Strength), aspirin, ibuprofen (Advil), and aspirin with caffeine (Anacin). The most common prescription medications used for headache were acetaminophen with codeine (Tylenol with Codeine); butalbital with aspirin and caffeine (Fiorinal); butalbital with aspirin, caffeine, and codeine (Fiorinal with Codeine); and isometheptene mucate with acetaminophen and dichloralphenazone (Midrin).

Headache in the elderly

Headache in the elderly (defined in these studies as age $\geq$ 65) is less prevalent than in younger adults. Cook et al.[7] found that 53% of women and 36% of men reported headache in the past year. Headaches occurring several times a month or more often were reported by 17% of their elderly population. The overall prevalence of migraine was 12% among women and 7% among men. The prevalence of migraine fell with advancing age from 14% in women aged 65 to 69 years to 6% in women over 90 years old. In men the prevalence fell from 10% in those aged 65 to 69 to 0% in men over 90 years old. Solomon et al.[37] found that older headache sufferers attending a referral medical center had more tension-type headache (27% versus 20%) and less migraine headache (15% versus 31%), when compared with younger headache patients.

To describe the magnitude and distribution of the public health problem posed by migraine Stewart et al.[38] sent a self-administered questionnaire to 15,000 households representative of the U.S. population. Each household member with severe headache was asked to respond to detailed questions about his or her headaches. Responses were obtained from 20,468 subjects between 12 and 80 years old. The large sample allowed the authors to evaluate migraine prevalence, frequency, and disability by gender, age, race, household income, and geographic factors. This study did not address headaches other than migraine.

In this study migraine was defined as at least one severe headache in the last 12 months in a patient not experiencing daily headaches with one of the following sets of symptoms associated with the severe headaches: unilateral or pulsatile pain and either nausea or vomiting or phonophobia with photophobia, or visual or sensory aura before the headache. These criteria are consistent with the IHS criteria[20] and are somewhat more broad than those used by Linet.[23]

Migraine prevalence was 5.7% of males and 17.6% of females. Black and white females had the same prevalence of migraine, but migraine was less common in black males than white males (3.3% and 6.1%, respectively). Migraine prevalence was highest in both men and women between the ages of 35 and 45 years. Migraine prevalence was strongly associated with household income; prevalence in the lowest income group was more than 60% higher than in the two highest income groups.

Projecting these data to the U.S. population Stewart[38] suggested that 8.7 million females and 2.6 million males suffer from migraine headache with moderate to severe disability. Of these 3.4 million females and 1.1 million males experience one or more attacks per month. Females between the ages 30 to 49 years from lower-income households are at especially high risk of having migraines and are more likely to use emergency care services for their treatment.

Stewart[38] proposed several theories to explain the higher prevalence of migraine in lower-income groups. Diet, stress, and other factors associated with poverty may have precipitated migraine attacks. Alternatively access to good health care by higher-income groups may have decreased the duration, and therefore the prevalence, of migraine. In some sufferers the frequency of debilitating headaches may have led to loss of job or income, resulting in a downward drift in socioeconomic status.

Prevalence and impact of chronic migraine

To determine recent trends in the prevalence of chronic migraine and the impact on disability and use of medical care the National Health Interview Survey (NHIS)[25] collected data through personal interviews, conducted with a representative sample of the U.S. population, to determine the prevalence of migraine. Interviews were conducted from 1979 to 1989 from population samples of 60,000 to 125,000 persons. This study compared migraine prevalence for 1980 and 1989.

In the NHIS study[25] migraine was defined by answering yes to the question, "During the past 12 months, did anyone in the family have (a) migraine headache?," or by reporting migraine headaches that restricted or limited activity or resulted in hospitalization. This definition of migraine was the most broad of the ones used in the four studies reviewed here; however, its utility was limited by patient self-diagnosis.

In contrast to Linet,[23] who showed that about three quarters of headache sufferers did not seek medical care for their headaches, the NHIS study showed that more than 80% of female and 70% of male migraine sufferers had at least one physician contact per year because of migraine headaches, and 8% of female and 7% of male migraine patients were hospitalized at least once per year for migraine. Long-term limitations in functional capacity caused by migraines were reported by 3% of female and 4% of males.

NHIS reported the prevalence of migraine in the United States in 1989 (previous year prevalence) to be 41/1000 persons (4.1%). This represented a 60% increase in prevalence from 10 years earlier (25.8/1000 in 1980). These figures are considerably lower than the 10% previous year prevalence reported by the Danish group.[30] The difference in prevalence rate likely represents the method used to diagnose migraine, rather than a difference in the populations studied. The NHIS study used self-diagnosis, whereas the Danish study used physician evaluation, to diagnose migraine. Patients often misdiagnose themselves as having "sinus headache" or "stress headache" when migraine is the appropriate medical diagnosis.

The NHIS report[25] found that most (71%) of the increase in migraine occurred among persons younger than 45 years of age. In each year of the study the prevalence of migraine was greater in women than in men, and the rate of increase in migraine was greater in women than in men, 77% and 64%, respectively.

Although recent studies[23,25,30,38] have clarified the epidemiology of migraine headache (see Table 53-1), much less information has been found on other types of headache. Tension-type headache was evaluated only in Rasmussen's study,[30] which used direct patient interviews and examinations. Since tension-type headache lacks the dramatic associated symptoms of migraine, and because it may be self-diagnosed as "sinus headache" or "stress headache," tension-type headache is more difficult to study by questionnaires and phone interviews.

Cluster headache

In contrast to migraine and tension-type headache, cluster headache is rare. At specialized headache clinics its incidence has been reported as ranging from 2% to 16% of headache patients.[10] In his review of 18-year-old male Swedish army conscripts Ekbom[14] reported a 0.9% prevalence of cluster headache. D'Alessandro[9] reported a ratio of 0.69 cluster cases/1000 population. These figures are comparable with Rasmussen's[30] figure of approximately 1 cluster case/1000 population. This contrasted with a migraine frequency of 41/1000 (NHIS).[25]

Cluster headache is the only major headache that is more common in males. Studies suggest a male/female ratio of 5 to 9 males to every 1 female cluster sufferer.[10] The average age at onset for cluster is 26 years. Cluster headache in children is unusual, and only isolated cases are reported. Although migraine is a hereditary disorder, familial cluster headache is unusual, reportedly occurring in only 3% of cluster patients. A family history of migraine is reported in 15% to 17% of cluster patients, a figure compatible with the frequency of migraine in the general population.[10]

There is a significant association between cluster headache and cigarette smoking. Diamond et al.[10] found that 71% of patients with episodic cluster and 93% of patients with chronic cluster smoked cigarettes at the time of initial presentation. This contrasted with the U.S. population, in which 25% were smokers. Sadjapour[31] found that, with few exceptions, cluster patients were chronic, heavy cigarette smokers who began smoking during adolescence. He suggested that cigarette smoking may be etiologically related to cluster headache. A small percentage of cluster headache patients have been lifelong nonsmokers, however.

ECONOMIC COST OF HEADACHE

The economic toll from headache is enormous. The expense of physician appointments, emergency room visits, laboratory and radiographic studies, and prescription and over-the-counter medications is staggering. In addition to the expense of treatment the high cost of headache includes the cost to society in lost productivity.

Estimated productivity losses attributable to migraine range from $6.5 to $17.2 billion/year in the United States. The lost productivity of females caused by migraine was conservatively estimated at $4.3 to $4.7 billion in 1990. These figures addressed only labor costs related to lost workdays and lost productivity. Extrapolated to 1 year, the annual cost of lost labor from migraine was $2,712 to $3,072/person ($256/person/month). From the employer's perspective incorporating benefits and wages, the annual cost of lost labor attributable to migraine was $4,752 to $5,112/employee/year ($396 to $426/employee/month). These costs did not include direct costs associated with treatment (physician visits, medications, increased insurance premiums).[27]

SCREENING

Headache is a symptom rather than a disease. Headache usually is categorized as organic, meaning that it is a symptom of an underlying disease (i.e., giant cell arteritis, meningitis), or benign. Benign headaches are classified on the basis of patterns and accompanying symptoms (i.e., migraine, cluster). Screening in headache disorders is performed primarily to separate organic from benign disease. Screening for likelihood of headache in asymptomatic persons is not generally done.

History

The first step in evaluating any patient with headache is to obtain a thorough headache history.[11] The history is the key to making the correct diagnosis. Because the results of physical and neurologic examination, laboratory tests, and radiographic studies are usually normal, the headache history determines whether a headache is migraine, cluster, or tension-type or whether it represents a symptom of underlying disease. This does not mean that one can dispense with the proper examination of the headache patient. Every patient who seeks medical attention for headache should undergo a thorough physical and neurologic assessment to rule out organic causes of head pain. Most often a careful and complete history will provide a presumptive diagnosis, which can then be confirmed by physical examination and laboratory or radiographic studies.

Evaluating factors such as age of onset, temporal pattern, quality and location of pain, and settings that trigger headaches usually allows the physician to diagnose the headache problem and initiate therapy.

Most important at the beginning is the determination of how many types of headache the patient suffers. For each type of headache that the patient describes (and many have two or more types) a detailed headache history should be obtained.

Duration of the headache problem, or age of onset, is often a key indicator of probable underlying cause. Severe headache of sudden onset, especially if associated with focal neurologic signs or changes in level of consciousness, suggests serious illness, such as hemorrhage or meningitis (which must be immediately ruled out by physical and laboratory evaluation).

Recurrent episodic headache dating back many years, on the other hand, more likely reflects a type of vascular headache—migraine or cluster. A long history of daily headaches without associated symptoms suggests chronic tension-type headache.

The patient's initial migraine headache, unless preceded by a characteristic aura, may be confused with serious neurologic problems, such as meningitis or intracerebral hemorrhage.

Among the most difficult headaches to interpret are those developing over weeks or months. These may be benign or arise from conditions as diverse as sinusitis, ocular disease, subdural hematoma, mass lesion, hydrocephalus, or—in the patient above age 60—giant cell arteritis.

After establishing the frequency and duration of the headache the timing with respect to other physiologic events can be crucial to correct diagnosis of the recurrent headache. One should inquire as to the time of day the headache occurs and its relationship to puberty, menses, pregnancy, menopause, or use of hormones.

Migraine often initially occurs during puberty and may resolve after menopause. It may occur irregularly for months to years or may follow a regular pattern of occurring with menses. An acute migraine attack can last from 4 to 72 hours, with headache-free intervals between attacks.

Episodic cluster headache follows a pattern of cyclic bouts of attacks, lasting 2 weeks to several months, often in the spring and fall. These bouts are separated by quiescent periods lasting months to years. During these bouts severe headaches lasting 15 minutes to 3 hours may occur one to four times a day, often awakening the patient from sleep at night.

The duration of the cluster headache attack distinguishes it from trigeminal neuralgia, which is characterized by recurrent jabs of pain lasting less than a minute.

Cluster variant headaches, such as chronic paroxysmal hemicrania, show a pain pattern similar to that of cluster headache, but attacks are more frequent and predominantly occur during the day.

Chronic tension-type headaches show no periodicity and have rare headache-free intervals: the patient typically describes a daily unrelenting headache. The mixed headache syndrome is characterized by intermittent paroxysms of severe, throbbing, "sick" (migraine) headache superimposed on a constant daily headache.

Location of the head pain can sometimes aid in diagnosis, as in cluster headache or trigeminal neuralgia, but also can be misleading. Although migraine is unilateral two thirds of the time, it is bilateral one third. Chronic tension-type headache is usually bilateral but may be unilateral. Cluster headache, trigeminal neuralgia, and headache linked to local disease of the eye, nose, sinuses, or scalp are always unilateral. Headaches arising from hemorrhage or space-occupying lesions may begin unilaterally but usually become bilateral. Migraine usually alternates sides with different attacks but may be predominantly unilateral throughout life. Cluster headache is invariably unilateral and affects only one side during a series of attacks.

The patient's description of the quality of the pain can be valuable. Migraine is usually throbbing or pulsatile, whereas a constant ache suggests tension-type headache, and deep, boring, intense pain points to cluster headache. Trigeminal neuralgia is marked by short, intense, shock-like jabs.

The intensity of pain in cluster headache and trigeminal neuralgia is invariably described as severe, so much so that the cluster headache patient usually cannot remain still. The migraine patient, by contrast, often seeks to rest in the stillness of a darkened room.

If the patient tells of an aura or warning signs, this generally indicates migraine with aura (classic migraine), the only type of headache with a recognizable prodrome. Visual or neurologic symptoms commonly precede the headache by 10 to 60 minutes (usually 20 minutes). Premonitory symptoms, which can include euphoria, fatigue, yawning, and craving for sweets, may occur 12 to 24 hours before an attack.

Associated symptoms that may accompany migraine include photophobia, phonophobia, anorexia, nausea, vomiting, and focal neurologic signs. Seen with cluster headache are partial Horner's syndrome, constricted pupils, injected conjunctiva, and unilateral lacrimation and rhinorrhea. Rhinorrhea and nasal congestion are also common in sinusitis.

Neck stiffness or other signs of meningeal irritation can signal meningitis, encephalitis, or hemorrhage. A mass lesion, hydrocephalus, or encephalitis may be suggested by decreased level of consciousness or obtundation. Seizures can reflect cortical irritation resulting from a mass lesion or arteriovenous malformation. Fever and sweating suggest an infectious process.

One also should consider precipitating factors (see box below). Fatigue, particularly loss of sleep, may trigger either migraine or tension-type headache. Stress may exacerbate tension-type headache, whereas migraine may follow a period of stress, often occurring on weekends or vacations. Migraine patients may associate their headaches with menses, missed meals, or foods rich in tyramine, such as red wine or aged cheese. Alcohol may trigger a cluster attack during a series but will have no effect during a quiescent period. Weather changes can be associated with migraine or exacerbation of sinusitis. Commonly associated with chronic tension-type headache are symptoms of depression, such as sleep and appetite disturbances.

One also should assess possible exposure to occupational toxins, chemicals, or infectious agents. Carbon monoxide poisoning, for example, often manifests as headache. Certain chemicals such as nitrates induce withdrawal and reintroduction headache. It should be emphasized that exposure to infectious agents in immunosuppressed or acquired immunodeficiency syndrome (AIDS) patients may induce encephalitis or meningitis unaccompanied by classic fever and stiff neck.

Family history

Reviewing the patient's family history may prove rewarding. Migraine is a familial disorder, with a positive family history in two thirds of cases. Three quarters of patients have a family history of migraine on the maternal side only, 20% on the paternal side only, and 6% on both sides. As indicated by a number of studies there is approximately a 70% risk of migraine in offspring when both parents suffer from migraine, 45% risk when only one parent is affected, and less than 30% risk when both parents are unaffected. The risk for siblings indicated by an affected child but with unaffected parents is estimated at 20%. The genetic basis for migraine is probably multifactorial: the genetic component is polygenic with an additive effect of a number of genes that render the individual more or less susceptible to the disorder in response to a number of environmental trigger factors.

Cluster headache is familial in only about 3% of patients.[10] In tension-type headache a family history of depression or alcohol abuse is common. This may reflect a hereditary abnormality of serotonin neurotransmission, which has been associated with tension-type headache sufferers, depressed patients, and alcohol and physical abusers.

Other related history

The patient's medical-surgical history and history of current and previous medications can aid in diagnosis. Head trauma, for instance, may suggest subdural hematoma or skull fracture. Certain medications can trigger the onset of headache or exacerbate headache in patients with an underlying headache disorder. Askmark and colleagues[1] evaluated data from the World Health Organization Collaborating Centre for International Drug Monitoring. Medication-induced headache was most frequently reported with the following medications: indomethacin, nifedipine, cimetidine, atenolol, trimethoprim-sulfamethoxazole, zimeldine, nitroglycerin, isosorbide dinitrate, ranitidine, isotretinoin, captopril, piroxicam, metoprolol, and diclofenac. When the frequency of headache was evaluated with respect to the amount of drug sold, the drugs most

---

Common triggers for migraine

Foods
  Aged cheese
  Alcohol
  Monosodium glutamate (MSG)
  Chocolate
  Caffeinated beverages
  Nitrites and nitrates (hot dogs, sausages, luncheon meats)
  Avocado
  Smoked or pickled fish or meats
  Yeast or protein extracts (brewer's yeast, marmite)
  Onions
  Nuts
  Dietary sweetener (Aspartame)
Medications
  Antibiotics: trimethoprim-sulfamethoxazole, griseofulvin
  Antihypertensives: nifedipine, captopril, atenolol, metoprolol, prazosin, reserpine, minoxidil
  Histamine-2 blockers: cimetidine, ranitidine

Hormones: Oral contraceptives, estrogens, clomiphene citrate, danazol
NSAIDs: indomethacin, diclofenac, piroxicam
Vasodilators: nitroglycerin, isosorbide dinitrate
Others: isotretinoin, erythropoetin
Life-style
  Fasting or skipping meals
  Sleeping late or changes in sleep patterns (shift changes or jet lag)
  Letdown following stress (weekends, vacations, after college examinations)
  Caffeine withdrawal
Others
  Weather changes
  High altitude (air travel, mountain climbing)

likely to cause headache were zimeldine, nalidixic acid, trimethoprim, griseofulvin, ranitidine, and nifedipine.

Certain medications were found to initiate migraine headaches. These included cimetidine, oral contraceptives, atenolol, indomethacin, danazol, nifedipine, diclofenac, and ranitidine. Medications that may aggravate existing migraine include vitamin A, its retinoic acid derivatives, and hormonal therapy, such as oral contraceptives, clomiphene, and postmenopausal estrogens (see box on p. 993).

Both migraine and cluster headaches may be exacerbated by vasodilators such as nitrates, hydralazine, minoxidil, nifedipine, and prazocin.

Reserpine depletes catecholamine and serotonin stores within the brain and can cause depression, migraine, and tension-type headaches. Indomethacin, although useful in treating cluster variant headaches, can cause a generalized headache. Chronic use of some drugs, including narcotics, barbiturates, caffeine, and ergots, can lead to rebound or withdrawal headaches.[34]

The final step in history taking includes assessment of psychological functioning. It is necessary to identify or rule out psychiatric disease or personality disorders. If these are present concomitant psychologic or psychiatric management must be considered. Second, the psychological reaction to pain should be recounted, because it reflects the underlying personality or coping style. Third, general health behavior (i.e., exercise, alcohol use, recreational drug use, sleep and eating habits, smoking) is reviewed. Such habits may reflect the patient's perceived locus of control for his or her health. Previous health behavior, as well as the patient's reaction to the suggestion that he or she modify current health behavior, can provide important data for predicting success with nonpharmacologic therapy for headache.

Differential considerations

In medical practice most headaches are not caused by underlying disease. It is important to recognize, however, that headache can be the presenting symptom of several diseases. Fever, regardless of cause, is probably the most common medical problem that causes headache. Less common causes include pheochromocytoma, chronic renal failure, hyperthyroidism, and malignant hypertension. Pheochromocytoma may be associated with a pounding headache associated with hypertension, diaphoresis, tachycardia, and palpitations.[34]

Rheumatologic diseases may have headache as an early manifestation. Headache is common in systemic lupus erythematosus, polyarteritis nodosa, and giant cell arteritis. About two thirds of patients with fibrositis/fibromyalgia report headache, usually tension-type headache. Many types of vasculitis are also accompanied by headache.[34]

Headache on awakening may be the initial symptom of sleep apnea syndrome. The headache often improves as the day progresses. Sleep apnea is most commonly observed in obese middle-aged males. Associated symptoms include snoring, daytime somnolence, hypertension, and arrhythmias.[34]

Physical examination

After evaluating the headache history the physician should perform a targeted physical examination. This should include a mental status examination (often performed as part of obtaining the history), blood pressure and pulse measurement, examination of the cranial nerves, funduscopic examination, palpation of the head and neck, auscultation of the carotid arteries and heart, evaluation of motor and balance, and palpation of peripheral pulses (particularly if vasoconstrictor medications are to be prescribed).

Diagnostic testing

Diagnostic testing of the headache patient should be based on the results of the history and physical examination. In a patient with a typical headache history of several years' duration and normal neurologic examination findings no further evaluation may be needed. All patients older than 60 years with new onset headache or change in headache pattern should have a sedimentation rate measurement to evaluate for giant cell arteritis. If the rate is elevated, a temporal artery biopsy should be obtained to confirm the diagnosis.

Screening laboratory studies should be obtained to rule out the diseases more likely to be associated with headache. Testing may be limited to measurement of thyroid stimulating hormone (TSH) and sedimentation rate (in patients with symptoms of rheumatologic disease and those above 60 years old). Patients suspected of sleep apnea should be evaluated by sleep study (polysomnography). "Routine" laboratory testing including complete blood count, urinalysis, and chemistry profile adds little diagnostic information but may be useful to monitor for potential complications of drug therapy.

Several commonly ordered tests have little or no value in the headache evaluation.[12] Electroencephalography (EEG) findings may be abnormal in some migraine patients, but EEG changes are neither specific for nor diagnostic of migraine. As a screening test to localize organic lesions EEG has been supplanted by more specific computed tomographic (CT) and magnetic resonance (MR) imaging. Evoked potentials (visual, auditory, and somatosensory) fail to show specific findings in migraine. Like EEG evoked potentials have no utility as a screening test for headache. Thermography has been touted by its practitioners as diagnostic for vascular headache and other pain states. Careful review of the medical literature[8] fails to support the use of thermography in generating a diagnosis, in guiding therapy, or in determining prognosis for headache disorders. The use of thermography in headache should be discouraged.

Neuroradiology has little role in the diagnosis of headache beyond ruling out occult lesions such as neoplasm, hemorrhage, vascular malformations, brain abscesses, hydrocephalus, or congenital malformations (i.e., Arnold-Chiari malformations). MRI and CT do not detect other organic causes of headache, such as idiopathic intracranial hypertension (pseudotumor cerebri), meningitis or other infections, glaucoma or eye disease, and metabolic or toxic causes of headache.[12] It is critical that the physician obtain a complete history and examination and not rely solely on MRI or CT to eliminate organic causes of headache.

Most patients suffering from acute severe headaches should undergo imaging with CT or MRI to rule out the organic causes listed. Because organic causes of headache are rare (estimated at less than 1% in headache clinics), these tests are generally unrevealing. The benefits of a normal CT or MRI result in reassuring the patient and doctor should not be overlooked, however. Patients (and physicians) may be unwilling to embark on a course of therapy for a benign headache disorder without the reassurance of a normal scan finding.

MRI detects differences in signal intensity emanating from tissues and is superior to CT in detecting tumors and changes in brain tissues. Vascular lesions such as arteriovenous malformations, cerebral venous thrombosis, and venous angiomas are more readily detected by MRI than CT. Magnetic resonance angiography (MRA) provides a noninvasive test for evaluation of aneurysms of the carotid and basilar systems and the circle of Willis.

Parenchymal brain lesions, described as well-defined, high-intensity T_2 foci in the periventricular white matter, have been reported on MRI in 12% to 46% of migraine patients.[33,26] These "unidentified bright objects" (UBOs) have also been reported in patients with demyelinating disease (multiple sclerosis) and small vessel atherosclerotic disease (lacunar infarcts). These white matter abnormalities increase in frequency with patient age and may reflect low-grade vascular insufficiency with resulting perivascular gliosis.[29] Neither multiple sclerosis nor atherosclerotic cerebrovascular disease typically has headache as a dominant clinical feature. Further evaluation for these conditions is not necessary if UBOs are noted on an MRI in a patient with symptoms of migraine.[33]

In the patient suspected of having a subarachnoid hemorrhage, CT scan (without enhancement) is superior to MRI in identifying subarachnoid blood. The CT scan result can be normal in from 5% to 10% of patients initially presenting with subarachnoid hemorrhage. Therefore, lumbar puncture is indicated whenever subarachnoid hemorrhage is strongly suspected, despite a normal CT scan result.[12]

CT scanning is preferred to MRI for detecting bony abnormalities. The advent of CT and MRI has replaced plain film radiography of the skull in evaluating headache patients. The use of cervical spine roentgenography is rarely useful in the diagnosis and management of headache patients.[12]

In summary the appropriate screening for the outpatient with recurrent headaches includes obtaining a complete headache history, assessing psychological functioning, conducting both physical and neurologic examinations, sedimentation rate, TSH, other laboratory tests if indicated by history and physical findings, and CT or MRI, if the headaches are of recent onset, if indicated by troubling neurologic symptoms in the history, or if associated with abnormalities detected on the neurologic examination. Consider obtaining a scan when needed to reassure the patient.

Expected outcome of screening

The stated goal of screening headache patients is to separate those rare patients with organic causes from those with a benign headache disorder. Once a primary (benign) headache diagnosis is made, the major role of the physician is to initiate a therapeutic plan.

Because headache is often a disorder of otherwise healthy young adults, the physician often is able to use the headache evaluation to encourage a healthy life-style. Patients are usually relieved when their headache evaluation shows no abnormalities, and this can open the door to a dialogue on maintaining health. This opportunity to reach young, health-conscious patients should not be overlooked.

One valuable intervention for the headache patient is smoking cessation. Cigarette smoking is associated with increased headache intensity.[28] One third of patients believe that smoking precipitates or aggravates their headache symptoms. The initial headache evaluation serves as an ideal time to initiate smoking cessation as part of the overall therapeutic plan.

Effectiveness of early detection

The purpose of early detection of headache is to diagnose the organic causes of headache, initiate therapy, and reduce the morbidity caused by chronic headache disorders.

The morbidity resulting from chronic headache can be financial as well as physical. Osterhaus reported that 55% of migraine sufferers missed 2 workdays/month and 88% worked 5.6 days/month with migraine symptoms that reduced their productivity.[27] Stewart found that migraine was more prevalent in the lowest income group.[38] This was postulated to be due to downward socioeconomic drift caused by disruption of function at school or work related to recurrent migraines. Early intervention may stop the downward economic spiral caused by recurrent migraine headaches.

The value of early intervention is largely determined by the effectiveness of therapy. Some therapies appear to be more effective if used early in treatment. Biofeedback therapy for headaches is more effective in younger subjects who are not chronically habituated to pain medications.[5] Patients older than 60 years had a poor response to biofeedback and relaxation therapy; only 18% noted clinical improvement.[3] Therefore, if headache patients are identified at a young age and before they become habituated to pain medications, biofeedback therapy has a 60% to 65% likelihood of inducing improvement.[5] The percentage of patients reporting continued significant improvement at 3 to 5 years post treatment with biofeedback ranges from 30% to 80%.

Prophylactic drug therapy of migraine (see Therapeutic Interventions) is effective in reducing headache frequency for about two thirds of patients. Because the efficacy of drug therapy, like that of biofeedback, is reduced in patients taking large amounts of habituating pain medication, early intervention with appropriate prophylactic therapy is quite valuable (see boxes below).

Because the efficacy of prophylactic therapy is reduced by excessive use of habituating medications, early intervention permits the selection of nonhabituating medications to treat acute headache attacks. Furthermore, early intervention may reduce the morbidity caused by frequent use of over-the-counter analgesics (peptic ulcer diseases, analgesic nephropathy).

Follow-up screening

Benign headache disorders tend to be chronic illnesses, offering the physician significant opportunities for follow-up care. The major questions in the continuing care of the headache patient are whether the prescribed intervention has been effective, whether the therapy has caused adverse effects, whether new medical problems that require treatment have developed, and an organic cause of headache has developed (or was overlooked on initial screening).

Therapy of headache and adverse effects of headache medications are discussed in the section Preventive and Therapeutic Interventions.

Certain medical illnesses are more common in the headache patient. Featherstone evaluated the prevalence of concomitant medical diseases in chronic headache sufferers by reviewing 1414 life insurance applications obtaining 200 headache cases with matched controls without chronic headaches.[16] The average age for study patients was 45

Prophylactic medications for migraine

β-Blockers

Propranolol (FDA approved)	60-160 mg/d
Timolol (FDA approved)	10-20 mg/d
Nadolol	20-120 mg/d
Metoprolol	100-200 mg/d
Atenolol	25-100 mg/d

Side effects may include fatigue, depression, sleep disorders, diarrhea, exacerbation of asthma, Raynaud's syndrome, and congestive heart failure.

Calcium channel blockers

Verapamil	120-480 mg/d
Diltiazem	90-360 mg/d
Nicardipine	40-90 mg/d
Nimodipine	60-120 mg/d
Flunarizine (not available in U.S.)	10 mg/d

Side effects may include constipation with verapamil; sedation, weight gain, and parkinsonism with flunarizine; flushing and edema with nicardipine; and gastrointestinal upset with diltiazem. Verapamil and flunarizine are the best studied calcium channel blockers in migraine.

Nonsteroidal antiinflammatory drugs

Aspirin	325 mg/d
Fenoprofen	600 mg tid
Flurbiprofen	100 mg bid
Ketoprofen	75 mg tid
Naproxen	250-500 mg bid

Side effects may include dyspepsia, heartburn, upper gastrointestinal bleeding, diarrhea, constipation, nausea, and vomiting. Renal effects may include decreased glomerular filtration rate (GFR) and analgesic nephropathy.

Others

Antidepressants (see box on p. 997)	Valproate (see box on p. 997)
Methysergide	Clonidine
Cyproheptadine	Angiotension converting enzyme inhibitors

years. The groups were equally divided by gender. Headaches were not classified by diagnosis (migraine, cluster, etc.). Six conditions were found to occur more often in the chronic headache group: hypertension, dizziness (or vertigo), gastroesophageal reflux, depression or anxiety, peptic ulcer disease, and irritable bowel syndrome. Three conditions were significantly more common in the nonheadache population: nephrolithiasis, alcohol abuse in men, and abdominal pain in women. Several conditions had the same prevalence in both headache and nonheadache groups: ischemic heart disease, mitral valve prolapse, cardiovascular disease, central nervous system ischemia, cigarette smoking, emphysema, and previous surgery.

Other investigators have found associations between specific headache diagnoses and medical diseases. To examine the association between migraine and other conditions, Merikangas reviewed the Health and Nutrition Examination Survey (HANES I), a study of 12,200 adults aged 25 to 74, which was used to estimate the health of the general population of adults in the United States.[24] Merikangas found the following conditions to be strongly associated with migraine: stroke (odds ratio 3.1), heart attack (odds ratio 2.4), bronchitis (odds ratio 2.3), colitis (odds ratio 2.3), nervous breakdown (odds ratio 2.2), urinary tract disorders (odds ratio 2.2), and ulcers (odds ratio 2.2). Migraine has also been associated with an increased prevalence of coronary vasospasm, Raynaud's phenomenon, aspirin-sensitive asthma, mitral valve prolapse, and hypertension.[34]

Cluster headache is associated with a threefold increase in the prevalence of peptic ulcer disease.[10] Chronic tension-type headache sufferers have an increased prevalence of depressive symptoms.

A controversy in headache management is the issue of repeated evaluations to look for organic causes of headache. Most physicians agree that repeating the pertinent headache history and the targeted physical examination is important to find clues for new diagnoses and diagnoses missed in initial evaluation. The issue of obtaining additional CT or MRI scans is unsettled. It is generally prudent to repeat neuroradiographic imaging in a patient whose condition is deteriorating or where history or physical examination has revealed new neurologic abnormalities. There appears to be little yield in obtaining repeated studies in patients whose headache course is stable, even if the patient is not responding well to treatment.

PREVENTIVE AND THERAPEUTIC INTERVENTIONS
Drug habituation and detoxification

Because drug habituation is a common accompaniment of many chronic headache syndromes, this is the first issue that must be considered in patient management. Medications that are known to cause habituation and rebound headaches include narcotics, barbituates, ergotamine tartrate compounds, benzodiazepines, and caffeine preparations.[35] There is no evidence that simple analgesics such as aspirin, acetaminophen, or nonsteroidal antiinflamma-

---

Prophylactic medications for tension-type headache

Tricyclic antidepressants

Nonsedating	**Sedating**
Protriptyline	Amitriptyline
Desipramine	Doxepin
	Nortriptyline
	Imipramine

Side effects may include constipation, dry mouth, weight gain, blurred vision, and urinary retention. Nortriptyline is the least sedating drug in its group.

Serotonin reuptake inhibitors (antidepressants)

Nonsedating	**Sedating**
Fluoxetine	Trazedone
Sertraline	

Side effects may include insomnia, agitation, sexual dysfunction, diarrhea, and nausea. Adverse effects are less common than those of tricyclic drugs.

Other antidepressants
Monoamine oxidase inhibitors
Buspirone
Bupropion
Alprazolam

Nonsteroidal antiinflammatory drugs (see previous box)

Others

Valproate	250-2000 mg/day

Side effects may include hepatic dysfunction, gastrointestinal upset, weight gain, and hair loss.

tory drugs cause rebound headaches with daily use.

Detoxification from habituating drugs is the initial step in the treatment of patients who are taking excessive pain medications (i.e., using daily or almost daily habituating pain medication or taking ergotamine more than twice weekly). Prophylactic medication is ineffective in patients suffering from rebound or withdrawal headaches. Frequently patients say that they "would stop taking pain medication if only the preventive medication prevented the headaches." Patients must be instructed that the "pain medication" is part of the cause of the headaches, and that headache therapy is futile until the rebound/habituation cycle is resolved.

Management of the habituated patient can be difficult, and the medical literature offers little insight into proper techniques of detoxification. Patients who are habituated to narcotics can benefit from clonidine to prevent physical signs and symptoms of withdrawal.[18] At the Cleveland Clinic Headache Center corticosteroids and phenothiazines are prescribed for outpatient detoxification from butalbital, ergotamine, or low doses of narcotics. Generally a 6- to 14-day tapering course of corticosteroids is given, with chlorpromazine suppositories prescribed for severe withdrawal headaches associated with vomiting. For patients with concomitant medical problems, a history of seizures, or prior unsuccessful outpatient detoxification inpatient detoxification is often required.

Trigger factors in migraine

It is important to understand how trigger factors work in precipitating migraine. Most migraines are precipitated only when several triggers occur in close temporal proximity, usually in the 12 hours preceding the migraine onset. The simultaneous elimination of several headache triggers has an additive effect in decreasing the probability that the migraine threshold will be crossed. Migraines are rarely induced 100% of the time on exposure to individual triggers. For example, alcohol exposure precipitates migraine 60% to 80% of the time in headache-prone individuals. The triggers may vary from migraine attack to migraine attack in the same patient, although patients may have their own typical triggers. The combination of trigger elimination with medication management improves headache control in more patients than either approach alone.[32]

Identification and elimination of triggers of headache have been found to constitute a highly effective and long-lasting migraine treatment. Blau reported a 50% reduction in migraine attacks in approximately 80% of previously intractable migraine conditions by the elimination of multiple triggers.[4] The key to treatment success was careful physician questioning and education about precipitating factors. Individuals were usually able to identify four to five trigger factors.[32]

The most common migraine trigger factors are alcohol and four food substances: tyramine (found in aged cheese, fermented foods), aspartame (found in many diet soft drinks), monosodium glutamate ([MSG], in Chinese restaurant food, flavor enhancers), and phenylethylamine (in chocolate)[32] (see box on p. 993). Additional common trigger factors are hormonal changes (menses, climacteric), alterations in sleep patterns (shift changes, jet lag, sleeping late on weekends), fasting, weather changes, and "letdown" after stress (weekends, vacations).

Medications for migraine

A wide variety of medications have been used in the prophylaxis of migraine, including methysergide, β-blockers, calcium channel blockers, nonsteroidal antiinflammatory drugs (NSAIDs), tricyclic antidepressants, and cyproheptadine. Methysergide is rarely used today for migraine prophylaxis because of the risk of serious complications such as retroperitoneal fibrosis. Cyproheptadine is generally used for migraine prophylaxis in children. Adults often find the side effects of fatigue and weight gain caused by this antihistamine/antiserotonin drug intolerable.

β-Blockers, along with calcium channel blockers and NSAIDs, are valued as first-line drugs for the prophylaxis of migraine. Because β-blockers also have anxiolytic effects, they are sometimes used to treat chronic tension-type headaches. Several β-blockers have been shown to be effective in migraine prophylaxis. Among these are propranolol and timolol (the only β-blockers approved by the U.S. Food and Drug Administration for migraine prophylaxis), nadolol, metoprolol, and atenolol. β-Blockers with intrinsic sympathomimetic activity, such as pindolol and acebutolol, have not been found useful in migraine prophylaxis (see boxes on p. 996 and p. 997).

Although generally well tolerated β-blockers are contraindicated in patients with congestive heart failure, bronchospastic disease (i.e., asthma, emphysema, chronic bronchitis), diabetes mellitus, and Wolff-Parkinson-White syndrome. β-Blockers may also exacerbate Raynaud's phenomenon, a condition found more commonly in migraine sufferers. Side effects include depression, fatigue, and sleep disorders. Depression is more commonly reported with propranolol than with other β-blockers. These side effects may worsen the tension-type headache component of the mixed headache syndrome.

Patients should not abruptly discontinue β-blocker therapy, since abrupt discontinuation may lead to myocardial infarction even in patients with no prior history of heart disease.[34]

Medications for multiple headache types

Calcium entry blockers are useful in the prophylaxis of migraine and cluster headache. Several calcium entry blockers have been shown to be effective in migraine prophylaxis, including verapamil, diltiazem, flunarizine, nimodipine, and nicardipine. Nifedipine is either weakly effective or ineffective for migraine prophylaxis and can exacerbate migraine in some patients through profound vasodilation. In the United States verapamil is considered the calcium channel blocker of choice for migraine and cluster prophylaxis.[15]

The calcium entry blockers constitute a diverse group of drugs with varying effects on the heart and peripheral vasculature. Verapamil and diltiazem have negative inotropic effects and slow conduction through the atrioventricular (AV) node. Therefore, these agents should be avoided in patients with congestive heart failure, advanced heart block, or sick sinus syndrome. The dihydropyradine calcium entry blockers—nifedipine, nicardipine, and nimodipine—have no effect on cardiac conduction but can cause marked vasodilation.

Adverse effects of calcium entry blockers include constipation with verapamil; sedation, weight gain, and parkinsonism with flunarizine; flushing and edema with nifedipine; and gastrointestinal upset and parkinsonism with diltiazem.

Nonsteroidal antiinflammatory drugs are widely prescribed in the treatment of arthritis and as analgesics and antipyretics. They are valuable both in prophylaxis of migraine headache and as adjunctive therapy for tension-type headache.[36] This dual effect on migraine and tension-type headache allows for NSAIDs to be used as single-drug therapy in some patients with the mixed headache syndrome.

Several NSAIDs have been reported to have prophylactic activity in migraine. Among these are aspirin, naproxen, flurbiprofen, ketoprofen, flufenamic acid, tolfenamic acid, and fenoprofen. At the Cleveland Clinic Headache Center naproxen and flurbiprofen are the most frequently prescribed NSAIDs for headache prevention.

Adverse effects of NSAIDs are relatively common and may include gastrointestinal symptoms such as dyspepsia, heartburn, nausea, vomiting, diarrhea, constipation, and generalized abdominal pain. Most NSAIDs can cause bleeding of the upper gastrointestinal tract. Renal effects of NSAIDs may include decreased glomerular filtration rate (GFR) with sodium, chloride, and water retention. These renal problems are most likely to occur in patients who are elderly, who are hypertensive, who have renovascular or advanced atherosclerotic disease, or who take diuretics. Indomethacin and fenoprofen appear to be more nephrotoxic than other NSAIDs. Analgesic nephropathy, the most common cause of drug-induced renal failure, has been associated with excessive use of NSAIDs along with phenacetin or acetaminophen.

Alternative medications

For the patient in whom conventional therapy has failed alternatives include monamine oxidase inhibitors or valproic acid. Because of the potential for serious toxicity prescription of these agents for headache should be limited to physicians experienced in their use.

For the abortive (acute) treatment of migraine headaches a NSAID or isometheptene/acetaminophen/dichloralphenazone (Midrin) compound is prescribed. The most effective NSAIDs to abort migraine attacks are naproxen sodium, flurbiprofen, and meclofenamate. Generally a dose is given at the onset of the headache (naproxen sodium 550 mg, flurbiprofen 100 mg, meclofenamate 200 mg) and repeated in 1 hour, if the headache is still present. Ergotamine tartrate is usually effective for the migraine component, but, because of the problem of ergotamine rebound with frequent use, is used only if the other medications are ineffective. When ergotamine is prescribed it should be given no more often than every 4 days to prevent rebound headaches. Sumatriptan, a serotonin agonist, has been found effective in the acute treatment of migraine. It acts very rapidly and is generally well tolerated. Limitations to its use include parenteral dosing formulation (oral formulation is undergoing evaluation), high cost, and the problem of recurrent headache in up to 40% of patients.

Antidepressants are the drugs of choice for chronic tension-type headache, and several of these agents are also effective in migraine prophylaxis. Of the antidepressants the tricyclic drugs and the newer serotonin reuptake inhibitors are usually the agents of first choice because of the lower incidence of side effects and less serious drug interactions compared with those of the monamine oxidase inhibitors (MAOIs).

The selection of a specific antidepressant drug should be based primarily on whether or not the patient has a sleep disturbance. Patients who begin and maintain sleep easily generally tolerate nonsedating drugs better than sedating agents. Those patients who have difficulty beginning or maintaining sleep respond better to sedating drugs. Patients often note improvement in headaches within 1 or 2 weeks after their sleep disturbance is corrected.

The nonsedating antidepressants include fluoxetine, sertraline, bupropion, protriptyline, and desipramine. The MAOIs are nonsedating and may induce insomnia.

The sedating antidepressants include amitriptyline, doxepin, nortriptyline, imipramine, trimipramine, and trazodone. Of these drugs nortriptyline appears to cause the least morning sedation.

The second consideration, after effect on sleep, is whether the patient is likely to be intolerant of anticholinergic side effects. The common anticholinergic side effects seen with tricyclic antidepressants are urinary retention (primarily in men with prostatic hypertrophy), dry mouth, blurred vision, and constipation.

All tricyclic antidepressants have anticholinergic side effects. Of the tricyclics doxepin appears to cause the least anticholinergic side effects. Serotonin reuptake inhibitors, such as fluoxetine, sertraline, bupropion, and trazodone, are generally free of anticholinergic effects.

Tricyclic antidepressants have several potential cardiac effects.[34] These drugs may cause orthostatic hypotension, although they do not have negative inotropic effects on the heart. The orthostatic hypotension is mediated through α_1-adrenergic receptor blockade and is most commonly reported with tertiary amines such as amitriptyline and imipramine. Cardiac conduction problems can occur with all tricyclic antidepressants but not with the nontricyclic drugs such as trazodone, fluoxetine, sertraline, and bupropion. Tricyclics slow the process of depolarization and prolong repolarization, a quinidinelike effect. On electrocardiogram there may be prolongation of PR, QRS, and QT intervals. This effect is only of clinical significance in patients with second-degree heart block, right or left bundle branch block, or intraventricular conduction delays (QRS width > 0.11 seconds). In patients with first-degree heart block treatment with tricyclics does not cause the development of higher degrees of heart block. Patients with advanced heart block or intraventricular conduction delays, who require therapy with antidepressant agents, should be treated with fluoxetine, sertraline, bupropion, trazodone, or monamine oxidase inhibitors.

Some antidepressants have unique adverse effects. Trazodone has been reported to cause priapism in some men. Fluoxetine and sertraline may cause anorexia and weight loss in a small percentage of patients. Although the medical literature does not support the contention, reports of suicide and violent behavior with fluoxetine have been widely heralded by the lay media.

Treatment of the daily, tension-type headache with abortive medications is difficult. Muscle relaxants such as chlorzoxazone, orphenadrine citrate, carisoprodol, and metaxalone, either alone or in combinations with aspirin, acetaminophen, and/or caffeine, are generally helpful. NSAIDs are also useful as analgesics for daily headache. Benzodiazepines, butalbital combinations, and narcotics should be avoided, or their use carefully controlled, because of the risk of habituation.

Prophylactic therapy of the mixed headache syndrome generally consists of treatment of both the daily tension-type headache and the migraine component. This often requires the use of more than one daily preventive medication.

Treatment of acute headache attacks is a major challenge in patients with mixed headache syndrome. Because headaches occur daily, with intermittent severe attacks, the patient may use abortive drugs quite frequently. Avoidance of habituating medications is critical.

Medications for cluster headache

Medications used in the prophylaxis of cluster headache include ergotamine, corticosteroids, methysergide, verapamil, and lithium carbonate. Verapamil, 240 to 480 mg/day, is useful in both episodic and chronic cluster headache and is generally considered the drug of choice for cluster prophylaxis. Corticosteroids and methysergide are used only in episodic cluster headache because of the potential adverse effects of long-term use. Lithium carbonate, 300 mg three times daily, is reserved for patients with chronic cluster headache.

The drug of choice for the acute treatment of cluster headache is oxygen, given at 8 to 10 L/min by mask for 10 minutes. Other useful abortive medications include ergotamine and dihydroergotamine, sumatriptan, and lidocaine nosedrops. The use of intranasal capsaicin for cluster therapy is being investigated.

Nonpharmacologic therapy also has an important role in the management of chronic headache syndromes. Biofeedback can help patients to change vasomotor tone and to relax tight muscles. Physical therapy is used to train patients to strengthen neck muscles, improve mobility, and correct poor posture. Physical therapy should not be limited to heat and massage. Although heat and massage provide short-term pain relief, only strengthening exercises provide long-term benefit.

Biofeedback

Biofeedback refers to a collection of techniques in which the physiologic activity of unconscious bodily functions is monitored and indicated instantly by audio or visual instruments in an attempt to permit the patient to gain control over these functions. The rationale underlying biofeedback is that the physiologic activity being monitored is causally related to a clinical problem and that alteration of the physiologic activity can lead to resolution of that problem.[21]

Biofeedback for tension-type headache primarily measures electromyographic (EMG) changes in the tension of the frontalis muscle or in the most tense muscle in the head or neck. The patient is instructed to use thoughts, feelings, or other strategies to reduce the muscle tension. Daily home practice of these skills is encouraged.[21] Metaanalysis of this technique showed posttreatment improvement of 61% (compared with placebo response of 35%). Relaxation training alone was statistically equivalent to biofeedback (59%), and the combination of relaxation training and EMG biofeedback was also equivalent (59%) in efficacy.[5]

Biofeedback for migraine also may use EMG but usually includes thermal biofeedback. Patients are taught to increase the surface temperature of their hands, causing a reduction in sympathetic tone.[21] The technique of thermal biofeedback is similar to that of EMG biofeedback. Metaanalysis of frontalis EMG biofeedback with relaxation training in migraine subjects showed posttreatment improvement of 65%, relaxation therapy showed posttreatment improvement of 53%, and thermal biofeedback showed posttreatment improvement of 52%.[5]

The appropriate role for biofeedback in headache remains uncertain. In their 1985 position paper on biofeedback for headaches the American College of Physicians concluded that there is insufficient evidence of the efficacy of biofeedback to recommend it for the treatment of mixed headaches.[21] They stated that it may be useful adjunctively in some patients with tension-type or migraine headaches to assist relaxation, or in patients whose headaches are refractory to other forms of therapy. They also concluded that biofeedback was no more effective than other relaxation techniques.[21] In Chapman's review of biofeedback for chronic headaches he concluded that biofeedback has a high degree of short-term efficacy, which has been maintained on long-term follow-up evaluation.[5] Comparisons of biofeedback with relaxation have shown similar effectiveness. He also concluded that there is little apparent benefit to repeating biofeedback for more than a maximum of 12 sessions.

The management of chronic headache disorders requires close follow-up observation and frequent physician visits until therapy is successful with a minimum of adverse effects. Although this requires commitment by both the practitioner and the patient, good results should be expected in the vast majority of cases.

COUNSELING AND COMPLIANCE

In an effort to evaluate the nature of consumer expectations, barriers to care, and levels of satisfaction Klassen and Berman surveyed subjects attending an educational seminar on headache.[22] Most subjects (86%) had seen physicians for headache, and 82% used prescription medications for it. Subjects desired one or more helpful outcomes of their visits to physicians: pain relief, 90%; medication and related advice, 66%; explanation of cause of the headache, 55%; being listened to, 43%; and reassurance of absence of serious disease, 40%.

Three of four subjects indicated the presence of factors that made it difficult to see physicians for headache. These included attitudes and actions of physicians ("doctors won't listen") by 27% of subjects and high cost or inconvenience by 18% of subjects.

A lack of satisfaction with treatments received from physicians for their headaches was indicated by 34% of subjects. The most frequently cited reasons for dissatisfaction were ineffectiveness of medications and physician behavior. The most frequent suggestion made by subjects to improve medical care for headache was to change physician behavior or performance ("know more," "listen more," or "try harder").

It is estimated that nearly half of all migraine sufferers have given up seeking help for their headaches from their physicians. Although patients sometimes find their headache medications to be ineffective, it is physician behavior toward the headache patient that discourages continuity of care. Counseling the patient on the mechanisms of headache, trigger factors, expected outcome of therapy ("control" of headaches and improvement in life-style without "cure" of disease), and reassurance of the absence of serious disease should help to cement the therapeutic relationship. Further discussion on the wide varieties of medications available to aid the headache sufferer should encourage the patient to continue care if the initial therapy is ineffective or poorly tolerated.

When the patient and physician have formed a relationship based on an understanding of the disease, the patient's response to her/his illness, and knowledge of the risks, benefits, and goals of therapy, compliance rarely is a problem. Limiting the dietary and life-style restrictions (reduction of trigger factors) to those that apply to a given patient improves compliance (see box on p. 993). For example, a woman who has migraines only with menses should not be asked to eliminate chocolate and cheese from her diet. Patients with cluster headache must eliminate alcohol during the cluster cycle, but abstinence between cycles will not influence the headache pattern. Smoking cessation, however, may benefit the headache patient.

The physician treating headache patients must be available to handle the episodic exacerbations of headache and the occasional headache that does not respond to usual medications. Additionally the patient and physician must forge a long-term relationship to deal with the chronic nature of headaches.

SUMMARY

Headache, one of the most frequent complaints in the outpatient setting, tends to be a recurrent, chronic medical problem. As physicians become more involved in the management of headache, they will find that headache medicine fits well within the long-term care ideals of preventive medicine. Physicians, hospitals, and, most important, patients can only benefit from physicians' assuming a preventive approach to the care of chronic headaches.

REFERENCES

1. Askmark H, Lundberg PO, Olsson S: Drug-related headache, *Headache* 29:441-444, 1989.
2. Bensemana D, Gascon AL: Relationship between analgesia and turnover of brain biogenic amines, *Can J Physiol Pharmacol* 56:721-730, 1978.
3. Blanchard EB et al: Biofeedback and relaxation treatments for headache in the elderly: a caution and a challenge, *Biofeedback Self Regul* 10:69-73, 1985.
4. Blau JN: Preventing migraine: a study of precipitating factors, *Headache* 28:481-483, 1988.
5. Chapman SL: A review and clinical perspective on the use of EMG and thermal biofeedback for chronic headaches, *Pain* 27:1-43, 1986.
6. Choi D: Glutamate neurotoxicity in disease of the nervous system. *Neuron* 1:623-634, 1988.
7. Cook NR et al: Correlates of headache in a population-based cohort of elderly, *Arch Neurol* 46:1338-1344, 1989.
8. Cotton P: AMA's council on scientific affairs takes a fresh look at thermography, *JAMA* 267:1885-1887, 1992.
9. D'Alessandro R et al: Cluster headache in the Republic of San Marino, *Cephalalgia* 6:152-162, 1986.
10. Diamond S, Solomon GD, Freitag FG: Cluster headache, *Clin J Pain* 3:171-176, 1987.
11. Diamond S, Solomon GD, Freitag FG: Differential diagnosis of

headache pain. In Tollison CD, editor: *Handbook of chronic pain management,* Baltimore, 1988, Williams & Wilkins.

12. Donohoe CD, Waldman SD: The targeted physical examination, *Intern Med Special* 12(5):30-39, 1991.

13. Duckro PN: Biofeedback in the management of headache, *Headache Q* 1(4):290-298, 1990.

14. Ekbom K, Ahlborg B, Schele R: Prevalence of migraine and cluster headache in Swedish men of 18, *Headache* 18:9-19, 1978.

15. Elkind AH: Interval therapy of migraine: the art and science, *Headache Q* 1(4):280-289, 1990.

16. Featherstone HJ: Medical diagnoses and problems in individuals with recurrent idiopathic headaches, *Headache* 25:136-40, 1985.

17. Gaucher A et al: Diffusion of oxphenbutazone into synovial fluid, synovial tissue, joint cartilage and cerebrospinal fluid, *Eur J Clin Pharmacol* 25:107-112, 1983.

18. Gold MS et al: Opiate withdrawal using clonidine, *JAMA* 243:343-346, 1980.

19. Groppetti A et al: Effect of aspirin on serotonin and met-enkephalin in brain: correlation with the antinociceptive activity of the drug, *Neuropharmacology* 27:499-505, 1988.

20. Headache classification committee of the international headache society: Classification and diagnostic criteria for headache disorders, cranial neuralgias, and facial pain, *Cephalalgia* 8(suppl 7):1-96, 1988.

21. Health and Public Policy Committee, American College of Physicians: Biofeedback for headaches, *Ann Intern Med* 102:128-131, 1985.

22. Klassen AC, Berman ME: Medical care for headache—a consumer survey, *Cephalalgia* 11(Suppl 11):85-86, 1991.

23. Linet MS et al: An epidemiolgic study of headache among adolescents and young adults, *JAMA* 261:2211-2216, 1989.

24. Merikangas KR: Comorbidity of migraine and other conditions in the general population of adults in the United States, *Cephalalgia* 11(Suppl 11):108-109, 1991.

25. *MMWR* 40:331-338, 1991.

26. Osborn RE, Alder DC, Mitchell CS: MR imaging of the brain in patients with migraine headaches, *Am J NeuroRadiology* 12:521-524, 1991.

27. Osterhaus JT, Gutterman DL, Plachetka JR: Labor costs associated with migraine headaches, *Headache* 30:302-303, 1990.

28. Payne TJ et al: The impact of cigarette smoking on headache activity in headache patients, *Headache* 31:329-332, 1991.

29. Prager JM et al: Evaluation of headache patients by MRI, *Headache Q* 2(3):192-195, 1991.

30. Rasmussen BK et al: Epidemiology of headache in a general population—a prevalence study, *J Clin Epidemiol* 44:1147-1157, 1991.

31. Sadjadpour K: Cluster headache, *Bergen Migraine Symposium* Bergen, Norway, (Suppl 1), 1975.

32. Scopp AL: Headache triggers: theory, research, and clinical application, *Headache Q* 3(1):32-37, 1992.

33. Soges LJ et al: Migraine: evaluation by MR, *Am J NeuroRadiology* 9:425-429, 1988.

34. Solomon GD: Concomitant medical disease and headache, *Med Clin North Am* 75(3):631-639, 1991.

35. Solomon GD: Management of chronic mixed headaches, *Curr Manage Headache* (in press).

36. Solomon GD: Pharmacology and use of headache medications, *Cleve Clin J Med* 57:627-635, 1990.

37. Solomon GD, Kunkel RS, Frame J: Demographics of headache in elderly patients, *Headache* 30:273-276, 1990.

38. Stewart WF et al: Prevalence of migraine headache in the United States, *JAMA* 267:64-69, 1992.

39. Willer JC et al: Central analgesic effect of ketoprofen in humans, *Pain* 38:1-7, 1989.

RESOURCES

National Headache Foundation, 5252 N. Western Ave., Chicago, IL 60625. A national nonprofit group dedicated to educating the public, promoting research, and serving as an information resource. They have a referral list of member physicians.

American Council for Headache Education (ACHE), 875 Kings Highway, West Deptford, NJ 08096. A nonprofit organization whose goal is to educate the public that headache is a valid and treatable disease.

American Association for the Study of Headache (AASH), 875 Kings Highway, West Deptford, NJ 08096. Professional and scientific organization dedicated to headache.

Chapter 54

ASTHMA AND THE ALLERGIC DISORDERS

William O. Wagner

PREVALENCE OF ALLERGIC DISEASES

Allergic diseases affect more than 15% of the general population of the United States and are an important part of the medical practice of all primary care physicians. Allergic rhinitis and asthma are the most common allergic diseases. The National Health and Nutrition Examination Survey (NHANES II) surveyed noninstitutionalized people age 12 to 74 years at 64 sites around the United States. The prevalence of allergic rhinitis was slightly higher among whites; the prevalence of asthma was slightly higher among blacks[50] (Table 54-1).

The prevalence of allergic rhinitis was highest in the 25- to 49-year-old group while the prevalence of asthma was highest in the 50- to 74-year-old group.

Allergic diseases are also common in childhood. Asthma is the most common chronic disease of childhood and is the most frequent cause of hospitalization of children. The development of respiratory allergy may be, but is not always, preceded by allergic diseases of infancy such as atopic dermatitis and food allergy. Two percent of children aged 1 to 5 years suffer from atopic dermatitis.[27] The incidence of food allergy in children is estimated to be between 0.3% and 7.5%.[57] The prevalence of food allergy is commonly overestimated as a result of failure to differentiate various forms of food intolerance or coincidence of symptoms from true food allergy. By the age of 20 years respiratory symptoms are the predominant form of allergic disease. Among college students 5.7% have a history of asthma, 16.6% have a history of allergic rhinitis, and 19.1% have a history of one or both diseases.[33]

PREVENTION OF ALLERGIC SYMPTOMS
Overview

Allergic diseases are the clinical manifestation of immunoglobulin E (IgE) mediated immune reactions. Three components must be present for the development of allergic disease: exposure to allergen, allergic sensitization, and target organ susceptibility.[49] In most cases allergens are extrinsic proteins that must come in contact with a body surface to trigger an allergic reaction. The body surface may be the respiratory mucosa, the intestinal mucosa, the conjunctiva, or the skin.

If all potential allergens could be avoided, allergic disease could be prevented. In practice avoidance of the offending allergen such as a food or drug is optimal management. In reality many allergens such as pollens and mold spores cannot be avoided, and primary prevention of allergic respiratory disease is impossible. Immunotherapy provides a secondary form of prevention to minimize the symptoms resulting from unavoidable allergen exposure. Primary prevention of food allergy in infants at high risk of development of allergic disease has been accomplished but is difficult. Secondary prevention of symptoms by avoidance of the sensitizing food is the basis of management of food allergies.

Risk factors

Development of IgE antibodies against environmental allergens is a prerequisite for manifestation of allergic disease. Atopy is the tendency to produce IgE antibodies against usually harmless environmental allergens. Predic-

Table 54-1. Prevalence of respiratory disease

	Race	
	White (n = 11,260)	Black (n = 1,482)
Allergic rhinitis	9.8%	8.1%
Asthma	6.9%	9.2%

From Turkeltaub PC, Gergen PJ: Second national health and nutrition exam survey, 1976-1980, (NHANES II), *Ann Allergy* 67:147-157, 1991.

tion of atopy is based primarily on genetic heritage. If both parents are atopic, there is a 40% to 60% risk of atopy in the child. If one parent is atopic, there is a 25% to 35% risk.[9]

Elevation of cord blood IgE level above 0.5 IU/ml has been correlated with subsequent development of atopic dermatitis in early childhood, but respiratory allergy, which frequently develops later in childhood, has not shown close association with cord blood IgE. A cord blood IgE level of less than 0.5 IU/ml has a negative predictive value of 94% for the development of atopic disease in the first 24 months of life. In contrast the positive predictive value of cord blood IgE level greater than 0.5 IU/ml is only 18%.[56] Maternal smoking influences cord blood IgE and increases the risk for subsequent infant allergy. In a report from Sweden newborn infants of nonallergic parents had more than a threefold higher incidence of elevated cord blood IgE level and a fourfold higher risk of atopic disease before 18 months of age if the mother smoked than if she did not.[26] The family history of allergic disease is more important than the measurement of an infant's serum IgE level in the estimation of allergic risk. Later in life a dramatically elevated serum IgE level above 1000 IU/ml may be helpful in confirming a diagnosis of severe atopic dermatitis. Except for the assessment of disease activity in allergic bronchopulmonary aspergillosis measurement of total serum IgE level is not usually needed in the management of allergic diseases.

FOOD ALLERGY AND ATOPIC DERMATITIS
Role of food allergy in atopic dermatitis

Atopic dermatitis is the form of atopy most likely to appear in infancy. Food hypersensitivity has been strongly implicated as a contributing factor in the severity of atopic dermatitis. In studies by Sampson, 24 of 26 children with atopic dermatitis had at least one positive food skin test result in 28 tests applied. Fourteen of the 26 children developed cutaneous symptoms on double-blind food challenge. Egg was by far the most common offending food (36% of positive challenges), followed by milk (14%), wheat (11%), and peanut (11%).[45] All cutaneous symptoms developed within 2 hours of the challenge. In 10 children gastrointestinal symptoms developed after food challenge, and respiratory symptoms developed in 7 children. With the demonstration of the contribution of food allergy to atopic dermatitis avoidance has become part of the management of atopic dermatitis, and avoidance of the commonly offending foods has been recommended as a means to reduce the risk of developing atopic dermatitis. Sampson has recommended avoidance of eggs, nuts, peanuts, and shellfish in the first 1 to 2 years for infants in the high-risk category (cord blood IgE level greater than 2 IU/ml and two immediate family members atopic).[42]

Attempts at primary prevention

Demonstration of prevention of atopic dermatitis has been difficult. Food proteins ingested by the mother appear in breast milk and may cross the placental barrier. Zeiger et al. studied the effect of combined maternal and infant food allergen avoidance on development of atopy in early infancy.[56] Infants of atopic parents were prenatally randomized to prophylactically treated and control groups. Dietary restrictions in the prophylactically treated group (n = 103) included maternal avoidance of cow's milk, eggs, and peanuts during the third trimester of pregnancy and during lactation. Breast-feeding was encouraged for at least 4 to 6 months in both the prophylactic and the control groups. In the prophylactic group Nutramigen, a casein hydrolysate formula with low sensitization potential, was used as a supplement and after weaning until 12 months of age. Solid food was introduced at 6 months. Cow's milk, wheat, soy, corn, and citrus were withheld until 12 months. Eggs were withheld until 24 months. Peanuts and fish were withheld until 36 months. The presence of atopic diseases was monitored at 12, 24, and 36 months of age. Atopic diseases included atopic dermatitis, urticaria/angioedema, gastrointestinal (GI) disease (vomiting or diarrhea after ingestion of specific food on at least two occasions with positive skin test result), asthma, and allergic rhinitis. The cumulative prevalance of atopy was lower at 12 months in the prophylactically treated group (16.2%) than in the control group (27.1%). Atopic dermatitis, urticaria, and GI food allergy were less frequent in the prophylactic group. The cumulative prevalance of allergic rhinitis and asthma was not affected by the prophylactic regimen. This study suggests that extremely rigid avoidance of commonly allergenic foods during pregnancy, during lactation, and during early infancy has a measurable benefit. However, the prevention of allergic disease is not complete, and most people find the restrictions too difficult to follow. Sampson's recommendation of avoidance of eggs, nuts, peanuts, and shellfish in the first 2 years of life for the infant at risk for atopic disease seems more reasonable. If atopic dermatitis or food intolerance develops, specific skin testing under the guidance of a pediatric allergy specialist is needed.

Label ingredients that indicate the presence of soy protein

Soy flour
Soy protein
Soy nuts
Soy sauce
Textured vegetable protein
Tofu

Adapted from Koerner CB, Sampson HA: Diets and nutrition. In Metcalfe KK, Sampson HA, Simon RA, editors: *Food allergy: adverse reactions to foods and food additives,* Boston, 1991, Blackwell Scientific Publications.

Skin testing for food allergy

The preceding recommendations aimed at the primary prevention of food allergy and atopic dermatitis are associated with incomplete patient compliance. The role of specific food avoidance in the setting of prior sensitization to the food is much more easily appreciated by patients. In many cases the role of the allergist is to help the patient limit the list of foods that really must be avoided. The clinical history of reaction to foods can be very misleading, and even a positive prick test result in response to the suspected food may not correlate with clinical disease. Screening for atopy with immediate hypersensitivity prick skin tests is very useful for limiting the number of foods to be considered for double-blind food challenge.[43]

In addition to atopic dermatitis food allergies are capable of triggering urticaria, gastrointestinal symptoms, and respiratory symptoms in children and adults. Fish, shellfish, nuts, peanuts, cow's milk, and eggs account for the majority of true allergic food reactions. Cross-reactivity is frequent among fish, such as codfish, halibut, bass, and trout. Among shellfish cross-reactivity to crustaceans (crab, crayfish, lobster, and shrimp) is also common. Although they are not closely related in the animal kingdom, allergic sensitivity is also common to mollusks: oysters, scallops, clams, and mussels. Almonds, brazil nuts, walnuts, and cashews are each in a different botanical family, yet it is common practice to warn patients to avoid all true nuts when sensitivity to one is demonstrated. Peanuts are not true nuts and are in the legume family with beans and peas. Recent studies have demonstrated that proven hypersensitivity to one legume does not necessitate elimination of the entire legume family.[3] Soybean products are used in numerous processed foods from infant formula to frozen dinners. Fortunately in the extraction of soybean oil the protein fraction is removed. Soy allergic patients have tolerated blinded oral challenge with soy oil.[10] Clinical soybean hypersensitivity is much less common than clinical peanut sensitivity, and a positive blinded oral challenge response to soy is needed before recommending the difficult

---

Label ingredients that indicate the presence of milk protein

Milk solids
Casein
Caseinates
Butter
Butter fat
Lactalbumin
Sour cream
Whey
Curds
Artificial butter flavor
Cheese
Yogurt

Adapted from Koerner CB, Sampson HA: Diets and nutrition. In Metcalfe KK, Sampson HA, Simon RA, editors: *Food allergy: adverse reactions to foods and food additives,* Boston, 1991, Blackwell Scientific Publications.

Label ingredients that indicate the presence of egg protein

Egg white
Egg yolk
Albumin
Eggnog
Mayonnaise
Ovalbumin
Ovomucoid

Adapted from Koerner CB, Sampson HA: Diets and nutrition. In Metcalfe KK, Sampson HA, Simon RA, editors: *Food allergy: adverse reactions to foods and food additives,* Boston, 1991, Blackwell Scientific Publications.

task of soy avoidance. The box above, left lists ingredients that need to be avoided in proven soy sensitivity. Cow's milk and egg sensitive patients need to avoid foods containing the ingredients listed in the boxes above.

The physician must keep in mind that allergy is only one of the many possible mechanisms of adverse reaction to foods.[41] Lactose intolerance is far more common in the general population than is true cow's milk allergy. Allergic reactions may be closely mimicked by toxic reactions to histamine in improperly handled scromboid fish, such as tuna and mackerel. The initial screening test for true food allergy is the prick skin test. If the prick test result is negative in most cases an IgE mechanism for induction of symptoms by that food can be eliminated. A positive double-blind challenge test result is required to prove a cause and effect relationship between a food and a symptom.[44] In cases of food allergy either proved by challenge test or accepted by both physician and patient on the basis of compatible history and positive skin test result the only treatment is avoidance of the specific food. This may require avoidance of related foods. As previously noted when one kind of true nut causes allergic reaction all true nuts are usually avoided. Similarly when one type of shellfish triggers reactions various forms of shellfish are usually avoided. In these examples and in most clinical situations it is easy to maintain a balanced diet despite the avoidance of the incriminated foods. In all situations requiring avoidance of cow's milk products an alternate calcium source needs to be recommended. In infancy the dietary impact is much more drastic. Human breast milk is the obvious choice for newborn babies; however, the presence of allergens in human breast milk must be recognized. In severe cases of allergy to cow's milk the only formula substitute tolerated is one in which protein fragments are small enough to be nonallergenic, such as Nutramigen.[57] Fortunately with avoidance of a food allergen the clinical hypersensitivity often resolves. The avoidance does not always have to be maintained throughout life.[6] Most infants sensitized to cow's milk outgrow this problem by 2 years of age. Children diagnosed with food allergy after 3 years of age are less likely to outgrow the allergy.[7]

ALLERGIC RHINITIS
Skin testing for aeroallergens

In the second National Health and Nutrition Examination Survey 20.2% of the population had at least one positive skin test result out of the eight inhalant allergens tested.[17] Peak reactivity occurred in the 12- to 24-year-old age group. Among whites males had higher rates of reactivity than females (22.0% versus 17.6%). Among blacks the sexes had equal reactivity (23.3%). People living at or above poverty level had significantly higher rates of reactivity than people living below poverty level. The Northeast had the highest prevalence of skin test reactivity (25.6%), and the South had the lowest (12.5%).

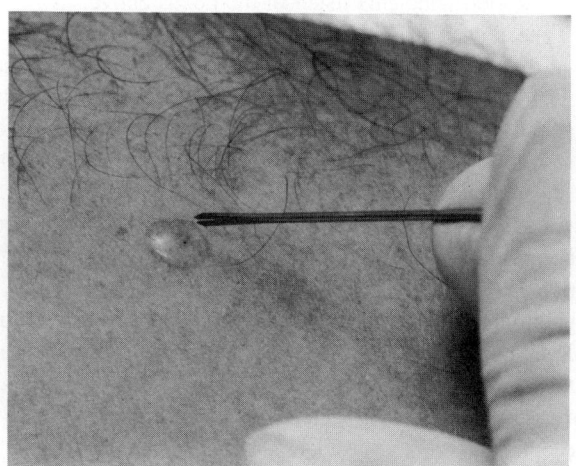

Fig. 54-1. Skin testing with a bifurcated needle.

The aeroallergens used in skin testing include grass pollens, ragweed and other weed pollens, tree pollens, house dust mites, molds, and animal danders. Prick skin testing is the standard type of testing used to identify the presence of specific IgE to allergens. Drops of extracts are applied in rows on the back or arm. The skin is pricked through the drop using a solid (nonhollow) needle (Fig. 54-1). Negative controls (diluent) and positive controls (histamine) are applied for comparison. The wheal and flare responses in positive test results are usually less than 2 cm in diameter, allowing a large number of skin tests to be applied to the back. If any systemic symptoms develop during the testing, the extracts can be wiped from the back before the usual observation time of 20 minutes. If prick test findings are negative, intradermal skin tests may be used to identify the more weakly reactive allergies.

Prick and intradermal skin testing allows the physician to determine the presence or absence of specific IgE to a wide variety of aeroallergens. There is a very small risk of systemic allergic reaction during skin testing, and the physician needs to be experienced in the interpretation of the skin test results, as well as be prepared to treat systemic allergic reactions if they occur. In many cases allergy skin testing is most appropriately carried out by specialists trained in allergy and immunology. Radioallergosorbent tests (RASTs) provide an in vitro method for detection of specific IgE. RAST is most useful when the skin is not suitable for testing. However, cost issues limit the number of allergens that can be practically tested by RAST.[53]

Geographic factors

Pollens are wind-borne and are carried for miles. Although specific pollens may be avoided (for example, ragweed is not found high in the Rocky Mountains), pollen grains of all types are potentially allergenic. Pollen seasons exist throughout the vegetated world, and in warm climates the pollen season may persist throughout the year. Geographic moves are rarely justified on the basis of pollen allergy, because in the atopic patient new allergies to the pollens encountered in the new environment can develop. Use of central or room air conditioners can reduce exposure to allergens, permitting the windows to be closed in the warm months, thus excluding outdoor particulate allergens.[46] Use of air-conditioning in the car is also important. Riding in a car with the windows open or on a motorcycle exposes the allergic rhinitis sufferer to tremendous volumes of air and large amounts of pollen. If possible the allergic rhinitis patient should not mow grass since this is another cause of very intense allergen exposure.

Indoor allergens

Pets are among the most important indoor allergens, and the prevalence of dander sensitivity among atopic cat and dog owners may be as high as 90%. Avoidance is the safest means of management of animal dander sensitivity.

Even if they do not own a pet, patients may be exposed to pets in the homes of family and friends. In selecting a house or apartment the animal dander sensitive patient needs to establish whether previous occupants owned pets.

House dust mites are the other common source of indoor year round allergens. In an Ohio study 25 of 26 homes screened yielded a positive finding for dust mites. The highest concentrations of mites were in heavily used fabric upholstered furniture and in carpets of living rooms, family rooms, and bedrooms.[2] Sensitivity to dust mites is especially common among asthmatic patients. In young asthmatic populations the prevalence of mite sensitivity may exceed 70%.[35] The quantity of dust mite allergen in the home has been identified as a risk factor for the development of asthma in prospective studies of children of atopic parents.[47] Dust mite exposure can be reduced by covering pillows and mattresses in airtight vinyl cases, removing carpets from the bedroom, and washing bed linen frequently. These steps have been shown to reduce asthmatic symptoms and bronchial histamine sensitivity in children.[31] In general the effort to reduce dust mite exposure is most intense in the bedroom. Measures that reduce the generation and collection of dust are desirable. Hardwood floors are better than carpeted floors. Simple furniture that can be damp wiped is better than fabric upholstered furniture. For the dust mite sensitive keeping the indoor humidity low helps reduce dust mite growth. These patients should not use humidifiers in the winter and should use dehumidifiers in the summer.

Symptomatic therapy

Antihistamines are the first line treatment of itching of the nose, eyes, and throat. The newer antihistamines, terfenadine and astemizole, have the advantage of being nonsedating and free of anticholinergic side effects. Both terfenadine and astemizole have been linked in rare instances with "torsades de pointes."[39] If an older antihistamine, such as chlorpheniramine, is well tolerated, it has the advantage of far lower cost than the nonsedating antihistamines. The anticholinergic side effects of the older antihistamines need to be avoided in patients with narrow angle glaucoma or prostatic hypertrophy. In addition the antihistamines may have an adverse effect on the mental status of elderly patients.

Antihistamines compete with histamine for receptors on target tissues. Therefore antihistamines work best when present in the tissue before any allergic reaction. During the peak of a pollen season antihistamines are taken daily. Oral decongestants may be used temporarily, but they may cause insomnia and are contraindicated in hypertension.[15] Over the counter decongestant nasal sprays are to be avoided because of the rebound congestion of the nose that develops with prolonged use. Nasal decongestion in allergic rhinitis is usually managed by nasal corticosteroid sprays (beclomethasone, flunisolide, or triamcinolone). In contrast to the decongestant sprays the corticosteroid nasal sprays, even with very prolonged use, do not cause rebound congestion. As with antihistamines nasal corticosteroids need to be used daily during the peak of pollen season. Nasal corticosteroid sprays are also used instead of decongestant sprays in chronic nonallergic vasomotor rhinitis, although the improvement is less dramatic. Nasal corticosteroids continue to be used in combination with antibiotics during episodes of sinusitis. Elimination of smoke exposure is important in control of nasal symptoms in allergic rhinitis, vasomotor rhinitis, and sinusitis.

Immunotherapy

Preventive avoidance is completely applicable to animal danders, partially applicable to dust mites, and minimally applicable to pollens. Fortunately immunotherapy is an additional intervention that reduces the symptomatic consequences of allergen exposure. Immunotherapy is most dramatically effective in pollen related allergic disease. Ragweed immunotherapy has been shown to reduce ragweed season nasal symptom scores, nasal challenge mediator release, and late phase cutaneous skin test response to ragweed.[22] Immunotherapy results in generation of allergen specific IgG antibody and allergen specific T suppressor cells and suppresses the seasonal rise in specific IgE.[38] In addition to ragweed immunotherapy has been shown to be effective in relieving allergic disease caused by grass pollen, house dust mites, and cat dander. In general immunotherapy is continued until the patient no longer experiences a seasonal increase in symptoms for 2 years. The average duration of immunotherapy is 3 to 5 years.[1]

As with allergy skin testing there is always a risk of systemic allergic reaction during immunotherapy. Patients whose symptoms cannot be adequately controlled by medications are selected to receive immunotherapy. The selection of patients for immunotherapy, and the planning of the course of immunotherapy, may be best supervised by a certified allergist. All medical facilities administering allergy shots must be prepared to treat anaphylaxis.

ASTHMA
Allergic factors

Asthma is a disease of hyperreactive airways with responsiveness to a variety of stimuli. Most asthma is not strictly limited to a pollen season. However the prevalence of atopy in asthma is high. In the pulmonary clinic at Rhode Island Hospital 58.3% of the adult asthmatic patients were found to be atopic by skin testing for 14 aeroallergens.[24] At the Hospital for Sick Children in Toronto 65% of the asthmatic children aged 6 to 17 years were skin test positive to three or more allergens of 16 tests applied. There was an increase in the number and size of the positive skin test results with increasing severity of asthma.[58]

Most clinicians are aware that even allergic asthmatic

Table 54-2. Agents causing occupational asthma

Agent	Occupation
Animal protein	Lab workers
	Veterinarians
Shellfish	Food processors
Plant dusts	Textile workers
Organic dyes	Printers
Wood dust	Carpenters
	Sawmill workers
Fungal allergens	Farmers
	Office workers
Enzymes	Drug industry
	Food handlers
Antibiotics	Drug industry
	Health workers
Metals	Chemical industry
	Metal refining
	Plating
Anhydrides	Plastic industry
	Food wrapping
Formaldehyde	Particle board
	Biomedical
Isocyanates	Plastic workers

From Butcher BT, Salvaggio JE: Occupational asthma, *J All Clin Immunol* 78:547-556, 1986.

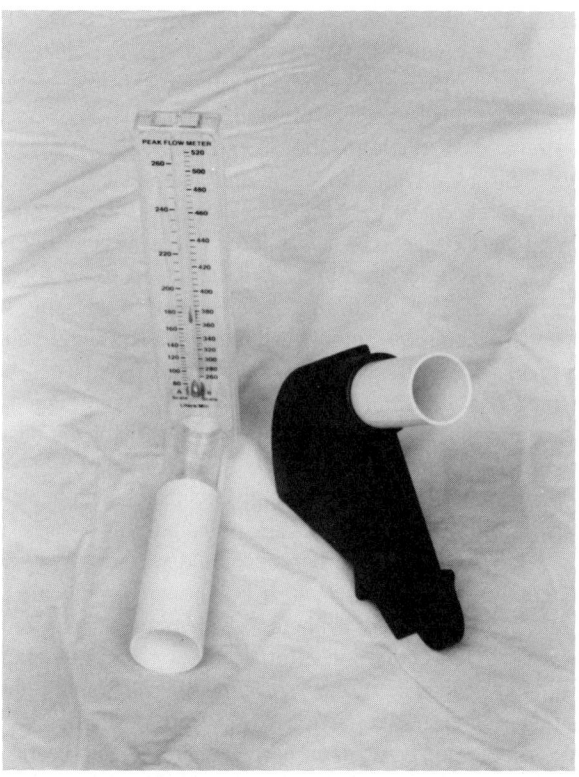

Fig. 54-2. Peak flow meters.

patients experience asthma attacks triggered by nonspecific stimuli such as cold air or smoke exposure. The gold standard proof of asthma is bronchial constriction after inhalation of histamine or methacholine. In addition to the immediate bronchospasm induced by allergen inhalation challenge increased nonspecific histamine and methacholine bronchial reactivity lasting up to 7 days after a single allergen exposure has been demonstrated in allergic asthmatic patients.[13] Ragweed sensitive asthmatic patients have been shown to have increased methacholine responsiveness sustained throughout the ragweed season.[8] Once contributing allergens are identified, their influence on the severity and frequency of asthma can be reduced by avoidance and immunotherapy.

In addition to natural environmental allergens occupational allergens may also trigger asthma. According to the National Jewish Center for Immunology and Respiratory Disease occupational asthma accounts for 2% to 15% of all adult onset asthma. The prevalence of occupational asthma is high among workers exposed to high molecular weight compounds such as proteins of animal or plant origin. More than 200 agents have been reported to cause occupational asthma[11] (Table 54-2).

Skin testing procedures have been described for 44 different agents implicated in IgE mediated occupational lung disease.[18] However, a positive skin test result is not sufficient to establish a diagnosis of occupational asthma, and not all occupational asthma is IgE mediated. The diagnosis of occupational asthma includes both symptoms of asthma

and significant work related changes in forced expiratory volume in 1 second, peak flow, nonspecific airway responsiveness, or specific positive response to inhalation challenge.[12] Identification of an allergic reaction to an occupational allergen permits prevention of future asthma attacks through avoidance or protection of workers.

Symptomatic therapy

Asthma is now treated as an inflammatory disease of the airways rather than just a bronchospastic disease. Although bronchodilators are still routinely used for the relief of bronchospasm, airway obstruction caused by inflammation is the main target of daily asthma therapy. Inhaled corticosteroids have moved to first-line therapy in all but the mildest asthma. Regular use of inhaled corticosteroids has been shown to reduce bronchial hyperreactivity.[23] In effect regular use of inhaled corticosteroids becomes preventive therapy in controlling the airway inflammation associated with asthma.

The other type of antiinflammatory drug currently available is cromolyn sodium, which is capable of blunting the asthmatic response to inhaled allergens. In the case of animal dander induced asthma cromolyn should be inhaled at least 30 minutes before anticipated exposure. Cromolyn needs to be inhaled on a daily basis during long-term exposure such as a pollen season.[4] For current management of chronic asthma an inhaled β_2 agonist is used as often as every 3 or 4 hours to control bronchospasm. The need for the bronchodilator may be determined by the presence of overt wheezing or by a fall in peak flow measured at home using a peak flow meter (Fig. 54-2). If the inhaled bronchodilator is needed as often as four times per day, either an inhaled corticosteroid (two to four puffs bid) or inhaled cromolyn (two puffs qid) is added to the daily therapy. An antiinflammatory agent is also indicated if the peak flow falls more than 20% below the patient's personal best measurement during symptomatic episodes.[32]

Immunotherapy

Because asthma is more commonly multifactorial than allergic rhinitis, demonstrating efficacy of immunotherapy in asthma has been more difficult. In a study of asthmatic patients predominantly sensitive to grass pollen the symptom/medication scores of patients treated with grass immunotherapy were significantly lower than those of patients receiving immunotherapy without grass pollen.[36] Evidence of improved control of asthma has also been demonstrated for *Alternaria* mold,[21] dust mite,[34] and cat.[20]

Every asthmatic patient should be asked questions aimed at detecting potential allergic factors contributing to the course of the disease. In younger patients and in patients with upper respiratory symptoms the yield of these questions will be high. Patients with personal or family histories of atopy should be referred to a specialist for allergy evaluation including skin testing. Identification of specific allergens guides the treating physician's decisions regarding environmental control, use of cromolyn sodium, and use of immunotherapy. Antiinflammatory agents and bronchodilators still have their place in the management of the allergic asthmatic patients, but the opportunity to prevent allergically triggered airway inflammation should not be overlooked.

The total direct and indirect cost of asthma in the United States in 1985 was estimated at nearly $4.5 billion. Fifty-three percent of this total was for direct medical expenditures. The largest category of medical expenditure was for hospitalization.[55] The goal of current asthma management is to use control of triggering factors (allergic and nonallergic) and antiinflammatory medications in a way that prevents the need for emergency room visits and hospitalization. Although expenditures for asthma medication will rise with this approach, the morbidity and cost for hospitalization for asthma should decline.

VENOM ALLERGY

Venoms from bees, yellow jackets, wasps, and hornets are potentially allergenic and are occasionally life threatening (Fig. 54-3). Yellow jackets and honeybees are the insects most commonly responsible for stings. Avoidance is the primary means of prevention of illness. The necessary measures include moving away from stinging insects encountered, eliminating scented sprays and beverages, wearing footwear outdoors, and removing any nests found around the home. Even the most cautious may be stung. Fortunately immunotherapy with venom has been proven effective in lowering the risk of anaphylactic reaction to stings. The number of deaths in the United States per year resulting from stinging insect allergy is thought to be less than 50. However, the number of people sensitized to insect venom is much larger. In a Baltimore survey 4% of a sample of employees at a manufacturing plant reported systemic reactions to insect stings, and more than 20% had either RAST or skin test evidence of sensitization to at least one Hymenoptera venom.[51] Protection against systemic reaction on subsequent sting is nearly complete during venom immunotherapy, in contrast to a 35% systemic reaction rate among patients who are sensitized and decline immunotherapy.[37] Immunotherapy is usually offered to adults who have had a systemic allergic reaction to an insect sting with a corresponding positive venom skin test result. Pain, swelling, and itching at the site of the sting are the natural consequences of venom toxicity. Even large local reactions are not an indication for venom skin testing or for venom immunotherapy.[29] Although children below 16 years of age may become sensitized to insect stings, they rarely experience systemic reactions, and immunotherapy is usually not needed.[52] The life-style of the patient is also an important consideration in selection of candidates for venom immunotherapy. Venom immunotherapy was first used on an allergic family member of a beekeeper. Any outdoor occupation or hobby increases the risk of stinging insect exposure. Sensitized patients who rarely encounter stinging insects may choose to manage the risk by carrying injectable epinephrine and oral antihistamines. All patients with stinging insect sensitivity, even those on immunotherapy, need to be prepared to begin medical management of a systemic reaction whenever there is a possibility of exposure to stinging insects. If they are stung, they should take the oral antihistamine. If systemic symptoms begin, they should inject epinephrine using a device such as the Epi-Pen and proceed to an emergency room for further treatment.

One of the most difficult aspects of venom allergy management has been determining when to stop shots. Evidence is beginning to accumulate that protection afforded by 3 to 5 years of immunotherapy may persist beyond the time shots are discontinued.[30]

DRUG ALLERGY

Adverse drug reactions occur frequently. Approximately 37,000 adverse drug reactions were reported to the Food and Drug Administration in 1985.[16] Surveys of hospitalized patients have reported a prevalence of adverse drug reactions between 6% and 15%. Most of the reactions are toxic; allergic reactions account for only 6% to 10% of the adverse reactions.[14] Many of the nonallergic adverse

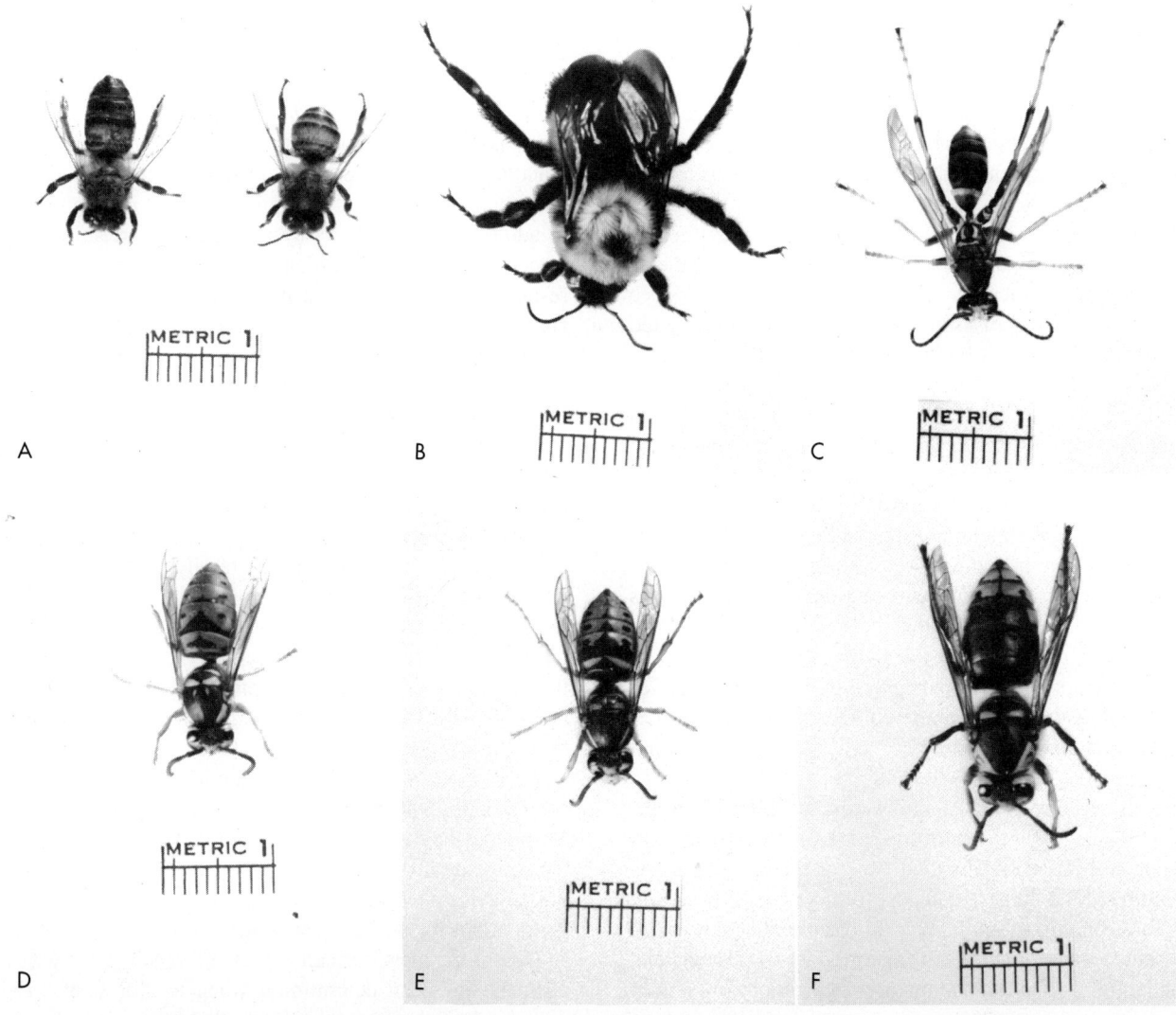

Fig. 54-3. Selected Hymenoptera insects. **A,** Honeybee *(Apis mellifera).* **B,** Bumblebee *(Bombus* sp.). **C,** Paper wasp *(Polistes fuscatus).* **D,** Yellow jacket *(Vespula maculifrons).* **E,** Yellow hornet *(Dolichovespula arenaria).* **F,** White-faced hornet *(Dolichovespula maculata).* (From Parker CW: *Clinical immunology,* Philadelphia, 1980, WB Saunders.)

reactions are predictable and some are preventable. The side effect of hypokalemia from diuretics is predictable. The secondary effect of vaginal candidiasis is preventable with concurrent use of vaginal antifungal therapy during systemic antibiotic treatment. Even some idiosyncratic reactions are highly predictable such as the rash associated with ampicillin therapy in a patient with mononucleosis. Prevention consists of choosing an alternate antibiotic.

True allergic reactions are usually unexpected and occur in the setting of prior tolerance of the same drug. Prior exposure and IgE sensitization are required to produce immediate hypersensitivity reactions. In most cases drugs associated with prior reaction in an individual are avoided. However, the number of patients claiming drug allergy is estimated to be three times the actual number.[14] In some cases patients suffer as a result of unnecessary avoidance of a drug they incorrectly think caused an allergic reaction. A large part of this problem is the unfortunate labeling of any adverse reaction as an "allergy." In a typical example a patient who has had a vagal reaction after local anesthetic injection may avoid further local anesthetic exposure because of the erroneous diagnosis of a drug allergy. In fact allergic reactions to local anesthetics other than procaine are very rare. Skin testing with nonallergenic local anesthetics such as lidocaine can be very reassuring to the fearful patient.

Antibiotics account for the largest portion of true allergic drug reactions. The β-lactam antibiotics and the sulfonamides are the most allergenic. The β-lactam group includes the penicillins, the cephalosporins, the cephamycins, the penems, and the monobactams. Penicillin cross-reactivity is greater than 50% for the first-generation cephalosporins and less frequent for the second- and third-generation cephalosporins.[54] The monobactams are not cross-reactive with penicillin. Although sulfonamide antibiotic sensitivity is common, allergic reaction to sulfonamide diuretics such as the thiazides is low. Tetracycline and erythromycin, although frequently responsible for gastric upset, are rarely responsible for true allergic reactions.

Fortunately the assumption of permanent persistence of drug allergy is erroneous. In patients more than 10 years past from a penicillin reaction the penicillin skin test reactivity falls to only 22%. In a study by Sullivan none of 83 skin test negative patients treated with β-lactam antibiotics experienced acute allergic reactions.[48] In these examples detailed histories of drug reactions and drug skin testing can prevent unnecessary avoidance of a needed drug.

Radiographic contrast dye reactions are often incorrectly labeled as allergic reactions. IgE has not been found to participate in such reactions, including urticaria, angioedema, and hypotension, even though they may have an anaphylactoid character. Fortunately pretreatment of these patients with systemic corticosteroids and antihistamines before planned radiographic dye study has been successful in preventing repeat systemic reactions.[19] Further progress

has been made with the introduction of nonionic low-osmolality contrast media, which have a lower rate of adverse reaction than the ionic contrast agents.[5] One of the possible reasons for reduced reactions may be reduced histamine release from basophils by the nonionic agents.[40] Either pretreatment with corticosteroids and antihistamines or nonionic dye may be used in preventing contrast dye reactions in selected patients.

The intraoperative anaphylactic event is one of the more difficult clinical situations to analyze. Usually several drugs are given in a short period of time. In addition the physical events of surgery may induce part of the picture of anaphylaxis, such as sudden hypotension. The importance of latex as an allergen has recently been recognized. A latex sensitive patient may develop anaphylaxis during surgery as a result of the latex in gloves and many other sites. Children with a history of several surgeries for neural tube defects constitute a group commonly sensitive to latex. Extensive precautions are needed to prevent intraoperative reactions in sensitized patients.[28]

Prevention of allergic drug reactions involves common-sense measures. The larger the number of drugs being taken, the greater the chance for an adverse reaction. Limit the number of drugs prescribed to the minimum necessary. Avoid drugs that have been associated with allergic reaction previously. Use skin testing in selected cases to determine current drug sensitivity. Administer drugs orally when possible since allergic reactions to oral drugs tend to be less severe than allergic reactions to parenteral drugs.[14]

SUMMARY

Immediate hypersensitivity skin testing essentially screens patients for atopy to foods, inhalants, and certain drugs. Clinical history, physical examination, oral challenge, inhalation challenge, rhinoscopy, and spirometry are needed to establish the presence of allergic disease. The development of atopy and the susceptibility of the target organ (skin, gut, nose, or lungs) are largely determined genetically, making primary prevention of allergic disease largely unattainable. Most of the practice of allergy is aimed at secondary prevention of symptoms induced by established sensitivity to ingested and inhaled allergens.

Once a clinically relevant allergen is identified, the patient can be advised to avoid the allergen when possible. In the management of food allergies and most drug allergies avoidance is the only intervention needed. In the management of allergic rhinitis and asthma usually more than one allergen can be identified, and the target organ responds to nonspecific irritants as well as the allergens. In pollen, mite, and mold allergy immunotherapy provides the opportunity to prevent symptomatic reaction to environmental allergens resulting in reduced need for medication. Many years of improved quality of life may follow recognition and treatment of allergic disease.

REFERENCES

1. AMA council report: In vivo diagnostic testing and immunotherapy for allergy, *JAMA* 258:1363-1367, 1987.
2. Arlian LG, Bernstein IL, Gallagher JS: The prevalence of house dust mites, Dermatophagoides spp, and associated environmental conditions in homes in Ohio, *J Allergy Clin Immunol* 69:527-532, 1982.
3. Bernhisel-Broadbent J, Sampson HA: Cross-allergenicity in the legume botanical family in children with food hypersensitivity, *J Allergy Clin Immunol* 83:435-440, 1989.
4. Bernstein IL: Cromolyn sodium in the treatment of asthma: coming of age in the United States, *J Allergy Clin Immunol* 76:381-388, 1985.
5. Bettmann MA, Higgins CB: Comparison of an ionic with a nonionic contrast agent for cardiac angiography, *Invest Radiol* 20:S70-S74, 1985.
6. Bock SA: Natural history of severe reactions to foods in young children, *J Pediatr* 107:676-680, 1985.
7. Bock SA: The natural history of food sensitivity, *J Allergy Clin Immunol* 69:173-177, 1982.
8. Boulet LP et al: Asthma and increases in nonallergic bronchial responsiveness from seasonal pollen exposure, *J Allergy Clin Immunol* 71:399-406, 1983.
9. Bousquet J, Kjellman NI: Predictive value of tests in childhood allergy, *J Allergy Clin Immunol* 78:1019-1022, 1986.
10. Bush RK et al: Soybean oil is not allergenic to soybean-sensitive individuals, *J Allergy Clin Immunol* 76:242-245, 1985.
11. Butcher BT, Salvaggio JE: Occupational asthma, *J Allergy Clin Immunol* 78:547-556, 1986.
12. CDC report: Occupational disease surveillance: asthma, *MMWR* 39:119, 1990.
13. Cockcroft DW et al: Allergen-induced increase in nonallergic bronchial reactivity, *Clin Allergy* 7:503-513, 1977.
14. Deswarte RD: Drug allergy-problems and strategies, *J Allergy Clin Immunol* 74:209-221, 1984.
15. Druce HM, Kaliner MA: Allergic rhinitis, *JAMA* 259:260-263, 1988.
16. Faich GA et al: National adverse drug reaction surveillance: 1985, *JAMA* 257:2068-2070, 1987.
17. Gergen PJ, Turkeltaub PC, Kovar MG: The prevalence of allergic skin test reactivity to eight common aeroallergens in the U.S. population: results from the second National Health and Nutrition Examination Survey, *J Allergy Clin Immunol* 80:669-679, 1987.
18. Grammer LC, Patterson R, Zeiss CR: Guidelines for the immunologic evaluation of occupational lung disease, *J Allergy Clin Immunol* 84:805-814, 1989.
19. Greenberger PA et al: Emergency administration of radiocontrast media in high-risk patients, *J Allergy Clin Immunol* 77:630-634, 1986.
20. Hedlin G et al: Immunotherapy with cat and dog dander extracts, *J Allergy Clin Immunol* 87:955-964, 1991.
21. Horst M et al: Double-blind, placebo-controlled rush immunotherapy with a standardized Alternaria extract, *J Allergy Clin Immunol* 85:460-472, 1990.
22. Iliopoulos O et al: Effects of immunotherapy on the early, late, and rechallenge nasal reaction to provocation with allergen: changes in inflammatory mediators and cells, *J Allergy Clin Immunol* 87:855-866, 1991.
23. Juniper EF et al: Effect of long-term treatment with an inhaled corticosteroid (budesonide) on airway hyperresponsiveness and clinical asthma in nonsteroid-dependent asthmatics, *Am Rev Respir Dis* 142:832-836, 1990.
24. Kalliel JN et al: High frequency of atopic asthma in a pulmonary clinic population, *Chest* 96:1336-1340, 189.
25. Koerner CB, Sampson HA: Diets and nutrition. In Metcalfe KK, Sampson HA, Simon RA, editors: *Food allergy: adverse reactions to food and food additives,* Boston, 1991, Blackwell Scientific Publications.
26. Magnusson CG: Maternal smoking influences cord serum IgE and IgD levels and increases the risk for subsequent infant allergy, *J Allergy Clin Immunol* 78:898-904, 1986.
27. Massicot JG, Cohen SG: Epidemiologic and socioeconomic aspects of allergic diseases, *J Allergy Clin Immunol* 78:954-958, 1986.
28. Mathew S, Melton A, Wagner W: Latex hypersensitivity: a case series, *Ann Allergy* 68:71, 1992.
29. Mauriello PM et al: Natural history of large local reactions from stinging insects, *J Allergy Clin Immunol* 74:494-498, 1984.
30. Muller U, Berchtold E, Helbling A: Honeybee venom allergy: results of a sting challenge 1 year after stopping successful venom immunotherapy in 86 patients, *J Allergy Clin Immunol* 87:702-709, 1991.
31. Murray AB, Ferguson AC: Dust-free bedrooms in the treatment of asthmatic children with house dust or house dust mite allergy: a controlled trial, *Pediatrics* 71:418-422, 1983.
32. *National asthma education program guidelines for the diagnosis and management of asthma,* NIH Pub No 91-3042, Bethesda, Md, 1991.
33. Nelson HS: The atopic diseases, *Ann Allergy* 55:441-447, 1985.
34. Price JP et al: A controlled trial of hyposensitization with adsorbed tyrosine Dermatophagoides pteronyssinus antigen in childhood asthma: in vivo aspects, *Clin Allergy* 14:209-219, 1984.
35. Platts-Mills TA, deWeck AL: Dust mite allergens and asthma—a worldwide problem, *J Allergy Clin Immunol* 83:416-427, 1989.
36. Reid MJ et al: Seasonal asthma in northern California: allergic causes and efficacy of immunotherapy, *J Allergy Clin Immunol* 78:590-600, 1986.
37. Reisman RE et al: Stinging insect allergy: natural history and modification with venom immunotherapy, *J Allergy Clin Immunol* 76:735-740, 1985.
38. Rocklin RE: Clinical and immunologic aspects of allergen-specific immunotherapy in patients with seasonal allergic rhinitis and/or allergic asthma, *J Allergy Clin Immunol* 72:323-334, 1983.
39. Safety of terfenadine and astemizole, *Med Lett* 34:9-10, 1992.
40. Salem DN et al: Comparison of histamine release effects of ionic and nonionic radiographic contrast media, *Am J Med* 80:382-384, 1986.
41. Sampson HA: Differential diagnosis in adverse reactions to foods, *J Allergy Clin Immunol* 78:212-219, 1986.
42. Sampson HA: Food allergies and the infant at risk, *JAMA* 260:3507, 1988.
43. Sampson HA: Immediate hypersensitivity reactions to foods: blinded food challenges in children with atopic dermatitis, *Ann Allergy* 57:209-212, 1986.
44. Sampson HA: Immunologically mediated food allergy: the importance of food challenge procedures, *Ann Allergy* 60:262-269, 1988.
45. Sampson HA: Role of immediate food hypersensitivity in the pathogenesis of atopic dermatitis, *J Allergy Clin Immunol* 71:473-480, 1983.
46. Solomon WR, Burge HA, Boise JR: Exclusion of particulate allergens by window air conditioners, *J Allergy Clin Immunol* 65:305-308, 1980.
47. Sporik R et al: Exposure to house dust mite, allergen and the development of asthma in childhood, *N Engl J Med* 323:502-507, 1990.
48. Sullivan TJ et al: Skin testing to detect penicillin allergy, *J Allergy Clin Immunol* 68:171-180, 1981.
49. Terr AI: *Basic and clinical immunology,* ed 7, Norwalk, Conn, 1991, Appleton & Lange.
50. Turkeltaub PC, Gergen PJ: Prevalence of upper and lower respiratory conditions in the US population by social and environmental factors: data from the second National Health and Nutrition Examination Survey, 1976 to 1980 (NHANES II), *Ann Allergy* 67:147-154, 1991.
51. Valentine MD: Insect venom allergy: diagnosis and treatment, *J Allergy Clin Immunol* 73:299-304, 1984.
52. Valentine MD et al: The value of immunotherapy with venom in children with allergy to insect stings, *N Engl J Med* 323:1601-1603, 1990.

53. VanArsdel PP, Larson EB: Diagnostic tests for patients with suspected allergic disease, *Ann Intern Med* 110:304-312, 1989.

54. Wedner HJ: *Drug allergy*. In Stites DP, Terr AI, editors: *Basic and clinical immunology,* Norwalk, Conn, 1991, Appelton & Lange.

55. Weiss KB, Gergen PJ, Hodgson TA: An economic evaluation of asthma in the United States, *N Engl J Med* 326:862-866, 1992.

56. Zeiger RS et al: Effect of combined maternal and infant food-allergen avoidance on the development of atopy in early infancy: a randomized study, *J Allergy Clin Immunol* 84:72-89, 1989.

57. Zeiger RS: Prevention of food allergy in infancy, *Ann Allergy* 65:430-441, 1990.

58. Zimmerman B et al: Allergy in asthma, *J Allergy Clin Immunol* 81:63-70, 1988.

RESOURCES

American Academy of Allergy and Immunology, 611 East Wells Street, Milwaukee, WI 53202.

American College of Allergy and Immunology, 800 East Northwest Highway, Suite 1080, Palatine, IL 60067.

Asthma and Allergy Foundation of America, 1125 15th Street NW, Suite 502, Washington, DC 20005.

Chapter 55

CHRONIC OBSTRUCTIVE LUNG DISEASE AND OTHER CONDITIONS OF THE CHEST

Thomas L. Petty

DEFINITIONS IN COPD

Chronic obstructive pulmonary disease (COPD) encompasses a broad spectrum of clinical labels. These labels include asthmatic bronchitis, chronic bronchitis, emphysema, and overlapping conditions. All components of COPD have various degrees of chronic airflow obstruction, but they often follow different clinical courses and demonstrate different responses to therapy.[11] In all some 20 to 30 million Americans suffer from some form of these related clinical disorders.

COPD is characterized by airflow obstruction (see Origins of Airflow and Fig. 55-2). Expiratory airflow limitation or obstruction may be caused by loss of elastic recoil or obstruction of the conducting airways, both small and large. Of course, both basic abnormalities may occur in the same patient. The cardinal symptoms of both acute and chronic airflow obstruction are cough, dyspnea, and wheeze. It must be emphasized that these are not specific symptoms and only allow a diagnosis to be made in the context of other clinical and laboratory information. For example, the same symptom complex can occur in acute and chronic bronchiolitis, bronchiectasis, tuberculosis, and lung cancer.

The discrimination of airflow obstruction from other conditions associated with these can sometimes be identified by experienced clinicians on the basis of the intensity and quality of breath sounds as assessed by auscultation. Marked prolongation of the expiratory time well beyond the normal 4 to 6 seconds also helps to indicate the degree of airflow obstruction in advanced stages of disease. But objective measurements are, by far, superior and critical to the evaluation of patients in pursuit of a diagnosis and necessary to monitoring of responses to therapy. Simple measurements by spirometry or even by simple peak flow meters and a vital capacity meter, can be useful in measuring expired airflow and air volume to be able to diagnose the disease states that are defined subsequently. For the purposes of this chapter airflow is judged by the simple forced expiratory volume in 1 second (FEV_1), which is obtained by spirometry, and total exhaled volume by the forced vital capacity (FVC), also obtained by spirometry.

Asthma

Asthma is a heterogenous disorder characterized by cough, wheeze, and dyspnea and variable degrees of reversible airflow obstruction. Asthma may be episodic or chronic. Acute intermittent or episodic asthma is easy to define and diagnose. Attacks are characterized by the sudden onset of dyspnea, cough, and wheeze caused by bronchospasm and reflected by mild, moderate, or severe airflow obstruction. These acute attacks are often followed by complete or nearly complete cessation of symptoms and a return to normal airflow after treatment or after removal from a hostile environment. Reversible airflow obstruction, which usually follows the use of bronchodilators, may sometimes occur spontaneously as in exercise-induced asthma. Acute, intermittent, and completely reversible asthma *should not be included in the COPD designa-*

tion. But even acute reversible asthma should be considered to be a chronic condition, because of the lifelong predisposition to the recurrence of acute attacks.

Asthmatic bronchitis

Asthmatic bronchitis, a term that is now reappearing, refers to a somewhat different clinical state.[10,42] The asthmatic symptoms of cough, dyspnea, and wheeze may occur throughout the year with varying degrees of airflow obstruction. *Asthmatic bronchitis* refers to chronic, persistent asthma, but the designation *bronchitis* is also appropriate because of significant airway inflammation in asthmatic bronchitis. Major reversibility cannot usually be achieved by bronchoactive drugs, even in conjunction with preventive therapy (e.g., avoidance of precipitating factors or use of drugs that inhibit the release of inflammatory mediators such as cromolyn sodium [Intal]). Asthmatic bronchitis *should* be included in the COPD spectrum (see subsequent discussion). Indeed a degree of fixed airflow obstruction, often with progressive features, commonly occurs in asthmatic bronchitis. It should be emphasized that asthmatic bronchitis is actually a form of chronic bronchitis.

Asthmatic bronchitis has been described histologically as hypertrophic and desquamative eosinophilic chronic bronchitis,[21] to refer to the eosinophilic inflammatory infiltrates of the conducting airways in protracted and chronic states of bronchial asthma. A polymorphonuclear cell infiltrate may also be present. In addition to chronic and variable airflow obstruction hyperinflation (see following discussion) may be present in asthmatic bronchitis, but not to the degree present in advanced emphysema. An increase in the residual volume is also common in asthmatic bronchitis, indicating expiratory air trapping from small airway obstruction. The diffusion test, which is a useful indicator of the integrity of the air-blood interface (alveolar-capillary membrane), is well preserved in asthmatic bronchitis. The test of carbon monoxide transfer known as the diffusion test often yields normal or near-normal results even in states of severe, protracted airflow obstruction from chronic asthmatic bronchitis.

Chronic bronchitis

So-called chronic bronchitis is very similar to asthmatic bronchitis. Cough and sputum for many months to several years are the hallmarks of chronic bronchitis. Historically chronic bronchitis has been defined as a chronic cough with expectoration for at least 3 months/year for at least 2 years.[15] But not all patients with chronic cough and expectoration have associated airflow obstruction.[4] Chronic bronchitis without airflow obstruction has been termed simple chronic bronchitis. Patients with this symptom complex have a good prognosis, as contrasted with the premature morbidity and mortality that characterize patients with chronic bronchitis with chronic airflow obstruc-

tion.[4] Although this subset of patients with chronic cough and airflow obstruction have sometimes been designated as having chronic *obstructive* bronchitis, the less specific term *chronic bronchitis* is still most commonly used.

The pathophysiology of chronic bronchitis is similar to that of asthmatic bronchitis and is characterized by varying degrees of airflow obstruction produced by a combination of inflammation and increased bronchomotor tone resulting from so-called nonspecific bronchial hyperreactivity.[48] Thus neither measurements of airflow obstruction nor lung compartments can be used to distinguish asthmatic bronchitis from chronic bronchitis. This distinction may not be important at all.[40,42] Air trapping (increased residual volume), without hyperinflation and with a normal or near-normal diffusion test result, is commonly present in both asthmatic bronchitis and chronic bronchitis; these states are often indistinguishable or mistaken for each other. Indeed they may be different names for the same pathophysiologic process.

Emphysema

Emphysema is characterized clinically by progressive dyspnea and variable cough. It is characterized physiologically by loss of elastic recoil and hyperinflation followed by chronic progressive airflow obstruction (limitation). The degree of hyperinflation exceeds that of other states of chronic airflow obstruction. In fact, an increased total lung capacity, associated with reduced elastic recoil, is found in the earliest stages of emphysema in studies of excised human lungs.[44] The gold standard for the diagnosis of emphysema is reduction of elastic recoil or loss of alveolar walls. This is a diagnosis founded on anatomic studies, usually post mortem.

More recently a consensus conference has redefined emphysema in more practical and clinical terms.[55] Loss of alveolar surface finally results in a reduction of carbon monoxide uptake, the basis of the single-breath diffusion test. Such reduction in the single breath diffusion test result correlates well with loss of alveolar walls.[19,61] Thus in advanced states of emphysema severe degrees of airflow obstruction, air trapping, marked hyperinflation, and a reduced diffusion test result are all present. By this stage of disease the chest roentgenogram shows hyperinflation and a flattened diaphragm, along with reduced pulmonary markings, signifying loss of lung parenchyma. Chest roentgenographic criteria for suggesting the diagnosis of emphysema have been offered.[47] But it must be emphasized that the chest roentgenogram is only accurate in indicating advanced states of emphysema. Some degree of reversibility of airflow obstruction may be expected in response to vigorous treatment, even in advanced emphysema.[20] Most recently chest computed tomographic scanning has been used to detect loss of alveolar walls in patients who have not yet developed expiratory airflow limitation.[31] Expiratory computed tomography offers a noninvasive method of assessing lung structure in the living human subject. The potential of performing serial studies to help shed light on the evolution from asymptomatic to symptomatic stages of emphysema is enormous.[31]

Inflammation of both small airways and surrounding alveoli is caused by the release of polymorphonuclear leukocyte elastases.[62] These pathogenetic processes are augmented by cigarette smoke, which can also inactivate the normal antielastase protective material at the air-blood interface.[27] Some of the same airway inflammatory mediators that are included in asthmatic and chronic bronchitis may also participate in the pathogenesis of emphysema.

The concept of COPD

It should be apparent from preceding comments that there are multiple pathways into the final state of COPD. These include untreated and unrelenting asthmatic bronchitis, chronic (obstructive) bronchitis, and emphysema. By the time the patient has advanced and irreversible airflow obstruction, particularly at an older age, there is little point in seeking a more specific diagnosis than COPD if airflow obstruction cannot be substantially reversed by systemic bronchodilators and corticosteroids. By contrast there is great importance in identifying those patients with major reversibility in response to therapy: the so-called hidden asthmatics. These individuals enjoy a much better prognosis with bronchodilator and corticosteroid therapy than those with fixed and progressive airflow obstruction.[11]

Table 55-1 lists the clinical and pulmonary function measurements that help to classify the various disease states that together constitute the spectrum of COPD. Patients with other disease states also characterized by chronic airflow obstruction—e.g., cystic fibrosis, bronchiectasis, bronchiolitis obliterans, and other interstitial disease states with airflow obstruction such as sarcoidosis, eosinophilic granuloma, and lymphangiomyomatosis (all rare)—should not be designated by the label COPD. These other states either have a different prognosis or sometimes require forms of therapy not appropriate for COPD (e.g., hormonal manipulations in lymphangiomyomatosis).

The definitions offered in this chapter appear useful as we approach the end of this century. And as we face an aging society, it is certain that a greater proportion of our population will suffer from chronic disorders of airflow obstruction. In fact, virtually everyone who achieves the age of 100 has some degree of emphysema as defined as loss of elastic recoil. The great majority of the "old old," that is, people older than 85, also have enlargement of alveolar ducts (previously termed ductectasia), which is not a specific disease state, but rather a result of an unfolding of the alveolar ducts produced by the reduced elasticity of the lung that is a normal consequence of aging.[64]

Emphysema and the broader concept of COPD have been considered premature aging of the lung. Thus premature losses of airflow can be an important signal of future clinical problems. This notion is embodied in the concept of "lung age" considered later.

RISK FACTORS AND EPIDEMIOLOGY

COPD is a family clustering disease caused by smoking in susceptible individuals. Other inhalant irritants and toxins, such as grain dust and industrial fumes, can also trigger the damaging mechanisms that result in airflow obstruction. COPD can thus be considered an interrelationship between inheritable and environmental factors that conspire to create airflow obstruction and its attendant

Table 55-1. Physiologic determinants of diseases characterized by acute and chronic airflow obstruction

Disease	Major symptoms complex	Pattern of airflow obstruction (FEV_1)	Trapping residual volume	Hyperinflation	Diffusion
Intermittent asthma	Acute wheezing, dyspnea with variable cough	Reversible airflow obstruction	Mild, intermittent	Transient	Normal
Asthmatic and chronic bronchitis	Chronic cough, wheeze with variable degrees of dyspnea	Partly reversible or irreversible airflow obstruction	Moderate, partly reversible	Mild to moderate	Normal and slightly reduced
Emphysema	Dyspnea, variable cough, and wheeze	Irreversible airflow obstruction	Moderate to marked; progressive	Moderate to marked	Reduced
COPD, advanced	Elements of asthmatic and chronic bronchitis and emphysema, most caused by emphysema and irreversible changes in the conducting airways	Varying degrees of reversibility or irreversible	Moderate to marked; progressive	Moderate to marked	Variable

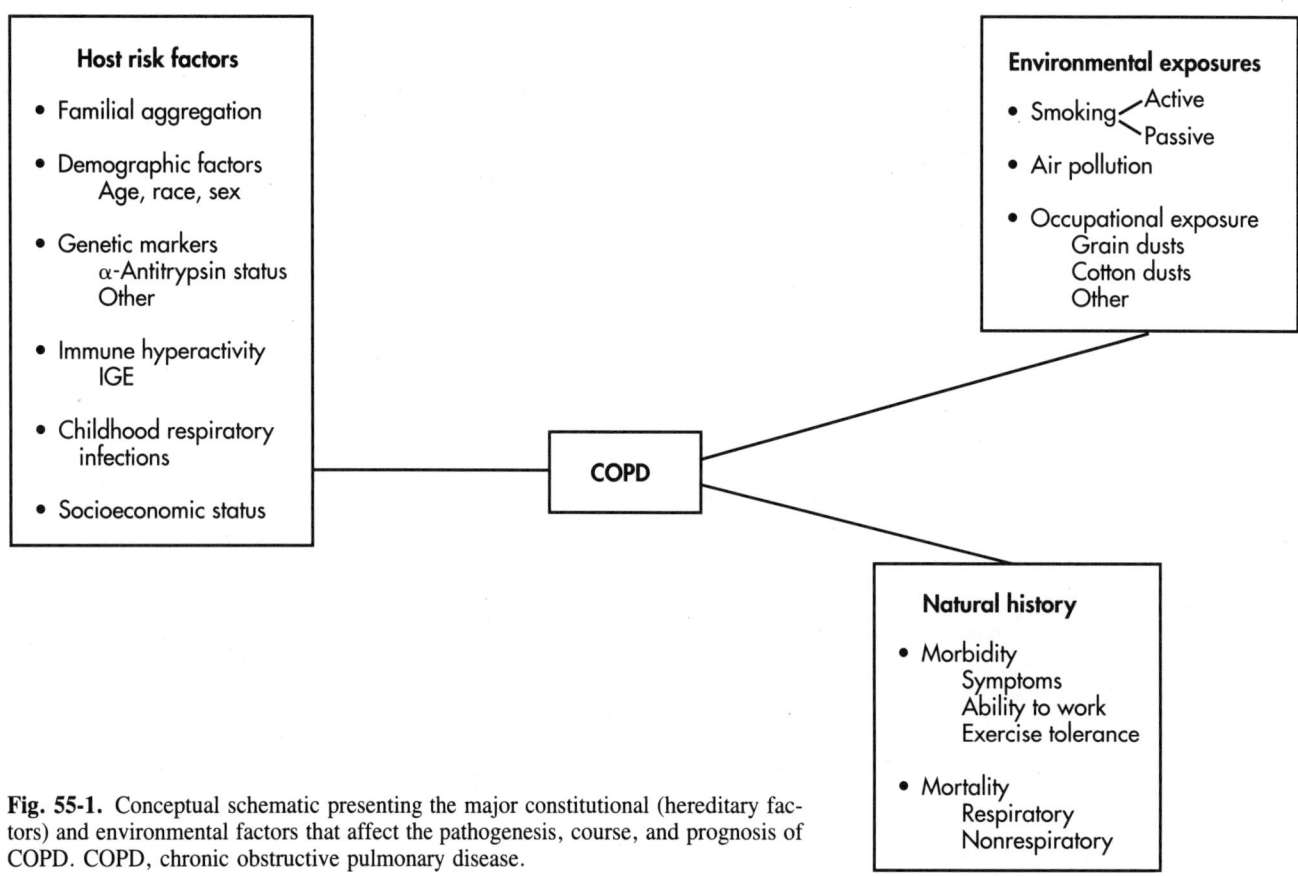

Fig. 55-1. Conceptual schematic presenting the major constitutional (hereditary factors) and environmental factors that affect the pathogenesis, course, and prognosis of COPD. COPD, chronic obstructive pulmonary disease.

symptoms (Fig. 55-1). Together both host and environmental factors affect the course of prognosis of COPD.

The symptoms of COPD that compel patients to consult their physician are dyspnea, cough, expectoration, wheeze, and impaired exercise tolerance. These are the consequences of inflammation, mucosal edema, mucus formation, and airflow obstruction.

ORIGINS OF AIRFLOW

The origins of expiratory airflow are depicted in simplified form in Fig. 55-2. Thus airflow abnormalities can result from either loss of elastic recoil (emphysema), compromise of conducting air passages (asthmatic or chronic bronchitis), or, as is the case in most patients, combinations of these fundamental factors in lung mechanics.

Assessment of airflow in COPD

COPD and its various components can only accurately be assessed by measures of airflow and air volume. The most practical and accurate method of measuring airflow and air volume is by spirometry. However, for a variety of reasons today spirometry is not commonly done in primary care physicians' offices, where the vast majority of patients with COPD are seen, either because of COPD symptoms or for some other medical reason.

It is an astonishing fact that the spirometer was invented by John Hutchinson, a surgeon, in 1846.[23] He believed that a device to measure air capacity, which he termed the "vital capacity," that is, the capacity for life, could be useful information for the insurance industry of London because it could predict premature morbidity and mortality. Hutchinson introduced his instrument, an inverted bell with a water seal, which is almost identical to the Collins type of laboratory instrument used up to the present time. Hutchinson's device and concept were originally accepted with considerable acclaim, "We have no hesitation in recording our deliberate opinion, that it forms one of the most valuable contributions to physiological science that we have seen for some time. In all future investigations the name of Mr. Hutchinson must achieve honorable notice."[6] However, neither his device nor his brilliant concept ever caught on in his era. He left England and died in Fiji, where a monument to his momentous discovery remains today.

A perspective on clinical medicine without technical guidance

Before further defining spirometry and commenting on its utility in diagnosing and monitoring COPD and other chronic pulmonary disorders plus documenting responses

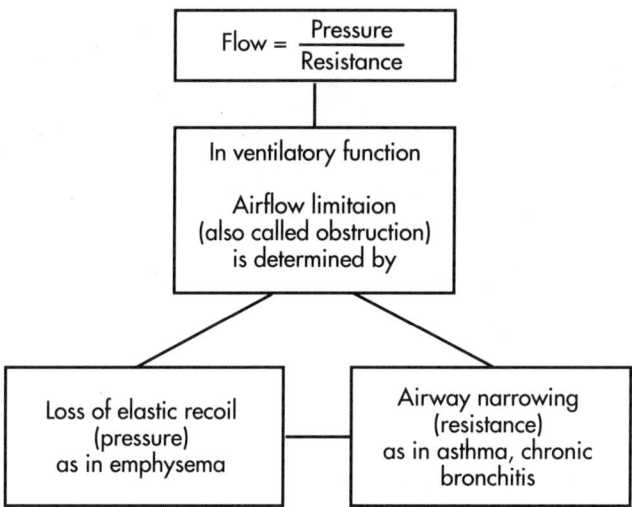

Fig. 55-2. Origins of airflow. Airflow is a function of alveolar pressure and airways resistance. Expiratory pressure is caused by elastic recoil and muscular effort. Airways resistance is caused by anything that compromises the conducting air passages, such as mucus, bronchospasm, inflammation, mucosal edema, dynamic airways collapse, or a combination. (Reproduced by permission of Thieme Medical Publishers, Inc., NY.)

to therapy let us consider how effective we would be as clinicians if we:

- Tried to diagnose and treat hypertension without a sphygmomanometer
- Attempted to diagnose and treat cardiac arrhythmias without an electrographic machine
- Attempted to diagnose and treat pneumonia without chest roentgenograms
- Tried to manage diabetes without measurements of serum or urine glucose level
- Attempted to diagnose and treat endocrinopathesis without any measures of end organ function

The essence of spirometry

When energy is applied to the chest, contracting the respiratory muscles (i.e., diaphragm and intercostals), and creating a full inspiratory effort the result is the movement of air through the branching airways and the stretching of the lungs and thorax.

Once the lungs are full reversing this maneuver results in the forced expiratory volume (Fig. 55-2). The air contained in the fully inflated lungs is forcibly expelled into a spirometer. This volume is recorded over time. Normal expiratory time is 6 seconds or less. A carefully recorded expiratory time listening to the sound of forced airflow over the manubrium can be a fairly accurate indicator of moderate to advanced states of airflow obstruction.[33] In obstructive states expiratory time is prolonged, and the

amount of air expelled in the first second is reduced. Thus the normal ratio of FEV_1 (the flow test) to FVC (the volume test) becomes less than the normal 70% to 75%. (In the examples cited later the lower limit of FEV_1 percentage of FVC is set at 71% by convention.)

Classic spirometry simply measures air volume over time. Volume per unit of time is flow. The total amount of air that can be exhaled from fully inflated lungs is the *vital capacity,* a term coined by Hutchinson. Because by convention it is also a function of the patient's effort it is properly termed the *forced vital capacity* (FVC).

The most useful flow test is that produced in the first second. This is the forced expiratory volume in 1 second (FEV_1). Other timing indices such as $FEV_{0.5}$; $FEV_{0.75}$; $FEV_{2.0}$; and $FEV_{3.0}$ have had their proponents, but they are not superior to FEV_1 in indicating airflow obstruction or limitation. At one time it was taught that the midportion of the expiratory flow curve (i.e., the $FEF_{25-75\%}$, also known as the maximum midexpiratory flow [MMEF]) would be a more sensitive indicator of airflow. It is not. It is only more variable because the $FEF_{25-75\%}$ or MMEF is largely a function of the degree of lung inflation. Thus a lung that is more fully inflated has greater elastic recoil and more widely open airways via radial traction than a lung that is less completely inflated. One way to deal with this fundamental fact of physiology is to measure $FEF_{25-75\%}$ from the same part of the lung volume, but this takes elaborate equipment and, in plain language, is *simply not worth doing.*

Needless to say many other tests have been devised to look at various aspects of airflow and airways structure and function. So-called tests of closing volume,[8,16] frequency dependency tests,[16,30] and tests using test gases of different density in relation to maximum expiratory flow volume curves[24] are not of any practical value. They have done nothing to promote the use of simple practical office spirometers in primary care physicians' offices for the purpose of diagnosing and treating common chronic lung disease states such as COPD.

I can be a little less critical of the advent of the flow-volume method of measuring airflow and air volume, but I continue to believe that this method only confuses some clinicians. I will illustrate the comparison of the volume over time curve compared with the flow-volume method of measuring airflow and air volume in the following section.

Flow volume and volume time curves

The figures that follow show a comparison of flow volume and volume time curves in different situations.

Fig. 55-3, *A* and *B*, presents both the flow volume (upper) and time volume (lower) expiratory airflow curves of a normal person. Note that the beginning of the flow volume curve is on the left lower corner. There is a rapid increase in the flow, which peaks near 10 L/sec, followed by a downward movement. This rapid and high peak flow in-

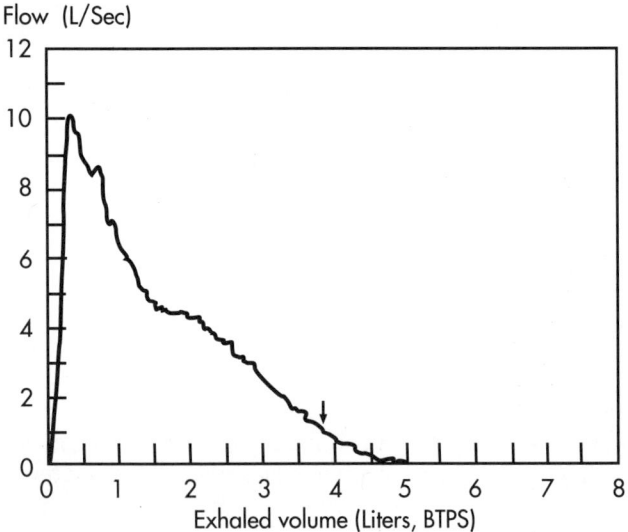

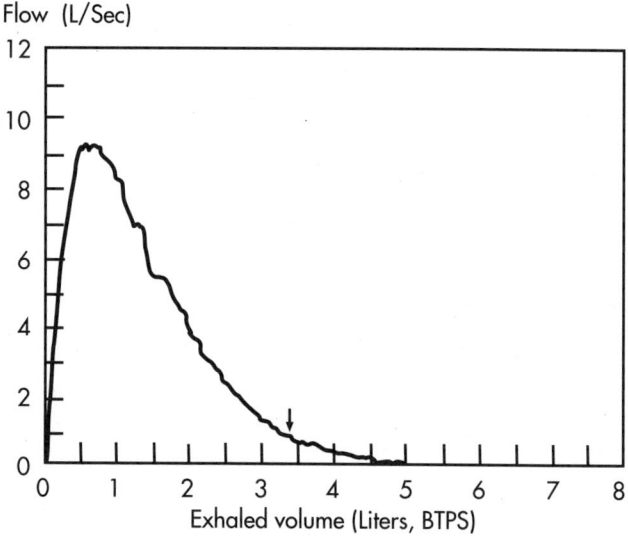

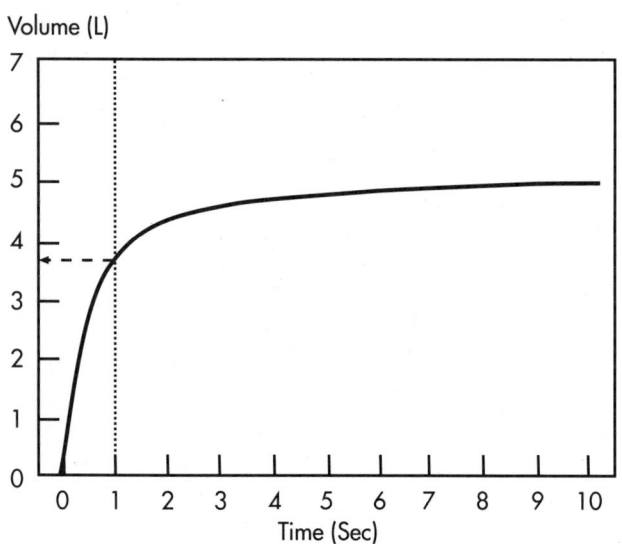

	Result	LLN
FVC	5.00	(3.88)
FEV₁	3.79	(3.12)
%FEV₁	76%	(71%)

	Result	LLN
FVC	4.98	(3.88)
FEV₁	3.37	(3.12)
%FEV₁	68%	(71%)

Fig. 55-3. Normal flow volume *(upper)* and volume over time curves *(lower)* of a normal individual. Notice that the expiratory time can be visualized from the volume over time curve, but the peak flow can only be visualized from the flow volume curve. Thus both curves are useful. LLN, lower limit of normal. (From Enright PL, Hyatt PR: *Office spirometry, a practical guide to the selection and use of spirometers,* Philadelphia, 1987, Lea & Febiger.)

Fig. 55-4. Flow volume curve (upper) and time volume curve (lower) of a patient with borderline airflow abnormalities. The only "abnormality" is a reduction of low volume flow as shown on the flow-volume curve (arrow). The FVC is above normal and the FEV₁ is also normal. Only the FEV₁/FVC is slightly reduced (68%). This patient has been dogmatically diagnosed as having "small airway disease," which is an incorrect concept. Note the degree of hyperinflation as suggested by the FVC (44) that occurs. This shows the earliest stages of emphysema. (From Enright PL, Hyatt PR: *Office spirometry, a practical guide to the selection and use of spirometers,* Philadelphia, 1987, Lea & Febiger.)

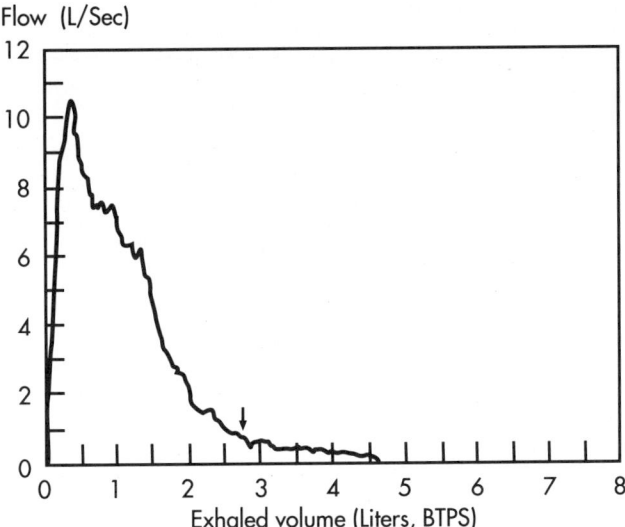

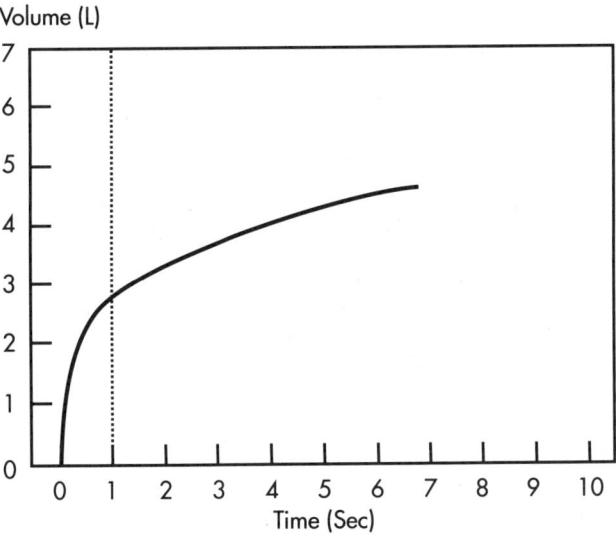

	Result	LLN
FVC	4.60	(3.88)
FEV$_1$	2.74	(3.12)
%FEV$_1$	59%	(71%)

Fig. 55-5. Flow volume and volume over time curves of a patient with mild obstructive airflow disorder. The FVC is again above normal and the FEV$_1$ is slightly low. This results in an FEV$_1$/FVC of 59%, which is clearly abnormal. (From Enright PL, Hyatt PR: *Office spirometry, a practical guide to the selection and use of spirometers,* Philadelphia, 1987, Lea & Febiger.)

dicates excellent effort. Continuing the expiratory effort for more than 6 seconds is standard practice; in this case the expiratory effort continues for 10 seconds. Lower limit of normal (LLN) is in parentheses. Note the rapid emptying of the lung with FEV$_1$ 3.79 L as indicated by the arrow on both the flow volume and volume time curves. A vertical dotted line is added at the 1-second time point on this and the following figures to indicate the time point from which the FEV$_1$ is taken.

Fig. 55-4 presents the flow volume curve with borderline reduced flow rates during the last two thirds of the expiratory maneuver. This phenomenon is more difficult to detect on the upward slope of the volume-time curves. *Slight* obstruction or limitation to airflow is suggested by the percentage FEV$_1$ of 68%. But any obstruction is at most borderline because the FEV$_1$ is still within the normal range. Note that the FVC is more than 1 L above the lower limit of normal and is consistent with early loss of elastic recoil and hyperinflation in the earliest stages of emphysema.[44]

Figs. 55-5 through 55-7 present both the flow volume and volume time curves of patients with progressive degrees of obstructive airflow disorders. Fig. 55-5 shows the pattern of mild airflow obstruction and reveals a concavity of the flow volume curve. Note that the FVC is above the lower limit of normal, but the FEV$_1$ is below normal. This makes the FEV$_1$ 59%, or well below the normal 71%. Thus there are actually two factors in the low FEV$_1$ percentage: an increased denominator, (volume) and a decreased numerator (flow). My own studies in whole excised human lungs have shown that in the earliest stages of emphysema total lung capacity increases along with decreased elastic recoil.[44] This is probably the best explanation for the increased FVC and low FEV$_1$/FVC ratio in the very earliest stages of emphysema.

Fig. 55-6 shows the flow volume and volume time curves of a patient with moderate airflow obstruction. The FEV$_1$ is clearly below the lower limit of normal and the FEV$_1$ percentage of FVC is also reduced (57%). Fig. 55-7 presents the expiratory airflow curves of a patient with severe airflow obstruction. Note the immediate drop-off in airflow after the peak flow. This is caused by collapse of the major conducting airways, a result of airway atrophy and loss of elastic recoil. This rapid drop in flow is also due to inward bulge of the post membrane and flattening of the cartilaginous "C" by increase in surrounding intrapulmonary pressure. Note that the patient is still attempting to empty his lungs at the end of 10 seconds. Finally Fig. 55-8 shows the expiratory flow curves of a patient with moderate ventilatory *restriction*. Note in this case that the expiratory time is shortened, but that peak flow is high as a result of excessive elastic recoil from pulmonary fibrosis. The FEV$_1$/FVC percentage is high, equaling 89% as a result of rapid lung emptying.

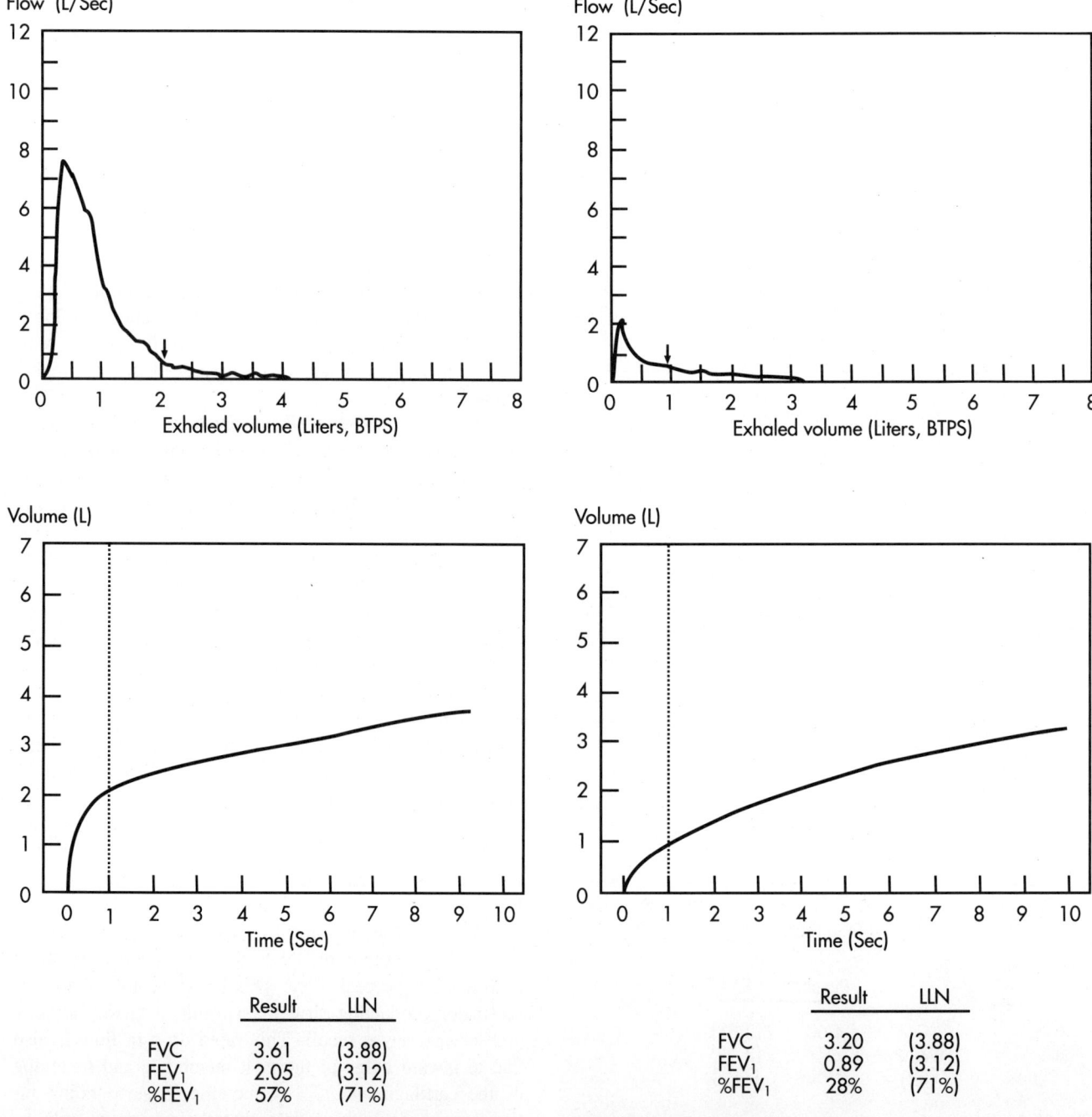

	Result	LLN
FVC	3.61	(3.88)
FEV₁	2.05	(3.12)
%FEV₁	57%	(71%)

Fig. 55-6. Flow volume and volume over time curves of a patient with moderate airflow obstruction. (From Enright PL, Hyatt PR: *Office spirometry, a practical guide to the selection and use of spirometers,* Philadelphia, 1987, Lea & Febiger.)

	Result	LLN
FVC	3.20	(3.88)
FEV₁	0.89	(3.12)
%FEV₁	28%	(71%)

Fig. 55-7. Flow volume and volume over time curves from a patient with advanced airflow obstruction caused by emphysema. (From Enright PL, Hyatt PR: *Office spirometry, a practical guide to the selection and use of spirometers,* Philadelphia, 1987, Lea & Febiger.)

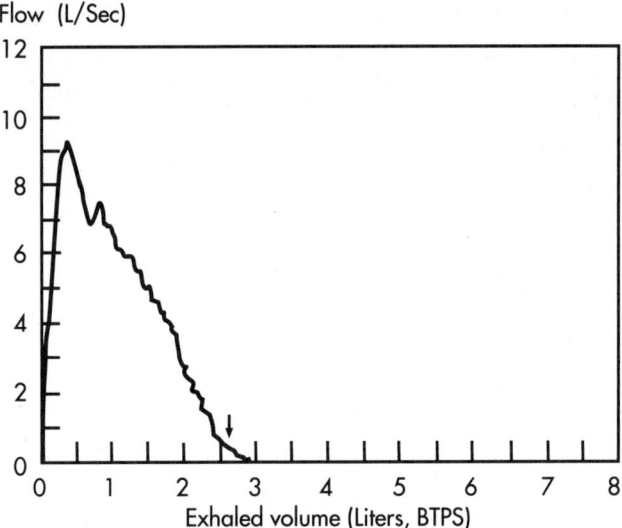

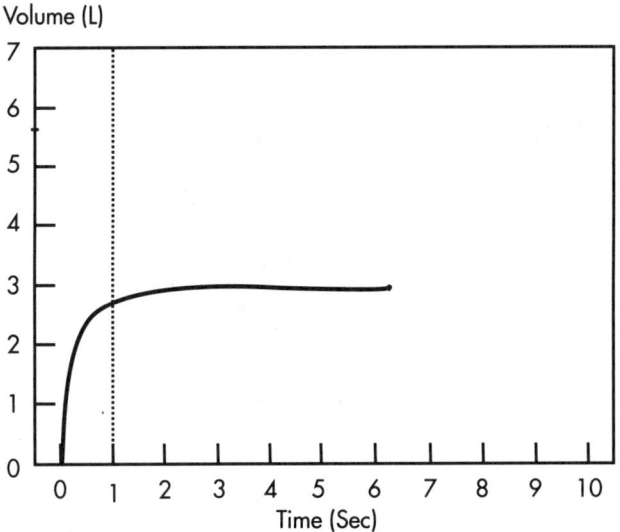

	Result	LLN
FVC	2.97	(3.88)
FEV$_1$	2.64	(3.12)
%FEV$_1$	89%	(71%)

Fig. 55-8. Flow volume and volume over time curves of a patient with a moderate restrictive ventilatory disorder. Notice that the percentage FEV$_1$ is nearly 90%, which often suggests a restrictive disorder when this ratio is high. However, normal individuals can often empty most of the lung in 1 second. (From Enright PL, Hyatt PR: *Office spirometry, a practical guide to the selection and use of spirometers*, Philadelphia, 1987, Lea & Febiger.)

In restrictive ventilatory defects the lung and thorax cannot be filled to the normal volume because of fibrosis of the lungs, thoracic deformities, or some space-preempting problem, such as massive heart failure, large pleural effusions, or major tumors. If little air can be put into the lungs, little can be expelled.

Elastic recoil is normal or above normal in many restrictive defects, and if airways are open the FEV$_1$ is more than 75% of the FVC. When the FEV$_1$ reaches 90% to 95% of the FVC, it becomes virtually certain that restrictive ventilatory defect is present.

Thus it is apparent that the flow-volume method gives the clinician exactly the same information available from the volume over time curve but is presented in a different way. The one advantage of the flow volume method is that the peak flow, that is, the instant of greatest flow, is readily visualized as a test of the patient's effort. Peak flow is only a "snapshot" of flow and thus it is scarcely visible on the volume over time curves. Another possible advantage is the ability to scrutinize certain qualitative features of the expiratory flow volume curve and this could have clinical utility in the future. Of course, ability to observe the inspiratory flow is valuable in diagnosing states of upper airway obstruction but these conditions are so rare as to be of little concern to primary care physicians.

Objections to flow volume curves are as follows: the FEV$_1$ cannot be seen, the expiratory time cannot be seen, and the transducer will also print out 20 to 30 more numbers beyond the FEV$_1$, FVC, and so on, and the ratio between the two, but these additional numbers have no established meaning or value above and beyond the FEV$_1$, the FVC, and the ratio between them. But for some unexplained reason, third-party reimbursement is greater for flow-volume tests than for time-volume measures: more pay for more extraneous "information" and for more nonsense!

Note: The FEV$_1$ is a very simple expression of a complex process of lung emptying. It measures elastic recoil, small airway function, and large airway function. This is because alveoli empty into small airways, which in turn empty into large airways, and finally into the spirometer, whether by the volume over time convention or the flow volume method. Most modern spirometers measure flow and volume *both ways*, for comparison and for possible teaching value. See Figs. 55-3 through 55-8 and the spirometer that produces this curve (Fig. 55-9). Some direct displacement spirometers are still preferred by many clinicians who adhere to the volume over time principle. These devices remain popular because of their practicality, reliability, and relatively low cost (see Fig. 55-10).

Normal values for FVC and FEV$_1$ and FEV$_1$/FVC ratio percentage

Normal values are based on age, sex, and height. Younger, taller individuals have better air volume and

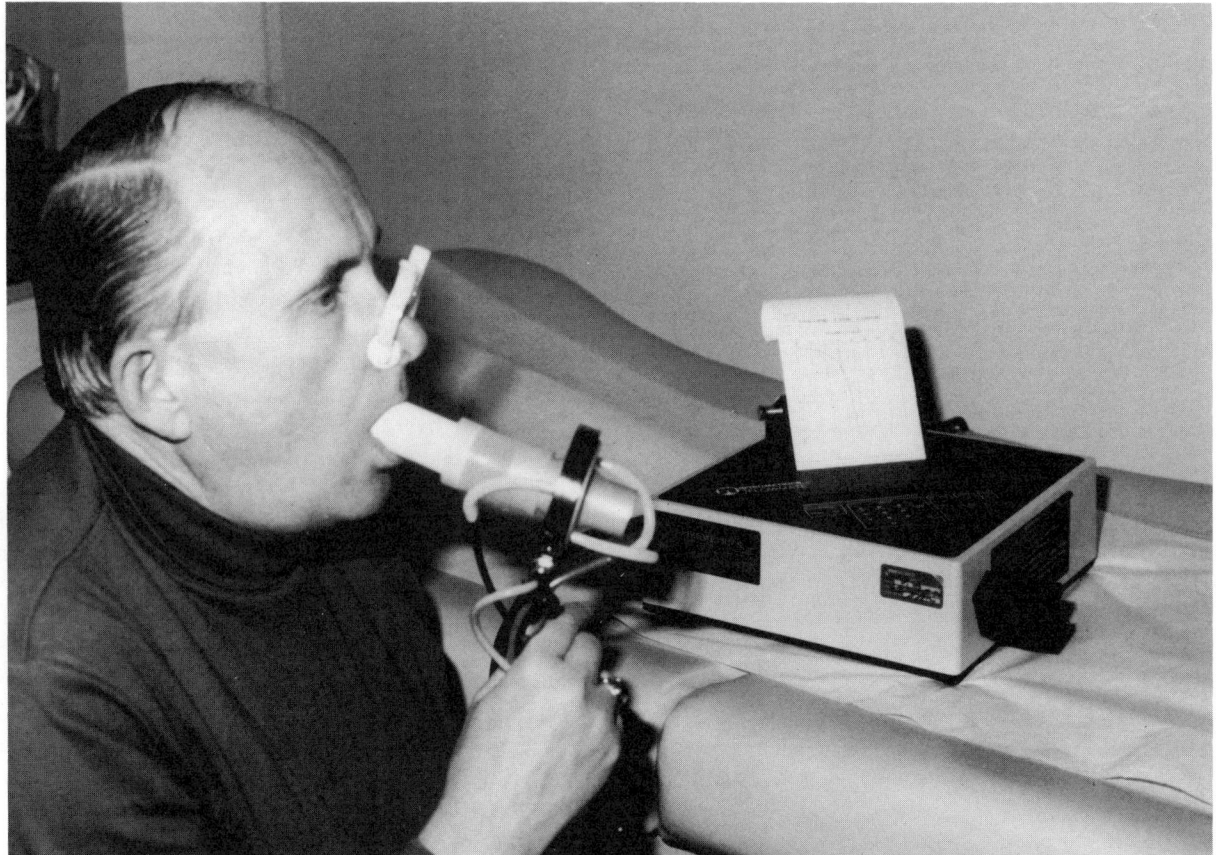

Fig. 55-9. Flow transducer device that accurately measures either flow volume or volume over time curves. Volume is on the vertical axis and time is on the horizontal axis. These devices are popular and convenient. They perform the calculations and give percentages of predicted normal values.

flow than shorter, older individuals. Men have slightly higher values than women. For some reason certain ethnic groups, such as blacks, have slightly lower normal values (but most athletes would deny that this is true).[50]

Figs. 55-11 and 55-12 present normal values for FEV_1, FVC, and FVC/FEV_1 percentage. A straight-edge to contact and height helps to determine normal values. A range of ± 20% is commonly taken as normal.

Needed: a revolution in spirometer teaching

For more than two decades I have tried to figure out a way to persuade all primary care physicians to practice spirometry in their offices and clinics. Some time ago I made an informal survey of primary care physicians in the Colorado and Wyoming region and found the following:

- 100% had an electrogram (ECG) machine
- 100% had a sphygmomanometer
- 100% had an ophthalmoscope
- 100% had a scale, equipped with a height measurement

- 100% had thermometers
- 27% had a spirometer

Ideally these statistics have changed in the interim, but I still doubt that even 50% of primary care physicians have and use a spirometer regularly in their offices or clinics. When I ask questions about the use of powerful broncho-active drugs such as bronchodilators and even corticosteroids, I get some amazing answers. "I go by the patient's symptoms" is the most common excuse, yet it has been well established that symptoms of breathlessness (shortness of breath is equivalent to a physiologic state), whereas breathlessness suggests a subjective state, or dyspnea, which is the feeling of being short of breath or inability to breath (e.g., in hyperventilation syndrome) are not accurately classified or quantified by the physical examination by physicians.[51] "I've gotten along without a spirometer all my life—why do I need one now?" One answer might be for medical legal reasons. I have been involved for the defense in two major malpractice suits

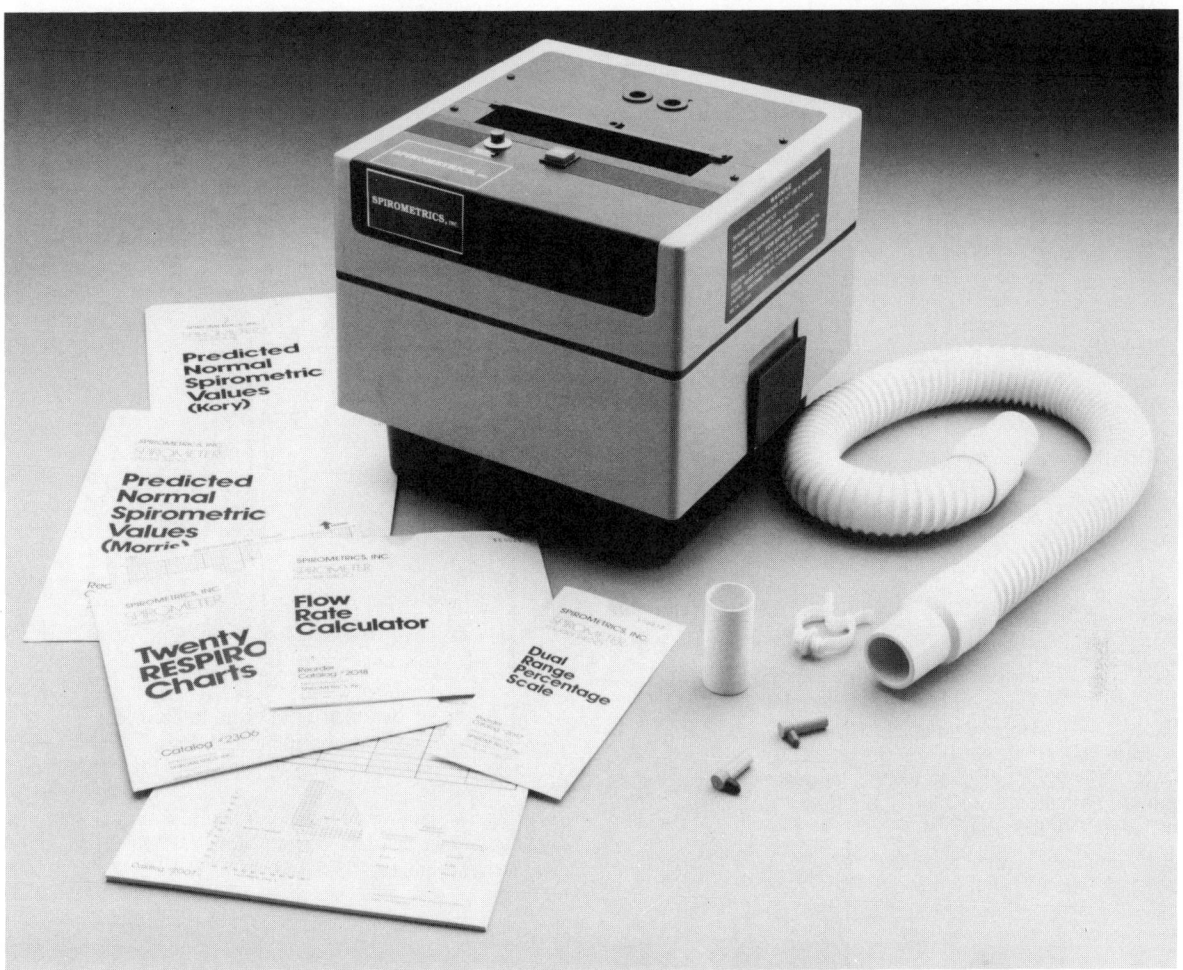

Fig. 55-10. Example of a simple dry direct recording spirometer suitable for clinic or office use. These devices have complete instructions, mouthpieces, nose clips, spirometer paper, and replacement pens, and calculations aids as illustrated.

against physicians for allegedly causing aseptic necrosis of the femoral heads because of the use of corticosteroids in asthma or COPD when the doctor had absolutely no documentation of the fact of airflow obstruction or its improvement with the use of corticosteroids by *any* measurement of airflow, not even by a peak flow meter!

It is well known that an ECG result can be entirely normal within minutes of a fatal heart attack. A sphygmomanometer is notoriously inaccurate, particularly when used by marginally trained individuals. But the indiscriminant use of the sphygmomanometer to detect occult hypertension, even labile hypertension, has probably done more to improve the health of people through the control of hypertension than the use of virtually any other medical instrument.

Could the same impact on health be achieved through the widespread use of spirometry? The following are possible reasons why it could:

- Abnormal spirometry results are highly predictive of fatal heart attack.[29,36]
- Abnormal spirometry findings are highly predictive of hypertension.[52]
- Abnormal spirometry results are highly predictive of fatal stroke.[58]
- Abnormal spirometry results are highly predictive of the presence of occult lung cancer.[32,34]
- Abnormal spirometry findings are highly predictive of decline in lung function and of its decline in middle-aged smokers who are progressing toward obstructive pulmonary disease. It is more useful than the so-called sensitive tests.[26]
- A reduction in FEV_1 combined with wheezing identifies a population of smokers at risk of premature morbidity and mortality caused by COPD.[26]
- Respiratory symptoms and FEV_1 are predictors of hospitalization and need for medication in COPD.[63]

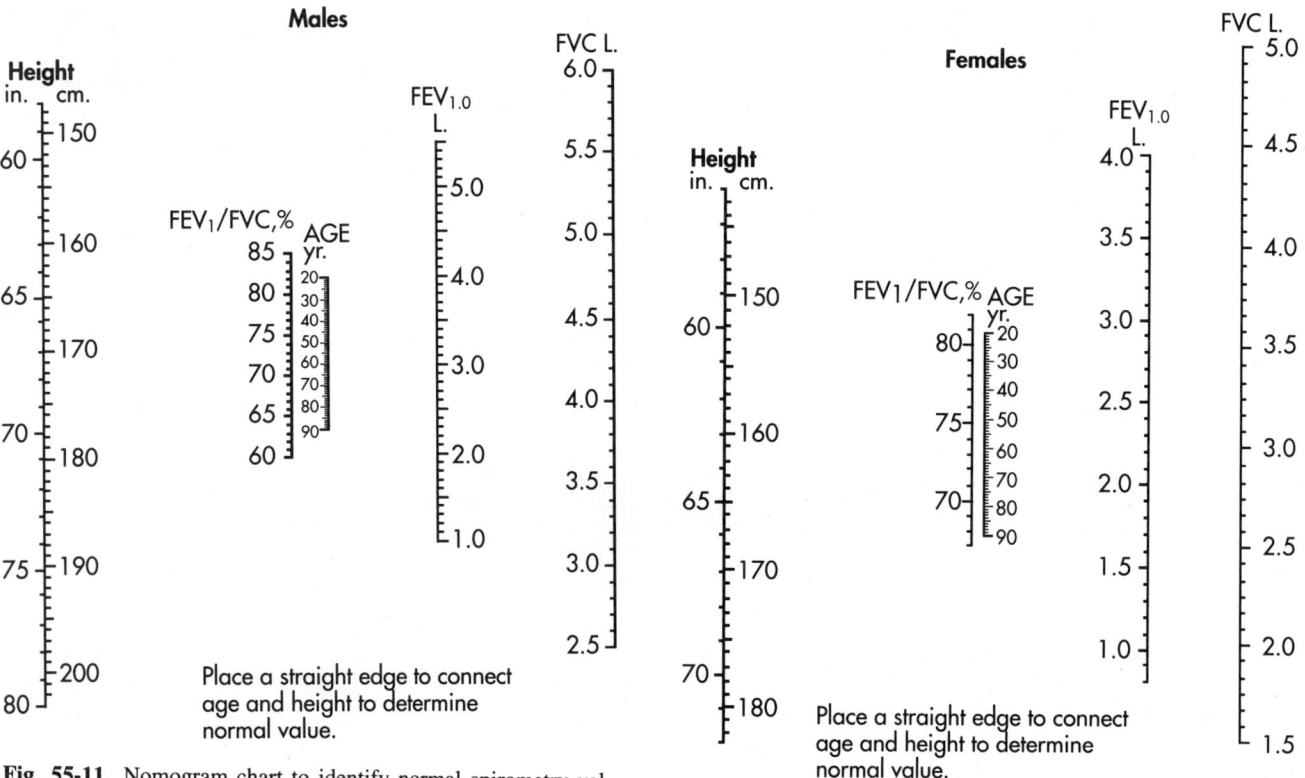

Fig. 55-11. Nomogram chart to identify normal spirometry values for men. (Adapted from Morris JF, Koski A, Johnson LC: *Am Rev Respir Dis* 153:57-67, 1971.)

Fig. 55-12. Nomogram chart to identify normal spirometry values for women. (Adapted from Morris JF, Koski A, Johnson LC: *Am Rev Respir Dis* 153:57-67, 1971.)

• Impaired pulmonary function is a predictor of total mortality caused by a variety of disease states.[5]

Thus an abnormal spirogram finding can help to identify most of the 450,000 excess deaths that result from tobacco abuse, because each of the disease states discussed is largely caused by the products of tobacco smoke.

How can we teach spirometry in our medical schools?

There is no question that physicians' thoughts and attitudes about health and disease are largely influenced by the 4 years of undergraduate medical school. There interviewing techniques, physical examination, and certain diagnostic techniques are taught. Nearly every doctor remembers his or her first venipuncture, arterial puncture, thoracentesis, and delivery of a baby. Performing preoperative urinalysis and an ECG is still considered important enough in a medical student's education to avoid the label "scut work."

What about spirometry? I believe this should be taught during physical diagnosis of the chest, just as the use of the ophthalmoscope is taught during the eye examination.

There are only 126 allopathic and 15 osteopathic medi-

cal schools in the United States today, and 16 allopathic schools in all of Canada. Thus we have 157 "doctor factories" in North America. It should be possible to teach the essence of spirometry with hands-on experience and the basics of interpretation in 1 to 2 hours as a minimum. A study by our group has shown that the physical examination can help identify moderate to advanced COPD,[3] but use of the peak flow meter (as part of the physical examination) was found to be the most accurate indicator of abnormality.[3] The peak flow meter must immediately become a key component of the medical students', interns', and residents' bags. A pocket-sized device that is accurate and can be cleaned in an ordinary dishwasher costs about $10 (see Fig. 55-13). But peak flow meters are not equal in value to the whole volume over time curve with FEV$_1$ (flow test) and FVC (volume test), even if it must be done by the flow over time method. Get rid of all those other extraneous numbers! Keep it simple, like determining systolic and diastolic blood pressure, and spirometry will probably become more widespread as this century ends. Perhaps the widespread use of spirometry will usher in a new era of preventive medicine. [John Hutchinson, are you smiling now?]

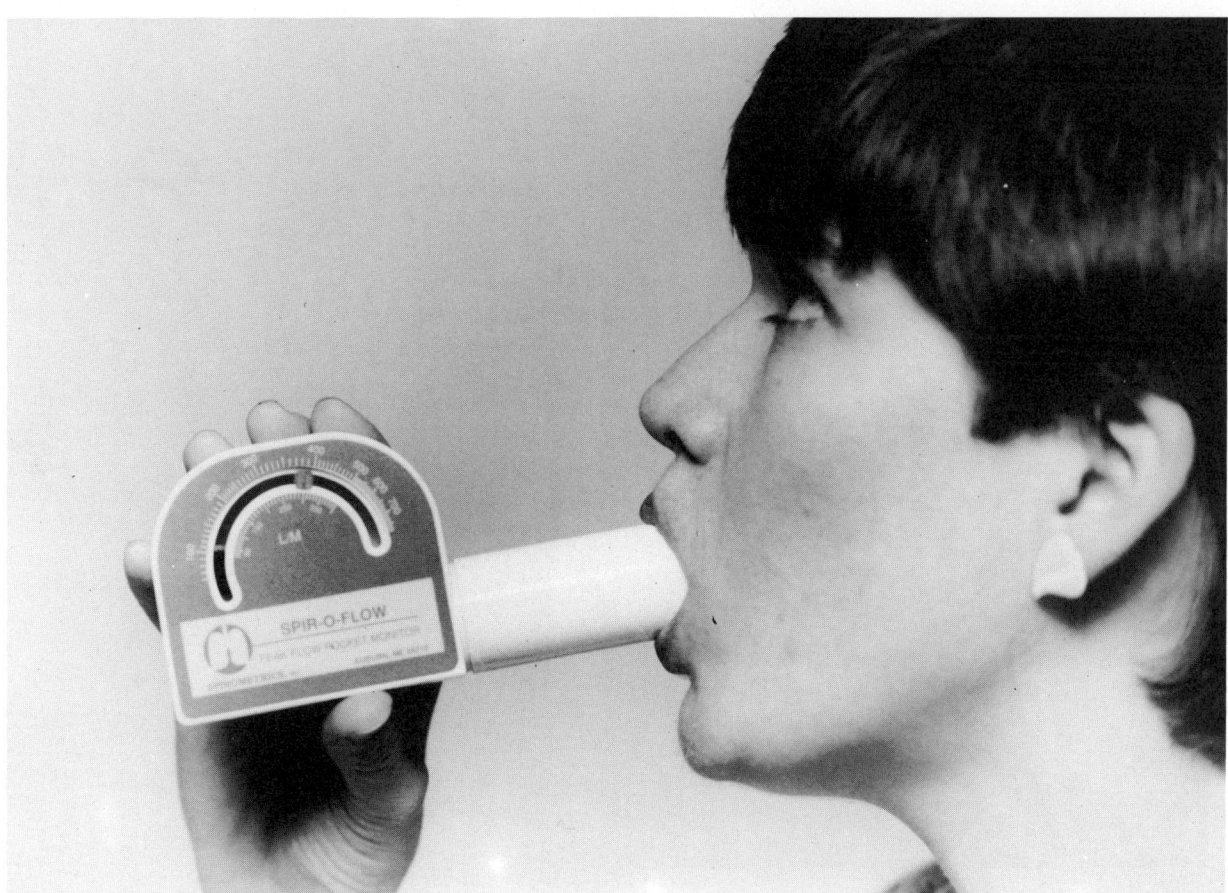

Fig. 55-13. Popular newly introduced peak flow meter. Flow meter measures a snapshot of expiratory airflow. A peak flow meter does not measure FEV$_1$ but tracks it in the individual so that conversion formulas can be used.

Alternatives to spirometry

There really are no true alternatives to spirometry. A hand-held spirometer possesses accuracy of 5% to 10% of that of standard laboratory devices (see Figs. 55-14, *A* and *B*).

A peak flow meter is practical and easy to use, and its findings are far better than no measurement at all. Most asthmatics regularly measure their peak flow at home to monitor responses to therapy and to detect periods of bronchial hyperreactivity, its ups and downs in morning and evening measurements, as a possible prelude to worsening asthma.

A simple volume device for FVC is accurate to within 5% to 10% of laboratory devices and can easily be used in the field, as can the peak flow meter.[1]

Practical spirometry

Today flow transducer devices that allow the physician to use either the flow-volume method of airflow measure-

ment or the volume over time expiratory flow curve, which I prefer, are both practical and reliable and are marketed at an acceptable price of $3500 to $4000, which is a bargain compared with the value of other diagnostic instruments. Figure 55-9 demonstrates such device. The time-honored volume displacement devices are still popular and highly accurate (see Fig. 55-10).

COURSE AND PROGNOSIS OF COPD

Classically COPD begins with cough and expectoration after about 20 years of smoking, in the early forties or fifties; dyspnea on exertion begins after 5 to 10 years of often subclinical inflammation within the lung; physical impairment begins in the late fifties or early sixties; and the need for oxygen and other supportive therapy begins after approximately 30 years of an inexorable process of damage to the conducting air passages of the lung and alveoli. Figure 55-15 depicts the time course in the evolution of COPD, beginning with damage of alveoli and small air-

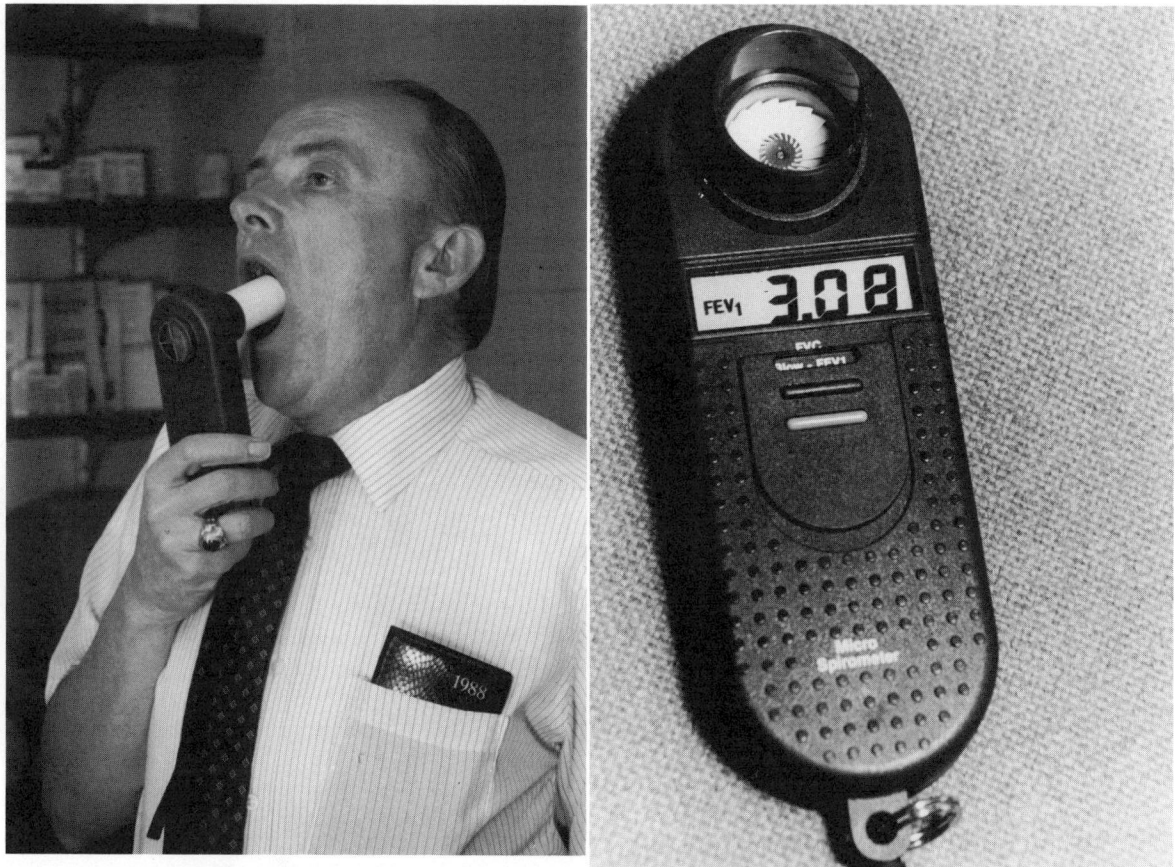

Fig. 55-14. A & B, Simple handheld microspirometers. These devices have accuracy within 5% to 10% of a standard spirometer. This is a very practical device for bedside, clinic, or office measurements of FVC and FEV_1. These devices are also used by some patients in the home, such as those who have received heart or lung transplantation, in order to identify early stages of infection or rejection.

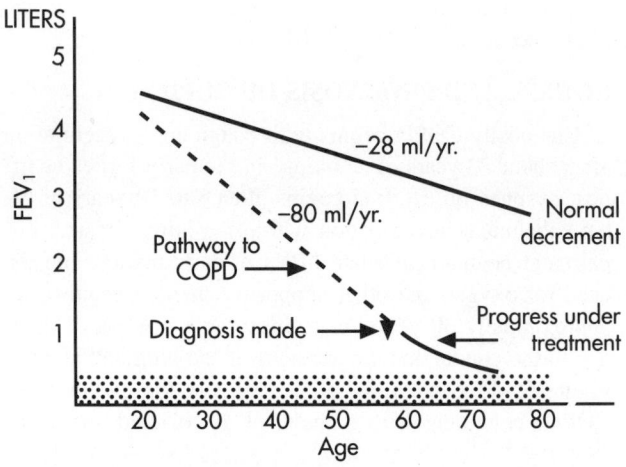

Fig. 55-15. Hypothesized loss of FEV_1 as a consequence of aging in a 6-foot male over his lifetime. An approximate reduction of -28 cm³ is noted. Ventilatory function losses are not necessarily linear *(solid line)* and may accelerate with advancing age. By contrast dotted line depicts the accelerated losses of FEV_1 over a lifetime from leukocyte elastase ṅ mediated lung injury in susceptible smokers. Unfortunately the diagnosis of COPD is usually made in the symptomatic later stages of the disease. The apparent slowing of the rate of deterioration *(curved extension of dotted line)* is derived from a prospective study of patients participating in a pulmonary rehabilitation program. COPD, chronic obstructive pulmonary disease.

ways in susceptible individuals. The reasons for susceptibility to the harmful effects of cigarette smoke are not entirely known. One subset of patients, those with α-antitrypsin deficiency, have a deficiency of a glycoprotein that protects the lungs against proteolytic injury. More commonly the oxidant effects of cigarette smoke can inactivate the normally produced α-antitrypsin and render it impotent in dealing with the release of leukocyte-derived elastases. The reason for susceptibility to the toxic effects of inhaled tobacco smoke and other products in some individuals but not others remains unknown. It is possible that antioxidant defense mechanisms, either in the lung or on red cells, may be the answer. Identifying factors associated with vulnerability to lung damage remain a high research priority. But even if this susceptibility factor becomes known, and further if it can be corrected, we face huge numbers of patients with various stages of COPD in need of *preventive therapy* now. A major portion of this chapter is devoted to stressing the importance of early identification and intervention in early stages of COPD.

PRIMARY PREVENTION
Early identification and intervention

The earliest stages of COPD are not symptomatic. Cough and expectoration are probably the earliest manifestations of clinically significant disease. Dyspnea on exertion is an indicator of moderate to severe impairment in lung mechanics, resulting in the increased work of breathing. Thus by the time the patient recognizes an impairment in activities of daily living, the disease is usually very far advanced.

The physical examination finding may be totally normal in early stages of airflow obstruction. However, normal lungs empty in 6 seconds, and in the case of airflow obstruction expiratory airflow is delayed. In addition, hyperinflation occurs in early stages of disease, even when airflow is normal. Thus identifying patients with a prominent chest, evident hyperinflation indicated by chest roentgenograms, and impaired expiratory emptying, as judged by timing forced expiration by listening with a stethoscope over the trachea or manubrium and employing a sweep second hand, can be valuable in identifying patients with airflow obstruction fairly early.

Spirometry remains the most valuable technique of identifying patients with all degrees of airflow abnormality.

The concepts of lung age and reversibility of airflow abnormalities are relevant. Lung age is that age at which a patient's measured pulmonary function is normal.[37] These concepts are illustrated in Fig. 55-16. Thus if a 48-year-old man has an FEV$_1$ of 2.8 L and is 6 foot tall, he may well be asymptomatic but this individual possesses the lung age of a man 85 years old (approximation). This concept can be used as a potent motivator in smoking cessation, by telling patients, "You are in generally good

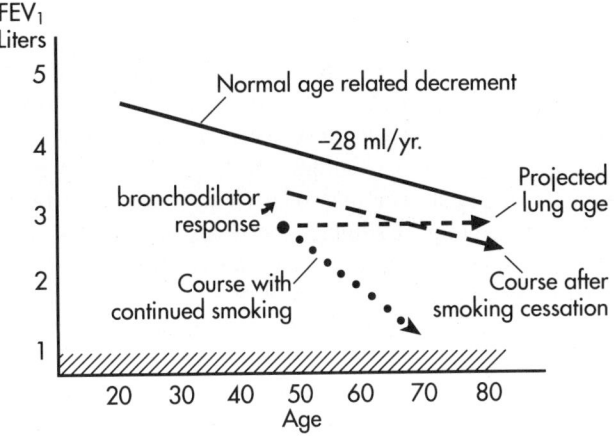

Fig. 55-16. Concept of lung age. In this example a 47-year-old patient has a measured FEV$_1$ of 2.5 L/sec, but this is the normal lung age for a patient age 85 *(see short dashed line)*. But this patient demonstrated a significant response to inhaled bronchodilators, i.e., a measurable reversible component of approximately 505 cm^3. Now a horizontal line *(not shown to the mark X)* projected to the normal estimate of FEV$_1$ reveals a lung age of approximately 72. The figure [also projects the bronchodilator response can be sustained and the patient stops smoking.] In most such patients the rate of decline parallels the age-related slope of decline *(see course-dashed line)*. By contrast if the patient continues to smoke and if the rate of deterioration is assumed to be equal to the patient's previous decline rate up to age 48, which resulted in an FEV$_1$ of 2.5 or a lung age of greater than 80, a much more rapid rate of decline is predicted as depicted by the dotted line.

health, but your lungs are more than 30 years older than you are." This can catch patients' attention. For example, this patient had a significant response to an inhaled β-agonist resulting in a FEV$_1$ of 3.05 L/sec. Now a projection to the line of normality reveals a calculated "lung age" of 72 (see Fig. 55-16). In this illustration the projected rate of deterioration on stopping smoking, which usually parallels the age-related loss of lung function, is shown on the course-dashed line with an arrow. But assuming that smoking continues at the rate that caused the abnormality (i.e., FEV$_1$ 2.8), the dotted line projects a much faster rate of decline.

Identifying reversibility of airflow abnormalities after inhalation of a bronchodilator aerosol, or, as is becoming more commonplace, after a trial of corticosteroids to deal with inflammatory processes within conducting air passages can identify patients with a much more favorable prognosis than if these reversible features were not present. In the case of reversibility, the patient's lung age is reduced. Further if the patient is able to stop the continuing damage to the lungs that results from inhaling of toxic tobacco fumes, both voluntarily and involuntarily in the case of passive smoking, the prognosis may be greatly improved.

Smoking cessation

The techniques of affecting smoking cessation are covered in detail in Chapter 16. In brief smoking cessation is the single most important action that can be accomplished in the prevention of premature morbidity and mortality of patients facing chronic airflow obstruction. By far most quitters simply stop on their own volition after some intellectual or emotional stimulus motivates them to abandon life's most threatening substance abuse. By contrast addicted smokers need additional help. Focus on behavioral modification, identifying factors that stimulate the urge to smoke (i.e., so-called cues to action); strategies to change the cycle of social reflexes; and selection of a "quit date" can be valuable. Use of nicotine replacement in the form of nicotine polarcrilex (nicotine-containing gum) or transdermal nicotine delivery can also be a valuable adjunct. How these techniques can be applied to given individuals is considered in Chapter 16. Now that the Environmental Protection Agency has wisely designated passive smoking as a carcinogen, it is likely "public" smoking will be further limited and individuals further motivated to abstain.

Vaccines

Patients with COPD and particularly those above the age of 50 are particularly vulnerable to influenza epidemics and to pneumonia caused by pneumococcus. Fortunately influenza virus vaccine is both safe and effective.[38] The duration of immunity and the antigenic shifts of the organisms that create epidemics require annual vaccination. In general this should be done in October or November or within 1 to 3 months before an anticipated epidemic. Approximate 80% protection is afforded. If a person has not had a vaccination or is one of the rare individuals who is allergic to egg products used in the production of the vaccine amantadine hydrochloride can be used as a preventive measure during epidemics, or at the first sign of symptoms, effective only against influenza type A. Although pneumococcal vaccine has been controversial, recent evidence strongly indicates that it is also effective in the majority of immunocompetent people who receive this vaccine. At present influenza vaccine is considered suitable for a single inoculum (i.e., once in a lifetime); however, more and more experts consider that boosters at 5-year intervals may be appropriate.[53]

SECONDARY PREVENTION

HOW TO FORESTALL MORBIDITY AND MORTALITY IN COPD
Treating reversible features of disease

The great majority of patients with early stages of COPD have nonspecific bronchial hyperreactivity. Most patients are responsive to an inhaled or oral bronchodilator. Inhaled β-agonists are most commonly used; oral β-agonists can also be valuable. Oral theophyllines may be useful.[59] Inhaled anticholinergics may well be the most useful bronchodilators available. A controlled clinical trial known as the Lung Health Study is currently studying a large population of patients with mild to moderate airflow obstruction: 5877 current cigarette smokers between the ages of 35 and 59. Thus a far higher prevalence in nonspecific airway hyperreactivity in response to inhaled methylcholine has been observed in women than in men. The longitudinal study is evaluating the effects of smoking cessation and the anticholinergic ipratropium bromide in randomized groups of patients within this major study.[60]

Because COPD has inflammatory components use of antiinflammatory agents in the form of corticosteroids is worth consideration. Studies of carefully observed populations in the Netherlands suggest that the use of systemic corticosteroids by the oral route can slow the rate of deterioration of airflow in both severe and moderate forms of COPD.[45,46] The use of corticosteroids today is the subject of controlled clinical trials.[13]

Infections and antibiotics

A growing body of evidence relates childhood respiratory infections to the later development of chronic bronchitis with airflow obstruction (COPD).[65] Repeated childhood infections may be a marker of inadequate natural antimicrobial defense mechanisms. An alternate hypothesis is that early and subtle injury of the lungs makes later infection more likely. Juvenile bronchial hyperreactivity may follow viral illnesses in children.[18] This bronchial hyperreactivity may persist into adult life and perhaps become a factor in the pathogenesis of progressive airflow obstruction.

The effect of repeated infections on the course and prognosis of adults with COPD is also not well known. Some patients suffer severe losses in ventilatory function after bronchopulmonary infections; this finding suggests that infection has a major impact on the progress of disease. However, it should be pointed out that these losses tend to be transient. Certainly the use of antimicrobials can shorten the symptomatic period of exacerbations of chronic bronchitis.[12,35] Some old evidence exists that the prophylactic use of antimicrobials reduces the frequency of winter exacerbations in patients who often have acute attacks of purulent bronchitis.[12,28] However, no controlled clinical trial has shown a favorable influence in the long-term course and prognosis of COPD treated with antimicrobial agents. Nonetheless, the weight of clinical experience and the high likelihood of improving the symptom complex of acute attacks have established the widespread use of antimicrobial agents for episodes of acute purulent bronchitis. It has become standard practice to institute a 7- to 10-day empiric course of broad-spectrum antimicrobials for each episode on empiric grounds. Sputum culture and sensitivity tests are not usually found useful in this context.[2]

Antiprotease replacement

Blood-derived human α-antitrypsin is currently under study as an antiprotease replacement for patients with inheritable forms of α-antitrypsin deficiency. These studies are predicated on the protease-antiprotease imbalance therapy of the pathogenesis of emphysema, including emphysema that occurs at early ages such as in the thirties and forties.[17] The normal α-antitrypsin phenotype is MM, resulting in circulatory blood levels of 150 to 350 mg %. Thus far approximately 75 alleles for the α_1-antitrypsin gene have been identified. The most lethal abnormality is the ZZ type, or null type, of allelic abnormality, which results in levels of 40 mg % or lower, even down to zero. Patients with the SZ type may be less vulnerable but may also be the subject of replacement therapy. It is estimated that approximately 20,000 to 40,000 Americans have significant α_1-antitrypsin deficiency.[22] The current dogma is that protection against leukocyte-related elastase injury occurs at a threshold level of 80 mg %. There is no scientific basis for this estimate. Therefore, patients with the MZ phenotype with blood levels higher than 100 mg % are not considered candidates for replacement therapy. Presently the most efficacious method of replacement therapy is the subject of study. Weekly infusions are most commonly employed.[66] Monthly infusions may also be protective.[22] Both methods of intravenous augmentation therapy have been well tolerated. Cost is a serious factor, however, as $12,000 to 20,000/year is a common reimbursement figure. Use of antiproteases by the inhaled route may offer advantages, inasmuch as only approximately 2% of the infused product actually reaches the alveolar surface.[54] Whether inhaled preparations will be effective in humans is also the subject of study. Use of synthetic antiproteases by the inhaled or oral route is also under study.

So far no randomized controlled clinical trials have been conducted to prove the efficacy and safety of augmentation therapy in α_1-antitrypsin deficiency states with emphysema. Rather a working group for the evaluation of elastase inhibitor therapy was organized[9,25] and plans for the careful follow-up care of treated patients focusing on the rate of decline of FEV_1 were made. Presently the National Heart, Lung and Blood Institute is funding a study to characterize the course and prognosis of approximately 1000 patients in a national registry.[57] Many answers about the efficacy or lack of efficacy of augmentation therapy will likely be produced by this registry in the next several years.[57]

Pulmonary rehabilitation

Today pulmonary rehabilitative techniques are considered the standard of care for motivated patients with advanced stages of airflow obstruction.[14] The details of pulmonary rehabilitation are outside the scope of this chapter. Preventing or forestalling premature morbidity or mortality is still a valid goal in the care of any patient with any form

of disease. Thus approaches to improve patient education and compliance to therapy and methods to improve breathing efficiency through training and systemic exercise may improve the quality of life, if not the length. Oxygen in selected patients with chronic stable hypoxemia also improves both the length and the quality of life.[43] But oxygen can hardly be considered for preventive therapy for the early or asymptomatic stages of disease.

The only realistic approach to early prevention is through smoking cessation, and this is where all efforts should be placed.[49] All smokers should be advised to quit on the basis of their personal health risk. Combining the results of spirometric tests with emphasis on lung age (discussed earlier), exhaled carbon monoxide monitoring, and serial recording of respiratory symptoms can offer powerful and practical feedback and enhance advice to stop smoking in the interest of better lung and general health.[7,49] *When patients are successful in stopping smoking when they have only mild pulmonary function abnormalities, the rate of decline of FEV_1 is slowest to the age expected rate.[39] Even patients who stop smoking at advanced stages of disease have a better prognosis than most who continue.[39]*

Future considerations

We know exactly what causes COPD in the great majority of patients. Smoking cessation, a clean workplace, and a healthy social environment could begin to end this disease process in 95% of individuals immediately. There should be no smoking at all in areas of recreation, including social events and restaurants, where smoking should be identified as an environmental health hazard. Fortunately, the Environmental Protection Agency has finally labeled tobacco smoke as a carcinogen equal to asbestos or benzene. Some locations have been quite successful in making their communities smoke free, such as Aspen, Colorado. For the small percentage of patients destined to develop chronic obstructive pulmonary disease because of congenital defects in the production or delivery of antielastases replacement therapy will continue to be studied and refined. Let us hope that COPD will become a rarity within the next century, as our society begins to embrace a more healthful life-style. But in the intervening years before the happy ideal of a smoke-free society finally arrives we as physicians can and must do better in the early identification and treatment of all forms of emerging COPD.[41]

REFERENCES

1. Anders AJ, Baidwan B, Petty TL: An evaluation of the vitometer, a simple device for measuring vital capacity, *Respir Care* 29:1144-1146, 1984. (Note: a modification of this device is now known as the Spir-O-Meter and is marketed by Spirometrics, Inc., Auburn, ME 04210.)
2. Anthonisen NR et al: Antibiotic therapy for exacerbations of chronic obstructive pulmonary disease, *Ann Intern Med* 106:196-204, 1987.

3. Badgett RG et al: Can chronic obstructive pulmonary disease be diagnosed by historical and physical findings alone? (*Am J Med* 94:188-196, 1993.

4. Bates DV: The fate of the chronic bronchitic: a report of the ten-year follow-up in the Canadian Department of Veterans Affairs Coordinated Study of chronic bronchitis, *Am Rev Respir Dis* 108:1043-1065, 1973.

5. Beaty TH, Newill CA, Cohen BH: Effects of pulmonary function on mortality, *J Chronic Dis* 8:703-710, 1985.

6. Bishop PJ: A biography of John Hutchinson, *Med Hist* 21:384-396, 1977.

7. Bosse R, Sparrow D, Garvey AJ: Cigarette smoking, aging, and decline in pulmonary function: a longitudinal study, *Arch Environ Health* 35:247-252, 1980.

8. Buist AS, Van Fleet DL, Ross BB: A comparison of conventional spirometric tests and the test of closing volume in an emphysema screening center, *Am Rev Respir Dis* 107:735-743, 1973.

9. Burrows B: A clinical trial of efficacy of antiproteolytic therapy: can it be done? *Am Rev Respir Dis* Suppl 127:S42-S43, 1983.

10. Burrows B: An overview of obstructive lung diseases, *Med Clin North Am* 65:455-471, 1980.

11. Burrows B et al: The course and prognosis of different forms of chronic airways obstruction in a sample from the general population, *N Engl J Med* 317:1309-1314, 1987.

12. Burrows B, Nevin W: Antibiotic management in patients with chronic bronchitis and emphysema, *Ann Intern Med* 77:993-995, 1972.

13. Callahan CM, Dittus RS, Katz BP: Oral corticosteroid therapy for patients with stable chronic obstructive pulmonary disease (a meta analysis), *Ann Intern Med* 114:216-223, 1991.

14. Casaburi R, Petty TL: *Principles and practice of pulmonary rehabilitation,* Philadelphia, 1993, WB Saunders.

15. Ciba Foundation Guest Symposium: Terminology, definition and classification of chronic pulmonary emphysema and related conditions, *Thorax* 14:286-299, 1959.

16. Cosio M et al: The relation between structural changes in small airways and pulmonary-function tests, *N Engl J Med* 298:1277-1281, 1978.

17. Gadek JE et al: Anti elastases of the human alveolar structure, *J Clin Invest* 68:889-898, 1981.

18. Garewitz D, Corey M, Levison H: Pulmonary function and bronchial reactivity in children after croup, *Am Rev Respir Dis* 122:95-98, 1980.

19. Gelb AF et al: Physiologic diagnosis of subclinical emphysema, *Am Rev Respir Dis* 107:50-63, 1973.

20. Guyatt GH et al: Bronchodilators in chronic airflow limitation, *Am Rev Respir Dis* 135:1069-1074, 1987.

21. Hogg JC: The pathology of asthma, *Chest* 87:152S-153S, 1985.

22. Hubbard RC et al: Biochemical efficacy and safety of monthly augmentation therapy for alpha-1 antitrypsin deficiency, *JAMA* 260:1259-1264, 1988.

23. Hutchinson J: On the capacity of the lungs and the respiratory function with a view of establishing a precise and easy method of detecting disease by the spirometer, *Med Chir Transactions (London)* 29:137-147, 1846.

24. Hutcheon M et al: Volume of isoflow: a new test in detection of mild abnormalities of lung mechanics, *Am Rev Respir Dis* 110:458-465, 1974.

25. Idell S, Cohen AB: Alpha-1-antitrypsin deficiency, *Clin Chest Med* 4:359-375, 1983.

26. Jaakkola MS et al: Ventilatory lung function in young cigarette smokers: a study of susceptibility, *Eur Respir J* 4:643-650, 1991.

27. Janoff A et al: The role of oxidative processes in emphysema, *Am Rev Respir Dis* 127:31S-38S, 1983.

28. Johnston RN et al: Five-year winter chemoprophylaxis for chronic bronchitis, *Br J Dis Chest* 4:265-269, 1969.

29. Kannel WB et al: The value of measuring vital capacity for prognostic purposes, *Trans Assoc Life Ins Med Dir Am* 64:66-83, 1980.

30. Kjeldgaard JM et al: Frequency dependence of total respiratory resistance in early airway disease, *Am Rev Respir Dis* 114:501-508, 1976.

31. Knudson RJ et al: Expiratory computed tomography for assessment of suspected pulmonary emphysema, *Chest* 99:1357-1366, 1991.

32. Kuller LH et al: Relation of forced expiratory volume in one second (FEV_1) to lung cancer mortality in the Multiple Risk Factor Intervention Trial (MRFIT), *Am J Epidemiol* 132:265-274, 1990.

33. Lal S, Ferguson AD, Campbell EJM: Forced expiratory time: a simple test for airways obstruction, *Br Med J* 1:814-817, 1964.

34. Lange P et al: Ventilatory function and chronic mucus hypersecretion as predictors of death from lung cancer, *Am Rev Respir Dis* 141:613-617, 1990.

35. Lead article: antimicrobial treatment of chronic bronchitis, *Lancet* 1:505-506, 1975.

36. Marcus E et al: Pulmonary function as a predictor of coronary heart disease, *Am J Epidemiol* 129:97-104, 1989.

37. Morris JF, Temple W: Spirometric "lung age" estimation for motivating smoking cessation, *Prev Med* 14:655-662, 1985.

38. Nichol K, Lofgren RP, Gapinski J: Influenza vaccination. Knowledge, attitudes, and behavior among high-risk out-patients, *Arch Intern Med* 152:106-110, 1992.

39. Peto R et al: The relevance in adults of airflow obstruction, but not of mucus hypersecretion, to mortality from chronic lung disease: results from 20 years of prospective observation, *Am Rev Respir Dis* 128:491-500, 1983.

40. Petty TL: Chronic bronchitis vs asthma—or what's in a name? *J Allergy Clin Immunol* 62:323-324, 1978.

41. Petty TL: Chronic obstructive pulmonary disease—can we do better? *Chest* Suppl 97:2S-5S, 1990.

42. Petty TL: Definitions in chronic obstructive pulmonary disease, *Clin Chest Med* 11:363-373, 1990.

43. Petty TL: Home oxygen therapy, *Mayo Clin Proc* 62:841-847, 1987.

44. Petty TL, Silvers GW, Stanford RE: Mild emphysema is associated with reduced elastic recoil and increased lung size but not with airflow limitation, *Am Rev Respir Dis* 136:867-871, 1987.

45. Postma DS et al: Moderately severe chronic airflow obstruction: can corticosteroids slow down obstruction? *Eur Respir J* 1:22-26, 1988.

46. Postma DS et al: Severe chronic airflow obstruction: can corticosteroids slow down progression? *Eur J Respir Dis* 67:56-64, 1985.

47. Pratt PC: Role of conventional chest radiology in diagnosis and exclusion of emphysema, *Am J Med* 82:998-1006, 1987.

48. Ramsdell JW et al: Bronchial hyperreactivity in chronic obstructive bronchitis, *Am Rev Respir Dis* 126:829-832, 1982.

49. Risser NL, Belcher DW: Adding spirometry, carbon monoxide, and pulmonary symptom results to smoking cessation counseling, *J Gen Intern Med* 5:16-22, 1990.

50. Rossiter CE, Weill H: Ethnic differences in lung function: evidence for proportional differences, *Int J Epidemiol* 3:55-61, 1974.

51. Russell NJ et al: Quantitative assessment of the value of spirometry, *Thorax* 41:360-363, 1986.

52. Selby JV, Friedman GD, Quesenberry CP: Precursors of essential essential hypertension: pulmonary function, heart rate, uric acid, serum cholesterol, and other serum chemistries, *Am J Epidemiol* 131:1017-1027, 1990.

53. Shapiro ED et al: The protective efficacy of polyvalent pneumococcal polysaccharide vaccine. *N Engl J Med* 325:1453-1460, 1991.

54. Smith RM et al: Pulmonary deposition and clearance of aerosolized alpha-1 proteinase inhibitor administered to dogs and to sheep, *J Clin Invest* 84:1145-1154, 1989.

55. Snider GL et al: The definition of emphysema (Report of the National Heart, Lung, and Blood Institute, Division of Lung Diseases Workshop), *Am Rev Respir Dis* 132:182-185, 1985.

56. Stanescu DC et al: "Sensitive Tests" are poor predictors of the de-

cline in forced expiratory volume in one second in middle-aged smokers, *Am Rev Respir Dis* 135:585-590, 1987.

57. Stoller J: Alpha-1-antitrypsin deficiency and augmentation therapy in emphysema, *Clev Clin J Med* 56:683-689, 1989.

58. Strachan DP: Ventilatory function as a predictor of fatal stroke, *Br Med J* 302:84-87, 1991.

59. Tandon MK, Kailis SG: Bronchodilator treatment for partially reversible chronic obstructive airways disease, *Thorax* 46:248-251, 1991.

60. Tashkin DP et al: The lung health study: airway responsiveness to inhaled methacholine in smokers with mild to moderate airflow limitation, *Am Rev Respir Dis* 145:301-310, 1992.

61. Thurlbeck WM: Overview of the pathology of pulmonary emphysema in the human, *Clin Chest Med* 4:337-350, 1983.

62. Travis J: *Alpha-1 proteinase inhibitor deficiency*. In Masarine G, editor: *Lung Cell Biology*, vol 41, New York, 1989, Dekker.

63. Vestbo J, Rasmussen FV: Respiratory symptoms and FEV$_1$ as predictors of hospitalization and medication in the following 12 years due to respiratory disease, *Eur Respir J* 2:710-715, 1989.

64. Vincent TN et al: Duct ectasia: an asymptomatic pulmonary change related to age, *J Lancet* 84:331-336, 1964.

65. Weiss ST et al: The relationship of physician diagnosed croup or bronchiolitis to the subsequent development of increased levels of airway responsiveness, *Chest* 85:95-105, 1984.

66. Wewers MA et al: Replacement therapy for alpha-1-antitrypsin deficiency associated with emphysema, *N Engl J Med* 316:1055-1062, 1987.

RESOURCES

Kay Bowen, Manuscript Assistant, 1719 East 19th Avenue, Denver, Colorado 80218. Three booklets for patients: Essentials of Pulmonary Rehabilitation: A "Do-it-Yourself" Program and Essentials of Pulmonary Rehabilitation, Part II: A "Do-it-Yourself" Program, Part III: Essentials of Pulmonary Rehabilitation: New Developments.

Chapter 56

PREVENTIVE ASPECTS OF HIV INFECTION

Gregory J. Forstall
David L. Longworth

In June 1981 the first cases of a disease subsequently termed *acquired immunodeficiency syndrome* (AIDS) were described.[20] By August 1989, 100,000 cases of AIDS had been reported to the Centers for Disease Control (CDC), and by December 1991 an additional 100,000 cases had been recognized.[27] An estimated 1 million persons in the United States are presently infected with the human immunodeficiency virus (HIV); of these, approximately 165,000-215,000 will die during 1991-1993.[17] AIDS is the second leading cause of death in men ages 25-44 years and the sixth leading cause of death in women of the same age group.[18]

Infection with HIV has become an epidemic of global proportion. An estimated 12 million adults are HIV-infected worldwide, including nearly 8 million in Africa. The prevalence of HIV infection is increasing rapidly in India and Southeast Asia.[77] Significant progress has occurred in the development of effective antiviral therapies and in the management of many of the complicating infections and neoplastic disorders associated with AIDS. A cure for AIDS is the ultimate goal of investigators and clinicians involved with this illness and is the hope of persons infected with HIV. However, until an effective vaccine or treatment to limit the spread of HIV is developed, prevention of infection remains the major weapon against this epidemic.

This chapter will review the epidemiology and risk factors predisposing to the acquisition of HIV infection, the screening strategies to identify those infected with the virus, the therapeutic and preventive interventions recommended for persons infected with HIV, and the infection control aspects of HIV infection for the health care worker.

CLASSIFICATION OF HIV INFECTION

Two different classification systems have been proposed for staging patients with HIV infection (Table 56-1 and see box). The Centers for Disease Control (CDC) system is more widely used (see box), but in its current form it does not take into account the degree of immunodeficiency.[13] Patients are classified into one of four groups. Group I consists of the acute, self-limited infectious mononucleosis syndrome that may occur in up to 92% of individuals.[93] This illness typically occurs within several weeks to several months following acquisition of infection. The most common symptoms include fever, lethargy, malaise, sore throat, anorexia, and myalgias, which occur in more than 50% of individuals. Other common signs and symptoms include headache, arthralgias, weight loss, lymphadenopathy, and retroorbital pain. A maculopapular rash occurs in about 25% of individuals. This illness may mimic acute infectious mononucleosis. Primary infection with HIV should be considered in patients at risk who present with "heterophile negative" infectious mononucleosis. The diagnosis is confirmed by documenting seroconversion to HIV.

Patients in CDC Group II consist of individuals who are asymptomatic, but seropositive for the virus, regardless of their quantitative CD4 cell count. By definition, patients with acute retroviral infection (Group I) progress to Group II as signs and symptoms of their primary infection resolve. Patients in CDC Group II represent a heterogeneous group of individuals in terms of their risk for opportunistic infections or malignancies, although all are asymptomatic. This represents the major problem with the CDC system; that is, Group II can comprise individuals with virtually no CD4 cells, who are asymptomatic but at considerable risk of opportunistic infections and malignancies, as well as individuals with normal CD4 counts, in whom the risk of such complications over the short term is negligible.

Patients in Group III have a syndrome of persistent generalized lymphadenopathy (previously termed AIDS-related complex). In addition to generalized lymph node enlargement, individuals in Group III often have persistent fever, weight loss, and oral thrush. These individuals usu-

ally have low CD4 counts or inverted CD4:CD8 lymphocyte ratios. Not all patients develop the syndrome of persistent generalized lymphadenopathy, and it is common for patients who are asymptomatic (Group II) to present with an AIDS-defining illness and therefore progress directly to Group IV.

In the current CDC classification system, patients in Group IV are considered to have AIDS. AIDS-defining ill-

Table 56-1. Walter Reed classification system for HIV infection

Stage	HIV Antibody or Culture	Chronic Lymphadenopathy	CD4+ Cell Count/ul	Cutaneous Anergy	Thrush	Opportunistic Infection
WRO	−	−	>400	None	−	−
WR1	+	−	>400	None	−	−
WR2	+	+	>400	None	−	−
WR3	+	±	<400	None	−	−
WR4	+	±	<400	Partial	−	−
WR5	+	±	<400	Complete/partial	+	−
WR6	+	±	<400	Complete/partial	±	+

From Redfield RR, Wright DC, Tramont ED: The Walter Reed staging classification for HTLV-III/LAV infection, *N Engl J Med* 314(2):131-132, 1986.

Centers for Disease Control (CDC) classification system for HIV infection

Group I. Acute infection

Mononucleosis-like syndrome associated with seroconversion.

Group II. Asymptomatic infection

Positive HIV antibody or viral culture.

Group III. Persistent generalized lymphadenopathy

Palpable lymphadenopathy (>1 cm) at two or more extrainguinal sites for more than three months in the absence of concurrent illness or infection to explain the findings.

Group IV. Other disease

SUBGROUP A. CONSTITUTIONAL DISEASE

One or more of the following: fever or diarrhea persisting more than one month or involuntary weight loss greater than 10% of baseline; absence of a concurrent illness or infection to explain the findings.

SUBGROUP B. NEUROLOGIC DISEASE

One or more of the following: dementia, myelopathy, or peripheral neuropathy; absence of a concurrent illness or condition.

SUBGROUP C. SECONDARY INFECTIOUS DISEASES

Infectious disease associated with HIV infection and/or at least moderately indicative of a defect in cell-mediated immunity.

Category C-1. Specified secondary infectious diseases listed in the CDC surveillance definition for AIDS
Pneumocystis carinii pneumonia, chronic cryptosporidiosis, toxoplasmosis, extraintestinal strongyloidiasis, isosporiasis, candidiasis (esophageal, bronchial, or pulmonary), cryptococcosis, histoplasmosis, nontuberculous mycobacterial infection, cytomegalovirus infection chronic mucocutaneous or disseminated herpes simplex virus infection, or progressive multifocal leukoencephalopathy.

Category C-2. Other specified secondary infectious diseases
Oral hairy leukoplakia, multidermatomal herpes zoster, recurrent Salmonella bacteremia, nocardiosis, tuberculosis, or oral candidiasis (thrush).

SUBGROUP D. SECONDARY CANCERS LISTED IN THE CDC SURVEILLANCE DEFINITION OF AIDS

Kaposi's sarcoma, non-Hodgkin's lymphoma (small, noncleaved lymphoma or immunoblastic sarcoma), or primary CNS lymphoma.

SUBGROUP E. OTHER CONDITIONS

Clinical findings or diseases that may be attributable to HIV infection and are indicative of a defect in cell-mediated immunity; symptoms attributable to either HIV infection or a coexisting disease not classified elsewhere; or clinical illnesses that may be complicated by HIV infection. These include chronic lymphoid interstitial pneumonitis and constitutional symptoms, secondary infectious diseases, and neoplasms not listed in other categories.

From CDC: Classification for human T-lymphotropic virus type III/lymphadenopathy-associated virus infection, *MMWR* 35:334-339, 1986.

nesses are summarized in the box on p. 1035 and include progressive constitutional disease, neurologic complications attributable to HIV, certain secondary infections and malignancies, and other conditions such as idiopathic thrombocytopenia, seen in association with HIV infection. The major flaw in the current CDC system is its failure to take into account a patient's CD4 count. An expansion of the AIDS surveillance case definition for adolescents and adults was implemented on January 1, 1993 to include CD4 counts less than 200/μl or a CD4 percentage less than 14.[26]

The Walter Reed Classification System is more cumbersome and less widely used but does take into account the patient's CD4 cell count (see Table 56-1).[87] This system requires documentation of the CD4 cell count, delayed hypersensitivity skin testing, as well as documentation of the presence or absence of oral thrush or an opportunistic infection. It does not take into account patients with opportunistic malignancies or neurologic syndromes attributable to HIV, which may be encountered in patients with advanced immunodeficiency.

When it comes to the pragmatic assessment and the risk stratification of patients with HIV infection, it is by no means clear that these classification systems are superior to simply measuring the CD4 cell count. Several recent studies have demonstrated that the absolute CD4 cell count is the best predictor of the risk of developing an AIDS-defining opportunistic infection or malignancy over a specified period of time.[42,50,74,82]

Recent studies suggest that the mean incubation period from acquisition of HIV infection to the development of an AIDS-defining illness is about 8 years in homosexual men and recipients of HIV-contaminated blood transfusions.[72,80]

EPIDEMIOLOGY

AIDS is now the eleventh leading cause of death in the United States.[18] Cases have been reported from all of the 50 states, the District of Columbia, and the US territories. By December 31, 1991, a total of 206,392 cases of AIDS had been reported to the CDC and the total number of deaths attributed to AIDS was 133,232.[27]

The major routes of HIV transmission include homosexual or heterosexual spread; exposure to HIV-contaminated blood by transfusion, needle sharing, or accidental needlestick injury; and prenatal or perinatal transmission from an HIV-infected mother to infant. Numerous studies have failed to demonstrate a risk of transmission by casual household or school contact to HIV-infected persons.[6,47,75]

A number of studies have examined the seroprevalence of HIV infection in different populations in the United States during the past decade (Table 56-2). In selected high-risk populations, such as male homosexuals and injecting-drug-users (IDUs), the prevalence of HIV infection has varied widely by geographic area. Infection is most

Table 56-2. Seroprevalence of HIV infection in different populations in the United States

Population	Year	Seroprevalence (%)
Household survey[19]	1989	0.4
Blood donors		
All[10]	1988	0.010
First time male	1988	0.067
First time female	1988	0.014
Adults with cardiac arrest in community[16]	1989-1990	0.8
Military recruits[7]	1985	0.15
Job Corps applicants[11,15]	1987	0.41
Female prostitutes[12]	1986	0-57
Intravenous drug users		
Bronx, NY[89]	1985-1986	39.4
Nationwide[56]	1984-1987	5-33
San Francisco[32]	1986-1987	12
Homosexual men[33]	1992	20-70
Pregnant women		
Massachusetts[63]	1986-1987	0.21
New York City[40]	1987-1988	0.66

prevalent in urban areas, especially New York City, Miami, San Francisco, and Houston. Among female prostitutes, seroprevalence rates are highly varied from one region of the country to another. Studies to assess the overall seroprevalence rate in the general population have been more difficult to perform. A study in 1985 examining military recruits documented a seroprevalence rate of 0.15%.[7] A more recent study of Job Corps applicants beginning in 1987 identified a seroprevalence rate of 0.41%.[11] Patients suffering out-of-hospital cardiac arrest in Seattle had a seroprevalence rate of 0.8%.[16] The seroprevalence rate in blood donors is approximately 0.01%.[10] First-time blood donors are more likely to be seropositive, with seroprevalence rates of 0.067% in males and 0.014% in females.[10]

GROUPS AT RISK

Most reported AIDS cases in the United States have occurred among homosexual or bisexual men and IDUs. However, during the period of September 1989 through November 1991, the proportion of reported cases associated with heterosexual transmission of HIV and the number of cases occurring in women increased.[27] AIDS has had a major impact on minority communities throughout the United States. Cases in children associated with perinatal (mother-to-infant) HIV transmission have continued to increase. A comparison of percentages of AIDS cases occurring in populations at risk in the first and second 100,000 cases is listed in Table 56-3. On a worldwide basis, heterosexual transmission is the leading mechanism of spread of the infection and may account for more than 80% of HIV transmission by the end of the decade.[62]

Table 56-3. Comparison of first 200,000 cases of AIDS

	First 100,000 Cases 1981-Aug. 1989	Second 100,000 Cases Sept. 1989-Nov. 1991
Homosexual/bisexual men (no history of IDU)	61%	55%
Injecting-drug-user	11%	12%
Heterosexual transmission	5%	7%
Women	9%	12%
Black/African American	27%	31%
Latino/Hispanic	15%	17%
Transfusions (adults/children)	2.5%/11%	1.9%/5.6%

Homosexual and bisexual men

AIDS was first described among homosexual men in 1981. Homosexual and bisexual men comprise the largest single population infected with HIV in the United States (59%).[27] Behavioral studies have demonstrated that the risk of HIV infection in these men increases with their number of male sexual partners and with the frequency with which they are the receptive partner in rectal intercourse.[97] The proportion of AIDS cases in this group has declined from 61% of the first 100,000 reported cases to 55% of the second 100,000 cases.[27] This decline may be related to the effects of "safe sex" campaigns to reduce the number of sexual partners and the practice of receptive anal intercourse.[62]

Women and heterosexual men

As of December 31, 1990, 10% of adults reported with AIDS in the United States were women.[40] Of these, 73% were women of color. The majority of women with AIDS have been IDUs; however, a significant number of cases have resulted from heterosexual transmission. Of all AIDS cases among women, 34% were the result of heterosexual transmission and women accounted for 61% of all cases attributed to heterosexual transmission.[27] The highest incidence rates of women with HIV infection occurred in Puerto Rico and in urban areas along the Atlantic coast, including New Jersey, New York, the District of Columbia, Florida, Connecticut, Maryland, Delaware, Massachusetts, and Rhode Island.

Women with AIDS who reported sexual relations only with a female partner since 1977 represented 0.8% of AIDS cases in women reported to the CDC through September 30, 1989.[35] Ninety-five percent of these women with AIDS were IDUs.

As of December 31, 1990, 24% of reported cases of AIDS occurred in heterosexual men. Of this group, 45% occurred in black males, while 27% occurred each in

white and Hispanic males. The incidence rates of AIDS cases in heterosexual men were highest in Puerto Rico, followed by New York, New Jersey, the District of Columbia, and Florida.[40] IDUs comprised the largest proportion of heterosexual men with AIDS, making up 66% of cases in 1990.

Most heterosexual transmission of HIV occurs during vaginal intercourse. Factors that increase the risk of heterosexual transmission of HIV include unprotected sexual contact, genital ulcer disease, and multiple sexual partners.[83]

Injecting-drug-users

Twenty-two percent of all cases of AIDS in the United States occur in IDUs.[27] Illicit drug use is the second most common risk behavior in the HIV epidemic in the United States and Europe. This population plays a crucial role in the spread of HIV infection because it represents the principal bridge to other adult populations through heterosexual transmission and to children through perinatal transmission. The importance in disease transmission of sharing unsterilized needles and syringes contaminated with HIV is supported by anecdotal and epidemiologic studies.[54] Other factors that determine the risk of HIV transmission with injecting-drug use include the number of persons with whom needles are shared, median number of injections in "shooting galleries," and residence in an area with a high prevalence of HIV infection.[34]

Blood and blood products

Persons who have acquired HIV infection through the transfusion of infected blood or blood products represent a small but important proportion of the total number of cases. Parenteral exposure to contaminated blood or blood products is a continuing problem, especially in developing countries.[33] Seroprevalence rates among blood donors in some AIDS-endemic areas of Africa remain as high as 5% to 18% because screening of donors for HIV is not yet universal. The proportion of AIDS cases in the United States related to transfusions declined in adults (2.5% to 1.9%) from the first to the second 100,000 cases.[27] The screening of donated blood and plasma for antibody to HIV, which began in April 1985, and heat treatment of clotting-factor concentrates coupled with donor screening have reduced the risk associated with transfused blood products. The risk of HIV transmission from screened blood has recently been estimated to range from 1 in 38,000 to 1 in 153,000.[8] However, individuals who receive an HIV-contaminated unit of blood have a 90% likelihood of seroconverting to HIV.[96]

Persons aged 50 years or older

AIDS is not just a disease of young persons. In 1990 there were 4148 cases of AIDS in individuals over the age of 50. More than 40% of persons with AIDS ages 60 and above were exposed by male homosexual contact.[90] In a study by Ship et al., 67.5% of individuals with AIDS ages 50-59 reported male homosexual contact.[90] In persons with AIDS over the age of 70, 64.2% acquired the infection through blood transfusion, whereas 18.7% became infected by male homosexual contact. About 4% of persons with AIDS above age 50 acquired the infection by heterosexual contact.[90]

Adolescents

Although only 604 cases of AIDS among adolescents ages 13-19 were reported to the CDC as of October 31, 1990, the adolescent age group is an important population to consider regarding AIDS prevention. Twenty percent of AIDS cases have occurred in adults ages 20-29. Many adults in this group acquired HIV during adolescence. As opinions and behaviors regarding sex and drug use are developing during this time, education regarding risk behaviors and AIDS prevention could have a major impact in limiting the spread of HIV in adolescents.[48]

Eighty percent of reported AIDS cases in adolescents have occurred in males. Blood product exposure accounted for the largest proportion of cases (38%), closely followed by homosexual or bisexual contact (37%).[48]

Infants

Perinatal transmission accounts for more than 80% of all reported cases of pediatric AIDS.[73] Infants become infected with HIV through the maternal circulation *in utero,* by inoculation or ingestion of blood and other infected fluid during labor and delivery, and through ingestion of infected breast milk shortly after birth.[5] It is estimated that 13% to 45% of infants born to women infected with HIV will acquire the virus.[73]

The major risk factors predisposing an infant to the acquisition of HIV infection *in utero* or at birth are women who have advanced HIV disease, women who are IDUs, or women who have sexual partners who are infected with HIV.[5] The diagnosis of HIV infection in infants is difficult because tests based on the detection of IgG antibody to HIV cannot distinguish maternally acquired IgG antibody to HIV (which can persist through 15 months of age in uninfected infants) and antibody produced by the infant.[86] Progress has been made in the development of strategies to allow for earlier detection of HIV infection in infants. These strategies include direct detection of HIV by culture, polymerase chain reaction, and detection of anti-HIV specific IgA antibodies, which do not cross the placenta and are of infant origin if present.[37]

SOCIO-MEDICO-ECONOMICS

AIDS has had a profound impact on the cost of health care in the United States. In 1991 national spending on HIV-related illness consumed about 1.6% of all health-related costs in the United States.[51] The Public Health Ser-

vice estimates the cumulative cost of treating people with HIV will increase from $10.3 billion in 1992 to $15.2 billion in 1995. The lifetime cost of treating a person with AIDS has increased from $57,000 in 1988 to $102,000 in 1992. Inpatient care represents an important and costly portion of the total medical care for HIV-infected individuals. Andrulis et al. estimated that the average hospital spent $948,028 in 1988 for inpatient AIDS care.[2] With earlier medical intervention occurring in patients with HIV infection and an increased ability to manage these patients effectively using fewer inpatient hospital resources, the economic demands are shifting from the inpatient setting to outpatient services.

However, the largest component of the cost of HIV-related illness is due to lost work rather than direct expenditures for medical care. Yelin et al. reported in a study of 193 persons with symptoms of HIV-related illness that 50% of those who worked before the onset of HIV infection had stopped working within two years and all had stopped within ten years after the onset of the first symptom of HIV infection.[98]

SCREENING
Expected outcome of screening

Because AIDS is a leading cause of death in men and women ages 25-44, it is of critical importance to identify individuals infected with HIV and those at risk to acquire the infection in an effort to prevent the continued spread of the virus. The availability of early medical treatment for asymptomatic HIV-infected individuals is also a major incentive to determine the HIV-antibody status of those at risk.

Individuals who undergo HIV testing and are found to be seronegative possess the opportunity to alter their behavior and reduce the risk of contracting HIV. Individuals who test positive for HIV may benefit from the implementation of prophylactic regimens and antiretroviral therapy that can retard the progression of the disease and reduce the occurrence of serious opportunistic infections. Early detection and prompt treatment of other infections such as tuberculosis or syphilis can further reduce the morbidity associated with HIV infection. Early recognition of HIV infection is of potential value in the prevention of viral transmission to other individuals through notification of sexual partners who may be infected.[94]

Utility of HIV screening

The screening tests to detect the presence of HIV are both sensitive and specific. The predictive value of these tests is greatest when they are applied to the population at highest risk for HIV seropositivity.[94] However, antibody testing alone is not an effective technique for reducing HIV transmission. HIV testing is only effective when it is used in conjunction with extensive counseling and assurance of confidentiality.

Groups for which screening for human immunodeficiency virus (HIV) infection should be offered

- Persons seeking treatment for sexually transmitted diseases
- Homosexual and bisexual individuals
- Injecting-drug-users
- Persons whose past or present sexual partners were HIV-infected, bisexual, or injecting-drug-users
- Persons with multiple sexual partners or a history of prostitution or having sex with a prostitute
- Persons with a history of blood transfusion between 1978 and 1985
- Women of childbearing age or pregnant women engaged in behaviors predisposing to the acquisition of HIV infection or who reside in a high-seroprevalence area

---

Questions to establish an individual's risk for HIV infection

- Do you have sex with men, women, or both?
- About how many sexual partners have you had in the past five years?
- Have any of your sexual partners been injecting-drug-users, homosexual or bisexual, developed AIDS, or lived in an area where many people have AIDS?
- Have you ever paid money or received money for sex?
- Have you ever had a sexually transmitted disease?
- Do you use condoms? If so, sometimes or always?
- Have you ever had a man put his penis in your rectum?
- Do you smoke cigarettes, drink alcohol, or use other drugs?
- (If the patient is an injecting-drug-user) Do you share needles, cookers, or other drug equipment?
- Have you ever used crack cocaine?
- (If the patient has used crack) Have you had sex in crack houses?
- Did you receive any blood transfusions or have surgery between 1978 and 1985?

Assessing patients for HIV testing

Individuals engaging in behaviors known to pose a risk for the acquisition of HIV should be offered serologic testing. The risk behaviors and groups for which screening for HIV infection is indicated are listed in the box above.

Health care providers must become proficient in determining the sexual orientation and the presence of risk behaviors for HIV infection in their patients. These inquiries must be nonjudgmental and communicate open-mindedness in order to achieve an accurate assessment of an individual's risk factors for HIV infection.[58] The box above, right lists questions helpful to identify behaviors predisposing to HIV infection.

Other aspects of general history-taking can offer clues to the presence of unrecognized HIV infection. These include the presence of unexplained fever, night sweats, cough, lymphadenopathy, prolonged diarrhea, and weight loss.[58] In women HIV infection should be considered in individuals with the following conditions: persistent recurrent vaginal candidiasis; severe genital herpes simplex lesions; genital ulcer disease such as syphilis or chancroid; recalcitrant or multifocal *Condyloma acuminatum;* Pap smear evidence of moderate to severe cervical dysplasia, carcinoma *in situ,* or squamous cell carcinoma; and persistent or recurrent pelvic inflammatory disease despite appropriate nonsurgical treatment.[79] Dermatomal varicella-zoster virus infection should prompt an inquiry regarding potential risk behaviors for HIV infection, since this sometimes may represent the first clinical clue to the diagnosis. As noted earlier, patients presenting with an infectious mononucleosis-like syndrome should be questioned regarding risk behaviors for HIV infection. In those at risk in whom another cause of the illness cannot be identified, serologic testing for HIV should be performed in an attempt to document seroconversion. Serologic tests may be negative at the time of the acute illness but usually turn positive within three months.

Informed consent must be obtained from all patients undergoing serologic testing for HIV and should be documented in the medical record. Pretest and posttest counseling should be offered, as will be discussed, to educate patients regarding the medical and psychologic implications of testing.

The initial screening test for the presence of HIV is the enzyme-linked immunoassay (ELISA), which is based on the detection of antibodies to HIV.[91] Antibodies to HIV normally develop 6 to 8 weeks after infection with the virus. The ELISA has a reported sensitivity of 99.7% and a specificity of 98.5%. A blood sample that tests positive for antibodies to HIV by ELISA undergoes repeat ELISA testing to reduce the chance of a false positive result. Two successive reactive ELISAs are then followed by a confirmatory test, such as the Western blot, before classifying an individual as HIV seropositive.[91] The combination of positive sequential ELISA tests followed by a positive Western blot has a false positive rate of <0.001%. Results of HIV serologic testing should be charted in the patient's medical record.

Baseline studies in HIV-infected patients

At initial diagnosis of HIV infection, a complete history and thorough physical examination should be performed along with a number of baseline laboratory tests (see box on p. 1040). A complete blood count can be repeated every 6 to 12 months in asymptomatic patients. A rapid plasmin reagin (RPR) test is important in identifying untreated

---

**Suggested baseline laboratory studies
in HIV-infected patients**

Complete blood count with differential
Chemistry panel
Urinalysis
RPR
Toxoplasma gondii IgG
HBsAg, HBsAb
Tuberculin skin test with anergy panel
T-lymphocyte subsets
DLCO
Chest x-ray examination
Baseline ophthalmology and dental examinations
Pap smear

---

cases of syphilis and should be repeated if new potential exposures occur or if a patient develops an illness consistent with syphilis. A baseline toxoplasma IgG titer is helpful in identifying previously exposed patients who may have up to a 30% chance of developing cerebral toxoplasmosis during the course of their HIV infection.[53] In patients without serologic evidence of prior exposure, the titer should be repeated if an illness subsequently develops that is compatible with central nervous system toxoplasmosis. In most patients with AIDS, toxoplasmosis represents a reactivation of latent infection and thus patients usually have a positive IgG titer to *Toxoplasma gondii*. Patients may sometimes be seronegative and nevertheless have central nervous system toxoplasmosis, but this usually occurs in patients with far advanced immunodeficiency and CD4 cell depletion, in whom antibody production is also impaired. In a healthier individual with a CD4 count of 100-200, a negative toxoplasma IgG would make less likely a diagnosis of central nervous system toxoplasmosis in a patient with a space-occupying lesion of the central nervous system.

A hepatitis B surface antigen and hepatitis B surface antibody should be performed to identify chronic hepatitis B carriers and nonimmune individuals requiring hepatitis B immunization. Purified protein derivative (PPD) skin testing identifies patients with prior exposure to *Mycobacterium tuberculosis*. An anergy battery should be performed to identify anergic individuals in whom a negative PPD does not exclude tuberculosis.[58] Five millimeters of induration or greater from a tuberculin skin test is considered positive in patients with HIV. A January 1992 report suggested a definition of 2 mm of induration or greater to indicate a positive tuberculin skin test,[52] but this requires validation in other studies. In fact, a recent population-based survey in Haiti suggested that 5 mm of erythema and induration was the most discriminating breakpoint for defining a positive tuberculin skin test in HIV-infected pa-

tients.[65] In patients without clinical evidence of pulmonary or extrapulmonary tuberculosis, a positive skin test represents an indication for isoniazid prophylaxis because of the significant risk of development of active tuberculosis in HIV-infected patients. Patients with evidence of pulmonary or extrapulmonary tuberculosis require therapy with at least two antituberculous drugs.

T-lymphocyte subset analysis provides a useful method to assess the degree of immunodeficiency and to decide when antiretroviral therapy and *Pneumocystis carinii* pneumonia prophylaxis should begin. These values should be repeated every 4 to 6 months for HIV-infected individuals with CD4 counts >500 cells/mm³. Patients with CD4 counts <500 cells/mm³ are candidates for antiretroviral therapy. Individuals with CD4 counts <200 cells/mm³ require prophylaxis against *Pneumocystis carinii* pneumonia. Individuals with CD4 counts between 200 and 500 cells/ml³ should have T-lymphocyte subset analyses performed every 3 to 4 months, especially as the count approaches 200 cells/mm³. Once the count falls below 200 cells/mm³, individual physician practice varies regarding T-lymphocyte subset testing. Some physicians continue to follow the CD4 cell count every 3 to 4 months and will alter antiretroviral therapy in those patients whose counts deteriorate while on zidovudine. Others take a more nihilistic approach and do not follow counts once they fall below 200 cells/mm³, but they will alter antiretroviral therapy on the basis of the patient's overall clinical condition.

A baseline chest radiograph and carbon monoxide diffusing capacity (DLCO) should be performed, even in asymptomatic individuals. These will often prove valuable for future comparison if the patient presents with an illness suggestive of mild *Pneumocystis carinii* pneumonia. Routine ophthalmologic and dental examinations should be performed every 6 to 12 months. Patients with CD4 counts <200 cells/mm³ should have formal ophthalmologic examinations every 6 months and whenever symptoms suggestive of CMV retinitis develop, such as blurry or decreased vision. The primary care of HIV-infected women should also involve routine semi-annual Pap smears and investigation by colposcopy if the smears are abnormal. A study by Maiman suggested that colposcopy is a more effective screening method for cervical intraepithelial neoplasia in women with HIV infection.[76]

THERAPEUTIC INTERVENTIONS
Antiviral therapy

Zidovudine at a dose of 250 mg every 4 hours has been demonstrated to decrease mortality and the frequency of opportunistic infections in patients with AIDS and AIDS-related complex.[46] A follow-up study demonstrated that zidovudine in a divided daily dose of 600 mg was as effective as high-dose therapy and was less toxic.[45] Asymptomatic seropositive individuals with fewer than 500 CD4 cells/mm³ have also been demonstrated to benefit from therapy with zidovudine in divided doses of 500 mg/day or 1500 mg/day.[95] As in the studies in patients with AIDS or AIDS-related complex, zidovudine at lower doses (500 mg/day) is less toxic and equally effective as higher dose therapy.

Therapy with zidovudine is therefore recommended for both symptomatic and asymptomatic HIV-infected individuals whose CD4 counts are consistently below 500 cells/mm^3. The currently recommended dose of zidovudine is 100 mg given 5 times daily; some practitioners give 200 mg every 8 hours to simplify the dosing schedule.[1] There is some evidence that doses as low as 100 mg tid are effective.[36] Follow-up contact should be scheduled every 2 weeks following initiation of therapy to identify possible drug side effects, the major ones being anemia and leukopenia.[88] Less common side effects include headache (which may sometimes remit despite continued therapy), myopathy, rash, and fatigue. Subsequent follow-up visits may be scheduled at 1- to 2-month intervals depending upon how well the patient tolerates the drug. The complete blood count should be monitored at each visit to assess for hematologic toxicity. In general, zidovudine may be continued as long as the absolute neutrophil exceeds 500 cells/mm^3. Patients with marginal granulocyte counts require closer follow-up and should have complete blood counts performed every 2 weeks. Neutropenia related to zidovudine often responds to temporary cessation of therapy, after which the drug may be cautiously reintroduced at a lower dose with careful monitoring of the neutrophil count.

Anemia is another common complication of zidovudine and is often partially reversible with temporary cessation of therapy. Anemia usually comes on slowly over weeks to months but occasionally may occur precipitously. Patients with more severe anemia requiring frequent transfusions may benefit from the administration of recombinant human erythropoietin if endogenous erythropoietin levels are less than 500 IU/L.[36] In a recent placebo-controlled study, doses of 100 U/kg 3 times per week were effective in reducing transfusion requirements of HIV-infected patients receiving zidovudine and were well tolerated.[43]

Zidovudine invariably produces megaloblastic indices. A normal mean corpuscular volume (MCV) in a patient on the medication suggests either noncompliance or occult iron deficiency. Vitamin B12 deficiency is occasionally encountered in patients with HIV infection, so megaloblastic indices in patients receiving zidovudine cannot automatically be ascribed to the drug.[57] Thrombocytopenia is a rare side effect of zidovudine and alternative explanations should be sought in patients with HIV infection.

Because of the toxicity associated with zidovudine as well as the emergence of viral resistance in patients on prolonged therapy, studies have examined the usefulness of several new antiviral agents alone or in combination with zidovudine. In open studies, didanosine (ddI) has demonstrated promise in patients with AIDS or AIDS-related complex.[38,68] A recent trial compared zidovudine and ddI in patients who previously had tolerated zidovudine for at least 16 weeks. Didanosine recipients of doses of 500 mg per day had fewer AIDS-defining events and deaths than patients who continued to receive zidovudine.[66] In addition, CD4 counts and p24 antigenemia improved in ddI recipients compared with patients who received zidovudine.[66] The beneficial effects of didanosine were primarily seen in asymptomatic HIV-infected patients or in those with AIDS-related complex. Didanosine recipients who entered the study with a prior AIDS-defining diagnosis had a similar outcome compared with those who remained on zidovudine. The most common toxic effects of ddI are pancreatitis and peripheral neuropathy, but abnormal liver function studies, hyperuricemia, rash, and myositis can occur.[38,68]

Dideoxycytidine (ddC) is another deoxynucleoside analog that inhibits HIV replication but demonstrates less hematologic toxicity. The combination of zidovudine 200 mg tid plus ddC 0.01 mg/kg tid is effective in improving CD4 cell counts, reducing p24 antigenemia, and improving weight in recipients.[81]

We believe that zidovudine remains the drug of choice for the initial therapy of HIV infection in patients with fewer than 500 CD4 cells/mm^3. Didanosine cannot be recommended as initial therapy at this time.[55] Sufficient data do not presently exist to recommend optimal therapy in patients who fail zidovudine or who cannot tolerate the drug. Current options include didanosine alone or combination therapy with zidovudine plus either ddI or ddC. Unpublished data suggest that ddC may also have a role as monotherapy in such individuals.[55]

Other prophylactic therapies

Pneumocystis carinii pneumonia (PCP) remains the most frequent initial opportunistic infection in AIDS patients. The risk of PCP rises when the CD4 count falls below 200 cells/mm^3, and this has become the criterion for initiating prophylaxis.[14] Trimethoprim-sulfamethoxazole (TMP-SMX) has been demonstrated to reduce the incidence of PCP.[44] A variety of doses may be employed, including one double-strength tablet daily, one double-strength tablet 3 times a week or every other day.[67] The major adverse reactions with TMP-SMX are skin rashes and other allergic reactions that occur in up to 50% of HIV-infected individuals. If TMP-SMX is not tolerated, aerosolized pentamidine may also be employed at a dose of 300 mg every month via nebulizer.[70] Aerosolized pentamidine is not well absorbed and cases of extrapulmonary pneumocystosis may occur in individuals receiving this type of prophylaxis. In addition, upper lobe PCP may also occur in such individuals because of the preferential delivery of the drug to the lung bases. Administration of the drug in the semi-recumbent position may alleviate this problem. Breakthrough episodes of PCP may occur despite prophylaxis with either TMP-SMX or aerosolized pentamidine. Alternative regimens in this setting include monthly parenteral pentamidine 4 mg/kg, dapsone 100 mg orally daily, or dapsone together with trimethoprim 100 mg orally tid.

The usefulness of chemoprophylaxis to prevent other opportunistic infections such as central nervous system toxoplasmosis or cryptococcosis is presently being investigated. A recent retrospective study suggested that patients receiving low-dose trimethoprim sulfamethoxazole (1 DS tab bid twice weekly) for pneumocystis prophylaxis had a lower incidence of toxoplasmic encephalitis compared with patients receiving pentamidine prophylaxis.[9] Recommendations regarding prophylaxis for CNS toxoplasmosis presently await the completion of well-designed prospective studies.[4]

Cryptococcal disease occurs in 5% to 10% of patients with AIDS.[39] Primary prophylaxis to prevent cryptococcosis in HIV-infected patients has not been studied. A recent controlled trial, however, demonstrated that fluconazole 200 mg po qd was superior to weekly amphotericin B in preventing relapses of cryptococcal meningitis in patients with AIDS who had previously completed a primary course of therapy with amphotericin B.[85] Fluconazole is generally well tolerated, although occasional adverse reactions such as rash, abnormal liver function studies, and nausea occur. In patients with prior cryptococcosis, suppressive therapy with fluconazole must be continued indefinitely.

Patients with HIV infection have an increased incidence of pneumococcal pneumonia and are more vulnerable to influenza, providing the rationale for yearly influenza vaccines and a pneumococcal vaccine. Patients with HIV infection are also at higher risk for serious infections caused by *Haemophilus influenzae*. A recent study assessed the immunogenicity of both polysaccharide polyribosylribitol phosphate (PRP) and protein-conjugated polysaccharide *Haemophilus influenzae* vaccines in men with HIV infection.[92] This study demonstrated that patients with asymptomatic and symptomatic HIV infection had a greater response to the protein-conjugate vaccine, whereas those with AIDS had a greater response to the PRP vaccine. Although the efficacy of immunization in preventing invasive *Haemophilus influenzae* infections in HIV-infected patients is not presently known, this study provided indirect support for the recommendation of immunizing all HIV-infected individuals with *Haemophilus influenzae* type B vaccines. We presently offer our patients immunization.

COUNSELING AND COMPLIANCE

One of the key preventive strategies for the HIV epidemic is the presence of publicly funded HIV antibody counseling and testing services for individuals at risk of acquiring or transmitting HIV.[61] Counseling and testing are initially offered to explain the limitations of the HIV antibody test and to provide information about risk reduction. The pretest counseling includes the nature of HIV infection, the meaning of a positive and negative HIV antibody test result, the accuracy of the test, the routes of HIV transmission and activities during which HIV transmission can occur.

During posttest counseling, if the antibody test was negative, high-risk patients are advised of their need for continued evaluation of their infection risk if they continue high-risk behavior. Posttest counseling for a positive test result includes psychosocial assistance, including access to local support groups. The patient is encouraged to inform previous sexual partners and any persons with whom needles may have been shared of the result of their test and to recommend that they also seek testing.[78]

It is important to identify as early as possible the patient's particular fears about HIV infection and AIDS, as well as the patient's coping strategies and available support groups. The health care provider should help in educating patients about safer sex practices, assist with patients having an ongoing problem with substance abuse, and be available to advise patients on notifying current or former sexual partners about the infection.[61]

Regarding sexual activity, abstinence or a mutually monogamous relationship with an uninfected partner are the major means of preventing acquisition of HIV. Individuals with several sexual partners should be encouraged to use proper barrier methods to decrease the risk of acquiring or transmitting HIV, such as latex condoms impregnated with nonoxynol-9, vaginal foams, or contraceptive sponges. None of these contraceptive methods are foolproof. Individuals who continue to abuse injecting drugs should be encouraged to avoid the sharing of needles and to sterilize used needles with effective, practical methods (bleach). HIV-infected women contemplating pregnancy, particularly those with low CD4 counts, should be informed about their increased risk of perinatal transmission.[41]

Studies have shown that sustained behavioral changes occur only after repeated counseling sessions as well as a variety of additional motivational interventions.[99] Higgins et al. reviewed 66 studies on the behavioral effects of HIV antibody counseling and testing.[61] In the homosexual population, dramatic reduction in risk behaviors occurred during the 1980s attributable either to counseling interventions or to changes in the homosexual community as a result of the AIDS epidemic. The studies on heterosexual couples show a substantial impact of counseling interventions on sexual risk reduction. Studies among IDUs do not provide compelling evidence for an effect of counseling on either drug or sexual risk reduction. Research on pregnancy decisions of women suggests that counseling does not have a significant impact on pregnancy rates or decisions whether to terminate pregnancy.[61]

HIV AND HEALTH CARE WORKERS

Since the beginning of the epidemic, health care workers have been concerned about potential occupational acquisition of HIV. Studies in the 1980s demonstrated that the incidence of AIDS in health care workers is comparable to the general population at large.[28] At least 95% of health care workers with AIDS have had other documented risk behaviors for acquiring HIV infection.[28] Nevertheless, there is a real but fortunately small risk of acquiring HIV infection in the health care setting.

Transmission of HIV from patients to health care providers may occur via percutaneous injuries with sharp instruments or by mucosal splashes with HIV-infected blood or body fluids. Transmission through accidental exposure of mucous membranes to contaminated body fluids has been reported but is exceedingly uncommon.[29] In a recent study, no seroconversions occurred in more than 1000 mucous membrane exposures to HIV-contaminated blood or secretions.[59] In the small number of documented seroconversions following nonparenteral occupational exposure, none have involved intact skin.[59]

The estimated risk of transmission of HIV infection to health care workers through percutaneous needlestick exposure to the blood of a seropositive patient is 0.3%.[23,59,71] However, not all needlestick injuries appear to carry the same risk of HIV transmission. Factors associated with HIV transmission through accidental needlestick injury include sustaining a deep intramuscular injection, injury with a hollow bore needle (presumably harboring a larger volume of infected blood than a solid needle), failure to wear gloves, and exposure to blood from patients with advanced HIV infection.[49]

Nurses and laboratory workers comprise the majority of individuals acquiring HIV in the health care setting. Needlesticks have been the most frequent mechanism of transmission, and one third of injuries are related to attempts at recapping used needles.[64] Steps to prevent injuries include education of health care workers, exercising universal blood and body fluid precautions on all patients with appropriate use of eye protection and gloves, avoidance of needle recapping, and the availability and use of needle and syringe disposal containers.[25]

Health care workers who sustain a percutaneous needlestick or mucosal splash exposure should be offered HIV testing. If the source patient can be identified, permission from that individual should be sought to perform HIV serologic testing. If the patient consents and is seronegative, further evaluation and testing of the health care worker for HIV is not mandatory. If the patient refuses serologic testing or is HIV seropositive, the health care worker should undergo periodic HIV testing every 3 to 4 months for 1 year. In addition, some authorities recommend prophylactic zidovudine for 4 to 6 weeks following significant percutaneous or mucous membrane exposures from HIV seropositive patients.[22,60] The efficacy of such prophylaxis has never been proven and anecdotal failures have been reported.[69] Our policy is nevertheless to offer prophylactic zidovudine at a dose of 200 mg po 5 times per day for 6 weeks to health care workers who sustain a deep percutaneous needlestick exposure from a known HIV-infected patient in accordance with published recommendations.[60]

The potential for transmission of HIV from infected health care workers to uninfected patients has been a cause of great concern to the lay public in view of recent reports of a cluster of HIV infections among patients of one dental practitioner with AIDS.[21,30,31] Studies analyzing the viral strains of HIV in the dentist and the patients suggested that transmission did in fact occur, although the precise mechanism remains unclear. Subsequent studies examining potential transmission of HIV from two infected surgeons to their patients failed to document transmission.[3,84] Although the potential exists for transmission from the health care worker to the patient, the risk appears to be very low. Nevertheless, the CDC has issued recommendations for preventing such transmission, which include adherence to universal precautions, appropriate use of protective barriers and handwashing, and prudence in the disposal and use of sharp instruments.[23] HIV-infected health care workers with exudative skin lesions or dermatitis are advised to refrain from direct patient care. HIV-infected health care workers are advised by the CDC to not perform exposure prone procedures that require digital palpation of a needle tip in a patient's body cavity or the simultaneous presence of a health care worker's fingers and a sharp instrument or needle in a confined and poorly visualized anatomic site of a patient's body.[23]

SUMMARY

AIDS is the eleventh leading cause of death in the United States. It is the second leading cause of death in men ages 25-44 years and the sixth leading cause of death in women of the same age group. Most reported cases of AIDS have occurred among homosexual or bisexual men and IDUs; however, the proportion of reported cases associated with heterosexual transmission of HIV and the number of cases occurring in women is increasing. IDUs play a critical role in the spread of HIV infection because this group represents the principal bridge to other adult populations through heterosexual transmission and to children through perinatal transmission.

The screening tests to detect the presence of HIV are both sensitive and specific. However, the predictive value of these tests is greatest when they are applied to the population at highest risk for HIV seropositivity. The availability of early medical treatment for asymptomatic HIV-infected individuals is a major incentive to determine the HIV-antibody status of those at risk. However, antibody testing alone is not an effective technique for reducing HIV transmission. It is effective only if used in conjunction with extensive counseling, assurance of confidentiality, and a variety of additional motivational interventions.

Effective antiviral therapy has been developed to retard the progression of HIV infection. In addition, prophylactic antimicrobials are effective in preventing certain opportunistic infections such as *Pneumocystis carinii* pneumonia. A cure for AIDS does not presently exist. Vaccines are in various stages of development. Prevention of acquisition of infection remains the major weapon to limit the spread of the AIDS epidemic at this time.

Acknowledgement

The authors gratefully acknowledge the excellent secretarial assistance of Diane M. Jeunnette in the preparation of the manuscript.

REFERENCES

1. *AIDS/HIV Treatment Directory*, St. Louis, 1991, American Foundation for AIDS Research.
2. Andrulis DP et al: Comparisons of hospital care for patients with AIDS and other HIV-related conditions, *JAMA* 267:2482-2486, 1992.
3. Armstrong FP, Miner JC, Wolfe WH: Investigation of a health-care worker with symptomatic human immunodeficiency virus infection: an epidemiologic approach, *Milit Med* 152:414-418, 1987.
4. Beamen MH, Luft BJ, Remington JS: Prophylaxis for toxoplasmosis in AIDS, *Ann Intern Med* 117:163-164, 1992.
5. Berkelman RL et al: Epidemiology of human immunodeficiency virus infection and acquired immunodeficiency syndrome, *Am J Med* 86:761-770, 1989.
6. Bertheir A, Chamaret S, Fauchet R et al: Transmission of human immunodeficiency virus in haemophiliac and non-haemophiliac children living in a private school in France, *Lancet* 2:598, 1986.
7. Burke DS et al: Human immunodeficiency virus infections among civilian applicants for United States military service, October 1985 to March 1986: Demographic factors associated with seropositivity, *N Engl J Med* 317:131-136, 1987.
8. Busch MP et al: Evaluation of screened blood donations for human immunodeficiency virus Type 1 infection by culture and DNA amplification of pooled cells, *N Engl J Med* 325:1-5, 1991.
9. Carr AC et al: Low-dose trimethoprim sulfamethoxazole prophylaxis for toxoplasmic encephalitis in patients with AIDS, *Ann Intern Med* 117:106-111, 1991.
10. Centers for Disease Control: AIDS and human immunodeficiency virus infection in the United States: 1988 update, *MMWR* 38(S-4):1-38, 1989.
11. Centers for Disease Control: AIDS and human immunodeficiency virus infection in the United States: 1988 update, *MMWR* 38(S-4):25, 1989.
12. Centers for Disease Control: Antibody to human immunodeficiency virus in female prostitutes, *MMWR* 36:157-161, 1987.
13. Centers for Disease Control: Classification system for human T-lymphotropic virus type III/lymphadenopathy-associated virus infection, *MMWR* 35:334-339, 1986.
14. Centers for Disease Control: Guidelines for prophylaxis against *Pneumocystis carinii* pneumonia for persons infected with human immunodeficiency virus, *MMWR* 38(S-5):1-9, 1989.
15. Centers for Disease Control: HIV prevalence estimates and AIDS case projections for the United States: report based upon a workshop, *MMWR* 39(RR16):1-31, 1990.
16. Centers for Disease Control: HIV seroprevalence among adults treated for cardiac arrest before reaching a medical facility—Seattle, Washington, 1989-1990, *MMWR* 41:381-383, 1992.
17. Centers for Disease Control: Mortality attributable to HIV infection/AIDS - United States, 1981-1990, *MMWR* 40:41-44, 1991.
18. Centers for Disease Control: Mortality patterns—United States, 1989, *MMWR* 41:121-125, 1992.
19. Centers for Disease Control: Pilot study of a household survey to determine HIV seroprevalence, *MMWR* 40:1-5, 1991.
20. Centers for Disease Control: Pneumocystis pneumonia—Los Angeles, *MMWR* 30:250-252, 1981.
21. Centers for Disease Control: Possible transmission of human immunodeficiency virus to a patients during an invasive dental procedure, *MMWR* 39:489-493, 1990.
22. Centers for Disease Control: Public health service statement on management of occupational exposure to human immunodeficiency virus, including considerations regarding zidovudine postexposure use, *MMWR* 39:(RR-1) 1-14, 1990.
23. Centers for Disease Control: Recommendations for preventing transmission of human immunodeficiency virus and hepatitis B virus to patients during exposure-prone invasive procedures, *MMWR* 40:(RR-8) 1-9, 1991.
24. Reference deleted in galleys.
25. Centers for Disease Control: Recommendations for prevention of HIV transmission in health care settings, *MMWR* 36(2S):1-18, 1987.
26. Centers for Disease Control: Review of draft for revision of HIV infection classification system and expansion of AIDS surveillance case definition, *MMWR* 40:787, 1991.
27. Centers for Disease Control: The second 100,000 cases of acquired immunodeficiency syndrome - United States, June 1981 - December 1991, *MMWR* 41:28-29, 1992.
28. Centers for Disease Control: Update: acquired immunodeficiency syndrome and human immunodeficiency virus infection among health-care workers, *MMWR* 37:229-234, 1988.
29. Centers for Disease Control: Update: human immunodeficiency virus infections in health-care workers exposed to blood of infected patients, *MMWR* 36:285-289, 1987.
30. Centers for Disease Control: Update: transmission of HIV infection during an invasive dental procedure—Florida, *MMWR* 40:21-27,33, 1991.
31. Centers for Disease Control: Update: transmission of HIV infection during invasive dental procedures—Florida, *MMWR* 40:377-381, 1991.
32. Chaisson RE et al: Cocaine use and HIV infection in intravenous drug users in San Francisco, *JAMA* 261:561-565, 1989.
33. Chaisson RE: Epidemiology of human immunodeficiency virus infection and acquired immunodeficiency syndrome. In Gorbach SL, Bartlett JG, Blacklow NR, editors: *Infectious diseases*, Philadelphia, 1992, WB Saunders.
34. Chamberland ME, Curran JW: Epidemiology and prevention of AIDS and HIV infection. In Mandell GL, Douglas RG, Bennett JE, editors: *Principles and practices of infectious diseases*, New York, 1990, Churchill Livingstone.
35. Chu SY et al: Epidemiology of reported cases of AIDS in lesbians, United States, 1980-1989, *Am J Public Health* 80:1380-1381, 1990.
36. Collier AC et al: A pilot study of low-dose zidovudine in human immunodeficiency virus infection, *N Engl J Med* 323:1015-1021, 1990.
37. Connor E: Advance in early diagnosis of perinatal HIV infection, *JAMA* 266:3474-3475, 1991.
38. Cooley TP et al: Once-daily administration of 2',3'-dideoxyinosine (ddI) in patients with the acquired immunodeficiency syndrome or AIDS-related complex: results of a phase I trial, *N Engl J Med* 322:1340-1345, 1990.
39. Dismukes WE: Cryptococcal meningitis in patients with AIDS, *J Infect Dis* 157:624-628, 1988.
40. Ellerbrock TV et al: Epidemiology of women with AIDS in the United States, 1981 through 1990—a comparison with heterosexual men with AIDS, *JAMA* 265:2971-2975, 1991.
41. European Collaborative Study. Risk factors for mother-to-child transmission of HIV-1, *Lancet* 339:1007-1012, 1992.
42. Fahey JL et al: The prognostic value of cellular and serologic mark-

ers in infection with human immunodeficiency virus type I, *N Engl J Med* 322:166-172, 1990.

43. Fischl M et al: Recombinant human erythropoietin for patients with AIDS treated with zidovudine, *N Engl J Med* 322:1488-1493, 1990.

44. Fischl MA, Dickinson GM, La Voie L: Safety and efficacy of sulfamethoxazole and trimethoprim chemoprophylaxis for *Pneumocystic carinii* pneumonia in AIDS. *J Am Med Assoc* 259:1185-1189, 1988.

45. Fischl MA et al: A randomized controlled trial of a reduced daily dose of zidovudine in patients with the acquired immunodeficiency syndrome, *N Engl J Med* 323:1009-1014, 1990.

46. Fischl MA et al: The efficacy of azidothymidine (AZT) in the treatment of patients with AIDS and AIDS-related complex: a double-blind, placebo-controlled trial, *N Engl J Med* 317:185-191, 1987.

47. Friedland GH et al: Lack of transmission of HTLV III/LAV infection to household contacts of patients with AIDS or AIDS-related complex with oral candidiasis, *N Engl J Med* 314:344-349, 1986.

48. Gayle HD, D'Angelo LJ: Epidemiology of acquired immunodeficiency syndrome and human immunodeficiency virus infection in adolescents, *Pediatr Infect Dis* 10:322-328, 1991.

49. Gerberding JL, Schecter WP: Surgery and AIDS: reducing the risk, *JAMA* 265:1572-1573, 1991.

50. Goedert JJ et al: Effect of T4 count and cofactors on the incidence of AIDS in homosexual men infected with human immunodeficiency virus, *JAMA* 257:331-334, 1987.

51. Goldsmith MF: Cost in dollars and lives continue to rise, *JAMA* 266:1055, 1991.

52. Graham NM et al: Prevalence of tuberculin positivity and skin test anergy in HIV-1 seropositive and seronegative intravenous drug users, *JAMA* 267:369-373, 1992.

53. Grant IH et al: *Toxoplasma gondii* serologies in HIV-infected patients: the development of central nervous system toxoplasmosis in AIDS, *AIDS* 4:519-521, 1990.

54. Griedland GH, Klein RS: Transmission of the human immunodeficiency virus, *N Engl J Med* 317:1125-2235, 1987.

55. Groopman JE, Molina J-M: Nucleoside therapy for HIV infection—some answers, many questions, *N Engl J Med* 327:639-641, 1992.

56. Hahn RA et al: Prevalence of HIV infection among intravenous drug users in the United States, *JAMA* 261:2677-2684, 1989.

57. Harriman GR et al: Vitamin B12 malabsorption in patients with acquired immunodeficiency syndrome, *Arch Intern Med* 149:2039-2041, 1989.

58. Hecht FM, Soloway B: *HIV infection—a primary care approach*, Waltham, Mass, 1992, Massachusetts Medical Society.

59. Henderson DK et al: Risk for occupational transmission of human immunodeficiency virus type 1 (HIV-1) associated with clinical exposures: a prospective evaluation, *Ann Intern Med* 113:740-746, 1990.

60. Henderson DK, Gerberding JL: Prophylactic zidovudine after occupational exposure to the human immunodeficiency virus: an interim analysis, *J Infect Dis* 160:321-327, 1989.

61. Higgins DL et al: Evidence for the effects of HIV antibody counseling and testing on risk behaviors, *JAMA* 266:2419-2429, 1991.

62. Holmes KK: The changing epidemiology of HIV transmission, *Hospital Practice* 26(11):153-178, 1991.

63. Hoff R et al: Seroprevalence of human immunodeficiency virus among childbearing women: estimation by testing samples of blood from newborns, *N Engl J Med* 318:525-530, 1988.

64. Jagger J et al: Rates of needle-stick injury caused by various devices in a university hospital, *N Engl J Med* 319:284-288, 1988.

65. Johnson MP et al: Tuberculin skin test reactivity among adults infected with human immunodeficiency virus, *J Infect Dis* 166:194-198, 1992.

66. Kahn JO et al: A controlled trial comparing continued zidovudine with didanosine in human immunodeficiency virus infection, *N Engl J Med* 327:581-587, 1992.

67. Kovacs JA, Masur H: Prophylaxis for *Pneumocystis carinii* pneumonia in patients infected with human immunodeficiency virus, *Clin Infect Dis* 14:1005-1009, 1992.

68. Lambert JS et al: 2',3'-dideoxyinosine (ddI) in patients with the acquired immunodeficiency syndrome or AIDS-related complex: a phase I trial, *N Engl J Med* 322:1333-1340, 1990.

69. Lange JMA et al: Failure of zidovudine prophylaxis after accidental exposure to HIV-1, *N Engl J Med* 322:1375-1377, 1990.

70. Leoung GS et al: Aerosolized pentamidine for prophylaxis against *Pneumocystis carinii* pneumonia: the San Francisco community prophylaxis trial, *N Engl J Med* 323:769-775, 1990.

71. Lo B, Steinbrook R: Health care workers infected with the human immunodeficiency virus, *JAMA* 267:1100-1105, 1992.

72. Lui K-J, Darrow WW, Rutherford GW: A model-based estimate of the mean incubation period for AIDS in homosexual men, *Science* 240:1333-1335, 1988.

73. MacDonald MG, Ginzburg HM, Bolan JC: HIV infection in pregnancy: epidemiology and clinical management, *J Acq Immun Def Synd* 4:100-108, 1991.

74. MacDonnell KB et al: Predicting progression to AIDS: combined usefulness of CD4 lymphocyte counts and p24 antigenemia, *Am J Med* 89:706-712, 1990.

75. Madhok R et al: Lack of HIV transmission by casual contact, *Lancet* 2:863, 1986.

76. Maiman M et al: Colposcopic evaluation of human immunodeficiency virus—seropositive women, *Obst Gyn* 78:84-88, 1991.

77. Mann JM: AIDS—the second decade: a global perspective, *J Infect Dis* 165:245-250, 1992.

78. Manzella JP et al: Impact of the counselor on rates of informed consent and pre and posttest HIV counseling, *AIDS Patient Care* 6:19-20, 1992.

79. Marte C, Allen MH: HIV infection in women: presentations and protocols, *Hosp Pract* 27(3):113-120, 1992.

80. Medley CF et al: Incubation period of AIDS in patients infected via blood transfusion, *Nature* 382:719-721, 1987.

81. Meng T-C et al: Combination therapy with zidovudine and dideoxycytidine in patients with advanced human immunodeficiency virus infection: a phase I/II study, *Ann Intern Med* 116:13-20, 1992.

82. Phillips AN et al: Serial CD4 lymphocyte counts and development of AIDS, *Lancet* 337:389-392, 1991.

83. Plummer FA et al: Cofactors in male-female sexual transmission of human immunodeficiency virus Type 1, *J Infect Dis* 163:233-239, 1991.

84. Porter JD et al: Management of patients treated with HIV infection, *Lancet* 335:113-114, 1990 (letter).

85. Powderly WG et al: A controlled trial of fluconazole or amphotericin B to prevent relapse of cryptococcal meningitis in patients with the acquired immunodeficiency syndrome, *N Engl J Med* 326:793-798, 1992.

86. Quinn TC et al: Early diagnosis of perinatal HIV infection by detection of viral-specific IgA antibodies, *JAMA* 266:3439-3442, 1991.

87. Redfield RR, Wright DC, Tramont EC: The Walter Reed staging classification for HTLV III/LAV infection, *N Engl J Med* 314:131-132, 1986.

88. Richman DD et al: The toxicity of azidothymidine in the treatment of patients with AIDS and AIDS-related complex: a double-blind, placebo-controlled trial, *N Engl J Med* 317:192-197, 1987.

89. Schoenbaum EE et al: Risk factors for human immunodeficiency virus infection in intravenous drug users, *N Engl J Med* 321:874-879, 1989.

90. Ship JA, Wolff A, Selik RM: Epidemiology of acquired immune deficiency syndrome in persons aged 50 years or older, *J Acq Immun Def Synd* 4:84-88, 1991.

91. Sloand EM et al: HIV testing—state of the art, *JAMA* 266:2861-2866, 1991.

92. Steinhoff MC et al: Antibody responses to *Haemophilus influenzae*

type B vaccines in men with human immunodeficiency virus infection, *N Engl J Med* 325:1837-1842, 1991.

93. Tindall B et al: Characterization of the acute clinical illness associated with human immunodeficiency virus infection, *Arch Intern Med* 148:945-949, 1988.

94. U.S. Preventive Services Task Force: Screening for infection with human immunodeficiency virus. In Fisher M, editor: *Guide to clinical preventive services,* Baltimore, 1989, Williams & Wilkins.

95. Volberding PA et al: Zidovudine in asymptomatic human immunodeficiency virus infections: a controlled trial in persons with fewer than 500 CD4-positive cells per cubic millimeter, *N Engl J Med* 322:941-949, 1990.

96. Ward JW et al: Risk of human immunodeficiency virus infection from blood donors who later developed acquired immunodeficiency syndrome, *Ann Intern Med* 106:61-62, 1987.

97. Wofsy CB: Prevention of HIV transmission. In Sande MA, Volberding PA, editors: *The medical management of AIDS,* Philadelphia, 1990, W.B. Saunders.

98. Yelin EH et al: The impact of HIV-related illness on employment, *Am J Public Health* 81:79-84, 1991.

99. Zenilman JM et al: Effect of HIV posttest counseling on STD incidence, *JAMA* 267:843-845, 1992.

RESOURCES

AIDS Clinical Trials Information Service (800) 874-2574.

American Foundation for AIDS Research (AmFAR), 733 3rd Avenue, 12th Floor, New York, NY 10017.

Asian and Pacific Islander Coalition on HIV/AIDS, 150 West 26th Street, #503, New York, NY 10001.

Centers for Disease Control, AIDS Activity, Bldg. 6, Room 274, 1600 Clifton Road, NE, Atlanta, GA 30333.

Gay Men's Health Crises, P.O. Box 274, 132 West 24th Street, New York, NY 10011.

National AIDS Clearing House, P.O. Box 6003, Rockville, MD 20849-6003.

National AIDS Hotline (800) 342-2437.

National Minority AIDS Council, 300 I Street NE, Suite 400, Washington, DC 20002.

The National Native American AIDS Prevention Center, 3515 Grand Avenue, Suite 100, Oakland, CA 94610.

People of Color Against AIDS Network, 1200 South Jackson, Suite 25, Seattle, WA 98144.

Project Inform, 1965 Market Street, Suite 220, San Francisco, CA 94110.

Women and AIDS Resource Network, 30 Third Avenue, Suite 212, Brooklyn, NY 11217.

Chapter 57

INFECTIOUS DISEASES
AND IMMUNIZATIONS

Arif Z. Chaudhry

Infectious diseases have played an immensely important role in the fate of humanity since earliest recorded history. However, only in the last several hundred years have we made any significant progress in understanding these conditions. After clarification of the etiologic and pathogenic mechanisms came the era of treatment of established disease. Although we have by no means found ways to treat all known infections, such as the acquired immunodeficiency syndrome, much progress has been made in this area. Today we are perhaps on the threshold of yet another change in emphasis. The extreme importance and potential effectiveness of preventive strategies to the population as a whole, rather than just the individual, seem to have caught the imagination of those at the forefront of medical research and practice. We are thus witnesses to the dawn of the exciting age of prevention. Our hopes in the decades to come will be pinned on eradication rather than just cure of established disease. Some infections, by virtue of their unique cause-and-effect nature, are particularly susceptible to preventive strategies. This chapter serves to highlight important aspects of infections alterable by preventive measures.

ADULT IMMUNIZATIONS
Overview

Vaccines are one of the most cost-effective methods of improving health today. In this country, childhood vaccinations have increased life expectancy more than all investments in tertiary care, and at a fraction of the cost. Although routine immunizations have become an accepted part of pediatric clinical practice and have markedly reduced the incidence of vaccine-preventable disease in children, the same is unfortunately not true in adults, and a substantial proportion of the remaining morbidity and mortality of these infections still occurs in adolescents, adults,

and the elderly. It is up to practitioners who care for adult patients to consider and discuss immunizations whenever possible. This is preferably done at the initial encounter, and then at appropriate intervals thereafter. Although such encounters primarily occur in the primary care setting, vaccination opportunities are often missed not only in the hospitals, emergency rooms, and other health care settings, but also in schools, colleges, and the workplace.

There are good data to recommend the routine use of vaccines against measles, rubella, tetanus, influenza, and pneumococcal infections in adults. Most adults should receive seven immunizations: influenza, pneumococcal and hepatitis B vaccines, tetanus and diphtheria toxoids, and measles and rubella vaccines.[112] Each year, there are more than 20,000 influenza-associated deaths during epidemics, pneumococcal disease claims 40,000 lives, and 300,000 new cases of hepatitis B infection occur, mostly in patients 15 to 29 years old. Despite the magnitude of the problem, and the clear need for and availability of vaccination programs in adults, most adult patients today remain inadequately immunized.

Some conditions affect children as well as adults. People who escape natural infection or immunization against measles, mumps, rubella, and polio as children are often at increased risk from these conditions. Tetanus and diphtheria childhood vaccination needs to be boosted periodically. In contrast, other immunizations are aimed primarily at adults rather than children. Elderly people and others with certain compromising medical conditions are at increased risk for hospitalization and death caused by pneumonia and influenza, both conditions that may be preventable by immunization. Certain occupations, lifestyles, environmental circumstances, and medical conditions are associated with an immunocompromised status and thereby place selected groups of adults at increased risk for other vaccine-preventable diseases. Table 57-1 summarizes immunization and prophylaxis recommendations for a few of these special groups. Lastly, travelers to areas with endemic diseases not found in developed countries often require special immunizations for adequate protection.

Vaccine administration. The recommended route of administration varies with each vaccine. Table 57-2 summarizes commonly used vaccines. Most adult vaccines are given by intramuscular or subcutaneous injection. The but-

tock is not recommended as a site for routine immunization in adults. Studies with immunogenicity after hepatitis B vaccination in adults have shown that the vaccine is far less effective when injections are given in the gluteal region. This consideration may also apply to other vaccines. The buttock can be used, however, for large-volume injections such as immunoglobulin. However, one must take care to give the injection in the upper outer quadrant to avoid a sciatic nerve injury.

Table 57-1. Immunization and prophylaxis recommendations for special groups

Population group	Intervention indicated
Pregnancy	Hepatitis A immune globulin indicated if exposed. HBV(hepatitis B virus) screening recommended; may vaccinate during pregnancy. Influenza vaccine and pneumococcal vaccination (pneumovax) in high-risk only. Polio vaccine only when exposure risk high. Tetanus, diphtheria vaccines at 0, 1, 6 mo in unimmunized only. VZIG (varicella zoster immune globulin) indicated only to reduce risk to neonate if disease develops from 5 days before to 48 hr after birth. MMR (measles-mumps-rubella) is live-virus vaccine therefore contraindicated. Yellow fever vaccine is live attenuated vaccine but not teratogenic. May be used in high-risk patients.
Family members, household contacts	*Hemophilus influenza* type b vaccine only for uninfected children under age of 4. Not protective short-term; provides long-term immunity. Hepatitis A immune globulin NOT recommended for casual contacts. HBV vaccine recommended for sex partners and intimate contact (1 dose HBIG [hepatitis B immune globulin] plus three-dose series of vaccine). Influenza vaccine indicated for ALL members of families with high-risk patients. Amantidine recommended for members of families without high-risk patients. Rifampin or a sulfonamide indicated for family members of an index case of meningococcal meningitis. Pregnant women in the first 20 weeks of pregnancy should be immediately tested for rubella antibody. If nonimmune and later shown to be infected, elective abortion should be considered. Immunocompromised family contacts of VZV (varicella zoster virus) patients need acyclovir treatment.
Nursing home residents	Influenza vaccine, pneumovax, tuberculin testing
Inmates of institutions for the mentally handicapped	HBV vaccine
Prison inmates	HBV vaccine
Homeless persons	Tetanus/diphtheria, MMR, influenza vaccine, HBV, tuberculin skin testing
Health care workers	HBV, influenza, rubella, mumps, measles, polio, tetanus/diphtheria vaccinations
Essential community service personnel	Influenza, HBV vaccinations (emergency medical personnel only)
Day care workers	MMR, polio vaccinations
Laboratory personnel	HBV vaccine for all; plague vaccine, rabies vaccine, live-attenuated tularemia vaccine, anthrax vaccine, and smallpox vaccine only for those involved in special handling.
Veterinarians, animal handlers	Rabies vaccine with boosters every 2 yr, plague vaccine, especially in southwestern United States, where it is transmitted by pet dogs and cats; anthrax vaccine only if there is frequent exposure to specimens involving *Bacillus anthracis*.
Homosexual, bisexual men	HBV vaccine
Intravenous drug abusers	HBV vaccine
Prostitutes and persons with multiple sexual partners	HBV vaccine

The simultaneous administration of the most widely used live-virus vaccines does not result in impaired antibody responses or increased adverse reactions. When feasible, live virus vaccines that need not be administered on the same day should be given at least 1 month apart because of the concern that the immune response to the second vaccine might be impaired if it is administered too soon. In most instances, inactivated and live attenuated virus vaccines can also be administered simultaneously at separate sites as long as the precautions that apply to each vaccine are followed. Exceptions are vaccines for cholera and yellow fever. Some data suggest that when these vaccines are given within 3 weeks of each other, possible interference with antibody production levels may occur.

Certain disease-specific immunoglobulins contain antibodies that can interfere with the response to certain live-attenuated vaccines. Therefore if live-attenuated vaccines such as those against measles, mumps, and rubella are given simultaneously or shortly after immunoglobulin administration, these passively acquired antibodies may interfere with the replication of the vaccine virus and thereby limit the antibody response of the patient. Therefore these vaccines should not be given until at least 6 weeks and preferably 3 months have elapsed since the administration of immunoglobulin. However, immunoglobulin does not appear to interfere with antibody responses to either oral polio or yellow fever vaccines. Such interference also does not occur with inactivated vaccines, which can be given anytime after or simultaneously with immunoglobulin. If a live-virus vaccine has already been given and immunoglobulin administration is then indicated, the minimal interval between these is 2 weeks. If these rules regarding the timing of immunoglobulin administration cannot be followed, the patient should be retested 2 to 3 months later to confirm seroconversion to the vaccine.

Contraindications. Severe hypersensitivity reactions to vaccines, including anaphylaxis, are rare. These reactions are listed in Table 57-2 for the commonly used vaccines and are almost invariably a result of hypersensitivity to one or more vaccine components. The most common allergic component is the egg protein found in vaccines prepared in embryonated chicken eggs or chicken embryonal cultures. These vaccines include those against measles, mumps, influenza, and yellow fever. Rarely, patients may have an anaphylactic hypersensitivity reaction to trace amounts of neomycin (MMR vaccine) and streptomycin (oral polio vaccine) present in some vaccines. Occasional rare systemic reactions after cholera, typhoid, or plague vaccines probably represent toxic rather than true hypersensitivity reactions. Nevertheless, revaccination of such people should if possible be avoided.

In general, immunizations with live-virus vaccines should be avoided in immunocompromised patients, in family households with one person known to have congenital immunodeficiency, and in patients on oral or topical steroid therapy likely to cause systemic effects. Other forms of steroid therapy are not contraindications to live-virus vaccine immunization because of their minimal systemic immunosuppression. These include short-course high dose therapy, low-dose therapy for less than 2 weeks, alternate-day treatment, and topical, intraarticular, and intrabursal administration. Oral polio vaccine is contraindicated until the immunocompetence of other household members is established. However, mumps, measles, and

Table 57-2. Summary of commonly used vaccines

Vaccine	Dose	Frequency	Contraindications
Influenza	0.5 ml IM	Annual	Egg hypersensitivity
Pneumococcal	0.5 ml IM	Once; may need repeating in 6 to 8 yr in some patient groups.	None
Hepatitis B	Three doses, 1.0 ml each at 0, 1, and 6 mo	Probably 10 yr in normal individuals, sooner in immunodeficient.	None
Tetanus, diphtheria	0.5 ml each at 0, 1, and 6 mo	Booster every 10 yr	Severe hypersensitivity or neurologic reaction
Measles	0.5 ml single antigen, MR* or MMR,† SC	See text	Febrile illness, recent immunoglobulin, blood products, pregnancy, immunodeficiency
Rubella	0.5 ml MMR† SC	Not recommended	Recent immunoglobulin, blood products, pregnancy, immunodeficiency, neomycin sensitivity
Mumps	0.5 ml MMR† SC	Not recommended	Recent immunoglobulin, blood products, pregnancy, immunodeficiency, anaphylactic reactions
Hemophilus influenza type b	0.5 ml IM	Not recommended	Not recommended

*MR, measles and rubella vaccination.
†MMR, measles, mumps, and rubella vaccination.

rubella vaccines can be given in such families because, although the recipients will shed vaccine virus, infection is not transmitted to others.

A history of reactions consisting of mild local tenderness, redness, swelling, or fever of less than 40.5° C, a mild acute upper respiratory or gastrointestinal illness with fever of less than 38° C, current antimicrobial therapy, convalescence from a recent illness, pregnancy in another household contact, recent exposure to an infectious disease, breast feeding, personal history of allergies unless there have been anaphylactic reactions to neomycin or streptomycin, and a family history of allergies to vaccination, or seizures are not valid contraindications to vaccination.

Socioeconomic issues. In the past decade, much attention has been given to the cost effectiveness and cost-benefit ratio of adult immunization. Influenza and pneumococcal vaccines have been studied most. Both have been found to be highly cost effective if given to persons 65 years of age or older, and to younger persons with high-risk conditions.[93] Other studies have analyzed the indications for serologic screening in hepatitis B vaccination programs for health care workers, and guidelines have been established identifying those groups in whom such screening is cost effective.[93] The cost effectiveness of other vaccines recommended for routine use in adults has not yet been studied. However, the high costs of controlling outbreaks of measles and rubella have been documented repeatedly. This, coupled with the continuing high mortality of rare cases of tetanus, suggests that even in the absence of formal cost-effective analyses, the benefits of vaccinating adults against these diseases are substantial.

In spite of the generally favorable physician attitudes toward adult vaccines and extensive data supporting their cost effectiveness, adult immunization is not widespread. In particular, influenza and pneumococcal vaccines are grossly underused. In the United States, nearly half of elderly people do not regard influenza as a threat to health and consider the vaccine unnecessary. An even greater proportion of this subgroup is unfamiliar with the importance of pneumococcal infections. Thus, only 20% of high-risk people receive influenza vaccine each year, and only 10% to 15% have ever received pneumococcal vaccine.

In addition to physicians, hospitals can also play important roles in immunizing adults against vaccine-preventable diseases. Although prenatal screening for rubella antibody has become routine, greater efforts are needed to ensure that pregnant women who are not immune are given rubella vaccine after they deliver. Serologic screening of all pregnant women for hepatitis B is now recommended to identify all carriers of the virus. Newborn infants of carriers can then be given hepatitis B immunoglobulin and hepatitis B vaccine. Similarly, ensuring that health-care workers themselves are adequately protected against hepa-

titis B, rubella, measles, and other diseases preventable through vaccine, especially influenza, requires an organized approach. The American College Health Association now recommends that all students have documented evidence of immunity against measles, mumps, rubella, tetanus, and diphtheria. Many colleges have successfully implemented these recommendations by requiring such evidence before students enroll. Regulations recently mandated by the Occupational Safety and Health Administration (OSHA) now require all health-care institutions to bear the cost of hepatitis B vaccination for their employees. Thus one hopes that the rate of vaccination will continue the upward trend that began when many institutions voluntarily instituted this policy. However, financial incentives do not always succeed in penetrating the veneer of complacency and misconception; unfortunately, Medicare reimbursement for pneumococcal immunization has had no discernible effect on the use of this important vaccine.

Influenza

Influenza attack rates often approach 20% to 30%. Outbreaks of influenza often disrupt community life and cause dramatic increases in the use of health care services. It is estimated that 172,000 hospitalizations at a cost of more than $600 million occur per epidemic. Estimates of the cost of a severe epidemic are greater than $12 billion.[16] During influenza epidemics from 1972 to 1981, total influenza-associated excess mortality was 200,000, with an average of more than 20,000 influenza-associated deaths per year.[139] Elderly people and those with certain underlying medical conditions, especially cardiopulmonary diseases, are at increased risk of experiencing more severe and complicated illness, usually secondary bacterial pneumonia. Such patients are also much more likely to require hospitalization. From 80% to 90% of influenza-associated mortality occurs in people 65 years of age and older. Influenza A viruses are classified into subtypes on the basis of their hemagglutinin (H) and neuraminidase (N) antigens into H1, H2, H3, N1, and N2 subtypes. These represent the antigenic variance of influenza A viruses that cause widespread human disease. These antigens also change with time, a phenomenon called *antigenic drift*. Therefore eventually infection or vaccination with one strain will not protect against infection with a distantly related strain of the same subtype. This antigenic drift and occasionally abrupt antigenic shift from one influenza virus subtype to another accounts for the continued recurrence of major outbreaks of this disease.

Indications. Influenza vaccine is indicated for all people who are at increased risk of influenza-related complications, and for those who are likely to transmit infection to high-risk persons. Therefore, at highest risk are adults and children 6 months of age or more with chronic cardiopulmonary disorders who have required medical care or hospitalization in the preceding year, as well as nursing home and chronic care facility residents. Next in priority are those with diabetes mellitus, renal disease, hemoglobinopathies, HIV infection or other immunosuppression, and otherwise healthy people 65 years of age and older. Children, adolescents, and young adults who are on long-term aspirin therapy also should be vaccinated because they are at risk of contracting Reye's syndrome if they develop influenza.

Healthy people capable of transmitting infection to high-risk individuals also need to be vaccinated. This category includes physicians, nurses, and other health-care workers, especially those who have regular contact with high-risk patients in hospitals and chronic care facilities. Families with high-risk members also should be vaccinated.

People without high-risk conditions can be given the influenza vaccine if they wish to reduce their risk of developing influenza. Such individuals include those who provide essential community services that might otherwise be disrupted during an outbreak, such as police and firefighters.

The vaccine is considered safe for the fetus. Pregnant women should be vaccinated if they have underlying high-risk medical conditions. Although vaccination can be delayed until after the first trimester, it should not be postponed if the high-risk pregnant women would be in her first trimester during the influenza season.

Vaccine. The influenza vaccine is made from egg-grown viruses that are highly purified and inactivated; it cannot cause infection. The vaccine contains two type-A strains (H1,N1 and H3,N2) and one type-B strain, representing the most recent influenza viruses. The vaccine is available in both whole-virus and split-virus (subvirion) preparations. In adults, the two preparations are generally similarly effective and tolerated. In children, split-virus vaccines are often better tolerated.

Administration. The vaccine should be administered intramuscularly only. The adult dose is 0.5 ml. Influenza vaccine can be administered simultaneously with pneumococcal vaccine as long as the two are given at separate sites. Although studies have not been conducted, it is reasonable to assume that this vaccine can also be given at the same time as other vaccines as long as separate sites are used. Optimally, the vaccine is administered in November but can be given in the period September through February each year.

Clinical effectiveness. The protection afforded by influenza vaccination is best correlated with serum antihemagglutinin antibodies. Vaccination of younger adults is associated with a 70% to 80% reduction in clinical illness. In older individuals the efficacy of the vaccine may be less. In nursing home residents, while the vaccine may be only 30% to 40% effective in preventing clinical illness, it is effective in preventing pneumonia, hospitalization, and

death. Moreover, in residential institutions, vaccination rates of greater than 80% can create herd immunity, with the result that only sporadic cases rather than outbreaks of influenza occur. Currently, it is estimated that approximately 22% to 32% of noninstitutional elderly patients and approximately 10% of younger high-risk patients receive the vaccine each year.

Revaccination. People for whom influenza vaccination is indicated should be revaccinated each year with the currently recommended vaccine. Physicians need to establish procedures to ensure that their high-risk patients are notified each year of the need to be revaccinated. Patients also should be encouraged to ask for influenza vaccination each year.

Adverse reactions, precautions, and contraindications. Influenza vaccine is an inactivated preparation and does not contain infectious virus. Therefore it is incapable of producing respiratory or other illness. Occasional anecdotal respiratory illnesses after vaccination represent coincidental unrelated infection.

The most frequent side effect of vaccination is transient injection site soreness. Two types of systemic reactions may be seen. Transient fever, myalgias, and malaise may be seen in younger first-time vaccinees. More severe immediate hypersensitivity reactions ranging from hives to anaphylaxis are extremely rare. These are probably caused by small amounts of residual egg protein in the vaccine, when given to persons with the severe egg allergy. In 1976, swine flu vaccination was associated with an increased incidence of the Guillain-Barré syndrome. Since then, no association between influenza vaccination and the Guillain-Barré syndrome or other serious neurologic conditions has been noted.

Contraindications include an anaphylactic hypersensitivity to influenza vaccine. Such reactions include hives, lip or tongue swelling, respiratory distress, or collapse after the ingestion of eggs. Asthma or other allergic responses after occupational exposure to egg protein are also contraindications. People who eat eggs or egg-containing foods without incident can be vaccinated safely.

Antiviral prophylaxis and therapy. Amantadine hydrochloride is an effective prophylactic and therapeutic agent against influenza A virus infection. It is not effective against influenza B. Rimantadine hydrochloride is a related drug with similar activity that may be licensed in the near future. Both of these drugs interfere with viral replication. They are 70% to 90% effective when given prophylactically to healthy adults. Amantadine prophylaxis is recommended as an adjunct to vaccination when vaccine is given after the onset of a community outbreak of influenza. It should be taken for 2 weeks to provide early protection until the appearance of vaccine-induced antibody. It is also recommended for unvaccinated household mothers and other caregivers who have close contact with high-risk individuals in the home, and for high-risk people for whom influenza vaccine is contraindicated. In addition, amantadine needs to be considered as supplemental protection for immunodeficient people, including those with HIV infection who can be expected to have a suboptimal antibody response to influenza vaccinations.

Amantadine prophylaxis is especially useful in controlling outbreaks of influenza among high-risk people in nursing homes, chronic-care facilities, and hospitals. When an outbreak is recognized, all patients should receive the drug regardless of whether they have previously received the vaccine. Amantadine also should be given to unvaccinated staff members who care for high-risk patients.

Treatment with amantadine can shorten the duration of fever and severity of other symptoms in healthy adults. It must be given within 24 to 48 hours of the onset of illness and continued until 48 hours after resolution of signs and symptoms.

Amantadine does not interfere with the normal antibody response to influenza A virus infection. The dosage recommendations for amantadine in adults have recently been revised. Because of reports of nausea, dizziness, insomnia, and difficulty with concentration with the earlier 200 mg/day dose, and the observation that side effects were fewer with the lower doses, the current recommendation is to give 100 mg/day after a single loading dose of 200 mg. Amantadine is excreted unchanged in the urine and may accumulate in persons who have reduced kidney function. For this reason, people 65 years of age and older should not be given more than 100 mg/day for either prophylaxis or treatment. Further reductions may be necessary in individuals with overt renal disease. Because high doses may be epileptogenic, patients with seizure disorders should not receive more than 100 mg/day.

Pneumococcal disease

Pneumococcal infection is the most common bacterial cause of mild lower respiratory tract infection, as well as severe life-threatening pneumonia. Approximately 150,000 to 570,000 cases of pneumococcal pneumonia, 16,000 to 55,000 cases of pneumococcal bacteremia, and 2,600 to 6,200 cases of pneumococcal meningitis occur annually. Of these cases, 5% of patients with pneumonia, 20% of patients with bacteremia, and 30% of patients with meningitis die, resulting in a total of 40,000 pneumococcal-related deaths annually. Mortality is highest among patients with underlying medical conditions and in older people despite therapy with antibiotics, presumably because of irreversible physiologic injury. In this country, the estimated incidence of pneumococcal pneumonia is 68 to 260 cases per 100,000 persons per year. The overall case fatality rate in treated patients is approximately 5%. Pneumococci are also an underrecognized cause of nosocomial pneumonia. Both the incidence of disease and the case fatality rate increase with age and with underlying medical

conditions such as chronic cardiac and pulmonary disease, hepatic and renal failure, alcoholism, anatomic and functional asplenia, multiple myeloma, and Hodgkin's disease. Approximately 5% to 20% of all pneumococcal pneumonia is associated with bacteremia. The case fatality rate of bacteremic disease is approximately 15% to 25%, but among patients with underlying medical conditions it is increased to 30% or more. In elderly patients with pneumococcal bacteremia, mortality can be as high as 60%. Pneumococcal meningitis is infrequent, with an incidence of 1 to 3 per 100,000 persons per year, but the overall mortality rate is 30%, and it rises to 65% in patients over 70 years of age.

Ironically, the mortality rates for pneumococcal infections have not improved substantially in recent decades, despite the prompt use of appropriate antimicrobial chemotherapy and intensive care support. Most deaths occur in patients irreversibly injured early in the course of their infections. Moderate penicillin resistance has been documented among pneumococcal isolates in several countries, but this is not an important factor in treatment failures in the United States.

Indications. This vaccine is indicated for all adult patients who have underlying conditions associated with either an increased susceptibility to infection or increased risk from serious disease caused by infection and its complications. These patients are usually healthy adults who are 65 years of age or older; those with chronic cardiac or pulmonary diseases, especially congestive heart failure, recurrent bronchitis, and chronic obstructive lung disease; and those with anatomic or functional asplenia, chronic liver disease, alcoholism, and diabetes mellitus. Patients with chronic renal failure, Hodgkin's disease, chronic lymphatic leukemia, or multiple myeloma and those receiving hemodialysis or chemotherapy for malignancies or organ transplantation should also be vaccinated but have diminished antibody responses and therefore diminished benefit from the vaccine. Patients with HIV infection should be vaccinated[181] because they are at high risk for pneumococcal disease. They too may suffer from decreased antibody responsiveness. Patients with cerebrospinal fluid (CSF) leaks (CSF rhinorrhea) caused by trauma or neurosurgery should also be vaccinated, because recurrent pneumococcal meningitis is frequent in this patient group.

Whenever possible this vaccine should be given before elective splenectomy and chemotherapy to maximize the antibody response.

Vaccine. The pneumococcal vaccine in use since 1983 contains capsular polysaccharide extracted from 23 pneumococcal types responsible for 85% to 90% of bacteremic infections. This vaccine replaced the earlier 14-valent vaccine that was licensed in 1977. Pneumococcal capsular polysaccharide antigens induce type-specific antibodies of the immunoglobulin G2 subclass that enhance the opsonization, phagocytosis, and killing of pneumococci by leukocytes and fixed phagocytic cells.

The 23-valent vaccine contains 25 mcg of each capsular polysaccharide antigen, as opposed to 50 mcg of each antigen in the 14-valent vaccine. After vaccination with either the 14- or 23-valent vaccine, 80% or more of healthy young adults develop a twofold or greater rise in antibody titer to each antigen. Antibody levels decline over the next few years, but in most subjects protective levels are maintained for 7 to 10 years. Among elderly subjects, antibody levels may decline below levels considered to be protective after 6 or more years. Compared with normal young adults, lower antibody responses are seen in the elderly and those with diabetes mellitus, chronic obstructive pulmonary disease, and alcoholic cirrhosis. However, these levels are considered adequate for protection. Antibody responses are also excellent in patients with splenectomy and sickle cell disease. In Hodgkin's disease, pneumococcal vaccination is effective if given before splenectomy, radiation, or chemotherapy. After treatment has begun these patients respond less well. In those with leukemia, lymphoma, multiple myeloma, and HIV infection, the antibody response to pneumococcal vaccination is suboptimal even before therapy. In hemodialysis patients, renal transplant recipients, and those with the nephrotic syndrome, the initial antibody response is lower, and antibody levels decline more rapidly than in normal subjects.

Administration. The pneumococcal vaccine is given as a single intramuscular dose of 0.5 ml. Hospital discharge is a convenient time for vaccination. Because the indications for pneumococcal and influenza vaccines are similar, annual influenza vaccination should serve as a reminder for this vaccination as well. These two vaccines can be given simultaneously, provided they are administered at different sites, with no decrease in the antibody response and also no increase in the adverse reaction rate. The cost of the vaccine and its administration is partially reimbursed by Medicare both in the hospital and in the office.

Clinical effectiveness. Pneumococcal vaccine has been found to be 60% to 95% effective in certain moderate- to high-risk clinical groups,[113] although somewhat lower efficacy figures of 60% to 82% are seen in low-, moderate-, and high-risk patients with bacteremic disease.[207]

Although several earlier randomized controlled trials around the world showed the vaccine to be protective in healthy young adults, three randomized placebo controlled trials in this country conducted in older adults have raised doubts about the universal efficacy of this vaccine. The CDC has compared the type distribution of pneumococci isolated from blood or cerebrospinal fluid obtained from 1635 vaccinated people with the type distribution of isolates obtained from unvaccinated people. These studies have indicated an overall protective efficacy of 64%. Moreover, protection was shown in patients with diabetes mellitus, heart disease, and lung disease, and in those

above 55 years of age, although it was not consistently seen in those with alcoholism. One can conclude from the various studies conducted to date that pneumococcal vaccination is effective in reducing the incidence of pneumococcal bacteremia and pneumonia among younger patients in whom rates of pneumococcal disease are high. Pneumococcal vaccination also appears to be useful in reducing the incidence of pneumococcal bacteremia among older high-risk patients who have good antibody responses to vaccination. The vaccine appears to have little efficacy in patients who are severely immunocompromised.[32]

Revaccination. Revaccination with the 23-valent pneumococcal vaccine is now recommended for all individuals who received the older 14-valent pneumococcal vaccine if they are at highest risk for serious or fatal pneumococcal infection (e.g., those with surgical or functional asplenia). Revaccination also should be strongly considered for high-risk individuals who were vaccinated 6 or more years earlier.[93] In patients with nephrotic syndrome and renal failure and in transplant recipients, antibody titers decline rapidly, and revaccination after 3 to 5 years is recommended. In these patient groups, adverse reactions after revaccination have not been a problem.

Adverse reactions, precautions, and contraindications. Side effects are usually minor and local, such as pain or redness at the injection site, which occurs in about 50% of people given the 14-valent vaccine. Although local Arthus-like reactions have been reported after revaccination with the 14-valent vaccine, they are very infrequent after revaccination with the current 23-valent vaccine. No neurologic disorders, such as Guillain-Barré syndrome, have been observed after pneumococcal vaccination. Adverse consequences to the fetus have not been reported in women vaccinated during pregnancy. Pregnant women with high-risk conditions, such as heart, lung, or sickle cell disease, can be vaccinated, although it is preferable to do so before pregnancy or after the first trimester.

Hepatitis B infection

Epidemiology. Hepatitis B virus (HBV) infection occurs worldwide with highly variable prevalence rates. The pool from which the infection originates is a human reservoir of persistently infected individuals that occurs in nearly all communities worldwide.

In those areas of the world where HBV infection is rampant and prevalence rates are high, infection typically occurs early in life and principally as a consequence of maternal-neonatal spread and horizontal spread among children. Most children are seropositive by the age of 10 to 15 years.[71] In contrast, in areas with moderate prevalence rates, infection does not occur until later, a substantial number having serologic markers by the age 25 years. Sexual activity may play a role in this pattern. In the United States and other low-prevalence areas, serologic markers of HBV infection are found in less than 5% of the general population. Parenteral drug abuse, sexual activity, occupationally acquired infection, and imported cases of HBV infection in immigrants or travelers returning from abroad may be the principal mechanisms of transmission in this subgroup. In the United States peak attack rates of HBV infection are seen in the age group 15 to 34 years, and the risk of infection in children appears to be low.[206]

Modes of transmission. The principal modes of transmission of the hepatitis B virus are contact transmission, maternal-neonatal transmission, and percutaneous transmission. Respiratory or airborne modes of transmission, and food and water-borne spread are not accepted transmission modes at present. The role of biting insects and other insects also remains open to question.

Contact transmission occurs via HBV-contaminated body secretions, including semen, vaginal secretions, blood, and saliva. This may occur between sexual contacts as well as between some household members who do not engage in sexual activity.

Less than 5% to 10% of neonatal HBV infections result from infection in utero.[240] This presumably occurs by transplacental leakage of HBV-contaminated maternal blood, resulting from uterine contractions and the disruption of placental barriers.[165] However, the vast majority of HBV infections in this setting occur as a consequence of exposure of the neonate to the virus during labor, delivery, or the early postpartum period. The available data on the efficacy of cesarean section in reducing the risk of intrapartum HBV infection are conflicting at present. Breast feeding, however, does not seem to increase the risk of transmission of this virus.

Percutaneous inoculation is the most efficient mode of HBV transfer. The infection is thus very common in intravenous drug abusers who share needles. It is also a common consequence among health-care workers who are accidentally exposed via needle stick injury. The HBV acquisition risk in this situation is about 5%. This risk increases to 20% if the source of exposure has definite serologic markers of HBV infection (i.e., HBsAg-negative and HBeAg-positive serologic status). Acupuncture needles, tattoo needles, and ear-piercing equipment may be responsible for sporadic cases as well as many outbreaks. Communal use of water for bathing also has been implicated in spread of this disease. Percutaneous transmission also may occur via transplantation of HBV-contaminated organs. Lastly, permucosal transfer may result when mucosal surfaces are accidentally splashed with contaminated biomaterials.

Serologic markers. The hepatitis B surface antigen (HBsAg) is the first readily identifiable serologic marker of this infection. This appears before ALT elevation and may be the only serum marker in those patients who manifest the HBV-associated prodromal serum-sickness–like syndrome. The HBsAg generally becomes undetectable within a few weeks to a few months after its appearance. In a mi-

nority of cases it may disappear before the onset of symptoms. In contrast, the persistence of HBsAg beyond 6 months suggests the development of the HBV carrier state. Pre-S proteins (pre-S1 and pre-S2) have been identified in the sera of HBV-infected patients during the period in which HBsAg is present and HBV replication is active. Both these proteins disappear while HBsAg is still present.[79] The corresponding IgM and IgG antibodies to the pre-S proteins develop shortly thereafter and may persist or may disappear with the development of circulating antibody to HBsAg (anti-HBs). These proteins and their antibodies are not commercially measurable.

The e antigen (HBeAg) is a derivative of the core antigen (HBcAg) and is usually detected days to weeks after the appearance of HBsAg in acute HBV infection. Hbcag, on the other hand, is generally not detectable in serum. HBeAg is a marker of active HBV replication, and in uncomplicated acute HBV infection it disappears before HBsAg. Shortly after the disappearance of HBeAg, its corresponding antibody, anti-HBe, becomes detectable and may persist for long periods.

HBV viral DNA is the single best marker of active viral replication during the early phase, generally becoming undetectable within weeks.[107] Its persistence indicates continued infection with continued infectivity.

Antibody to the core antigen (anti-HBc) is detected shortly after HBsAg is detected and before anti-HBs becomes detectable. Initially most of the anti-HBc is of the IgM type, and this peaks within several weeks after the onset of infection. It remains detectable after the disappearance of the HBsAg. *The IgM anti-HBc is the single most sensitive test for acute HBV infection.* In most patients IgM anti-HBc disappears by 4 to 8 months after its appearance. However, the results for anti-HBc remain positive, being predominantly due to IgG anti-HBc during the late convalescence from HBV infection. The levels of this antibody decline slowly over a long period of time.

Antibody to HBs (anti-HBs) usually becomes detectable as the titer of HBsAg declines, and this antibody reaches peak levels within a few months. This antibody is believed to be neutralizing and protective in nature. During very late convalescence the titer of anti-HBs begins to drop and in very rare cases may eventually become undetectable.

Diagnosis. The serologic diagnosis of acute HBV infection requires assays for HBsAg and IgM anti-HBc. Even though HBsAg may have become undetectable by the time testing is done in a minority of patients, IgM anti-HBc testing will identify all infected patients.

Prevention. Limiting sexual activity, practicing "safe sex," and avoiding other means of percutaneous exposure to body fluids is desirable for the prevention of this infection. The effect of these interventions may be limited, however, by the fact that for as many as 30% to 40% of acute HBV infections, the route of transmission and source remain uncertain. Therefore the key to the control of this infectious disease lies in the induction of preinfection immunity (i.e., immunoprophylaxis).

Vaccine. The protective antibody is the anti-HBs neutralizing antibody. This may be administered preformed exogenously in the form of hepatitis B immunoglobulin (HBIG) prepared from patients who have recovered from active HBV infection, although this is rarely used alone. Preferred approaches involve the combined use of HBV vaccine and HBIG. HBsAg is the active immunogenic element of both the original plasma-derived and the more recent yeast-recombinant HBV vaccine. The latter recombinant vaccines contain HBsAg particles without HBV DNA, HBcAg, HBeAg, and pre-S sequences. They are safe, immunogenic, and effective. A successful immune response to active immunization by vaccination is the appearance of anti-HBs alone. This is in striking contrast to the markers of natural HBV infection, which induces the production of both anti-HBc and anti-HBs. Protection is usually life-long, although anti-HBs levels may diminish with time. Specific values below which immunity is uncertain have not yet been established. The timing and necessity of booster doses also remain controversial.

Administration. HBV vaccine is injected into the deltoid muscle in children and adults and into the anterolateral muscle of the thigh in infants. A three-dose schedule is given at 0, 1, and 6 months. The usual adult dose is 1 ml, and 0.5 ml is used for infants. Intragluteal injections are avoided because of reports of suboptimal immune response when this site is used. Although accelerated schedules with shorter intervals may provide more rapid induction of protective levels of HBs, the long-term protection afforded by these regimes is still open to question. Under normal conditions of the regimen of 0, 1, and 6 months, anti-HBs levels peak 7 to 10 months after the first dose.

Indications. Preexposure prophylaxis with HBV vaccine is recommended for homosexual or bisexual men; people with a history of STDs; medical personnel exposed to body fluids, such as surgeons, pathologists, medical technicians, blood bank technologists, dialysis workers, OR, ICU, and ER staff, dental professionals, and other first responders; parenteral drug-users; inmates and staff of institutions for the mentally retarded; frequent recipients of blood products; and prison inmates. HBV vaccine also should be given to travelers to HBV-endemic areas who anticipate intimate contact with the local population.

All unvaccinated health workers who are exposed to HBV via needle sticks, lacerations, or splashing accidents should be given combined passive-active immunization with HBIG and HBV vaccine. The dose of HBIG is 0.06 ml/kg body weight as soon as possible after exposure, given along with the first of three 1 ml doses at a different site in the deltoid muscle. Subsequent doses of the HBV vaccine are given 1 and 6 months later. Sexual contacts of patients with acute HBV infection require a single dose of 0.06 ml/kg body weight of HBIG within 14 days of expo-

sure. With the exception of male homosexuals and promiscuous heterosexuals, HBV vaccine is not indicated in this setting. In contrast, HBV vaccine alone is recommended for intimate and household contacts of index case patients with chronic HBV infection. Neither form of immunoprophylaxis is recommended for casual contacts of HBsAg-positive patients, whether acute or chronic.

Screening of all pregnant women to determine carrier status or the universal immunization of all neonates is required for the prevention of maternal–neonatal transmission of this disease. Neonates of HBsAg-positive mothers should be given 0.5 ml of HBIG within a few hours of birth, followed by 0.5 ml of HBV vaccine in the contralateral thigh a week later and again at 1 and 6 months. The protective efficacy of the combined program exceeds 90%.[239]

Tetanus and diphtheria

Tetanus is caused when spores of *Clostridium tetani* contaminate a wound, germinate, and produce a powerful toxin, tetanospasmin, which in turn is responsible for the dramatic findings associated with the disease.

The incidence of tetanus has declined dramatically in the United States in the last few decades, with only 50 to 90 cases now reported each year. During 1985 and 1986, 147 cases were reported in the United States.[77] Virtually all disease occurs in unimmunized or inadequately immunized patients. Adults 60 years of age or older make up 60% of all tetanus cases. The overall mortality is 31% but rises to 42% in persons 50 years of age or older.

Indications and administration. Most adolescents and young adults have completed a three-dose primary series of tetanus and diphtheria toxoids, usually in combination with pertussis vaccine during childhood. If there is doubt regarding the completion of this primary series, two doses of 0.5 ml each of combined tetanus-diphtheria toxoid should be given intramuscularly at least 4 weeks apart, followed by a third dose at 6 to 12 months. The combined tetanus-diphtheria toxoid should be used to enhance immunity against both diseases simultaneously. Booster doses should be given at 10-year intervals thereafter.

Adverse reactions and contraindictions. Mild reactions of erythema and induration may occur. The only contraindication is a history of a hypersensitivity reaction to a prior dose.

Measles

Measles is usually a benign illness unless complications arise. Most common among these are otitis media and pneumonia. Encephalitis or death may ensue in 1 out of 1000 reported cases. The risk of encephalitis is greater in adults, but the highest case fatality ratio occurs in infants. Measles during pregnancy increases the risk of spontaneous abortion, premature labor, and low birth weight. Although indigenous transmission of measles has been eliminated from most of the United States through widespread vaccination, it is estimated that 100 cases per year are imported, and there is a continuing risk of exposure, particularly for young adults attending college abroad or traveling abroad.

Indications. Measles vaccine is indicated for all adults born in or after 1957 who lack documentation of immunization with live measles vaccine on or after their first birthday, physician-diagnosed measles, or laboratory evidence of immunity. Those who received live measles vaccine before their first birthday, received killed measles vaccine alone or killed measles vaccine followed within three months by a live vaccine, or received a measles vaccine of unknown type between 1963 and 1967 should receive another dose of live measles vaccine.

All college and university students need immunity to this disease because outbreaks have occurred in these settings. The immunity of health-care workers is also important, and especially so when the risk of exposure to natural disease is increased such as during foreign travel. Because long-term protection is not assured after one dose of the measles vaccine, revaccination is recommended for students entering institutions of higher learning and for health-care workers at the time of employment. Many international travelers also will need to be revaccinated. Recently revised recommendations for child immunization also call for a second dose of measles vaccine at school entry (i.e., at 4 to 6 years of age).

In general, susceptible adults who are exposed to measles should be vaccinated. The vaccine is protective only if it is administered within 72 hours of exposure. If exposure does not result in infection, vaccination will protect against subsequent infection. An acceptable alternative is to use immunoglobulin, which can prevent or modify infection if given within 6 days of exposure. Immunoglobulin is particularly indicated if patients have contraindications to measles vaccination. It should not be used, however, in an attempt to control measles outbreaks. The recommended dose is 0.25 ml/kg intramuscularly, not to exceed a total of 15 ml.

Vaccine and clinical effectiveness. The measles vaccine is a live attenuated virus vaccine that is prepared in chick embryo cell culture and is available as monovalent (measles only), as measles and rubella (MR), and as measles, mumps, and rubella (MMR) vaccines. In most circumstances, MMR is the preferred vaccine. A single dose of measles vaccine induces protection in approximately 95% of recipients that in most is probably lifelong.

Administration. Measles vaccine, 0.5 ml as a single antigen, MR vaccine, or MMR vaccine should be given subcutaneously. Whenever two doses are required, they should be separated by no less than 1 month.

Revaccination is not routinely recommended for all adults born after 1956. However, revaccination should be strongly considered for students entering colleges or other institutions of higher learning, and for health-care workers

at the time of employment. If a measles outbreak occurs in an educational or health-care institution, all younger adults should be revaccinated. Adults born after 1956 who plan to travel to areas where measles is highly endemic also should be revaccinated. In individuals with either natural or vaccine-induced immunity, revaccination is not associated with adverse effects.

Adverse reactions, precautions, and contraindications. Adverse reactions do not appear to be age related. A fever greater than 103° F may develop in 5% to 15% of recipients. This reaction generally occurs 5 to 12 days after vaccination and lasts 1 to 2 days. Transient rashes have been reported. The incidence of encephalitis after measles vaccination is lower than the observed background incidence of encephalitis of unknown cause and is much lower than that observed after natural measles itself.

About half of those who previously received killed measles vaccine develop reactions after live measles vaccination. Most are local reactions lasting 1 to 2 days. Such reactions are considerably milder than atypical measles, the illness that follows exposure to natural measles in individuals who have received the killed measles vaccine.

In those with severe febrile illnesses, measles vaccination should be postponed until after recovery. Vaccinations should not be given for at least 6 weeks and preferably 3 months after a person has received immunoglobulin, whole blood, or other antibody-containing blood products.

Because of the theoretical risk to the fetus, measles vaccine should not be given to pregnant women or to women who are considering becoming pregnant within 3 months of vaccination. The vaccine also should not be given to immunocompromised patients. There are no data available on the use of measles vaccine in adults with HIV infection, but it is unnecessary to undertake serologic testing for HIV infection for the purpose of making a decision regarding measles vaccination. In immunocompromised individuals, including those with HIV infection, especially those who are symptomatic, postexposure prophylaxis with immunoglobulin should be strongly considered regardless of the history of measles or measles vaccination.

Measles has no effect on clinical tuberculosis. If tuberculin skin testing is needed, it should be done on the day of vaccination and the result read 48 to 72 hours later. In recent vaccinees, it is prudent to wait 4 to 6 weeks after giving measles vaccine before administering a tuberculin skin test because measles vaccination may temporarily suppress tuberculin reactivity.

People with a history of anaphylactic reactions after ingesting eggs or to neomycin should be vaccinated with extreme caution and only under strict protocols that have been developed for this purpose.

Rubella

Rubella was once a common childhood disease, the transmission of which has been almost totally interrupted by universal immunization. Because of failure to vaccinate adolescents and adults, the reported decrease in incidence has been primarily seen in children. Therefore an estimated 10% to 15% of young adults remain susceptible to rubella, and limited outbreaks continue to be reported, primarily in congregated settings such as universities, colleges, and employment venues, most notably hospitals.

Rubella infection in early pregnancy, especially in the first trimester, results in abortions, miscarriages, still births, and other fetal abnormalities. Therefore one of the primary objectives of rubella immunization is to prevent fetal infection and consequent congenital rubella syndrome.

Vaccination of children has prevented epidemics of rubella and congenital rubella syndrome and, one hopes, will lead to the elimination of this syndrome as vaccinated people reach childbearing age. However, increased efforts to ensure that all women of childbearing age are vaccinated can hasten the elimination of this disorder.

Indications. The rubella vaccine is recommended for adults, particularly women, unless there is proof of immunity (documented rubella vaccination on or after their first birthday, or a positive serologic test), or the vaccine is specifically contraindicated. In particular, susceptible women of childbearing age who are not pregnant should receive a rubella vaccine. Ideally, every step should be taken to vaccinate women whenever they have contact with the health care system. Evidence of rubella immunity should be required for all people in colleges and universities. Programs in the workplace and other settings where women of childbearing age congregate should ensure that the rubella-immune status of every female employee is ascertained and that vaccination is made available to those who are not immune. All health-care workers, men and women alike, who might be at risk of exposure to patients infected with rubella virus or who might have contact with pregnant women also should be immune.

Serologic testing can be used to determine immunity; however, routine testing of all women of childbearing age has not been found to be cost-effective, and the rates of follow-up immunization have been low. However, vaccination of women who are not pregnant and have no known history of vaccination is justifiable without serologic testing.

Vaccine and clinical effectiveness. Rubella vaccine is a live attenuated vaccine that is prepared in human diploid cells (RA 27/3). It is available as a monovalent vaccine (rubella only) as well as in combinations: measles and rubella (MR), and mumps, measles, and rubella (MMR). In most circumstances, MMR is the preferred vaccine.

A single dose of live attenuated rubella vaccine provides long-term, probably lifetime immunity to over 90% of recipients. Protection is effective against both clinical disease and asymptomatic viremia.

Although some vaccine recipients may shed small amounts of vaccine virus from the pharynx, more than 15 years of experience provides no evidence that transmission occurs from vaccinated individuals. Thus there is no contraindication to immunizing contacts of pregnant women.

Administration and revaccination. A single dose, 0.5 ml of reconstituted vaccine, preferably MMR, should be administered subcutaneously. Revaccination is currently not recommended because immunity after single dose vaccination is thought to be lifelong. However, MMR is the preferred vaccine if measles or mumps vaccines are to be given. The administration of rubella vaccine to a person with either naturally acquired or vaccine-induced immunity is not associated with an increased risk of adverse reactions.

Adverse reactions, precautions, and contraindications. Adverse reactions occur only in susceptible vaccinees; those already immune to rubella are at no risk of developing untoward reactions. Up to 40% of these persons may develop joint pain, usually in the small peripheral joints. Frank arthritis is infrequent. When joint symptoms occur, they generally begin within 1 to 4 weeks of immunization and rarely last for more than 10 days. Transient peripheral neuritis, parasthesias, and extremity pain may occur rarely.

Because of the theoretical risk to the fetus, women of childbearing age should receive this vaccine only if they are not pregnant. They should also be counseled not to become pregnant for 3 months after vaccination. If a pregnant woman is vaccinated or becomes pregnant within 3 months of vaccination, she needs to be counseled on the theoretical risks to the fetus. Studies by the CDC of such women who carry their pregnancies to term have found no cases of malformations compatible with congenital rubella syndrome. The risk of rubella-vaccine–associated malformations appears to be so small that it is negligible. Although the final decision must be made individually, rubella vaccination during pregnancy is generally not a reason to recommend termination of pregnancy.

The rubella vaccine does contain trace amounts of neomycin, to which the rare patient may be allergic. Therefore patients with a history of anaphylaxis after receipt of neomycin should not be given the rubella vaccine.

Ideally, rubella vaccine should be given at least 14 days before the administration of immunoglobulin, whole blood, or other blood products that contain antibody, or vaccination should be deferred for at least 6 weeks, or preferably 3 months, after their administration. However, previous administration of such blood products is not a contraindication to postpartum vaccination. In such cases, serologic testing should be done 6 to 8 weeks after vaccination to ensure that seroconversion has occurred and revaccination is not necessary.

The vaccine should not be given to immunocompromised patients. It is not known whether this vaccine can be given safely to adults with HIV infection.

Mumps

Although mumps is generally a self-limited disease in the pediatric population, in adults it can be associated with complications. The most notable of these is orchitis, which is seen in up to one fifth of postpubertal males with this infection. Mumps orchitis is usually unilateral and rarely results in sterility. Meningeal signs can appear in up to 15% of cases, with nerve deafness occurring in 1 per 15,000 cases.

Indications. The vaccine is indicated for adults who are believed to be susceptible to the infection. People born before 1957 are considered naturally immune because of the lack of vaccination and subsequent natural immunity after infection in the general population before this date. Those born after 1957 are usually considered susceptible unless they can document physician-diagnosed mumps, have a record of prior adequate vaccination, or have laboratory evidence of immunity. Therefore special efforts need to be made to ensure that all college and university students are in fact immune to mumps because outbreaks have occurred in these settings.

Vaccine. Mumps vaccine is a live attenuated virus vaccine that is prepared in chick embryo culture. It is available as a monovalent (mumps only) vaccine and in combinations as MR (mumps, rubella) and MMR (mumps, measles, rubella) vaccines. In general, the preferred vaccine is the MMR vaccine.

Administration. A single dose of 0.5 ml of the reconstituted vaccine (preferably MMR) should be administered subcutaneously.

Clinical effectiveness. A single dose of the vaccine results in protective levels of antibody in about 90% of recipients. The duration of immunity is long, and in epidemic situations vaccine efficacy rates have ranged from 75% to 90%.

Revaccination. Revaccination is not currently recommended because immunity after a single dose is thought to be long lasting. However, if the vaccine is administered to a person who already has natural immunity or vaccine-induced immunity, such an event is not associated with adverse affects.

Adverse reactions, precautions, and contraindications. Parotitis after mumps vaccination has been reported rarely. Allergic reactions including rash, pruritus, and purpura have been temporarily associated with vaccination, but they are uncommon and usually mild and transient. Central nervous system dysfunction may rarely occur after mumps vaccination.

Hemophilus influenzae type B

Hemophilus influenzae type B is an unusual cause of invasive disease in adults. When it is pathogenic, the source of which is usually organisms that colonize the respiratory tract, it usually causes otitis media and bronchitis, and such disease is not preventable by *Hemophilus influenzae* type B vaccination. In contrast, however, more than 85% of pediatric cases in children less than 5 years of age are caused by *Hemophilus influenzae* type B, which is the leading cause of bacterial meningitis in this age group.

Indications. There are no data to support routine immunization of adults or children above the age of 5 with *Hemophilus influenzae* type B vaccine. This includes those with splenectomy, sickle cell disease, Hodgkin's disease, and other hematological malignancies as well as other immunosuppressed patients on the basis of their increased susceptibility to infection with encapsulated microorganisms. However, because of the safety of the vaccine and the fact that is well tolerated, there appear to be no contraindications to its use on an individual basis. There is no rationale, however, for the use of this vaccine to prevent recurrent sinusitis and bronchitis in adults because these infections are usually associated with nontypeable Hemophilus influenzae organisms that are not affected by antibody levels to *Hemophilus influenzae* type B. The vaccine is also not necessary for health care personnel and day-care workers who frequently come in contact with children with invasive *Hemophilus influenzae* type B disease. In such situations, vaccination against the bacteria is not effective in preventing secondary cases of invasive disease. Instead, rifampin prophylaxis is recommended, and the reader is referred to the section on preventive antibiotics. The dose of rifampin is 20 mg/kg once daily for 4 days, the maximum daily dose being 600 mg.

Vaccine. The first vaccine was licensed in the United States in 1955. This was composed of *Hemophilus influenzae* type B capsular polysaccharide polyribosylribitolphosphate (PRP). Subsequently, two conjugated vaccines were licensed in December 1987.

There are, however, not much data available about the antigenicity of *Hemophilus influenzae* type B vaccine in adults, or of the efficacy of this vaccine in subgroups of adults who might be at risk for invasive *Hemophilus influenzae* disease.

Administration. *Hemophilus influenzae* type B vaccine or conjugate vaccine should be administered as a single dose of 0.5 ml given intramuscularly.

Clinical effectiveness. As mentioned previously, there are no studies of vaccine efficacy in the subgroup of adults who might be at risk for invasive disease. However, the conjugate vaccines licensed in December 1987 are more antigenic than the PRP vaccine in children under the age of 2. Clinical trials in Finland have shown that the PRP vaccine is effective in preventing disease in children 2 years of age and older, whereas conjugate vaccines have also been found to be protective when given to infants 3 to 6 months of age.

Revaccination. Revaccination of children and adults with the conjugate vaccine is not currently recommended.

Adverse reactions, precautions, and contraindications. In children, mild local side effects occur infrequently, usually appear within 24 hours, and subside rapidly. More severe febrile reactions are uncommon. Reaction rates with *Hemophilus influenzae* type B conjugate vaccines are similar to those with the PRP vaccine.

THE COMMON COLD (VIRAL URI)

Viral infection of the upper respiratory tract is one of the most common human conditions. There is currently no specific therapy for most of its causes.

Although the common cold is mentioned in medical writings since earliest recorded history,[96] it was not until early this century that experiments involving the inoculation of volunteers with filtered nasal secretions from patients with colds led to the theory that a nonbacterial, nonfilterable, etiologic agent was probably responsible for this syndrome.[130] During most of these studies in the middle part of this century, the specific agents responsible were not identified. Not until much later were rhinoviruses identified in the filtered nasal secretions used to inoculate volunteers. These studies did, however, describe important conditions that favored the transmission of cold viruses and host factors related to susceptibility and resistance. The induction of immunity to reinfection with the same secretion pool,[15] the lack of effect of moderate cold and dampness on the risk of infection,[65] and the increased susceptibility of women in the middle third of the menstrual cycle[64] were all described during this period.

Virology

More than 200 viruses have been associated with the common cold syndrome. These include adenoviruses, coronaviruses, influenza viruses, parainfluenza viruses, respiratory syncytial viruses, rhinoviruses, and enteroviruses. The rhinoviruses of the picornaviridae family are by far the most important etiologic agents of the common cold, being responsible for up to one half of all colds. More than 89 distinct serotypes have been accepted and more than 100 have been described. Antigenic variation, driven by immunity, leads to the emergence of new strains. Rhinoviruses are extremely acid labile, a characteristic that separates them from enteroviruses. They are relatively stable in the environment and can survive for long periods on surfaces and fomites. This stability is important for their dissemination in human populations.

Also important causes of the common cold, but about which less is known, are human coronaviruses. At least two distinct serotypes are known to cause human upper respiratory illnesses and reinfections. These viruses are less stable in the environment compared with rhinoviruses.

Adenoviruses, specifically types 1, 2, 5, and 6, are common causes of febrile undifferentiated upper respiratory illness in children. Types 3 and 7 cause pharyngoconjunctival fever in civilians, and types 4, 7, and 21 are associated with disease in military recruits. Type 8 is less associated with epidemic keratoconjunctivitis, and all the above as well as type 11 have been associated with viral pneumonia.

Parainfluenza and respiratory syncytial viruses both belong to the paramyxoviridae family and are more noted for their ability to cause lower respiratory illness in infants and children. They are important etiologic agents of upper respiratory illness in this age group, exemplified by the fact that by the age of 3 years, virtually all children have been infected with parainfluenza type 3 and respiratory syncytial viruses, more than one half of these involving only the upper respiratory tract. Reinfections by these agents, manifesting as the common cold syndrome, are common.

Influenza viruses, commonly considered only in the context of lower respiratory tract disease, also must be considered important causes of the common cold. The influenza C virus is probably an especially important cause of upper tract illness.

Epidemiology

Respiratory infections are among the commonest acute conditions experienced in the United States. An average of three illnesses a year, with a range of six per year for infants to about one per year for people over 60 years of age, has been described in one study.[151] In 1987 data from the National Center for Health Statistics,[160] one fourth of the population reported a common cold that altered their usual activities or caused them to seek medical care. An estimated 62 million colds met that definition and resulted in almost 170 million days of restricted activity, 22 million episodes of seeking medical attention, and 23 and 21 million days lost from work and school respectively. From these statistics the economic burden imposed by viral upper respiratory tract disease in the United States is estimated to be greater than $1 billion each year.

Most respiratory infections are spread by direct contact with the respiratory secretions of infected people.[104] This usually results from hand-to-hand transmission or hand-to-environmental-surface-to-hand transmission, with inoculation of the recipient's eye or nose. The mouth is usually a less effective portal of entry. Direct spread explains the high rate of secondary infection within households. The stability of rhinoviruses facilitates contact spread; virus particles may remain infectious on environmental surfaces for hours or even days. Although there is some experimental evidence to support aerosol transmission of picornaviruses,[52] most studies favor spread by direct contact. Preventive efforts are best directed at reducing secondary infection. Careful hygiene to reduce direct spread of the infection is the mainstay of reducing secondary infection.

The role of climate and temperature change on the transmission of upper respiratory viruses is not completely understood. Cooler temperatures, which promote congregation of people indoors, may thus result in more effective contact. Indeed, in cooler climates respiratory viruses spread more during the cooler months of the year. Each autumn, as enterovirus activity declines, that of rhinoviruses increases. Increasing virus activity also always accompanies the return of children to school. Several studies have demonstrated the importance of school children in the spread of respiratory viruses in the community and in the introduction of these agents into the home.[85] Humidity also may be an important factor, the survival of rhinoviruses being possibly favored by relative humidities in the 40% to 50% range, which are common in the autumn and spring.

Clinical manifestations

A prodrome of feeling cold and vague symptoms of non–well-being are usually seen. This is commonly followed by a dry, scratchy, sore throat and, later, sneezing, nasal stuffiness, and rhinorrhea. Feverishness, malaise, myalgias, headache, hoarseness, and a dry, nonproductive, annoying cough may be seen. Fever, if present, is usually low grade.

Mucosal inflammation can result in occlusion of the ostia of the paranasal sinuses and eustachian tubes, leading to acute sinusitis and otitis media.[9] The resulting entrapment of bacteria may cause suppuration. Sinusitis and otitis media are therefore the most common complications of upper respiratory illnesses. Most children will have an average of about one episode of otitis media per year during the early years of life. Such complications should be suspected if the patient develops fever 3 to 5 days after the onset of a cold. Ear pain or facial pain over the involved sinus may be seen. The most common secondary bacterial invader is *Streptococcus pneumoniae,* followed by *Hemophilus influenzae* and *Branhamella catarrhalis.* Less common complications include bacteremias, bacterial meningitis, and other distant foci of infection, presumably seeded by bloodstream invasion of the secondary bacterial pathogens. Upper respiratory illnesses have also been described as a triggering event for Guillain-Barré syndrome.[132] In children with hyperreactive airways disease, respiratory viral infections are common initiators of asthma attacks,[86] possibly by stimulating the production of chemical mediators of bronchospasm.

Diagnosis

The diagnosis of the common cold syndrome is presumptive and based on the clinical presentation. Identification of the specific etiologic agent is not usually warranted. In patients with a sore throat, one must rule out group A streptococcal infection by means of a culture or rapid antigen detection technique. This is perhaps the only uncomplicated upper respiratory infection that warrants antibiotic treatment. Presumptive etiologic diagnosis can be made on the basis of knowledge of the seasonality of the various viruses. Rhinoviruses are more common in the autumn and early spring. Parainfluenza viral infection with types 1 and 2 has been an autumn disease of odd-numbered years since 1973.[87] Parainfluenza reinfection often manifests as hoarseness, and croup and laryngotracheobronchitis are often signal illnesses for the presence of these viruses. Epidemics of the respiratory syncytial virus and influenza virus are epidemic in mid-winter. The respiratory syncytial virus produces bronchiolitis and pneumo-

nia in infants, manifesting as annual epidemics, during which time much of the acute respiratory disease of older children and adults is also caused by this agent. Influenza often first appears as a sudden febrile respiratory illness in groups of school-aged children.

In the case of mid-winter upper respiratory epidemics, rapid diagnosis may be warranted for epidemiologic reasons. Influenza A infections can be aborted with amantadine, which also reduces virus shedding and therefore the risk of spreading the infection to vulnerable contacts.

The differential diagnosis of the common cold syndrome includes allergic rhinitis and hay fever. The presence of eosinophils on a nasal smear is indicative of allergic rhinitis. As mentioned previously, group A streptococcal infection must always be ruled out in the presence of a sore throat. The finding of hoarseness has a negative correlation with group A streptococcal infection. In addition continuous rhinorrhea may be the result of a spontaneous cerebrospinal fluid leak, and in such situation the nasal secretions should be tested for glucose, which is present in cerebrospinal fluid.

Management and preventive concepts

Nonspecific therapy. Over-the-counter remedies are usually sufficient in providing relief for most of the nonspecific symptoms of the common cold syndrome. Although aspirin may be symptomatically effective, studies have demonstrated prolonged excretion of rhinoviruses from patients given aspirin.[227] Aspirin has also been associated with an increased risk of Reye's syndrome and is therefore contraindicated for influenza infections in children. While acetaminophen is a better choice, this too should be used only when necessary because antipyretic use probably does not favor early recovery from infection. Oral decongestants such as pseudoephedrine are effective. Topical decongestants are also effective but are often associated with a distressing rebound phenomenon. Antihistamines may also be useful in decreasing secretions. A chronic, lingering, nonproductive cough is a common occurrence and usually can be treated easily with a cough suppressant such as dextromethorphan. This should be used with caution in children, however, because here cough may be an important mechanism of keeping the airways patent.

Specific therapy. There is no specific treatment for the common cold. Several drugs have been investigated for rhinoviral infections, however. Enviroxime, a benzimidazole derivative with potent in-vitro antirhinoviral activity, is one of the most extensively studied compounds. The mechanism of action of enviroxime is not completely understood, but the drug is believed to inhibit the formation of the viral RNA-polymerase replication complexes. Noncytotoxic concentrations of enviroxime are associated with complete inhibition of replication of 83 rhinovirus serotypes.[170] In a prophylactic role, studies have shown significant benefit when intranasal administration four times a day was combined with low-dose oral administration.[178] Other initial limited in-vitro data also suggest that this may be a promising approach.[80,272] In contrast, several studies of enviroxime intranasal administration after rhinoviral challenge have failed to demonstrate any therapeutic benefit.[134,148] Chemically related derivatives with improved oral bioavailability, such as enviradene,[245] and the use of alternative topical delivery methods, such as incorporation into liposomes, remain under investigation. Although specific therapy for rhinoviral infection is not yet available, viral structure as well as the cell attachment site have been completely described,[194] and this should in time allow the development of antiviral drugs able to block attachment of the virus to human epithelial cells.

In influenza A epidemics, amantadine should be considered for health-care workers and household contacts of high-risk patients, the purpose being to reduce risk and abort early clinical disease. Recommended doses are 0.2 gm/day for adults and 2.2 to 4.4 mg/kg every 12 hours for children. Amantadine has been shown, however, to have no direct effect on the virus particle, and to exert its effect by interfering with the uncoating of the virus instead. The drug is secreted into the nasal epithelium after oral dosage. Although the agent has important central nervous system toxicity, it is clearly indicated in certain specific circumstances for the prophylaxis and treatment of influenza A infection. Rimantadine is probably marginally better clinically[63] but is otherwise very similar. Recommended rimantadine dosing is 0.2 gm/day for adults and 3 mg/kg every 12 hours for children.

There is no role for routine conventional antimicrobial chemotherapy in viral upper respiratory disease.[217] Antibiotics have not been shown to alter the frequency of bacterial complications. They may change the bacterial flora, however, allowing the emergence of more virulent and resistant organisms.

Vaccines

The only vaccines currently available against respiratory viral disease are the inactivated influenza vaccines and a live-virus vaccine for adenovirus types 4 and 7, the latter administered as an enteric-coated capsule to military recruits. Unfortunately, if used routinely these vaccines would be preventive for only a small proportion of colds in the adult civilian population and are therefore not generally recommended. The indications for influenza vaccine are covered earlier in this chapter.

The large number of rhinovirus serotypes as well as the lack of effective postinfection cross-protection make it unlikely that immunoprophylaxis will work in this setting. Additionally, because of antigenic variation and the emergence of new serotypes, which seem to be driven by immunity, a vaccine approach is even more unlikely to be feasible.

Preventive therapy

Natural and recombinant interferons have received attention as possible prophylactic and therapeutic agents for the common cold. Their protein nature makes them ineffective when given orally. Intranasal recombinant interferon alpha-2 has been shown to be effective in preventing experimental rhinoviral infection.[103,200] Long-term administration, however, has been associated with lymphocyte infiltration and nasal blockage. The mechanism of action of interferons has not been completely defined, but it involves the intracellular production of antiviral proteins that in turn inhibit viral replication. This activity allows potential use against a broad spectrum of respiratory pathogens, including rhinoviruses, influenza A and B viruses, parainfluenza viruses, adenoviruses, and coronaviruses. Resistant viral strains after therapy have not been observed. Systemic toxicity does not occur except with extremely large doses. When doses of 10 million units per day or greater are used, transient leukopenia has been reported. However, the major limiting factor that still stands in the way of routine use and general acceptance is the occurrence of irritating local nasal symptoms, such as bleeding, dryness, ulceration, erosion, and blockage. Although interferons appear to be very efficacious in preventing rhinovirus colds, they have not been effective in treating established infections.[151] In contrast to interferon alpha, studies of recombinant interferon beta serine as a nasal spray did not show this to be effective in the prophylaxis of natural colds.[218] Interferons have no effect on the other viruses associated with the common cold syndrome.

Vitamin C (ascorbic acid) has frequently been touted to offer benefits in the prevention and treatment of the common cold. Preliminary studies that suggested this were flawed by inadequate design,[46] and subsequent trials have not supported the earlier reports.[180]

An interesting, nondrug avenue that has been repeatedly explored in the management of common colds has been the application of hot air to the nasal mucosa. Because rhinoviruses grow optimally at 33° C and their growth is markedly inhibited at normal body temperature (i.e., 37° C), it seemed plausible that temperature of the nasal mucosa may be an important factor in the pathogenesis of colds. Early unsuccessful experiments involved blocking the anterior nares, and there was doubt whether the cure was better than the disease. Steam inhalation and various types of devices delivering hot, humidified air to the nasal passages have been tried, mostly without consistently reproducible benefits. One such device, developed and tested both in South Africa and the United Kingdom, has provided what appear to be promising initial results. This apparatus, named the Virotherm, delivers 40 liters/min^{-1} of fully humidified air at 43° C through an anesthetic mask. In British trials carried out in Andover, Hants,[257] symptoms were markedly reduced at day 4, compared with the placebo group. Supporting evidence has been presented in a recent Israeli trial using an improved version of an earlier similar device, the Rhinotherm.[168]

Meanwhile, intensive research continues in an effort to develop an effective agent for the prophylaxis of common cold infections.

URINARY TRACT INFECTION

The recorded history of urinary tract infection dates to 400 BC when Hippocrates devoted a book to the study of urine that recognized stone, hematuria, and suppuration. In 1851, George Owen Rees, FRS, delivered the first Lettsomian lecture at the medical society of London on "some pathological conditions of the urine." Roberts in 1881 noted the occurrence of postinstrumentation cystitis and the presence of rod-shaped bacteria in the urine. Escherich, a well-known pediatrician and bacteriologist, described the clinical features "pyelitis" in childhood in 1884 and in 1885 discovered the bacterium *Coli commune*.

Definitions

With infections of the urinary tract, one must be clear about some basic definitions and use these terms consistently and accurately. Bacteriuria literally means bacteria in the urine, and significant *bacteriuria* is used to describe voided urine containing bacteria that exceed the numbers usually seen caused by contamination from the anterior urethra (i.e., equal to or greater than 10^5 bacteria/ml). The implication here is that this infection is more likely to be serious, and therefore should be viewed as such. Asymptomatic bacteriuria refers to significant bacteriuria in a patient without symptoms. Urinary tract infection may involve the upper tract, lower tract, or both. Cystitis describes the syndrome of dysuria, frequency, urgency, and occasionally suprapubic tenderness. These symptoms may be related to noninfectious inflammation of the lower tract and may also be due to the urethritis seen in gonorrheal and chlamydial infections. The mere presence of lower tract symptoms does not exclude upper tract involvement. Acute pyelonephritis describes the clinical syndrome characterized by flank pain and/or tenderness, and fever, often with dysuria, urgency, and frequency. Renal infarction or renal stone symptoms may cause similar symptoms in the absence of infection.

Urinary infection may occur de novo or as a recurrent infection. Recurrences may be relapses or reinfections. Relapse refers to recurrence if infection is with the same organism as was present before the start of therapy. This is due to the persistence of the organism within the urinary tract. Reinfection, on the other hand, is a recurrence of infection with an organism different from the original infecting bacterium. It is by definition a new infection. Occasionally reinfection may occur with the same organism that may have persisted in the vagina or feces and be thus mistaken for a relapse. The diagnosis of chronic urinary tract infection strictly requires multiple relapses after treatment.

Reinfections do not qualify for classification as chronic. Chronic pyelonephritis is a somewhat ambiguous term and to most authors refers to the pathologic changes seen in the kidney.

There are three possible routes by which bacteria can invade and spread within the urinary tract. These are ascending, hematogenous, and lymphatic pathways. The pathology of upper tract involvement includes acute pyelonephritis, chronic pyelonephritis or chronic interstitial nephritis, and papillary necrosis caused by infection.[244] The first is characterized by discrete yellowish raised abscesses on the renal surface along with histologic evidence of suppurative necrosis within the renal substance. Gross scarring, interstitial fibrosis, and periglomerular fibrosis are seen in chronic pyelonephritis. Because several studies[74,75,155] have found little correlation between these pathologic changes and evidence for urinary tract infection, a better term for this pathologic entity is chronic interstitial nephritis. In papillary necrosis, involvement is frequently bilateral with involvement of one of more pyramids. Yellow necrotic tissue eventually sloughs to produce a calyceal deformity and results in a radiologic filling defect. Urinary tract obstruction may ensue.

Epidemiology

The prevalence of urinary tract infection is 1% under the age of 1 year. Anatomic or functional urologic abnormalities are the main risk factor in this age group, and boys are much more commonly affected.[24] From ages 1 through 5, the prevalence is 4% to 5% in females and 0.5% in males,[185] the main risk factors being congenital abnormalities in both sexes, vesicourethral reflux (VUR) in females, and noncircumcision in males. In this age group boys appear to be affected only when serious congenital anomalies are present. Infections during this period are often symptomatic, and much of the renal damage that occurs from urinary tract infection is believed to take place at this time.[111,213] The same prevalence rates persist until the age of 15 in both sexes. Several studies have found that bacteriuria is common in school-going girls, is often asymptomatic, and frequently recurs;[82,183,184] thus the presence of bacteriuria in childhood defines a population at higher risk for the development of bacteriuria in adulthood. In the age group 16 to 35 years, women acquire a prevalence of 20%, but men remain at 0.5%. The risk factors for women in this group are sexual intercourse and diaphragm use, and for men homosexuality is considered important. Although diaphragms can cause urinary obstruction, their main effect is probably a change in the vaginal flora.[72] From ages 36 to 65, the prevalence is 35% and 20% in women and men respectively. Gynecological surgery and bladder prolapse in women, and prostatic hypertrophy, obstruction, catheterization, and surgery in men are risk factors. In patients above the age of 65, the differential in the prevalence between the sexes is again narrowed, being 40% and 35% in women and men respectively. In addition to the previously mentioned risk factors, the loss of bactericidal activity of prostatic secretions, poor emptying of the bladder because of prolapse in women, perennial soiling from fecal incontinence in demented women, neuromuscular disease, increased instrumentation,[28] urinary incontinence, and long-term catheterization also become important in this age group.[222] There are high rates of spontaneous cure and reinfection in both elderly women and men.[27]

In acute infection and in the outpatient setting, *Escherichia coli* is by far the most frequent infection organism.[88] In so-called chronic infection, especially in the presence of structural abnormalities of the urinary tract such as obstructive uropathy, congenital anomalies, neurogenic bladder, and fistulous communication involving the urinary tract, the relative frequency of infection caused by *Proteus, Pseudomonas, Klebsiella,* and *Enterobacter* species, and by the enterococci and staphylococci increases greatly. The hospital environment also favors the isolation of the these organisms. Anaerobic organisms are rarely pathogens in the urinary tract.[73] Other bacteria may be found in specific clinical settings. *Salmonella* species are found in Salmonella bacteremia.[150] Fungi, particularly of the *Candida* species, occur commonly in patients with indwelling catheters who are on antimicrobial therapy. *Staphylococcus saprophyticus* is isolated in young, sexually active females.[109,120] Coagulase-positive staphylococci often hematogenously seed the kidney, resulting in intrarenal or perirenal abscesses.[49] Using serotyping techniques on *E. coli,* researchers have demonstrated that only a relatively small number of serologically distinct strains (e.g., 04, 06, 075, and secondarily 01, 02, and 07) are responsible for most *E. coli* urinary tract infections. Adenoviruses, particularly type 11, have been strongly implicated in the causation of hemorrhagic cystitis in pediatric patients, especially boys.[152,163]

Clinical manifestations

The manifestations of urinary tract infection in children differ depending on the age of the child. Symptoms in neonates and children under 2 years of age are nonspecific.[89,143,146] Failure to thrive, vomiting, and fever are the major symptoms. Children above the age of 2 years, and more consistently those above the age of 5, are more likely to show typical localizing symptoms such as frequency, dysuria, and abdominal or flank pain.

In adults, urinary tract infection is usually easy to recognize. Dysuria, frequency, suprapubic discomfort, continuous or terminal hematuria, and the absence of a fever tend to typify lower tract involvement. Fever, often with chills; and flank pain, along with lower tract symptoms, constitute upper tract symptomatology. Various patterns of referred pain may be seen, often resulting in difficulties in differential diagnosis.

In the elderly, most urinary tract infection is asymptomatic, and pyuria may be absent.[124,197] When symptoms are present, they are often not diagnostic, because many noninfected elderly patients often experience frequency, dysuria, hesitancy, and incontinence. However, urinary tract infection tends to be a more serious disease in the elderly, often resulting in life-threatening illness over a relatively short period of time. One study found a much higher frequency of bacteremia associated with pyelonephritis (61%) in the elderly than is found in the young, and shock commonly supervened.[84] No association has been found between asymptomatic bacteriuria on the one hand, and well-being, appetite, and urinary continence in the elderly on the other.[27]

Diagnosis

Confirmation of urinary tract infection requires documentation of bacteriuria by culture. The finding of more than 10^5 bacteria/ml of voided urine was shown by Kass, et al. to differentiate infected from contaminated urine of women with asymptomatic bacteriuria or acute pyelonephritis.[221] However, despite this widely used criterion, a third of women with acute cystitis do indeed have colony counts in midstream urine between 10^2 and 10^4 colony-forming units (CFU)/ml.[224] Similarly, acute pyelonephritis has been reported in association with low bacterial counts in voided urine.[25] Therefore, in acutely symptomatic women, a more appropriate value for defining significant bacteriuria is more than 10^2 CFU/ml of a known uropathogen.[223]

As alternatives to standard culture techniques, several more rapid methods for the detection of bacteriuria have been developed in recent years, the discussion of which is beyond the scope of this chapter.[34] Although very sensitive above counts of 10^5 CFU/ml, they are of limited value between bacterial loads of 10^2 and 10^5 CFU/ml.

From a practical standpoint in the outpatient setting, urine needs to be examined microscopically to diagnose and treat urinary tract infection, a procedure that is usually 80% accurate. Rapid noncultural diagnostic tests other than microscopy involve the use of dipsticks. These measure the transformation of nitrites to nitrates or leukocyte-esterase and further increase the clinician's accuracy when used with microscopic examination.[153]

Management

The management of urinary tract infections is an involved and extensive topic. This section will review the general principles involved in the care of patients with urinary tract infections.

Maintaining adequate hydration is important, and indeed forcing fluids has been shown to reduce bacterial counts rapidly at least transiently.[164] However, there is currently no evidence to support the view that hydration improves the results of appropriate antimicrobial therapy.

The antibacterial activity of urine results mainly from the high urea concentration and is pH-dependent, being greater at a lower or more acidic pH.[125] Most antimicrobial agents exhibit adequate antibacterial activity at usual urinary pH levels. The major exceptions are mandelic and hippuric acids and methenamine, which require maintenance of low urinary pH, as can be accomplished by the administration of ascorbic acid or methionine. To acidify the urine, often one must restrict those dietary constituents that tend to cause urinary alkalinization, such as milk, fruit juices other than cranberry juice, and sodium bicarbonate. Caution is advisable in attempting acidification in patients with renal insufficiency, because systemic acidosis may ensue. Acidification for long-term antimicrobial therapy should be used only with concomitant use of organic acids.

Urinary analgesics such as phenazopyridine hydrochloride (Pyridium) have little place in the routine management of symptomatic infections. Dysuria is usually responsive to antimicrobial therapy and, if severe or accompanied by flank pain, usually requires systemic analgesia. However, phenazopyridine hydrochloride may indeed be useful in the management of certain patients with dysuria without infection.

Symptomatic urinary tract infection may involve the upper tract, the lower tract, or both. Upper tract involvement when acute is termed acute pyelonephritis. Most patients with acute pyelonephritis require hospitalization and intravenous antimicrobial therapy. In uncomplicated cases, there should be a marked decrease in bacterial titers in the urine within 48 hours of onset of the treatment, and in general a course of 14 days of antimicrobial therapy is required.[226] When upper tract infection is complicated, longer antimicrobial courses may be required. All patients with acute pyelonephritis should have an ultrasound examination to evaluate for obstruction and stones. Follow-up urine cultures are mandatory within 2 weeks of completion of therapy in pregnant women, children, and patients with recurrent symptomatic pyelonephritis. Although optional in the majority of nonpregnant adults who remain asymptomatic, this remains a desirable practice.

In lower tract infection, in the past, 7 to 10 days of oral therapy was routinely recommended. In recent years, however, this view has changed significantly. Single-dose therapy versus 3-day therapy has emerged as the treatment of choice for most female patients with suspected lower tract infection, and studies in pediatric populations have shown similar good results.[208] Short-course therapy has not been adequately evaluated in men and is not recommended at present. It is also not appropriate for women with a history of infection with antibiotic-resistant organisms or more than 7 days of symptoms.[118] In these patients with an increased likelihood of upper tract involvement and in males, 7 to 10 days of therapy are recommended. Symptomatic response followed by recurrence after the discontinuation of therapy indicates the probability of upper tract infection and the need for a urine culture and at least 2 weeks of therapy. Preferred agents for presumptive short-course therapy include trimethoprim-sulfamethoxazole, trimethoprim, cephalexin, amoxicillin-clavulanic acid, norfloxacin, or ciprofloxacin. The choice of therapy in more complicated cases should always be tailored to the antimicrobial susceptibilities of the infecting microorganism isolated by sterile urine culture. Short-course therapy for urinary tract infections is summarized in Table 57-3.

The selection of an appropriate antimicrobial agent is a complex process because of the increasing number of compounds available, each with its own antimicrobial spectrum and toxicity. In most cases, several choices are perfectly satisfactory, and the agent with the least toxicity should be used. Currently no evidence supports the use of bactericidal drugs over bacteriostatic agents in urinary tract infections. There is generally a poor correlation between blood levels of the antibiotic and the response of the bacteriuria. This is because at the dosages commonly employed for this purpose, most antimicrobial agents do not achieve serum levels above the minimal inhibitory concentration (MIC) for most urinary pathogens. Disappearance of bacteriuria, on the other hand, is closely correlated with the sensitivity of the microorganism to the concentration of the antimicrobial achieved in the urine.[145,219,220] Although blood levels may not be important in the treatment of most urinary infections, they are probably critical in patients with bacteremia and may well be important in the cure of patients with renal parenchymal infection who relapse.

In patients with renal insufficiency, dosage modifications are necessary for those agents that are excreted primarily by the kidneys and cannot be cleared by other mechanisms. In renal failure the kidney may additionally not be able to adequately concentrate antimicrobial agents in the urine, thus resulting in difficulty in eradicating the infection. This may be an important factor in urinary tract infection treatment failures with aminoglycosides. In addition, high concentrations of magnesium and calcium, as well as a low pH, may raise the minimal inhibitory con-

Table 57-3. Short-course therapy for urinary tract infections

Antimicrobial agent	Dose
Trimethoprim	100 mg PO BID for 1-3 days
Trimethoprim-sulfamethoxazole	1 double-strength tablet PO BID for 1-3 days
Amoxicillin-clavulanic acid	250-500 mg amoxicillin PO TID for 1-3 days
Norfloxacin	400 mg PO BID for 1-3 days
Ciprofloxacin	500 mg PO BID for 1-3 days

Adapted from Mandell: *Principles and practice of infectious diseases,* ed 3, New York, 1990, Churchill Livingstone.

centrations of aminoglycosides for gram-negative bacilli to levels above those achievable in the urine of patients with renal failure.[149] In general, the penicillins and cephalosporins retain adequate urinary concentrations despite severely impaired renal function and therefore are the agents of choice in renal insufficiency.

The objective of antimicrobial therapy is to eliminate bacteria from the urinary tract. Because symptoms usually abate spontaneously even in the absence of chemotherapy, despite the persistence of bacteriuria, follow-up urine cultures are essential in evaluating the effects of therapy. There are four patterns of response of bacteriuria to antimicrobial therapy: cure, persistence, relapse, and reinfection. Quantitative bacterial counts in urine should decrease within 48 hours after initiation of appropriate therapy. If this does not occur, the therapy almost invariably will be unsuccessful. Cure is defined as negative urine cultures on therapy and during the follow-up period, which is usually 1 to 2 weeks. However, some of these patients will become reinfected. Persistence is used both to describe the presence of significant bacteriuria after 48 hours on therapy and to denote the persistence of low numbers of the infecting organisms in the urine after 48 hours. Relapse usually occurs within 2 weeks of cessation of chemotherapy and is often associated with concurrent upper tract or renal infection, obstructive uropathy, or chronic bacterial prostatitis. After initial sterilization of urine, reinfection may occur during treatment, also termed *superinfection,* or anytime thereafter.

SEXUALLY TRANSMITTED DISEASES
Overview

The emergence and phenomenal growth within the last decade of human immunodeficiency virus (HIV) infection and disease have afforded HIV an ominous and unparalleled importance the like of which modern medicine has never seen before. The subject of HIV infection has become tremendously complex and ever-changing, and is considered independently elsewhere in this text. This discussion of sexually transmitted diseases therefore will be limited to non-HIV entities.

One of the trends that we saw in the 1980s is the rapid increase in the spectrum of sexually transmitted diseases. Changes within the past 2 decades in the epidemiology of sexually transmitted diseases and an increasing awareness of the consequences of such infection make it essential that primary care physicians be well equipped to deal with this disease group. In few areas of infectious disease have the changes in our understanding of the clinical manifestations been as profound. At least 50 distinct clinical syndromes caused by more than 25 pathogenic organisms and viruses have been identified. In each of these the common denominator is that sexual contact is an important mode of transmission but not necessarily the only one.

The major sexually transmitted diseases are more seri-

ous for women and their offspring than for men. Many are transmitted far more efficiently from male to female than the reverse, probably because the vagina serves as an efficient reservoir that prolongs the exposure of the host to infectious secretions. Women also are more likely to be asymptomatic or minimally symptomatic early in the clinical course. This fosters delay in seeking health care and thus promotes transmission. Third, the diagnosis of sexually transmitted diseases is more difficult in women, because of both the limited specificity of symptoms and the inadequate sensitivity of the microbiologic tests. Finally, infected women and their offspring are at greater risk than men for severe or permanent sequelae such as infertility, malignancy, and serious disorders of the fetus or newborn. New frontiers in the known spectrum of sexually transmitted diseases over the past 2 decades have largely involved the recognition of new viral pathogens. These include the human immunodeficiency virus (HIV), type 2 herpes simplex virus (HSV), hepatitis B virus (HBV), human papillomavirus (HPV), and cytomegalovirus (CMV). The rising prevalence of these syndromes probably reflects true incidence as well as enhanced recognition.

This section will highlight the epidemiologic principles, public health considerations, and control and prevention strategies of this disease group. The major sexually transmitted diseases include gonorrhea, chlamydial infections, syphilis, and genital herpes. Less common entities are chancroid, lymphogranuloma venereum, granuloma inguinale, and human papilloma virus infections.

It is convenient and more manageable to think of STDs in several distinct disease groups—vaginal and pelvic infections, male urethritis, genital ulcer disease, and disseminated STD syndromes. Vaginitis and vaginal discharge is probably the most common symptom leading to consultation with physicians.[171] Vulvovaginal candidiasis, trichomoniasis, and bacterial vaginosis make up over 90% of these cases, bacterial vaginosis being the most common form of vaginal infection. Other miscellaneous causes of vaginitis include atrophic vaginitis, puerperal vaginitis, the presence of a foreign body, ulcerative vaginitis associated with toxic shock syndrome, desquamative inflammatory vaginitis, streptococcal vaginitis, and vaginitis associated with collagen diseases. Chlamydial infections are the most common cause of endocervicitis in sexually active women. Other important pelvic pathogens include *Neisseria gonorrhea* and primary genital herpes. Male urethritis is often considered the male counterpart of mucopurulent cervicitis. Causes of this include *Neisseria gonorrhea, Chlamydia trachomatis,* genital mycoplasmas, HSV, and *Trichomonas vaginalis.* Of the genital ulcer syndromes, only syphilis and chancroid are reportable. Other causes of ulcers include HSV infections. Disseminated STD in an immunocompetent host encompasses entities such as gonorrhea and syphilis.

Epidemiology

Despite improvements in diagnosis and treatment, sexually transmitted diseases remain endemic in virtually all societies. They are a prime example of the influence that behavioral and demographic factors can have on an infectious disease, despite the availability of effective therapy and other technological advances.[7,39]

The principal risk factor for the acquisition and transmission of STD is sexual behavior favoring exposure to a specific sexually transmitted pathogen. The number and selection of partners, as well as specific sexual practices, in turn predict the probability of such exposure. Secondary risk factors include coinfection with other STDs, male circumcision, contraceptive practices, health care behavior such as the timeliness of medical care, and the continuation or cessation of sexual activity. These risk factors are distinct from risk markers that are considered indirect indicators of sexual behavior. These are primarily demographic and social characteristics such as race, marital status, sexual orientation, socioeconomic level, urban vs. rural residence, and substance abuse. Variables such as gender and age, which influence both behavior and susceptibility to infection, are more difficult to classify.

All STDs are transmitted with considerably less than 100% efficiency. Most infections are treated or resolve spontaneously over weeks to months. Most viral STDs, although permanent insofar as they commonly persist for the life of the host, are also transmissible only intermittently. For these reasons, a minimal frequency of sexual partner changes is necessary for STD propagation in a given population. People whose sexual behavior is sufficient to sustain the epidemic are termed core transmitters and make up the core population.[273] Others commonly acquire infection by sexual contact with this core group but do not themselves cause indefinite propagation outside the core. The core transmitter hypothesis was initially developed as a model for gonorrhea, and several studies have supported this theory. In the United States, the characteristics of the core transmitters for gonorrhea and syphilis are similar.[196] The core group for chlamydial infections is larger and probably includes most sexually active young adults. For genital herpes and other persistent sexually transmitted viral infections, the core group is larger still and probably includes most of the adult population. An understanding of the core transmission hypothesis is invaluable in assessing patients' STD risk and targeting facilities appropriately.

It is interesting to note that in the last 2 decades, the number of reported cases of gonorrhea has declined in the United States. This probably reflects both a reduced infection rate in whites of higher socioeconomic strata and stable or rising rates in disadvantaged ethnic minority populations.[191] Rapidly rising rates of syphilis are due to an increasing incidence in the latter population. Moreover, it is likely that the expansion of the gonorrhea-syphilis core is being driven largely by illicit drug use and inner-city socioeconomic conditions. Interestingly, this pattern of gonorrhea and syphilis represents a return to that seen in the preantibiotic era, when most cases were associated with prostitution and low socioeconomic level.

Most people with genital symptoms cease sexual activity and seek health care. Therefore infected individuals who transmit STDs are likely to have no symptoms or to have mild symptoms that they ignore. To identify this large group of asymptomatic or minimally symptomatic patients who do not themselves seek health care, health care providers absolutely must actively screen populations at high risk. After these individuals are identified, the partners of patients with STDs must be notified, regardless of gender of specific infection.

Clinical and public health considerations

Because of the effect of sexually transmitted diseases not only on the individual but on large groups of people, there are certain unique aspects to its management. Risk assessment requires above all a complete social and sexual history, including an assessment of secondary factors such as illicit drug use. A forthright approach is usually best and also sets the stage for risk-reduction counseling later. The latter should emphasize abstinence, judicious selection of sexual partners, the use of condoms and spermicides, and periodic screening examinations for high-risk groups.

Immediate access to tests for HIV antibody (including confirmatory assays by Western blot), syphilis serology, culture for *Neisseria gonorrhea,* culture or antigen detection tests for *Chlamydia trachomatis,* and microscopy to examine gram-stained smears and wet mounts of vaginal secretions should be available. Viral isolation or antigen-detection tests for herpes simplex are also desirable, as is darkfield microscopy for detection of *Treponema pallidum,* in the appropriate setting.[101] Cases of gonorrhea always should be confirmed by isolating the organism, because the emergence and spread of resistant strains makes it necessary that isolates be tested for antimicrobial resistance. Chlamydia infections, because of their nonspecific patterns of clinical presentation, also require culture or immunochemical identification for successful detection and treatment. Although genital herpes is usually reliably diagnosable on clinical grounds, atypical presentations do occur, and isolation of the virus should be attempted in all ulcers that are not typical of herpes or syphilis. The most common causes of vaginal discharge in sexually active women—mucopurulent cervicitis, bacterial vaginosis, trichomoniasis, and candidiasis—may be difficult to distinguish clinically and usually require laboratory identification.

The principal components of disease control as they apply to the sexually transmitted diseases are education and counseling on the one hand, and screening on the other. Counseling and education have a role not only in infected or at-risk patients, but also for primary prevention before the onset of sexual activity in all young people in primary health care settings. Ideally, prevention is best achieved through sexual abstinence and the maintenance of permanent, mutually monogamous relationships. Coupled with this are measures aimed at preventing the spread of disease, such as condoms and spermicides in the setting of all nonmonogamous sexual encounters involving penile penetration of any orifice.

The occurrence of a sexually transmitted disease should always be taken as an event that is indicative of unprotected sexual activity and should prompt screening for other STDs. Screening has a central role in the control of gonorrhea, syphilis, chlamydial infections, and HIV infection. Its value in controlling HSV infections, HPV infections, and other STDs remains to be determined.

Principles of management

Because STD patients traditionally have been thought unlikely to comply with prolonged therapeutic regimens, an emphasis has been placed on single-dose treatment. In practice, the compliance of many STD patients has been found to be similar to that of other young adults, if given appropriate and thorough counseling. Pharmacists and physicians both have important roles in this process. In any case, the commonest STDs are not usually amenable to single-dose treatment.

The choice of the antimicrobial agent also should consider its activity against other possible concurrent infectious agents. Gonorrhea, chlamydial disease, and syphilis often coexist. The anatomic site of infection, for example, the pharynx or rectum in gonorrhea and the nervous system in syphilis, also will affect the choice of the antimicrobial agent. Other important considerations include toxicity and cost.

Because of the risk of reinfection, sexually transmitted diseases are unique in that failure to examine and treat the partner is often tantamount to not treating the index case. Therefore all physicians treating STD patients must take specific steps to examine the partner or partners personally or to ensure specific referrals elsewhere. In rare situations, it may also be necessary to treat partners without examining them, but such treatment, which is usually devoid of counseling, often meets with limited success. In addition, because blind prescribing carries a very real medicolegal risk, this practice is better avoided even in apparently monogamous settings.

TRAVELERS' DIARRHEA

It is said that travel expands the mind and loosens the bowel.[87a] Although this may not be universally true, most travelers from temperate climates do experience some debilitating gastrointestinal dysfunction, most commonly diarrhea, when traveling to more tropical parts of the world. This affliction is commonly known as travelers' diarrhea and is a common and well-recognized disease entity. Other more colorful synonyms include "Delhi belly," "Turkey trots," "Montezuma's revenge," "Aztec two step," "Aden gut," "Backdoor sprint," "Hong Kong dog," "tourist trots," "la tourista trots," and several others.[92] The diversity of euphemisms emphasizes the global nature of this disorder.

Epidemiology

Although travelers' diarrhea is seldom a life-threatening disorder, the economic and social consequences of this disease are highly significant. Each year, nearly 350 million individuals cross the worlds' geographic frontiers, and thus this population is susceptible to travel-related illness.

Risk factors for travelers' diarrhea include compromised immune status, advanced age, general ill health, the absence of gastric acid, and geographic location. Those at the highest risk of acquiring travelers' diarrhea are residents of industrialized countries visiting a developing country.[50] The attack rate usually depends on the country being visited and ranges from 10% to 50%. North America, Northern and Central Europe, Australia, and New Zealand are considered low-risk areas, with attack rates of less than 8%. Intermediate-risk areas include the Caribbean, North Mediterranean, Israel, Japan, and South Africa. High-risk areas are Central and South America, Africa, and Asia, with prevalence rates between 20% and 50%.[237]

Travelers' diarrhea is more common in young adults compared with older people. This difference may relate to the less prudent eating habits of the young or their relative lack of acquired immunity. There is no difference, however, in attack rates between the sexes.

Clinical manifestations

The composition of the intestinal flora changes during travel, regardless of whether a diarrheal illness develops. Travelers acquire "new" serotypes of *Escherichia coli* as those previously resident decrease in concentration. This "new" population includes commensals as well as enteropathogens and is acquired from the local fecally contaminated environment.

The typical manifestations of travelers' diarrhea include the sudden onset of malaise, anorexia, and colicky abdominal pain. This is closely followed by watery diarrhea, typically with the passage of four to five stools per day. A minority of patients may also have nausea and vomiting. Dysentery occurs in less than 10%, with the presence of fever, blood in the stools, or both. The usual incubation period ranges between 5 and 15 days, and the median duration of untreated illness is usually between 3 and 5 days. Illness lasts longer than a week in 10% of cases, and only 2% persist longer than a month.

Microbiology

Travelers' diarrhea is usually acquired by the ingestion of fecally contaminated food, water, or both. In microbiologic surveys of food in hotels in countries with traditionally high rates of travelers' diarrhea, high levels of contamination with fecal organisms have been consistently found.[254] Studies of antimicrobial prophylaxis show that more than 90% of all travelers' diarrhea is bacterial in origin, rather than from other noninfective causes such as jet lag, dietary changes, and fatigue. Foods that are of particular risk include raw or improperly cooked food, seafood, tap water, unpasteurized milk, and unpeeled fruit. Even properly cooked food can be infectious if it is improperly handled and thereby contaminated after the cooking process. Bottled, carbonated drinks, beer, wine, hot coffee, tea, and water that has been boiled or treated appropriately with chlorine or iodine are all generally considered safe for consumption.

Although the infectious agents responsible for causing travelers' diarrhea vary in importance from country to country, the overall list remains surprisingly constant, no matter where one visits. The responsible organisms and their frequency are as follows: *Escherichia coli,* 50%; *Shigella* species, 5% to 10%; *Giardia,* 5% to 10%; *Campylobacter jejuni,* 15%; rotaviruses, 10%, and miscellaneous organisms, 5% to 15%. The last group includes *Salmonella* species, *Vibrio* species, *Yersinia* species, parvoviruses, *E. histolytica,* and other parasites.[167] No recognized pathogen can be found for 20% to 40% of cases.[199]

Enterotoxigenic *E. coli* (ETEC) have emerged as the most important pathogens in all countries where surveys have been conducted. These organisms adhere to the cells of the small intestine, where they multiply and produce an enterotoxin (which may be heat stable or heat labile) that causes fluid secretion and diarrhea. Adults who live in tropical climates often harbor ETEC without symptoms. This is in contrast to travelers from temperate zones, who are nearly all susceptible to the organism upon arriving in the area. ETEC is involved in a median of 42% of episodes in Latin America, 36% in Africa and 16% in Asia.[22] The likelihood of acquiring the infection seems also to be greater in the summer months. The organism is not invasive, causing diarrhea through the effect of enterotoxins. Typically, ETEC-associated diarrhea is usually mild and painless, and no inflammatory exudate is seen. An occasional episode may be severe enough, however, to resemble cholera.

Diarrhea resulting from enteroinvasive *E. coli* (EIAC) infection clinically resembles *Shigella* infection. As is suggested by the name, this organism does indeed cause invasion of the colonic mucosa. Abdominal pain, fever, and an inflammatory exudate are seen. In one Mexican study, EIAC organisms were responsible for up to 5% of cases.[259]

Enteropathogenic *E. coli* (EPEC) is a more common pathogen in children and is usually not an important cause of travelers' diarrhea. Other forms of E. coli include enterohemorrhagic *E. coli* (EHEC), associated with undercooked hamburger meat in North America, and enteroadherent *E. coli* (EAEC), which made up 15% of cases in Mexico in another recent survey.[144] Despite the many

types of E. coli organisms, by far the most important in travel-related diarrhea illness is the ETEC variety. Current data suggest that, by comparison, the other organisms play only a minor role.

Shigellosis is a highly contagious infection, showing a 75% attack rate with an inoculum as low as 10^5 organisms. Consequently infection spreads very rapidly. The *Shigella* species include four major groups of gram-negative rods that closely resemble *E. coli: S. dysenteriae, S. flexneri, S. boydii,* and *S. soneii.* These organisms invade the colonic and occasionally the ileal mucosa, and adhere to the mucosal surface via the elaboration of an enterotoxin. These organisms are very sensitive to heat and drying. *Shigella soneii* is the most common species, and fortunately also causes the mildest disease of the four types. Although responsible for only a small proportion of cases of travelers' diarrhea, *Shigella* species and *Campylobacter jejuni* are probably responsible for most of the severe or dysenteric forms of the syndrome. These organisms are also more important in Asia. In India, members of the *Shigella* family make up 6% to 11% of the episodes of travelers' diarrhea,[249] but they are rarely seen in Africa.

Salmonella organisms are flagellated, nonencapsulated, nosporulating, gram-negative, aerobic and facultatively anaerobic bacilli. The O cell-wall antigen defines the group to which the organisms belong, and the H antigen determines the specific serotype within a group. The two main clinical categories of *Salmonella* illness are typhoidal and nontyphoidal. Typhoidal disease is caused by *Salmonella typhi* and some strains of *S. paratyphi.* Of all the potential pathogens that are capable of causing travel-related diarrhea, the *salmonellae* have the greatest potential for severe disease, disastrous complications, and a fatal outcome. Strains that originate in the United States are almost all nontyphoidal, and are endemic in animals that are consumed for food. Potential sources include hamburger, chicken, eggs, and other foods. In developing countries, particularly Mexico and India, *salmonella* infections reflect poor sanitary conditions and are nearly all typhoidal in type. The transmission of infection is human-to-human, and the destinations the traveller visited can provide powerful clues to the cause of the diarrhea. Like members of the *Shigella* family, the *salmonellae* are also commonest in India and other parts of southwest Asia, may be encountered in Latin America, and are rare as a cause of travelers' diarrhea in Africa.

Vibrio parahemolyticus has been associated with the consumption of raw or poorly cooked seafood and has been a particular problem in Japanese tourists to Southeast Asia. *Vibrio cholerae,* however, is an exceedingly uncommon cause of travel-related illness.

Other causes of travelers' diarrhea include *Aeromonas hydrophila, Plesiomonas shigelloides,* and *Yersinia enterocolitica*—the latter often with lower abdominal discomfort that may be confused with acute appendicitis.

Campylobacter jejuni infection can cause acute enteritis and colitis. It may mimic many disorders, including idiopathic colitis, toxic megacolon, hemorrhagic and pseudomembranous colitis, mesenteric adenitis, and appendicitis. Geographically, it is most common in Asia, occurring in up to 15% of cases, but is found in only 1% of Latin American cases.[250]

The role of parasitic pathogens in travelers' diarrhea depends primarily on the area of travel. *Giardia lamblia*, although an important pathogen in the republics of the former Soviet Union, is less common in Asia and Central America.[251] Where symptoms last beyond 2 weeks, the likelihood of giardiasis becomes much greater. *Cryptosporidium*, a recently recognized pathogen that has achieved widespread recognition with the AIDS epidemic, has also been reported as a cause of travel-related illness. *Entamoeba histolytica*, the organism responsible for amebic dysentery and related syndromes, although an important endemic pathogen in the developing world, is an uncommon cause of travel-related illness.

Viral agents most often implicated in travelers' diarrhea are the rotavirus and the Norwalk virus. They are more likely to infect water than food but are probably not a major cause of travelers' diarrhea worldwide.

Helminth infections are found in fewer than 1 per 1000 travelers per month. *Trichuris, Ascaris lumbricoides,* and *Strongyloides stercoralis* together are thought to account for less than 1% of all cases of travelers' diarrhea and usually cause mild symptoms. Infection with *Strongyloides stercoralis* can remain dormant for several decades after initial exposure but causes pulmonary symptoms and overwhelming disease as the hyperinfection syndrome.[261] Other organisms that have been linked to diarrhea in travelers are *Blastocystis hominis, Endolimax nana, Sarcocystis,*[269] *Isospora belli,*[173] and *Dientamoeba fragilis.*[243] Food poisoning caused by preformed staphylococcal enterotoxin is more often reported in association with long-distance air travel than with actual residence in a tropical location.[17]

Finally, other less common but more severe primarily nongastrointestinal illnesses acquired in tropical locations may initially present with gastrointestinal symptoms. These include *falciparum malaria*, typhoid fever, melioidosis, legionellosis, and others. Not all travelers' diarrhea is infectious in origin. Food intolerance and natural laxatives found in local fruits may contribute to travelers' diarrhea. Induced lactose-intolerance and the subsequent ingestion of dairy products and other foods rich in lactose may result in persistent diarrhea.[106]

Diagnosis

For otherwise healthy adults, mild diarrhea usually requires no work-up and is usually a self-limited disorder. Moderate to severe disease, or disease that lasts more than 10 days, requires a stool culture and examination for ova and parasites, and in some cases treatment may be necessary before results are available.

Those with prolonged diarrhea are likely to be infected with *G. lamblia, E. histolytica, Campylobacter, Salmonella, Yersinia,* or *Cryptosporidium* species. In most cases selection of the antimicrobial agent can usually await identification of the infecting organism.

Management

For mild diarrhea, usually only reassurance and perhaps the replacement of fluids is needed. Despite the fact that travelers' diarrhea usually does not result in significant dehydration, adequate hydration remains the cornerstone of therapy for all patients with diarrheal diseases, especially children. The ingestion of soft drinks and salted biscuits is usually adequate. Oral rehydration salts or intravenous fluids may be needed in severe cases.

Despite the many drugs used and recommended for the treatment of established travelers' diarrhea, there appears to be little evidence to support the use of the vast majority of these. Some agents are useful, however, when used appropriately.

Diphenoxylate (Lomotil), loperamide (Imodium), and bismuth subsalicylate are perhaps the nonantimicrobial agents used most frequently in travelers' diarrhea. In moderate to severe disease, antimicrobials are usually indicated, although many authorities also recommend their use in milder forms.

The antimotility agents, diphenoxylate (Lomotil) and loperamide (Imodium) provide prompt effective symptomatic relief. Loperamide is as effective as antimicrobial agents provided the diarrhea is nondysenteric. Contraindications to their use include the presence of bloody stools, persistence of the symptoms more than 48 hours after initiation of therapy, or age of less than 2 years.[137]

The only agent found to be effective both for immediate treatment and as prophylaxis of acute travelers' diarrhea is bismuth subsalicylate (Pepto-Bismol). In a recent report summarizing four clinical field trials,[236] this agent was found to decrease stool frequency in the total study population, as well as in subgroups divided according to etiology, including shigellosis. In two studies in which bismuth subsalicylate was compared with loperamide, the loperamide exerted a more rapid effect. Bismuth subsalicylate is not as effective, however, as antimicrobial agents. In general, therefore, when rapid control of symptoms is needed, loperamide is preferred over bismuth subsalicylate. The mechanism by which bismuth subsalicylate protects is not entirely clear, although in the animal model it appears to reduce the secretory effects of enterotoxins.[69]

The early administration of antibiotics is generally effective in reducing the severity and duration of illness. Doxycycline, cotrimoxazole, trimethoprim, norfloxacin, and ciprofloxacin have all been found to be equally effective, and 3 days of therapy is usually recommended.[238]

Table 57-4. Travelers' diarrhea: treatment regimens

Agent	Dose
Diphenoxylate (Lomotil)	Two 2.5 mg tablets after each loose stool to a maximum of 8 tablets per day.
Loperamide (Imodium)	4 mg, then 2 mg after each unformed stool, to not more than 8 mg/24 hrs.
Bismuth subsalicylate (Pepto-Bismol)	60 ml PO QID
Doxycycline	100 mg PO BID
Co-trimoxazole	160 to 800 mg TMP-SMX PO BID
Trimethoprim	200 mg PO BID
Norfloxacin	400 mg PO BID
Ciprofloxacin	300 mg PO BID

Doses are specified in Table 57-4. Tetracyclines are contraindicated in children younger than 12, and the antimotility agents are contraindicated in children under the age of 2 years.

In general, self-administration of antimicrobials is not desirable. If prompt medical care is not likely to be available to a patient at high risk for developing travelers' diarrhea, however, self-treatment may be a reasonable alternative if symptoms persist longer than 2 days or if fever and bloody stools are present.

In children, antibiotic therapy without consultation with the physician should generally be avoided, especially if the stools are bloody or the illness severe. In mild illness, however, the administration by parents of trimethoprim-sulfamethoxazole in a dose of 4 to 20 mg to infants above the age of 2 months and children may be appropriate.[119] If bloody diarrhea, fever greater than 103° F, moderate to severe dehydration, or duration of the illness for more than 3 days are present, medical care should be sought.

Travelers to developing countries, where standards of drug prescription are less stringent than in the West, need to be cautioned against the use of iodochlorohydroxyquin, commonly known as Enterovioform or Clioquinol. Not only is this agent ineffective, but it has real potential to cause severe subacute myelooptic atrophy. Its use is thus extremely hazardous.

Prevention

Prevention is the key to controlling travelers' diarrhea. In general, precautionary measures include dietary discretion, water purification, and chemoprophylaxis or preventive medications.

Dietary discretion. Because most cases of travelers' diarrhea are caused by bacterial pathogens that are ingested via food or water, strategies aimed at avoiding or neutralizing the source have been recommended. The potential advantages of these approaches include the benefi-

cial effect on other similarly transmitted disorders such as hepatitis A, typhoid fever, and polio.

The chances of acquiring travelers' diarrhea can be markedly reduced by consuming only well-cooked food, peeled fruit, and boiled or chlorinated drinks, and by avoiding all salads and shellfish.[128] The traveler also should avoid the use of ice, which may be contaminated. Water is consumed not only while drinking, but also during other activities such as brushing teeth and swimming. Swimming in a man-made lake near Los Angeles has been implicated in an outbreak of shigellosis.[216] Cryptosporidiosis in the United Kingdom also has been described after a similar swimming episode.

It has also been shown, however, that most travelers do not or cannot strictly adhere to these rules to produce the desired effects. Recent evidence also suggests that even strict adherence to such dietary advice may not prevent the occurrence of all travel-related diarrhea. The commonly implicated enteropathogens commonly survive at refrigerator temperature, room temperature, and 50° C, which is too hot to touch.[14] The temperature of tap water has to be raised to above 65° C to ensure reliable killing of enteropathogens.

Water disinfection. Water is disinfected with chlorine or iodine. Chlorine, however, does not kill cysts of *Giardia lamblia,* amoebae, and other parasites. Water purification techniques include the adding 0.1 ml of 5% household bleach (hypochlorite) or 0.25 ml (10 drops) of 2% tincture of iodine per liter of water and allowing it to stand for 30 minutes before drinking. Turbid water needs to be first filtered and requires double the dose of hypochlorite or iodine. Other forms of water purification include tablets and portable water purifiers based on filtration and iodine-containing resins. Because the pores used in portable filtration systems are usually not small enough to ensure entrapment of all microbes, these can be considered only partial purifiers. Water also can be rapidly rendered safe to drink by bringing it to a boil, even transiently. The commonly considered 5 to 10 minutes of boiling is probably not necessary.

In infants, breast-feeding is the best prevention of travelers' diarrhea. Data about the use of antidiarrheal drugs in children are limited. Although recent evidence might suggest a role for the nonsedating opioid loperamide (Imodium), the CDC recommends against the use of antiperistaltics in children.[60] The box on p. 1071 provides a simple summary of recommendations for patients.

Chemoprophylaxis

Chemoprophylaxis of adult travelers' diarrhea continues to provoke controversy. Most authorities remain unenthusiastic about the prospect of routinely prescribing these agents. A recent National Institutes of Health consensus panel did not in general recommend preventive medication, antimicrobials or other, for travelers' diarrhea.[255]

Traveler's diarrhea: dietary dos and don'ts

Do	*Dont's*
Drink only boiled, chlorinated, or bottled water. Even ice must be made from boiled water.	Do not drink unboiled water even though it may look clean.
Eat only freshly cooked food and peeled fruit.	Avoid salads. Avoid shellfish.
Any fruit to be eaten with the skin must be washed thoroughly.	Avoid brushing teeth with obviously dirty water.
Warming food is usually insufficient to kill most enteropathogens; it must be boiled.	Avoid swimming in obviously dirty water.
	Avoid any foods exposed to flies, etc.

The use of prophylactic medication should be reserved for high-risk patients. These include the immunosuppressed, the frail elderly, and those with gastric achlorhydria gastrectomy. Younger, immunologically naive travelers, on a first visit to high-risk areas, are also more likely to succumb than are expatriates living in endemic areas. In contrast, visitors from one developing country to another are less at risk than those from temperate countries.

Because of the high percentage of cases that are due to enterotoxigenic *E. coli* (ETEC), most preventive and therapeutic modalities have targeted this organism. When appropriate, preventive antibiotics may be given for up to 3 weeks, with 70% to 90% protection against diarrheal disease.[66,198] Agents found to be effective include doxycycline, trimethoprim-sulfamethoxazole, cotrimoxazole, norfloxacin, trimethoprim, and bismuth subsalicylate. Doses are specified in Table 57-5. Doxycycline and trimethoprim-sulfamethoxazole are begun on the first day of travel and continued until 2 days after returning home. Bismuth subsalicylate is administered from 1 day before leaving until 2 days after returning from the journey.

The problem with routine prophylactic antimicrobial use for travelers's diarrhea is twofold. First, all such agents have important and potentially serious side effects. Bismuth subsalicylate may blacken the tongue and feces or cause the ears to ring. Patients also must be questioned about aspirin sensitivity or intolerance before bismuth-subsalicylate is prescribed. Skin rashes are common with trimethoprim-sulfamethoxazole, and photosensitivity may occur with doxycycline. Other more serious complications of sulfonamide therapy include the potentially fatal Stevens-Johnson syndrome. Tetracyclines are contraindicated in pregnant women and in children under 10 years of age because of their discoloring effect on dental enamel. The 4-fluoroquinolones also must not be used in infants

Table 57-5. Travelers' diarrhea: prophylactic regimens

Agent	Dose
Doxycycline	100 mg PO QD
Cotrimazole	160 to 800 mg TMP-SMX PO QD
Norfloxacin	400 mg PO QD
Trimethoprim	200 mg PO QD
Bismuth-subsalicylate	60 ml PO QID

and children because of their adverse effects on developing cartilage. Any antibiotic therapy also may be complicated by fungal superinfection and antibiotic-associated diarrhea.

Second, and more important, resistance to these agents may be induced. Resistance to doxycycline occurs particularly rapidly, resistant organisms being detectable in the feces within 2 weeks of the onset of therapy. Drug-resistant shigellosis and enteric fever are already a problem in the developing world. *Shigella* serotypes have been found to be 87% resistant to ampicillin in Thailand, and 80% to 91% resistant to trimethoprim-sulfamethoxazole in India and Mexico.[154] Fortunately, resistance has not yet been a major problem with the 4-fluoroquinolones.

Despite the presence of dissenting views, the consensus still appears to argue against the routine use of prophylactic antibiotics for all travelers to the tropics. Another argument to support this view is that such routine medication may give the traveler a false sense of security, resulting in less precautions while in travel. Despite this generally valid view, it is probably not appropriate to deny some form of prophylaxis to selected high-risk, short-term travelers when their activities in the foreign locale would be severely and significantly affected by even a transient illness. Patients should be counseled, however, about the risks, benefits, and shortcomings of such treatment. Travelers' diarrhea chemoprophylaxis should not be used when the anticipated length of stay is greater than 3 weeks.

Vaccines

A vaccine against ETEC, although still some time away from widespread use, may offer the best hope for relief. Studies seeking a vaccine for ETEC-mediated illness are in progress at several laboratories. The major impediment to the development of a successful ETEC vaccine is the variety of antigens involved. The vaccines currently under development contain live attenuated strains of ETEC. Researchers hope that these will colonize the small bowel without causing symptoms and stimulate the local secretory immune system of the gut. The newly tested, oral cholera vaccine,[48] which contains the B-subunit of the cholera enterotoxin, has also been shown to be protective against diarrhea caused by ETEC. Given that the two enterotoxins are antigenically closely related, this is not an unexpected finding. Although *Shigella* species are not common causes of travelers' diarrhea, the vaccines being developed, which would involve the oral administration of live-attenuated strains, will afford protection against all four *Shigella* species.

GIARDIASIS

Giardia was probably first seen through a hand lens made by Anton van Leeuwenhoek in the late seventeenth century while examining his own feces during a diarrheal illness.[62] He named this organism *pissabed,* which in old Dutch means woodlouse. It was Vilem Lambl who first formally discovered the parasite in 1859 and named it *Ceromonas intestinalis.* Kunstler identified a similar amphibian parasite 2 decades later and named it *Giardia agilis,* after his mentor professor Giard. The term *Giardia lamblia* was later introduced by Stiles in 1915. Although the parasite was initially thought to be a normal inhabitant of the upper intestinal tract,[176] a series of experiments in the 1950s established its infectivity.[189] Awareness of this infection increased in the United States in the 1970s, with several reports of disease in travelers returning from the Soviet Union.[260]

Epidemiology

In the United States, *Giardia lamblia* is currently the most frequently isolated parasite.[40] Prevalence rates are as high as 16% in certain areas of this country. In the developing world, *Giardia lamblia* is among the first enteric pathogens to infect infants, with peak prevalence rates of 15% to 20% occurring in children under 10 years of age.[83] The infection usually occurs in the settings of day-care centers, institutions for the mentally retarded, and nursing homes, and in male homosexuals and patients with compromised humoral immunity.

Transmission of this organism is particularly common in certain high-risk groups, such as children and employees in day-care centers, male homosexuals, consumers of contaminated water, and those exposed to certain animals.[53,67] The major reservoir and vehicle for the spread of *Giardia* appears to be water contaminated with the cyst form of the organism.[29,31,108,209] During the period 1965 to 1984, *Giardia lamblia* was the most commonly identified pathogen in outbreaks of water-borne diarrheal illness and accounted for 90 outbreaks affecting more than 23,000 people. Common to most of these outbreaks was the use of surface water treated by a faulty purification system or by inadequate chlorination and not subjected to flocculation, sedimentation, and filtration.[116] Untreated wilderness water has also been known to transmit this infection. As occurs in most waterborne outbreaks of disease, the common factor is the ingestion of inadequately purified surface water. In addition, drinking untreated mountain stream water also presents a risk of giardiasis for hikers. Recently, however, food-borne transmission has also been documented with increasing frequency.[177]

Because the inoculant dose for the transmission of this

infection has been found to be between 10 and 100 cysts, person-to-person spread has been identified and occurs frequently.[23,126] Such person-to-person transmission is now the second-most-commonly identified mode of acquisition and occurs in groups with poor fecal-oral hygiene, such as small children in day-care centers, sexually active male homosexuals, and persons in custodial institutions. Sexually active gay men have cyst passage rates as high as 20%.[127] Risk factors that predispose to the transmission of enteropathogens such as *Giardia lamblia* include individual susceptibility, lack of toilet training, crowding, and fecal contamination of the environment.

Increasing evidence suggests that giardiasis may well be a zoonosis.[252] Many wild and domestic animals carry a parasite indistinguishable from the human organism. Genetic analysis data of *Giardia* isolates obtained from mammalian species,[159] cross-transmission experiments,[270] and epidemiologic data linking at least one waterborne outbreak of giardiasis to beavers, imply that many mammalian species serve as reservoirs of *Giardia lamblia.* Although the circumstantial evidence is impressive, as yet there are no concrete data to support direct infection from animals to humans. However, these observations undoubtedly have important implications with regard to protecting public water supplies from contamination.

Life cycle. There are three traditionally recognized morphological species: *G. muris* in rodents, birds, and reptiles; *G. agilis* in amphibians; and *G. lamblia* in humans. The life cycle of *Giardia lamblia* comprises two stages: the trophozoite or free-living stage, and the cyst. The acquisition of the parasite requires oral ingestion of *Giardia* cysts, most often via fecally contaminated water. After ingestion each *Giardia* cyst produces two trophozoites. These are flat forms with a convex dorsal surface and a ventral surface containing a flat disc by which the organism attaches to the intestinal epithelium of the duodenum and proximal jejunum. As detached trophozoites pass down the intestinal tract under intestinal influences that are not fully understood, these encyst to form smooth, oval-shaped, thin-walled cysts, which are then passed in the feces. Cysts are the infective stage of the organism and are the form most commonly found in the feces. Encystation may be enhanced by multiple factors, including the presence of secondary bile salts.[81] As the cyst matures, trophozoite division may occur, resulting in two daughter trophozoites. In patients with profuse watery diarrhea and rapid intestinal transit times, trophozoites may be found in stool specimens as well. Although the incubation period between the ingestion of *Giardia lamblia* cysts and the appearance of symptoms is usually about 2 weeks, the time from cyst ingestion to the detection of cysts in the stool may well be longer than the incubation period.[158] Thus a negative stool examination at the time of onset of symptoms does not reliably argue against infection with *Giardia lamblia.*

Clinical manifestations

Infection with the protozoan *Giardia lamblia* encompasses a wide spectrum of symptoms. These range from asymptomatic cyst passage, through acute, usually self-limited, diarrhea, to a chronic syndrome of diarrhea, malabsorption and weight loss. Of 100 people ingesting *Giardia* cysts, 5% to 15% will become asymptomatic cyst passers, 25% to 50% will develop an acute diarrheal syndrome, and the remaining 35% to 70% will have no trace of infection. Of those who do have symptoms, most will spontaneously clear their infection within several weeks, but the remainder will go on to develop a chronic diarrheal syndrome or come to antimicrobial therapy. The stage of asymptomatic cyst passage may indeed last as long as 6 months.[179]

Symptomatic giardiasis is usually characterized by acute diarrhea, abdominal cramps, bloating, and flatulence. The patient also usually complains of fatigue, malaise, nausea, and loss of appetite. Sulfuric belching may be noted. Vomiting, fever, and tenesmus are infrequent. The severity of symptoms triggered by *Giardia lamblia* depends on the number of organisms ingested.[189]

In giardiasis, the stool is commonly greasy and foul smelling, and characteristically floats in the toilet bowl. Less commonly, profuse watery diarrhea may be seen. Gross blood, pus, and mucus are usually absent, and stool examination for polymorphonuclear cells is usually negative.

Chronicity of the diarrhea is an important distinguishing feature of giardiasis. When initially seen, most patients have usually been symptomatic for several days to weeks. Weight loss of up to 10 lb may occur in about half the patients. Rarely a reactive arthritis also occurs.[210]

The chronic diarrhea syndrome is characterized by profound malaise, lassitude, headache, and diffuse abdominal discomfort, often exacerbated by eating. Weight loss is usually seen, and periods of diarrhea may be interrupted by periods of constipation or normal bowel function. The syndrome continues to wax and wane for months until spontaneous resolution ensues or appropriate therapy is given. Intestinal malabsorption is one of the principal physiologic consequences of chronic giardiasis. Children may present with a failure to thrive or with a spruelike illness.[37]

Diagnosis

Giardiasis should be entertained as a diagnostic possibility in all patients who present with prolonged diarrhea or malabsorption of unknown etiology. The suspicion is heightened in the presence of any of the risk factors, such as travel to an endemic area, contact with children or workers of day-care centers, an institutionalized setting, or a homosexual lifestyle.

Using standard microscopy methods, including those that involve concentration techniques, most studies indicate that even after examination of three consecutive stool specimens on different days, only about 80% of infections are detected.[122] The usual method of diagnosis is a stool examination for *Giardia lamblia* trophozoites or cysts. A saline wet mount of liquid stool may yield motile trophozoites because of rapid intestinal transit times. More often, however, the stool is semiformed and trophozoites are not seen. Such a specimen may be examined fresh, or after preservation in formalin or polyvinyl alcohol (PVA) and subsequent trichrome or iron-hematoxylin staining.[253] With these commonly employed methods, cysts are usually identified in 50% to 75% of cases after single stool examination, and in up to 90% of cases after three stool examinations.[157] Purging does not increase yield. Contrast material such as barium will mask the presence of parasites in stool. In addition, medications such as antibiotics, antacids, antidiarrheal compounds, and certain enema and laxative preparations can also interfere with the identification of the organism by altering morphology or by causing the temporary disappearance of the organism from stool specimens.[267]

When stool examination is negative, duodenal contents may be sampled. The three principal methods include the string test (Entero-Test, Hedeco, Palo Alto, California),[192] duodenal aspiration, and duodenal biopsy. The string test involves swallowing a nylon string contained in a gelatin capsule, the free end of which is secured at the mouth. The capsule dissolves in the stomach while the rest of the string is propelled by peristaltic movement into the duodenum. After several hours, the string is pulled out through the mouth and its bile-stained mucus is squeezed on to microscope slide for examination. Some studies have reported a slightly higher yield by this method compared with stool microscopy.

Although stool microscopy is currently the gold standard for the diagnosis of *Giardia lamblia,* it is inherently a laborious process, dependent to a considerable degree on observer expertise. Because giardiasis may be encountered in sporadic outbreaks among susceptible population groups, alternative diagnostic strategies for screening a large number of specimens are actively being developed. Most of these involve immunologic techniques applied to fecal specimens. Several commercially available enzyme linked immunosorbent assay (ELISA) kits have been developed. The ProSpect/Giardia kit from Alexon Inc., Mountain View, California, was evaluated to have a sensitivity and specificity of 96% and 100% respectively, compared with 74% and 100% for microscopic examination.[193] A second ELISA test, the Trend *Giardia lamblia* Direct Detection System (Trend Scientific Inc., St. Paul, Minnesota) uses anti-*Giardia* cyst and trophozoite polyclonal antibodies to detect *Giardia lamblia* antigens in stool. On concentrated stool specimens, this technique was found to have a sensitivity and specificity of 94% and 98% respectively.[47] Another study evaluating the same system found comparable results with a sensitivity and specificity of 94% and 97% respectively.

Serologic testing for *Giardia lamblia* antibodies is currently available only on a research basis. In addition, because of the time required for a detectable serum antibody response after infection, this method is not useful for the rapid detection of infection.

Management

There are several drugs with excellent efficacy against *Giardia lamblia*.[57] Most authorities consider the acridine dye derivative quinacrine to be the drug of choice.[268] The adult dose is 100 mg tid, and that for children is 6 mg/kg/day in three divided doses, given for 5 to 7 days. Although it has an efficacy of 90%, it may be poorly tolerated in children, requiring interruption of therapy. Side effects are prominent, and include yellow discoloration of the skin, sclerae, exfoliative dermatitis, and rarely toxic psychosis.

The nitroimidazole metronidazole is usually better tolerated, and although not approved for this indication in the United States, is the much more commonly used agent for giardiasis. The dose is 200 mg tid in adults and 15 mg/kg/day in three divided doses in children. Its efficacy is in the range of 80% to 95%.[133] Concerns remain about its potential mutagenicity, and these make its routine use debatable. Side effects include a metallic taste, nausea, dizziness, a disulfiram-like reaction with alcohol, headache, and, rarely, reversible neutropenia.

The nitrofuran and monoamine oxidase (MAO) inhibitor, furazolidine, is an alternative for use in children because of its availability in the liquid suspension form. Given in a dose of 8 mg/kg/day in divided doses for 10 days, it has an efficacy of 80%. Side effects include brown discoloration of the urine and mild hemolysis in glucose-6-phosphate dehydrogenase (G6PD)-deficient individuals. The nitroimidazole tinidazole is also highly effective against *Giardia lamblia*. A single dose of 2 gm, and a dosage of 150 mg bid for 7 days were found to be equally effective in eradicating this organism from the gut, with restoration of absorptive function within 1 to 3 weeks.[94,211] This agent, along with the closely related agent ornidazole, is not currently available in the United States.

For those patients who fail to respond to a single course, a second course of the same agent or an alternative usually succeeds in eradicating the infection.

There is no consensus on the therapy for pregnant women with giardiasis. This caution stems from the theoretical teratogenicity of the agents involved. In mild disease, therapy should be delayed until after delivery, if at all possible, or at least until after the first trimester. The oral aminoglycoside paromomycin has been used[129] and is attractive because of its lack of intestinal absorption. A 5- to 10-day course of 25 to 30 mg/kg/day in three divided doses is usually employed.[195] Further testing is required before more definitive recommendations can be made.

Prevention

The prevention of giardiasis includes measures to interrupt the fecal-oral transmission route. These include the proper handling and treatment of water used for communities and good individual hygiene.

Although chlorination is usually sufficient to kill *Giardia lamblia* cysts, several important variables such as water temperature, turbidity, Ph, and contact time may alter the efficacy of chlorine and result in a need for higher chlorine levels.[41] Thus supplemental flocculation, sedimentation, and filtration also should be employed routinely.

In the setting of back country traveling, all water should be considered suspect because of the wide animal reservoir of giardiasis, and boiling for 1 minute should be routinely employed, with longer durations at higher altitudes. When boiling is not possible, halazone (5 tabs/liter for 30 min), a solution of saturated crystalline iodine (12.5 ml/liter for 30 min), or other chlorine or iodine preparation may be used.[117]

Endemic foci of giardiasis in day-care centers continue to be a major problem. Some authorities recommend that initially only symptomatic children be treated. If this along with strict hand-washing does not succeed in controlling the outbreak, consideration may be given to treating all infected children. The venereal transmission of *Giardia* can be decreased by the avoidance of oral-anal and oral-genital sex.

SCABIES

Scabies is an arthropod-borne infectious disease caused by the mite *Sarcoptes scabiei*. Although the clinical disease has been known for more than 2,500 years,[5] it was not until 1687 that Giovan Cosimo Bonomo described the causative mite in his famous letter to the naturalist Francisco Redi.

Epidemiology

Although precise figures for the prevalence of this very common infection in temperate countries are not available, estimates vary from 2% to 5%.[90] Because scabies infection is not a reportable condition in the United States and in most other countries, exact estimates in a given population are usually not available.[258] In developing nations, the incidence is similar for both genders and all ages.[38] Worldwide prevalence is in the range of 300 million cases.[188] Scabies affects all ages and both sexes, but its prevalence decreases after the age of 40, and blacks appear to be less susceptible than whites.[3]

Nosocomial infections are common in nursing homes,[175] mental institutions, and other settings of overcrowding coupled with poor personal hygiene. Although scabies is certainly more common in persons subjected to overcrowding, such as refugees, disaster victims, and the poor, this infestation afflicts all strata of all races worldwide and is not limited to the impoverished or those with poor hygiene. It is said of *Sarcoptes scabei* that it is "notorious for its lack of respect for person, age, sex, or race, whether it be in the epidermis of an emperor or a slave, a centurian or a nursling, it makes itself perfectly at home with indiscriminating impudence and equal obnoxiousness."[76] Despite extensive studies, the incidence of this disease has not been equated with personal hygiene or the availability of running water in countries where this disease is an issue. By far, the most important factor in influencing the incidence and distribution of this disease is the extent of physical contact with an infected source. Thus in decreasing order of risk are children, mothers, older mother-role female siblings, other family members, and, finally, adult males. Although they do not appear to contribute to the risk of acquiring the infection, standards of personal hygiene, living conditions, and climate certainly do seem to play a role in the likelihood of secondary bacterial infection.[246]

The transmission of scabies is primarily by way of direct contact with the infested patient, as opposed to via fomites such as contaminated clothing and bedding. This is directly as a result of the inability of mites to survive for more than 2 days away from an animate host. Crowded conditions thus promote the spread of this infection. Cattle, horses, mules, sheep, goats, pigs, dogs, and cats have all been reported as reservoirs of Sarcoptes mites for man.[45] Zoonotic scabies can be a problem in those who come into contact with animals in poor hygiene conditions, and transmission of mites that usually infest domestic animals and pets does occur.[18] Dogs are most commonly infected, but cats, horses, pigs, and pigeons have been implicated as well.[44,187]

Clinical manifestations

Careful historical inquiry will usually reveal evidence of contact with an infected case, often 4 or more weeks earlier. All varieties of scabies other than Norwegian scabies has a 4- to 6-week latent period without pruritus. During this period the female mite burrows into the skin, presenting antigen to the host immune system.[4,70,95,169] Although these patients are asymptomatic, they are fully infective to others, so contacts must be treated effectively to control spread.

The mite *Sarcoptes scabei* is oval, less than 1 mm long, and colorless, and can move at up to 2.5 cm in an hour[147] (see Fig. 57-1). It causes an infection limited to the skin, in which the mites characteristically burrow in the stratum corneum. Because mites cannot survive away from a host for more than 2 days, direct contact with an infested person during this period is far more important than is transmission via contaminated beddings or clothes. Any circumstance that includes or promotes overcrowding thus favors the outbreak of this infestation. A secondary attack rate of 38% among household members provides the rationale for presumptive community treatment.

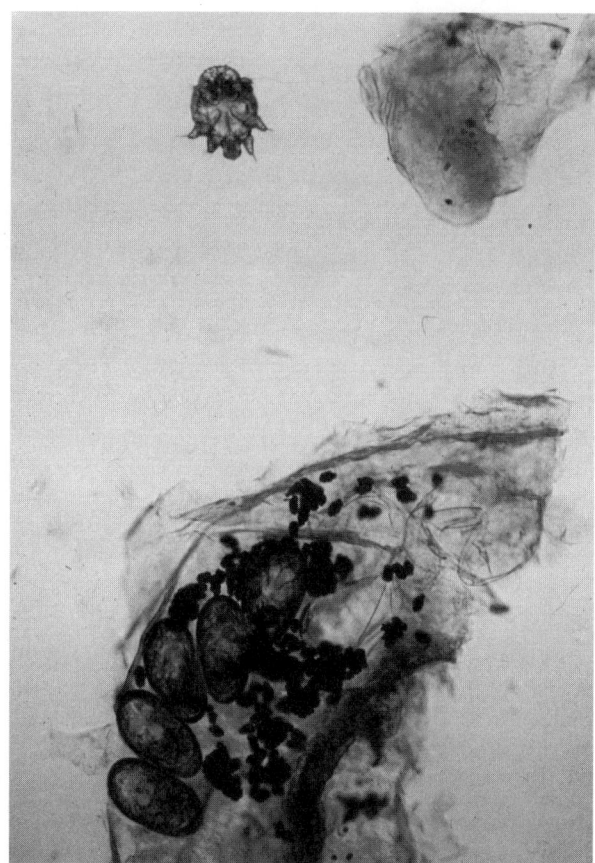

Fig. 57-1. *Sarcoptes scabiei* mite. (Courtesy Babar K. Rao.)

The clinical manifestations of scabies are highly variable; thus it is also known as the great imitator, a title once reserved for syphilis.[8] It should be suspected in any patient presenting with pruritus, particularly if more than one person of the same household has the symptom. The itching is typically nocturnal or is exacerbated after a hot shower.

The early lesions are characteristically 1 to 2 mm, highly pruritic, red papules, which may become lichenified, erythematous, or hyperpigmented when chronic. The burrows themselves measure 3 to 15 mm and are fine, irregular, threadlike, and often difficult to find. Slightly larger papulovesicular, macular, pustular, or scaly plaque-like lesions also may be seen. Depending on the degree of sensitization of the individual, localized or generalized erythema, severe scaling, vesicles, or even bullae may occur. Chronic cases may develop nodular lesions. Scabies lesions are most common on the flexor surfaces of the wrists and dorsal interdigital spaces. Other affected areas include the breasts, periumbilical area, belt line, buttocks, thighs, penis, scrotum, elbows, feet, ankles, and anterior axillary folds. In children the disease may involve any part of the skin, and bullous lesions may be seen.

Atypical forms of the disease may occur in groups that may not appear to be at high risk. Patients with a high

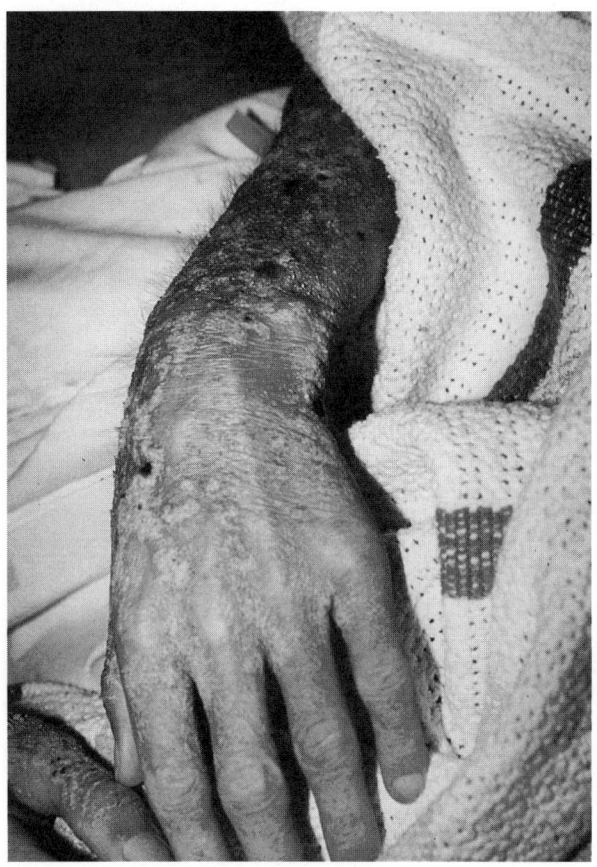

Fig. 57-2. Rash of Norwegian scabies. (Courtesy Babar K. Rao.)

level of hygiene may develop "scabies of the cultivated." Burrows are found only in a minority of such patients, and other findings also may be scant, but they continue to be infectious.

Norwegian scabies is characterized by erythema, hyperkeratosis, and crusting, but little or no itching[21,61,266] (see Fig. 57-2). It is particularly hazardous because it lacks the typical pruritus and is extremely infectious.

Patients infected with the human immunodeficiency virus tend to develop papulosquamous lesions in skin cleavage lines, findings that are similar to those in pityriasis rosea. Norwegian scabies has also been described in patients with HIV disease[98,114,121] and with acquired selective IgA deficiency.[212]

Diagnosis

Definitive diagnosis requires identification of the mites, their eggs, and fecal pellets or scybala. Microscopic examination of a mineral oil and skin scraping under a cover slip (the mineral oil scrape), is the most common method used to directly visualize mites and has largely replaced the older method of picking out a mite on the point of a needle.

Burrows should be sought diligently at the appropriate

anatomic sites and can be made to fluoresce yellow-gray to Wood's lamp with the topical application of liquid tetracycline followed several minutes later by alcohol.[174] The burrow-ink test (BIT) is also useful. Blue or black ink or a felt-tipped pen is applied over the lesions, and the excess ink is then wiped away with an alcohol pad. The dark ink retained in the burrows renders them easily visible.

The diagnosis of scabies does not preclude the presence of other skin conditions. Pediculosis is an often coexistent dermatosis.

Management

Good hygiene serves as little protection against scabies outbreaks, even though it probably plays a role in successful treatment and prevention in the individual.

In the United States, the most commonly used scabicide is the gamma isomer of benzene hexachloride, gamma benzene hexachloride, or lindane 1%, in a vanishing cream formulation marketed under the brand name Kwell.[156] Lindane in a concentration greater than 1% is used as an insecticide. It can be applied to all areas of the body except the face and scalp, and is left in place for 6 to 8 hours before washing off. Concurrent treatment with a topical corticosteroid for the severe accompanying pruritus and psychological support to the patient are other important aspects of scabies management. The best-known toxicity is that to the nervous system.[215] Considering the enormous amounts of Kwell used to treat lice and scabies in this country, the reports of toxicity are relatively few. Most toxicity usually occurs when the medication is misused, overused, or ingested.[20] Although aplastic anemia and other blood dyscrasias have long been known to be associated with the use of lindane as an insecticide,[136,271] recently aplastic anemia secondary to the scabicidal concentration of lindane in Kwell has also been reported.[186] Patients should be instructed not to exceed recommended doses, and prescriptions should not be refilled. Multiple treatments are often initiated by patients, in many cases without knowledge of the physician. Persistent pruritus, reinfestation from untreated contacts, and failure to adequately treat all body areas are the most common causes for overtreatment. Thus patients should be warned that pruritus may persist for up to 2 weeks or more after treatment. In recent years, multiple reports of lindane-resistant scabies have appeared. In 1983, Hernandez-Perez first reported scabies in El Salvador that was apparently unresponsive to 1% lindane. Similar treatment failures have been reported from Panama[247] and several states in the United States.

Topical 5% permethrin cream appears to be a highly effective and a relatively nontoxic alternative to lindane.[248] In one double-blind study, 91% of patients treated with 95% permethrin were free of lesions at 1 month, compared with only 45% of those treated with 1% lindane.

Alternative scabicides, including benzyl benzoate, crotamotion cream (Eurax), or sulfur ointment, may be used for infants or pregnant women, or for unsupervised mass treatments. In infants, monosulfiram is applied at diagnosis and then at 1 day and 1 week. Sulfur dermatitis may result, and with all sulfur preparations, alcohol ingestion must be avoided because an antabuse-like reaction may occur.

Calamine lotion and antihistamines usually suffice for the urticarial manifestations, but occasionally corticosteroids may be required.

The treatment of infected people does not in any way prevent reinfestation. This is particularly common in homeless people, where treating all contacts simultaneously is usually impractical and impossible.

For Norwegian scabies and for all cases with nail involvement, a keratolytic agent such as salicylic acid may be required before a scabicide is applied, and repeated treatments may be necessary.

LYME DISEASE
History

Borrelia burgdorfori was isolated as the agent of Lyme disease in 1982.[36] Subsequently it became evident that many prior descriptions of similar clinical syndromes, both in Europe and North America since the beginning of this century, were probably also a result of infection with this pathogen. The earliest sign of Lyme disease, erythema migrans (EM), was first recognized by Afzelius in 1909.[1] He hypothesized that the skin lesion was the result of a tick bite that transmitted the causative organism from animals to humans. Later, in 1921, the tick *Ixodes ricinus* was identified as the vector for the disease.[35] The first well-documented human case of erythema migrans in the United States was reported in 1970.[204] In 1975, Steere et al. named the entity *Lyme arthritis* after observing an association between erythema migrans and arthritis in a group of patients living near Old Lyme, Connecticut.[233] These cases bore a marked clinical resemblance to juvenile rheumatoid arthritis. After it became obvious that this was a multisystem disorder not limited to the skin and joints, the name was changed to Lyme disease.

The pathogen

Borrelia burgdorferi is a motile spirochete from the family Spirochaetaceae, genus *Borrelia*. It is usually difficult to see this organism under bright field conditions, but it is readily visible by phase-contrast or darkfield microscopy. It is not easily demonstrated in tissue sections, especially after the disease has entered the chronic phase. Thus histopathologic identification is not used routinely in the diagnosis of this infection. The organism itself is microaerophilic and can be grown in a modified Kelly medium (Barbour-Stoner-Kelly) at 33° C.[15] Although it is easily isolated from the tick vector, *Borrelia burgdorferi* is difficult to culture from human body fluids. Its fastidious

nature and doubling time of 8 to 24 hours make it difficult to use routine culture for diagnosis, and only rarely has the organism been isolated from blood, CSF, or synovial tissue. In contrast, the yield rate from cultures of skin biopsies of erythema migrans lesions is as high as 50%.[11]

Epidemiology

Lyme borreliosis is currently the most common tick-borne infectious disease in the United States.[42] Ixodes ticks are the principal vector of the illness throughout the world, and cases of the disease are indeed limited to areas where these species of tick are endemic.[19] In this country, Lyme disease has been reported in 47 states.[256] The vast majority of cases have occurred in three main regions: coastal areas of the upper Northeast extending from Maryland to Massachusetts; the upper Midwest, predominantly Wisconsin and Minnesota; and the far West, in California and western Nevada. These geographic areas correspond to the distribution of the tick vector in the United States; *Ixodes dammini* in the east and *Ixodes pacificus* in the west. Lyme borreliosis also occurs throughout Europe, Scandinavia,[203] and Australia.[241] It also has been reported recently from China,[2] Japan,[123] and extensive areas of the former Soviet Union.[59]

The three developmental stages of the tick are the larva, nymph, and adult. Immature *Ixodes dammini* larvae and nymphs feed primarily on rodents, particularly the white-footed mouse, whereas adult ticks usually feed on larger mammals, especially deer. Tick feeding patterns influence the distribution of the disease worldwide. Larvae or first-stage ticks are usually born uninfected, and become infected only after feeding on an infected animal. Infected nymphs usually transmit the infection to rodents. Uninfected larvae usually feed on these rodents and become infected, and subsequently molt to form nymphs, which go on to infect other rodents. Thus *B. burgdorferi* is maintained in nature by such horizontal transmission. Each successive stage of ticks feeds on progressively larger mammals. The intermediate or nymphal stage of the tick is the most frequent vehicle for transmission of this disease to humans. It has been estimated that a feeding period of at least 24 hours is required for a tick to transmit the infection to humans.[19]

The risk of acquiring the infection seems to be the same in all age groups and is related more to the risk of exposure and the endemicity of infection within a given area. Males and females are equally affected. Because of scarcity of the requisite tick vector in severe winter, most cases of Lyme disease occur between the months of May and November. Asymptomatic infection has been shown to occur in endemic areas.[235]

Clinical features

Lyme disease is a multisystem disorder with protean manifestations involving several organ systems. As with other spirochetal diseases, Lyme borreliosis generally occurs in stages, with exacerbations, remissions, and varying clinical manifestations at each stage.

From a conceptual point of view it is helpful to consider the clinical features of Lyme disease in three chronological stages. Stage I consists of erythema chronicum migrans along with various constitutional signs and symptoms to be described here. In stage 2, which occurs weeks or months later, neurologic and cardiac manifestations, musculoskeletal abnormalities, and intermittent attacks of arthritis occur. In stage 3, seen months to years later, there is chronic involvement of the skin, nervous system, and joints. Despite this artificial division, in any given patient the clinical course of this infection tends to be highly variable, with significant overlap between these stages in most cases.[12] The clinical spectrum ranges from mild, almost asymptomatic infection to simultaneous involvement of the skin, nerves, heart, and joints. Indeed the disease may begin in any organ system, following a transient, recurrent, or chronic course. During its course the disease will typically disseminate to many organs in the body, often so in the early or acute phase of the infection. A disease-free interval may occur between the acute and chronic phases of the disease, during which time the infection remains dormant.

Skin lesion and accompanying symptoms. The earliest and most easily recognized sign of the infection is erythema chronicum migrans, the characteristic skin lesion. This is found in 50% to 75% of cases and usually follows an often-unnoticed tick bite by 14 to 23 days. Although warm to touch, the lesion is not often painful. It may be accompanied by nonspecific systemic symptoms such as fever, malaise, headache, stiff neck fatigue,[232] regional lymphadenopathy,[228] sore throat, nonproductive cough, or testicular swelling. Such signs and symptoms often herald the systemic spread of the infection. As dissemination progresses, other signs also may develop, often within the first few weeks, such as smaller multifocal EM lesions, which occur in almost half the patients in the United States, arthralgias, myalgias, conjunctivitis, and meningismus. Multiorgan involvement, although typical of a later stage in the disease, may occur in the acute or subacute phase as well. When this occurs, acute meningitis, myocarditis, conduction system defects, hepatitis, myositis, and much less commonly, arthritis, may also be seen. Because some patients may indeed present with such nonspecific systemic findings even in the absence of a rash, Lyme disease needs to be considered in the differential diagnosis of any vague flulike illness. In addition, the fatigue and lethargy may persist for months after the skin lesions have disappeared.

Erythema migrans is an expanding annular erythematous skin lesion, which characteristically shows central clearing. Variations with scaling, vesicles, purpura, or erythema without central clearing are commonly seen. When a skin lesion is present, the organism can be cultured from skin biopsy specimens in up to 50% of cases.

Another dermatologic manifestation of this disease, *Borrelia* lymphocytoma, occurs in the form of bluish red nodules found mainly in the earlobes of children and over the skin of the nipple in adults. These lesions may occur in the acute phase or later.[110] When present on the breast, this disease can be confused with a malignancy. Histologically, differentiation from lymphoma can be difficult.

A third dermatological manifestation of the infection, acrodermatitis atrophicans, is a chronic, insidious skin disorder that occurs primarily in elderly women and is seen a decade or so after the initial infection. Bluish discolored areas with a doughy consistency have been described, typically over the distal extremities, but with sparing of the palms, soles, and face. Rheumatologic and neurologic signs may be present along with acrodermatitis atrophicans.[10]

Musculoskeletal symptoms. Musculoskeletal manifestations may be seen from within a few weeks to 2 years after the onset of infection. Overall, about 80% of patients develop some evidence of joint involvement, the ranging in severity from arthralgias to full-blown arthritis.[234] In acute cases, arthralgias may be seen within days to weeks of initial infection with *Borrelia burgdorferi*. Other early signs include myalgias and tendon and bone pain. Multiple joints may be involved in succession. Large-joint arthritis, with joint swelling and other signs of inflammation, is uncommon in the early stage. Such involvement tends to be episodic, and although other large joints also can be affected, the knee is the most commonly involved joint.

Nervous system manifestations. Data suggest that *Borrelia burgdorferi* invades the nervous system early in the course of infection. Thus signs and symptoms of meningeal irritation may occur early in the illness when ECM is present.[229] Patients with erythema migrans have frequent complaints referable to the nervous system. These are most commonly malaise, fatigue, lethargy, headaches, and neck stiffness.[232] Cranial neuritis, painful radiculitis, and even meningitis may occur within the first 3 months of infection. CSF abnormalities such as pleocytosis, moderate elevations of CSF protein in the face of a normal CSF glucose concentration, serve to distinguish patients with meningitis from those with meningismus. Cranial neuropathy may occur with or without accompanying meningitis and most frequently involves the seventh cranial nerve in a unilateral or bilateral distribution.

Chronic infection with *Borrelia burgdorferi* is associated with nervous system dysfunction in about 15% of patients. These abnormalities include meningitis, encephalitis, cranial neuritis, motor and sensory radiculoneuritis, mononeuritis multiplex, myelitis, or chorea, alone or in various combinations.[172] Symptoms involving the central nervous system range from subtle impairment of cognitive function to full-blown focal neurological abnormalities. In some respects chronic neuroborreliosis may resemble multiple sclerosis, but the two disorders usually can be differentiated. Lyme borreliosis also may involve the peripheral nervous system.[99] The spectrum of involvement here ranges from the severe, painful, and debilitating meningopolyneuritis (Garin-Bujadoux-Bannwarth syndrome) to more common milder neuropathy in patients with chronic infection. The single most useful test in the diagnosis of CNS infection with *Borrelia burgdorferi* is measurement of anti-*Borrelia burgdorferi* antibodies in the CSF.[232]

In cases of nervous system involvement with this infection, unifocal and multifocal areas of inflammation have been demonstrated in the brain and the spinal cord.[242] It is yet unknown whether this inflammation is due to vasculitis, immune mechanisms, or direct infection.

Cardiac manifestations. Acute cardiac involvement, within several weeks of the infection, is a recognized feature that may occur in up to 8% of adults and a lower proportion of children.[230] Most commonly, fluctuating conduction system abnormalities, ranging from atrioventricular block to complete heart block, are seen. Atrioventricular block is almost always a localized abnormality that occurs proximal to the bundle of His but can fluctuate and cause syncope. The complete heart block associated with Lyme disease is self-limited in the majority of cases. Diffuse cardiac involvement with acute myopericarditis also may occur. Left ventricular dysfunction is demonstrable in up to half of the cases, but this is usually transient and not severe.[190] T-wave changes and ST-segment depression are frequently observed on the electrocardiogram. Chest pain or shortness of breath may occur because of myopericarditis. Heart murmurs are not a feature of cardiac involvement in Lyme disease. Endomyocardial biopsy may demonstrate spirochetes.[190]

Other organs. The eyes may be involved, most commonly manifesting as a conjunctivitis.[232] Ischemic optic neuropathy,[201] iritis, panophthalmitis, and blindness[231] also have been described. During the acute phase of the infection, hepatitis,[232] myositis, osteomyelitis, and pneumonitis also have been reported.[138]

Congenital infection. Congenital infection can occur as a result of maternal-fetal transmission. Premature birth and fatal congenital heart disease, with wide dissemination of the organism in fetal tissues, was demonstrated in one case.[202] Other adverse fetal outcomes include syndactyly, blindness, and intrauterine death.

Diagnosis

The protean manifestations of Lyme disease and the infrequently obtainable history of a tick bite can make the diagnosis of this disease challenging. Serological tests for *Borrelia burgdorferi* are currently the most accurate and widely used method for diagnosis. Their diagnostic accuracy is improved when dealing with symptomatic patients living in endemic areas.[214] The indirect fluorescent antibody (IFA) and the enzyme-linked immunosorbent assay (ELISA) are the tests most commonly used to diagnose Lyme disease. The ELISA method is considered more sensitive and more specific than the IFA.[141] False positives can be seen with other spirochetal diseases, such as *Treponema pallidum* infection, infectious mononucleosis, autoimmune disorders, and Rocky Mountain spotted fever.[228] False-negative reactions can be seen in early disease within the first 2 weeks, infection localized to the skin, or cases of partially treated infection. The Western blot, flegellin antigen, and polymerase chain reaction (PCR) are experimental assays that are more sensitive than the IFA and ELISA tests but are not in widespread use at this time.[91]

Management

A complete discussion of the various factors that influence treatment and the agents used to treat Lyme disease is beyond the scope of this chapter. Tetracycline, phenoxymethyl penicillin, and erythromycin, in descending order of preference, are the agents of choice for early disease. Intravenous penicillin G or ceftriaxone is the therapy of choice in those with frank meningitis or significant cardiac conduction system involvement.

Prevention

The tick. The prevention of Lyme disease ultimately depends on how effectively one is able to control its vector, the Ixodes tick. Despite the number of possibilities being investigated, there is currently no proven method to totally eliminate the tick vector from the environment.[6] Chemical insecticide sprays, although possibly effective in reducing tick numbers, are also unlikely to result in eradication. Long-acting sprays also may pose safety hazards to the environment.

Where acceptable in residential and selected areas, clearing of bush by mowing is effective in controlling the tick population. Mechanical clearing followed by use of a herbicide can result in a 90% reduction in larval tick population and a 50% reduction in adult and nymphal tick forms.[100] Where environmentally acceptable, controlled burning of edge habitat also has been shown to reduce tick populations for up to 1 year.

The use of an acaricide or any other pesticide must be consistent with the EPA requirements stated on the label and the Environmental Pesticide Control Act of 1972, as well as any local or state regulations governing such use. The use of agents specifically designed to eliminate ticks has generally met with disappointing results because of the difficulty in penetrating the foliage where ticks are usually found on their animal hosts. *Ixodes dammini* adults, which quest in shrubbery in the fall after the leaves are shed and again in the spring before the leaves appear, are an exception to this rule and are thus susceptible to chemical sprays. Diazinon (e.g., Spectracide), carbaryl (e.g.,

Sevin) and chlorpyrifos (e.g., Dursban) all have been used successfully outdoors.[100] Diazinon and chlorpyrifos also are labeled for spot treatment of cracks and crevices indoors and for use in pet bedding to control brown dog ticks but are not considered safe to use on pets directly.

The deer. The explosive increase in the number of deer in the United States from 300,000 in 1900 to 15 million today seems to account in large part for the pandemic status of Lyme disease. One approach is to limit the number of deer, which is unlikely to be successful short of complete eradication of all deer. Indeed, a study that involved eliminating the deer population showed a slow decline in the number of ticks.[263] However, other studies that involved only reduction in the number of deer failed to demonstrate any significant reduction in tick numbers. In addition, when the number of deer is reduced, ticks tend to be found in greater density on the remaining animals, or alternatively, move to other hosts.[100]

The individual. Patient education is of paramount importance. It is helpful to teach patients what the involved ticks look like in their local area. If actual ticks are unavailable, photos or slides can be used for this purpose. On an individual level, some exposure to ticks is unavoidable in most endemic areas. Personal protection is the single most effective measure in avoiding Lyme disease and is appropriate in all habitats and situations. The incidence of Lyme disease in a given endemic area is determined largely by the extent to which the public knows and practices personal protection measures. A number of measures are available for individuals to limit tick exposure and the risk of Lyme disease.[6]

Protective clothing should be worn at all times and should be tucked in at the ankles, wrists, and waist. Light-colored clothing also makes the dark-colored ticks easier to spot, thus facilitating removal. One also should inspect clothing for ticks before coming indoors.

Tick repellents are divided into those applied to skin and those applied to clothing. Skin-applied repellents include N,N-diethyl-meta-toluamide (DEET), 2-ethyl-1, 3-hexanediol, and dimethyl phthalate. Permethrin is the most effective clothing-applied repellent. In states where this ingredient has Environmental Protection Agency registration, Permethrin-containing compounds (e.g., Permanone) have been shown to be highly effective in killing and repelling ticks. However, these repellents should be applied to clothing only, and never to bare skin.[100] The use of DEET along with a Permethrin-containing repellent for clothing offers the best overall protection.[51] The adverse effects of these repellents are minimal, but cases of hypersensitivity have been reported, especially in children.[51] DEET may also cause both contact urticaria and a bullous eruption.[142] In addition, DEET is also associated with a toxic encephalopathy that is characterized by seizures and coma.[182] This complication has been observed after both ingestion and routine application of products containing DEET. Because of these potential problems, products containing high concentrations of DEET should be avoided in children. In addition, if possible, body parts likely to have contact with the eyes or mouth, such as parts of the hands, should be avoided. After the person is indoors, repellent-treated skin should be washed immediately.

Because at least 24 hours of continuous feeding are required for the transmission of infection, even if a tick bite does occur, removing the tick significantly reduces the likelihood of acquiring the infection. The tick must be removed in a proper manner. The tick should be grasped with tweezers behind the head, as close to the mouth parts as possible, because the grasping and squeezing of the tick's body may inject its fluids into the wound. Pulling slowly but steadily encourages the tick to withdraw its mouth parts. If the head is accidentally detached during this process, the wound should not be probed with a needle. The tick should be saved in a sealed bottle and sent to appropriate testing centers for determining the presence of spirochetes. An antiseptic should be applied to the wound and the site monitored. If a rash develops at the site or other constitutional symptoms develop up to 8 weeks after the tick bite, immediate medical attention should be sought.

To reduce disease-induced morbidity in endemic areas, secondary prevention of Lyme disease after presumed infection via a tick bite assumes great importance. In endemic areas, the probability of Lyme disease after a tick bite ranges from 0.012 to 0.05. Early treatment of this infection has been shown to prevent most complications of Lyme disease. However, in most instances, antimicrobials are not prescribed until a rash or some other symptoms develop. A recent study found that empirical treatment of patients with tick bites is indicated when the probability of *B. burgdorferi* infection after a bite is 0.036 or higher, and that empirical treatment may be the preferred option when the probability of infection ranges from 0.01 to 0.035. However, empirical treatment was not found to be warranted when the probability of infection with *Borrelia burgdorferi* in a given area was below 0.01.[140]

In a vector-borne disease such as Lyme borreliosis, public health education is also extremely important. One such program conducted in an endemic area from 1983 to 1989 targeted three major segments of the community—the general public, health care providers, and elected officials. Within the general public, school children and teachers participated particularly enthusiastically in the educational campaign. The media also were particularly helpful in disseminating information about this important, largely preventable infection.[56]

In summary, the main prevention strategies for Lyme disease are the avoidance of heavily wooded areas or tall grasses in endemic areas from May through October; the wearing of light-colored clothing outdoors to facilitate easy recognition of attached ticks; the use of protective clothing to minimize the chance of tick bites; the use of DEET-type insect repellents on the skin coupled with Permethrin-containing products applied to clothing; the frequent visual examination of skin, clothing, bedding, and pets after being outdoors; the proper and judicious removal of ticks within 24 hours of attachment; and finally increasing vigilance for any signs or symptoms compatible with Lyme disease[173] so that consideration can be given to empirical treatment in the appropriate epidemiological setting.

PREVENTIVE ASPECTS OF ANTIBIOTICS

Prophylactic antibiotics refers to the use of antimicrobial agents to prevent the occurrence of a morbid condition. Prophylaxis can be primary (i.e., that given before the onset of some condition with the aim of preventing it from occurring), or secondary (i.e., treatment that is implemented after the onset of the initiating disease or condition, to prevent recurrences or further complications and morbidity). Preventive antibiotics may be employed for surgical conditions or nonsurgical conditions, or to prevent infection of prosthetic material in the body.

Prophylaxis for surgical infections

Postoperative wound infection remains the primary source of infectious morbidity in the surgical patient.[161] The type of operative procedure, that is, whether the wound is clean, clean contaminated, contaminated, dirty, or infected, has traditionally been considered the best predictor of wound infection. The often-quoted infection rates for these are: clean wounds, 1% to 5%; clean contaminated wounds, 3% to 11%; contaminated wounds, 10% to 17%; and dirty wounds, more than 27%.[78] Although not proven, evidence appears to be increasing that the most important risk factor for postoperative infection, rather than the type of wound, is the patient's physical status at the time of procedure. Weight loss of more than 10% along with physiologic dysfunction of at least two organ systems has been associated with significantly higher postoperative complications.[265] The incidence of major complications, pneumonia, and longer hospital stays similarly has been shown to be greater for protein-depleted as opposed to protein-replete patients.[264]

Immunocompetence, as measured by degree of hypersensitivity response, is also important in the postoperative period. Anergic patients are found to have more postoperative septic complications than those with intact immune systems. Other evidence of individual patient risk indicates a lower infection rate for operative procedures of all types in children compared with adults, probably because younger patients have a better overall health status than older individuals. The first studies[97] of risk factors for surgical wound infections described a model containing four risk factors: abdominal operation, operation lasting longer

than 2 hours, contaminated or dirty infected wound by the traditional wound classification system, and presence of three or more diagnoses. This approach was found to predict surgical wound infection approximately twice as well as the traditional classification of wound contamination mentioned previously. Most recently, investigators from the CDC have reported on a composite risk index used in the National Nosocomial Infections Surveillance System (NNIS).[55] In this, host variables are identified as risk factors for infection instead of the number of discharge diagnoses. In addition, in this report the definition of *prolonged surgery* is procedure-specific, thus making this index more discriminating.

Many perioperative factors have been proven to have a significant influence on the development of postoperative wound infection, especially in clean procedures. Higher infection rates are associated with longer preoperative hospital stays, preoperative razor shaving 1 day before surgery,[54] absence of preoperative showering or bathing with an antiseptic, presence of remote infections at the time of elective surgery,[68] longer duration of the operative procedure itself, and use of prophylactic abdominal drains.[43]

The timing and choice of agent for preoperative antimicrobial prophylaxis depend on the type of procedure being performed. Preoperative antibiotics are routinely employed in gastroduodenal procedures, cholecystectomy, elective colon resection, small intestinal resection, appendectomy, penetrating abdominal trauma, vaginal or abdominal hysterectomy, cesarean section, abortion, and prostatectomy (see Table 57-6). Because of the limited duration of uncomplicated preoperative prophylaxis, it is useful to have limited-time orders with automatic stop dates or other automated mechanisms to ensure timely discontinuation of the antibiotics.

Prophylaxis for nonsurgical infections

In the nonsurgical setting, antibiotics are often employed to prevent infection of the host by exogenous pathogens or to prevent the host's resident flora from infecting a normally sterile site. The term *prophylaxis* also is often used to describe attempts to prevent disease by a dormant pathogen that has infected the host in the remote past, or to prevent disease from a recently acquired infection that has not yet become clinically manifest, as in isoniazid prophylaxis for tuberculosis. Table 57-7 lists selected medical conditions and the recommended antibiotic prophylaxis.

Intramuscular benzathine penicillin is used to prevent streptococcal pharyngeal infections in patients with previous rheumatic fever. In the early days of meningococcal prophylaxis, sulfadiazine was extremely effective in epidemic outbreaks in military installations in World War II, but the subsequent development of sulfadiazine resistance has made this agent useful only when the epidemic strain is known to be susceptible to the drug. Prophylaxis is

Table 57-6. Prophylaxis for surgical infections

Procedure	Regimen recommended
Clean surgical procedures (not involving prostheses or other foreign material)	Controversial at present
Clean surgical procedures (utilizing foreign materials, grafts, or prosthetic devices)	No clear evidence of efficacy Cefazolin 1 g IV q6h until 48 hr postop usually used
Gastroduodenal	Cefazolin 1 g IV 30 min before incision
Cholecystectomy	Cefazolin 1 g IV 30 min before incision
Elective colon resection	Neomycin-erythromycin base, 1 g each PO at hours 0, 1, and 10 on day before surgery *plus* single dose of appropriate IV antibiotic(s) just before incision (e.g., imipenem-cilastatin 1 g IV)
Small intestine resection	Neomycin-erythromycin base, 1 g each PO at hours 0, 1, and 10 on day before surgery *plus* single dose of appropriate IV antibiotic(s) just before incision (e.g., imipenem-cilastatin 1 g IV)
Appendectomy	Cefoxitin 1 g IV q6h *or* ceftizoxime 1-2 g IV q8h for 2 doses
Penetrating abdominal trauma	Cefoxitin 1 g IV q6h for 2 doses beginning shortly before incision
Vaginal or abdominal hysterectomy	Cefazolin 1 g IV q6h shortly before incision
Cesarean section	Cefazolin 1 g IV q6h shortly before incision
Abortion	Cefazolin 1 g IV q6h shortly before incision
Prostatectomy	Cefazolin 1 g IV q6h shortly before incision

Modified from Nichols RL: Prophylaxis for surgical infections. In: Gorbach SL, Bartlett JG, Blacklow NR, editors: *Infectious diseases,* Philadelphia, 1992, WB Saunders.

nowadays directed mainly at household contacts of patients with meningococcal disease, in whom the medication used, usually oral rifampin, functions mainly to eradicate asymptomatic colonization, rather than to prevent acquisition of the organism. Similarly, the administration of antibiotics to household or day-care contacts of children with invasive *Hemophilus influenzae* type B infections serves to eradicate the organism from asymptomatic carriers who are at high risk of developing serious disease.[33] In children, prophylaxis with sulfisoxazole or ampicillin is generally recommended in those who have at least three episodes in 6 months, or four within a year.[135] In contrast, several studies have shown no benefit of antimicrobial prophylaxis in viral upper respiratory diseases such as colds and influenza.[58] Immunosuppressed patients, such as those with the acquired immunodeficiency syndrome, with hematologic malignancies, or receiving certain forms of cancer chemotherapy, are at particularly high risk for developing opportunistic infections such as *Pneumocystis carinii* pneumonia, and prophylaxis with oral trimethoprim-sulfamethoxazole or intravenous pentamidine has been found to be beneficial in reducing these infections.

Recurrent urinary tract infections in women often require antimicrobial prophylaxis. Trimethoprim-sulfamethoxazole three times a week is as effective as daily doses of the agent[102] and appears worthwhile for women who have three or more urinary tract infections per year.[225]

Neutropenic patients are particularly susceptible to infection. Most such infections are thought to originate from the indigenous aerobic flora of the gastrointestinal tract in the face of altered immunity. Many studies have been done to evaluate the efficacy of total decontamination of the gut using combinations of nonabsorbable oral antibiotics, as well as of more selective regimens directed primarily at enteric gram-negative organisms. Despite unchanged survival rates, some reduction in the frequency of infection has been noted with these methods.[105] The agents most commonly used for selective decontamination have been trimethoprim-sulfamethoxazole and the quinolones. Their use is based on the assumption that anaerobic bowel flora help prevent colonization by potential pathogens and should not be eradicated. There has been much diversity in the results shown by the various studies evaluating the efficacy of prophylactic antimicrobials in neutropenic patients have produced diverse results. Nevertheless, antimicrobial prophylaxis does not seem to work when the neutropenia is short-lived,[262] with benefit rarely being seen with granulocytopenia of less than 3 weeks duration. Another consistent finding is that even where antimicrobial prophylaxis reduces infectious mortality, it does not have any effect on the overall fatality rate.

Monthly injections of intramuscular benzathine penicillin or daily oral doses of penicillin or erythromycin for 1 week each month have been found to be beneficial in patients with lymphedema and recurrent cellulitis,[13] as has oral daily clindamycin for recurrent staphylococcal skin abscesses.

In hemodialysis patients who are nasal carriers of *Staphylococcus aureus,* topical bacitracin in combination with oral rifampin has been effective in reducing the frequency of *S. aureus* infections, including bacteremia, cutaneous abscesses, and access site infections.[274]

Table 57-7. Medical antimicrobial prophylaxis

Condition	Indication	Regimen
Recurrent streptococcal pharyngitis	Recent rheumatic fever or rheumatic heart disease	Benzathine PCN G IM, 1.2 million units every 4 wk *or* PCN V 250 mg PO BID
Meningococcal disease	Household contact with meningococcal disease	Rifampin PO: adults 600 mg BID for 2 days, children 5-10 mg/kg BID for 2 days
H. influenzae disease	Household or day-care center contact with under 2 yr old with systemic H. flu type b disease	Rifampin PO 20 mg/kg QD for 4 days
Recurrent otitis media	At least 3 episodes in 6 months or 4 in 1 year	Ampicillin 125-250 mg QD *or* sulfisoxazole 500 mg PO BID
Pneumocystis carinii pneumonia	Cancer chemotherapy in certain high-risk patients	SMX-TMP PO 150/750 mg/m^2 in 2 doses per day for 3 consecutive days per week
	AIDS	SMX-TMP PO 800/160 mg BID
Recurrent urinary tract infections in females	At least 3 infections per year	SMX-TMP PO 200/40 mg three times a week or nitrofurantoin PO 100 mg QHS
Neurogenic bladder	Intermittent catheterizations; bladder re-training	Methenamine mandelate PO 1 g Q6H *or* doxycycline PO 100 mg QD *or* Noroxin PO 400 mg QD
Travelers' diarrhea	Controversial: see text	See text
Granulocytopenia	Absolute neutrophil count < 500 with neutropenia expected to last more than 3 weeks	SMX-TMP PO 800/160 mg BID *or* noroxin PO 400 mg QD *or* ciprofloxacin 500 mg PO BID
Recurrent cellulitis	Multiple episodes, especially with lymphedema	Benzathine PCN G IM, 1.2 million units every month *or* PCN V or erythromycin PO 250 mg QD 1 week per month
Recurrent staph skin infections	Multiple episodes	Clindamycin PO 150 mg QD
Group B streptococcal disease in neonates	Maternal colonization at delivery	PCN V or erythromycin PO 500 mg QD from 38 weeks' gestation to delivery or ampicillin IV 500 mg Q6H during labor
Staph aureus infection in patients undergoing long-term hemodialysis	Recurrent infections and nasal colonization	Rifampin PO 600 mg BID for 5 days plus topical bacitracin to nares QD for 7 days every 3 months if nasal cultures positive for *Staph aureus*

Modified from Hirschmann JV: Antimicrobial prophylaxis for non-surgical infections. In Gorbach SL, Bartlett JG, Blacklow NR, editors: *Infectious disease*, Philadelphia, 1992, WB Saunders.

Prophylaxis for prosthetic devices

Prosthetic devices are particularly vulnerable to infection (see Table 57-8). Whenever a patient with a prosthesis presents with signs or symptoms of infection, or evidence of prosthetic dysfunctio periprosthetic inflammation, the possibility of an infected device must always be entertained. In general, every attempt must be made to obtain microbiologic data before the initiation of broad-spectrum antimicrobial therapy, so that the likelihood of identifying the causative microorganism is maximized. Often the prosthetic device may need to be removed for the infection to be adequately treated, many instances requiring its reinsertion later. In such cases, the need for the device must be weighed against the hazard of the infection. Other factors such as the role and relative importance of the prosthesis, as well as the availability of alternatives, must also taken into account. Devices may be essential for life, such as

prosthetic heart valves; essential for life but with convenient alternatives, such as hemodialysis shunts; necessary for important activities, such as prosthetic hip joints; an aid in performing nonessential activities, such as penile prostheses; or primarily cosmetic, such as breast implants.

Because of the potentially catastrophic effects of infection of prosthetic devices, one must make every attempt at primary prophylaxis. Factors predisposing to infection and bacteremia, such as pyogenic dentogingival conditions, obstructive uropathy, and skin infections, should be especially avoided or controlled before the insertion of prosthetic joints. Perioperative antibiotic prophylaxis has been shown to effectively reduce deep wound infection in total joint replacement surgery.[162] For patients with artificial joints, early recognition and prompt treatment of infection are critical in reducing the risk of seeding the joint implant hematogenously. Any situation likely to cause bacteremia

Table 57-8. Prevalence and microbiology of prosthetic device infections

Prosthetic device	Prevalence of infection	Usual pathogens
Cardiac valves	3% at 1 yr 4%-6% at 4-5 yr	S. epidermidis S. aureus
Joints	Hip 0.5%-1.3% Knee 1.3%-2.9%	S. aureus S. epidermidis
Transvenous perma- nent pacemaker	Pocket sepsis 1%-7% Lead only <1%	S. aureus S. epidermidis
Arterial graft	Aortoiliac <1%- 1.5% Femoropopliteal 2%-7%	S. aureus S. epidermidis
Intraocular lens	<1%	S. epidermidis
CSF shunt	1.5%-15%	S.epidermidis S. aureus
CAPD catheter	60% first yr; 0.5-1.0 episodes/patient/yr	S. epidermidis S. aureus Streptococci
Breast implant	Augmentation 2%-3% Reconstruction >3%	S. aureus S. epidermidis
Penile prosthesis	1%-5%	S. epidermidis enterobacteriaceae

Modified from Karchmer AW: Approach to the patient with infection in a prosthetic device. In Gorbach SL, Bartlett JG, Blacklow NR, editors: *Infectious disease,* Philadelphia, 1992, WB Saunders.

should be avoided. Using the same rationale as for infective endocarditis prophylaxis, the use of prophylactic antibiotics before anticipated bacteremic events such as dental surgery, cystoscopy, or colonoscopic biopsy in patients with artificial joints has also been suggested.[30,131] Currently, no available data are available to determine the adequacy or cost effectiveness of such measures, and clinical decisions in such situations still must be made on an individual basis.

SUMMARY

The choice of subjects covered in this discussion serves to highlight the protean nature of preventable infections. From the superficial pruritic eruptions of scabies, to the deep cardiac damage inflicted by rheumatic fever; from the commonplace urinary tract infections, to the worldwide sexually transmitted infections; from the common cold and giardiasis to travelers' diarrhea; infections that are inherently alterable by preventive strategies appear in all spheres of disease and affect us in our interaction with the world within which we live. Apart from specific measures aimed at these disorders, perhaps the most important weapons at our command today are the appropriate but aggressive use of vaccines, coupled with prophylactic antimicrobial agents in those situations where they are of benefit.

Acknowledgments

This manuscript was transcribed by my wife Mateen, without whose support, encouragement, and indulgence this chapter would simply not have been possible. My gratitude also goes to Judy Shapiro and Lisa Dute for their patient secretarial assistance.

REFERENCES

1. Afzelius A: Verhandlungen der dermatologischen Gesselschaft zu Stockholm, *Arch Dermatol Syphilol* 101:405, 1910.
2. Ai C et al: Clinical manifestations and epidemiological characteristics of Lyme disease in Hailin County, Heilongjiang Province, China, *Ann NY Acad Sci* 539:302, 1988.
3. Alexander AM: Role of race in scabies infestation, *Arch Dermatol* 114:627, 1978.
4. Alexander JO: Scabies and pediculosis, *Practitioner* 200:632, 1968.
5. Alexander JO: *Arthropods and human skin,* Berlin/New York, 1984, Springer-Verlag.
6. Anderson JF: Preventing Lyme disease, *Rheum Dis Clin North Am* 15:757, 1989.
7. Aral SO, Holmes KK: Epidemiology of sexual behavior and sexually transmitted diseases. In Holmes KK, et al, editors: *Sexually transmitted diseases,* ed 2, New York, 1990, McGraw-Hill.
8. Arlian LG: Biology, host relationships and epidemiology of Sarcoptes scabei, *Ann Rev Entomol* 34:139, 1989.
9. Arola M, et al: Rhinovirus in acute otitis media, *J Pediatr* 113:693, 1988.
10. Asbrink E, Brehmer-Andersson E, and Hovmark A: Acrodermatitis chronica atrophicans—a spirochetosis, clinical and histopathological picture based on 32 patients; course and relationship to erythema chronicum migrans Afzelius, *Am J Dermatopathol* 8:209, 1986.
11. Asbrink E, Hovmark A: Successful cultivation of spirochetes from skin lesions of patients with erythema chronicum migrans Afzelius and acrodermatitis chronica atrophicans, *Acta Pathol Microbiol Immunol* (B) 93:161, 1985.
12. Asbrink E, Hovmark A: Early and late cutaneous manifestations in Ixodes-borne borreliosis (Erythema migrans borreliosis, Lyme borreliosis), *Ann NY Acad Sci* 539:4, 1988.
13. Babb RR et al: Prophylaxis of recurrent lymphangitis complicating lymphedema, *JAMA* 195:871, 1966.
14. Bandres JC, Mathewson JJ, and Du Pont HL: Heat susceptibility of bacterial enteropathogens, *Arch Intern Med* 148:2261, 1988.
15. Barbour AG: Isolation and cultivation of Lyme disease spirochetes, *Yale J Biol Med* 57:521, 1984.
16. Barker WH: Excess pneumonia and influenza associated hospitalization during influenza epidemics in the United States, 1970-78, *Am J Public Health* 76:761, 1986.
17. Beers KN, Mohler SR: Food poisoning as an in-flight safety hazard, *Aviat Space Environ Med* 56:594, 1985.
18. Beesley WN: Arthropod, oestridial, myiasis and acarines. In Soulsby EJL, editor: *Parasitic zoonoses,* New York, 1964, Academic Press.
19. Benach JL et al: Adult *Ixodes dammini* on rabbits: a hypothesis for the development and transmission of *Borrelia burgdorferi, J Infect Dis* 155:1300, 1987.
20. Billstein SA, Mattaliano VJ: Molluscum contagiosum, scabies and crab lice, *Med Clin North Am* 74:1487, 1990.
21. Binford CH, Connor DH, editors: *Pathology of tropical diseases II,* Washington, DC, 1976, Armed Forces Institute of Pathology.
22. Black RE: Epidemiology of travelers' diarrhea and relative importance of various pathogens, *Rev Infect Dis* 8:S122, 1986.
23. Black RE et al: Giardiasis in day care centers: evidence of person to person transmission, *Pediatrics* 60:486, 1977.

24. Boineau FG, Lewy JE: Urinary tract infection in children: An overview, *Pediatr Ann* 4:515, 1975.
25. Bollgren I et al: Low urinary counts of P-fimbriated *Escherichia coli* in presumed acute pyelonephritis, *Arch Dis Child* 59:102, 1984.
26. Boscia JA, Kaye D: Asymptomatic bacteriuria in the elderly, *Infect Dis Clin North Am Dec* 1(4):893, 1987.
27. Boscia JA et al: Lack of association between bacteriuria and symptoms in the elderly, *Am J Med* 81:979, 1986.
28. Boscia JA et al: Epidemiology of bacteriuria in an elderly ambulatory population, *Am J Med* 80:208, 1986.
29. Brady PG, Wolfe JC: Waterborne giardiasis, *Ann Intern Med* 81:498, 1974.
30. Brause BD: Infections associated with prosthetic joints, *Clin Rheum Dis* 12:523, 1986.
31. Brodsky RE, Spencer HC Jr, and Schultz MG: Giardiasis in American travelers to the Soviet Union, *J Infect Dis* 130:319, 1974.
32. Broom CV, Facklam RR, and Fraser DW: Pneumococcal disease and pneumococcal vaccination: an alternative method to estimate the efficacy of pneumococcal vaccine, *N Engl J Med* 303:549, 1980.
33. Broome CV et al: Use of chemoprophylaxis to prevent the spread of *Hemophilus influenzae* B in day-care facilities, *N Engl J Med* 316:1226, 1987.
34. Brumfitt W, Hamilton-Miller JMT: Urinary infection in the 1990's: the state of the art, *Infection* 18:34, 1990.
35. Burgdorfer W: Discovery of the Lyme disease spirochete: a historical review, *Zentralbl Bakteriol Mikrobiol HYG [A]* 263 (1-2):7, 1986.
36. Burgdorfer W et al: Lyme disease: a tick-borne spirochetosis? *Science* 216:1317, 1982.
37. Burke JA: Giardiasis in childhood, *Am J Dis Child* 129:1304, 1975.
38. Burkhart CG: Scabies: an epidemiological reassessment, *Ann Intern Med* 98:498, 1983.
39. Cates W Jr: Epidemiology and control of sexually transmitted diseases: strategic evolution, *Infect Dis Clin North Am* 1:1, 1987.
40. Centers for Disease Control: Intestinal parasite surveillance annual summary 1978, issued August, 1979.
41. Centers for Disease Control: Waterborne giardiasis—California, Colorado, Oregon, Pennsylvania, *MMWR* 29:121, 1988.
42. Centers for Disease Control: Lyme disease—United States, 1987 and 1988, *MMWR* 38:668, 1989.
43. Cerise EJ, Pierce WA, and Diamond DL: Abdominal drains: their role as a source of infection following splenectomy, *Ann Surg* 171:764, 1970.
44. Chakrabarti A: Human notoedric scabies from contact with cats infested with *Notoedres cati, Int J Dermatol* 25:646, 1986.
45. Chakrabarti A: Pig handler's itch, *Int J Dermatol* 29:205, 1990.
46. Chalmers TC: Effects of ascorbic acid on the common cold: an evaluation of the evidence, *Am J Med* 58:532, 1975.
47. Chaudhry AZ, Rutherford I, and Stinson W: Evaluation of an ELISA immunoassay technique for the detection of *Giardia lamblia* in stool specimens, unpublished data, 1992.
48. Clemens JD et al: Field trial of oral cholera vaccines in Bangladesh, *Lancet* 2:124, 1986.
49. Cluff LE et al: Staphylococcal bacteremia and altered host resistance, *Ann Intern Med* 69:859, 1968.
50. Consensus Development Conference Statement. In Gorbach SL, Edelman R, editors: Travelers' diarrhea: National Institutes of Health Consensus Development Conference, *Rev Infect Dis* 8:S227, 1986.
51. Couch P, Johnson CE: Prevention of Lyme disease, *Am J Hosp Pharm* 49:1164, 1992.
52. Couch RB et al: Airborne transmission of respiratory infection with Coxsackie virus A type 21, *Am J Epidemiol* 91:78, 1970.
53. Craft JC: Giardia and giardiasis in childhood, *Pediatr Infect Dis* 1:196, 1982.
54. Cruse PJE, Foord R: A five-year prospective study of 23,649 surgical wounds, *Arch Surg* 107:206, 1973.
55. Culver DH, Horan TC, Gaynes RP et al: Surgical wound infection rates by wound class, opoerative procedure and patient risk index, National Nosocomial Infections Surveillance System, *Am J Med* 91(3B):1525,1991.
56. Curran AS: Lyme disease: prevention and control, *N J Med* 87:541, 1990.
57. Davidson RA: Issues in clinical parasitology: the treatment of giardiasis, *Am J Gastroenterol* 79:256, 1984.
58. Davis SD, Wedgwood RJ: Antibiotic prophylaxis in acute viral respiratory diseases, *Am J Dis Child* 109:554, 1965.
59. Dekonenko EJ et al: Lyme borreliosis in the Soviet Union: a cooperative US-USSR report, *J Infect Dis* 158:748, 1988.
60. Diarrheal Disease Study Group: Loperamide in acute diarrhea in childhood: results of a double-blind, placebo controlled multicenter clinical trial, *Br Med J* 289:1263, 1984.
61. Dick GF, Burgdorf WHC, Gentry WC Jr: Norwegian scabies in Bloom's syndrome, *Arch Dermatol* 115:212, 1979.
62. Dobell CA: The discovery of intestinal protozoa in man, *Proc R Soc Med* 13:1, 1920.
63. Dolin R et al: A controlled trial of amantadine and rimantidine in the prophylaxis of influenza infection, *N Engl J Med* 307:543, 1982.
64. Dowling HF, Jackson GG, and Inouye T: Transmission of the experimental common cold in volunteers. II. The effect of certain host factors upon susceptibility, *J Lab Clin Med* 50:516, 1957.
65. Dowling HF et al: Transmission of the common cold to volunteers under controlled conditions. III. The effect of chilling of the subjects upon susceptibility, *Am J Hyg* 68:59, 1958.
66. Du Pont HL: Non-fluid therapy and selected chemoprophylaxis of acute diarrhea, *Am J Med* 78:81, 1987.
67. DuPont HL, Pickering LK: *Infections of the gastrointestinal tract,* New York, 1980, Plenum.
68. Edwards LD: The epidemiology of 2056 remote site infections and 1966 surgical wound infections occurring in 1865 patients: a four-year study of 40,923 operations at Rush-Presbyterian-St. Luke's Hospital, Chicago, *Ann Surg* 184:758, 1976.
69. Ericsson CD et al: Bismuth subsalicylate inhibits activity of crude toxins of *Escherichia coli* and *Vibrio cholerae, J Infect Dis* 136:693, 1977.
70. Magnarelli LA, Meegan JM, Anderson et al: Comparison of an indirect fluorescent antibody test with an enzyme-linked immunosorbent assay for serological studies of Lyme disease, *J Clin Microbiol* 20:181, 1984.
70a. Felman YN, Nickolas JA: Scabies, *Cutis* 33:270, 1984.
71. Feret E et al: Epidemiology of hepatitis B virus infection in the rural community of Tip, Senegal, *Am J Epidemiol* 125:140, 1987.
72. Fihn SD et al: Diaphragm use and urinary tract infections: analysis of urodynamic and microbiological factors, *J Urol* 136:853, 1986.
73. Finegold SM et al: Significance of anaerobic and capnophilic bacteria isolated from the urinary tract. In Kass EH, editor: *Progress in pyelonephritis,* Philadelphia, 1965, FA Davis.
74. Freedman L: Chronic pyelonephritis at autopsy, *Ann Intern Med* 66:697, 1967.
75. Freedman LR: Natural history of urinary tract infection in adults, *Kidney Int* 8:S96, 1975.
76. Friedman R: In: *The story of scabies,* New York, 1947, Froben Press.
77. Furste W, Skudder PA, and Hampton OP: The evolution of prophylaxis against tetanus from the Civil War to the present, *Bull Am Coll Surg* 8:I, 1967.
78. Garner JS: CDC guidelines for the prevention and control of nosocomial infections: guideline for prevention of surgical wound infections, 1985, *Am J Infect Control* 14:71, 1986.
79. Gerken G et al: Pre-S encoded surface proteins in relation to the

major viral surface antigen in acute hepatitis B virus infection, *Gastroenterology* 92:1864, 1987.

80. Gilbert BE et al: Small particle aerosols of enviroxime-containing liposomes, *Antiviral Res* 9:355, 1988.

81. Gillen FD et al: Encystation and expression of cyst antigens by *Giardia lamblia* in-vitro, *Science* 235:1040, 1987.

82. Gillenwater JY, Harrison RB, and Quinin CM: Natural history of bacteriuria in school girls: a long-term case-control study, *N Engl J Med* 301:396, 1979.

83. Gilman RH et al: Epidemiology and serology of *Giardia lamblia* in a developing country: Bangladesh, *Trans R Soc Trop Med Hyg* 79:469, 1985.

84. Gleckman R et al: Acute pyelonephritis in the elderly, *South Med J* 75:551, 1982.

85. Glezen WP: Consideration of the risk of influenza in children and indications for prophylaxis, *Rev Infect Dis* 2:408, 1980.

86. Glezen WP: Reactive airway disorders in children: role of respiratory virus infections, *Clin Chest Med* 5:635, 1984.

87. Glezen WP et al: Parainfluenza virus type 3: seasonality and risk of infection and reinfection in young children, *J Infect Dis* 150:851, 1984.

87a. Gorbach, personal communication, 1982.

88. Gould JC: The comparative bacteriology of acute and chronic urinary tract infection. In O'Grady F, Brumfitt W, editors: *Urinary tract infection,* London, 1968, Oxford University Press.

89. Govan D: Investigation and management of urinary tract infections in children, *Urol Clin North Am* 1:397, 1974.

90. Green RW: Infestations: scabies and lice. In Brickner P, et al, editors: *Health care of homeless people,* New York, 1985, Springer-Verlag.

91. Grodzicki RL, Steere AC: Comparison of immunoblotting and indirect enzyme-linked immunosorbent assay using different antigen preparations for diagnosing early Lyme disease, *J Infect Dis* 157:790, 1988.

92. Guerrant RL, Hughes JM: Nausea, vomiting and noninflammatory diarrhea. In Mandell GL, Douglas RG, and Bennett JE, editors: *Principles and practices of infectious diseases,* New York, 1985, John Wiley and Sons.

93. *Guide for adult immunization,* ACP Task Force on Adult Immunization and Infectious Diseases Society of America, ed 2, Philadelphia, 1990, American College of Physicians.

94. Gupta JP, Jain AK, and Nanivadekar AS: Efficacy of tinidazole (Fasigyn) in giardiasis by parasitologic, biochemical, and gut transit studies, *Indian J Gastroenterol* 8:103, 1989.

95. Gurevitch AW: Scabies and lice, *Pediatr Clin North Am* 32:987, 1985.

96. Gwaltney JM Jr: Rhinoviruses. In Evans AS, editor: *Viral infections of humans,* ed 2, New York, 1982, Plenum Medical Book.

97. Haley RW et al: Identifying patients at high risk of surgical wound infection, *Am J Epidemiol* 121:206, 1985.

98. Hall JC, Brewer JH, and Appl BA: Norwegian scabies in a patient with acquired immunodeficiency syndrome, *Cutis* 13:325, 1989.

99. Halperin JJ et al: Nervous system abnormalities in Lyme disease, *Ann NY Acad Sci* 539:24, 1988.

100. Hamilton DR: How can I avoid Lyme disease? What to say to the patient who asks, *Postgrad Med* 87:167, 1990.

101. Handsfield HH: Asymptomatic gonorrhea in men: diagnosis, natural course, prevalence and significance, *N Engl J Med* 290:117, 1973.

102. Harding GKM et al: Prophylaxis of recurrent urinary tract infections in female patients. Efficacy of low-dose, thrice-weekly therapy with trimethoprim-sulfamethoxazole, *JAMA* 242:1975, 1979.

103. Hayden FG: Use of interferons for prevention and treatment of respiratory viral infections. In Mills J, Corey L, editors: *Antiviral chemotherapy: new directions for clinical application and research,* New York, 1986, Elsevier Science Publishing.

104. Hendley JO, Gwaltney JM Jr: Mechanisms of transmission of rhinovirus infections, *Epidemiol Rev* 10:242, 1988.

105. Henry SA: Chemoprophylaxis of bacterial infections in granulocytopenic patients, *Am J Med* 76:645, 1984.

106. Holtz TH, Nettleman MD: Emporiatrics: diarrhea in travelers, *Infect Control Hosp Epidemiol* 11:606, 1990.

107. Hoofnagle JH, Schafer DF: Serologic markers of hepatitis B virus infection, *Semin Liv Dis* 6:1, 1986.

108. Horowitz MA, Hughes JM, and Craun GF: Outbreaks of waterborne disease in the United States, *J Infect Dis* 133:588, 1974.

109. Hovelius B, Mardh P: *Staphylococcus saprophyticus* as a common cause of urinary tract infections, *Rev Infect Dis* 6:328, 1984.

110. Hovmark A, Asbrink E, and Olsson I: The spirochetal etiology of lymphadenosis benigna cutis solitaria, *Acta Dermatol Venereol (Stockh)* 66:479, 1986.

111. Huland H, Bush R: Pyelonephritic scarring in 213 patients with upper and lower tract infections: long term follow-up, *J Urol* 132:936, 1984.

112. Immunization Practices Advisory Committee: Adult immunization, *MMWR* 33S:1S, 1984.

113. Immunization Practices Advisory Committee: Update: Pneumococcal polysaccharide vaccine usage—United States, *MMWR,* 33:273, 1984.

114. Inserra DW, Bickley LK: Crusted scabies in acquired immunodeficiency syndrome, *Int J Dermatol* 29:287, 1990.

115. Jackson GG, Dowling HF: Transmission of the common cold to volunteers under controlled conditions. IV. Specific immunity to the common cold, *J Clin Invest* 38:762, 1959.

116. Jakubowski W: Purple burps and the filtration of drinking water supplies (editorial), *Am J Public Health* 78:123, 1988.

117. Jarroll EL, Bingham AK, and Meyer EA: Giardia cyst destruction: effectiveness of six small-quantity water disinfection methods, *Am J Trop Med Hyg* 29:8, 1980.

118. Johnson J, Stamm W: Diagnosis and treatment of acute urinary tract infection, *Infect Dis Clin North Am* 1:773, 1987.

119. Johnson PC, Du Pont HL, and Ericsson CD: Chemoprophylaxis and chemotherapy of travelers' diarrhea in children, *Pediatr Infect Dis* 4:620, 1985.

120. Jordan PA et al: Urinary tract infections caused by *Staphylococcus saprophyticus, J Infect Dis* 142:510, 1980.

121. Jucowies P et al: Norwegian scabies in an infant with acquired immunodeficiency syndrome, *Arch Dermatol* 125:1670, 1989.

122. Kamath KR, Murugasu R: A comparative study of four methods for detecting *Giardia lamblia* in children with diarrheal illness and malabsorption, *Gastroenterology* 66:16, 1974.

123. Kawabata M, et al: Lyme disease in Japan and its possible incriminated tick vector, *Ixodes persulcatus, J Infect Dis* 156:854, 1987.

124. Kaye D: Urinary tract infection in the elderly, *Bull NY Acad Med* 56:209, 1980.

125. Kaye D: Antibacterial activity of human urine, *J Clin Invest* 47:2374, 1968.

126. Keystone JS, Krajden S, and Warren MR: Person-to-person transmission of *Giardia lamblia* in day care nurseries, *Can Med Assoc J* 119:241, 1978.

127. Keystone JS, Keystone DL, and Proctor EM: Intestinal parasitic infections in homosexual men. Prevalence, symptoms, and factors in transmission, *Can Med Assoc J* 123:512, 1980.

128. Kozicki M, Steffen R, and Schar M: "Boil it, cook it, peel it, or forget it", does this rule prevent travelers' diarrhea? *Int J Epidemiol* 14:169, 1985.

129. Kreutner AK, Del Bene VE, and Amstey MS: Giardiasis in pregnancy, *Am J Obstet Gynecol* 140:895, 1981.

130. Kruse W: Die Erregen von Husten und Schupfen (the etiology of cough and nasal catarrh), *Munch Med Wochenschr* 61:1574, 1914.

131. Lattimer GL et al: Hematogenous infection in total joint replacement, *JAMA* 242:2213, 1979.

132. Leneman F: The Guillain-Barré syndrome, *Arch Intern Med* 118:139, 1966.

133. Lerman SJ, Walker RA: Treatment of giardiasis: literature review and recommendations, *Clin Pediatr* 21:409, 1982.

134. Levandowski RA, et al: Topical enviroxime against rhinovirus infection, *Antimicrob Agents Chemother* 22:1004, 1982.

135. Liston TE, Foshee WS, and Pierson WD: Sulfisoxazole chemoprophylaxis for frequent otitis media, *Pediatrics* 71:524, 1983.

136. Loge JP: Aplastic anemia following exposure to benzene hexachloride (lindane), *JAMA* 193:110, 1965.

137. Looke DFM: Traveller's diarrhea, *Austral Fam Phys* 19:194, 1990.

138. Luft BJ, Dattwyler RJ: Lyme borreliosis: problems in diagnosis and treatment, *Curr Clin Top Infect Dis* 11:56, 1989.

139. Lui KJ, Kendal AP: Impact of influenza epidemics on mortality in the United States from October 1972 to May 1985, *Am J Public Health* 77:712, 1987.

140. Magid D et al: Prevention of Lyme disease after tick bites: a cost-effective analysis, *N Engl J Med* 327:534, 1992.

141. Magnarelli LA et al: Comparison of an indirect fluorescent antibody test with an enzyme-linked immunosorbent assay for serological studies of Lyme disease, *J Clin Microbiol* 20:181, 1984.

142. Maibach HL, Johnson HL: Contact urticaria syndrome. Contact urticaria to diethyltoluamide (immediate-type hypersensitivity), *Arch Dermatol* 111:726, 1975.

143. Margileth AM et al: Urinary tract bacterial infections: symposium on pediatric nephrology, *Pediatr Clin North Am* 23:71, 1976.

144. Matthewson JJ et al: A newly recognized cause of travelers' diarrhea: enteroadherent *Escherichia coli, J Infect Dis* 151:471, 1985.

145. McCabe WR, Jackson GG: Treatment of pyelonephritis: bacterial drug and host factors in success or failure among 252 patients, *N Engl J Med* 272:1037, 1965.

146. McCracken GH: Diagnosis and management of acute urinary tract infections in infants and children, *Pediatr Infect Dis* 6:107, 1987.

147. Mellanby K: *Scabies,* Hampton, England, 1972, E W Classey.

148. Miller FD et al: Control trial of enviroxime against natural rhinovirus infections in a community, *Antimicrob Agents Chemother* 27:102, 1985.

149. Minuth JN, Masher DM, and Thorsteinsonn SB: Inhibition of antibacterial activity of gentamicin by urine, *J Infect Dis* 133:14, 1976.

150. Mitchell RG: Urinary tract infections caused by salmonellae, *Lancet* 1:1092, 1965.

151. Monto AS, Schwartz SA, and Albrecht JK: Ineffectiveness of postexposure prophylaxis of rhinovirus infection with low-dose intranasal alpha 2-b interferon in families, *Antimicrob Agents Chemother* 33:387, 1989.

152. Mufson MA et al: Adenovirus infection in acute hemorrhagic cystitis: a study in 25 children, *Am J Dis Child* 121:281, 1971.

153. Mulholland SG: Urinary tract infection, *Clin Ger Med* 6:43, 1990.

154. Murray BE: Resistance of Shigella, Salmonella and other enteric pathogens to antimicrobial agents, *Rev Infect Dis* 8:S172, 1986.

155. Murray T, Goldberg MD: Etiologies of chronic interstitial nephritis, *Ann Intern Med* 82:453, 1975.

156. Mussen JE: Lindane: a prudent approach, *Arch Dermatol* 123:1008, 1987.

157. Naik SR, Rau NR, and Vinayak VK: A comparative evaluation of three stool samples, jejunal aspirate and jejunal mucosal impression smears in the diagnosis of giardiasis, *Ann Trop Med Parasitol* 72:491, 1978.

158. Nash TE et al: Experimental human infections with *Giardia lamblia, J Infect Dis* 156:974, 1987.

159. Nash TE et al: Restriction endonuclease analysis of DNA from 15 Giardia isolates obtained from humans and animals, *J Infect Dis* 152:64, 1985.

160. National Center for Health Statistics: *Current estimates from the National Health Interview Survey, United States, 1988,* DHHS Publication No. (PHS) 88-1594.

161. Nichols RL: Postoperative wound infection, *N Engl J Med* 307:1701, 1982.

162. Norden C: A critical review of antimicrobial prophylaxis in orthopedic surgery, *Rev Infect Dis* 5:928, 1983.

163. Numazaki YN et al: Further study on acute hemorrhagic cystitis due to adenovirus 11, *N Engl J Med* 289:344, 1973.

164. O'Grady F et al: In vitro models simulating conditions of bacterial growth in the urinary tract. In O'Grady F, Brumfitt W, editors: *Urinary tract infection,* London, 1968, Oxford University Press.

165. Ohto H et al: Intrauterine transmission of hepatitis B virus is closely related to placental leakage, *J Med Virol* 21:1, 1987.

166. Onto AS, Ullman BM: Acute respiratory illness in an American community, *JAMA* 227:264, 1974.

167. Opal SM, Wiest PM, and Olds CR: Travelers' diarrhea: methods of prevention and treatment, *RI Med J* 73:199, 1990.

168. Ophir D, Elad Y: Effect of steam inhalation on nasal patency and nasal symptoms in patients with the common cold, *Am J Otolaryngol* 3:149, 1987.

169. Orkin M, Mailbach HI: Current views of scabies and pediculosis pubis, *Cutis* 33:85, 1984.

170. O'Sullivan DG et al: Protective action of benzimidazole derivatives against virus infections in tissue culture and in-vivo, *Lancet* i:446, 1969.

171. Paavonen J: General sexually transmitted diseases, *Curr Opin Gyn Obstet* 3:715, 1991.

172. Pachner AR, Steere AC: The triad of neurologic manifestations of Lyme disease: meningitis, cranial neuritis and radiculoneuritis. *Neurology* 35:47, 1985.

173. Palmer SM, Small RE: A review of Lyme disease: its prevention and treatment, *Am Pharm* NS31:36, 1991.

174. Parish LC, Nutting WB, and Schwartzman RM: *Cutaneous infestations of man and animals,* New York, 1983, Praeger.

175. Parish LC, Witkowski JA, and Millikan LE: Scabies in the extended care facility, revisited, *Int J Dermatol* 30:703, 1991.

176. Paulson M, Andrews J: The incidence of human intestinal protozoa in duodenal aspirates, *JAMA* 94:2063, 1930.

177. Petersen LR, Cartter ML, and Hadler JL: A food-borne outbreak of *Giardia lamblia, J Infect Dis* 157:846, 1988.

178. Phillpotts RJ et al: The activity of enviroxime against rhinovirus infection in man, *Lancet* i:1342, 1981.

179. Pickering AK et al: Occurrence of *Giardia lamblia* in day-care centers, *J Pediatr* 104:522, 1984.

180. Pitt HA, Costrini M: Vitamin C prophylaxis in marine recruits, *JAMA* 241:908, 1979.

181. Polsky B et al: Bacterial pneumonia in patients with the acquired immunodeficiency syndrome, *Ann Intern Med* 104:38, 1986.

182. Prose NS, Abson KG, and Berg D: Lyme disease in children: diagnosis, treatment and prevention, *Semin Dermatol* 11:31, 1992.

183. Quinin CM: The natural history of recurrent bacteriuria in school girls, *N Engl J Med* 282:1443, 1970.

184. Quinin CM: Urinary tract infections in children, *Hosp Pract* 11:91, 1976.

185. Randolph MF, Greenfield M: The incidence of asymptomatic bacteriuria and pyuria in infancy, *J Pediatr* 65:57, 1964.

186. Rauch AE et al: Lindane (Kwell)—induced aplastic anemia, *Arch Intern Med* 150:2393, 1990.

187. Regan AM, Metersky ML, and Craven DE: Nosocomial dermatitis and pruritus caused by pigeon mite infestation, *Arch Intern Med* 147:2185, 1987.

188. Reid AF, Poonking T: Epidemic scabies and associated acute glomerulonephritis in Trinidad, *Bull Pan Am Health Org* 22:103, 1988.

189. Rendtorff RC: The experimental transmission of human intestinal protozoan parasites. II. *Giardia lamblia* cysts given in capsules, *Am J Hyg* 59:209, 1954.

190. Reznick JW et al: Lyme carditis: electrophysiologic and histopathologic study, *Am J Med* 81:923, 1986.

191. Rice RJ: Gonorrhea in the United States, 1975-1984: is the giant only sleeping? *Sex Transm Dis* 14:83, 1987.

192. Rosenthal P, Liebman WM: Comparative study of stool exams, duodenal aspiration, and pediatric Entero-Test for giardiasis in children, *J Pediatr* 96:278, 1980.

193. Rosoff JD et al: Stool diagnosis of giardiasis using a commercially available enzyme immunoassay to detect Giardia-specific antigen 65 (GSA-65), *J Clin Microbiol* 27:1997, 1989.

194. Rossman MG et al: Structure of a human common cold virus and functional relationship to other picornaviruses, *Nature* 317:145, 1985.

195. Rotblatt MD: Giardiasis and amebiasis in pregnancy, *Drug Intell Clin Pharmacol* 17:187, 1983.

196. Rothenberg RB: The geography of gonorrhea: empirical demonstration of core group transmission, *Am J Epidemiol* 117:688, 1983.

197. Rumano JM, Kaye D: UTI in the elderly: common yet atypical, *Geriatrics* 36:113, 1981.

198. Sack RB: Antimicrobial prophylaxis of travelers' diarrhea: a selected summary, *Rev Infect Dis* 8:S160, 1986.

199. Sack RB: Travelers' diarrhea: microbiologic basis for prevention and treatment, *Rev Infect Dis* 12:S59, 1990.

200. Samo TC et al: Efficacy and tolerance of intranasally applied recombinant leukocyte A interferon in normal volunteers, *J Infect Dis* 148:535, 1983.

201. Schechter SL: Lyme disease associated with optic neuropathy. *Am J Med* 81:143, 1986.

202. Schlesinger PA et al: Maternal-fetal transmission of the Lyme disease spirochete, *Borrelia burgdorferi, Ann Intern Med* 103:67, 1985.

203. Schmid GP: The global distribution of Lyme disease, *Rev Infect Dis* 7:41, 1985.

204. Scrimenti RJ: Erythema chronicum migrans, *Arch Dermatol* 236:859, 1970.

205. Shaffer N, Moore L: Chronic travelers' diarrhea in a normal host due to *Isospora belli, J Infect Dis* 159:596, 1989.

206. Shapiro ED: Lack of transmission of hepatitis B in a day-care center, *J Pediatr* 110:90, 1987.

207. Shapiro ED, Clemens JD: A controlled evaluation of the protective efficacy of pneumococcal vaccine for patients at high risk for serious pneumococcal infections, *Ann Intern Med* 101:325, 1984.

208. Shapiro ED, Wald ER: Single-dose amoxicillin treatment of urinary tract infection, *J Pediatr* 99:989, 1981.

209. Shaw PK et al: A community-wide outbreak of giardiasis with evidence of transmission by a municipal water supply, *Ann Intern Med* 87:426, 1977.

210. Shaw RA, Stevens MA: The reactive arthritis of giardiasis. A case report, *JAMA* 258:2734, 1987.

211. Sheehe TW, Holley HP: Giardia-induced malabsorption in pancreatitis, *JAMA* 233:1373, 1975.

212. Shindo K et al: Crusted scabies in acquired selective IgA deficiency, *Arta Derm Venereol* (Stoekh) 71:250, 1991.

213. Smellie JM, Normand ICS: Bacteriuria reflux and renal scarring, *Arch Dis Child* 50:581, 1975.

214. Smith LG Jr et al: Lyme disease: a review with emphasis on the pregnant woman, *Obstet Gynecol Surv* 46:125, 1991.

215. Solomon LM, Fahrner L, and West DP: Gamma benzene hexachloride toxicity: a review, *Arch Dermatol* 113:353, 1977.

216. Sorvillo FJ et al: Shigellosis association with recreational water contact in Los Angeles county, *Am J Trop Med Hyg* 38:163, 1988.

217. Soyka LF et al: The misuse of antibiotics for treatment of upper respiratory tract infections in children, *Pediatrics* 55:552, 1975.

218. Sperber SJ et al: Ineffectiveness of recombinant interferon-beta serine nasal drops for prophylaxis of natural colds, *J Infect Dis* 160:700, 1989.

219. Stamey TA et al: Serum versus urinary antimicrobial concentrations in case of urinary tract infections, *N Engl J Med* 291:1159, 1974.

220. Stamey TA, Govan DE, and Palmer JM: The localization and treatment of urinary tract infections: the role of bactericidal urine levels as opposed to serum levels, *Medicine* 44:1, 1965.

221. Stamm WE: Recent developments in the diagnosis and treatment of urinary tract infections, *West J Med* 137:213, 1982.

222. Stamm WE: Approach to the patient with urinary tract infection. In Gorbach SL, Bartlett JG, and Blacklow NR, editors: *Infectious diseases,* Philadelphia, 1992, WB Saunders.

223. Stamm WE: Quantitative urine cultures revisited (editorial) *Eur J Clin Microbiol* 3:279, 1984.

224. Stamm WE et al: Diagnosis of coliform infection in acutely dysuric women, *N Engl J Med* 307:463, 1982.

225. Stamm WE et al: Is antimicrobial prophylaxis of urinary tract infections cost effective? *Ann Intern Med* 94:251, 1981.

226. Stamm WE, McKevitt M, and Counts GW: Acute renal infection in women: treatment with trimethoprim-sulfamethoxazole or ampicillin for two or six weeks. A randomized trial, *Ann Intern Med* 106:341, 1987.

227. Stanley ED et al: Increased virus shedding with aspirin treatment of rhinovirus infection, *JAMA* 231:1247, 1975.

228. Steere AC: Lyme disease, *N Engl J Med* 321:586, 1989.

229. Steere AC et al: The early clinical manifestations of Lyme disease, *Ann Intern Med* 99:76, 1983.

230. Steere AC, et al: Lyme carditis: cardiac abnormalities of Lyme disease, *Ann Intern Med* 93:8, 1980.

231. Steere AC et al: Unilateral blindness caused by infection with the Lyme disease spirochete, *Borrelia burgdorferi, Ann Intern Med* 103:382, 1985.

232. Reference deleted in proofs.

233. Steere AC et al: Lyme arthritis: an epidemic of oligoarticular arthritis in children and adults in three Connecticut communities, *Arthritis Rheum* 20:7, 1977.

234. Steere AC, Schoen RT, and Taylor E: The clinical evolution of Lyme arthritis, *Ann Intern Med* 107:725, 1987.

235. Steere AC et al: Longitudinal assessment of the clinical and epidemiological features of Lyme disease in a defined population, *J Infect Dis* 154:295, 1986.

236. Steffen R: Worldwide efficacy of bismuth subsalicylate in the treatment of travelers' diarrhea, *Rev Infect Dis* 12:S80, 1990.

237. Steffen R, Boppart I: Travelers' diarrhea. In *Tropical gastroenterology, Balliere's clinical gastroenterology,* London, 1987, Balliere Tindall.

238. Steffen R et al: Efficacy and side-effects of six agents in the self-treatment of travelers' diarrhea, *Trav Med Intern* 6:153, 1988.

239. Stevens CE et al: Yeast-recombinant hepatitis B vaccine. Efficacy of hepatitis B immune globulin in prevention of perinatal hepatitis B virus transmission, *JAMA* 257:2612, 1987.

240. Stevens CE et al: Perinatal hepatitis B virus transmission in the United States. Prevention by passive-active immunization, *JAMA* 253:1740, 1985.

241. Steward A et al: Lyme arthritis in Hunter Valley, *Med J Aust* 1:139, 1982.

242. Stierntedt G et al: Clinical manifestations and diagnosis of neuroborreliosis, *Ann NY Acad Sci* 539:46, 1988.

243. Strum WB: Update on travelers' diarrhea, *Postgrad Med* 84:163, 1988.

244. Susin M, Becker EL: The pathology of pyelonephritis. In Kaye D, editor: *Urinary tract infection and its management,* St Louis, 1972, CV Mosby.

245. Swallow DL, Kampfner GL: The laboratory selection of antiviral agents, *Br Med Bull* 41:322, 1985.

246. Taplin D, Meinking TL: Scabies, lice and fungal infections, *Primary Care* 16:551, 1989.

247. Taplin D et al: Permethrin 5% dermal cream: a new treatment for scabies, *J Am Acad Dermatol* 15:995, 1986.

248. Taplin D et al: A comparative trial of three treatment schedules for the eradication of scabies, *J Am Acad Dermatol* 9:550, 1983.

249. Taylor DN, Echeverria P: Etiology and epidemiology of travelers' diarrhea in Asia, *Rev Infect Dis* 8:S136, 1986.

250. Taylor DN et al: Polymicrobial etiology of travelers' diarrhea, *Lancet* 1(8425):381, 1985.

251. Taylor DN et al: Etiology of diarrhea among travelers and foreign residents in Nepal, *JAMA* 260:1245, 1988.

252. Thompson RCA, Meloni BP, and Lymbery AJ: Humans and cats have genetically identical forms of Giardia: evidence of a zoonotic relationship (letter), *Med J Aust* 148:207, 1988.

253. Thorton SA et al: Comparison of methods for identification of *Giardia lamblia, Am J Clin Pathol* 80:858, 1983.

254. Tjoa WS et al: Location of food, consumption and travelers' diarrhea, *Am J Epidemiol* 106:61, 1977.

255. Travelers' diarrhea, *Consensus Dev Conf Summ Natl Inst Health* 5, 1985.

256. Tsai TS, Bailey RE, and Moore PS: National surveillance of Lyme disease 1987-1988, *Conn Med* 53(6):324, 1989.

257. Tyrrell DAJ: Hot news on the common cold, *Ann Rev Microbiol* 42:35, 1988.

258. Van Neste DJ: Human scabies in perspective, *Int J Dermatol* 27:10, 1988.

259. Wagner AR et al: Enteroinvasive *Escherichia coli* in travelers with diarrhea, *J Infect Dis* 158:640, 1988.

260. Walzor PD, Wolfe MS, and Schultz MG: Giardiasis in travelers, *J Infect Dis* 124:235, 1971.

261. Weinke T et al: Prevalence and clinical importance of *Entamoeba histolytica* in two high-risk groups: travellers returning from the tropics and male homosexuals, *J Infect Dis* 161:1029, 1990.

262. Weiser B et al: Prophylactic trimethoprim-sulfamethoxazole during consolidation chemotherapy for acute leukemia: a controlled trial, *Ann Intern Med* 95:436, 1981.

263. Wilson ML et al: Reduced abundance of immature *Ixodes dammini* (acarixodidae) following elimination of deer, *J Med Entomol* 25:224, 1988.

264. Windsor JA, Hill GL: Protein-depletion and surgical risk, *Aust N Z J Surg* 58:711, 1988.

265. Windsor JA, Hill GL: Weight loss with physiologic impairment: A basic indicator of surgical risk, *Ann Surg* 207:290, 1988.

266. Wolf R, Krakowski A: Atypical crusted scabies, *J Am Acad Dermatol* 17:434, 1987.

267. Wolfe MS: Giardiasis, *N Engl J Med* 298:319, 1978.

268. Wolfe MS: Symptomatology, diagnosis and treatment. In Erlandsen SL, Meyer EA, editors: *Giardia and giardiasis,* New York, 1984, Plenum Press.

269. Wolfe MS: Acute diarrhea associated with travel, *Am J Med* 88:S34, 1990.

270. Woo PK: Evidence for animal reservoirs and transmission of *Giardia* infection between animal species. In Erlandsen SL, Meyer EA, editors: *Giardia and giardiasis,* New York, 1984, Plenum Press.

271. Woodliff HJ, Cannon PM, and Scopa J: Aplastic anemia associated with insecticide, *Med J Aust* 1:628, 1966.

272. Wyde PR et al: Activity against rhinoviruses, toxicity, and delivery in aerosol of enviroxime in liposomes, *Antimicrob Agents Chemother* 32:890, 1988.

273. Yorke JA et al: Dynamics and control of the transmission of gonorrhea, *Sex Transm Dis* 5:51, 1978.

274. Yu VL et al: Staphylococcal aureus nasal carriage and infection in patients on hemodialysis. Efficacy of antibiotic prophylaxis, *N Engl J Med* 315:91, 1983.

--------- **RESOURCES** ---------

Adult immunization

Guide for Adult Immunization, ACP Task Force on Adult Immunization and Infectious Diseases Society of America, ed 2, Philadelphia, 1990, American College of Physicians. Available from: American College of Physicians, Division of Scientific Affairs, Health and Public Policy, 4200 Pine St, Philadelphia PA 19104.

Health Information for International Travel 1992, US Department of Health and Human Services, Public Health Service, Centers for Disease Control. Available from: Centers for Disease Control, 1600 Clifton Rd NE, Atlanta GA 30333.

Foreign Travel & Immunization Guide, ed 13, Dardick KR, Neumann HH, editors. Available from: Medical Economics Company, Oradell, NJ 07649.

Sexually transmitted diseases

1989 Sexually Transmitted Diseases. Treatment Guidelines. *MMWR* 38(suppl 8) 1989. Centers for Disease Control, 1600 Clifton Rd NE, Atlanta GA 30333.

Lyme disease

Lyme Disease Foundation, PO Box 462, Tolland CT 06084.

Chapter 58

OTOLOGIC DISORDERS

Gordon B. Hughes

This chapter reviews nine common otologic problems that collectively illustrate important principles of preventive medicine in otology: physician awareness, diagnostic screening tests, early detection and treatment, appropriate monitoring, careful follow-up observation, and patient education. Each problem commonly involves a specific part of the ear but is not necessarily limited to that part. Moreover general principles apply regardless of specific disease or symptom. All patients who have unilateral hearing loss without obvious cause (earwax, middle ear fluid) on examination should have a hearing test. Progressive, unexplained unilateral sensorineural hearing loss should be evaluated for possible acoustic neuroma. The audiologist can determine how extensive the hearing assessment should be. All patients with hearing loss are potential candidates for hearing aids. The otologist determines whether some alternate treatment is required or preferred. Inner ear dizziness and tinnitus can indicate serious disease but are otherwise benign symptoms. Treatment depends on the underlying disorder and severity of symptoms.

Ear anatomy can be divided into three parts: external, middle, and inner (Fig. 58-1). The external ear includes the pinna and external auditory canal. The external and middle ears are separated by the eardrum (tympanic membrane). The middle ear contains the eustachian tube, tympanic cavity, mastoid air cells, and ossicles. The inner ear contains the auditory and vestibular end-organs and eighth cranial nerves.

EXTERNAL EAR
Cerumen impaction

Wax is formed from the ceruminous glands of the cartilaginous canal.[13] Together with lubrication and pH provided by ear wax migration of the wax from medial to lateral mechanically cleanses the canal and promotes resistance to infection. Normal wax production varies consider-

ably, but some ear canals tend to self-cleanse less well then others.

On routine otologic examination most normal individuals have a small amount of wax, predominantly in the lateral half of the canal. The consistency is usually soft. Chronic Q-Tip impaction, previous mastoid surgery, and other factors can predispose to wax accumulation. Many individuals do not perceive wax buildup so long as a small opening through the wax provides sound conduction to the drum. With nearly complete obstruction of the canal, however, a small drop of water introduced by shower or shampoo may produce "abrupt" hearing loss. The patient may experience a sensation of pressure and fullness, or mild irritation if secondary inflammation is present.

Wax impaction can be prevented by periodic cleaning of the ears by a physician, usually as part of an annual physical examination. Small amounts of wax can be dissolved by mild peroxide solutions that can be purchased without prescription (a pharmacist can indicate which ones are available). Once established wax impaction can be removed by curettage, occasionally requiring the use of a microscope and special instruments. All methods are equally effective when performed delicately, but the Water-Pik should not be used because it can perforate the drum.[2] The chosen method for each patient depends on the firmness of the wax. If the wax is quite soft, the easiest removal is by suction; if firm, by curette (loop). Ideally if a hard plug can be loosened gently from the circumferential canal skin, then grasped at its apex, it sometimes can be withdrawn from the canal in one or two pieces.

The most difficult wax to remove is that which is neither soft nor firm as it may both plug the suction equipment or slip from the curette. A combination of both techniques, and even lavage of the canal, usually works. Sometimes firm wax trapped near the drum must be softened with topical peroxide (Debrox), two drops twice

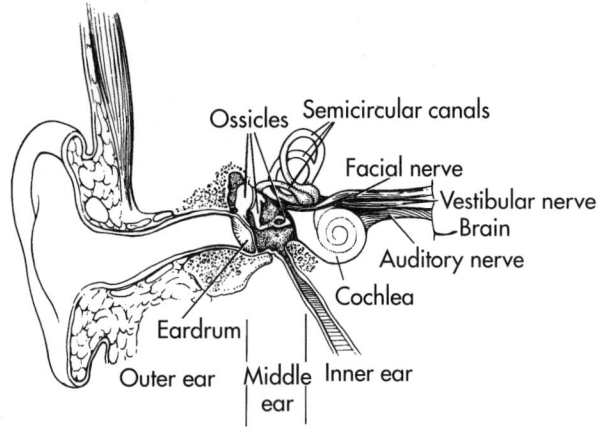

Fig. 58-1. Ear anatomy can be divided into three parts: external, middle, and inner.

daily for several days. Then the patient can return for completion of wax removal.

External otitis

External otitis is diffuse, circumferential bacterial infection of the external auditory canal. Infections are more common in hot, humid climates; in summer months in the United States; in adolescents; and in people who frequently swim or use hot tubs. The most common pathogen is *Pseudomonas aeruginosa*, followed by *Staphylococcus aureus* and *S. albus*, *Proteus*, coliforms, and other gram-negative organisms.

The cartilaginous canal becomes erythematous and edematous. Glandular function is disrupted with loss of normal cerumen and lipid protection. Maceration of the canal skin follows, and exfoliated epithelial cells are trapped in the canal. The canal may remain open or swell shut, with infection spreading to adjacent soft tissue structures. In diabetic and immunosuppressed patients infection can invade bone (necrotizing external otitis).

The patient complains of pain, hearing loss, and/or canal drainage. Examination reveals diffuse redness and swelling of the lateral canal. Localized swelling more often is a sebaceous gland furuncle, which specifically requires antistaphylococcal antibiotics and occasional incision and drainage. In both external otitis and furuncle the medial canal, eardrum, and middle ear are normal.

Treatment of mild external otitis consists of topical antibiotics. Canal cleaning may not be necessary in early cases. The most commonly used topical antibiotics (Cortisporin otic, Coly-Mycin otic, Otocort) combine polymyxin (for pseudomonas), neomycin (for staphylococcus), and hydrocortisone (for canal swelling).[7] Three or four drops are placed into the canal three times daily. The patient should leave the drops in the canal for a full 5 minutes. Treatment of mild cases requires only 5 to 7 days. A

follow-up appointment is not required if symptoms disappear quickly.

Treatment of severe external otitis with canal obstruction and adjacent soft tissue infection requires careful canal cleaning, placement of a canal wick impregnated with topical antibiotic and cortisone (e.g., Cortisporin), oral ciprofloxacin hydrochloride 250 to 500 mg bid for pseudomonas, and frequent follow-up observation. These severe cases should be referred to an otolaryngologist if possible. The wick usually is removed in 2 days, at which time the canal is cleaned again. The patient is seen once or twice weekly as needed, and treatment is continued at least 10 days. Hospitalization and intravenous antibiotics are required if associated auricular perichondritis does not quickly improve. Cultures of canal drainage should be taken in refractory cases, to ensure that the choice of antibiotic is correct.

Persistence of pain and drainage, granulation tissue at the bony-cartilaginous canal junction, pseudomonas on culture, and (rarely) facial palsy are the hallmarks of necrotizing external otitis in a diabetic or immunosuppressed patient. The canal biopsy specimen shows no malignancy, computed tomography (CT) scan shows bone destruction, and technetium bone scan shows bone invasion. These patients usually require 6 weeks of intravenous antibiotic therapy, often by an otolaryngology-infectious disease team.

During and after treatment the patient continues "dry ear" precautions: doing no swimming or other water sports, putting no water into or near the ear, and inserting cotton or lamb's wool (often covered with petroleum jelly) into the concha and lateral canal during bathing. After the infection resolves the patient continues some of these precautions: avoiding unnecessary water and drying the ear carefully when wet. If infections recur from swimming the patient should wear earplugs. Whatever plugs stay in and are comfortable are the best. Swimmers' custom-fitted earmolds can be made by a hearing aid specialist or other professional. Alcohol or acetic acid eardrops can be used prophylactically, but their role is relatively less important.

MIDDLE EAR
Otitis media

Otitis media is perhaps the most common disorder of childhood, with highest incidence in children 6 to 11 months. The earlier the first infection the higher the risk of recurrent and chronic disease in later childhood.[3] The incidence is higher in winter months, higher in whites than blacks, and higher with antecedent upper respiratory infections. The incidence probably is higher in children with allergic and immunologic disease, although reports are conflicting. Otitis media is more common in American natives (American Indians and Alaskan Eskimos), Australian aborigines and New Zealand Maori, and children with Down's syndrome, cleft palate, and related craniofacial disorders. Breast-feeding may provide some protection compared with bottle feeding.[3] The incidence of otitis media drops sharply after age 6 or 7 years.

The child complains of pain. Fever may be present. On examination the drum is hyperemic and the middle ear contains cloudy effusion or pus. The light reflex can be preserved until late in the disease, or the drum may rupture from pus under pressure. The physician should remember that clinical signs can be very subtle, and the disease can be subclinical (silent otitis media) but still active. Fortunately complications of otitis media are rare in the post-antibiotic era.

The most common pathogens are *Streptococcus pneumoniae* (pneumococcus), *Hemophilus influenzae,* and *Branhamella catarrhalis.* β-Lactamase-producing strains of *H. influenza* and *B. catarrhalis* are increasingly common. Amoxicillin, erythromycin-sulfisoxazole, cefaclor, sulfamethoxazole-trimethoprim, and similar antibiotics usually are the first line of choice; amoxacillin-clavulinic acid, cefixime, and other "third-generation" antibiotics are used in resistant cases.[7] Treatment is given for 10 days. Failure to improve clinically in 2 days warrants a change in treatment or referral to an otolaryngologist.

After antibiotics have sterilized the middle ear, effusion can persist for 1 month in 40% of otherwise normal children, 2 months in 20%, and 3 months in 10%.[23] Failure to resolve fluid by 3 months (sooner in selected cases) or frequent recurrent infections warrant referral to an otolaryngologist. Antibiotic prophylaxis can be given (usually two thirds of the daily treatment dose is given as a single daily dose during the high-risk winter months) if the child tolerates antibiotics well, clears the effusion, and has no "breakthrough" infections. Ventilation (pressure equalization [PE]) tubes should be placed by an otolaryngologist if effusion persists for 3 months, if three infections occur within 6 months, or if four infections occur within 1 year (the indication varies somewhat from patient to patient).

If infections are severe or frequent or if behavior suggests hearing loss, a hearing test should be ordered. Failure to recognize and treat chronic middle ear fluid is one of the most common causes of chronic childhood hearing loss and can delay development of verbal communication and other intellectual skills. Fortunately these skills mature promptly to normal when hearing is restored.

Increased clinical observation of high-risk patients, early recognition, prompt treatment, appropriate follow-up care, newer antibiotics, and timely placement of ventilation tubes significantly control otitis media in childhood and prevent many complications later in adolescence and adulthood.

Barotrauma

The eustachian tube passes air to the middle ear from the nasopharynx. Closed most of the time to prevent autophony and aural pressure the tube opens momentarily during swallowing, yawning, and certain other activities. Only a fraction of a second is required to equilibrate air pressure between the middle and outer ear (ear canal). This equilibrium is vital to maintain normal function.

When circumstances combine to prevent tubal opening, air pressure equilibrium is not maintained. Most often ambient pressure in the ear canal exceeds that in the middle ear, producing a middle ear "vacuum." The eardrum retracts inward, producing aural pressure and muffled hearing. As negative pressure builds, a transudate from small blood vessels within the middle ear mucosa produces effusion, which can fill the entire middle ear with clear or amber colored fluid. Severe negative pressure that builds rapidly can rupture middle ear vessels, inner ear membranes, and the eardrum itself. The results are extreme ear pain, hemotympanum, bleeding from the canal, severe hearing loss, and/or vertigo.[8]

Usually barotrauma heals spontaneously with no residual impairment. The tympanic membrane heals within several days or weeks (occasionally within several months), middle ear fluid and hemorrhage resorb, and inner ear function recovers. Particularly severe injury, however, can produce permanent drum perforation and total sensorineural hearing loss. Fortunately even in severe barotrauma vertigo usually resolves spontaneously as compensatory mechanisms take over balance control, despite permanent loss of vestibular function in the injured ear.

Children and adults (if without upper respiratory disease) should fly, swim, and dive without concern for barotrauma. If symptoms develop after these recreations, the ear can be examined and hearing tested. Normal individuals with marginal eustachian tube function—who are therefore predisposed to middle ear barotrauma—will learn quickly whether they can fly and dive comfortably. They should avoid activities that produce ear pain and hearing loss. Mild ear pressure without other symptoms usually does not indicate injury.

If the upper respiratory mucosa is diseased, however, air flight and diving should be avoided. The most common disease is viral infection, but any active nasal, sinus, or middle ear disease can adversely affect eustachian tube function. Thus many patients with upper respiratory allergy, acute or chronic sinusitis, and chronic middle ear inflammation should fly with caution and avoid diving altogether. If air travel is unavoidable, nasal decongestants may improve eustachian tube function temporarily. Most nasal decongestants last for hours and can be used even before flight begins. The critical time is during aircraft descent, when cabin pressure increases faster than middle ear pressure (producing a relative decrease in middle ear pressure). Nasal decongestants should be used 30 minutes before descent begins to allow maximum effect. Chewing, yawning, and swallowing then may allow air to enter the middle ear.

If a patient complains of mild ear pressure and muffled

hearing after barotrauma, nasal and systemic decongestants often help. As soon as the patient can gently "pop" the ear (force air up the eustachian tube against a closed glottis), he or she should continue this Valsalva's maneuver periodically daily until symptoms improve. A patient who suffers middle ear hemorrhage, drum perforation, profound hearing loss, or vertigo should have hearing tested and be promptly referred to an otolaryngologist.

Sometimes an individual with marginal or poor eustachian tube function must fly frequently for professional or personal reasons, and decongestants seemingly do not help. In these patients an otolaryngologist can provide months of relief by placing a small ventilating (PE) tube across the drum. The tube can be inserted in several minutes under local anesthesia in the office as an outpatient procedure. It does not interfere with hearing, equalizes pressure instantly through the canal, and extrudes spontaneously after 6 to 9 months with good drum healing.

Mild middle ear barotrauma is very common when individuals must fly during acute upper respiratory infections. Fortunately common sense and decongestants almost always prevent severe injury.

INNER EAR
Childhood hearing loss

Verbal communication skills are developed virtually from birth, especially through 4 years of age. Failure to recognize infantile and childhood hearing loss can irreversibly and significantly handicap a child for the rest of his or her life. Not only are these individuals socially ostracized, they also are more often physically and sexually abused.[22] Because so many infants and young children can be well rehabilitated if treated early in life, prompt recognition of childhood hearing loss is critical.[10]

Between 2000 and 4000 "deaf" infants are born each year in the United States, 35% to 50% of whom have genetic hearing loss.[14] Of these one third are syndromal and usually are bilateral but can be unilateral. Of those children born deaf in the United States no cause can be identified in 30%. Of those cases that are genetic two thirds are autosomal recessive, one third are autosomal dominant, and 2% are X-linked. Just recently two deafness genes have been discovered—Usher's type I on chromosome 1 and Waardenburg's type I on chromosome 2. The next decade should witness explosive growth in our understanding of human genetics and the molecular basis of disease.[19]

In 1982 the Joint Committee on Infant Hearing updated seven infant groups with a combined incidence of moderate to profound hearing loss of 2.5% to 5%, much higher than among healthy infants (see the box above). In addition to children who have these inherited, maternal infectious, and developmental factors, all those who require intensive medical care after birth are at increased risk.

A careful family, prenatal, gestational, and postnatal history is mandatory in suspected hearing loss. The clini

---

Infants at high risk for hearing loss

A. Family history of childhood hearing impairment
B. Congenital perinatal infection
   1. TORCH: toxoplasmosis, rubella, cytomegalovirus, herpes simplex
   2. Syphilis
C. Anatomic malformations of the head and neck
   1. Syndromal and nonsyndromal
   2. Cleft palate
   3. Abnormalities of the pinna
D. Birth weight less than 1500 g
E. Hyperbilirubinemia requiring exchange transfusion (or greater than 20 mg %)
F. Bacterial meningitis, especially *Hemophilus influenzae*
G. Severe asphyxia with Apgar scores 0 to 3, no spontaneous respiration by 10 minutes, and/or hypotonia persisting to 2 hours of age

---

cian must remember that recessive inherited conditions, more common than dominant, may not yield a positive family history. The majority of familial disorders are not expressed until later in life. In selected patients, however, many aspects of the history can be almost diagnostic: night blindness of retinitis pigmentosa, syncope of Jervell-Lange-Nielsen syndrome, multiple fractures of osteogenesis imperfecta, perinatal jaundice of erythroblastosis fetalis, maternal rash in the first trimester of pregnancy in congenital rubella, and family history of early cardiovascular disease in familial hyperlipidemia.[18]

The general physical examination may be diagnostic: xanthomas of hyperlipidemia, thyroid enlargement (at age 8) of Pendred's syndrome, parrot nose of craniofacial dysostosis, white forelock or different colored irides of Waardenburg's syndrome, albinism, enlarged liver of mucopolysaccharidosis, blue sclerae of osteogenesis imperfecta, dwarfism of Cockayne's syndrome, and characteristic facies of Treacher-Collins syndrome.[18]

In "normal" babies and children developmental milestones should be checked. For babies failure to startle or awaken to loud noises, to babble at about 3 months, or to begin to use words at 1 to 1.5 years of age may indicate hearing loss. Older children with hearing loss may turn the television or radio to louder than normal volume, ask the parent to repeat words too often, or not "pay attention" in school.

Speech development should be investigated, as normal speech is delayed in the hearing-impaired child. The parent's assessment of the child's hearing behavior is particularly important. If the parent suspects hearing loss, the physician must be equally suspicious until complete auditory and otologic evaluation has been completed. Underlying factors (e.g., middle ear fluid) may be intermittent; however, the history will suggest chronic hearing impair ment despite normal examination findings on any given day.

Particularly if middle ear disease is suspected, an otoscope with adequate illumination should be used to evaluate the appearance and mobility of the tympanic membrane. The normal eardrum is translucent and pearly gray. The light reflex may be present even with significant middle ear disease. Although most of the eardrum may appear normal, small pockets of infection can lie superiorly to the short process of the malleus. A small amount of wax may cover a pocket of deep-seated infection (cholesteatoma). Uncooperative children should be appropriately restrained to permit adequate examination. By positive and negative pressure through the otoscope head eardrum mobility can be evaluated. The eardrum may appear to move freely if only a small amount of fluid is present. Impaired mobility indicates a significant abnormality of the middle ear.

If hearing loss is suspected, the child should be tested by an audiologist. Infants and older children who are uncooperative or mentally handicapped should be tested with both behavioral and evoked potential audiometry.[4] The Ohio Department of Health Infant Screening and Assessment Program (and those of most other states) requires retesting and/or referral to an otolaryngologist if the infant does not respond consistently to 35 decibel signals presented to either ear.

Early identification of hearing loss, prompt detection of cause, appropriate binaural amplification of residual hearing, prompt enrollment in an education-habilitation program, and ongoing audiologic monitoring and medical treatment can provide gratifying results.[17]

Acoustic trauma (noise-induced hearing loss)

We live in a very noisy world (Table 58-1). Noise can damage inner ear function profoundly and irreversibly. Prevention is mandatory. In 1973 the American Academy of Otolaryngology—Head and Neck Surgery recommended that a hearing conservation program (noise avoidance or protection) be *initiated* if there were difficulty communicating by speech in the presence of noise, tinnitus after working in noise several hours, or temporary loss of hearing after exposure to noise.[6] In 1981 the Occupational Safety and Health Administration, Department of Labor, required that noise exposure not exceed 90 decibels for 8 hours per day. In 1990 the limit was reduced to 85 decibels.[15] For each additional intensity of 5 decibels the exposure time must be halved, up to a maximum of 115 decibels. In other words the potential for damage is related to both noise intensity and duration of exposure. One must bear in mind that these sound intensity levels do not correlate precisely with audiometric measurements, in that a series of octave band audiometric measurements are reduced to a single equivalent number (decibel average) for simplicity.

Because environmental sounds are often multiple and

Table 58-1. Approximate noise levels for common daily events

Sound/noise	Average sound pressure level (decibels)
Faintest audible sound	0
Whisper, quiet library	30
Normal conversation, typewriter, sewing machine	60
Lawnmower, shop tools, truck traffic (8 hours per day is maximum safe exposure without hearing protection)	90
Jackhammer, pneumatic drill, snow mobile (2 hours per day is maximum safe exposure without hearing protection)	100
Sandblasting, loud rock concert, automobile horn (15 minutes per day is maximum safe exposure without hearing protection)	115
Gun muzzle blast, jet engine (maximum allowable noise *with* hearing protection; even brief exposure injures unprotected ears)	140

From American Academy of Otolaryngology—Head and Neck Surgery: *Noise, ears and hearing protection,* Alexandria, Va, 1992.

complex, and because the pathogenesis of noise-induced hearing loss is often multifactorial, the exact pathophysiologic mechanism remains controversial. Noise can biochemically alter inner ear function to produce temporary hearing impairment or can anatomically damage inner ear function to produce permanent hearing impairment. The patient also may complain of tinnitus and aural pressure. The ear examination result is normal unless massive impact trauma (140+ decibels) ruptures the eardrum.

Audiometric testing of early noise-induced hearing loss reveals symmetric high-pitched loss in a notched configuration centered at 4000 Hz. Additional noise exposure reduces hearing in adjacent frequencies. Verbal communication is significantly impaired when loss extends into the speech frequencies (500, 1000, 2000, and 3000 Hz) or when other factors such as age-related loss are superimposed on preexistent noise-induced loss.

The Medical Aspects of Noise Committee of the American Council of Otolaryngology in 1979 established audiologic and referral criteria for occupational hearing conservation programs.[5] Workers should undergo screening audiometry by approved personnel on properly calibrated equipment, preferably yearly. Workers should be referred if hearing in the speech range is worse than 30 dB, if there is significant difference in hearing between ears, if there is a significant change from previous hearing test results, or if responses are inconsistent. Workers also should be referred if otologic symptoms are significant, persistent, or

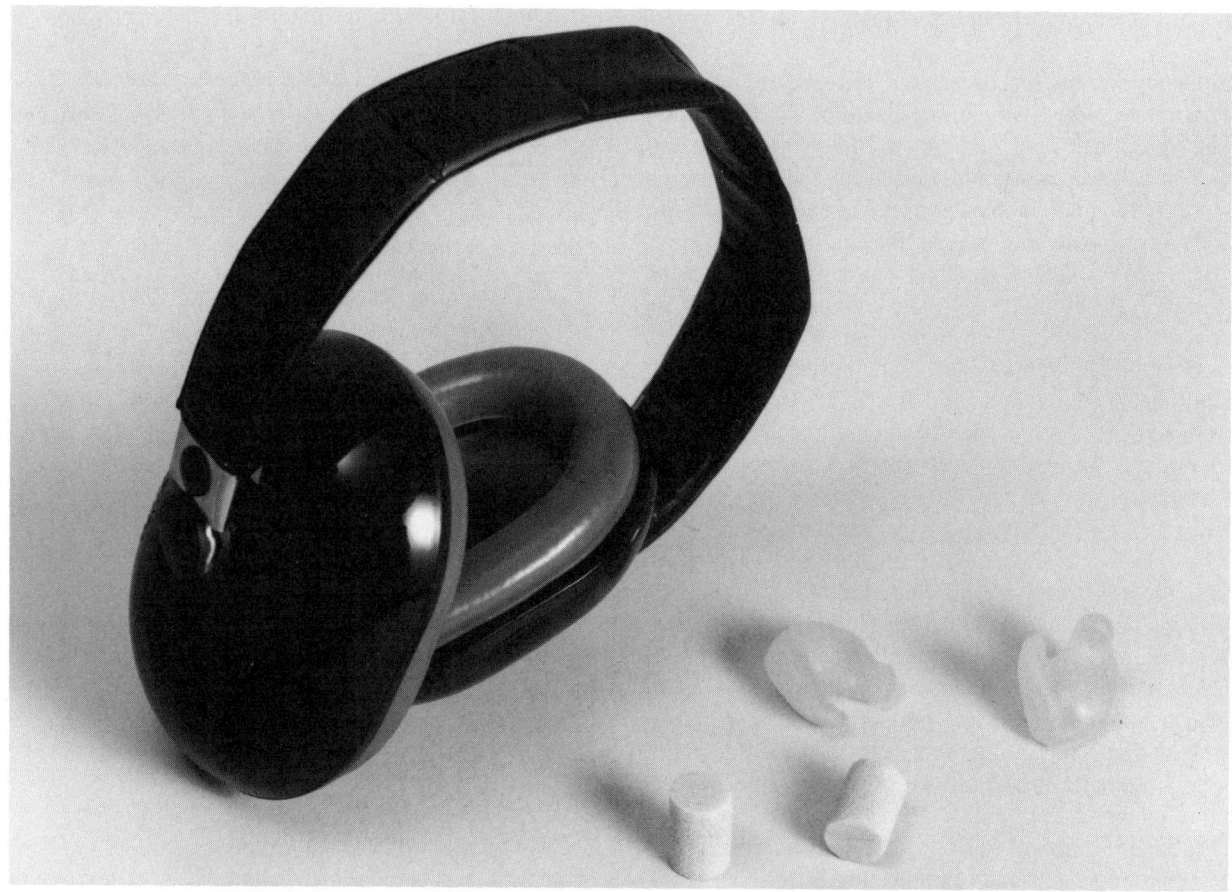

Fig. 58-2. Ear protection may consist of muffs, molds, or plugs, depending on the intensity of the noise.

recurrent. For practical purposes *any* change in auditory function after *any* noise exposure warrants an audiogram, ear examination, and discussion of preventive measures.

Potentially harmful noise should be either reduced at the source or shielded from the work area. Otherwise work assignments should be rearranged to reduce the duration of exposure, or the patient should wear ear protection. Ear protection may consist of ear muffs, plugs, or molds (Fig. 58-2). Appropriate protection is selected on the basis of the noise intensity. The best protector is one that is worn properly and constantly.

Recreational noise is an equally damaging cause of hearing loss. Sources include stereo headphones; music concerts; sporting events; hunting, particularly with a shotgun; power tools; outboard motors; lawnmowers—the list is endless. Even classical musicians are exposed to chronic noise at peak levels varying from 83 to 112 dB, depending on the instrument.[9]

Age and sex also influence hearing measurements in patients who have noise-induced hearing loss. Usually the configuration of the audiogram with a high-frequency "notched recovery" suggests noise trauma. Also normative hearing data for men and women of varying ages (Fig. 58-3) can be compared.

Each individual must balance enjoyment against risk if recreational or professional noise is intense and frequent. Normal hearing is one of the miracles of life. We take it for granted every day.

Tinnitus

By some estimates 40 million Americans suffer from tinnitus and 8 million find that it significantly impairs their quality of life.[14b] Tinnitus can result from abnormalities of the external, middle, or inner ear; the brain; and the cardiovascular system. So widespread is tinnitus, it is surprising our ability to treat this symptom is so limited.

First the physician should identify any easily treated cause. Ototoxic drugs, particularly aspirin, should be stopped if possible, especially if tinnitus began when the medication was started. When in doubt, check the *Physician's Desk Reference*. Cerumen impaction should be removed. Middle ear fluid should be treated. When these contributing factors are resolved, tinnitus may disappear or greatly improve.

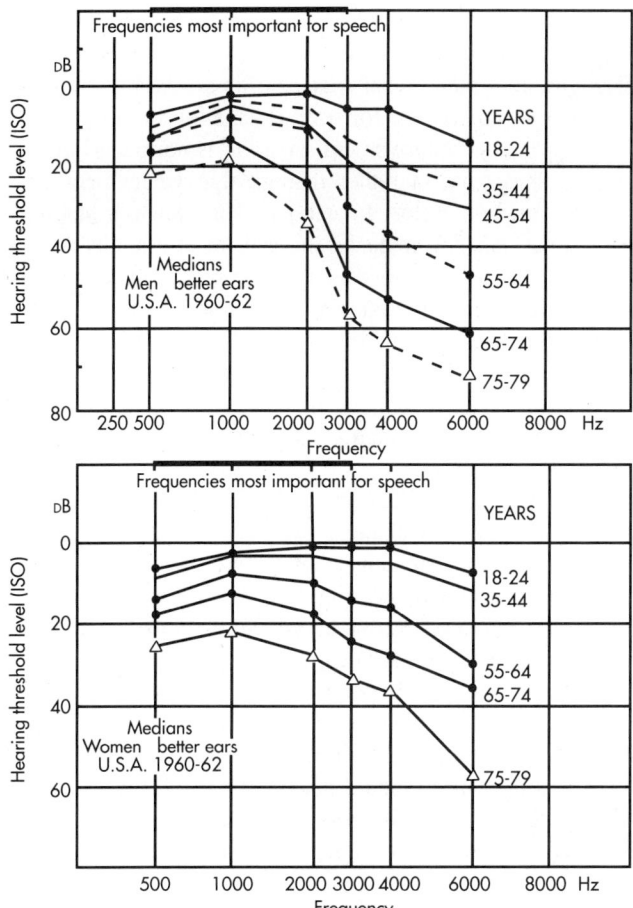

Fig. 58-3. Effects of age and sex on hearing. Composite audiograms for the better ear are presented for both men *(above)* and women *(below),* by age groups. Data recalculated to the ISO zero reference level. (From United States National Health Survey, Hearing Levels of Adults by Age and Sex, Public Health Service Publication, No 1000, Series 11, No 11, 1960-1962.)

Second, a hearing test should be obtained if tinnitus persists. The patient should be referred to an otolaryngologist if the ear examination result remains abnormal, conductive hearing loss is present, sensorineural hearing loss is asymmetric, or sensorineural hearing loss is progressive. Unilateral tinnitus, whether accompanied by sensorineural hearing loss or not, warrants brain stem auditory evoked potential (BAEP) testing or magnetic resonance imaging (MRI) with contrast to rule out acoustic tumor. Bilateral, rapidly progressive sensorineural loss can be caused by ototoxicity, Meniere's disease, immune inner ear disease, and inner ear syphilis. Most often a tinnitus patient has normal hearing or bilateral, symmetric, stable sensorineural hearing loss consistent with age or prior noise exposure. No obvious underlying cause is present, and the ear examination result is normal.

Third the physician should determine whether tinnitus is objective and pulsatile or subjective and nonpulsatile. Ob-

jective tinnitus can be heard by the examiner by using a Toynbee tube in the canal or stethoscope near the ear. Pulsatile tinnitus usually is synchronous with the pulse and implies a cardiovascular cause. Objective, pulsatile tinnitus warrants more detailed evaluation to rule out serious underlying abnormality: radiating heart murmur, carotid artery bruit, vascular tumor of the brain or skull base, and benign intracranial hypertension (pseudotumor cerebri syndrome).[20] Most of these patients should be seen by a specialist. Magnetic resonance imaging (MRI) with gadolinium enhancement, magnetic resonance angiography (MRA) if available, intraarterial digital subtraction angiography (IA-DSA), carotid Doppler study, or lumbar puncture with spinal fluid pressure measurement may be necessary. Generally intravenous digital subtraction angiography (IV-DSA) of the head and neck is not sufficiently detailed to be helpful. IA-DSA is invasive and may require overnight hospitalization; therefore, it should be reserved for highly suspicious cases, for example, when a vascular tumor or "blush" is present behind the eardrum. Benign intracranial hypertension is most common in middle-aged, obese females with headache and blurred vision. If appropriate testing yields normal findings, at least the patient can be reassured that pulsatile tinnitus results from a benign cause such as blood flow through a tortuous but normal artery.

Much more often tinnitus is subjective and nonpulsatile. The most common cause is sensorineural hearing loss from presbycusis or acoustic trauma. The most common conditions that aggravate tinnitus are noise exposure, a quiet setting, emotional stress, loss of sleep, and physical exhaustion.[21] There is no immediate cure and tinnitus can be extremely frustrating. Several very simple suggestions can greatly help the patient cope with tinnitus. These recommendations collectively represent the fourth step in managing severe tinnitus. First, reassure the patient that tinnitus is a symptom, not a disease, and will not cause deafness or any other serious problem. The patient should avoid nervous anxiety, which only aggravates the tinnitus. Second, remind the patient to have adequate rest and eat a well-balanced diet. Occasionally medication for sleep is required to break a vicious cycle of tinnitus-anxiety-insomnia-exhaustion-tinnitus. At bedtime a fan or FM radio detuned on "white noise" can mask the tinnitus and permit sleep. Third, tell the patient to avoid caffeine, nicotine, and other stimulants that aggravate tinnitus. Finally advise the patient that he or she will have to live with tinnitus and begin to deal with it. The treating physician should be honest and straightforward, to minimize false hopes and unrealistic expectations.

Antidepressant medication may significantly lessen tinnitus in depressed patients, but no scientific evidence has proved that any medication has definite benefit in nondepressed patients. Hearing aids for hearing-impaired patients, tinnitus maskers, or non-hearing-impaired patients, and biofeedback for depressed/anxious patients can be provided by audiologists, psychologists, and other professionals.

Tinnitus is a difficult, frustrating, albeit benign, symptom that requires a direct approach. Treatment can help some patients, but not all. The sooner the patient accepts the symptom, the sooner he or she can begin to cope with it.

Dizziness

The vestibular system maintains normal posture and balance by the interaction and coordination of impulses received from the inner ear, visual system, and proprioceptive system. Dizziness—disorientation in space—encompasses a wide variety of disorders, including lightheadedness, imbalance, giddiness, and vertigo. Although any of these sensations can be produced by inner ear disease, true vertigo—the perception that the patient or the environment is spinning—generally indicates a disturbance of the inner ear.[11]

Dizziness can be functional (psychosomatic) or organic. The latter results from central (brain) or peripheral (inner ear) vestibular dysfunction. Psychoneurosis may cause giddiness and loss of balance, but not vertigo. Often such symptoms are accompanied by anxiety and hyperventilation, almost never by aural symptoms (hearing loss, tinnitus), nausea, or nystagmus. Diagnosis is based on the lack of physical findings and on psychological evaluation.

Central vestibular dysfunction arising in the brain often produces lightheadedness rather than true vertigo. Underlying conditions include vascular disease, posterior fossa tumor, cerebellar hemorrhage, temporal lobe epilepsy, atypical migraine, multiple sclerosis, and head trauma. These disorders can produce weakness, diplopia, dysarthria, headache, and memory loss. Nystagmus, best seen with Frenzel glasses, may be direction-changing and is not suppressed by staring at an object in the examination room.

Peripheral vestibular dysfunction arising in the labyrinth or vestibular nerve more often produces true vertigo, which lasts at least several minutes and is worsened by head movement. It is frequently accompanied by hearing problems, nausea, past-pointing, and nystagmus that is direction-fixed and suppressed by visual fixation. The most common peripheral vestibular disorders are paroxysmal positional vertigo, Meniere's disease, vestibular neuritis (labyrinthitis), ototoxicity, and temporal bone trauma.

Paroxysmal positional vertigo is positional, short-lived, and relieved by holding the head still. Hearing is normal. Nystagmus and dizziness are pronounced when the head is placed in a provocative position, such as lying flat with the head turned back and to one side (Hallpike's maneuver). Recovery usually is spontaneous within a few weeks or months. Meniere's disease produces spontaneous episodic vertigo with hearing loss, tinnitus, and/or aural pressure.

Dizziness improves when vestibular function stabilizes with treatment or "burns out" after some years but can be disabling until then. Vestibular neuritis (viral labyrinthitis) produces severe vertigo for several days followed by gradual spontaneous improvement. Hearing is normal. Ototoxicity produces ataxia rather than vertigo when inner ear balance function is lost bilaterally. The patient's hearing can remain normal or he or she can be profoundly deaf. Rarely does deafness or dizziness improve although the patient learns coping strategies with time. Temporal bone trauma can produce a wide variety of vestibular and auditory symptoms resulting from fracture through the inner ear, concussion of the inner ear, perilymph fistula, and/or central vestibular dysfunction. Management and prognosis vary with each case.

A careful, detailed history of dizziness usually prompts a diagnosis. The ear examination result usually is normal except in trauma. An audiogram should be obtained in patients with subjective hearing loss, unilateral tinnitus, or persistent dizziness. An otolaryngologist should be consulted if unilateral sensorineural hearing loss or tinnitus is present, or if vertigo is persistent and severe. A neurologist, cardiologist, or psychiatrist can be consulted if other causes are suspected. Electronystagmography (ENG) and other vestibular tests should not be performed during acute vertigo; the patient will not tolerate testing. ENG can be obtained if dizziness persists and consultation is required. *Enhanced* magnetic resonance imaging or computed tomography of the head with special attention to the internal auditory canal (for acoustic tumor) should be obtained if sensorineural hearing loss is unilateral or neurologic disease is suspected.

For medical and legal reasons virtually all dizzy patients should *drive at their own risk* or not at all and should *refrain from any activities that place them or others at increased risk for injury*. These two points should be documented in the chart. Although the large majority of dizzy patients can drive and work safely, the burden of proof is deliberately placed on them to use appropriate caution. Determination of work disability usually requires vestibular testing, consultation with a specialist, and arbitration by a court of law. With these exceptions in mind patients otherwise should be encouraged to be as active as they can, to increase their confidence and promote self-care.

Motion sickness (motion intolerance) is one of the most common cause of dizziness; however, it is not a disease. Many normal persons cannot ride comfortably in a boat or the back seat of a car. Most give up amusement park rides early in life. Others are uncomfortable when they simply look at tidal currents, waves, and moving water. Some cannot comfortably walk down grocery store aisles where bright, colorful sales products distract peripheral vision.

Motion sickness results from a disparity of vestibular, visual, and proprioceptive input. In normal persons without motion intolerance the central vestibular system (cerebellum and brain stem) integrates this input to reflect orientation in space, change of posture, or movement relative to environment. In motion sickness, however, excessive stimulation of vision or proprioception even at rest or exaggerated movement compared with "normal" can produce lightheadedness, usually without vertigo. For example, motion intolerant patients can drive a car comfortably but feel uneasy in the passenger seat and uncomfortable in the back seat. Driving requires holding onto the steering wheel, which provides excellent proprioception. Moreover, sitting in the front seat provides maximum frontal and peripheral vision. With excellent proprioception and vision the patient remains comfortable despite stimulation of the vestibular system caused by bumps and curves in the road. In the back seat, however, adequate integration of information is lost. Sitting in a car seat provides minimal proprioception; sitting in the rear provides minimal vision. Both conspire to overwhelm vestibular input. The patient knows he or she is stationary relative to the car but feels a sense of motion. The result is motion sickness.

Because motion intolerance is a variation of normal—an exaggerated response to normal stimulation—it cannot be simply cured like a disease. It usually persists throughout life and may become worse as the patient grows older. Thus the best treatment is common sense: avoid activities or circumstances that tend to produce lightheadedness and disorientation. Sit in the front seat of the car or next to a window in an airplane. Avoid reading while traveling, and do not sit facing backward. If uncomfortable in a ship cabin, go out on deck and stare at the horizon. Avoid heavy meals while traveling. Also, when getting up at night turn on a light to avoid walking in darkness and use a night light in the bathroom. When getting up in the morning sit on the edge of the bed for several minutes before trying to stand or walk. Patients should change positions carefully and deliberately and have a stable object nearby to hold onto if needed. Some patients, particularly older ones with impaired vision or proprioception, should use a cane, a four-prong cane, or walker as needed. Patients should continue medications and diet prescribed for other medical problems to keep them under optimal control.

Vestibular suppressants can be given if dizziness is frequent or severe, or not at all if dizziness is infrequent and mild. Meclizine 12.5 to 25 mg tid or diazepam 2 to 5 mg tid is very helpful but does not cure the underlying disorder, which resolves spontaneously over time or responds to more specific treatment by a specialist. Diazepam 10 mg intravenously can be given for acute vestibular crisis. For prophylaxis during a cruise or air travel the patient can take these medications as needed or can use transdermal scopolamine. The latter controls vegetative symptoms of nausea and vomiting (seasickness) well but does not actually sedate the vestibular system. In other words transder-

mal scopolamine helps motion sickness more than vertigo. Medication is given transcutaneously from a patch, requires 3 hours to take effect, reaches plateau at 12 hours, and wears off at 3 days, at which time a new patch can be used. Patients who use transdermal scopolamine chronically, however, become "addicted" to it. Although inner ear function can remain stable and normal, as scopolamine wears off on the third day, these patients feel that their problem is returning. They replace the patch, feel better, and repeat the cycle for another 3 days. Some patients continue to use scopolamine for months! They should be reassured and the patch removed "cold turkey." Other suppressants can be given if needed.

Specialized care of the dizzy patient can be sophisticated and complex; however, preventive medical care can be summarized in four simple points: Rule out more serious nonvestibular causes. Prevent the patient from hurting himself or herself or others. Expect spontaneous improvement. Refer to a specialist if dizziness persists.

Ototoxicity

Ototoxicity is medication-induced functional impairment of the auditory and/or vestibular system of the inner ear. The box below lists some of these medications. Recognition of potentially ototoxic medication, pharmacokinetic dosing of medication, and early recognition of ototoxicity illustrate well the practice of preventive medicine in otology. A vast amount of literature has been published on the subject; however, within the context of this chapter prevention and recognition are emphasized rather that specific drug pharmacologic effects.[12]

Partial list of potentially ototoxic medications

A. Aminoglycosides
1. Streptomycin
2. Gentamicin
3. Tobramycin
4. Amikacin
B. Loop diuretics
1. Furosemide
2. Ethacrynic acid
3. Bumetidine
4. Piretamide
5. Azosemide
6. Triflocin
7. Indapamide
C. Erythromycin
1. Oral stearate ester
2. Intravenous lactobionate and gluceptate esters
D. Vancomycin
E. Salicylates
F. Quinine
G. *Cis*-platinum

First, the treating physician should recognize that a drug is potentially ototoxic. Some have effects that are reversible (aspirin, quinine, and erythromycin) and audiovestibular testing and intervention are less critical. Effects of others usually are not reversible (aminoglycosides, loop diuretics) and pharmacokinetic dosing and constant monitoring are vital in selected patients. Physicians are responsible for any medication they prescribe. When in doubt the treating physician should consult the *Physician's Desk Reference,* although drug manufacturers often overstate potential for ototoxicity to protect themselves. A medication with known potential for ototoxicity should be used if benefits outweigh risks and there are no better treatment alternatives.

Second, the physician should adjust medication dosage according to individual patient needs, particularly with aminoglycosides. Renal function, use of coexistent ototoxic medications, and peak/through serum levels all interact to determine potential for toxicity. In selected patients with several medical problems and prolonged need for treatment a specialist in pharmacokinetic dosing can be consulted to monitor day-to-day changes in drug levels.

Third, the treating physician or otolaryngology consultant should monitor auditory and vestibular function in patients who are at higher risk for developing ototoxicity. When possible baseline audiometric and vestibular testing should be obtained. Obviously some patients cannot undergo auditory and caloric testing: comatose, mentally handicapped, and medically debilitated patients. A patient who can communicate reliably, however, should report each day whether he or she perceives a change in hearing or dizziness. In addition periodic testing of selected high-risk patients is advisable: those with impaired renal function, higher drug levels, previous sensorineural hearing loss from ototoxicity, age greater than 65, treatment longer than 2 weeks, and multiple ototoxic drug therapy (especially aminoglycoside combined with loop diuretic). Monitoring will vary with each patient.

Finally if the patient perceives a change in hearing or balance function or if auditory or vestibular testing indicates a subclinical change of function, the treating physician should recognize that severe, permanent damage can occur if treatment is continued. Immediately the patient must be informed of the imminent risk, alternative therapy considered, and a definitive treatment decision made on the basis of available information, disease prognosis, and physician/patient preferences. The decision should be documented carefully in the chart.

Ototoxicity can be reversible, especially if detected early. Such cases may require no treatment. Permanent sensorineural hearing loss, however, may require hearing aid amplification. Ataxia from bilateral absent vestibular function does not respond to medicine or surgery. These patients should use a cane or walker if necessary, avoid ambulation in darkness, and avoid activities that place them at risk for injury. For example, they should not swim in water more than several feet deep because they can be disoriented if their head is below water. Shallow water allows them to stand instantly if needed. Although inner ear damage from ototoxicity can be severe and permanent, most patients eventually learn to compensate for their handicap.

REFERENCES

1. American Academy of Pediatrics, Joint Committee on Infant Hearing: Position statement 1982, *Pediatrics* 70:496-497, 1982.
2. Bailey BJ: Removal of cerumen, *JAMA* 251(13):1681, 1984.
3. Bluestone CD et al: Workshop on epidemiology of otitis media, *Ann Otol Rhinol Laryngol* 99(suppl 149):1-60, 1990.
4. Brookhouser PE et al: Auditory brainstem response results as predictors of behavioral auditory thresholds in severe and profound hearing impairment, *Laryngoscope* 100:803-810, 1990.
5. Cantrell RW et al: The otologic referral criteria for occupational hearing conservation program. Medical aspects of noise committee, American Council of Otolaryngology, *Otolaryngol Clin North Am* 12(3):635-636, 1979.
6. Catlin FI et al: Guide for conservation of hearing in noise, *Trans Am Acad Ophthalmol Otolaryngol* suppl, 1973.
7. Fairbanks DNF: *Antimicrobial therapy in otolaryngology—head and neck surgery,* ed 6, Alexandria, Va, 1991, American Academy of Otolaryngology—Head and Neck Surgery.
8. Farmer JC Jr: Otologic barotrauma. In Britton BH, editor, *Common Problems in Otology,* St. Louis, 1991, Mosby–Year Book.
9. Folprechtova A, Miksovska O: The acoustic conditions in a symphony orchestra, *Practov Lek* 28:1-2, 1978.
10. Hughes GB: Clinical evaluation of hearing loss. In Hughes GB, editor, *Textbook of clinical otology,* New York, 1985, Thieme Medical Publishers.
11. Hughes GB: Clinical evaluation of the dizzy patient. In Hughes GB, editor, *Textbook of clinical otology,* New York, 1985, Thieme Medical Publishers.
12. Hughes GB, Koegel L Jr: Ototoxicity. In Hughes GB, editor, *Textbook of clinical otology,* New York, 1985, Thieme Medical Publishers.
13. Hughes GB, Levine SC: Disorders of the external ear. In Hughes GB, editor, *Textbook of clinical otology,* New York, 1985, Thieme Medical Publishers.
14. Konigsmark BW: Hereditary deafness in man, *N Engl J Med* 281:713-720, 774-778, 827-832, 1969.
14b. Neher A: Tinnitus: the hidden epidemic: a patient's perspective, *Ann Otol Rhinol Laryngol* 100:327-330, 1991.
15. NIH consensus conference: noise and hearing loss, *JAMA* 263:3185-3190, 1990.
16. Occupational Safety and Health Administration, Department of Labor: Occupational noise exposure: hearing conservation amendment, *Fed Regist* 46:4078, 1981.
17. Pappas DG, Banyas JB: Hearing loss in the infant. In Britton BH, editor, *Common problems in otology,* St. Louis, 1991, Mosby–Year Book.
18. Proctor C: Diagnosis, prevention and treatment of hereditary sensorineural hearing loss, *Laryngoscope* 87(suppl 7):1-60, 1977.
19. Ruben RJ: Otolaryngology and head and neck surgery in the twenty-first century, *Otolaryngol Head Neck Surg* 104:775-779, 1991.
20. Sismanis A et al: Objective tinnitus in benign intracranial hypertension: an update, *Laryngoscope* 100:33-36, 1990.
21. Stouffer JL et al: Tinnitus as a function of duration and etiology: counselling implications, *Am J Otol* 12:188-194, 1991.

22. Sullivan PM et al: Patterns of physical and sexual abuse of communicatively handicapped children, *Ann Otol Rhinol Laryngol* 100:188-194, 1991.

23. Teele DW et al: Epidemiology of otitis media in children, *Ann Otol Rhinol Laryngol* 89(suppl 68):5-6, 1980.

RESOURCES

The American Academy of Otolaryngology—Head and Neck Surgery, Inc., offers patient education pamphlets on the following topics:

Cochlear implants
Doctor, what causes the noise in my ears?
Earache and otitis media
Ears, altitude and airplane travel
5-Minute hearing test
Is my baby's hearing normal?
Noise, ears and hearing protection
Travel tips for hearing impaired persons
These can be obtained by sending a stamped, self-addressed envelop, specifying the pamphlet title, to American Academy of Otolaryngology—Head and Neck Surgery, Inc., One Prince Street, Alexandria, VA 22314. The academy also will send patients a list of appropriate specialists in their area.

Information on tinnitus treatment, research, self-help groups, and related topics can be obtained from American Tinnitus Association, PO Box 5, Portland, OR 97207.

Chapter 59

OPHTHALMOLOGIC DISORDERS

Gary A. Varley

In the twentieth century significant advances have been made in the recognition and treatment of ocular disease. Of the four leading causes of blindness (glaucoma, cataract, age-related macular degeneration, and diabetic retinopathy) each has seen landmark progress toward this end. New medications, improved surgery, and use of lasers have preserved vision for many glaucoma patients. With technical advances in cataract surgery, vision of approximately 95% of cataract patients will improve after surgery. Because of smaller incision surgery and the new intraocular lens design visual recovery is faster and the resulting optical correction approaches the natural adult state. Laser surgery has proved to be pivotal in preserving vision for patients with diabetic retinopathy and for some patients with age-related macular degeneration. However, despite these successes little progress has been made in the prevention of these disease states. I suspect ophthalmology, much like the rest of medicine, will see great strides in the prevention of disease in the next few decades.

Everyday scores of patients' eyes are examined by different eye care providers with the goal of preserving ocular health and preventing visual impairment. The majority of this eye care in the United States is provided by optometrists and ophthalmologists. Optometrists are licensed eye care providers who have 4-year optometric training after at least 2 years of college. Their training focuses on the nonsurgical correction of refractive disorders as well as the recognition of ocular disease. In some states they have been licensed to prescribe a limited number of therapeutic medications for the treatment of some ocular disorders. An ophthalmologist completes 4 years of college and 4 years of medical school to graduate as a licensed doctor of medicine (M.D.). He or she then completes a 1-year medicine or surgical internship before starting a 3- or 4-year oph-

thalmology residency. After completion of the ophthalmology residency they are licensed to provide comprehensive ophthalmic care including surgical and nonsurgical correction of refractive disorders, as well as diagnosis and medical and surgical treatment of eye disease.

EPIDEMIOLOGY
Prevalence of blindness

Studies attempting to define the prevalence of blindness in the United States are fraught with technical difficulties. To overcome population sample biases large sample sizes are needed. This correspondingly limits the age range of the sample size. In addition even the definition of blindness is not uniform and complicates comparisons between studies. Two definitions have become popular. Legal blindness in the United States is considered when the corrected visual acuity is 20/200 or worse in the better eye, or the visual field is constricted to less than 20 degrees. Visual impairment in the United States is defined as visual acuity less than 20/40 in the better eye. The World Health Organization has proposed a standard definition for blindness and visual impairment as vision worse than 20/400 and worse than 20/60, respectively, in the better eye. Early data from *Statistics on Blindness* in the *Model Reporting Area (1969-1970)* were based on a blindness registry maintained in 16 states and therefore probably underestimated the true prevalence of blindness.[17] In 1980 the Framingham Eye Study reported the prevalence of binocular blindness to be 0.6% for persons aged 55 to 84 years old. The prevalence of blindness in at least one eye was 5.2%.[19] The major cause of blindness was senile cataract. It was also noted that the prevalence of blindness increased with increasing age. Recent data from the Baltimore Eye Survey studied blindness and visual impairment in an

American urban population.[34] The primary aim of this study was to compare the prevalence of ocular disease in black and white urban populations. This study confirmed the increasing prevalence of blindness and visual impairment with increasing age. Although no difference in the prevalence of blindness was found in the different sexes, blacks on average had a twofold excess prevalence of blindness and visual impairment than whites. For blindness this difference lessened with increasing age. On the basis of 1985 national census population for persons 40 years or older the Baltimore Eye Survey group estimated that more than 3 million people are visually impaired (vision worse than 20/40) and 890,000 people are bilaterally blind (vision worse or equal to 20/200).[34] More conservative figures from the American Foundation for the Blind estimate 620,300 blind residents of the United States.[5]

Cause of visual loss in the United States

The Framingham Eye Study found that 16% of the United States population 55 years or older had at least one of four leading causes of blindness found in the United States:[19] senile cataracts, age-related macular degeneration, diabetic retinopathy, and glaucoma. The most common, cataract, was found in 12.3% of study patients. Age-related macular degeneration was seen in 5.7%. However, it must be remembered that the Framingham Eye Study group is a select sample population and is thus subject to sample errors.

Socioeconomic impact of eye disease

Accurate figures demonstrating the socioeconomic impact of visual impairment or blindness are not available. Direct cost, such as special education and tax benefits, must be added to the indirect cost of decreased revenue, such as lost wages and lost taxes if the person is not productive. It has, however, been estimated that a year of blindness in the United States cost the U.S. government approximately $13,607 per blind person.[24] Using the conservative U.S. blindness figures blindness in the United States costs nearly $8.5 billion annually. Certainly for a motivated patient who has special training a visual handicap need not mean irrevocably lost production.

ROUTINE EYE CARE AND THE PREVENTION OF VISUAL LOSS
Recommendations for routine eye examinations

Unfortunately with present technology prevention of the four common diseases that lead to blindness in the United States is not possible. For many ocular disorders the only symptom is reduced vision, which may occur late in the course of the disease, and in some cases visual loss is irreversible. Therefore since ophthalmic care may prevent blindness resulting from each of these diseases, the most important preventive measure is early diagnosis. As such routine comprehensive eye examinations do play a role in

Table 59-1. Routine eye examination

Age (years)	Frequency
65 or older	Every 1-2 years
40-64	Every 2-4 years
20-39	Because of the high incidence and more aggressive course of glaucoma in blacks, even in the absence of visual or ocular symptoms, they should receive a comprehensive examination every 3-5 years.
	Other asymptomatic, otherwise normal, patients require a comprehensive evaluation less frequently.

From American Academy of Ophthalmology, *Comprehensive Adult Eye Evaluation, Preferred Practice Pattern*, San Francisco, 1992, American Academy of Ophthalmology.

the prevention of blindness. After considering the incidence of ocular disease related to age and race the American Academy of Ophthalmology has recommended routine comprehensive examinations (Table 59-1).[3] Of course symptoms or risk factors of ocular disease would indicate the need for more frequent examinations. The American Academy of Ophthalmology and the American Academy of Pediatrics have recommended that normal children have their eyes evaluated in the newborn nursery, at age 6 months, at 3½ years, and yearly starting at 5 years.[4] Unlike the adult examination screening of asymptomatic children can be performed by pediatricians or family physicians rather than ophthalmologists. The complexity of the examination is based on the age and development of the child. The most important aspects of visual screens for children less than 10 years of age are the presence of a good red reflex, ocular alignment, and visual acuity. Often yearly vision screens are provided at school.[4]

Glaucoma

Glaucoma is a leading cause of blindness in the United States and is the number one cause of blindness in blacks.[25] The distribution of the type of glaucoma differs in different races. For whites approximately 90% of primary glaucoma is due to open-angle glaucoma. In this population angle-closure glaucoma is responsible for only 0.1% of the glaucoma seen. Among Eskimos, however, angle-closure glaucoma is much more common, contributing to up to 8% of the glaucoma seen.[8] Open-angle glaucoma in its early stages is an asymptomatic disease and approximately half of the 3 million affected Americans are unaware of their blinding condition. This is particularly devastating because glaucoma damage and subsequent visual loss are irreversible. Early diagnosis is mandatory to prevent blindness. Medical and/or surgical treatment is aimed at the prevention of further damage. Although intraocular pressure is often used as a screening examination, not all glaucomatous patients have elevation of this value. These screens are acceptable for annual checks for low-risk patients, but they are not a substitute for a periodic comprehensive eye examination as previously outlined. In addition they are not adequate screens for high-risk patients such as those who have a significant family history for glaucoma.

Three common tools for measuring intraocular pressure (IOP) include a Schiotz tonometer, a noncontact air-puff tonometer, and Goldman applanation tonometry. The Schiotz tonometer has the advantage of being relatively inexpensive, very portable, and easy to use. However, as it is subject to a number of sources of error, its clinical usefulness is primarily as a screening device for the nonophthalmologist. The noncontact air-puff tonometer has reasonable accuracy for IOP close to the normal range, but this accuracy falls off at higher levels of IOP. Disadvantages of the air-puff tonometer include expense, requirement for precise technique, and abnormal readings caused by corneal abnormalities. Most ophthalmologists rely on the Goldman applanation tonometer, which has become the standard by which other instruments are measured. However, it must be remembered that the diagnosis of glaucoma does not rest on the value of the IOP. Critical stereoscopic evaluation of the optic nerve, sometimes supplemented with visual field testing, is required when considering the diagnosis of glaucoma. Therefore, although screening IOP evaluations are important and may indicate possible glaucoma, they are no substitute for periodic comprehensive eye examinations by an ophthalmologist.

Diabetic retinopathy

Diabetes affects approximately 14 million Americans. It is estimated that approximately half of these patients have at least early signs of diabetic retinopathy. Annually it is thought that 8000 people become blind as a result of this disorder.[24] Type I diabetic patients are more likely to develop retinopathy, but the prevalence of retinopathy increases with duration of diabetes for both type I and type II. Unfortunately prevention of diabetic retinopathy is not possible, but the incidence may be reduced with "good" control of the blood sugar. "Tight" control of blood sugar has not shown additional benefit.

Early diabetic retinopathy, so-called background diabetic retinopathy or nonproliferative retinopathy, does not generally require treatment. At this stage retinal hemorrhages, microaneurysms, hard exudates, and nerve fiber layer infarcts occur (see Plate 7 after page 16). If these changes lead to retinal edema in the macular area, so-called macular edema, visual acuity can be significantly reduced. In fact it is estimated that up to 20% of the visual loss associated with diabetes results from diabetic maculopathy. The most severe form of diabetic retinopathy is called "proliferative diabetic retinopathy." In this form new vessels proliferate on the surface of the retina and into the vitreous (see Plate 8 after page 16). Complications caused

Table 59-2. Diabetic eye examinations

Type of diabetes	First eye examination after diagnosis	Follow-up examination
Type I	5 Years	Annual
Type II	Within months	Annual

From Newsome DA et al: Arch Opthalmol 106:192-198, 1988; Kahn H, Moorhead HB: Statistics on blindness in the model reporting area 1969-1970, Washington, DC, 1973, Department of Health, Education, and Welfare.

by these vessels such as retinal detachment and vitreous hemorrhages severely reduce visual acuity. In 1978 a landmark study performed by the Diabetic Retinopathy Study Research Group demonstrated a 60% reduction of severe visual loss when panretinal photocoagulation is performed in high-risk eyes.[9] High-risk characteristics include vitreous hemorrhage, presence of new vessels, presence of new vessels on the disc (optic nerve head), and severity of new vessels. It is best to treat these eyes as soon as they demonstrate high-risk characteristics. A recent study failed to demonstrate the advantage of treating before the development of high-risk characteristics so long as close follow-up observation is possible.[11] In a related study aspirin did not alter the course of diabetic retinopathy.[13] Focal macular laser photocoagulation for clinically significant macular edema can reduce visual loss in 50% of patients with diabetic maculopathy.[12]

In short significant advances have been made in the treatment of diabetic retinopathy to reduce the incidence of visual loss. Since severe diabetic retinopathy remains easier to prevent than treat, the National Eye Health Education Program, coordinated by the National Eye Institute and the American Academy of Ophthalmology, has recommended annual routine dilated eye examinations (Table 59-2) for diabetic patients.[1,24] Patients who have "poor" glycemic control, uncontrolled hypertension, or significant renal disease should be seen more frequently. If high-risk characteristics are found during the eye examination, the ophthalmologist may recommend more frequent follow-up examinations. As pregnancy can worsen diabetic retinopathy, diabetic patients who are planning to conceive should have a dilated eye examination before conception and follow-up care during the pregnancy.

PREVENTION OF SPECIFIC OCULAR DISEASES
Cataract

Despite extensive and ongoing research on the pathogenesis of cataracts we are still unable to prevent the natural aging changes of the human lens. Cataracts remain the major cause of blindness worldwide with an estimated 15 million affected persons. When visual acuity is significantly affected, cataract surgery remains the only method of improving vision. In 1988 an estimated 1.25 million cataract operations were performed in the United States alone. The economic impact of this surgery is staggering, costing approximately $2.5 billion per year in the United States. Since many of these patients are elderly, this economic burden in the United States falls on the Medicare system, thus straining already limited resources. Fortunately modern microscopic cataract surgery, using smaller incisions and posterior chamber intraocular lenses, has made this surgery highly successful. Typically more than 95% of patients see an improvement in their visual acuity after cataract surgery. For the patient who may lose his or her driver's license or the patient no longer able to read this improved vision can significantly enhance independence and enjoyment of life.

The most common cataract is a natural consequence of aging. Nearly all patients above the age of 60 have some degree of lenticular opacity (see Plate 9 after page 16). Other causes have been identified: intraocular disease such as uveitis, as well as intraocular surgery. Trauma, ocular and systemic medications, and metabolic and endocrine abnormalities are also associated with early cataract formation (see the box). The most common drug-induced cataract results from topical or systemic use of corticosteroids. Corticosteroids produce a dose-related posterior subcapsular cataract. Since this cataract is aligned with the visual axis, it can significantly affect visual acuity. It has been suggested that 15 mg or more of prednisone given daily for 1 year will probably cause a cataract sufficient to affect visual acuity.[2] However, more important than the daily dose of corticosteroids is the cumulative dose. Using the lowest possible cumulative dosage is the best way to delay this complication. However, in all patients on long-term corticosteroids lenticular change eventually develops. Of course, if the medication is needed to sustain life, as in renal or cardiac transplantation patients or steroid-dependent asthmatics, this ocular complication is tolerated. When the vision is adversely affected, cataract surgery can restore visual acuity.

Studies evaluating risk factors for the development of cataracts have implicated dietary factors, medications, exposure to sunlight, race, level of education, metabolic abnormalities, smoking, body mass, handgrip strength, and family history.[15,22] With such a large list it is obvious that cataractogenesis is multifactorial. Considerable interest has focused on the effect and prevention of sunlight-induced lenticular changes. Several studies have demonstrated an increased prevalence of cataracts in persons with a high ultraviolet (UV) light exposure history.[6,32] One such study demonstrated that high cumulative levels of ultraviolet B (UVB) light exposure increased the risk of cortical lens changes in the watermen of Chesapeake Bay.[32] If oxidative damage is thought to cause or hasten the progression of age-related cataracts, then it follows that antioxidative nutrients may be beneficial. A host of elements, including riboflavin, proteins, amino acids, vitamin C, vitamin E,

---

Selected list of conditions associated with cataracts

Aging
Intraocular diseases
  Uveitis
  Intraocular neoplasms
  Retinitis pigmentosa
  Chronic retinal detachment
Trauma
Mendelian inheritance
  Autosomal dominant
  Autosomal recessive
  X-linked
Drugs
  Corticosteroids
  Phenothiazines
  Phosphaline iodide eyedrops
Endocrine and metabolic dysfunction
  Diabetes mellitus
  Hypoglycemia
  Hypothyroidism
  Hypoparathyroidism
  Galactosemia
Congenital/intrauterine infection
  Rubella
  Chickenpox/herpes zoster
  Herpes simplex
  Cytomegalovirus
Systemic syndromes
  Hallermann-Streiff syndrome
  Myotonic dystrophy
  Stickler's syndrome
  Marinesco-Sjögren syndrome
  Smith-Lemli-Opitz syndrome
  Meckel's syndrome
Dermatologic disorders
  Poikiloderma atrophicans
  Congenital icthyosis
  Ectodermal dysplasia
  Incontinentia pigmenti
  Atopic dermatitis
Chromosomal disorders
  Trisomy 21 (Down's syndrome)
  Trisomy 13
  Trisomy 18

Modified from Tasman W: *Duane's clinical ophthalmology*, Philadelphia, JB Lippincott.

---

carotene, selenium, calcium, and zinc, have been investigated. Supporting this concept are reports of lower cataract prevalence in persons with high serum levels of antioxidants such as vitamin E, vitamin C, and carotenoids.[16] However, other reports have not demonstrated the association of sunlight exposure and age-related cataracts.[10] The data linking sunlight exposure and age-related cataracts are extrapolated from either animal research or observational human studies. Research animals may differ significantly in their absorption and metabolism of antioxidative elements. In addition, animal studies have severely restricted or massively oversupplemented these elements, practices that may also lead to false conclusions. Since cataract formation is no doubt multifactorial, confounding variables are difficult to control in the observational human studies.

Therefore, lacking nonrefutable scientific evidence for the benefit of nutritional supplementation to prevent or retard the progression of cataracts, megadose supplementation is not recommended. If a well-balanced diet is not practical for a particular patient, use of a daily multivitamin supplement is not unreasonable. However, it must be understood that definitive proof of its efficacy is not yet available. Certainly avoidance of UVB light is supported by the skin damage studies alone. It is reasonable to advocate the use of sunglasses when high exposure to sunlight is anticipated. In this case the expense of a UV filter is reasonable.

Age-related macular degeneration (ARMD)

The National Eye Institute estimates that by 1995 10 million Americans will have some visual impairment caused by age-related macular degeneration (ARMD) (see Plate 10 after page 16). The most devastating form of this disease results in rapid deterioration of vision when abnormal vessels proliferate under the retina. This severe so-called exudative form accounts for almost 10% of the visual loss in this disease. If exudative ARMD is discovered when the damage to the foveal area of the retina is limited and not involved with these new vessels, laser photocoagulation may slow and in some cases prevent further visual loss. Therefore, patients must know they have macular degeneration and monitor their vision for new changes. Monitoring is best accomplished by viewing an Amsler grid daily with each eye (Fig. 59-1). Patients are asked to look at the central "black dot" and notice the lines in the periphery. Any new distortion (metamorphopsia) or loss of these lines (scotoma) may indicate new subretinal vessel growth (choroidoneovascularization).

Many epidemiologic associations have been linked with ARMD. Some include a positive family history of hypertension, a hyperoptic refractive error, light colored irides and hair, short stature, a weak hand grip, and severe elastic degeneration. The association between cigarette smoking and ARMD has been inconsistent. It has been speculated that oxidative stress associated with sunlight exposure contributes to the development and progression of ARMD. Certainly there is no doubt that sunlight can adversely affect the retina. Solar retinopathy is a well-known toxicity that occurs from viewing the sun. Numerous reports of this phenomenon occur when people attempt to view a solar eclipse directly. However, implicating sunlight as a cause of ARMD is more difficult. In the normal adult eye the lens and other ocular media filter out most

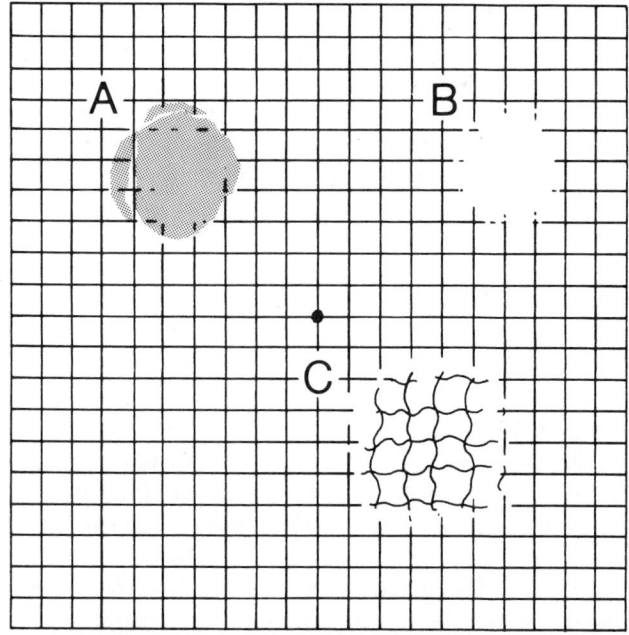

Fig. 59-1. The Amsler grid is viewed at 35.5 cm (14 inches), using the central dot for fixation. Regions of metamorphopsia, scotoma, and blur are noted. (From Ryan SJ: *Retina*, vol 1, St. Louis, 1989, Mosby–Year Book.)

light below 400 nm. The original analysis of the data studying the watermen at Chesapeake Bay failed to demonstrate an association with UV light exposure and ARMD.[36] However, a reanalysis of the data linked exposure to visible light with an increased risk for ARMD.[33] As with cataracts it is reasonable to advocate the use of sunglasses when high exposure to sunlight is anticipated. For the retina it is preferable to limit all light below 510 nm. This includes blue and violet light in addition to the ultraviolet range. Many sunglasses do not limit this high-energy spectrum of visible light. If the sunglasses allow pupillary dilatation without absorbing this spectrum, they may actually increase retinal exposure to the potentially harmful light. Therefore, individuals who spend a significant amount of time outdoors should be encouraged to wear sunglasses that block 100% of UV light and preferably blue and violet light of the visible spectrum. Also, wraparound sunglasses protect the eye and adnexa from lateral UV light.

If oxidative damage contributes to ARMD, then it follows that nutritional factors may limit this harmful effect. Theoretically antioxidants may prevent cellular damage by acting as free-radical scavengers. A small randomized trial has suggested a possible benefit of zinc supplementation.[26] However, these investigators point out the pilot nature of their study and suggest that because of "the possible toxic effects and complications of oral zinc administration, widespread use of zinc in macular degeneration is not now warranted."[26] Even so zinc preparations are being advertised for macular degeneration. Sales of vitamins and mineral supplements continue to grow rapidly and now exceed $2 billion a year. It seems prudent that if a balanced diet is not maintained, then a multivitamin tablet is reasonable, but pending the results of further studies, megadose supplementation is not recommended.

Trauma

Although ocular trauma is not a leading cause of blindness in the United States, its economic impact is enormous since it typically affects persons below the age of 30.[28] In many cases these injuries are very preventable. The incidence of ocular trauma varies with the method and location of the study. In 1979 the number of hospital-treated eye injuries in Dane County, Wisconsin, was 423/100,000 residents.[18] Others have found that 1.3% of all emergency room visits were related to eye and adnexal injuries.[23] The most common causes of eye injuries are assaults, work-related accidents, sports-related accidents, recreational activities, and motor vehicle accidents. The geographic area of any study analyzing the cause of traumatic injuries must be considered. Whereas alkali corneal burns in a large metropolitan city are often the result of assault, in the rural farm belt this same injury is typically work-related. Blunt trauma that results from assault is inherently difficult to prevent, but many other causes, such as accidental gunshot injuries, work-related accidents, and sports-related injuries, are preventable.

In a study conducted in Boston eye injuries in the workplace accounted for 48% of the total eye injuries studied. More significantly 50% of these resulted in ruptured globes with an inherently poorer prognosis for visual recovery. Only 66% of injured persons reported that protective eye wear was available on the job. Of even more concern was that only 10% stated that they were using protective eye wear.[28] Clearly it is the responsibility of the employer to provide and require the use of protective eye wear, and the employee must comply with these guidelines. Since serious eye injuries in the workplace typically result in legal action against the employer, the employer would be wise to demand the use of protective eye wear. This is critically important in automobile-repair and construction-related work as these occupations have a higher incidence of serious ocular injuries.[28]

Sports-related accidents are thought to be responsible for 33,000 eye injuries each year and are unrelated to the expertise of the participant. A year-long study found that nearly 14% of these injuries required hospital admission and almost 6% necessitated intraocular surgery. Over 12% will sustain permanent ocular sequulae, including loss of vision in 3.5%. Sports most commonly leading to eye injuries are basketball, baseball/softball, and racquetball.[21] A racquetball striking the cornea with a velocity of 65 mph can raise the intraocular pressure of the eye 10-fold to 240

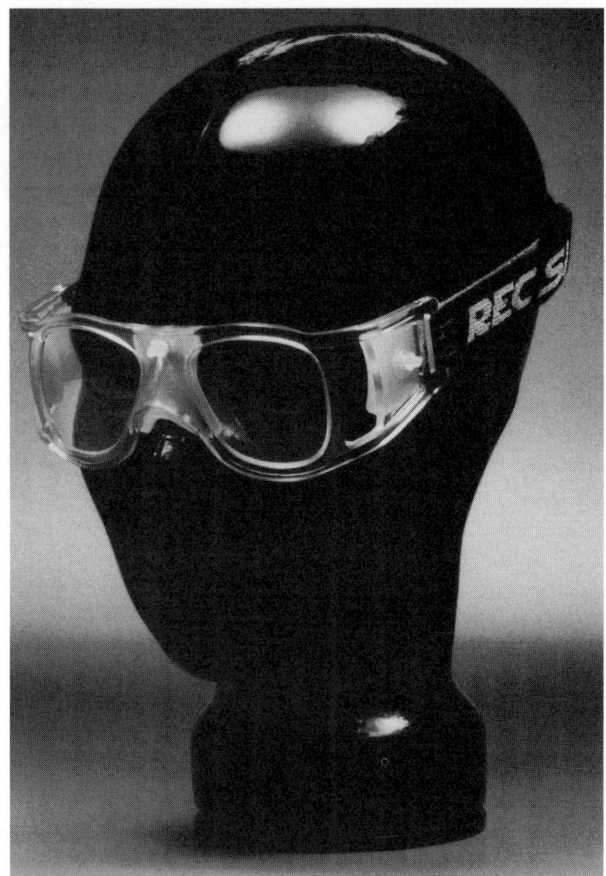

Fig. 59-2. Safety glasses.

millimeters of mercury (mm Hg). The tragedy of these injuries is that many are preventable. It is of great concern that sports participants still commonly do not wear protective eye wear. In one study only 5% of such patients had worn protective eye wear. In addition, in a follow-up study only 31% of these same persons previously injured were using eye protection for subsequent sporting activities.[21] Ocular injuries caused by sporting events include hyphemas, orbital fractures, ruptured globes, and vitreous hemorrhages with or without retinal detachment, as well as simple contusions and abrasions. Effective sports goggles can prevent many of these injuries. A well-devised study in 1983 demonstrated that all standard dress spectacles studied failed to provide ocular protection. In addition if the dress-spectacle lenses or frames break, their components can do more harm than the projectile itself. Safety lenses made of polycarbonate did not shatter but were dislodged if the frame was not adequate. Lenses made of polycarbonate provide effective eye protection. The frame must be a one piece unit without hinges and made of polycarbonate or stronger material. Fortunately these safety glasses are available with prescriptions.[14] (Fig. 59-2). Lensless eye guards should never be used for racquet

---

Partial list of sporting events requiring protective eyewear

Squash	Baseball/Softball	Boxing (helmet)
Racquetball	Badminton	Ice hockey (helmet)
Tennis	Fishing	Football (helmet)
Paddleball	Shooting/archery	
Handball	Running/jogging	

From Burke MJ et al: Soccerball-induced eye injuries, *JAMA* 249:2682-2685, 1983.

---

sports as the small balls used can deform through the guard and strike the cornea. Larger balls can also cause serious eye injuries. A series of 24 contusion injuries resulting from a soccer ball found 12 hyphemas and 7 vitreous hemorrhages. These authors confirmed that protective eye wear should be worn in any competitive sport involving large or small projectiles (see the box).[7]

Finally an all too common source of severe ocular injury is air-powered guns. Despite the significant morbidity and mortality associated with these weapons they continue to find their way into the hands of children. In 1981 it was estimated that 22,800 injuries related to air-powered guns were treated in U.S. emergency rooms. Of these 1255 were eye injuries.[31] A study in a children's hospital found that 7% of children's ocular injuries were associated with BB guns. Even more worrisome is the degree of these injuries. When a projectile from this weapon strikes the eye, its blunt nature causes severe ocular damage. Of 22 penetrating injuries from BB guns Sternberg found that 19 (86%) eyes were enucleated and that in the remaining 3 vision was worse than 5/200.[31] Part of this problem stems from the perception that these guns are harmless and therefore children are allowed to play with them unsupervised. Even in states that restrict the sale of these guns parents must be taught the danger and must not allow children to fire these weapons unsupervised.

Ocular injuries by gunshot wounds are not restricted to those by air-powered guns. In each hunting season accidental facial gunshot wounds occur. In this case not only eyes but even lives may be lost when the pellet gains entry into the central nervous system through the orbit. It has been demonstrated, however, that polycarbonate protective eye wear with integral side shields and a secure headband can virtually eliminate injuries from shotguns fired at more than 25 yd.[35]

Ocular infections

Ocular infections range from mild viral conjunctivitis, which is as difficult to prevent as the common cold but resolves without treatment, to severe endophthalmitis with loss of the eye. One particular infection, however, is partially preventable and can result in profound visual loss. Over 13 million Americans wear soft contact lenses for re-

fractive correction. A recent study determined that the annual incidence of ulcerative keratitis in patients wearing extended-wear contact lenses for refractive correction was 20.9/10,000 persons. For daily-wear soft contact lenses wearers the annualized incidence is 4.1/10,000 persons.[27,29] This suggests that 12,000 corneal ulcers related to soft contact lenses occur annually. In addition, persons wearing their lenses overnight have a 10 to 15 times increased incidence of ulcerative keratitis. Therefore, many ophthalmologists believe patients should be discouraged from sleeping with contact lenses in, and if they choose to, they must understand the risk and remove the lenses at the first sign of trouble. Although it has never been definitively proved that proper lens hygiene (i.e., cleaning and disinfecting) reduces this complication, most corneal specialists feel this to be the case. As such it is disappointing to discover that as many as 50% of successful contact lens wearers do not disinfect their lenses daily.[29]

To reduce the risk of contact-lens-related ulcerative keratitis the wearer should have specific instructions that must be reviewed and reinforced regularly. The lenses must be cleaned and disinfected daily for the daily contact lens wearer and no less than weekly for extended contact lens wearers. An appropriate schedule for enzyming should be maintained. Soft contact lenses should be rinsed only in sterile saline solution before insertion into the eye. They should never be rinsed in tap water or homemade saline products. No lens should ever be moistened with saliva. Regular routine follow-up consultation with the eye care provider should be maintained as the comfort of the lens does not preclude problems. Finally if the eye becomes irritated or red or the vision worsens, the lens should be removed immediately and the eye care provider contacted if the symptoms do not subside.

OCULAR MEDICATIONS

A variety of ocular medications are available both over-the-counter and with a prescription at any pharmacy. Most over-the-counter preparations are restricted to artificial tears and related products. In general I prefer artificial tears without medications designed to "get the red out." The tetrahydrozoline found in these preparations can result in "rebound" redness after the drops wear off. Artificial tear preparations can be broadly divided into those with and without preservatives. Although preservative-free drops are necessitated by sensitivities for some patients, they are significantly more expensive. Artificial tears ointments are useful at bedtime for dry eye patients. As they blur the vision, their usefulness during the day is limited.

SUMMARY

An estimated 47,000 persons become legally blind each year. Although many of these cases are not preventable, certainly some are, simply by earlier detection of disease and common sense to prevent injuries. Since an eye disor-

---

Occupations and household activities requiring protective eye wear

Machine operators
   Grinders
   Metal workers
Welders
Use of a hammer
   Carpenters
   Metal workers
   Construction workers
Use of almost any power tool
   Home shop
   Grinders
Automotive repair
Gardening
   Lawn mowing
   Lawn trimming
   Shrub/tree trimming

---

der develops in 6.4 million people in the United States each year, routine eye care is needed to treat these conditions. Most of these (50%) are conditions with significant symptoms such as infections and inflammatory disease; however, many (33%) are chronic disorders that appear with little warning such as cataracts, glaucoma, and retinopathy.[30] Visual loss secondary to glaucoma is irreversible and therefore to prevent it, early diagnosis is mandatory. Although, diabetic retinopathy is treatable in its advanced stages, prevention of visual loss is easier and more successful. Therefore, routine eye examinations are critical to prevent some blinding ocular diseases. More frequent examinations are necessary for those at increased risk such as diabetics or patients with a strong family history for glaucoma. Glaucoma screens and preschool vision testing are a step in this direction and must be supported. Unfortunately 20% of the 6.4 million eye disorders occurring annually are the result of trauma. Although assault is difficult to prevent, a great number of these injuries are work- or sport-related. Many are preventable with protective eye wear. Despite this knowledge it is not uncommon to hear many excuses for not wearing eye protection. Employers and directors of sports complexes must mandate the use of protective eye wear. In addition public awareness of the risk of visual loss associated with common household chores must be heightened. For example, as nylon line lawn trimmers became available, so did injuries associated with this new gardening equipment.[20] In short protective eye wear needs to be a common item in every household and must be worn when performing any activity that could result in injury by an uncontrolled projectile (see box above). Prevention of cataracts and age-related macular degeneration by the use of sunglasses and antioxidant supplements is still not clear. It seems reasonable at this time to encourage the use of sunglasses that filter light below 510 nm. The use of a multivitamin especially for a patient not eating a well-balanced diet should not be discouraged. However, pending the results of additional studies additional nutritional supplementation does not seem warranted.

REFERENCES

1. The American Academy of Ophthalmology, *At first sight: Diabetic retinopathy,* 1990.
2. The American Academy of Ophthalmology, *At first sight: Drugs that are toxic to the eyes,* 1989.
3. The American Academy of Ophthalmology, *Preferred practice pattern: Comprehensive adult eye evaluation,* 1992.
4. The American Academy of Ophthalmology, At First Sight: *Children's vision screening,* 1988.
5. The American Foundation for the Blind, Department of Social Research, January 1992.
6. Bochow TW et al: Ultraviolet light exposure and risk of posterior subcapsular cataracts, *Arch Ophthalmol* 107:369-372, 1989.
7. Burke MJ et al: Soccerball-induced eye injuries, *JAMA* 249:2682-2685, 1983.
8. Congdon N, Wang F, Tielsch JM: Issues in the epidemiology and population-based screening of primary angle-closure glaucoma, *Surv Ophthalmol* 36(6):411-423, 1992.
9. The Diabetic Retinopathy Study Research Group: Photocoagulation treatment of proliferative diabetic retinopathy: the second report of Diabetic Retinopathy Study findings, *Ophthalmology* 85:82-106, 1978.
10. Dolezal JM, Perkins ES, Wallace RB: Sunlight, skin sensitivity, and senile cataract, *Am J Epidemol* 129(3):559-568, 1989.
11. Early Photocoagulation for diabetic retinopathy: ETDRS Report Number 9, *Ophthalmology* 98:766-785, 1991.
12. The Early Treatment of Diabetic Retinopathy Study: Photocoagulation for diabetic macular edema, *Arch Ophthalmol* 103:1796-1805, 1985.
13. Effects of aspirin treatment on diabetic retinopathy: ETDRS Report Number 8, *Ophthalmology* 98:757-765, 1991.
14. Feigelman MJ et al: Assessment of ocular protection for racquetball, *JAMA* 250:3305-3309, 1983.
15. The Italian-American Cataract Study Group: Risk factors for age-related cortical, nuclear, and posterior subcapsular cataracts, *Am J Epidemiol* 133(6):541-53, 1991.
16. Jacques PF et al: Antioxidant status in persons with and without senile cataract, *Arch Ophthalmol* 106:337-340, 1988.
17. Kahn H, Moorhead HB: *Statistics on blindness in the model reporting area, 1969-1970.* Washington, DC: Department of Health, Education, and Welfare, 1973.
18. Karlson TA, Klein BEK: The incidence of acute hospital-treated eye injuries, *Arch Ophthalmol* 104:1473-1476, 1986.
19. Leibowitz HM: The Framingham Eye Study Monograph, *Surv Ophthalmol* Suppl 24:335-610, 1980.
20. Lubniewski A, Olk RJ, Grand MG: Ocular dangers in the garden: a new menace—nylon line lawn trimmers, *Ophthalmology* 95:906-910, 1988.
21. Larrison WI et al: Sports-related ocular trauma, *Ophthalmology* 97:1265-1269, 1990.
22. Leske MC, Chylack LT, Wu SY: The lens opacities case-control study: risk factors for cataract, *Arch Ophthalmol* 109:244-251, 1991.
23. Liggett PE et al: Ocular trauma in an urban population: review of 1132 cases, *Ophthalmology* 97:581-584, 1990.
24. National Eye Institute, National Eye Health Education Program: *Facts about diabetic eye disease,* 1991.
25. National Eye Institute, National Eye Health Education Program: *Facts about open-angle glaucoma,* 1991.

26. Newsome DA et al: Oral zinc in macular degeneration, *Arch Ophthalmol* 106:192-198, 1988.

27. Poggio EC et al: The incidence of ulcerative keratitis among users of daily-wear and extended-wear soft contact lenses, *N Engl J Med* 321:779-783, 1989.

28. Schein OD et al: The spectrum and burden of ocular injury, *Ophthalmology* 95:300-305, 1988.

29. Schein OD et al: The relative risk of ulcerative keratitis among users of daily-wear and extended-wear soft contact lenses, *N Engl J Med* 321:773-778, 1989.

30. Springer M: In focus: sight-saving month calls attention to eye care, *Arch Ophthalmol* 106:593, 1988.

31. Sternberg P et al: Ocular BB injuries, *Ophthalmology* 91:1269-1277, 1984.

32. Taylor HR et al: Effect of ultraviolet radiation on cataract formation, *N Engl J Med* 319:1429-1433, 1988.

33. Taylor HR et al: Visible light and risk of age-related macular degeneration, *Trans Am Ophthalmol Soc* 138:163-178, 1990.

34. Tielsch JM et al: Blindness and visual impairment in an American urban population, *Arch Ophthalmol* 108:286-290, 1990.

35. Varr WF III, Cook RA: Shotgun eye injuries: ocular risk and eye protection efficacy, *Ophthalmology* 99:867-872, 1992.

36. West SK et al: Exposure to sunlight and other risk factors for age-related macular degeneration, *Arch Ophthalmol* 107:875-879, 1989.

RESOURCES

American Academy of Ophthalmology, P.O. Box 7424, San Francisco, CA 94120-7424.

American Foundation for the Blind, 15 West 16th Street, New York, NY 10011.

National Eye Health Education Program, National Eye Institute, Box 20/20, Bethesda, MD 20892.

National Society to Prevent Blindness, 500 East Remington Road, Schaumburg, IL 60173.

Chapter 60

DIABETES AND OTHER
ENDOCRINE DISORDERS

John P. Campbell

This chapter is devoted to selected endocrine disorders and possible interventions to prevent these diseases or their associated complications. Prevention of these disorders can be facilitated by

- Delineation of the pathophysiologic processes of the disorder
- Identification and screening of high-risk populations
- Availability of specific laboratory markers associated with susceptibility, presence, and progression of these disease states
- Research and development of treatments with high benefit to risk ratios
- Astute physicians and allied health workers
- Education of affected individuals and the general population about warning signs of the diseases or their complications

This chapter focuses on aspects of diabetes mellitus and thyroid and adrenal gland disorders.

DIABETES MELLITUS

Diabetes mellitus is a disturbance in the metabolism of carbohydrates, lipids, and protein that can affect the circulation and all organ systems in the body. Table 60-1 lists the various types of diabetes mellitus and glucose intolerance. Further discussion of additional characteristics of the various types of diabetes mellitus and glucose intolerance follows.

Since diabetes mellitus is a heterogenous disease, the incidence and prevalence rates can vary with types of diabetes mellitus, geographical areas, age groups, ethnic groups, environmental factors, and methods of data collection (medical records versus patient surveys). Despite these limitations the federal government estimates that 6%

of the US population, or 14 million Americans, have diabetes mellitus. Only 7 million of these Americans have been diagnosed with diabetes; the other 7 million are not aware of having the disease. Most of the undiagnosed diabetics have non-insulin-dependent diabetis mellitus (NIDDM), which has a slow, insidious course and may be present up to several years before diagnosis. Only 10% of the entire diabetic population have insulin-dependent diabetes mellitus (IDDM). Diabetes mellitus is a leading cause of death in the United States and kills more than 150,000 each year. It is the leading cause of blindness and accounts for up to 12,000 new cases each year. In 1987 approximately 56,000 foot or leg amputations were performed on diabetics in the United States. Approximately 10% of all diabetics develop significant renal disease. Diabetics account for 25% of all new renal dialysis patients each year. Diabetics are two to four times more likely to die of coronary artery disease and two to six times more likely to have strokes than the nondiabetic population. Diabetes also increases the risks of unsuccessful pregnancies, complicated deliveries, and birth defects. Direct and indirect costs of diabetes have been estimated at more than $20.4 billion annually and account for almost 5% of the total US health care costs.[2] As the population ages, number of diabetics, use of medical resources, and medical expenses will increase unless effective strategies are identified to prevent diabetes and its complications.

Type I diabetes mellitus

Type I diabetes mellitus or insulin-dependent diabetes mellitus (IDDM) has a prevalence of 1/600 and incidence of 15/100,000 per year in the United States.[21] The peak age of onset of IDDM is age 11 to 13 years, which usually coincides with puberty. The next peak age of onset occurs

Table 60-1. Types of diabetes mellitus and other categories of glucose intolerance

Clinical classes	Distinguishing characteristics
Diabetes mellitus (DM)	
Type I Insulin-dependent diabetes mellitus (IDDM)	Patients may be of any age, are usually thin, and usually have abrupt onset of signs and symptoms with insulinopenia before age 40. These patients often have strongly positive urine glucose and ketone test results and are dependent upon insulin to prevent ketoacidosis and to sustain life.
Type II Non-insulin-dependent diabetes mellitus (NIDDM) (obese or nonobese)	Patients usually are older than 40 years at diagnosis, obese, and have relatively few classic symptoms. They are not prone to ketoacidosis except during periods of stress. Although not dependent upon exogenous insulin for survival, they may require it for stress-induced hyperglycemia and hyperglycemia that persists in spite of other therapy.
Secondary or other types of diabetes mellitus	Patients with secondary diabetes mellitus associated with infiltrative, surgical, or radiation damage to the pancreas; endocrinopathies such as Cushing's syndrome and acromegaly; and medications such as high-dose steroids, thiazides, and nicotinic acid.
Impaired glucose tolerance (IGT) (obese or nonobese)	Patients with impaired glucose tolerance have plasma glucose levels that are higher than normal but not diagnostic for diabetes mellitus.
Other types of impaired glucose tolerance	Patients with other types of impaired glucose tolerance associated with emotional stress or factors capable of eventually producing secondary diabetes mellitus.
Gestational diabetes mellitus (GDM)	Patients with gestational diabetes mellitus have onset or discovery of glucose intolerance *during* pregnancy.
Statistical risk classes*	
Previous abnormality of glucose tolerance (PrevAGT)	Persons in this category have normal glucose tolerance and a history of transient diabetes mellitus or impaired glucose tolerance.
Potential abnormality of glucose tolerance (PotAGT)	Persons in this category have never experienced abnormal glucose tolerance but have a greater than normal risk of developing diabetes mellitus or impaired glucose tolerance.

Adapted from American Diabetes Association: *The physician's guide to Type II diabetes mellitus (NIDDM): diagnosis and treatment,* New York, 1984, American Diabetes Association.
*Used for epidemiologic and research purposes.

at age 6 to 8 years around the start of grade school.[51] Although the incidence rate of IDDM markedly falls off by the third decade, IDDM can occur at any age. It is more common in nonobese white populations or populations with a substantial white genetic mixture such as American blacks. IDDM is most common in Nordic populations, particularly in Finland and Sweden, with rates of 28.6 and 22.7/100,000.[52] It is rare in Japanese, Chinese, American Indians, and African blacks.[69]

Type I diabetes mellitus can be diagnosed with two fasting plasma glucose levels of 140 mg % or more *or* a random plasma glucose level of 200 mg % or greater with an elevated hemoglobin A1c level or overt hyperglycemic symptoms.

Type I diabetics develop progressive insulinopenia, which usually results in rapid onset of hyperglycemic symptoms particularly polydipsia, polyuria, polyphagia, and weight loss over several weeks with fasting and random blood sugar levels well above 250 mg %, low to zero insulin levels, and ketoacidosis. With the exception of a transient honeymoon period type I diabetics have the permanent need of lifelong insulin replacement. The omission of daily insulin therapy can result in ketotic acidosis, coma, and death. The honeymoon or temporary remission period usually occurs within 4 months of the initial diagnosis of IDDM. This honeymoon period is the result of

partial recovery of islet cell function and associated with a decreased or absent requirement of daily exogenous insulin. Within 2 years all of these individuals lose all islet cell function and develop total diabetes mellitus requiring exogenous insulin at approximately 1 U/kg/day.[25]

IDDM appears to develop in a genetically predisposed individual exposed to some environmental stimuli such as a virus or chemical agent. These agents appear to produce an autoimmune response with infiltration of killer lymphocytes and macrophages in the islets of the pancreas resulting in destruction of β-cells and loss of insulin production necessary to maintain life.

The mode of inheritance of IDDM is unknown. Monozygotic twin studies have demonstrated a concordance rate of less than 50% for IDDM whereas it approaches 100% in NIDDM.[6] Studies have shown that familial transmission of IDDM is uncommon. Table 60-2 estimates the risk of development of IDDM in first-degree relatives of type I diabetics.

Siblings appear to have almost a twofold increased risk of IDDM if the onset of IDDM in the proband occurs before age 10 years rather than after age 10 years.[15] In approximately 1.9% of offspring of type I diabetics IDDM develops.[71] Offspring of type I diabetic fathers are at higher risk for IDDM than offspring of type I diabetic mothers.[72]

Predisposition to IDDM appears to be polygenic. Several different and possibly linked genes may increase susceptibility to IDDM. The major histocompatibility complex (MHC) is on the short arm of the sixth chromosome and produces gene products including human leukocyte antigen (HLA) found in the plasma membranes of cells. HLA-DR3 and/or DR4 is present in more than 90% of white type I diabetics and 80% of black type I diabetics. Approximately 55% to 60% of white type I diabetics have both HLA-DR3 and DR4.[20] However, HLA susceptibility to IDDM appears to vary in different ethnic groups. Approximately 30% to 35% of the nondiabetic population are positive for HLA-DR3 or DR4.[20] Therefore, widespread HLA typing for screening of IDDM is not a consideration.

Although HLA alleles do not cause IDDM, they may be linked to genes directing specific immune responses at islet β-cells. Lymphocytes from type I diabetic children can destroy more insulinoma cells in culture than nondiabetic lymphocytes. Newly diagnosed type I diabetics have increased numbers of killer T lymphocytes and increased antibody dependent cytotoxicity than controls.[55] Interleukin I (IL1) and tumor necrotic factor (TNF) have been shown to have destructive effects on islet β-cells.[69] Since the destructive effects of IL1 on β-cells may be mediated by oxygen derived free radicals, antioxidants such as vitamin E and vitamin C could theoretically have some protective role against islet β-cell damage in IDDM.

Islet cell cytoplasm antibodies (ICA-cyt) are found in 60% to 90% of newly diagnosed type I diabetics compared to 0.5% of nondiabetic controls. Islet cell antibodies disappear in 85% to 90% of type I diabetics within 2 years of onset.[40] The 10% to 15% of type I diabetics who continue to have positive islet cell antibodies for more than 3 years after onset of IDDM are characterized by being predominantly female and having increased frequency of HLA-DR3/B-8 and antibodies to the thyroid and parietal cells. The immediate relatives of these type I diabetics with chronically positive ICA have an increased risk of development of any type of autoimmune disease.[41] Unfortunately assays for surface and cytoplasmic islet-cell antibodies are relatively crude and poorly standardized. Furthermore cytoplasmic islet cell antibodies now appear to represent a mixture of different antibodies to distinct antigens. Not all of these subtypes of antibodies confer increased risk of IDDM. Unfortunately isolated insulin autoantibodies have less predictability of future IDDM than ICA-cyt. One of the newest and most promising markers for IDDM is an antibody to an immunoprecipitate islet cell protein with molecular mass of 64,000 (64K) identified as glutamic acid decarboxylase. This 64K enzyme is found in other tissues and can promote the synthesis of the inhibitory neurotransmitter γ-aminobutyric acid (GABA).[5] The antibody to 64K is most predictive of IDDM in individuals less than age 34 years and is often found before the development of islet cell antibodies or insulin autoantibodies. In

Table 60-2. Risk for diabetes in those with affected relatives

Proband(s) with type I diabetes	Diabetes risk
Identical twin	30%-50%
Mother and father	30%
Parent and sibling	20%
Father	6%
Sibling	5%
Mother	3%

From Eisenbarth GS, Pietropaolo M: Prediction and prevention of type I diabetes mellitus, *Contemp Intern Med* 4(3):27, 1992.

one study, antibodies to 64K were present in 82% of 28 individuals, 2 to 75 months before the eventual clinical onset of IDDM.[4] Unfortunately, the assay for antibodies to 64K is not routinely available. Currently the battery of studies most predictive of future IDDM includes individuals with positive islet cell antibodies, positive insulin autoantibodies, and loss of first-phase insulin secretion after the administration of intravenous (IV) glucose. The cost yield and use of medical resources limit the practicality of these methods for general screening. They are used for research and evaluation of potential renal transplant donors at some medical centers.

IDDM has been arrested with the institution of cyclosporin therapy within 6 weeks of the onset of diabetic symptoms, which is before the irreversible destruction of islet β-cells. During cyclosporin therapy in new onset IDDM there appear to be preservation and enhancement of β-cell function for up to 3 years. One study demonstrated remission of insulin requirement in 24% of a cyclosporin treated group compared to 9% in a placebo group at 12 months. The results were statistically significant and made it unlikely that the "honeymoon phenomenon" could account for the lost requirement of exogenous insulin between the two groups. Unfortunately the calculated creatinine clearance fell by 20% in the cyclosporin treated group.[12] Since the non-insulin-requiring state in these type I diabetics depends on chronic cyclosporin therapy, the risks of cyclosporin-related nephropathy, infections, and possible lymphomas in these young individuals are major drawbacks. In addition almost all patients achieving metabolic remission require insulin within 3 years despite continuation of cyclosporin A.[27] Trials with azathioprine, prednisone, and plasmapheresis have been unable to produce remissions of IDDM.

Early detection of developing IDDM might be facilitated by screening high-risk siblings or children of type I diabetics for antibodies to 64K along with periodic fasting blood sugar tests. These children or young adults with a fasting glucose above 108 mg % are at high risk of development of overt IDDM within the next 12 to 24 months.[9] Intervention therapies to induce remission of IDDM might include (1) use of antioxidants to prevent free radical induced islet cell damage; (2) development of vaccines to interfere with antigen presentation to or recognization by macrophages and lymphocytes, or activation of killer T cells by IL2 or interferon; and (3) refinement of immunosuppressive drugs to provide increased potency with fewer side effects. Development of an internal glucose monitor to function with an insulin pump and/or perfection of pancreatic and islet cell transplant techniques may help limit the progression or severity of complications often associated with IDDM.

Type II diabetes mellitus

Type II diabetes mellitus has also been labeled non-insulin-dependent diabetes mellitus (NIDDM). Type II diabetics are not ketosis prone and do not require diet, insulin, or oral hypoglycemic agent therapy to live but to maintain a sense of well-being and metabolic balance. Approximately 90% of all individuals with diabetes mellitus have NIDDM. Eighty percent of type II diabetics are obese. NIDDM is usually diagnosed after 40 years of age. It is 10 times more prevalent in developing or developed countries. This parallels the observation of increasing incidence of NIDDM in populations with marked and rapid changes in diet and life-style.[8] NIDDM is often characterized by many months or years of asymptomatic hyperglycemia, i.e., fasting blood sugar (FBS) concentration greater than 140 mg/dl. The diagnosis of NIDDM can be made if two fasting plasma glucose levels are 140 mg/dl or greater *or* if a random plasma glucose concentration greater than 200 mg/dl is associated with an elevated hemoglobin A_{1c} level. In type II diabetics, eventually symptomatic hyperglycemia with some or all of the following signs or symptom develops: generalized fatigue, polydipsia, polyuria, polyphagia, weight loss, blurring of vision, frequent correction of visual refraction errors, leg cramps, paresthesias in the face and extremities, sexual dysfunction, chronic periodontal problems, refractory tinea pedis, recurrent carbuncles, chronic vaginal infections, peripheral vascular disease, and cardiovascular or cerebrovascular insults. Their hyperglycemia is usually associated with fasting and random blood sugar concentrations over 200 mg/dl, normal to elevated serum C-peptide levels, and elevated Hgb A_{1c} levels without ketotic acidosis. Concomitant hypertriglyceridemia, hypercholesterolemia, hypertension, or hyperuricemia often is present. In this setting of chronic hyperglycemia associated with borderline dehydration, calcium oxalate or uric acid renal stones are not uncommon.

Reaven labeled the constellation of impaired insulin stimulated glucose uptake, impaired glucose tolerance, hyperinsulinemia, hypertriglyceridemia, low high-density lipoprotein (HDL) cholesterol, and hypertension as Syndrome X.[56] He attributed all of these findings to insulin resistance. His studies revealed resistance to insulin stimulated glucose uptake in not only individuals with impaired glucose tolerance or NIDDM but 25% of the control population without any evidence of diabetes mellitus or impaired carbohydrate metabolism. This theory postulates a causative role of insulin resistance in development of hyperlipidemia and hypertension with or without diabetes mellitus possibly leading to accelerated atherosclerosis with premature vascular complications and death. Since insulin resistance with high endogenous or exogenous insulin levels may be an aggravating factor for diabetic vascular complications, physicians will have to reevaluate the use of high-dose insulin therapy and specific oral antidiabetic agents directed at increasing insulin levels. Oral agents such as metformin, which is used in Canada but not FDA-approved in the United States, work by increasing peripheral use of glucose without raising insulin levels. This group of oral antidiabetic agents help ameliorate insulin resistance and possible acceleration of diabetic vascular complications.

NIDDM differs from IDDM in many other aspects besides average age of onset and body build. Monozygotic twin studies have revealed almost a 100% concordance rate for NIDDM. Unlike IDDM, NIDDM is not associated with an autoimmune cause, specific HLA phenotypes, increased frequency of islet cell antibodies, or other autoimmune diseases such as Addison's disease. There appear to be significant ethnic differences in the susceptibility to NIDDM. A study in the Pacific region between 1975 to 1980 found the prevalence rate of NIDDM to vary from 0.8% in rural Melanesians to 30.3% in Westernized Micronesians.[22] The prevalence of diagnosed and undiagnosed NIDDM in the US population varies among different groups as follows:

Pima Indians	50.0%
Puerto Ricans	13.4%
Mexicans	13.0%
Blacks	10.2%
Cubans	9.3%
Non-Hispanic Whites	6.2%

The highest rates of NIDDM in these groups were associated with increasing age, obesity, and family history of NIDDM but not with sex, physical activity, or education.[37,52]

The exact mode of inheritance is uncertain. Lean as opposed to obese type II diabetics have an increased familial aggregation of NIDDM.[42] Lean type II diabetics also have increased frequency of islet cell antibodies and conversion to IDDM. A study from India estimated the prevalence of NIDDM in offspring of both parents with NIDDM to approach 63% by age 60 years.[70] The prevalence of NIDDM in siblings and offspring of individuals with NIDDM has been as high as 38% by age 80 compared to 11% in control groups.[71] A study of 52 type II diabetic subjects found restriction fragmentation length polymorphism in the insulin gene to be three times greater than in the control group. Nondiabetic individuals with insulin receptor gene polymorphism had hyperinsulinemia and/or a nondiagnostic glucose tolerance test result suggesting a link between insulin resistance and insulin receptor gene polymorphism.[48] Studies have also found defective tyrosine kinase activity in the insulin receptor in skeletal muscle of obese and type II diabetic individuals, which may account for some resistance to insulin stimulated glucose uptake in this tissue.[48]

NIDDM appears to start with resistance of insulin to stimulate glucose uptake in insulin sensitive tissues such as muscle and adipose cells. The pancreas tries to compensate by producing and secreting supranormal amounts of insulin to maintain normal blood sugar levels. Increasing body weight associated with obesity causes a progressive decrease in cellular insulin receptors and compensatory increase in insulin levels. The elevated insulin levels have been implicated in retaining salt and increasing plasma catecholamines, which may lead to or aggravate hypertension. During this process the pancreatic β cells slowly require higher levels of blood sugar to signal the secretion of insulin, resulting in impaired glucose tolerance. At some future time the pancreas may not be able to maintain these compensatory high levels of insulin secretion and burn out. An amyloid protein called amylin associated with a strong inhibitory effect on the action of insulin activity in β-cells has been identified in islet β-cells of individuals with long-standing NIDDM and irreparable β cell damage.[18] As insulin levels progressively fall, there is a gradual increase in serum free fatty acids (FFAs), leading to increased hepatic glucose production and progressive elevation of the fasting blood sugar. The slow, continued elevations of blood sugar level eventually produce overt symptoms of NIDDM. Despite regular exercise and reduction to ideal body weight, individuals with NIDDM convert to IDDM at 1% to 2% per year.[19] The rare maturity onset diabetes mellitus of the young (MODY) or childhood onset NIDDM converts to IDDM at a slower rate of 10% over 17 years. MODY has an autosomal dominant mode of inheritance and is the only form of diabetes mellitus with a clear mechanism of transmission. Individuals with MODY have not demonstrated any HLA patterns or polymorphic sequence in DNA near the insulin gene.[65]

The prevalence of NIDDM and obesity increases with advancing age and body mass. The prevalence of obesity is greater in females than males, white males than black males, and black females than white females. There is a greater incidence of NIDDM in black than white females. This racial difference in the incidence of NIDDM can be eliminated by studying only black and white females at ideal body weight (IBW). A follow-up study demonstrated that the progressive increase in the black to white female ratio for the incidence of NIDDM paralleled the amount of excess body weight in the two groups. These findings suggest that the racial disparity in NIDDM in black and white

females can be eliminated by reducing to and maintaining IBW.[22]

Obesity is identified by body mass index (BMI) greater than 27.8 kg/m² or body fat composition greater than 30% in females, and BMI greater than 27.3 kg/m² and body fat composition greater than 20% in males.[22] One large study observed the degree of weight change in different age groups between the ages of 25 to 74 years in American adults over a decade. The findings revealed that young women overweight at the start of the study had the highest incidence of major weight gain, black females below age 45 years gained more and were more likely to become overweight than white females, and the highest incidence of obesity in individuals not obese at the start of the study was similar in both sexes and greatest between the ages of 35 and 44 years.[73]

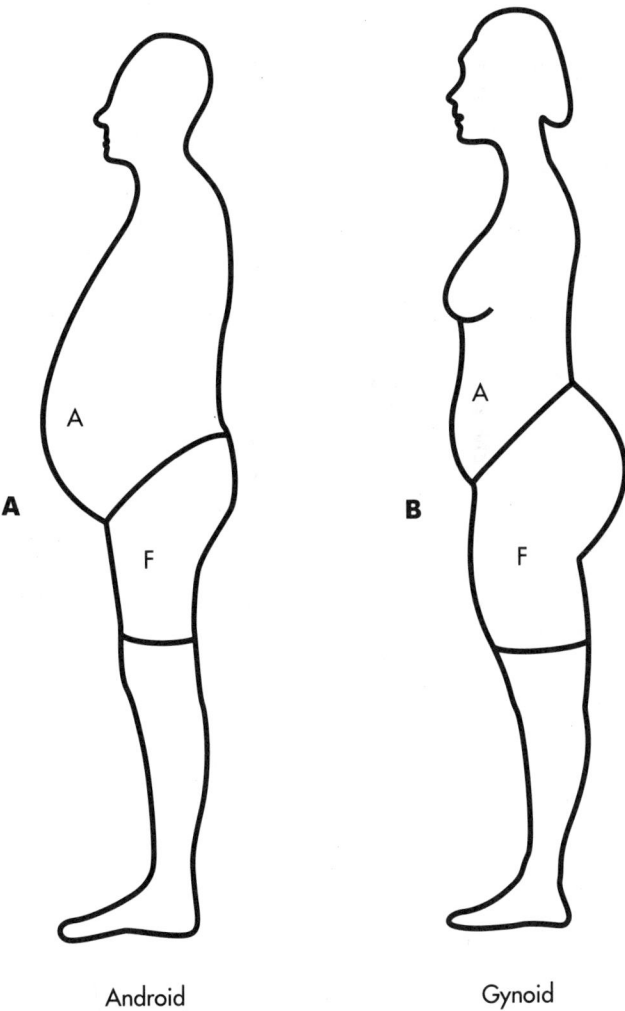

Fig. 60-1. Different types of body fat distribution. **A,** Android, abdominal or upper body pattern of body fat distribution. **B,** Gynoid, femoral or lower body pattern of body fat distribution. (From Davidson J, DiGirolamo M: Non-insulin depended diabetes mellitus. In *Clinical diabetes mellitus,* New York, 1991, Thieme Medical Publishers.)

Two types of body fat distribution are identified by profiles in Fig. 60-1. The android (abdominal) or upper body distribution of body fat is associated with an increased incidence of insulin resistance, NIDDM, hypertension, hypercholesterolemia, and coronary artery disease. This android body habitus can be identified by a simple waist (smallest circumference of the abdomen) to hip (widest circumference of the hips) ratio greater than 1.0 in females and 1.1 in males. The metabolism in adipose tissue located centrally seems to differ from that in adipose tissue located elsewhere by releasing more free fatty acids in proximity to the liver. These increased free fatty acids cause decreased insulin clearance, increased insulin levels, and interference with peripheral glucose use. Abnormal FFA or carbohydrate metabolism does not develop in all obese patients. Factors that are important in preventing obese individuals from developing NIDDM are absence of a genetic disposition, limited duration of obesity, size and location of adipose mass, insulin secretory capacity of the pancreas, diet content, and amount of exercise. For example, individuals with a gynoid (femoral) or lower body fat distribution have a lower incidence of diabetes mellitus and hypertension than those who have android body habitus. In an 8-year study of nondiabetic Mexican Americans in whom NIDDM eetually developed, individuals in whom diabetes developed had higher BMI, central obesity indices, and fasting blood sugar and insulin levels than those in whom NIDDM did not develop. However, a multivariate analysis revealed the lack of significance of BMI and central obesity indices after adding glucose and insulin levels, suggesting that all of the variables might be mediated by insulin resistance.[36] Individuals with acanthosis nigricans, particularly young females with hirsutism and polycystic ovaries, often have decreased cellular insulin receptors associated with insulin resistance and increased frequency of NIDDM.

Many children and adults acquire the habit of skipping breakfast. Since the brain can only use carbohydrates for fuel and requires this fuel 24 hours a day, skipping breakfast places individuals at risk of inadequate carbohydrate fuel, resulting in possible attention or memory deficit, chronic fatigue, headaches, blurring of vision, or lightheadedness. Progression of this fuel deficit or hypoglycemia can reach a critically low level, resulting in the release of the stress hormones epinephrine and norepinephrine from the adrenal gland. Although these stress hormones are helpful in releasing needed fuel or glucose from the liver, they also can speed up the heart, causing increased oxygen demand, and increase the potential for cardiac arrhythmias; elevate blood pressure; and lower the pain threshold. The intake of caffeinated beverages can be additive in producing similar symptoms. After being on emergency glucose fuel from the liver there will be maximal absorption of glucose in the stomach after the next meal, resulting in supranormal blood sugar levels. Since

the body in the absence of diabetes is programmed not to tolerate high blood sugar levels, the pancreas quickly releases insulin and often overshoots the amount of insulin needed to normalize blood sugar level. The resultant high insulin level can induce (1) a hunger sensation shortly after eating a normal sized meal; (2) salt retention, possibly raising the blood pressure; and (3) another lowering of the blood sugar level 3 to 4 hours after the meal, producing recurrent symptoms of hypoglycemia. This roller coaster pattern of insulin and glucose swings can be perpetuated after the supper meal. Although these swings in the insulin and glucose levels have not been shown to produce diabetes mellitus, they may hinder school or work performance, aggravate blood pressure problems, cause inefficient metabolism of calories and thus hinder weight reduction or maintenance of ideal body weight, and produce strain on a disturbed pancreas. Therefore, all individuals should be encouraged to eat three to four small feedings a day consisting of less than 30% of fat (no more than one third of the total consisting of saturated fat), 15% to 20% of protein, and 50% to 55% of carbohydrates as recommended by the American Diabetes Association and the American Heart Association.

Ideal body weight for adults can be estimated by the following formula: medium frame woman: start with 100 pounds for a height of 60 inches and add 5 pounds for each additional 1 inch increment; medium frame man: start with 106 pounds for a height of 60 inches and add 6 pounds for each additional 1 inch increment; for both men and women: the calculated ideal body weight (IBW) can be increased by 10% for a large frame or decreased by 10% for a small frame.[19]

Prevention of NIDDM should start by

- Initiating proper eating habits in preschool and school age children
- Promoting the avoidance of junk foods high in refined sugars and saturated fats
- Encouraging the maintenance of ideal body weight as early as childhood
- Stressing the importance of regular exercise.[38]

Impaired glucose tolerance

The significance of the classification of impaired glucose tolerance (IGT) is unclear. IGT in a nonpregnant adult is identified by a fasting 2 hour glucose tolerance test using an oral 75 g glucose load with a fasting plasma glucose level less than 140 mg/dl, a 2-hour plasma glucose level between 140 and 200 mg/dl and an intervening plasma glucose level of 200 mg/dl or higher at the 30-, 60-, or 90-minute test points. Studies have shown that in anywhere from 2% to 35% of adults with IGT diabetes mellitus have developed during 20-year follow-up observation.[51]

Several conditions should be observed to standardize the test. The patient should be prepared with at least 150 g of dietary carbohydrate/day for 3 days before the test. The 75 g of oral glucose should be totally consumed within 5 minutes, which is difficult for some individuals. The validity of the oral glucose tolerance test (GTT) has been questioned because of the frequent finding of a change from an abnormal to a normal test result during a short time span without any obvious intervention. A false positive GTT result can be related to age; sex; race; amount of recent carbohydrate intake; amount of exercise; recent weight change; certain medications, such as diuretics, antidepressants, anticonvulsives, nicotinic acid, pain pills, or estrogen; chronic disease involving any major organ system; and stress, particularly in a hospitalized patient. With these limitations there is little utility in using oral glucose tolerance tests in nonpregnant adults to screen for IGT or NIDDM. In addition, the lack of cost effectiveness of indiscriminate mass blood sugar screening after a glucose load has been verified in several studies.[39] Discriminate screening of high-risk populations with random blood sugar levels still has a place because of the increased morbidity and mortality associated with chronic complications of NIDDM. Ideally these diabetic complications can be reduced or eliminated by early detection and appropriate treatment. Even innocuous treatment such as diet, weight reduction, and exercise can help blood sugar level control and improve lipid and cardiovascular status. Discriminate diabetic screening should include

- Individuals requesting the test
- Pregnant women
- Individuals above age 40
- Obese individuals
- Individuals with a history of gestational diabetes mellitus or birth of term babies weighing more than 9 pounds
- Individuals with refractory hyperlipidemia
- Individuals with a family history of diabetes mellitus

A good, safe, and cost-efficient diabetes screening program should include close supervision by a physician or trained medical personnel; preliminary screening with a verbal interview or written questionnaire for symptoms, risk factors, and pertinent family history; referral mechanism for symptomatic individuals without a personal physician; written follow-up observation of abnormal results (fasting plasma glucose level greater than 140 mg/dl or random plasma glucose level greater than 160 mg/dl) to the patient and their physician; and proper human immunodeficiency virus (HIV) and viral hepatitis precautions at screening sites.[54,14]

Gestational diabetes mellitus

Approximately 3% of all pregnant women have gestational diabetes mellitus (GDM), which develops during pregnancy and usually resolves at the baby's birth. Unfortunately in up to 40% of these women diabetes mellitus develops over the following 10 to 15 years.[3] Gestational diabetes mellitus most likely represents a transient post-insulin-receptor disturbance. High maternal blood sugar levels cross the placenta without accompanying maternal insulin and stimulate fetal pancreatic insulin production resulting in macrosomia and possibly a difficult and complicated labor and delivery. These babies are also at increased risk for neonatal hypoglycemia, hypocalcemia, and hyperbilirubinemia. Congenital birth defects are not increased in babies of mothers with GDM as they are in babies of poorly controlled type I diabetic mothers. Congenital defects in the fetus can occur with poor diabetic control during a critical period in the first 8 to 12 weeks of pregnancy.[44] Gestational diabetes mellitus does not develop until well into the second trimester of pregnancy. Women with gestational diabetes and term babies weighing more than 9 pounds are at high risk of development of GDM in subsequent pregnancies. In most mothers gestational diabetes mellitus can be controlled with a calorie-controlled diet of 30 to 35 kcal/kg of ideal body weight. However, weight loss and ketonuria secondary to inadequate caloric intake must be avoided to prevent adverse effects on the fetus.

To prevent the possible complications of undiagnosed gestational diabetes, all pregnant women should be screened with a simple glucose loading test between the 24th and 28th weeks of pregnancy. This screening test entails giving a nonfasting pregnant woman a 50-g oral glucose load and drawing a plasma glucose level 1 hour later. If the 1-hour plasma glucose level is greater than 150 mg/dl, the patient should have a fasting 3-hour glucose tolerance test with a 100-g glucose load. Gestational diabetes is diagnosed when two of the following values are met or exceeded: fasting plasma glucose level ≥105 mg/dl, 1-hour plasma glucose level ≥190 mg/dl, 2-hour plasma glucose level ≥165 mg/dl, and 3-hour plasma glucose level ≥145 mg/dl.[51]

An evaluation of the simple glucose screen of pregnant women with a 50-g oral glucose load by Carpenter et al. found a sensitivity of 83% and specificity of 87% when compared to the 3-hour GTT with a 100-g challenge.[13] The screening of all pregnant women with a simple 50-g glucose challenge is advocated because of the potential benefits of decreasing birth complications and identifying women at increased risk for NIDDM in the future.

Diabetic screening

Table 60-3 lists normal plasma glucose values. The box on p. 1118 contains recommendations for diabetic screening. The box on p. 1119 summarizes the criteria for diagnosis of the various types of diabetes mellitus.

Diabetic complications

Both IDDM and NIDDM can be associated with the same types of complications, such as retinopathy, neurop-

Table 60-3. Normal plasma glucose values*

Nonpregnant adults	
Fasting plasma glucose	<115 mg/dl
Plasma glucose values following 75-gram oral glucose dose	30 minutes <200 mg/dl
	60 minutes <200 mg/dl
	90 minutes <200 mg/dl
	120 minutes <140 mg/dl

Children	
Fasting plasma glucose	<130 mg/dl
Plasma glucose value following glucose dose of 1.75 g/kg ideal body weight up to a maximum of 75 grams	120 minutes <140 mg/dl

Modified from American Diabetes Association: *The physician's guide to Type II diabetes mellitus (NIDDM): diagnosis and treatment,* New York, 1984, American Diabetes Association.
*Note: Glucose values above these concentrations but below the criteria for diabetes mellitus or impaired glucose tolerance should be considered nondiagnostic.

Indications and criteria for diabetes screening tests

Indications

Screening tests for diabetes mellitus are indicated when the individual:
- has a strong family history of diabetes mellitus.
- is markedly obese or has abdominal obesity.
- has a morbid obstetric history or a history of babies over 9 pounds at birth.
- is pregnant (between 24 and 28 weeks).
- has hypertension, hyperlipidemia, or hyperuricemia.
- is in a high-risk ethnic adult group, including American Indians, Puerto Ricans, Mexicans, Black females, and Cubans.

Criteria for screening tests

Nonpregnant Adults: A fasting plasma glucose level determination should be used for screening. A fasting plasma glucose level of 115 mg/dl or greater is considered as indication for diagnostic testing (see box on p. 1119).

Children: A fasting plasma glucose determination should be used for screening. A fasting plasma glucose level of 130 mg/dl or greater is considered an indication for diagnostic testing (see box on p. 1119).

Pregnant Women: An oral glucose tolerance test with a 50-g glucose load is recommended for screening. A fasting plasma glucose level above 105 mg/dl or a plasma glucose level of 150 mg/dl or greater 1 hour later is considered an indication for diagnostic testing (see box on p. 1119)

Adapted from American Diabetes Association: *The physician's guide to Type II diabetes mellitus (NIDDM): diagnosis and treatment,* New York, 1984, American Diabetes Association.

---

athy, coronary artery disease, renal disease, impotency, and bladder or bowel dysfunction. Although the exact cause of these complications has not been elucidated, many mechanisms are proposed, such as glucose toxicity,[60] glycation of proteins,[69] polyol pathway,[69] and hemodynamic changes.[69] Tight control of blood sugar levels has been proved to be beneficial in reducing birth defects along with labor and neonatal complications. However, tight blood sugar level control in IDDM and NIDDM has not been definitively shown to prevent, retard, or reverse microvascular or macrovascular diabetic complications. These complications are thought to be associated with the severity and duration of diabetes along with possible genetic predisposition toward certain types of diabetic complications. For example, there is an increased incidence of retinopathy in diabetics with a positive family history of hypertension in a parent. Ideally, the current large multicenter prospective study called the Diabetic Control and Complications Trial will provide better insight into the effect of blood sugar level control on diabetic complications.[23] Interestingly in individuals with secondary diabetes diabetic complications do not seem to develop. This may reflect the fact that their diabetes often is short-lived and resolves with correction of the underlying nondiabetic disease state.

Physicians must make a major effort to prevent iatrogenic problems, particularly in the elderly, caused by overzealous attempts to achieve tight blood sugar level control. Hypoglycemia is not uncommon in patients treated with oral hypoglycemic agents or insulin when associated with irregular or changing eating or exercise patterns, weight loss, or progressive renal, hepatic, pulmonary, gastrointestinal, or cardiac dysfunction.[63] This *hypoglycemia* can result in altered memory or pseudodementia; decreased coordination associated with falls or other accidents at home, at work, or while driving; increased appetite associated with weight gain; precipitation of angina or transient ischemic attacks; and possible depression.

The goal should be to keep diabetic patients functional while minimizing the risk of microvascular or macrovascular complications aggravated by hypertension and/or hyperlipidemia. An initial consultation with the dietitian may help the patient and family adjust to lifelong diet restrictions. Attendance in a formal diabetic education program is encouraged to lay down a good foundation for prevention or early detection of possible diabetic complications. The availability of hemoglobin A_{1c} (Hgb A_{1c}) levels and home glucose monitoring help to provide adequate information regarding blood sugar control in most diabetics. Diabetics should be encouraged to follow a good daily foot

Diagnostic criteria for diabetes mellitus, impaired glucose tolerance, and gestational diabetes.

Nonpregnant adults

Criteria for Diabetes Mellitus: Diagnosis of diabetes mellitus in nonpregnant adults should be restricted to those who have *one* of the following:
- A random plasma glucose level of 200 mg/dl or greater *plus* classic signs and symptoms of diabetes mellitus including polydipsia, polyuria, polyphagia, and weight loss
- A fasting plasma glucose level of 140 mg/dl or greater on at least two occasions
- A fasting plasma glucose level of less than 140 mg/dl *plus* sustained elevated plasma glucose levels during at least two oral glucose tolerance tests. The 2-hour sample and at least one other between 0 and 2 hours after the 75-g glucose dose should be 200 mg/dl or greater. Oral glucose tolerance testing is not necessary if the patient has a fasting plasma glucose level of 140 mg/dl or greater.

Criteria for Impaired Glucose Tolerance: Diagnosis of impaired glucose tolerance in nonpregnant adults should be restricted to those who have *all* of the following:
- A fasting plasma glucose of less than 140 mg/dl
- A 2-hour oral glucose tolerance test plasma glucose level between 140 and 200 mg/dl
- An intervening oral glucose tolerance test plasma glucose value of 200 mg/dl or greater

Pregnant women

Criteria for Gestational Diabetes: Following an oral glucose load of 100 grams, the diagnosis of gestational diabetes may be made if two plasma glucose values equal or exceed the following:

Fasting	**1 Hour**	**2 Hour**	**3 Hour**
105 mg/dl	190 mg/dl	165 mg/dl	145 mg/dl

Children

Criteria for Diabetes Mellitus: Diagnosis of diabetes mellitus in children should be restricted to those who have *one* of the following:
- A random plasma glucose level of 200 mg/dl or greater *plus* classic signs and symptoms of diabetes mellitus, including polyuria, polydipsia, ketonuria, and rapid weight loss
- A fasting plasma glucose level of 140 mg/dl or greater on at least two occasions *and* sustained elevated plasma glucose levels during at least two oral glucose tolerance tests. Both the 2-hour plasma glucose and at least one other between 0 and 2 hours after the glucose dose (1.75 g/kg ideal body weight up to 75 grams) should be 200 mg/dl or greater.

Criteria for Impaired Glucose Tolerance: The diagnosis of impaired glucose tolerance in children should be restricted to those who have *both* of the following:
- A fasting plasma glucose concentration of less than 140 mg/dl
- A 2-hour oral glucose tolerance test plasma glucose level of greater than 140 mg/dl

Adapted from American Diabetes Association. *The physician's guide to Type II diabetes mellitus (NIDDM): diagnosis and treatment*, New York, 1984, American Diabetes Association.

care program (see Chapter 44) and to see an ophthalmologist once a year.[1]

Since diabetes mellitus is often complicated by multisystem disease, asymptomatic diabetics should be monitored by their primary physician at 3- to 6-month intervals. These assessments should include the following:

- Review of pertinent body systems, diet, medications, exercise, smoking status, and results of home glucose monitoring
- Monitoring of body weight and blood pressure in sitting and standing positions
- Physical examination assessment for retinopathy, glaucoma, periodontal disease, cardiovascular dysfunction, bruits or compromise in carotid or peripheral circulation, altered deep tendon reflexes, altered sensation to pinprick and vibration, and skin changes
- Fasting blood sugar level, Hgb A_{1c} level, and urinalysis determinations at 3- to 6-month intervals

- Serum creatinine and potassium levels at 6- to 12-month intervals
- Fasting serum lipid levels at 12-month intervals

All diabetics on insulin or oral hypoglycemic agents should be encouraged to do home glucose monitoring at weekly to monthly intervals as indicated. Symptomatic diabetics should be monitored more frequently as indicated.

Because of the increased frequency of silent and nonsilent cardiovascular disease in both IDDM and NIDDM, a treadmill or cycle exercise stress test should be considered after 20 years of IDDM or 10 years of NIDDM or earlier for cardiac symptoms or unexplained fatigue. The treadmill test also assists the physician in determining arrhythmia potential and tolerance for exercise programs.[30,50] The high cost and high number of false-positive thallium exercise study results limit its use in screening for asymptomatic coronary artery disease in the diabetic population.[43]

Diabetes mellitus will continue to be a major health

problem until research provides further interventional techniques to prevent this complex disease and its complications.

THYROID DISEASES AND MULTIPLE ENDOCRINE NEOPLASIA II AND III SYNDROMES

Prevention of thyroid diseases or their complications depends on recognition of any of the following:

- Enlargement or nodules in the thyroid gland
- Symptoms or signs of excess or deficient thyroid hormone production
- Increased risk factors for thyroid disease such as history of prior external neck irradiation, familial thyroid cancer, and presence of other nonthyroidal autoimmune diseases.

Possible iatrogenic thyroid disease must also be considered in patients on thyroid supplement particularly in the elderly population.

It is estimated that 2% to 3% of the US population have either hyperthyroidism or hypothyroidism. Congenital hypothyroidism occurs in 1 of every 3500 to 4000 newborns each year. Thyroid cancer accounted for at least 11,300 new cases and 1000 deaths in the United States in 1989.[58]

Screening for thyroid dysfunction

Thyroid screening blood tests for hyperthyroidism are indicated in patients reporting or exhibiting any of the following: thyroid enlargement or nodule, heat intolerance, increased sweating, unexplained weight loss, diarrhea, anxiety, insomnia, fatigue, generalized muscle weakness, bilateral hand tremors, new menstrual changes, infertility, palpitations, cardiac arrhythmia, cardiac failure, new or changing angina, hypertension, prominence of one or both eyes, unexplained elevation of serum alkaline phosphatase level, anemia, or decreased duration of medication effect.

Thyroid screening blood tests for hypothyroidism should be considered for individuals reporting or exhibiting any of the following: thyroid enlargement, cold intolerance, unexplained weight gain, severe constipation, depression, hypersomnia, generalized fatigue, muscle cramps, menstrual changes, infertility, galactorrhea, generalized skin dryness, carotenosis, vitiligo, alopecia, dementia, ataxia, progressive hearing loss, carpal tunnel syndrome, hypercholesterolemia, hypertension, bradycardia, persistent hoarseness, unexplained pleural or joint effusions, unexplained hyponatremia, unexplained elevations of serum glutamic-oxaloacetic transaminase (SGOT) and creatine phosphokinase (CPK) levels, anemia, or increased duration of medication effect. Any unexplained change in diabetic control should also trigger thyroid testing.

Since various autoimmune diseases tend to cluster in individuals or their family members, screening tests for autoimmune thyroid disease should be considered in individuals with a personal or family history (first-degree relative) of autoimmune thyroid disease, type I diabetes mellitus, Addison's disease, systemic lupus erythematosus (SLE), pernicious anemia, multiple sclerosis, inflammatory bowel disease, rheumatoid arthritis, myasthenia gravis, or other connective tissue diseases. In addition, any individual with a tender thyroid gland, history of prior radioactive iodine therapy, unexplained anemia, or chronic intake of kelp or medications containing iodides should have a screening test of thyroid function.

The development of a highly specific thyroid stimulating hormone (TSH) assay has simplified the screening evaluation for primary hypothyroidism and hyperthyroidism. Serum pituitary TSH level is elevated most often with a failing thyroid gland or primary hypothyroidism. Elevated serum TSH levels are rarely associated with a pituitary TSH secreting tumor, pituitary resistance to peripheral thyroid hormone, or in euthyroid patients, recovery from subacute thyroiditis or severe caloric deprivation or illness. Minimally elevated serum TSH levels can be seen in asymptomatic elderly men and women.[46] Although a minimally elevated serum TSH level does not guarantee the development of primary hypothyroidism, a study revealed that 5% per year of these individuals with coexistent thyroid antibodies go on to develop primary hypothyroidism.[67] In fact, it is estimated that in up to 1 of 20 elderly individuals primary hypothyroidism eventually develops.[46]

If the screening serum TSH level is elevated, a follow-up free thyroxine index (FTI) and thyroid antimicrosomal antibody level should be drawn. If the FTI is low in this clinical setting, it is indicative of primary hypothyroidism except for the rare exceptions of resolving subacute thyroiditis or severe nonthyroidal illness. Elderly patients with an elevated serum TSH level should have a yearly thyroid evaluation by palpation along with an FTI to detect chemical hypothyroidism.

The most common cause of hypothyroidism is Hashimoto's thyroiditis, which is associated with positive thyroid antibodies in 95% of cases. Hashimoto's thyroiditis is four to five times more frequent in women than men. There is an increased frequency of atrophic Hashimoto's thyroiditis in individuals with HLA-B8 or DR3. Approximately 10% of females and 3% of males in the general population have positive thyroid microsomal antibodies without obvious thyroid disease. However, in 10% to 20% of these individuals chemical or clinical signs of hypothyroidism will develop. Individuals with Hashimoto's thyroiditis have an increased frequency of other autoimmune disease, such as Sjögren's syndrome, SLE, and Addison's disease.[45] Additional difficulty in the evaluation of possible Hashimoto's thyroiditis arises from the presence of false-positive thyroid antibody test results in individuals with nonthyroidal autoimmune diseases.

Other causes of primary hypothyroidism include thyroid dyshormonogenesis, use of high-dose steroids or lithium, chronic intake of iodides in cough medication or amino-darone, high-dose irradiation of the neck for cancer or lymphoma, thyroidectomy, or radioactive iodine treatment.

Primary hypothyroidism requires lifelong thyroid supplement. The goal of the thyroid replacement is to relieve the symptoms of hypothyroidism and to raise the serum TSH level to the normal range. Most hypothyroid patients require the equivalent of 0.075 to 0.15 mg of L-thyroxine each day. It is important to avoid giving hypothyroid patients supranormal doses of thyroid supplement, which can produce subclinical or clinical hyperthyroidism with a significant loss of cortical bone density (osteopenia) particularly in postmenopausal women.[59] In occasional elderly hypothyroid patients with compromised cardiac status, doses of thyroid supplement needed to normalize the serum TSH may not be tolerated because of angina or congestive heart failure.[34] In these patients L-thyroxine should be started at 0.025 mg/day and gradually increased at 2- to 4-week intervals until the serum TSH level is normal or adverse cardiac signs or symptoms appear, limiting any further increase in thyroid dosage. Since the bioavailability of generic forms of L-thyroxine can vary widely, the maintenance dosage may vary with any change in generic companies.[57] Avoiding the use of generic thyroxine products minimizes this problem.[24] If there is a question of the lifelong need for thyroid supplement and the patient has been on thyroid replacement for many years without documented history of a goiter, thyroid surgery, radioactive iodine therapy, or low thyroid test results, baseline serum TSH level and thyroid antimicrosomal antibody screen should be obtained. If the thyroid antibody results are positive, continued thyroid supplement will most likely be beneficial in preventing hypothyroidism. If the serum TSH level is normal, and thyroid antibody test results are negative, the L-thyroxine dosage can be cut by 50% and a serum TSH level determination and clinical examination of thyroid status should be repeated in 6 to 8 weeks. If the repeat examination and TSH level findings are normal, the L-thyroxine can be discontinued and a repeat serum TSH level and clinical examination of thyroid status should be repeated in 3 months. If those results are normal, the patient most likely will never require thyroid replacement again.

Low serum TSH levels in the absence of pituitary or hypothalamic disease are highly suggestive of hyperthyroidism. The serum TSH level may also be suppressed during the first trimester of pregnancy, psychiatric illness, critical life-threatening illnesses, or treatment with dopamine, phenytoin (Dilantin), or high-dose steroids.[64,26]

Hyperthyroidism

If the suppressed serum TSH level is subsequently associated with an elevated serum T_3 level by radioimmunoassay (RIA), elevated serum T_4 level by RIA, or elevated FTI, hyperthyroidism is confirmed. Autoimmune hyperthyroidism or Graves' disease is the most common type of hyperthyroidism. It is 10 times more common in women than men. There is a 50% concordance rate of Graves' disease in monozygotic twins and 30% concordance rate in dizygotic twins.[49] There is increased risk of Graves' disease with HLA-B8 and DR3 in whites, HLA-B 35 in Japanese, and HLA-Bw 45 in Chinese.[45]

Three possible treatments for hyperthyroidism of Graves' disease are radioactive iodine therapy, antithyroid medication, or near-total thyroidectomy. Regardless of the type of therapy used for Graves' disease, in a high percentage of patients, especially those with positive thyroid antimicrosomal antibody findings, primary hypothyroidism associated with coexisting Hashimoto's thyroiditis develops, necessitating lifelong thyroid supplementation. The presence of thyroid antimicrosomal antibodies and/or thyroid stimulating immunoglobulins (TSIs) in pregnant patients with a history of Graves' disease is associated with increased risk of fetal or neonatal thyrotoxicosis.[7]

Less than 5% of Graves' disease patients develop significant exophthalmopathy that involves the extraocular muscles and sometimes damage to the cornea or optic nerve.[49] Patients with hyperthyroidism should have baseline Hertel exophthalmometry and periodic follow-up examinations by an ophthalmologist.

Subacute thyroiditis

Painful or painless subacute thyroiditis can cause transient clinical and laboratory findings of either hyperthyroidism or hypothyroidism. This illness is most often caused by a viral attack on the thyroid, producing inflammation of the thyroid and unregulated release of thyroid hormones into the blood, inducing a transient picture of hyperthyroidism that can last up to 3 months. After release and use of all stored thyroid hormone transient primary hypothyroidism develops. It may last up to 3 months before the patient spontaneously returns to an euthyroid state. During the viral damage to the thyroid gland, cellular debris is released and can initiate the transient production of thyroid antibodies simulating Hashimoto's thyroiditis during the hypothyroid phase.

Subacute thyroiditis is a self-limiting illness. Aspirin may be helpful for thyroid pain and β-blockers may alleviate other bothersome symptoms in the hyperthyroid phase. No treatment is needed for the hypothyroid phase. The proper diagnosis of this entity can be aided by obtaining a history of an antecedent viral infection such as a pharyngitis 2 to 4 weeks before the onset of thyroid tenderness or enlargement and abnormal thyroid laboratory findings. An important chemical finding during the hyperthyroid phase is a zero to low normal (<8%) 24-hour radioactive iodine thyroid uptake, which is completely opposite to the supranormal 24-hour thyroid uptake (>50%) associated with hyperthyroidism of Graves' disease in the absence of concomitant intake of iodine in medications or radiographic dyes. The only other clinical entities associated with laboratory findings of hyperthyroidism and a zero to low 24-hour thyroid uptake are factitious hyperthyroidism associated with excess intake of thyroid supplement and thyrotoxicosis associated with stroma ovarii. It is important to recognize these entities to prevent possible adverse side effects of use of unnecessary antithyroid medications or lifelong thyroid supplement.

Thyroid nodules and thyroid cancer

Thyroid nodules are common, whereas thyroid cancer is uncommon. Approximately 4% of the population has thyroid nodules.[66] Solitary thyroid nodules are found twice as often in females as males. Thyroid nodules can be found in up to 90% of females above age 70 years and 60% of males above age 80 years.[46] Autopsy studies have found nodules in up to 50% of thyroid glands. Although histologic findings of cancer in these nodules are not uncommon, clinically significant thyroid cancers are uncommon. The incidence of thyroid cancer indicated by mortality studies is low, at 0.4 to 0.8/100,000.[11]

After detection of a thyroid nodule or nodules through physical examination the clinical challenge of determining the risk of an underlying thyroid malignancy and the appropriate follow-up plan arises. If a suppressed TSH level is associated with an elevated serum T_3 level by RIA and an I^{123} thyroid scan displaying a hot thyroid nodule, the findings are indicative of a toxic nodule associated with hyperthyroidism and almost zero incidence of thyroid cancer in the hot nodule. Treatment of this toxic nodule consists of surgical excision or moderate dose of radioactive iodine, which usually results in a permanent cure without the subsequent need for lifelong thyroid supplement.

If the thyroid nodule or nodules are associated with an elevated serum TSH level and/or positive thyroid antimicrosomal antibody findings along with a follow-up low FTI associated with hypothyroidism or normal FTI associated with a failing thyroid gland, the individual will require lifelong thyroid supplement. Treatment with adequate doses of thyroid supplement often induces partial or complete shrinkage of thyroid nodules associated with elevated serum TSH level or positive thyroid antibody findings. Autonomous or adenomatous thyroid nodules do not suppress or benefit from lifelong thyroid supplement.

The risk of thyroid cancer is extremely low in the cases of thyroid nodules associated with a suppressed serum TSH level described. It is important to remember that circulating TSH can stimulate growth of both sensitive benign and malignant thyroid tissue. A difficult diagnostic challenge is the evaluation of a nodular thyroid with a normal serum TSH level and negative thyroid antibody result. An immediate aggressive clinical evaluation should begin with determination of the presence of any of the following: progressive enlargement of the nodule; hard, rocklike consistency of the nodule; persistent cervical adenopathy; persistent hoarseness, or dysphagia; inhabitation of an iodine deficit region; Cowden's syndrome or familial polyposis; remote history of irradiation of the face and neck areas; and positive family history of thyroid cancer, pheochromocytoma, or unexplained premature sudden death syndrome (<age 50). A thyroid needle aspiration biopsy with multiple and adequate sampling of the suspicious nodule or nodules performed by an experienced thyroidologist and pathologist with special training in thyroid disease is the most productive and cost-efficient method to rule out a cancerous thyroid nodule. A biopsy result showing malignancy requires consideration of surgery, except for most large lymphomas or anaplastic cancers of the thyroid where other treatment modalities are indicated. Because of sampling variability, a negative biopsy result does not exclude cancer, and lifelong monitoring for any new changes in the nodule or neck is required at 6- to 12-month intervals. If the thyroid nodule biopsy result is indeterminate for malignancy or the nodule continues to enlarge or develop other suspicious features mentioned, a repeat thyroid needle aspiration biopsy or definitive surgical excision of the thyroid nodule should be considered. Large studies have revealed a 1% false-positive rate and 4% false-negative rate for aspiration needle biopsies for thyroid malignancies.[31,47]

There are significant limitations to the use of either thyroid scans or ultrasound studies for evaluation of thyroid malignancies. Although ultrasound studies revealing thyroid cysts less than 4 cm are rarely malignant, any sized thyroid cyst may be the result of a degenerative thyroid cancer. Although a solitary hot nodule on a thyroid scan has a low risk of malignancy, it does not exclude it. Since up to 20% of cold solitary thyroid nodules on scan can be malignant, they will require further evaluation with a needle aspiration biopsy or surgical excision. Only up to 1% of cold areas on scan in a multinodular goiter are malignant.[16] Some thyroid cancers can trap Tc^{99} pertechnetate and may not demonstrate a cold nodule that would be apparent on an I^{123} or I^{131} thyroid scan.[62] If a physician prefers to use a scan for evaluation of a thyroid malignancy, it should only be done with I^{123} or I^{131}. The intake of oral or intravenous iodine by an euthyroid patient within 3 months can interfere with obtaining an acceptable thyroid scan image.

For at least three decades starting in the 1920s physicians often used low-dose external irradiation to treat facial acne, ringworm, and enlargement of tonsils, adenoids, or thymus gland. In approximately 40% of individuals with a history of external neck irradiation, a nodular goiter may develop and in 5% thyroid cancer develops.[33] Low-dose neck irradiation of 6.5 to 2000 rad may change the growth pattern of thyroid cells and induce an atypical or malignant cell line.[33] The incidence of thyroid nodules and cancer increases linearly as radiation exposure increases to

2000 rad. With 6000 rad or more to the thyroid gland, thyroid cells are often destroyed and primary hypothyroidism develops. A patient with a thyroid nodule and history of remote neck irradiation has a 40% risk of development of thyroid cancer. These cancers are often multicentric. Approximately 60% are found in the index thyroid nodule and 40% are found elsewhere in the thyroid gland.[16] For this reason patients with a thyroid nodule and history of external neck irradiation may be best served with an open thyroid biopsy and exploration of both thyroid lobes rather than random needle aspiration biopsies of the thyroid nodule. Since nonhomogeneous, cold areas can be seen on thyroid scanning of the general population with no obvious thyroid disease, routine scanning of individuals without palpable enlargement of the thyroid or nodules is not recommended. These high-risk individuals should be followed at yearly intervals with palpation of the neck area. Some studies in humans have suggested that suppression of serum TSH levels with chronic thyroid supplement may decrease the development of thyroid nodules or cancers in these high-risk individuals.[28]

There is an increased risk of lymphoma of the thyroid in individuals with Hashimoto's thyroiditis.[17] It is sometimes difficult to differentiate lymphoma from Hashimoto's thyroiditis on small samples obtained during needle aspiration biopsies. A tru-cut or open thyroid biopsy may be more helpful if the needle aspiration biopsy is not diagnostic. Early detection of a lymphoma of the thyroid may help limit the treatment to localized neck irradiation and thyroid supplement.

Multiple endocrine neoplasia II and III

Although medullary thyroid carcinoma only makes up 7% of all thyroid cancers, it is an extremely interesting cancer, which can occur sporadically or be inherited as an autosomal dominant trait associated with multiple endocrine neoplasia (MEN) II or III. The MEN II syndrome consists of medullary thyroid carcinoma, pheochromocytoma, and hyperparathyroidism. On the other hand, the MEN III syndrome includes medullary thyroid carcinoma and pheochromocytoma along with neurofibroma and neuromata of the tongue, lips, and eyelids. MEN III is not associated with hyperparathyroidism.

Medullary thyroid carcinoma has almost equal occurrence in males and females. The familial form usually occurs before age 35 years; the sporadic form usually occurs after age 50 years. There is a 50% chance that any child of a proband will inherit medullary thyroid cancer. Other individuals at high risk for this type of thyroid cancer are first-degree relatives, particularly those who have neurofibromas or café au lait spots; individuals with a pheochromocytoma; and family history of thyroid medullary cancer, pheochromocytoma, or premature sudden death syndrome (before age 50 years).

This unique cancer secretes excessive amount of calci-

tonin, which provides an excellent tumor marker that can be obtained from blood samples. Since at least 20% of patients with medullary thyroid cancer have a normal baseline serum calcitonin level, all suspects at high risk for this type of thyroid cancer should have an intravenous pentagastrin stimulation test. This test requires determining a baseline serum calcitonin level; this is followed by an intravenous push of pentagastrin (0.5 μg/kg) in normal saline solution and subsequent blood samples for serum calcitonin levels at 2 and 5 minutes after pentagastrin administration.[61] In individuals who have premalignant medullary C-cell hyperplasia or medullary thyroid cancer the pentagastrin stimulation produces a 2.5- to 5.3-fold rise in plasma calcitonin level, pushing it well above the normal range. If pentagastrin stimulation test results from two different laboratories are abnormal on two separate occasions, these individuals have C-cell hyperplasia or medullary thyroid cancer and should be advised to have a total thyroidectomy. The screening pentagastrin tests should start in high-risk individuals at age 6 years and continue yearly until abnormal test results are found or the patient reaches age 35 years. If there is no evidence of an abnormal pentagastrin test result by age 35 years, the individual has most likely escaped the disease.[53] Any person suspected of having the MEN II or MEN III syndrome should also have screening for a pheochromocytoma. If the individual is hypertensive, the screen can consist of a 24-hour urine collection for metanephrines or a clonidine suppression test.[10] If the adult suspect is normotensive, a glucagon, histamine, or tyramine stimulation test under close monitoring with availability of phentolamine can be considered. If any of the test results are positive or not available, magnetic resonance imaging (MRI) of the adrenals could be considered to rule out pheochromocytoma.

SELECTED ADRENAL PROBLEMS
Cushing's syndrome

Cushing's syndrome consists of a variety of disease states manifested by excess corticosteroid effects on the body. Signs and symptoms of excess endogenous or exogenous corticosteroids include round facies, plethora, acne, thinning of the skin, purple stria, recurrent skin ulcers, easy bruisability, centripetal obesity, female hirsutism, menstrual irregularities, proximal muscle weakness, osteoporosis, hypokalemia, diabetes mellitus, hypertension, generalized fatigue, and mental changes. Children may also show growth retardation.

Approximately two thirds of all cases of Cushing's syndrome can be attributed to Cushing's disease. Cushing's disease is caused by excess production and secretion of pituitary adrenocorticotropic hormone (ACTH), resulting in bilateral adrenal hyperplasia and excess plasma cortisol levels. Although a hypothalmic lesion, pituitary hyperplasia, or pituitary adenoma can usually be identified, the initial stimulus producing hypothalmic or pituitary disease has not been elucidated. The incidence of Cushing's disease is difficult to ascertain; it is five times more frequent in females than males and has its highest incidence between the ages of 20 and 40 years.[68]

Approximately 15% of cases of Cushing's syndrome represent adrenal adenomas or carcinomas, which are more prevalent in women than men and are most commonly diagnosed around 40 years of age. The remaining 15% of cases are due to ectopic ACTH secreting tumors and chronic excessive use of topical or oral steroid preparations. The ectopic ACTH secreting tumors are most commonly associated with oat cell lung cancer in men and most frequently diagnosed between the ages of 40 to 60 years.[68] These patients often have extremely high levels of serum ACTH associated with generalized bronze hyperpigmentation.

The 24-hour urine collection for free cortisol by RIA is the best screening test for Cushing's syndrome. Normal individuals excrete less than 90 μg/dl of free cortisol/day.[66] If a 24-hour urine collection is inconvenient or unobtainable, an overnight decadron suppression test can be performed. This test entails giving decadron 1 mg orally at 11 p.m. and drawing a subsequent 8 a.m. plasma cortisol level on the next day. In individuals without Cushing's syndrome the 8 a.m. plasma cortisol level can be suppressed to less than 5 μg/dl. Unfortunately 1 mg of decadron may not be able to suppress the 8 a.m. plasma cortisol level in moderately obese or depressed individuals. Individuals suspected of the syndrome who have abnormal 24-hour urinary cortisol level or overnight decadron level suppression results would benefit from a referral to an endocrinologist for selection of the best and most cost-effective second-line diagnostic studies, which might include multiple determinations of plasma ACTH and cortisol levels, low- and high-dose decadron suppression, metyrapone stimulation, corticotropin-releasing hormone stimulation, computed tomographic (CT) or MRI studies of the pituitary and/or adrenal glands, CT study of the lungs, or venous sampling of the adrenal veins or inferior petrosal sinuses.[35]

Adrenal insufficiency

Adrenal insufficiency is a rare disease with an incidence of 50 per million in Western countries. Approximately 80% of all cases of primary adrenal insufficiency in the United States can be attributed to autoimmune destruction of the adrenal glands. Autoimmune adrenal insufficiency or Addison's disease is two to three times more common in females than males. It usually develops between the third and fifth decades of life. These individuals have an increased frequency of HLA-B8 and DR3. Addison's disease is often associated with other autoimmune diseases, such as type I diabetes mellitus, hyperthyroidism of Graves' disease, Hashimoto's thyroiditis, pernicious anemia, and hypothyroidism. Interestingly approximately 40% of addisonians have first- or second-degree relatives with some type of autoimmune disease.[68]

Other causes of adrenal insufficiency include tuberculosis, sepsis, bilateral adrenal hemorrhage associated with anticoagulation therapy or seat-belt accidents, sarcoidosis, hemachromatosis, amyloidosis, lymphoma, arteritis, metastatic tumors, particularly from the lung, and inappropriate discontinuation of chronic steroid therapy.

Symptoms and signs of adrenal insufficiency irrespective of the cause include chronic fatigue, anorexia, weight loss, nausea, vomiting, hiccups, abdominal pain, confusion, psychosis, hypotension, orthostatic problems, syncope, coma, generalized bronze hyperpigmentation, hypoglycemia, hyponatremia, and hyperkalemia.

A simple screening test for adrenal insufficiency consists of drawing a plasma cortisol level before and 60 minutes after a challenge with intramuscular synthetic ACTH (Cortrosyn) 250 μg. Because of the increased risk of a suboptimal test result caused by poor or delayed absorption of Cortrosyn in individuals with low to low normal blood pressures (systolic <110 mm Hg), an intravenous Cortrosyn test should be done. This entails drawing a plasma cortisol level before and 30 minutes after the challenge with IV Cortrosyn 250 μg. A normal response is demonstrated by an increment in the plasma cortisol level of more than 7 μg % and a maximal plasma cortisol level of at least 18 μg %.[29] A blunted test result can be seen in patients with pituitary disease or recent use of exogenous steroid preparations. A flat response during the Cortrosyn test is highly indicative of adrenal insufficiency. If the patient is stable, the presence of adrenal insufficiency should be confirmed by a 48-hour IV ACTH stimulation test. To prevent complete depletion of the limited storage supply of adrenal steroids during the 48-hour ACTH test and precipitation of an adrenal crisis, the patient should be maintained during the test with adequate infusion of 5% dextrose and normal saline (D5/NS) along with decadron 0.5 mg every 12 hours.

In a critically ill patient with hypotension, tachycardia, confusion, generalized hyperpigmentation, hypoglycemia, hyponatremia, and hyperkalemia, an immediate plasma cortisol level and ACTH level can be determined and therapy started with large volumes of D5/NS and IV steroids. If the patient has a subnormal plasma cortisol level and supranormal plasma ACTH level, the diagnosis of adrenal insufficiency is confirmed and lifelong steroid maintenance is required. If the results of the immediate blood evaluations are not indicative of adrenal insufficiency, further studies will be needed when the patient is stable. Supporting findings would be presence of adrenal antibodies and small adrenal glands indicated on a CT scan. Almost all causes of adrenal insufficiency are associated with enlarged adrenal glands, with the exception of Addison's disease and in patients previously treated with chronic high-dose steroids where steroids are acutely withdrawn.

Patients diagnosed with adrenal insufficiency should wear a medical alert bracelet or necklace and be instructed to double or triple their steroid doses with any febrile illness or excessive stress until feeling better and receiving further recommendations from their physician. In addition the patient and a family member should be instructed in the emergency use of intramuscular injections of hydrocortisone when patients vomit and are unable to keep down their oral steroids. It is critical to check the emergency supply of steroids periodically to ensure that they are not out of date. Ideally these measures will prevent any adrenal crisis and increased risk of death.

Doses of the various steroid preparations are roughly equivalent to the normal daily body glucocorticoid requirements (Table 60-4). Some patients with complete adrenal insufficiency such as in Addison's disease also require the addition of a mineralocorticoid (Florinef) 0.05 to 0.1 mg daily to maintain electrolyte balance and adequate blood pressure. After the daily intake of the steroid equivalent of 10 mg of prednisone for 3 to 6 months the intrinsic adrenal and/or pituitary gland function can become temporarily suppressed. The daily intake of the steroid equivalent of 20 mg of prednisone or more can cause adrenal suppression within 1 to 4 weeks.[29] The higher the daily dose of steroids the quicker the suppression of the adrenals and/or pituitary gland. Any individual who may have suppressed adrenal or pituitary gland function should be given a steroid preparation before any elective surgery, before stressful procedures such as cardiac catheterization, or during a highly stressful situation such as trauma. One example of a steroid preparation would be hydrocortisone sodium succinate (Solu Cortef) 100 mg IM on call and 100 mg IV in the operating room. If the patient is not stable and has hypotension in the recovery room, IV Solu Cortef 100 mg should be given at 2- to 4-hour intervals along with adequate D5/NS until he or she is stable. An additional safety precaution would be to also give IM Solu Cortef 50 to 100 mg at 6- to 8-hour intervals in case of any lapse in the timed regularity of the IV steroid administration. Intravenous hydrocortisone has a rapid onset of action and lasts up to 4 hours, whereas intramuscular hydrocortisone is dependent on an adequate systolic blood pressure for absorption, has a slow onset of action, and lasts up to 6 to 12 hours. The combined use of IV and IM steroids for preparation or maintenance of a critically ill patient provides some of the theoretical advantages indicated. When stable the patient can be converted to oral steroids at two to three times the normal daily steroid requirements for 3 to 10 days or as required by his or her medical status. As the patient is recuperating the oral steroids can be tapered to the preoperative levels.

If a patient has had any chronic steroid therapy within 12 months, a steroid preparation is recommended for any significant invasive procedure requiring general anesthesia. Although the pituitary gland usually recovers faster than

Table 60-4. Equivalent doses of oral glucocorticoids mimicking daily requirements in unstressed patients.

Prednisone	7.5 mg/24 hr
Hydrocortisone	30 mg/24 hr
Cortisone acetate	37.5 mg/24 hr
Dexamethasone	0.75 mg/24 hr

the adrenal gland from chronic steroid suppression, this is not always the case. Since the short Cortrosyn stimulation test challenges the integrity of only the adrenal glands and not the integrity of the hypothalamus or the pituitary gland's responsiveness to stress, this test should not be used as the basis for determining the need for a steroid preparation. The adrenal and/or pituitary gland can take as long as 9 to 12 months to recover fully from exogenous steroid suppression, depending on the amount and duration of the past steroid use.[32]

In patients not requiring lifelong corticosteroid maintenance the steroid regimen can be switched to an alternate day program with rapid tapering of the steroid dose to the equivalent of prednisone 25 mg every other day. The dose of prednisone may then be tapered by 2.5 mg/week until the patient is off all steroids. If the speed of tapering steroids is too fast for the patient's body, withdrawal symptoms or signs, such as chronic fatigue, hiccups, anorexia, nausea, vomiting, abdominal discomfort, headaches, low-grade fever, electrolyte imbalance, hypoglycemia, hypotension, or shock, may develop.

SUMMARY

This overview of selected endocrine problems and possible interventions for their prevention has emphasized the importance of the following:

- Elicitation of pertinent personal and family history to identify high-risk individuals
- Discriminate use of screening tests
- Patient education about the disease, its possible complications, and his or her responsibilities
- Avoidance of traps leading to iatrogenic disease
- Need for further research for better diagnostic and therapeutic techniques

REFERENCES

1. American College of Physicians: Screening guidelines for diabetic retinopathy, *Ann Intern Med* 116(8):683-685, 1992.
2. American Diabetes Association: *Diabetes facts and figures,* Alexandria, Va, 1988, American Diabetes Association.
3. American Diabetes Association: *The physician's guide to type II diabetes mellitus (NIDDM): diagnosis and treatment,* New York, 1984, American Diabetes Association.
4. Atkinson MA et al: 64000M, autoantibodies as a predictor of insulin-dependent diabetes, *Lancet* 335:1357-1360, 1990.
5. Baekkeskov S et al: Identification of the 64K autoantigen in insulin-dependent diabetes as the GABA-synthesizing enzyme glutamic acid decarboxylase, *Nature* 347:151-156, 1990.

6. Barnett AH et al: Diabetes in identical twins: a study of 200 pairs, *Diabetologia* 20:87-93, 1981.

7. Becks GP, Burrows GN: Thyroid disease and pregnancy, *Med Clin North Am* 75:121-150, 1991.

8. Bennett PH: Diabetes in developing countries and unusual populations. In Mann JI et al, editors: *Diabetes in epidemiological perspective,* London, 1983, Churchill Livingstone.

9. Bleich D et al: Analysis of metabolic progression to Type I diabetes in ICA$^+$ relatives of patients with Type I diabetes, *Diabetes Care* 13:111, 1990.

10. Bravo EL et al: Clonidine—suppression test: a useful aid in the diagnosis of pheochromocytoma, *N Engl J Med* 305:623, 1981.

11. Burrow GN: The thyroid: nodule and neoplasia, In Felig PF et al, editors: *Endocrinology and metabolism,* New York, 1987, McGraw-Hill.

12. Canadian-European Diabetes Study Group: Cyclosporin-induced remission of IDDM after early intervention: association of 1 year of cyclosporin treatment with enhanced insulin secretion, *Diabetes* 37:1574-1582, 1988.

13. Carpenter W, Coustan DR: Criteria for screening for gestational diabetes, *Am J Obstet Gynecol*:144:768-773, 1982.

14. Centers for Disease Control: Recommendations for prevention of HIV transmission in health care settings, *MMWR* 36(Suppl 2):3-18, 1987.

15. Chern MM et al: Empirical risk for insulin-dependent diabetes (IDD) in sibs: further definition of genetic heterogenicity, *Diabetes* 31:1115-1118, 1982.

16. Clark OH, Dul Q-Y: Thyroid cancer, *Med Clin North Am* 75:211-234, 1991.

17. Compagno J, Oertel JE: Malignant lymphoma and other lymphoproliferative disorders of the thyroid gland: a clinical pathologic study of 245 cases, *Am J Clin Pathol* 74:1-11, 1980.

18. Cooper GJ et al: Amylin found in amyloid deposits in human type 2 diabetes mellitus may be a hormone that regulates glycogen metabolism in skeletal muscle, *Proc Natl Acad Sci USA* 85:7763-7766, 1988.

19. Davidson J: Diet therapy for non-insulin-dependent diabetes mellitus. In Davidson J, editor: *Clinical diabetes mellitus,* New York, 1991, Thieme Medical Publishers.

20. Davidson J: Genetic factors in diabetes mellitus. In Davidson J, editor: *Clinical diabetes mellitus,* New York, 1991, Thieme Medical Publishers.

21. Davidson J: Screening for Diabetes Mellitus. In Davidson J, editor: *Clinical diabetes mellitus,* New York, 1991, Thieme Medical Publishers.

22. Davidson J, DiGirolamo M: Non-insulin dependent diabetes mellitus. In Davidson J, editor: *Clinical diabetes mellitus,* New York, 1991, Thieme Medical Publishers.

23. DCCT Research Group: Diabetes control and complications trial (DCCT)—update, *Diabetes Care* 13:20-26, 1990.

24. Dong BJ, Brown CH: Hypothyroidism resulting from generic levothyroxine failure, *J Am Board Fam Pract* 4(3):167-170, 1991.

25. Drash AL: The child with diabetes mellitus. In Rifkin H, Raskin, editors: *Diabetes mellitus,* vol 5, Bowie, Md, 1981, RJ Brady.

26. Ehrmann DA et al: Limitations to the use of a sensitive thyrotrophin in the assessment of thyroid states, *Arch Intern Med* 149:369, 1989.

27. Eisenbarth GS, Pietropaolo M: Prediction and prevention of type I diabetes mellitus, *Contemp Intern Med* 4(3):27, 1992.

28. Forgelfeld L et al: Recurrence of thyroid nodules after surgical removal in patients irradiated in childhood for benign conditions, *N Engl J Med* 320:835-840, 1989.

29. Fujimoto WY: Disorders of glucocorticoid homeostasis. In Metz R, Larson EB, editors: *Blue book of endocrinology,* Philadelphia, 1985, WB Saunders.

30. Gerson MC et al: Prediction of coronary artery disease in a population of insulin requiring diabetic patients: results of an 8-year follow-up study, *Am Heart J* 116(3):820-826, 1988.

31. Ghabrib H et al: Fine needle aspiration biopsy of the thyroid, *Ann Intern Med* 101:25-28, 1984.

32. Graber AL et al: Natural history of pituitary-adrenal recovery following long-term suppression with corticosteroids, *J Clin Endocrinol* 25:11, 1965.

33. Greenspan FS: Radiation exposure and thyroid cancer, *JAMA* 237:2089-2091, 1976.

34. Gregerman RI et al: Thyroxine turnover in euthyroid men with special reference to changes with age, *J Clin Invest* 41:2065, 1962.

35. Grua JR, Nelson DH: ACTH-producing pituitary tumors, *Endocrinol Metab Clin North Am* 20:319-362, 1991.

36. Haffner SM et al: Incidence of type II diabetes in Mexican Americans predicted by fasting insulin and glucose levels, obesity and body-fat distribution, *Diabetes* 39:283-288, 1990.

37. Harris MI: Epidemiological correlates of NIDDM in Hispanics, whites and blacks in the U.S. population, *Diabetes Care* 14(7):639-648, 1991.

38. Helmrich SP et al: Physical activity and reduced occurrence of non-insulin dependent diabetes mellitus, *N Engl J Med* 325:147-152, 1991.

39. Houser HB et al: A three year controlled follow-up study of persons identified in a mass screening program for diabetes, *Diabetes* 26:619-627, 1977.

40. Irvine WV et al: Islet cell antibody as a marker for early stage Type I diabetes mellitus. In Irvine WV, editor: *Immunology of diabetes mellitus,* Edinburgh, 1980, Tevcot Scientific Publications.

41. Irvine WJ et al: Pancreatic islet cell antibodies in diabetes mellitus correlated with duration and type of diabetes, coexistent autoimmune disease and HLA type, *Diabetes* 26:138-147, 1977.

42. Kobberling J: Studies on the genetic heterogenicity of diabetes mellitus, *Diabetologia* 7:46-49, 1971.

43. Koistinen MJ et al: Evaluation of exercise electrocardiography and thallium tomographic imaging in detecting asymptomatic coronary artery disease in diabetic patients, *Br Heart J* 63(1):7-11, 1990.

44. Landon MB, Gabble SG: Diabetes and pregnancy, *Med Clin North Am* 72:1493-1511, 1988.

45. Larsen PR: The thyroid. In Wyngaarden J, Smith L, Jr, editors: *Cecil textbook of medicine,* Philadelphia, 1985, WB Saunders.

46. Levy EG: Thyroid disease in the elderly, *Med Clin North Am* 75:151-167, 1991.

47. Lowhagen T et al: Aspiration biopsy cytology (ABC) in nodules of the thyroid gland suspected to be malignant, *Surg Clin North Am* 59(1):3-18, 1979.

48. McClain DA et al: Restriction-fragmentation-length polymorphism in insulin-receptor gene and insulin resistance in NIDDM, *Diabetes* 37:1071-1075, 1988.

49. McDougall R: Grave's disease, *Med Clin North Am* 75:79-95, 1991.

50. Naka M et al: Silent myocardial ischemia in patients with non-insulin-dependent diabetes mellitus as judged by treadmill exercise testing and coronary angiography, *Am Heart J* 123(1):46-53, 1992.

51. Olefsky J: Diabetes mellitus. In Wyngarden J, Smith L, Jr, editors: *Cecil textbook of medicine,* Philadelphia, 1985, WB Saunders.

52. Olson OC: Classification and epidemiology. In Olson OC, editors: *Diagnosis and management of diabetes mellitus,* New York, 1988, Raven Press.

53. Ponder BA et al: Risk estimation and screening in families of patients with medullary thyroid carcinoma, *Lancet* 1:397-401, 1988.

54. Position statement of the American Diabetes Association: Screening for diabetes, *Diabetes Care* 12:588-590, 1989.

55. Pozzilli P et al: Evidence for raised K-cell levels in type I diabetes, *Lancet* 2:173-175, 1979.

56. Reaven G: Role of insulin resistance in human disease, *Diabetes* 37:1595-607, 1988.

57. Rees-Jones RW et al: Hormonal content of thyroid replacement preparations, *JAMA* 243:549, 1980.

58. Report of the U.S. Preventive Services Task Force: *Guide to clinical preventive services,* Baltimore, 1989, Williams & Wilkins.

59. Ross RS et al: Subclinical hyperthyroidism and reduced bone density as a possible result of prolonged suppression of the pituitray-thyroid axis with L-thyroxine, *Am J Med* 82:1167-1170, 1987.
60. Rossetti L et al: Glucose toxicity, *Diabetes Care* 13:610-630, 1990.
61. Sizemore G, Go V: Stimulation tests for diagnosis of medullary thyroid carcinoma, *Mayo Clin Proc* 50:53-56, 1975.
62. Steinberg M et al: Uptake of technetium 99-pertechnetate in a primary thyroid carcinoma: need for caution in evaluating nodules, *J Clin Endocrinol* 31:81-84, 1970.
63. Sugarman JR: Hypoglycemia associated hospitalization in a population with a high prevalence of non-insulin-dependent diabetes mellitus. *Diabetes Res Clin Pract* 14(2):139-147, 1991.
64. Taft AD: Use of sensitive immunoradiometric assay for thyrotropin in clinical practice, *Mayo Clin Proc* 63:1035, 1988.
65. Tattersall RB, Fagans SS: A difference between the inheritance of classical juvenile-onset and maturity-onset type diabetes of young people, *Diabetes* 24:44-53, 1975.
66. Thompson NW et al: Thyroid carcinoma: current controversies, *Curr Probl Surg* 15(11):1-67, 1978.
67. Tunbridge WMG et al: The spectrum of thyroid disease in a community: the Whickham survey, *Clin Endocrinol (Oxf)* 7:481, 1977.
68. Tyrrell JB, Baxter JD: Disorders of the adrenal cortex. In Wyngaarden J, Smith L, Jr, editors: *Cecil textbook of medicine,* Philadelphia, 1985, WB Saunders.
69. Unger R, Foster D: Diabetes mellitus. In Wilson J, Foster D, editors: *Williams textbook of endocrinology,* Philadelphia, 1992, WB Saunders.
70. Viswanathan M et al: High prevalence of type 2 (non-insulin dependent) diabetes among the offspring of conjugal type 2 diabetic parents in India, *Diabetologia* 23:907-910, 1985.
71. Wagener DK et al: The Pittsburgh study of insulin-dependent diabetes mellitus: risk for diabetes among relatives of IDDM, *Diabetes* 31:136-144, 1982.
72. Warram VH et al: Differences in risk of insulin-dependent diabetes in a offspring of diabetic mothers and diabetic fathers, *N Engl J Med* 311:149-152, 1984.
73. Williamson DF et al: The 10 year incidence of overweight and major weight gain in US adults, *Arch Intern Med* 150:665-672, 1990.

RESOURCES

American Diabetes Association, Diabetes Information Service Center, 1660 Duke Street, Alexandria, VA 22314. Provides information to physicians and patients.

The Thyroid Foundation of America, Inc., Massachusetts General Hospital, ACC 630, Boston, MA 02114. Provides information to physicians and patients.

Chapter 61

PREVENTION OF DENTAL DISEASE AND COMMON ORAL SOFT-TISSUE CONDITIONS

Salvatore J. Esposito
Geza T. Terezhalmy

DENTAL DISEASES: DIAGNOSIS AND PREVENTION
Dental caries

Dental caries (Fig. 61-1) is one of the most common diseases in humans. It is caused by the acid demineralization of tooth enamel by the cariogenic bacteria *Streptococcus mutans, Streptococcus sobrinus, Lactobacillus,* and gram-positive filamentous rods. These microbes act on monosaccharides and disaccharides of food to produce a strong lactic acid, which decalcifies enamel and begins the carious process. Dental plaque containing these cariogenic bacteria strongly adheres to tooth surfaces and is the ideal environment for caries formation. In addition, several predisposing factors contribute to caries activity. A high-carbohydrate diet predisposes to caries; irregular tooth morphology and enamel defects make teeth more susceptible to caries; and most important, poor oral hygiene is a major contributing factor.

Caries can easily be identified by the presence of a white decalcification on the smooth surfaces of teeth or dark brown stains on either the occlusal surfaces or areas between posterior teeth. Carious lesions have been classified as follows[3]:

1. Occlusal—lesions that occur in the deep pits and fissures of the biting surfaces of posterior teeth.
2. Smooth surfaces—lesions that generally occur at the gum line of teeth, usually adjacent to the cheek.
3. Interproximal—lesions that develop between posterior teeth.

4. Nursing bottle caries—lesions that involve deciduous teeth, usually upper anteriors and deciduous first molars. This type of caries is generally the result of prolonged bottle feeding and/or putting a child to bed with a bottle of juice or milk.

Epidemiologic studies have shown that caries has declined in children and adolescents in the past 25 years.[11] Not only has the incidence decreased, but patterns of caries production have changed from smooth tooth surfaces to pits and fissures of the teeth. Even with this demonstrated decline, the incidence remains greatest in children and tends to taper off after adolescence and into adulthood. Children in poorer urban areas have significantly more problems with caries than children from middle class socioeconomic families. The highest incidence occurs in the first few years after the eruption of teeth because of the deep pits and fissures present in newly erupted dentition.[22] The longer teeth are exposed to abrasive foods, salivary flow, and good hygiene habits, the more caries resistant teeth become.

Prevention. To prevent dental caries, it is important to alter the predisposing factors that contribute to its formation. Prevention strategies can be directed at protecting or increasing the resistance of the teeth, improving hygiene regimens, and decreasing the cariogenicity of the diet.

Fluorides. Altering the enamel matrix of developing teeth with the use of *fluoride* has proven to be a most effective way of minimizing dental caries. Fluoride's multi-

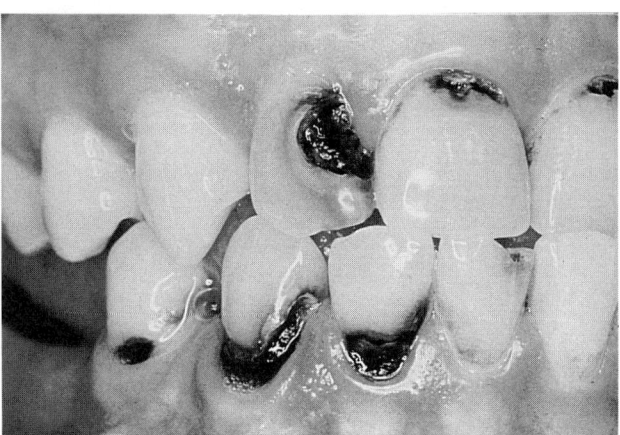

Fig. 61-1. Dental caries.

faceted process consists of (1) the reduction of enamel solubility, (2) its effect on microbial action in plaque, and (3) the enhancement of remineralizations.[24] When fluoride is available systemically during the dental calcification process, the hydroxyapatite crystalline matrix of the enamel of a tooth is altered, changing it to a fluorapatite structure and reducing its solubility. Enamel formation for some permanent teeth begins at or shortly after birth and continues throughout the fourteenth year. Therefore the use of fluoride during this period is important. Systemic fluoride is available by means of fluoridated drinking water, chewable fluoride tablets, or fluoride drops. It can also be administered topically with controlled treatments by the dentist and with fluoride rinses and fluoridated toothpaste. After fluoride is incorporated within the enamel matrix (either systemically or topically administered), it is released whenever a lesion develops, aiding in the remineralization process and thereby resisting the acid solubility of the caries process. In addition, fluoride in contact with the plaque tends to be bactericidal to the microbes in the plaque, reducing their virulence.

Communal water fluoridation continues to be the basis for any dental health promotion program. It is important to assess the fluoride content of a family's drinking water. The recommended optimal level of fluoride ranges from .7 to 1.2 parts per million. Although 87% of the U.S. population is served by community water supplies, only 55.8% of the total population receives optimally fluoridated water.[4,12] In communities where water fluoridation cannot be properly implemented, other forms of systemic fluoride supplementation are indicated. These can be fluoride tablets in the form of sodium fluoride (NaF) 2.2 mg and 1 mg of fluoride, or fluoride drops with each drop equivalent to .25 mg.

Fluoride acts both systemically and topically. The efficacy of topical therapy is based on two premises: fluoride uptake by enamel is proportionate to the duration of application, and the degree of caries prevention is proportionate to the concentration of fluoride in the agent and the frequency of its use. Self-applied fluoride includes mouth rinses, tray-applied gels, and dentifrices. Mouth rinses contain either 226 or 904 parts per million fluoride, depending on whether they are used daily or weekly. Brush-on gels contain 1000 parts per million as .4% stannous fluoride (SnF) and tray-applied gels contain 5000 parts per million fluoride as 1.1% NaF. Dentifrices range from 1000 to 2000 parts per million fluoride in the form of NaF or mono fluoro phosphate (MFP).[26]

Occlusal sealants. The use of occlusal sealants has proved to be a very effective means of reducing dental caries on the posterior teeth of children. The posterior teeth, with their deep pits and fissures, are prime targets for the caries process. Where fluorides are very effective on smooth surfaces, occlusal sealants protect the more susceptible occlusal surfaces of posterior teeth when applied after the teeth erupt.

Sealants are thin layers of composite acrylic resin that are applied to tooth surfaces without grinding away any tooth surfaces. This material is brushed into the pits and fissures of the teeth and then hardened by exposure to ultraviolet light for 30 seconds. Sealants create a mechanical barrier and prevent the accumulation of debris on the occlusal surfaces of teeth. When properly placed, sealants may last up to 5 years and, along with the use of fluorides, give optimum resistance to dental caries. Occlusal sealants are indicated when there are deep, narrow pits and fissures on the occlusal surfaces, when there is modest caries activity, and when teeth are recently erupted.

Oral hygiene. Clearly a good oral hygiene regimen is imperative if the incidence of dental caries is to be reduced. When deciduous teeth erupt, parents should be cautioned about bottle caries. Tooth brushing by the parents at an early age is vitally important. At the age of 2 to 3, children should be seen by a dentist for their first professional visit. By the age of 6, the child should be able to perform normal oral hygiene procedures, namely, tooth brushing two to three times daily, with occasional supervision by the parents.

During adolescence and later, maintaining a plaque-free environment is important. This is achieved through good tooth brushing with a soft-bristle brush and fluoride dentifrice approved by the American Dental Association, combined with the use of dental floss. This regimen should be done three times daily.

Periodic examinations by a dentist are important to detect new carious lesions. Although the frequency of these visits is very patient specific, an examination every 6 months is generally recommended as appropriate to maintain good dental health. High-risk patients, such as those who live in nonfluoridated areas or those with decreased salivary flow (e.g., head and neck radiation patients or patients using medications that dry mucous membranes),

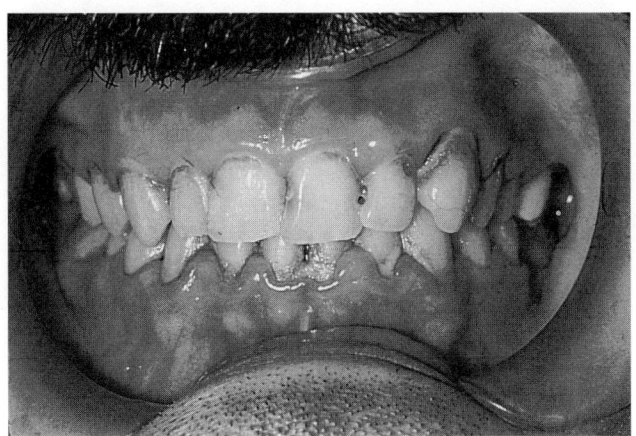

Fig. 61-2. Gingivitis.

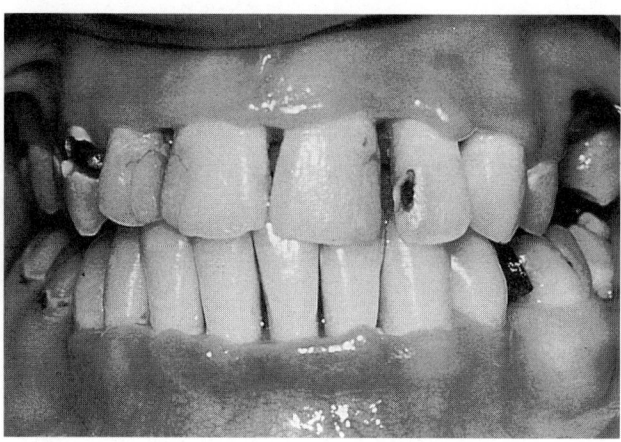

Fig. 61-3. Moderate periodontitis.

should seek professional help more often. This category of patient generally should be seen at least every 3 months.

Periodontal disease

Unlike dental caries, where the incidence decreases with advancing age, periodontal diseases are the leading causes of tooth loss in adults. The periodontium is composed of gingival tissues (gums), periodontal ligament, cementum, and alveolar bone. When healthy, the gingiva is uniformly pink, firm, and nonmobile. The surface texture may be smooth or stippled, depending on the degree of keratinization, pigmentation, and thickness. Healthy periodontal tissue is not inflamed and does not bleed when gently probed or brushed.

The basic pathologic process in periodontal diseases are inflammation and related immunopathological variations.[10,18] The primary cause of periodontal disease is bacterial plaque. The disease manifestation is the classic host-bacterial interaction, with the clinical signs being those involved in the inflammatory process. The primary pathogens identified in periodontal disease are *Actinobacillus actinomycetem-comitans*, *Bacteroides gingivalis*, and *Bacteroides intermedius*.[8,32]

Classification of periodontal disease. The classification of periodontal disease is as follows[2]:

Gingivitis. Symptoms are inflammation of the gingiva (Fig. 61-2), generally characterized by changes in color and texture of the tissue with associated bleeding. Gingivitis may sometimes be seen in children from the time teeth erupt.

Slight periodontitis. This results from the extension of the inflammatory process of gingivitis into the supporting periodontal tissues. Some mild alveolar bone loss usually is associated with this stage. The disease may be localized to a single tooth or present as a generalized condition throughout the mouth.

Moderate periodontitis. This is a more advanced stage (Fig. 61-3) of the condition previously mentioned. There is generally more bone loss, tooth mobility, and greater visible destruction of the periodontal tissues. Pain usually is not associated with this stage, except for some minor thermal changes and discomfort associated with the wedging of food into periodontal pockets.

Advanced periodontitis. Symptoms are further progression of the disease with major loss of alveolar bone support, significant tooth mobility, shifting of teeth, and destruction of the periodontal ligament combined with vascular, degenerative, and necrotic changes of the ligament.

Prevention. Periodontal diseases can be prevented by keeping teeth free of bacteria-containing plaque. This requires time and motivation to brush thoroughly and clean between the teeth with floss at least two to three times daily. In addition to impeccable home care, periodic cleanings and scalings by a dentist are needed. The thoroughness of plaque removal is more important than the frequency of cleaning.

If periodontal disease develops, therapy involves scaling and root planing, instruction in oral hygiene procedures, and possible periodontal surgery to remove pockets to facilitate good hygiene and allow for removal of dental plaque. The combined personal and professional approach to plaque control for the prevention of periodontal disease has proved to be the most effective. As with dental caries, the frequency of professional cleaning varies with the patient. In general, every 6 months is recommended.

In addition to the preventive measures mentioned, the use of the antimicrobial rinse, chlorhexidine gluconate, has proved to be effective in many randomized studies. However, it has some undesirable side effects, such as an unpleasant taste and the staining of teeth and tongue. Therefore it has not been recommended for routine use and should be prescribed only when deemed necessary.

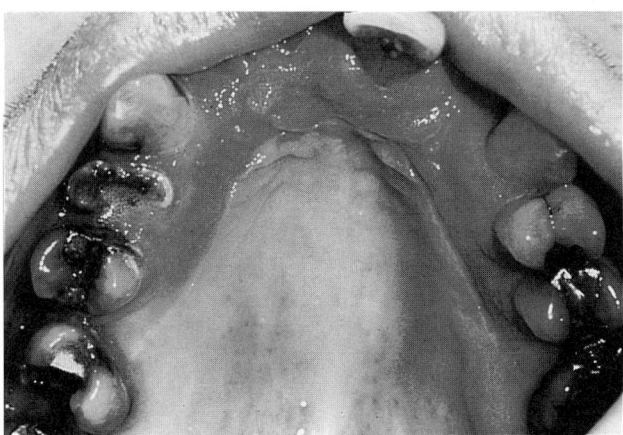

Fig. 61-4. Candidiasis.

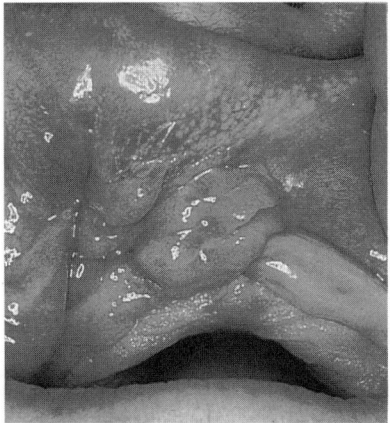

Fig. 61-5. Epulis fissuratum.

Oral problems associated with dental prostheses

Approximately 7 million Americans wear dental prostheses to replace missing teeth, and approximately half of them are completely edentulous. Although clearly important for both functional and cosmetic reasons, dental prostheses must be considered alternatives to having no teeth but not substitutes for real teeth. Because of this, a variety of problems may result from the use and abuse of dental prostheses.

Denture sore mouth. Traumatic injuries or irritation to the soft tissues supporting denture bases are the most frequent causes of denture sore mouth. Unstable denture bases, be they new or old prostheses, are generally the cause of the problem. The longer patients wear removable dental prostheses, the more soft- and hard-tissue changes occur. Although quite patient specific, patients who have been edentulous, or partially edentulous, for long periods of time clearly experience significant alveolar bone loss. As resorption occurs, the dental prosthesis becomes ill-fitting. The more ill-fitting a prosthesis becomes, the greater is the soft-tissue irritation secondary to alveolar resorption, creating an obvious vicious circle.

Other causes of denture sore mouth may be associated with systemic diseases. Any disease that lowers the resistance of the oral tissues may be primarily or secondarily responsible for the development of denture sore mouth. The systemic diseases that are associated with denture sore mouth may vary widely and, in most instances, they represent only one of several etiologic factors. Some of the more common systemic conditions with potential intraoral complications are latent or chronic nutritional deficiencies (in particular vitamin B complex deficiency); diabetes, both controlled and uncontrolled; immunosuppression; and xerostomia related to medications or after head and neck radiation therapy.

In addition to the aforementioned causes of denture sore mouth, superimposed *Candida albicans* infections (Fig. 61-4) are common in patients with older, poorly fitting dentures who may or may not also have associated systemic diseases.

Paresthesia associated with denture wearing. The edentulous patient may complain of paresthesia of the denture-bearing area and/or the lower lip and chin. This is usually related to pressure on the mental nerve as it exits the mental foramen. It is generally seen only in patients exhibiting severe alveolar ridge atrophy resulting in the foramen being immediately on the crest of the denture-bearing area. Clearly, one must also rule out malignant disease in cases where the denture is not in contact with the mental nerve.

Chronic lesions associated with denture borders. Occasionally the edges (flanges) of a denture may be extended beyond the physiological limits of the musculature and soft tissue attachments. This may occur because of excessive bone loss and longstanding use of a denture or simply improper techniques during impression making by the dentist.

The lesions that result, often called epulis fissuratum (Fig. 61-5) or prosthetic ulcers, may pose diagnostic problems for the untrained person. These lesions generally appear as ulcerations with varying degrees of hypertrophy and hyperplasia. They often become secondarily infected. These lesions generally closely follow the outline of the denture. The margins are not indurated or hyperkeratotic, which differentiates them from malignant disease.

Prevention. Virtually all denture-related problems are associated with ill-fitting prostheses. It is imperative that patients wearing removable dental prostheses remove the dentures for several hours during the course of the day. This gives the soft tissues a chance to rest and recover from the trauma of their use. The ideal time would be during sleep; however, many patients find this difficult to do. They should be encouraged, nonetheless, to rest the mucosa at least 4 to 6 hours daily. Failure to allow the tissues to rest may be a contributing factor in the development of serious oral lesions.

Any ulceration, either under the denture or associated with the flanges of the prosthesis, requires immediate attention. Patients should be encouraged to make regular recall appointments with their dentist even though they are completely edentulous. This category of patient is generally advised to visit their dentist every 6 months to a year. Dental prostheses require occasional modifications in the form of adjustments or relines. Dentures should be relined to keep them well fitting every 2 to 3 years and remade every 5 to 10 years. This clearly is patient specific and can be determined only based on sound clinical judgment.

In addition to professional intervention, patients should be told that dentures must be thoroughly brushed at least twice daily. The denture should be removed and cleaned with a soft brush and a mild dishwashing detergent. Patients are also advised soak dentures in water containing a mixture of 1 teaspoon of Calgon and 1 teaspoon of bleach for 30 minutes once a week to remove stains and disinfect the prosthesis.

TRAUMATIZED TEETH

Traumatic injury of the teeth is a common dental problem. The majority of injuries are minor and consist of cracked and chipped teeth; however, some injuries are more severe.[1] Endodontic emergency situations involve avulsion, luxation (dislocation) injuries, and fractures.[1,16] Although management of these conditions falls clearly in the purview of dental practitioners, avulsion in particular requires urgent measures to save the tooth, and physicians are particularly well poised to educate parents about preventive intervention.

An avulsed tooth is one that has been completely displaced from the alveolus. In both primary and permanent dentitions, the maxillary central incisors are most frequently avulsed. Time is an important factor in saving an avulsed tooth; the sooner the tooth can be returned to its alveolar socket after avulsion, the better the prognosis. Treatment of avulsed teeth includes replantation, possibly some form of stabilization and, in most cases, root canal therapy.

Primary prevention

The damage to the teeth and oral tissues that can be caused by sustaining a sudden impact to the front or side of the face while participating in a contact sport can be effectively prevented in most cases by the use of mouthguards. Three types of mouthguards may be used by athletes: (1) stock protectors, (2) mouth-formed protectors, and (3) custom-fitted mouth protectors. Stock mouth protectors may be purchased from any sporting goods store in a variety of sizes and shapes. These mouthguards can be held in place only while the mouth is closed. They make breathing and talking difficult, and provide only minimal protection. Mouth-formed protectors are also available from sporting goods stores. Made from a thermoplastic material, they must be immersed in boiling water for 15 to 45 seconds, allowed to cool sufficiently, and then placed in the mouth for adaptation. These mouthguards are reasonably priced but should be processed by a dentist to minimize bulk and ensure optimal fit. Custom-made mouth protectors are fabricated on dental casts of the athletes' maxillary dental arch under the supervision of a dentist. These color-tinted, polyvinyl acetate-polyethylene mouthguards are acknowledged as the best type of mouthguard.

Preventive intervention in tooth avulsion

Because an avulsed tooth should be replanted as soon as possible, it may at times be feasible to have the patient or someone with the patient replant the tooth by following your telephone directions: (1) rinse the tooth gently in tap water, (2) do not scrub the tooth, (3) insert the tooth gently into the socket as close to the original position as possible—seating the tooth into the socket can be accomplished by having the patient bite down on a piece of cloth such as a handkerchief, and (4) instruct the patient to go directly to the family dentist for follow-up care.[1,16]

If it is not feasible or practical to replant the tooth at the place of accident, the patient and the tooth should be brought to the office of the family dentist as rapidly as possible. The tooth may be transported by either (1) keeping the tooth in the mouth, bathed in saliva—under the tongue or in the vestibule are good locations, but the patient must be old enough to not be at risk of accidental ingestion; or (2) carrying the tooth in a cup or plastic bag filled with milk, saline, or ice water.

Replanted teeth invariably undergo some form of external resorption. The rate of resorption determines the prognosis; the slower the resorption, the longer the tooth may be useful. In those fortunate cases in which a tooth can be replanted immediately after avulsion, complete recovery may take place.

COMMON ORAL SOFT-TISSUE CONDITIONS: DIAGNOSIS AND PREVENTION

Although most common oral lesions are self-limiting, they do produce enough discomfort and embarrassment to cause many affected patients to seek some form of preventive intervention. In addition, the epidemiologic association of some of these conditions with neoplasia has placed health care professionals under increased pressure to treat such lesions to reduce not only the discomfort, but also the potential risk of neoplastic changes and in some instances the likelihood that the patient will transmit an infection to others.

Actinic cheilitis

Diagnosis. Ultraviolet (UV) radiation of the vermilion border of the lips can precipitate recurrent herpetic infec-

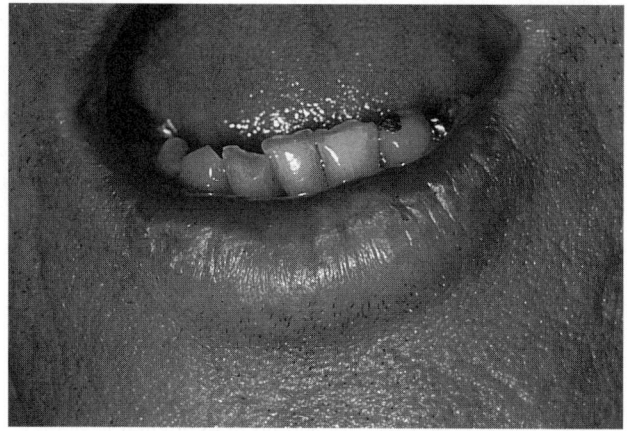

Fig. 61-6. Actinic cheilitis.

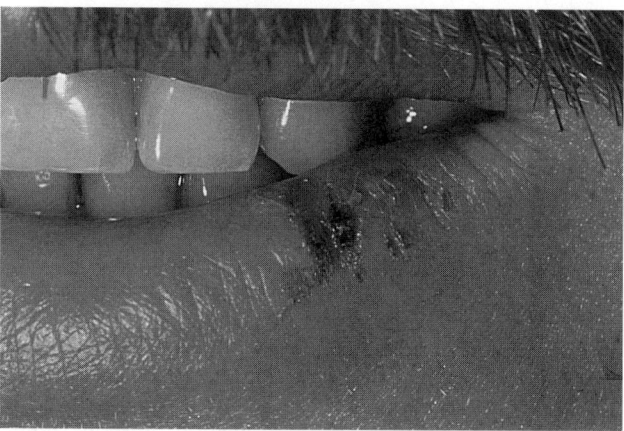

Fig. 61-7. Dysplasia.

tions, varying degrees of dysplasia, and squamous cell carcinoma. The short-term effects of exposure to UV light are transient, but the cumulative long-term effects produce irreversible damage to the lip in all patients.[19,20] Although degenerative changes have been observed predominantly in men after age 40, the condition now is increasingly recognized in younger men. The patients will present to the clinician with a history of chronic or recurrent crusting, scaling, and occasional ulceration of the lower lip. A history of long-term exposure to direct sunlight usually can be elicited. Clinically, the lip appears dry, mottled, and opalescent, with white or gray plaques that are slightly elevated and cannot be stripped off (Fig. 61-6). Isolated areas of hyperkeratosis may also be evident, as well as loss of elasticity and definition of the vermilion border. Other clinical signs include erythematous or hemorrhagic areas, parallel marked folds, and an unobtrusive "chapped lip" appearance. Malignant change is manifested clinically by areas of more intense hyperkeratosis surrounded by diffuse cheilitis and ulcerations of relatively long duration (Fig. 61-7).

Prevention. Prevention of actinic damage to the lips centers on avoidance of long-term exposure to direct sunlight. Occupational and environmental factors often preclude this. An effective alternative is to apply a chemical or physical sunscreen[19,20] (see Chapter 49, Skin Cancer and Protection of the Skin). Chemical sunscreens absorb potentially harmful UV light, whereas physical sunscreens reflect it. Of the chemical sunscreens, those containing para-aminobenzoic acid (PABA) and certain of its esters provide superior protection. Physical sunscreens include such active agents as titanium dioxide, talc, or zinc oxide.

Petroleum-based and cream sunscreens are the most durable, but can be difficult to keep on the lips because people tend to lick off the residual coating, which lessens the effectiveness of the sunscreen. For this reason, liquid or gel sunscreens provide significantly greater protection for

the lips. Sunscreen preparations should be applied uniformly and generously to the lips. Two applications 1 hour before exposure to sunlight may be necessary for maximum protection. Reapplication every hour is required to provide adequate continuous protection.

Herpetic infections

Diagnosis. Seroepidemiologic studies indicate that 80% to 90% of the adult population has been exposed to Herpesvirus hominis type I (HVH-1), and 40% of those with serologic evidence of primary infection may experience recurrent lesions. Although most herpetic infections are localized and self-limiting,[9] disseminated primary and recurrent HVH-1 infections are potentially fatal. The epidemiologic association of Herpesvirus hominis type 2 (HVH-2) with neoplasia has placed health care professionals under increased pressure to diagnose and treat herpetic infections. The late cytopathogenic effects of herpetic infections are characterized by general disintegration of the host cell membrane and expulsion of infectious viral units into the extracellular space. Thus the viral organisms may infect nearby cells or may be seeded in other tissues, particularly in sensory ganglia, establishing latent infections via the hematogenous route. Latent infections may be reactivated, and recurrences may be caused by a number of different stimuli, such as ultraviolet light, mechanical trauma, fever, emotional stress, and dietary factors.

Acute herpetic gingivostomatitis is the most common form of primary invasion by HVH-1. In young children the infection may be only transient or subclinical. In adults, however, it is often more dramatic. After an incubation period of 4 to 5 days, the patient complains of malaise, irritability, headache, fever, and lymphadenopathy, and within a day or two the mouth becomes uncomfortable. Examination shows widespread inflammation of the marginal and attached gingivae, characterized by erythema, edema, and capillary proliferation (Fig. 61-8). Nu-

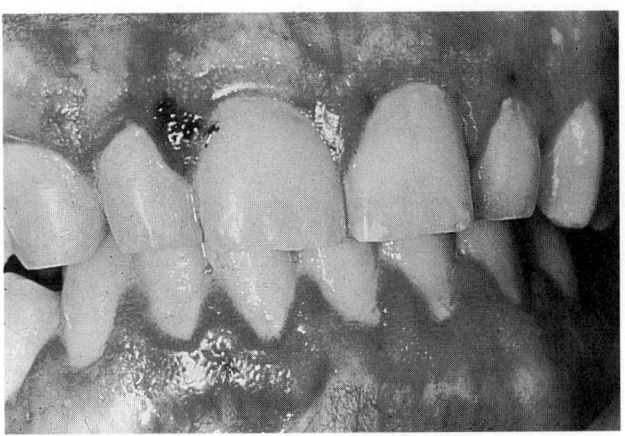

Fig. 61-8. Acute herpetic gingivostomatitis.

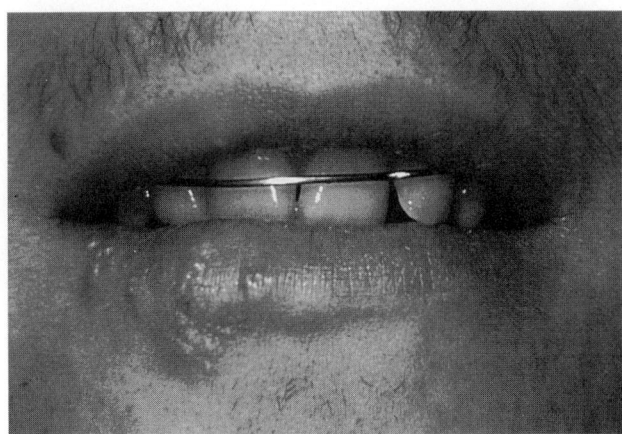

Fig. 61-9. Herpes labialis.

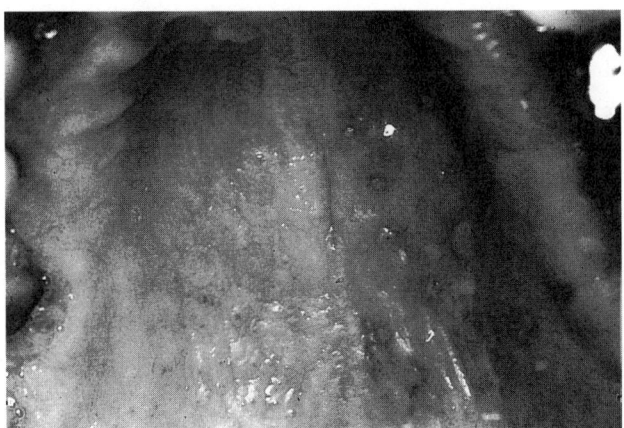

Fig. 61-10. Recurrent intraoral herpes.

merous small vesicles may develop anywhere on the oral mucosa and lips. The vesicles soon ulcerate and may become secondarily infected. The ulcers on the lips become crusted, and if saliva dribbles from the mouth, similar lesions may develop on the face. The symptoms begin to subside about the sixth day of fever, and the oral lesions and lymphadenopathy take 10 to 14 days to resolve.

Herpes labialis, the most frequent type of recurrent herpetic infection, is characterized by marked local symptoms unaccompanied by systemic illness. Prevalence apparently increases with age, and the lesions tend to recur in a similar site in a particular individual, most commonly on or adjacent to the vermilion border of the lip. The clinical course is marked by a prodromal period of hyperesthesia or altered sensation, and erythema and edema at the site of involvement. Prodromata are followed by the eruption of clusters of vesicles, which coalesce and crust (Fig. 61-9).

Recurrent intraoral infections. The typical features of recurrent intraoral herpetic infections include single or small clusters of vesicles, which rapidly break down into ulcers (Fig. 61-10). These lesions occur on the keratinized mucosa of the hard palate or gingivae and may at times be associated with herpes labialis.

Prevention. Orolabial herpetic infections are usually self-limiting. Preventive measures should be primarily supportive and directed toward controlling the signs and symptoms of the particular condition under consideration. Successful management consists of controlling fever, dehydration, and pain; preventing secondary infections; and monitoring closely for evidence of visceral viremia.

Acyclovir therapy, topical and systemic, shows significant therapeutic efficacy in the management of HVH infections.[14,15] Although it does not appear to eliminate latent infection, it can provide effective prophylaxis against reactivated mucocutaneous infections. However, any protocol must consider well-documented evidence of drug resistance in HVH-1 isolated from the oral cavity of patients treated with acyclovir. This observation may have far-reaching implications for the clinical use of acyclovir for the treatment of orolabial herpetic infections.

Lysine hydrochloride is an HVH-1 antagonist when added to culture media. In one clinical trial it was demonstrated to have no effect on the rate of healing in recurrent herpes labialis. The same investigators further evaluated the effect of prophylactic lysine, 1000 mg per day for 12 weeks, and concluded that, although it has no significant effect on the healing of existing lesions, it does appear to prevent recurrence during therapy.[23] Lysine hydrochloride is generally recognized as safe for over-the-counter use in a dosage of up to 3000 mg daily.

Water-soluble bioflavonoid ascorbic acid complex (Peridin-C) presents an antipodal approach to antiviral chemotherapy. The complex is directed primarily at supporting cell physiology and function in the host cell by preserving cellular integrity. The complex has been observed

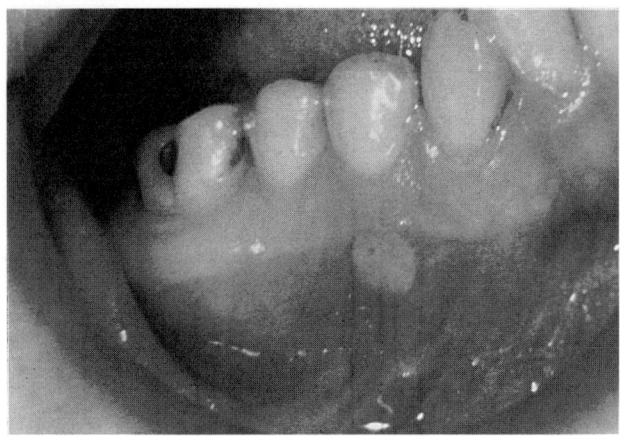

Fig. 61-11. Minor aphthous.

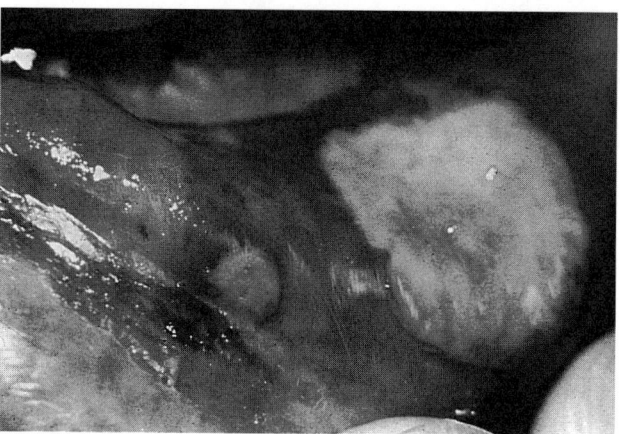

Fig. 61-12. Major aphthous.

to shorten the duration of pain and reduce vesiculation and disruption of the vesicular membrane.[35] The preventive regimen, 200 mg three times a day, is most effective when instituted in the early prodromal stage of the disease.

Aphthous stomatitis

Diagnosis. Recurrent aphthous stomatitis is one of the most common oral ulcerative lesions.[37] Pleomorphic alpha-hemolytic streptococcus, *Streptococcus sanquis,* has been isolated from early lesions, and when inoculated into laboratory animals, has produced lesions consistent with aphthous stomatitis. Cell-mediated and humoral immunity may also be an important factor because lymphocytes and antibody complexes from patients with recurrent aphthous stomatitis are cytotoxic to mucosal epithelium. Recurrent aphthae may be the first clinical evidence of celiac disease and are commonly associated with tropical sprue and gluten-sensitive enteropathy. The condition may also be due to deficiencies of vitamin B_{12}, folic acid, and iron; however, reports dealing with these possibilities are conflicting. Increased incidence of ulcerations has also been noted in some women during the luteal phase of the menstrual cycle, with complete remission during pregnancy. The role of stress is less specific, but at least in some instances may also be a valid contributing factor.

Minor aphthae, by far the most common type, are characterized by recurrent crops of ulcers less than 1 cm in diameter. Prodromata associated with localized altered sensation are followed by the appearance of erythematous papules. Consequently, a painful erosion with a grayish-yellow pseudomembranous crater is accentuated by an erythematous halo (Fig. 61-11). The patients are afebrile but may present with discrete submandibular lymphadenopathy. Complete resolution without scarring may take 7-14 days.

Major aphthae are chronic, solitary ulcers greater than

1 cm in diameter. Prodromal nodules enlarge to destructive craterlike lesions with an indurated, raised border (Fig. 61-12). Persistent necrosis suggests vascular damage and infiltration of microorganisms into the underlying connective tissue. Associated signs and symptoms include severe pain and submandibular and cervical lymphadenopathy. Complete resolution with extensive scarring may take weeks or even months.

Behçet's syndrome. Both minor and major aphthae may be accompanied by ulcers of the genital mucosa and the eyes that are suggestive of Behçet's syndrome. Ulceration of the soft palate and fauces is an ominous sign (Fig. 61-13). In many cases multisystemic involvement may include arthritis, skin lesions, thrombophlebitis, arteritis, and neuropathy.

Herpetiform ulceration, a less common type of recurrent problem, is characterized by shallow, pinpoint ulcers not necessarily confined to the nonkeratinized tissues of the oral cavity (Fig. 61-14). There may be 20 or more ulcers at a time superficially resembling but unrelated to herpetic infections.

Prevention. It has been suggested that 80% to 90% of the treatment for recurrent aphthous stomatitis is less than effective. Therefore palliative and supportive care should be directed to reducing precipitating factors, controlling pain, shortening the duration of the lesions already present, and preventing new ulcers.[6,28,29,37] Precipitating factors vary from patient to patient, but self-induced trauma is by far the most common factor. Foods to avoid during an episode of exacerbation include citrus fruits, melons, vinegar, spices, chocolate, walnuts, sour substances, and tomatoes. If the patient does not respond to conservative treatment, further diagnostic workup should extend to hematology screening, including a complete blood count; a determination of serum iron, folic acid, and B_{12} levels; and other appropriate consultations.

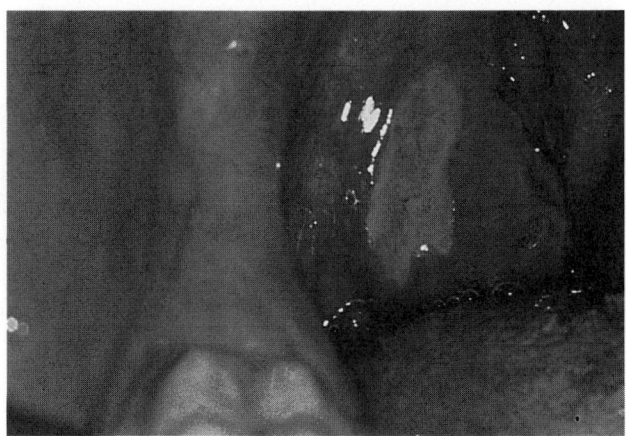

Fig. 61-13. Behçet's syndrome.

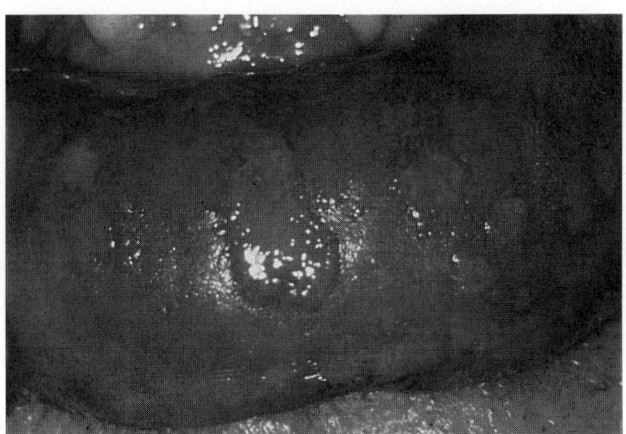

Fig. 61-14. Herpetiform ulceration.

Stomatitis

Diagnosis. Stomatitis is inflammation and ulceration of the oral mucosa caused by local or systemic factors.[33] The degree of mucosal involvement in stomatitis varies greatly depending on the predisposing and precipitating factors. The clinical signs may range from discrete ulcerations to generalized erythematous or pseudomembranous involvement of the tissues. The ulceration is associated with mild to moderate pain, and carries the potential for secondary bacterial and fungal infections. Some of the common factors producing stomatitis are trauma from sharp, fractured teeth or restorations, problems related to prosthetic and orthodontic appliances, toothbrush abrasions, and factitious injury. Aspirin or other agents used as local obtundents, pizza burns, excessive smoking, accidental aspiration of chemicals such as gasoline, and systemic administration of gold salts or other drugs are other possible etiologic factors.

The aspirin tablet or the hot pizza will cauterize the tissues, causing a white, sloughing epithelial layer that leaves a raw, bleeding, painful surface (Fig. 61-15). Heat and chemical irritants produced by excessive smoking cause erythema of the hard palate and a consequent grayish-white, thickened papular appearance with small red spots representing the dilated orifices of minor salivary glands. Gasoline and similar agents may cause small bullae or generalized swelling of all tissues contacted. Stomatitis caused by gold therapy may range from superficial erosions to pronounced ulcerations covered with fibrin and at times surrounded by an erythematous halo.

Ill-fitting removable dental prostheses may traumatize the oral mucosa, producing erythema, erosion, or ulceration, or predisposing to chronic erosive candidiasis. Prostheses may also cause chemical or thermal burns, and the acrylic resin and its monomers may provoke an allergic reaction. Diabetes mellitus may also present with symptoms

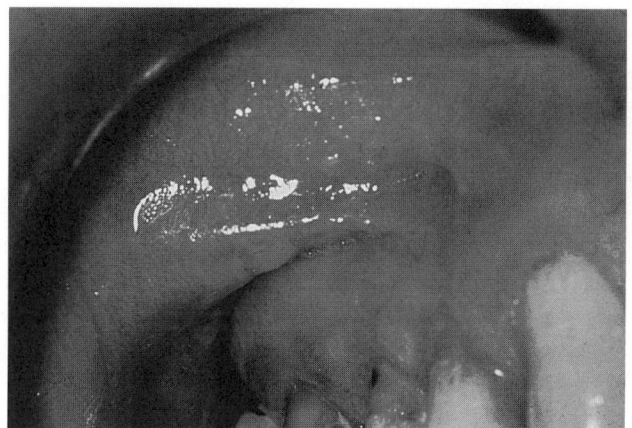

Fig. 61-15. Aspirin burn.

of stomatitis caused by associated vascular changes and candidiasis. In patients with removable dental prostheses, this response may be exaggerated.

Perhaps the most dramatic form of stomatitis is seen in the response of the oral tissues to chemotherapy and head and neck radiotherapy. The therapeutic value of both these modalities lies in their ability to interfere with cellular activity (Fig. 61-16). On this basis, it would seem that one could selectively damage cancer cells by exploiting simple differences in cell cycle kinetics. This, however, is not entirely the case. Tumor cells do not necessarily proliferate faster than normal cells, and there may be further differences in the fraction of cycling cells and the rate of cell loss. Consequently, drugs and radiation used to eradicate malignant lesion may also destroy certain normal cells, resulting in clinically expressed adverse effects such as stomatitis.

Prevention[33]. Individuals should be informed that topical application of medicaments such as aspirin that are

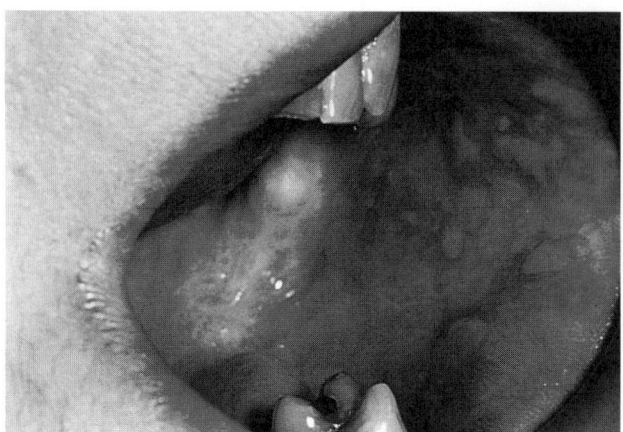

Fig. 61-16. Chemotherapy-induced stomatitis.

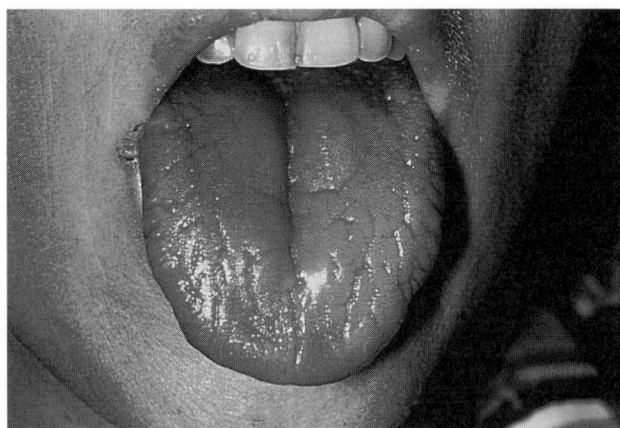

Fig. 61-17. Folic acid deficiency resulting in beefy red tongue and angular cheilosis.

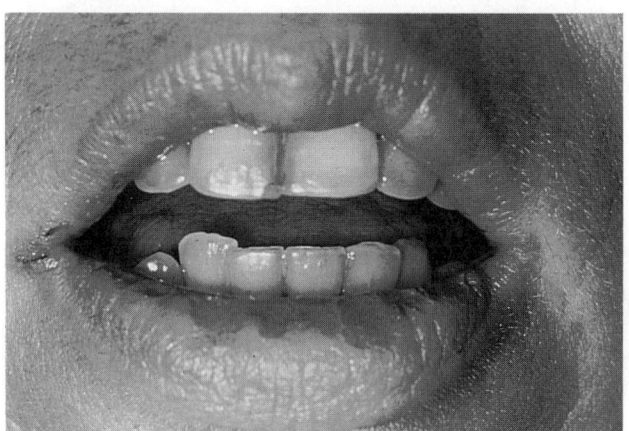

Fig. 61-18. Angular cheilosis.

compounded for systemic use is ill-advised. The severity of nicotine stomatitis may be reduced and regression of the lesions may be affected if the patient stops smoking. Oral lesions associated with the accidental aspiration of gasoline and other chemicals generally are not severe, but they may require supportive treatment. Complete healing usually occurs within 7 days. The treatment of stomatitis caused by ill-fitting removable dental prostheses may require only minor denture adjustment—or complete refabrication of the prostheses. The importance of meticulous oral hygiene cannot be overemphasized as an effective preventive and therapeutic modality in the management of stomatitis.

The painful inflammatory response to the oral mucosa may be minimized if the patient uses a topical anesthetic and rinses with an alkaline-saline solution. Diphenhydramine hydrochloride elixir is the recommended topical an-

esthetic and should be applied before meals and at bedtime. This agent is preferred to lidocaine hydrochloride viscous because it does not interfere with the pharyngeal phase of swallowing. Lidocaine hydrochloride can be used but should be diluted to one-third or one-half strength, especially when prescribed for young or debilitated patients. Frequent rinses with the alkaline-saline solution provide considerable mechanical debridement. Some patients, however, have a lowered resistance to infection, especially patients with diabetes mellitus and those undergoing chemotherapy or radiotherapy. Such patients should rinse with the alkaline-saline solution and with chlorhexidine gluconate, 0.12%.

Glossodynia

Diagnosis. Glossodynia or painful tongue is often a symptom of a complex systemic disease rather than a pathologic entity. The clinician must look for deficiency states such as iron deficiency anemia, pellagra, achlorhydria, and pernicious anemia; metabolic problems such as diabetes mellitus; hypersensitivity reactions; psychogenic or idiopathic factors; and local conditions such as benign migratory glossitis, candidiasis, lichen planus, xerostomia, and oral cancer.[34]

Deficiency states may produce signs and symptoms involving the tongue. In iron deficiency anemia the patient's tongue may cause the loss of filiform papillae. Early manifestations are noted on the lateral margins and tip of the tongue. A deficiency of folic acid and vitamin B_{12} may cause generalized atrophy of the lingual papillae. The patient usually presents with a painful, beefy-red tongue (Fig. 61-17), in many instances accompanied by angular cheilitis (Fig. 61-18).

Diabetes mellitus is often associated with glossodynia concomitant with xerostomia and candidiasis. Diabetic neuropathies may also be manifested in the head and neck

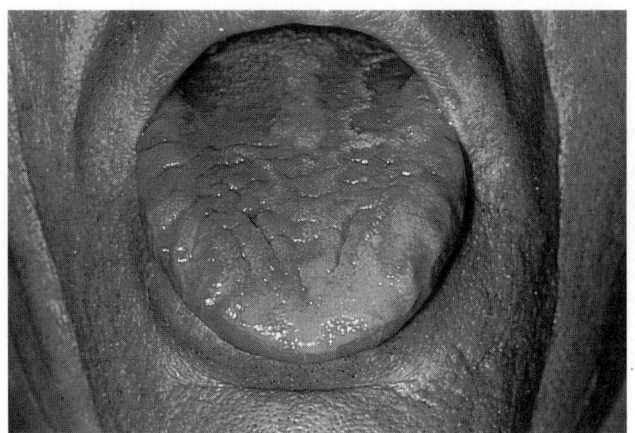

Fig. 61-19. Benign migratory glossitis.

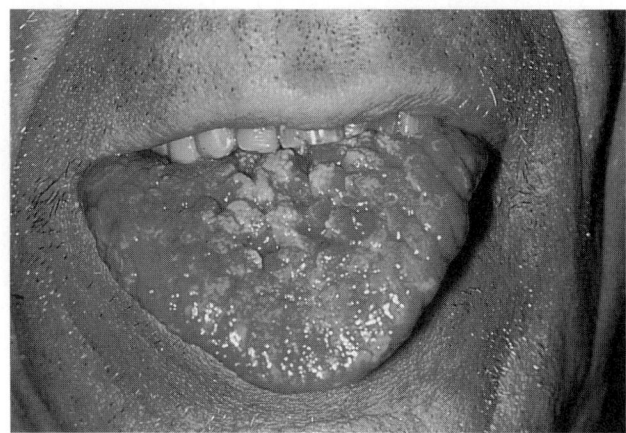

Fig. 61-20. Acute pseudomembranous candidiasis.

and may contribute to the symptoms. *Neurotic glossodynia* has been described in typical postmenopausal women and is often accompanied by cancerphobia. A painful tongue may be the first indication of depression, and glossodynia, the complaint of a metallic taste, and pruritus (often of the scalp) may be associated with stress and anxiety. *Benign migratory glossitis* is a commonly recurring condition in which there is a loss of filiform papillae in an irregular pattern (Fig. 61-19). This condition is usually asymptomatic, although patients may present with glossodynia caused by mild irritation from spicy foods. Factors predisposing to *candidiasis* include diabetes mellitus, nutritional deficiencies, cytotoxic drugs, radiotherapy, corticosteroids, xerostomia, and pregnancy (with secondary infection to the infant). Poor oral hygiene, especially in a patient with dental prostheses, is a significant predisposing factor. Clinical manifestations include acute pseudomembranous, chronic hyperplastic, or chronic atrophic forms of candidiasis and may contribute significantly to symptoms of glossodynia (Fig. 61-20). *Oral lichen planus* is usually associated with asymptomatic, hypertrophic Wickham's striae. However, erosive oral lichen planus with painful, eroded ulcerations up to several centimeters in size must be considered in the differential diagnosis of the burning tongue syndrome. Glossodynia may also be the initial symptom of Sjögren's disease, primarily as a complication of xerostomia.

Prevention. *The pain, itching, and stinging* are appropriately treated with topical anesthetic agents.[34] *Xerostomia,* regardless of the etiology, is treated symptomatically with artificial saliva.[17] Because qualitative and quantitative changes in the saliva contribute significantly to the incidence of caries, a fluoride regimen is added to the therapeutic approach. The clinician should provide palliative and supportive care and initiate appropriate evaluation of the patient's physical status. Once the precipitating systemic disease is adequately managed, the oral manifestations will resolve.

Xerostomia

Diagnosis. Dry mouth is not a specific disease entity but may be secondary to a number of significant local and systemic factors.[17,31] A reduction in salivary flow has been attributed to such factors as heavy smoking and alcohol intake, aging, altered psychic states, and idiopathic conditions. Specific local factors may include the rare congenital absence or aplasia of one or more major salivary glands or ducts; glandular hyperplasia seen in mumps, sialolithiasis, and sialoadenitis; and neoplasias, which usually affect an isolated gland (although there may be infiltration of multiple glands in leukemia and lymphoma).

Systemic conditions associated with xerostomia include diabetes mellitus and Sjögren's syndrome, a relatively common condition in women between the ages of 40 and 60 characterized histologically by lymphocytic infiltration of the salivary glands. Xerostomia may also be associated with collagen vascular or connective tissue disorders, such as systemic lupus erythematosus, scleroderma, mixed connective tissue disease, and polydermatomyositis.

The most dramatic form of xerostomia is seen secondary to external irradiation of the head and neck (Fig. 61-21). Implants produce more localized, less destructive structural changes because effective irradiation drops off at the periphery. Medications from such varied categories as hypnotics, antispasmodics, decongestants, diuretics, antihistamines, amphetamines, tranquilizers, and neoplastic inhibitors have all been implicated in xerostomia.

Chronic xerostomia may result in painful oral soft-tissue problems, a high incidence of rampant caries (Fig. 61-22), and poor tissue adaptation to prostheses. Furthermore, the reduced buffering capacity of the saliva leads to a more acid oral environment, altering the sensitivity of taste buds and precipitating the development of hairy tongue. The increased acidity contributes significantly to the alteration of the oral ecology, producing predictable, dramatic changes in the oral microflora.

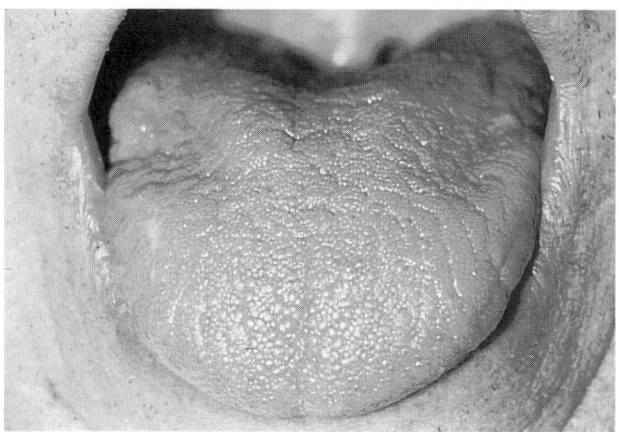

Fig. 61-21. Radiation-induced xerostomia.

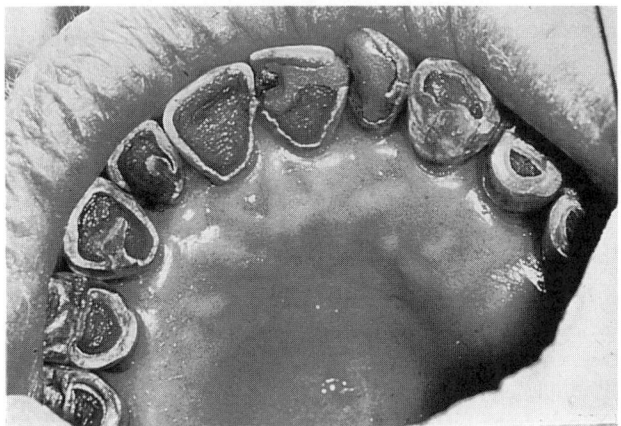

Fig. 61-22. Caries secondary to xerostomia.

The virulence of the resultant cariopathogenic microorganisms is responsible for the logarithmic increase in the caries incidence of xerostomic patients. This type of caries characteristically involves the dentin and cementum exposed at the cervical areas of the teeth and affects cusp tips and incisal edges, in contrast to the traditional carious penetration of the enamel noted interproximally and in pits and fissures of occlusal surfaces.

Tooth loss, a predictable sequela of advanced carious lesions, presents further difficulties for both the patient and clinician. Xerostomia contributes to decreased retention of tissue-borne prostheses, which may in turn contribute to the development of traumatic ulcerative lesions on already compromised tissue. In irradiated patients, such lesions take on added significance because they allow oral bacteria to penetrate to deeper osseous areas, with a potential for the development of markedly morbid osteoradionecrosis.

Prevention. Symptomatic and supportive care of the xerostomic patient should include good oral hygiene pro-

cedures, proper dietary control, and the use of saliva substitutes.[17] The substitutes should have a pleasant taste, contain electrolytes in concentrations normally found in saliva, and have the viscosity adjusted with the addition of sodium carboxymethylcellulose. The use of supplemental fluoride agents to promote remineralization of the enamel is recommended. Fluoride delivery systems that provide optimal protection are now available.

Saliva substitutes. Systemic management directed at the underlying cause of xerostomia in most instances is within the purview of the physician. Saliva substitutes are palliative. They are used primarily to compensate for the deprivation of salivary flow and relieve intraoral symptoms without significant accumulation of mucosal plaques.

Stannous fluoride gel. Saliva substitutes do not constitute a total chemical approach to the problem of rampant caries. A fluoride self-application program for caries prevention in the irradiated patient has shown excellent results. A daily application of 0.4% SnF_2 gel in conjunction with a comprehensive oral hygiene program is advocated. Although these programs were implemented initially for the benefit of irradiated patients, their applicability is readily apparent for many patients with xerostomia.

TRANSIENT BACTEREMIAS: PROPHYLAXIS FOR THE HIGH-RISK PATIENT

The human fetus is bacteria free. However, at birth the oral cavity of human infants is invaded by microorganisms, and the dynamic process of colonization begins. After initial exposure, most organisms are soon eliminated, but others, such as *Streptococcus salivarius, Veillonellae,* and *Actinomyces,* that have the ability to attach to oral epithelium, become part of the permanent oral flora. *Streptococcus mutans* can be cultured after the eruption of teeth, and other species soon populate the newly formed gingival sulcus. The adult oral cavity harbors a dense, diverse, indigenous flora that include protozoa, yeasts, viruses, and at least 20 identified genera of bacteria. A dynamic interaction between the various microbial ecosystems, such as dental plaque, gingival sulcus, tongue, oral mucosa, and saliva will determine the normal flora. The microorganisms of the oral flora establish symbiotic relationships (commensalism, mutualism, or parasitism) with their human host until age, altered anatomy, diet, dental caries, periodontal disease, certain systemic problems, and antibiotic therapy modify or shift the balanced environment of the microbial flora and the organisms become pathogenic. Transient, usually asymptomatic, bacteremias occur in a wide variety of dental manipulations, particularly those associated with mucous membranes. These bacteremias can cause serious complications and even death. Physicians are often consulted by other health care providers, especially dental practitioners, requesting guidance to minimize morbidity and mortality in high-risk patients.

Prevention. Although there is no concrete evidence that antibiotics given before bacteremia-causing dental procedures prevent infections in humans, experimental data in rabbits supports their use to prevent bacterial endocarditis. Similarly, laboratory tests in which asplenic mice were exposed to pneumococci showed that asplenic mice on prophylactic penicillin had a significantly reduced mortality rate when compared with asplenic mice not receiving penicillin. In situations where bacteremia is highly predictable, administering prophylactic antibiotics to patients at high risk seems wise to minimize morbidity and mortality.

Infective endocarditis. The historical association of dental procedures and subsequent infective endocarditis has prompted the American Heart Association to recommend antibacterial prophylaxis with *all* dental procedures that are likely to cause gingival bleeding[7] (see also Chapter 42, Other Cardiac Conditions).

Total joint replacement. Among the many potential complications after total joint replacement, infection is one of the most serious. There have been several reports of infections at sites remote from the hip, such as the kidney, lungs, and gastrointestinal tract, causing bacteremia with possible seeding to the hip prosthesis. Therefore the circumstantial association reported between dental therapy and metastatic infection of hip prostheses should be a point of concern.[5]

If such seeding of a prosthetic implant can occur from transient bacteremia, the paramount question is the role of antibiotic prophylaxis in preventing such seeding: Should patients with total joint replacement who are undergoing dental care be treated with antibiotics as are patients with prosthetic heart valves? Data is insufficient to answer these questions definitively. But the point remains that metastatic infection of total joint replacement is a definite possibility. Morbidity associated with such infections is so devastating that the risks of antibiotic prophylaxis for dental therapy seem small in comparison.

The granulocytopenic patient. Infections are a major cause of morbidity and mortality during periods of granulocytopenia often associated with cancer chemotherapy, acute leukemia, aplastic anemia, and immunosuppression. The risk of developing an infection is the greatest when the polymorphonuclear leukocyte count falls below 1000 per mm^3; and when the granulocyte count is less than 100 per mm^3 for more than a few days, bacteremia and severe infection become virtually inevitable. Primarily because of invasion by environmentally-acquired organisms that have colonized the alimentary canal and upper respiratory passage, nearly 80% of infections are caused by five organisms: *Pseudomonas aeruginosa, Klebsiella pneumoniae, Escherichia coli, Staphylococcus aureus,* and *Candida albicans.* In dental situations in granulocytopenic patients in which nosocomial colonization and bacteremia from foci of oral infections and soft-tissue manipulations are highly

predictable, prophylactic preoperative and postoperative antimicrobial therapy seems appropriate.

The asplenic patient. Removal of the spleen predisposes a patient to the development of overwhelming sepsis characterized by the onset of high-grade bacteremia without a primary site of infection. Characteristically, the bacteremia is followed by the sudden onset of nausea and vomiting, meningitis, disseminated intravascular coagulation, adult respiratory distress syndrome, shock, and death in less than 72 hours. Although primarily infants and children are affected, the risk extends to teenagers and adults. The period of heightened susceptibility to infections is 1 to 2 years after splenectomy. However, fulminant infections have been reported 5 and even 25 years after the surgical procedure.

The organism responsible for about half of these cases of fulminant septicemia is *Streptococcus pneumoniae* (pneumococcus). The remaining infections are due to *Neisseria* species, *Hemophilus influenzae, Staphylococcus aureus,* group A Streptococci and, rarely, *Escherichia coli, Klebsiellae, Salmonellae,* and *Pseudomonas aeruginosa.* Streptococcal and staphylococcal bacteremias, as well as those associated with *Hemophilus* organisms, have been documented secondary to dental treatment and even after such daily functions as toothbrushing. Pneumococci, staphylococci, and *Hemophilus* organisms are also commonly associated with infections of the ear, nose, and throat and therefore, at least under certain circumstances, are found in the oral cavity.

Prophylactic penicillin has significantly reduced the mortality of asplenic mice exposed to pneumococci. Therefore, in dental situations in which bacteremia is highly predictable, prophylactic preoperative and postoperative antimicrobial therapy seems appropriate[36] (see also Chapter 57 regarding pneumococcal and *Hemophilus influenza* vaccinations in the asplenic patient.)

CANCER THERAPY: PREVENTION OF ORAL COMPLICATIONS

Oral complications of cancer therapy include mucositis, infection, hemorrhage, xerostomia, neurologic disorders, and nutritional disorders.[21,25] The severity of these conditions may be affected by patient- and therapy-related variables. Patient-related variables include the patient's oral health status before and during therapy. Therapy-related variables include the type of agent(s) used, dosage, and frequency of treatment. The clinician absolutely must recognize and anticipate the conditions that predispose patients to complications.

Preventive measures before cancer therapy

The prevention of oral complications from cancer therapy is the oral health care provider's primary goal. Oral complications that are not prevented should be treated carefully and eliminated by following a protocol of dental evaluation and preventive treatment before, during, and after chemotherapy.

All patients with cancer who will receive chemotherapy or head and neck radiotherapy should have a thorough oral examination, which should include a clinical and radiographic analysis.[21,25] Even if therapy has to begin immediately or has already begun, this examination will provide a basis for comparison and assist in the monitoring and treatment of oral complications. At the least, the patient should be instructed in proper oral hygiene. Frequently, many patients become highly motivated to increase their oral health care to minimize oral complications.

If time permits, optimal dental treatment should include prophylaxis, restoration of carious teeth, replacement of faulty restorations, smoothing of rough enamel or restored surfaces, elimination of ill-fitting prostheses, and fabrication of fluoride trays. Any teeth that are unrestorable or have severe periodontal involvement should be extracted, which may require a radical alveolectomy to provide primary closure. If a dental abscess is present, endodontic therapy is necessary. Most of these procedures can be performed during the week before therapy begins. However, when surgical treatment is done to eliminate an infection, chemotherapy and head and neck radiotherapy should be delayed for at least 1 week, but 2 weeks are preferred.

If dental treatment would delay chemotherapy, and the patient's condition is grave, the hemoncologist may begin the chemotherapeutic regimen immediately. Any necessary dental treatment may be delayed until the patient is between courses of chemotherapy and hematologic values permit. If a potential source of infection is present, prophylactic antibiotics may be administered to decrease the chance of infection in the patient who is myelosuppressed.

Prevention of oral complications during cancer therapy

Proper oral health care is important for patients undergoing cancer treatment. When oral health is neglected, the oral complications resulting from chemotherapy will be more severe and may compromise the treatment and prognosis of the patient.

Good oral hygiene and elimination of existing or potential sources of infection or irritation will minimize mucositis, infection, hemorrhage, xerostomia, neurologic disorders, and nutritional problems.[21,25] When oral complications from chemotherapy and head and neck radiation therapy are minimized, the clinician can help patients by prolonging and improving the quality of their lives.

Prevention for patients who have received cancer therapy

Posttreatment dental management of the patient is essential. Normally, the dental procedures that were postponed can now be performed and function can be restored.

Posttreatment management should be directed at minimizing recurrent disease, providing palliation, and improving the patient's quality of life.[21,25]

HIV INFECTION: PREVENTION OF ORAL COMPLICATIONS

For optimal preventive oral health care, the physician should recommend dental consultation after HIV infection has been determined.[30] Because many of the orofacial manifestations of HIV infections are treatable, dental consultation should also be sought promptly when these conditions develop.

The HIV-infected patient should have a comprehensive dental evaluation that includes complete radiographic data. Particular attention should be given to detecting the presence of orofacial manifestations associated with HIV infection. The most common of these HIV-related oral diseases are candidiasis, hairy leukoplakia, Kaposi's sarcoma, oral warts, HIV-related gingivitis and periodontal diseases, xerostomia, chronic recurrent *Herpes simplex* infections, *Varicella zoster,* bacterial infections, and nonspecific oral ulcers.[13,38]

Timing or extent of the treatment plan may need to be modified according to the immunologic and hematologic status and general medical condition of the patient. Appropriate emergency treatment should be rendered and pain relieved at all times.

All existing acute and chronic infection, as well as all potential sources of infection, should be eliminated where possible. Gingivitis and periodontal disease should be expeditiously treated in an attempt to prevent the rapid form of periodontal destruction that often occurs in HIV-infected individuals.

HIV-infected patients should be told about the necessity of continued dental care, with particular emphasis on the possibility of acceleration of dental disease because of their immunocompromised state. Patients or their caregivers may be taught to perform periodic orofacial examinations and be encouraged to contact the dentist whenever signs and symptoms of HIV-associated oral disease occur.

REFERENCES

1. Antrim DD, Bakland LK, Parker MW: Treatment of endodontic urgent care cases, *Dent Clin North Am,* 30(3):549-572, 1986.
2. Barrington EP, Nevins M: Diagnosing periodontal diseases, *J Am Dent Assoc* 121:460-464, 1990.
3. Blain SM, Trask PA: Dental caries. In Hudson TW, et al, editors: *Clinical preventive medicine: health promotion and disease prevention,* Boston, 1988, Little, Brown.
4. Centers for Disease Control: Fluoridation census—1985, Washington, DC, 1988, Center for Preventive Services.
5. Cioffi GA, Terezhalmy GT, Taybos GM: Total joint replacement: a consideration for antimicrobial prophylaxis, *Oral Surg Oral Med Oral Pathol* 66:124-129, 1988.
6. Colvard M, Kuo P: Managing aphthous ulcers, *J Am Dent Assoc* 122:51-53, 1991.
7. Dajani AS et al: Prevention of bacterial endocarditis: recommendations by the American Heart Association, *J Am Dent Assoc* 264(22):2919-2922, 1990.

8. Dzink JL, Socransky SS, Haffajee AD: The predominant cultivable microbiota active and inactive lesions of obstructive periodontal disease, *J Clin Periodontol* 15:316-322, 1988.

9. Ferguson CD, Terezhalmy GT: Orolabial herpetic infections, *US Navy Med* 73(6):22-24, 1982.

10. Genco RJ: Pathogenesis of periodontal disease: new concepts, *J Can Dent Assoc* 5:391-396, 1984.

11. Glass RL: The First International Conference on the Declining Prevalence of Dental Caries, *J Dent Res* 61:1301, 1982.

12. Green JC, Louie R, Wycolf SJ: Preventive dentistry. In Lawrence RS, Goldbloom RB, editors: *Preventive disease—beyond the rhetoric,* New York, 1990, Springer-Verlag.

13. Greenspan D, Greenspan JS: Management of the oral lesions of HIV infection, *J Am Dent Assoc* 122:26-32, 1991.

14. Hirsch MS, Schooley RT: Treatment of herpesvirus infections (first of two parts), *N Engl J Med* 309(16):963-970, 1983.

15. Hirsch MS, Schooley RT: Treatment of herpesvirus infections (second of two parts), *N Engl J Med* (17):1034-1039, 1983.

16. Kawashima Z, Pineda LFR: Replanting avulsed primary teeth, *J Am Dent Assoc* 123:90-92, 1992.

17. Konzelman JL, Terezhalmy GT: Xerostomia: diagnosis and treatment, *US Navy Med* 74:16-18, 1983.

18. Listgarten MA: Pathogenesis of periodontitis, *J Clin Periodont* 13:418-422, 1986.

19. Lundeed RC, Langlais RP, Terezhalmy GT: Sunscreen protection for lip mucosa: a review and update, *J Am Dent Assoc* 111:617-621, 1985.

20. MacFarlane GE, Terezhalmy GT: Actinic cheilitis: diagnosis, prevention, and treatment, *US Navy Med* 73(6):22-24, 1982.

21. Marciani RD, Ownby HE: Treating patients before and after irradiation, *J Am Dent Assoc* 123:108-112, 1992.

22. McDonald RE, Avery DR: *Dentistry for the child and adolescent,* ed 3, St Louis, 1978, Mosby.

23. Milman N, Scheibel J, Jessen O: Lysine prophylaxis in recurrent herpes simplex labialis: a double-blind controlled crossover study, *Acta Derm Venereal (Stockh)* 60:85-87, 1980.

24. Mintzer MA: Mechanism of fluoride action: effect on microbes. In *A symposium: insights into the caries process and the role of fluorides,* 1982, Procter & Gamble.

25. Naylor GD, Terezhalmy GT: Oral complications of cancer chemotherapy: prevention and management, *Special Care in Dentistry,* July-August:150, 1988.

26. Newburn E: Preventing dental caries: current and prospective strategies, *J Am Dent Assoc* 123:68-73, 1992.

27. Otis LL, Terezhalmy GT: The granulocytopenic patient: another consideration for antimicrobial prophylaxis, *Oral Surg Oral Med Oral Pathol* 60(1):125-129, 1985.

28. Rodu B, Mattingly G: Oral mucosal ulcers; diagnosis and management, *J Am Dent Assoc* 123:83-86, 1992.

29. Rosenstein DI, Chiodo GT, Bartley MH: Treating recurrent aphthous ulcers in patients with AIDS, *J Am Dent Assoc* 122:64-68, 1991.

30. Schulten EAJM, ten Kate RW, van der Waal I: The impact of oral examination on the Centers for Disease Control classification of subjects with human immunodeficiency virus infection, *Arch Intern Med* 150:1259-1261, 1990.

31. Ship JA, Fox PC, Baum BJ: How much saliva is enough? "Normal" function defined, *J Am Dent Assoc* 122:63-69, 1991.

32. Slots J et al: The occurrence of actinobacillus actinomycetemcomitans, bacteroides intermedius in destructive periodontal disease in adults, *J Clin Periodontol* 13:570-579, 1986.

33. Taybos GM, Terezhalmy GT: Clinical diagnosis and treatment of stomatitis, *US Navy Med* 73:17-19, 1982.

34. Taybos GM, Terezhalmy GT: Glossodynia: diagnosis and treatment, *US Navy Med* 74:18-19, 1983.

35. Terezhalmy GT, Bottomley WK, Pellen GB: The use of water-soluble bioflavonoid-ascorbic acid complex in the treatment of recurrent herpes labialis, *Oral Surg Oral Med Oral Pathol* 45(1):56-62, 1978.

36. Terezhalmy GT, Hall EH: The asplenic patient: a consideration for antimicrobial prophylaxis, *Oral Surg Oral Med Oral Pathol* 57(1):114-117, 1984.

37. Tyler MT, Terezhalmy GT: Diagnosis and treatment of recurrent aphthous stomatitis, *US Navy Med* 72:26-28, 1981.

38. Wolford DT, Miller RL: Acquired immune deficiency syndrome (AIDS): disease characteristics and oral manifestations, *J Am Dent Assoc* 111:258-261, 1985.

━━━━━━━━━━ **RESOURCES** ━━━━━━━━━━

University of California at San Francisco, School of Dentistry, Division of Oral Medicine, Box 0432, San Francisco, CA, 94143.

Indiana University, School of Dentistry, Graduate Division, Department of Dental Diagnostic Science, 1121 West Michigan St, Indianapolis, IN, 46202.

National Institute of Dental Research, Building 31, Room 2C35, NIH, Bethesda, MD, 20892. Chief, Public Information and Reports Section, Office of Planning, Evaluation and Communication.

University of Pennsylvania, School of Dental Medicine, Department of Advanced Dental Education, 4001 Spruce St, Philadelphia, PA, 19004-6003.

University of Washington, School of Dentistry, Department of Oral Medicine, SC-63, Seattle, WA, 98195.

University of Iowa, College of Dentistry, Dental Science Building, Iowa City, Iowa, 52242.

University of Texas at San Antonio, Graduate Division, School of Dentistry, Department of Dental Diagnostic Science, 7703 Floyd Curl Drive, San Antonio, TX, 78284.

The Cleveland Clinic Foundation, Department of Dentistry, Section of Oral Medicine, 9500 Euclid Ave, Desk A-70, Cleveland, OH, 44195.

Part XII

PREVENTION IN THE HOME AND WORKPLACE

Chapter 62

INDUSTRIAL HYGIENE AND SAFETY IN THE WORKPLACE

Peter L. Lubs

OVERVIEW OF INDUSTRIAL HYGIENE AND SAFETY

Industrial hygiene (IH) and safety are a combination of science and art that involves anticipation, recognition, evaluation, and control of workplace stresses and behavioral stresses that may cause injury, illness, impaired health and well being, or significant discomfort and inefficiency to workers or the community.

Overall, accidents were the fourth leading cause of death in 1988. In 1990 workplace accidents caused some 10,500 deaths and 1.8 million disabling injuries and cost $63.8 billion dollars.[1] Some 280,000 workplace illnesses were reported in 1989. The most common illnesses were repeated trauma disorders, skin diseases, respiratory conditions caused by toxic agents, physical agent disorders, and poisonings.[1] Although these figures are a major improvement over the last 50 years, they are still a very significant concern because of the suffering and cost, which warrant continuing improvement in systems and programs to further reduce workplace injuries and illnesses.

An industrial hygienist is a person with a college or university degree or degrees in industrial hygiene, engineering, chemistry, physics, medicine, or related physical and biological sciences who, by virtue of special studies and training, has acquired competence in industrial hygiene. In addition, to become a Certified Industrial Hygienist, applicants must have at least 5 years of full-time employment in the professional practice of industrial hygiene and successfully complete written examinations in both core knowledge and either comprehensive practice or a specialized industrial hygiene aspect, such as engineering or toxicology. Each Certified Industrial Hygienist must maintain his or her professional qualifications in a continuing program of certification maintenance.[5]

The industrial hygiene and safety role is filled most effectively through an interdisciplinary or team approach. At larger companies this involves communication and discussion of concerns with management and employees as well as with other professions including medicine, health physics, engineering, toxicology, epidemiology, chemistry (IH laboratory), and training/communication. Although these relationships may vary depending on the specific project, interaction of the team is important not only in resolving specific problems, but also in developing improved health and safety programs and systems.

Industrial hygiene and safety process

The industrial hygiene and safety process involves anticipation and recognition of stresses and accidents, evaluation or analysis of the magnitude of the stress as well as the causes of the accidents, and then the development of corrective measures to control health and safety hazards by either reducing or eliminating the exposures.

The typical IH and safety process includes consideration of chemical, physical, biologic, and ergonomic stresses. Chemical stresses include gases, vapors, dusts, mists, fibers, and other chemical agents. Physical stresses include, most commonly, noise, radiation, and heat stress. Biological stresses include bacteria and viruses, such as *Legionnella,* hepatitis B, and human immunodeficiency virus, that might be encountered in the workplace. Ergonomic stresses involve human considerations such as workplace design, biomechanics, fatigue, shift work, and repetitive motion.

Recognition. Stresses are recognized by a combination of techniques. Approaches may include a chemical and physical inventory of the facility, an initial inspection or walk-through survey, consideration of available hazard communication information, discussions with employees and management, and a review of previous injuries and illnesses.

Evaluation. Once the hazards have been identified, a qualitative workplace evaluation is performed to assess risk. In addition, this step may include quantification of the hazard as well as analysis of the causes of injuries and illnesses. Quantification may be accomplished by both area and personal monitoring in the workplace.

Once the concentration has been determined, many companies computerize their data to facilitate further analysis of the information as well as to help in communication of the data to employees and management.

The desired evaluation approach is to develop a routine preventive industrial hygiene sampling schedule for most facilities, rather than monitoring only during emergencies or when employees complain or are ill. In this manner, elevated exposures may be reduced before illnesses or other medical complaints or symptoms arise.

Accident data is analyzed to determine information about injuries and illnesses, such as the nature of the injury/illness, the body part affected, the job being performed, the accident description, contributing factors, the employee's experience performing the job, and the time and date of the accident. The analysis also provides information to determine what actions should be taken to eliminate or reduce the number and severity of similar accidents.

Control. If the exposures and analysis do indicate excessive levels of a material, attempts are made to reduce and thereby control the hazard. Many different control methods are employed to reduce or eliminate the exposure, including substitution of another less hazardous material, isolation of the process, local or general ventilation or other engineering improvements, and personal hygiene and sanitation.

Industrial hygiene and safety reviews of new plant or process designs or modifications are excellent opportunities to incorporate good control techniques before the facility is built or redesigned. Once the control strategy has been implemented and integrated into operating plans, a follow-up evaluation is conducted to ensure that the control techniques are effective.

Regulatory agencies and standards

The regulatory agency responsible for oversight of safety and health activities in the workplace is the Occupational Safety and Health Administration (OSHA) in Washington, D.C. Its purpose is to ensure, as far as possible, that every working man and woman in the nation has safe and healthful working conditions. OSHA was established by the Occupational Safety and Health Act of 1970 and is part of the Department of Labor. It is responsible for setting and enforcing workplace safety and health standards. Although OSHA has promulgated specific standards for

specific issues and chemicals, the General Duty Clause of the OSH Act requires that each employer furnish a place of employment that is free from recognized hazards that are causing or are likely to cause death or serious physical harm to its employees.

Recently, the OSHA maximum penalty has increased from $10,000 to $70,000 per violation, and OSHA has proposed numerous penalties that have exceeded $1 million and have increased the interest and concern of business.

In addition to its national headquarters in Washington, D.C., OSHA has established 10 regional offices throughout the country (see the box on p. 1149), with area offices in each region. OSHA also encourages the states to assume responsibility for safety and health. Many states have chosen to submit a state plan to OSHA for approval and, as of December, 1991, some 23 states and territories have approved plans, as listed in the box on p. 1149.

These states administer their own safety and health programs and receive funding of up to 50% from the federal government. If the programs in these states become ineffective, OSHA has the right to withdraw its approval and assume jurisdiction for safety and health concerns. General OSHA requirements for employers include the information in the box on p. 1149.

The National Institute for Occupational Safety and Health (NIOSH) was established by the OSH Act of 1970 and is currently part of the Department of Health and Human Services. It is responsible for research on the health effects of exposures in the workplace and provides training and information to workers and employers. NIOSH also conducts workplace health hazard evaluations upon request by management or labor.

Professional associations

The national professional association of industrial hygienists is the American Industrial Hygiene Association (AIHA), with over 11,000 members. It publishes the *AIHA Journal* and various publications, cosponsors a yearly conference, and offers numerous IH-related courses. Similarly, the American Society of Safety Engineers (ASSE) is the national professional organization of safety engineers, with over 20,000 members. It publishes *Professional Safety* as well as other publications and offers related educational courses. There are numerous local AIHA sections and ASSE councils throughout the United States and in several additional countries. These sections and councils normally meet on a routine basis to hear speakers on IH and safety-related topics.

The American Board of Industrial Hygiene conducts certification examinations for industrial hygiene and provides for maintenance of the certificate. There are more than 3000 certified IHs who may use the Certified Industrial Hygienist or CIH designation. The Board of Certified Safety Professionals conducts certification examinations

---

Regional OSHA offices

Region I: Connecticut, Maine, Massachusetts, New Hampshire, Rhode Island, Vermont

133 Portland St., First floor, Boston, MA 02114.

Region II: New York, New Jersey, Puerto Rico

201 Varick St., Room 670, New York, NY 10014.

Region III: Delaware, District of Columbia, Maryland, Pennsylvania, Virginia, West Virginia

Gateway Bldg., Suite 2100, 3535 Market St., Philadelphia, PA 19104.

Region IV: Alabama, Florida, Georgia, Kentucky, Mississippi, North Carolina, South Carolina, Tennessee

1375 Peachtree St., N.E., Suite 587, Atlanta, GA 30367.

Region V: Illinois, Indiana, Minnesota, Michigan, Ohio, Wisconsin

Room 3244, 230 S Dearborn St., Chicago, IL 60604.

Region VI: Arkansas, Louisiana, New Mexico, Oklahoma, Texas

525 Griffin St., Room 602, Dallas, TX 75202.

Region VII: Iowa, Kansas, Missouri, Nebraska

911 Walnut St., Room 406, Kansas City, MO 64106.

Region VIII: Colorado, Montana, North Dakota, South Dakota, Utah, Wyoming

Federal Office Bldg., Room 1576, 1961 Stout St., Denver, CO 80294.

Region IX: Arizona, California, Hawaii, Nevada, Guam, American Samoa, Trust Territories of the Pacific Islands

71 Stevenson St., Fourth floor, Suite 420, San Francisco, CA 94105.

Region X: Washington, Oregon, Idaho, Alaska

1111 Third Ave., Suite 715, Seattle, WA 98101-3212.

OSHA approved state and territory plans

Alaska	Michigan	Tennessee
Arizona	Minnesota	Utah
California	Nevada	Vermont
Hawaii	New Mexico	Virginia
Indiana	North Carolina	Virgin Islands
Iowa	Oregon	Washington
Kentucky	Puerto Rico	Wyoming
Maryland	South Carolina	

General OSHA requirements for employers

1. Posting of the OSHA job safety and health protection poster (#2203) in the workplace.
2. Maintaining occupational injury and illness records, including the OSHA Form 200 annual summary (this must also be posted in the workplace beginning no later than February 1 and continuing until March 1 of the following year) and the supplementary record (on OSHA Form 101 or equivalent) for each case. OSHA recordable cases include workplace:
   - Fatalities
   - Illnesses
   - Injuries, if they
     - Require medical treatment or
     - Involve loss of consciousness or
     - Involve restriction of work/motion or
     - Involve transfer to another job[22]

   Physicians or medical personnel may be involved in the determination of recordability of workplace injuries as well as the maintenance of such records.
3. Notifying OSHA within 48 hours of an employment accident that is fatal to one or more employees or that results in the hospitalization of five or more employees. OSHA has recently proposed that this be reduced to notification within 8 hours for either case above and has also proposed that notification be required for hospitalization of three or more employees, although these new requirements have not yet been finalized. Physicians and medical personnel may be involved in notification of OSHA in such cases.

In addition, employers must also comply with the OSHA safety and health regulations (general industry, agriculture, construction, or maritime standards) specific to their workplace.

---

for safety. There are more than 9000 certified safety professionals who may use the Certified Safety Professional or CSP designation.

The American Conference of Governmental Industrial Hygienists is composed of IHs with government or educational institution affiliation. They sponsor the committee that publishes the Threshold Limit Values (TLVs). In addition, they cosponsor a yearly conference with AIHA and publish the *Applied Occupational and Environmental Hygiene Journal*.

The National Safety Council, with more than 20,000 members, is a nonprofit organization involved in accident prevention. In addition to sponsoring the yearly National Safety Congress and Exposition, it also offers numerous safety-related services and publications.

Industrial hygiene and safety assistance

Industrial hygiene assistance may be obtained through the American Industrial Hygiene Association consultants listing that is published in the *AIHA Journal* twice a year. Safety assistance may be obtained through the *National*

Directory of Safety Consultants, which is published by the American Society of Safety Engineers. In addition, the National Safety Council provides a consulting service in safety and health management.

Also, free on-site safety and health consultation is available in all states. This service is generally delivered by state government agencies and funded substantially by federal OSHA. They typically do not issue citations, propose penalties, or provide information about the workplace to the federal inspection staff unless imminent danger conditions are discovered, in which case the condition must be resolved immediately. Those interested in this approach should contact the local, area, or regional OSHA office for direction to the nearest OSHA consultative program.

In addition, many workers compensation carriers and insurance companies conduct safety and health inspections and provide related services for their customers. A university or college in the area also may have a health or safety program that may provide consulting services.

HAZARD COMMUNICATION

Environmental stresses are recognized through a combination of techniques. Approaches may include:

- Chemical and physical inventory of the facility
- General description of the operation or process
- Review or description of the various jobs and activities
- Initial inspection or walk-through survey
- Review of previous injuries and illnesses (such as the OSHA 200 log and supplemental record)
- Review of available hazard communication information
- Discussions or interviews with employees and management

The Occupational Safety and Health Administration Hazard Communication Standard[12] was published in 1983 and became effective in November of 1985. It requires chemical manufacturers and importers to evaluate the hazards of the chemicals they produce or import and to forward information on hazardous materials to their customers. This information must be communicated to affected employees by the use of container labels, material safety data sheets, and employee training.

OSHA has classified hazardous materials into two categories—health hazards and physical hazards. These health and physical hazard classes are listed in the box above.[12] OSHA health hazards are those chemicals for which there is statistically significant evidence, based on at least one study conducted in accordance with established scientific principles, that acute or chronic health effects may occur in exposed workers. Likewise, OSHA physical hazards are chemicals for which there is scientifically valid evidence that they meet the criteria for any of the specific classes shown in the box above. The specific health hazard defini-

OSHA health and physical hazard classes[12]	
Health hazards	*Physical hazards*
Carcinogen	Combustible liquid
Corrosive	Compressed gas
Highly toxic	Explosive
Toxic	Flammable
Irritant	Organic peroxide
Sensitizer	Oxidizer
Hepatotoxin	Pyrophoric
Nephrotoxin	Unstable (reactive)
Neurotoxin	Water-reactive
Hematopoietic system agent	
Reproductive toxin	
Lung toxin	
Skin hazard	
Eye hazard	

tions given in the OSHA Hazard Communication Standard[12] are less precise and more subjective than the physical hazard definitions.

The regulation automatically includes as hazardous chemicals those materials that appear on the OSHA Permissible Exposure Limit[11] and the ACGIH Threshold Limit Values[4] listings. Also, carcinogens that are listed in the National Toxicology Program Annual Report on Carcinogens,[19] the International Agency for Research on Cancer Monographs,[16] or OSHA 29CFR 1910.1000 Subpart Z[11] are automatically included as health hazards. The OSHA carcinogen standards are listed in Table 62-1. Other chemicals or mixtures that do not appear on these lists must be evaluated by criteria in the regulation to determine whether they are hazardous.

The National Toxicology Program Annual Report on Carcinogens is published by the U.S. Department of Health and Human Services. The evaluation and listing of chemicals as carcinogens in the annual report are performed by scientists from the National Toxicology Program and other federal health research and regulatory agencies. The report categorizes substances into two groups: known carcinogens (human studies) or substances reasonably anticipated (human or animal studies) to be carcinogens. Many of the National Toxicology Program substances have been chosen from the International Agency for Research on Cancer (IARC) monographs. IARC is part of the World Health Organization, and the monographs constitute a program beginning in 1969 to evaluate the carcinogenic risk of substances to humans. As of 1992, some 52 IARC monographs have been published. Each monograph is the product of a working group of experts (usually international) in chemical carcinogenesis and related fields. Although industry experts do participate, the primary participants are individuals with government and uni-

Table 62-1. OSHA cancer regulations

CFR 29 reference	Material
1910.1001	Asbestos
1910.1003	4-Nitrobiphenyl
1910.1004	Alpha-Naphthylamine
1910.1006	Methyl chloromethyl ether
1910.1007	3,3'-Dichlorobenzidine (and its salts)
1910.1008	Bis-chloromethyl ether
1910.1009	Beta-naphthylamine
1910.1010	Benzidine
1910.1011	4-Aminodiphenyl
1910.1012	Ethyleneimine
1910.1013	Beta-propiolactone
1910.1014	2-Acetylaminofluorene
1910.1015	4-Dimethylaminoazobenzene
1910.1016	N-nitrosodimethylamine
1910.1017	Vinyl chloride
1910.1018	Inorganic arsenic
1910.1028	Benzene
1910.1029	Coke oven emissions
1910.1044	1,2-Dibromo-3-chloropropane
1910.1045	Acrylonitrile
1910.1047	Ethylene oxide
1910.1048	Formaldehyde

Information required in material safety data sheet[12]

- Identity of material used on the label
- Chemical and common name of hazardous ingredients above 1% or 0.1% for carcinogens
- Physical and chemical characteristics (e.g., vapor pressure, flash point)
- Physical hazards (e.g., potential for fire, explosion, reactivity)
- Health hazards (including signs/symptoms of exposure and medical conditions aggravated by exposure)
- Primary route(s) of entry into the body
- Recommended exposure limits (OSHA, ACGIH, etc.)
- Safe handling procedures
- Control measures (e.g., engineering controls, work practices, and personal protective equipment)
- Emergency and first aid procedures
- Preparation date
- Responsible party identification (name, address, telephone number)

---

versity affiliation. The IARC monographs currently categorize substances into the following groups:

Group 1—Human carcinogens
Group 2A—Probable human carcinogens
Group 2B—Possible human carcinogens
Group 3—Not classifiable as to human carcinogenicity
Group 4—Probably not a human carcinogen

Substances falling into Groups 1, 2A, and 2B are automatically considered carcinogens under the OSHA Hazard Communication Standard.

Material safety data sheets

Chemical producers must develop a material safety data sheet (MSDS) on every hazardous chemical they manufacture. This must be distributed to each customer, and each employer must make them readily accessible to all employees. No one form or format is required, although OSHA has issued a nonmandatory sample material safety data sheet, form 174.[20] However, each MSDS must contain the components listed in the box above.[12]

Although the OSHA nonmandatory MSDS sample is a two-page form, many companies generate their MSDSs by computer, and some now exceed six pages.

Trade-secret provisions enable manufacturers, importers, or employers to withhold the specific chemical identity from the MSDS if the company can support a trade-secret claim. However, in a medical emergency, the company must immediately submit the specific chemical identity to the treating physician or nurse, regardless of the existence of a written statement of need of a confidentiality agreement. In nonemergency situations, the company must disclose the chemical identity, on request, to a health professional (physician, industrial hygienist, toxicologist, nurse, epidemiologist, etc.) if the request is in writing and describes the occupational health reason for the information. In this case, the health professional would need to sign and comply with the company's written confidentiality agreement restricting the use of the information to occupational health purposes only.

Because every employer must provide an MSDS and all the required information listed in the box above on each hazardous chemical to their affected employees, physicians can obtain them from the employee or company if they suspect possible occupational exposure of a patient. Because MSDSs summarize the available health information on the chemical and list the ingredients of the material, it is a worthwhile document for physicians or health professionals to review in an attempt to determine whether certain materials may be linked to certain symptoms or conditions in patients. Often, the employee can obtain the MSDSs in question. If not, the physician should contact the company to obtain the MSDS and related information. As previously explained, even trade-secret information is available to a health professional. When the company resists sending the MSDS to the treating physician or health professional, the local area OSHA office should be contacted for assistance.

The new draft American National Standards Institute (ANSI) Standard Z400.1 for the Preparation of Material

Safety Data Sheets[9] explains in detail how to prepare an MSDS. The Chemical Manufacturers Association served as the secretariat to ANSI for the development of this voluntary standard. It is currently being reviewed, and the final standard is expected to be available by ANSI in mid-1992.[9]

Labels

OSHA requires that each container of hazardous chemicals leaving the workplace be labeled with the following:

- Identity of the hazardous chemical
- Appropriate hazard warning
- Name and address of the chemical manufacturer, importer, or responsible party[12]

The name on the container may be the chemical, common, or trade name. However, the name used on the container must be the same as the name used on the MSDS to enable an employee to locate the MSDS for a material he or she encounters in the workplace.

The type of hazard warning information and the label format are not specified by OSHA. The purpose of the label is to identify the container and provide a summary of hazard information for employees or users of the material. Detailed information can be found in the MSDS. Guidance for labeling is given in the American National Standards

Institute Standard for Hazardous Industrial Chemicals— Precautionary Labeling Z129.1,[6] which was sponsored by the Chemical Manufacturers Association. The ANSI Z129.1 standard uses signal words (Danger, Warning, Caution), statements of hazards, precautionary measures, and instructions in case of contact or exposure, and includes numerous examples of each. This voluntary standard is the basis for most labeling in use in the United States.

In addition, two numerical warning or labeling systems are used widely. These systems are the National Fire Protection Association (NFPA) Recommended System for the Identification of the Fire Hazards of Materials #704[15] and the National Paint and Coatings Association Hazardous Materials Information System (HMIS).[18] HMIS materials are copyrighted by the National Paint and Coatings Association and are available from Labelmaster/American Labelmark Company. These both use an easily visible color-coded warning system. The NFPA system is in the form of a diamond (Fig. 62-1), and the HMIS uses bars (Fig. 62-2). Each has a blue health section, a red fire or flammability section, and a yellow reactivity section. Warnings are presented using numbers from 0 to 4, with 0 presenting no hazard and 4 presenting the worst or highest hazard. The NFPA rating represents the health, fire, and reactivity hazards in the case of a fire, and the HMIS rating represents

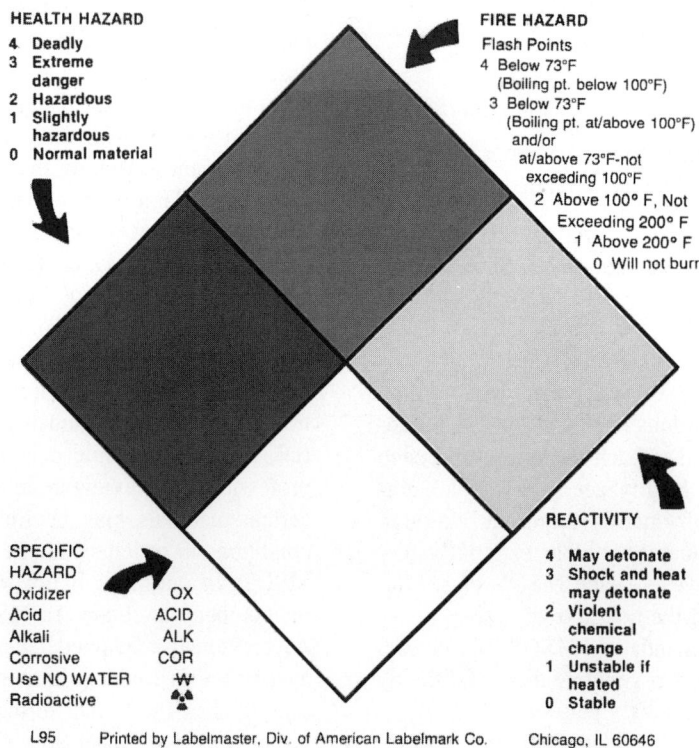

Fig. 62-1. NFPA warning label. The label contains a blue health hazard section, a red fire hazard section, and a yellow reactivity section to which numbers from 0 to 4 are added corresponding to the hazard of the specific chemical. (From Labelmaster, American Labelmark Co.)

normal-use conditions. The HMIS health rating represents acute toxicity, and use of an asterisk indicates that a chronic health hazard may be present. The NFPA system, however, does not attempt to identify chronic health hazards. The NFPA label warning system is widely available through most chemical supply companies and label/sign supply companies, and the HMIS system is available through Labelmaster/American Labelmark Company.

Employee training

The third component of a hazard communication program is to provide routine employee training on the hazardous chemicals in use in the workplace. This should include information about:

- OSHA Hazard Communication Standard
- Labeling system used
- MSDS system (location, how to access, terminology, etc.)
- Specific hazardous chemical information in the employee's work area
- Methods to detect the presence or release of a hazardous chemical (such as odor or an industrial hygiene monitoring technique)

- Safe work practices
- Emergency procedures
- Personal protective equipment

EVALUATION

Evaluation is the process resulting in a decision about the hazard existing in a process or operation. The evaluation phase may involve various assessments of employee exposure ranging from a simple qualitative evaluation to a comprehensive industrial hygiene monitoring strategy.

Exposure assessment

To develop an industrial hygiene monitoring scheme, the qualitative information may be prioritized to determine which chemicals or employees should be monitored. This process typically considers the toxicity of the chemical, the employee exposure to the chemical, and the frequency of use of the material. The toxicity factor describes the health hazard of a chemical, incorporating both acute and chronic effects. The exposure factor describes the employee exposure to each chemical and can be gathered by reviewing previous industrial hygiene data or by the use of models. When no data are available, a professional industrial hygienist and/or a survey of employees can produce

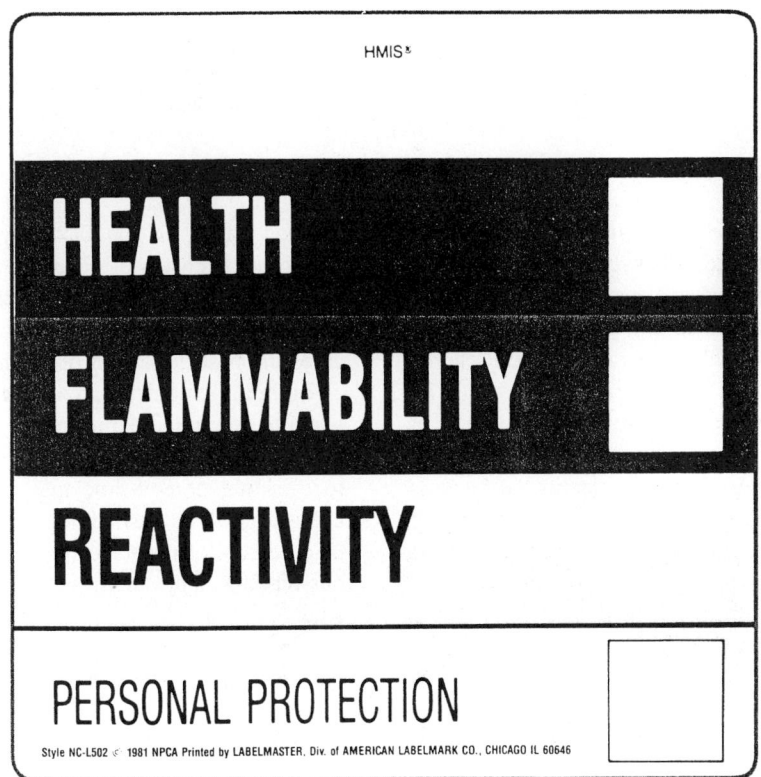

Fig. 62-2. HMIS warning label. The label contains a blue health section, a red flammability section, and a yellow reactivity section to which numbers from 0 to 4 are added corresponding to the hazard of the specific chemical. (From Labelmaster, American Labelmark Co.)

Table 62-2. Hazard prioritization scheme

Exposure factor × toxicity factor × frequency factor = hazard rating*

Exposure factor	Toxicity factor	Frequency factor
1 No exposure (e.g., less than 1% of exposure limit**) 1	Minimal (e.g., no risk to health) 1	No use (e.g., used less than 1 day per year) 1
2 Minimal exposure (e.g., 1%-10% of exposure limit) 2	Slight (e.g., irritation or minor reversible effect) 2	Minimal use (e.g., infrequent contact, such as once per month) 2
3 Moderate exposure (e.g., 10%-75% of exposure limit) 3	Moderate (e.g., minor effect may occur) 3	Moderate use (e.g., moderate contact, such as once per week) 3
4 High exposure (e.g., 75%-125% of exposure limit) 4	High (e.g., major effect) 4	High use (e.g., frequent contact, such as once per day) 4
5 Extreme exposure (e.g., greater than 125% of exposure limit) 5	Extreme/severe (e.g., dangerous to life/health from single exposure) 5	Maximum use (e.g., very frequent contact, such as greater than once per day) 5

Score	Rating
1-25	Minimal hazard
26-50	Slight hazard
51-75	Moderate hazard
76-100	High hazard
101-125	Extreme hazard

*Hazard rating is the product of exposure, toxicity, and frequency, which may range from 1 to 125:
**Exposure limit is the exposure limit used as a reference, for example, either the OSHA permissible exposure level or the ACGIH threshold limit value.

information that may be used to estimate various exposures. The frequency factor describes the frequency of employee exposure to a chemical and may be listed in number of days per year the chemical is used. One example of a formal simplified hazard ranking or prioritization scheme is shown in Table 62-2. A separate hazard rating would be determined for each chemical and for each employee or employee grouping.

The result of this process is a prioritization of hazards that will help to determine the necessity to perform IH monitoring and, if performed, the degree of attention and resources to assign to the chemical. For example, a chemical with a moderate hazard might be monitored within a year, but an extreme hazard would be monitored within a month.

When a formal prioritization is not performed, an informal determination should be made by a health professional based on such factors as employee complaints, housekeeping, and odors that may become obvious during a walk-through inspection or by reviewing previous IH data.

An industrial hygiene monitoring program is then de-

veloped based on the hazard prioritization/rating or the subjective decision of a health professional based on the qualitative assessment. Both area and personal monitoring techniques may be selected, although personal monitoring gives the best indication of an individual's exposure.

In area monitoring, area industrial hygiene samples are taken to determine exposures in various locations throughout the workplace (Fig. 62-3). This approach may use direct-reading or real-time methods in which the exposure concentration is given immediately. These may be hand-held devices or permanently mounted, fixed-point continuous-reading units with recording capability that alarm when exposure levels reach preset limits. One disadvantage of this technique is that the exposures measured do not necessarily reflect a worker's exposure because he or she may move throughout the whole workplace. Area monitoring is most useful in identifying the source of a leak or upset conditions.

Personal industrial hygiene samples are taken to determine employee exposures and are worn by the employee for the period of interest. The monitor is attached to the

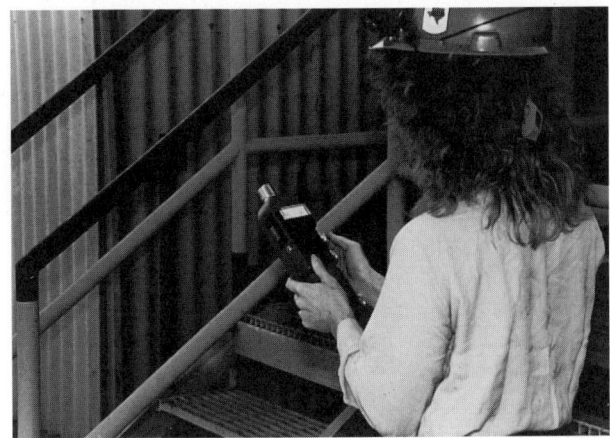

Fig. 62-3. Area industrial hygiene monitoring for noise.

worker near the employee's breathing zone to estimate the concentration of the contaminant being breathed by the worker. Personal monitoring techniques typically include a battery-operated pump worn on the worker's belt and a sample device such as a sorbent (a material used to collect gases or vapors during air sampling by the process of adsorption or absorption) tube to collect gases or vapors or a filter to collect particulates (a particle of solid matter [such as dusts, fumes, or smokes] or liquid matter [such as fogs or mists]) attached to the worker's shirt lapel (Fig. 62-4). The most common sorbent is charcoal, but many others are available, such as silica gel and Tenax. Certain monitoring devices give direct results, but most sampling media are forwarded to an industrial hygiene laboratory for analysis. Laboratories should be selected from those accredited by the American Industrial Hygiene Association and published in their *AIHA Journal*.

Other common personal monitoring devices include charcoal badges for gases (a state of matter in which the material diffuses to distribute itself throughout any container) and vapors (the gaseous form of a substance that is normally a solid or liquid at standard temperature and pressure) (Fig. 62-5) and long-term dosimeters, which may be worn for extended periods and from which the exposure concentration may be directly calculated.

Analytical techniques include gas chromatography for gases and vapors, atomic absorption for metals, and gravimetric analysis for particulates.

Exposure limits

Once the monitoring data have been collected, they are compared with the specific exposure limit to properly evaluate and analyze the exposure. Overexposures require that control measures be implemented or modified to reduce the hazard. The two exposure limits most commonly used in the United States are the OSHA Permissible Exposure Limits (PELs)[11] and the ACGIH Threshold Limit Values

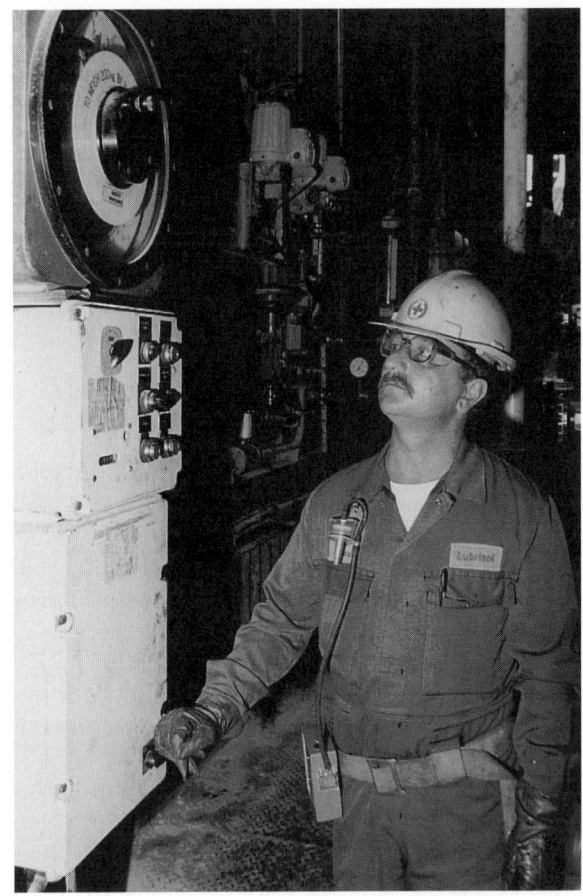

Fig. 62-4. Personal industrial hygiene sampling of particulate in which air is drawn by a battery-operated pump worn on the belt through a cyclone/filter attached to the employee's shirt lapel.

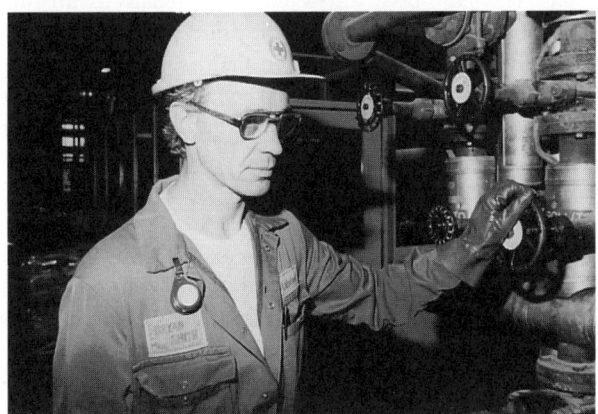

Fig. 62-5. Personal industrial hygiene monitoring using 3M organic vapor badge connected to the employee's shirt lapel.

Table 62-3. Categories of TLVs/PELs[*,4,11]

Category	Name	Definition
TWA	Time-weighted average	Concentration for a normal 8-hour workday (40-hour workweek) to which nearly all workers can be repeatedly exposed without adverse effect TWAs permit excursions above the TLV provided they are compensated by equivalent exposures below the TLV during the workday
STEL	Short-term exposure limit	Concentration to which workers can be exposed continuously for a 15-minute period without suffering an adverse effect; it supplements the TWA for certain chemicals
C	Ceiling	Concentration not to be exceeded during any part of the working exposure

*TLVs, American Conference of Governmental Industrial Hygienist's Threshold Limit Values; PELs, Occupational Safety and Health Administration Permissible Exposure Limits.

(TLVs).[4] The PELs are legally enforceable standards that were first adopted by OSHA in 1971 (from the 1968 TLVs). They have rarely been revised or updated. However, they received a major revision in 1989. The Threshold Limit Values were first adopted in 1946 and are guidelines or recommended limits that are revised and updated periodically by the Chemical Substances TLV Committee of the American Conference of Governmental Industrial Hygienists.[4] This committee is made up of health professionals with government and university affiliation. Industry professionals may participate as consultants to the committee. The TLV booklet is published annually, with supporting documentation for each limit published in the "ACGIH Documentation of Threshold Limit Values and Biological Exposure Indices."[3] Therefore the TLVs have been revised more frequently than the PELs. More than 600 materials have assigned limits, which are typically given in parts per million for gases and vapors and in milligrams per cubic meter for particulates. After the major 1989 updating of the PELs, many of the PEL and TLV concentrations became the same. In addition, some companies have created internal limits for some materials that may differ from their assigned TLV/PEL limit. They may also have limits for materials that have no assigned TLV or PEL. NIOSH has also developed recommended exposure limits for certain materials, and many other bodies (inside and outside the United States) are also involved in development of exposure limits.

Limits are concentrations of materials under which it is believed that nearly all workers may be repeatedly exposed without adverse effect. However, because of wide variation in human susceptibility, a small percentage of workers may experience discomfort and suffer adverse health effects or aggravate preexisting diseases at concentrations below the limit. Therefore some individuals may not be adequately protected even though chemical exposures are at concentrations at or below their assigned limit. The typical categories of limits are defined in Table 62-3, which include time-weighted averages, short-term exposure limits, and ceiling limits.[4]

None of the limits are used universally, and some professionals debate which limits should be used. OSHA inspectors must use their PEL limits for compliance and regulatory purposes. They are probably the least conservative. Most industrial hygiene professionals use the ACGIH TLVs because they have been updated more frequently. The NIOSH RELs and several of the foreign limits are perhaps the most conservative in terms of the actual chemical concentration. The health professional may find it useful to consider several of the limits in his or her evaluation.

Accident analysis

Although a good health and safety process is designed to minimize or prevent accidents, systems must be developed to investigate injuries and illnesses when they do occur. In addition, accidents should be analyzed periodically on a plant-wide and company-wide basis to determine trends and problem areas and to enable management to take corrective actions.

Accidents are defined as unplanned events that can lead to personal injury or illness, property damage, product loss, or environmental release. To evaluate the causes of accidents, they must be promptly and thoroughly investigated to determine the details of the incident. The investigation should be conducted by the local health/safety professional and a member of line management. More serious accidents will include additional members in the investigation, such as the plant engineer, plant manager, and corporate representatives. The information included in the box on p. 1157 is typically gathered during the accident investigation and is used to take corrective actions or institute control measures to prevent similar occurrences.

Information gathered during accident investigations will then be included in a periodic analysis of incidents. Many companies now computerize this information to facilitate the accident analysis. The purpose of the analysis is to provide a systematic formal review of the accident experience to determine accident trends over time and to then assist the business division or plant in setting safety and health goals and in providing guidance in taking proper corrective actions. Typical health/safety analysis of accidents include those factors highlighted in the box on p. 1157.

Many companies measure and report their accident ex-

Information included in accident investigations

Accident type/classification
Department where incident occurred
Accident location
Nature of injury
Date/time of accident, date accident reported
Occupation when injured
Experience on occupation
Regular occupation
Job being performed
Accident sequence
Unsafe act or practice(s)
Unsafe condition(s)
Supervisor's action(s) to prevent similar accident

Accident analysis factors

Severity of accidents
Nature of injury/illness
Body parts affected
Accident type
Occupation of injured
Accident cause
Contributory accident cause
Number of accidents/year of experience
Number of accidents/year in occupation
Injury/illness rates by corporation/division/plant

Control measures

Substitution of less-hazardous materials or equipment
Engineering controls:
    Ventilation
    Process modification
    Isolation of the process
    Wet methods (to reduce dust)
    Process automation or remote control
Work practice/administrative controls:
    Modification of work schedules/rest periods
    Rotation of employees/jobs
Personal hygiene
Personal protective equipment

---

perience in terms of injury/illness rates internally as well as for OSHA recordkeeping purposes. The accidents that result in OSHA-recordable injury and illness cases (previously discussed in Regulatory Agencies and Standards section) and that are placed on the OSHA 200 log are the most serious incidents. For example, fatalities and injuries requiring days away from work for recuperation represent the tip of the iceberg in terms of accidents. Every fatality or serious injury may be preceded by less severe incidents such as first-aid cases, near misses, or property damage incidents that may represent the hidden base of the iceberg. If a company is to evaluate its accident experience accurately and thoroughly, it must also include these less-serious incidents in both its accident-investigation and accident-analysis programs. Companies also report their accident experience to industry associations, such as the Chemical Manufacturers Association, which enables rates to be compared throughout industries.

PERSONAL PROTECTIVE EQUIPMENT AND CONTROLS

The exposure data and accident information is analyzed and is compared with the specific exposure limit of interest. Overexposures warrant application of controls to reduce the exposures to acceptable levels. Other factors, in addition to the monitoring results, should be used to determine whether controls are needed, including employee complaints, injury and illness rates, medical surveillance results, adverse health symptoms, results of accident investigations, and new toxicology information. Once controls have been implemented or modified, the evaluation is performed again periodically to verify that the control measures are effective.

Workplace controls

Several methods of control are commonly used, including engineering controls, work practice or administrative controls, and personal protective equipment as shown in

the box above. The preferable solution to reducing exposures and accidents is to engineer the hazard out of the operation during the design stage before the process is built, or to reengineer the process to reduce the hazard at the source. Work practice or administrative measures control exposures by limiting the time employees spend in the exposure and/or by modifying the job to reduce exposures.

Personal protective equipment is typically used as a last resort to control exposures. This would be used where engineering or other control techniques are not feasible, during the period when engineering controls are being installed, during maintenance operations for which engineering solutions are not possible, and during emergency response operations. Their disadvantage is that removal or failure of the device causes immediate exposure to the hazard.

Respiratory protection

A respirator is a device that covers the mouth and/or the nose to prevent inhalation of hazardous substances.

Respiratory protective device approvals in the United States are issued jointly by the National Institute for Occupational Safety and Health (NIOSH) and the Mine Safety and Health Administration (MSHA). Each approved respi-

---

Components of an effective respirator program[13]

- Written standard operating procedures
- Assignment of a program administrator
- Use of NIOSH/MSHA-approved respirators
- Respiratory selection based on nature of the hazard
- Industrial hygiene monitoring to determine the hazard concentration
- Respirator user training
- Periodic medical surveillance/evaluation[8]
- Proper storage
- Regular inspection/maintenance/cleaning
- Fit testing of users
- Use of type I, grade D breathing air[14]
- Periodic program review/audit

Table 62-4. Color code for cartridges and gas mask canisters*

Atmospheric contaminants to be protected against	Color assigned
Acid gases	White
Organic vapors	Black
Ammonia gas	Green
Carbon monoxide gas	Blue
Acid gases and organic vapors	Yellow
Acid gases, ammonia, and organic vapors	Brown
Acid gases, ammonia, carbon monoxide, and organic vapors	Red
Other vapors and gases not listed above	Olive
Radioactive materials (except tritium and noble gases)	Purple
Dusts, fumes, and mists (other than radioactive materials)	Orange

*Adapted from ANSI K13.1-1973[7]

Notes:

1. A purple stripe shall be used to identify radioactive materials in combination with any vapor or gas.
2. An orange stripe shall be used to identify dusts, fumes, and mists in combination with any vapor or gas.
3. Where labels only are colored to conform with this table, the canister or cartridge body shall be gray, or a metal canister or cartridge body may be left in its natural metallic color.
4. The user shall refer to the wording of the label to determine the type and degree of protection the canister or cartridge will afford.

---

rator will carry the NIOSH/MSHA approval in the form of a label or attachment to the device.

Components of an effective respirator program are listed in the box above.[13]

There are two major types of respiratory protective devices—air purifying and atmosphere supplying. Air-purifying devices simply filter or remove contaminants from the air, and atmosphere-supplying devices supply breathing air to the users.

In choosing the proper respirator, the nature and concentration of the hazard should be assessed. The two types of respiratory hazards are a deficiency of oxygen and the presence of a toxic contaminant (gas/vapor or particulate). Only atmosphere-supplying devices would be used in oxygen-deficient atmospheres, but atmosphere-supplying or air-purifying devices would be used for toxic contaminants, depending on the type and concentration of the contaminant.

Respirator facepieces consist of either a tight-fitting or loose-fitting covering. Tight-fitting facepieces create a tight seal between the facepiece and the user's face and come in the following configurations:

- Quarter mask—covers nose/mouth with lower sealing surface between the mouth and chin.
- Half mask—covers nose/mouth with lower sealing surface under the chin.
- Full mask—seals from hairline to below the chin.

Loose-fitting facepieces such as hoods and helmets do not have a tight seal between the facepiece and the user's face. Loose-fitting facepieces include paint or abrasive blasting hoods. Attached to the facepiece are elements for removing contaminants from the air or hoses to supply respirable air.

Air-purifying devices remove the contaminant by the use of filters or sorbents, but, because they do not supply oxygen, they cannot be used in oxygen-deficient atmospheres. They also cannot be used when the contaminant has poor warning properties (such as odor), because it would not give adequate warning to the user in case of respirator breakthrough or failure. The most common type of respirator is the dust filter, which is a particulate-removing air-purifying device. Air-purifying respirators for gas and vapors typically use either smaller cartridge-sized (Fig. 62-6) or larger canister-sized (Fig. 62-7) sorbents to remove the contaminant by absorption or adsorption. These both come in single-use/disposable or reusable types. A standard color code is used for respirator cartridges and canisters (Table 62-4), which is adopted from ANSI K13.1-1973.[7]

Air-supplying respirators provide breathing air from a source independent of the surrounding atmosphere and deliver the air through a tube or hose to the facepiece. Types of air-supplied respirators include air-line respirators (Fig. 62-8), in which the air is supplied from a remote source (bottled air or a breathing air compressor) through an air line; and self-contained breathing apparatuses (Fig. 62-9), which are carried by the wearer. Compressed air used in air-supply respirators must meet the requirements of the Compressed Gas Association specification CGA G-7.1-1989, grade D air.[14]

Respirator fit testing is a method used to determine the ability of each respirator wearer to obtain a satisfactory fit. Fit testing can be either qualitative or quantitative. Quali-

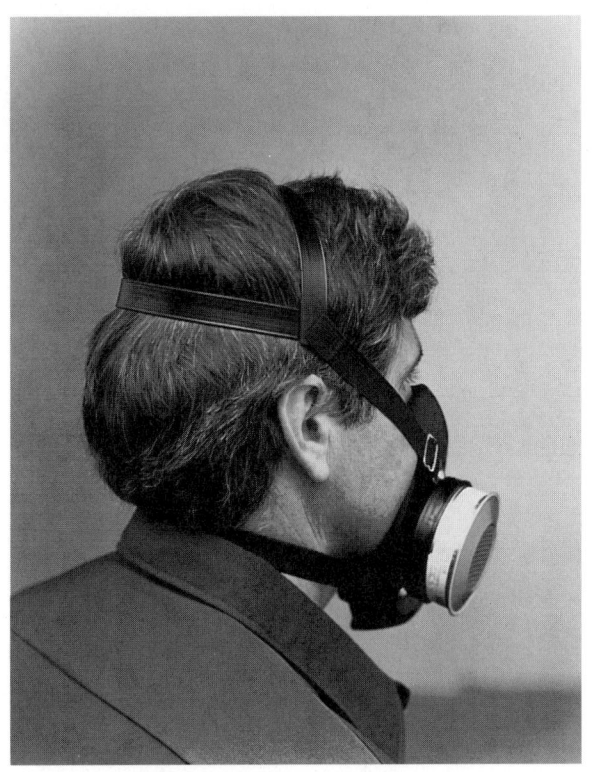

Fig. 62-6. Half-mask cartridge air-purifying respirator. (Courtesy of Mine Safety Appliances Co.)

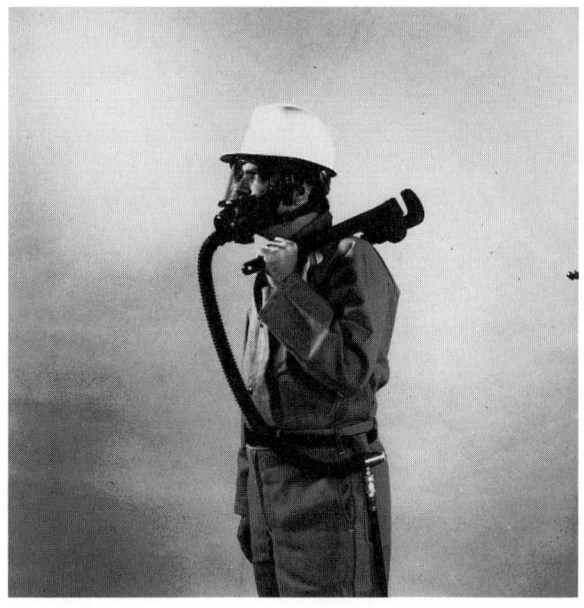

Fig. 62-8. Full facepiece air line atmosphere-supplying respirator. (Courtesy of Mine Safety Appliances Co.)

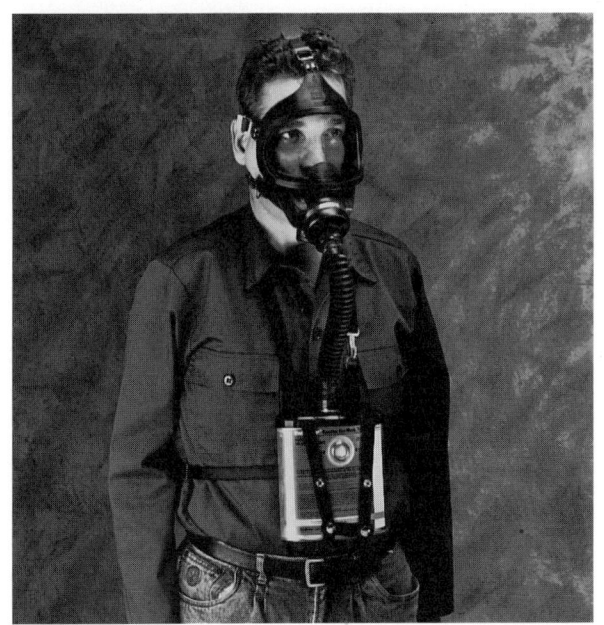

Fig. 62-7. Full facepiece canister (gas mask) air-purifying respirator. (Courtesy of Mine Safety Appliances Co.)

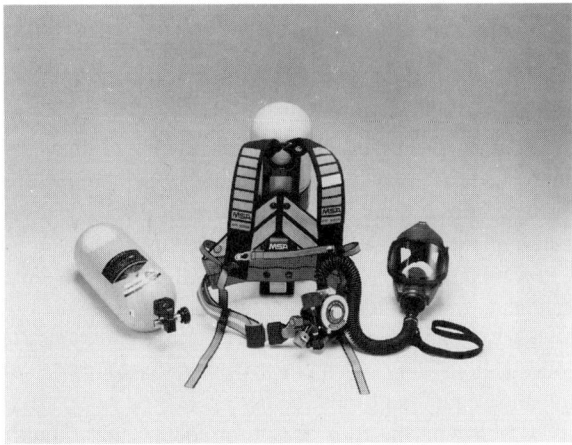

Fig. 62-9. Self-contained breathing apparatus atmosphere-supplying respirator. (Courtesy of Mine Safety Appliances Co.)

tative fit tests generate a test atmosphere around the respiratory protective device sealing surface. If a leak develops, the wearer should be able to sense the presence of the test agent inside the respirator. If the test agent is not detected inside the respirator, the respirator is presumed to have provided satisfactory protection.

The most common agents used are irritant smoke, an odorous vapor (such as isoamyl acetate or banana oil), or saccharin. The most effective of these is irritant smoke, because it may cause a cough reflex in the wearer if a leak is present.

Quantitative fit testing generates actual measurements of leakage. In this case, the respirator user wears a special probed respirator in a test atmosphere (usually a portable booth) in which a test agent is generated. Instrumentation measures any penetration of the agent from the test atmosphere into the respirator inlet covering through the probe in the facepiece. During the testing, the respirator wearer carries out a series of exercises that may partially simulate work movements. Common quantitative test agents used are dioctyl phthalate aerosol, sodium chloride aerosol, and Freon gas. Although more costly and time consuming, quantitative fit testing is usually more repeatable and reliable than qualitative techniques.

The larger respirator manufacturers listed in the box at right provide guidance and training in the use of respiratory protection. In addition, local safety/respirator supply companies may be a source of information.

Skin protection

Protective clothing would be used after other control techniques have been considered but are determined not to be feasible. For example, substitution of a less-hazardous dermatological agent as a coolant in a machine tool operation, use of a prilled or pelletized material in place of a powder, use of an automated handling system in place of manual addition to a chemical process vessel, frequent and effective housekeeping in the workplace, and good personal hygiene are desired control techniques.

In cases where skin contact is still a concern during maintenance operations that cannot be automated or improved by engineering controls, during emergency response actions, and when corrosives are handled, personal protective equipment must be used.

To determine the type of skin protection that should be worn, one must properly evaluate the workplace, including a review of the job task and chemicals in use. In addition, the duration of chemical contact, the part of the body in potential contact with the chemical, and the other physical requirements of the clothing, such as temperature extremes, abrasion resistance, and flexibility, must be known or anticipated.[17]

Once the job task, the chemicals being used, and the other physical requirements have been determined, the possible skin-protection materials or coatings should be re-

---

Respirator manufacturers

E.D. Bullard Co.
Rte. 7, Box 596
Cynthiana, KY 41031-8822

Glendale Protective Technologies
130 Crossways Park Dr.
Woodbury, NY 11797

Mine Safety Appliance
121 Gamma Drive
Pittsburgh, PA 15238

3M Company
OH & ES Division
Building 220-3E-04
St. Paul, MN 55144

National Draeger
101 Technology Dr.
P.O. Box 120
Pittsburgh, PA 15230-0120

North Safety Equipment
2000 Plainfield Pike
Cranston, RI 02920

Racal Airstream
7505 Executive Way
Frederick, MD 21701

Scott Aviation
A Figgie International Company
225 Erie St.
Lancaster, NY 14086

Survivair
Division of Comasec Inc.
3001 S. Susan
Santa Ana, CA 92704

Willson Safety Products
P.O. Box 622
Reading, PA 19603

This list is not all inclusive. In addition, local safety supply companies may be contacted for assistance.

---

viewed. Protective clothing or glove manufacturers and local safety supply companies should be contacted for assistance in selecting the proper protective clothing for specific uses. Several protective clothing/glove manufacturers are listed in the box on p. 1161. Fig. 62-10 provides guidance on choosing the correct glove and lists commonly used glove materials and coatings.[21]

Protective clothing and glove manufacturers and vendors

Allied Glove and Safety Products Corp.
P.O. Box 2126
Milwaukee, WI 53201

Ansell Edmont Industrial
1300 Walnut St.
Coshocton, OH 43812

Best Manufacturing Co.
Edison St.
Menlo, GA 30731

Comasec Inc.
P.O. Box 1219/8
Niblick Rd.
Enfield, CT 06082

E.I. du Pont de Nemours & Co.
Textile Fibers Dept.
Spunbonded Products Div.
Centre Road Bldg. Room 1144
Wilmington, DE 19898

Durafab Inc.
Subsidiary of Scott Paper Company
Box 658
Cleburne, TX 76033

Encon Manufacturing Co.
6825 W. Sam Houston Pkwy. North
Houston, TX 77041

W.L. Gore & Associates, Inc.
297 Blue Ball Rd.
P.O. Box 1130
Elkton, MD 21922-1130

Kappler Inc.
P.O. Box 218
5000 Grimes Drive
Guntersville, AL 35976

Mine Safety Appliance
121 Gamma Drive
Pittsburgh, PA 15238

North Hand Protection
4090 Azalea Drive
Charleston, SC 29405

Pioneer Industrial Products Co.
512 East Tiffin St.
Willard, OH 44890

Protech Safety Equipment Inc.
37 E. 21st St.
P.O. Box 4280
Linden, NJ 07036

Safety Supply America Corp.
6230 Cochran Rd.
Solon, OH 44139

Willson Safety Products
P.O. Box 622
Reading, PA 19603

This list is not all inclusive. In addition, local safety supply companies may be contacted for assistance.

ERGONOMICS

Ergonomics is the science of designing the job and the workplace to fit the worker. It involves designing equipment, operations, procedures, and work environments to make them compatible with the capabilities, limitations, and needs of workers. The objective of an ergonomics program is to teach managers and supervisors the interrelationships among people, machines, and tasks so that plant operations are designed that adapt the job and workplace to the worker by keeping the job tasks within the worker's abilities.

Without the consideration of ergonomics in the design of operations, the probability of human error is increased, with results ranging from excessive cumulative trauma injuries such as carpal tunnel syndrome and tenosynovitis to major process accidents. Ergonomics focuses on reducing human error by matching operator tasks with the operator's capabilities and limitations.

Successful ergonomic programs contain the basic elements outlined in the box on p. 1163. In addition, the box on p. 1163 lists some of the principles of ergonomics.[2]

RADIATION

Radiation is a form of energy that may be transferred from a source or emitter to matter or a receiver. There are both ionizing and nonionizing forms of radiation, as sum-

Glove material	Chemical resistance chart							
	Mineral acids	Organic acids	Caustics	Alcohols	Aromatic solvents	Petroleum solvents	Ketonic solvents	Chlorinated solvents
	Hydrochloric (38%	Acetic	Sodium hydroxide (50%)	Methanol	Toluene	Naphtha	Methyl ethyl ketone	Perchlor-ethylene
Natural rubber	G	E	E	E	NR	F	E	NR
Neoprene	E	E	E	E	F	E	G	P
Polyvinyl chloride	G	G	G	G	P	F	NR	NR
Polyvinyl alcohol	P	NR	NR	F	E	E	F	E
NBR	E	G	E	G	G	E	F	G

Glove material	Miscellaneous							
	Lacquer thinner	Benzene	Formaldehyde	Ethyl acetate	Vegetable oils	Animal fats	Turpentine	Phenol
Natural rubber	F	NR	E	F	F	P	F	F
Neoprene	G	P	E	G	G	E	G	E
Polyvinyl chloride	F	P	E	P	F	G	G	G
Polyvinyl alcohol	E	E	P	P	E	E	E	F
NBR	G	G	E	G	E	E	E	G

Coating	Physical performance chart*							
	Abrasion resistance	Cut resistance	Puncture resistance	Head resistance	Flexibility	Ozone resistance	Tear resistance	Relative cost
Natural rubber	E	E	E	F	E	P	E	Medium
Neoprene	E	E	G	G	G	E	G	Medium
Chlorinated polyethylene (CPE)	E	G	G	G	G	E	G	Low
Butyl rubber	F	G	G	E	G	E	G	High
Polyvinyl chloride	G	P	G	P	F	E	G	Low
Polyvinyl alcohol	F	F	F	G	P	E	G	Very High
Polyethylene	F	F	P	F	G	F	F	Low
Nitrile rubber	E	E	E	G	E	F	G	Medium
Nitrile rubber/Polyvinyl chloride (Nitrile PVC)	G	G	G	F	G	E	G	Medium
Polyurethane	E	G	G	G	E	G	G	High
Styrene-butadiene rubber (SBR)	E	G	F	G	G	F	F	Low
Viton	G	G	G	G	G	E	G	Very High

This figure shows the relative resistance ratings of various glove materials to some industrial solutions. **NOTE:** the purpose of gloves is to eliminate or reduce skin exposure to chemical substances. NEVER IMMERSE the hands, even with gloves rated E (excellent).

   KEY TO CHARTS: E=excellent; G=good; F=fair; P=poor; NR=no rating (ratings are subject to variation, depending on formulation, thickness, and whether the material is supported by fabric).

   The listings were taken from various glove manumgacturers and NIOSH, and are ONLY A GENERAL GUIDE. When selecting gloves for any application, contact the manufactureer, giving as much detailed information as possible, according to the following:
1. Ability of glove to resist penetration of the chemical, thus ensuring the protection of the wearer
2. Chemical composition of the solution
3. Degree of concentration
4. Abrasive effects of materials being handled
5. Temperature conditions
6. Time cycle of use
7. Specify in purchase order what materials are to be handled
8. Cost

*Grip/slip is related to glove surface and is enhanced when the glove surface is rough. Dexterity/tactility is related to glove thickness and decreases as the glove thickness increases.

Fig. 62-10. Choosing the right glove. (Modified from Plog BA: *Fundamentals of industrial hygiene,* ed 3, Chicago, 1988, National Safety Council.)

Elements of successful ergonomic programs

Identification of ergonomic hazards
- Analysis of injuries/accidents from cumulative trauma
- Review of risk factors in current and new jobs for ergonomic concerns
- Review of current and new equipment and processes for proper ergonomic design

Hazard prevention and control
- Engineering control (workstation design, equipment design, tool design, material handling, material flow, etc.)
- Work practice controls (proper lifting and other work techniques, exercise/conditioning)
- Personal protective equipment
- Administrative control (reduce duration and/or severity of exposure, provide additional work breaks, increase number of employees)

Training
- Ergonomic awareness
- Job-specific training
- Management training

Medical management
- Early identification
- Treatment
- Rehabilitation

Principles of ergonomics[2]

1. Design the workplace and tasks to minimize awkward postures.
2. Minimize static muscular loading.
3. Minimize the force requirements of the task.
4. Minimize nonneutral body movements.
5. Minimize routine, repetitive motions.
6. Design equipment to provide adequate access and clearance.
7. Provide adequate floor surfaces.
8. Design or select equipment and tools to fit the hand and the task.
9. Keep equipment and tools clean and properly maintained.
10. Minimize the need for personal support devices.
11. Provide mechanical assists.
12. Design job procedures to maximize the comfort, health, safety, and efficiency of the worker.
13. Train the workers in their assigned work procedures.
14. Eliminate the need for heavy manual materials handling.
15. Decrease the job demands.

This list is not all inclusive.

Excerpted from *A manager's guide to ergonomics in the chemical and allied industries.*

marized in Table 62-5. This classification is based on whether the specific type of radiation has the ability to form ions when transferred to matter. Nonionizing types of radiation include visible and ultraviolet light, infrared, radiowave, microwave, and lasers. Overexposure to many of the nonionizing forms of radiation can lead to ocular and skin problems. Ionizing radiation includes alpha rays, beta rays, gamma rays, x-rays, and neutrons. Both ionizing and nonionizing radiation are found in the electromagnetic spectrum and exhibit wave motion that can be described in terms of frequency of vibration and wavelength. Nonionizing types of radiation exhibit longer wavelengths and lower frequencies than ionizing types.

Health physics is the profession involved with radiation physics and the recognition, evaluation, and control of radiation hazards. Occupational uses or exposures of ionizing radiation include medical x-ray, radioisotopes, gauging devices for tanks and metals (to determine thickness of metals or levels of liquids in tanks), analytical devices (electron capture detectors used on gas chromatographs), well-logging devices, electron microscopes, nuclear reactors, and uranium miners. Radioactive materials can be naturally occurring, such as uranium, or may be produced artificially by exposing stable materials to high energies from devices such as x-ray machines or nuclear reactors. A listing of common ionizing radiation exposures is shown in Table 62-6.

The principal types of ionizing radiation include alpha (helium nucleus, mass, +2 charge), beta (electron, small mass, −1 charge), gamma (emitted from nucleus, no mass, 0 charge), x-rays (emitted from electrons, no mass, 0 charge), and neutrons (emitted from nucleus, mass, 0 charge). Those types that have no mass or charge (x-rays, gamma) may penetrate deeply before interacting with tissue, in comparison with particles, which have mass and a charge (alpha, beta, neutrons). However, alpha radiation, which has the greatest charge (+2), has the greatest potential for transfer of energy (or ionization) to the tissues and, therefore, damage. This is an important consideration in the control of ionizing radiation.

The basic measurement of radioactivity is the number of disintegrating nuclei per second. The conventional unit of radioactivity is the curie. Curies do not reflect either mass or the number of particles. The basic unit of radiation exposure is the roentgen, and radiation dose is expressed as a rad (radiation absorbed dose). Rads describe the amount of energy actually absorbed by tissue. Rads multiplied by quality factors for the biological effectiveness of the specific radiation are expressed as a rem (radiation equivalent man). Radiation exposure limits are typically given in rems.

Biological effects from radiation occur as a result of energy transfer to human tissues and the formation of free radicals and excited molecules at the molecular and cellular level. Genetic effects may occur if the testes or ovary are involved. Somatic effects may occur in any affected

Table 62-5. Ionizing/nonionizing radiation types and health effects

Radiation category	Radiation type	Radiation health effect
Ionizing	Alpha Beta Gamma X-ray Neutron	Acute radiation syndrome: anorexia, vomiting, diarrhea, intestinal cramps, fatigue, leukopenia, dermatitis, hemorrhage, infection, hair loss, convulsions, death Carcinogenesis: leukemia, bone, thyroid, liver, lung, breast, kidney, bladder, stomach Sterility Teratogenesis

Nonionizing	Ultraviolet (U)/Visible (V)
	  Sunlight
	  Artificial sources (e.g., tanning booths, mercury vapor lamps, welding)
	Infrared (I)
	Microwave (M)
	  Security systems
	  Door opening systems
	  Radar
	  Ovens
	Radio frequencies (R)
	  Radio
	  Mobile radio/phone systems
	  Television
	  Satellite communication
	Extremely low frequency (E)
	  Electric power generation/transmission
		Thermal effects: erythema, edema, etc.; U, V, I, M, R,
		Ocular effects
		  Conjunctivitis (welder's flash); U, V
		  Cataract formation; U, V, I
		Photosensitivity: Phototoxic and allergenic reactions; U
		Other skin effects:
		  Benign and malignant skin lesions; U

Table 62-6. Summary of common ionizing radiation exposures

Source	Approximate dose
Natural/environmental	**Millirem/year**
Radon	200
Fallout	4
Cosmic (highest at higher elevations)	25-100
Terrestrial (depends on concentrations of uranium in soil and groundwater)	15-100
Nuclear power	<1
Air travel (12 flights)	<1
Consumer products	**Millirem/year**
Television	1
Video display terminals	1
Tobacco (smoker)	1500
Building materials	5
Airport security x-ray	<1
Medical	**Millirem/procedure**
Chest x-ray	6
Barium enema x-ray series	400
CAT scan	110
Nuclear medicine	100-1000

tissue. The tissues or systems with the most reproductive activity are the most sensitive to radiation. These include the reproductive, hematopoietic, lymph, and gastrointestinal systems.

Acute radiation effects such as acute radiation syndrome are the result of high exposures, typically exceeding 100 rems. Symptoms may include anorexia, vomiting, diarrhea, intestinal cramps, fatigue, leukopenia, dermatitis, hemorrhage, infection, and hair loss, and are summarized in Table 62-7.

Chronic radiation effects occur over longer periods and may include sterility and carcinogenesis. Cancers produced by ionizing radiation include leukemia and cancers of bone, thyroid, liver, lung, breast, kidney, bladder, and stomach. Latency periods for these cancers range from 2 years (leukemia) to over 30 years.

Regulatory agencies and exposure limits

Several regulatory agencies are involved in radiation protection. The Nuclear Regulatory Commission (NRC) is responsible for licensing and regulating nuclear facilities and nuclear materials and for conducting research in support of the licensing and regulatory process.[10] The NRC headquarters is at 1717 H St, NW, Washington, D.C. 20555. It also has five regional offices throughout the United States: King of Prussia, Pennsylvania; Atlanta,

Table 62-7. Summary of effects of acute whole-body dose of ionizing radiation

Whole-body dose (REM)	Biological effect
10-25	Asymptomatic, normal blood results, may detect genetic effects (e.g., chromosomal aberrations)
100	Possible vomiting within 1 day, slight to moderate leukopenia, nausea, fatigue
500	Vomiting within 1-2 hours, severe leukopenia, diarrhea, hemorrhage, infection
1000	Vomiting within 30 minutes, diarrhea, fever, death within 2 weeks
5000	Vomiting immediately, convulsions, death within 1-2 days

Georgia; Glen Ellyn, Illinois; Arlington, Texas; and Walnut Creek, California. They conduct inspections to enforce their regulations.

OSHA covers employee exposures for all radiation sources not regulated by the NRC, including x-ray equipment, electron microscopes, and naturally occurring radioactive materials such as radium.

Both NRC and OSHA use the same exposure limit for ionizing radiation. Whole body, gonads, active blood forming organs, head and trunk, and lens of the eye are limited to 1.25 rems per quarter (3-month period), with higher doses allowed for other body areas (e.g., hands and skin). Both also restrict ionizing radiation to those individuals under 19 years of age. The limits provide a maximum dose of $5(N - 18)$ rems where N is the individual's age.

In addition, the Environmental Protection Agency is involved in the regulation of nuclear waste, and the Food and Drug Administration, Bureau of Radiological Health is involved in regulation of radioactive medical devices (e.g., x-ray machines) and electronic products such as microwave ovens and lasers.

Evaluation

Radiation measurement includes the use of both area and personal monitoring techniques. The most commonly used portable instruments for conducting area surveys are ionization chambers and Geiger-Müller meters. They are used to measure beta, gamma, and x-ray radiation. They can be calibrated to read in counts per minute as well as milliroentgens or millirads per hour.

Personal monitoring most commonly employs the use of pocket dosimeters, film badges, and thermoluminescent detectors (TLDs). The pocket dosimeter is a direct-reading small ionization chamber the size of a large pencil, typically worn in the shirt pocket. Both film badges and TLDs

require processing and reading after the exposure and are not direct-reading devices. Film badges use special photographic film to measure radiation dose, and TLDs are crystals of different salts (usually lithium fluoride). They both report results in millirad or millirem and are used for measuring beta, gamma, and x-ray radiation. In addition, TLDs can be used for neutron measurement.

The NRC requires periodic area surveys that include physical inventories of the location of radioactive materials and equipment as well as measurements of levels of radiation. The NRC also requires personal monitoring when an individual is likely to exceed an exposure of 0.3 rem per quarter or if he or she works in a restricted (exceeds an hourly dose of 2 millirem), radiation (exceeds an hourly dose of 5 millirem), or high-radiation (exceeds an hourly dose of 100 millirem) area. In certain cases, surface testing and leak testing of sealed sources by wipe testing techniques are also required.

Protection

Basic prevention of exposure to external radiation is provided by time, shielding, and distance. Time is directly related to radiation dose. For example, reducing the exposure time by one fourth reduces the dose by one fourth. Radiation dose decreases by roughly the inverse square law as one moves away from the source. For example, if the distance from the source is doubled, the dose decreases by a factor of four, and when the distance from the source is tripled, the dose decreases by a factor of nine. Shielding is a common method for reducing radiation from sources. The material to be used as a shield depends on the type of radiation and the source strength. Usually, the denser the shield, the more effective it is (lead is denser than concrete), and the thicker the shield, the more effective it is.

When radioactive materials are used or when exposures to radiation are possible, a formal written radiation control program should be developed and in many cases may be required. A radiation safety officer should supervise the radiation control activities.

WORKPLACE HEALTH AND SAFETY COMPONENTS

The major components of a workplace health and safety management system are listed in the box on p. 1166 and are essential in developing and maintaining a good health and safety effort. Many companies use a quality management activity, a management process, to continuously improve these health and safety components or elements. Health and safety auditing should find that improvements continue and deficiencies are corrected over time.

Health and safety should not be considered a program separate and distinct from the rest of a business. It should be viewed as an integral component of the business and incorporated into the organization at all levels of responsibility. In the past, the health/safety function may have been

---

Major components of a workplace health and safety management system

- Health/safety corporate policy, approved by senior management
- Defined responsibilities for health/safety management
- Health and safety organization and administration
- Health and safety training for health and safety professionals, plant supervisors, employees
- Accident investigation procedure
- Accident/illness reporting and analysis
- Plant inspection and hazard control
- Emergency response
- Health and safety management audit
- Occupational health
    Industrial hygiene
    Epidemiology
    Medical surveillance
    Hazard communication
    Ergonomics
    Employee assistance
- Occupational safety
    Employee safety
        Observations/contacts
        Permits
    Process safety
        Process hazard reviews
        Job safety analysis
    Loss control
- Contractor health and safety management
- Health and safety due diligence; acquisition/divestiture
- Health and safety regulatory compliance/monitoring
- Health and safety promotion
    Off-the-job
    Wellness

---

organized as a staff function only, with all health and safety responsibilities falling on the health and safety professional. Today, in addition to using health and safety professionals as resources, coaches, and auditors, health and safety is most effective when it is also integrated into the line management of each business or division within a company. In this manner, all managers and employees are intimately involved in and responsible for their own individual and group health and safety performance. This is one of the best approaches for constantly improving the health and safety process.

EVALUATION OF PATIENT EXPOSURES

Much of the health and safety process is preventive, rather than in response to overexposure incidents. However, there are times when patients must be evaluated for possible workplace exposures. Although many of the pertinent questions for patients would be covered in a medical questionnaire and history conducted by the medical professional during an examination, a thorough occupational history should also be collected from the patient where workplace exposures are suspected or possible. A good occupational or work history will include questions about the patient's current and previous jobs, including:

- The patient's job title
- A description of his or her job duties, including any chemical exposures
- The length of time on the jobs
- Whether personal protective equipment (e.g., respirators, gloves, other clothing, hard hats) was supplied, worn, and effective
- Whether uniforms were supplied and laundered
- Whether ventilation was used and effective
- Whether there was a workplace medical program
- Whether the patient consumed food or beverages or smoked at his or her work station or had a lunch room separate from the work environment
- Whether a washroom and shower facility was present and used
- Whether industrial hygiene monitoring had been conducted (and, if so, what were the results)
- Whether the employer had an effective hazard communication program and whether the patient had access to material safety data sheets
- Whether the employer conducted safety or health training
- Whether the employer had an individual assigned to safety/health

In addition, several related questions should be asked to determine whether problems and symptoms have arisen from possible exposures at home or from off-the-job activities:

- Whether the patient has any hobbies or part-time jobs that require chemical use
- Whether other family members have chemical exposure
- Whether the patient has exposure to chemicals at home
- Whether the patient has had new carpeting or insulation installed recently in the home
- The type and condition of the home insulation
- Whether the patient has pets at home
- Whether the patient has farm animals or visits farms routinely
- The type of furnace in the home and whether it is serviced routinely
- Whether the patient has a humidifier in the home

The responses to the occupational and off-the-job questions should be integrated into the medical history to arrive at an overall evaluation to determine whether the patient's workplace or home may be causing, contributing to, or aggravating the medical problem.

SUMMARY

Workplace industrial hygiene and safety involve anticipation, recognition, evaluation, and control of workplace stresses that may cause injury, illness, and impaired health and well-being to workers. Workplace accidents are still a significant concern in suffering and cost and are managed by a comprehensive health and safety process that is most effective when it is integrated into the line management organization.

Health and safety assistance in the workplace is provided by the following professional associations: the American Industrial Hygiene Association, the American Society of Safety Engineers, the American Board of Industrial Hygiene, the American Conference of Governmental Industrial Hygienists, and the National Safety Council. Several of these groups provide listings of industrial hygiene and safety consultants. In addition, state government agencies provide free on-site safety and health consultation services. In addition, many workers' compensation and insurance carriers provide related consultative services.

A good workplace health and safety program is preventive and attempts to constantly improve the health and safety management process.

REFERENCES

1. *Accident Facts, 1991 edition,* Chicago, 1991, National Safety Council.
2. Adams E, Marcotte A: *Managers guide to ergonomics in the chemical and allied industries,* Washington, DC, 1992, Chemical Manufacturers Association.
3. American Conference of Governmental Industrial Hygienists: *Documentation of the threshold limit values and biological exposure indices,* ed 5, Cincinnati, 1986, ACGIH.
4. American Conference of Governmental Industrial Hygienists: *1991-1992 Threshold limit values for chemical substances and physical agents and biological exposure indices,* Cincinnati, 1991, ACGIH.
5. American Industrial Hygiene Association: *1991-1992 Membership directory of the AIHA,* Akron, 1991, AIHA.
6. American National Standards Institute: *American national standard for hazardous industrial chemicals—precautionary labeling (ANSI Z129.1),* New York, 1988, ANSI.
7. American National Standards Institute: *Identification of air-purifying respirator canisters and cartridges (ANSI K13.1-1973),* New York, 1973, ANSI.
8. American National Standards Institute: *American national standard practices for respiratory protection—respirator use—physical qualifications for personnel (ANSI Z88.6-1984),* New York, 1984, ANSI.
9. American National Standards Institute: *American national draft standard for the preparation of material safety data sheets (ANSI Z400.1),* New York, expected 1993, ANSI.
10. Code of Federal Regulations: *10 CFR section 20 (standards for protection against radiation),* Washington, DC, 1991, US Nuclear Regulatory Commission, Superintendent of Documents.
11. Code of Federal Regulations: *29 CFR section 1910.1000 (air contaminants),* Washington, DC, 1991, US Department of Labor, OSHA, Superintendent of Documents.
12. Code of Federal Regulations: *29 CFR section 1910.1200 (hazard communication),* Washington, DC, 1991, US Department of Labor, OSHA, Superintendent of Documents.
13. Code of Federal Regulations: *29 CFR 1910.134 (respiratory protection),* Washington, DC, 1991, US Department of Labor, OSHA, Superintendent of Documents.
14. Compressed Gas Association: *Commodity specification for air (CGA G-7.1-1989),* Arlington, Va, 1989, CGA, available from American National Standards Institute, New York.
15. *Fire protection guide on hazardous materials,* ed 9, Quincy, Mass, 1986, National Fire Protection Association.
16. *International Agency for Research on Cancer monographs on the evaluation of the carcinogenic risk to humans,* multivolume work, Lyon, France, 1972-present, World Health Organization.
17. Johnson JS, Anderson KJ, editors: *Chemical protective clothing,* vol 1, Akron, 1990, American Industrial Hygiene Association.
18. National Paint and Coatings Association: *Hazardous materials information system* (HMIS), Chicago, available from Labelmaster/American Labelmark Co., Chicago.
19. National Toxicology Program: *Sixth annual report on carcinogens,* Research Triangle Park, N.C., 1991, National Toxicology Program, US Public Health Service.
20. *OSHA material safety data sheet form 174,* Washington, DC, US Department of Labor, OSHA.
21. Plog B, editor: *Fundamentals of industrial hygiene,* ed 3, Chicago, 1988, National Safety Council.
22. *Recordkeeping guidelines for occupational injuries and illnesses,* Washington, DC, 1986, US Department of Labor, Bureau of Labor Statistics.

RESOURCES

General industrial hygiene

Brief RS: *Basic industrial hygiene, a training manual,* Akron, Ohio, 1975, American Industrial Hygiene Association.

LaDou JL, editor: *Introduction to occupational health and safety,* Chicago, 1986, National Safety Council.

Peterson JE: *Industrial health,* revised ed 2, Cincinnati, 1991, American Conference of Governmental Industrial Hygienists.

Plog B, editor: *Fundamentals of industrial hygiene,* Chicago, 1988, National Safety Council. Comprehensive industrial hygiene text.

General occupational safety

Accident prevention manual for industrial operations, two-volume set, ed 9, vol 1, "Administration and programs" and vol 2 "Engineering and technology," Chicago, 1988, National Safety Council. Comprehensive occupational safety textbooks.

Ferry T: *Safety and health management planning,* New York, 1990, Van Nostrand Reinhold. Safety/health management text.

Regulatory agencies/standards

Code of Federal Regulations, Occupational Safety and Health Administration, Department of Labor, CFR 29 Part 1900 through 1910, latest revision. For sale from Superintendent of Documents, U.S. Government Printing Office, Washington, DC 20402. Contains OSHA regulations.

National Institute for Occupational Safety and Health, 1600 Clifton Rd., N.E., Atlanta, GA 30333.

Occupational Safety and Health Administration, 3rd and Constitution Avenues, N.W., Washington, DC 20210.

Occupational Safety and Health Reporter, Bureau of National Affairs, 1231 25th St, N.W., Washington, DC 20037. Weekly newsletter on occupational safety and health.

Professional associations

American Board of Industrial Hygiene, 4600 W. Saginaw, Suite 101, Lansing, MI 48917.

American Conference of Governmental Industrial Hygienists, 6500 Glenway Ave., Bldg. D-5, Cincinnati, OH 45211-4438. Publishes ACGIH TLVs and related documentation of TLVs.

American Industrial Hygiene Association, Suite 201, 2700 Prosperity Ave., Fairfax, VA 22031.

American National Standards Institute, 1430 Broadway, New York, NY 10018.

American Society of Safety Engineers, 1800 E Oakton St, Des Plaines, IL 60018-2187.

Bureau of Certified Safety Professionals, 208 Burwash Ave., Savoy, IL 61874.

National Safety Council, 444 N Michigan Ave., Chicago, IL 60611.

Trade associations

Chemical Manufacturers Association, 2501 M Street, N.W., Washington, DC 20037. *Managers guide to ergonomics in the chemical and allied industries,* also secretariat for ANSI MSDS document.

National Paint and Coatings Association, 1500 Rhode Island Ave., N.W., Washington, DC 20005. Hazardous Material Information System (HMIS).

Industrial hygiene sampling/analysis

Hering S, editor: *Air sampling instruments for evaluation of atmospheric contaminants,* ed 7, Cincinnati, 1989, ACGIH. Comprehensive summary of air sampling equipment.

NIOSH manual of analytical methods, ed 3, Cincinnati, 1984, US Department of Health and Human Services, NIOSH (1990 supplement). Analytical methods for industrial hygiene samples.

SKC comprehensive catalog and air sampling guide, 1992, SKC, Inc., RR 1, Box 334, Eighty Four, PA 15330-9614. Summary of industrial hygiene sampling and analytical methods.

Respiratory protection

American National Standards Institute: *American national standard practices for respiratory protection (ANSI Z88.2-1980),* New York, 1980, American National Standards Institute.

American National Standards Institute: *American national standard practices for respiratory protection—respirator use—physical qualifications for personnel (ANSI Z88.6-1984),* New York, 1984, American National Standards Institute.

Colton E, Birkner LR, and Brosseau LM, editors: *Respiratory protection, a manual and guideline,* ed 2, Akron, 1991, American Industrial Hygiene Association.

NIOSH respirator decision logic (DHHS/NIOSH Pub. No 87-108), Washington, DC, 1987, U.S. Department of Health and Human Services/NIOSH.

Rajhaus GS, Blackwell DSL: *Practical guide to respirator usage in industry,* Stoneham, Mass, 1985, Butterworth.

Ergonomics

Ergonomics: a practical guide, Chicago, 1988, National Safety Council.

Ergonomics guide series, Akron, 1970-1983, American Industrial Hygiene Association.

Making the job easier/an ergonomics idea book, Chicago, 1988, National Safety Council.

Occupational health and safety products/vendors

Labelmaster/American Labelmark Company, 5724 N. Pulaski Rd, Chicago, IL 60646. HMIS and NFPA label materials.

Occupational health and safety purchasing sourcebook, Waco, Texas, 1991, Occupational Health and Safety, PO Box 2573, Waco, TX 76702-2573. Lists of companies selling occupational health and safety equipment.

Chapter 63

WELLNESS IN THE WORKPLACE

Bill Zuti

This chapter is written for the physician who has an interest in starting a wellness program or has been given the responsibility of developing one. This chapter presents the information and procedures needed to develop and manage a worksite wellness program.

TERMINOLOGY

Wellness program is the currently popular term for what used to be called a prevention program for health and fitness. It is thought that the name *wellness* became popular because it is the opposite of illness. The more correct terms are *wellness behavior, wellness lifestyle,* or *wellness activities.* " All of these terms are really synonymous with health promotion or health/fitness.

HISTORY

Only a very limited interest in the preventive aspects of health and fitness activities existed before the 1960s. Dr. Ken Cooper published *Aerobics* in 1968,[11] which seemed to be the start of the fitness boom. Subsequently, in the 1970s, jogging and running were almost the only activities of those who wanted to be healthy. Health professionals also then began encouraging people to evaluate their lifestyles and develop complete health behaviors. Professional organizations such as the American College of Sports Medicine (ACSM) and the President's Council on Physical Fitness and Sports (PCPFS) were reexamining their goals and programs to determine what new directions should be taken. A few companies saw the potential benefits of fitness and developed on-site programs for employees.

In 1973, under the direction of the President's Council on Physical Fitness and Sports, the group that would become the Association for Worksite Health Promotion (AWHP) was formed. The group then was known as the Association of Fitness Directors in Business and Industry (AFDBI) and the Association for Fitness in Business (AFB). AWHP now has 3500 members, which reflects how much these programs have grown and how strong the interest is in worksite wellness. As the programs evolved through the 1980s, they expanded from the "for profits," who had extensive resources to develop such services, to all types of employers.

Many of the early programs were limited in both scope of offerings and those who were entitled to participate. The corporations that started wellness programs in the 1970s offered only fitness activities and often only to executives. The programs developed in the 1980s provided the models for the comprehensive and cost-effective programs that can now be offered to all employees at facilities of all sizes.

The cost-benefit aspects of these programs have been shown to be of real value, which helps to justify their implementation (see Justification section of this chapter). However, some employers also have offered the programs as an employee benefit and/or used them as a recruiting device. The philosophy behind this is that the program can improve retention and recruitment and that a healthy, fit, and happy employee is a more productive worker. This is particularly true if employees think the company really cares about them as individuals.

JUSTIFICATION
Economic effect

When one considers establishing a wellness program, cost is always a consideration. However, based on research conducted by a broad range of companies, we now have data to demonstrate that properly managed programs can be cost effective. That is, they provide a significant return on investment. The Association for Worksite Health Promotion (AWHP) has been the leader in this field, conducts conferences on this subject, and in August of 1991 published a "white paper" on this subject. This document, *Economic Impact of Worksite Health Promotion,*[21] focuses on four major areas of research:

1. Risk reduction/behavior change
2. Health (medical) costs
3. Absenteeism
4. Productivity.

In the area of risk reduction/behavior change, evidence suggests that wellness programs can be effective within employee groups. Published studies of health promotion programs of companies such as Control Data,[1] Johnson and Johnson,[32,34] Blue Cross/Blue Shield of Indiana,[15,19] Canadian Life Insurance Company,[30] and NASA,[10] with some limitations, have shown positive health behavior changes for those who participated. Because these studies were not always the same and had inadequate control groups, the findings from a true research standpoint must be evaluated in a general way. These studies did not restrict themselves to "at-risk" patients, which may have enhanced the beneficial effect of the program. When these programs are evaluated for their practical worth, there is little doubt of their effectiveness.

For those interested in starting wellness programs, the cost-benefit data have been of the greatest interest. Studies reported by Prudential Insurance Company,[10] Kimberly Clark,[5] Control Data,[1] Mesa Petroleum,[14] and others previously cited[6,9,30] have shown positive effects. Even with the limitations of small samples that were not randomly selected, these relatively short-term studies showed that both utilization and costs of health care were less for program participants. The primary limitation is that these are volunteer programs, and it can be argued that those who are more interested in a healthy lifestyle will elect to participate. However, the professionals involved with these programs point out that after the initial start-up of a program, others are recruited by friends or staff, and therefore are more representative of the employee population.

In 1989 Roy Shepard's review[29] of 20 available studies reported that 14 showed a reduction in absenteeism. The vast majority of these studies involved employees participating in physical activity rather than a complete wellness program. The absentee rates from these studies ranged between one and two fewer days missed per year than average. A more carefully controlled study by DuPont Corporation[6] showed an average reduction of 0.4 day/year for those in the health promotion programs compared with those employees in the control groups.

The area of productivity has been evaluated from two directions: the physical output and the mental capacity or attitude of those involved in wellness. Studies*

have reported that fit and healthy employees consistently receive higher work performance ratings than those who are less fit and healthy. Companies that offer stress management and other mental health programs have demonstrated the benefit of early intervention on productivity.†

To summarize the cost-benefit argument, the literature reports that worksite health promotion programs can show a return on investment. As yet, these numbers are not absolutely scientific, but more companies are reporting that their worksite wellness programs are producing gains. Unpublished data from one major Ohio employer reported a return of $8 for every $1 invested in health promotion. In light of these data, it is difficult for management to argue against having a worksite wellness program.

MEDICAL DIRECTOR
Role of the medical director

The implementation and continued success of the worksite wellness program often depends on the medical director being the driving force behind it. Good leadership is essential to getting employees involved in health and fitness programs. The physician must understand the needs and wants of the employees, and how scientifically sound principles must be used to develop a complete wellness program. However, the physician also must remember that most people participate in programs for enjoyment, not because the programs are good for them.

The medical director must use his or her knowledge and training to oversee the program. Oversight includes assessing the health and fitness needs of the employees, determining the general program content, selecting a program director or wellness manager, and continuing to supervise the operation to ensure quality.

Leadership

The medical director provides an essential part of the leadership for the program. However, he or she need not manage the program directly. Almost without exception, worksite wellness programs are not directly administered by a physician. In most cases the medical director will assign or hire someone to serve as wellness manager. The job requirements for this person will be covered in the Staff section of this chapter.

In the primary leadership role, the medical director not only must believe in health promotion, but he or she also should have a wellness lifestyle. This is usually not a problem, because most physicians practice, as well as promote, this type of positive health behavior. The greater challenge in this leadership role is to enlist the help of top management of the corporation to also serve as role models. Years of experience have shown that, without the solid visible support of top management, in particular the emphasis and commitment of the CEO, the program will

---

*References 3,12,13,15,21,25,26,31,33.

†References 4,8,17,18,20,27,28.

not succeed. For example, PepsiCo was an early leader in developing a corporate fitness program because of the commitment of the chairman, Don Kendall.

THE PROGRAM
Program organization system

A comprehensive health and fitness or wellness program for a corporation is intended to include all components that affect a person's health and well being. The organizational system presented in this section allows all wellness offerings to be placed into a systematic organizational structure, to determine whether all areas of health and fitness are included or whether any area is being overemphasized. This system can provide the medical director and wellness management with a tool for understanding the interrelationships among all health, fitness, medical, and benefits-cost-containment programs and also help them to evaluate these programs.

Components of wellness. A corporate wellness program should provide programs and information that deal with all aspects of an individual's health and fitness. These components include the following:

- *Physical activity:* This area includes all physical activities that provide the means for developing and maintaining the physiological fitness of the individual.
- *Behavioral health:* This area includes all programs that are intended to improve quality of life by developing personal behavior that improves health and reduces the risk of disease.
- *Emotional health:* This area includes all programs and services that help maintain emotional and/or mental health, which will also enhance quality of life.
- *Medical health:* This area includes all programs that provide information and education on diseases, illnesses, rehabilitation, and medical services.

Interrelation of components. All components of a good health and fitness program must be integrated to reinforce a positive lifestyle. Total wellness must include all of the components that influence the health and well-being of the individual. One cannot make up for poor nutrition or substance abuse by running extra miles. All areas of wellness must be addressed for a person to be healthy and fit. The program must be designed so that it provides the employee with the opportunity to participate in a wide variety of activities and programs of physical activity, behavioral health, emotional health, and medical health.

Specific programs and courses. Programs and courses to be offered in each component area include:

I. Physical activity
   1. Fitness assessment/profile
   2. General physical conditioning/training
      a. Aerobic
      b. Muscular strength and endurance
      c. Flexibility
      d. Others
   3. Recreational programs and sports activities
II. Behavioral health
   1. Substance abuse education and intervention
   2. Nutrition education/weight management
   3. Stress management
   4. Safety education and implementation
III. Emotional health
   1. Personal development
   2. Relating to others
   3. Marriage/divorce
   4. Family, children, and parents
   5. Aging/aged
   6. Preparation for retirement
IV. Medical health
   1. Rehabilitation
   2. Prenatal
   3. Prevention/screening
   4. Disease education
   5. Emergency care
   6. Selection of medical services

Departments involved. A comprehensive approach can involve several corporate departments in the delivery of these programs and services. These could include:

- Medical department
- Fitness center (if separate from medical)
- Benefits
- Safety/security
- Public affairs
- Employee relations
- Management development
- Human resources
- Counseling (if separate from medical)
- Cafeteria services
- Legal

Examples of programs that could be offered

I. Physical fitness
   1. Wellness and fitness profiles and interpretations
   2. General physical conditioning/training
      a. The fitness center provides a continuous opportunity for physical activity and training for all employees.
      b. Specific classes in physical conditioning/training are:
         Aerobic low impact
         Aerobic advanced
         Step aerobics
      c. Muscular strength and endurance
         FUN (For Unfit Newcomers) exercise class

Exercise Plus
Leg workout/upper-body workout
d. Flexibility
Basic stretching
Included as part of total fitness
e. Others
Self-defense
3. Recreational programs and sports activities
a. Basketball
b. Bowling
c. Golf
d. Olympic days
e. Racquetball
f. Running
g. Skiing
h. Soccer
i. Softball
j. Swimming
k. Tennis
l. Volleyball
II. Behavior health
1. Substance abuse: alcohol, drug, and tobacco
a. Stop-smoking clinic
b. Reasons For stopping smoking
c. Driving and drinking
d. Substance abuse awareness
2. Nutrition/weight management
a. Weight Watchers
b. Diet directions
c. Eating and stress
d. Cooking nutritious meals
e. Conscious eating, conscious living
f. Prenatal nutrition
g. Understanding cholesterol
h. Salt and blood pressure
3. Stress management
a. Time stress
b. Managing expectations
c. Time management: time and priorities
d. The creative energy within stress
e. Relaxation
f. Daily physical exercise
4. Safety education and implementation
a. Defensive driving
b. "Street-proofing" your child
c. Commonsense approach to personal safety
d. Exercising in high heat
III. Emotional health
1. Personal development
a. Personal appearance
b. Secrets of being well dressed
c. Art of makeup and color
2. Relating to others
a. How to have better relationships
b. Relationship planning

c. Interpersonal communications
d. Singles
3. Marriage/divorce
a. The challenges of the two-career couple
b. Blended family
4. Family/children
a. The working parent
b. Talking to your children about sex
c. Healthy mothers, healthy babies
d. Communicating with your adolescent
e. Adolescent sexuality
f. Parenthood after 30
g. Families and children
5. Aging/aged
a. You and your aging parent
b. Elder care
c. Planning for your retirement
IV. Medical health
1. Rehabilitation is provided as a continuous offering
to all employees
a. Spinal care
b. Postural analysis
c. Injury prevention
d. Massage therapy
e. Cardiac rehabilitation
f. Sports rehabilitation
2. Prevention/screening
a. Breast cancer
b. Testicular cancer
c. Skin cancer
d. Exercising in high heat
e. Pulmonary function testing
f. Health fair
g. Medical department tapes on prevention
h. Cholesterol and its fractions
3. Disease education
a. AIDS: health care issue of the 1990s
b. Blood pressure education
c. Cholesterol
d. Osteoporosis
e. Cancer risk
f. Preventing birth defects
g. Medical Department: individual instruction
h. Medical Department: disease education
4. Emergency care
a. CPR/first aid
b. Medical department: emergency service
5. Selection of medical services
a. Hot lines
b. Medical department: individual instruction
c. What you need to know about second opinions

Examples of how this system can be used are shown in Tables 63-1 and 63-2. Table 63-1 shows a template for a comprehensive program, and Table 63-2 shows the same template with sample programs added and scheduled.

Table 63-1. Wellness program template

Workout series	First quarter	Second quarter	Third quarter	Fourth quarter
I. Physical fitness				
1. Fitness assessment/ profiles				
2. General physical conditioning/ training*				
* A = aerobic				
B = strength				
C = flexibility				
D = sports				
3. Recreational programming and sports activities:				
II. Behavioral health				
1. Substance abuse				
2. Nutrition/weight management				
3. Stress management				
4. Safety education				
III. Emotional health				
1. Personal development				
2. Relating to others				
3. Marriage/divorce				
4. Family/children				
5. Aging/aged				
IV. Medical health				
1. Rehabilitation (ongoing)				
2. Prenatal				
3. Prevention/ screening				
4. Disease education				
5. Emergency care				
6. Medical services				

Developing the program

Assessing needs. A review of the Program Organizational System (POS) shown in Tables 63-1 and 63-2 can give the impression that developing a wellness program could get overwhelming. However, with needs assessments completed and goals developed, a clear pattern of sequential steps can be established that will lead to a comprehensive program. If a program is planned, this program plan becomes the basis for building decisions. The steps in building a comprehensive program, including facilities, are:

1. Assess needs
2. Establish goals
3. Determine the program that will meet the goals
4. Develop the construction plan.

Goal setting. The first step in this process is goal setting. As the old expression says, You must know where you want to go in order to get there. To the corporate medical director, goal setting is nothing new. Set goals to start

the program and then draft a master plan that will develop the program through the next 3 years. This will give you and management the means to determine where and how to start and what it will cost.

The determination of needs before goal setting should include:

1. An assessment of corporate medical records
2. Comprehensive analysis of the records of medical benefits
3. Survey of employee interests in health and fitness programs
4. Analysis of the work tasks of the company
5. Interpretation and tempering of these data with data from existing programs of other similar companies in the same geographic area.

The assessment of corporate medical records can reveal a wealth of wellness needs and health problems. The most common method of evaluating uses the last 3 years of

Table 63-2. Wellness program sample

	First quarter	Second quarter	Third quarter	Fourth quarter
I. Physical fitness				
1. Fitness assessment/profiles			ON — GOING	
2. General physical conditioning/training*				
ABC	Fun exercise class	Fun exercise class	Fun exercise class	Fun exercise class
A	Jazz aerobics	Jazz aerobics	Jazz aerobics	Jazz aerobics
A	Aerobic fever	Aerobic fever	Aerobic fever	Aerobic fever
BC	Bottom line	Bottom line	Bottom line	Bottom line
ABC	Exercise plus	Exercise plus	Exercise plus	Exercise plus
ABC	Aerobic eye opener	Aerobic eye opener	Aerobic eye opener	Aerobic eye opener
BC	Upper body workout			
* A = Aerobic				
B = Strength				
C = Flexibility				
D = Sports				
3. Recreational programs and sports activities				
	Golf (twice)	Golf		
	Tennis	Tennis	Tennis (twice)	
		Swimming	Swimming	
				Self-defense
				Ski conditioning
II. Behavioral health				
1. Substance abuse	Drinking and driving	Breaking the smoking habit	Abusive substance awareness	Feel like quitting
2. Nutrition/weight management	Weight Watchers	Weight Watchers	Weight Watchers	Weight Watchers
	Current diet programs	Current diet programs	Current diet programs	Current diet programs
		Compulsive eating	Sport nutrition	Weight control tips for special occasions
3. Stress management	Interpersonal communication	Time management	Time management	Keeping the happy in your holidays
		Living with "hurry sickness"		
	Improving your memory			
4. Safety education	Defensive driving	Personal defense	Defensive driving	Home safety
III. Emotional health				
1. Personal development			Skin care	Secrets of being well dressed
2. Relating to others	Creating, believing, and selling your image	Making relationships better		Single life
	Balancing your life			
3. Marriage/divorce	The marriage game	Parenthood after 30		Balancing both worlds
		Blended family		The working parent
4. Family/children/ parents	Communicating with your family	Healthy mother-healthy baby	The working parent	Healthy mother-healthy baby
5. Aging/aged	Elder care	Planning for your retirement	Elder care	You and your aging parent
IV. Medical health				
1. Rehabilitation (ongoing)				
2. Prenatal	Prenatal education	Prenatal education		
3. Prevention/ screening	Breast cancer	Testicular cancer	Skin cancer	
4. Disease education	Current health issues	Communicating with your physician	PMS	Osteoporosis
5. Emergency care				
6. Medical services			CPR	

data. First, the primary reason for corporate medical care, as stated by the employee, is compiled. Next, the actual diagnosis by the attending physician is compiled. These data are best represented as a summary of listings for the last 3 years, starting with the current month and working backward. This method allows one to stop compiling information when data is sufficient; it also permits one to add data from additional months to obtain a clear pattern of illness and injury.

The company's insurance carrier can provide a detailed analysis of claims filed by employees over a similar time period. This analysis can be done in several ways, but the two that will probably be most valuable are an analysis of the type of claim by cost and an analysis by the number of incidents, accidents, or cases of illness. This will show whether particular types of claims are occurring at a disproportionate rate.

As an example of how these data can help identify methods of reducing clinic visits, consider a report from the medical clinic at the hypothetical XYZ Corporation. The analysis showed that more than one third of all patient visits to the clinic in the summer months were related to softball. Management's reaction was to consider canceling this league. However, the medical director and the wellness manager determined that eliminating sliding and changing the pitching rules could eliminate most of the injuries. The savings in reduced sick time were probably greater than the budget for the league.

The third step toward the establishment of goals is to survey the employees to determine their interest in health and fitness programs. The key to conducting a good survey is to ask the right questions. The best resource is the personnel department. Nearly any personnel professional can get valid information from a list of questions about program interests. More important, these professionals will do it in a way that will generate interest in this new program.

The fourth step is to examine the demands of the company as a whole to determine the nature of the work tasks and to assess the possible effect on employee health of various jobs. For example, loading and warehousing should include preemployment evaluation of the back and instruction in lifting, whereas those working all day with word processors would need screening and education on carpal tunnel syndrome.

The final step in this process is one that medical directors already use to gain other information. Networking is one of the most effective means of obtaining accurate, valid, reliable, and relevant data. Other professionals working in existing programs in similar companies are likely to have already encountered and solved many problems and are willing to share this information. This information is usually easy to obtain and reliable, because these colleagues want to make a positive impression and may need help at some time themselves.

After completing all of the above steps, one is now ready to develop general goals and specific objectives for the wellness program. A general goal for the program might be, "To provide the employees of the XYZ corporation and their families with the knowledge, skills, and programs necessary to keep them healthy and fit." This would be followed by specific goals and measurable objectives, such as, "Give employees an understanding of prevention, identification, and treatment of cancer." Specific measurable objectives might include, "Provide the opportunity for all female employees, age 40 and older, to obtain a mammogram at 50% of cost." If this program were offered, early detection and subsequent treatment of cancer will probably offset the reduced cost of screening. Innovative programs such as this are to be monitored for cost-effectiveness. Associated improvement in employee morale is more difficult to measure but it is certainly an appreciable spinoff.

Designing the program. The program organization system was described in detail previously in this chapter. With this system (Table 63-1) and the goals and objectives that have been established, a comprehensive program can be designed. However, the nature of the company, workforce, and budget will influence the final product.[2]

The most successful worksite wellness programs have been employee based. Employees can be formally or informally involved in the development and implementation of the program. The formal involvement is usually a structured committee with appointed or elected members. If there is an existing employee leadership system, such as a union, it can be incorporated into the process. Informal systems involve employees on an as-needed basis. In general, a formal committee can be involved during the development phase, and the informal process can be used when needed for the ongoing program. These are only advisory committees, and final decisions must be the responsibility of the medical director and the wellness manager. Employee leaders can provide information on how their coworkers feel, what their interests are, or how they may react to the program, but they rarely have the technical knowledge to make informed program decisions.

Type of company

Implications. The size and type of business will affect the program. The larger for-profit businesses can usually offer more programs because they have more people to participate and often more money.

Large or small. Companies with fewer than 500 employees will have difficulty supporting an on-site fitness facility. Their programs most often focus on health education, with staffing limited to one professional who contracts with outside vendors for special services. If interest becomes great, supporting a small fitness center may be possible.

Locations with 500 to 2000 employees will need to start small and expand as the program grows. This is enough people to support an on-site fitness center with a dedicated staff, but interest in the program must be developed and maintained to justify this expenditure. This size of company is best advised to start with health education programs and nonfacility fitness programs before choosing to build.

An employee population of 2000 or more is large enough to support a fitness center and health education program with a professional staff. With the current interest in health, fitness, and wellness, one can assume that at least 10% of employees are presently involved in these activities and will participate on site. This is only the beginning; the program goals should be set to grow by 10% per year, until 50% or more of the employee population is involved. The fitness center for this operation can include an aerobic dance area, weight training area, cardiovascular training area, and more. The staff will consist of a wellness manager, fitness leaders (and/or health educators), and support personnel (See Staffing and Construction sections of this chapter).

Not-for-profit. Government programs at the federal and state level are managed through their respective headquarters at the capitals. Programs for local government agencies fall into the guidelines previously discussed for small businesses. The primary difference in not-for-profit programs is that the program costs are covered by tax dollars, which usually keeps the program at a minimum level.

Health/fitness programs in the education sector (both public and higher education) have the unique advantage of having access to physical education facilities and the in-house expertise of the health and physical education faculty. This can reduce the program start-up costs. However, this does not mean that programs in education are always easy to start. A university may have a gym, but getting to use it for an employee fitness program might be a major problem because it is scheduled for classes, athletics, and special events. The faculty has general knowledge in health and fitness but may lack the expertise and interest in developing a program. Faculty members also might not have the time to devote to it.

Hospital-based programs. Hospital-based programs differ significantly from other worksite wellness programs in that they are operated for their employees *and* can be marketed to others. Medical facilities have entered the wellness center business for three main reasons. The first is that properly managed centers can produce significant revenue. With their staff expertise, program development will usually take less effort and cost less. The public views hospitals as a resource for health information, which makes marketing wellness programs to the public and other employers much easier. Hospitals will develop a program and facility for their employees and then, using their program as a model, offer to develop a similar program for others in their service area. If the hospital develops a fitness center, it can be opened to the public on a fee basis.

The second reason for developing and marketing wellness programs to the community is the positive image this projects for the hospital. Those residing within the immediate area of the hospital will feel good about a medical institution that helps them get healthy and fit. This positive image will affect their choice of major medical services when needed. In summary, the wellness program is part of the feeder system for all other medical services the hospital offers.

The third and most obvious reason for developing a wellness program is the hospital employees. The program will reduce medical costs, and more important, the employees will view it as an additional benefit. In some cases, the wellness program has been a real morale booster. If presented in the right way, the program can say that the hospital cares about the employee as an individual and wants to help the employee live a healthier life.

STAFFING
Wellness manager

Probably the most critical decision affecting the success of the program is the selection of the wellness manager. The medical director obviously must hire someone to manage the program. It is unrealistic to expect this physician to manage the program and the budget and recruit participants. Having the right person in this job can make the program a success; the wrong person can ensure failure.

Participants usually see the wellness manager as the direct leader of the program. In essence, he or she is an extension of the medical director's leadership and authority. The manager should supervise the staff in addition to being the main leadership figure for the program participants. The typical program manager qualifications include: a BS at minimum, MS preferred, in some area of health, fitness, wellness, exercise science, exercise physiology, or a related field; at least 5 years (with more than one company preferred) experience in worksite wellness; and, probably most important, the ability to get along with, motivate, and lead people. In addition to these three qualifications, the wellness manager should have a good fitness image, be well organized, be able to manage a budget, have the skill and experience of recruiting people to become program participants, and have all the other traits that one would expect of a good manager. The American College of Sports Medicine (ACSM) is the only professional organization that is currently certifying people in this area. The details of these requirements are listed in the *Guidelines for Exercise Testing and Prescription.*[7] The certification level of health/fitness leader should be a minimum, with the health/fitness director preferred.

The wellness manager should have total responsibility for the day-to-day operation of the program and should report directly to the medical director. All major program decisions are the responsibility of the wellness manager. Thus he or she has the responsibility to: hire and fire staff, manage the budget, select and schedule program offerings, and be the direct link to the participants, both by recruiting them into the program and servicing their special needs. This person must pull all other staff members together as a team to make the program operate efficiently.

Health/fitness instructors

The positions of health educator, fitness specialist, or health/fitness leader are the next level of staffing. Depending on the program and the size of the company, the responsibilities and duties of this position will vary greatly. Staff for a small program might be only one health educator. In contrast, a large, well-established program can have several staff members at this level, with each having specific responsibilities.

Qualifications of the health/fitness leaders include: BS minimum in health and physical education/fitness or related field; ability to work well with and motivate people; a wellness lifestyle and a good professional image; and other abilities and traits that one would expect of any other employee at this level.

The American College of Sports Medicine (ACSM) certifies health/fitness instructors.[7] Its requirements will meet or exceed the requirements for these types of positions. The Institute for Aerobics Research offers a health/fitness leader short-course certification, which is not as thorough as ACSM but is an excellent program for exercise leaders.

Aerobics instructors

Most programs that offer any physical activity will usually include aerobics, aerobic dancing, step aerobics, and/or some similar program. These classes can be offered in-house or contracted out to a vendor. In general, large programs manage their aerobic activities, and small programs contract these services with specialty vendors.

Several "aerobics" organizations (American Council on Exercise [ACE], Aerobic and Fitness Association of America [AFAA], International Dance Exercise Association [IDEA], and Nike Inc.) offer certifications that are excellent for this type of instructor and should be required of anyone working in this area. Those who have contracted for services with an established "aerobics" vendor may find these vendors do their own training and do not participate in these national programs. However, this level of instructor must understand the principles of exercise, and the program must provide good, safe exercise at the appropriate level. A poorly trained but enthusiastic instructor may do more harm than good.

Vendors and consultants

Almost all programs, regardless of size, will need to use a consultant or outside vendor at some time. These firms provide a valuable resource to solve problems that cannot be managed by the staff and can solve them in a cost effective manner. The key is knowing how to select the proper vendor or consultant for the job. Harris, McKenzie, and Zuti,[16] developed a checklist in which they listed multiple items in six areas to assist in vendor selection. The areas they included were:

1. Initial experience
2. Product quality
3. Service providers
4. Delivery and services
5. Cost
6. General concerns

Finally, the best advice is to hire those with a track record of getting the job done right. One should talk to their costumers, not just listen to what the firms say.

Other staff

Depending on the size and type of the program, other staff members such as secretaries or locker room attendants may be needed. These individuals fill essential roles within the team and should be hired not only for their ability to do the job but more important for their ability to get along with people.

CONSTRUCTION
The construction plan

Before construction starts one must have detailed program plans that are based the company's needs, goals, and objectives. Only then can one address the issue of floor space. It is important to do as much long-range planning as possible, considering corporate growth. Most important is to plan so that future projects can be added easily and with the least cost. One example would be to determine the proposed site for a swimming pool that will be added only if the program grows and funds are available. Even though this is only a hope, planning for plumbing, support walls, and traffic flow at the start will reduce both costs and other problems if the pool is added, and the cost of planning is minimal.

When the medical director and the wellness manager have finalized the program plan and corporate management has approved it, the next step is the selection of the architect. If the company uses a particular firm regularly, this step is easy. One may need only to secure a consultant to help the firm with the detailed specifics of fitness center construction. If the company does not have a preferred architectural firm, one should contact those who have experience in fitness center construction, and evaluate them as one would any other consultant or vendor. Patton et al.[23,24] have described in detail the what, how, and why of fitness center design with examples. Reviewing these texts before selecting the architect could provide considerable insight into the specifics of design and construction and facilitate the selection.

The equipment

The equipment and supplies needed for health education are minimal. Educational videos and models will be the majority. These are relatively inexpensive to obtain, will last for several years, and are easy to store. In contrast, physical fitness equipment is expensive and requires regular maintenance and a well-designed center to house it. A detailed plan with budget should be developed at the same time and in the same way the construction plan is developed.

The physical fitness equipment needed for a full-service center is considerable and expensive. Items must be carefully evaluated based on interests and needs of the employees as determined in the survey. The climate and the company's location can affect equipment like treadmills.

Computer equipment will be needed for general office use as well as for specific functions for health and fitness. When selecting software, one should be sure to select computer programs that will deliver what is wanted. Second, and most important, select standard, proven software, and avoid custom software and/or programs that have not been tested.

BUDGET
Program costs

The cost-benefit material cited in this chapter justifies developing a worksite wellness program. However, starting a program will require one budget and maintaining the operation will require another. When developing the budget, one should consider start-up costs and operational costs. Most programs keep the wellness budget as a separate line item within the medical department's budget. This allows for better cost tracking and also permits the wellness manager to be assigned the responsibility for the budget.

As with any budget, the start-up costs are for the one-time initial costs that occur within the first year or two of the program. Most of these initial costs are for construction and equipment. Ongoing operational costs are treated the same as in any other annual budget, with most of the expenses being in salaries for the professional staff.

If the strategy is to start small to determine whether there is an interest in wellness, the plan should start with health education programs and *no* physical fitness programs. This saves or delays the start-up cost for the construction of a fitness center and the salaries of full-time professionals to staff it. The health education components of wellness are very effective and with a little effort can be done at very low cost. This is possible because those providing wellness services are usually fee-for-service providers, not full-time staff members with salary and benefits.

One can start a wellness program with no cash outlay by the company, only the investment of time of one staff member to manage the scheduling and paperwork. Employees can pay the cost for the programs offered by organizations such as "Weight Watchers"; the company does the promotion, handles registration, and provides the location for the class. When employees pay for part of the wellness program, they show that they have a commitment and some ownership.

Other programs can be obtained at no cost through agencies such as the American Cancer Society. Their education and screening programs are offered free to any company that requests them and will do the promotion and scheduling and provide the meeting space. Organizations that can provide health education services at minimal or no cost include: American Cancer Society, American Heart Association, American Lung Association, American Red Cross, other voluntary health agencies, YMCA, YWCA, Jewish community centers, and federal, state, and local agencies.

Construction costs

Those interested in developing a physical fitness program will probably need to do some major construction. The size and cost of the facility will depend on the goals and the amount of money the company is willing to invest. Depending on the part of the country, the cost of commercial construction will vary from $80 to $150 per square foot. The department responsible for facilities at the company can give an estimate of the costs of recent work, which can give the medical director an idea of what to expect. These approximations are only educated guesses. Two or more formal bids will give the exact dollar cost. In *Developing and Managing Health/Fitness Facilities,* Patton et al.[24] describe in detail what items should be considered when developing facilities.

It is possible to start a fitness program with only minor alterations in an existing facility. However, when planning major construction, experience has shown that building to meet the projected *future* need will be more cost effective. This is particularly true for the building or shell of the facility. Equipment and other interior designs can be altered as the program develops, but if one does not have the space, the program cannot grow.

Annual budget

The annual budget for the operation of the wellness program must be set up the same way as the operating budgets for the company. Items such as salary, benefits, office supplies, telephone, and travel will be standard. Unique items in the wellness budget might include:

- Fees paid to vendors and consultants who provide classes and other services
- Service contract fees on major equipment, such as treadmills and stairsteppers
- Promotion or participant incentives, including awards
- Sport equipment that requires regular replacement
- Staff uniforms
- Chemicals for the swimming pool and Jacuzzi

- Toiletries for the locker room
- Landscaping supplies for sport fields, and other similar items.

PROGRAM EVALUATION AND REVISION
Class evaluation

Every class that is offered should be evaluated by the participants, the instructor, and the wellness manager. Formal written information should be obtained from the participants describing the benefits of the class, the positive and negative aspects of the method of presenting the material, and suggestions for improving or changing the class. Recommended changes could include changing instructors or dropping the class.

The instructors' evaluation is usually presented to the wellness manager in a brief written form describing strengths and weaknesses. This report usually concludes with recommendations for revision that will improve the offering. The wellness manager's evaluation is often in the form of an executive summary based on the other evaluations and is sent to the medical director. These evaluations should be kept on file for later use in determining future staff and program planning.

Program evaluation

At least once a year, all participants should complete a written evaluation of the goals and objectives of the entire program.[22] This type of feedback is more difficult to obtain and interpret than the class evaluations because it is less specific. However, employees must be given an opportunity to comment and make suggestions as to how the program could be improved. A user survey, much like a "customer satisfaction surveys" would be appropriate for evaluating the program.

Program revision

A successful wellness program is dynamic. It must be flexible and responsive to the ever-changing needs and interests of the participants. However, the program need not be changed just for change sake. When program revisions are made, they must be based on the current interests of the employees. The classic trap occurs when management wants a change and the employees will not support it. One of the best ways to evaluate is by results. If a class or particular aspect of the program is well attended, then do *not* change it. On the other hand, when participation begins to drop, that is the time to revise and move on to other areas or interests.

SUMMARY

One reason for developing a wellness program is the cost justification data that attests to employee as well as employer benefit. This and the fact that employees perceive these program as benefits, or even perks, make the decision to develop a program easier. The medical director must provide strong leadership in the program, but the day-to-day operation should be delegated to an experienced wellness manager. Based on a survey of employee needs and interests, the goals and objectives must be established. With these, the program plan can then be developed. With this plan in place, a budget can be developed and, if necessary, construction started. As the program grows, it must be regularly reexamined and revised to meet the ever-changing needs and interests of the employees. All of this is to make it possible for employees to develop the knowledge and skills to keep themselves healthy and fit. And by doing so, they will be happier and more productive.

REFERENCES

1. Anderson DR, Jose WS: Employee lifestyle and the bottom line, *Fitness Bus* 2(3):86, 1987.
2. Association for Fitness In Business: *Guidelines for employee health promotion programs,* Champaign, Ill, 1992, Human Kinetics Books.
3. Bernacki EJ, Baun WB: The relationship of job performance to exercise adherence in a corporate fitness program, *J Occup Med* 26(7):529, 1984.
4. Bensinger A, Pilkington C: An alternate method in the treatment of alcoholism: The United Technologies Corporation day treatment program, *J Occup Med* 300, 1983.
5. Berry CA: An approach to good health for employees and reduced health care costs for industry, *Health Insurance Association of America,* p 9, 1981.
6. Bertera RL: The effects of workplace health promotion on absenteeism and employment costs in a large industrial population, *Am J Pub Health* 80(9):1101, 1990.
7. Blair SN et al: *Guidelines for exercise testing and prescription,* ed 3, Philadelphia, Penn, 1986, Lea & Febiger.
8. Blum T, Roman R: Alcohol, drugs, and EAPs: new data from a national study, *Almacan* 16:20, 1986.
9. Bly J, Jones RC, and Richardson RE: Impact of worksite health promotion on health care costs and utilization, *J Am Med Assoc* 256:3235, 1986.
10. Brown DW et al: Reduced disability and health care costs in an industrial fitness program, *J Occup Med* 26:809, 1984.
11. Cooper KH: *Aerobics,* New York, 1968, Bantam Books.
12. Cristina J: GTE: Florida's in-house physical therapy program, *Corporate Fitness* 65, 1987.
13. Fitzler SL, Berger RA: Chelsea back program: one year later, *Occup Health Safety* 52(7):52, 1983.
14. Gettman LR: Cost/benefit analysis of a corporate fitness program, *Fitness Bus* 1(1):11, 1986.
15. Gibbs JO et al: Worksite health promotion: five-year trend in employee health care costs, *J Occup Med* 27:826, 1985.
16. Harris JH, McKenzie JF, and Zuti WB: How to select the right vendor for your company's health promotion program, *Fitness Bus* 1(3):53-56, 1986.
17. Manuso JSJ: The Equitable Life Assurance Society program, *Prev Med* 12:658, 1983.
18. McGaffey TN: New horizons in organizational stress prevention approaches, *Personnel Administrator* 11:26, 1978.
19. Mulvaney DE et al: Staying alive and well at Blue Cross and Blue Shield of Indiana. In Opatz JP, editors: *Health promotion evaluation: measuring the organizational impact,* Stevens Point, Wisc, 1987, National Wellness Institute.
20. Norris E: Alcohol: companies are learning it pays to help workers beat the bottle, *Business Insurance* Nov. 16, 1981.
21. Opatz J, Chenoweth D, and Kaman R: *Economic impact of worksite health promotion,* Indianapolis, Ind, 1990, Association of Fitness in Business.

22. Parkinson RS et al: *Managing health promotion in the workplace: guidelines for implementation and evaluation,* Palo Alto, Calif, 1982, Mayfield Publishing.

23. Patton RW et al: *Implementing health/fitness programs,* Champaign, Ill, 1986, Human Kinetics Books.

24. Patton RW et al: *Developing and managing health/fitness facilities,* Champaign, Ill, 1989, Human Kinetics Books.

25. Pender NJ, Smith LC, and Vernoff JA: Building better workers, *Am Assoc Occup Health Nurs J* 35(9):386, 1987.

26. Rhodes EC, Dunwoody D: Physiological and attitudinal changes of individuals involved in an employee fitness program, *Can J Publ Health* 71:331, 1980.

27. Rudman WJ: Do onsite health and fitness programs affect worker productivity? *Fitness in Bus* 2(1):2, 1987.

28. Schrier JW: A survey on drug abuse in organizations, *Personnel Journal* 16:478, 1983.

29. Shephard RJ: Current perspectives on the economics of fitness and sport with particular reference to worksite programs, *Sports Med* 7:286, 1989.

30. Shephard RJ, Corey P, and Cox MH: Health hazard appraisal—the influence of an employee fitness programme, *Can J Pub Health* 73:183, 1982.

31. Shephard RJ, Cox M, and Corey P: Fitness program participation: its effects on worker performance, *J Occup Med* 23:359, 1981.

32. Shipley RH et al: Effect of the Johnson & Johnson Live for Life Program on employee smoking, *Prev Med* 17:25, 1988.

33. Tsai SP, Bernacki EJ, and Baun WB: Injury prevalence and associated costs among participants of an employee fitness program, *Prev Med* 17(4):475, 1988.

34. Wilbur CS: The Johnson & Johnson Program, *Prev Med* 12:672, 1983.

RESOURCES

Aerobics and Fitness Association of America (AFAA), 15250 Ventura Blvd., Suite 310, Sherman Oaks, CA 91403.

American College of Sports Medicine (ACSM), P.O. Box 1440, Indianapolis, IN 46202.

American Council on Exercise (ACE), 5820 Oberlin Dr., Suite 102, San Diego, CA, 92121.

Association for Worksite Health Promotion (AWHP), 60 Revere Dr., Suite 500, Northbrook, IL 60062.

International Dance Exercise Association (IDEA), 6190 Cornerstone Ct. East, Suite 202, San Diego, CA 92121.

Institute for Aerobics Research, 12330 Preston Rd., Dallas, TX 75230.

Nike Inc., 3900 Southwest Murray Blvd., Beaverton, OR 97005.

President's Council for Physical Fitness and Sports (PCPFS), 450 Fifth St., Suite 7103, Washington, DC 20001.

Chapter 64

SAFETY IN THE HOME
AND AUTOMOBILE

Jack T. Collins
Roslyn S. Collins

SAFETY IN THE HOME

As the twentieth century draws to a close, it is becoming increasingly clear that being "safe" within our homes is no longer as simple as it used to be. Industrial growth and urbanization have taxed our environmental resources, threatening the quality of the water we drink and the air we breathe. Poverty and the breakdown of the family have presented us with a scenario of increasing violence. The aging of our population, a happy byproduct of our increased medical knowledge, now confronts us with new challenges in safer product design for a burgeoning senior population.

At the same time, much has been accomplished in solving these problems. In the last 20 years we have seen a proliferation of good legislation designed to address these challenges; to clean up our air, to keep our waters safe, and to ensure the safety of the products that come into our homes. Many of our health statistics already reflect benefits from these efforts.

The role of the physician, then, has expanded to include being a proponent of those environmental controls and legislation, as well as product improvement, that will lead to better health for patients.

ENVIRONMENTAL FACTORS AFFECTING THE HOME
Water quality

The availability of safe drinking water has always been a primary health concern to all households, and throughout time, the lack of such has been responsible for plagues, numerous diseases, and infant mortality. In this industrial era, a safe supply of potable water appears to increasingly depend on governmental regulation.

An understanding of what is happening in the environment and how legislation has affected the quality of water entering the home is important in deciding whether to recommend testing or treatment of the home water supply. (In rural areas, this is usually accomplished in cooperation with the health officer.) A knowledge of current trends in water quality is also important if one is seeking public support for protection of our water resources.

The Safe Drinking Water Act. The current governmental strategy for protection of the domestic water supply began in 1974 with the passage of the Safe Drinking Water Act (SDWA). This legislation established nationally consistent water standards and gave responsibility for compliance with the law to state health and environmental agencies (Indiana and Wyoming were exceptions by opting to employ the federal Environmental Protection Agency [EPA] to run their programs). Under the SWDA, all systems serving more than 25 people or having more than 15 service connections are required to comply with the national guidelines. Smaller systems are under the jurisdiction of state regulations.[44]

In 1986 the number of contaminants regulated by the SWDA was expanded from 26 to 83. The amended law also required filtration of surface water and expanded the monitoring of unregulated contaminants.

Safety of the home water supply. How safe has this made our water? In 1988 more than 80% of Americans were receiving drinking water from systems conforming with SDWA standards. Compliance problems were found mostly in small rural systems serving 25 to 3300 people.[44]

Recent studies have linked sporadic cases of community-based Legionnaire's disease with household water supplies harboring Legionella pneumophila, especially those in large multidwelling residences with large storage tanks. The growth of these microbial agents may be encouraged by hosting conditions that are found in these large storage tanks, such as low temperatures, microbial flora, scale, and sediment. Because of epidemiological uncertainty concerning diagnosed cases of community-based Legionnaire's diseases, the culturing of water sources associated with these diagnosed cases had not been recommended by the Centers for Disease Control. These new findings, however, may open the possibility that the water of a patient's residence may be the source of exposure.[72]

The current focus of federal drinking water regulation has been shifting from a preoccupation with total coliform levels, which are the most common violation but also the easiest to correct, to the control of contaminants, such as pesticides, which pose long-term health threats.[44] These are difficult and expensive to monitor, placing a harsh financial burden on smaller water supply systems and their customers. Prevention of contamination of the water supply, therefore, becomes not only a health and environmental issue, but also an economic concern.

Safety of groundwater supplies. Approximately one half of the population of the United States, including 34 of the largest cities and over 85% of rural households, receives its drinking water from groundwater, or water found in aquifers and layers of sand and rock underlying the earth's surface. Once it is polluted, slow-moving groundwater is expensive and difficult to clean. Left alone, the cleansing process could take as long as 250 years.[17]

Hazardous waste disposal is now highly regulated near underground water sources. The injection of chemical wastes, municipal sewage, and brine used to force oil and gas into wells near the groundwater sources demanded control, and this was given to the EPA in 1974.

However, many injection wells used in the oil and gas industry continue to present challenges. Because of an economic downturn in the industry, improper plugging of abandoned wells is reported on the increase in Texas, Oklahoma, Kansas, and other petroleum-producing states. Brine fluids containing high levels of chlorides and other dissolved solids flow upward through these wells to damage local water supplies or ruin crops.[17]

Agrichemical and pesticide contamination of water. Agrichemical contamination of groundwater is increasing, matching the 15% growth in the use of commercial fertilizers and pesticides between 1974 and 1985. In 1986, pesticides were applied by approximately 57% of American farms, and 75% used commercial fertilizers.[8]

In 1988, 46 pesticides were documented by the EPA in the groundwater from 26 states. A 1989 study by the United States Geological Society (USGS) reported that 90% of streams tested in 10 Midwestern agricultural states showed detection of pesticides shortly after spring application. Although quantities were small, numerous samples exceeded health advisory limits for the restricted-use chemicals atrazine and alachlor.[8]

Pesticides are less dangerous in drinking water than exposure to the pure compound on food or in handling; however, minute quantities of chemicals in the water can cause concern. Exposure risks depend on the concentration levels, length of exposure, and the ingestor's body weight, age, and health. Health effects range from mild headaches and skin rashes to long-term damage to internal organs, cancer, and death. The EPA has developed technical guidance documents that provide detailed assessments for particular pesticides, as well as nitrates/nitrites.[56]

Farm families can take steps to reduce exposure to agrichemical pollution of the home water supply. Some of these include the relocation away from wells of holding and mixing facilities for agrichemicals. Improved storage, handling, and treatment techniques can also reduce potential groundwater contamination from livestock wastes (Fig. 64-1).

Agrichemical applications can also be timed to meet crop needs more closely, pest scouting can result in fewer chemical applications, and agrichemical applications can be avoided during weather conditions that are conducive to leaching.[8]

Testing and treatment of home water supplies. Testing of water in drinking wells for pesticides is more complex and costly than examinations for minerals or bacteria. State or county officials are the best source of information on contamination problems experienced in the area; state or county officials, state university laboratories, or EPA regional offices can advise on certified testing services or laboratories. If pesticide levels are above the EPA's Health Advisory levels, retesting is advised. State or county health officials can recommend appropriate action for polluted wells, such as treatment of the water, digging a new or deeper well, or switching to alternative water supplies, including bottled water.[56]

Some home water-treatment devices may effectively remove particular pesticides and impurities, and the EPA has issued Health Advisory Summaries that provide guidelines for selection of the proper system for removing the pollutant. Current technologies for home systems include use of carbon filters, reverse osmosis or distillation, and anion exchange. All home treatment systems require periodic monitoring and maintenance for optimum performance.[56]

Air quality in the home

The air inside homes is a potential harbinger of pollution, and with it some important disease states. These include Radon 222 and its decay products (with the late sequelae of lung carcinoma), asbestos, carbon monoxide, dust pollution, sulfur dioxide and, on the farm, nitrogen dioxide (silo-filler's disease) and farmer's lung.

The Environmental Protection Agency has indicated

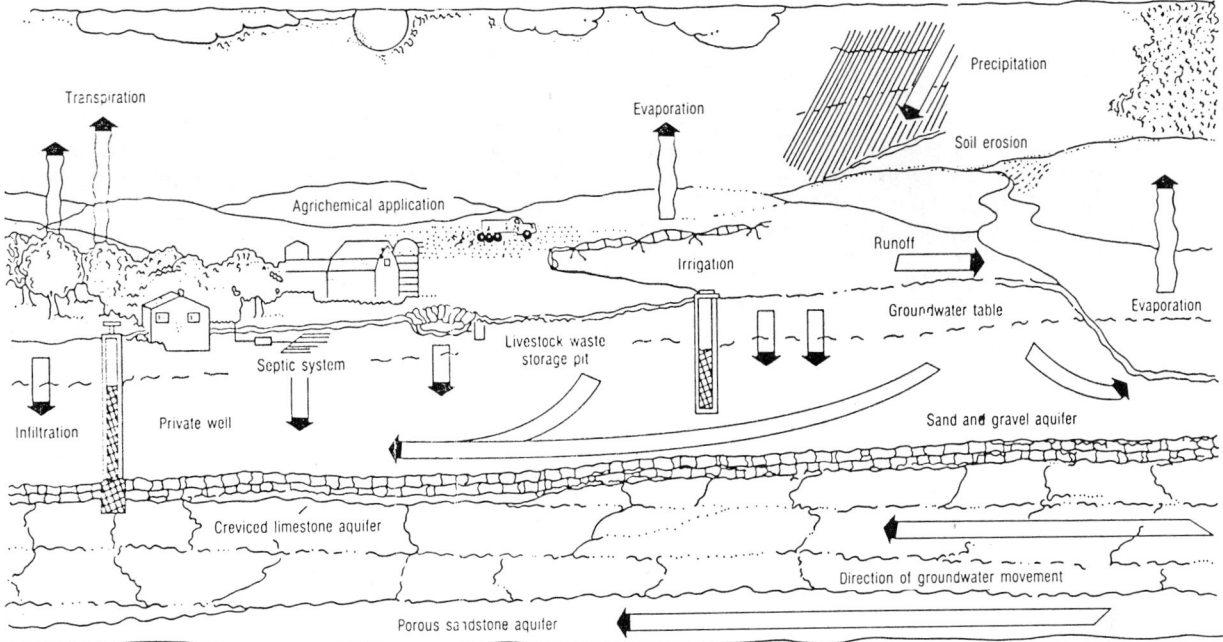

Fig. 64-1. Primary on-farm pathways of agrichemical contamination of ground water. (Adapted from Soil and Water Conservation Society: *Treasure of abundance or Pandora's box?: a guide for safe, profitable fertilizer and pesticide use,* Washington, DC, 1989, US Congress, Office of Technology Assessment; *Beneath the bottom line: Agricultural approaches to reduce agrichemical contamination of ground water.*)

that in the last several years scientific evidence has been accumulating that the air within homes and other buildings can be more seriously polluted than the outdoor air in even the largest and most industrialized cities. Most people spend approximately 90% of their time indoors. Thus the risks to health may be greater because of exposure to air pollution indoors, and the persons most likely to be affected are those spending the most time indoors, namely, the young, the elderly, the chronically ill, and especially those suffering from respiratory or cardiovascular disease.[75] A substantial amount of this indoor pollution is related to radon.

Radon

Radon 222. Radon 222 is an inert gas with a half-life of 3.8 days. Although it does not deposit or decay within the respiratory tract to any significant extent, its progeny are particulates attached to other aerosol particles that do deposit on the surfaces of the respiratory tract.[27]

As early as the sixteenth century a high incidence of lung disease was recognized among certain underground mine populations in eastern Europe, particularly in Schneeberg and in the Erz mountains. The disease was later identified as lung cancer. Fairly recent research has shown that the cause was high radon concentrations in mine air. Other affected populations have included both uranium miners and other hard rock miners. After these

discoveries came safety standards for the air in mines, resulting in a marked reduction in radon pollution.

However, the dangers of the radon progeny inhalation became a major public concern with the discovery of high levels of radon within domestic dwellings. Regulatory agencies from many countries set standards for exposure levels within domestic environments, with the standards based on epidemiological studies of populations of miners.

Nationally the EPA has stated that the level of radon in the home should be less than 4 pCi/L of air. The national average is estimated at 1.5 pCi/L. Levels as high as 200 pCi/L have been found.[27]

Indoor radon, a colorless, odorless gas, originally comes from uranium in the soil and rock on which homes are built. With the natural breakdown of the radon into its daughters (progeny), radon gas enters homes through dirt floors, cracks in concrete walls and floor drains, and sumps (Fig. 64-2).

In rural areas and some other areas radon can be found in well water. In addition, according to the EPA, some houses are made of radon-containing construction materials, with resultant release of radon into the indoor air. Studies have reported that as many as 10% of all U.S. homes may have elevated levels of radon. These levels can be detected only by the use of measurement instruments called radon detectors.

The only known health effect related to radon exposure

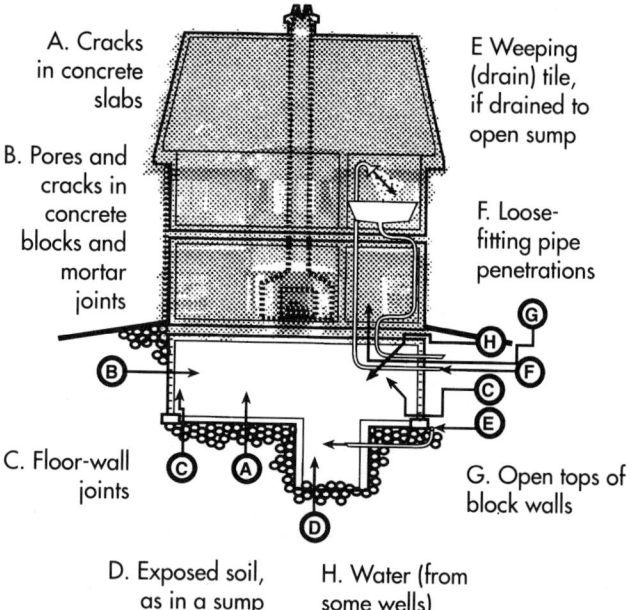

A. Cracks in concrete slabs

B. Pores and cracks in concrete blocks and mortar joints

C. Floor-wall joints

D. Exposed soil, as in a sump

E Weeping (drain) tile, if drained to open sump

F. Loose-fitting pipe penetrations

G. Open tops of block walls

H. Water (from some wells)

Fig. 64-2. How radon enters the home. (From Environmental Protection Agency and the American Medical Association: *Radon, the health threat with a simple solution, a physician's guide,* AMA15:90-594, 1990.)

is lung carcinoma; the EPA estimates 8000 to 40,000 lung cancer deaths annually in the United States may be attributed to radon (total lung cancer deaths in 1988 from all causes estimated at 139,000).[13,31,53]

Reducing exposure to radon in homes[13,75]

Measuring radon levels. Two types of radon detectors are most commonly used in homes: charcoal canisters that are exposed for 2 to 7 days, and alpha track detectors that are exposed for 1 month or longer. (Some states recommend that residents use only the alpha track monitors.)

Action to reduce radon levels. An effective radon mitigation plan may include one or more of the following actions: sealing cracks and other openings in basement floors, ventilating crawl spaces, installing subslab or basement ventilation, or installing air-to-air heat exchangers.

Increasing ventilation can be an effective means of reducing exposure to many indoor air pollutants. In homes with elevated concentrations of radon, however, increasing ventilation incorrectly may increase infiltration through the foundation and draw even larger amounts of radon into the home. The problem of ventilation can be solved by opening windows evenly on all sides of the home. Opening windows is particularly important when using outdoor-vented exhaust fans.

The EPA suggests that all but the most experienced "do-it-yourselfers" get professional help in selecting and installing radon reduction measures. The EPA booklet *Radon Reduction Methods: A Homeowner's Guide* offers advice about how to evaluate proposals for radon mitigation.

Lead. "Lead toxicity is the most common illness of environmental origin in American children today, with well over one-sixth of the nation's children affected." This was one of the statements made at hearings on the Lead Ban and Lead Exposure Reduction Acts of 1990, which contained stringent proposals for eliminating additional sources of lead from the U.S. environment.[76]

Lead paint remains in at least 30 million homes in the United States. Lead continues to seep into the water supply of both homes and schools from leaded plumbing, and is still present in product packaging, food cans, cosmetics, and gasoline in urban areas, leaving long-term effects on the health of U.S. children.[52] In addition, U.S. manufacturers use 1.4 million tons of lead annually, three fourths of this in storage batteries. In 1990, 20% of these batteries were still ending up in trash heaps.[76] A thorough discussion on lead screening of the pediatric patient and prevention can be found in Chapter 27.

Patients concerned about lead in the paint of their homes may choose to take a sample to a testing laboratory for analysis. HUD recommends action be taken to reduce exposure if lead in the paint is greater than 0.5% by lab testing, or greater than 1.0 milligrams per square centimeter by x-ray fluorescence, and especially if the paint is deteriorating or when infants, children, and pregnant women are present. Removing lead-based paint of more than one square foot should be done by qualified professionals.[81]

Where chronic lead exposure is discovered in the home or thought to be present, lead per se can be sampled from body tissues. In the blood, it is confined to the red cells, and whole blood must be analyzed. Long-term exposure may be assayed by determination of the level of zinc protoporphyrin (ZPP) in blood, a good screening test.

In this age of intercontinental travel, when medical centers often see patients from all over the globe, the physician must be aware of patients' cultures and living conditions (see section on Prevention of home accidents in this chapter). Chronic low-grade lead exposure in the adult may be difficult to detect, and the patient may present only with lab findings of mild anemia and a slight increase in serum bilirubin (which are nonspecific findings). Other signs such as "failing health," irritability, decrease in concentration, anorexia, dysphagia, and change in bowel character may be present. Some houses in use hundreds of years, as in the eastern Mediterranean, may contain lead piping or lead-lined water storage tanks.

Similar to the other potential toxins in this chapter, the key treatment remains the removal of the source of exposure.

Asbestos. Asbestosis is the most frequent inorganic dust-related chronic pulmonary disease. Not only is the pulmonary disease disabling, but the end result is often adenocarcinoma or squamous cell carcinoma of the lung, (potentiated by cigarette smoking) and mesothelioma (incidence not affected by smoking).[51,74]

Asbestos was introduced to industry in the 1940s and was noted for its excellent thermal qualities, its ability to resist fire, and other properties. It was used widely in construction of buildings and homes. In the 1970s the toxic effects of asbestos fibers became widely known, and the material has been undergoing a long period of replacement with man-made mineral fibers, such as fiberglass or slag-wool. Brake linings are still being made with asbestos, and the material probably will remain to some extent in insulation both in homes and industry.

Because the patient may be eligible for compensation, the physician must keep an accurate history of the rate of occupational exposure and assist the patient in making a prompt application for compensation. Because of the high risk of lung cancer, if that patient is a smoker, every effort should be made to stop this practice as soon as possible. (Smoking in an asbestos worker produces much more than a simple additive effect.)

What to do about asbestos in the home[3]

Steps taken by the EPA. In 1973 the EPA prohibited the spraying of asbestos-containing materials for insulation, fire protection, and soundproofing. In 1975 the EPA prohibited the use of asbestos for pipe covering if the material crumbles easily after it dries. In 1977 the Consumer Product Safety Commission (CPSC) banned two asbestos-containing products: patching compounds and artificial fireplace emberizing materials (ash and embers) containing respirable asbestos. In 1986 the CPSC required labeling of products containing asbestos. In 1989 the EPA announced a phased-in ban of most asbestos products, culminating in 1996.

Action by homeowners. Generally, the homeowner should leave asbestos-containing materials undisturbed. Expert advice and assistance should be obtained for major renovating. For more complete information, contact the nearest EPA office or the EPA Toxic Substance Control Act (TSCA) assistance line (see Resources at end of this chapter).

Formaldehyde. An important chemical used widely by the building industry, especially in pressed wood products, formaldehyde is also a byproduct of combustion and certain other natural processes. A colorless, pungent-smelling gas, it can cause irritation of eyes, nose and throat, skin rash, and severe allergic reactions and has been shown to cause cancer in animals.

Formaldehyde emissions generally decrease as products age. Therefore, in older homes, formaldehyde levels are generally below 0.1 ppm, whereas homes with large amounts of pressed wood products can reach 0.3 ppm.

During the 1970s, urea-formaldehyde foam insulation was widely used until high concentrations of formaldehyde were measured in homes in which it had recently been installed. Most of this insulation has aged and no longer continues to give problems unless it is damp or there are cracks in interior walls that expose the foam. In addition,

the formaldehyde emission limits on plywood and particleboard used in construction of prefabricated and mobile homes have been restricted since 1985 by the U.S. Department of Housing and Urban Development (HUD).

Steps to reduce exposure include using exterior-grade pressed wood products, using air conditioning and dehumidifiers to reduce humidity levels and maintain moderate temperatures, and increasing ventilation after bringing new sources of formaldehyde into the home.[75]

Sulfur dioxide. In an article entitled "The Environment and the Lung," Samet and Utell describe the relationship of sulfur dioxide/particulate matter pollution and the pollution disasters in Donora, Pennsylvania in 1948 and during the London fog of 1952; high levels of acid aerosols and sulfur dioxide were involved. During the London fog an estimated 4000 deaths occurred, primarily among the elderly and those with a chronic respiratory disease.[64]

Passage of the Clean Air Act in the United States in the early 1970s under the EPA has resulted in local reduction of air pollution. However, because of the new employment of tall smoke stacks, particularly for power plants, the pollutants were now being emitted high into the atmosphere, allowing them to be transported long distances and to remain in the air for a long time. Prolonged residence time at this high altitude permitted their transformation into acid chemicals, particularly sulfuric acid. According to Samet and Utell's report, an "emerging concern about the effects of these acidic aerosols has now extended beyond environmental effects on trees and lakes to human health."

The effects of elevated levels of acid aerosols/sulfur dioxide are primarily pulmonary (i.e., exacerbation of asthma and chronic obstructive pulmonary disease and irritation by sulfuric acid).

Nitrogen dioxide. *Silo-filler's disease* refers to the hazards associated with silos resulting from nitrogen-dioxide–induced injury to the lung (the gas formed by the silage). This is a fully preventable disease and, if it is diagnosed early and treated with corticosteroids right away, a great deal of the alveolar damage can be avoided, unlike the toxicity of sulfur dioxide.[16]

Douglas et al. at the Mayo Clinic describe four phases of silo-filler's disease:

1. Physical collapse and possible sudden death
2. Acute alveolar injury and pulmonary edema
3. Early and reversible bronchiolitis obliterans
4. Late scarring and irreversible bronchiolitis obliterans

Because of corticosteroid use scarring seldom takes place as in phase 4. Prevention is essential for the elimination of silo-filler's disease. With the naming of this entity as silo-filler's disease in 1956, the following steps were outlined:

1. Allow no one to enter the silo for any purpose from the time of filling until 7 to 10 days thereafter

2. Provide good ventilation above the base of the silo during this dangerous period
3. Provide fencing or other barriers to prevent children or animals from straying into any space adjoining the silo
4. Always activate the blower fan before entering the silo

The major pathogenic manifestations of silo-filler's disease are alveolar damage and broncholitis obliterans, which may have either acute or delayed onset. In addition, the physician needs to be aware that the sudden collapse of a person near a silo may be from nitrogen dioxide asphyxiation. Prompt CPR should be instituted until a rescue team arrives. One hopes that the design of future silos will eliminate the development of toxic gas conditions.

Farmer's lung. In the same category as silo-filler's disease is farmer's lung and organic dust syndrome, both of which can occur in the same farmer. The provoking stimulus of farmer's lung is moldy hay, which contains the spores of thermophilic actinomycetes, which produce a hypersensitivity pneumonitis. Although the 2 million farmers in the United States and the half million workers in grain elevators are potentially at risk, exact figures on incidence are difficult to obtain because of the wide variety of grain dusts that are capable of producing a similar picture.

The usual picture is that of an acute flu-like illness starting 4 to 8 hours after exposure and characterized by rapid onset of fever and malaise, chills, cough, and dyspnea with absence of wheezing. Repeated episodes can lead to a chronic phase of illness. In addition like most of the other respiratory diseases, the condition is greatly worsened by prior cigarette smoking, and, although usually confined to adults, there have been some scattered reports of farmer's lung in children.[54]

Prevention of farmer's lung still rests on the avoidance of moldy hay. The use of a breathing mask has reportedly greatly reduced the severity of the illness and may possibly act as a preventive in the future.[43]

Approximately two dozen other organic dusts are involved in hypersensitivity pneumonitis besides farmer's lung, any of which can cause an acute flu-like illness. A careful inventory will usually reveal the offending agent (e.g., mushroom worker's disease, woodcutter's disease).

RADIATION EXPOSURE EFFECTS ON HEALTH

The physician plays an important role in treating people injured by ionizing radiation. The partial core meltdown at Three Mile Island in 1979 sounded the alarm throughout the United States that nuclear power plants were in danger of emitting ionizing radiation that would affect the health of the employees of the plant as well as whole communities nearby. No new applications for a nuclear power plant have been filed since 1977. At the same time, many measures have been adapted to make nuclear reactors safer.

The steam-hydrogen explosion at Chernobyl in Russia in 1986 resulted in many lost lives from the immediate effects of radiation. Bone marrow transplants saved some lives. Long-term effects will probably be leukemia and other neoplastic diseases.

According to the report of the Council on Scientific Affairs, American Medical Association, 1989, if an emergency occurs physicians should know how to find out how much radiation was released "and be able to offer appropriate advice to patients and the public." For additional information on nuclear power and the physician, see the council report.[12]

NOISE POLLUTION

One of the characteristics of civilization is noise pollution, with continuous noise being more dangerous than interrupted noise. Numerous studies have reported that a decibel level above 115 for a duration of perhaps 30 minutes will result in hearing deficit if it persists for a period of time. This level is achieved when standing close to jet aircraft or with simultaneously running the dishwasher and vacuum cleaner in the home.

This danger is also present when listening to uninterrupted rock music rather than intermittent rock, and the danger is greater when higher decibels are directed at the ears with use of the Walkman-type stereo listening devices that are turned up too high.

The family physician must be aware of this increasing noise in our environment, with its increase in numbers of persons with high-tone nerve deafness. The family needs to be advised about the importance of reducing the number of noise-producing gadgets in the household and especially of avoiding their simultaneous use. Ear plugs should be worn when operating garden or lawn equipment, chain saws, and any device that puts out similar sound intensities.

The development of low-noise home equipment, such as dishwashers, lawnmowers, and power saws, is important to preventive medicine. Surely silence must be an active ingredient in the health program.

PREVENTION IN NATURAL DISASTERS

"Then to the elements be free, and fare thou well!"
William Shakespeare, from "The Tempest"

Natural disasters and the accompanying injury and death have usually been considered outside the realm of preventive medicine. Recent reports from the National Weather Service, however, have demonstrated that adequate warnings and preparedness can significantly decrease morbidity and mortality in storms and other natural hazards. The physician, therefore, may need to assume a leadership role in counseling for potential disasters common to his or her geographic area. Such a role might include such tasks as stressing the importance of preparedness, promot-

ing family disaster plans and an awareness of safer home-
steads, and supporting government policies that provide
for protection in natural disasters.

The most significant and gradual decline in U.S. fatalities during the last 50 years from violent storms has been
recorded in those associated with lightning storms. In addition, in 1990 only 53 people died from tornadoes despite
an increase in tornado frequency and a new annual record
of 1121 tornadoes. Both of these statistics reflect improvements in watch and warning systems and public compliance with awareness and preparedness activities.[4,6]

Floods, flash floods, and hurricanes

On average more than 300,000 U.S. citizens are driven
out of their homes by floods each year, with 200 people
killed. Flood warnings can be issued hours before the
flood peak for major river basins, but flash floods, sometimes producing a "wall of water," give little warning and
require fast action. The time between detection of flood
conditions and the arrival of the flood crest may be short.
No area is immune from flash floods, which may arise on
small streams, near mountainous areas, and in urban areas.[24] In desert states, floods resulting from heavy storms
in the mountains have occured even when skies are clear at
the point of flooding.

Reacting within seconds to flash flood warnings for the
area (or on the observation of rising stream water) by seeking higher ground is a vital life-saving maneuver. Cars
should not be driven through flooded areas because they
may stall and be carried away. Campers should avoid
campsites near streams and washes, particularly during
threatening conditions.

Storm surges, or great domes of water often 50 miles
wide and up to 35 feet high that sweep across coastal areas
in hurricanes, are the most devastating part of a hurricane,
causing 9 out of 10 hurricane fatalities. During hurricane
watches for the area, one should stress the importance of
keeping abreast of National Weather Service announcements, being prepared to leave if local authorities recommend evacuation, securing mobile home tie downs, windows, and loose objects outside, and stocking up with containers of drinking water, canned food, and necessary
medicines.[71]

To prevent disease after floods, fresh food and medicines that have come in contact with flood waters should
be destroyed. Until the public water system has been declared safe, drinking water should be boiled for 10 minutes
or disinfected with ½ teaspoon of commercial liquid laundry bleach to 2½ gallons water.[32]

Tornadoes and severe thunderstorms

Tornadoes occur in all 50 states and can develop at any
time of the year, but are more common in the continental
plains and Gulf Coast of the United States in April, May,
and June. In an average year, tornadoes claim 100 lives.[77]

Seniors aged 60 and over are seven times more likely to be
injured than people under age 20. This can be attributed to
the effects of medical illnesses, decreased mobility, slower
reaction times, and greater susceptibility to injury.[6]

The National Severe Storms Forecast Center in Kansas
City, Missouri has developed a Severe Thunderstorm and
Tornado Watch and Warning System that is broadcast on
NOAA Weather Radio, television, and commercial radio.
Watches indicate that atmospheric conditions are conducive to violent storms and call for preliminary plans for action. Warnings are issued by local weather service offices
when severe storms have been spotted in the area by radar,
trained spotters, or other reliable sources.

The key to survival in nature's most violent storm may
depend on having a tornado emergency plan. All members
of a household should know where the safest areas are,
i.e., in the basement or interior part of the lowest level of
the home (which could include interior bathrooms, closets,
or halls) and should move to such areas at the first sign of
danger. People in mobile homes should leave and take
shelter in a substantial structure or the nearest ditch or ra-
vine with hands shielding the head.[80]

In populated areas, automobiles should not be used for
fleeing from tornadoes. More than half of the deaths in the
1979 Wichita Falls tornado were attributed to people trying to escape in motor vehicles. Driving vehicles away
from tornadoes may be safer in open country, but it is still
usually best to seek or remain in a sturdy shelter.[80]
Schools should not dismiss students if a tornado warning
has been issued, because buses, like other vehicles, provide no protection. If caught in a tornado, bus drivers
should look for nearby shelter, including ditches and ra-
vines.[5]

Lightning

There are at least 100,000 thunderstorms each year in
the United States, spawning lightning that kills an average
of 100 Americans per year and injures approximately 250
more.

The chance of injury from lightning strikes can be lessened if weather warnings are heeded and shelter is chosen
wisely in emergencies. Safer choices include getting off or
away from open water, metal farm equipment, and small
metal vehicles such as motorcycles, bicycles, and golf
carts. Golfers should put down their clubs and remove golf
shoes. Groups caught in the open should spread out and
keep persons several yards apart. Tall isolated trees, telephone poles, wire fences, pipes, rails, and telephones
should be avoided, as well as standing above the surrounding landscape, such as on a hilltop. Feeling the hair "stand
on end" may mean that lighting is about to strike, and an
immediate drop to the knees, bending forward with hands
on the knees, may prevent injury, as lightning takes the
shortest path to the ground. Do not lie flat, as the lightning
charge may spread through the wet ground.[77] Hikers on

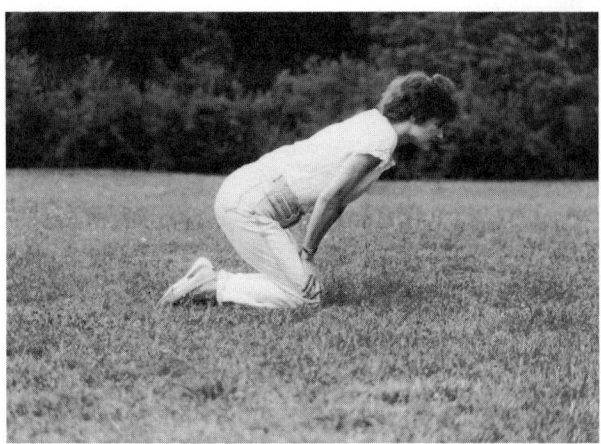

Fig. 64-3. Low, "prayer-like" crouching position to assume in a thunder or lightning storm. (Photo by Mark NeuCollins.)

mountains who cannot get to lower levels should not seek shelter in caves, which are usually wet, but should assume the low crouching position described (Fig. 64-3). Vehicles remain one of the safest places to be in thunderstorms, as few cases have been reported of lightning striking automobiles.[5]

Earthquakes

The United States has had five devastating earthquakes in the last 200 years. Geologists claim that 37 states and more than 150 million people across the land are at risk from earthquakes.[18] The western states, particularly Alaska, California, Washington, Oregon, Nevada, Utah, and Montana, experience them more frequently, but major quakes have occurred in widely scattered locations.

Loss of life in earthquakes can be reduced by attention to special construction techniques for homes, public buildings, highways, and utilities in seismically active areas. This point is emphasized by the fact that 20,000 lives were lost in the Armenian earthquake in December of 1988, and fewer than 100 in the San Francisco Bay area quake during the 1989 World Series. In government hearings on reducing earthquake hazards after the California quake, Robert Hanson, engineering directorate of the National Science Foundation, said, "Recent earthquakes have demonstrated that man-made systems designed and constructed in accordance with current resistant knowledge and techniques have not collapsed," while other structures not designed with such detail have resulted in major loss of life.[18]

Most earthquake-related casualties can be attributed to falling objects and debris as shocks demolish buildings and other structures.[19,25,63] The best prevention of injury from earthquake begins long before the quake occurs, especially in the consideration of earthquake hazard when decisions are made on structure design and land and building use in quake-prone areas. Citizens and physicians must encour-

age this, as well as advocate the adoption and enforcement of local building codes for housing, public buildings, and utilities that help to reduce earthquake injuries.[19]

Homeowners in the quake areas can prepare by checking their homes for earthquake hazards. Gas appliances and water heaters should have strong support and flexible connections wherever possible, as fire damage can result when gas lines are broken. Large, heavy objects should be placed on lower shelves and shelves fastened to walls. High or top-heavy objects should be braced or anchored.[63]

Conducting family earthquake drills, as well as knowing what to do and where to go regardless of whether the individual is at home or elsewhere, is important in preventing injury and panic. At home, responsible family members should know how to turn off electricity, gas, and water at main switches and valves.[25]

Wildfires and the home

Proper site selection for homes in forested areas of the United States that are susceptible to wildfires, as well as good planting and storage techniques, is vital in protecting life and property from this hazard. In addition, fire plans should be developed that include normal and alternate escape routes, communication areas to "ride out fires" if evacuation is not possible, and decisions on when to evacuate and who is to do what in an emergency.

Narrow canyons and saddles should be avoided for homesites, as uphill fires rage dangerously fast. The most level areas of a site are the safest and provide easier access for firefighting equipment. The size and number of windows facing the normal carrying wind or downhill side, or both, should be minimized.

Planting fire-resistant plant species and providing green zones 30 feet around the home, as well as regularly trimming trees, shrubs, and weeds and disposing of the brush, will help to impede the fire's progress. Homeowners remaining behind to fight the fire should have protective clothing ready; cotton clothing is necessary as synthetics can melt on the skin.[82]

Heat waves

Nearly 20,000 people died in the United States in the 40-year period from 1936 to 1975 from the effects of heat and solar radiation. Approximately 175 die of summer heat in a normal year. The deadly 1980 heat wave claimed the lives of 1250.[30]

Heat is most severe on the health of the elderly, small children, chronic invalids, people on certain medications or drugs (especially tranquilizers and anticholinergics), and people with weight and alcohol problems. In addition, stagnant atmospheric conditions often trap pollutants in urban air, compounding the health problems of these at-risk populations living in cities.

The National Weather Service initiates alerts when the heat index is expected to exceed 105° to 110° F for 2 consecutive days in normally temperate areas. Prevention advice should include reduction of strenuous activity, less ingestion of proteins, increase of nonalcoholic fluid intake, avoidance of sun, and an increase in time spent in air-conditioned places. Air-conditioned homes markedly reduce the health dangers from heat.[30] Proper dress is also important. During periods of high heat (as well as in desert areas) clothing should be light colored to reflect the sun and loose fitting for ventilation. Work in desert areas should be accomplished in early morning, early evening, or at night to avoid physical distress from the heat. One must be aware of the dangers assumed on hiking in desert areas. In desert states, pamphlets and brochures may be obtained from sources such as various state and federal park services and the Department of Natural Resources. In addition to proper dress, one should carry water, a compass, and maps, and prepare for the unexpected, such as getting lost.

PREVENTION OF HOME FIRES

Fires were the fourth leading cause of accidental deaths in 1988.[2] There were 454,500 home fires in the United States in 1990, causing 4050 civilian deaths and 20,225 civilian injuries, and resulting in over $4 billion in property damage.

From 1985-1989, the major causes of these fires, listed in order of frequency, were heating systems, cooking equipment, incendiary or suspicious causes, other equipment, electrical distribution systems, and smoking materials.

During these years, the greatest percentage of home fires transpired between 4 and 8 PM with the peak occurring from 6 to 7 PM. The kitchen was the most common site of origin. Small extinguishers suitable for grease fires are available at hardware stores and should be kept accessible in the kitchen. Most fatal home fires occur between midnight and 4 AM, with the peak hours for fire-associated deaths being from 2 to 3 AM.[15]

Cigarette fires

The leading cause of death from fire is cigarette-ignited fires. In 1987, 1492 lives were lost in such fires. There were also 3809 serious injuries, as well as $395 million in property damage.[23]

If a smoking habit cannot be altered, or if there are smokers in the home, one should emphasize the importance of taking steps to reduce the risk from cigarette-ignited fires. These include the safe disposal of cigarettes, cigars, and matches (not in wastebaskets), checking for smoldering cigarettes in chairs and sofas before retiring, keeping matches and lighters in areas inaccessible to children, and refraining from smoking in bed.

Recent studies funded by the government have addressed some of the problems of cigarette-ignited fires and have found it technically feasible, and probably commer-

cially feasible, to develop a cigarette that is less likely to ignite furniture. Final reports on this subject are due in the early 1990s.[23]

Smoke alarms

The installation of smoke detectors is an inexpensive and reliable action for reducing the risk for fire injuries and deaths. An estimated 75% of American homes have smoke detectors, and their presence is estimated to have prevented 3000 fire deaths annually since the late 1970s.[55] Unfortunately, people living in low-income, high-risk fire areas have not always recognized the importance of smoke alarms in preventing fire deaths and injury or cannot afford them.

Several community-based studies have identified higher education as the most predictive aspect of smoke detector ownership, which also related closely to higher income and home ownership. The use of smoke detectors was also positively correlated with the patient's knowledge that a community smoke detector law was in effect and with the practice of other safety behaviors in the home (such as locking up poisons and using child-restraint seats in automobiles). Groups that most resisted efforts to increase smoke detector usage in give-away programs were those who lived in public housing, apartment dwellers, and teenage mothers. Few of these families reported hearing about smoke detectors from their primary physicians, pointing out a need for clinical preventive intervention.[67]

Types of smoke alarms. Two basic types of residential smoke alarms are currently marketed, ionization and photoelectric. Ionization smoke alarms respond more quickly to smoke originating from flaming fires; photoelectric alarms generally respond faster to smoke from smoldering fires. Both have two main components, the smoke sensor and the alarm device. If either of these does not work, the alarm system is ineffective. The alarm should be cleaned and maintained according to the manufacturer's directions.

In brief, ionization smoke alarms use a weak radiation source to ionize the air in the ionization chamber, which is then electrically charged. Smoke particles entering this chamber cause a reduction in the flow of electric currents between electrodes, causing an alarm to sound. Photoelectric smoke alarms operate on the principle of light obscuration. The smoke alarm chamber houses a smoke sensor consisting of a light source and a special photosensitive cell. In normal operation, a beam of light falling on the photocell establishes a small current of electricity, a process that is interrupted when smoke enters the chamber, causing the alarm to sound.[73]

Placement of smoke alarms. The number and placement of smoke alarms depend on the configuration and size of the home. Smoke alarms may be installed on either the ceiling or upper portion of a wall but should never be placed in "dead-air" spaces where the ceiling meets the wall, behind obstructions such as doors or draperies, or within 3 feet of an air supply register that may prevent smoke from reaching the unit.[59]

For best all-round protection, smoke detectors should be installed on every level of a house. As fires that occur at night are the most lethal, the most important alarm is one installed in the corridor outside the bedroom door.[73]

Fire alarms for the hearing-impaired. About 21 million U.S. citizens are hearing impaired, creating a need for smoke alarms that provide other than auditory warnings. The most common fire alarm device used to alert this group is the flashing strobe light. The effectiveness of this mechanism may depend on its placement. Currently most of these strobe-light alarms are wall-mounted and viewed directly; however, Underwriters Laboratories Inc. (UL) proposes that an indirect flashing system that bounces off walls and ceilings may be more effective in waking the hearing-impaired.

Vibration devices that warn of fire are already extensively used in the deaf community. Other warning systems currently being researched for their feasibility are air-movement alarms and odor-releasing devices.[55]

The importance of assigning a responsible adult to wake the hearing-impaired should not be overlooked.

Escape routes

Rehearsing for fires is exceptionally important for reducing deaths and injuries. Families should have alternate escape routes from every room in the house. Fire exits should be kept clear, and fire ladders or other means of escaping from upper-story windows should be available in every bedroom. Fire extinguishers should be kept in crucial areas—the kitchen, workroom, and near stairways—and family members should know how to use them.

The most important rule to stress in home fire drills should be to get family members out safely first before summoning help. Individuals should be designated to assist children or handicapped people in escaping. If a smoke-filled room must be used for an exit, this should be accomplished on hands and knees to avoid smoke inhalation. An appointed meeting place should be set where the safety of family members can assessed. The importance of not returning into a burning building to rescue possessions or pets should be stressed.

Home inspections

Defective home electrical systems are estimated to be the cause of 46,000 fires annually, taking 440 lives and inflicting 1420 injuries. Electrical systems wear out, as do other parts of the home, and need to be checked and repaired when deficiencies are found. Many homes that are 40 to 100 years old, especially those in lower-income neighborhoods, have not had adequate electrical inspections since they were built.[14] This contributes to the high risk for residential fires of low-income populations.

The U.S. Consumer Product Safety Commission offers these guidelines for judging when an electrical inspection of a home is needed: It is overdue for houses that have not been checked for 40 years. If it has been 10 to 40 years since the last inspection, inspection is advisable, especially if appliances, lights, or receptacle outlets have been added or if there are warning signs of electrical distress. If it has been less than 10 years, the electrical system may not need to be checked unless there are indications of problems or temporary wiring has been added. If there are no current, dated records of inspection or service by an electrician on the electrical service panel door, the age of the house should be used as a guide to the probable need for an expert inspection.

Warnings of potential hazards include frequent power outages; dim, flickering lights; arcs, sparks, and unusual sounds from the electrical system; overheating of plates, cords, and plugs (plugs may be warm but should never be hot or discolored from heat); or the odor of hot insulation or any shocks, even mild tingles.

The electric panel should not be "overfused" or equipped with fuses or circuit breakers rated at higher currents than the capacity of the branch circuits. Insulation on wires should not be cut, broken, or cracked, plugs should not wobble in the receptacle, and extension cords are not recommended for permanent access to a receptacle outlet. Defects in the system should be fixed immediately.

Other home fire precautions

Home owners should also be told of other steps to take to reduce the risk of home fires. These steps include proper maintenance and use of heating systems, such as periodically checking chimneys and flues, proper installation of coal and wood stoves, cautious use of portable heaters (never leaving them unattended), the use of fireplace screens, and extinguishing fires before leaving the house.

Extra precautions should be taken in the kitchen, with attention paid to avoiding dropping grease and drippings on sources of heat or leaving food that is cooking unattended. Ideally, a class B fire extinguisher (for fires involving flammable liquids and gases, oil, grease, tars, or oil-base paints) should be mounted on the wall near the stove. It is possible to extinguish stove-top fires by placing a large lid over the pot or applying baking soda, but if the fire begins to spread, it is essential to evacuate immediately.

Home fires caused by improper storage can be reduced by storing combustibles away from heat and children, removing unnecessary items from attics, basements, and garages, and keeping flammable cloth and paper away from light fixtures.

PREVENTION OF HOME ACCIDENTS

Accidents are the leading cause of death in the United States for those aged 1 to 37 and the fourth leading cause of death for all ages. The largest number of these occur in motor vehicles; the other leading causes, in decreasing order, are falls, poisonings from liquids and solids, and burns, all of which are endemic to the home setting.

On the positive side of the ledger, accidental home deaths showed a steady decrease between 1912 and 1990, with fatalities declining 68% during this period, or from 28 to 9 per 100,000 population.

In 1990 accidental home injuries disabled 3.2 million people for one or more days, or one person in 78. About 90,000 of these injuries resulted in some permanent impairment.[2]

Prevention of falls

There were 6500 fatalities from home falls in 1990; 6050 of these were people age 45 and older, and 4400 of that number were 75 years of age and over.[2] Falls are a major health problem for the elderly and are the sixth leading cause of death for that age group. They are also responsible for nonfatal injuries such as fractures, hematomas, sprains, joint dislocations, and serious and minor soft-tissue injuries. Falls may also precipitate psychological consequences (a fear of falling may contribute to a self-imposed reduction in activity) or social outgrowths (falls and instability are mentioned as a contributing factor in 40% of nursing home admissions).[78,79]

The risk of falling is compounded by a variety of physical conditions that affect sensory, cognitive, neurological, or musculoskeletal functions.[79] Appropriate diagnostic evaluation of the patient, including use of medications and alcohol, has been addressed in other chapters of this text. The concern of this chapter is prevention of falls in the home setting.

Most falls occur during the routine activities of the elderly, such as walking or changing position. Only about 5% of the falls occur during precarious activities such as climbing chairs or ladders or participating in sports. About 10% of the falls are on stairs, but elderly people who use stairs regularly are at a lower risk for falls. Descending stairs is more hazardous than ascending.[79]

Home safety evaluations to prevent falls should assure that lighting is adequate without glare or shadows; night lights are in the bedroom, hall, and bathrooms; floors have nonskid wax; throw rugs have nonskid backing or are tacked down; carpets are shallow-piled; floors are free of small objects; stairways are well lighted, in good repair, not too steep, have securely fastened handrails, and are clear of hazards; bathrooms are equipped with safety features for tub, shower, and toilets; yards and entrances have even pavements, well-lit walkways, and are free of hazards.

Involving elderly patients in the hazard assessment in the home is recommended to encourage them to modify these hazards and to make them aware of changes in their habits and behavior that could make them less susceptible to falling.[79] Falls in this population can be lessened by modifying even a few of the factors that predispose them

to falls; one of the most important of these changes is to improve the safety of the home environment.

Prevention of accidental poisonings

Accidental deaths from solid and liquid poisoning increased by 21% in 1987, with the precipitating factors having changed dramatically over the last 30 years. The number of deaths from drugs, medications, and biological products has increased steadily over the last 7 years, but the number of deaths from other solid and liquid poisons, including household chemicals, has decreased. Protective packaging, improved household storage, poison prevention centers, and education have helped dramatically reduce the number of poisoning fatalities in infants and toddlers.[57] This information is covered in detail in Chapter 27.

Currently, 18 categories of household products are required to be distributed in child-resistant packaging, pursuant to the Poison Prevention Act of 1974, which is administered by the Consumer Product Safety Commission (CPSC). They can be sold in noncomplying packaging only if they are single size and are clearly labeled with warnings that the package is only for households without young children.[57]

Disposal of household toxic wastes

Household hazardous waste is defined as any material discarded from a home that may pose a threat to human health. Motor oil is the most common household hazardous waste; community-based studies have recorded that up to 60% of used motor oil was disposed of improperly on the ground, in sewers, or at ordinary landfills.[2]

The Federal Hazardous Substances Act of 1960 mandated warning labels on toxic products, including indoor, outdoor, workshop, automotive, and personal care products, but household hazardous waste was specifically exempted from the 1976 EPA Resource Conservation and Recovery Act, which regulates disposal of other toxic wastes.

Disposal and storage of household toxic waste creates complex challenges to the safety of the home environment. Household chemicals dumped into backyards and storm sewers can leach into ground-water supplies or pollute nearby lakes and rivers. Cautious disposal (diluting with water, not mixing chemicals) into household drains that are serviced by biological and chemical sewage treatment systems is a solution for getting rid of some of the least noxious of these household toxic chemicals (used antifreeze should not be handled this way because it contains heavy metals). Inquiries should be made to local water authorities about the capabilities for handling specific household toxic chemicals. Home septic systems are not safe disposal sites (an estimated 40% of these are already not working properly); chemicals can cause the system to fail, releasing contaminants into drinking water supplies.[66]

In 1989, 600 communities addressed this problem with periodic toxic waste collections; 36 communities had permanent toxic waste collection programs or facilities.[2] Toxic wastes that cannot be immediately disposed of safely may need to be stored. In this case, they should be rendered as harmless as possible, sealed tightly, labeled carefully (original containers preferred), and placed in a cool, dry place away from direct sunlight, flames, or sparks, in locked storage areas away from pets and children. Regular monitoring for disintegration of containers is advised.[66]

Poisonous plants in the home

There are 700 species of plants, ferns, horsetails, and fungi that can cause toxic reactions in humans and animals. Although only a small number of domestic plants are highly toxic (plants in the wild tend to be more dangerous), because of their ubiquitous nature in U.S. homes and yards, the problem of plant ingestion by small children remains a safety concern.

Dieffenbachia and philodendron are responsible for more cases of symptomatic distress (although not serious poisoning) in preschool children in the United States than all other plants combined and should probably be removed from homes with very young children.

Other common plants that can cause toxic reactions are jimson weed, castor bean (extremely toxic), golden chain tree, nightshade, coyotillo (a deadly plant; muscle weakness and paralysis appear after several weeks), poison hemlock, pokeweed, rhododendron, tree tobacco, water hemlock, wisteria, and yew. The ingestion of one well-chewed seed of rosary pea (found in Florida, Hawaii, and the West Indies) can be fatal. Some common plants affecting cardiac function are foxglove (digitalis), monkshood, lily of the valley, and oleander.

A sample of the offending plant, with flowers and seeds, should be requested for identification. Treatment may include observation, induced vomiting, or additional emergency medical assistance. If there is question, vomiting (unless spontaneous), should be induced with ½ oz of syrup of ipecac for children (adult dose, 1 oz). After emesis, 1 oz of activated charcoal (3 oz for adults) in water should be ingested to absorb poisons. Some pediatricians recommend that these remedies be kept in medicine cabinets of families with preschool children, especially in areas where medical help is not readily available.[38]

Household plants should be put out of the reach of toddlers, leaf debris should be picked up, and children should be taught never to use plants as "play foods."

Poison ivy and poison oak are responsible for more cases of allergic contact dermatitis than all other substances combined, usually causing more intense reactions in adults than children. Plant resin on the hands can be distributed to all parts of the body. It can also be carried on the fur of dogs and cats, and as it remains stable for a "considerable period of time," tools, fishing rods, and camping equipment cannot be overlooked as contact points

for acquiring the dermatosis. Smoke from burning poison ivy is harmless unless the smoke carries unburned plant particles.[38]

Carbon monoxide poisoning

During a 10-year study period from 1979-1988, there were 11,547 unintentional deaths from carbon monoxide reported in the United States (this excludes carbon monoxide fatalities from burns, fires, suicides, homicides, and deaths classified as intent undetermined). Of these, 57% were caused by motor vehicle exhaust.[11]

Carbon monoxide is the leading cause of death from poisonings in the United States, and carbon monoxide poisoning causes an estimated 10,000 people to seek medical attention or to miss 1 day of normal activity each year.[11,29] The typical symptoms (dizziness, nausea, and headache) may mask the precipitating cause. Universal screening of patients arriving in emergency departments with flu-like illnesses found 3% to 5% had elevated carbon monoxide levels.[29]

New drivers, males, and older people are candidates for programs that stress prevention of carbon monoxide intoxication and poisoning. The first rule to stress is not to run engines in enclosed spaces. If available, carbon monoxide monitors should be installed in garages, as well as automobile repair shops.

The dangers of cars with defective exhausts and holes in the body should be stressed, as should be the folly of parking with the motor running for long periods of time. In a review of 68 pediatric cases treated for carbon monoxide poisoning with hyperbaric oxygen between 1986 and 1991, it was found that 20 of these children had been riding in the back of pickup trucks in rigid closed canopies or under tarpaulins. In all cases exhaust from a leaking exhaust system or tail pipe was found to be exiting beneath the rear bumper of the pickup truck.[29] Sleepiness when driving should also be suspected as a symptom of low-level carbon monoxide intoxication.

Inside the home, gas appliances should be checked for proper flame adjustment and venting. Flues and chimneys should be kept cleaned and checked for leaks. The safety of heating and cooking appliances, a major source of home-based carbon monoxide poisonings, has already been improved through efforts of the Consumer Product Safety Commission (CPSC), Underwriters Laboratories, and private industry.[11]

Finally, the physician should be alert to the possibility of carbon monoxide poisoning when nonspecific, flu-like symptoms or coma are present.

Drowning

The incidence of drowning has already been discussed in Chapter 27, especially as this problem relates to the pediatric patient.

A recent 5-year study on the incidence of immersion injuries in an east coast state noted some interesting statistics for the adult population that are applicable for prevention consideration. These include the relatively high rate of bathtub drownings for the elderly (37% of the drownings age 75 and over were in bathtubs), which suggests a need for greater safety precautions in this activity for this age group.

Other statistics from this study show that drowning rates are highest in warm, rural areas and, as might be expected, in areas abutting large bodies of water. Fatalities from immersion injuries leading to hospital admission appear to increase with age. (In this study, fatalities for infants from these incidents were 20%, whereas the rate was 65% for persons 65 and older.[21])

The physician concerned with reducing injuries from recreational swimming will encourage the acquisition of swimming skills for children and adults, safer swimming areas, and boating safety.

FIREARMS

Firearm deaths in the home have shown steady increases every year from 1953 to 1988, years for which we have accurate statistical information, with the death rate per 100,000 blacks being over twice that for whites. Blacks account for 25% of all firearm deaths, but only 12% of the U.S. population. According to the National Safety Council, accidental deaths have decreased by about one third, but suicides have more than doubled, and homicides have more than tripled.[2]

The family physician can no longer take a passive role in this disturbing trend. As important, costly, and time consuming is the treatment of gun-related injuries, real improvement in this grim scenario will come only with prevention. As reported in the editorial, "Firearms and the killing threshold," by Jerome P. Kassirer, editor of the New England Journal of Medicine, we now have data showing that controlling handguns in communities reduces firearm deaths. Nothing short of legislation limiting private ownership of handguns and automatic rifles will achieve this.[35]

PREVENTING VIOLATION OF THE HOME

In the quarter of a century from 1969 to 1984, serious crimes in the United States have increased by 40% and violent crimes by more than 60%. This trend is continuing to accelerate, as noted in later statistics from 1985 to 1987, when a 13% increase is recorded.[42] Homeowners at all income levels are at risk, and there is a greater demand than ever for advice on protection within the home.

The high cost of arming the home with firearms that are misused by children and adolescents and in domestic quarrels is addressed in Chapter 27. This chapter will deal mostly with advice the physician can give on securing the homestead from without.

Elderly citizens are frequently targets of crime, and fear of crime can make them virtual prisoners in their homes. This group is especially vulnerable on the delivery day for government checks, and the use of direct deposit can reduce that risk. Senior citizens should be discouraged from carrying a lot of cash or purses that can be snatched. Doors should not be opened to people who do not identify themselves. The elderly person should have daily telephone contact with a safety network of family and neighbors, and emergency numbers, including 911, should be clearly posted.

Owning a dog can provide some effective protection from crime, particularly as a warning device and a deterrent to the criminal.

Preventing entry into the home

The easiest way for someone to enter the home is through an unlocked door, and although locks do not guarantee protection from the hardened criminal, they obviously must be used to provide any protection. Three quarters of the burglaries victimizing older people involve unlocked doors and windows.[42]

Doors to the outside should be sturdy and fit properly in the frame. Locksmiths can provide L-shaped metal strips that can be attached to door frames of inward-swinging doors; this will help prevent jimmying with a crowbar. The dead-bolt lock is the best security buy for all doors to the outside, and for high-risk applications, a multilock dead-bolt lock is available that bolts into all four edges of the door frame. Entrances should be well lighted and windows locked. Grates on main floor and basement windows may be an advisable precaution.

Apartment dwellers with security concerns should look for these features in their buildings: security guards, attended elevators, properly secured interior fire stairwells and garages, remotely operated door-opening systems, adequate lighting, and closed circuit TV. Knowing one's neighbors and working together for crime prevention and mutual security is highly recommended. Single women should not indicate their gender on the mailbox.

Alarm systems

Alarm systems are designed to detect and communicate, and are based on the principal of point protection (intrusion though a specific location) and space protection (which detects movement within a particular area). There are many simple as well as sophisticated systems on the market, and objective advice should be sought when planning home alarm systems. Many police crime-prevention units and fire departments have alarm system specialists; impartial advice may also be available from casualty insurance carriers and master locksmiths.

FOOD SAFETY IN THE HOME

Dietary strategies in clinical preventive medicine have been extensively covered in Chapters 22 through 24; however, the safety of the food supply in the home is another concern to be addressed here. As in most other areas covered in this chapter, both governmental protection and individual action are important in this matter.

The government has regulated the food supply since 1906, when the Pure Food and Drugs Act passed, allowing the government to condemn foods that had been adulterated with chemicals that were hazardous to public health. As knowledge of the complexity of this issue increased, so did the extent of government participation in protecting foods. In 1938, the Food, Drug, and Cosmetic Act allowed consideration of the extent to which contaminants, such as aflatoxins and polychlorinated biphenyls (PCBs), could be controlled in food.

The Food and Drug Administration (FDA) now sets guidelines or establishes formal rulings for the maximum amounts of these contaminants allowed in food, while the Environmental Protection Agency (EPA) sets maximum legal limits for chemical residues, such as pesticides. Monitoring of domestic and imported foods is by the FDA and the U.S. Department of Agriculture (USDA), with the Food Safety and Inspection Service (FSIS) of the USDA testing for more than 130 animal drugs and pesticides in meat and poultry.[47]

Food safety is a highly emotional and publicized issue, as seen in the recent controversies over Alar-treated apples and cyanide-laced Chilean grapes (the latter, a terrorist activity, presented a totally different and uncontrollable danger to the food supply).

Consumer surveys show that the public is afraid of pesticides in foods, more than any other chemicals, and often erroneously assumes that "man-made" is dangerous and "natural" is safe. Plants, especially those under stress, manufacture toxins for defense against insects, birds, and grazing animals. Aflatoxin, a natural carcinogen that is produced by a mold that attacks crops such as corn and peanuts, is under intensive study by the FDA as a potential carcinogen. The most urgent threat to the safety of the food supply, however, comes from familiar microorganisms that contaminate poultry, eggs, dairy products, and meat.[83]

Sulfites

America's 10 million asthmatics are at the greatest risk from allergic reactions to sulfites, which are used to reduce or prevent spoilage and discoloration of many foods and some intravenous and drug products.

From March, 1985 to January, 1990, 1000 alleged allergic reactions to sulfites were reported, with 27 deaths. FDA epidemiologists say 10 were probably sulfite related, although direct evidence of sulfites as the cause of death is elusive. Of the 1000 reactions, 40% occurred after consumption of fresh fruits and vegetables, 13% from restaurant foods, 12% from wine and beer, and 9% from seafood.

In 1986 the use of sulfites on raw produce was banned, and labeling was required if the sulfite levels are 10 or more parts per million, or if sulfites are used as a preservative.[39]

Sensitive individuals should read labels carefully. The presence of sulfiting agents on foods can be identified on labels as sulfur dioxide, potassium bisulfite, potassium metabisulfite, sodium bisulfite, sodium metabisulfite, or sodium sulfite. Some major food categories in which these are found are avocado dips, beer, cider, dried cod, fruits and juices, gelatins, potatoes, dry salad dressings and relishes, canned or dried sauces, sauerkraut, shellfish, canned or dried soup, vegetables, wine vinegar, wine, and wine coolers.

Microbiological hazards in food

In recent years, an outburst of diseases from food-borne microorganisms has been noted. More than 81 million cases of diarrheal diseases are reported from this source each year in the United States. In 1985, there were 16,000 cases of salmonella food poisoning, with two fatalities from contaminated, pasteurized milk. Also recorded were 47 deaths and 187 illnesses caused by a Mexican-style soft cheese, as well as 3 patients requiring ventilator management because of botulism poisoning from a prepared garlic-in-oil product.[83]

Egg-borne *Salmonella enteritidis* infections (once confined primarily to the northeastern United States) are becoming a major public health problem. Recent illnesses in the Midwest have been traced to chicken breeder farms where *S. enteriditis* is transmitted through infected chicken ovaries, especially where hens have been stressed by food and water deprivation. *S. enteriditis* has been demonstrated in intact grade A shell eggs that have been disinfected and inspected. Special groups are at risk for this infection: the very young, pregnant women, elderly people, and immunocompromised people. These people should avoid raw or lightly-cooked foods that contain eggs or use pasteurized egg products.[50]

Another human pathogen, *Yersinia entercolitica,* a major cause of diarrhea in much of the industrialized world, has also been reported on the increase in the United States, although its epidemiology is poorly understood. Ingestion of contaminated foods and contact with sick dogs have been implicated. Pigs and pork products have been demonstrated to be an important reservoir for this organism, and an outbreak in the South in 1989 produced febrile, diarrheal illnesses in 15 black infants where chitterlings (a pork intestine food) were being prepared in a household. None of the infants had direct contact with raw chitterlings, but all were in contact with a person cleaning the pig intestines, suggesting an indirect route for infection and emphasizing the importance of good hygiene during preparation of this product.[40]

Precautions for pesticide exposure from food

Although the EPA does limit dietary pesticide exposure by setting tolerances or standards for the amount of residue that may be left on foods, extra home precautions can be taken. These include rinsing fruits and vegetables, brushing and peeling, trimming fat from meat and poultry, and discarding fats and oils in broths and pan drippings because residues of some pesticides concentrate in fat.[10,47]

Home garden sites should be planned on land that has had suitable previous usage and is free from run-off from chemical applications. The process of recovering pesticide-contaminated land can be accelerated with good agricultural practices. Food collected from the wild, such as fish and game, should be harvested from areas where pesticide contamination is not present.

Correct storage of pesticides on the farm or in the home requires that they never be stored with or near foods, nor be put into soft drink bottles or other containers that children may associate with something to eat or drink.

Safe food handling in the home

The USDA estimates that 7 million U.S. citizens will have food-borne illness each year and that 85% of these food poisoning cases could be prevented with proper handling of food in the home [1] (see the box at right).

SAFETY IN THE AUTOMOBILE

Motor vehicle accidents took the lives of 37,800 U.S. citizens in 1990.[2] They are the most common fatal accident for older Americans ages 55 to 79 and youth ages 1 to 24, especially teens.[65] Reducing the number of these highway casualties should be a major concern to the physician, who is in the position to encourage responsible behavior by both drivers and passengers, to advocate the selection of safer cars and equipment, and to encourage support for legislation that helps reduce the number and severity of automobile accidents.

High-risk behaviors of drivers

Several high-risk behaviors have been shown to increase the incidence of motor vehicle accidents and the accompanying morbidity and mortality for both driver and passengers. Three of these that have proven especially dangerous are drinking and driving, speeding, and failing to wear seat belts.

Alcohol use and driving. The combination of alcoholic beverage use and driving has consistently been identified with the increased likelihood of a motor vehicle accident. Blood alcohol concentrations over .05 g/dl by weight have been found in 8% of drivers involved in property damage crashes, 17% of those with all types of nonfatal injuries, 29% of those with serious injuries, and almost half of those in fatal crashes.[37]

About 35% of the drivers in the high-risk age group of

Summary of USDA safe food handling rules

When shopping: Buy cold food last; watch use-by dates; select food in good condition. Canned goods should be free of dents or bulging lids, which can indicate a serious threat of food poisoning or contamination.

When storing food: Keep refrigerator at 40° F and freezer at 0° F. Freeze meat, fish, and poultry if not using within a few days. Do not allow raw bacteria-laden juices to drip onto other food.

When preparing food: Keep hands, implements clean. Thaw foods in microwave or refrigerator.

When cooking: Cook thoroughly: red meat to 160° F, poultry to 180°, and check visually for doneness. When microwaving, cover and rotate foods, observe standing times.

When serving: Never leave perishable food out over 2 hours. Carry picnic foods and lunches in insulated containers.

When handling leftovers: Cool in small, shallow containers; separate stuffings from poultry or meat. Reheat sauces to a boil, other leftovers to 165° F. Avoid moldy or strange-looking or smelling food. Discard if in doubt.

---

21 to 24 who were involved in fatal accidents in 1989 were intoxicated (blood alcohol concentrations, or BAC, greater than .10%). The percentages of intoxicated drivers involved in this kind of accident decrease after age 25.[2]

On the positive side, alcohol involvement in fatal traffic crashes has dropped 8% since 1982, when 57% of all traffic crashes involved drinking. Alcohol-related fatalities in the 15-to-17 age group have shown the biggest decline during this period.[2] These statistics attest to the combined effects of legal sanctions, media campaigns and reduced alcohol consumption.[84]

Speed of driving. After a 1987 federal repeal of the 55-mile-per-hour speed limit, 40 states returned to the 65 mph speed limit on interstate highways passing through areas of 500,000 or less population by 1991. Of these 40 states, 28 have shown fatality increases on rural interstates, and 12 have shown decreases. Eight states have shown increase of more than 30% (Fig. 64-4).

One recent study concluded that the increase to 65 mph had dissimilar effects on different states; however, more states had increases in fatalities than decreases after speed limits were raised. In addition, there were more fatalities on rural noninterstate roads, which could suggest a spillover from the interstate speed increases.[2]

Use of seat belts

The National Highway Traffic Safety Administration (NHTSA) has estimated that using seat belts has reduced the risk of death 40% to 50% for front seat occupants and

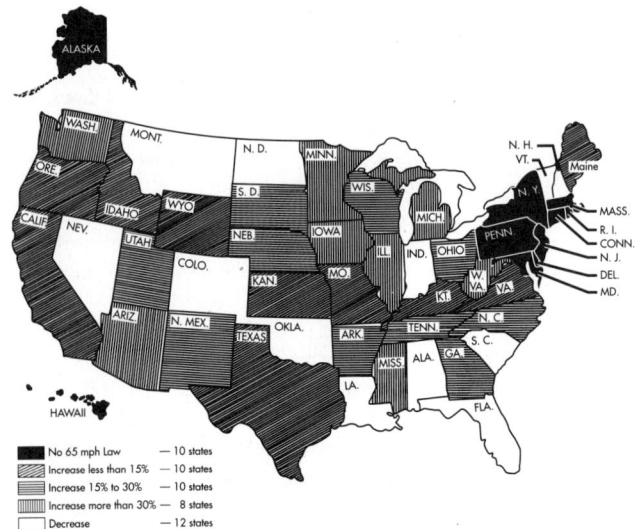

Fig. 64-4. Changes in rural interstate fatalities associated with 65 mph speed laws. (From National Safety Council: *Accident facts,* Chicago, 1991.)

reduced injury to the same by 45% to 55%.[41] Seat belts combined with the shoulder harness have proven almost 50% effective in preventing injuries from collision inside the car and from ejection from the vehicle.

Of the unrestrained occupants of passenger cars that were involved in fatal traffic accidents in 1989, 50% were killed; the statistic drops sharply to 27% for restrained passengers.[2] Seat belts also play a major role in preventing the ejection of occupants from an auto in a roll-over crash (mortality rates are 25% higher for ejected individuals than for those who are restrained in the vehicle).[34]

As of July, 1991, 40 states had seat belt laws. Regional analysis has noted the decrease in the severity of injury to front-seat occupants and fewer head and face injuries in accidents after the enactment of seat belt use laws.[41]

The NHSTA, in a 19-city observation survey, estimated overall usage of seat belts at 49% in 1990, an increase of 3% from 1989.[2] Recent statistical surveys record the greatest increase in belt use was in the nine states with primary seat belt laws (those that permit police to stop vehicles whose occupants are not wearing seat belts). The second highest gain was reported in states with secondary seat belt laws (vehicles must be stopped for another violation before the occupants are charged with failure to use seat belts), and the least use was reported in states with no seat belt laws. Young adults and people who drink and drive, two high-risk groups, were less likely to use seat belts, even when mandated.[20]

Motorized shoulder belt systems had the highest usage rate in 1990 (93%), but only 28% of vehicles so equipped were using the accompanying lap belts. Another recent study found that belt usage in 1628 cars that were equipped with manual belts and air bags was slightly

higher than a group of cars with manual belts only, suggesting that drivers may not rely on air bags alone for their total protection.[2] This is a wise decision, as in a diagonal-impact crash and deceleration, the occupant could be displaced, losing the protective cushioning of the air bag.[34]

General recommendations for seat belt use include using belts for trips of any distance (statistics show that most accidents happen within 25 miles of home and that the greatest number of serious injuries and deaths occur at speeds of less than 40 mph).[65] Seat belts should be positioned snugly over the bony parts of the body, as low on the hips as possible. No more than one person should be placed in a restraint system, regardless of age.

Seat belts are recommended for all passengers including pregnant women, with the exception of infants and small children. Automobile safety restraints that are appropriate for children's safety are discussed in Chapter 27.

Selection of safer vehicles

Safety features have been incorporated into contemporary cars by both mandated and voluntary means. Minimum performance standards for passenger cars are set by the U.S. Department of Transportation to help prevent vehicle crashes, as well as to protect occupants from injury from trauma and postcrash fires.[68] The insurance industry and consumer groups have also persuaded the automobile industry to modify designs by stimulating customer demands for more effective safety features.

In 1984 the Transportation Secretary ruled that by 1990 the automobile industry would be required to install automatic crash devices (either air bag or automatic seat belts) in all new model cars. This deadline was recently extended to 1994 for manufacturers that intended to provide driver-side air bags rather than automatic seat belts.[34]

Air bags

About one half of all hospitalized brain injury cases are result from vehicular accidents. Air bags, designed to protect the occupants of a vehicle from colliding with the interior of a vehicle in a crash, offer specific protection to the brain, face, and cervical spine, which lap and shoulder belts alone do not provide. They are triggered by sensors to deploy in about a twentieth of a second (faster than an eye blink). Expectations are high for this new passive restraint system, and several insurance companies are lowering insurance rates for owners of air bag-equipped autos, some reducing premiums up to 30%.[34] Driver-side and passenger-side air bags are now being offered as optional or standard equipment on many new car models.

Air bags inflate in frontal and front-angle crashes (52% of collisions), which account for the most serious injuries and fatalities. They do not deploy in lateral crashes (where 28% of the serious injuries and deaths are sustained) or rear-end impacts (accounting for 4% of the major injuries or deaths).[34]

Field data on the effectiveness of air bags has not been adequately assembled because of their newness in mass markets. One study suggests that traffic fatalities might be reduced by 6.5% if all cars had air bags; however, shoulder belts would also have to be worn. Without the latter, the fatality risk would increase by 41%.[61] Contusions of the eyes, chemical keratitis, and ocular trauma have been reported during air-bag inflation, which may be one of the tradeoffs for this important new safety product.[33,60,61]

Head restraints

Head restraints to protect occupants from neck or cervical sprains are currently required on the driver and right front seats of cars (but not passenger vans). Nonadjustable head restraints, or adjustable ones that provide a wide range of protection even in the "down" position, are recommended.[68] Steering wheels, one of the most frequent sources of injury, are now being designed to distribute crash forces in an accident more widely on the body, reducing chest and abdominal injuries.[49]

Crash avoidance features in cars

Antilock brakes. Originally developed for airplanes in the 1950s, this technology holds great promise in automobile accident prevention. By automatically pumping brakes many times per second, antilock brakes prevent wheels from locking when brakes are suddenly applied. Antilock brakes give the driver more steering control during braking, making the car less likely to skid, especially on wet and slippery roads, and allow for shorter-distance braking. Once available exclusively on luxury cars, these brakes are gradually being introduced into the popularly-priced passenger car line.[49]

Future trends. Research on the use of yellow rear-turn signals, rather than red rear-turn signals, which can be confused with brake lights or emergency flashers, is proving that yellow is safer. These, too, will probably be introduced on domestic cars in the near future.[68] Shift interlock devices, requiring drivers to press the brake before they can shift out of park, should eliminate accidents caused by hitting the gas pedal during starting.[49]

Size of car and safety

Controversy rages over the relationship of car size to the safety of its occupants, with insurance and auto industry analysts differing with conservationists on the interpretation of statistics.

Injuries occurring in accidents in 200 popular U.S. car models have been recorded by the insurance industry. Some of their findings are: Passengers involved in accidents are more likely to be injured in small cars than in large cars. Nearly half the small cars showed 24% to 85% more occupant injury in crashes than the norm; large cars, station wagons, and passenger vans were 25% to 51% below the average.[70]

Small sports/specialty cars recorded the highest number of deaths per 10,000 reported vehicles.[9] In single-vehicle crashes, the death rate for occupants of small cars is double the rate for people in larger cars. The passenger occupant death rate per 10,000 registered vehicles in 1989 ranged from 1.3 for large cars with wheel bases larger than 114 inches to 3 for small cars with wheelbases less than 95 inches.[68] Exceptions to this rule do arise, however, indicating, as conservationists argue, that critical variables of design can compensate for small size and light weight.[28]

The effect of emission controls on health

From 1979 through 1988, the number of deaths from carbon monoxide (at a rate of 63 per year) has consistently declined each year, especially those that are related to motor vehicle exhaust. This is a new finding and may be explained by several interventions that have occurred during this period.

Engineering changes in automobile design made to comply with the Clean Air Act have reduced carbon monoxide emissions in new vehicles by 90% since controls began in 1968. It now takes longer for carbon monoxide to build up to toxic levels when a car is producing exhaust in an enclosed space. California's low death rate from motor vehicle exhaust (.09 per 100,000) may be related to its stringent pollution controls, despite a high rate of automobiles-to-people and a high number of passenger miles traveled. The mortality statistics may be reduced even further as the effect is felt from additional amendments to the Clean Air Act made in 1990 that mandate the use of oxygenated fuels and improved emission control systems.[11]

Incidence of accidents

More fatal automobile crashes were reported in cars that had drivers under age 30, with lower death rates being recorded in cars that were driven by female drivers.[9]

In both urban and rural driving, death rates for night driving are triple the rate for daytime driving. Fatalities are more likely in automobile accidents occurring in rural areas at any time of day, whereas injuries are more common in auto accidents in urban areas. Weekend driving is more dangerous than mid week (Saturdays are the most dangerous), and May through October are more risky months to be on the highways.[2]

Older drivers, less able to cope with driving challenges, should be encouraged to begin trips or run errands during less congested times and in daylight hours.

Older drivers

By the year 2000, one out of every three drivers in the United States will be 55 years of age or older.[45] In proportion to their numbers, older drivers have fewer accidents and fatalities; however, when accidents and fatalities are compared with the number of miles driven by the senior driver, the accident rate is disproportionately high, second only to the highest-risk 16-to-24-year-olds.[46]

Despite the fact that physical abilities needed for driving are reported to begin to deteriorate after age 55 (for example, at age 45, four times more light is required for driving than at age 19), the skills of aging drivers vary widely. According to the AAA Foundation for Traffic Safety, age alone is not an indication of an older person's ability to maneuver an automobile safely. The driver may deny the loss of driving aptitude; in this case, a self-assessment driving test (available through this foundation) may help senior drivers recognize problems in their driving abilities.

A comprehensive medical examination is recommended to identify health problems that could affect driving performance; that is, diseases that might cause loss of consciousness (diabetes), inattention (Alzheimers, dementia, depression), and vision problems.[46] Recent reports on the driving performance of untreated obstructive sleep apnea have also recorded a high automobile crash rate in this population, indicating an additional reason for treatment of this condition.[22]

Patients should be told the effects of prescription and over-the-counter drugs, as well as alcohol, on their driving. Selection of the right car and its options is essential for the senior driver. Sizing the car to the driver is important; 50% of the elderly female population falls outside the design range of automobile manufacturers in matching height to vision capabilities.[45] This problem may be solved by the simple solution of providing a seating pad, or pedal extenders.

Highly tinted windows are not recommended for the senior driver, and all glass, including eye glasses, should be kept clean. Mirrors that distort distances can be confusing. Gauges should be easy to read and well lit. Options that compensate for loss in muscle strength and flexibility, such as power steering, power brakes, and automatic transmissions, should be considered. Safety options should have a high priority in car selection, and the physician should strongly encourage the use of seat belts, especially because older drivers in accidents are highly susceptible to death and injury.

At least three organizations, AAA, the American Association of Retired Persons (AARP), and the National Safety Council (NSC), offer courses to improve the driving ability of seniors, Insurance companies offer discounts in some states, and the number of infraction "points" on the driver's record may be reduced, upon completion of the course. Graded licensing, which can limit the use of vehicles and require safety features for high-risk drivers, is already used in some states and may become more common as our driving population ages.

Teen-age drivers

Prevention of accidents related to teen-age driving is addressed in Chapter 28.

OTHER VEHICLE ACCIDENTS
Motorcycles

Motorcycles accounted for about 2% of the vehicles registered in 1990 and about 8% of the occupant deaths in motor-vehicle accidents. Of motorcycle injuries reported, 57% were due to collisions with other vehicles, 21% were due to noncollision accidents, and 15% were due to collisions with fixed objects.

Three states do not require helmet use; 24 other states require passenger helmet use or possession of a helmet for those under a specific age. Another 23 states and the District of Columbia require helmet usage by all motorcycle riders.[2]

The physician should actively promote such legislation and should advise the use of helmets for all motorcyclists, even if law does not require it.

Pedestrian and bicycle accidents

Because the largest number of these accidents occur in the pediatric subject, these are discussed in Chapter 27.

The number of bicycles in the United States has increased thirteenfold since 1940, and bicycle-related injuries and death are on the rise.[2] Head injuries cause 62% of all bicycling deaths. Between 1984 and 1988, there were an estimated 2500 deaths and 757,000 head injuries (i.e., one death per day and one head injury every 4 minutes). Many of these could have been avoided with the universal use of bicycle helmets for both children and adults.[62] Here is another area for preventive action by the health practitioner.

Farm vehicle safety

Agriculture has one of the highest fatal accident rates of any occupation,[36] with 1300 deaths recorded in 1990.[2] Tractors are associated with about half of the fatal agricultural accidents, and overturns on tractors were responsible for about half of these.[2,36] The other leading causes of tractor accidents were runovers (33%), other (12%), and power take-off (a mechanical function on tractors that allows extra power for specific jobs but is also highly dangerous) accidents (3%). Recent studies have shown that rollover protective structures (ROPS) could prevent most of these deaths. ROPS are now standard equipment on all new tractors. Mandating the retrofit of older tractors with ROPS has been proposed by agricultural groups oriented toward safety, with opponents debating the cost effectiveness of compliance.[36]

REFERENCES

1. *A quick consumer guide to safe food handling*, USDA Food Safety and Inspection Service, Home and Garden Bulletin 248, Sept, 1990.
2. *Accident Facts*, Chicago, 1991, National Safety Council.
3. *Asbestos in the home*, US Consumer Product Commission & US Environmental Protection Agency, Washington DC, August, 1989.
4. *AWARE*, National Weather Service/Warning Coordinator & Hazard Awareness Report, U.S. Dept of Commerce, National Oceanic and Atmospheric Administration, Spring 1991.

5. *AWARE*, Oct., 1990.

6. *AWARE*, Winter, 1990.

7. Beaches Environmental Assessment, Closure and Health Act of 1990, Hearing before the Subcommittee on Superfund, Ocean and Water Protection of the Committee on Environment and Public Works, June 25, 1990, Washington, DC, US Senate.

8. *Beneath the bottom line: agricultural approaches to reduce agrichemical contamination of groundwater*, Washington, DC, 1990, US Congress, Office of Technology Assessment.

9. Car safety: size counts, *Consumers' Research* 73(3):27, 1990.

10. *Citizen's guide to pesticides*, Washington, DC, 1990, US Environmental Protection Agency.

11. Cobb N, Etzel RA: Unintentional carbon monoxide-related deaths in the United States, 1979 through 1988, *JAMA* (266)5:659, 1991.

12. Council on Scientific Affairs: Medical perspective on nuclear power, *JAMA* 262(19):2724, 1989.

13. Council on Scientific Affairs: Radon in homes, *JAMA* 258(5):668, 1987.

14. *CPSC guide to home wiring hazards*, Washington, DC, 1990, U.S. Consumer Product Safety Commission.

15. Current statistics provided by National Fire Protection Association, Quincy, Mass, 1992.

16. Douglas WW, Hepper NGG, and Colby TV: Silo-filler's disease, *Mayo Clin Proc* 64:291, 1989.

17. Drinking water safeguards are not preventing contamination from injected oil and gas wastes, US General Accounting Office: Report to the Chairman, Environment, Energy & Natural Resource Subcommittee, Committee of Government Operation, House of Representatives, July, 1989.

18. Earthquake Hazards Reduction, Hearing before Subcommittee on Science, Technology and Space of the Committee on Commerce, Science and Transportation, US Senate, 101st Congress, second session, March 29, 1990.

19. *Earthquakes and volcanoes*, USGS, 22(6):230, 1989.

20. Escobedo LG et al: State laws and the use of car safety belts, *N Engl J Med* 325(22):1586, 1991.

21. Fife D, Scipio S, and Crane GL: Fatal and nonfatal immersion injuries among New Jersey residents: *Am J Prev Med* 7(4):189, 1991.

22. Findley LJ, Weiss JW, and Jabour ER: Drivers with untreated sleep apnea, a cause of death and serious injury, *Arch Intern Med* 151:1451, 1991.

23. Fire Safe Cigarette Act of 1990, Public Law 101-352, 101st Congress, August 10, 1990.

24. *Flash floods and warnings*, US Department of Commerce, National Weather Service, NOAA/PA 81010, 1981.

25. Gates GO: Safety and survival in an earthquake, *Earthquakes and Volcanoes*, 22(1):26, 1990.

26. Grandjean P: *Last JM's public health and preventive medicine*, ed 12, Norwalk, Conn, 1986, Appleton-Century-Crofts.

27. Guilmette RA et al: Risks from radon progeny exposure: what we know, and what we need to know, *Ann Rev Pharmacol Toxicol* 31:569, 1991.

28. Hamilton J: Safe by design, *Sierra* 76(6):36, 1991.

29. Hampson NB, Norkool DM: Carbon monoxide poisoning in children riding in the back of pickup trucks, *JAMA* 267(4):538, 1992.

30. *Heatwave*, US Department of Commerce, National Weather Service NOAA/PA 85001.

31. Hendee WR: Radon and the family physician, *J Fam Pract* 33(1):95, 1991.

32. *In the event of a flood*, Federal Emergency Management Agency, US GPO 1991-0-521-753.

33. Ingraham HJ, Perry HD, and Donnenfeld ED: Air-bag keratitis, *N Engl J Med* 324(22):1599, 1991.

34. Jagger J, Vernberg K, and Jane JA: Air bags: reducing the toll of brain trauma, *Neurosurgery* 20(5):815, 1987.

35. Kassirer JP: Firearms and the killing threshold, *N Engl J Med* 325(23):1647, 1991.

36. Kelsey TW, Jenkins PL: Farm tractors and mandatory roll-over protection retrofits: potential costs of the policy in New York, *Am J Public Health* 81(7):921, 1991.

37. Knight KK, Fielding JE, and Goetzel RZ: Correlates of motor-vehicle safety behaviors in working populations, *J Occup Med* 33(6):705, 1991.

38. Lampe KF: *Common poisonous and injurious plants*, Washington, DC, 1981, US Department of Health & Human Services.

39. Lecos C, Blumenthal D: Reacting to sulfites, reprint *FDA Consumer Mag*, DHHS Pub (FDA) 90-2209, Jan, 1986.

40. Lee LA et al: *Yersina entercolictica* 0:3, infections in infants and children, associated with the household preparation of chitterlings, *N Engl J Med* 322(14):984, 1990.

41. Lestina DC et al: Motor vehicle crash injury patterns and the Virginia seat belt law, *JAMA* 265(11):1409, 1991.

42. Lipman IA: *How to protect yourself from crime*, ed 3, Chicago, 1990, Contemporary Books.

43. Muller-Wening D, Repp H: Investigation on the protective value of breathing masks in farmer's lung using an inhalation provocation test, *Chest* 95(1):100, 1989.

44. *Maintaining safe drinking water*, 1990, Washington, DC, US EPA Office of Water.

45. Malfetti JL, Winter DJ: *Drivers 55 plus: test your own performance*, 1986, Safety Research and Education Project, Teachers College, Columbia University and AAA Foundation for Traffic Safety.

46. Malfetti JL, Winter DJ: *Concerned about an older driver? A guide for families and friends*, 1991, Safety Research and Education Project, Teachers College, Columbia University and AAA Foundation for Traffic Safety.

47. *Meat and poultry safety, questions and answers about chemical residues*, Washington, DC, 1990, US Department of Agriculture, FSIS.

48. Meredith T, Vale A: Carbon monoxide poisoning, *Br Med J* 296:77, 1988.

49. Merline J: Special report, part I, what's new from Detroit for 1992, *Consumers' Research* 74(11):11, 1991.

50. Misu B et al: *Salmonella enteritidis* gastroenteritis transmitted by intact chicken eggs, *Ann Intern Med* 115(3):190, 1991.

51. Mossman BT, Gee JBL: Asbestos-related diseases, *N Engl J Med* 320(26):1721, 1989.

52. Needleman HL et al: The long-term effects of exposure to low doses of lead in childhood, *N Engl J Med* 322(2):83, 1990.

53. Nero AV et al: Distribution of airborne radon-222 concentrations in US homes, *Science* 234:992, 1986.

54. O'Connell EJ et al: Childhood hypersensitivity pneumonitis (farmer's lung): four cases in siblings with long-term follow-up, *J Pediatr* 114(6):995, 1989.

55. Oversight on the National Fire Academy and fire safety equipment for hearing-impaired individuals, Hearing before subcommittee on Science, Research and Technology of the Community on Science, Space and Technology, US House of Representatives, 101st Congress, second session, Sept. 13, 1990.

56. *Pesticides in drinking water*, Washington, DC, revised Sept 1990, US EPA.

57. *Poison prevention packaging: a text for pharmacists and physicians*, Washington, DC (revised) Sept. 1990, Consumer Product Safety Division.

58. *Radon, a physician's guide*, American Medical Association, AA15:90, 1990.

59. Reisinger KS: Smoke detectors; reducing deaths and injuries due to fire, *Pediatrics* 65(4):718, 1980.

60. Rimmer S, Shuler JD: Severe ocular trauma from a driver's-side air bag, *Arch Opthamol* 109:774, 1991.

61. Rosenblat M, Freilich B, and Kirsch D: Air bags: trade-offs, *N Engl J Med* 325(21):1518, 1991.

62. Sacks JJ et al: Bicycle-associated head injuries and deaths in the United States from 1984 through 1989, *JAMA* 266(21):3016, 1991.

63. *Safety and survival in an earthquake,* US Geological Survey, Department of Interior, USGPO 1990-0-253-830.

64. Samet JM, Utell MJ: The environment and the lung, changing perspectives, *JAMA* 266(5):670, 1991.

65. *Seat belts and the family,* a pamphlet by General Motors Corp and the AMA.

66. Sharp D: What a dump! Your home is a toxic waste site. Here's how to clean it up without messing up the rest of the planet, *Hippocrates* 6(1):62, 1992.

67. Shaw KN et al: Correlates of reported smoke detector usage in an inner-city population: participants in a smoke detector give-away program, *Am J Public Health,* 78(6):650, 1988.

68. *Shopping for a safer car,* a pamphlet by Insurance Institute for Highway Safety, Oct, 1990.

69. Special report, part 3, how safe is your car? What insurance data say, *Consumers' Research* 74(11):16, 1991.

70. Special report, part 5, safety comparisons: insurance statistics, *Consumers' Research* 73(11):25, 1990.

71. *Storm surge and hurricane safety,* US Department of Commerce, National Oceanic and Atmospheric Administration, National Weather Service, NOAA/PA 78019, US GPO:1991-293-054.

72. Stout JE et al: Potable water as a cause of sporadic cases of community-acquired legionnaire's disease, *N Engl J Med,* 326(3):151, 1992.

73. Sultan MA, Feldman WM: Smoke alarms in the home: what every physician should know, *Can Med Assoc J* 133(12):1207, 1985.

74. Talcott JA et al: Asbestos-associated diseases in a cohort of cigarette-filter workers, *N Engl J Med* 321(18)1220, 1989.

75. *The inside story, a guide to indoor air quality,* Washington, DC, 1988, United States EPA and CPSC.

76. The Lead Ban Act of 1990 and the Lead Exposure Reduction Act of 1990, hearing before the Subcommittee on Toxic Substances, Environmental Oversight, Research and Development of the Committee on Environment and Public Works, US Senate, June 27, 1990.

77. *Thunderstorms and Lightning,* US Department of Commerce, National Weather Service, revised 1985. US GPO 1990-254-050.

78. Tinetti ME, Speechley M, and Ginter SF: Risk factors for falls among elderly persons living in the community, *N Engl J Med* 319(26):1701, 1988.

79. Tinetti ME, Speechley M: Prevention of falls among the elderly, *N Engl J Med* 320(16):1055, 1989.

80. *Tornado safety, surviving nature's most violent storms,* US GPO, 1991, 281-617/42729.

81. *What you should know about lead-based paint in your home,* Consumer Product Safety Alert, Washington, DC, Sept, 1990, Consumer Product Safety Commission.

82. *Wildfire protection, a guide for homeowners and developers,* Ogden, Utah, 1990 USDA, Forest Service, Intermountain Region.

83. Young FE: Weighing food safety risks, FDA *Consumer Magazine,* DHHS Pub (FDA) 90-2231, Sept, 1989.

84. Zador PL: Alcohol-related relative risk of fatal driver injuries in relation to driver age and sex, *J Stud Alcohol* 52(4):302, 1991.

85. Ziperman HH, Cromack JR, and Clark JM: Airbags and seatbelts in injury amelioration, *J Trauma* 16(9):686, 1976.

◼◼◼ RESOURCES: ◼◼◼

Environmental factors affecting home safety

United States Environmental Protection Agency

EPA's Safe Drinking Water Hotline provides information on health effects of pesticides and pesticide poisoning.

TSCA Assistance Information Service provides information on regulations under the Toxic Substances Control Act and EPA's asbestos programs.

National Pesticides Telecommunications Network provides information to the public and medical and professional communities on pesticides.

The EPA Hotline number for Radon provides information on radon testing.

Numerous publications are available from the Consumer Information Agency, PO Box 100, Pueblo, CO 81002, including *Radon reduction methods: a homeowners guide,* (also available through state radon offices of the EPA); *The inside story, a guide to indoor air quality,* an EPA and CPSC consumer handbook on home air-quality, September, 1988; and *Citizen's guide to pesticides, 1990.*

US Consumer Product Safety Commission, Washington, DC 20207. The CPSC hotline handles questions on manufacturer's recalls and unsafe products.

Many CPSC publications, including *CPSC guide to home wiring hazards,* 1990, and *Asbestos in the home,* 1989 (USPC and EPA) are available through Consumer Information Center, Pueblo, CO 81009.

National Weather Service

Provides latest information on safety in storms pertinent to geographical areas; 1325 East Highway, Rm. 14360, Silver Spring, MD 20910 or regional weather services, under US Department of Commerce in local directories.

Sierra Front Wildfire Cooperators. Provides planning assistance to prevent wild fire damage to homes in California and Nevada. Located at Toiyabe National Forest, Sparks, Nevada; Lake Tahoe Basin Management Unit, S. Lake Tahoe, California, and Tahoe National Forest, Nevada City, California.

Safety and Survival in an Earthquake, US Department of the Interior/Geological Survey, Federal Center, Box 25425, Denver, CO 80225. A general interest pamphlet on earthquake safety.

Food safety

US Department of Agriculture, USDA Meat and Poultry Hotline. Home economists and registered dietitians answer questions on the proper handling of foods.

Fire safety

National Fire Protection Association, P.O. Box 9101, Quincy, MA 02269-0910. To place bulk orders for fire safety brochures, posters, films, children's coloring books.

Automobile safety

American Automobile Association and National Safety Institute, 1000 AAA Drive, Heathrow, FL 32746; and local AAA chapters. See local phone books. A source for up-to-date information and pamphlets on car safety, driving programs for seniors, etc.

General consumer publications

Consumer information center, PO Box 100, Pueblo, CO 81002; free or low-cost federal publications of consumer interest. New catalogs published seasonally.

Chapter 65

PREVENTION AND THE TRAVELLER

Richard N. Matzen, Sr.

This chapter shall address those illnesses that may result by the physical circumstances of travel *per se,* environments that may be experienced and toxins that could be ingested by eating certain foods. Infectious diseases to which the traveller might be exposed are discussed in Chapter 57 (e.g., traveller's diarrhea) and two resources on this subject at listed at the end of this chapter.

HISTORICAL PERSPECTIVE

It is very useful to consider the history of travel to better appreciate our current travel risks and possible future risks.

D.J. Bradley of the London School of Hygiene and Tropical Medicine opened the First Conference on International Travel Medicine in Zurich, Switzerland in April, 1988 with a presentation on travel medicine including a fascinating recount of the travel experiences of his great-grandfather, grandfather, father, and himself.[2] These four generations' travels are illustrated on maps of the town of Kettering and its vicinity, southern England, Western Europe, and the world (Fig. 65-1). He reports that his great-grandfather's life was encompassed in a square area 40 km to a side, that his grandfather, by visiting London once from Northamptonshire enlarged his travelled area to 400 km to the side, that his father, before WW II, extended his forays into Western Europe and his area measured 4000 km to the side, and that he himself has travelled worldwide. The four generations thus increased their "world" by factors of 10 linearly and 100 in area in each generation. Bradley thus has reached the ultimate in travel, and there will be no chance of his children carrying on the family tradition, unless one or more of them become space travellers.

My own father was born in the town of Fredericia, Denmark located on an arm of the Kattegat—the strait between Denmark and Sweden. (The permanence of families in those times is attested to by our tracing his mother's family to the late 1500s as all residents of the same town.) The women of the family never left the area, apparently, but each male member is described under occupation as "boatman" and was likely a fisherman and/or travelling seafarer. At age 13, he went to Hamburg to serve as cabin boy on one of his uncle's three masted ships of the sea. At midnight on March 24, 1890, the bark Lina left the dock, cleared the estuary of the Elbe to the North Sea, and set sail for Sydney, Australia. Lina returned to Hamburg by way of Chile and Cape Horn on October 9, 1891 after 1 year, 4 months, and 15 days at sea. The same trip (Hamburg-Australia-Santiago, Chile-Hamburg) now takes a few days by air!

My father's first voyage likely corresponds to the time when Bradley's grandfather's "world" measured 400 km a side. His example is one of very limited and circumscribed travel typical of the vast majority of people who were inland natives. Few people travelled 100 years ago, and when they did, they went most often by foot or post coach and not far. As Bradley states, there has been roughly a tenfold increase in area covered by travel in each of the last four generations. In the case of people "born to the sea" on coastal waters, distant travel was not uncommon, but it was basically a male pursuit, the trips were infrequent, and they were extraordinarily long in duration. Today's traveler is as likely to be female as male and can circumnavigate the globe in days rather than years.

At the same time, the average distance travelled per trip has increased, and the amount of time required to do so

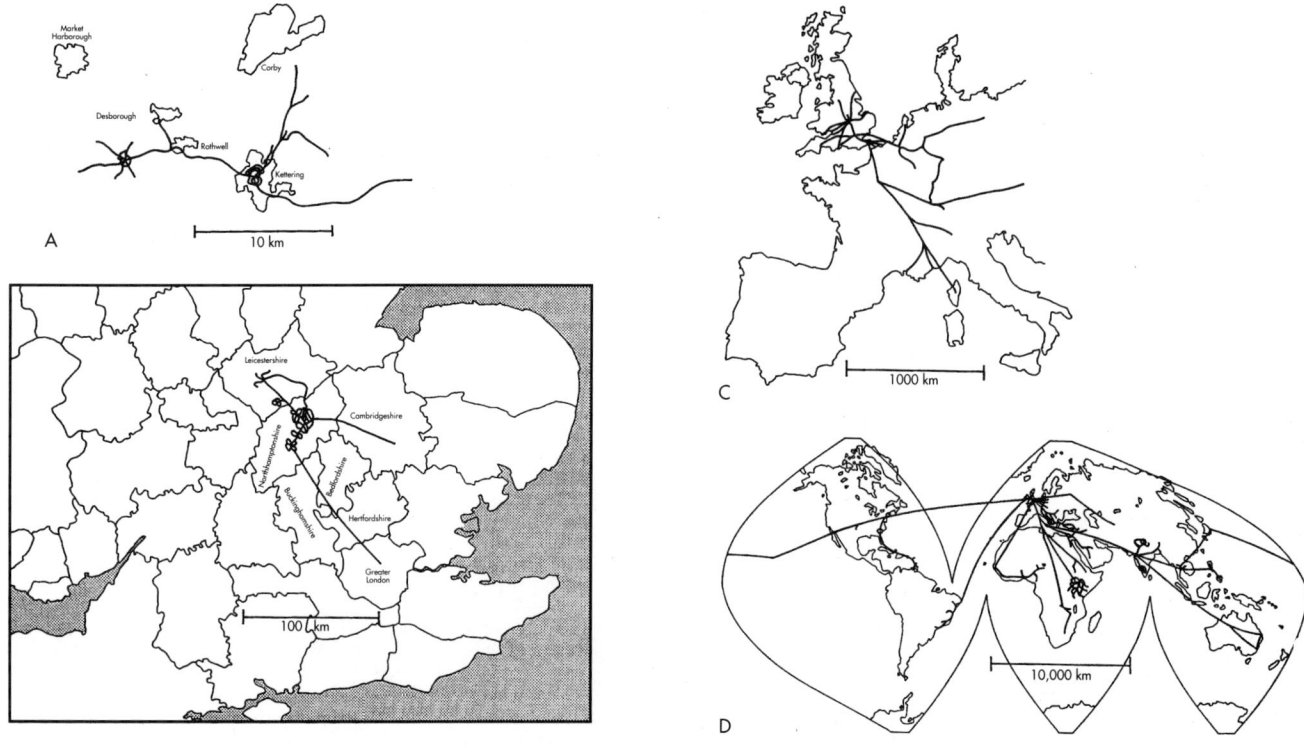

Fig. 65-1. A-D, Maps of the lifetime track of four generations of the same family. The linear scale increases by a factor of 10 and the map area by a factor of 100 between each pair of adjacent figures. **A** represents the track of the author's great-grandparent, **B** that of the grandparent, **C** the parent, and **D** the author's own movements. (From Bradley DJ: The scope of travel medicine: an introduction to the conference on international travel medicine. In Steffen R et al, editors: *Travel medicine,* New York, 1989, Springer Verlag.)

has decreased disproportionately. Jet travel to the citizen of the 1890s would have been a miracle. We have good reason to see our world as too hurried, for travel and communications have accelerated enormously.

The problems addressed in this chapter, especially those connected to travel by air and to stress, are directly related to the speed of travel (see Chapter 11 regarding jet lag). The balance are indirectly related to the speed of travel, because speed permits more trips per unit of time. Increased carrier capacity decreases the cost of travel so that most people, regardless of income, can and do travel longer distances and more frequently with consequent enormous growth in traffic volume.

People travel for five basic reasons:

1. Exploration, adventure
2. War
3. Commerce, business
4. To avoid travail
5. Pleasure, vacation

One hundred years ago the first four were dominant by a large margin. In the last decade the last four have domi-

nated. Leisure travel 100 years ago might have been an overnight or fortnight in London, or summer at the nearby beach or mountains. Today it is a huge and growing business that knows no season or destination too remote. In a compilation of the various tourist countries' statistics, Keller and Koch[23] found that, in the 37 years between 1950 and 1987, arrivals per annum grew from 25 million to 355 million (a factor of 13) in the tourist countries, and that tourist receipts in the same countries grew from $2.1 billion (U.S.) to $150 billion (U.S.) (a factor of 70). Add to that the fantastic growth in business travel related to international commerce, and we arrive at a still larger figure for number of miles travelled and people transported.

THE CAUSES OF MORTALITY IN TRAVELLERS

Epidemiologic data show that more than half of those travelling abroad suffer some ailment, and respiratory and gastrointestinal ailments are the two leading causes of the largest category of problems, infectious diseases. Traveller's diarrhea is probably the single greatest complaint and reaches its greatest incidence in warm and tropical countries.[36] Some diseases have more serious consequences,

Table 65-1. Injury deaths of American travelers—1975, 1984

Cause of death	No. of deaths 1975 and 1984	% of total
Motor vehicle crash	163	27.1
Drowning	96	16.0
Plane crash	43	7.2
Homicide	52	8.7
Poisoning	39	6.5
Suicide	20	3.3
Burns	21	3.5
Electrocution	3	0.5
Others	164	27.2
Totals	**601**	**100.0**

From Hargarten SW, Baker T, and Guptill K: Injury deaths and American travellers. In Steffen R et al, editors, *Travel medicine*, New York, 1989, Springer Verlag

Injury control strategies for American tourists

1. Avoidance of motorcycles and small, less protective vehicles or at least use of helmets when using these vehicles
2. Use of seat belts, where available, including taxicabs
3. Use of larger in preference to smaller vehicles and not riding in the back of open trucks
4. Avoidance of small, nonscheduled aircraft
5. Careful selection of swimming areas, avoidance of alcohol while swimming
6. Avoidance of travel at night
7. Encouragement of travel in groups or pairs
8. Require rental agencies of cars, motorcycles, and bicycles to provide seat belts for cars, car seats for infants, and helmets for cyclists and motorcyclists
9. Require usage of protective equipment as a condition of rental
10. Review toxins to which the patient might be exposed by way of foods, particularly if travel is to an area of high incidence or exposure

From Hargarten SW, Baker T, and Guptill K: Injury deaths and American travellers. In Steffen R et al, editors: *Travel medicine*, New York, 1989, Springer Verlag.

such as amebiasis, hepatitis, malaria, cholera, and poliomyelitis. However, in terms of mortality, the infectious diseases fall far down the list, and death from infectious diseases represent only 1% of all recorded travel deaths (S.W. Hargarten, et al.)[17]

Hargarten, Baker, and Guptill[17] investigated the causes of all deaths in Americans abroad in the years 1975 and 1984 and found that there were 2,463. Of these, 78.4% occurred in people over the age of 45, with the highest incidence in the two decades between 55 and 75. The leading cause of death was found to be cardiovascular disease, much as would be the case in the population at home. In travel the risk of a cardiovascular death would presumably be increased considering the stress of travel, overindulgence of many kinds, such as physical exertion and alcohol, and long days on the go. But this is not the case.

The figures these authors give for males are surprising. The death rates per 100,000 for men in the age group 55 to 64 years are 793.2 for travellers and 808.9 for all of the United States. (A similar pattern is seen in all the age groups over 45 years of age.) A second surprise is that in those under the age of 45, where one would expect the least susceptible and most fit people unlikely to die of cardiovascular disease, the reverse is true, where the rates are increased by factors of 11.4, 2.9, and 1.3 in the age groups 15 to 24, 25 to 34, and 35 to 44 respectively.

Cardiovascular deaths make up 49% of the total deaths during travel, and intentional and unintentional injuries are a strong second at 25%. As previously noted, only 1% of deaths are caused by infection.

This chapter will address the preventive steps regarding previously known conditions and where to get help should any illness, in this instance, cardiovascular disease, occur for the first time and without warning.

The authors noted found that, unlike cardiovascular disease, injuries were increased in travel in all age groups up

to the age of 75. Those over 75 were a little less than half as likely to sustain an injury as those ages 25-34. Women older than 75, however, were more prone to injury than all younger groups. Males older than 65 have between approximately one third to one half the number of injuries as those ages 15-64. The highest incidence occurs in the age group 35 to 44, where risk overseas increases threefold. These authors present in Table 65-1 the causes of injury, the first being motor vehicle crashes and the second drowning. In the box above they present a list of precautions, which includes those for preventing such accidental motor vehicle injuries.

There were 601 deaths resulting from injury in the 2 study years presented by Hargarten et al.[18] Of these, Mexico alone accounted for 205. In 1975, the Americas and the Caribbean accounted for 43% of the total deaths. By 1984, 74% of the total foreign deaths by trauma occurred in this same area, a foreboding trend. The risk of injury is increased in less developed nations.

PROBLEMS COMMON TO AIR TRAVEL
General statistics of air travel and the environment

Air travel differs from other modes of travel in that with increasing altitude, the oxygen content and air pressure decrease. This was literally true in the day of piston-driven aircraft; the higher the airplane flew, the lower was the oxygen content and the atmospheric pressure of the cabin air. These aircraft flew at lower altitudes than modern jet-powered craft, however. Greater speed is possible at higher altitudes, so jets utilizing the altitude-speed advantage needed a cabin atmosphere that would sustain life and mental acuity. This atmosphere was produced through the use of engine-driven superchargers that compressed the air into the cabin to create an atmosphere as close to that of sea level as possible. Above an altitude limit that is determined by the type and age of aircraft, the superchargers are unable to meet the ideal of sea level atmosphere and slightly decompensate; that decompensation increases as the aircraft ascends.

Experienced altitude refers to the cabin pressure, in contrast to the absolute altitude (above sea level) of the aircraft itself. The former can affect the health of the traveller. For example, at the cruising altitude of 35,000 to 42,000 feet, someone in a DC-9 (an older aircraft) will experience an altitude of 8000 feet, or about the height above sea level of Aspen, Colorado. The same person in a B-747 at the same altitude will be at an experienced altitude of 4700 feet, or somewhat lower than Albuquerque, New Mexico (Table 65-2).

Shesser[35] points out that during the era of piston-driven aircraft, there were fewer in-flight emergencies than in the jet age, despite the fact that, without compressors, the experienced altitude of the passenger was higher than today's passenger. He postulates that this is due to longer flights, less healthy passengers, and data reporting and collecting differences, or some other unrecognized factor in the jet age.

His article presents data to support the hypothesis that longer flights have an effect. He analyzes the experience of long-distance carriers vs. short-distance carriers and notes that the longer flights have an increased risk of about a factor of a third, at least as measured by in-air deaths. He also notes that there are known factors that predispose one to symptoms in flight (not necessarily serious), and these are persons with prior myocardial infarction, pulmonary emphysema, and simply poor exercise tolerance.

Dan[10] notes that 550 million travellers pass through the 25 busiest U.S. airports and that "more people enplane, deplane and transfer through Chicago's O'Hare International Airport annually than live in Australia, New Zealand, Sweden, Finland, Norway, Denmark, Switzerland, Ireland, Greece, and the Congo combined." He likens the incidence of in-flight medical emergencies to that found at a football game or rock concert. In-flight requests for medical aid are most likely for one of three things: gastrointestinal symptoms, an episode marked by cardiac symptoms, or respiratory symptoms.

Flying is safer than driving and actually has less morbidity and mortality than everyday existence. One must not presume, however, that simply because one is in flight all will be well. Flight predisposes to or exacerbates several conditions.

Of the 120 carriers of the International Air Transport Association, only 42 reported deaths onboard between the years 1977 and 1984, for an average of 72 per year[8] (to put the problem in perspective, note the figure given previously for domestic passengers). This was a death rate of .31 per million passengers. The average passenger was a man 66% of the time, and his mean age was 53.8 years. Of in-flight emergencies, 77% occurred in people who reported no health problems before departure; 56% seemed to be cardiac problems; and of the "healthy" people, the cause of death was unexpected sudden cardiac death in 63%.

Whereas most figures are gathered retrospectively, one study[9] of the experience at a single airport (Seattle-Tacoma) with a traffic of 14 million arriving and departing passengers was done prospectively over 1 year and is unique. This study can be related to one's own airport and in general corresponds to other data on the magnitude of travel and the occurrence of emergency incidents not only in the air but at the airport. In this year, the emergency personnel at the airport evaluated 1107 people; 21% were employees, 11% were area residents, and 68% (754) were travellers. Only 25% of these travellers had their emergency (something requiring medical assistance) in flight, and 75% had theirs on the ground within the terminal! Of those on the ground, the great majority (68%) were effectively handled by persons trained as emergency medical technicians. The in-flight emergencies occurred at a rate of one per 753 inbound flights or one per 39,600 inbound passengers. The most common complaints in the group studied were abdominal pain, chest pain, shortness of breath, syncope, and seizures. Seven flights were diverted for emergency landing elsewhere, and this was thought to be probably unnecessary. They were not all, as one might assume, due to cardiac crises. There were episodes of angina resolved by nitroglycerine, abdominal pain, minor scalp laceration, seizure in a known epileptic, an acute asthma attack that resolved with self-administered bronchodilator, syncope in an intoxicated youth, and irregular heart rhythm. Of these, only two, possibly three, could conceivably be related to the environs of flight (altitude), and that assumption would be greater or lesser depending on the experienced altitude, which was not reported.

The economy class syndrome

For many years physicians have recognized that holding a limb still for a prolonged period will lead to venostasis and predispose to the formation of a thrombus that does not adhere to the vessel wall (phlebothrombosis) by virtue of associated inflammation, as is the case with thrombophlebitis. Virchow first pointed this out in 1856.[38] It appears not uncommonly in postoperative immobilized patients with pulmonary emboli, and all surgeons have guarded against it routinely for decades. This has been emphasized in driver education classes in high schools (on long trips travellers should get out, stretch, and walk about every 30 to 60 minutes). Embolization after long auto trips has been reported. It has occurred even in situations of

Table 65-2. Recommendations for unescorted air travel

Condition	American Medical Association*	American College of Chest Physicians†	Aerospace Medical Association‡
Heart disease			
Acute myocardial infarction	No air travel for 4 weeks after attack	8-24 weeks: no travel above 6000 feet; 0-8 weeks: no travel above 2000 feet	Can travel with oxygen unless cyanotic, in shock, or unstable rhythm
Heart failure	Can travel 2 weeks after decompensation	No travel above 2000 feet while in failure; no travel above 10,000 feet after stabilization	Can travel only if oxygen is available
Lung disease			
Obstructive pulmonary disease	No travel if vital capacity <50% predicted	No travel above 6000 feet if cyanosis, cor pulmonale, or respiratory acidosis; no travel above 4000 feet if two or three above conditions; no travel above 2000 feet if all three above conditions	No cabin altitude above 5000 feet if vital capacity <50% predicted
Pneumothorax	Contraindicated	No recommendation	No flight for 10 days if stable
Asthma	No recommendation	If symptomatic, no ascent above 10,000 feet	No restriction
Neuropsychiatric			
Seizure disorders	May fly if: (1) well controlled; and (2) flight <8000 feet	No recommendation	May fly if: (1) accompanied by a companion; (2) preflight sedation; and (3) flight <8000 feet
Recent skull fracture	Contraindicated	No recommendation	Contraindicated
Gastrointestinal			
	No travel for 10-14 days after abdominal surgery	No recommendation	No air travel for 10 days
	Travel contraindicated for acute diverticulitis, acute ulcerative colitis, acute esophageal varices, acute gastroenteritis	No recommendation	
Obstetric/gynecologic			
Pregnancy	No travel beyond 240 days	No recommendation	Can travel in 7th or 8th month; physician certification required for nineth month
Hematologic			
Anemia with normal hemoglobins	Contraindicated if hemoglobin < 8.5 gm/100 ml	No recommendation	Travel with oxygen if hemoglobin < 8.5 gm/100 ml
Abnormal hemoglobins	Travel contraindicated for atmospheric altitudes > 22,000 feet in pressurized aircraft	No recommendation	Patients with SS and SC hemoglobin should be advised not to fly
Ophthalmologic			
Recent eye surgery	Air travel contraindicated	No recommendation	Cabin altitude not to exceed 4000-5000 feet
Retinal disease	No recommendation	No recommendation	Cabin altitude not to exceed 10,000 feet

(From Shesser R: Medical aspects of commercial air travel, *Am J Emerg Med* 7(2):216, 1989.)
*From American Medical Association: Medical aspects of transportation aboard commercial aircraft, *JAMA* 247:1007-1011, 1982.
†From American College of Chest Physicians: Air travel in cardiorespiratory disease, *Chest* 37:579-588, 1960.
‡From Aerospace Medical Association: Medical criteria for the flying passenger, *Aerospace Med* 32:124-137, 1961.

prolonged confinement in air raid shelters in London during the "blitz" until cots were provided.[34]

In travelers, this syndrome has been called *traveller's thrombosis,* and lately its occurrence in air travel has produced the name *economy class syndrome.* Although this phenomenon should not be considered unique to travelling economy class by air, the name is descriptive as it immediately conjures the picture of cramped quarters conducive to immobility, which can lead to thrombosis. All physicians should educate their travelling patients about it and the preventive measures; all travellers should be knowledgeable about it. Reported cases, and those with which I am familiar, seem to have the embolus originating in the leg, but some have pointed out that the same phenomenon can occur in the immobile cramped upper extremity.

A discussion of the apparent pathophysiology will illustrate the prevention of the problem. In the dependent limb, blood flow through the veins back to the right atrium is passive, wherein blood is pushed by more blood coming through the capillary system and to the greatest extent by muscle contraction about the veins, which milks the fluid along and upward. Intact venous valves act as lift stations in this process and guard against an even greater intravascular pressure at the lowest or most distal point, which would occur if the valve were incompetent, as in the varicose vein. Any proximal restriction, such as a band of elastic at the top of hose, will retard venous flow. The more dependent the extremity, the lower the rate of flow and the greater the risk. Warm ambient temperature also increases the arterial circulation to the part and thus increases the venous load. If conditions cause intravenous pressure to increase, the pressure will overcome the colloid osmotic pressure of the blood, which holds fluid within the vessel, and cause extravasation of fluid into the surrounding tissue. This causes an increase in the hematocrit locally and further predisposes to clot; this risk is highest during dehydration of the individual. Carruthers, Arguelles, and Mosovich[4] reported a study of 15 passengers and crew on a 20-hour flight from Buenos Aires to London in which they found "the subjects passed small volumes of highly concentrated urine during the flight, though urine volume and osmolality returned to normal on the 2 postflight days." Moyses[29] reported 14 experiments on seven subjects sitting quietly with the foot a meter below the heart. At the beginning of the experiment the hematocrit was 42.1% mean and the plasma protein concentration 6.53 g/dl as drawn from the arm. He reported an increasing rise in both during 1 hour of dependency to a hematocrit of 53.8% (mean) and a protein concentration of 9.34 g/dl (mean) after 1 hour, with several subjects exceeding 10 g/dl.

The more passengers a flight carries, the more profitable is the flight. Deregulation and increased competition have produced a trend toward decreasing seating space to fit more seats in the plane, compared with the era of regulation and the propeller-driven aircraft. Unfortunately, over the past 4 decades, the average height and build of the traveller has increased. The result is less chance to change body position and move about in the seat. The increased number of fliers has resulted not only from the increasing population but also the lower air fares, which resulted not only from increased competition but the same increased seating capacity per flight (larger aircraft and increased "efficiency" of seating). Therefore, regardless of the incidence of the problem, the sheer number of fliers will result in an increase in the number of cases.

It should be pointed out that both deep venous thrombosis and pulmonary embolism (PE) are difficult diagnoses to make under the best of circumstances and under diagnosis and occurrence without symptoms is a surety. Monreal et al.[27a] recently have shown that in a prospective study of patients with deep venous thrombosis in whom all received lung scans, only 54% of patients with PE had symptoms. They estimate that, as a preexisting condition, those with previous thrombosis were likely to have more than a twofold increase risk of recurrence. It is interesting in the traveler's context that they suggest that simple immobilization DVT (vs., e.g., postoperative DVT) seems to be associated with considerable less risk of PE and theorize this could be due to the thrombus being rich in fibrin and trapped erythrocytes. These patients (N = 434) were not travelers, but the implications apply.

Figures on the incidence of thrombosis resulting from flights of any distance are unfortunately lacking. Reports of the so-called economy class syndrome or traveller's thrombosis are largely of a case or a cluster of cases, and the experience of physicians is largely anecdotal, but nonetheless real.[3,14,20,26,37] Physicians involved with the air carrier industry would agree that we need well-designed prospective controlled studies to determine under flight conditions of some length the number of thromboses per thousand travellers and the number of resultant emboli. The thrombus itself is silent and, unless an embolus results, often remains undiagnosed. The pulmonary embolus problem is also difficult to estimate, for the embolus that occurs can be in flight but also may occur as long as an estimated 10 to 14 days or longer after the trip. Even at several days later the patient may not associate the event to the preceding trip.

One study has attempted to gauge the problems of long-duration (over 3 hours) flights. At the Aerospace Medical Association Annual Meeting in Cincinnati, May 8, 1991, a panel on "Current Concerns in Passenger Health" in part addressed this issue. Dawson, speaking for Thompson of Air New Zealand,[11] reported on a preliminary study of the question. This preliminary study sought to determine whether there was a problem and the size of the problem, and to lay the basis for a future study. The investigators sent questionnaires to all people who had been hospitalized in the Auckland area during 1988 to 1989 with the discharge diagnosis of deep vein thrombosis and/or pulmonary embolus. There were 502 such cases, and there were 257 replies (51%). The questionnaire asked whether the patient recalled long-distance travel (air or ground) within the 2 months preceding the illness. Of the respondents, 10 recalled a long-distance flight, and 13 recalled a long-distance road trip. The total of 23 was 8.6% of the respondents. Dawson noted that, even if all of the nonrespondents replied in the negative, the positives would represent about 4% of cases, and he thought this was significant. This study had known defects: (1) There were no controls. (2) The staff relied on recall going back 1 to 2 years—difficult for anyone but perhaps more so in the older population represented. (3) Only in-hospital patients were addressed, and a significant number of area residents could have been treated as outpatients during the study period. The division of diagnoses in this group was 127 with pulmonary emboli, 121 with deep vein thrombosis, and 9 with both diagnoses.

Dawson suggested that the aircraft seat itself could play a part in compromising venous circulation, because over the past 20 years the seat had gradually been elevated, the support of the cushion often had been converted from a webbed support to an aluminum pan that made it stiffer, and the seat cushion itself had been made harder to wear longer and to provide flotation through close-cell foam, which also causes it to be firmer. As a result, the leading edge of the seat impinges with less give on the posterior thigh.

Dawson thought that the study certainly suggested a risk, that further research was indicated, and that passengers should be advised of potential risk. Air New Zealand should be complimented, in my opinion, on its reported policy of showing a videotape on all overseas flights, regardless of length, on ways a passenger may prevent venous thrombosis. The tape includes instruction on isometric exercise of the legs and thigh muscles, getting up to walk about, and changing position. The airline also advises at-risk passengers to consider low-dose aspirin use in travel.

At this same panel discussion, Landgraf[25] of the Department of Internal Medicine at the University Hospital in Frankfurt commented on a study he had done on the coagulation parameters and rheological measurements in the systemic veins and the dorsal foot veins of healthy volunteers in aircraft seats for three hours. He reported that he found no significant changes, in contrast to Moyses' study, previously cited. He also commented on a study presented at the same meeting[24] in which he participated with the Lufthansa Medical Department. This study was of 24 healthy volunteers divided into two groups and seated in a 747 for a 12-hour simulated flight. One group got up every 3 hours only, the second hourly. They were crossed over for one daytime flight and one nighttime flight. Although there was a statistically significant increase in leg volume

at the end of the flight, rheological and hemodynamic changes were only slight. The conclusion was that the changes noted did not seem to be important factors in the development of a thrombus. Nonetheless, he noted Lufthansa was also developing an audiovisual tape to teach passengers in-seat isometric exercises in-flight. Perhaps more studies, ideally prospective and under flight conditions, will be reported soon, for as noted, the Lufthansa study was in a simulator and involved healthy younger persons, and the cabin humidity was 40% rather than the experienced 10% in actual flight.

Cruickshank, Gorlin, and Jennett[7] present six cases of economy class syndrome with thrombosis and embolus. There were five cases in men and one in a woman. Three were very healthy, and three had a predisposing medical history. The ages were 48, 60, 43, and 51, 79, and 31, respectively, in the two groups. The embolus occurred 4 hours into a flight in the case of the female, and in the men, a few hours after the flight and 1, 2, 7, and 10 days after the trip. In the one case where the patient sustained two separate episodes, an embolus occurred 7 days after a flight from England to the Far East; after a return trip 3 weeks later, the embolus appeared 1 day after returning home. Only in the first instance was the embolus preceded by calf symptoms. In all other episodes (six) the presenting symptom was chest pain (five) and hemoptysis with cough (one). Sarvesvaren[33] reported on 104 sudden deaths occurring in Heathrow Airport from Feb. 1979 to Jan. 1982. The deaths were divided into three categories. The first were spectator/staff (15 cases); the second were "would-be passengers" (28 cases); the third group were 61 cases of passengers on incoming flights. There were no emboli found at postmortem in the group of spectator/staff, and only one such case in the "would-be passengers" (3.6%). Of the deaths of passengers on arriving flights however, there were 11 pulmonary embolisms determined to be the cause of death, (all cases underwent postmortem examination) or 18%. Of these 11 deaths, 9 were females. In one, the flight was less than 12 hours duration. In the other 10, the flight was 12 to 18 hours long. The author felt it was reasonable to conclude, as 72.7% of the cases of emboli due to deep venous thrombosis were in persons with no preexisting illness, healthy air passengers confined for a long period of time are at risk for venous thrombosis and possible secondary sudden death by embolization. Females might be more susceptible to this problem.

Unfortunately, sudden death syndrome may be due to this cause, as embolus is exceedingly difficult to determine even in postmortem autopsied cases, and the number of these cases resulting from this cause, more specifically, from traveller's thrombus, is unknown. That this disease is not restricted to the coach or economy class passenger is supported by a recent report of a case involving a business class passenger. Flight duration is most important.

The circumstances of air travel probably predispose to

the risk more than train or bus. One unique feature of the environment in aircraft is that the humidity is very low, and the constant air flow further exacerbates evaporation. In addition, travelers tend to indulge in alcohol on these trips, which induces diuresis. Many passengers also reduce fluid intake to avoid having to use the restroom. The result is some degree of dehydration and presumably consequent increase in hematocrit. There is also more room in the bus seat, private car, and train in which to move about and to get out.

In summary, we face a potentially lethal condition of unknown magnitude but undoubted existence that is amenable to primary prevention.

Prevention, or at least risk reduction, is possible through a number of techniques aimed at increasing limb motion/muscle use, increasing hydration, and decreasing the tendency to clot formation. These are:

1. Use aspirin beginning the day before the trip as required to reduce platelet stickiness and clotting ability. Consult your doctor.
2. Drink fluids (nonalcoholic) liberally throughout the trip.
3. Opt for seats that allow the maximum room when possible.
4. Do not wear clothes or assume positions that have a tourniquet effect.
5. Consider use of support hose.
6. Alternately contract and relax muscles in the extremities during the trip and occasionally get up and move about.
7. Where a predisposing condition exists, travel first class if it is affordable and sit with the legs elevated as much as possible.
8. In short persons, or in the case of certain seats with hard leading edges, place the feet up on some object a few inches high or invent some other way to relieve the pressure on the posterior upper leg. Recline the seat back.
9. As smoking increases blood viscosity, abstain.

Problems in low humidity

Some patients seem very sensitive to the low (approximately 10%) humidity of aircraft; they report symptoms of an annoying, dry or sore throat or nose. This increases with the duration of flight and the number of consecutive days flying, and possibly because many hotel rooms have closed heating/cooling units and windows that cannot be opened. I do not know of a way to totally relieve these complaints, but they seem to be alleviated by using nasal saline, coating the membranes with ointment, hanging wet towels in the bathroom of the hotel, running the shower or leaving some water in the bathtub at night, or selecting a hotel that allows windows to be opened, allowing air of increased humidity to enter.

Problems common to air travel

Stress. Several factors over the past decade seem to have caused increased stress in travel for chief executives, upper managers, and middle managers. They report that these are exclusively related to air travel and are:

- My company will no longer send me by first class.
- The seats are becoming more cramped, and they seem more uncomfortable.
- There is greater crowding not only in the plane but also in the airport.
- More travel is necessary now that our plants and/or customers are less regional and more national/international.
- With increasing competition we are expected to do more with less, and this means more business stops per trip and a tighter itinerary.
- My itinerary goes as planned in one trip in four or five (the causes of disruption are various but appear to be late takeoffs, late arrivals, missed connections, lost luggage, last-minute changes caused by business needs, late arrival at the airport because of traffic, etc.)

The root cause of all this frustration and stress is the "bottom line." Corporations apply pressure to produce more with less and reduce overhead, because our economy is not robust and competition has increased, not just from domestic companies but from overseas as well. These factors also affect the airlines as corporations, and the sheer volume of traffic, demand for their services, and often limited facilities (a problem not of their own making, airport capacity), they too are under pressure. The chances for an interrupted schedule increase accordingly. However, we can suggest some preventive measures to reduce stress in individual patients.

Harry Truman's adage, "If you can't stand the heat, get out of the kitchen" is not an option for most of our patients. However, two CEOs of midsize healthy corporations told me that they were opting out even though each was in his 50s, was not ready to retire, and basically liked what he did. The reason was purely that they could not or were not willing to put up with the "hassle" of travel anymore. For them the decision was a very appropriate and good one. For those who cannot afford to get out, the problem is much more difficult. In many cases where the patient does control his own itinerary, he or she should not expect too much of himself or herself, allow for a looser schedule, allow adequate time to reach the airport, schedule an overnight stay, anticipate prolonged meetings, and so on. Many people who must reduce stress for health's sake find they can avoid a trip, delegate some travel to others, and even opt for a lateral transfer to a position that requires less travel.

Not all people required to travel find it stressful; indeed, some seem to thrive on it and are not bothered by the delays and other problems that one encounters. For the rest, who suffer to a greater or lesser degree, the reader should refer to several chapters in this book that deal with stress (see Chapters 11, 12, 17, 18) to better advise the patient. A notable release from stress for countless business travellers is daily exercise, and it is surprising how many place this 30- to 60-minute period in their daily schedule and carry it out whether at home or on the road. They report that if they have a week when their exercise is impossible, they definitely do not feel as well.

Heber[19] notes in a presentation that spiritual stress occurs in those who have no control over their destiny, or who think they have no such control. Their response will often be meditation or self-preoccupation, and they can be helped by relaxation techniques. Second, he notes that those who travel often experience culture shock, but that this can be avoided by taking pretrip classes in the culture of the destination. Many companies send employees to such courses for several weeks before overseas assignments. The casual traveller is more likely to experience this stress when the cultures rapidly change (e.g., "five countries in 14 days") and may well respond with longing for home or depressed feelings. In the latter instance, the traveller must realize that one trades a lower stress level for the privilege of seeing more countries. When the physician knows that this is not compatible with the patient's personality or needs, the physician should suggest alternative plans.

PREEXISTING CONDITIONS AND AIR TRAVEL

All physicians who care for patients with preexisting conditions that may be exacerbated by air and ground travel should advise their patients (particularly those with unstable seizure disorder, heart disease, and advanced COPD) about travel in general and suggest an office visit a week or two before embarking to assess the patient's status at the time of the trip.

Shesser covered several conditions in the American Journal of Emergency Medicine (see Table 65-2).[35] A discussion of several common and potentially serious conditions follows.

Advanced chronic obstructive pulmonary disease (COPD)

As noted previously, experienced cabin altitude on modern airliners may be 5000 to 8000 feet above sea level, depending on the altitude, aircraft type, and age. The Federal Aviation Agency (FAA) has mandated that aircraft maintain a cabin environment of 8000 feet or less, although this is subject to exception under certain conditions. Because oxygen is required above 10,000 feet, this altitude is not exceeded. In advising patients who may need supplemental oxygen, the practitioner can assume the experienced altitude will be 8000 feet and base advice on that assumption. The altitude is clinically important in that

each 1000 feet of higher experienced altitude causes a corresponding drop in Pa_{O_2} and hence presents potential risk to those who already have a decreased arterial oxygen pressure or in whom the coronary circulation is seriously compromised. Most authorities suggest that supplemental oxygen be advised if flight will result in a Pa_{O_2} of as low as 50 mm Hg. The normocapnic patient (barring illness, e.g., respiratory infection) with a resting sea level Pa_{O_2} of about 72 mm Hg can be projected to have a Pa_{O_2} of 50 mm Hg or better at 8000 feet.[6] In turn, a resting preflight level of less than 70 mm Hg would require supplemental oxygen during flight.

Gong et al.[16] have described a hypoxia/altitude-simulation test that can be used with fair precision to determine the response of the individual patient to altitude. When a patient's response to flight conditions is in doubt, the patient should be placed in simulated flight conditions, as the authors describe. This may include a pressure chamber, which is available at many hospitals and university laboratories. Dillard et al.[12] confirmed the reliability of Pa_{O_2} as a predictor of altitude response, but they thought their studies showed that preflight measurement of the $FEV_{1\ sec}$ improved the prediction of Pa_{O_2} at altitude. Both these reports are highly recommended.

When supplemental oxygen is indicated, alternatives may be considered, and at times are preferable, such as air ambulance or ground transportation. Airlines are not obligated to accept all passengers. Because airlines are required to furnish the oxygen, each may have a different system of delivery, so the patient must be aware of the practical consequences of such factors as tube diameters. All arrangements must be made in advance, the earlier, the better. A physician's letter to an airline must contain all pertinent case data. This includes not only the diagnosis and statement of need, but also other requirements such as stability and safety to travel at an experienced altitude of 8000 feet. The more information provided, including altitude simulation testing, the better. The airline will give or deny clearance.

Gong[15] presented an excellent summary of this subject in a recent article that covered the physiology of these patients, altitude, and practical questions of in-flight oxygen therapy, prescription, oxygen vendors, and personal equipment for use in connection points.

The patient with cardiovascular disease

The rules for flying for cardiovascular patients are more difficult to establish. With the COPD patient, one is considering a relatively simple system whose function is to transfer oxygen into the blood and whose efficiency can be objectively measured by the Pa_{O_2}. The cardiac patient's problem is much more complex, and the risks are often hidden. General rules apply less and the conservative judgment of the physician experienced in this discipline should be applied on an individual basis. For example, people who have sustained a stroke and recovered fully can generally fly without a problem. However, a person who has been undergoing transient ischemic attacks could be put at increased risk. In the recovered heart-attack patient, flight after 8 weeks is usually no problem. However, those suffering postinfarct angina, who are prone to dysrhythmia, or who have experienced failure are unique cases who must be evaluated on a case-by-case basis.

As previously noted, cardiovascular death rates are lower than expected in travel.[17] In fact, the cardiac patient under the care of a physician may be safer than the traveller who has an unknown risk, such as heart disease that is asymptomatic until the occurrence of a heart attack or sudden death. In reporting on in-flight deaths among commercial air travellers, Cummins, et al.[8,9] found that during the study period, sudden cardiac death occurred in 253 of 399 cases (63%) in passengers with no known health problems but only in 32 of 124 passengers (26%) with known health problems. These authors point out that this has an important implication for prevention of death, because "well" persons who suffer sudden cardiac episodes are more likely to respond to resuscitation.

The physician must practice primary prevention of the sudden cardiac event in the asymptomatic person at the periodic health examination to uncover occult heart disease with fatal potential. Although imperfect, the treadmill stress test is the only screening tool that is noninvasive and that offers a reasonable chance of uncovering such disease. The cost effectiveness of this tool is a concern. The physician should select the subset of patients who are more likely to have this disease to increase yield and efficiency. Accepting that age increases risk of occult disease and that the symptom of chest discomfort increases yield, the candidate subsets are those with a significant family history and those with abnormal blood lipids.[13] In dealing with many executives who are under stress, experience long working hours, and travel a great deal, we tend to extend these screening guidelines. One should not abandon clinical judgment, part of the art of medicine, and rely solely on general rules for the use of treadmill testing as a screen.

Screening for occult heart disease is not directly related to travel, but as discussed is important in reducing travel risk among those with unknown heart disease. The hypoxia altitude simulation test described by Gong may determine the known heart patient's tolerance to altitude just as it does with the COPD patient and should be used in appropriate cases where tolerance is in doubt.

Patients who have sustained a stroke and paralysis or decreased motion in an extremity have a limb that is normally moved and repositioned less than a healthy limb. In restrictive seating conditions or long trips in any conveyance, the limb is less likely than usual to be moved, and isometric exercises are impossible. All this, added to dependency of the lower extremities, produces a predisposition to traveller's thrombosis. These patients should be educated in the associated risk of both thrombosis and embolism, and preventive measures should be used. This also applies to situations other than stroke, such as poliomyelitis and peripheral edema of any cause.

Barotitis media

We have all experienced the ear "popping" that occurs with changes in altitude. This process for equalizing air pressure on both sides of the tympanic membrane is remarkably efficient in most people. Those who have inner ear discomfort or pain with air pressure change should consult an otolaryngologist. With moderate congestion of the nasal membranes, as may occur during a trip, decongestant nasal sprays and oral decongestants often reduce or prevent symptoms. The person who flies frequently who has significant nasal allergy must maintain a prophylactic program of desensitization or use of nasal cromolyn or steroids, which have been proven with experience. The modified Valsalva maneuver with a closed nares is folk medicine that works in minor cases.

Motion sickness

Almost all seamen under certain conditions are prone to transient "mal de mer." The traveler may experience it as well. People especially susceptible to motion sickness may wish to consult an ear specialist. Scopolamine patches are in vogue and apparently are effective in many. However, one should observe the "warnings" for use. Others have found that commonly recommended remedies work; whether this is from a placebo effect or real, one should use what works. The more central one is in the craft, the less motion is experienced. In a ship, a cabin amidship experiences less pitch and roll. In an aircraft, aisle seats over the wing area likewise experience less motion. Patients should be advised to close their eyes and recline rather than attempt to distract themselves from the problem by reading.

The ideal preventive for motion sickness would be a medication that prevents the malady and has few, if any, side effects. The predominant side effect of scopolamine, reportedly the best of the anti-motion sickness medications, is severe dryness of the mouth and drowsiness, both obviously undesirable and of particular concern in pilots, navigators, stewardesses and space flight air crew. Such a medication may be in the offing if an initial report holds up under further investigation. It is of interest too, because of its very recent reporting, ancient origins, the unavailability of the source to most readers, and its apparent efficacy. This medication, called Pingangdan, was a secret prescription for the treatment of nausea and vomiting to the emperors and the court of the Qing dynasty of China (circa 200-100 BC). It has recently been "rediscovered" and investigated for use in air and space travel by Jing-shen Pei, Bo-lun Tong and associates in China and was reported at the 62nd Annual Scientific Meeting of the Aerospace

Medical Association (abstract 99) May 5-9, 1991 in Cincinnati, Ohio. This paper has since been published.[31a] The principle active ingredients of Pingandan are reported to be Rhizoma Atractalodis, Pericarpium Citri Reticulatae, Fructus Amomi Rotundus Crataegi and Lignum Aguilariae Resinatum. The medication was compared with scopolamine hydrobromide 1 mg, Dramamine[R] 25 mg, and placebo in cats. Both slow and fast components of nystagmus were suppressed by scopolamine and Pingandan to a greater degree than other agents and the latter was nearly as efficacious as scopolamine. Pingandan resulted in less symptoms than all other agents in alluding to human experiments (unreported in detail). The authors state that the side effects of Pingandan in experiments in humans were few. In comparing it with a scopolamine/dextroamphetamine mixture, dry mouth was a side effect in 9% and 20% of subjects, respectively. Perhaps there is promise in one or a combination of these biologic constituents of Pingandan.

CHEMICAL OR TOXIN ILLNESSES BY INGESTION

Illness secondary to the ingestion of foodstuffs and water can be divided into four types: *bacterial, parasitic, viral* and *chemical.* Infectious diseases are considered in Chapter 57, and the reader is referred to other common available sources on the subject of food poisoning of infectious nature. Those caused by the chemical agents (see box above) will be discussed here for several reasons. First, among all "food poisonings," the illnesses caused by the toxins are least likely to be associated to the ingestion of food as these chemicals produce symptoms that are not predominately gastrointestinal. Schatz[33a], in a paper entitled "Ciguatera Fish Poisoning, A Jet Age Peril," writes a very thorough discussion of the subject and introduces the description of the poisoning by describing a case in a physician seen by a number of specialists in whom the diagnosis remained unsuspected until some weeks after the exposure. This emphasizes how easily the true nature of the illness may be missed even in the most knowledgeable of persons. Second, these illnesses are not rare by any means, even in the United States, and are both common and endemic in certain areas often visited by tourists who may suffer an exposure and incidence of illness similar to the resident population, particularly in the South Pacific. Finally, with increased travel, there is increased exposure that may produce symptoms *in situ,* in transit, or even after arrival at a secondary destination or return. In similar fashion, the speed of travel by air has provided a way to transport the source to the individual, predominately fish flown in to inland sites. Exposure to fish-borne toxins are no longer confined to coastal areas but must be suspected usually by a primary care or emergency physician in patients seen in the interior.

In the years between 1973 and 1987, there were 7458

Food-borne diseases due to toxic chemicals of noninfectious origin

Scromboid (histamine) fish poisoning
Ciguatera fish poisoning
Paralytic shellfish poisoning
Neurotoxic shellfish poisoning
"Chinese restaurant syndrome"—monosodium glutamate ingestion
Mushroom poisoning
Heavy metals
Miscellaneous toxins in vegetables and grains

---

outbreaks of food-borne disease reported in the United States to the CDC.[1a] They were caused by a bacterial agent 66% of the time and chemical agents 25% of the time, with 5% due to virus and 5% to protozoa and parasites. Of all cases in these outbreaks, 87% were due to bacteria and 4% to chemical agents, with scromboid fish poisoning (1216 cases) and ciguatera (1052 cases) by far the most common. As has been noted, in individual cases where the symptomatology is misleading as to the food source, under reporting must be a factor taken into account in estimating occurrences. In addition, the chemical group of food poisonings will be far more common in those endemic regions of the Pacific and the West Indies or Japan.

Those toxic disorders to be considered here are scromboid fish poisoning, ciguatera, paralytic and neurotoxic shellfish poisoning, ergot poisoning, monosodium glutamate, heavy metals, mushroom poisoning, and miscellaneous toxins found in vegetables and grains (see box above).

Because of the emphasis in this text on risk during travel and that they are the most common, the first four will be discussed in more detail.

Scromboid fish poisoning

Scromboid fish poisoning usually results from the ingestion of "spoiled" fish of two families, *Scrombidae* and *Scromberesocidae,* which includes the tuna, mackerel, skipjack and bonito.[28b] However, other fish, such as the mahi-mahi, bluefish, amberjack, herring, sardines, and anchovies (as well as cheese) have been cited as transmitters.[36a] The toxic agent is almost surely histamine as recently shown by Morrow and co-workers[28b] who showed that not only is histidine content high in scromboid fish, but in spoiled fish causing poisoning, the histamine content is high as well, and histamine and N-methyl-histamine excretion by the patients studied also was high (up to 20 times the norm) compatible with the ingestion of toxic amounts of histamine. If these species of fish are allowed to stand at room temperature for any significant time, the histidine can be decarboxylated to form histamine by enteric bacteria present in the fish. The ingested histamine-laden fish either cause the direct absorption of histamine through the gut (previously thought not possible) or some substances in the fish lead to pharmacologic enhancement of the histamine, facilitate its absorption, or inhibit its inactivation allowing absorption. The symptoms produced are those of histamine itself, which has given rise to the synonym "histamine fish poisoning." The symptoms, in terms of dominance, will vary by degree from case to case but always seem to include intense flushing and heat especially in the blush area, as well as some degree of headache, sweating, palpitations, hives, dizziness, bronchospasm, nasal stuffiness, and some gastrointestinal symptoms of diarrhea and nausea possibly with emesis. Hypotension and a feeling of decreased mental acuity can occur as well. These symptoms probably are not only dose dependent, but perhaps, as with the atopic person, vary with target organ predisposition. Time of onset probably varies with several factors including dose. Generally it is an hour or more but can be quite prompt. The symptoms persist in some cases as long as 12 or more hours but are generally less. Ingested fish may be described as having tasted spicy or peppery but this could be attributed to condiments; generally no difference in taste in noted. The relationship of the illness to histamine has always been highly suspected because of the symptoms and that the administration of antihistamines, corticoids, and adrenaline, as with allergies, often brought prompt relief.

The ultimate prevention is twofold, namely the avoidance of all fish of the species known to be high in histidine and/or proper handling of these (and all) fish from the time of catching to consumption. This makes refrigeration or freezing to the time of cooking mandatory. Unfortunately, there is no way to know that proper handling has been followed; even though the restaurant at which the meal is taken has an impeccable reputation and follows correct procedure, the history of the fish before purchase is unknown. Certainly once bitten, twice wary. In the United States, Hawaii and California are cited as areas of higher incidence,[21b] but wherever the species are served, there is a risk and it is a year-round possibility. Once the scrombotoxin is produced, cooking does not cause risk or dose reduction as the responsible element(s) are heat stable.

Ciguatera poisoning

In a review article on food poisoning from fish and shellfish, it is stated that the most commonly reported fishborne illness worldwide is ciguatera fish poisoning.[13a] Morgan and Fenwick[28a] state that the toxin can be found in as many as 400 different species of fish from 60 different families. The common denominator among the affected fish is that they are usually large reef predators native to tropical subtropical waters. This belt circles the globe between 35 degrees south latitude and 35 degrees north latitude and is considered endemic in most of the Caribbean basin and the tropical islands of the South Pacific. In the states, reefs are found in Hawaii and Florida, and it is here that the concentration of U.S. cases are found.[25a] The season for the disease is said to be May through September; however, cases are known to occur year round in areas such as the Caribbean. The ciguatera toxins are produced by the dinoflagellate gambiediscus toxicus, a photosynthetic species that attaches to epiphytic microalgae and enters the food chain via their consumption by herbivores and scavenger fish about reefs where the algae are found.[33a] These heat-stable fat-soluble toxins are then passed on to the large carnivore population feeding about the reefs where fish life is highly concentrated.[28a] Ruff[32a] has closely studied the incidence of ciguatera in Micronesia, Melanesia, and Polynesia and found a dramatic incidence in disease with any human disturbance of the reef in building docks, dredging, shelling, missile and atomic bomb testing. The disease had not occured at Hao atoll until 1966 when the French converted it to a nuclear testing base. The disease then spread to nearby undisturbed atolls over 2 years. From 1966 to 1968 herbivores became toxic, followed by the reef feeding carnivores. By mid-1968 43% of the population was affected; only after 10 years did the toxicity in herbivorous fish after the initial reef disturbance occurred begin to fall. This disturbance of the ecology of the reef dispersing the dinoflagellate G. toxicus into the waters may occur from natural forces such as hurricanes, storms, and earthquakes. Ruff cites many other episodes, but the Hao story alone clearly demonstrates the relation to reef trauma and the biologic chain culminating in human disease. Cases are underreported, but still the incidence in some areas is staggering, as his citation of 22,700 cases/100,000 pop. in the Gambier Archipeligo (1960 to 1984).

Despite the noted variation of the species involved, it appears that, of those identified in most cases, red snapper, amberjack, barracuda, Hawaiian snapper (mahimahi), jackfish, surgeon fish, mullet and grouper predominate.

The symptoms usually develop about 6 hours after ingestion and are ushered in by gastrointestinal complaints of nausea, emesis, diarrhea and abdominal cramps that may not be extreme. Shortly thereafter (several hours), neurologic symptoms appear and are variable in type but include paresthesias of the digits and face with increased sensitivity of touch, reversal of heat and cold sensation, even stupor and coma.[33a] Weakness and psychologic disturbances occur as well. Mild poisoning may be associated with myocardial irritability, and in more severe cases, frank arrhythmia can occur, often involving various blocks and bradycardia. Postural hypotension has been described (Geller and Benowitz) and shock can occur. Lange et al.[25a] reviewed 23 cases and also reports the occurrence of myalgia, arthralgia, headache, dental pain, and pruritus in these cases, with an indication there is an increase in symptoms with alcohol use and sexual intercourse, also noting that chronic symptoms may persist. Relief of severe symptoms occurred in 45 percent of their cases in 2 weeks. Hughes and Tauxe[21b] describe the acute illness as a few days to a few months, with pain in the extremities occurring intermittently for a few years in some. Second attacks may be more severe and sensitization may occur such that symptoms are recalled by ingestion of nontoxic fish, alcohol, and other foods and illness.[32a]

Since the toxins (ciguatoxin, maitotoxin, palytoxin) of ciguatera are heat stable and tasteless, cooking is not a preventive step nor is recognition of affected fish by taste or smell. The avoidance of ingestion of affected fish, notably the commonly affected and served barracuda, mahi-mahi and other snappers, amberjack and grouper is a logical step. When on site, natives may know of "safe reefs" where fish may be taken,[33a] if one cannot resist fresh fish. For the fish industry, testing before marketing would be the ultimate answer to certify safe fish of these species. Such a test based on immunologic assay has been developed and tested at the University of Hawaii[19a] and could be in commercial use.

Paralytic shell fish poisoning (PSP): neurotoxic shellfish poisoning (NSP)

Several neurotoxins that cause PSP and NSP originate in dinoflagellates and plankton, some of which have the characteristic of producing toxic substances. Evidence of the presence of these tiny water organisms is the well-known "red tide" that is a visible expression of a massive population growth, which may occur under ideal conditions of sunlight, nutrients, temperature and water currents. The "tides" or "blooms" may not be red necessarily nor should it be assumed that all red tides are necessarily harmful in any of their characteristics.[14a] When these marine organisms are of the type that produce the neurotoxins under consideration if they are ingested by bivalve mollusks such as scallops, mussels, clams or oysters, the host mollusk is not harmed but will harbor the poison that, on ingestion by humans, will produce the symptoms of PSP and NSP. NSP differs from PSP in that the particular toxin involved does not produce respiratory paralysis but is otherwise symptomatically similar. In these milder forms, the illness may last a few hours to several days only.[21b] These symptoms may be both of the central and peripheral nervous systems, initial symptoms appearing in 30 to 60 minutes (although this varies in outbreaks and individuals) generally of peripheral paresthesias—tingling and numbness. There may be muscular incoordination and even respiratory paralysis in 12 to 24 hours and death.[28a] Perl et al.[31b] describe a bloom off Prince Edward Island in Canada in 1987 that caused mussels harvested at that time to produce an unusual epidemic of gastrointestinal and respiratory symptoms associated with encephalopathy. In this case the toxin was found to be the amino acid *domoic*

acid. Subsequent to this outbreak, harvest of clams have been tested for the presence of domoic acid before marketing.

These toxins also are heat stable and undestroyed by cooking and the distribution is worldwide from 30° north latitude to 30° south latitude. The season of high incidence in the United States is May to November and primary sites are New England and the West Coast, but there are other seasons and times of incidence at other global locations.

As with ciguatera and scromboid, the preventive steps a traveller may take are to avoid eating these sea foods. The ultimate preventive measure is to screen the product at the source as was done in the case of the Prince Edward Island mussels. These preventive steps, of course, cannot be taken without the accumulation and documentation of cases as well as outbreaks and underlines the importance of all physicians reporting them to the CDC. Some states, such as California, place a quarantine on the harvesting of potentially offending mollusks at the time of year when plankton blooms are likely to appear.

Other toxins

There are many other toxins, some of which will be briefly discussed here with the notation that they individually, and as a group, are less likely to be encountered in travels than those four already addressed. Of this miscellaneous group, perhaps the one most commonly experienced is the infamous "Chinese restaurant syndrome," which is caused by exposure to foods with a high monosodium-L-glutamate content and is expressed by headache, flushing, diarrhea with nausea and cramps. It resolves in a few hours. The prevention of symptoms is avoidance of the exposure; this product is found in breads and, of course, restaurants other than Chinese. Questioning restaurant personnel may help.

There is one toxin, found in the pufferfish locally called *Fugu* in Japan.[13a] Exposure in the Japanese islands is notorious but the geographic location is practically isolated to this group. The symptoms are basically those of PSP and the preventive measure—avoid Fugu!

Mushroom poisoning,[21b] of course, can occur anywhere. There are five or more syndromes that may follow ingestion: symptoms of alcoholic intoxication, those of parasympathetic overactivity, acute psychotic reactions (including hallucinations), symptoms of disulfiram reaction, acute gastroenteric reaction only, and finally, a syndrome of bradycardia, miosis, and bronchospasm. The clinical expression is determined by the particular toxin in that mushroom species. The safeguard is to stick to those mushrooms that are commercially marketed as safe, if a sophisticated "mushroom picker" to harvest only those you are confident of, and if overseas, depend on the "starred" restaurants and avoid local uncertain picking even though you feel yourself to be sophisticated in that art. The symptoms are generally over in 24 hours, at the most 48 hours.

Nausea, vomiting, and cramps subsiding in 2 to 3 hours after emesis, with rapid onset of 5 to 15 minutes, is experienced from the acute gastric irritation of the heavy metals copper, zinc, tin, and cadmium.[21b] Approximately 16% to 17% of cases of chemical poisoning are from heavy metals.[1a] These exposures are likely to be encountered when a liquid such as juice is dispensed through a dispenser of corroded metal parts where the beverage has stood some time. The answer is to stick to licensed canned beverages or avoid poorly maintained or older dispensing units of questionable origin.

There is a host of toxins associated with produce, plant toxicants and grains,[28a] none of which are likely to be encountered in usual travel. Some are the cause of historic pandemics such as the gangrenous ergotism that occurred in Russia after the war from the fungal growth on poorly stored or old grains. Such outbreaks are known to have occurred as far back as the ninth and tenth centuries. Potatoes contain glycoalkoloids that at times can be present in toxic levels. This is most likely to occur in green potatoes, and the toxin is concentrated in the skin. Peeled potatoes adequately cooked are likely safe. The illness produced has symptoms such as apathy, restlessness, drowsiness, and visual symptoms. Cassava, common as a staple in South America, Southeast Asia and Africa, is rich in cyanogenic glycosides that yield hydrogen cyanide on hydrolysis. Symptoms of acute poisoning are dyspnea, paralysis, coma, and death. Lower doses produce optic, auditory, and peripheral nerve lesions. For travellers, the practical preventive is "don't go native." Cyanogenic glycosides are also contained in some legumes and this has led to a ban in the importation and cultivation of some species of lima beans in the United States. Overseas, some severe cases are reported from apple seeds, bitter almonds and peach pits (laetrile). Thiocyanates can be found as a breakdown product in cruciferous vegetables (e.g., cabbage and brussel sprouts). *Jamaican vomiting sickness,* a syndrome of vomiting, somnolence, muscular weakness, and even coma and death, is caused by breakdown products of two hypoglycins in the unripe fruit ackee in which they are contained. Onset is from 4 to 10 hours. Another staple, fava beans, used heavily in North Africa, and the Middle and Far East, can be hazardous to those persons with glucose-6-phosphate dehydrogenase deficiency. Initial symptoms of "favism" are headache, back pain, nausea with emesis and fever. Blood in the urine occurs in 5 to 30 hours, with jaundice thereafter and (in some cases) death in 48 hours. Nonfatal cases will cause illness for 5 to 7 days.

Prevention. To review, prevention of these toxic diseases can occur in a number of ways at different levels. First, the well-informed person can avoid eating those foods that offer a chance of disease in preference for substitutes, as in fish. Second, prevention can occur at the producer's level in many cases such as the cited seasonal harvesting by law of sea food products in California and the assaying of muscles for demoic acid in Nova Scotia. Third, preparation has some role such as choice of potatoes and skinning of same. In the traveller's case, the knowledge of risk and avoidance of such foods is probably the option on which to rely.

Other conditions

Other preexisting conditions listed in Table 65-2 should be addressed. In addition to these, Shesser has addressed scuba diving.[35] After a dive that requires no stopping for decompression, a diver can fly after 6 to 12 hours on the surface. The risk is in going from a hyperbaric environment to a hypobaric environment, in which case the increased amount of nitrogen dissolved in the tissues may form N_2 gas bubbles.

Ikeda et al.[21c] found that bubbles in the bloodstream may first be seen at about a dive to a depth of 19 feet (6 m) after surfacing. At 26 feet (8 m) symptomatic decompression sickness will occur, requiring recompression. The traveler would be wise to confine dives to a maximum of 18 feet on the basis of this study.

PROBLEMS ASSOCIATED WITH ALTITUDE

The ills discussed in this section, although all caused by altitude, do not directly relate to flight, but to those people who are acclimated to a lower altitude and ascend to altitudes of 8000 feet or more above sea level on vacation or for temporary residence. With an increasingly mobile population and the growing popularity of sports such as skiing, mountain climbing, and camping, the number of people at risk and symptomatic has increased greatly over the last 4 decades. Chronic mountain sickness, or Monge's disease, will be considered not as a part of the travel experience, but as a hazard of living at high altitude.

Acute mountain sickness

Some authors have applied this term to all the syndromes of altitude. The syndromes might never exist in a pure form but present with a dominant feature that typifies them. Their common physiologic feature is the extravasation of fluid into the tissue spaces from the vascular compartment. For the purposes of this discussion, these syndromes will be called respectively:

1. Acute mountain sickness (AMS), or "Saroche," a mild constellation of symptoms that seems not to correlate well with the degree of hypoxia, thus altitude
2. High altitude peripheral edema, more likely to occur in warm weather
3. High altitude cerebral edema (HACE)
4. High altitude pulmonary edema (HAPE), most likely to occur in cold weather.

The last three occur generally at altitudes of 8000 feet above sea level or higher.

A mild form of AMS may be mimicked by psychologic or transient factors. Many of the tourists who ascend Pike's Peak to 14,000 feet by auto or cog railway also suffer similar symptoms that may be a little of both AMS and psychological factors. Breathlessness, giddiness, and nausea seem to be common psychological reactions to heights and are symptoms found in true AMS as well. When a patient is susceptible, the prevention is simply enjoying the mountain from base level.

All of us practicing at an altitude of less than 1000 feet above sea level have seen patients that have had syncope associated with hyperventilation with or without the sensation of dyspnea. The hyperventilation may or may not have been precipitated by an emotional event. At altitude, the sea level resident may experience lightheadedness or syncope, and when associated with dyspnea, it might be on the basis of either relative (to sea level saturation) hypoxia or the psychologic experience of being at altitude, or both. Thus it is often difficult to determine in any one individual having one or two of the symptoms of AMS, whether these symptoms are truly altitude related, might have occurred at sea level in the same circumstance, or are a psychologic phenomenon of altitude or an effect of travel per se. I think most physicians would agree that if there are three of the five symptoms of AMS present, it is likely that this diagnosis is a true one.

A recent study done by Nicholas, O'Meara and Calonge[30] from the Colorado Altitude Research Center sheds light on this gray area, at least regarding syncope and near syncope experienced at an intermediate altitude (2770 m). Their study of persons presenting with this symptom was divided into three groups: (1) the natives of the area; (2) Colorado natives of a lower resident altitude; and (3) persons who resided at near sea level. They found that the incidence in this group of persons who had no reason for the syncope (it was not cardiac, vasovagal or of obvious neurologic origin) was 65% of area residents with the syndrome, 88% of the Colorado residents of lower altitude and 98% of those persons of low altitude residence. Likewise, the oxygen saturation of each group was highest in the resident group (97%) and 93% and 92% in the low Colorado and near sea level groups, respectively. As might be expected, the resident group had a correspondingly higher hematocrit. At 18 to 24 months after the event, 34% of the sea level group was contacted and in no case was there a recurrence or any subsequent cardiovascular event. This suggests an excellent prognosis in contrast to those who have syncope due to an identifiable cause who may experience a fatal event (20% to 30% of those due to cardiac cause may die within one year usually due to sudden death). The authors propose the name of "high altitude syncope" for this syndrome as the evidence supports its common occurrence in recent arrivals to moderate altitude, the number of persons with "unidentifiable cause of syncope" far exceeds the occurrence in residents, and there is a correlation of syncope with a decrease in saturation of the blood with oxygen. The mechanism is not known but the authors conjecture on the possibilities of a reflex bradycardia or hyperventilation with secondary hypocapnia and reflex cerebral vasoconstriction. It would seem appropriate to identify this syndrome with a name to assist in delineating a specific group of syncopal patients of good prognosis.

Montgomery et al.[28] suggest that AMS might be fairly common and occur at even more moderate altitudes, as in skiing from base facilities of approximately 2000 m (6560 feet), for they found in a retrospective poll by questionnaire that one of four or five of 454 individuals experienced at least moderate symptoms of AMS, namely headache, insomnia, dyspnea, anorexia, and fatigue. All symptoms occurred in the first 72 hours and were brief. Symptoms were most likely to occur in those who ascended from sea level rather than from a higher altitude, suggesting that the latter group was partially acclimatized and that the higher the absolute ascent, the more prone the individual.

Maggiorini et al.[27] conducted a study in the Alps to determine the prevalence of AMS (the authors include all manifestations of high altitude under the umbrella of AMS) among healthy hikers at various higher altitudes. Their method was to question all hikers who participated for symptoms (headache, anorexia or nausea, vomiting, dizziness, shortness of breath, and insomnia). The subjects were also physically examined for vital signs; periorbital, hand, and pedal edema; pulmonary rales; and ataxia. By use of an established scoring system, subjects were judged free of symptoms (zero), showing some effect of altitude (one to two points), or suffering from AMS (three or more points). The study was conducted at four hiking huts at increasing altitude. The results were: (1) at 2850 m (9350 feet), 9%, or 4 of 47 subjects, had AMS, and 18 showed some effect of altitude; (2) at 3050 m (10,000 feet), 13%, or 16 of 128 subjects, had AMS, and 47 showed some effect; (3) at 3650 m (12,000 feet), 34%, or 28 of 82 subjects, had AMS, and 33 had some effect; and (4) at 4559 m (15,000 feet), 53%, or 110 of 209 subjects, had AMS, and 39 had some effects. Mild AMS, high-altitude cerebral edema, and the feeling of the effects of altitude all increased with increased elevation. Periorbital and peripheral edema appeared at relatively lower altitude but also increased with altitude. Pronounced pulmonary rales were heard in five (2%) at 10,000 feet and 12,000 feet and in eight (4%) at 15,000 feet. There is general agreement that exertion at altitude predisposes to both AMS and HAPE as well as the other syndromes of altitude, and the climbers certainly would be meeting the definition of considerable exertion at these altitudes.

One would not expect as high an incidence at 8000 feet, or in skiers who start from a base of 6000 to 8500 feet and ski from as high as 12,500 feet or in people who are relatively passive in reaching and being at these higher altitudes.

Dr. Ben Honigman of the University of Colorado Health Sciences Center in Denver states in a personal communication that of 3900 individuals studied by their team, 25% suffered from AMS in travelling to altitudes between 7000 and 10,000 feet. Individual symptoms of the syndrome occurred more frequently with headache as the most common single symptom being experienced by 60% of participants. Honigman feels that, generally, data are soft as to whether or not a stopover at an intermediate altitude will prevent AMS or not, but the study did show that persons staying in Denver 2 or more days had a lower incidence even though the ultimate destination was of moderate elevation. Of the nearly 100 patients who had prior HAPE, only 10% suffered a recurrence. This figure is lower than that shown in other studies; however, one must always take into account the elevation achieved (e.g., under or over 10,000 feet). This recently completed series of observations has just been submitted for publication.

Nonetheless, the three studies cited, as do others, suggest that in any one patient going for vacation to altitudes of 8000 feet or higher, there is a fairly good chance they will at least suffer some symptoms of AMS if not AMS per se.

In addition to exercise at altitude, predisposing factors are rapid ascent without acclimation, the absolute amount of ascent, and history of prior episodes. Although ensuring adequate fluid intake is appropriate, avoidance of alcohol appears helpful in preventing symptoms, and therefore alcohol must be considered predisposing. The young generally are considered most susceptible, and those at or above early middle age are less susceptible. On the other hand, Maggiorini et al.[27] demonstrated an increased incidence of AMS in those under age 20 but also in those age 41 and older. Gender is not a predisposing factor, with male and female at equal risk. Physical fitness per se does not prevent illness at altitude.

HAPE

HAPE is the more common and better known of the serious effects of high altitude. It occurs with relative frequency, even at altitudes often visited by travellers, such as the ski resorts in the Rockies with bases of 8000 feet. It *can* be fatal. This syndrome of noncardiac pulmonary edema may also occur subtly so that the early symptoms (e.g., a dry, nonproductive, hacky cough) do not alert the victim to the potential seriousness of the situation. In addition, as Maggiorini et al. noted in their study of climbers, HAPE may occur early (as detected by significant pulmonary rales) without other symptoms. As treatment is mandatory at the earliest possible time in the development of

HAPE, the physician advising a patient about a trip that involves ascent should educate him or her about the symptoms of the malady and the necessity to seek medical aid early. The keystones of treatment are (1) descent to lower altitude and (2) supplemental oxygen, with or without pressure. Where the patient might be hiking or camping in high mountains isolated from medical aid, the patient must be advised that, with the first symptoms of HAPE, he or she should move to a lower altitude with the least expenditure of energy possible, then seek medical help as soon as possible. Even descending several hundred meters is helpful. Other treatments of this condition are mainly dexamethasone and nifedipine.

HACE

HACE also can be fatal and should not be ignored. The cardinal early symptom of *severe* headache that cannot be relieved must be considered indicative of this problem and must lead to appropriate treatment. Severe headache associated with ataxia makes the diagnosis certain. As with HAPE, the keystones of treatment are descent and oxygen. The same predispositions and preventive measures apply.

HARH

High altitude retinal hemorrhage (HARH) is a syndrome of altitude that is rarely recognized without fundoscopic examination, as it is usually without symptoms unless the macular hemorrhage occurs. When HARH is present, one might suspect coexistent HACE. The predisposing factors are the same as for the other syndromes described. Jacobson[22] states that it occurs in 50% of subjects ascending to 16,500 feet and almost 100% of those above 21,000 feet. Prevention is much the same as with the other syndromes. and is perhaps less certain.

Prevention of altitude illness

Of the nonpharmacologic preventive measures, the most reliable seems to be acclimation. For example, one might plan a pleasant stay at an intermediate point (preferably at least 2 days) before proceeding to a high altitude. If one drives to a ski resort, slow acclimation is fairly well assured. Oelz[31] suggests a 2- to 4-day sojourn at 4900 to 8200 feet before ascending, and that the rate of ascent above 10,000 feet be limited to 1000 feet per 24 hours.

Houston[21] in an article on trekking at high altitude suggests the following preventive measures:

1. Gradual ascent, taking 1 day for each 2000 feet above 5,000 feet
2. Acetazolamide, 250 mg twice a day (or an alternative dosage of 125 mg twice a day beginning a day before and continuing through the first day at altitude)
3. Additional fluid intake (not alcoholic) and only gradual increase in effort the first few days at altitude

4. Avoidance of sedatives that depress respiration in sleep, also noting that anticoagulants may convert minor trauma to major trauma and birth control pills may increase thrombotic illness.

Coote[5] gives a good review of the physiological changes that cause these syndromes. He too suggests acetazolamide in similar dosage. He compares the use of dexamethasone and its pharmacologic action but advises that, with a dose of 4 mg each 6 hours, the side effects and its lack of effect on respiratory control make it an inferior choice. Spironolactone has been shown to be effective as well, but it is active in prophylaxis only in the presence of aldosterone, which is reduced by hypoxia. Coote discusses progesterone as an agent that apparently stimulates ventilation centrally rather than through any effect on the peripheral chemoreceptors. Furosemide as a powerful diuretic will draw fluid from the lungs, but the resultant hypovolemia must be watched. Finally, he suggests nifedipine might be useful, as it reduces pulmonary hypertension.

The evolution of HAPE, a noncardiac pulmonary edema, starts with pulmonary hypertension, a response to altitude and hypoxia. (This is somewhat simplified, and the reader is referred to Resources at the end of this chapter to further understand the physiologic changes that occur at altitude.) With the hypothesis that reducing the increase in pulmonary arterial pressure could prevent HAPE, Bartsch et al.[1] studied mountaineers with a history of radiographically documented HAPE. A group of 21 received either placebo (11) or nifedipine (10), with both patient and doctor blinded. The diagnosis of HAPE was based on radiography. The group was taken to 4559 m (14,953 feet) from low altitude (490 m) and remained there 3 days. Seven of 11 who received placebo developed HAPE, but only one of 10 who received nifedipine did. The treated group also demonstrated a lower mean systolic pulmonary artery pressure, alveolar-arterial pressure gradient, and symptom score of AMS. Their conclusion was that nifedipine was effective in preventing HAPE in susceptible subjects and that the rise in pulmonary artery pressure has an important role in its development.

Reeves and Schoene,[32] both of whom have spent much time in remote mountain laboratories in the study of altitude sickness, wrote a commentary on this article in the same journal and issue with the intriguing title of "When Lungs on Mountains Leak." They discuss in some detail the physiology or pathophysiology of HAPE and the effect of nifedipine, especially as shown in the article. Not only does pulmonary artery pressure increase, but pulmonary membrane permeability and inflammation also increase. They suggest that there appear to be factors other than pulmonary hypertension alone that cause HAPE (cases of HAPE have been described without pulmonary hypertension) and that, "If an increase in neither pressure nor permeability can account for all the findings, it is probably because pressure and permeability are mutually reinforc-ing." They suggest that nifedipine "not only lowered pressure but may also have acted to decrease permeability by blunting an inflammatory response" (via its effect on calcium). Despite its side effects of possible hypotension, headache, nausea, vomiting, dizziness, fatigue, and leg edema (paradoxically, all symptoms seen in AMS), taking the medicine in advance of ascent is appropriate in people known to be susceptible to HAPE. Once HAPE is experienced, there is about a 60% chance (this figures varies between studies) of a recurrence, a statistic that justifies the use of nifedipine. It appears to be a good preventive agent in this group of people, who often are in a situation in which rapid descent is limited and oxygen is unavailable.

Environment and temperature

Extremes of heat and cold, as might be experienced in the tropics or at altitude, have their own effects on the body's physiology and must be considered when advising a patient about travel at these extremes. The individual's health must be evaluated to determine whether he or she is fit to endure short or intermediate stays in a hostile environment, and whether under favorable conditions (e.g., good transport, air conditioned housing, accessible medical care) or unfavorable conditions (e.g., remote areas, unalleviated environmental conditions, poor infrastructure as in third world countries). Problems can occur even in the young, healthy individual (e.g., heat stroke), and thus all must be aware of the potential risks and be prepared. The spectrum of patients is infinite and advice must be tailored to each case; thus the physician practicing prevention must consider the patient's unique health status and the proposed exposure (see Resources at the end of this chapter).

A PRETRAVEL CHECKLIST

The traveller and the physician may use this checklist to evaluate the traveller's preparation.

1. Visit your physician for pretravel consultation, including immunizations needed, medications currently being taken, and medications that might be carried to meet contingencies.
2. Visit your dentist. Is there a problem that might "worsen" during travel?
3. Carry an extra pair of glasses.
4. Check your charge cards. Do these companies have overseas offices that can help in financial, travel, and medical emergencies? Where are they in relation to your itinerary?
5. Carry health identification prominently if you suffer from a preexisting illness (e.g., diabetes, epilepsy) and carry a current history and physical summary, for reference by a consulting doctor.
6. If you are taking medication carry two supplies if possible, in case one is lost carry a complete set in carry-on luggage.

7. Are you allergic? Again, health identification should make this easily obvious to an examiner.

8. Are there embassies or consuls on your route that could be consulted if need be?

9. If you need medical help, the following resources can be indexed:
   1. Your hotel or travel agent representative
   2. Telephone directory
   3. Local U.S. corporation medical departments or executive offices for referral
   4. Red Cross or Traveller's Aid Societies
   5. Mission stations
   6. An airport authority
   7. Local hospital
   8. A "hot line" for aid at home

10. Review chemical toxins in foods that might be found in an area the patient is to visit.

Check with a large local medical facility near your home. For example, our clinic has a staff member who can often advise travellers about competent local or regional care, and arrange medical air transport by a proven carrier should transportation home be necessary for hospital care.

SUMMARY

All the health risks of travel cannot be covered in one chapter. This chapter has highlighted the common and less-known risks, not including infectious diseases, to emphasize the environmental and physical risks in travel.

REFERENCES

1. Bartsch P et al: Prevention of high altitude pulmonary edema by nifedipine, *N Engl J Med* 325(18):1284, 1991.
1a. Bean NH, Griffin PM: Food-borne disease outbreaks in the United States, 1973-1987: pathogens, vehicles and trends, *J Food Prot* 53:801-817, 1990.
2. Bradley DJ: The scope of travel medicine: an introduction to the conference on international travel medicine. In Steffen R et al, editors: *Travel medicine,* New York, 1989, Springer Verlag.
3. Burki U: Economy class syndrome, *Schweiz Med Wschr* 119(9):287, 1989.
4. Carruthers M, Arguelles AE, and Mosovich A: Biochemical and physiological changes during intercontinental flights, *Lancet* 1:977, 1976.
5. Coote JH: Pharmacological control of altitude sickness, *Trends Pharmacol Sci* 12(12):450, 1991.
6. Cotrell JJ: Altitude exposure during aircraft flight: flying higher, *Chest* 92:81, 1988.
7. Cruickshank JM, Gorlin R, and Jennett B: Air travel and thrombotic episodes: the economy class syndrome, *Lancet* 2(8609):497, 1988.
8. Cummins RO et al: In-flight deaths during commercial air travel, *JAMA* 259(13):1983, 1988.
9. Cummins RO, Schubach JA: Frequency and types of medical emergencies among commercial air travellers, *JAMA* 261(9):1295, 1989.
10. Dan BB: The accidental tourist: medical emergencies in the air, *JAMA* 261(9):1328, 1989.
11. Dawson S, Thompson L: Panel: current concerns in passenger health, Aerospace Medical Association Meeting, Cincinnati, Ohio, May 8, 1991 (as recorded by Audiotranscripts, Ltd, no 37-633-91).
12. Dillard TA et al: Hypoxia during air travel in cases with chronic obstructive pulmonary disease, *Ann Intern Med* 111(5):362, 1989.
13. Dunn RL, Matzen RN, and Vanderbrug-Mendendorf S: Screening for the detection of coronary artery disease by using the exercise tolerance test in a preventive medicine population, *Am J Prev Med* 7(5):255, 1991.
13a. Eastaugh J, Shepherd S: Infectious and toxic syndromes from fish and shellfish consumption, a review, *Arch Int Med* 149:1735-1740, 1989.
14. Ernst E: Air travel, DVTs and pulmonary embolism (letter), *N Z Med J* 104(912):213, 1991.
14a. Garrison DL: Red tide. World Book Encyclopedia 16:192-193, Chicago, 1989, World Book.
15. Gong H: Air travel and oxygen therapy in cardiopulmonary patients, *Chest* 101(4):1104, 1992.
16. Gong H et al: Hypoxia altitude simulation test, evaluation of patients with chronic airway obstruction, *Am Rev Respir Dis* 130:980, 1984.
17. Hargarten SW, Baker T, and Guptill K: Fatalities of American travellers—1975, 1984. In Steffen R et al, editors: *Travel medicine,* New York, 1989, Springer Verlag.
18. Hargarten SW, Baker T, and Guptill K: Injury deaths and American travellers. In Steffen R et al, editors: *Travel medicine,* New York, 1989, Springer Verlag.
19. Heber L: Mental stress as international hazard. In Steffen R et al, editors: *Travel medicine,* New York, 1989, Springer Verlag.
19a. Hokoma Y: A rapid simplified enzyme immunoassay stick test for the detection of ciguatoxin and related polyethers from fish tissues, *Toxicon* 23(6):939-946, 1985.
20. Homans J: Thrombosis of the deep leg veins due to prolonged sitting, *N Engl J Med* 250(4):148, 1954.
21. Houston CS: Trekking at high altitudes. How safe is it for your patients? *J Postgrad Med* 88(1):56, 1990.
21a. Hughes JM, Potter ME: Scromboid fish poisoning from pathogenesis to prevention, *N Engl J Med* 324:766-768, 1991.
21b. Hughes JM, Tauxe RV: Food-borne disease. In Mandell GL, Douglas G Jr, Bennett JE, editors: *Principles and practice of infectious diseases,* ed 3, New York, 1990, Churchil Livingstone.
21c. Ikeda T et al.: Bubble formation and decompression sickness on direct ascent from shallow air saturation diving, *Aviat Space and Environ Med* 64(2):121-125, 1993.
22. Jacobson ND: Acute high-altitude illness, *Am Fam Phys* 38(3):135, 1988.
23. Keller P, Koch K: World tourism: facts and figures. In Steffen R et al, editors: *Travel medicine,* New York, 1989, Springer Verlag.
24. Landgraf H et al: The economy class syndrome: studies during a 12 hour simulated flight in a Boeing 727 mockup, Abstract #120, Aerospace Medical Association Scientific Program, A21, May, 1991.
25. Landgraf H: Panel: current concerns in passenger health, Aerospace Medical Association Meeting, Cinncinnati, Ohio, May 8, 1991 (as recorded by Audiotranscripts, Ltd, no 37-633-91).
25a. Lange WR, Snyder FR, Fudala PJ: Travel and ciguatera fish poisoning, *Arch Intern Med* 152:2049-2053, 1992.
26. Lederman JA, Keshavarzian A: Acute pulmonary embolism following air travel, *Postgraduate Med J* 59:104, 1983.
27. Maggiorini M et al: Prevalence of acute mountain sickness in the swiss alps, *Br Med J* 301:835, 1990.
27a. Monreal M, Ruiz J, Olazabal A, et al.: Deep venous thrombosis and the risk of pulmonary embolism, *Chest* 102(3):677-681, 1993.
28. Montgomery AB, Mills J, and Luce JM: Incidence of mountain sickness at intermediate altitude, *JAMA* 261(5):732, 1989.
28a. Morgan MR, Fenwick GR: Natural foodborne toxicants, *Lancet* 336:1492-1495, 1990.
28b. Morrow JD et al.: Evidence that histamine is the causative toxin of scromboid-fish poisoning, *N Engl J Med* 324:716-720, 1991.
29. Moyses C: Economy class syndrome (letter), *Lancet* 2(8619):1077, 1988.
30. Nicholson R, O'Meara PD, Calonge N: Is syncope related to moderate altitude exposure, *JAMA* 268(7):904-906, 1992.

31. Oelz O: Prophylaxis and treatment of acute mountain sickness. In Steffen R, et al, editors: *Travel medicine,* New York, 1989, Springer Verlag.

31a. Pei J et al: Experimental research on anti-motion sickness effects of Chinese medicine "Pingandan" pills in cats, *So Chin Med J China* 105(4):322-327, 1992.

31b. Perl TM et al.: An outbreak of toxic encephalopathy caused by eating mussels contaminated with demoic acid, *New Engl J Med* 322(25):1775-1780, 1990.

31c. Pei J, Tong B, Chen K, Li C, and Zhang G. Experimental research on antimotion sickness effects of Chinese medicine "Pingandan" pills in cats, *Chin Med J* 105:322-327, 1992.

32. Reeves JT, Schoene RB: When lungs on mountains leak, *N Engl J Med* 325(18):1306, 1991.

32a. Ruff TA: Ciguatera in the Pacific: a link with military activities, *Lancet* 1:201, 1989.

33. Sarvesvaran R: Sudden natural deaths associated with commercial air travel, *Med Sci Law* 26(1):35-38, 1986.

33a. Schatz IJ: Ciguatera fish poisoning. A jet age peril, *Hosp Pract* 24:79-86, 1989.

34. Simpson K: Shelter deaths from pulmonary embolism, *Lancet* ii:744, 1940.

35. Shesser R: Medical aspects of commercial air travel, *Am J Emerg Med* 7(2):216, March, 1989.

36. Steffen R: Health risks for short-term travellers. In Steffen R et al, editors: *Travel medicine,* New York, 1989, Springer Verlag.

36a. Taylor SL, Stratton JE, Nordlee JA: Histamine poisoning (scromboid fish poisoning): an allergy-like intoxication. *J Clin Toxicol* 27(4,5):225-240, 1989.

37. Trubuhovich RV: Air travel, DVTs and pulmonary embolism, *N Z Med J* 104(908):126, 1991.

38. Virchow R as cited by Cruickshank JM, Gorlin R, and Jennett B: Air travel and thrombotic episodes: the economy class syndrome, *Lancet* 2(8609):497, 1988.

RESOURCES

Directory of preventive medicine residency programs in the United States and Canada, general preventive medicine, occupational medicine, public health, aerospace medicine. American College of Preventive Medicine, 1015 15th Street, NW, Washington, DC, 20005.

Health information for international travel. U.S. Department of Health and Human Services, Public Health Service, Centers for Disease Control, Center for Preventive Services, Atlanta, GA 30333. For sale by the superintendent of documents, US Government Printing Office, Washington, DC 20402. This document details infectious disease risks and pinpoints the distribution of such diseases. Details on required vaccinations are given.

International Association for Medical Assistance to Travellers (IAMAT), 736 Center Street, Lewiston, NY 14092. A list of English-speaking doctors in foreign countries is available through this office.

International travelers' handbook (revised edition). Department of Infectious Disease, The Cleveland Clinic Foundation, 9500 Euclid Avenue, Cleveland, OH 44195. A general pamphlet on travel risks other than infection.

Travel medicine, Steffen R et al, editors. 1989, Springer Verlag. A record of the presentations at the First Conference on International Travel Medicine, Zurich, Switzerland, April 5-8, 1988. A comprehensive reference covering most aspects of travel and health, both infectious and physical. Easy to read and use.

Tso E: High altitude illness, *Emerg Med Clin North Am* 10(2):231, 1992.

Vogel JHK, editor: *Advances in cardiology: hypoxia, high altitude and the heart,* vol 5, Basel, Switzerland, 1970, S. Karger AG. This volume records the presentations at the First Conference on Cardiovascular Disease at Snowmass-at-Aspen, Colorado, in January, 1970 shortly after the Olympic Games at Mexico City. Although dated, much of the data presented is not. These papers address not only the compensatory changes that occur at altitude, but also the pathophysiology (such as HAPE), and human performance at altitude. An excellent basic text from which to move forward to date.

Weil JV: Lessons from high altitude, *Chest* 97(3 suppl):70S, 1990. A fairly recent review of high-altitude physiology and adaptation to height, Med 227:1, 1988. An extremely readable, informative history of the study of the physiology of man at altitude. A classic account with many amusing anecdotes.

West JB: High points in the physiology of extreme altitude, *Adv Exp Med Biol* 227:1-15, 1988. A fascinating review of the history of man's attempts to climb ever higher from Jose de Costa, a Jesuit missionary in 16th century Peru, to the American Medical Research Expedition to Everest in 1981.

Chapter 66

THE PERFORMER

Richard J. Lederman
Harvey M. Tucker
L. Sunday Homitz

Performing artists represent a special and in some ways unique occupational group. Less than 0.1% of the population of the United States earn its living in the performing arts. However, this does not include the large number of performers-in-training and serious amateurs, all of whom are at risk for the development of health problems that may affect their ability to perform. Many of the problems that do arise are common to the general population, resulting from genetic and environmental factors common to all of us. Many of the ailments that afflict performers, however, can be considered performance-related, that is, arising as a direct result of the performing art itself. In this sense, they are true occupational disorders.

One of the unique features of the performing arts is that preparation for such a career most often begins in the first or early second decade of life. Thus a young adult performer may have been seriously pursuing his or her art for 15 or more years. Therefore efforts to design programs for prevention of performance-related injuries must of necessity begin at an early age, and parents and teachers, as well as health care providers, must be an integral part of a preventive medicine program.

All human beings face potential injury from daily activities and the environment, and we vary greatly in the attention we pay to avoiding or preventing these deleterious effects. Basic nutrition, a reasonable exercise program, annual physical examination, maintenance of immunizations, and wearing seatbelts are all examples of the types of activities that healthy individuals carry out in the interest of self-preservation and general well-being. The successful professional athlete usually spends a good deal of time in a planned program to maintain those special abilities that permit continued excellence and performance at the high level required by the particular sport. The performing artist is in many ways similar to the athlete and must actively strive to protect the equipment that provides his or her livelihood. As the violinist not only masters the use of his or her Stradivarius, but also cares for and protects it, so the professional voice user and the dancer must train their respective "instruments."

This chapter will, by necessity, present a restricted view of the performing arts community. We will focus on instrumental musicians, vocalists, and dancers. Although a more global view of the performing arts may rightfully include many other groups (e.g., actors), the information regarding performance-related problems and health care issues in these groups is so sparse as to make a fruitful discussion virtually impossible. One hopes that as the field of performing arts medicine, currently in its infancy, develops and expands, much more information will become available.

EPIDEMIOLOGY AND RISK FACTORS
Instrumentalists

Interest in the special health problems of instrumentalists has largely developed in the last 10 years, although earlier efforts can be identified.[29] Initial attempts to gather information regarding the prevalence of playing-related problems of musicians began to appear in the mid-1980s, and a sobering if not alarming pattern emerged. Some of the larger surveys are summarized in Table 66-1. Virtually all of these studies can be criticized for epidemiological and statistical inadequacies, but a brief perusal of the results shows a surprising consistency. Despite differences in populations surveyed as well as methods of survey, playing-related pain was identified in 40% to 65% of in-

Table 66-1. Surveys of playing-related problems in musicians

Author, year	Population studied	Number	Instrument(s)	Survey method	% with playing-related symptoms
Fry et al, 1988[13]	Secondary school	98	All	Questionnaire	56
Lockwood, 1988[18]	Secondary school	113	All	Questionnaire	49
Fry, 1987[12]	College/conservatory	116	All	Student report of problem	9.3
Grieco et al, 1989[15]	Conservatory	117	Piano	Questionnaire	62
Revak, 1989[23]	College/conservatory	71	Piano	Questionnaire	42
Caldron et al, 1986[7]	Conservatory	145	All	Questionnaire	59
	Professional	103	All		
Fry, 1986[11]	Professional	485	Orchestral	Interview	64
Fishbein et al, 1988[9]	Professional	2212	Orchestral	Questionnaire	76 (Overall)
					58 (Musculoskeletal)

strumental musicians, from secondary school students in their teens to major professional orchestra musicians, most in their fifth to seventh decades of life.

In our Medical Center for Performing Artists, 85% of instrumentalists seeking consultation for a playing-related problem report pain as the most prominent symptom. The average age of instrumentalists referred to our center is 32 years; this information, coupled with the prevalence studies listed in Table 66-1, suggest that patterns of playing-related pain are established relatively early.

Data regarding incidence of playing-related problems among instrumentalists are both more difficult to obtain and less readily available. Manchester reported an incidence rate of 8.5 episodes of performance-related hand problems per 100 performance majors per year at a major music conservatory.[19] In all of these studies, women are consistently more likely to be affected than men; keyboard and string players are at higher risk to develop playing-related pain than others; and the left upper extremity of string instrumentalists and the right arm/hand of keyboard players are particularly prone to be affected.

Many sources suggest that multiple risk factors contribute to the development of playing-related problems among instrumentalists. In the box at right, these are divided for convenience into two general categories, intrinsic and extrinsic. Intrinsic factors are those relating to anatomical and physiological characteristics of the instrumentalist, such as body habitus, level of conditioning, and presence of disease that may increase susceptibility. Extrinsic factors include various aspects of playing technique as well as the amount of playing. Despite some contrary views, no single technique of playing an instrument can be considered "proper" or correct. What is important medically is that the technique be suited to the individual performer and that it be ergonomically efficient and practical. Many observers have commented on the apparently unphysiologic position required to play certain instruments, such as the violin. While this observation may well be true, the most frequent contributors to the development of playing-related

---

Risk factors for development of playing-related disorders in instrumentalists

Intrinsic	*Extrinsic*
Body size and build	Inefficient ("faulty") technique
Conditioning	Change in technique
Strength	New instrument
Flexibility (both excessive and inadequate)	Increase (abrupt) in practice, playing time, or intensity
Endurance	"Excessive" total playing time
Muscular tension	New or inappropriate repertoire
Underlying disease or condition (e.g., arthritis, scoliosis)	Economic or social stresses
	Unrelated activities (job, athletic, recreational)
	Substance abuse

---

problems appear to be superimposition of inefficient or unduly stressful muscle activity, attempts to alter the existing technique by a new teacher or the instrumentalist himself or herself, and the abrupt and often inordinate increase in playing time or intensity (a rather vague and poorly quantified term that implies elements of effort, concentration, repetition, and emotional investment). The effects of emotional stress, socioeconomic factors, and lifestyle issues are more difficult to identify and quantitate, but these are probably no less important.

Professional voice users

It can be said that vocal performers call on the voice to do things for which the mechanism was not really designed. Primitive man did not often find it necessary to sing an aria or to perform rock music for several hours in a smoky and noisy environment. It is small wonder then that even gifted singers must train, both vocally and physi-

---

General health issues in professional voice users

1. Allergy
2. Age
3. Upper respiratory infections
4. Respiratory tract dysfunction
5. Reflux and other gastrointestinal dysfunction
6. Obesity
7. Endocrine dysfunction
8. Neurological disorders
9. Emotional factors and stress

Special risk factors in professional voice use

1. Smoking
2. Voice abuse
3. Poor or absent voice training
4. Alcohol abuse
5. Drug abuse
6. Vocal nodules

---

cally, if they are to perform successfully on a regular basis. General health maintenance is of paramount importance to the professional voice user, inasmuch as his or her vocal instrument requires the support of the entire body to function well. Even when illness or injury does not directly affect the vocal tract or its respiratory support, any health aberration will influence the singer's ability to perform to some degree. The general health issues that are likely to have particular negative effect on the voice are listed in the box above, and special risk factors are in the box above, right.

In a sense, *voice abuse* is the single common denominator for most special risk factors for the professional singer. Almost all of the epidemiological factors leading to vocal problems are the result of such intemperate voice usage, with the possible exception of *direct trauma*. *Smoking* and even secondary exposure to smoke is probably the most prevalent form of voice abuse. Any professional voice user who chooses to bathe his or her larynx and lungs in cigarette smoke at best is foolish and at worst does not wish to have a long career.

Upper respiratory infections are among the most common special problems for professional voice users. They are also among the most important, because they directly affect the vocal folds and the resonators of the upper vocal tract and also impair the lungs, which must drive the entire mechanism. Moreover, if the vocalist tries to perform or even practice in the face of such an infection, further and more permanent injury (e.g., vocal nodules) is likely to ensue. In general, the professional voice user is unwise to attempt to perform if he or she has any significant health problem, because this will of necessity put the vocal tract under unnecessary stress and therefore at risk for further injury.

Dancers

In 1983 Reid conducted a survey on injury patterns of young amateur dancers. Results showed that 18% of the injuries were to the knee, 16% were to the ankle, 14% had shin splints, 13% experienced foot problems, 12% had lumbar spine problems, and 8% had nondescript hip problems.[22]

Schafle et al. recently studied the injuries of company dancers, including ballet, modern, and aerobic dancers.[28] They evaluated 3251 injuries occurring from January, 1979 to April, 1988. Of the dancers studied, 55% were in ballet, 30% were aerobic dancers, and 15% were in modern dance. Of the injured dancers, 79% were women. Most ballet dancers suffering injuries were 13 to 18 years of age; modern and aerobic dancers were generally in the older age groups (26 to 39 years). In this study, the knee was again found to be the most common injury site, followed by the foot and toes.

The most frequent disorders in Schafle's study were due to overuse, followed by strains and fractures. Of the injuries sustained by ballet dancers, 40% were secondary to overuse, compared with the 25% suffered by modern and aerobic dancers. Strains accounted for 30% of the injuries sustained by ballet and modern dancers.

In a 3-year injury survey of Cleveland Ballet dancers (unpublished data), 70% were foot and ankle injuries, 25% involved knee, hip, and lower back, and 10% were fractures or dislocations.

Health risk factors of the dance profession are many. Long, painstaking hours of rehearsal, classes, and choreographic demands cause overuse injuries, including tendinitis, bursitis, and stress fracture. Traveling company dancers suffer injuries caused by poor flooring and facilities encountered while "on the road." Improper foot protection, even with a properly sprung floor, can damage soft tissues, nerves, and bones of the feet. Nutritional and psychological stresses are also risk factors in dancers in all stages of their training and careers.

The problem of "turn-out" has been treated extensively in the dance medicine literature.[26] Dancers are trained from a very early age to turn out (externally rotate) the lower extremity from the hip joint. Sacrificing proper alignment by attempting to compensate at the foot, ankle, or knee for inadequate hip turn-out predisposes young dancers to twisting injuries, such as torn ligaments in the affected joints.

Dancers who received inadequate early training can encounter disastrous problems when they begin a grueling apprenticeship or enter a company. Problems created over time, if left uncorrected, may set up a pattern of complex negative interrelationships between bony structures and their associated musculature.

Other risk factors are related to specific age groups. The younger dancer aged 13 to 20 may be still adapting to special footwear and isolations (dissociations) of various muscle groups. The dancer must develop a very keen proprioceptive sense and strong technical knowledge to understand and use consistently the appropriate muscle groups to "pull up," "release," "lengthen," and "turn-out."

With regard to nutritional and psychological stresses, dancers, particularly those who must meet "contract weights," need to pay close attention to proper nutritional principles when trying to lose and maintain weight. Brownell et al.[5] theorize that when athletes attempt to lose or gain weight, lowered fat levels increase the body's efficiency to utilize food, serving as a self-protective adaptation. When the body is taken through repetitive weight loss and gain cycles ("yo-yo" syndrome), food efficiency is increased so that future losses will require greater caloric restrictions.[2]

As the athlete or dancer goes through weight gain and loss cycles, redistribution of body fat can occur, and the reproductive system can be negatively affected. In females, menstrual function depends on both fat deposition and level of physical activity.[6,32] In male athletes, decreased testosterone production parallels menstrual dysfunction in females. Increased exercise levels, e.g., weight lifting and possibly endurance work, may lead to diminished testosterone in males, as well as decreased menstrual activity in females.

SOCIO-MEDICO-ECONOMICS
Instrumentalists

The concept of the "poor starving artist" is one firmly entrenched in our collective perception. Certainly the great and "near-great" among performing artists are often admirably compensated for their efforts. Musicians in major professional ensembles, although clearly not rewarded financially at the same level as the rock star or top classical soloist, are generally able to pursue a comfortable lifestyle. However, these make up only a relatively small percentage of professional musicians; a larger number are self-employed freelancers and teachers, often with unpredictable and sometimes inadequate sources of income. Further, many musicians are underserved by federal, state, and local programs when disabled or unemployed.[27] Musicians, even those in relatively high-level ensembles, may have no insurance or may be underinsured when health problems or disability threaten their capacity to perform on a daily basis.[8] Many segments of the performing arts community have limited access to health care providers or facilities. This problem has only occasionally been discussed in the medical literature.[3] Finally, even those who have had access to medical care when confronted with a playing-related problem may have been underserved by those

of us who provide health care. Too often in the past, but perhaps less so recently, the special needs of the instrumental performer have been poorly understood, and all too commonly the instrumentalist with a playing-related problem has simply been advised to stop playing or change careers. Increased awareness of the specific needs and problems of instrumental musicians and the development of centers for performing arts medicine have begun to affect these issues. Nonetheless, musicians and other performing artists tend to be wary of physicians and other health care professionals even if they have the resources to obtain medical care.

Professional voice users

Professional singers (particularly opera singers) tend to be very sensitive to even slight imbalances in their voices. This is because they recognize both the great socioeconomic value and the delicacy of the instrument that they use. Many have demanded the contractual right to refuse to perform if they do not feel that everything is "right" with their voices. Some female performers, for instance, feel that they can detect slight nuances of roughness during certain times in their monthly cycles.

Because the singing voice is much more sensitive to slight physical imbalances than the speaking voice, singers who are in the early stages of some type of vocal fold problem may have difficulty convincing theater managers that they are really unable to perform. Both social and economic pressures may lead to injudicious vocal use and eventually result in both greater damage and longer periods of recovery. Less well-trained voice users are much more likely to be willing to "push" their vocal capabilities, even when they are not at their physical best, so that "the show can go on." This, along with the nature of the music and the unconducive environment in which it is often performed, probably accounts for the much higher incidence of abuse-related vocal injuries in those with less formal voice training (typically pop and rock singers).

Dancers

When dealing with dancers' injuries, documentation is extremely important for medical insurance. In the past 3 years, Homitz has worked with the accounting, insurance, and legal departments at the Cleveland Clinic Foundation to formulate policy and procedures for all contractually covered salaried dancers. Dance students who are not employees, and therefore nonsalaried, are responsible for their own medical insurance coverage, which is often through their parents' insurance.

Full-time dancers usually have automatic coverage through their companies, but this is not universally true.[8] Other avenues of possible assistance for the disabled performer need to be explored. Whether they be actors, dancers, or musicians, performers need help in career planning and training, and upon retirement, they need help with lifestyle orientation. Our Canadian counterparts have been more successful in this regard.[14] Major areas where retired performers have proven very successful include arts management, allied health careers, education, and private business relative to the arts.

SCREENING
Instrumentalists

Little attention has been paid to the subject of health screening in instrumental musicians, certainly less than has recently been paid to the subject in young dancers. Some consideration, primarily in the dental literature, has been given to the pattern of dental occlusion in the choice of a wind instrument, with the suggestion that choosing certain instruments might aid in orthodontic treatment. For instance, the youngster with an overjet and/or overbite might benefit from playing a brass instrument such as the trumpet rather than the clarinet, which would have the opposite effect of increasing overjet and overbite.[16] Because of the young age at which instrumental lessons begin, effective screening programs are unlikely ever to have wide applicability. Music teachers who are the first to see and judge the beginning musician are more likely to focus on musical talent and aptitude than on specific physical characteristics or skills, although there are some exceptions.[1]

One potential area of screening might be hand size or flexibility as an indicator of the likelihood for success or failure in musicians.[31] Extreme caution is required in this area, however. While there might be an "ideal" hand configuration for a pianist, there are many examples of outstanding concert artists with very small as well as very large hands. To have steered one of the former group away from the piano would have been a great disservice not only to the artist but to the concert audience as well. These studies, along with those relating the biomechanics of the hand to subsequent development of focal dystonia, are of great interest and may potentially help us to understand the factors that contribute to the development of musculoskeletal problems, but await considerable further investigation and confirmation.[33]

Several investigators have observed that joint hyperextensibility may have a deleterious effect on the instrumental musician.[4,17] There are some discrepancies in the results of these analyses and, at the moment, no recommendations can be made regarding the potential usefulness of screening for joint hypermobility in young music students. Certainly more studies are needed to identify the positive and negative factors in the very young and the more advanced instrumental student in the hope of predicting and preventing future physical problems related to playing.

Professional voice users

Screening of patients with incipient voice problems is really not possible in most settings. If the performer has a good voice coach (as all of them should), the coach may be able to detect problems in the early stages before serious damage is done. Usually, however, the performer must be aware of small changes in vocal status so that medical evaluation can be sought.

If early voice changes *are* detected and treated, most longer-term and more serious difficulties can be avoided. Usually a period of relative voice rest or at least avoidance of singing will prevent further damage and permit resolution of the problem. An otolaryngologist can not only examine and document any physical changes, but also usually prescribe treatment appropriately to achieve early return to normal vocal status.

Dancers

It is essential to evaluate dancers for preexisting injuries or problems.

The screening method developed for the dance population by Plastino is time consuming, yet comprehensive and well thought out.[21] The plan requires the participation of physicians, therapists, trainers, kinesiologists, exercise physiologists, and others, as available. The purpose is to protect both the individual performer and the company.

The screening procedure includes evaluation of vital statistics, posture, genetic history, general medical history including chronic illnesses and medications, flexibility, body composition, blood lactate, and biomechanics. Any needed specific adjunctive equipment should be specified and used.

Additional diagnostic movement analysis classes to screen for alignment can be incorporated into a dancer's program, such as floor barre work. Equipment such as the Pilates Reformer (an apparatus used for body conditioning consisting of a moveable spring-loaded carriage on a platform) can also be used in a variety of settings.[10]

Although extensive research has not been conducted on the statistical effectiveness of early detection of problems in dancers, the integration of total functional body movement through sound applied kinesiological principles appears to have intuitive benefit. Length/strength relationships need to be analyzed, and muscle imbalances associated with the dancer's pain syndrome(s) should be examined.

The Cleveland Clinic has incorporated a trial-and-error system, (i.e., based on patient response) to produce a comprehensive prescription for exercise. The plan is aimed to combine muscle balance and coordinated function with appropriate flexibility, using the Sahrmann technique.[25] Included in Sahrmann's manual is a kinesiopathological model of the elements of movement based on the following areas:

- Base (musculoskeletal)
- Modulation (nervous system)
- Biomechanics (kinematics)
- Support (cardiopulmonary system)

Sahrmann's system can also be applied to postscreening situations. It focuses to some degree on the outcomes of correct vs. faulty posture and balanced vs. unbalanced movement patterns. If the dancer continues with faulty posture and unbalanced movement patterns over a period of time, dysfunction will be the outcome, followed ultimately by pathological problems within one or more of the body's systems. The goal of these studies is to develop a workable, measurable system that coordinates the efforts of all the dancer's healthcare practitioners. With this system, personalized, organized, and balanced functional movement patterns can be developed for the dancer.

Throughout the performance season, specific problems can be addressed through observation of the dancers in class. Close observation of the dancer's technique at the barre is an essential part of this concept.

THERAPEUTIC INTERVENTIONS
Instrumentalists

As in any field of medicine, the first step in treatment is to analyze the problem and make an accurate diagnosis. For the instrumental musician with a playing-related problem, this requires a careful and thorough medical history as well as some musical history. The physician should obtain a detailed description of the playing-related symptoms and the setting in which these symptoms arose. The degree of detail regarding practice and playing schedules, recent changes in technique, repertoire, and other relevant activities is tailored to the individual situation. Similarly, the extent of physical examination is also geared to the specific problem. In most cases, observation of the instrumentalist while playing is desirable if not mandatory. Some of the disorders encountered, such as the occupational cramps or focal dystonias, can only be identified in this manner, but valuable information is often gained regarding many other problems as well.

Because pain is a major complaint in about 85% of instrumentalists and musculoskeletal disorders represent about 60% of the diagnoses in our practice, the treatment discussion will focus on this general category. Therapy can be considered in two phases, as outlined in the box on above. The cornerstone of acute treatment is rest for the affected part. For most problems, this consists of a general reduction in activity, sometimes with 1 to 2 weeks of abstinence from playing. Most often, a reduction in playing time is all that is required. Occasionally, for more severe or prolonged pain episodes, a more radical rest period is required, including not only the prohibition of playing but also the discontinuation of *any* stressful hand or limb activities. Splinting the affected part can sometimes achieve a greater degree of immobilization. Unless the period of splinting is relatively brief, it should be accompanied by some gentle stretching exercises, with few exceptions. A variety of modalities are utilized as adjuncts, such as icing, massage, ultrasound, and electrical stimulation. Medications during this acute phase can be helpful, including

---

Treatment of playing-related disorders

Acute phase

Rest: relative vs. total ("radical")
Splinting
Gentle stretching
Modalities (icing, heat, massage, ultrasound, electrical stimulation)
Medication (analgesic, antiinflammatory, muscle relaxants)
Injections (trigger point, nerve block, steroid)
Surgery

Rehabilitation phase

Gradual increase in playing
Modification of playing schedule (total time, rest breaks)
Modification of technique
Improvement in playing posture
Warm-up and cool-down
Decrease static/dynamic muscle load (support device, alter instrument)
Playing aids/protective devices (dental prostheses, orthoses, modify instrument)
Body awareness and movement education

---

analgesics, antiinflammatory medications, and muscle relaxants. Trigger-point injections, nerve blocks, and one or two corticosteroid injections for acute tendon inflammation may also be useful in selected circumstances. Surgery is rarely required for any of these disorders except in cases of nerve entrapment that have not responded to more conservative measures and the occasional tendinitis that has similarly failed to respond to other methods.

The rehabilitation phase begins when the pain subsides. Here the physician may well recede into the background as therapists and teachers begin to assume a more important role. The patient returns to playing slowly and gradually with increasing segments of playing punctuated by rest breaks. The physician offers advice regarding overall modification of the playing and practice schedule; in general we recommend that a break of 10 to 15 minutes be taken every 25 to 30 minutes if possible, even after complete recovery has occurred. If total playing time has been considered excessive, this can also be reduced; clearly each situation must be approached individually.

Technical modifications are carried out largely in conjunction with the teacher. The physician's advice may focus on efficiency of muscle activity and methods of reducing static and dynamic loads. These methods may include a variety of support devices (Fig. 66-1) and methods of modifying the instrument. The size and position of thumb rests may be altered on wind instruments, the size or position of a chin rest or shoulder pad may be changed for the violin, or the shape of an instrument may even be modified (e.g., angulating the head of a flute). Warm-up and cool-

Vocal hygiene

1. Do not speak unless you get paid for it.
2. Speak only to people who are within arm's reach.
3. Speak in the most quiet, least effortful voice you can manage.
4. Avoid telephone use as much as possible.
5. No singing, shouting, coughing, throat clearing, or vigorous laughing.

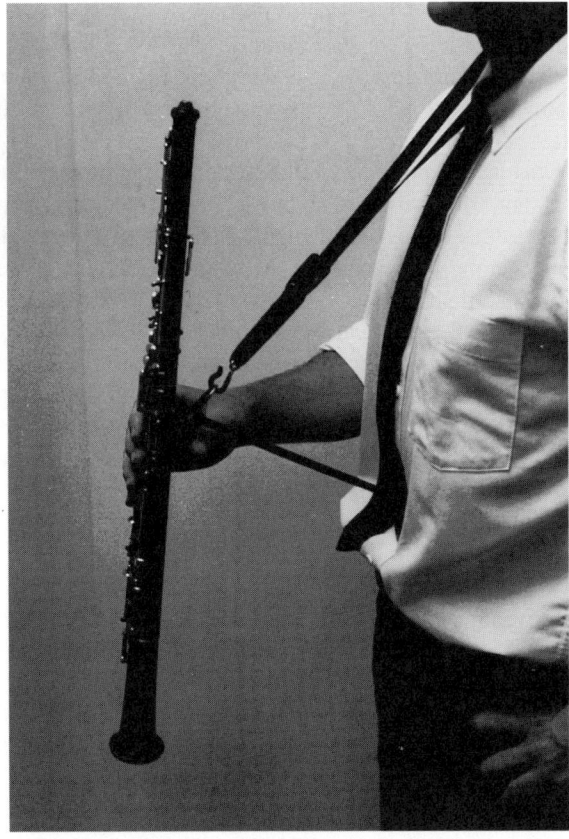

Fig. 66-1. A support device for the oboe, with neck strap and support post. (Courtesy Steven I. Reger, Ph.D.)

down exercises are performed before and after practice sessions respectively. A comprehensive exercise program is individually designed, geared toward improving overall conditioning, restoring disordered muscle balance, stretching and strengthening, and improving endurance. Our experience suggests that improving posture, enhancing the proximal supporting muscles of the upper trunk, neck, and shoulders, and promoting aerobic conditioning are among the most important things we can do to reduce the chances of relapse or worsening, even for hand, wrist, and forearm pain. Along with these therapeutic modalities must be a program of education about the susceptibility of the human musculoskeletal system to injury. A variety of techniques for enhancing body awareness and promoting efficient movement are available and have been applied to the musician population.[20,24]

Professional voice users

Depending on the exact nature of the vocal problem discovered, voice rest, vocal hygiene (see the box above), medication, and/or surgery may be indicated. Because the great majority of vocal problems in singers are due to viral upper respiratory infections or other mild inflammatory changes, simple voice rest will be adequate in many cases. Once the problem has resolved, however, it is important that, like any athlete, the singer undertake a period of nonperformance reconditioning (voice coaching, speech therapy).

Antihistamines, systemic decongestants, and even steroids can be helpful in managing the underlying physical cause for the performer's vocal problems, but these *should seldom be used* to permit performance ("I've just got to get through tonight") when the patient's physical condition does not justify it. Just as the professional football player who has sprained his ankle can finish the game if the ankle is anesthetized, so can the vocal performer "get through" one or two performances on steroids. However, neither of these performers is likely to be at his or her best under these circumstances, and both run the significant risk that performing under medication will result in further injury and longer recovery periods than would have been the case if they had been "taken out of the game." When medication is necessary to relieve such an illness, the performer should recognize that he or she also should not try to perform until completely recovered.

Surgery, such as removal of polyps or vocal nodules, is highly successful in restoring normal speaking voices in most patients. The ability to achieve the presurgical level of performance in a professional singer, however, is much less certain, because the fine "tuning" of a superb voice is often related to reestablishment of Reinke's space and the free "flow" of mucous membrane over the underlying musculature. Neither of these can be achieved in every case. Therefore, *no surgical intervention* should be considered in a professional voice user unless he or she cannot continue his or her career with the best voice that can be achieved with nonsurgical means. In this situation, the singer has nothing to lose, because he or she cannot expect to advance or maintain his or her career if surgery is not done.

Dancers

When working with dancers in more acute situations, for instance when providing assistance in the theater, one uses modalities such as ice packs or cups (heat is rarely used), ultrasound, phonophoresis, fluoromethane spray, massage, and electrotherapy. Sahrmann's technique is applicable where a preprogramming or deprogramming is needed for therapeutic exercise regimens.[25] Adaptive foot and ankle padding for posturing, skin lesions, such as blisters, and complications of infection may be applied in the treatment room. Pool therapy may be added, when available.

Less acute conditions, such as chronic tendinitis, fracture, and dislocation/subluxation seldom require or respond to modalities such as those listed above and usually need ongoing aggressive rehabilitation in the clinical setting. The emphasis here is on attainment of normal range of motion, strength, and body alignment to decrease musculoskeletal dysfunction from second- and third-degree overuse, poor technique, and overly repetitive activity. Dance training should be supplemented by other muscle reeducation techniques such as Pilates, Alexander, or Feldenkreis, among others.

COUNSELING AND COMPLIANCE
Instrumentalists

Prevention obviously is preferable to treatment. There is very little if any data in the medical literature regarding prevention of playing-related problems among instrumentalists. Most of what we assume to be sound advice for preventing these disorders is derived from our successful therapeutic approaches. All of this must ultimately be validated in longitudinal studies to show whether this advice in fact is effective in reducing the frequency or severity of problems associated with performance. All that we can say at the moment is that clinical experience indicates that the preventive programs we institute in those who have had problems seem to work in the majority.

Some general principles seem applicable. The total amount of time spent in playing should be limited. This will obviously vary, depending on the individual and the instrument. Clearly some instrumentalists, particularly younger professionals and students, can play for 8 or 10 hours per day without any apparent ill effects. Others have much lower tolerance but may be able to play effectively for 2 or 3 hours daily. Instrumentalists may never have considered that the effort expended to play softly and slowly may be less than that required for consistently loud and fast playing, and the simple expedient of playing fortissimo passages mezzoforte except during dress rehearsal and performance may be a revelation to even an advanced professional. Insisting on frequent rest breaks, although not always feasible, particularly in ensemble players who do not have a choice, can go a long way toward reducing playing-related discomfort and overuse. The instrumentalist should be counseled to maintain a good general exercise program, including aerobics. General conditioning has obviously been a major focus of attention in athletics and in dance but not in music and is only recently finding its way into some conservatory curricula. Strength of the proximal muscles that bear the brunt of the static load for supporting the instrument is important. Even more important is the effective use of muscle, as can be taught through multiple disciplines. The techniques of physical and occupational therapy as well as body and movement awareness techniques can all improve the chances for maintaining pain-free playing.

The instrument teacher or coach must be an integral part of the counseling team. We have emphasized so far the need for efficient playing technique, creating the minimum of stress on the muscles used. At the same time, the technique must serve the musical master as well, providing the desired sound and musical result. Too often in the past the teacher has been interested in the latter to the exclusion of the former, and the health care professional has had the opposite goal. These approaches must be consolidated. The teacher must further provide advice and expertise in choosing repertoire that is appropriate to the skill level and physical characteristics of the performer. Singers and voice teachers have been much more careful in tailoring the repertoire to the individual voice than have instrumentalists, who have largely been expected to play everything equally well.

The influence of emotional state on the development of physical performance-related problems has not been particularly emphasized in the preceding discussion but has been implicit in almost every aspect. Emotional stress has a direct effect on muscle tension and function, and no successful preventive program can ignore the effect of stress on the student or professional performer. Most musicians develop their own techniques for controlling the influence of stress, but continuing support of the teacher, the physician, and the therapist is of critical importance to some. Stress management techniques, psychological counseling, and in some cases psychiatric consultation and treatment are important components of the preventive program.

The instrumental musician tends to be an extremely compliant and at times overcompliant patient. As a group, they are extraordinarily dedicated and motivated, at times to a fault. The treating physician and therapist must be careful to advise against overzealous adherence to the prescribed program. Just as they may be likely to practice a difficult passage for hours at a time, they may believe that if 20 repetitions of an exercise are therapeutic, 200 must be that much more helpful. However, as with all patients, the compliance with a preventive program is likely to be less faithful than with a treatment program, when the injury from which they are recovering is recent. In our experience, many of the relapses after successful treatment have been the result of gradual discontinuation of the prescribed maintenance regimen.

As was noted previously, no data exist regarding the effectiveness of these preventive measures. Spaulding has described a preventive program in a Norwegian conservatory.[30] The program is only briefly outlined and consists of courses teaching posture, ergonomics, relaxation techniques, and stress management. Although the author implies that the program successfully reduces the risk of injury, no data are supplied. One hopes that this institution and other similar institutions will publish further reports.

Professional voice users

As previously discussed, counseling is the major intervention for most professional voice users with vocal problems. Even the voice coaching and/or speech therapy that most will require as part of recovery can be regarded as counseling. If the patient is unwilling or unable to comply with the advice given, little progress can be expected. Emotional overlay is a critical part of what separates the brilliant performer from the individual with a "nice voice." Therefore it should not be surprising that many vocal performers are temperamental and sometimes hypochondriacal, at least regarding their singing. The physician who seeks to deal with this group of patients must be prepared to provide the special emotional support that they often require.

Dancers

Inefficient techniques used by the dancer because of faulty programming methods are continually analyzed and reevaluated to decrease oversubstitution by synergistic muscles. An example is the overuse of the sartorius muscle, hip flexors, back muscles, and gluteals to lift the leg with the hips flexed. Dancers using improper technique will rely less on external rotators, psoas, and lower abdominals, which are better able to perform these specific maneuvers. The muscles of the middle and lower back are also frequently misused.

The dancer must dissociate the hip, lower back, and abdominal muscle groups for the dancer to continually identify his or her "center." Then he or she can begin working from that point. The Pilates system can be used to reinforce correct movement patterning by the performer via use of the Reformer and matte-work exercise system.[10] Each individual can be fully counseled and instructed in the technique as applied to his or her body structure. Dancers should be advised to keep logs of their work, continually advance and update their exercise plans, and review long-term and short-term goals. Additionally, the physician can offer further instruction through assigned readings, videotapes, or studio work, incorporating some or all of the many movement-awareness and body-conditioning techniques.

Many of these techniques or instructions involve variable resistance work with verbal and manual cues to re-strengthen specific areas. Because of the strong work ethic among the dance population, compliance is generally in the range of 90% to 95%. Dancers tend to have a high level of physical and mental stamina; their desire for continuing reeducation is often limited only by time and funding. The remaining 5% to 10% have often appeared to be persons who prefer alternative healing methods, based on their own philosophy of health care.

SUMMARY

Performing artists represent a relatively small and in some ways unique occupational group, with a predilection to specific problems related to their art. Understanding the special characteristics of performing artists, their needs and goals, and the factors contributing to the development of performance-related health problems is required to provide adequate advice for treatment and prevention. The body of medical knowledge available in this area has been sparse but is expanding rapidly. Increasing our understanding of these performance-related problems, increasing the ability of the performer to gain access to adequate health care, and improving our ability to treat and prevent these disorders will ensure that this precious commodity will be preserved for future generations.

REFERENCES

1. Birkedahl N: Identification, prevention, and remediation of medical problems in very young violin students, *Med Probl Perform Art* 4:176-178, 1989.
2. Blackburn GL, Brownell KD: Weight cycling: the experience of human dieters, *Am J Clin Med* 49:1104-1109, 1989.
3. Brandfonbrener AG: The jazz musician: a challenge to arts medicine, *Med Probl Perform Art* 3:iii, 1988.
4. Brandfonbrener AG: Joint laxity in instrumental musicians, *Med Probl Perform Art* 5:117-119, 1990.
5. Brownell KD, Steen SN, and Wilmore JH: Weight regulation products in athletes: analysis of metabolic and health effects, *Med Sci Sports Exerc* 19:546-556, 1987.
6. Calabrese LH et al: Menstrual abnormalities, nutritional patterns and body composition in female classical ballet dancers, *Phys Sports Med* 11:86-98, 1983.
7. Caldron PH et al: A survey of musculoskeletal problems encountered in high-level musicians, *Med Probl Perform Art* 1:136-139, 1986.
8. Chmelar RD: Health insurance and workers' compensation issues for performing artists I, II, *Med Probl Perform Art* 5:67-71, 101-105, 1990.
9. Fishbein M et al: Medical problems among ICSOM musicians: overview of a national survey, *Med Probl Perform Art* 3:1-8, 1988.
10. Friedman P, Eisen G: *The Pilates method of physical and mental conditioning*, New York, 1980, Doubleday and Company.
11. Fry HJH: Incidence of overuse syndrome in the symphony orchestra, *Med Probl Perform Art* 1:51-55, 1986.
12. Fry HJH: Prevalence of overuse (injury) syndrome in Australian music schools, *Br J Indust Med* 44:35-40, 1987.
13. Fry HJH, Ross P, and Rutherford M: Music-related overuse in secondary schools, *Med Probl Perform Art* 3:133-134, 1988.
14. Greben SE: The Dancer Transition Centre of Canada: addressing the stress of giving up professional dancing, *Med Probl Perform Art* 4:128-130, 1989.
15. Grieco A et al: Muscular effort and musculo-skeletal disorders in piano students: electromyographic, clinical and preventive aspects, *Ergonomics* 32:697-716, 1989.
16. Howard JA: Temporomandibular joint disorders, facial pain, and dental problems in performing artists. In Sataloff RT, Brandfonbrener AG, and Lederman RJ, editors: *Textbook of performing arts medicine*, New York, 1991, Raven Press.
17. Larsson L-G, Baum J, and Mudholkar GS: Hypermobility: features and differential incidence between the sexes, *Arthritis Rheum* 30:1426-1430, 1987.
18. Lockwood AH: Medical problems in secondary school-aged musicians, *Med Probl Perform Art* 3:129-132, 1988.

19. Manchester RA: The incidence of hand problems in music students, *Med Probl Perform Art* 3:15-18, 1988.

20. Nelson SH: Playing with the entire self: the Feldenkrais method and musicians, *Semin Neurol* 9:97-104, 1989.

21. Plastino JG: Physical screening of the dancer: general methodologies and procedures. In Solomon R, Minton S, and Solomon J, editors: *Preventing dance injuries: an interdisciplinary perspective,* Reston, Va, 1990, American Alliance for Health, Physical Education, Recreation, and Dance.

22. Reid DC: Prevention of injuries to the dancer. In Horvell ML, Bullock MT, editors: *Physiotherapy in sports,* St Louis, 1983, Queensland University.

23. Revak JM: Incidence of upper extremity discomfort among piano students, *Am J Occup Ther* 43:149-154, 1989.

24. Rosenthal E: The Alexander technique—what it is and how it works, *Med Probl Perform Art* 2:53-57, 1987.

25. Sahrmann S: *Diagnosis and treatment of muscle imbalances and associated regional pain syndromes,* St Louis, 1991, Washington University.

26. Sammarco GJ: The hip in dancers, *Med Probl Perform Art* 2:5-14, 1987.

27. Saxon J: Cost constraints on health care access to some performing artists, *Med Probl Perform Art* 2:105-107, 1987.

28. Schafle M, Requa R, and Garrick J: A comparison of patterns of injury in ballet, modern, and aerobic dance. In Solomon R, Milton S, and Solomon J, editors: *Preventing dance injuries: an interdisciplinary perspective,* Reston, Va, 1990, American Alliance for Health, Physical Education, Recreation, and Dance.

29. Singer K: *Diseases of the musical profession: a systematic presentation of their causes, symptoms, and methods of treatment,* translated by Lakond W, New York, 1932, Greenberg.

30. Spaulding C: Before pathology: prevention for performing artists, *Med Probl Perform Art* 3:135-139, 1988.

31. Wagner C: Success and failure in musical performance: biomechanics of the hand. In Roehmann FL, Wilson FR, editors: *The biology of music making: proceedings of the 1984 Denver Conference,* St Louis, 1988, MMB Music.

32. Warren MP: Reproductive disorders in female dancers. In Sataloff RT, Brandfonbrener AG, and Lederman RJ, editors: *Textbook of performing arts medicine,* New York, 1991, Raven Press.

33. Wilson FR, San Ramon CA, and Wagner C: Interaction of biomechanical and training factors in musicians with occupational cramp/focal dystonia, *Neurology* 41(suppl 1):291-292, 1991.

SUPPLEMENTAL READING

Lockwood AH: Medical problems in musicians, *N Engl J Med* 320:221-227, 1989.

Ryan AJ, Stephens RE, editors: *Dance medicine: a comprehensive guide,* Chicago, 1987, Pluribus Press.

Sataloff RT: *Professional voice: the science and art of clinical care,* New York, 1991, Raven Press.

Sataloff RT, Brandfonbrener AG, and Lederman RJ: *Textbook of performing arts medicine,* New York, 1991, Raven Press.

Tucker HM: *The larynx,* ed 2, New York, 1992, Theime Medical Publishers.

RESOURCES

International Association of Dancemedicine and Science, 4510 W. 77th St., Minneapolis, MN 55435; Attention: Allan J. Ryan, MD.

Dancemedicine/Health Newsletter, 7922 Oceanus Drive, Los Angeles, CA 90046; Attention: Dr. Ernest Washington.

Dancemedicine Resource Directory, 27 Filley Rd, Haddam, CT 06438; Attention: Jan Dunn; gives listings of Dancemedicine Centers in the USA.

Center for Safety in the Arts, 5 Beekman St., New York, NY 10038; brochures and other information on hazards associated with the performing and creative arts.

International Arts Medicine Association, 3600 Market St., Philadelphia, PA 19104; publishes a newsletter and fosters interdisciplinary communication among healthcare workers and performing/creative artists.

The Singer Support Group, The American Institute for Voice and Ear Research, 1721 Pine St., Philadelphia, PA 19103; information and support for the professional voice user.

INDEX